Medical-Surgical Nursing Across the Health Care Continuum

Donna D. Ignatavicius, MS, RNC, Cm

Clinical Nurse Specialist, Calvert Memorial Hospital,
Prince Frederick, MD
Former Professor, Charles County Community College, La Plata, MD

M. Linda Workman, PhD, RN, FAAN

Associate Professor of Nursing, Frances Payne Bolton School of Nursing,
Case Western Reserve University, Cleveland, OH

Mary A. Mishler, MSN, RNCS, CNN

Adjunct Faculty, Helene Fuld School of Nursing in Camden County,
Blackwood, NJ
Adjunct Faculty, Gloucester County College, Sewell, NJ
Faculty, American Health Care Institute, Silver Spring, MD

VOLUME 1

3rd
EDITION

W.B. Saunders Company
A Division of Harcourt Brace & Company
Philadelphia London Toronto Montreal Sydney Tokyo

W.B. SAUNDERS COMPANY
A Division of Harcourt Brace & Company

The Curtis Center
Independence Square West
Philadelphia, Pennsylvania 19106

Library of Congress Cataloging-in-Publication Data

Medical-surgical nursing across the health care continuum / [edited by] Donna D. Ignatavicius, M. Linda Workman, Mary A. Mishler. — 3rd ed.

    p.   cm.

  Rev. ed. of: Medical-surgical nursing. 2nd ed. c1995.
Includes bibliographical references and index.

  ISBN 0-7216-6981-6. — ISBN 0-7216-6980-8 (2 v. set)

  1. Nursing. 2. Surgical nursing. I. Ignatavicius, Donna D.
II. Workman, M. Linda. III. Mishler, Mary A. IV. Medical-surgical nursing.
  [DNLM: 1. Perioperative Nursing. 2. Nursing Process.
WY 161M489 1999]
  RT41.I36 1999   610.73—dc21

  DNLM/DLC   98-38329

MEDICAL-SURGICAL NURSING ACROSS THE HEALTH CARE CONTINUUM, 3rd edition
    Single Volume 0-7216-6981-6
    Volume 1 0-7216-999714370-1
    Volume 2 0-7216-999714371-x
    (set) 0-7216-6980-8

Printed in the United States of America.

Last digit is the print number: 9   8   7   6   5   4   3   2   1

To Stephanie and Charles, who continue through the years to tolerate my unending hours of travel, computers, and phone calls—I love you both so very much for your support; and to Lee Henderson, whose mentoring helped me grow and develop as a writer—thank you for your patience and guidance.

DDI

To my father, Homer D. Workman, the gentle giant who was my first, best, and most inspiring teacher; and to the other men in my life, my husband John and sons David and Gregory, for their love, patience, and humor.

MLW

To Laura Vogel, my daughter, a sophomore at Boston University School of Communication, and to Aaron Vogel, my son, a sophomore at Ithaca College School of Music; you have made my life more interesting and fulfilling than you can possibly imagine—love you always!

MAM

About the Authors

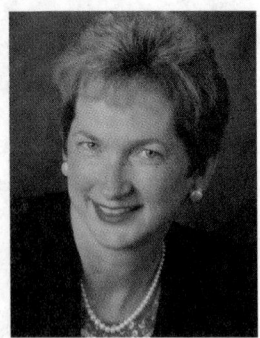

Donna D. Ignatavicius received her diploma in nursing from the Peninsula General Hospital School of Nursing in Salisbury, Maryland, in 1969. After working as a staff and charge nurse in medical-surgical nursing, she became Instructor in Staff Development at the University of Maryland Medical Center. In 1976 she received her BSN from the University of Maryland School of Nursing. For 5 years she taught in several schools of nursing while working toward her MS in nursing, which she received in 1981. Ms. Ignatavicius then taught in the baccalaureate program at the University of Maryland School of Nursing for 6 years, after which she pursued her interest in gerontology by becoming Director of Nursing at a skilled nursing facility. She has been a certified gerontological nurse since 1989 and was certified in nursing case management in 1998. Through her consulting and seminar business, Ms. Ignatavicius has gained national recognition in case management, including an appointment as the national Education Chair for the Case Management Society of America. She is currently employed as a clinical nurse specialist in medical-surgical/gerontological nursing at the Calvert Memorial Hospital in Prince Frederick, Maryland.

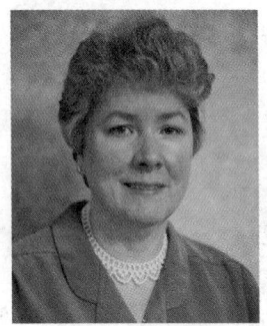

M. Linda Workman received her BSN from the University of Cincinnati College of Nursing and Health. After serving in the U.S. Army Nurse Corps and working as an Assistant Head Nurse and Head Nurse in civilian hospitals, Dr. Workman, a native of Canada, earned her MSN from the University of Cincinnati College of Nursing and Health and a PhD in developmental biology from the University of Cincinnati College of Arts and Sciences. Dr. Workman's 18 years of academic experience include teaching at the diploma, associate degree, baccalaureate, and master's levels. Her areas of teaching expertise include physiology, pathophysiology, genetics, oncology, and immunology. She is a former American Cancer Society Professor of Oncology Nursing and currently is an Associate Professor of Nursing at the Frances Payne Bolton School of Nursing at Case Western Reserve University, Cleveland.

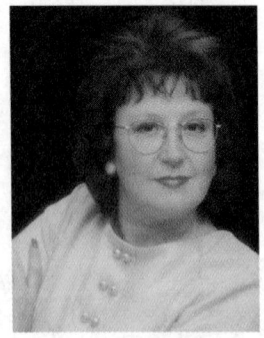

Mary A. Mishler has practiced medical-surgical nursing throughout her entire nursing career. She has worked as a staff nurse, staff development coordinator, clinical nurse specialist, nursing supervisor, and assistant director of nursing as well as a consultant. She has also served as senior-level course coordinator at a school of nursing. A 1971 graduate of Temple University Hospital School of Nursing in Philadelphia, Ms. Mishler received her BSN in 1973 and her MSN in 1977 from the University of Pennsylvania. A member of Sigma Theta Tau, Ms. Mishler is a faculty member at the Helene Fuld School of Nursing in Camden County and at Gloucester County College, both in New Jersey. She is certified both as a Clinical Specialist in Medical-Surgical Nursing and as a Nephrology Nurse. In 1993 she received a Certificate for Excellence in Nursing from the New Jersey State Department of Health. She has served as a member of the Standard Setting Panel for the NCLEX-RN examination and on the Editorial/Advisory Board of *Nursing Spectrum*. She also teaches continuing education seminars throughout the United States.

Contributors

Barbara Diebold Ahlheit, MSN, RN, CS; Adjunct Faculty, Vanderbilt School of Nursing, Nashville, Tennessee; Family Nurse Practitioner, Veterans Administration Medical Center, Nashville, Tennessee

Suzanne Cushman Beyea, PhD; Co-Director, Perioperative Nursing Research, Association of Operating Room Nurses, Denver, Colorado

Marilyn Booker, RN, MS, CRNI; Infusion Consultant, Sunnybrook Services; Case Manager, Diversified Health Services, Inc., Baltimore, Maryland

Marcia Sue DeWolf Bosek, DNSc, RN; Associate Professor, Department of Adult Health Nursing, College of Nursing, Rush University, Chicago, Illinois

Janice Cuzzell, MA, RN; Vice-President of Service Development/Business Models, Clinical Service Consultant, Island Health Care, Inc., Savannah, Georgia

Lucille Sanzer Eller, PhD, RN; Assistant Professor, College of Nursing, Rutgers University, Newark, New Jersey

Kathleen Ellstrom, MS, RN, CS; Pulmonary Clinical Nurse Specialist, Pulmonary and Critical Care Division, UCLA Medical Center, Los Angeles, California

Cynthia Gerrett, MSN, RNC; Women's Health Clinical Nurse Specialist, University of North Carolina Hospital, Chapel Nill, North Carolina

Kathy Hausman, PhD, RNC; Instructor, University of Maryland, Baltimore County, Baltimore, Maryland; Director of Education Services, Harbor and Franklin Square Hospitals, Baltimore, Maryland

Donna D. Ignatavicius, MS, RNC, CM; Clinical Nurse Specialist, Calvert Memorial Hospital, Prince Frederick, Maryland; Former Professor, Charles County Community College, La Plata, Maryland

Ann Putnam Johnson, EdD, MSN, BSN; Associate Dean, College of Applied Sciences, Associate Professor, Department of Nursing, Western Carolina University, Cullowhee, North Carolina

Kathleen J. Jones, MS, RN, ANP; Adult Nurse Practitioner, Hematology/Oncology Clinic, Walter Reed Army Medical Center, Washington, D.C.

Mary K. Kazanowski, PhD, RN, CS, OCS, CRNH; Associater Professor, Department of Nursing, Saint Anselm College, Manchester, New Hampshire; Hospice Nurse, Optima VNA Hospice, Manchester, New Hampshire

Anne Keane, MSN, EdD, FAAN; Associate Director, Program Direction, Acute/Tertiary Nurse Practitioner Program, University of Pennsylvania School of Nursing, Philadelphia, Pennsylvania

Deitra Leonard Lowdermilk, PhD, RNC, FAAN; Clinical Professor, Department of Community, Family, Mental, and Women's Health, School of Nursing, University of North Carolina, Chapel Hill, North Carolina

Judy Malkiewicz, PhD, RN; Professor, School of Nursing, University of Northern Colorado, Greeley, Colorado

Tina M. Marrelli; MA, MSN, RNC; Editor, Home Care Nurse News; President, Marelli and Associates, Inc., Boca Grande, Florida

Jan Hoot Martin, PhD, RN, GNP; Associate Professor, School of Nursing, University of Northern Colorado, Greeley, Colorado

Margaret Elaine McLeod, MSN, RNCS, CDE; Clinical Nurse Specialist/Diabetes Educator, VA Medical Center, Nashville, Tennessee

Mary A. Mishler, MSN, RNCS, CNN; Adjunct Faculty, Helene Fuld School of Nursing, Camden County, Blackwood, New Jersey; Adjunct Faculty, Gloucester County College, Sewell, New Jersey; Faculty, American Health Care Institute, Silver Spring, Maryland

Phyllis Naumann, MA, MSN, CRNP; Coordinator, Undergraduate Program; Assistant Professor, The Johns Hopkins University School of Nursing, Baltimore, Maryland

Kathleen Ouimet Perrin, MS; Associate Professor, Nursing, Saint Anselm College, Manchester, New Hampshire

Carmen J. Petrin, RN; Cardiac Services Educator, Catholic Medical Center, Manchester, New Hampshire

Charon A. Pierson, RN, PhD, GNP, CS; Instructor, Advanced Practice Nursing, University of Hawaii School of Nursing, Honolulu, Hawaii; Geriatric Nurse Practitioner/Clinical Nurse Specialist, Kaiser Permanente Long-Term Care Team, Honolulu, Hawaii

Rosemary Polomano, MSN, PhD, FAAN; Pain Clinical Nurse Specialist, Department of Surgical Nursing, University of Pennsylvania Medical Center, Philadelphia, Pennsylvania

Lynn Rew, EdD, RNC, FAAN; Associate Professor, and Graduate Advisor, School of Nursing, The University of Texas, Austin, Texas

Denise A. Sadowski, RN, MSN; Independent Burn and Wound Care Nurse Consultant and Educator, Cincinnati, Ohio

Theresa A. Savage, PhD, RN; Adjunct Assistant Professor, Maternal–Child Nursing; Postdoctoral Research Fellow in Primary Health Care/Social Ethics, College of Nursing, University of Illinois, Chicago, Illinois

Susan M. Schneider, PhD, CS, OCN; Assistant Professor, Frances Payne Bolton School of Nursing, Case Western Reserve University, Cleveland, Ohio; Pediatric Oncology Nurse, Ireland Cancer Center, University Hospitals of Cleveland, Cleveland, Ohio

Susan N. Shelton, RD, LD, MA; Consultant Dietitian, Arnold, Maryland

Deborah Shpritz, PhD, RN, CCRN; Assistant Professor, Department of Adult Health, School of Nursing, University of Maryland, Baltimore, Maryland

Ann E. Furiel Sievers, MA, RN, CORLN; Clinical Associate, Department of Physiological Nursing, School of Nursing, University of California, San Francisco, San Francisco, California; Otolaryngology Clinical Nurse Specialist, University of California, Davis Health System, Sacramento, California

Karen M. Stanley, MS, RN, CS; Psychiatric Consultation Liaison Nurse, Medical University of South Carolina, Charleston, South Carolina

Georgeanne V. Stilley, RN, MSN, OCN; Clinical Nurse Specialist, Pain Management/Oncology, Our Lady of Lourdes Medical Center, Camden, New Jersey

Judith Sturgis, RN, BSN, CIC; Director of Infection Control, Calvert Memorial Hospital, Prince Frederick, Maryland

Debera Jane Thomas, DNS, ANP; Associate Professor, Florida Atlantic University College of Nursing, Boca Raton, Florida

Connie Visovsky, RN, MS, ACNP; University Hospitals of Cleveland, Cleveland, Ohio

M. Linda Workman, PhD, RN, FAAN; Associate Professor of Nursing, Frances Payne Bolton School of Nursing, Case Western Reserve University, Cleveland, Ohio

Reviewer List

Marianne Adam, RN, MSN; St. Luke's Hospital, Bethlehem, Pennsylvania

Jeanette Adams, ADCN, APN, DrPH; University of Texas–Houston, Houston, Texas

Janice Allen, RN, MS, CNOR; University of Arizona College of Nursing, Tucson, Arizona

Lisa K. Anderson-Shaw, RNC, MSN, MA; University of Illinois at Chicago, Chicago, Illinois

Linda Craig Baker, RNC, MSN, FNP; Scottsdale Community College, Phoenix Children's Hospital, Phoenix, Arizona

Sharon Beasley, RN, MSN; Rend Lake College, Ina, Illinois

Barbara J. Benz, RN, MS; Roswell Park Cancer Institute, Buffalo, New York

Madalyn A. Biggs, RN, BSN; Johns Hopkins Hospital, Baltimore, Maryland

Phyllis Ann Bonham, RN, MSN, CCRN; University of North Carolina; North Carolina Jaycee Burn Center, Chapel Hill, North Carolina

Kennith Culp, PhD, RN, CS; University of Iowa, College of Nursing, Iowa City, Iowa

Maria Piccolo-Cvach, RN, MS, CCRN, ACLS; Johns Hopkins Hospital, Baltimore, Maryland

Sharon L. Daut, RN, MS; Erie Community College–North, Williamsville, New York

Karen Keady Davis, RN, MS, CCRN; Johns Hopkins Hospital, Baltimore, Maryland

Carrie Dowdy, MSN, RNC; Piedmont Virginia Community College, Charlottesville, Virginia

Julie Doyon, BScN, MScN; University of Ottawa, Ottawa, Ontario, Canada

Cathy Eddy, MSN, RN, CCRN; University of South Dakota; Rapid City Outreach, Rapid City, South Dakota

Barbara Fitzsimmons, RN, MS, CNRN; Johns Hopkins Hospital, Baltimore, Maryland

Nancy Nightingale Gillespie, PhD, PHN II, RN; Saint Francis College, Fort Wayne, Indiana

Mary Ann Goetz, MS, BSN, RN, CANP; Ohio University, Zanesville, Ohio

Margaret J. Greene, EdD, RN; Fairleigh Dickinson University, Teaneck, New Jersey

Elisabeth Greenfield, RN, MSN, CCRN; U.S. Army Institute of Surgical Research, Fort Sam Houston, Texas

Susan J. Hart, MSN, RN, CS, CCRN; Seton Hall University College of Nursing, South Orange, New Jersey

Janie Heath, MS, RN, CS, CCRN, ANP, ACNP; Veterans Administration Medical Center; Medical College of Georgia School of Nursing, Augusta, Georgia

Gale Hess, RN, MS; Mayo Medical Center, Rochester, Minnesota

Robin R. Higley, RN, MS, CNA; Fairview Hospital, Cleveland, Ohio

Sr. Esther Holzbauer, BS, MSN, RN, ANAC; Mount Marty College, Yankton, South Dakota

Renée S. Hyde, RN, MSN, CNRN; Carolinas College of Health Sciences, Charlotte, North Carolina

Mary Jane Jones, RN, BSN, MN; Henderson Community College, Henderson, Kentucky

David R. Johnson, DNSc, RN, CS; Saint Francis College, Fort Wayne, Indiana

Lorene M. Kimzey, RNC, MEd; National Institutes of Health, Bethesda, Maryland

Donna Lee Kistler, RN, MS; University of California–Davis Medical Center, Sacramento, California

Pamela Sue Laughlin, RN, AD; W.S. Major Hospital, Shelbyville, Indiana

Jean Marie Lucas, RN, BSN, CEN; Johns Hopkins Hospital, Baltimore, Maryland

Suzanne K. Marnocha, RN, MSN, CCRN; University of Wisconsin, Oshkosh, College of Nursing, Oshkosh, Wisconsin

Michel S. Martin, RN; Mayo Medical Center, Rochester, Minnesota

Lisa J. Massarweh, RN, MSN, CCRN; Kent State University, Ashtabula, Ohio

viii Reviewer List

Eileen McMyler, RN, MS; Mayo Medical Center, Rochester, Minnesota

Wilma Kathleen Mechsner, MN, RN, CFNP; Molina Medical Center, Palmdale, California

Christine Cloutier Mihal, RN, MS; Fairleigh Dickinson University, Teaneck, New Jersey

David K. Miller, RNC, BSN, MSEd; W.S. Major Hospital, Shelbyville, Indiana

Liana Marie Mosier, RN, BSN, MS; Evergreen Valley College, San Jose, California

Carla L. Mueller, MS, RN; Saint Francis College, Fort Wayne, Indiana

Erin E. Mullins-Rivera, PhDc, RN; Saint Francis College, Fort Wayne, Indiana

Kay B. O'Neil, MSN, RN; El Centro Community College, Dallas Texas

Patricia A. O'Neill, RN, MSN, CCRN; De Anza College, Cupertino, California

Ann Marie Palatnik, MSN, CS; Our Lady of Lourdes Medical Center, Camden, New Jersey

Kathleen M. Parsons, RN, MS, CCRN, CS; Physicians Memorial Hospital, La Plata, Maryland

Diana Lee Reding, RN, BS, MS, ACLS; Dallas County Community College District; El Centro College, Parkland Memorial Hospital, Dallas, Texas

Beverly M. Reynolds, RN, BSN, MBA; Johns Hopkins Hospital, Baltimore, Maryland

Anne G. Russo, RN, MSN, DNSc; University of Alabama at Birmingham, Birmingham, Alabama

Margaret Skulnick, ANP, CDE; Durham Technical Community College, Durham, North Carolina

Cynthia C. Small, RN, MSN; Lake Michigan College, Benton Harbor, Michigan

Carol J. Stockinger, RN, MS, BSN, ACLS; St. Mary's Hospital, Mayo Foundation, Rochester, Minnesota

Martha E. Summers, RN, MSN, FNPc; West Virginia University, Morgantown, West Virginia

Kay I. Swiger, RNc, MN; University of South Carolina–York Technical College, Rock Hill, South Carolina

Tina Tiburzi, RN, BSN, MBA; Johns Hopkins Hospital, Baltimore, Maryland

Kuei-Shen Tu, RN, MSN; University of Alabama at Birmingham, Birmingham, Alabama

Marilyn J. Vontz, RN, BS, MA, MSN, PhD; Bryan Memorial Hospital, Lincoln, Nebraska

Judith P. Warner, BSN, RN; Crawford County Practical Nursing Program, Meadville, Pennsylvania; Forestview Skilled Nursing Center, Erie, Pennsylvania

Meg Wilson, MS, RN; Saint Francis College, Fort Wayne, Indiana

Cynthia B. Wolfer, RN, MSN, ONC; Tacoma Community College, Tacoma, Washington

Preface

The first edition of this text, titled *Medical-Surgical Nursing: A Nursing Process Approach,* found widespread acclaim as the medical-surgical nursing text of the 1990s. The second edition built on that achievement and further solidified the text's position. Now, with the publication of the third edition, a title change signals the text's focus on the changing nature of nursing and health care as we prepare to enter the 21st century.

The title *Medical-Surgical Nursing Across the Health Care Continuum* was carefully chosen to reflect an emphasis on collaborative care and continuing care that extend beyond the hospital setting into the community and home. Our goal has been to ensure that the book you hold today is as current and as accessible as possible to help nursing students provide state-of-the-art health care in today's—and tomorrow's—rapidly evolving health care system.

Medical-Surgical Nursing Across the Health Care Continuum embraces collaborative, interdisciplinary client care in a variety of health care settings. This revision provides expanded coverage of women's health issues, transcultural care, and special needs of the elderly. Case management and managed care concepts are interwoven throughout to help the reader understand these new emerging roles and variables. Simple, but effective, complementary therapies that nurses can use to relieve pain and manage chronic illness are also discussed. Finally, critical thinking is promoted through case studies with questions provided at the end of most chapters.

Clinical Currency and Comprehensiveness

To ensure the text's currency, accuracy, and comprehensiveness, we listened to the readers of the first two editions—their impressions of and experiences with the text. We also listened to experts' opinions on the current state of nursing and the health care system and trends that are driving change. Based on this input, we formulated our revision plan. We assembled a team of clinical experts to revise, rewrite, and in some cases draft entirely new chapters. We then commissioned in-depth reviews of each chapter by clinicians and instructors from across the United States and Canada, using their reviews to guide us in revising the chapters into their final form.

The results are reflected in the third edition's strong, consistent focus on pathophysiology, collaborative care, and continuing care; foundation of relevant nursing research; and emphasis on the critical "need to know" information that nurses must master to provide safe, effective care.

Ease of Access

To make the text as easy to use as possible, we maintained the second edition's approach of smaller chapters of more uniform length. The third edition now has 80 chapters, including new chapters on complementary therapies, continuing care, managed care and case management, and infusion therapy. We also maintained the second edition's unit structure, with vital body systems (cardiovascular, respiratory, and neurologic) appearing earlier in the book. In these three units, we also maintained the approach of providing critical care content in separate chapters on managing critically ill clients with coronary artery disease, respiratory problems, and neurologic problems. Within each chapter, we carefully edited to ensure maximum readability for all levels of students. To help break up long blocks of text and also highlight key information, we included numerous headings, bulleted lists, tables, charts, and in-text highlights. We end each chapter with Selected Bibliography (with classic sources noted by an asterisk*) and Suggested Readings lists.

One of the most obvious changes in the third edition is the new full-color design. Color is used not only in the photographs and drawings, enhancing their usefulness as learning tools, but also in the design of the text itself to help distinguish key features and clarify chapter organization.

A Collaborative Approach

As in the previous two editions, we take a collaborative approach to client care. We believe that in the real world of health care, nurses, clients, physicians, and other health care providers share responsibility for the management of client problems. Thus, we present client care in a *collaborative management* framework. In this framework, we make no artificial distinctions between medical treatment and nursing care—instead, we cover the entire range of approaches that health care providers of all disciplines take in dealing with client problems.

Nonetheless, because this text is first and foremost a *nursing* text, we organize discussion of client problems and their management using a *nursing process* approach. Discussions of key disorders follow the full nursing process format, with the following structure:

DISORDER

Overview
   Pathophysiology
   Etiology
   Incidence/Prevalence

Collaborative Management

 Assessment

 Analysis
   Common Nursing Diagnoses/Collaborative
      Problems
   Additional Nursing Diagnoses/Collaborative
      Problems

 Planning and Implementation
   Nursing Diagnoses/Collaborative Problems
   Planning: Expected Outcomes
   Interventions

 Continuing Care
   Health Teaching
   Home Care Management
   Health Care Resources

 Evaluation

Discussions of other disorders, while not given this complete subhead structure, nonetheless follow the same basic format: a discussion of the disorder itself, including pertinent pathophysiology, etiology, and incidence information, followed by a section on collaborative management of clients with the disorder.

Integral to this collaborative management approach is a clear delineation of just who is responsible for what. When a responsibility is primarily the nurse's, the text says so. When a decision must be made jointly by the client, nurse, physician, and therapist, this is clearly stated. When different health care providers in different care settings might be involved in the client's care, this is stated, too.

Multinational, Multicultural, Multigenerational Focus

Reflecting the increasing diversity of our society in general and the health care system in particular, *Medical-Surgical Nursing Across the Health Care Continuum* includes a number of special features.

To address the needs of American and Canadian readers, we have included examples of trade names of drugs available in the United States and drugs available in Canada. A maple leaf icon identifies the Canadian trade names.

To help nurses provide quality care for clients whose race, culture, or ethnic background differs from their own, numerous *Transcultural Considerations* throughout the text highlight important aspects of culturally competent care.

Increased life expectancy means a steadily increasing elderly population. To help nurses prepare for this trend, the third edition features expanded coverage of the care of elderly clients. This edition includes a greater number of *Nursing Focus on the Elderly* charts and highlights laboratory values and drug dosages typical for elderly clients. Charts specifying normal physiologic changes to expect in the elderly are included in each assessment chapter. In addition, highlighted *Elderly Considerations* presented throughout the text emphasize key points to consider when caring for these clients.

Also appearing throughout the text, *Women's Health Considerations* address topics of concern to female clients and their health care providers. Specifically, this feature highlights gender-related differences in assessment parameters and in the incidence, severity, treatment, or expected client responses to health problems.

Organization

The 80 chapters of *Medical-Surgical Nursing Across the Health Care Continuum* are grouped into 16 distinct units. Unit 1, Health Promotion and Illness, lays the groundwork for the health care concepts incorporated throughout the text. It includes new chapters on integration of care across the health care continuum (Chapter 2), case management and managed care (Chapter 3), and complementary, holistic therapies (Chapter 4). Unit 2 covers specific biopsychosocial concepts, including pain, stress, and sexuality. Unit 3 comprises six chapters on the management of clients with fluid, electrolyte, and acid-base imbalances. This unit includes a new chapter on infusion therapy (Chapter 17).

Unit 4 presents the perioperative nursing content that medical-surgical nurses need to know. This content provides a solid foundation to help the student better understand the coverage of specific surgeries throughout the remainder of the text. Unit 5 provides core content on health problems related to immune system function. This content includes normal inflammation and the immune response, altered cell development and growth, and interventions for clients with connective tissue disease, AIDS, and other immunologic disorders, cancers, and infections.

The remaining 11 units cover medical-surgical content by body system. Each of these units begins with a chapter on assessment and then continues with one or more chapters on interventions for clients with specific health problems related to the subject body system.

Pedagogical Features

The third edition includes various features to help the student quickly identify and retain key information and to serve as study aids:

- At the beginning of each chapter, a list of *Chapter Highlights* provides a guide to the chapter's contents and organization.
- *Nursing Care Highlight* charts emphasize important "hands-on" nursing care.
- *Nursing Focus on the Elderly* charts highlight normal age-related changes that affect nursing care and specify the individualized care that nurses need to provide to elderly clients with specific conditions or undergoing specific procedures.
- Written in "client-friendly" language, *Education Guide* charts provide the kind of instructions that nurses must learn to provide to clients and their families to help them cope with life changes caused by illness.
- *Health Promotion Guide* charts, also written in client-oriented language, give examples of instructions that nurses can provide to help clients and their families prevent illness and maintain optimum health.
- *Laboratory Profile* charts summarize important information on laboratory tests commonly ordered to evaluate health problems. Information typically includes normal ranges of laboratory values (including differences for elderly clients, when appropriate) and the possible significance of abnormal findings.
- *Drug Therapy* charts summarize important information about commonly used drugs. These charts include U.S. and Canadian trade names, usual dosages (including dosages for elderly clients, as appropriate), and nursing interventions with rationales.
- *Key Features* charts highlight the clinical manifestations of important disorders.
- *Research Applications for Nursing* boxes, provided in nearly every chapter, give synopses of recent nursing research articles and other scientific articles applicable to nursing. Each box provides a summary of the article, a brief critique, and a summary of possible implications for nursing practice. The goal of this feature is to help the student identify the strengths and weaknesses of the research and see how research can help guide nursing practice.
- A selection of representative *Client Care Plans* provides detailed plans of nursing care for specific client problems.
- Various *Clinical Pathways* provide examples of how hospitals are implementing a collaborative approach to client care.
- Included at the end of most chapters, a *Case Study* presents a brief clinical scenario and poses pertinent questions designed to stimulate critical thinking.
- To further guide students in locating important information, a list of *Resources*—including Internet resources—is included in an appendix.

Complete Teaching and Learning Package

A full complement of companion, or ancillary, publications accompany *Medical-Surgical Nursing Across the Health Care Continuum,* providing a complete teaching and learning package for both instructors and students.

Every effort has been made to correlate content among these ancillary publications and to focus the content on a set of core concepts developed specifically for this purpose. An editor of this text has been involved in writing each of the ancillaries to ensure consistency and cohesion with the text itself.

Resources for instructors include an *Instructor's Manual, Test Manual, ExaMaster,* and *LectureView.* The *Instructor's Manual,* written by Elaine Kennedy, an expert in cooperative learning, and Donna Ignatavicius, is a truly groundbreaking educational ancillary. It provides content on how to promote collaborative or cooperative learning with features never before presented in any comparable instructor's manual, including critical learning outcomes, suggested learning activities, and a list of supplemental resources arranged in a unique three-column format. Learning activities that involve group work are included, as are time frames for learning and strategies for promoting active learning, including aspects of teaching/learning via distance education. Supplemental resources, which foster independent exploration, include transparency masters, Internet resources, and materials from community organizations. Numerous graphic organizers are provided, including concept maps, algorithms, team concept maps, and sequence chains to assist students in making connections among isolated pieces of information and to encourage them to assemble the puzzle of today's complex health care system. The focus of content is on the Core Concepts Grids, which are provided for each unit and serve as the basis for material presented therein. Also provided are answer guidelines for the questions posed in the case studies that appear in the text.

A printed *Test Manual* and a computerized *ExaMaster* provide instructors with more than 1,500 completely new test questions coded for correct answer, rationale, and cognitive level. These questions, prepared by M. Linda Workman, have been written in response to feedback from the market to be both more challenging and reflective of the scope of questions on the NCLEX examination. Most are application-based questions, and only about 10 percent are knowledge-level or comprehension-level questions. Questions were written focusing on the Core Concepts Grids presented in the *Instructor's Manual* and the *Critical Thinking Study Guide.* The *ExaMaster,* now on CD-ROM, allows the instructor to generate comprehensive tests by selecting questions based on instructor-chosen criteria.

Representing a quantum leap from the former acetate transparencies, *LectureView,* a new CD-ROM presentation program, includes 500 full-color images from the text with slide copy for projection in the classroom. This PowerPoint-compatible ancillary allows the instructor to provide lecture material and key illustrations, using powerful new classroom presentation software.

For students, the *Critical Thinking Study Guide* provides material to enhance learning in various formats to promote mastery of the text. Echoing one of the text's themes, the study guide emphasizes questions aimed at enhancing critical thinking skills. The guide was written by Elaine Kennedy and Donna Ignatavicius in conjunction with the *Instructor's Manual* to ensure consistency. Its focus is also on the Core Concepts Grids in the *Instructor's Manual,* which are also included here for student review.

The *Pocket Companion for Medical-Surgical Nursing,* authored by Donna Ignatavicius and Kathy Hausman, retains the alphabetical format that proved so popular in the first two editions. It also includes extensive cross-referencing to help the student access vital information quickly.

In summary, we feel that *Medical-Surgical Nursing Across the Health Care Continuum* and its teaching-learning package provide all of the resources needed by students preparing to meet the challenge of practicing nursing in the 21st century.

Donna D. Ignatavicius
M. Linda Workman
Mary A. Mishler

Acknowledgments

Publishing a textbook of this depth and breadth would not be possible without the combined efforts of many people. Our contributors provided consistently excellent manuscripts in a timely fashion. Our reviewers, expert clinicians and instructors from around the United States and Canada, provided invaluable suggestions and encouragement throughout the book's development.

The staff of the W.B. Saunders Company once again provided us with crucial guidance and support throughout the planning, writing, revision, and production of the third edition. In particular, two Senior Editors—first Barbara Nelson Cullen, followed by Robin Carter—kept us on schedule and encouraged us every step of the way. Senior Developmental Editor Kevin Law—with the invaluable assistance of Senior Developmental Editor Lee Henderson; Assistant Developmental Editors Rachel Hubbs and Marie Pelcin; Editorial Assistants Beth Dean, Ross Landy, and Amelia Cullinan; and freelance developmental editors Neal Fandek, Marian Sandmaier, and Debra Osnowitz—helped us translate our conceptual vision into a consistently formatted and pedagogically sound reality.

W.B. Saunders Copy Editors Blair Davis and Scott Filderman, aided by freelance copy editors Mary McCoy and Debra Adleman, assumed the monumental task of checking all of the text's editorial details and ensuring consistency throughout. They did an outstanding job. Other W.B. Saunders staff deserving special thanks include Production Managers Laurie Sanders and Peter Faber, Illustration Coordinator Lisa Lambert, Marketing Manager Jean Rodenberger, and Marketing Assistant Linda Lee.

Creating a new, full-color design and art program for a major textbook is a enormous undertaking. Our thanks go to W.B. Saunders Designer Gene Harris for the text's clean yet visually arresting design; Academy Artworks for the hundreds of wonderful line drawings; and Rick Williams and John Workman for the clear, instructive color photographs.

Contents

UNIT 7: Problems of Cardiac Output and Tissue Perfusion: Management of Clients with Problems of the Cardiovascular System 713

35. Assessment of the Cardiovascular System 715
Kathleen Ouimet Perrin
Anatomy and Physiology Review 715
History 724
Physical Assessment 728
Psychosocial Assessment 735
Diagnostic Assessment 736

36. Interventions for Clients with Dysrhythmias 753
Carmen J. Petrin
Review of Cardiac Electrophysiology 753
Cardiac Conduction System 755
Electrocardiography 756
Normal Rhythms 763
Dysrhythmias 764

37. Interventions for Clients with Cardiac Problems 807
Kathleen Ouimet Perrin
Heart Failure 807
Valvular Heart Disease 821
Mitral Stenosis 821
Mitral Regurgitation (Insufficiency) 822
Mitral Valve Prolapse 822
Aortic Stenosis 822
Aortic Regurgitation (Insufficiency) 822
Inflammations and Infections 827
Infective Endocarditis 827
Pericarditis 830
Rheumatic Carditis 832
Cardiomyopathy 832

38. Interventions for Clients with Vascular Problems 837
Suzanne Cushman Beyea
Arteriosclerosis and Atherosclerosis 837
Hypertension 843
Peripheral Arterial Disease 852
Acute Peripheral Arterial Occlusion 860
Aneurysms 866
Aneurysms of the Peripheral Arteries 870
Aortic Dissection 870
Buerger's Disease 870
Subclavian Steal 871
Thoracic Outlet Syndrome 871
Raynaud's Phenomenon 872
Popliteal Entrapment 872
Venous Thrombosis 872
Venous Insufficiency 876
Varicose Veins 878

Phlebitis 878
Vascular Trauma 879

39. Interventions for Clients with Shock 881
M. Linda Workman
Overview 881
Collaborative Management of Hypovolemic Shock 888
Collaborative Management of Sepsis-Induced Distributive Shock 893

40. Interventions for Critically Ill Clients with Coronary Artery Disease 901
Kathleen Ouimet Perrin
Angina Pectoris 902
Myocardial Infarction 902

UNIT 8: Management of Clients with Problems of the Hematologic System 933

41. Assessment of the Hematologic System 935
M. Linda Workman
Anatomy and Physiology Review 935
History 942
Physical Assessment 943
Psychosocial Assessment 945
Diagnostic Assessment 946

42. Interventions for Clients with Hematologic Problems 951
Susan M. Schneider
Red Blood Cell Disorders 951
Anemia 951
Anemias Resulting from Increased Destruction of Red Blood Cells 951
Sickle Cell Disease 951
Glucose-6-Phosphate Dehydrogenase Deficiency Anemia 957
Immunohemolytic Anemia 957
Anemias Resulting from Decreased Production of Red Blood Cells 958
Iron Deficiency Anemia 958
Vitamin B$_{12}$ Deficiency Anemia 958
Folic Acid Deficiency Anemia 959
Aplastic Anemia 960
Polycythemia 960
Polycythemia Vera 960
White Blood Cell Disorders 961
Leukemia 961
Malignant Lymphoma 978
Hodgkin's Lymphoma 978
Non-Hodgkin's Lymphoma 979
Coagulation Disorders 980
Platelet Disorders 980
Autoimmune Thrombocytopenic Purpura 981

Guide to Special Features

TRANSCULTURAL CONSIDERATIONS

WOMEN'S HEALTH CONSIDERATIONS

NURSING FOCUS ON THE ELDERLY CHARTS

FOCUSED ASSESSMENT CHARTS

LABORATORY PROFILE CHARTS

DRUG THERAPY CHARTS

EDUCATION GUIDE CHARTS

HEALTH PROMOTION GUIDE CHARTS

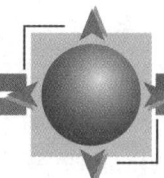

UNIT 1

Health Promotion

and Illness

Chapter 1

MEDICAL-SURGICAL NURSING AND THE ROLE OF THE MEDICAL-SURGICAL NURSE

CHAPTER HIGHLIGHTS

Medical-surgical nursing is a quickly changing specialty practice that is influenced by increasing knowledge about disease etiology, rapid advances in technology, reform of the health care system, and trends in health promotion and protection. A major focus of medical-surgical nursing is to promote well-being and prevent complications of illness and disease.

HEALTH

Beliefs about health and illness are a major feature of every known culture. How one views himself or herself as a person and as a part of the environment affects how health is defined. Health is often viewed as a continuum on which optimal wellness, at one end, is the highest level of function, and illness, at the other end, results in death (Fig. 1–1). Every person is somewhere on the continuum. As one's health state changes, the location on the continuum changes.

Although the term *health* is used every day, no universally accepted definition has been established. Over time, the focus and expression of health have varied, depending on knowledge, theories, and beliefs. Some people have

viewed health and disease as reward or punishment for their actions. Others have considered health as a soundness or wholeness of the body.

Definitions of Health

A typical dictionary may define health in terms of a person's ability to function in society. Some definitions also describe health as a disease-free state or condition. Definitions such as these do not make clear what constitutes health and illness and seem to present an "either/or" situation—that is, a person is either healthy or ill.

World Health Organization Definition of Health

As science has progressed, the definition of health has evolved. One of the most frequently quoted definitions is the one presented in 1947 by the World Health Organization (WHO). WHO stated that health is "a state of complete physical, mental, and social well-being and not merely the absence of disease or infirmity" (WHO, 1947, p. 1). Thus, according to WHO, to be healthy a person

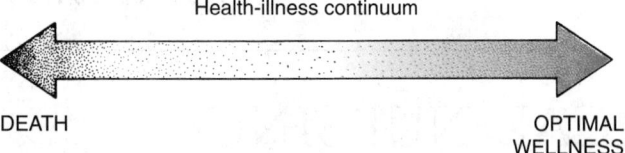

Health-illness continuum

DEATH   OPTIMAL WELLNESS

Figure 1–1. Common concept of health as a continuum ranging from optimal wellness at one end to illness culminating in death at the other end.

must be in a state of well-being physically, mentally, and socially. Health professionals have found this concept problematic because achieving a state of "health" seems to be an unrealistic goal. This definition does not allow for degrees of health or illness, and it fails to reflect the dynamic, ever-changing nature of health.

A concept related to health is *homeostasis,* or internal equilibrium or balance. When a person experiences a disturbance in homeostasis, he or she is considered to be "unhealthy." Like the WHO definition of health, this concept is losing popularity because "stasis" implies an unchanging state, and most theorists today believe that health is always changing.

Sociologic Definitions of Health

Sociologists view health as a condition that allows for the pursuit and enjoyment of desired cultural values. Studies that have polled laypeople for their definitions of health concur that health is the absence of symptoms and a feeling of well-being. "Good health" includes the ability to carry out "normal," daily activities, such as going to work and performing household chores.

Holistic Health

A term frequently used when health and wellness are discussed is *holistic health.* The holistic view considers the body, mind, and spirit as interrelated parts of a person's being. The concept of high-level wellness, which consid-

ers the needs of the whole person, has led to the growth of holistic health care. Holistic health focuses on promoting health and preventing illness, with emphasis on the person's responsibility to achieve high-level wellness. There is also concern with bringing the person's mind, body, and spirit into harmony with the environment. Various complementary therapies, sometimes referred to as alternative medicine practices, have been used for many years to promote mind-body-spirit harmony. Chapter 4 describes some commonly used therapies and how they can be incorporated into medical-surgical nursing practice.

Definition of Health Used in This Book

In this text, health is defined as a person's level of wellness. This level of wellness is a process in which a person is striving to attain his or her full potential. Health reflects one's biological, psychological, and sociologic state (Fig. 1–2). The *biological* (physical) state refers to the structure of body tissues and organs as well as to the biochemical interactions and functions within the body. The *psychological* state includes a person's mood, emotions, and personality. The *sociologic* (social) state involves the interaction between a person and the environment. *Spiritual health* is sometimes considered as part of sociologic health but may be described as a separate aspect of one's overall health state.

Factors that affect a person's biological, psychological, or social well-being require additional energy and thus alter the level of wellness. Therefore, a high level of wellness is achieved when one's biopsychosocial needs are met.

One of nursing's primary functions is to assist clients in reaching a high level of wellness. Understanding the concept of health and high-level wellness is therefore essential. As nurses assess clients, they must be aware of factors that affect a person's health state and must use nursing interventions to promote and maintain an optimal level of wellness (Fig. 1–3).

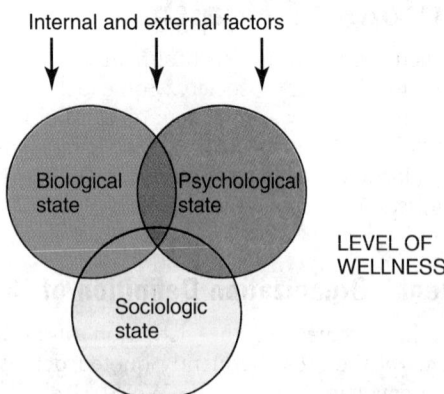

Figure 1–2. Textbook definition of health—one's biological, psychological, and sociologic state. Internal and external factors affect a person's level of wellness.

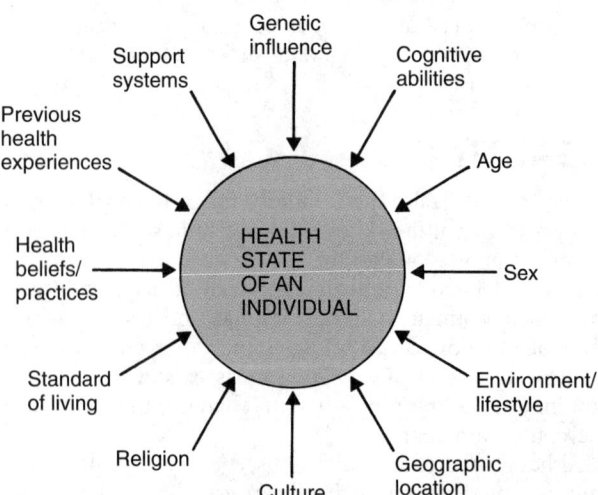

Figure 1–3. Multiple variables influence health and illness.

HEALTH PROMOTION

Health promotion refers to activities that are directed toward developing a person's resources to maintain or enhance well-being as a protection against illness. Reversing the emphasis from curing a disease to promoting health provides a more positive orientation for health care. Illness no longer needs to be the primary focus of health care. In addition, illness care is much more expensive than promoting health.

The U.S. Department of Health and Human Services (1990) joined the world mission to promote health in its "Healthy People 2000" campaign. The expectation was that by the year 2000 people would be healthier and practicing healthier lifestyles. In particular, the agenda calls for health care access for everyone, a longer life expectancy, and equal life expectancy for people of all cultures. At present, some ethnic groups in the United States (especially Hispanics, African/Americans, and Asian Americans and Pacific Islanders) have shorter life expectancies than others.

TRANSCULTURAL CONSIDERATIONS

The demographic profile of the U.S. population is rapidly changing. Whereas the African-American population is currently the largest nonwhite ethnic group in the country, by the year 2010 the Hispanic population will outnumber African-Americans. The Census Bureau projects that by the year 2000, 11% of the population will be Hispanic, for a total of 31 million people. People of Mexican origin make up the largest subgroup. Access to health care, lifestyle, and environmental factors affect the health of Hispanics. Among adults, heart disease, diabetes mellitus, cancer, and liver disease are much higher in Hispanics than in non-Hispanic whites (Castillo & Torres, 1995). Many Hispanics use "folk healing" remedies because they are more available, affordable, and user friendly. Chapter 4 describes some of these nontraditional health practices.

Nearly a third of African-Americans live in poverty, compared with 11% of Caucasians. Cancer, heart disease, and acquired immune deficiency syndrome (AIDS) lead to higher mortality rates among African-Americans compared with Caucasians. This is partly because many African-Americans lack access to health care and have a reluctance to seek health promotion care, especially primary prevention and early detection (Douglas, 1995).

Asian-Americans and Pacific Islanders (AAPIs) presently represent between 3% and 4% of the U.S. population, but that number is expected to jump to 11% by the year 2050 (Louie, 1995). Chen and Hawks (1995) reported that the mortality rates for AAPIs with lung cancer and cardiovascular disease will probably exceed those of other ethnic groups in 20 years. In addition, the prevalence of hepatitis B and tuberculosis is higher among AAPIs than among any other ethnic group. Like Hispanics, many AAPIs lack access to health care and have lifestyle and environmental factors that influence their health status. Beliefs about health and illness for AAPIs are strongly guided by religion (Louie, 1995).

WOMEN'S HEALTH CONSIDERATIONS

Historically, women's health issues have not been studied, especially for women of color (non-Caucasian). Recent interest in women's health has shown that many women in the United States do not receive necessary health care; have many undetected, treatable problems; and experience long-lasting effects of abuse. Women of color are more likely to be poor and uninsured when compared with Caucasian women. All women are at serious risk of heart disease, lung cancer, and osteoporosis, and they lack the knowledge about how to prevent these health problems (Allen & Phillips, 1997).

Today, the National Institutes of Health strongly support research on women's health. Throughout this book, women's health considerations are highlighted, as appropriate, and research on women's health issues is included when possible.

Several nursing theorists have developed nursing health promotion models. One of the best-known models is that advocated by Pender. In her model, Pender (1987) makes a distinction between health promotion and illness prevention: Health promotion is not "health problem–specific," but prevention (sometimes called health protection) is. In addition, Pender believes that health promotion is a positive activity, whereas illness prevention is an avoidance activity.

Although this text integrates illness prevention with health promotion, it recognizes that the two concepts are somewhat different. The goal of both types of activities, explained later, is to improve or maintain the client's health. Throughout this text, Health Promotion Guide charts help the nurse in teaching clients about health promotion activities.

Part of the health promotion movement in nursing is reflected in the use of the term *client* rather than *patient*. Whereas the word *patient* is associated with a dependent position in a hospital, the word *client* suggests an active partnership in the process of health care delivery and maintenance in any setting. *Client* is therefore the term used for the health care consumer in this text.

Practices to Promote Health

Researchers have found certain health practices to have a positive correlation with health promotion in adults. Some of these general health practices include

- Eating well-balanced meals that incorporate foods from the food pyramid, as recommended (see Fig. 64–1)
- Moderate eating to maintain ideal weight and prevent obesity
- Moderate exercising on a routine schedule
- Sleeping regularly, about 7 to 8 hours each day
- Limiting consumption of alcohol to a moderate amount
- Not smoking
- Keeping exposure to the sun to a minimum

These practices have been associated with high-level wellness regardless of sex, age, or economic status. The greater the number of these practices followed in a consistent, routine manner, the better the health state.

Practices to Prevent Illness

Illness prevention is related to health promotion and maintenance. In an effort to decrease the occurrence of illness, prevention is essential. Preventive health behavior is described as voluntary action taken by a person or group to decrease the potential or actual threat of illness and its harmful consequences. As mentioned earlier, some ethnic groups are not focused on health promotion activities, especially prevention and early detection. Throughout this text, where appropriate, these transcultural considerations are discussed.

People must be motivated and educated to make health-related changes. Three levels of illness prevention are summarized in Table 1–1: primary, secondary, and tertiary.

Primary Prevention

Primary prevention is used to avoid or delay the actual occurrence of a specific disease. Strategies for health maintenance raise the general level of health and well-being of a person, family, or community. Smoking cessation clinics, immunizations, use of seat belts, and use of helmets by motorcyclists are examples of primary prevention strategies.

Secondary Prevention

The purpose of secondary prevention is early detection of a disease or condition, sometimes before the signs and symptoms are evident. Emphasis is on early diagnosis and treatment as well as on intervention to prevent or limit permanent disability or death. Screening procedures such as the Papanicolaou (Pap) smear for cervical cancer and the purified protein derivative (PPD) skin test for tuberculosis are examples.

Tertiary Prevention

Tertiary prevention involves rehabilitation and begins when the disease or condition has stabilized and no further healing is expected, such as cardiac rehabilitation after a myocardial infarction. The goal is to return the person to the highest level of function and to prevent severe disabilities.

Consumer Education and Awareness

Consumer education and awareness have been the major focus in an attempt to influence people and promote wellness. Information about nutrition, exercise, stress management, and routine health examinations is available at schools, work sites, and community centers and in the media. This abundance of information and materials is a major resource for increasing public awareness of the need for health promotion. The Internet also provides access to a vast amount of public health information. (See Appendix for a list of commonly used web sites.)

ROLE OF THE MEDICAL-SURGICAL NURSE

Medical-surgical nursing is one of the many specialties in nursing, yet its scope is much broader than other specialties such as cardiovascular or orthopedic nursing. In 1991, the Academy of Medical-Surgical Nurses (AMSN) was formed as the first specialty organization for this group of nurses. AMSN has published standards for medical-surgical nursing and a core curriculum. The official journal of the AMSN is *MEDSURG Nursing*.

The focus of medical-surgical nursing is on the adult client with acute or chronic illness in any health care setting. Nurses who specialize in medical-surgical nursing need a broad knowledge of the biological, psychological, and social sciences because of the range of clients for whom they care. The overall outcome of care is similar to that for any other specialty—the achievement of an optimal level of wellness and prevention of illness, as discussed earlier in this chapter.

Medical-surgical clients range in age from 18 years to more than 100 years, and their health problems are usually complex. Because the typical client is usually older than 65 years, medical-surgical nurses need a strong background in *gerontology*, or care of the elderly. In this text, charts entitled Nursing Focus on the Elderly highlight the special nursing interventions that this group of clients requires.

As medical-surgical nursing meets changing health care needs, the expectations for providing client care have expanded and increased. Medical-surgical nurses assume various roles and functions within a number of health

TABLE 1–1

Examples of Health Behaviors for the Three Levels of Illness Prevention	
Level	**Examples of Behaviors**
Primary prevention	• Wearing seat belts, helmets • Eating well-balanced meals • Not smoking • Consuming no or minimal alcohol • Being immunized • Maintaining ideal body weight
Secondary prevention	• Having yearly Papanicolaou (Pap) smear tests • Doing monthly breast or testicular self-examination • Having mammograms as recommended • Getting skin tests for tuberculosis screening • Having routine tonometry tests to detect glaucoma
Tertiary prevention	• Following a cardiac rehabilitation program • Pursuing rehabilitation programs for stroke, head injury, or arthritis

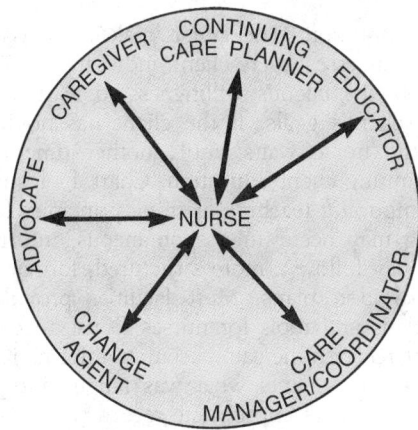

Figure 1–4. Major roles of the medical-surgical nurse.

care settings (Fig. 1–4). Although each role is associated with specific responsibilities, some aspects of each role are interrelated and are common to all nursing positions and specialties.

Care Manager or Coordinator

As a result of health care reform during the 1990s, *managed care* has become the predominant health care delivery system in the United States and other countries. Simply defined, managed care is a system to contain health care costs through a case management process.

Case management targets high-risk, high-cost, complex-problem clients and aims to improve their care by meeting cost-effective clinical outcomes. Most case managers are nurses. Although nurses are not typically taught how to become case managers in their basic education programs, they should learn how to manage and coordinate care. As a *care manager*, the medical-surgical nurse coordinates client care through collaboration with the health care team: The nurse does not provide all of the direct care. Chapter 3 discusses case management, care management, and managed care in more detail.

Caregiver

Another role commonly associated with the medical-surgical nurse is *caregiver*. In this role, nurses assess clients, analyze collected information to determine clients' needs, develop nursing diagnoses and collaborative problems, plan care and carry out the plan with the health team, and evaluate the care given. This process, referred to as the *nursing process* and discussed later, is used throughout this text as an organizational and practice framework.

As a caregiver, the nurse provides physical care through skills such as administering medications and performing comprehensive assessments. Some nursing tasks and activities may be delegated to unlicensed assistive personnel. Throughout this textbook, activities that the nurse may delegate are indicated. The nurse also implements psychosocial interventions, such as encouraging the client to discuss concerns or offering measures to reduce the client's anxiety.

The activities performed by the nurse caregiver are often categorized as *collaborative* (interdependent) or *independent. Collaborative* functions include

- Those mutually determined by the nurse and the physician or other health care team member, such as setting activity limitations or providing a special diet
- Those directed or prescribed by the health care provider (physician, nurse practitioner, or physician's assistant) but requiring nursing judgment to perform, such as giving medications

Independent nursing functions are those initiated and carried out by the nurse without direction from the health care provider. Examples include

- Weighing a client
- Listening to bowel sounds
- Testing blood glucose with a fingerstick

This text discusses both types of functions—collaborative and independent—in an interrelated framework under the heading *Collaborative Management*. Charts entitled Nursing Care Highlights identify the most important nursing care for clients with selected health problems.

Continuing Care Planner

Because health care continues to emphasize early discharge from the hospital, nursing home, and home care, the role of the medical-surgical nurse as continuing care planner has become increasingly important. This process involves an assessment of the client's health needs across the health care continuum. A large part of this process is health teaching and assessment of the home or other setting to which the client is discharged for available resources, support systems, and equipment, if needed.

Continuing care planning may be coordinated by a designated discharge planner employed by the agency in collaboration with the staff nurse, or by a case manager. The discharge planner or case manager is usually a nurse or social worker. If the agency does not employ designated discharge planners, the staff nurse caring for the client is typically responsible for the continuing care planning process. Throughout this text, a section entitled Continuing Care is included to facilitate planning.

Educator

Client education is a major component of medical-surgical nursing care. In collaboration with the interdisciplinary health team, the nurse tries to improve health by providing information on health promotion, disease and illness, and specific treatment. As educators, nurses work with individual clients as well as with family members or other caregivers. The role of education has become increasingly important because clients are discharged "quicker and sicker" from the hospital, subacute unit, or nursing home to their homes. Nurses often become frustrated when they feel that they do not have as much time as they need to teach in these fast-paced settings.

Nursing Care Highlight: Principles of the Adult Teaching-Learning Process

- Assess the client's goals and willingness to learn.
- Before beginning teaching, assess how the client is feeling (e.g., a client in acute pain is unlikely to learn)
- Include family and significant others in teaching as appropriate
- Assess factors that may influence the client's ability or motivation to learn, such as educational level, socioeconomic status, and cultural background
- Provide pictures or other types of visual aids to reinforce learning
- Break complex information or skills into small parts until the client learns them
- Provide the client with "hands-on" experience for psychomotor skills, and request a return demonstration by the client (e.g., insulin administration, dressing change, colostomy care)
- Provide the client with a health resource contact for follow-up questions or concerns

The Teaching-Learning Process

Before educating clients, the nurse, in collaboration with members of the health care team, assesses the client's learning needs. A client with a disease of 20 years' duration may need as much teaching as one who has a newly diagnosed condition. The nurse makes no assumptions but instead assesses each client individually. The nurse also assesses the client's willingness to learn and determines the client's goals. If the client has no interest in learning, the nurse waits until another time or setting before beginning client education. Chart 1–1 summarizes the most important teaching-learning principles for adults.

Teaching may occur in a spontaneous, informal manner, or it may follow a more structured, formal approach based on written plans. Most facilities provide written teaching plans and tools for nurses to use to ensure that every client receives the same accurate information.

The nurse documents what was taught and what the client learned on the appropriate record (Fig. 1–5). Some health care agencies use a lay version of the clinical pathway (discussed later in this chapter), which outlines care in a sequential manner for the client. A summary of the teaching-learning process for each client generally becomes a part of the client's medical record. A copy is also given to the client or family member or significant other at the time of discharge. Each Continuing Care section within this text includes a section entitled Health Teaching. Education Guides for teaching clients are also included as appropriate throughout the text.

Factors Affecting the Teaching-Learning Process

As interdisciplinary team members assess the teaching-learning needs of each client, they evaluate many factors.

Teaching-Learning Record for Insulin Self-Administration			
Client Steps	Taught/Demonstrated (Initial)	Date	Return Demonstration (Initial)
1. Selects correct insulin type.			
2. Selects correct syringe.			
3. Cleans top of vial.			
4. Draws up correct insulin amount(s).			
5. Selects appropriate site for injection.			
6. Cleans skin with alcohol swipe.			
7. Uses 90-degree angle when injecting insulin.			

Figure 1–5. A sample teaching-learning record for self-administration of insulin.

Some of the most important factors include the client's educational level, socioeconomic level, support system, age, and transcultural considerations.

Educational Level

The client's educational level directly affects the nurse's plans for teaching. In the United States, it is estimated that more than a third of adults do not have a high school diploma. Consequently, illiteracy in the United States is quite widespread. Information written for the public should therefore not be above the eighth-grade reading level and often needs to be lower. Albright et al. (1996) found that most health education materials are typically written at a level between the 8th and 13th grades (see the Research Applications for Nursing box).

For illiterate clients and those with limited reading skills, the nurse uses other types of visual aids, such as pictures and symbols. When possible, the nurse explains and interprets information for clients rather than merely offering them a booklet or instruction sheet.

▷ Research Applications for Nursing

Reading Level of Education Materials Too High for Most Clients

Albright, J., de Guzman, C., Acebo, P., et al. (1996). Readability of patient education materials: Implications for clinical practice. Applied Nursing Research, 9, 139–143.

The purpose of this nursing study was to examine the readability of education materials at one medical center across four units as well as hospital-wide. A government study reported that 47% of people in the United States lack basic reading skills. Other studies have shown that reported grade completion level is higher than actual reading level.

The results showed that mean readability scores (grade level) ranged from 8.62 for diabetes education materials to 11.37 for surgery education materials. Many of the materials were commercially prepared by manufacturers. Recommendations for the hospital where this study was conducted include

- Provide verbal explanation as well as written materials
- Begin to write new education materials at a sixth-grade reading level
- Inform manufacturers of the high readability levels
- Build a bank of education materials for use in a variety of areas
- Assess the reading level of clients who receive health care at the hospital

Critique. The researchers reviewed a wide variety of educational materials from various suppliers of educational tools. Although they limited their study to one setting, many health care agencies use these same materials and can benefit from the study findings.

Possible nursing implications. Nurses must augment the written client education materials with verbal teaching and provide answers to client questions. For nurses involved in writing educational materials, a fifth- or sixth-grade reading level is most appropriate.

Socioeconomic Level

When teaching clients how to care for themselves at home, the nurse must consider their financial resources. For example, if the client needs to perform muscle-strengthening exercises using small weights, the nurse cannot always expect the client to purchase expensive commercial weights. Instead, the nurse suggests the use of 1- or 2-pound coffee cans or bags, bags of sugar or flour, or similar available household items.

Another concern for the nurse is the cost of required medication, equipment, or supplies. For instance, clients who do not qualify for medical assistance but work for an employer that does not provide group health insurance may not be able to afford the necessary medical items or follow-up care. As part of continuing care planning, the nurse attempts to locate resources, such as community health organizations like the American Cancer Society, that can provide the necessary resources. In addition, clinics that specialize in providing care for working uninsured clients are available in some parts of the United States. Some of these clinics are nurse-managed community centers.

Support Systems

The nurse assesses the client's support systems and should include part or all of these systems in client education. Examples of support systems include families, significant others, churches, and social community clubs and organizations. In general, people tend to be more compliant with their health regimen if they have the encouragement of others. Support is particularly important if the client must follow many lifestyle restrictions. For instance, a farmer who may be accustomed to eating fried foods and red meat may find it difficult to change to a low-fat, low-sodium diet. If the farmer's wife has always been the cook in the home, the nurse includes her in the teaching process to help to ensure compliance with the new dietary restrictions.

Age

Age affects the teaching-learning process as well. An elderly client may take longer than a younger person to process information or may have visual or hearing deficits (Chart 1–2). The nurse provides small amounts of information at one time and checks with the client before proceeding to make sure that he or she has understood. Too much information is difficult to comprehend and absorb and usually results in the client's frustration and noncompliance.

TRANSCULTURAL CONSIDERATIONS

The nurse considers the client's cultural background before teaching. If the client does not clearly understand the nurse's language, the nurse locates resources that can help with the teaching process. For example, many people who emigrated to the United States in the 1940s have attempted to retain their language and culture and not become too "Americanized." As a result, when

---

Chart 1-2

Nursing Focus on the Elderly: Teaching the Older Adult

- Ensure that the client wears glasses or hearing aids if needed
- Be sure that the area for teaching has ample lighting and minimal distraction
- Provide most of the teaching in the morning (after breakfast), before the client becomes too fatigued
- Speak slowly, and provide small amounts of new information at a time
- Ask the client to repeat the information to make sure that he or she has learned it
- Provide written information so that the client can refer to it later if needed

---

they interact with health care professionals, they often cannot understand and need someone to interpret for them.

Another factor to consider during health teaching is the health practices of various cultures. For example, Mexican-Americans, particularly those living near the Mexican border, often use *curandismo,* or folk medicine, because they cannot afford Westernized health care or prefer their own medical traditions. Another reason that these clients avoid the health care system is that they may have limitations in speaking, reading, or writing English or Spanish. The nurse needs to know this information so that she or he can incorporate cultural beliefs and practices into the teaching-learning process.

The nurse also considers spiritual and religious differences. A client whose spiritual beliefs forbid taking medication is not likely to comply with instructions about drug therapy.

Advocate

As a client advocate, the medical-surgical nurse assists the client and family in interpreting information from other health care team members. The nurse offers additional information that the client needs to make decisions about health care. This assistance may include explanations about the implications of the client's decisions about health and ensuring that the client receives appropriate care. For example, a client scheduled for a total knee replacement may not understand that the knee joint will be removed and replaced with a prosthesis. If the nurse determines that the client does not fully understand the operative procedure, he or she notifies the surgeon of the need for additional preoperative education. The nurse reinforces the information even if another health team member has provided it.

Client advocacy is closely associated with the field of ethics. Chapter 7 discusses ethics in detail and illustrates examples of ethical dilemmas that medical-surgical nurses encounter in their practice.

Change Agent

The medical-surgical nurse serves as a change agent within the work setting and within the profession. The role of change agent involves planning and implementing a system to change the client's health-related behaviors. In the work setting, the nurse assesses health behaviors of the client and family to identify those that need altering. The most important factor in this process is to assess the client's readiness to change. If the client is not ready, he or she will not comply with the change and the nurse will be ineffective in this role.

Within the community, medical-surgical nurses serve as role models and assist consumers in bringing about changes to improve the environment, work conditions, or other factors that affect health. Nurses also work together to bring about change through legislation. For example, nurses provide and support bills for legislation that can affect a person's health status, such as those mandating increased hospital stays for clients having mastectomies.

PRACTICE SETTINGS FOR MEDICAL-SURGICAL NURSES

Medical-surgical nurses have opportunities to provide health care in a variety of settings, including hospitals, long-term care facilities, and community-based settings. The hospital setting is described in this chapter. Chapter 2 discusses community-based settings.

Hospitals, or acute care facilities, are the largest employers of nurses; approximately 57% of all nurses work within hospitals. However, this number is declining.

In the United States, the cost of hospital care is usually paid for by third-party payers, or insurers. Medicare Part A (in-hospital coverage), a federal program, pays for most of the care given to people older than 65 years and to any client who is disabled. Private insurers and managed care organizations pay for most or part of the care provided to clients with insurance. State medical assistance programs pay for some of the health care provided for clients of any age who are indigent.

In Canada, all people are entitled to free comprehensive health care for life. In the 1960s, the Canadian government started this system with the belief that health care should be accessible to all Canadian citizens.

There are three general types of inpatient units in most hospital settings:

- Critical care units
- Intermediate care units
- Long-term care units (including subacute units)

Critical Care Units

Critical care units are areas for the intense care of critically ill clients. Examples are surgical or medical intensive care units, shock trauma and "step-down" units, and neurosurgical intensive care units. Emergency and operating departments are also considered critical care areas because of the acute and intense nature of the care provided in these parts of the hospital. Critical care areas require nurses who thrive in crisis situations and work effectively under high stress. Nurses must be highly skilled in making accurate observations of clients' conditions and interpreting findings quickly and correctly. The nurse-to-client ratio in critical care units is typically 1:2.

Intermediate Care Units

Intermediate care units have changed dramatically over the past decade. The clients on these units today are much sicker than those in the past. Examples of intermediate care areas are neuroscience (neurology) units, urology units, and orthopedic units. In hospitals that are too small to separate clients by specialty, intermediate care units provide treatment for a combination of medical and surgical health problems.

Nurses in intermediate care areas must be able to adapt to caring for various types of illness and must be interested in health teaching and discharge planning. As in critical care areas, nurses must also be highly skilled in making accurate assessments and performing technical procedures.

Long-Term Care Units

Long-term care (LTC) units are areas within or adjacent to the hospital in which clients have chronic illnesses or health problems requiring constant care and rehabilitation. Examples are rehabilitation and chronic disease units. Some hospitals also offer a skilled nursing facility (SNF) or subacute unit as part of the in-hospital system. Chapter 2 describes long-term care in detail.

Overview of the Nursing Process

The nursing process is an organized, systematic approach used by medical-surgical nurses to meet the individualized health care needs of their clients, families, and communities. The term *nursing process* emerged in the mid-1960s. As nursing became more recognized and respected as a profession, there was a growing need to define more clearly what nurses do.

Comparison of the Nursing Process with the Scientific Method

The nursing process is a decision-making approach that promotes critical thinking. Critical thinking exercises are found in this text at the end of the body system interventions chapters and in the accompanying *Student Study Guide*.

Many books compare the nursing process with the scientific method of solving problems. The steps are similar in the two approaches as they proceed from identification of the problem to evaluation of the solution. However, one difference is that the scientist identifies the problem first and then collects the data. In contrast, the nurse collects the data first and then determines the problem.

Intuitive Judgment in Nursing Practice

Over the past 20 years, research has shown that nurses sometimes use (and should use) intuitive judgment in clinical practice (Benner & Tanner, 1987). *Intuition* is the ability to understand immediately without using formal analysis and is based on experience and knowledge. Intuition helps the nurse act quickly if necessary, particularly in critical care settings or emergency situations in which he or she must assess the client and intervene at once.

The authors of this book use the nursing process as the organizing framework for its content. We do not believe that the nursing process is merely a technical skill with rules that apply in all situations but rather that nurses need to use intuition as well as a scientific basis for nursing care.

Steps of the Nursing Process

Most literature citations list five steps of the nursing process: assessment, analysis (nursing diagnosis), planning, implementation, and evaluation.

The steps initially are followed in sequence, from assessment to evaluation. However, once the nursing process begins, it is continuous or cyclic (Fig. 1–6). For example, if the client's outcomes are not met on the basis of the initial evaluation, the nurse may need to reassess the client or implement new actions to help the client achieve the desired outcomes. To understand the nursing process as a whole, it is first necessary to briefly review each step and its associated activities. A more detailed discussion of the nursing process may be found in basic nursing textbooks.

 Assessment

Assessment, the first step of the nursing process, is a systematic method of collecting data about the client, family, or community for the purpose of identifying actual and potential health problems. The data base is the organization of assessment data and frequently refers to the tool or chart form used to record the data.

Types of Data Bases. Jarvis (1996) names four kinds of data bases: complete; episodic, or problem-centered; follow-up; and emergency.

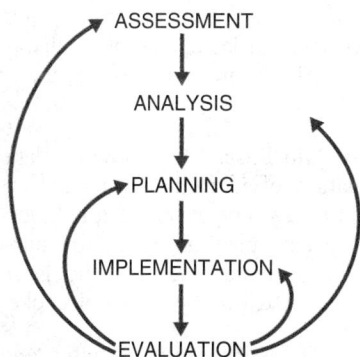

Figure 1–6. The nursing process cycle.

Complete Data Base. The complete, or total, data base includes a thorough health history and physical assessment. In the acute care setting, the data base is usually completed during the first 8 hours after a client's admission to the hospital. In the home, the nurse completes the data base during the first visit. In the nursing home, the nursing assessment is documented within the first 24 hours; the federally mandated interdisciplinary Minimum Data Set (MDS) requires completion within 14 days of admission. For Medicare A residents, the MDS must be completed and electronically transmitted to the Health Care Finance Administration (HCFA) within 7 days of admission. A copy of the MDS is located in the Appendix.

The information collected by the nurse is *not* a repetition of the medical history that the health care provider records. Rather, the nurse collects additional data regarding the client's response to health problems, functional ability, ability to perform activities of daily living, usual health behaviors, coping patterns, health goals, and support systems.

Episodic, or Problem-Centered, Data Base. An episodic data base is collected for a limited or short-term problem. It focuses on one problem, and data collected are associated with the problem. For example, an elderly hospitalized woman falls when trying to get out of bed and complains of hip pain. The nurse's history focuses on how the fall occurred, which parts of the client's body made contact with the floor, and what position she assumed after she fell. The physical assessment is centered on the neurologic and musculoskeletal systems, especially the head, hip, and knee. These data are usually not recorded on a data base form as such, but the information is documented according to agency policy.

In other situations, the nurse documents assessment findings frequently during the day on a flow sheet. For example, the client who is receiving patient-controlled analgesia (PCA) for pain control must be monitored carefully to determine whether the intervention is successful. The Daily Pain/PCA Flow Sheet shown in Figure 1–7 is an episodic data base that requires the nurse to assess and document the client's level of pain and sedation.

Emergency Data Base. The emergency data base is similar to the episodic data base in that the nurse focuses on the immediate problem. However, the assessment must be more rapid to prevent life-threatening consequences. For example, a hospitalized client begins to choke on a piece of meat. The nurse quickly assesses whether there is a partial or complete airway obstruction before selecting the appropriate emergency nursing intervention.

Follow-Up Data Base. The follow-up data base is simply an evaluation of identified problems at regular and appropriate intervals. For example, for the client who was choking in the example just given, the nurse checks on him frequently to make sure that he is still breathing without difficulty and that he does not choke again.

Sources of Data. The nurse obtains and documents data from several sources in the client's medical record according to the policies of the health care agency.

Client. The client is the primary source of data. This information is direct and firsthand and is collected by interview. Interviewing is a communication skill by which a nurse can explore the thoughts, feelings, and perceptions of the client. As in the teaching-learning process, the interview process is affected by many variables, including timing, environment, and demographic factors such as age. Chart 1–3 provides tips for interviewing an elderly person.

A medical history differs from a nursing history. A *medical* history is taken by the health care provider to determine the presence of a pathologic condition and to provide a basis for planning medical care. A *nursing* history is obtained by the nurse and focuses on the meaning of the illness and/or hospitalization to the client and family. It is used as a basis for planning nursing care.

Family and Significant Others. The client's family members or significant others are secondary sources of data. They can often supplement or verify information provided by the client. They may also be able to offer information about the client before the illness, provide family history related to health and illness, and describe the client's home environment.

Records. Previous medical histories, laboratory records, vital signs, and diagnostic reports provide pertinent data.

Chart 1–3

Nursing Focus on the Elderly: Interviewing

- Review old records and the medical history, if available, before interviewing the client
- Provide privacy as much as possible
- Ask the client whether family or significant others should be present during the interview
- Refer to the client by his or her last name (e.g., Mrs. Brown) unless the client prefers another name
- Make sure that eyeglasses, contact lenses, and hearing aids are available and working properly, if the client wears these devices
- Conduct the interview when the client is not experiencing pain and after basic comfort needs have been met
- Before conducting the interview, allow the client to adjust to a new environment
- Sit at the client's eye level during the interview
- Speak clearly, slowly, and in a low-pitched voice; do not shout
- Be aware that the client may not be able to distinguish soft consonant blends, like "sh" or "ch"
- Interview in the morning, after breakfast, or in the early afternoon, after the client has rested
- Use open-ended questions, when possible, to gather more information; avoid questions that can be answered "yes" or "no"
- Consider the client's education, culture, and age when phrasing questions, especially about sensitive or controversial issues
- Observe the client's nonverbal behavior as well as what he or she says

MEMORIAL HOSPITAL AT EASTON, MD. INC.

DAILY PAIN / PCA FLOW SHEET

Initial Assessment & Plan

1. Has MD told pt. about PCA?

___ YES ___ NO

2. Does patient verbalize understanding?

___ YES ___ NO

3. BP: _____ PULSE: _____

NOTE: Actual settings in Blue/Black ink.

Nurse Initials & Signature

Init.	Signature	Init.	Signature

ASSESSMENT INFORMATION

DATE/TIME	DRUG NAME & CONC.	PCA DOSE (ML)	LOCKOUT INTERVAL (MIN.)	4 HR LIMIT (ML)	PAIN LEVEL 0-5	SEDATION LEVEL 1-5	RESPIRATORY RATE	INITIALS	I.E. AMOUNT WASTED, WITNESS, ETC. INJECTOR VIAL CHANGED COMMENTS

LEVEL OF PAIN   **SEDATION LEVEL**

0 - ASLEEP AT TIME OF CHARTING
1 - COMFORTABLE
2 - MILD DISCOMFORT
3 - IN PAIN
4 - IN BAD PAIN
5 - IN VERY BAD PAIN

1 - ALERT AND AWARE
2 - DROWSY
3 - DOZING INTERMITTENTLY
4 - MOSTLY SLEEPING
5 - DIFFICULT TO AROUSE

REVISED 1/90

FORM# 140265

Figure 1–7. An example of an episodic data base: a Daily Pain/PCA Flow Sheet. (Courtesy of Memorial Hospital at Easton, Easton, MD.)

These data validate information identified in the current history and physical examination or serve as a comparison to indicate changes in the client's health condition. Records from previous admissions to the hospital also supply additional pieces of information. The client's health care provider usually requests the old records from the agency's medical records department or other health care facility where the client has sought health care.

Collaboration. A nurse may gather client information in collaboration with other health care team members. The physician or nurse practitioner is a key source of information. A social worker or home care nurse who has worked with the client can also contribute valuable information.

When a client is admitted to the hospital from another health care facility, such as a nursing home, the hospital nurse should contact the nurse who cared for the client in the facility for specific client information. Most nursing homes supply a nursing transfer form that accompanies the client to the hospital or other facility. The transfer form describes the client's abilities and limitations, drug therapy, diet therapy, and past and current health state. This information is particularly helpful when the client cannot communicate and if no family is available.

 Analysis

The second step of the nursing process is the analysis of data. In this phase, the nurse summarizes and analyzes the data and draws conclusions to determine what health problems the client may have or is at risk for. Client data are compared with "normal" findings and behaviors for the client's age, education, and cultural background. Abnormal data are reviewed to determine patterns of altered functioning. Client health problems are identified and categorized as potential problems requiring prevention or actual problems being managed or requiring interventions.

In a classic book, Aspinall and Tanner (1981) state that nurses make two types of judgments or conclusions about the health state of a client: (1) those health problems that nurses, "by virtue of their education and experience, are licensed and able to treat" (p. 4) (nursing diagnoses) and (2) those problems that are diagnosed and treated by other members of the health team but require continued nursing assessment and implementation of therapeutic interventions (collaborative problems).

This textbook uses nursing diagnoses and collaborative problems that incorporate both types of client health problems.

Nursing Diagnoses. The nursing profession's acknowledgment and endorsement of the term *nursing diagnosis* began in 1973, when the American Nurses' Association (ANA) published its first *Standards of Nursing Practice.* Since then, other countries have also adopted nursing diagnoses as a way to describe client health problems.

In the early 1980s, the North American Nursing Diagnosis Association (NANDA) was formed to serve as the official organization for the development and dissemination of nursing diagnoses. Nurses from all over the world belong to this organization, although most are from countries within North America. The official journal of

NANDA is *Nursing Diagnosis,* which is published quarterly. Other countries or continents such as Europe have formalized nursing diagnosis associations.

Although many definitions of nursing diagnosis have been proposed by various nursing leaders, the authors of this book recognize the official definition approved by NANDA at its Ninth Conference in 1990: "A nursing diagnosis is a clinical judgment about an individual, family, or community response to actual or potential health problems/life processes which provides the basis for definitive therapy toward achievement of outcomes for which the nurse is accountable" (Carpenito, 1995, p. 65).

Unlike medical diagnoses, which identify illness, nursing diagnoses identify the *responses* to health problems and life processes, such as aging or death. A medical diagnosis is the basis for medical interventions; a nursing diagnosis is the basis for nursing interventions. Nursing diagnoses are not diagnostic tests, medical treatments, or problems experienced by the nurse while caring for the client. Table 1–2 differentiates medical and nursing diagnoses. The current nursing diagnosis list is located on the inside back cover of this text.

Collaborative Problems. Collaborative problems, as identified in this text, are potential health problems for which the nurse monitors. The nurse then reports on these problems, if they occur, to the health care provider. Measures that help prevent the problem are implemented. Through keen assessment skills, the nurse detects the health problem as early as possible if it occurs. Then, in collaboration with members of the interdisciplinary care team, he or she carries out interventions to resolve the problem. An example of a collaborative problem is Potential for Hemorrhage following a vaginal hysterectomy.

 Planning

The planning step follows the analysis step of the nursing process. Throughout the planning process, the nurse performs several important functions: setting priorities and expected outcomes, selecting nursing interventions, and determining resources.

TABLE 1–2

Differentiation Between Medical and Nursing Diagnoses	
Medical Diagnosis	**Nursing Diagnosis**
Identifies the pathologic basis for an illness	Identifies a response to illness
Focuses on the physical condition of the client	Focuses on the physical, psychosocial, and spiritual needs of the client
Addresses actual, existing problems	Addresses actual and potential problems
Is not validated with the client	Is validated with the client if possible
Uses standardized goals and treatments	Uses individualized outcomes and intervention
May not be resolvable	Is usually resolvable

Setting Priorities and Outcomes. After analyzing the needs of the client to identify client health problems, the nurse decides on the urgency of the problems. This step is vital because some problems are more critical than others. Problems of higher priority require more immediate intervention than problems of lower priority. Setting priorities helps the nurse organize and plan care that solves the most urgent problems first.

Establishing Priorities. In determining the priority of the problems, the nurse must consider the impact on the client. Several classic theorists have presented hierarchies that are still used today to assist in determining priorities.

Bower (1972) offers a three-level approach, in descending order of priority:
- First priority—problems that threaten life, dignity, and integrity of the client
- Second priority—problems that destructively change the client
- Third priority—problems that affect normal growth and development

Maslow's hierarchy of needs can also serve as a useful guide for establishing priorities. These needs form five levels. The client progresses up the hierarchy when attempting to satisfy needs. As shown in Figure 1–8, physiologic needs are of greatest priority and must be met first. Once they are met, the client is more willing and able to seek fulfillment of higher-level needs.

Priorities may fluctuate as the client's level of wellness changes. The nurse should consider both actual and high-risk problems when establishing priorities. Actual problems are usually more important than high-risk problems; at times, however, high-risk problems may be more important. For example, in a client who is asthmatic, the high-risk problem of Ineffective Airway Clearance is more life-threatening than an actual problem of constipation.

The establishment of priorities reflects an agreement between the client and nurse when possible. In addition to the guidelines for priorities that theorists have offered, the nurse must be aware of factors such as the client's health goals, the availability of resources, and the client's knowledge of the problem. The priorities of the client are often more important to the client than the priorities outlined by theoretical guidelines.

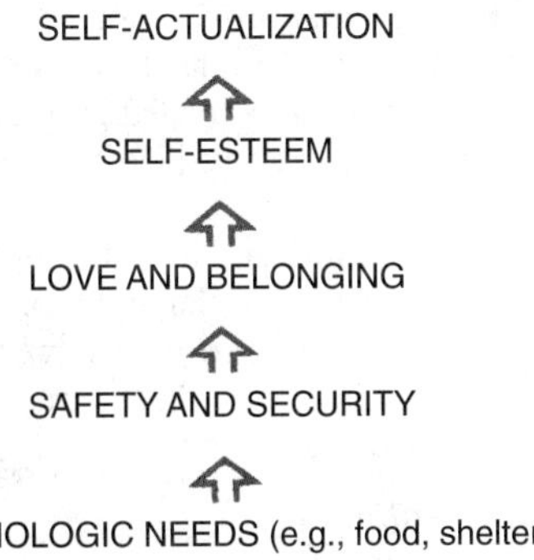

SELF-ACTUALIZATION

⇑

SELF-ESTEEM

⇑

LOVE AND BELONGING

⇑

SAFETY AND SECURITY

⇑

PHYSIOLOGIC NEEDS (e.g., food, shelter)

Figure 1–8. Maslow's hierarchy of needs. Needs must be met in ascending order. For example, safety and security must be achieved before love and belonging.

Establishing Outcomes. After establishing priorities, the client and nurse mutually try to decide on expected outcomes on the basis of identified nursing diagnoses and collaborative problems. Outcomes serve as guides in selecting nursing interventions and in determining criteria for evaluating nursing interventions. The purpose of writing expected outcomes is to assist in the evaluation of the client's progress and to determine resolution, if possible, of the client's problem.

Expected outcomes should be
- Client-centered
- Realistic in terms of the client's potential for achievement and the nurse's ability to help the client achieve them
- Specific and measurable to the extent possible

When writing outcomes, the nurse should state them in a clear, concise manner that can be understood and measured by all health care team members. Any health care professional caring for the client should be able to determine whether the outcomes have been achieved. For example, "The client will state that pain is reduced within 45 minutes after interdisciplinary intervention" is a specific outcome for one client that can be measured easily. If after 45 minutes the client states that pain is reduced, the outcome has been met.

Selecting Nursing Interventions. After determining the outcomes, the nurse develops strategies to accomplish them. Nursing interventions, also known as nursing actions or measures, are designed to assist the client in achieving goals. They are based on the client's health problems and define activities required to promote, maintain, or restore the client's health.

Bulachek and McCloskey (1989) define nursing interventions as "any direct care treatment that a nurse performs on behalf of a client. These treatments included nurse-initiated treatments resulting from nursing diagnoses, physician-initiated treatments resulting from medical diagnoses, and performance of the daily essential functions for the client who cannot do these" (p. 25).

Although the definition of nursing interventions proposed by these experts seems to imply that a nurse performs only treatments or technical skills, these authors have broadened their definition. In a more recent book, Bulechek and McCloskey (1992) discuss interventions that range from physical interventions (positioning, feeding) to psychosocial interventions (therapeutic touch, reminiscence therapy). In 1992 they also published the results of the first phase of the Iowa Intervention Project. This research produced a Nursing Interventions Classification (NIC) system of 336 standardized nursing interventions. Like the development of nursing diagnoses, NIC is intended to help nurses standardize their terminology and practice. Most recently, the authors have developed a Nursing Outcomes Classification (NOC).

Nurse-initiated interventions, also called nurse-prescribed interventions or *nursing orders,* are independent activities that address nursing diagnoses. In the North American Nursing Diagnosis Association (NANDA) definition of nursing diagnosis, "definitive therapy" refers to nurse-initiated interventions. For example, the nurse teaches relaxation techniques for a client experiencing the nursing diagnosis of Ineffective Coping.

For some of the currently approved nursing diagnoses, the nurse may implement health care provider–initiated interventions. For example, the nurse gives analgesic medication to relieve pain. The health care provider prescribes the medication, but the nurse uses clinical judgment about when and how to administer the medication. The nurse may also use non-drug interventions, like imagery or massage, to help reduce the client's pain. Thus, the nurse and health care provider *collaborate* in an effort to resolve the client's problem of pain.

Developing the Collaborative Plan of Care. The collaborative plan of care (POC) is an interdisciplinary document that outlines the essential aspects of client care, often across a time sequence. The format commonly used is a clinical pathway, which is also called a critical path, care map, or coordinated POC.

The clinical pathway delineates what care must be provided, who will provide the care, and when the care will be provided. It is a guideline for care that can be individualized if needed. Most pathways also list expected outcomes for the client, which may be hourly, daily, or weekly, depending on the nature of the health care setting. This textbook provides samples of clinical pathways. When possible, one pathway may view care across the health care continuum.

This text also includes Client Care Plans. Although these plans of care are not interdisciplinary, they are necessary for beginning students to help them follow the steps of the nursing process and to identify the rationale for selected nursing interventions. In most clinical practice settings, this format is no longer used because the accrediting agency for hospitals and other health care facilities, the Joint Commission on the Accreditation of Healthcare Organizations (JCAHO), does not require the use of columnar care plans. Instead, JCAHO requires evidence that nurses plan and implement care based on identified client health problems in collaboration with the interdisciplinary team.

To save time and duplication, a number of computer programs and books have been developed to create standardized plans of care or clinical pathways that can be individualized as needed. As technology advances, these programs should be more widely available to nurses in all health care settings.

Determining Resources. While planning the nursing interventions, the nurse determines which resources are necessary to implement them. The client is a valuable source of information about health care resources that were successful in the past. For example, the client with an irritated stoma may mention that an enterostomal therapist was helpful with previous problems with an ileostomy. Including the client and family in planning care often promotes their cooperation during the implementation phase.

Other nurses and health care team members are valuable resources. An interdisciplinary conference or "walking rounds" during which health care team members

identify problems and resources to solve them may be very helpful, especially for continuing care planning.

When the financial feasibility of the plan is explored, the nurse takes into account the availability of other resources for the client, such as equipment, time, personnel, and money. The client's value system is also considered. For instance, if the client requires dialysis in the home, the type of system implemented depends on the home water supply, electrical capability, space, available money, spiritual beliefs, and personal support system.

 ## Implementation

Implementation involves the actual carrying out of a specific, individualized POC. This step of the nursing process is the action phase, in which the nurse assumes the responsibility for implementing the POC based on the nursing diagnosis and collaborative problems. Interventions are based on scientific principles and, at times, intuitive judgment.

Because planning and implementation are closely related, this book discusses them under one heading: Planning and Implementation. However, expected outcomes and interventions are clearly labeled.

 ## Evaluation

Evaluation, the fifth step of the nursing process, is a cognitive activity that completes the nursing process by indicating the degree to which the client's goals have been met.

Although evaluation is given as the final step of the nursing process, it is an ongoing and integral part of each step of the process (see Fig. 1–6). The nurse reviews the data to determine whether sufficient information was collected and whether the behaviors identified were appropriate. Client health problems are evaluated for their accuracy and completeness. The nurse examines the expected outcomes and interventions to determine whether they were realistic, achievable, and effective.

The outcome of evaluation may be one or a combination of the following:

- The client responded as expected and the problem is resolved. No additional nursing actions are needed.
- Client behaviors indicate that the client's problem has not been resolved. Outcomes have been accomplished, but the overall long-term goal has not been achieved. Re-evaluation will continue.
- Client behaviors are similar to those present initially. Little or no evidence is available to show that the problem has been resolved. Reassessment and re-planning are needed.
- Client behaviors indicate a new problem. Assessment, planning, and implementation of an additional plan of action are needed to resolve the problem.

In this book, expected outcomes are listed under the planning and evaluation sections.

Documentation

Documentation of each phase of the nursing process is essential and is accomplished by various means. Two gen-

Date/Time	Focus/Problem	Notes

4/18/98
 	
2:15 P.M.
	Fever	D: T = 102.2° (R); face
		        flushed; diaphoretic
		A: Give Tylenol 2 tab as
		        ordered. Recheck temp.
		        in 1 hr.
		                    R. Jones, RN

4/18/98
 	
3:15 P.M.
	Fever	R: T = 100.2° (R); face not
		        flushed; not diaphoretic
		                    D. Ignas, LPN

4/19/98
 	
3:30 A.M.
	Impaired skin	D: 2-cm reddened area
		        over coccyx; blanches
		A: Positioned on (L) side
		                    N. Smith, RNC

Figure 1–9. A sample of focus charting.

eral, traditional methods of documentation are still used in many health care settings: (1) source-oriented charting, which usually includes narrative notes that organize varied data that are entered into the medical record by health care professionals (e.g., nurses' notes, physicians' progress notes, dietary notes) and (2) the problem-oriented record (POR), in which a master health problem list is developed. Each problem is numbered, and all chart entries refer to one of the problems identified on the list.

The notes may be recorded in a SOAP, SOAPIER, or PIE format (or one of its many variations) on the same progress note form in the chart by all health profession-

als. The initials represent **S**ubjective data, **O**bjective data, **A**nalysis, **P**lan of action, **I**nterventions, **E**valuation, and **R**evision of the plan. This technique of documentation is systematic and limits data to only pertinent information related to the identified problem. Although this system assists the nurse in addressing each step of the nursing process, it is very time-consuming and promotes duplication of record-keeping. Many physicians, social workers, and dietitians still use the SOAP format, but new systems for nursing documentation have been and are being developed.

Documentation Systems

Focus Charting. A commonly used format in documentation is focus charting. Focus charting is not limited to specific client health problems but, rather, encourages nurses to document any significant changes in the client's condition, any client concern, or any significant client event. As seen in Figure 1–9, the record has three columns. The actual notes are divided into **D**ata, **A**ction, and **R**esponse information. An **E** may be added for documenting client **E**ducation. This technique helps locate desired information but still uses the familiar narrative approach to recording pertinent data.

Charting by Exception. Another system is charting by exception (CBE). CBE was started at St. Luke's Hospital in Milwaukee, Wisconsin, in an attempt to save nursing time. It incorporates three basic components (Burke and Murphy, 1988):
- Comprehensive flow sheets that list normal findings and require the nurse to initial them if they are present. If the findings are not present, the nurse writes an entry into the notes.
- Reference to pre-established nursing standards. The nurse initials the appropriate space when they are completed.

Chart 1–4

Nursing Care Highlight: Legal Tips for Nursing Documentation

- Write clearly and legibly
- Do not erase or "white-out" any part of the client's record
- To correct an error, use one line to cross out the incorrect entry, then initial the change
- Use only standard and facility-approved abbreviations and symbols
- Document significant information as close as possible to the time it is collected instead of waiting until the end of a shift
- Transcribe physicians' orders carefully and correctly
- If using nurses' notes or progress notes, do not leave blank spaces between entries
- Time and date each entry on the client's record
- Use only blue or black ink (it visualizes best for copies or microfilm)
- Document like a reporter: State facts objectively and avoid judgment or criticism
- Do not state that "an incident report has been completed" or refer to any unusual occurrence or special event as an "incident"
- Follow all facility policies for documentation
- To add one or two words, use a caret (^) and insert the words, then initial the change; if agency policy does not allow this practice, write a late entry
- To make a late entry, begin by stating that it is a "Late entry for (date and time);" if the entry is more than a day late, state the reason for the late entry (e.g., "on vacation for 3 days")
- If an order is discontinued on the record as indicated by a highlighter, be sure that the original can still be read, especially on copies

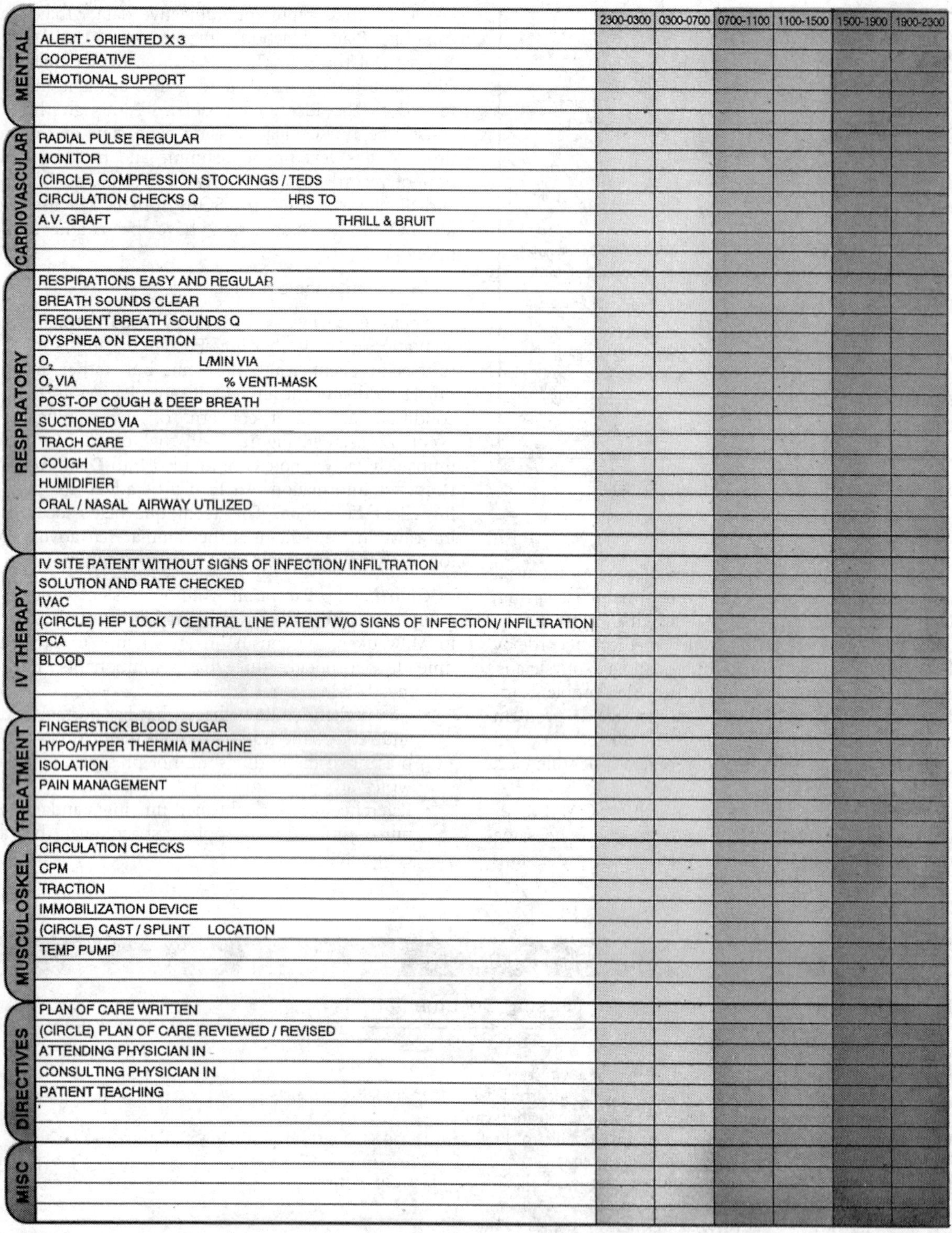

		2300-0300	0300-0700	0700-1100	1100-1500	1500-1900	1900-2300
MENTAL	ALERT - ORIENTED X 3						
	COOPERATIVE						
	EMOTIONAL SUPPORT						
CARDIOVASCULAR	RADIAL PULSE REGULAR						
	MONITOR						
	(CIRCLE) COMPRESSION STOCKINGS / TEDS						
	CIRCULATION CHECKS Q HRS TO						
	A.V. GRAFT THRILL & BRUIT						
RESPIRATORY	RESPIRATIONS EASY AND REGULAR						
	BREATH SOUNDS CLEAR						
	FREQUENT BREATH SOUNDS Q						
	DYSPNEA ON EXERTION						
	O_2 L/MIN VIA						
	O_2 VIA % VENTI-MASK						
	POST-OP COUGH & DEEP BREATH						
	SUCTIONED VIA						
	TRACH CARE						
	COUGH						
	HUMIDIFIER						
	ORAL / NASAL AIRWAY UTILIZED						
IV THERAPY	IV SITE PATENT WITHOUT SIGNS OF INFECTION/ INFILTRATION						
	SOLUTION AND RATE CHECKED						
	IVAC						
	(CIRCLE) HEP LOCK / CENTRAL LINE PATENT W/O SIGNS OF INFECTION/ INFILTRATION						
	PCA						
	BLOOD						
TREATMENT	FINGERSTICK BLOOD SUGAR						
	HYPO/HYPER THERMIA MACHINE						
	ISOLATION						
	PAIN MANAGEMENT						
MUSCULOSKEL	CIRCULATION CHECKS						
	CPM						
	TRACTION						
	IMMOBILIZATION DEVICE						
	(CIRCLE) CAST / SPLINT LOCATION						
	TEMP PUMP						
DIRECTIVES	PLAN OF CARE WRITTEN						
	(CIRCLE) PLAN OF CARE REVIEWED / REVISED						
	ATTENDING PHYSICIAN IN						
	CONSULTING PHYSICIAN IN						
	PATIENT TEACHING						
MISC							

Figure 1–10. A portion of a daily flow sheet used for charting by exception. (Courtesy of Dorchester General Hospital, Cambridge, MD.)

- Bedside accessibility of forms. All flow sheets are kept at the bedside, which prevents wasting the nursing time in looking for a client's chart. Bedside charting also prevents transcription of data from one form to another, which can lead to errors as well as wasted time. The information is available for any health care professional to read.

Like all charting systems, variations of the concept are being implemented. A portion of a flow sheet used in a CBE system is found in Figure 1–10.

Computerized Nursing Information Systems. A major advantage of documentation systems, such as CBE, is the ability to transfer the concept to computerization. Bedside computer charting, also known as point-of-care charting and online documentation, is beginning to appear in hospitals, nursing homes, home care agencies, and ambulatory care settings.

The literature suggests that the major advantages of point-of-care documentation are accuracy and time savings. Electronic charting at the bedside also increases the time that the nurse spends in the client's room. Kirk (1995) noted that in addition to improving the quality of care, handheld documentation devices decreased costly nursing overtime. The goal of any system should be to streamline or diminish paperwork and save valuable nursing time, giving nurses more time for direct client care.

The Methodist Hospital in Arcadia, California, established criteria for point-of-care technology, including the following (Gianni, Beasley, & Linson, 1996):

- It must take the same time as or less time than manual charting.
- Radio frequency must be reliable, with no lost data.
- Charting cannot be redundant.
- Hardware must be standardized on all units.
- Assistance is readily available.

Legal Aspects of Documentation. Regardless of the type of documentation system used, the nurse remembers that the client's chart is a legal document. Chart 1–4 lists basic charting guidelines that all nurses should follow.

SELECTED BIBLIOGRAPHY

Albright, J., de Guzman, C., Acebo, P., et al. (1996). Readability of patient education materials: Implications for clinical practice. *Applied Nursing Research, 9,* 139–143.

Allen, K. M., & Phillips, J. M. (1997). *Women's health across the lifespan: A comprehensive perspective.* Philadelphia: Lippincott-Raven.

*Aspinall, M. J., & Tanner, C. (1981). *Decision-making for patient care.* Norwalk, CT: Appleton & Lange.

Barry, R., & Burggraf, V. (1996). Healthy people: Objective look at the elderly. *Journal of Gerontological Nursing, 22*(10), 9–11.

*Benner, P., & Tanner, C. (1987). How expert nurses use intuition. *American Journal of Nursing, 87,* 23–31.

*Bower, F. (1972). *The process of planning nursing care.* St. Louis: C. V. Mosby.

*Bulechek, G., & McCloskey, J. (1989). Nursing interventions: Treatments for potential nursing diagnoses. In R. M. Carroll-Johnson (Ed.), *Classification of nursing diagnoses: Proceedings of the eighth conference* (pp. 23–30). Philadelphia: J. B. Lippincott.

*Bulechek, G. M., & McCloskey, J. C. (1992). *Nursing interventions: Essential nursing treatments* (2nd ed.). Philadelphia: W. B. Saunders.

*Burke, L. J., & Murphy, J. (1988). *Charting by exception: A cost-effective, quality approach.* New York: John Wiley.

Bush, A. M. P., & Ebel, C. A. (1996). Testing an electronic documentation system. *Nursing Management, 27*(7), 40–42.

Carpenito, L. J. (1995). *Nursing care plans and documentation: Nursing diagnoses and collaborative problems.* Philadelphia: J. B. Lippincott.

Castillo, H., & Torres, S. (1995). Cultural considerations: Providing quality nursing care to Hispanics. *Imprint, 42*(5), 52–55.

Chen, M. S., & Hawks, B. L. (1995). A debunking of the myth of the healthy Asian Americans and Pacific Islanders. *American Journal of Health Promotion, 8,* 261–268.

Clay, J. C., Wyatt, L. K., & Norris, G. M. (1996). Patient and family education: An interdisciplinary process. *MEDSURG Nursing, 5*(5), 333–338, 354.

Cordell, B. (1994). Streamlined charting for patient education. *Nursing94, 24*(1), 57–59.

Douglas, C. Y. (1995). Cultural considerations for the African-American population. *Imprint, 42*(5), 57–59.

*Dunn, H. L. (1980). *High level wellness.* Thorofare, NJ: Charles B. Slack.

Eggland, E. T. (1995). Charting smarter—Using mechanisms to organize your paperwork. *Nursing95, 25*(9), 35–41.

Gianni, N., Beasley, E., & Linson, D. (1996). Online documentation: Making it work with POC technology. *Health Management Technology, April,* 46–50.

Gruber, M. (1995). Documentation is communication. *Gastroenterology Nursing, 18*(3), 107–108.

Ignatavicius, D. D., & Hausman, K. (1995). *Clinical pathways for collaborative practice.* Philadelphia: W. B. Saunders.

Jarvis, C. (1996). *Physical examination and health assessment* (2nd ed.). Philadelphia: W. B. Saunders.

Johnson, D., & Martin, K. (1996). Preparing for electronic documentation. *Nursing Management, 27*(7), 43–44.

Jones, M., & Nies, M. A. (1996). The relationship of perceived benefits of and barriers to reported exercise in older African American woman. *Public Health Nursing, 13,* 151–158.

King, C., & Macmillan, M. (1994). Documentation and discharge planning for elderly patients. *Nursing Times, 90*(20), 31–33.

Kirk, T. (1995). On the front lines of patient care. *Healthcare Informatics, June,* 50, 54.

Krause, C. R., Westdorp, J. M., Coonen, D. A., & Jenks, D. L. (1996). Forming an integrated documentation system. *Nursing Management, 27*(8), 25–26.

Leddy, S. K. (1996). Development and psychometric testing of the Leddy Healthiness Scale. *Research in Nursing and Health, 19,* 431–440.

Louie, K. B. (1995). Cultural considerations: Asian-Americans and Pacific Islanders. *Imprint, 42*(5), 41–46.

*Maslow, A. (1970). *Motivation and personality.* New York: Harper & Row.

Maidwell, A. (1996). The role of the surgical nurse as a health promoter. *British Journal of Nursing, 5*(15), 898–904.

*McCloskey, J. C., & Bulechek, G. M. (1992). *Nursing interventions classification (NIC).* St. Louis: Mosby-Year Book.

Northam, S. (1996). Access to health promotion, protection, and disease prevention among impoverished individuals. *Public Health Nursing, 13,* 353–364.

*Pender, N. J. (1987). *Health promotion in nursing practice* (2nd ed.). Norwalk, CT: Appleton & Lange.

Rasmussen, N., & Gengler, T. (1994). Clinical pathways of care: The route to better communication. *Nursing94, 24*(2), 47–49.

Schielke, C. (1997). Patient advocacy: The shield that empowers. *Continuing Care, 16*(3), 22–26.

*U.S. Department of Health and Human Services, Public Health Service. (1990). *Healthy people 2000: National health promotion and disease prevention objectives.* Washington, D. C.: U.S. Government Printing Office.

Weiler, K. (1994). Legal aspects of nursing documentation for the Alzheimer's patient. *Journal of Gerontological Nursing, 20*(4), 31–40.

*World Health Organization. (1947). *Constitution of the World Health Organization: Chronicle of the World Health Organization.* Geneva: Author.

Zander, K., & McGill, R. (1994). Critical and anticipated recovery paths: Only the beginning. *Nursing Management, 25*(8), 34–40.

Zink, M. R. (1994). Nursing diagnosis in home care: Audit tool development. *Journal of Community Health Nursing, 11*(1), 51–58.

SUGGESTED READINGS

Castillo, H., & Torres, S. (1995). Cultural considerations: Providing quality nursing care to Hispanics. *Imprint, 42*(5), 52–55.
This article begins with a thorough description of the demographic characteristics of the Hispanic population in the United States. The authors then discuss health care beliefs and health status of Hispanics. Finally, they make suggestions regarding how to use the nursing process with this growing subgroup of the population.

Clay, J. C., Wyatt, L. K., & Norris, G. M. (1996). Patient and family education: An interdisciplinary process. *MEDSURG Nursing, 5*(5), 333–338, 354.
This article describes an interdisciplinary education and discharge

plan developed in a 404-bed teaching hospital. The Learner Assessment, Education Plan, and Discharge Plan forms are included in the article to demonstrate the necessary documentation.

Louie, K. B. (1995). Cultural considerations: Asian-Americans and Pacific Islanders. *Imprint, 42*(5), 41–46.

The author points out that there are 23 subgroups of Asian-Americans and a number of subgroups of Pacific Islanders living in the United States. The article disputes a 1985 report that concluded that the AAPI population is at a lower risk of early death than the Caucasian population. Newer findings show that this fast-growing minority group has higher mortality rates when compared with other groups, especially for lung cancer and cardiovascular disease. The remainder of the article describes specific characteristics of some of the Asian-American subgroups.

CONTINUING CARE

Continuing care for medical-surgical clients can be provided in a number of settings. Continuing care may be needed after a hospital or nursing home stay or as an alternative to inpatient hospital care. Although the majority of health care currently occurs in the hospital, the trend is rapidly moving toward care in alternative settings, such as ambulatory care, home care, and long-term care in rehabilitation centers, nursing homes, and chronic care facilities. This chapter provides a brief description of each of these settings.

This textbook covers care for clients in all settings in which medical-surgical nurses practice. Continuing Care sections after discussions of major health problems highlight the most important aspects of care in nonhospital environments.

AMBULATORY CARE

Ambulatory health care is a general term for client care provided in myriad community settings, such as physician offices, hospital or freestanding outpatient clinics, freestanding surgicenters, and health maintenance organizations, a type of managed-care organization (see Chap. 3). The purpose of ambulatory care is health promotion, health protection (illness prevention), short-term treatment, and follow-up for existing health problems.

Client visits to ambulatory care settings are episodic and based on need. For example, clients may visit their health care provider for annual physical examinations (health promotion). Alternatively, they may seek out providers for acute health care problems or selected surgeries, such as cataract removal or laparoscopic cholecystectomy (removal of the gallbladder). Still others are monitored periodically for chronic health conditions, such as diabetes mellitus and hypertension.

Clients discharged from the hospital are frequently followed in one or more ambulatory care settings. The cost of ambulatory care is typically far less than that provided by a nursing home or home care agency.

Role of the Nurse in Ambulatory Care

One of the major roles of the nurse working in an ambulatory care setting is health promotion activities, including client education, health screening, and comprehensive assessment. In a surgicenter, for example, the nurse provides preoperative teaching to prepare clients for the surgical procedure and postoperative expectations. Clients' vital signs and general condition are assessed to ensure that clients are ready to have the surgery.

Some physician offices employ nurses to assist in their practice. These nurses often triage clients who call; that is, the nurse decides which clients need priority care and intervenes accordingly. In some parts of the country, large physician practices employ nurse case managers who monitor high-risk, high-cost, problem-prone clients throughout the continuum of health care in all settings. Case management is discussed in Chapter 3.

Nursing Community Centers

Nursing community centers are ambulatory care settings operated by nurses. Although the organizational structure and services provided vary among centers, most centers are affiliated with large university schools of nursing. The primary health care providers are typically nurse practitioners, nurse midwives, clinical nurse specialists, and students preparing to become one of these advanced-practice specialists. Funding for nursing community centers also varies. Some monies come from city, state, and federal governments, whereas others come from grants obtained by university faculty.

HOME CARE

Home care in the United States is a diverse and rapidly growing industry. For many clients, the home is the lowest-cost health care setting.

History of Home Care Nursing

Modern home care nursing has its roots in public health nursing and community health nursing models. In the mid-1880s, visiting nurse associations evolved in Philadelphia, Boston, and Buffalo, New York. The traditions of Lillian Wald, regarded as the founder of public health nursing, began with the Henry Street Settlement in New York City in 1893.

Home care, however, was a small entity until the passage of the Medicare Law in 1965. At that time, Medicare required agencies to provide a minimum of nursing services plus one additional service, such as physical or occupational therapy, speech-language pathology, medical social services, or home health aide services. The advent of Medicare began the trend toward and basis for reimbursement of home care services. In 1963, 3 years before Medicare became law, it has been estimated that there were only 1100 home care programs. Today, more than 16,000 home care organizations provide some kind of

service or product to clients in their homes. About one half of these are Medicare certified and provide skilled nursing services.

Many factors have contributed to the growth and acceptance of home care, including the following:

- The continued shift from inpatient-based care to community-based and home care
- The increasing need for health care for the elderly
- Technology, such as mobile x-ray machines, apnea monitors, electrocardiography (ECG) machines, and others that help clients remain at home
- The increased general acceptance of home care as a care site
- The generally lower cost of home care (compared with inpatient care)
- The hospitals' continuing incentives to reduce lengths of stays in a managed-care environment
- The growth of hospital-based home health agencies

Types of Home Care

The term *home care* can be confusing and can refer to different kinds of products or services. There are different specialty areas within the home care industry, and nurses may work in any of these segments (Fig. 2–1). In addition, some companies may provide all or just one of these home care segments. There are generally four markets or segments of the home health care industry.

1. The home medical equipment (HME) market, which can also include durable medical equipment (DME) (such as hospital beds and wheelchairs). HME companies provide products to clients such as walkers, beds, wheelchairs, oxygen equipment, and other equipment. Medicare and other insurers pay for products that are "covered" (reimbursed) based on the insurance programs rules.
2. The home infusion or intravenous (IV) company. These companies deliver and administer infusion therapies in the client's home. Home infusion includes antibiotic therapies, hyperalimentation, blood and blood products, and other infusion therapies. Nursing services may be covered under Medicare or

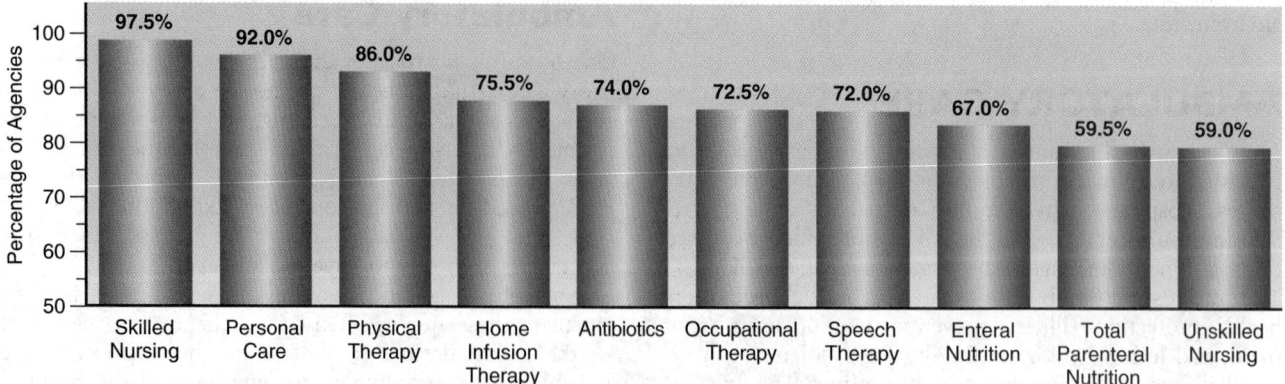

Figure 2–1. Ten most commonly offered home care services. (Courtesy of Marion Merrell Dow, Inc., Managed Care Digest Series, *Institutional Digest*, 1995, and SMG Marketing Group, Inc.)

other insurers for such services as IV site care and observation and assessment. The medications may or may not be reimbursed based on the insurance or managed-care company's rules.

3. Personal care or private duty services. These agencies may provide "shifts" of nurses or home health aides or private duty nurses to clients in their homes. They may provide other services such as respite for caregivers, homemakers, and meal preparation, among others. Usually these services are paid for privately by the client or family. Some insurance programs may pay for limited services related to health care based on medical necessity.

4. Skilled home care services (the largest type). These agencies employ most of the home care nurses as well as other health professionals to provide care as needed. Skilled home care services are provided by home care organizations that are usually Medicare certified and provide the six services of nursing, physical and occupational therapy, speech-language pathology services, medical social services, and home health aides. They may also provide dietitian services and have specialists such as enterostomal therapist nurses or others based on the program's mission. The interdisciplinary aspects of home care make it truly client centered.

Role of the Nurse in Home Care

Home health nursing is a synthesis of community health nursing and selected skills from other specialty nursing practices. In 1986 the American Nurses' Association (ANA) published its *Standards of Home Health Nursing Practice*, identifying home care nursing as a component of community health nursing that incorporates public health principles and practice. The standards include both health promotion and care of the sick and are targeted toward communities, families, and individuals. Activities necessary to achieve goals may warrant preventive, maintenance, and restorative emphasis to avoid potential deficits from developing (ANA, 1986).

Home care has come to mean a variety of specialized and generalized nursing care provided to clients whose primary health care site is their home. Adult health (medical-surgical) care, child care, perinatal care, elder care, mental health care, and many other specialties are practiced routinely in the community setting by home care nurses. Effective home care nursing incorporates aspects of comprehensive assessment skills of community health with technology and "hi-touch" care of skilled, caring nursing intervention, planning, and evaluation (Table 2–1).

Home care nursing incorporates the client care plan with effective care coordination and ongoing communication, also called *case management*. In addition, in home care, collaborative communication among team members, along with active and ongoing client participation, ensures that clients are truly equal partners in their health care.

TABLE 2–1

Major Differences Between Nursing Care in the Home and Inpatient Settings	
Home Setting	**Inpatient Setting**
Nurse is more autonomous.	Nurse relies heavily on physician directives.
Environment is controlled by the client.	Environment is controlled by the facility and its staff.
Nurse must be knowledgeable about care of all types and ages of clients.	Nurse is typically knowledgeable about care of specific types of clients, often based on diagnosis.
Nurse must know reimbursement for home care and document care accordingly.	Financial officer and accounting department usually handle reimbursement.
For elderly clients, only selected skilled services are reimbursed by Medicare.	For elderly clients, hospital care is largely reimbursed by Medicare.
There is limited direct supervision of assistive staff, such as home health aides.	There is continuous direct supervision of assistive staff. Nurse and staff work on a single unit.

Home Visits

Home care is usually provided in "visits," not shifts or hours as in the inpatient area. A visit is usually composed of preparation time for the client's visit, such as telephone calls to the physician for clarification of orders for the client's care, obtaining and organizing needed supplies (e.g., wound dressings, catheters, venipuncture supplies), and equipment or insurance authorization of care. There is also travel time, such as driving to clients' homes, and the actual visit time spent in the home for the provision of ordered care. In addition, there is the time for completion of assessment findings, analysis, and care planning and the completion of required, often lengthy documentation.

The usual number of visits per day can vary from four to seven. Clearly, the range is based on the geographic location of the clients and the distance between them, the unique needs of the clients (examples of long visits would be the admitting visit or those involving very ill or terminally ill clients), as well as other factors. The actual client assignments are usually based on the diagnosis and the nurse's expertise as well as physical location.

Client Plan of Care

Like other care settings, a physician's order is needed for care interventions and care plan changes. Because home care nursing practice is more autonomous than in many traditional inpatient settings, it is imperative that orders are obtained from physicians for care and care changes. Sometimes physicians do not see the home care client for months and rely on the home care nurse's judgments and reports. Therefore, verbal or telephone orders are a large

Department of Health and Human Services
Health Care Financing Administration

Form Approved
OMB No. 0938-0357

HOME HEALTH CERTIFICATION AND PLAN OF CARE

1. Patient's HI Claim No.	2. Start Of Care Date	3. Certification Period		4. Medical Record No.	5. Provider No.
		From:	To:		

6. Patient's Name and Address

7. Provider's Name, Address and Telephone Number

8. Date of Birth	9. Sex ☐ M ☐ F	10. Medications: Dose/Frequency/Route (N)ew (C)hanged

11. ICD-9-CM	Principal Diagnosis	Date

12. ICD-9-CM	Surgical Procedure	Date

13. ICD-9-CM	Other Pertinent Diagnoses	Date

14. DME and Supplies

15. Safety Measures:

16. Nutritional Req.

17. Allergies:

18.A. Functional Limitations

1 ☐ Amputation	5 ☐ Paralysis	9 ☐ Legally Blind
2 ☐ Bowel/Bladder (Incontinence)	6 ☐ Endurance	A ☐ Dyspnea With Minimal Exertion
3 ☐ Contracture	7 ☐ Ambulation	B ☐ Other (Specify)
4 ☐ Hearing	8 ☐ Speech	

18.B. Activities Permitted

1 ☐ Complete Bedrest	6 ☐ Partial Weight Bearing	A ☐ Wheelchair
2 ☐ Bedrest BRP	7 ☐ Independent At Home	B ☐ Walker
3 ☐ Up As Tolerated	8 ☐ Crutches	C ☐ No Restrictions
4 ☐ Transfer Bed/Chair	9 ☐ Cane	D ☐ Other (Specify)
5 ☐ Exercises Prescribed		

19. Mental Status:

| 1 ☐ Oriented | 3 ☐ Forgetful | 5 ☐ Disoriented | 7 ☐ Agitated |
| 2 ☐ Comatose | 4 ☐ Depressed | 6 ☐ Lethargic | 8 ☐ Other |

20. Prognosis: 1 ☐ Poor 2 ☐ Guarded 3 ☐ Fair 4 ☐ Good 5 ☐ Excellent

21. Orders for Discipline and Treatments (Specify Amount/Frequency/Duration)

22. Goals/Rehabilitation Potential/Discharge Plans

23. Nurse's Signature and Date of Verbal SOC Where Applicable:	25. Date HHA Received Signed POT

24. Physician's Name and Address	26. I certify/recertify that this patient is confined to his/her home and needs intermittent skilled nursing care, physical therapy and/or speech therapy or continues to need occupational therapy. The patient is under my care, and I have authorized the services on this plan of care and will periodically review the plan.
27. Attending Physician's Signature and Date Signed	28. Anyone who misrepresents, falsifies, or conceals essential information required for payment of Federal funds may be subject to fine, imprisonment, or civil penalty under applicable Federal laws.

Form HCFA-485 (U-4) (02-94)

Figure 2–2. Health Care Financing Administration Form 485.

part of home care practice and communication with physicians. For Medicare clients, physicians must sign HCFA Form 485, which is the client's home health certification and plan of care (Fig. 2–2).

Medicare pays for 15 skills that are attributable to nursing knowledge and licensure. Medicare coverage is predicated on the client meeting defined eligibility criteria (e.g., the client is a Medicare beneficiary, Medicare is the correct payer, the client is homebound [see Homebound Consideration]), and other rules. These 15 skills are

1. Observation and assessment of the client's condition when only the specialized skills of a medical professional can determine a client's status
2. Management and evaluation of a client care plan
3. Teaching and training activities
4. Administration of medications
5. Tube feedings
6. Nasopharyngeal and tracheostomy suctioning
7. Catheters
8. Wound care
9. Ostomy care
10. Heat treatments
11. Gas administration, such as oxygen
12. Rehabilitation nursing
13. Venipuncture
14. Nursing visits
15. Psychiatric evaluation and therapy

Documentation Systems

Reimbursement for home health care relies heavily on the documentation of care. In many home care and other community-based settings, the Omaha Problem Classification System is used instead of the nursing diagnoses from the North American Nursing Diagnosis Association (see Chap. 1). The Omaha system delineates four general areas that represent community and home health practice and provide organizational groupings for client problems: environmental, psychosocial, physiologic, and health-related behaviors. More than 40 nursing diagnoses with modifiers, such as potential deficit, deficit, and health promotion, are then listed within their appropriate domains (Martin & Scheet, 1992). The Omaha Problem Classification System may be found in the Appendix.

NURSING HOME CARE

Long-term care (LTC) has become synonymous in clinical practice with nursing home or chronic care. However, LTC for adult clients with medical-surgical problems occurs in either the home or in facilities such as nursing homes, subacute units, or rehabilitation centers. In general, LTC implies that clients receive care for a prolonged period of time, usually weeks or months. A small percentage of clients may remain in a facility indefinitely, perhaps a lifetime.

Nursing homes in the United States provide care for clients with physical and cognitive impairments as well as those with chronic illness. Clients admitted to a nursing home are called *residents* because the facility is considered their home. The majority of residents are female and older than 65. However, nursing homes are experiencing an increase in the number of younger residents as people live longer with debilitating chronic illnesses, such as multiple sclerosis and muscular dystrophy.

Nursing homes are undergoing another major change. If Medicare certified, most facilities increasingly admit short-term (1–3 weeks) residents for rehabilitation or recovery from an illness or injury. Many of these clients are discharged from hospitals "quicker and sicker," and these individuals often require complex care.

Types of Nursing Homes

Nursing homes can be divided into residential care homes, nursing facilities, and skilled nursing facilities. Some nursing homes are part of retirement communities, and others have specialty units, such as dementia, ventilator, or subacute units.

Residential facilities include domiciliary homes, care homes, rest homes, assisted-living facilities, and group homes. Most of these facilities are small and much like boarding homes before the advent of Medicare (Ignatavicius, 1998). The typical resident in a residential facility is fairly independent and able to perform most or all self-care activities.

Formerly called intermediate care facilities, *nursing facilities* (NFs) provide an intermediate level of care. Certified, licensed NFs receive Medicaid funding for the care of residents who cannot independently perform activities of daily living. Each state has specific guidelines for reimbursement.

Skilled nursing facilities (SNFs, pronounced "snifs") provide care that requires licensed health care professionals, such as nurses and therapists. Only a small portion of most nursing home residents are categorized as skilled and are, therefore, eligible for Medicare reimbursement. Examples of skilled care include tube feedings, daily rehabilitation for postoperative fractured hips, and care of stage 3 and 4 wounds.

Role of the Nurse in Nursing Home Care

Nurses employed by nursing homes are generally more autonomous than those working in hospitals. Physicians are usually not present in the LTC facility on a continuous basis, because residents are considered to be more medically "stable" than those in acute care. However, with early discharge, nursing home nurses are caring for sicker residents than in the past.

Most nurses are placed "in charge" of a unit or shift, because there are more unlicensed personnel (geriatric nursing assistants) than professional nurses. Therefore, the nursing home or LTC nurse needs leadership, management, and clinical competencies to function in this interdisciplinary care environment. One nurse may be the only nurse on that unit in charge of 30 to 35 residents.

SUBACUTE CARE

Subacute care (SAC), one of the newest concepts in health care, is designed for clients who are too ill to be discharged from the hospital to a traditional nursing

TABLE 2-2

Categories of Subacute Care	
Definition of Category	**Examples of Services**
Transitional Subacute Care	
A substitute or alternative for continued hospital stays	Deep wound management Stroke rehabilitation Vascular or cardiac surgery Oncology surgery with chemotherapy Medically complex care Complicated orthopedic surgery
Medical-Surgical Subacute Care	
A setting for stable residents who require moderate level of care	Uncomplicated orthopedic surgery Individuals with human immunodeficiency virus Intravenous therapy Uncomplicated tracheostomy care Stroke rehabilitation
Chronic Subacute Care	
A setting for residents with little or no hope of recovery	Long-term comatose residents Ventilator-dependent residents Progressive neurologic diseases
Long-Term Transitional Subacute Care	
A setting for medically complex conditions with residents	Acute ventilator support Medically complex residents requiring an extended stay

Data from Stahl, D. A. (1994). Subacute care: The future of health care. *Nursing Management, 25*(10), 34–40. Used with permission from Ignatavicius, D. D. (1998). *Introduction to long term care nursing: Principles and practice.* Philadelphia: F. A. Davis.

home or the client's own home. SAC "fills the gap" between the hospital and LTC. Most SAC units are located in freestanding nursing home settings; a smaller percentage are located in hospital settings.

The American Health Care Association (AHCA), which represents the long-term care industry, defines subacute care as a "comprehensive inpatient program designed for the individual who has an acute event as a result of an illness, injury or exacerbation (flare-up) of a disease process; has a determined course of treatment; and does not require intensive diagnostic and/or invasive procedures" (AHCA, 1994). About one third of health care provided by SA units are rehabilitation services; the remainder are medical-surgical services (Stahl, 1994).

Types of Subacute Care

Most SAC units are part of traditional nursing homes. Some units are diagnostic specific, whereas others admit clients with a variety of health problems. Health problems for SAC can be divided into four broad categories: transitional, general medical-surgical, chronic, and long-term

transitional SAC (Stahl, 1994). Table 2–2 lists examples of services provided by each type.

Role of the Nurse in Subacute Care

Little has been published about the role of the nurse in SAC. Nurses who work in SAC must be knowledgeable about LTC and have medical-surgical, critical care, or rehabilitation skills, depending on the type of unit in which they work.

Few nurses have a background that encompasses all of the necessary SAC skills. Nursing homes and hospitals employing nurses for their units are responsible for educating them to ensure that clients' needs are met.

REHABILITATIVE CARE

Rehabilitation is designed for clients who have experienced an acute injury or illness or for those coping with chronic conditions. Rehabilitation services may be provided in the home setting, nursing home, or rehabilitation unit or center. Chapter 13 discusses rehabilitation of individuals with chronic or disabling health problems in detail.

SELECTED BIBLIOGRAPHY

American Health Care Association. (1994). *Blueprint for the future vision.* Washington, DC: Author.

American Nurses' Association. (1986). *Standards of home health nursing practice.* Washington, DC: Author.

Anderson, A. (1996). Nursing clinics in urban settings. *Home Healthcare Nurse, 14,* 542–546.

Bradley, P. J., & Alpers, R. (1996). Home healthcare nurses should regain their family focus. *Home Healthcare Nurse, 14,* 281–288.

Brown-Goebler, S. (1994). Subacute care: Nursing for the next century. *MedSurg Nursing, 3,* 497–499.

Erickson, G. P. (1996). Clinical pearls for home health nursing: Recollections from an oral history. *Home Healthcare Nurse, 14,* 907–913.

Hyatt, L. (1995). *Subacute care: Redefining healthcare.* Burr Ridge, IL: Irmin Professional.

Ignatavicius, D. D. (1998). *Introduction to long term care nursing: Principles and practice.* Philadelphia: F. A. Davis.

Jones, A. M., & Foster, N. (1997). Transitional care: Bridging the gap. *MedSurg Nursing, 6*(1), 32–38.

Marrelli, T. (1994). *Handbook of home health standards and documentation guidelines for reimbursement.* St. Louis: C. V. Mosby.

Marrelli, T., & Hilliard, L. S. (1996). *Home care and clinical paths.* St. Louis: C. V. Mosby.

Marrelli, T., & Whittier, S. (1996). *Home health aide: Guidelines for care.* Westerville, OH: Marrelli.

Martin, K. S., & Scheet, N. J. (1992). *The Omaha system: Applications for community health nursing.* Philadelphia: W. B. Saunders.

Stahl, D. A. (1994). Subacute care: The future of health care. *Nursing Management, 25*(10), 34–40.

Walsh, G. G. (1995). How subacute care fills the gap. *Nursing95, 25*(3), 51.

SUGGESTED READINGS

Anderson, A. (1996). Nursing clinics in urban settings. *Home Healthcare Nurse, 14,* 542–546.
   This article examines the roots of nurse-managed clinics and describes the experience of the Regis College School of Nursing as they developed and implemented two nursing clinics in elderly housing establishments in Boston. The school collaborated with a large medical center in creating the clinics to provide care as well as excellent practice for both students and faculty.

Brown-Goebler, S. (1994). Subacute care: Nursing for the next century. *MedSurg Nursing, 3,* 497–499.
This article emphasizes the growth of subacute care and the corresponding opportunities in the 21st century. It describes the purpose and components of subacute care as well as the roles and skills of nurses working in subacute units.

Ignatavicius, D. D. (1998). *Introduction to long term care nursing: Principles and practice.* Philadelphia: F. A. Davis.

This concise reference focuses on care in the nursing home, the largest component of the long-term care industry. The first half of the book explores clinical issues, such as common health problems, comprehensive assessment, and medication use. The second half discusses the role of nurses as leaders in the nursing home (e.g., the charge nurse, the survey process, and total quality management).

Chapter 3

INTRODUCTION TO MANAGED CARE AND CASE MANAGEMENT

Until the 1980s, health care costs in the United States escalated at a much greater rate than the general inflation rate. Duplication and fragmentation of health care services, as well as advanced technology, have contributed to rising costs.

Since the late 1980s, managed care has grown to be the largest provider system for health care in the United States. Managed health care is a system that "seeks to control the cost of health care by using a select group of providers, who have agreed to a predetermined payment, with the clinical intervention being managed via utilization and/or a case management process" (Owens, p. 1). In other words, the managed care concept integrates providing health care with paying for health care in an attempt to control costs while ensuring the quality of care.

MANAGED CARE

The managed care system is very different from the traditional way of paying for health care. Prior to the managed care movement, hospitals, physicians, and other health care providers were paid by health insurance companies on the basis of what the providers billed for their services. Under this *fee-for-service* arrangement, two physi-

cians could perform identical services but could bill at their own rates. For example, one physician might bill $3000 for a surgical procedure, and another might bill $1800 for the same service. Therefore, under the fee-for-service system, the "risk" was largely taken by the insurance companies.

Purpose of Managed Care

Managed care organizations (MCOs) seek to standardize costs and keep them reasonable. Under the managed care payment system, health care providers receive a uniform amount of money for each client; this is referred to as a *capitated reimbursement system* (Table 3–1).

Balancing costs with quality is an important concept for managed care. Health care providers have been concerned that some MCOs may be too focused on saving money rather than providing high-quality client care (Powell, 1996). The National Committee for Quality Assurance (NCQA) reviews and accredits MCOs that demonstrate high-quality care.

As discussed in Chapter 1, an important role for the nurse is to advocate for clients to ensure that they receive necessary and appropriate care. As a client advocate, care manager, and consumer, nurses need to know about

TABLE 3–1

Glossary of Terms Related to Managed Care	
Authorization	The process used by managed health care organizations to grant authorization of services for a specified period for reimbursement of specific services
Capitation	A managed care reimbursement arrangement that prepays the physician or other health care provider a set dollar amount on a per-member–per-month basis for the delivery of services to a specified group of members
Deductible	The amount of money that an insured person must pay toward health care costs before the insurance company begins reimbursement for health care
Fee-for-service	A reimbursement arrangement in which health care services are paid for as billed by the provider
Indemnity	An arrangement in which benefits are paid in a predetermined amount in the event of a covered loss
Integrated delivery system (IDS)	A system created to manage or provide health care services ranging from primary to tertiary inpatient care and all other settings for care
Risk sharing	A mechanism that provides incentives to physicians and other health care providers to deliver cost-effective and efficient services

managed care and the need for collaborative management of client care.

Role of Nurse Practitioners

Nurse practitioners (NPs) have become more predominant health care providers in the managed care environment because they can deliver more cost-effective health care. In addition, NPs work from a wellness model, with a focus on empowering clients to stay well and care for themselves. Several studies are underway to compare the outcomes from care provided by nurse practitioners with that provided by physicians.

As a result of the increased demand for this advanced practice role, many schools of nursing now offer graduate programs to prepare nurses to become NPs.

Types of Managed Care Organizations

Health care costs have become a national concern to consumers, employers, and health care providers in the United States. Many employers have contracted with a variety of MCOs to reduce health benefit costs. Govern-

ment reimbursement systems have also entered into managed care arrangements to control escalating costs. For example, Medicare, a federal program for the elderly and qualified disabled, is expected to become a managed care system by the year 2000. Many states' Medicaid programs, which pay for health services for the poor, have entered managed care agreements as well.

The oldest and most common type of MCO is the health maintenance organization (HMO), sometimes referred to as a membership organization. Many models for HMOs are used, but all either employ health care professionals to serve subscribing members (enrollees) in an ambulatory setting or contract with physicians and other providers to treat clients in their private offices. The enrollee usually pays a small copayment, typically $5 or $10, for each physician visit.

Another popular type of MCO is the preferred provider organization (PPO). PPOs provide contractual arrangements with physicians, hospitals, and other providers who meet their criteria. In other words, they are the "preferred" providers who render care to a group of subscribers in the health plan.

A point of service (POS) plan is actually an HMO that lets enrollees receive care outside of its network but at a higher copayment or deductible.

COLLABORATIVE MANAGEMENT

As the United States has been moving forward with the managed care system, health care professionals have realized that they must work together as an interdisciplinary team to provide comprehensive care. Although this idea is not new in certain settings, such as rehabilitation, home care, and long-term care, health care professionals in hospitals have not always worked as well as a team. One of the constraints in acute care is the short-term stay. However, the Joint Commission on Accreditation of Healthcare Organizations (JCAHO) mandates that *all* JCAHO-accredited agencies must provide collaborative, interdisciplinary care for their clients.

This text has advocated collaborative management of care since its first edition was published in 1991. This edition continues to discuss client care under "Collaborative Management" headings. Nurses often take the lead role in the interdisciplinary team because they tend to be with the clients for longer periods as they coordinate comprehensive, holistic care.

Focus on Outcomes

The primary focus of collaborative management is on the outcomes of care. The interdisciplinary team identifies expected outcomes for the client and provides interventions to help the client meet those outcomes. Both clinical and cost outcomes are established. This text identifies common clinical outcomes for clients with a number of diseases and illnesses. However, each client is an individual with unique problems and circumstances that may require modification of the commonly identified expected outcomes.

From Collaborative Care Management to Case Management

Whereas all clients need to have their care managed in a collaborative manner, not all clients need to be case managed. *Case management* is not a new concept. Since the turn of the 20th century, social workers, psychologists, and others have "carried a case load" of clients in the community for a variety of purposes. For instance, social workers have worked with at-risk elderly to keep them at home rather than admitted to a nursing home.

In the mid-1980s, Karen Zander and her colleagues at New England Medical Center introduced a nursing case management (NCM) model. The case managers followed up on high-risk, high-cost clients during their hospital stay to coordinate resources and ensure quality outcomes. Physician-nurse collaboration was a primary focus in this model.

The Carondolet integrated health system in Arizona expanded on the NCM model by using case managers across the health care continuum. Sometimes referred to as "beyond the walls" case management, this model incorporated the ethnic values and culture of the community.

Process of Case Management

Case management is "a collaborative process which assesses, plans, implements, coordinates, monitors, and evaluates services and options to meet an individual's health needs through communications and available resources to promote quality, cost-effective outcomes" (Case Management Society of America [CMSA], 1995, p. 8). Sometimes case managers may meet the health needs of a population, rather than a single individual (e.g., all diabetic clients in a given community).

The case management process is reserved for clients who have complex health problems (high risk) and incur a high cost to the health care system. An example of a client who could benefit from case management is an elderly woman with pulmonary emphysema and congestive heart failure who has had repeated admissions to the hospital for pneumonia and lives alone at home. The *Study Guide* and *Instructor's Guide* that accompany this text provide clinical scenarios to show how the case management process is used.

Part of the definition of case management endorsed by CMSA is similar to the steps of the nursing process (Chart 3–1). The individual who practices case management is called a *case manager*. In some agencies, the case manager is referred to as the care coordinator or care manager. Most case managers are nurses, although some are social workers or mental health workers. A few case managers have little or no clinical health background.

In general, case managers can be considered as internal or external. *Internal* case managers are employed by a health care agency and are usually nurses or social workers. Although these individuals manage resources, the primary focus of internal case managers is clinical care. *External* case managers are either employed by an MCO or traditional insurance company or are self-employed and

contract with the MCO or traditional insurance company. The primary focus of external case managers is the utilization of resources for insurance companies.

Standards for Case Management Practice

As the largest professional case management organization, CMSA published standards that specify the recommended preparation for a case manager (Table 3–2). As listed in these criteria, the recommended educational preparation is a baccalaureate degree in a health or human service. Although most case managers today are approximately 40 years of age and are nurses prepared at the associate degree level, it is likely that new case managers in the 21st century will be at least baccalaureate prepared. A number of graduate nursing programs offer masters' preparation as a case manager. The developers of these programs believe that case management is an advanced practice role for nurses.

According to CMSA, the criteria for preparation as a case manager also includes working toward obtaining a certified case manager degree (CCM). This certification process requires that the experienced case manager (with at least 2 years experience) successfully complete a na-

---

Chart 3–1

Nursing Care Highlight

The Process of Case Management

Needs Assessment

- Assesses/collects data
- Conducts case screening
- Identifies client's support systems and care providers
- Reviews history and determines current health care needs
- Obtains approvals for contracts

Plan Development

- Identifies services and funding options
- Reviews plan for consensus
- Advocates for client as needed
- Develops plan, including life care needs, if indicated

Implementation and Coordination

- Communicates regularly with clients and support systems
- Coordinates treatment plan
- Promotes coordinated and efficient care
- Identifies needs for additional services

Outcomes Monitoring and Evaluation

- Assesses benefit value to cost and value to quality of life
- Reviews plan for continuity of care
- Evaluates client satisfaction and compliance with treatment plan

Documentation

- Records services and outcomes
- Submits reports and other documentation as needed

TABLE 3-2

Recommended Preparation for a Case Manager
• Maintain current professional licensure or national certification in a health and human services profession or both
• Have a baccalaureate or higher degree for health and human services personnel
• Complete training and experience with the health needs of the population served
• Have knowledge of health, social service, and funding sources
• Maintain continuing education appropriate to case management and professional licensure
• Work toward and maintain case management certification

Adapted from the Case Management Society of America. (1995). *Standards of Practice for case management*. Little Rock, AR: Author.

tional standardized examination. The CCM designation is a valued credential in the field of case management for any discipline. A new certification is available for nurses who want to be credentialed by their professional organization as a nursing case manager. In October 1997, the first nursing case management examination was given by the American Nurses Credentialing Center (ANCC).

Other certifications may also be acquired by case managers, such as the CRRN for case managers in rehabilitation nursing. Resources in the book's appendices list the names and addresses of certifying organizations.

Roles of Case Managers

Although models for case management vary, all case managers assume a common set of roles and functions. The CMSA *Standards of Practice* outlines the major case manager roles, including assessment, planning, facilitation, and advocacy. For nurses, many of the skills needed to fulfill these roles can be learned as part of basic nursing education.

Case management is being used in a number of countries around the world, including Australia and Singapore. Nursing educators are revising curricula to better prepare their graduates for functioning in a managed care environment.

From Case Management to Disease State Management

Some parts of the United States are practicing disease state management, sometimes called disease management. Put simply, disease state management is a focus on care of clients with chronic disease or illness, such as asthma, diabetes, or congestive heart failure. The purpose of this care approach is to keep clients with chronic conditions as well as possible in the community. If successful, health management would be the goal and health care professionals would be reimbursed for wellness care rather than illness care.

The Role of Clinical Pathways

As mentioned in Chapter 1, the clinical pathway (CP) is a commonly used format for delineating the client's plan of care. It is an interdisciplinary guideline for care that optimally sequences interventions and expected outcomes for a client. Other names for the pathway include the collaborative plan of care (POC), multidisciplinary action plan (MAP), critical pathway, and care path.

The CP is developed by clinical experts for diagnoses, treatments, procedures, or symptoms that are costly, complex, and variable. The health team follows the pathway in managing the client's care. If expected outcomes are not met, the nurse or other health professional records variances, or deviations, on a data collection tool. These variances are then analyzed to identify actual or potential problems needing improvement. An action plan is then implemented and followed up to determine if the infection rate decreases. This entire sequence of data collection, problem identification, action plan, and follow-up is part of the continuous quality improvement (CQI) process that every health care agency uses to monitor and improve the care that it provides.

This textbook provides a number of examples of CPs with varying formats. Traditional client care plans are also included in the book to help students see the difference between a nursing focused care plan and an interdisciplinary plan of care, the CP.

SELECTED BIBLIOGRAPHY

Case Management Society of America. (1995). *Standards of practice for case management*. Little Rock, AR: Author.

Cohen, E. L. (1996). *Nurse case management in the 21st century*. St. Louis: Mosby-Year Book.

Hogan, T. D. (1997). Case management in a wound care program. *Nursing Case Management, 2*(1), 2–15.

Howe, R. S. (1996). *Clinical pathways for ambulatory care case management*. Gaithersburg, MD: Aspen.

Ignatavicius, D. D., & Hausman, K. (1995). *Clinical pathways for collaborative practice*. Philadelphia: W. B. Saunders.

Lee, S. S. (1996). Hospital-home care critical pathways in disease management: Improving case management and patient outcomes in postoperative cardiothoracic surgical patients. *The Journal of Care Management, 2*(3), 42–54.

Marrelli, T. M., & Hilliard, L. S. (1996). *Home care and clinical paths: Effective care planning across the continuum*. St. Louis: Mosby-Year Book.

Mullahy, C. M. (1995). *The case manager's handbook*. Gaithersburg, MD: Aspen.

Owens, M. (1997). Hi, I'm your case manager. *Home Care Provider, 2*(6), 307–310.

Pacala, J. T., & Boult, C. (1996). Factors influencing effectiveness of case management in managed care organizations: A qualitative analysis. *The Journal of Care Management, 2*(3), 29–35.

Powell, S. K. (1996). *Nursing care management: A practical guide to success in managed care*. Philadelphia: Lippincott-Raven.

Romaine, D. S. (1995). Case management challenges: Present and future. *Continuing Care, 14*(1), 24–31.

Siefker, J. M., Garrett, M. B., Van Genderen, A., & Weis, M. J. (1998). *Fundamentals of case management: Guidelines for practicing case managers*. St. Louis: Mosby-Year Book.

SUGGESTED READINGS

Hogan, T. D. (1997). Case management in a wound care program. *Nursing Case Management, 2*(1), 2–15.
This article uses a case study approach to show how case managers make a difference in care of clients with various types of wounds

being cared for at home. A complete plan of care with expected outcomes is also included in the article. A quiz at the end of the article can be completed for continuing education credit or practice.

Lee, S. S. (1996). Hospital-home care critical pathways in disease management: Improving case management and patient outcomes in post-operative cardiothoracic surgical patients. *The Journal of Care Management, 2*(3), 42–54.

This article is from the official journal of the Case Management Society of America. The author describes the development and implementation of a pathway for a cardiothoracic client across the health care continuum, from the hospital through home care.

COMPLEMENTARY THERAPIES

Health problems can no longer be separated into solely "physical" or "mental" categories. Research has clearly demonstrated that healing is successful when the mind, body, and spirit are integrated (Dossey et al., 1995). Complementary therapies, sometimes called complementary modalities or alternative medicine, allow clients to integrate the mind, body, and spirit, and make them active participants in their health care and healing.

Despite the increasing use of complementary therapies in the United States, the concept of "alternative" medicine remains controversial. Physicians have shown a growing openness to the possibility that these therapies can be effective. Younger physicians tend to be more receptive than older ones (American Health Consultants, 1997). Nurses have contributed a great deal to the acceptance and use of therapies that help promote healing.

HOLISTIC NURSING

Holistic nursing practice is a rapidly growing specialty field. According to the American Holistic Nurses' Association, the goal of holistic nursing is about healing the whole person (Dossey, 1997). Therefore, the role of the holistic nurse is to incorporate mind-oriented modalities to treat the physiologic as well as the psychological and spiritual results of illness. Holistic nurses specialize in supplementing traditional medical therapies with mind therapies to augment (not replace) the effects of drugs, surgery, and technology.

All nurses can use aspects of holistic care to enhance

healing. Medical-surgical nurses in a variety of settings care for clients who are physically ill, but have psychological and spiritual effects associated with their conditions as well.

Traditional medical therapies, sometimes referred to as the allopathic approach, focus on the body to treat illness. Complementary therapies, many of which have been used for thousands of years, focus on the mind-body-spirit connection. Examples of complements to conventional medical therapies include relaxation, imagery, biofeedback, prayer, humor, music therapy, and touch. Table 4–1 lists and defines some of the most common complementary therapies. Resources from which more information can be obtained are listed in the Appendix.

OFFICE OF ALTERNATIVE MEDICINE

In their classic study, Eisenberg and his colleagues (1993) found that one third of all adults in the United States used some type of alternative health care in their lifetime. This finding translates into 425 million visits to practitioners of alternative medicine, such as acupuncturists and chiropractors, at a cost of almost $14 billion. The authors divided alternative therapies into high-risk and low-risk groups. Examples of high-risk therapies are certain herbal preparations and some types of spinal manipulation (usually performed by chiropractors). Examples of low-risk therapies are relaxation, imagery, massage, and hypnosis. Not surprisingly, most of the money spent on

TABLE 4–1

Definitions of Common Complementary Therapies

Acupressure	Use of pressure from the fingers and hands to stimulate the energy points in the body, thereby removing energy blocks that are believed to produce health problems
Acupuncture	Use of needles to stimulate certain points on the surface of the body to treat pain, diseases, or dysfunctions of the body; the World Health Organization currently lists a number of medical conditions that may be effectively treated, including migraine, asthma, and arthritis (practitioners are usually licensed by the state)
Aromatherapy	Use of medicinal properties of essential oils extracted from plants and herbs; may be administered via inhalation, topically, or through ingestion
Biofeedback	Use of an electrical device to help the client become aware of certain body functions, such as heart rate, blood pressure, and muscle activity
Chiropractic medicine	Use of adjustments to realign the spine and nervous system so that the body can heal (practitioners are usually licensed by the state)
Imagery	Use of a technique in which a client experiences memories, dreams, and fantasies to relieve stress, decrease pain, and promote healing
Hypnotherapy	Use of hypnosis, posthypnotic suggestion, or any similar process in which the client is susceptible to suggestion or direction
Massage therapy	Manipulation of skeletal muscle to relieve stress or muscle tension; includes stroking, kneading, or stretching on muscles
Naturopathy	A system of prevention, diagnosis, and management of health problems using natural medicines and therapies to stimulate the client's healing process
Osteopathy	Use of body mechanics and manipulative techniques to detect faulty body structure and function

complementary therapies was not reimbursed by health insurance companies. Eisenberg et al. also found that consumers of alternative medicine tended to be educated, upper-income Caucasians in the 25- to 49-year age group.

TRANSCULTURAL CONSIDERATIONS

More recent studies have shown that ethnicity and culture may play a part in determining who seeks complementary therapies. For example, Arcury at al. (1996) found that rural clients in North Carolina used a variety of conventional and alternative remedies for arthritis. Prayer was the most common modality used (92% of the sample used it). African-Americans used alternative methods more often than Caucasians.

Another transcultural study revealed that 44% of Mexican-Americans in the Texas Rio Grande Valley visited an alternative practitioner one or more times during the study year (Keegan, 1996). The most commonly sought therapies were herbal medicine, spiritual healing and prayer, relaxation, and massage.

Paramore (1997) attempted to update national estimates of the use of complementary therapies using the 1994 Robert Wood Johnson Foundation National Access to Care Survey (N = 3450). The results showed that 10% of the U.S. population, or almost 25 million people, saw a professional in 1994 for at least one of the following therapies: chiropractic, relaxation, therapeutic massage, or acupuncture. The researcher concluded that alternative, or complementary, therapies could have a larger role in the health care system of the future.

Recognizing the growing trend toward complementary modalities, the National Institutes of Health created the Office of Alternative Medicine (OAM) in 1992 to evaluate therapies that hold the most promise in treating illness and disease. The ultimate goal of the OAM is to integrate validated complementary therapies into current conventional medical practice. At this time, a number of studies are being conducted around the country by physicians, nurses, and others interested in holistic health practice to determine which therapies are the most effective for which conditions. Many of the studies are focusing on mind-body control therapies, such as biofeedback and imagery; structural and energetic therapies, such as acupressure and therapeutic touch; and ethnomedicine, such as homeopathic medicine and herbal medicine. The safety, efficacy, mechanism of action, and cost effectiveness of individual therapies are being examined.

In 1996, the OAM cosponsored the first conference on medical and nursing education in complementary therapies. Schools of medicine and nursing were encouraged to continue to include content on complementary modalities in their curricula.

MANAGED CARE AND THE HOLISTIC APPROACH

As discussed in Chapter 3, the health care system in the United States has become managed care. Whereas traditional health insurance companies have not typically paid for complementary care, health maintenance organizations (HMOs) around the country are adding alternative medicine practitioners to their list of preferred providers. A study of HMOs in 13 states showed that subscribers are requesting alternative care therapies as part of the health plan. Many HMOs reported that they will offer a blend of conventional and alternative therapies, especially for clients with chronic illness (American Health Consultants, 1997; Eisenberg, 1997).

COMMONLY USED COMPLEMENTARY THERAPIES

It is beyond the scope of this chapter to describe all of the many therapies used by consumers and health care professionals. Some of the most common, low-risk therapies are briefly discussed here. In addition to this chapter's description, complementary therapies are found throughout the text as part of discussions related to management of health problems, such as pain (Chap. 9), fibromyalgia (Chap. 24), acquired immunodeficiency syndrome (Chap. 25), cancer (Chap. 27), and burns (Chap. 71). Many of these interventions can be independently used by nurses in medical-surgical nursing practice settings.

Prayer

Spirituality and religion are not the same. Spirituality gives meaning to a person; that is, it is an aspect of humanity that simply exists. Religion, on the other hand, is not essential for existence and is chosen by an individual. Religion refers to a belief system and practices of worship that are related to that system (Dossey, 1997).

Prayer is an activity related to religion. It has many forms and expressions, but can be generally defined as "a representation of one's longing for communion or communication with God or the Absolute" (Dossey, 1997, p. 45).

Research has demonstrated that faith and prayer can positively affect healing. For example, a qualitative study of adults undergoing coronary artery bypass grafting showed that spiritual-religious issues become very important when a person is faced with a crisis or potentially life-threatening event (Camp, 1996) (see Research Applications for Nursing).

Because religion and prayer take many forms, the medical-surgical nurse explores the way that clients express these beliefs. For instance, the nurse can help clients reflect on the meaning of prayer in their lives as well as other expressions of spirituality and religion, including inspirational readings and music. Questions that a nurse might ask clients to help them find meaning in spiritual or religious activities are listed in Chart 4–1.

Relaxation

Relaxation is one of the simplest and easiest complementary therapies to use. The purpose of relaxation techniques is to reduce physical, mental, and emotional tension, resulting in changes opposite to those of the fight-or-flight mechanism (Dossey, 1997). The physiologic effects of relaxation involve the autonomic, immune, and endocrine systems as summarized in Table 4–2. Com-

▷ Research Applications for Nursing

Meeting the Spiritual Needs of Clients

Camp, P. E. (1996). Having faith: Experiencing coronary artery bypass grafting. Journal of Cardiovascular Nursing, 10(3), 55–64.

Clients perceive coronary artery bypass grafting (CABG) as a potentially life-threatening event. The purpose of this qualitative study was to explore the spiritual needs of 17 clients (ages 34–83 years) who recently had CABG surgery (4–7 days postoperatively). The major findings from the client interviews were that spiritual needs centered around faith in their decision making, faith in the hospital staff (especially the nurses), and an overwhelming faith in God.

Critique. Although the sample size in this study was limited, the information obtained by a qualitative research methodology provides insight into the spiritual needs and resources of clients who are stressed by potential life-threatening events or illnesses. Few studies investigating spirituality have been conducted.

Possible Nursing Implications. Because nurses are with clients on a consistent basis, they are in the unique position of assessing and identifying spiritual needs of their clients. Nurses should be educated about how to assess these needs and provide the necessary spiritual resources for clients.

monly used relaxation techniques include progressive muscle relaxation (PMR), hypnosis, and biofeedback.

Progressive Muscle Relaxation

Progressive muscle relaxation is based on the tenet that stress increases skeletal muscle tension. Intentional tensing and releasing of successive muscle groups promotes relaxation and decreases anxiety. PMR has been used successfully for clients with hypertension, asthma, and panic attacks.

Chart 4–1

Nursing Care Highlight

Questions That Can Be Used as Part of a Spiritual Assessment

- What gives your life meaning?
- What brings you joy and peace in your life?
- What helps you cope when you are troubled or worried?
- How do you feel about yourself?
- Who are significant people in your life?
- Are worship and religion important to you?
- Do you believe in God or a higher power?
- Do you pray?
- Is faith important in your life?
- What is the most important or powerful thing in your life?

TABLE 4–2

Physiologic Effects of Relaxation
Increased peripheral blood flow
Decreased respiratory rate and volume
Decreased heart rate
Decreased blood pressure
Decreased epinephrine level
Decreased gastric acidity and motility
Increased activity of killer cells
Decreased oxygen consumption
Decreased sweat gland activity

Hypnosis

Hypnosis also relaxes skeletal muscles and enhances the clients' ability to use images through suggestions made when the clients are in an altered state of consciousness. In many cases, hypnosis has been successful for smoking cessation.

Biofeedback

Biofeedback is a technique in which clients learn to become aware of certain body functions, such as heart rate, blood pressure, and muscle activity. It involves instrumentation that allows clients to alter these functions using various relaxation techniques.

Biofeedback can also be used for muscular or neuromuscular retraining. For example, Jackson at al. (1996) successfully used biofeedback to help clients achieve continence after radical prostatectomy by increasing their ability to contract pelvic floor muscles. Twenty of 27 clients studied improved: 13 had complete success and 7 had significant improvement. The researcher also found that client motivation is an important factor for success.

The medical-surgical nurse can easily use PMR without special training. Hypnosis and biofeedback are more advanced relaxation techniques that require special training.

When caring for a client who is tense or anxious, the nurse assesses the client's (1) perception of the need for relaxation, (2) readiness and motivation to learn relaxation strategies, and (3) past experience, if any, with relaxation techniques. The nurse also determines whether the client can remain still for a short period of time and assesses his or her ability to see and hear.

To begin PMR, with eyes closed, the client takes several deep breaths, in through the nose and out through the mouth. Then the client tenses and releases each muscle group for several seconds, starting with the head and progressing to the toes. The entire procedure can be completed in a few minutes. The nurse evaluates the success of relaxation strategies by asking the client how he or she feels before and after the intervention.

ELDERLY CONSIDERATIONS

Muscle relaxation can also help promote sleep. Richards (1996) found that caring interventions that focus on the body-mind connection, such as muscle relaxation, back rubs, music, and imagery, promote sleep in the hospitalized elderly.

Imagery

Imagery is a technique in which a person experiences memories, dreams, and visions as a bridge for making the body-mind-spirit connection. Images can occur spontaneously or be induced deliberately. All senses may be involved, but most images are visual; that is, people see positive "mental pictures," such as a beautiful sunset or magnificent ocean. Herbs and aromas, sometimes referred to as aromatherapy, can enhance the formation of images.

Imagery produces physiologic effects that affect healing. Images and thoughts are transmitted through the hypothalamus and limbic system of the brain by neurotransmitters, especially norepinephrine and acetylcholine. These substances affect both the peripheral and autonomic nervous systems to promote relaxation. Clients with cancer or severe pain often use imagery as a complementary therapy.

The nurse assesses the client's history of using imagery and his or her readiness to participate actively in the imagery session. Each session should begin with a relaxation exercise, described in the last section. Sessions may last from 10 to 60 minutes depending on the desired outcomes. Scripts can be used to facilitate the process. Table 4–3 describes several types of imagery that can be employed. The nurse facilitates imagery sessions until the client feels comfortable with the technique and can induce images without assistance.

TABLE 4–3

Commonly Used Types of Imagery	
Interactive guided imagery	Uses a client's own images, both positive and negative; is facilitated by a practitioner
Receptive imagery	Occurs spontaneously when daydreaming and immediately on wakening
Active imagery	Occurs when a client intentionally focuses on forming an image
End-state imagery	Occurs when the client rehearses about being in a healed state
Packaged imagery	Uses tapes, such as relaxation or hypnosis tapes, to create images
Symbolic imagery	Occurs when a client creates images of people, objects, or events to achieve a desired result (e.g., cancer cells are mentally destroyed by a bomb)

Music

Soothing music produces a hypometabolic response in which the autonomic, immune, and endocrine systems are affected. Music also establishes a means of communication between the right and left sides of the brain. Because music is nonverbal, it appeals to the right side of the brain; traditional verbalization appeals to the left side of the brain.

Music can complement conventional medical therapy by reducing pain, anxiety, isolation, and stress. For example, music has been used for surgical clients in both the preoperative and postoperative phases of care. After listening to music of their choice, preoperative clients have reported less anxiety than those who did not. Music can also lower heart rates, blood pressures, and respiratory rates of preoperative clients (Augustin & Hains, 1996). Another nursing study showed that music in the immediate postoperative period helped clients relax and functioned as a distractor (Heiser et al., 1997).

Music can also reduce anxiety in clients receiving chemotherapy. Sabo and Michael (1996) found that music significantly reduced anxiety associated with chemotherapy treatment for cancer.

Like prayer, relaxation, and imagery, music therapy can be used in any health care setting or in the client's home. The nurse assesses the types of music that the client prefers and how it makes him or her feel. Recorded tapes can be played for several daily sessions, each lasting between 20 and 30 minutes. The nurse then evaluates the client's response to the therapy, including vital signs and the client's description of the experience (if possible) and its effects, such as decreased insomnia, pain relief, or decreased agitation.

ELDERLY CONSIDERATIONS

For elderly clients who are confused and restless, the calming effect of music may improve behavioral manifestations, such as agitation and combativeness (Ragneskog et al., 1996). Music causes a variety of experiences for the client, including imagery, sensory stimulation, and relaxation.

Touch

The use of touch for healing was documented more than 5000 years ago. All cultures have developed some form of touch therapy. The Oriental world view is founded on energy. Examples of touch therapies based on energy are acupressure and reflexology (see Table 4–1). The Western world view is based on reduction of matter; examples are massage and therapeutic touch.

Research has demonstrated that touch slows heart rate, decreases diastolic blood pressure, and reduces anxiety. Yet most nurses do not frequently use touch as a comfort or healing measure.

Many types of touch therapies are available, including therapeutic massage, therapeutic touch, acupressure, reflexology, and healing touch. Nurses have been administering back rubs for most of the 20th century, but time constraints have limited this intervention in most settings.

Yet back rubs are a type of therapeutic massage. Back rubs and massage of other parts of the body can promote relaxation and sleep and provide a distraction for clients with anxiety or pain.

Therapeutic touch is more involved. It is a healing modality that involves touching with the intent to help or heal. Therapeutic touch decreases anxiety, facilitates healing, and relieves pain. This modality works by mobilizing areas in the client's energy field that are not flowing and directing one's excess body energies to assist the client to repattern his or her own energies (Dossey et al., 1995).

Acupressure is based on the Oriental energy system of meridian lines and points. The application of the healer's finger and/or thumb to one or more of 657 energy points that run along 12 pathways, or meridian lines, releases congestion and promotes energy flow.

In the early 1900s, Dr. William Fitzgerald noted that pressure applied to certain parts of the hands caused anesthesia in other parts of the body. His work was used by others to explore the field of reflexology, based on the theory that there are 10 equal, longitudinal zones running the length of the body. Like acupressure, applying pressure to certain points releases congestion and promotes energy flow. The other major goal of this therapy is relaxation. Figure 4–1 shows a foot reflexology chart and the location of some of the pressure points.

Healing touch is an advanced group of touch therapies. It is a collection of noninvasive energy-based techniques to make energy available to the client and requires specialized training.

Like the previously described complementary therapies, the nurse can use touch in any health care setting or in the client's home. Massage or simple touching are most commonly used by medical-surgical nurses. Before using touch, however, the nurse assesses the client's feeling about touching, including cultural and age considerations. The nurse also evaluates the client's response to touch.

ELDERLY CONSIDERATIONS

Older clients are likely to receive the least amount of touch; these clients need touch as much as or more than any other age group. Elderly clients often have no family members or significant others. In addition, some elderly cannot communicate and need touch as an effective communication tool (Dossey et al., 1995).

Severely agitated elderly clients may not want to be touched; indeed, touch can cause an increase in aggressive behaviors. The severely cognitively impaired elderly may view touch as an invasion of their personal space.

Laughter and Humor

Laughter and humor have been shown to have physiologic effects on the body by strengthening the immune system, increasing circulation, and stimulating the cortex of the brain. Laughter decreases serum cortisol levels (which increases during stress), increases the numbers of helper T cells and natural killer cells (to destroy tumor cells), and increases salivary immunoglobulin A (to protect against upper respiratory and oral infections) (Berk & Tan, 1993). The physical activity of laughter dilates pe-

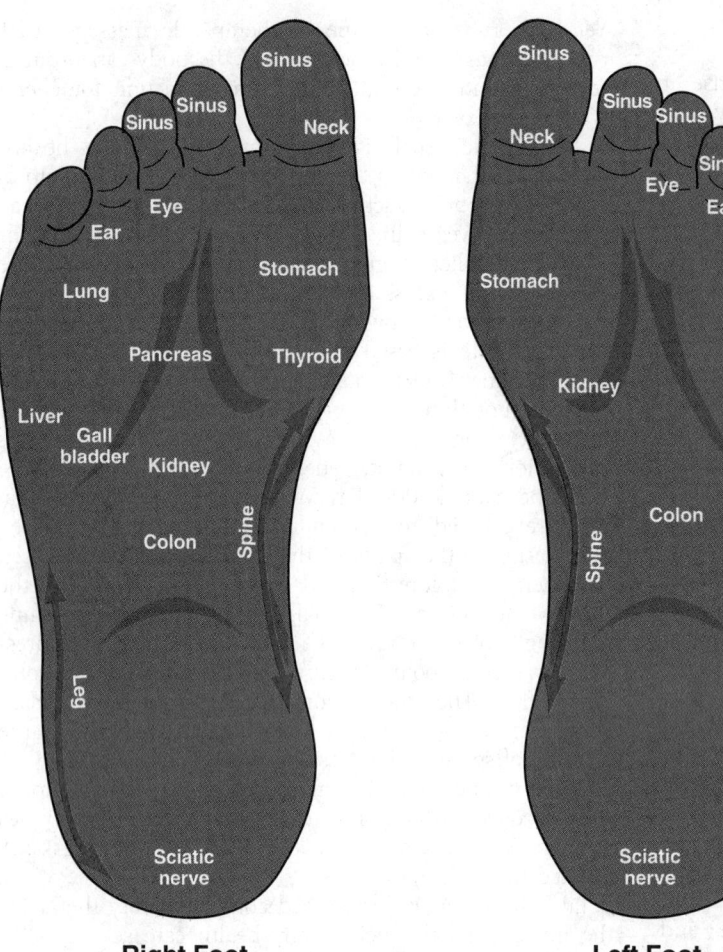

Right Foot   **Left Foot**

Figure 4-1. Reflexology chart of the foot. (From Dossey, B. M. [1995]. Using imagery to help your patient heal. *American Journal of Nursing, 95*[6], 41–46. Used with permission.)

ripheral blood vessels, increasing blood flow to extremities (Dossey, 1997).

Humor is a cognitive skill that involves both the logical left brain and the creative right brain. For example, the left side of the brain is active during joke telling, but the right side perceives the humor.

Laughter and humor also have psychological effects, resulting in relaxation, stress reduction, and distraction. Individuals who have a strong sense of humor generally deal better with stress than those who do not.

Nurses often use laughter and humor when caring for clients. Before using this therapy with clients, the nurse assesses the client's sense of humor as well as his or her own level of comfort with humor therapy. Humor can be very therapeutic for both the client and the nurse.

Some health care agencies use therapeutic, mobile comedy carts, humor rooms, or clown visitation programs. All of these techniques help distract the client, relieve pain, and promote stress reduction.

Nutrition

It has long been established that nutrition plays a major part in the healing process. The importance of trace elements, such as zinc, has been shown to impact healing,

especially of skin lesions. Chapter 64 discusses the role of nutrition as well as nutritional assessment and interventions that the nurse can use.

IMPLICATIONS FOR HEALTH CARE PROVIDERS

Physicians, nurses, and other health care professionals need to learn more about complementary therapies as research becomes available. As discussed earlier in the chapter, healing requires a body-mind-spirit approach.

Eisenberg (1997) suggested that physicians should incorporate the use of complementary therapies into their practices. He recommended that physicians discuss safety and efficacy issues with their clients and help them identify suitable licensed providers of alternative medicine. He further suggested that a follow-up visit after treatment by a practitioner of alternative therapies be made to review response to treatment.

Medical and nursing education programs should incorporate low-risk therapies into their basic curricula. Practicing health care providers need continuing education to keep up with the public's demand for alternative care. Continued nursing research is needed to better delineate the nurse's role in the use of complementary therapies.

CHAPTER 4 ■ Complementary Therapies **41**

SELECTED BIBLIOGRAPHY

American Health Consultants. (1997). HMOs moving more toward alternative care coverage. *Case Management Advisor, 8*(1), 18–19.

Arcury, T. A., Bernard, S. L., Jordan, J. M., & Cook, H. L. (1996). Gender and ethnic differences in alternative and conventional arthritis remedy use among community-dwelling rural adults with arthritis. *Arthritis Care Research, 9,* 384–390.

Augustin, P., & Hains, A. A. (1996). Effect of music on ambulatory surgery patients' preoperative anxiety. *AORN Journal, 63, 750,* 753–758.

*Berk, L. S., & Tan, S. A. (1993). Eustress of humor associated laughter modulates specific immune system components. *Annals of Behavioral Medicine, 15,* S111.

Bryant, J. P. (1996). Therapeutic touch in home healthcare: One nurse's experience. *Home Healthcare Nurse, 14,* 580–586.

Camp, P. E. (1996). Having faith: Experiencing coronary artery bypass grafting. *Journal of Cardiovascular Nursing, 10*(3), 55–64.

Collins, J. A., & Rice, V. H. (1997). Effects of relaxation intervention in phase II cardiac rehabilitation: Replication and extension. *Heart and Lung, 26,* 31–44.

Corley, M. C., Ferriter, J., Zeh, J., & Gifford, C. (1995). Physiologic and psychologic effects of back rubs. *Applied Nursing Research, 8*(1), 39–42.

Dossey, B. M. (1995). Using imagery to help your patient heal. *American Journal of Nursing, 95*(6), 41–46.

Dossey, B. M. (1997). *Core curriculum for holistic nursing.* Gaithersburg, MD: Aspen.

Dossey, B. M., Keegan, L., Guzzetta, C. E., & Kolkmeier, L. G. (1995). *Holistic nursing: A handbook for practice.* Gaithersburg, MD: Aspen.

Eisenberg, D. M. (1997). Advising patients who seek alternative medical therapies. *Annals of Internal Medicine, 127,* 61–69.

*Eisenberg, D. M., Kessler, R. C., Foster, C., et al. (1993). Unconventional medicine in the United States—Prevalence, costs, and patterns of use. *New England Journal of Medicine, 328,* 246–252.

Fascione, J. (1995). Healing power of touch. *Elder Care, 7*(1), 19–21.

Fawcett, J., Sidney, J. S., Riley-Lawless, K., & Hanson, M. J. (1996). An exploratory study of the relationship between alternative therapies, functional status, and symptom severity among people with multiple sclerosis. *Journal of Holistic Nursing, 14,* 115–129.

Ferrara-Love, R., Sekeres, L., & Bircher, N. G. (1996). Nonpharmacologic treatment of postoperative nursing. *Journal of Perianesthesiology Nursing, 11,* 378–383.

Heiser, R. M., Chiles, K., Fudge, M., & Gray, S. E. (1997). The use of music during the immediate postoperative recovery period. *AORN Journal, 65,* 777–778, 781–785.

Jackson, J., Emerson, L., Johnston, B., et al. (1996). Biofeedback: A noninvasive treatment of incontinence after radical prostatectomy. *Urology Nurse, 16*(2), 50–54.

Keegan, L. (1996). Use of alternative therapies among Mexican Americans in the Texas Rio Grande Valley. *Journal of Holistic Nursing, 14,* 277–294.

Mackey, R. B. (1995). Discover the healing power of therapeutic touch. *American Journal of Nursing, 95*(4), 26–33.

Maxwell, J. (1997). The gentle power of acupressure. *RN, 60*(4), 53–56.

McCain, N. L., Zeller, J. M., Cella, D. F., et al. (1996). The influence of stress management training in HIV disease. *Nursing Research, 45,* 246–253.

Paramore, L. C. (1997). Use of alternative therapies: Estimates from the 1994 Robert Wood Johnson Foundation National Access to Care Survey. *Journal of Pain and Symptom Management, 13*(2), 83–89.

Ragneskog, H., Kihlgren, M., Karlsson, I., & Norberg, A. (1996). Dinner music for demented patients: Analysis of video-recorded observations. *Clinical Nursing Research, 5*(3), 262–277.

Richards, K. C. (1996). Sleep promotion. *Critical Care Clinics of North America, 8*(1), 39–52.

Rimmer, L. (1998). The clinical use of aromatherapy in the reduction of stress. *Home Healthcare Nurse, 16*(2), 123–126.

Sabo, C. E., & Michael, S. R. (1996). The influence of personal message with music on anxiety and side effects associated with chemotherapy. *Cancer Nursing, 19,* 283–289.

Skinner, S. (1996). How homeopathy works. *RN, 59*(12), 53–56.

Turkosis, B., & Lance, B. (1996). The use of guided imagery with anticipatory grief. *Home Healthcare Nurse, 14,* 878–888.

Wallace, K. G. (1997). Analysis of recent literature concerning relaxation and imagery interventions for cancer pain. *Cancer Nursing, 20*(2), 79–87.

SUGGESTED READINGS

Bryant, J. P. (1996). Therapeutic touch in home healthcare: One nurse's experience. *Home Healthcare Nurse, 14,* 580–586.

This article describes how one nurse used therapeutic touch with 27 home health clients. It describes the technique she used and the positive results she obtained. The author believes that the clients recovered quicker than they would have without this important intervention.

Corley, M. C., Ferriter, J., Zeh, J., & Gifford, C. (1995). Physiological and psychological effects of back rubs. *Applied Nursing Research, 8*(1), 39–42.

This nursing study examined the benefits of back rubs on elderly residents living in nursing homes. The significant physiologic effects were increased skin temperature and relaxation of the trapezius muscle. However, change in mood (improved) was the most significant finding of the study.

Dossey, B. M. (1995). Using imagery to help your patient heal. *American Journal of Nursing, 95*(6), 41–46.

The author describes types of imagery that can be used with a variety of clients. She discusses how the nurse should conduct an imagery session, including client assessment and evaluation. At the end of the article, a continuing education quiz is available for contact hours.

ADULT DEVELOPMENT

The medical-surgical nurse needs an understanding of each stage of adult development because it affects the client's response to illness and other stressors. However, nurses must also remember that each person is unique and, therefore, may not follow all expected patterns of the developmental stage.

THEORIES OF ADULT DEVELOPMENT

The developmental stage of adolescence seems to fade gradually into adulthood. Adulthood is commonly described as having its onset at some point after a person achieves physical maturity. In contrast to earlier periods of the life cycle, adulthood has no established landmarks that precisely characterize its onset or its stages.

People share certain traits with respect to age and the rate of maturation. Age in years may indicate that several social milestones have passed. Designating arbitrary ages for the onset of maturity, middle age, and old age, however, may promote a stereotypic view of the stages of adulthood. The nurse should remember that there are many individual differences that result from factors such as heredity, gender, health history, and life experience.

A single theory explaining changes during adulthood has been difficult to construct. Thus, many theories have

been developed, each representing a different view. Theories of adult development can be divided into two broad areas: developmental theories and theories of aging.

Developmental Theories

Developmental theories imply that certain psychosocial growth mechanisms can be assigned to various ages. The classic theories expressed by Erikson, Peck, and Havighurst are the most commonly cited. However, these theories were constructed more than 30 years ago and may not reflect the developmental patterns of all adults in the 21st century.

Erikson's Eight "Stages of Man"

Erikson (1968) proposed that personalities continue to evolve throughout adult life in a gradual, continuous manner. The first five stages of Erikson's theory largely expand on Freud's stages of childhood development. The last three stages provide a useful model for understanding some general issues of adult developmental changes during the adult years. Table 5–1 explains these adult stages and related nursing assessment.

For example, the task of the older adult is ego integrity versus despair. If older adults cannot adjust to the physical, psychological, and sociologic changes that may occur

TABLE 5–1

Erikson's Adult Developmental Tasks		
Developmental Stage	**Developmental Task**	**Nursing Assessment**
Young adulthood	• Intimacy versus isolation	• Assess whether the client has meaningful, intimate relationships. • If the client has no intimate relationships, ask whether he or she has had one or more in the past. • Assess other support systems that the client may have.
Middlescence	• Generativity versus stagnation	• Assess whether the client is employed. • Ask the client what he or she does for leisure or recreation. • If the client is not employed or has no regular leisure activity, ask the client what he or she does during a 24-hour day. • Assess for signs of depression, such as excessive sleeping and decreased appetite.
Older adulthood	• Ego integrity versus despair	• Assess what the client does each day. • Ask about the client's family and other relationships. • Ask the client if he or she feels lonely; if so, assess for signs of depression.

as they age, they are at risk for despair. The result may be depression. The nurse assesses the older adult to determine whether this task has been accomplished successfully or whether the person is at a high risk for depression or is already depressed.

Peck's Developmental Tasks of Adulthood

The last two of Erikson's stages encompass all the middle adult and late years of the life cycle. This view of adulthood may be too simplistic and general. Using Erikson's model as a foundation, many developmental psychologists have expanded his theory to more realistically represent adulthood. Peck (1968) identified seven crucial developmental tasks for the last two periods of the life cycle: middlescence (middle adulthood) and late adulthood (Table 5–2). Peck believed that there are four major tasks in middlescence and three tasks in late adulthood that must be confronted for healthy adjustment. If these tasks

are not accomplished, a person's state of health may decline.

For example, in the period of "old age," one task is body transcendence versus body preoccupation. Peck included this task because he observed many older adults beginning to focus on the declines in their physical functioning, resulting in a preoccupation with their body. Peck said that to age successfully, older adults need to accept these body changes and adapt to them as well as possible. When caring for an older adult, the nurse assesses the person's view of body changes and how he or she has coped with them.

Havighurst's Theory of Adult Developmental Tasks

Havighurst's (1972) ideas have also contributed to the understanding of adult development. His theory has a

TABLE 5–2

Peck's Developmental Tasks of Adulthood		
Period of Life Cycle	**Developmental Task**	**Clinical Applications**
Middlescence	• Valuing wisdom vs physical powers • Socializing vs sexualizing in human relationships • Cathectic flexibility vs cathectic impoverishment • Mental flexibility vs mental rigidity	• The client is likely to have strong relationships with family or significant others. • The client is likely to be more flexible in his or her lifestyle if necessary. • The client is able to make and adapt to changes as needed.
Old age	• Ego differentiation vs work role preoccupation • Body transcendence vs body preoccupation • Ego transcendence vs ego preoccupation	• The client is able to have a meaningful life after retirement from work. • The client accepts and adapts to changes in body structure and function without difficulty. • The client accepts the inevitability of death and approaches it in a positive manner, feeling that he or she has lived a "good" life.

TABLE 5-3

Havighurst's Developmental Tasks of the Adult

Stage	Developmental Task
Early adulthood	• Selecting a mate • Learning to live with a marriage partner • Starting a family • Rearing children • Managing a home • Getting started in an occupation • Assuming civic responsibility • Finding a congenial social group
Middle age	• Achieving adult civic and social responsibility • Establishing and maintaining an economic standard of living • Assisting teenage children to become responsibile and happy adults • Developing leisure activities • Accepting and adjusting to the physiologic changes of middle age • Adjusting to the aging of parents
Later maturity	• Adjusting to decreasing physical strength and health • Adjusting to the death of a spouse • Adjusting to retirement and reduced income • Establishing an explicit affiliation with one's age group • Meeting social and civic obligations • Establishing satisfactory physical living arrangements

broad definition of successful aging that addresses social competency and adaptation to new roles. He viewed developmental tasks as a continual discovery of new and meaningful roles. This positive view of aging helps people "successfully age." He divided the life cycle into six age periods, each containing 6–10 developmental tasks. The tasks for the adult periods are summarized in Table 5–3.

A major criticism of Havighurst's ideas is his stereotypic presentation of the tasks in each age period (which were perhaps appropriate for the 1960s and 1970s). For example, he stated that people typically marry and start a family in young adulthood. Today, it is increasingly common for young adults to postpone marriage or not marry at all. Many couples choose to have children later in life or not at all. In addition, Havighurst did not acknowledge same-sex relationships.

Theories of Aging

In addition to theories of adult development, numerous theories are associated with the aging process. These include biological (physiologic), sociologic, and psychological theories. Several of the most commonly cited theories are briefly presented here.

Biological Theories of Aging

Biologists exploring the aging process concluded that aging can be viewed as a progression through a continuum of events that occur from birth to death. From this perspective, the aging process has been defined as the sum total of all changes that occur in a person over the life span. On the basis of this broad definition, it has been proposed that aging can best be understood by studying physiologic development. Over the years, many biological, or physiologic, theories have emerged, including exhaustion theories, genetic theories, single-organ theories, the free radical theory, and the immunity theory.

A number of very large studies are being conducted across the country to follow people as they age and learn more about the normal aging process.

Exhaustion Theories

Early theorists on aging proposed that there is a fixed store of energy available to the body. As time passes, the energy available is depleted, and, because it cannot be restored, the person dies.

Later, other related theories emerged. The *wear and tear theory* stated that the body is like a machine that wears out its parts with repeated use and comes to a grinding halt. Today, the concept of wear and tear is not widely accepted as an explanation for the aging process. However, this theory may explain the development of certain diseases, such as degenerative joint disease, in which the joint cartilage degenerates with prolonged use.

A more popular theory is the *stress theory,* which focuses on the physical and psychological wear and tear from sudden and unexpected stressors over which a person has no control. This theory maintains that a person copes with stressors through a three-stage process of alarm, resistance, and exhaustion (see Chap. 8). This process eventually leaves the person weakened because of the accumulation of successive stressful events over the life span. Stress theory suggests that as people age they are no longer capable of fighting off the various stressors as a result of the accumulation of wear and tear.

Genetic Theories

A major breakthrough to help explain biological development was the identification of deoxyribonucleic acid (DNA) molecules as the information center of the cell. This discovery led to the theory that cellular death results from DNA damage. The possibility that biological aging results when the wrong information is provided for normal cell function has been considered and is called *error theory*.

Several theories suggest that aging changes may occur as a result of an alteration in cellular genetic information. For example, the *cross-link theory* proposes that a chemical reaction occurs that produces irreparable damage to DNA and consequent cell death (Matteson et al., 1997).

In clinical practice, it is interesting to note the trend for similar life expectancies in families. It is not unusual for a person of advanced age to state that he or she had parents who also lived to be very old.

Single-Organ Theories

Other physiologic theories of aging have attempted to explain aging and the life span on the basis of changes in a single organ or in terms of impairments in control mechanisms. One theory suggests that aging results primarily from lowered oxygen supply delivered to crucial body tissue, such as brain tissue. Other theories suggest that thyroid gland function might be responsible for the slowing of metabolic processes at the cellular level (because cellular metabolism is regulated by the thyroid gland). The slowing of metabolic processes would then promote aging.

Free Radical Theory

Free radicals are highly reactive cellular components that replace genetic information at the cellular level. Lipofuscin is a material that is associated with free radicals and is rich in lipids and protein. This abnormal substance has been found in large quantities in body organs as they age. Some researchers suggest that the accumulation of lipofuscin interferes with cellular metabolism and may play an important role in the aging process (Matteson et al., 1997).

Immunity Theory

According to the immunity theory, as people age, mutations occur in some cells, resulting in the formation of proteins that the body does not recognize. The immune system then produces antibodies against these new proteins and attempts to destroy them, causing an autoimmune response (Matteson et al., 1997). With increasing age, there would then be a reduction in the function of the immune system. The antibodies fail to recognize abnormal cells, allowing them to divide and multiply. Immune system failure might then promote such late-life diseases as cancer, diabetes, and emphysema.

Sociologic Theories of Aging

The concept of socialization during adulthood refers to the process by which people, over the course of their adult lives, acquire ways to perform new roles. Several theories are relevant to how adults learn which roles bring rewards and which roles are considered undesirable and how they adjust to changing roles and role losses in society. These include Rosow's role theory and the activity theory.

Rosow's Role Theory

Rosow (1974) maintained that socialization for roles is a continuous and cumulative process that corresponds to the developmental stages of the life cycle. Socialization for roles begins in infancy and extends through adolescence. However, the actual learning of specific role demands begins and continues as a person moves through the stages of adulthood.

The concept of role continuity suggests that role demands of the previous stage prepare the person for the responsibilities associated with the next status or position

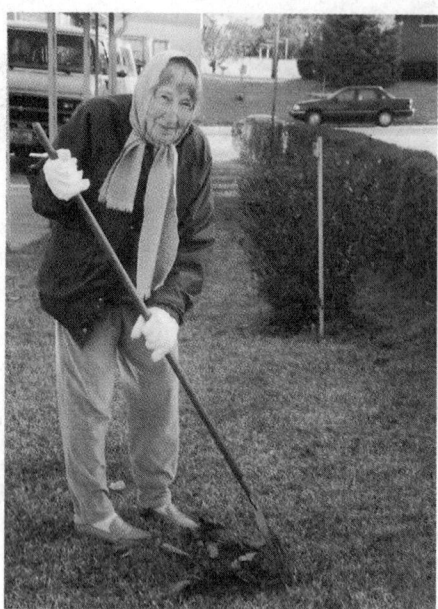

Figure 5–1. An active elderly woman.

that the adult assumes. Thus, role transitions through the life span progress in a smooth manner from one age level to the next.

Activity Theory

The activity theory holds that the maintenance of activities is important to most people as a basis for obtaining satisfaction, self-esteem, and health. Most research has shown the importance of activity as the basis for the promotion of vigor and satisfactory adjustment in the elderly (Fig. 5–1). People who restrict their activities as they age may tend to experience a reduction in overall life satisfaction. The significance of this theory to nurses is that they should encourage older adults to remain active to the extent they are able. Continued activity includes both physical actions and cognitive stimulation.

Psychological Theories of Aging

Psychological theories of aging are often the extension of sociologic and developmental theories. Personality theories usually consider the human needs and forces that motivate thought and behavior within a physical and social environment. The problem with studying personality changes throughout adulthood is that, as people pass through life, they become increasingly different rather than more similar. Theorists who have addressed adult personality development have primarily focused on one central issue: whether adult personality is characterized by continuity or by change.

Jung (1928/1971) was one of the first psychologists to consider that the latter half of life has a purpose of its own, quite apart from that of survival: namely, the development of self-awareness through reflective activity. He strongly believed in the importance of the latter half of life. This phase is characterized by inner discovery, as opposed to the first half of life, which is oriented toward biological and social goals. Jung's work regarding the life review process clearly defined the growth potential for aged adults. A review of past events, or reminiscence, helps with personal growth and evolving identity.

STAGES OF ADULTHOOD

Adulthood can be divided into three broad categories: young adulthood, middle adulthood, and older adulthood. In general, experts in adult development do not agree on the age span for each category. Therefore, differences in the professional and popular literature are common.

The medical-surgical nurse should know about normal adult development as a basis for physical and psychosocial assessment. A review of normal development and associated health issues follows.

Young Adulthood

Young adulthood is generally designated as the period between the 18th and 35th year. Many young adults are able today to postpone the tasks of adulthood, to experiment, and to prolong their own transition from childhood by exploring the many choices available to them. This period offers the time needed for the person to grow and make the necessary and complex linkages with adult society.

Physiologic Changes
Musculoskeletal Changes

Even though growth essentially ceases at adolescence, minimal growth can continue. Fusion of the epiphyses of long bones occurs approximately at age 18 to 25 years. Muscular efficiency is at its peak level between ages 20 and 30 years. Thereafter, muscular strength declines. Regular exercise is important to maintain a healthy body. People often become more sedentary in the postadolescent years as a result of the lack of a regular exercise plan, changes in work and leisure activities, and alterations in eating patterns.

Cardiopulmonary Changes

Physical development of the heart, blood vessels, and lungs stops in adolescence. Maintaining cardiopulmonary functioning and preventing pathologic changes during the second half of life largely depend on the young adult's lifestyle practices that are carried into middle age and late life.

Although arteriosclerotic disease becomes clinically evident in middle adulthood, it represents the result of progressive changes in the arterial walls that began in childhood. Studies are currently under way to examine the lifestyles of children and to find ways to improve health during childhood to prevent later problems.

TRANSCULTURAL CONSIDERATIONS

Although heart disease is not usually associated with the young adult age group, heart-related mortality for young Native Americans is about twice that for all other young adults living in the United States (Jarvis, 1996).

Integumentary Changes

The abundance of skin care and hair-coloring products attests to the aging changes that begin in young adulthood. These changes are often traumatic if a young adult has accepted the youth-oriented value system in Western countries like the United States and Canada.

Wrinkling of the skin occurs with aging and is markedly increased by exposure to the sun. Facial wrinkling becomes obvious in most adults in their 20s and tends to be progressive thereafter. Early wrinkling is usually related to habitual facial expressions, such as frowning and smiling. The skin loses its moisture and gradually dries. In later years, the atrophy of fat accelerates and increases the appearance of wrinkles.

The onset of graying hair and baldness often begins in young adulthood as well. Graying of hair results from the inability of melanocytes to provide hair with pigment granules over time. Hair loss with aging results from a number of factors. Although it is more common in men, it also occurs in women. Early balding is a result of genetic factors and is related to the amount of androgens, such as testosterone, that are produced (Fig. 5–2).

Dental Changes

The third molars, or wisdom teeth, normally erupt in an adult's early 20s. There are four third molars, although in some adults all four may not develop fully. Wisdom teeth frequently present problems and require dental care.

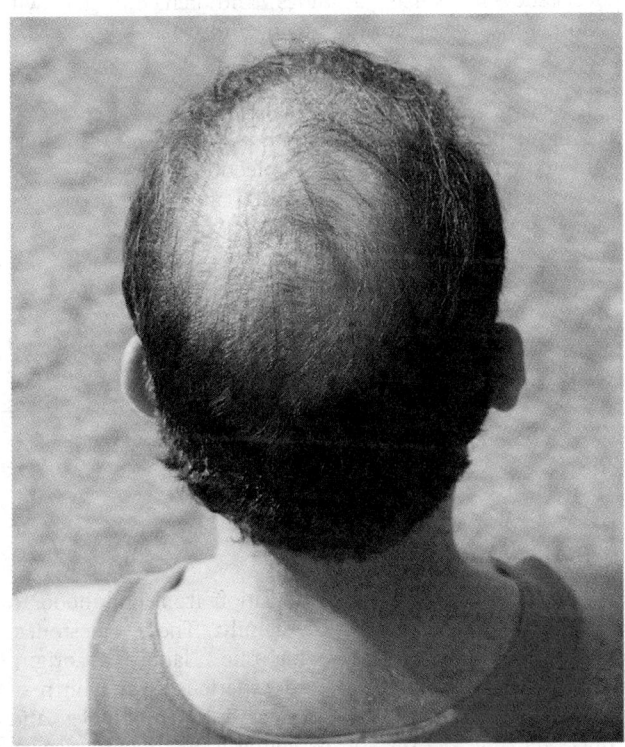

Figure 5–2. Early balding. This man is in his early 30s.

Their eruptions are unpredictable, and it is not uncommon for them to be malaligned or to remain impacted in the gums.

Psychosocial Development

The central issues of psychosocial development in young adulthood are related to the final resolution of the identity crises begun in adolescence. People work through these issues rather slowly. By the time the adolescent reaches young adulthood, some of these issues are nearing resolution.

The young adult struggles with expanding a sense of self in determining who he or she is within various social roles. In this stage of identity development, the prime concern is the relationship between the person and the social system. Young adults seek to resolve several psychosocial issues in their quest for maturity.

Self-Identity

In young adulthood, the sense of self usually becomes sharper and clearer, more consistent, and less influenced by others. This identification is quite different from that in the adolescent, who is self-conscious and concerned with seeing the self from the viewpoint of others.

Young adults become increasingly more comfortable with making decisions when faced with unexpected life events. In the mature young adult, coping with the unexpected does not easily disrupt the sense of continuity and integration.

As young adults participate in adult roles, they select lifestyle patterns and role combinations that endure through later life. These decisions solidify their self-identity and enable the young adult to develop a sense of consistency in beliefs, attitudes, and behavior that will continue to develop through their adult years.

Sexuality

The development of contraceptive pills, the fear of human immunodeficiency viral (HIV) infection, and changes in sexual mores have resulted in a dilemma for many young adults. Much conflict and confusion occur when one is questioning values related to sexuality.

Change in the sexual aspects of young adulthood relates to more than just sexual behavior. Relationships become increasingly more responsive to understanding and accepting others as they are. Interpersonal relationships depend more on appreciating the uniqueness of others and less on a projection of one's adolescent fantasies, physiologic needs, and a search for a sense of identity. Chapter 11 describes sexuality in detail.

Family Structure

The major milestones of the transition from childhood to adulthood largely involve the family. These milestones, which typically include leaving one's family of origin, selecting a mate, marrying, and experiencing the birth of the first child, mark the entrance into adult roles and functions (Fig. 5–3). Not all young adults experience all of these milestones. Not everyone marries or has chil-

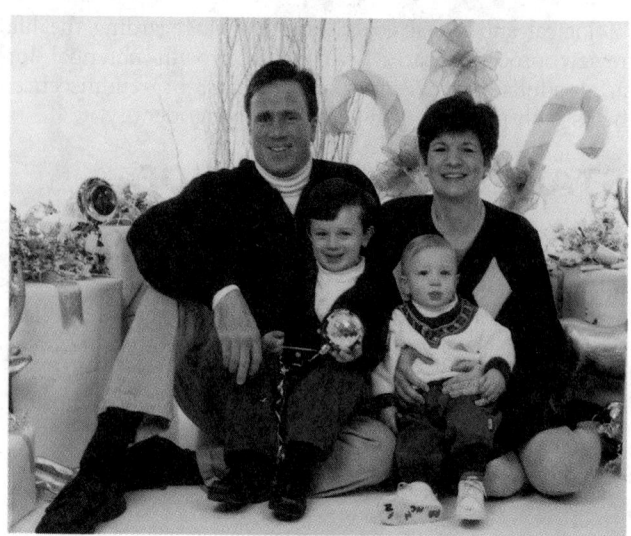

Figure 5–3. A young family.

dren. Some adults select homosexual rather than heterosexual relationships.

In the United States, two general types of family structures exist: patriarchal (headed by men) and matriarchal (headed by women).

TRANSCULTURAL CONSIDERATIONS

About half of all African-American families are matriarchal, in contrast to one fourth of Hispanic families and one sixth of Caucasian families (Giger & Davidhizar, 1995).

Patriarchal Family Structure

If the young adult marries and has children, the event of marriage and the establishment of the family bring about many changes and crisis points. The birth of a child requires a major shift from a primarily spousal role to the demands and responsibilities of a parental role. This resocialization requires not only the learning of a new role but also the ability to combine this new role into a set pattern with other roles. The addition of a dependent, demanding third person may disrupt the established couple relationship as well as one's routine patterns of living.

Matriarchal Family Structure

In the United States, one of every two marriages ends in divorce. More often than not, children of divorced parents live with their mother, which can place a physical, financial, and emotional burden on the single parent. Some single mothers have never been married or may not have ongoing contact with the father of their children. Financial or child care support may not be available, and the mother is left with the total responsibility of childrearing. The single mother often ignores personal needs to balance child care, work, and home responsibilities. This family structure, rather than the traditional patriarchal structure described by Havighurst (1972), is becoming increasingly more common in the late 1990s and into the 21st century.

Work

Entrance into the work world for the young adult involves a twofold process. The first aspect is the choice of an occupation, followed by socialization into the role demands of the job. The process of selecting and maintaining an occupation is characterized by more flexibility than in years past. The traditional factors of social class, culture, intelligence, gender, aptitudes, role models, and experiences that once operated to limit the range of choices have lost much, but not all, of their impact.

Both partners in a relationship may work outside the home. Not infrequently, one person may need to work at two jobs. Over the past decade, unemployment in the United States has dramatically increased as a result of restructuring and re-engineering of most major businesses. Finding jobs has become more difficult and has greatly increased stress for many adults. Homelessness has increased, and an increasing number of people have no health insurance or are underinsured.

Many young adults see prolonged or continuous education as the means to obtain desired standards of living. This often means postponing intimate relationships or combining the roles of student, temporary worker, partner, and parent. Balancing these responsibilities at a time when young adults are still acquiring basic knowledge and skills needed to resolve their developmental tasks can create considerable stress.

Leisure

Leisure in adulthood is often a difficult concept to define. Most adults consider their work to be the most meaningful activity in their lives. Work provides the necessities of life. It is also the major aspect of one's identity and status. Therefore, to many people, leisure is a negative concept rather than a potentially positive, healthful experience in its own right.

Health Issues

The young adulthood years are usually the healthiest years in the life cycle. Most young adults are not seriously ill or incapacitated. As a result, young adults often feel a sense of immunity to illness and neglect health promotion and maintenance activities. The greatest potential for improving health is in what people do and do not do for themselves. Young adults' decisions about diet, exercise, smoking, and drug use are of critical importance to their health status in middle age and later life.

Health Promotion

For young adults to maintain optimal health, the nurse should encourage them to have regular physical examinations, with more frequent visits if there are particular problems. For early detection of cancer, young women should have routine Papanicolaou (Pap) tests and perform breast self-examination (BSE) once a month. The nurse teaches BSE to women and teaches testicular self-examination (TSE) to young men. Young adults should schedule annual dental examinations to avoid dental and periodontal disorders. In addition, young adults should have

---

Chart 5–1
Health Promotion Guide: Activities to Promote Health and Prevent Illness

- Have regular (yearly) physical examinations.
- For women, have regular Pap tests and perform breast self-examination monthly.
- For men, perform testicular self-examination on a regular basis.
- Have annual dental examinations and prophylaxis.
- Have regular eye examinations (every 1–2 years).
- Exercise regularly at least three times a week for 30 minutes.
- Do not smoke; avoid second-hand (passive) smoke.
- Avoid alcohol and so-called recreational drugs.
- Decrease fat and increase fiber in the diet.

---

regular eye examinations every 1 to 2 years (Chart 5–1). Despite a general state of good health, young adults are susceptible to a few major health concerns.

Accidents

In the United States, accidents are the most frequent cause of death among young adults. Injuries occur as a result of work-related incidents, thrill-seeking pleasures, violent crimes, automobile accidents, and war. Men are consistently more frequently involved in accidents throughout the life cycle than women. Between the ages of 15 and 34 years, the death rate among males is more than three times that among females, largely because of the high rate of accidental deaths.

The everyday lives of young adults present stressful experiences, such as driving in city traffic and caring for small children, that contribute to accidents. Excessive fatigue occurs in young adults who attempt to balance too many roles. Stress overload combined with excessive fatigue can lead to accidents as well as psychosomatic illnesses.

Young adults should be especially aware of maintaining good health care practices, such as well-balanced diets, regular exercise, and adequate sleep. Because accidents and their consequences present major threats to their health, young adults should take care when engaging in potentially hazardous activities. This care includes using seat belts, avoiding drinking when driving, following speed limits, and observing caution around machinery. In many states in this country, nurses have advocated for legislation that mandates the use of seat belts and motorcycle helmets to help prevent serious injuries from accidents.

Homicide and Suicide

After accidents, the leading causes of death in young adults are homicide and suicide. The highest incidence of homicide is associated with young African-Americans living in urban areas (Giger & Davidhizar, 1995). Some of the deaths are related to substance abuse, such as drugs and alcohol, and the formation of gangs.

Drug and Alcohol Use and Misuse

Few issues have received as much recent attention as drug and alcohol abuse. Use of alcohol and other illicit drugs has increased significantly in the last two decades. Even though the use of tobacco has declined, the use of potentially addictive agents in young adulthood has not decreased, despite the numerous efforts to control this problem. Many law enforcement agencies have united in an effort to identify and prosecute drug dealers, buyers, and users. Clinics and programs have also been established to help people wean themselves from drugs. National prevention and awareness programs like DARE (Drug Awareness Resistance Education) have been conducted in elementary and middle schools across the United States for a number of years.

Regardless of the health care setting, the role of the nurse is affected by the growing problem of substance abuse. In the medical-surgical setting, the nurse often provides care for the client who is or has been a substance abuser. As a result, the planning of nursing interventions is typically more difficult and complicated. For example, the client in pain from a fractured tibia may want pain medication by injection on a regular basis. If the nurse's assessment does not validate that the client is in severe pain, the nurse is faced with an ethical dilemma as well as a care management decision.

Even though alcohol and drug problems are often associated with young adults, this age group is not the only one affected by these addictive agents. Middle-aged and older adults often use addictive agents, but the nurse may have more difficulty in assessing this problem in these groups.

Middle Adulthood

The time between 35 and 64 years of age is generally considered the period of middle age. This period has been described as the "best years" in the life cycle. During this span of time, adults refer to being in the "prime of life." If healthy development has occurred, the struggles of young adulthood are past and have been resolved, and middle-aged adults should be able to enjoy the results of their labor as established, mature, social, and personally valued people. Yet this time is fraught with its own difficulties.

Middlescence (middle age) is recognized as the midpoint in the life cycle. Most people reflect on and evaluate their lives during this period. Evaluation is not an unusual experience, but it takes on special meaning at this time. The accomplishments of young adulthood shape the life of the middlescent. At this point, people may suddenly realize that this transitional period is the last chance to change life's direction. Many middlescents begin to examine the results of their life work against what they want to do with the rest of their lives. Most of the young adulthood years were spent in working toward achieving goals set in youth. Middlescents reassess their choices and wonder if their chosen directions will progress toward realizing their life goals or desires. This examination may result in massive lifestyle changes for some. This often unsettling time of life, which entails the transition to old age, is often referred to as the midlife crisis.

Physiologic Changes

From young adulthood through the middle years, physiologic changes occur gradually.

Sensory Changes
Visual Changes

All people eventually experience a change in visual acuity. The decreased ability of the eyes to accommodate for close and detailed work (presbyopia) becomes evident at about age 35 and continues throughout the rest of one's life. Pupil size becomes smaller, which decreases the amount of light that reaches the retina. This change limits the ability of the pupil to constrict and dilate and affects the ability to adapt one's vision in dim light and darkness.

Toward the end of middlescence, the eyes are less able to detect the blues, violets, and greens of the color spectrum and more easily adapt to reds, yellows, and oranges. This change in color perception is linked to the yellowing of the lens with advancing age, but it is not actually a color vision impairment (Matteson et al., 1997).

People in their 50s need about twice as much light to see things as they did when they were in their 20s. There is a need for more light for all visual perception with advancing age. The nurse teaches middle-aged and older adults to use extra lighting at home to prevent falls. In the health care setting, the nurse provides adequate lighting, especially at night.

Hearing Changes

Hearing loss typically begins in late middlescense. Changes in the efficiency of the cochlea and the hair cells of the organ of Corti are responsible for the impaired transmission of sound waves along the nerve pathways of the brain. These changes are considered to be the most common cause of presbycusis, which is progressive hearing loss associated with aging (Ney, 1993). Presbycusis primarily affects the ability to hear high-pitched sounds and soft consonants or consonant blends. For example, the "s," "sh," and "ch" sounds are difficult for people with presbycusis to differentiate in conversations. Vowels that have a low pitch are more easily heard. Background noise interferes with conversation, so that it is difficult to hear what is being said.

The abilities to see and to hear are major contributors to communication. Age-related changes in these abilities are not only frustrating but also threatening to security and self-esteem. Yet many middlescents are reluctant to wear eyeglasses or hearing aids, even when vision or hearing problems significantly affect functioning. Many seem to want to deny the problem rather than to admit to age-related changes. The nurse teaches middle and older adults the importance of wearing assistive devices if needed to help prevent falls or other accidents.

Neuromuscular Changes

For many middlescents, sedentary or slower paced lifestyles result in loss of muscle strength and mass. This loss of muscle tone is noticed as the waistline thickens, the abdomen protrudes, and facial tissue sags.

There is a gradual decline in motor and sensory functioning from its peak during a person's 20s to lower levels in the middle years. Reflexes that entail responses to sudden changes in the environment may be slowed, but for the most part the alterations in function occur gradually and go unnoticed.

Middle-aged adults view neuromuscular changes as relatively insignificant because their progress is so gradual that most people have learned to compensate for them. For example, driving ability is considered to be *better* in middle-aged adults than in younger people, despite declines in coordination, increased reaction time, and sensitivity to glare. It seems that the improvements in judgment and caution compensate for the physical declines. The same is true for manual workers. Middle-aged people usually have fewer disabling injuries and are more conscientious and careful than their younger counterparts.

Cardiopulmonary Changes

Coronary and pulmonary diseases are among the leading causes of morbidity and mortality in middlescence. These problems are more probably related to lifestyle and genetic factors than to aging per se.

Heart function, rate, and rhythm usually remain unchanged in middlescence. However, when lifestyles become sedentary, anatomic and physiologic changes may occur. Lack of regular exercise over time causes the heart muscle to lose its tone, and changes in rate and rhythm result. Among the most significant factors implicated in atherosclerosis and heart disease are poor nutrition, lack of physical exercise, smoking, and stress.

Pulmonary changes in middlescence are largely related to whether the person is or has been a smoker. Smoking decreases respiratory efficiency and increases the risk of lung disease. Smoking and chronic lung disease largely account for the loss of functioning in lung tissues seen in middlescence. These risk factors, coupled with environmental or occupational pollution, inactivity, and altered cardiac status, can result in decreased breathing capacity. The nurse assesses for risk factors and provides health teaching, such as smoking cessation and regular exercise, to reduce them.

Dental Changes

Dental problems tend to be a major concern throughout middlescence. Many people older than 55 years have lost some of their teeth. This problem is related to lack of dental care throughout the earlier years rather than to the aging process. The nurse teaches the importance of proper dental health care to prevent further problems.

Endocrine Changes

Throughout the adult life span, there is a progressive decrease in a person's ability to metabolize glucose efficiently. In fact, this deterioration in performance is so great that nearly all older adults are thought to have increased glucose levels.

The levels of male and female sex hormones decrease in middlescence. Reduced hormone levels result in atrophy of the ovaries, uterus, and vaginal tissues in women. Women lose their ability to have children, but men can father children well into their 70s.

Women are also highly predisposed to osteoporosis, which can lead to painful fractures and heart disease. The decrease in estrogen production after menopause is associated with these health problems. In men, a tendency for benign prostatic hypertrophy occurs during the middle years.

Psychosocial Development

Middlescence (middle age) is an often unsettling time of questioning former goals, determining what a person wants for the future, and making decisions or changes that will influence the second half of life. It is the time when most people acknowledge that they have begun to grow older. Although middle-aged adults recognize that they are in their prime of life, they also realize that time is limited, and many accept that they cannot achieve all that they had once hoped. For many people, middlescence is the last chance to identify and pursue new goals and interests. For others, it is merely a plateau into old age.

Self-Concept

If the maturing years of young adulthood have been handled successfully, middlescents usually have the wisdom and skills to see themselves and their world more realistically. Awareness of their future assists them to see middlescence as a point in the life cycle when they must make changes, if changes are to be made at all. Typically, middle-aged adults are assessing what they have achieved in the second half of life regarding their careers, marriages or other intimate relationships, families, lifestyles, social roles, and friendships. For some, this reassessment can result in drastic changes in any or all of these aspects. Others may elect to continue with their established patterns for the remainder of their lives.

Sexuality

Biologically, the most significant milestone in middlescence is the so-called change of life. This change is signaled by the *climacteric* in both women and men, but it is far less dramatic in men. Climacteric in women, or *menopause,* refers to the process during which menses (menstrual periods) cease, ovaries stop producing ova and female sex hormones, and the genitals atrophy. Other possible signs are sweats, hot flashes, palpitations, dizziness, and emotional changes, such as irritability and depression.

Climacteric for men involves a decrease in the levels of the male sex hormones. This decline is so gradual that most men can produce sperm until well into old age. The male climacteric is not as abrupt or intense as menopause.

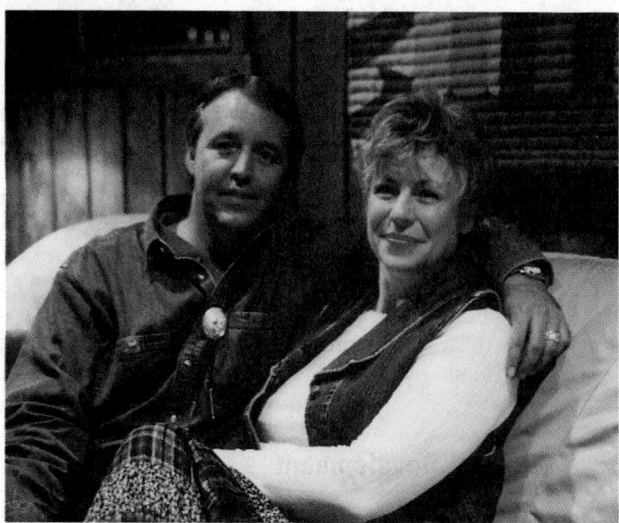

Figure 5–4. A middle-aged couple whose relationship is stronger after active parenting.

Family Structure

Changes within family relationships, such as children leaving home, separation and divorce, aging of parents, and death of a spouse or partner, are often experienced in the middle years. Coping adequately with these changes is a major task of middlescense. Ideally, people should deal with these considerable changes in a manner that helps them grow toward emotional maturity and feel secure and independent rather than depressed, ill, or dependent.

Child Launching

The child-launching phase begins when the first child leaves the parental home and ends when the parents face each other again as a couple. Because of their usually greater emotional and time investments in childrearing, readjustment tends to be more critical and profound for women than for men. The arrival of this change often coincides with menopause, and for family-oriented women the combination of these events may be very stressful. Some women seem unable, for a time, to develop an alternative workable identity, find new ways of nurturing, or find new interests and goals to fill empty time.

Reactions to child launching depend on individual differences and life situations. Women who have combined the work role with motherhood may find it a time of freedom from family responsibilities and financial pressures. Other women may continue to find satisfaction through the roles of wife, partner, or grandmother or through work or other activities. Other women may find their lives lonely, frustrating, and generally unsatisfying. To cope effectively, a strong sense of self-identity and an ability to shift roles are crucial.

Change in Intimate Relationships

The stage after active parenting in the family life cycle also greatly influences the marital or intimate relationship.

The couple must learn to divert the energy and feelings that flowed to their children back to each other. For many couples, the happiest years of the relationship are those before the children are born and after the children are on their own. In these latter years, the couple often experiences a sense of freedom and privacy they have not had for years. This freedom provides an opportunity to get to know each other as people. Divorce or dissolution of an intimate relationship may occur during this time if the relationship has been shaky over the childrearing years. If the relationship has been good, however, it is likely to improve at this time (Fig. 5–4).

If divorce has occurred, a middle-aged adult may remarry and begin a second family. It is not unusual for a middlescent to have several adult children and preschool children from a second or third marriage.

Caring for Aging Parents

During middlescence, a drastic change seems to occur in the relationship between middle-aged children and their parents. Parents suddenly seem old. Aged parents begin to seek their children's help in making decisions and may become dependent for physical and financial support. Middlescents may have to make tough decisions about their parents' living arrangements. Strain is often placed on married middlescents as they weigh their responsibilities toward their parents against those toward their spouse and children. When parents move in with their children, conflict can occur. There may be competition for existing family roles, financial strains, space constraints, or anger over increased responsibilities if the aged person is ill. If the decision to institutionalize the elder is made, the adult child often experiences guilt about the perceived abandonment of the parent. The middle-aged adult who has to care for an older parent while continuing to rear children is sometimes referred to as belonging to the "sandwich generation" (Fig. 5–5).

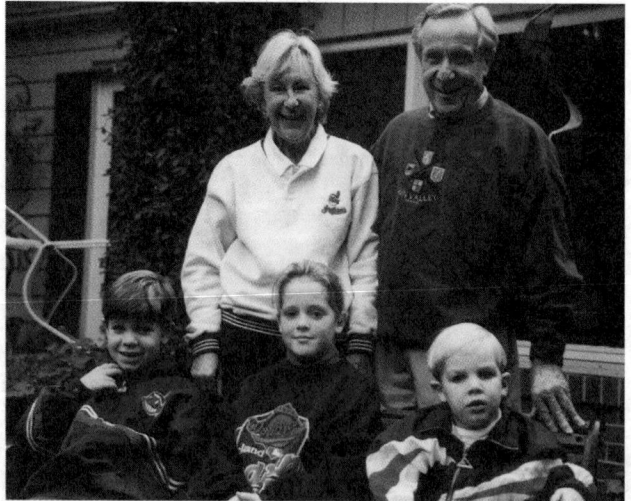

Figure 5–5. Grandparenting roles vary, but everyone involved may benefit from the relationships regardless of the roles.

TRANSCULTURAL CONSIDERATIONS

The overall institutionalization rate for elderly African-Americans is less than that for Caucasians. A greater number of African-Americans and other minorities choose to care for their elders themselves as a result of a greater sense of responsibility to their older family members and strong religious beliefs (Ignatavicius, 1998).

The medical-surgical nurse needs to be aware that families often are or will be the caregivers after a hospitalized older adult is discharged. The caregivers are usually wives or daughters. Chapter 8 discusses the caregiver stress experienced by these family members.

Work

For almost all adults, the work role provides a major source of esteem, satisfaction, happiness, and identity. It is a frequently observed phenomenon that career-oriented men and women become increasingly preoccupied with their work as they grow older. This preoccupation with work is a common phenomenon, tending to exclude leisure activities and other roles.

Most adults peak in their careers during middlescence and continue in their chosen fields until retirement. However, there is a new tendency toward changing occupational directions in the middle years. Seeking a second career is an emerging trend within some groups. One such group comprises people who are forced to find new directions because of technological or economic factors, such as unemployment. Another group includes women who, after devoting their adulthood years to marriage and children, seek a career as an avenue of financial gain and personal growth and satisfaction. Similarly, many people who joined the work force in early adulthood and are eligible for early retirement seek a second career rather than face retirement, which they perceive as boring, idle, and wasteful. Yet another group includes those who made career choices in young adulthood that did not provide them with a sense of satisfaction.

Leisure

During the later middle adult years, most people find themselves with more time on their hands than their experience or interests can accommodate. Settling into careers, launching children, and retiring result in much unstructured time. Adjustment to this free time is largely related to the person's attitudes toward these events. If the person perceives these losses negatively, fears the loss of accustomed roles or friends, or is uncertain about the future, adjustment may be difficult.

People seek to enhance a positive self-concept through numerous pursuits and interests beyond those of the work and family roles. These alternatives can make the pending loss of roles a means for greater involvement in challenges that are equally important. It is vital for all middlescents to sustain feelings of self-worth by having several alternative life pursuits as the means for achieving a continuing sense of personal growth.

Health Issues

Although there are inevitable physical changes and an increasing incidence of chronic conditions as one passes through the middle years, most of the changes from young adulthood are minor ones. Few middlescents are affected by conditions or diseases that necessitate a change in lifestyle or that have a substantial effect on their future. The most common causes of death during the middle years are heart disease, cancer, strokes, and respiratory tract disease. People who smoke, drink alcohol, are obese, have high cholesterol levels, and are inactive are at high risk for these health problems.

General health during middlescence is better than most people expect. Yet it is important for middlescents to engage in preventive and health promotion practices to retain optimal health. The nurse encourages middle-aged adults to schedule annual physical and eye examinations and semiannual dental examinations to detect and treat any significant changes. Because of the relationship of smoking and cardiopulmonary diseases, the nurse encourages smokers to limit or stop their habit. The nurse may refer clients to a smoking cessation program, if available. A regular exercise program and sound nutritional practices, such as reducing the intake of cholesterol and saturated fats, are also effective preventive health measures.

Marital state appears to influence health maintenance as well; married people often live longer than single or widowed people. When roles are lost in middlescence, it is important for one's mental health to move into another lifestyle that will be satisfying. Prolonged psychological stress throughout these transition periods can cause injury, illness, and physical and emotional threats.

Late Adulthood

Over the past century, the elderly population (those 65 years of age and older) has increased at rates far higher than those for other segments. The proportion of elderly people in the United States is expected to increase. In 1990, there were 30.1 million older adults, making up 13.3% of the U.S. population. By the year 2030, that proportion is expected to double. Advances in health care and improved health maintenance habits have resulted in a healthier aged population, with greater numbers of elderly living longer.

The aged person has unique attributes that can be either used or allowed to remain dormant. Many societies neglect or fail to activate the potential of these people because of stereotypic beliefs about older people. Gerontological research has indicated that there is a systematic stereotyping of and discrimination against people who are old. This is also called *ageism*. It is clear that an accurate understanding of the aged is often lacking.

Physiologic Changes

As in every other age cycle, there is no arbitrary dividing line to mark when middle age ends and old age begins. The most popular dividing point is 65 years of age, but some theorists use 55 or 60 years as a division point.

Chart 5-2

Nursing Focus on the Elderly: Effects of Aging on Body Systems

System/Function	Normal Changes	Abnormal Changes and Diseases
Cardiovascular	• Increase in the size of the heart • Increase in collagen • Increase in the thickness of valves and blood vessels • Decrease in cardiac output • Decrease in cardiac reserve • Decrease in blood flow to organs	• Hypertension • Coronary artery disease • Congestive heart failure • Peripheral vascular disease • Varicose veins
Endocrine		
Pancreas	• Decreased ability to metabolize glucose • Reduced insulin secretion • Delayed insulin response	• Diabetes mellitus
Gonads	• Decreased hormone levels • Atrophy of the ovaries, uterus, and vagina • Development of firmer testes • Benign prostatic hypertrophy	• Cancer of the uterus, ovaries, or vagina • Cancer of the prostate gland
Integumentary	• Thinning of epithelial cells and subcutaneous fat layers • Lines and wrinkles in the skin • Age spots • Roughness or dryness of the skin • Thinning and loss of color of the hair • Thickening and brittleness of the nails	• Infections: viral, bacterial, fungal • Abnormal cell growth • Tumors: benign and malignant • Skin ulcerations
Musculoskeletal	• Loss of flexibility in the joints • Cartilage degeneration • Bony growths at the edges of joints • Decreased muscle mass	• Osteoporosis • Rheumatoid arthritis • Fracture • Loss of height as a result of spinal column changes
Neurologic	• General slowing of reaction time • Slow responses to heat and cold • Changing sleep patterns • Decreased cerebral blood flow	• Cerebrovascular disease • Parkinson's disease • Senile dementia and Alzheimer's disease

Physical changes take place at different rates in different people. However, all the body systems are affected somewhat by the aging process. Although some changes become apparent in earlier stages, old age seems to be the time in the life cycle when the progressive changes become more readily apparent and degenerative changes occur more rapidly (Chart 5-2).

In each body system assessment chapter in this text, Nursing Focus on the Elderly charts list major physiologic changes in older people and the nursing implications associated with each change. In addition, normal laboratory values that differ in the elderly are included in Lab Profile charts when appropriate.

Integumentary Changes

Of all body tissue, the fatty tissue layer fluctuates the most throughout life and with aging is subject to the greatest change. Peripheral body parts display the most striking examples of this alteration. For example, veins and bones of the hand become prominent under a parchment-like, thin layer of skin, and deep hollows appear in the clavicular and axillary areas of the body. The elderly person is susceptible to skin tears, which heal slowly as a result of decreased blood flow to the skin and soft tissues. Breasts sag and become pendulous, and the eyes seem to sink, because of the disappearance of the fat layer around the orbit and decreased skin elasticity.

Subcutaneous tissue has a significant role in the body's adjustment to temperature change. The natural insulation that subcutaneous fat provides is lost. It is not uncommon to hear elderly people say that they are cold, nor is it uncommon to see them wearing a sweater or sitting with a lap blanket when environmental temperatures are comfortable for younger people.

Although subcutaneous tissue does not affect the aged person's tolerance of heat, problems with heat tolerance do exist. Changes in the sweat glands, which diminish in size, number, and activity, cause a decline in the efficiency of the body's cooling mechanism. The elderly do not perspire freely, leaving them at high risk for heat exhaustion. They need to be aware of these changes and learn how to compensate. The nurse teaches them to avoid extreme heat conditions. Sudden changes in room temperature or exposure to overly heated bath water causes the blood vessels in the skin and muscles to dilate.

Chart 5–2

Nursing Focus on the Elderly: Effects of Aging on Body Systems *Continued*

System/Function	Normal Changes	Abnormal Changes and Diseases
Pulmonary	• Increase in the diameter of the chest • Decrease in coughing ability • Decrease in vital capacity and tidal volume • Increase in the production of mucus • Progressive kyphosis • Calcification of the cartilage connecting the ribs to the spinal column and sternum • Decreased strength of the expiratory muscles • Thickening of the alveolar walls, decreased recoil	• Asthma • Bronchitis • Emphysema • Pneumonia • Tuberculosis
Sensory		
Sight	• Presbyopia • Lowered acuity • Altered accommodation to light and dark • Difficulty in color discrimination • Decreased lens clarity	• Cataracts • Glaucoma • Senile ocular degeneration
Hearing	• Decreased discrimination of pitch and acuity • Decreased sensitivity to higher frequency sounds • Excessive cerumen	• Deafness
Touch	• Decreased receptors • Lowered ability to distinguish temperature and feel pain	• Total loss of feeling
Taste	• Decreased number of taste buds • Diminished ability to distinguish specific tastes	• Total loss of taste
Smell	• Decreased olfactory function • Diminished sensation to distinguish specific odors	• Total loss of smell
Urinary	• Diminished kidney function • Decreased glomerular filtration rate • Decreased number of nephrons • Decreased muscle tone to bladder • Decreased bladder capacity • Decreased sphincter control	• Urinary retention • Urinary tract infection

This can result in temporary slowing of blood to the brain, leading to a temporary changes in mental status or to dizziness.

Sleep Changes

The aged take longer to move through the relaxation stages of non–rapid eye movement (non-REM) sleep. The number of awakenings and their duration increase. When asked about the quality of sleep, the aged often respond that they hardly slept all night. Typically, their sleep is more fragmented than that of the young. These interruptions are often caused by nocturia (urination at night), leg cramps, and mental stimulation through worry, bereavement, or extraneous noises (Johnson, 1991). It was thought at one time that the elderly needed more sleep, but this is not usually true. The aged seem to sleep less. If one sleeps more, it is usually because of boredom, depression, sedation, or symptoms of disease.

The aged who are not aware that these changes are normal may worry, and the more they worry, the less they sleep. Noisy environments, unresolved fears, worries, and concerns also disrupt sleep quality and patterns. Health care providers often attempt to address the problem by prescribing sleep medications. However, few hypnotic drugs have been found to promote the entire sleep cycle. Instead, these drugs depress REM sleep, or deep sleep, which is necessary for intellectual functioning and for the relief of tension and anxiety. When medications are discontinued, normal sleep patterns usually return but not until fully re-established dreaming patterns emerge.

Neurologic and Sensory Changes

With aging, the central nervous system loses neurons, has a decreased blood supply, and undergoes a decrease in electrical activity. Short-term memory may be affected, but long-term memory is usually intact. For the older adult, these changes may cause altered sensory perception and decreases in reaction time and movement time. It often takes the elder a longer time to respond and initiate action in a given situation.

Visual and hearing changes that started in a person's 30s become much more pronounced in old age. Vestibular (inner ear) functioning decreases, causing dizziness and poor balance. As a result, the elderly person is more prone to falls and accidents.

According to Ney (1993), 25% to 40% of all adults older than 65 are hearing impaired. Ninety percent of people in their 80s have a hearing handicap. Several anatomic changes contribute to hearing loss in the elderly. The cartilage of the auditory canal loses its elasticity and may become narrowed or collapse. In men, stiff coarse hairs in the auditory canal can block the outward flow of cerumen (Ney, 1993). Cerumen impaction sometimes results and can cause hearing impairment.

Cardiopulmonary Changes

All of the body systems and organs change with age, but the most serious changes affect the heart and lungs. The output of the heart is decreased, and the volume of oxygen-carrying blood to all parts of the body is reduced. The continuation of the arteriosclerotic process in the blood vessels ("hardening of the arteries") accentuates this problem.

Respiratory movements of the chest decrease as a result of reduced chest wall muscle activity and deterioration of the alveoli, which alters inspiratory and expiratory volumes. Less oxygen is consumed, and lower respiratory tract infections occur more frequently in older adults. The activity of the cilia diminishes, which allows pathogens and other foreign matter to enter the respiratory tract more easily. The cough reflex, another protective mechanism, is also diminished.

Musculoskeletal Changes

Musculoskeletal problems are very common in old age. The most frequent conditions are

- Degenerative joint changes
- Osteoporosis resulting from increased bone resorption
- Extra-articular pathologic changes of obscure origin, including fibrositis and bursitis
- Fractures caused by trauma and osteoporosis (bone loss)

In addition to these changes, posture and gait changes put the older person at risk for falls. The nurse teaches the older person how to prevent falls at home (e.g., by removing scatter rugs, wearing supportive shoes, and using ambulatory devices if needed).

A complete discussion of osteoporosis can be found in Chapter 53.

Urologic and Renal Changes

As a person ages, bladder capacity and muscle tone decrease, sometimes causing urinary retention and frequency. As a result, the older adult is prone to urinary tract infections and calculi. The older person typically has to wake in the middle of the night to void (nocturia).

Urinary incontinence is not a normal change associated with aging. However, many elderly people are incontinent. Because the urinary sphincter tone also decreases with age, stress incontinence, particularly in women, is fairly common. Stress incontinence, or urine leakage, occurs when the woman coughs, sneezes, or laughs. Although this can be very embarrassing, many lightweight protective products are available. If the condition worsens, treatment with exercises, medication, or surgery may be necessary.

Older men often experience benign prostatic hypertrophy, which causes overflow incontinence. Overflow incontinence is the constant dribbling of urine that results from an overly distended bladder. The enlarged prostate gland causes urine to be retained in the bladder.

The kidneys are also affected by the aging process. Renal nephrons decrease in number, resulting in a decreased ability to concentrate urine. Blood urea nitrogen (BUN) also increases as a result of a decreasing glomerular filtration rate.

Gastrointestinal Changes

In older people, the entire gastrointestinal tract undergoes atrophic changes that may interfere with the efficiency of its function. The capacity of the stomach may decrease, and gastric secretions may diminish. The nurse encourages the older adult to eat small, frequent meals. Digestion and absorption of nutrients from the small intestine are also slower. Constipation is a common complaint, usually caused by decreased peristalsis, decreased appetite, inadequate fluid consumption, and lack of exercise. Chronic laxative abuse over the years worsens the problem.

Nutritional Changes

As a result of a lack of proper dental care in earlier years, loss of teeth, gum disease, and bone degeneration may make eating more difficult for the elderly person. Chewing may become more difficult. Poor muscle tone, loss of digestive juices, and impaired circulation often create problems with digestion and elimination. Atrophy of the taste buds, coupled with problems related to dentition and digestion, diminishes the pleasure of eating for many older adults.

Changes in eating patterns often lead to anemia, malnutrition, and increased susceptibility to infections. The medical-surgical nurse should be aware that these problems can lead to serious complications when the client is ill or has had surgery.

Psychosocial Development

The last years of a person's life cycle constitute the final stage of development in which adults can grow and change. It is the phase in which the person has the opportunity to make final revisions. How well adults adapt to old age depends in part on how well they have resolved the tasks of the previous stages. People who enter old age with many unresolved crises from prior years experience a difficult time. For others, old age is a time to pass on the wisdom of one's experiences, continue fulfilling productive roles, and enjoy a sense of fulfillment for a life well lived.

Self-Concept

The way people regard themselves determines their life satisfaction. Self-concept is developed by a continuous interaction between a person and the environment. Loss of a significant other and loss of roles such as parent, spouse, and worker often affect the elder's sense of self and psychological well-being. The need to be creative and productive is particularly important in old age to gain attention and approval from others.

Other people may attempt to maintain a positive self-concept in several ways. These include such reactions as denial of illness, regression, or retreat into fantasy. Reminiscence may also be used as a defense against present threats to self-esteem. These reactions, although adaptive to conditions or events outside the control of the older person, do not help people to develop their personal potentials. Good health, adequate income, a useful role, opportunities for social interactions, and lively interests are the main determinants of a happy old age. An estimated 10% to 15% of the elderly population in the United States are in poor health and do not have adequate financial support to meet basic needs. (See Research Applications for Nursing.)

Sexuality

Studies of sexual behaviors and interest in these behaviors among the elderly have been limited and inconsistent in their findings. Many studies suggest that elders retain an interest in sexual function and are sexually active. Other studies conclude that there is a decline of sexual interest and behavior among the aged. Reported declines are largely the result of social, cultural, and psychological factors rather than biological and physical factors. Factors that determine sexual activity include present health status, past and present life satisfaction, and the status of marital or intimate relationship. For example, many older women are widowed or divorced and lack available sexual partners, which probably accounts for their decline in sexual interest.

Physiologic changes associated with the aging process occur in both men and women. In women, vaginal secretions diminish and the vagina atrophies. In men, the time required to attain an erection increases. With age, men are also able to maintain an erection for an extended period of time without ejaculation. After ejaculation, the older man often cannot have a subsequent erection for 12 to 24 hours. Despite these physiologic changes, both elderly men and women are capable of sexual activity, including intercourse.

▷ Research Applications for Nursing

Culture Influences Functional Health Status of Older Women

Gale, B. J., & Templeton, L. A. (1995). Functional health status of older women. Journal of the American Academy of Nurse Practitioners, 7, 323–327.

Two groups of elderly women were studied to determine differences in functional health status. Participants in the first group were 98% Caucasian and well educated, and reflected the profile of middle-class older women. The second group consisted of multiethnic women with lower socioeconomic indicators, including low income and less than high school preparation. As assessed by the Sickness Impact Profile tool, measuring physical, independent, and psychosocial health, the second study group had a poorer functional health status than the first group.

Critique. Most of the volunteers in the sample came from churches and volunteer community agencies. However, even though the study used a convenience sample, there was a total of 211 participants.

Possible Implications for Nursing. There has been a growing concern for the health of older women, who comprise most of the elderly population. All older women, especially non-Caucasians, need to be educated more about health promotion activities. The prescription of drugs that decrease functional ability should be discouraged among health care providers.

Family Structure

Three principal factors affect family structure and function in late life:

- Health status and expected life span
- Social changes, such as industrialization and urbanization
- Normal aging processes

Many married couples see their last child leave home when the couple are in their 40s or 50s and can expect to live another 30 or more years. This long period that follows active parenting responsibilities presents a variety of problems that elders have not had to deal with in previous generations, such as widowhood.

Widowhood

Although most elderly men are married, two thirds of all elderly women are widowed. Even when men have been widowed, their chances for remarriage are twice those of women (Matteson et al., 1997).

The elderly widowed person may confront the prospect of becoming socially isolated. The ability to prevent social isolation may be related to advanced level of education, residence in a small town or a rural area, or, most important, the presence of friends and neighbors with whom one can relate. Older widowed people may adjust better to bereavement because of anticipatory grieving and the tendency to view death as one of the developmental tasks of old age.

Factors other than choice frequently operate to isolate the widowed person. Those who lack skills, money, health, and transportation for engaging in society encounter more difficulties in adjusting to a change in role status. The isolated status of widows may be related to the socialization of women in past generations as dependent on men. Like any other life crisis, the loss of a spouse affects people in various ways. Adjustment is related to the person's previous lifestyle and coping patterns.

Family Support

The relationship between adult children and their elderly parents depends on a variety of factors, such as distance, economics, health, and emotional health. Relationships are often taxed by a complex mixture of conflicts. Pulls between love and resentment, duty to parents and obligations for others, and wanting to do what is right and not wanting to change one's lifestyle are not unusual in families. Yet, from the literature available, most families seem able to resolve problems in a way that provides the elder with a sense of support, belonging, and love.

Most older people live within an hour's traveling distance of their children and manage to see them often. There are, however, some differences according to social class. Upper- and middle-class adults are likely to live greater distances from their parents than are lower-class adults. This difference is more a result of professional career patterns than a desire to be separated. Although patterns of aid and contact vary among the socioeconomic classes, there is no difference in caring. Greater distance results in fewer visits, but the quality of the visits and frequent long-distance communication may compensate for periods of absence. Distance between family members also alters the type of support exchanged. Families living close to one another tend to exchange services, such as shopping and household maintenance tasks, whereas family members who live some distance apart tend to confine their assistance to monetary support.

Fewer than one third of the elderly live with their children. Many elders want their privacy, independence, and freedom rather than having to adjust to their children's lifestyle.

There is a growing proportion of frail, dependent elders. For this group, several options are available. They can live in a retirement community or other group setting or can remain in the community, sustained by families and friends. Most elders prefer to reside in their own communities, but there are problems that make realization of this preference difficult. Families generally attempt to help but may be limited in their ability. Most adult couples are active members of the work force and still have dependent children at home or in school.

Grandparenting

Grandparenting is often the most important role in the life of the elderly, providing them with a sense of purpose, value, and esteem. A relationship with grandparents often brings a sense of stability and perspective to the

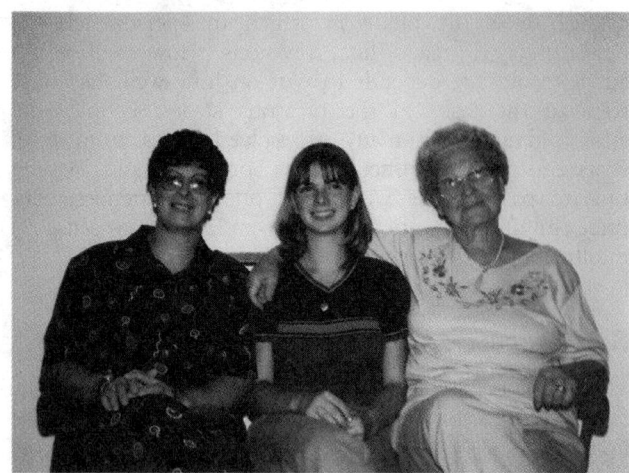

Figure 5–6. The woman on the left is in the "sandwich generation."

children and grandchildren (Fig. 5–6). Grandparents provide the young with advice, affirmation, and a sense of roots and continuity. In addition, grandparents may relieve some of their children's parenting burden by assuming actual caretaking responsibilities, especially when both parents are working.

Regardless of the type of role assumed, grandparenting benefits the older adult, the adult child, and the grandchild. Through the role of grandparent, the elder can maintain ego integrity (Erikson) and approach death with a sense of fulfillment and a feeling of extension of his or her influence into future generations. Many schools and senior citizen centers have joined forces to help children appreciate the pleasure of relationships with older adults other than their grandparents. This intergenerational visiting has also helped the elderly feel wanted and useful (MacPhail, 1993).

Work and Retirement

In 1900, every two out of three older men were employed. In recent years, retirement has become less a matter of choice, with only one of six older men employed. Because women were less likely to be working outside the home earlier in the century, the numbers of older female workers were less and have remained stable. This picture may change as the increased numbers of younger women who have entered the labor force become older. Adjustment to retirement remains a significant crisis for a working person. One survey of retirees revealed that one third of all retirees would prefer to work (Ferraro, 1990).

To most elderly people, it comes as a grim surprise that their income may be less than adequate. For those who depend solely on Social Security benefits, their incomes may fall below the poverty levels established by the U.S. government. For some people, therefore, one of the most serious problems retirement creates is inadequate financial resources.

Some older people prefer to work rather than retire. Some need to work to supplement income from other sources. One common emerging pattern is re-entry into the work force with part-time employment. Between 10% and 25% of retirees in the United States follow this pattern. Most of the time, these retirees take jobs for wage cuts, change industry or occupation, or become self-employed. Older adults who re-enter the labor force after retirement usually have retired early, whereas late retirees rarely return to the work force.

Leisure

Adjustment to time freed from work, family, and social responsibilities in old age depends, to a significant degree, on such factors as prior attitudes toward work, aging, and retirement; health; income; geographic location; and family situation. Favorable adjustment to old age is characterized by a tendency toward substitution. To adequately adjust to the acquired status of retiree, the individual must replace or find substitutes for those satisfactions relinquished with lost roles.

People tend to continue the same patterns of leisure established earlier in life. Some of the most popular activities before and after role losses include visiting friends, watching television, performing odd jobs at home, traveling, and reading. There do not seem to be changes in activities but rather an increase in the frequency of customary activities.

TRANSCULTURAL CONSIDERATIONS

In a study by Chin-Sang and Allen (1991), the researchers found that African-American women increased their involvement in their churches as they entered late adulthood. They also frequently attended senior citizen centers to form relationships and provide service to others.

How people use leisure time depends on their occupation or work role, education, gender, and family status. The success of transitions to retirement and old age relates to educational and occupational background. More highly educated people seem able to structure free time more easily. Similarly, people with higher income status tend to view leisure time more positively and believe that they have a greater degree of control over their lives. A number of studies have reported that life satisfaction in retirement is nearly always higher among professionals or among workers who manifested a positive preretirement attitude, although more professionals than other workers continue working.

Women consistently report an easier adjustment to leisure time in late life than men. Women generally have consistently developed more social relationships, been more involved with their children and grandchildren, and developed more hobby interests throughout their life spans than men.

Health Issues

Because the population of older adults is growing more rapidly than any other age group, an entire chapter is devoted to health care for the elderly (see Chap. 6). Specific diseases or disorders that commonly occur in the

elderly, such as arthritis, heart disease, and chronic lung disease, are discussed throughout the text.

SELECTED BIBLIOGRAPHY

Burke, M. M., & Walsh, M. B. (1997). *Gerontologic nursing: Wholistic care of the older adult* (2nd ed.). St. Louis: C. V. Mosby.
*Chin-Sang, V., & Allen, K. R. (1991). Leisure and the older black woman. *Journal of Gerontological Nursing, 17*(1), 30–34.
*Erikson, E. H. (1968). *Identity: Youth and crisis.* New York: W. W. Norton.
*Ferraro, K. F. (1990). Group benefit, orientation toward older adults at work. *Journal of Gerontology: Social Sciences, 45,* S220–S227.
Gale, B. J., & Templeton, L. A. (1995). Functional health status of older women. *Journal of the American Academy of Nurse Practitioners, 7,* 323–327.
Giger, J. N., & Davidhizar, R. E. (1995). *Transcultural nursing* (2nd ed.). St. Louis: Mosby-Year Book.
*Havighurst, R. (1972). *Developmental tasks and education.* New York: David McKay.
*Heriot, C. S. (1992). Spirituality and aging. *Holistic Nursing Practice, 7*(1), 22–31.
*Hines-Martin, V. P. (1992). A research review: Family caregivers of chronically ill African-American elderly. *Journal of Gerontological Nursing, 18*(2), 25–29.
Ignatavicius, D. D. (1998). *Introduction to long term care: Principles and practice.* Philadelphia: F. A. Davis.
Jarvis, C. (1996). *Physical examination and health assessment* (2nd ed.). Philadelphia: W. B. Saunders.
*Johnson, J. E. (1991). Progressive relaxation and the sleep of older noninstitutionalized women. *Applied Nursing Research, 4,* 165–170.
*Jung, C. (1971). The stages of life. In J. Campbell (Ed.), *The portable Jung.* New York: Viking. (Original work published 1928)
*MacPhail, J. (1993). Intergenerational caring in professional and family life. *Geriatric Nursing, 14,* 104–107.
Matteson, M. A., McConnell, E. S., & Linton, A. D. (1997). *Gerontological nursing: Concepts and practices* (2nd ed.). Philadelphia: W. B. Saunders.
*Ney, D. F. (1993). Cerumen impaction, ear hygiene practices, and hearing acuity. *Geriatric Nursing, 14,* 70–73.
*Olshansky, S. J. (1993). The human life span: Are we reaching the outer limits? *Geriatrics, 48*(3), 85–88.
*Peck, R. C. (1968). Psychological developments in the second half of life. In B. L. Neugarten (Ed.), *Middle age and aging.* Chicago: University of Chicago Press.
*Resnick, B. (1993). Wound care for the elderly. *Geriatric Nursing, 14,* 26–29.
Ringsven, M. K., & Bond, D. (1997). *Gerontology and leadership skills for nurses* (2nd ed.). Albany, NY: Delmar Publishers.
*Rosow, I. (1974). *Socialization to old age.* Berkeley: University of California Press.
*Sheehy, G. (1976). *Passages: Predictable crises of adult life.* New York: Bantam Books.
*Sheehy, G. (1992). *The silent passage: Menopause.* New York: Random House.
*Urinary Incontinence Panel. (1992). *Urinary incontinence in adults: Clinical practice guideline* (Agency on Health Care Policy and Research [AHCPR] Pub. No. 92-0038). Rockville, MD: AHCPR, Public Health Service, U.S. Department of Health and Human Services.

SUGGESTED READINGS

Burke, M. M., & Walsh, M. B. (1997). *Gerontologic nursing: Wholistic care of the older adult* (2nd ed.). St. Louis: C. V. Mosby.
The second edition of this reference book on gerontology is more comprehensive than the first. The initial chapters present demographic information followed by a number of clinical chapters. The last four chapters discuss issues related to care of elders such as ethics and legal issues.
Ringsven, M. K., & Bond, D. (1997). *Gerontology and leadership skills for nurses* (2nd ed.). Albany, NY: Delmar Publishers.
This small reference book is an excellent resource for nursing students and practicing nurses who work with the elderly in any setting. Nursing care of well elders and dependent elders is described in a concise, yet thorough manner.

HEALTH CARE OF OLDER ADULTS

Nurses have frequent contact with the elderly in both their professional and personal lives. Because much of their professional contact is through health care settings such as hospitals, nursing homes, and community health agencies, nurses sometimes have a tendency to stereotype the typical older adult as a confused, dependent person.

This chapter describes major health issues associated with late adulthood. The care of older adults with specific health problems, such as diseases and the need for surgical procedures, is discussed throughout this text under each body system as appropriate. In addition, Nursing Focus on the Elderly charts and Implications for the Elderly headings highlight the most important information related to care of the elderly client with a selected health problem.

SUBGROUPS OF LATE ADULTHOOD

Late adulthood, consisting of people older than 65 years, can be divided into four subgroups:

- Age 65–74 years: the young old
- Age 75–84 years: the middle old
- Age 85–99 years: the old old
- Age 100 years or more: the elite old

The fastest growing subgroup is the old old, sometimes referred to as the advanced elderly population. Their needs and problems are generally different from those of adults between 65 and 74 years old. The incidence of

chronic disease increases markedly when a person is older than 80. At any age, the older adult has specific needs and problems.

DISTRIBUTION OF OLDER ADULTS IN THE HEALTH CARE SYSTEM

About 80% to 85% of older adults are relatively healthy and living in the community at home, in assisted-living facilities, or in retirement complexes. Five percent are in long-term care facilities (nursing homes), and another 10% to 15% are ill but are being cared for at home (Matteson et al., 1997). The elderly from any setting usually experience one or more hospitalizations in their lifetime. Seventy percent to 90% of clients on most medical-surgical units in hospitals are older than 65.

ADMISSION OF THE OLDER ADULT TO A HOSPITAL OR NURSING HOME

Being admitted to a hospital or nursing home is often a traumatic experience for anyone, especially for the older adult. Many elders suffer from *relocation stress,* also known as relocation trauma or relocation syndrome. Most of the early studies on this syndrome examined the increased mortality rate associated with moving elderly people from their own homes to a nursing home or hospital

Chart 6-1

Nursing Care Highlight: Minimizing the Effects of Relocation Stress in the Elderly

- Provide opportunities for the client to assist in decision making.
- Carefully explain all procedures and routines to the client before they occur.
- Ask the family or significant others to provide familiar or special keepsakes to keep at the client's bedside (e.g., family picture, a favorite hairbrush).
- Reorient the client frequently to where he or she is.
- Ask the client what his or her expectations are during hospitalization or nursing home placement.
- Encourage the client's family and friends to visit often.
- Establish a trusting relationship with the client as early as possible.
- Assess the client's usual lifestyle and daily activities, including food likes and dislikes and preferred time for bathing.
- Avoid unnecessary room changes.
- If possible, have a family member, significant other, staff member, or volunteer accompany the client when leaving the unit for special procedures or therapies.

(Coffman, 1981). Other studies have investigated other effects of relocation on behavior and health. Few studies have examined the negative impact of relocation on health status and function, although physical and mental changes have been noted (Matteson et al., 1997).

In some cases, the elderly person who is admitted to the hospital or nursing home from the community can become disoriented, confused, agitated, or abusive. Risk factors thought to contribute to relocation syndrome are the lack of choice or preparation time and the major environmental change. Men older than age 75 who are physically and mentally impaired are at a very high risk for relocation syndrome. Chart 6-1 lists interventions that may help minimize the effects of relocation for the elderly client.

HEALTH ISSUES

This book presents many discussions of health problems that are experienced by the elderly, particularly in the institutional health care setting. Most of this chapter focuses on health issues and problems that may not warrant hospital or nursing home admission.

Health Promotion

Health is a major concern of most elderly people. Elderly clients' health status can affect their ability to perform basic activities of daily living and to participate in social roles. Failure in the performance of these activities may increase their dependence on others and may have a negative effect on morale and life satisfaction.

The health problems most frequently observed among older clients tend to be chronic and degenerative rather than acute. Further, the health problems of the aged are frequently the result of multiple causes, including physical, psychological, and social components, in a complex mixture.

For both middle-aged and older adults, heart disease and cancer are the most frequent causes of death. Most fatalities among older adults are due to disorders resulting from diminished physiologic defenses, such as a severe infection related to cancer or cancer treatment.

Like younger adults, older adults need to practice health promotion and prevention of illness to maintain or achieve a high level of wellness (Chart 6-2). The nurse working with the elderly in any setting needs to teach them the importance of promoting wellness and strategies for accomplishing this goal.

Health is related to a person's level of functioning. In assessing older people's level of functioning, the nurse considers self-responsibility and self-management, nutritional awareness, physical fitness and mobility, stress management, and environmental factors.

Self-Responsibility and Self-Management

The elderly's ability to maintain a positive self-concept and self-control may be hampered by the loss of re-

Chart 6-2

Health Promotion Guide: Lifestyles and Practices to Promote Wellness

Health-Protecting Behaviors
- Have yearly influenza vaccinations.
- Obtain pneumococcal vaccinations.
- Wear seat belts when you are in an automobile.
- Use alcohol in moderation or not at all.
- Avoid smoking.
- If you smoke at home, do not smoke in bed.
- Install and maintain working smoke detectors.
- Create a hazard-free environment to prevent falls; eliminate hazards such as scatter rugs and waxed floors.
- Use medications according to your physician's orders.
- Avoid over-the-counter medications unless your physician directs you to use them.

Health-Enhancing Behaviors
- Have a yearly physical examination; see your physician more often if health problems occur.
- Reduce dietary fat to not more than 30% of calories; saturated fat should provide less than 10% of your calories.
- Increase your dietary intake of complex carbohydrate– and fiber-containing food to five or more servings of fruits and vegetables and six or more servings of grain products daily.
- Allow at least 10 to 15 minutes of sun exposure two to three times weekly for vitamin D intake.
- Exercise regularly three to five times a week for 30 minutes per session.
- Manage stress through coping mechanisms that you have used successfully in the past.
- Get together with people in different settings.
- Reminisce about your life.

sources in the late years of life. The elderly may also experience a number of losses that can affect their sense of control over their lives: the death of a spouse and significant others, the loss of social and work roles, and a decrease in physical mobility. The nurse can support older clients' self-esteem and feelings of competency by encouraging them to maintain as much control as possible over their lives, participate in decision making, and perform as many tasks as possible.

Regardless of the situation, it is important that elderly clients direct their lifestyle in a manner that encourages them to feel capable and valued. The elderly need to find opportunities to be productive and take care of themselves as well as others.

The nurse in the community health setting often has the opportunity to assess older adults' self-care or self-management ability. A number of assessment tools are available for this, but most are too long and complex to be used in a hospital setting. When elderly clients are admitted, the nurse also needs to assess their self-management capabilities for discharge planning.

Nutritional Awareness
Nutrition Needs in the Community

A person's need for adequate nutrition remains constant throughout the life span, yet many elderly people eat an inadequate diet. Inflation, reduced income, and the lack of transportation are factors that may contribute to inadequate nutrition among older adults. Elderly people whose diets consist of inappropriate or unbalanced foods (e.g., an excess of carbohydrates) may also be poorly nourished. Some elders reduce their intake of food to near-starvation levels, even with the availability of assistive programs, such as food stamps, free food, and Meals on Wheels. The lack of transportation, the necessity of traveling to obtain such services, and the inability to carry large quantities of groceries prohibit some elders from taking advantage of food programs.

Poor nutrition among the elderly may also be related to loneliness. Elders may respond to loneliness, depression, and boredom by not eating, which can lead to malnutrition. Many elderly who live alone have lost the incentive to prepare or eat balanced diets. Still others respond to stress by overeating, which leads to obesity.

Nutritional Requirements

The human body's minimal nutritional requirements from youth through old age remain consistent, with a few exceptions. Older adults need increased dietary intake of calcium, vitamin C, and vitamin A because alterations with age disrupt the ability to store, use, and absorb these substances. Sedentary lifestyles and reduced metabolic rate require a reduction in total caloric intake to maintain ideal body weight.

Physical Changes Affecting Nutrition

Other physical aging changes influence the older adult's nutritional status or ability to consume needed nutrients. Diminished senses of taste and smell often result in a loss

of appeal of food. Elderly people experience a greater decline in the ability to taste sweet and salt than in the discrimination of bitter and sour. This phenomenon often results in the elder's overuse of table sugar and salt to compensate. The nurse teaches the elderly client to use herbs and spices to season food or to vary the textures of food substances to achieve satisfaction from food rather than increase the intake of sugar and salt.

The loss of teeth and poorly fitting dentures from inadequate dental care can also cause the elderly to avoid important foodstuffs. The extensive use of prescribed and over-the-counter drugs may affect one's appetite, food tolerances, and food absorption and utilization. Older people with dentition problems frequently resort to eating soft, high-calorie foods, like ice cream and mashed potatoes, which lack roughage and fiber. Unless the person carefully chooses more nutritious soft foods, vitamin deficiencies, constipation, and other disorders can result.

The aged person sometimes responds to problems associated with mobility, prescribed diuretics, and limited bladder capacity by limiting fluid intake, especially in the evening. The nurse teaches older adults that fluid restrictions make them prone to dehydration and electrolyte imbalances that can cause serious illness or death.

Nutrition Needs in the Hospital and Nursing Home

In addition to the nutritional needs that have been described for older adults living in the community, those who are in the hospital or nursing home have special needs related to their illness and general health state. For example, an elderly client with a pressure ulcer needs additional protein, vitamin C, and zinc to heal the open skin lesion. The health care provider, nurse, and dietitian collaborate to determine the best sources of these nutrients. The health care provider may prescribe a multivitamin tablet with zinc to be given every day. The dietitian may recommend a high-calorie, high-protein supplement like Ensure Plus to be given several times a day. The nurse encourages the client to select and eat high-protein foods to promote healing. (See Chapter 64 for further discussion of nutrition in the elderly.)

Physical Fitness and Mobility

Exercise and activity are important to older adults as a means of promoting and maintaining health (Fig. 6–1). Physical activity can help keep the body in shape and maintain an optimal level of functioning. In addition, regular, moderate exercise typically results in feelings of well-being. Numerous studies have shown a lower incidence of coronary artery disease in individuals who engage in regular physical activity compared with those who do not. Karper and Boschen (1993) found that moderate exercise in the elderly also helped to strengthen the immune system and, therefore, prevent the high incidence of acute respiratory infections that are common in this age group.

Without exercise, muscles, organs, and tissues tend to atrophy, and motor, sensory, and cognitive functions can become impaired. It is estimated that 50% of the physical

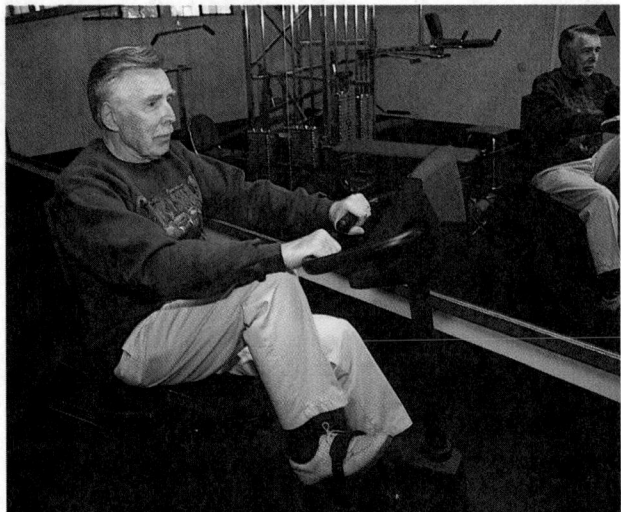

Figure 6-1. Exercise is important to the elderly for health promotion and maintenance.

decline of the elderly is caused by disuse rather than by the aging process or illness. A study by Mills (1994) showed the beneficial effects of low-intensity aerobic exercise on flexibility and balance (see Research Applications for Nursing).

The benefits and purposes of regular exercise are to improve circulation, improve blood pressure, improve respiratory function, maintain muscle tone throughout the body, reduce muscle tension, reduce muscle pain, and promote relaxation. One of the best exercises for older adults is to walk three to five times a week for at least 30 minutes each session (Karper & Boschen, 1993). Swimming is also recommended but does not offer the weight-bearing advantage of walking. Elders who have been sedentary should start their exercise programs slowly and gradually increase the frequency and duration of activity over time.

When older adults are hospitalized, the opportunity for continuing a program of physical fitness is interrupted, at least temporarily. During severe or prolonged illness, older adults are at high risk for complications of decreased physical mobility, such as pneumonia, skin impairment, contractures, muscle atrophy, constipation, and renal calculi. These problems are addressed elsewhere in this text.

Stress Management
Factors Contributing to Stress in the Elderly

According to many physiologic and psychological theories of aging, stress and disease play significant roles. Stress can speed up the aging process over time, or it can lead to diseases that increase the rate of degeneration (see Chap. 8). Stress can impair the reserve capacity of the elderly and lessen their ability to respond and adapt to changes in their environment.

Although no period of the life cycle is free from stress, the later years can be a time of especially high risk. Frequently observed sources of stress for the older popu-

lation include rapid environmental changes that require immediate reaction, changes in lifestyle resulting from retirement or physical incapacity, acute or chronic illness, loss of significant others, financial hardships, and relocation. How people react to these stresses depends on their personal coping skills and support networks. The loss of roles experienced by the elderly often limits the availability of external support networks. For instance, for a number of elderly, successive role losses have left them without friends to whom they can turn for support and help. As a result, many elderly have to rely solely on their personal resources to maintain their mental health. When poor physical health is combined with social problems, older people are susceptible to stress overload, which can result in illness and premature death.

Coping with Stress

The ways in which people adapt to old age largely depend on the personality traits and coping strategies that have characterized them throughout their lives. Establishing and maintaining relationships with others throughout life are especially important to the elderly's happiness. Even more important than having friends at all is the nature of the friendships. People who have close, intimate, stable relationships with others in whom they confide are more likely to maintain integrity in times of crises.

Environmental Factors

Most older adults live in and own their own homes. Physical incapacity or economic problems may force some to relocate (Matteson et al., 1997). If an older person

---

▷ Research Applications for Nursing

Does Exercise Help to Increase the Mobility of Sedentary Elders?

Mills, E. M. (1994). The effect of low-intensity aerobic exercises on muscle strength, flexibility, and balance among sedentary elderly persons. Nursing Research, 43(4), 207–211.

In this small experimental study, 20 sedentary elders were monitored for 8 weeks during a program of stretching and strengthening chair exercises. The control group consisted of 27 older adults who performed their usual activity level. At the end of the 8 weeks, there was a significant difference in flexibility but not in muscle strength or balance. However, balance among the experimental group was 22% better than among the control group at the end of the study period.

Critique. This was a very small study, but it used an experimental research design. The study needs to be replicated using a larger sample size and a random sample. It is an attempt, however, to show the importance of health promotion among the elderly population.

Possible Nursing Implications. Nurses need to teach the importance of exercise to their elderly clients as part of a comprehensive wellness program. Exercise does improve mobility in this population.

must move to a retirement center or a long-term care facility, family members and facility staff need to be aware that the older person needs personal space in the new surroundings. Older people need to participate in deciding how the space will be arranged and what they can keep in the new environment. Such participation helps to offset the feelings of powerlessness and depersonalization that often accompany relocation to a group setting. The nurse suggests that the client or family bring in personal items, such as pictures of relatives and friends, favorite clothing, and valued knickknacks to assist in making the new setting seem more familiar and comfortable. The same intervention can be carried out in a hospital setting.

Changes in vision, touch, and motor ability can create difficulties for the elderly in functioning in any environment. For example, decreased vision in old age, especially the poor perception of distance, may make walking more difficult; the person is less aware of where each step is. The reduced sense of touch gives the older person a decreased awareness of body orientation (e.g., whether the foot is squarely on the step). Decreased reaction time that commonly results from age-related changes in the neurologic system may also impair the older adult's ability to recognize or move from a dangerous setting.

Accidents

Accidents in the Community

The nurse teaches older adults about the need to be aware of safety precautions that should be taken to prevent accidents. The prevention of injury to muscles, bones, and other body parts that have grown fragile with age not only is critically important but also is probably the area in which aging people can do the most to preserve their fitness. Incapacitating accidents are a primary cause of restricted physical fitness and decreased mobility in old age.

Safeguards such as installing and holding onto hand rails when using steps and getting into and out of the shower or bathtub, securing rugs with slip-proof underpads, and making sure treacherous places are well lighted are essential. To minimize sensory overload in the elderly, the nurse advises the older person to concentrate on one activity at a time. If needed, the nurse encourages the use of visual, hearing, or ambulatory assistive devices. High costs and fear of appearing old sometimes prevent the elderly from obtaining or using hearing aids, eyeglasses, walkers, or canes.

Accidents in the Hospital and Nursing Home

The most common accident among elderly clients in a hospital or nursing home setting is falling. Many falls result in serious injuries such as fractures and head trauma. The nurse should be aware that these injuries are potentially life threatening and should take action to prevent them.

Risk Assessment for Falls

The nurse assesses the client for risk for falls. Many risk assessment tools have been developed to help the nurse

---

Chart 6-3

Nursing Care Highlight: Risk Factors and Measures for Preventing Falls in the Elderly

Assess for the presence of these risk factors:
- History of falls
- Advanced age (>80 years)
- Multiple illnesses
- Generalized weakness or decreased mobility
- Disorientation or confusion
- Use of drugs that can cause increased confusion, mobility limitations, or orthostatic hypotension
- Urinary incontinence
- Communication impairments
- Major visual impairments or visual impairment without correction
- Substance abuse
- Location of client's room away from the nurses' station (in the hospital or nursing home)
- Change of shift or mealtime (in the hospital or nursing home)

Implement these nursing interventions:
- Monitor the client's activities and behavior as often as possible, preferably every 30 to 60 minutes.
- Remind the client to call for help before getting out of bed or a chair.
- Help the client to get out of bed or a chair.
- Provide, or remind the client to use, a walker or cane for ambulating.
- Remind the client to wear eyeglasses or a hearing aid if needed.
- Toilet the incontinent client every 1 to 2 hours.
- Clean up spills immediately.
- Arrange the furniture in the client's room or hallway to eliminate clutter or obstacles that could contribute to a fall.
- Provide adequate lighting at all times, especially at night.
- Observe for side effects and toxic effects of drug therapy.

---

focus on factors that increase an older person's risk of falling. Chart 6-3 lists some of the common risk factors that the nurse should assess and measure to help prevent falls.

Once an elderly client has been identified as being at a high risk for falls, the nurse chooses interventions that help to prevent falls and possible serious injury. One of the most controversial issues in fall prevention is the use of side rails on the bed, and physical and chemical restraints, especially in the hospital setting.

Nursing Interventions to Prevent Falls

As a result of being in an unfamiliar environment and because of increased nocturia (urination at night), the elderly client commonly gets out of bed at night to go to the bathroom. In the darkness and disorientation of the room, the client may forget to ask for assistance to the bathroom and subsequently fall. In some cases, the client may crawl over the bed rail, which can make the results of a fall more serious. Because of this, side rails are used less often in both hospitals and nursing homes.

Similar considerations are being given to the use of physical and chemical restraints. A restraint is any device or medication that prevents the client from moving freely. The federal government enforced a law in 1990 that gives residents in nursing homes the right to be restraint-free. In a nursing home, bedside rails are classified as restraints. Although the majority of hospitals have not adopted this policy, most have policies that limit the use of restraints and require careful nursing assessment. The Joint Commission on Accreditation of Healthcare Organizations (JCAHO) has specific standards that limit the use of restraints in hospitals.

Physical Restraints

Experts agree that elderly clients should not be placed in a Posey vest or be sedated just because they are elderly. However, if all other interventions, such as reminding clients to call for assistance when needed or asking a family member to stay with the clients, are ineffective in fall prevention, the nurse may need to use a physical restraint for a specified period of time. Applying a restraint is a serious intervention and should be analyzed for its risk versus benefit (Wilson, 1996). The nurse checks the client in a restraint every 30 to 60 minutes and releases the restraint every 2 hours for turning, repositioning, and toileting. Physical restraints like cloth vests have caused serious injury and even death. If restraint is needed, the least restrictive device should be used.

Chemical Restraints

Chemical restraints, or psychoactive drugs, are often overused in hospital settings. Clients who are noisy, agitated, abusive, or combative may have an "as needed" order for a psychoactive drug. Such medications include

- Antipsychotic drugs, such as haloperidol (Haldol, Peridol✦)
- Antianxiety drugs, such as alprazolam (Xanax)
- Antidepressant drugs, such as nortriptyline (Pamelor)
- Sedative-hypnotic drugs, such as chloral hydrate

These drugs produce serious side and toxic effects and should, therefore, be reserved for clients who cannot be managed in any other way. Clients receiving these medications must be closely monitored for therapeutic and adverse effects.

The most potent group of psychoactive drugs is the antipsychotics. These drugs may be appropriate for the control of certain behavioral symptoms, such as hallucinations, delusions, and violent episodes. However, fewer than half of clients respond to these drugs.

If a psychoactive drug is used as a last resort, a low dose should be given. Table 6–1 lists some of the drugs commonly used as chemical restraints.

TABLE 6–1

Drugs Commonly Used as Chemical Restraints
Low Potency (High Sedation, High Anticholinergic Effects)
Chlorpromazine (Thorazine)
Thioridazine (Mellaril)
Chlorprothixene (Taractan)
Mesoridazine (Serentil)
Medium Potency (Medium Sedation, Medium Anticholinergic Effects)
Triflupromazine (Vesprin)
Acetophenazine (Tindal)
Loxapine (Loxitane)
Molindone (Moban)
High Potency (Low Sedation, Low Anticholinergic Effects)
Trifluoperazine (Stelazine)
Thiothixene (Navane)
Fluphenazine (Prolixin)
Haloperidol (Haldol)
Pimozide (Orap)

From Ignatavicius, D. D. (1998). *Introduction to long term care: Principles and practice.* Philadelphia: F. A. Davis. Used with permission.

Drug Use and Misuse

Drug therapy for the elderly population in general is another major health issue. Because of the multiple chronic and acute illnesses that occur in this age group, drugs for elderly people account for about a third of all prescription drug costs.

Older adults also frequently use nonprescription drugs, such as analgesics, antacids, cold and cough preparations, laxatives, and vitamins, often without consulting a physician. The occurrence of adverse drug reactions is directly related to the number and frequency of drug exposures. Elders are, therefore, at high risk for adverse drug reactions or interactions and are often admitted to the hospital for these problems.

Physiologic Changes Affecting Drug Use

It has been recognized only recently that older adults may not tolerate the standard dosage of medications traditionally prescribed for younger adults. The physiologic changes related to aging make drug therapy more complex and challenging. These changes affect the absorption, distribution, metabolism, and excretion of drugs from the body.

Age-related changes that can potentially affect drug absorption from an oral route include an increase in gastric pH, a decrease in gastric blood flow, and a decrease in gastrointestinal motility. Despite these changes, most elderly do not have difficulty with absorption because of age-related changes alone. Age-related changes that affect the distribution of a drug include smaller amounts of total body water, an increased ratio of adipose tissue to lean body mass, a decreased albumin level, and a decreased cardiac output. Increased adipose tissue in proportion to lean body mass can cause increased storage of lipid-soluble drugs. This leads to a decreased concentration of the drug in plasma but an increased concentration in tissue.

Drug metabolism most often occurs in the liver. Age-related changes affecting metabolism include a decrease in liver size, a decrease in liver blood flow, and a decrease in liver enzyme activity. These changes can result in increased plasma concentrations of a drug. Changes in the kidneys can also result in high plasma concentrations of drugs. Excretion of drugs most often involves the renal system. Age-related changes of the renal system include a decrease in renal blood flow and reduced glomerular filtration rate. These changes result in a decreased creatinine clearance and thus a slower excretion time for medications (Matteson et al., 1997)

Effects of Drugs in the Elderly

Because of age-related physiologic changes, older adults are at a high risk for side and toxic effects from drugs. In 1991, the Geriatric Drug Therapy Research Institute was established to study and make recommendations for drug therapy in the elderly. Currently, the institute is developing tools that physicians and other health care professionals can use when caring for the older adult.

When chronic disease is added to the physiologic changes of aging, drug reactions have a more dramatic effect and take a longer time to correct. This is because elders have less reserve capacity in most organ systems. Often a lower dose of medication is necessary to prevent adverse effects. The policy of "start low, go slow" is appropriate when health care providers prescribe drugs for the elderly. However, the physiologic changes of aging are highly individual. Thus, alterations in drug therapy should always be individualized according to the actual physiologic changes present and the occurrence and severity of chronic disease.

Common adverse drug reactions in elders include edema, nausea, vomiting, anorexia, dry mouth, fatigue, weakness, dizziness, urinary retention, diarrhea, constipation, and confusion. Many of these signs and symptoms can be mistakenly attributed to a concurrent illness clients might be experiencing or may be assumed to be part of the aging process. The nurse assesses all elderly clients with such symptoms for possible adverse reactions to medications.

Self-Administration of Medication

Most people older than 65 years live at home and are responsible for taking their own medications. Because the risk of drug toxicity is considerably increased in the elderly population, the nurse should assist elderly clients in assuming this task responsibly. The nurse helps prevent problems by educating clients and their caregivers, providing clear and concise directions, and developing ways to assist elders in overcoming self-administration handicaps or difficulties.

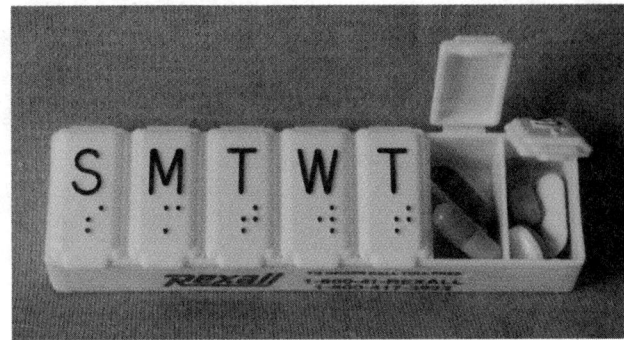

Figure 6–2. A medication system for safe self-administration.

Older adults make errors in self-administration for several reasons. First, they may simply forget. In the rush of daily activities, they may not take the drug at all or may take it too often because of an inability to remember when or whether medications have been taken. It can be helpful if clients associate pill taking with daily events, such as meals, or keep a simple chart or calendar. Pill boxes have been devised so that a daily, weekly, or monthly supply of medicine can be placed in appropriate compartments (Fig. 6–2). Large print on the drug label assists those clients with poor visual acuity. Writing the drug regimen on the top of the bottle with large letters and numbers is also helpful.

A second reason that elderly people frequently commit errors in taking medications is poor communication with health care professionals. These difficulties stem from such sources as inadequate explanations to elderly clients or explanations they cannot understand because of educational limitations or language barriers. Health care professionals frequently presume that if they tell the elder about the drugs, the elder has acquired the knowledge. The nurse or other health care provider needs to help older adults plan their medication schedules.

A third reason for medication errors is one's attitude and long-ingrained feelings about taking medicine. Some people are chronic pill takers; they think no physician can help them unless he or she is the one who prescribed the medication. These people often add to their drug regimen by taking over-the-counter drugs that can interact with prescription drugs and cause serious problems. For example, a client receiving warfarin (Coumadin, Warfilone♣) for anticoagulation may take aspirin (Ancasal♣) regularly for arthritis. Aspirin is also an anticoagulant, which can cause overt or occult bleeding.

Conversely, other elderly people avoid taking medication whenever they can. The fear of drug dependency or the cost of the drugs may cause many to discontinue medications too soon. In addition, the action or side effects of some drugs may not be desirable. For example, diuretics may cause incontinence when clients cannot get to the bathroom quickly enough. Others think that two pills will be twice as effective as one; some elders take medication that is left over from a previous illness or a drug that has been prescribed for someone else.

Health care providers can influence the attitudes of

elders toward their medication and their health problems. Laypersons of the same socioeconomic or cultural background as that of the elder can be effective instructors. A method that is being tried in some hospitals and nursing homes is supervised drug self-administration. Clients are allowed to take their own medications under supervision. In this way, the nurse can be sure of a client's understanding and ability to self-administer medications at home or in another health care setting.

Mental Health

A few changes in cognition have been identified as age-related. These changes are linked to specific functions of cognition as opposed to intellectual capacity. They include a decreased reaction time to stimuli and an impairment of memory of recent events. It is certain, however, that gross cognitive impairment, depression, hallucinations, and delusions are not part of the normal aging process. Most elders are mentally sound.

Losses in income and physical health, lack of comprehensive health care and social services, loss of social roles, and death of significant others may affect a person's emotional stability. It is not surprising that mental illness occurs among the aged population. Elders are often unaware of early symptoms of emotional or mental impairments. Symptoms may go unnoticed by family and friends and thus are allowed to progress until crisis results. The three most common cognitive problems among the elderly are depression, dementia, and delirium.

Depression

Depression, as a response to multiple life stresses, a single situation (situational depression), or a problem associated with dementia, is one of the major disturbances in cognitive functioning in elders. It is often underdiagnosed by physicians and, therefore, undertreated. Without treatment, depression can result in suicide.

Elderly people with the early clinical manifestations of depression may experience early morning insomnia, excessive daytime sleeping, poor appetite, a lack of energy, and an unwillingness to participate in social and recreational activities. The treatment for depression usually includes drug therapy and psychotherapy. Electroconvulsive therapy (ECT) may also be used, either as a last resort or when drugs are not effective. Table 6–2 lists commonly used drugs for depression. Most of these drugs take 2 to 3 weeks to become effective. More information on this disorder is available in mental health nursing textbooks.

TRANSCULTURAL CONSIDERATIONS

Caucasian males older than 70 years are at the highest risk for suicide during older adulthood. Older adults contemplating suicide usually do not talk about their plans and choose a method, such as gunshot, that will ensure death.

Dementia

Dementia is a broad term used for a syndrome that is characterized by a disturbance in cognition in elders. For-

TABLE 6–2

Medications Commonly Used for Depression in the Elderly and Their Adverse Effects

Medication	Adverse Effects
***Tricyclic Antidepressants**	
Amitriptyline (Elavil, Endep)	Cardiac dysrhythmias, orthostatic hypotension, weight gain, drowsiness, anticholinergic effects (dry mouth, constipation, urinary retention, visual disturbances) (amitriptytine has the most anticholinergic effects of any in this group)
Clomipramine (Anafranil)	
Desipramine (Norpramin)	
Doxepin (Sinequan, Adapin)	
Imipramine (Tofranil)	
Nortriptyline (Pamelor)	
Protriptyline (Vivactil)	
Trimipramine (Surmontil)	
†Heterocyclic Antidepressants	
Amoxapine (Asendin)	Drowsiness (maprotiline has the longest half-life in this group)
Bupropion (Wellbutrin)	
Maprotiline (Ludiomil)	
Trazodone (Desyrel)	
†Selective Serotonin Reuptake Inhibitors (SSRIs)	
Fluoxetine (Prozac)	Insomnia, agitation, gastrointestinal distress, weight loss (fluoxetine has the longest half-life in this group)
Paroxetine (Paxil)	
Sertraline (Zoloft)	
Monoamine Oxidase Inhibitors	
Isocarboxazid (Marplan)	Weight gain, insomnia, agitation
Phenelzine (Nardil)	
Tranylcypromine (Parnate)	Hypertensive crisis (avoid foods containing tyramine)

*Do not give with antidysrhythmics or monoamine oxidase inhibitors.
†Do not give with monoamine oxidase inhibitors.
Data compiled from *Depression in Primary Care: Volume 2. Treatment of major depression. Clinical Practice Guideline. Number 5.*
From Ignatavicius, D. D. (1998). *Introduction to long-term care: Principles and practice.* Philadelphia: F. A. Davis. Used with permission.

merly called organic brain syndrome (OBS) and chronic brain syndrome (CBS), dementia represents global impairment of intellectual function and is generally chronic and progressive. There are many types of dementia; the most common is Alzheimer's disease (senile dementia, Alzheimer type). Multi-infarct dementia, the second most common dementia, is a vascular disorder and accounts for 20% to 25% of all dementias. Chapter 44 discusses dementias in detail, with a focus on Alzheimer's disease.

Delirium

Whereas dementia is a chronic, progressive disorder, delirium is an acute state of confusion. Delirium is also different from dementia in that it is usually short-term and reversible. Delirium is often seen in the hospital setting or in a setting with which the client is unfamiliar. The client may try to climb out of bed, pull out invasive

TABLE 6-3

Differences in the Characteristics of Delirium and Dementia

Variable	Dementia	Delirium
Description	• A chronic, progressive cognitive decline	• An acute confusional state
Onset	• Slow	• Fast
Duration	• Continuous	• Usually 1 month or less
Cause	• Unknown, possibly familial, chemical	• Multiple, such as surgery, infection, drugs
Reversibility	• None	• Usually
Treatment	• Treat signs and symptoms	• Remove or treat the cause
Nursing interventions	• Reorientation not effective in the late stages; use validation therapy (acknowledge the client's feelings and don't argue); provide a safe environment; observe for associated behaviors, such as delusions and hallucinations	• Reorient the client to reality; provide a safe environment

catheters (e.g., oxygen or intravenous cannulas), or become quite agitated and combative.

The nurse should use a calm voice in reorienting the client and try to divert attention away from devices or tubes. A number of innovative nursing interventions have been used with some success. For example, playing tapes of soothing music in the client's room may have a calming effect. Giving the client a doll or stuffed animal to "fidget" with may prevent the client from removing important medical instrumentation. Some nurses believe that providing dolls and stuffed animals is treating the adult like a child, but, when used for therapeutic purposes, this intervention can be very effective with some clients. If the client already has a favorite item, such as an afghan or picture, the nurse asks the client's family or significant others to provide it for the same purpose.

There are multiple causes of delirium, including

- Medication (especially anticholinergic drugs)
- Metabolic disturbances
- Infections
- Surgical operations
- Circulatory, renal, and pulmonary disorders
- Nutritional deficiencies
- Major loss

Table 6-3 briefly differentiates delirium and dementia and the major nursing considerations for each. The most difficult challenge is caring for a client with both problems at the same time.

Elder Neglect and Abuse

Another problem that is sometimes encountered by the elderly is neglect and abuse, both verbal and physical. Some elders are very vulnerable to this problem, especially widowed women, who may have difficulty being assertive. Studies have shown that older persons who are neglected or abused are often physically dependent. The abuser may be a family member who becomes frustrated or distraught over the burden of caring for the elder (Greenberg, 1996; Lynch, 1997).

Role theorists propose that prolonged caregiving by a family member is a new, unexpected role for adult children, most often women. This new role may result in role fatigue and role conflict. Caregiver Role Strain and High Risk for Caregiver Role Strain have been added to the list of North American Nursing Diagnosis Association (NANDA)–approved nursing diagnoses (NANDA, 1992). From their research, McCloskey and Bulechek (1992) identified Caregiver Support as a major nursing intervention (Chart 6-4). Chapter 8 discusses caregiver stress in more detail.

The nurse carefully assesses the elderly client for signs of abuse. If the older adult is too weak or has no other resources or support system, the client may not acknowledge that the abuse is occurring. If physical abuse is suspected, the nurse notifies the physician and social

---

Chart 6-4

Nursing Care Highlight: Interventions for Family Caregiver Support

- Determine the caregiver's preparation and acceptance of his or her new role.
- Assess the caregiver's level of knowledge about the role and the client's health status.
- Teach stress management techniques to the caregiver (see Chap. 8).
- Monitor for signs of caregiver stress.
- Help the caregiver identify sources of respite care.
- Teach the caregiver health promotion practices for his or her own health.
- Help the caregiver identify caregiver support groups, and encourage participation in them.
- Teach the caregiver about the grieving process.
- Help the caregiver identify financial and other health care resources.
- Encourage the caregiver to share responsibilities with other members of the family or significant others.

worker to investigate the situation. Many states in the United States and some Western countries have laws requiring health care professionals to report suspected elder abuse.

ECONOMIC ISSUES
Income

Most adults hope that throughout their life cycle they can provide for their own needs. One of the greatest fears many adults have related to aging is becoming dependent on family, friends, or society. In many cases, older adults have not achieved economic self-sufficiency. One fifth of the total population of the United States is poor, and one fifth of the poor are older than 65 (Brock, 1992).

Most people expect financial resources to decline in their retirement years compared with their working years. However, they also expect that the level of their expenses will decline as well, and this may not occur. In the United States, for example, the inflation that began in the 1970s reduced the value of financial assets. The elderly were especially hard hit because most rely on Social Security benefits or pension funds for the bulk of their income. These assets are usually fixed and cannot be altered by the person. Therefore, many elders are unable to adjust their income to changing economic circumstances and hence are powerless to combat declining real income. Health care purchases are paid for in substantial part by private insurance and federal health and social programs. Yet the rising cost of these programs contributes substantially to rising government costs and may result in more out-of-pocket costs for the aged health care consumer.

Housing

The popular belief that the elderly are frail, dependent, senile people living out their last years in an institution has no factual basis. Only about 5% of the aged population reside in institutions providing long-term care (Ignatavicius, 1998). Many elders live in their own homes and have paid off their mortgages. Yet living arrangements are a major problem for some people as they age. The nurse needs to be aware of this issue because it can increase the client's stress level and have an impact on health care planning.

Rising energy and housing costs in many countries have joined the high costs of food and health care as factors that contribute to the economic hardship of aging people. In addition to financial difficulties, housing for the aged may be a problem because environmental supports that would help them to remain residing and participating in the community are lacking.

Deterioration of property, escalation of property taxes, and maintenance service costs create many problems for elder homeowners wishing to keep their homes. In some areas, elderly renters are extremely vulnerable to high rent fees, real estate speculation, and loss of living quarters because of removal of substandard, low-rent apartment or hotel buildings. Physical impairments and a lack of available, affordable support services, such as household help, transportation, home health care, and assistance with meals, prevent some aged people from being able to manage adequately in their own homes.

The need for special housing for the aged has long been recognized. Numbers of government and privately funded experiments in alternative housing for the aged have been tested. These projects incorporate such variables as personal care services, special health and safety remedies, and recreation and leisure plans. Although most of these projects provide security, improve life satisfaction, and prove cost effective, in many countries there is no overall plan for alternative living arrangements for the elderly.

RESOURCES FOR THE ELDERLY

In the United States, Canada, and other countries, a broad range of government benefits and services is available to assist older people with problems related to income, health insurance, housing, and social services. The nurse informs older adults and their families about the types of services available to help them achieve a higher quality of life.

Government Resources
Income

In the United States, the major portion of federal funds supporting programs for the elderly is devoted to the Social Security programs. The Social Security Act was passed in 1935, after the Depression, when many elderly were economically impoverished. Since that time, there has been a gradual shift from a program that was intended to provide a minimal supplement to retirees' sources of income to one that is the primary source of retirement income for many people. Other provisions of this act that are significant for people younger than 65 years are the disability and survivors' insurance provisions.

Health Insurance

Medicare was enacted as part of the amendments to the Social Security Act of 1965. This program was created to help older people meet the cost of health care. Despite its deficiencies, Medicare has provided a means for elders to obtain needed health care in times of escalating costs without decimating their total personal savings.

Medicare provides health insurance to people 65 years of age and older and to qualified disabled people of any age. Medicare A primarily pays for most of in-hospital care and is paid for by the federal government. It covers only a very small portion of care required in long-term care and minimal home health services. Currently, traditional Medicare requires a 3-day qualifying hospital stay before admission to a nursing home. Medicare B is an optional insurance and requires payment of a monthly premium. Medicare B pays most of the outpatient costs associated with physicians' visits, medication, and home health services. This traditional Medicare program is changing to managed care. It is predicted that all of

Medicare will be managed care shortly after the turn of the century. (See Chapter 3 for information on managed care.)

Medicaid (medical assistance) is a program designed to provide payment for medical services for the poor, including the poor elderly. For eligible people who are age 65 or older, it supplements the Medicare insurance program. Eligibility is related to determination of poverty level, and each state program determines its own criteria for eligibility. A number of states have completed the transition to managed care for their Medicaid recipients.

Housing Programs

In the United States, Congress has passed a number of legislative acts designed to alleviate housing problems for older citizens. Among these programs is rental assistance for lower-income families, the elderly, and the disabled. Direct low-interest loans are available to individuals to construct special rental housing facilities for the handicapped and the elderly. The federal government supports construction and rehabilitation of nursing homes. It subsidizes rental facilities, which can be rented by the aged at rates below the existing market price. For information related to these housing programs, nurses can contact the local public housing authority or the Housing and Urban Development area office in most communities.

Social Services

The Older Americans Act of 1965 provided social services to the aged. Under this legislation, each state created an office to provide leadership in the coordination and development of services for the elderly (Office on Aging). Some of the more significant programs and services carried out under this legislation are described in Chart 6–5.

Chart 6–5

Nursing Focus on the Elderly: Social Services Provided by the Older Americans Act of 1965

- Senior centers to meet the need for a central place for older people to congregate, develop new interests, and socialize.
- Nutrition programs to provide nutritious meals in a centralized setting as well as to the homebound elderly. Recreation, education, and health activities are incorporated in many sites as a regular part of the program.
- Transportation services to accommodate the elderly via special fares on existing public transportation systems and the operation of specially equipped vehicles for the frail and the handicapped elderly.
- Information and referral services to direct the elderly to the appropriate agency that provides needed services.
- In-home services, such as household help, telephone reassurance, chore maintenance, and visitation by home health aides, to enable the impaired elderly to remain living in the community.

Research Agencies

The National Institute on Aging was established in 1974. Its purpose is to conduct research on the biological, population-related, and sociologic aspects of aging at its Gerontology Research Center in Baltimore. It also supports research by others at universities and laboratories across the United States.

Within the National Institute for Mental Health, one division is devoted exclusively to problems of the aged: the Center for Studies of the Mental Health of the Aging. Its major role is to stimulate, coordinate, and support research training and to offer technical assistance relating to aging and mental health. Although it provides no monies for programs of service delivery to older people, it significantly affects the training of those working with elderly clients in community mental health centers and other service settings.

Community Resources

Over the years, it has become evident that government programs cannot provide all services needed by the aged. In many areas, private efforts can supply the same services at lower costs and without the red tape that some government programs involve. Transportation is an area in which the private sector and local, state, and federal governments all have roles.

In many urban areas, governments have provided Dial-A-Ride or similar services that provide free transportation. The federal government has subsidized the development and operation of transit systems, but its aid has been focused mainly on high-use systems and routes. For occasional travel, particularly in rural areas, the best solution may be for the elder to rely on a friend or a neighbor. Churches and community groups often help organize this approach by using sign-up sheets and recruiting volunteers to drive 1 day a week.

Education, recreation, and cultural activities help maintain a person's physical condition, mental alertness, and social contact. Education helps older people keep up with a rapidly changing world. Although advances in cable and satellite television systems, as well as the Internet, provide a broad range of new educational experiences at home, the value of person-to-person discussion and the need to focus some educational activities on local issues means that community discussion groups and other informal education will remain important.

Recreation and cultural activities are best managed on a local, nongovernment basis because personal preference plays such a large role in determining individual participation. A variety of activities run by different organizations or informal groups is more likely to please more people than a large program run by a government agency. For example, in the Midwest, elders have formed square dance groups and gourmet groups that meet frequently for socialization and compete with similar local, regional, and state groups.

Churches and other religious institutions serve the elderly in many ways. In addition to their primary role of providing organized worship, they sponsor many activities that bring the elderly together with their peers as well as with younger people. Clergypersons and other spiritual leaders are often excellent counselors, and other members of the congregation or religious group are sometimes willing to help older members in time of trouble.

Many communities have access to community resource books (e.g., those published by the United Way). Area agencies on aging are excellent referral centers. Some of these agencies publish directories of services that are specifically geared to the elderly. The nurse can help to inform elderly clients about community resources that they may need, depending on their specific life situation.

THE FUTURE OF GERONTOLOGICAL NURSING

Nurses in most adult health care settings encounter the challenges of caring for both well and ill older adults. In view of the rapidly increasing elderly population, especially the over-85 group, nurses in many settings are specializing in gerontological nursing or geriatric case management. Nurses can practice these specialties in acute care, long-term care, and community-based settings. Just as nurses can achieve certification in medical-surgical nursing, they can become certified in gerontological nursing or case management. The American Nurses Credentialing Center (ANCC) provides three gerontology examinations for certification for those who qualify: gerontological nurse, gerontological clinical specialist, and gerontological nurse practitioner. The ANCC also offers a nursing case management examination, which is broad-based and not specific for geriatric case management. Other professional organizations also certify case managers, including geriatric case managers (see Chap. 3).

SELECTED BIBLIOGRAPHY

All, A. C. (1994). A literature review: Assessment and interventions in elder abuse. *Journal of Gerontological Nursing, 20*(7), 25–32.

Baldwin, R. L., Craven, R. F., & Dimond, M. (1996). Falls: Are rural elders at greater risk? *Journal of Gerontological Nursing, 22*(8), 14–21.

Bradley, L., Siddique, C. M., & Dufton, B. (1995). Reducing the use of physical restraints in long-term care facilities. *Journal of Gerontological Nursing, 21*(9), 21–34.

*Brock, A. M. (1992). Economics and the aged. In E. Baines (Ed.), *Perspectives on gerontology nursing*. Boston: Sage.

Broussard, M. C., & Pitre, S. (1996). Medication problems in the elderly: A home healthcare nurse's perspective. *Home Healthcare Nurse, 14*(6), 441–443.

Burke, M. M., & Walsh, M. B. (1997). *Gerontologic nursing: Wholistic care of the older adult* (2nd ed.). St. Louis: C. V. Mosby.

*Coffman, T. L. (1981). Relocation and survival of institutionalized aged: A re-examination of the evidence. *Gerontologist, 21*, 483–500.

Commodore, D. I. (1995). Falls in the elderly population: A look at incidence, risks, healthcare costs, and prevalence strategies. *Rehabilitation Nursing, 20*(2), 84–89.

*Department of Health and Human Services. (1990). *Healthy people 2000*. Rockville, MD: Author.

Dunning, S. (1994). Elder abuse is our fight, too. *RN, 57*(8), 76.

Frost, M. H., & Willette, K. (1994). Risk for abuse/neglect: Documentation of assessment data and diagnoses. *Journal of Gerontological Nursing, 20*(8), 37–45.

Greenberg, E. M. (1996). Violence and the older adult: The role of the acute care nurse practitioner. *Critical Care Nursing Quarterly, 19*(2), 76–84.

Ignatavicius, D. D. (1998). *Introduction to long-term care: Principles and practice*. Philadelphia: F. A. Davis.

*Karper, W. B., & Boschen, M. B. (1993). Effects of exercise on acute respiratory tract infections and related symptoms. *Geriatric Nursing, 14*(1), 15–18.

Kuehn, A. F., & Sendelwick, S. (1995). Acute health status and its relationship to falls in the nursing home. *Journal of Gerontological Nursing, 21*(7), 41–49.

Lange, M. (1996). The challenge of fall prevention in home care: A review of the literature. *Home Healthcare Nurse, 14*(3), 198–206.

Lay, T. (1994). The flourishing problem of elder abuse in our society. *AACN Clinical Issues in Critical Care Nursing, 5*(4), 507–515.

Loughran, S. (1996). Medication use in the elderly: A population at risk. *MedSurg Nursing, 5*(2), 121–124.

Lynch, S. H. (1997). Elder abuse: What to look for, how to intervene. *American Journal of Nursing, 97*(1), 26–32.

Matteson, M. A., McConnell, E. S., & Linton, A. D. (1997). *Gerontological nursing: Concepts and practice* (2nd ed.). Philadelphia: W. B. Saunders.

*McCloskey, J. C., & Bulechek, G. M. (1992). *Nursing interventions classification (NIC)*. St. Louis: Mosby-Year Book.

Mills, E. M. (1994). The effect of low-intensity aerobic exercises on muscle strength, flexibility, and balance among sedentary elderly persons. *Nursing Research, 43*(4), 207–211.

*North American Nursing Diagnosis Association. (1992). *Definitions and classification 1992*. St. Louis: Author.

Rosen, S. L. (1994). Managing delirious older adults in the hospital. *MedSurg Nursing, 3*(3), 181–189.

Wilson, E. B. (1996). Physical restraint of elderly patients in critical care: Historical perspectives and new directions. *Critical Care Nursing Clinics of North America, 8*(1), 61–70.

SUGGESTED READINGS

Bradley, L., Siddique, C. M., & Dufton, B. (1995). Reducing the use of physical restraints in long-term care facilities. *Journal of Gerontological Nursing, 21*(9), 21–34.
    This article presents the findings of a longitudinal study that documented the positive outcomes of a structured restraint education program in reducing the use of physical restraints and promoting nonrestrictive alternatives. The researchers showed that restraint-free elder care can be attained in a cost-effective manner and without an increase in resident falls and injuries.

Lange, M. (1996). The challenge of fall prevention in home care: A review of the literature. *Home Healthcare Nurse, 14*(3), 198–206.
    This article provides an extensive review of the literature regarding falls and outlines successful clinical nursing strategies that can be used to prevent falls in the home. These interventions address primary, secondary, and tertiary activities.

Lynch, S. H. (1997). Elder abuse: What to look for, how to intervene. *American Journal of Nursing, 97*(1), 26–32.
    This comprehensive article examines the four types of elder abuse: physical, psychological, and financial abuse and neglect by self or others. The author describes detection and interventions for abuse as well as strategies to prevent abuse in long-term care settings. Resources are also presented in a chart. A continuing education quiz is available at the end of the article.

UNIT 2

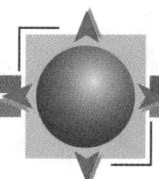

Biopsychosocial Concepts

Related to Health Care

ETHICS

Medical-surgical nurses in all settings experience a variety of ethical issues every day. These ethical issues vary in intensity from seemingly minor issues, such as whether a nurse should tell a client a "white lie," to extremely emotional issues about euthanasia or how to allocate scarce health care resources. Frequently, nurses realize that they are in the midst of an ethical dilemma when two or more equally unfavorable options exist (Curtin & Flaherty, 1982). At other times, however, the nurse may not recognize that an ethical issue has occurred until after the situation is over.

WHAT IS ETHICS?
Definition

Ethics is the study of what is right or what people ought to do in a specific situation. The nurse decides "what is right" by consulting a variety of resources, including

- Ethical theories and principles
- Legal statutes
- Decision-making models
- The values of the persons involved
- Professional codes
- Policies
- Nursing and ethics consultants

Thus, a nurse cannot learn the one correct answer for resolving any specific ethical issue because each clinical ethical issue is unique.

Ethical Theories

Ethical theories are a way of approaching ethical problems and determining what is the right action to implement. The two most common ethical theories are utilitarianism and deontology.

Utilitarianism

The guiding rule in utilitarianism is the greatest happiness principle, in which decisions are based on whatever action would bring about the greatest happiness for the greatest number of people. Recently, this principle has been expanded beyond happiness to include other intrinsic values, such as close relationships, success, personal freedom, good health, and beauty (Beauchamp & Childress, 1994). The consequences of the possible options are evaluated regarding their ability to promote group happiness or good rather than individual happiness. Utilitarians believe that rules such as "never lie" can be broken if the consequence of lying will bring about the most happiness. For example, if an unstable myocardial infarction client voices concern that his spouse has not visited, a utilitarian would justify not telling the client his spouse had been killed in an automobile accident if telling would cause a setback in recovery (Beauchamp & Childress,

1994; Beauchamp & Walters, 1982; Curtin & Flaherty, 1982; DeWolf, 1989b).

Deontology

In contrast, deontologists believe that actions are right or wrong despite their consequences and that a person's intentions to do good should be praised. Deontology emphasizes the importance of the individual person, not the group. Rules are rarely broken. In addition, a deontologist would agree that answers for an ethical issue can be identified and generalized to similar ethical issues (Beauchamp & Childress, 1994; Beauchamp & Walters, 1982; Curtin & Flaherty, 1982; DeWolf, 1989b). To return to the example given for utilitarianism, a deontologist would tell the unstable myocardial infarction client that his spouse had been killed because truth-telling is always the right action. However, rarely are people purely utilitarian or purely deontological in their approach to ethical decision-making. Generally, ethical decisions reflect a combination of theoretical approaches and ethical principles.

Ethical Principles

Ethical principles can also help the nurse determine what a correct action is for resolving an ethical issue. Four major ethical principles are nonmaleficence, beneficence, justice, and autonomy. However, one difficulty with using ethical principles is that no criteria exist for choosing between competing or conflicting principles (Beauchamp & Childress, 1994).

Nonmaleficence

The principle of nonmaleficence requires that no matter what other outcomes are achieved during an ethical issue, the nurse must prevent harm. "Do no harm" is the minimal standard of behavior for health care professionals. The principle of nonmaleficence is supported when a nurse follows the "five rights" of medication administration or helps a postoperative client to turn, cough, and deep breathe.

Beneficence

Beneficence builds on the principle of nonmaleficence. Besides doing no harm, the nurse must benefit the client by promoting good. Thus, the principle of beneficence requires the nurse to perform an action. For example, a nurse is acting beneficently when he or she relaxes visitation rules in a hospital to allow a family member to spend the night with a confused elderly client.

Justice

The principle of justice is concerned with how resources are divided among individual people and/or groups in the society. Typically, justice is concerned only with resources that are in short supply, such as financing for specialized health care services like organs for transplantation. How-

ever, little agreement exists whether resources should be allocated by a person's effort, need, merit, or social contribution or by free market exchange. Nurses make decisions based on justice when they decide how to allocate their time among clients.

Autonomy

The principle of autonomy requires that a person be involved in decisions that affect his or her life. Making a decision for a person when he or she could have made the decision is paternalistic and negates the person's autonomy. A nurse promotes client autonomy by advising the client of options in care, ensuring that the client has adequate information to make a decision, and supporting the client's decision.

Ethical Versus Legal Actions

Actions determined to be ethical for a given situation may not be considered legal actions. For example, it may be ethically justifiable to facilitate a client's death based on the principle of beneficence and utilitarian theory. However, assisted suicide is not a legal option in most countries. Typically, legal statutes reflect the ethical mindset held by society 10 to 15 years ago. Thus, new technology can create conflicts between current ethical reasoning and the law.

Because of conflicts between ethical and legal opinions, people may bring suit in the hopes of overturning current law and establishing a new legal precedent. For example, *Cruzan v. Director, Missouri Department of Health* (1990) addressed the right of a family to have a client's treatment—in this case, gastrostomy tube feedings—removed.

Values

A value is a way of looking at life that ultimately directs the person's behavior and gives life meaning. Values are beliefs that have been freely chosen, communicated to others, and acted on repeatedly throughout life. The development of values is influenced by one's family, religion, culture, interpersonal relationships, and activities. Despite being of long standing, values do change and are never stagnant (Steele & Harmon, 1983). Examples of personal values include a comfortable life, world peace, happiness, salvation, and love.

A nurse's personal values serve as the foundation for the development of professional values. Thus, nurses sometimes have difficulty in balancing their personal and professional values. Examples of professional values include promoting health, being truthful with clients, providing client advocacy, and having a nonjudgmental attitude.

Values serve as rationale for determining whether an action is right or wrong. The nurse may experience an ethical quandary when personal and professional values conflict. For example, when a client requires a valve replacement because of endocarditis caused by intravenous

TABLE 7–1

An Exercise for Clarifying Personal and Professional Values

- Step 1. Choosing freely
  - a. Am I sure I've thought about this value and have chosen to believe it for myself?
  - b. Who first taught me this value?
  - c. How do I know I'm "right"?
- Step 2. Choosing from among alternatives
  - a. What other alternatives are possible?
  - b. Which alternative has the most appeal for me and why?
  - c. Have I thought much about this value alternative?
- Step 3. Choosing after considering the consequences
  - a. What consequences do I think might occur as a result of my holding this value?
  - b. What price will I pay for my position?
  - c. Is this value worth the price I might pay?
- Step 4. Complement to other values
  - a. Does this value "fit" with other values, and is it consistent with them?
  - b. Am I sure this value doesn't conflict with other values I deem important?
- Step 5. Pride and esteem
  - a. Am I proud of my position and value? Is this something I feel good about?
  - b. How important is this value to me?
  - c. If this were not my value, how different would my life be?
- Step 6. Public affirmation
  - a. Am I willing to speak out for this value?
- Steps 7 and 8. Action
  - a. Am I willing to put this value into action?
  - b. Do I act on this value? When? How consistently?
  - c. Is this a value that can guide me in other situations?
  - d. Would I want others who are important to me to follow this value?
  - e. Do I think I'll always believe this? How committed to this value am I?
  - f. Am I willing to do anything about this value?
  - g. How do I know this value is "right"? How do I know? Are my values ethical?

Reprinted with permission from Fowler, M. D. M., & Levine-Ariff, J. (1987). *Ethics at the bedside: A source for the critical care nurse.* Philadelphia: J. B. Lippincott (pp. 160–161).

drug abuse, the nurse may experience conflict between professionally believing everyone deserves high-quality health care and personally believing that a person who uses illegal intravenous drugs does not deserve aggressive treatment.

Values clarification is a process of analyzing alternatives and exploring the associated feelings and beliefs (Table 7–1). The process serves to identify the conscious and unconscious values that guide behavior. When clarifying values, people ask themselves, "What is important to me?" or "What are my beliefs?" Values clarification can facilitate the nurse's understanding of competing values displayed by other health care professionals and clients.

ETHICAL DECISION-MAKING
Variables Influencing Ethical Decision-Making

Many variables can influence a nurse's ethical decision-making in any medical-surgical setting. The nurse's ethical decision-making can become more complex, depending on the variety and number of variables involved. These variables can be described as nurse, task, or environmental (Simon, 1978).

Nurse Variables

Variables that can influence ethical decision-making processes include those inherent within the nurse, such as values and beliefs, gender, age and maturity, assumptions, and self-image. A nurse's knowledge, education, moral reasoning, and communication skills and previous experiences can also influence how the nurse perceives an ethical issue (DeWolf, 1989a).

Task Variables

Task variables influence the process used to resolve ethical issues. Ethical decision-making is influenced by the amount of time available to make a decision. The complexity of the decision to be made also influences the decision-making task. Often nurses attempt to use a "rule of thumb," such as "Never give pain medication early," to simplify the decision task. Another variable influencing a decision task is the perceived costs and benefits associated with a possible option (DeWolf, 1989a).

Environmental Variables

Environmental variables can be classified as either institutional (health care agency) characteristics or community variables.

INSTITUTIONAL CHARACTERISTICS. Institutional characteristics identified by hospital-based nurses during a study by Crisham (1981) include

- Hospital policies
- Time limitations created by work shifts
- Conflicting loyalties between client, profession, and institution
- Difficulties applying knowledge in the clinical setting
- Diversity of expectations of clients, supervisors, and other health care professionals
- Limited awareness by nurses regarding their responsibilities and authority during clinical ethical decision-making

Other institutional characteristics that influence ethical decision-making are philosophy, tolerance for ethical questions, staffing patterns, client acuity, available technology or equipment, economic stability of the health care agency, the nurse's job description and associated responsibilities, overall quality of working relationships between nurses and other health care professionals, and accessibility of ethics resources (DeWolf, 1989a). Additional variables may enter into the decision-making process depending on the setting (e.g., home, clinic, nursing home, or ambulatory surgical center).

COMMUNITY VARIABLES. The ethical decision-making environment is also influenced by changing community variables. For example, the lay public is becoming more informed about health care issues, and community groups are involved in health care reform. Health care decisions are influenced by laws, public beliefs about how resources should be allocated, and current events in the media. Because communities are generally heterogeneous, each community reflects a specific mix of ethnic, religious, and cultural perspectives. Thus, these factors may influence how an ethical issue is resolved.

Normative Ethical Decision-Making Models

A variety of ethical decision-making models have been created to assist the nurse with clinical ethical decision-making. In each model, a specific concept is emphasized, such as rights (Curtin & Flaherty, 1982), biblical principles (Shelly, 1980), or the application of bioethical stan-

dards (Husted & Husted, 1994). Each model requires the decision-maker to

- Identify the ethical problem
- Identify and consider alternatives
- Implement a choice
- Evaluate the decision-making process and its outcome

Thus, normative decision-making models parallel the nursing process even though some models may require extra steps, such as values clarification or application of ethical principles. Frequently, nurses do not perceive these normative decision-making models as helpful. Nurses have difficulty considering a variety of options and their associated consequences during urgent, time-limited situations. Therefore, these normative models are more useful for retrospective or hypothetical case analysis. The more often nurses use a normative model for retrospective or hypothetical case review, the more apt they will be to use a logical decision-making process to resolve real clinical ethical situations.

Descriptive Ethical Decision-Making Models

The process nurses use to resolve clinical ethical situations in an acute medical-surgical setting has been investi-

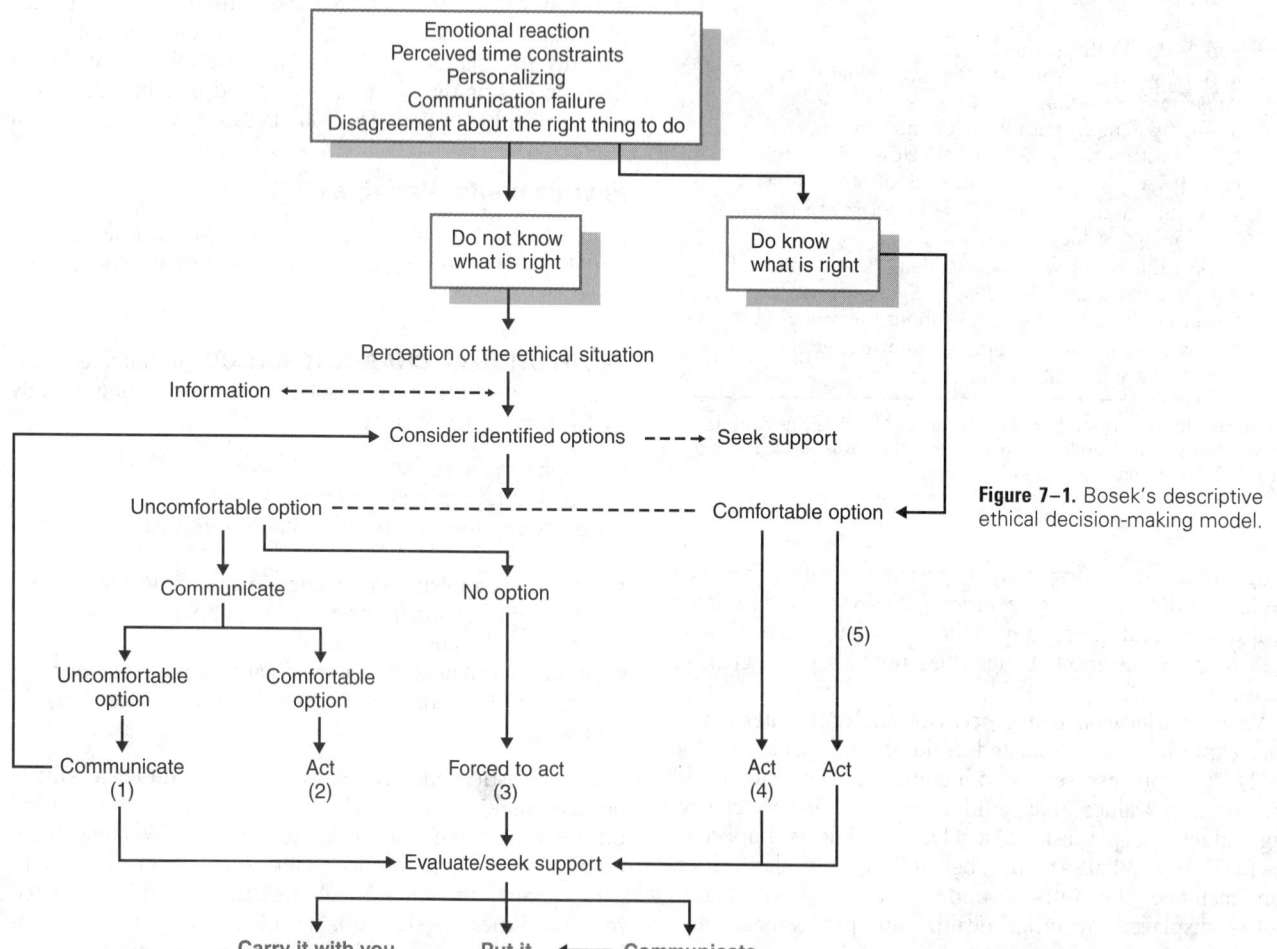

Figure 7–1. Bosek's descriptive ethical decision-making model.

gated and is described in the Descriptive Ethical Decision-Making Model (Fig. 7–1). From this model, several difficulties with the nurses' ethical decision-making process have been identified (DeWolf, 1989a).

First, the nurses did not perceive that an ethical situation was occurring until after they

- Experienced an emotional reaction
- Perceived a limited amount of time available to make a decision
- Considered what they would want done if they were the client
- Experienced a communication failure
- Did not know what was the right thing to do to resolve the ethical situation

Second, the nurses did not identify possible options; instead, they considered options identified by others. The nurses evaluated all possible options on a comfortable-uncomfortable continuum. Comfort was defined as the nurse's personal psychological comfort and the amount of physical comfort the client would experience as a result of implementing the option. If nurses were forced to choose between their own psychological comfort and the client's physical comfort, they always favored their own psychological comfort (DeWolf, 1989a).

Third, nurses often had difficulty putting the ethical issue behind them. Some nurses described their need to keep discussing the ethical issue and the fact that they continued to experience the same emotional reactions years after the issue occurred. Thus, for some nurses, the ethical issue was never resolved.

ETHICAL RESOURCES

Various ethical resources exist that may facilitate a nurse's ethical decision-making in a medical-surgical setting. These resources may vary among health care agencies. Nurses need to learn what resources are available in their practice setting. These resources may include professional codes, policies and procedures, nursing administrators, and institutional ethics committees or consultants.

Ethical Codes for Nurses

In Canada and the United States, major nursing associations have codes of ethics. The *Code for Nurses,* developed by the American Nurses' Association (1976; 1985) (Table 7–2) is undergoing revision. One of the requirements for a profession is the existence and adherence to an ethical code to regulate professional conduct. Each code signifies the profession's acknowledgment of the responsibility and faith entrusted by society to the nursing profession. Nurses are expected to follow the code in their daily practice.

Policies and Procedures

Ethical codes represent standards for ideal behavior. However, the codes do not tell nurses the exact actions to take in specific ethical situations. One way that health care agencies have addressed this lack of specificity is

TABLE 7–2

The American Nurses' Association Code for Nurses

1. The nurse provides services with respect for human dignity and the uniqueness of the client, unrestricted by considerations of social or economic status, personal attributes, or the nature of health problems.
2. The nurse safeguards the client's right to privacy by judiciously protecting information of a confidential nature.
3. The nurse acts to safeguard the client and the public when health care and safety are affected by the incompetent, unethical, or illegal practice of any person.
4. The nurse assumes responsibility and accountability for individual nursing judgments and actions.
5. The nurse maintains competence in nursing.
6. The nurse exercises informed judgment and uses individual competence and qualifications as criteria in seeking consultation, accepting responsibilities, and delegating nursing activities to others.
7. The nurse participates in activities that contribute to the ongoing development of the profession's body of knowledge.
8. The nurse participates in the profession's efforts to implement and improve standards of nursing.
9. The nurse participates in the profession's efforts to establish and maintain conditions of employment conducive to high-quality nursing care.
10. The nurse participates in the profession's efforts to protect the public from misinformation and misrepresentation and to maintain the integrity of nursing.
11. The nurse collaborates with members of the health professions and other citizens in promoting community and national efforts to meet the health needs of the public.

Reprinted with permission. American Nurses' Association. (1976; 1985). *Code for nurses with interpretive statements.* Kansas City, MO: Author.

through the development of policies and procedures that reflect the intents found in the codes.

Nurses have a responsibility to participate in the development and ongoing review of policies and procedures that facilitate ethical practice in their agency. For example, a preoperative policy requires that consent for surgery be obtained before the client receives preoperative sedation. This policy reflects the need to respect the client's autonomy and legal right to informed consent. At times, a nurse may experience intense pressure from others to "keep on schedule" and send the client to the operating suite although consent has not yet been obtained. In this situation, the policy provides legal and ethical support for a nurse's refusal to send the client to surgery before informed consent is obtained.

Nursing Administrators

Nursing administrators, including unit nurse managers, can be valuable resources when ethical issues arise. Most administrators have had experience as staff nurses and are also familiar with available agency resources and applicable policies and procedures that may assist in resolving an ethical issue. Nurses sometimes hesitate to consult a nursing administrator because of fears that they will be perceived as incompetent. However, the opposite is usually true. Nurses should keep nursing administrators informed of any potential or actual ethical situations and should seek an administrator's advice, because administrators have the authority to mobilize resources, redistribute responsibilities, and use discipline, if necessary, in resolving an ethical situation.

Institutional Ethics Committees

Ethical issues arise when a nurse does not know what is a correct course to follow. The Joint Commission on Accreditation of Healthcare Organizations (JCAHO) (1997–1998, 1998, 1998–1999a, b) requires all agencies to have a mechanism for dealing with ethical issues. Health care agencies may provide specific ethics resources through institutional ethics committees (IECs), ethics consultants, or a combination of both.

Most health care agencies have an interdisciplinary ethics committee that serves as an advisory group for ethical deliberation. In long-term care agencies, this committee is called the patient care advisory committee (PCAC). This committee has three functions:

- Providing agency and community education about ethical issues and ethical analysis
- Developing policies relevant to ethical decisions, such as resuscitation, refusal of treatment, or informed consent
- Deliberating on cases

Depending on agency policy, referral of an ethical issue to an ethics committee may be optional or mandatory. In addition, whether a health care professional must follow the recommendations of the IEC may be considered optional or mandatory.

Ethics committees may be composed of administrators, physicians, nurses, occupational therapists, physical therapists, dietitians, social workers, lay people, and someone with an extensive background in ethics (e.g., a philosopher, theologian, and/or clinician with advanced education in bioethics). The group process of analyzing a problem reflects the opinions and advice that many minds can contribute on a case. However, ethics committees can be bureaucratic and unwieldy with outspoken members who intimidate quieter members (Savage, 1994).

The following is an example of a home health case referred to an agency's ethics committee: A 78-year-old man with gangrenous feet was refusing amputation. He was legally competent, but the home health team was uncomfortable with his refusal. They referred his case to the committee. After considering relevant data, the committee concluded that if the client is determined to be competent, his wishes must be respected and the health care team should not amputate his feet. If he is determined to be incompetent, then a legal guardian should be appointed to decide what treatment is in the client's best interest. The committee also found that the client's refusal for amputation was consistent with earlier expressions of

valuing his independence. The home health team considered the committee's conclusions and recommendations. After the home health team followed the protocol to determine the client's competency, they believed that the client was competent to refuse amputation. Although the home health team regretted the client's decision, the committee's recommendation fortified their resolve to respect the client's right to make this difficult decision.

Ethics Consultants

An ethics consultant may be a health care professional, such as a physician, nurse, chaplain, or philosopher. This consultant gathers and reviews data and offers an ethical analysis. An ethics consultant model overcomes the bureaucratic problem of coordinating an agency ethics committee meeting, but the interdisciplinary perspectives of a committee are lacking. Nurses should be aware of the various ethics resources in their practice settings.

SELECTED ETHICAL ISSUES
Futility

One of the major ethical issues to be faced in the future is the concept of futility. Technology can extend human life beyond the point when a person cares to live, has consciousness, or has the possibility of recovery. The determination of futile treatment is made by analyzing the cost of treatment (financial, physical, emotional) and the likely outcome (cure, recovery, prolongation of life, death). The value of the costs and outcomes should be determined by the client or, if the client is unable, by the family and friends closest to the client. This is a gross oversimplification, however. Even if a client requests futile treatment (e.g., resuscitation in terminal disease), such requests are not automatically honored. The determination of futility also relies on the clinical judgment of health care professionals. Although treatment is thought to be futile, it may be continued because the health care agency may fear a lawsuit. However, discussion and education must occur to learn the client's values, goals, fears, and motives. A request for futile treatment may represent a client's fear of dying.

Do Not Resuscitate Orders

Cardiopulmonary resuscitation (CPR) was originally designed to treat witnessed cardiac arrests. Based on the principle of beneficence, the use of CPR has expanded. However, initiating CPR for persons with terminal illnesses, such as acquired immunodeficiency syndrome or cancer, or the severely ill or aged elderly may be perceived as causing harm. Discussions about the client's wishes and the benefits and burdens of CPR should occur periodically during any acute, chronic, or terminal illness. However, the presence of a written advance directive does not translate into an automatic do not resuscitate (DNR) order.

The agency DNR policy should be available in a prominent place so that health care professionals are familiar with the policy. The policy should stipulate how the DNR

TABLE 7–3

Components in a Do Not Resuscitate Order

Specify	Examples
Resuscitative measures	Cardiopulmonary arrest Pulmonary arrest Hypotensive event Life-threatening cardiac event Dysrhythmia
Measures to be withheld	External cardiac massage Endotracheal intubation Cardiotonic medications Vasopressors Cardioversion Ventilator or changes in ventilator settings
Measures to be continued	All current therapies Pain medications Oxygen Comfort medications (e.g., antibiotics, diuretics, steroids, chemotherapy)
Measures to be initiated	Artificial ventilation with a mask Cardiotonic drug trial Increased ventilator rate setting Increase oxygen to 100%
Who to notify in case of cardiac arrest	Attending physician House officer Nurse practitioner Consultant

order must be written (Table 7–3), how frequently the order must be reviewed, and under what conditions it is suspended. For example, DNR orders are frequently suspended when a client needs surgery requiring ventilator support, based on the principle of beneficence at the risk of violating client autonomy (Clarke et al., 1994; Langslow, 1995; Rhodes, 1994; Rosner et al., 1994).

Quality of Life

Quality of life (QOL) remains an elusive concept; no single definition exists. According to studies by Ferrans and Powers (1985), QOL is determined by the client's judgment about the importance of certain elements in his or her life and satisfaction with those elements. A client who is confined to a wheelchair, for example, may believe that mobility is very important. Although being in a wheelchair is not as good as walking, using a wheelchair may be better than being immobilized, according to this client. However, other people who believe that walking is crucial for happiness may perceive the client's QOL as being poor. If clients are unable to communicate, whether they never had this ability or have irreversibly lost this ability, it is impossible to know how they view their QOL.

Utilitarian Versus Deontological Approach

From a utilitarian standpoint (for the good of *all*), two perspectives can be taken when evaluating QOL. First, a person warrants resources on the basis of real or potential productivity that that person offers society. Second, humanity is served by protecting vulnerable individuals in society because one never knows when one may be in the vulnerable group. This perspective does not offer guidance in determining the quantity resources one should expend.

The deontological approach to QOL is based on respect for an *individual* person's life. Deontologists maintain that human life has intrinsic value and should be preserved at all costs.

When conflict exists in a specific case of whether to continue treatment for someone lacking decisional capacity and the client's wishes are unknown, the health care system turns to the legal system.

Legal Perspective

Through the legal system, society has grappled with how best to preserve the autonomy of incompetent clients, as in the cases of Nancy Cruzan and Karen Ann Quinlan (Weir, 1989), who were in irreversible comas. In these cases, the central issue was the incompetent person's right to refuse treatment and how this right is exercised. If the person's wishes are unknown, the law presumes that a person, even an incompetent person, prefers to live. While the state has an interest in preserving life, society is not in agreement on whether the financial burden of preserving life at all costs is justifiable.

The current health care system in the United States forces allocation based on accessibility to services and ability to pay. The uninsured and underinsured forego treatment except in emergency care, and then they may receive services only after a lengthy wait. Similarly, some people often must wait for appointments or referrals to specialists when they are in health maintenance organizations (HMOs). In Canada, however, clients are not limited by ability to pay, but they may have to wait for certain procedures or surgeries or they may not have access to some procedures available in the United States. Many groups, especially nursing associations, have worked tirelessly for universal access to health care and believe the health care system should be revamped to focus on preventive care and health maintenance rather than acute inpatient care.

The state of Oregon proposed an allocation of health care dollars based on a quality-of-life-year (QOLY) and probability of medical benefit. A prioritized list of more than 700 treatments was compiled as a method of determining what treatments would be supported and what treatments would not be funded with state dollars (Hadorn, 1991). The Bush administration (1989–1993) opposed this plan, arguing that it potentially discriminated against disabled clients. Thus, by 1993, the Oregon Health Plan was still not fully implemented. After making changes mandated by the federal government, Oregon was $83.6 million short of funding the plan, was losing

```
┌─────────────────────────────────────────────────────────────────┐
│            DECLARATION UNDER ILLINOIS LIVING WILL ACT             │
│                                                                   │
│        This declaration is made this _____ day of _____ 19___.│
│   I, _____, being of sound     │
│   mind, willfully                                                 │
│   and voluntarily make known my desires that my moment of death   │
│   shall not be                                                    │
│   artificially postponed.                                         │
│                                                                   │
│        If at any time I should have an incurable and irreversible │
│   injury,                                                         │
│   disease, or illness judged to be a terminal condition by my     │
│   attending                                                       │
│   physician who has personally examined me, and has determined    │
│   that my death is                                                │
│   imminent except for death delaying procedures, I direct that    │
│   such procedures                                                 │
│   which would only prolong the dying process be withheld or       │
│   withdrawn, and that                                             │
│   I be permitted to die naturally with only the administration    │
│   of medication,                                                  │
│   sustenance, or the performance of any medical procedure deemed  │
│   necessary by my                                                 │
│   attending physician to provide me with comfort care.           │
│                                                                   │
│        In the absence of my ability to give directions regarding  │
│   the use of                                                      │
│   such death delaying procedures, it is my intention that this    │
│   declaration shall                                               │
│   be honored by my family and physician as the final expression   │
│   of my legal                                                     │
│   right to refuse medical or surgical treatment and accept the    │
│   consequences from                                               │
│   such refusal.                                                   │
│                                                                   │
│   Signed _____                            │
│                                                                   │
│   City, County and State of Residence                             │
│                                           _____  │
│                                                                   │
│                                           _____  │
│                                                                   │
│                                           _____  │
│                                                                   │
│        The declarant is personally known to me and I believe the  │
│   declarant to                                                    │
│   be of sound mind.  I did not sign the declarant's signature     │
│   about, for or at                                                │
│   the direction of the declarant.  At the date of this instrument,│
│   I am not                                                        │
│   entitled to any portion of the estate of the declarant          │
│   according to the laws                                           │
│   of intestate succession or, to the best of my knowledge and     │
│   belief, under any                                               │
│   will of declarant or other instrument taking effect at          │
│   declarant's death, or                                           │
│   directly financially responsible for the declarant's medical    │
│   care.                                                           │
│                                                                   │
│                 Witness _____          │
│                                                                   │
│                 Witness _____          │
└─────────────────────────────────────────────────────────────────┘
```

Figure 7–2. An example of a living will.

support of the business community, and faced cutting the education budget to fund health care (Campbell, 1993).

Palliative Versus Curative Care

There may come a point in the course of a disease when a cure may not be possible. For example, clients with cardiomyopathy, neoplastic diseases, or degenerative diseases may no longer respond to treatment; thus, they might perceive continued treatment with poor probability of cure unbearable. These clients may opt for treatment that provides symptom management but does not cure the condition. Palliative care—aimed toward comfort, not cure—may involve radiation, chemotherapy, or surgery to reduce tumor mass; administration of analgesics in high and frequent doses; and/or variation in nutrition routes.

Nurses often have an opportunity to practice the art as

well as the science of nursing in palliative care. During palliative care, nurses make a commitment to provide relief for the client until death. A client's comfort is often related to the tenacity of the nurse in advocating and providing client care.

Intentionality

The doctrine of the "double effect" (Garcia, 1995) is moral reasoning presented by some Catholic theologians in defending the use of analgesics in terminal illness. The double effect doctrine holds that it is morally permissible to medicate a client to relieve pain even if there is a risk that the medication may suppress respirations and cause the client to stop breathing. If the *intent* is to relieve pain, the action is permissible. If the *intent* is to kill the person, it is not permissible. For example, a nurse gives morphine sulfate to a client dying of lung cancer. The nurse realizes that morphine can depress respirations, which are already compromised by the cancer. Nevertheless, the nurse intends to provide pain relief and is aware that an untoward side effect may be death due to apnea. The nurse is ethically justified in giving the morphine because the intent is to relieve pain, not to cause death.

Competency

Two forms of competency exist: legal and clinical competency. A person is considered to be *legally* competent if he or she is

- 18 years of age or older
- Pregnant or a married minor
- A legally emancipated minor who is self-supporting
- Not declared incompetent by a court of law

If a court determines that a person is legally incompetent, a guardian is appointed to make health care and/or financial decisions.

A person is considered to be *clinically* competent if he or she is legally competent and possesses decisional capacity. Decisional capacity is determined by the person who is the most knowledgeable about the issue. Decisional capacity is determined by assessing the client's ability to

- Identify the problem
- Recognize options and their potential consequences
- Make a decision
- Provide rationale supporting the chosen option

Thus, a surgeon would determine a client's decisional capacity related to surgery, an internist would assess capacity related to medical treatment, and a nurse would determine the client's ability to make decisions about nursing activities (Bosek, 1993).

Written Advance Directives

Written advance directives are "legal documents which provide a mechanism for individuals to indicate their decisions about future medical care" (Bosek & Fitzpatrick, 1992, p. 33). The U.S. Patient Self Determination Act of 1990 requires health care professionals to inform each client who is admitted to a hospital or nursing home about the availability of advance directives. If the client has a written advance directive on admission, a copy is placed with the medical record so that the directive will be available if needed.

There are two common types of written advance directives: living wills and durable power of attorney for health care.

Living Wills

Living wills, sometimes referred to as "death with dignity" documents, allow persons to document their wishes regarding life-sustaining treatment in case they are ever unable to speak for themselves and are imminently dying of a terminal illness (Fig. 7–2). Some states in the United States and provinces in Canada do not recognize living wills as legal documents. Nurses must investigate whether living wills are legally recognized in their state or prov-

ince. This information can be obtained from an ethicist or their agency's legal consultant or department. In most states, "imminent death" refers to when death is expected within a few hours or days according to best medical estimates (Kilner, 1990). In some states, imminent death may be defined as death that is expected to occur within a few months.

Durable Power of Attorney for Health Care

A durable power of attorney for health care (DPOA), sometimes called a durable medical power of attorney, is a legal document in the United States. This document allows people to

- Identify someone to make decisions for them if unable to speak for themselves
- Identify how aggressive treatment should be if they should ever be in a coma or a persistent vegetative state (PVS)
- List any medical treatments they would never want performed (Fig. 7–3)

Each state in the United States has legislation that describes the scope and execution of a DPOA.

The following example illustrates the use of advance directives: A client who sustained head trauma in an accident is now in a PVS and requires ventilator support. The spouse presents a copy of the client's living will and DPOA to the hospital staff and requests that the ventilator be discontinued. The living will does not apply in this situation because the client is not considered terminally ill. The DPOA, however, does apply and identifies the spouse as the agent to make the health care decisions. In addition, the client has documented the desire to forego artificial life support in the event of irreversible coma. The health care team respects the client's autonomy, as exercised by the spouse and the written advance directive, and discontinues the ventilator. Nurses should become familiar with applicable laws on advance directives in their state or province as well as remember that written advance directives are not to be implemented until the person has lost decisional capacity.

Verbal Advance Directives

Occasionally, family members, friends, or health care professionals are able to remember conversations with the client when specific comments were made about life-sustaining treatments. These comments may be considered verbal advance directives when the client has no written directives and is unable to communicate his or her wishes. A common myth is that the physician is obligated to follow the next-of-kin consent when the client cannot participate in decision-making. In most cases, next-of-kin do not have legal authority to consent or refuse treatment for an adult relative without becoming declared the legal guardian or the agent in a DPOA. Traditionally, however, health care professionals have obtained next-of-kin approval to minimize the chance of being sued.

If a client tells a nurse or other health care professional about his or her wishes regarding health care and life-sustaining treatment, the professional should encourage

DURABLE POWER OF ATTORNEY FOR HEALTH CARE

Power of Attorney made this _____ day of _____, 19 ____
    1. I, the undersigned hereby appoint (insert name and address of agent)

_____

as agent to act for me and in my name to make any and all decisions for me concerning my personal care, medical treatment, hospitalization and health care and to require, withhold or withdraw any type of medical treatment or procedure, even though my death may ensue. My agent shall have the same access to my medical records that I have, including the right to disclose the contents to others. My agent shall also have full power to make a disposition of any part or all of my body for medical purposes, authorize an autopsy and direct the disposition of my remains. (Neither the attending physician nor any other health care provider may act as your agent.)

    2. The powers granted above shall be subject to the following rules or limitations (if none, leave blank):

_____

_____

(The subject of life-sustaining treatment is of particular importance. For your convenience in dealing with that subject some general statements concerning the withholding or removal of life-sustaining treatment are set forth below. If you agree with one of these statements, you may initial that statement; but do not initial more than one.)

    (I do not want my life to be prolonged nor do I want life-sustaining treatment
    (to be provided or continued if my agent believes the burdens of the treatment
    (outweigh the expected benefits. I want my agent to consider the relief of
    (suffering the expense involved and the quality as well as the possible extension
_____(of my life in making decisions concerning life-sustaining treatment.

    (I want my life to be prolonged and I want life-sustaining treatment to be
    (provided or continued unless I am in a coma which my attending physician
    (believes to be irreversible, in accordance with reasonable medical standards at
    (the time of reference. If and when I have suffered irreversible coma, I want
_____(life-sustaining treatment to be withheld or discontinued.

    (I want my life to be prolonged to the greatest extent possible without regard to
_____(my condition, the chances I have for recovery or the cost of the procedures.

    3. This power of attorney shall become effective on _____

_____

Figure 7–3. An example of a durable power of attorney for health care.

the client to specifically elaborate on vague phrases, like "do everything" or "when my time comes, let me go." The health care professional helps the client to document these directives in written form when possible. In addition, the nurse should document the conversation in the medical record (Fig. 7–4). All health care professionals should refer to agency policies and procedures about the use of verbal advance directives for guiding clinical ethical decision-making.

Euthanasia

Euthanasia means "good death" (Bandman & Bandman, 1995, p. 308). Although this concept is an ethical issue,

in the United States it is dealt with more from a legal perspective. Chapter 12 includes a complete discussion on euthanasia.

Placebo Administration

A placebo is an inert substance or benign action intentionally administered as a treatment, usually as a modality for pain relief. For instance, a client may receive a normal saline injection for a complaint of pain. When prescribing a placebo, the physician is intentionally attempting to deceive the client and thus is limiting the client's autonomy. When clients are deceived, they are unable to make

4. This power of attorney shall terminate on _____

_____

5. If any agent named by me shall die, become legally disabled, resign, refuse to act or be unavailable, I name the following (each to act alone and successively, in the order named) as successors to such agent:

_____

_____

6. If a guardian of my person is to be appointed, I nominate the following to serve as such guardian (if same as agent, leave blank):

_____

7. I am fully informed as to all the contents of this form and understand the full import of this grant of power to my agent.

Signed _____
                                              Principal

The principal has had an opportunity to read the above form and has signed the form or acknowledged his or her signature or mark on the form in my presence.

_____ Residing at _____
Witness

(You may, but are not required to, request your agent and successor agents to provide specimen signature below. If you include specimen signature in this Power of Attorney, you must complete the certification opposite the signatures of the agents.)

Specimen signatures of agent   I certify that the signature of my agent
(and successors)   (and successors) are correct.

_____   _____
        (agent)   (principal)

_____   _____
   (successor agent)   (principal)

_____   _____
   (successor agent)   (principal)

Figure 7–3. *Continued*

informed decisions. In addition, the use of placebos denies that the client is experiencing pain and jeopardizes client trust in both the physician's and nurse's motives. When clients seek health care assistance, they are assuming that health care professionals will act in their best interest; thus, the use of a placebo threatens this assumption (Elander, 1991).

When a nurse cannot ethically implement a placebo order, he or she is obligated to explain this position to the physician. If the physician continues the placebo order after this discussion, the nurse is obligated to work toward a resolution of this ethical issue by seeking ethics consultation. When a nurse cannot follow a physician's

order, the nurse must follow the health care agency's policy and lines of nursing authority precisely while documenting each communication. Fox (1994) described the arduous but satisfying task of getting the policy on use of placebos changed in one health care agency.

Many nurses have no moral opposition to using placebos if a client expresses pain relief after receiving the placebo. Often, clients do experience increased comfort because of personal attention and associated nursing interventions, such as repositioning or relaxation techniques, provided with the placebo (Beauchamp & Childress, 1994; Elander, 1991).

When administering a placebo, the nurse has a basic

Nursing Focus Note

5/1/97   12 noon   Focus: HIV with lymphadenopathy

D: C/O cheek and neck swelling. R=20 and easy. Denies dysphagia.

A: Initiated discussion regarding use of emergency treatment for respiratory distress or arrest. Instructed on purpose and use of advance directives. Dr. Jones notified of swelling.

R: Stated: "I won't live much longer...I want all the usual emergency treatments...I wouldn't want a machine continued if there was no hope that I'd get better. I'm not sure if my Mom could actually carry out this request. I'll talk to her this afternoon."

A: Client discussed wishes with mother.

R: Durable Power for Attorney completed with mother as agent.

A: Dr. Jones notified of DPOA. Is a full code. *Marcia Bosek, RN*

Nursing Narrative Note

8 am	C/O neck swelling. Left cheek and entire neck obviously swollen. No C/O dysphagia. R = 20 and easy. Lungs clear bilaterally. *Marcia Bosek, RN*
8:30 am	Dr. Jones notified of cheek and neck swelling. *Marcia Bosek, RN*
10 am	Informed of O_2 saturation tests q shift, instructed to notify nurse of respiratory distress. Discussion initiated by RN regarding wishes about emergency treatment for respiratory arrest. Stated: "I won't live much longer. I want all the usual emergency treatments. I wouldn't want a machine continued if there was no hope that I'd get better. I'm not sure if my Mom could actually carry out this request. I'll talk to her this afternoon." Provided with copy of DPOA and instructed on use. Verbalized understanding of process. *Marcia Bosek, RN*

Figure 7–4. Sample documentation of verbal directives.

obligation to prevent harm. The nurse needs to conduct a thorough client assessment before and after administering a placebo. When a client does not experience pain relief, the nurse must notify the physician and request other treatment options. With the patient's permission, alternating pain medication with a placebo as a trial to determine the extent of genuine pain is ethically acceptable.

Restraints

Restraints are interventions that limit a person's freedom to move. Restraints can be physical (e.g., vest, limb, or geri-chair with lap table in place) or chemical (e.g., haloperidol [Haldol, Periodol♣]). Because restraints limit movement, they also limit autonomy. Before deciding whether to restrain a client, the nurse needs to identify the desired outcome and consider the related risks and benefits of all possible options.

When planning client care, the nurse may desire a variety of outcomes, such as preventing harm to the client and to the other clients, and/or maintaining the client's autonomy. However, balancing these two outcomes may be difficult when a client's autonomy is compromised by an illness such as Alzheimer's disease. A client with Alzheimer's disease may be free from harm if he or she has a steady gait, yet wandering may cause harm to other clients. Therefore, on the basis of nonmaleficence (preventing harm to others), the nurse in a case such as this would be justified in limiting the client's autonomy by preventing the wandering (Reigle, 1994).

When using a restraint, nurses must always consider both the risks and benefits (Table 7–4) and use the least restrictive method possible (Robbins, 1986). For instance, a waist restraint is less restrictive than a vest restraint, and a vest restraint is less restrictive than limb restraints. Chemical restraints (drugs) are the most restrictive be-

TABLE 7–4

Potential Benefits and Risks of Physical Restraints

Potential benefits
- Prevention of falls, which might result in injury
- Protection from other accidents or injuries
- Allowing medical treatment to proceed without client interference
- Protection of other clients or staff from disturbances or physical harm
- Increased client feelings of safety and security

Potential risks
- Injury from falls
- Accidental death by strangulation
- Functional decline
- Skin abrasions or skin breakdown
- Biochemical, physiologic, and psychological sequelae of prolonged immobilization
- Cardiac arrest
- Reduced appetite and dehydration
- Disorganized behavior
- Emotional desolation
- Possible increased mortality

Reprinted with permission from Evans, L. K., & Strumpf, N. E. (1989). Tying down the elderly: A review of the literature on physical restraint. *Journal of the American Geriatrics Society, 37,* 65–74.

cause they affect the client's physical and mental abilities.

As always, a nurse follows both state statutes and the health care agency's policies and procedure when using restraints. A client's mental and physical condition is routinely re-evaluated and documented along with justification for continued use of restraints (also see Chapter 6). Restraints should be discontinued as soon as possible or when an alternate intervention has been implemented (Bosek, 1993). Miles and Meyers (1994) suggest a restraint reduction program that includes "reviewing medications, allowing for naps to prevent fatigue, social stimulation, using nonrestraining postural supports, treating pain or Parkinson's disease or other debilitating conditions, physical therapy, and providing a safe and enclosed area for ambulating or wandering" (p. 522).

Personal Rights

A right is a justifiable claim that all persons can make (Curtin & Flaherty, 1982). In the past, health care was acquired through bartering. However, in the late 20th century, health care has evolved into a business industry. When health care is a right, every citizen will be able to access health care services and society will have an obligation to provide health care.

In Canada and several other countries, health care is recognized as a right. National health care programs have been implemented to guarantee that every citizen has equal access to health care; however, not all treatments and procedures are available.

In the United States, many people believe that health care is a right, but no universal health care system exists at this time. At present, health care is available to those who can afford to pay, have insurance, or qualify for Medicare and Medicaid. Emergency care is available to the uninsured, but access to other forms of health care is limited. A growing segment of the U.S. population is uninsurable or unemployed or does not have access to insurance through an employer. There has been much debate about how to deal with this access issue. Many advocate a two-tiered system that would provide basic health care to all while allowing each person to purchase additional "high-tech" medical treatment. Others propose a universal, single-payer system emphasizing health promotion and disease prevention.

Obligation

If a person has a specific right to health care, that person also has an obligation to maintain and protect his or her health. Rights and their associated responsibilities are inherently in conflict with autonomy. Life insurance companies often compensate for high correlations between voluntary behavior and disease by charging higher premium rates to people who smoke, drink alcoholic beverages, or engage in high-risk activities, such as auto racing.

Confidentiality

Confidentiality is a major ethical issue. Confidentiality requires that a person can expect that personal information will be kept in confidence and not shared without consent (Winslade, 1995). Some information may be perceived as sensitive and thus should be shared only on a "need-to-know" basis. For example, release of genetic test results could have long-reaching consequences for job and insurance discrimination. Thus, nurses must be ever vigilant to protect client information from any person without expressed permission from the client (McLure, 1995).

The nursing codes of the American Nurses' Association and the Canadian Nurses Association require nurses to maintain client confidentiality. Too often, nurses and other health care professionals discuss client cases in elevators, cafeterias, and other public places. Although they do not intend to breach a client's confidentiality, others may overhear the conversations.

Cultural and Spiritual Practices

Values are critical in ethical issues and are shaped by many influences—family, experiences, culture, and spirituality. Health care decisions involve clarification of values and interpreting the meaning that a client places on illness (see Table 7–4). Clients often interpret the meaning of their illness through the tenets of their faith. For example, they may view illness as a punishment for wrongdoings or lack of faith and may refuse pain medication because of the belief that suffering leads to redemption.

How clients cope with illness is also affected by their faith. When addressing ethical issues, the nurse assesses the client's spirituality. Often clients are asked to list their religious preference when admitted to a health care agency, but religion is only a part of the broader concept of spirituality. A nurse discusses the client's spiritual needs to learn how the client relies on spirituality during major life changes. Often clients share thoughts and feelings with the nurse, who can help them clarify questions and fears to discuss with family, physician, or others.

At times, a conflict can occur between the medical treatment plan and a client's spiritual beliefs. For example, consider a client who is a Jehovah's Witness and has multiple trauma injuries that necessitate blood transfusions. This is an ethical issue because the client requires blood but his religion prohibits accepting a blood transfusion. Facing this conflict can be emotionally taxing for the client and health care team. Strategies for dealing with similar issues can be developed to prepare for future challenging clients. Nurses and health care providers may also need to consult the hospital chaplain or other religious leaders to understand spiritual practices. These resources may also help health care professionals to deal with the dissonance created when they must implement acts contrary to their own personal beliefs.

Tube Feeding

Certain conditions prevent clients from taking food and fluids orally. For example, a client may have had extensive treatment for cancer of the head and neck or may have a neurologic disorder, such as PVS or permanent unconsciousness. For clients who hope to recover and take oral feedings again, tube feedings are a temporary intervention to ensure adequate nutrition and hydration. The ethical issue occurs when recovery is unlikely and tube feeding becomes death-delaying instead of life-prolonging treatment. Controversy exists over whether tube feeding (nasogastric, gastrostomy, or jejunostomy) is considered a medical treatment or a basic need that must be met. The American Academy of Neurology views artificial nutrition and hydration as medical therapy that competent patients or surrogate decision makers may refuse (Bernat et al., 1996).

Ethical Debate

Some ethicists (Weir, 1989) argue that feeding, whether oral or tube, is a basic need, like oxygen, that must be met regardless of prognosis. One is obligated to feed the client if the client would die of starvation and dehydration rather than of the underlying disease or disorder. The exception is if the client's condition would actually worsen if feedings were given, as with pulmonary edema, aspiration pneumonia, or renal failure. Other ethicists believe that tube feedings are a medical procedure that can be withheld or withdrawn if no medical benefit (improvement or recovery) is foreseen. For clients in a PVS who will not regain consciousness, tube feedings maintain but do not alter their condition.

If the client has expressed wishes in the form of an advance directive stating that tube feedings should not be initiated if there is no hope of recovery, then tube feedings should not be started or they should be discontinued

on presentation of this advance directive. However, if a client has no advance directive, the decision to initiate and continue tube feedings becomes more difficult, as in the Cruzan case (*Cruzan v. Director, Missouri Department of Health,* 1990). Tube feedings may have been started before the prognosis was certain (a diagnosis of a PVS is usually made 1 to 6 months after an initial injury). Hodges and Tolle (1994) defend the use of quality of life (QOL), medical goals, and patient preferences as criteria to consider when making decisions regarding tube feedings in the elderly.

Nursing Dilemma

Nurses often express ethical discomfort in caring for clients in a PVS who are receiving tube feedings. Nurses may respect the right to life of such clients but also may question what purpose is being served by expending resources for those who probably will not benefit. Alternatively, nurses may believe that all clients deserve basic comfort measures—food, warmth, protection from harm—and may resist withdrawing feedings. Deeper issues of respect for life, spirituality, QOL, and allocation of resources are involved in the question of whether to use tube feedings (see the Research Applications for Nursing box).

Nurses must first examine their feelings and beliefs about tube feedings and then participate in a team conference that explores the benefits and burdens of this treatment for a particular client. Decisions on whether to tube feed rest with the client (by advance directive) or family and the physician with input from other health care professionals who know the client and family. Legal requirements may necessitate obtaining a court order to withdraw feedings. In some states, the living will statute specifically mandates that nutrition, hydration, and medication must be provided, although all other treatments may be discontinued.

In some states of the United States, laws exist that allow a family and health care team to make the decision to withhold or withdraw feedings without obtaining a court order, provided that specific steps are taken and documented in the medical record. When the nurse does not personally agree with the decision that is made, two courses can be pursued: (1) even if the nurse would not make the same decision, he or she should respect the client's autonomy and the process that produced this decision and believe that the best decision was made under these circumstances; or (2) if the nurse morally objects to this decision, he or she can state the objection and rationale to the nursing supervisor and request to be reassigned to another client if necessary.

Unethical Professional Conduct

In the American Nurses' Association Code for Nurses (1976; 1985), the third plank addresses the responsibility of nurses to uphold the highest standards and protect clients from health care professionals who engage in illegal, unethical, or incompetent practice. The *Code of Ethics for Nursing* by the Canadian Nurses Association (1991)

⊳ Research Applications for Nursing

Level of Moral Certainty Influences View of Artificial Nutrition

Wurbach, M. W. (1996). Long-term care nurses' ethical convictions about tube feeding. Western Journal of Nursing Research, 18(1), 63–76.

Using a descriptive exploratory design, Wurbach interviewed 25 long-term care nurses about their experiences when artificial nutrition was withheld or withdrawn from elderly patients at the end of life. The interview data were analyzed, and five categories of moral conviction were identified from the interview data.

Moral conviction is the "willingness to act on strong beliefs, sometimes assuming risk to oneself personally or professionally" (p. 68). The nurses described experiencing absolute moral conviction (20%), strong moral conviction (16%), moderate moral conviction (48%), moral uncertainty with conviction (12%), and moral uncertainty (4%). Those nurses experiencing moral certainty described significant positive and negative experiences with artificial nutrition; however, the nurses experiencing moral uncertainty had little or no direct experiences with providing artificial nutrition. Morally certain nurses had a negative opinion regarding the use of artificial nutrition and took actions, such as education, to stop or prevent the use of artificial nutrition for elders in the last stage of life. In contrast, nurses with moral uncertainty rarely acted. Despite the level of moral certainty experienced, each nurse subject described making decisions on "gut feeling" rather than by a problem-solving approach.

Critique. The researcher investigated a frequently occurring yet little researched phenomenon. Actions were taken to ensure the trustworthiness of the data analysis, such as evaluation of the findings by subjects and process trail auditing by a second person. The convenience sampling method may have resulted in a skewed proportion of nurses with moral certainty participating because morally uncertain nurses may have been reluctant to discuss their uncertainty.

Possible Nursing Implications. The findings from this study appear to support Benner's (1984) theory described in *From Novice to Expert.* Nurses with practical experience with artificial nutrition described higher levels of moral certainty. Thus, nursing administrators and educators need to establish decision-making resources to facilitate the novice nurse's decision-making abilities regarding the withdrawing or withholding of artificial nutrition. Safeguards must also be in place to prevent nurses with high levels of moral certainty from using their beliefs to coerce clients or family members to refuse artificial nutrition. Further research is needed to describe whether the nurse's level of moral certainty changes when a written advance directive is present.

lists "Value VIII: Protecting Clients from Incompetence. Value: The nurse takes steps to ensure that the client receives competent and ethical care" (p. 15). In the health care system, however, it is not very easy to report another's unethical conduct ("whistleblowing") without suffering unpleasant and sometimes devastating consequences.

The nurse who observes or discovers an act that jeopardizes a client's safety (e.g., seeing a medication error or witnessing another health care professional verbally or physically abusing a client) has an obligation to take steps to protect the client. This includes notifying the physician if a medication error was made, verifying information as thoroughly as possible, and documenting each incident according to agency policy. Next, the nurse follows the lines of authority for reporting the incident. Some nurses may wish to discuss the incident with other professionals involved, advising them that an incident was discovered and giving them an opportunity to take corrective action or clarify their behavior. In the spirit of collegiality and peer review, nurses can assist each other in keeping the standards of practice of nursing at the highest level.

Some nurses, however, have found themselves in situations in which they are made a party to unethical practices and have been threatened with loss of their job or license and even bodily harm when they followed channels of communication (Witt, 1983). Nurses must realistically evaluate the consequences of their actions in whistleblowing. The American Nurses' Association published guidelines on reporting incompetent, unethical, or illegal practices (1994). To maintain the public's trust and to self-regulate, nurses must continue to monitor their practices and the practices of others.

Chart 7–1

Nursing Focus on the Elderly

Myths and Ethical Issues Related to Care of the Elderly

Myths
- The older the client, the less likely he or she is to be competent.
- Adult children have the right to know their parent's medical status or to make health care decisions for their parents.
- The elderly are more likely to have articulated their beliefs about death and life-sustaining treatment than are younger clients.
- When a client can no longer control his or her bodily functions, he or she is also unable to make informed decisions about health care.

Ethical Issues
- How should health care resources be allocated for the frail and terminally ill elderly?
- Should health care services be rationed by age?
- Should elderly clients be able to choose the time to die?
- Does society have an obligation to provide for the elderly?
- Should health care treatment decisions be influenced by the elderly client's ability to pay? by the type of payment (private insurance/Medicare/Medicaid)?
- What is "the best interest" standard for the elderly?
- What constitutes elder abuse?
- Do the elderly have clearly defined values because of life experiences?
- When is it appropriate to provide comfort care for the elderly, versus using all available technology?

OTHER ETHICAL ISSUES THAT MEDICAL-SURGICAL NURSES FACE

Some of the ethical issues that nurses in medical-surgical settings face have been described in this chapter, but many others also exist, especially in the care of the elderly (Chart 7–1). Other ethical issues that occur include

- Use of fetal tissue for Parkinson's disease treatment
- Allocation of organs for transplantation
- Mandatory direct observed therapy for tuberculosis or drug abuse treatment
- Health care professional whose judgment is impaired by alcohol, drugs, or lack of knowledge
- Confidentiality of computerized records
- Disclosure of the health care professional's human immunodeficiency virus (HIV) status to clients
- Mandatory genetic screening for insurance or employment
- Maintaining quality of care during downsizing
- Conflict between client advocacy and financial responsibility in managed care

Many of these issues are presented and discussed elsewhere in this text.

SELECTED BIBLIOGRAPHY

* American Nurses' Association. (1976, 1985). *The Code for Nurses with Interpretive Statements*. Kansas City, MO: Author.
American Nurses' Association. (1994). *Guidelines on reporting incompetent, unethical, or illegal practices*. Washington D. C.: American Nurses Publishing.
Bandman, E. L., & Bandman, B. (1995). *Nursing ethics through the life span* (3rd ed.). Norwalk, CT: Appleton-Lange.
* Beauchamp, T. L., & Childress, J. F. (1994). *Principles of biomedical ethics* (4th ed.). New York: Oxford University Press.
* Beauchamp, T. L., & Walters, L. (1982). *Contemporary issues in bioethics* (2nd ed.). Belmont, CA: Wadsworth.
* Benner, P. (1984). *From novice to expert: Excellence and power in clinical nursing practice*. Menlo Park, CA: Addison-Wesley.
Bernat, J. L., Goldstein, M. L., & Viste, K. M. (1996). The neurologist and the dying patient. *Neurology, 46*, 598–599.
* Bosek, M. S. D. (1993). Ethical issues with the use of restraints. *MEDSURG Nursing, 2*(2), 154–156.
* Bosek, M. S. D., & Fitzpatrick, J. (1992). A nursing perspective on advance directives. *MEDSURG Nursing, 1*(1), 33–38.
* Campbell, C. S. (1993). Gridlock on the Oregon Trail. *Hastings Center Report, 23*(4), 6–7.
*Canadian Nurses Association. (1991). *Code of ethics for nursing*. Ottawa: Author.
Clarke, D. E., Goldstein, M. K., & Raffin, T. A. (1994). Ethical dilemmas in the critically ill elderly. *Clinics in Geriatric Medicine, 10*(1), 91–101.
* Corley, M. C., & Selig, P. M. (1992). Nurse moral reasoning using the Nursing Dilemma Test. *Western Journal of Nursing Research, 14*, 380–388.
* Crisham, P. (1981). Decision analysis: A step by step guide for making clinical decisions. *Nursing & Health Care, 7*, 148–154.
* *Cruzan v. Director, Missouri Department of Health*. 110 S. Ct. 2841 (1990).
* Curtin, L., & Flaherty, M. J. (1982). *Nursing ethics: Theory and pragmatics*. Bowie, MD: Robert J. Brady.
* DeWolf, M. S. (1989a). *Clinical ethical decision-making: A grounded theory method*. Chicago: Rush University.
* DeWolf, M. S. (1989b). Ethical decision making. *Seminars in Oncology Nursing, 5*(2), 77–81.
* Elander, G. (1991). Ethical conflicts in placebo treatment. *Journal of Advanced Nursing, 16*, 947–951.

* Evans, L. K., & Strumpf, N. E. (1989). Tying down the elderly: A review of the literature on physical restraint. *Journal of the American Geriatric Society, 36*, 65–74.
* Ferrans, C. E., & Powers, M. J., (1985). Quality of life index: Development and psychometric properties. *Advances in Nursing Science, 8*, 15–24.
* Fowler, M. D. M., & Levine-Ariff, J. (1987). *Ethics at the bedside: A source book for the critical care nurse*. Philadelphia: J. B. Lippincott.
Fox, A. E. (1994). Confronting the use of placebos for pain. *American Journal of Nursing, 94*(9), 42–46.
* Fromer, M. J. (1981). *Ethical issues in health care*. St. Louis: C. V. Mosby.
Garcia, J. L. A. (1995). Double effect. In W. T. Reich (Ed.), *Encyclopedia of bioethics* (Rev. ed., Vol. 2, pp. 636–641). New York: Simon & Schuster Macmillan.
* Hadorn, D. C. (1991). The Oregon priority-setting exercise: Quality of life and public policy. *Hastings Center Report, 21*(3, Suppl), 11–16.
Hodges, M. O., & Tolle, S. W. (1994). Tube-feeding decisions in the elderly. *Clinics in Geriatric Medicine, 10*(3), 475–488.
Husted, G. L., & Husted, J. H. (1994). *Ethical decision making in nursing* (2nd ed). St. Louis: Mosby-Year Book.
Joint Commission on Accreditation of Healthcare Organizations. (1997–1998). *Comprehensive accreditation manual for home care*. Oakbrook Terrace, IL: Author.
Joint Commission on Accreditation of Healthcare Organizations. (1998). *Comprehensive accreditation manual for hospitals*. Oakbrook Terrace, IL: Author.
Joint Commission on Accreditation of Healthcare Organizations. (1998–1999a). *Comprehensive accreditation manual for ambulatory health care*. Oakbrook Terrace, IL: Author.
Joint Commission on Accreditation of Healthcare Organizations. (1998–1999b). *Comprehensive accreditation manual for long term care*. Oakbrook Terrace, IL: Author.
* Kilner, J. F. (1990). *Who lives? Who dies? Ethical criteria in patient selection*. New Haven: Yale University Press.
Langslow, A. (1995). "Not for CPR" orders: Current developments. *Australian Nursing Journal, 2*(10), 36–38.
McLure, H. (1995). The insurance industry's use of genetic information: Legal and ethical concerns. *Journal of Health and Hospital Law, 28*(4), 231–242.
Miles, S. H., & Meyers, R. (1994). Untying the elderly: 1989 to 1993 update. *Clinics in Geriatric Medicine, 10*(3), 513–525.
* Newell, A., & Simon, H. A. (1972). *Human problem solving*. Englewood Cliffs, NJ: Prentice-Hall.
Parkman, C. A., & Carfee, B. E. (1997). Advance directives: Honoring your patient's end-of-life wishes. *Nursing '97, 27*(4), 48–53.
Pinch, W. J. E. (1996). Feminism and bioethics. *MEDSURG Nursing, 5*(1), 53–56.
* Ratzan, R. M. (1987). The use of physical force. *Postgraduate Medicine, 81*(1), 125, 128.
Reigle, J. (1994). HealthCare Ethics Forum '94: Ethical challenges in the critically ill: Use of restraints. *AACN Clinical Issues, 5*(3), 329–332.
Rhodes, R. (1994). An alternate opinion: Do-not-resuscitate orders in the operating room. *Mount Sinai Journal of Medicine, 61*(6), 498–499.
* Robbins, L. J. (1986). Restraining the elderly patient. *Clinics in Geriatric Medicine, 2*(3), 591–597.
Rosner, F., Bennett, A. J., & Sechzer, P. H. (1994). Do-not-resuscitate orders in the operating room. *Mount Sinai Journal of Medicine, 61*(6), 493–496.
*Rushton, C. H., & Lynch, M. E. (1992, June). Dealing with advance directives for critically ill adolescents. *Critical Care Nurses*, 31–37.
Savage, T. (1994). The nurse's role on ethics committees and as an ethics consultant. *Seminars for Nurse Managers, 2*(1), 41–47.
*Shelly, J. A. (1980). *Dilemma*. Downers Grove, IL: InterVarsity Press.
*Simon, H. A. (1978). Information-processing theory of human problem solving. In W. K. Estes (Ed.). *Handbook of learning and cognitive processes* (Vol. 5, pp. 271–295). Hillsdale, NJ: Lawrence Erlbaum Associates.
*Steele, S. M., & Harmon, V. M. (1983). *Values clarification in nursing* (2nd ed.). Norwalk, CT: Appleton-Century-Crofts.
*Thompson, J., & Thompson, H. O. (1985). *Bioethical decision-making for nurses*. Norwalk, CT: Appleton-Century-Crofts.
*Veatch, R. M. (1980). Voluntary risks to health. *Journal of the American Medical Association, 243*(1), 50–55.
*Weir, R. F. (1989). *Abating Treatment with Critically Ill Patients: Medical*

and Legal Limits to the Medical Prolongation. New York: Oxford University Press.

*Wicclair, M. R. (1991). Differentiating ethical decisions from clinical standards. *Dimensions of critical care nursing, 10*(5), 280–288.

Winslade, W. (1995). Confidentiality. In W. T. Reich (Ed.) *Encyclopedia of bioethics* (Rev. ed., Vol. 1, pp. 451–459). New York: Simon & Shuster MacMillan.

*Witt, P. (1983). Notes of a whistleblower. *American Journal of Nursing, 83,* 1649–1651.

Wurbach, M. E. (1996). Long-term care nurses' ethical convictions about tube feedings. *Western Journal of Nursing Research, 18*(1), 63–76.

SUGGESTED READINGS

Bandman, E. L., & Bandman, B. (1995). *Nursing ethics through the life span* (3rd ed.). Norwalk, CT: Appleton-Lange.

Individual chapters are devoted to the various stages in the life span. In each of these chapters, the authors present selected cases with related ethical principles and identify nursing judgments and actions. Traditional and contemporary theories of ethical decision-making and the pitfalls that can occur in moral reasoning are also discussed.

Keffer, M. J. (1996). Nurse advocate: Advocate for whom? *MEDSURG Nursing, 5*(2), 125–126.

Nurses are taught to be patient advocates; however, this advocacy role can be undermined by agency policy or politics. Three categories of influence (persuasion, manipulation, and coercion) are described. Policies should be evaluated to identify potential situations in which the nurse may be coerced to place agency issues before the patient's best interests. Nurses need to be involved in creating and revising policies that keep the patient's interests as top priority.

STRESS, COPING, AND ADAPTATION

When laypeople speak of stress, they may say that it is an actual feeling of being overwhelmed. To others, stress is the cause of this feeling. In the social sciences, including nursing, the concept of stress has evolved to include both the feeling and the event.

OVERVIEW
Definitions
Stress

Stress is a relationship between a person and the environment that the person perceives as taxing or dangerous (Lazarus & Folkman, 1984). The cognitive evaluation, or thought process, through which a person determines that an event is stressful is called an "appraisal" of stress. A *stressor* is the taxing or dangerous physical, psychological, social, or environmental event that leads to the appraisal of stress. Following are some examples of stressors:

- *Physiologic:* Injuries; infectious, viral, or fungal agents; radiation; drugs; and alcohol
- *Psychological:* Frustrations, loss of control, and anger
- *Social:* Losses of social support, problems in living arrangements, and the difficulties associated with low economic status
- *Environmental:* Pollution, the hazards of the workplace, and extremes of temperature

Coping

To deal with stress effectively, people try to cope by using specific strategies. Coping strategies are the ways by which people try to control the causative problem or stress-related feelings. Some examples of coping strategies are denial, use of social supports, confrontation of the problem, and consideration of the positive aspects of the situation. These strategies are described later in this chapter.

Adaptation

Adaptation occurs when a person has mastered, changed, or accepted the stressful event. Adaptation implies that a sense of equilibrium is restored to the person disordered by stress. Adaptation is reflected in one or more changes in a person's psychological, social, or physical health.

THE IMPORTANCE OF STRESS IN MEDICAL-SURGICAL NURSING PRACTICE

Stress is particularly important in the practice of medical-surgical nursing for adults because its presence may cause, prolong, or aggravate a client's illness. Stress can interfere with other aspects of clients' lives because it may contribute to family, spiritual, and social crises.

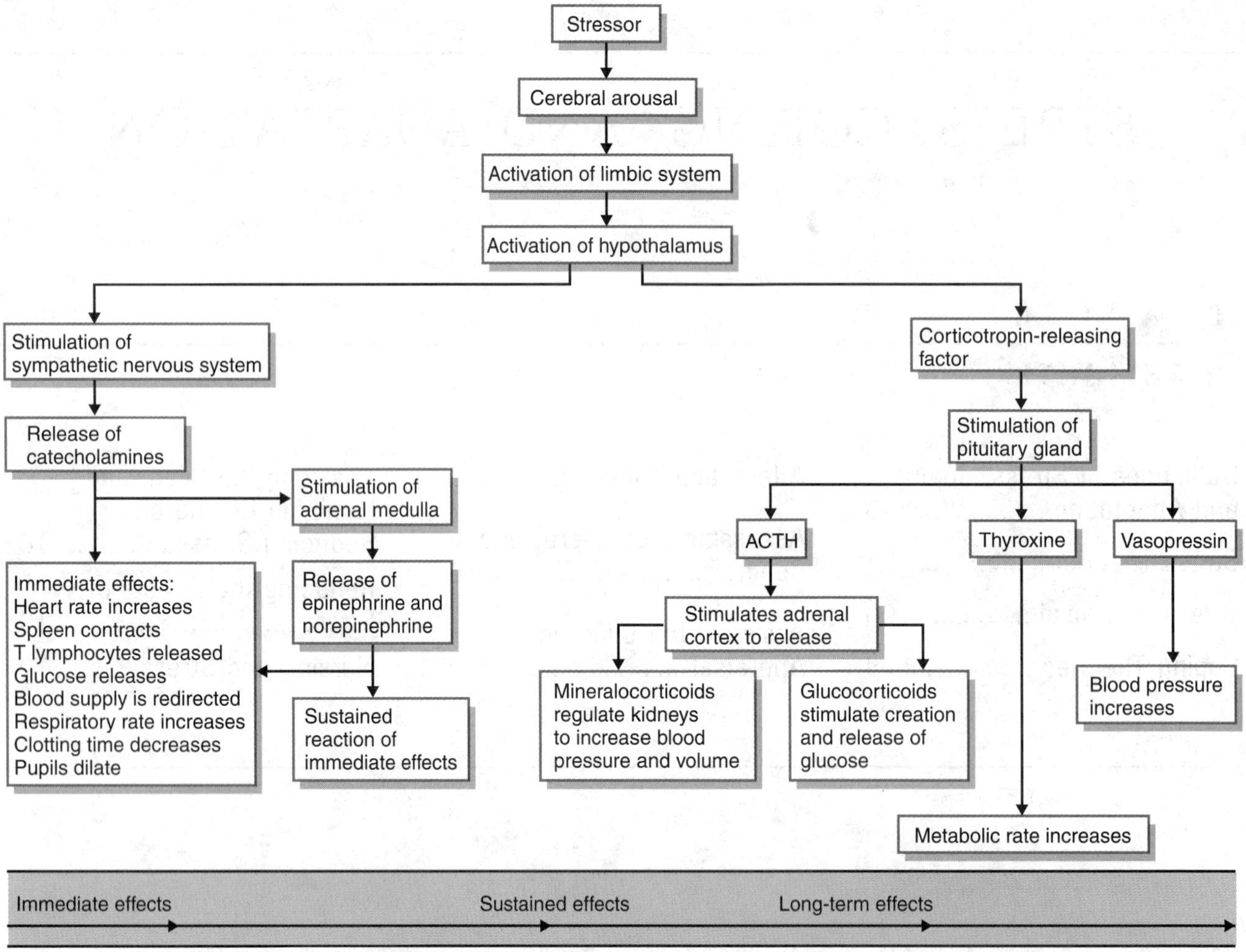

Figure 8–1. The general adaptation syndrome.

Clients use a variety of strategies to deal with stress. Nurses are commonly in positions in which they can aid the clients' coping, either through assisting the clients' self-initiated efforts or by suggesting alternatives. Successful coping and adaptation are the goals of both the client and the nurse. All clients want stress to be reduced to manageable levels or eliminated.

Theories About Stress

Stress has been studied from three major viewpoints. First, researchers have viewed stress as the body's physical response to threat. Second, stress has been considered to be a stimulus, or outside force, that causes a reaction. Third, stress has been examined as a transaction between the person and the event.

Stress as a Response

The biological and medical sciences have traditionally viewed stress as the body's response to an event; that is, stress is the physiologic response or change that occurs within the body. The idea of stress as a response gained prominence through the classic work of Hans Selye, who defined stress as "the nonspecific response of the body to any demand made upon it to adapt, whether that demand produces pain or pleasure" (1946, p. 230).

From Selye's definition, three phenomena are immediately apparent. First, Selye thought that the body's response to stress is nonspecific: The body reacts as a whole organism. Second, stress is considered a physiologic response, not a psychological one. Third, Selye believed that it is not just the "bad" things in life that cause stress but the "good" things as well. From Selye's viewpoint, a wedding can cause the same physiologic response as a funeral. Selye called the body's generalized response to a stressor the *general adaptation syndrome* (GAS) (Fig. 8–1). This syndrome has three distinct stages:

1. The alarm stage
2. The stage of resistance
3. The stage of exhaustion

In addition to recognizing the body's *generalized* response, Selye noted a *localized* response. He labeled the body's limited, localized response as the *localized adaptation syndrome* (LAS). Inflammation at a surgical site is an example of the LAS.

THE ALARM STAGE. The physiologic response to a stressor begins with the alarm stage, in which the body prepares itself for survival. Cannon (1931) called this initial physiologic response the "fight-or-flight response." As outlined by Cannon, this response process prepares all animals, including humans, for survival. When faced with danger, the body prepares to either fight the danger or flee from it. Either reaction is thought to cause the same changes in the body.

The stress-related changes are coordinated by the central nervous system (CNS). Within the CNS, the limbic system is the emotional response center that triggers the fight-or-flight response. The limbic system then activates the hypothalamus. The hypothalamus in turn initiates the stress response and directs the activities of the autonomic nervous system (ANS), composed of the sympathetic and parasympathetic systems. The ANS controls the body's involuntary responses, such as hormone secretions, metabolism, and fluid regulation.

The sympathetic system of the ANS is responsible for dynamic change, and the parasympathetic system is responsible for restoring the body to its normal resting state. In response to stress, the sympathetic nervous system stimulates the adrenal medulla, which in turn secretes the catecholamines norepinephrine and epinephrine. The adrenal cortex is also stimulated by the pituitary gland's release of adrenocorticotropic hormone (ACTH). The circulating ACTH causes the adrenal cortex to release glucocorticoids (cortisol, corticosterone, and cortisone) and mineralocorticoids (aldosterone and deoxycorticosterone). As a result of the CNS and adrenal activity, seven major changes occur within the body:

- *Increase in heart rate,* to ensure that adequate oxygen and nutrients are available to the muscles and organs
- *Contraction of the spleen,* to reduce the amount of blood lost from the spleen in case of injury and to release T lymphocytes into the bloodstream for defense
- *Release of glucose,* to fuel the body for response to danger
- *Redirection of blood supply,* to ensure blood flow to the vital organs, such as the brain
- *Changes in the respiratory system* (increased respiratory rate and depth), to provide for effective oxygen–carbon dioxide exchange
- *Decrease in blood clotting time,* to decrease blood loss in case of body injury
- *Dilation of pupils,* to enhance vision

These major changes, plus minor changes, such as increased perspiration and piloerection (hairs standing on end), appear to occur whenever a person is threatened. Selye called these collective processes the alarm stage in the body's preparation for survival. Although these preparations may have been useful to human beings in the past, they have limited utility in most of today's threat situations. It is unfortunate that these reactions persist, because they result in tremendous wear and tear on the body. If these reactions occur frequently or are sustained, a person may experience damage to the body's systems or illness, such as heart disease and diabetes mellitus.

THE STAGE OF RESISTANCE. The second stage in the GAS is called the stage of resistance. When the body recognizes continued threat, physiologic forces are mobilized to maintain an increased resistance to stressors. This resistance begins with a decrease in the production of ACTH. The body concentrates its activities on those organs or organ systems that are most involved in the specific stress response. Successful adaptation implies positive growth toward a return to or improvement in physical health. The efforts of the body to resist stress may be ineffectual, leading to a state of maladaptation in which deterioration occurs in levels of physical functioning. Chronic resistance eventually causes damage to the involved systems.

THE STAGE OF EXHAUSTION. The body enters the stage of exhaustion when organs or organ systems show evidence of deterioration. Selye determined that the overwhelmed body exhibits a triad of symptoms: hypertrophy of the adrenal glands, ulcerations in the gastrointestinal tract, and atrophy of the thymus gland. In this final stage, all energy for adaptation has been used, ACTH secretion increases, and a more generalized response is seen once again. This third stage can also result in what health care professionals call the diseases of adaptation, or stress-related diseases, and even death. Conditions and diseases in Table 8–1 represent examples thought to be related to or worsened by stress.

Stress as a Stimulus

Realizing that people do not react to all stressors as threats, theorists and researchers began to explore the stress associated with a stimulus. In the stimulus theory,

TABLE 8–1

Conditions and Diseases Thought to Be Stress-Related
• Cancer
• Hypertension
• Myocardial infarction
• Cerebrovascular accident
• Peripheral vascular disease
• Asthma
• Tuberculosis
• Emphysema
• Gastrointestinal ulcers
• Irritable bowel syndrome
• Sexual dysfunctions
• Obesity
• Anorexia nervosa
• Bulimia nervosa
• Connective tissue disease
• Ulcerative colitis
• Crohn's disease
• Infections
• Allergic and hypersensitivity diseases

stress is seen as the event itself, or the stressor, not as the response to the event.

With the advent of the stimulus concept of stress, research efforts were directed toward determining which life events were stressful and how stressful they were. Scales were developed by researchers, such as Holmes and Rahe (1967), to quantify the stress associated with different life events. These stress scales listed events such as death, divorce, and monetary and health concerns. Each event was assigned a score that reflected its relative stressfulness. The idea behind the scales was that the accumulation of a certain number of "stress points" would result in a reaction, such as illness. Despite the popularity of these scales in both the scientific and the lay literature, they have not proved to be valid as predictors of stress, especially in relation to illness. No research has been able to show more than a limited predictive relation between stressful life events and illness, hospitalization, and mortality.

Although the usefulness of stress scales has not proved valid, common sense indicates that certain events can and do provoke physiologic manifestations and feelings of stress. It seems, however, that the events that provoke stress symptoms may not always be life's major events but, rather, the minor annoyances of everyday life. These daily stresses, or "hassles," have shown more relation to illness than have the major life events (DeLongis et al., 1982). Within the hospital setting, there are many potential hassles that can increase stress. Table 8–2 presents examples of environmental and psychological hassles common to hospitalization and illness.

Stress as a Transaction Between a Person and the Environment

Gradually, nurse researchers and others have come to realize that all events have different meanings for different people. The perception of stress appears to be related to the person and event within a certain environment. The view of stress as a relation between the person and the environmental event is called the *transactional model of stress* (Lazarus & Folkman, 1984).

In this model, people are more than passive recipients of stress and are not merely unthinking reactors to the events around them. The person's interpretation of the event is important to consider, and the meaning given to the event by the person determines the perception of stress. Stress occurs only when a person appraises a situation as stressful.

In the transactional model of stress, there are few universal stressors because of the differences in individual appraisal. *Appraisal* is the cognitive evaluation of events (primary appraisal) and available coping resources (secondary appraisal). No event can be considered inherently stressful—not even tornadoes, hurricanes, and other disasters that are generally thought of as stressful. The transactional model states that there is no way of predicting how a person will respond to events. Although some people experience a stress reaction to these major events, many others do not. These differences are a result of individual appraisal.

Several factors contribute to a person's perception that an event is stressful. These include factors specific to the person, the environment, or the event itself. Effective nursing care must include an understanding of the many factors that enter into a client's decision that an event is stressful.

Appraisal Factors Related to the Person
Depth of Feeling

One important factor in an appraisal of stress is the depth of feeling that the event arouses in a person. Events about which people feel strongly are more likely to produce stress than events that arouse little or no feeling. For example, if hospitalization interferes with an important life event, such as marriage, the client's appraisal of hospitalization may result in a perception of stress.

Beliefs

Along with commitments, beliefs also influence the appraisal of stress. For example, a person with a strongly held religious belief that God can influence the course of life's events may appraise events differently from someone with other spiritual beliefs.

Control

Control is also important to the stress-coping response. Many researchers have reported that most people want to maintain a sense of control over their world. For that reason, not having control can be appraised as a stressor. The key to understanding control is the recognition that control means different things to different people and in different situations. Although it is obvious that ill or hos-

TABLE 8–2

Potential Stressors Common to Hospitalization and Illness

- Eating different foods at different times
- Having a stranger for a roommate
- Sleeping in a different bed
- Using a different pillow
- Being awakened at odd hours
- Feeling too hot or too cold
- Smelling hospital odors
- Hearing strange hospital noises
- Having movement restricted
- Being unable to obtain desired objects
- Having too many, no, or few visitors
- Worrying about bills, job, or family concerns
- Being uncertain of one's diagnosis
- Not understanding medical language
- Being dependent on others for bathing or toileting
- Being embarrassed about revealing body parts or intimate details
- Having to deal with large numbers of health care workers

pitalized clients cannot control situations such as the course of illness, research has identified a list of areas in which most people seek control even when they are sick (Moos & Tsu, 1977). These areas include

- Avoidance of pain and incapacitation
- The immediate hospital environment
- Treatments and procedures
- Relationships with hospital personnel
- Emotional balance
- A satisfactory self-image
- Relationships with family and friends
- Preparing for an uncertain future

This list is important for three reasons. First, it alerts nurses to the fact that people may seek control over most aspects of their lives, whether they are ill or not. Second, the loss of a sense of control, which is stressful to many people, can occur because of the nature of the hospital environment. Third, some people do not want active control. People who do not desire control may experience stress when they are given control. Nurses should ascertain how much control clients want before insisting or recommending that they take control.

Environmental Event Factors Related to Stress Appraisal

Differences in the appraisal of environmental event factors influence whether a person perceives an event as stressful.

Unpredictability of Events

One factor that can make a difference in the appraisal of events is their unpredictability. People generally believe that a predictable event is less stressful than a similar unpredictable event. This is partly because with time, people can prepare. Being able to prepare for events appears to be related to a reduction in stress. Without the necessary time or information needed for preparation, events may appear more stressful than they need to be. If possible, the nurse should give a client sufficient information and time to comprehend a potentially stressful event, such as an uncomfortable procedure, before he or she experiences it.

Uncertainty of Events

The client's uncertainty about an event can also increase its potential stressfulness. It appears that most people like to know what to expect. Although this is true of life events in general, people especially like to know the odds about health-related events. The key to understanding much of the stress experienced by clients with chronic disease may lie in their uncertainty about the disease course. Not knowing how a disease will evolve or the chances of recovery can be very stressful. For example, clients with cancer often experience such uncertainty. Despite such treatments as extensive surgery, chemotherapy, and radiation, many clients with cancer can never be

completely sure of a cure. Thus, the uncertainty of the event enhances its appraisal as stressful.

Timing of Events

The timing of events also has an impact on the level of stress. Events that are considered to be in the distant future are usually perceived as less stressful than events that are closer in time. The time that elapses between the client's hearing about an event and its occurrence can also influence appraisal. Although the stress may be manageable for a period of time, the longer a person is kept waiting, the harder it is to control the thoughts about what is to come. Thus, the appraisal of threat can build up when too much time elapses. People need sufficient time to prepare for events. However, too long a period of anticipation can have a negative effect. Unfortunately, there are no set guidelines as to timing for nurses who prepare clients for tests and procedures.

The timing of an event in relation to one's stage of life is also important. Having a heart attack at age 25 may be more stressful than at age 80. Any life event that occurs at an unexpected time can be more stressful than one occurring at a time of life when it is expected.

Duration of Events

Another factor related to timing is the duration of events. Chronic, long-term events can sometimes wear down a person's ability to cope. As in Selye's stage of exhaustion, constant demands over a long time can have massive psychological as well as physical effects. However, people can also become accustomed to long-term events. The difference between the two reactions may lie in a person's appraisal or in the coping strategies used.

Ambiguity of Events

Knowing what will happen, when it will happen, and how long it will last is important in the appraisal of stress. Yet, even with this information, unknown elements of an event always are present and contribute to the ambiguity, or vagueness, of the experience. Ambiguity is important to appraisal. Generally, the more vague a situation, the more stressful. Ambiguity can also influence what coping strategies are used. People usually choose their coping strategies on the basis of the information that they have. If information is missing, however, the planning of specific and appropriate coping strategies is not possible.

According to Lazarus and Folkman's theory (1984), the effectiveness of coping mechanisms depends on the accuracy of the appraisal of a stressful situation. Because people may not correctly appraise a situation and because no one can predict the future, misappraisals cannot be avoided—they are part of life. It is the degree of difference between the appraisal of what will happen and the reality of what occurs that makes a difference in coping effectiveness. Because situations are constantly changing, coping effectiveness also depends on the person's ability to reappraise and change strategies as necessary (Fig. 8–2).

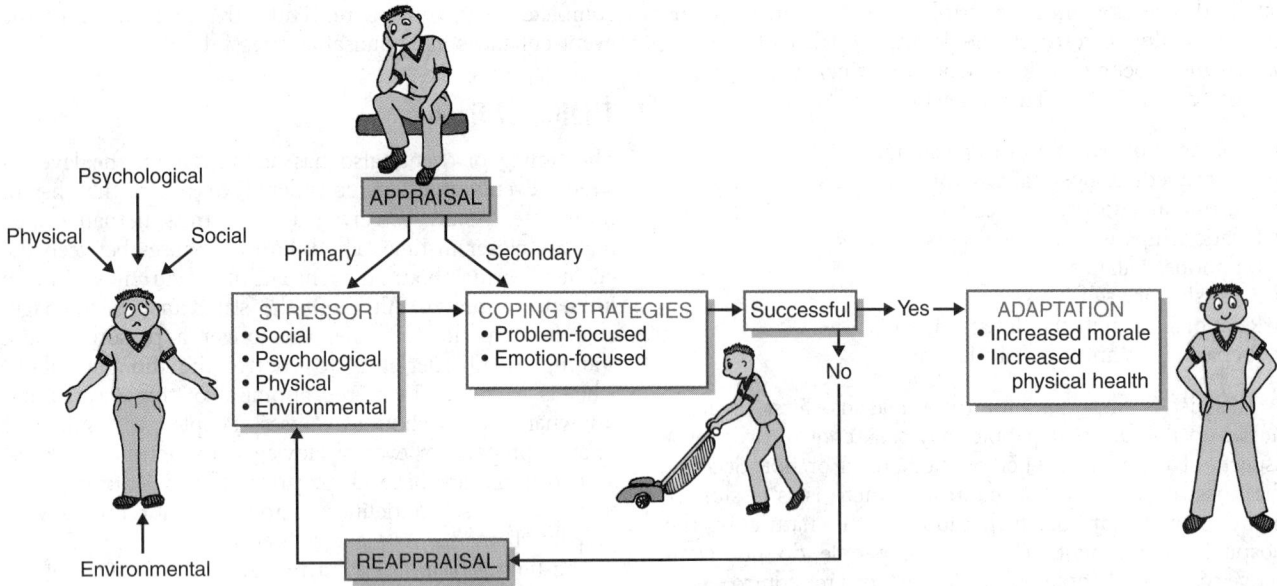

Figure 8–2. Appraisal and coping mechanisms.

THEORIES ABOUT COPING

Coping is any behavioral or cognitive activity that is used to deal with stress. If an event is perceived as taxing or dangerous, coping should occur. The concept of coping implies that most people do not remain passive and allow events to happen; rather, they react. The reactions to a stress-provoking event can be either to use the problem-solving approach to change the event (problem-focused coping) or to change emotional reactions to the event (emotion-focused coping). Coping strategies vary from person to person and event to event. It is thought that people generally use coping strategies that they have found successful in the past. If a strategy is not successful in the current situation, others may be considered.

Problem-Focused Coping

Problem-Solving

In many cases, the best way to deal with a causative stressor is to try to change or eliminate the problem. A major coping strategy is problem-solving.

Problem-solving as a coping strategy involves the same skills that are used in the nursing process. In problem-solving coping, a person defines the problem, lists alternatives, chooses the best alternative, and applies it to the problem. When asked about problem-solving coping, people may state that they try to find out more about the problem at hand, analyze the problem, make a plan, and follow it.

Some problem-solving activity is also directed inward. In this case, the coping activity is directed at how the problem is faced. Inward-focused problem-solving solutions might include learning new skills, changing aspirations, or finding other avenues of personal reward.

When people use problem-solving, they need accurate information and accurate appraisal so that their plans to deal with the stressor are based on reality. Nurses can ask clients if they have made any plans, on what the plans are based, and what is involved in these plans. When plans are unrealistic, the nurse helps the client by sharing his or her expertise and information.

Confrontive Coping

Many people cope by confronting the problem that is causing the stress. Confrontive coping is often used successfully in dealing with life's problems, such as those in the workplace. In addition, confrontive coping may be used when less forceful coping strategies have failed to alleviate the perception of stress. Clients in health care situations may use confrontive coping by aggressively seeking information, refusing treatments, and expressing their anger. Many times anger is the primary indicator that the client feels stressed and is attempting to cope. However, not all confrontive-type coping activities reflect aggression; sometimes the expressions of anger in confrontive coping reflect feelings of anxiety and powerlessness in the client.

Although these two problem-focused coping strategies are commonly used, they are not the only ways to cope. Nurses who are interested in supporting the client should find out how the client has coped in the past, how he or she plans to cope with the new stresses, and how other clients with the same problem have coped.

Emotion-Focused Coping

Some people are more skilled at problem-solving than others, and some problems are easier to resolve than others. When problem-focused strategies are not appropriate or are not sufficient, emotion-focused strategies are used. In some cases, a person may use both problem-focused and emotion-focused coping. Emotion-focused strategies reduce the emotional manifestations of stress, such as anxiety and anger.

Distancing Strategies

A vast array of distancing strategies are frequently used for coping in health-related situations. Some people deny a problem or blame others, and some people accept responsibility for their contribution to the occurrence of stress—they appear to be seeking a sense of control over life events. The refusal of a person who has had a motor vehicle accident while drinking alcohol to accept some blame is an example of distancing.

Drawing Strength from Adversity

A related coping strategy is drawing strength from adversity by growing as a person, finding new faith, and rediscovering what is important in life. At other times, strategies that emphasize the positive aspects of an event can be effective. Trying to have a positive outlook, looking on the bright side, and telling oneself that things could be worse are examples of this form of coping.

Tension Reduction

Coping strategies aimed at tension reduction can also be used to deal with stress. Some healthy means of reducing tension may include meditation, yoga exercises, biofeedback, and physical exercise. Other ways of coping, although not healthy, are to reduce tension through the use of alcohol or other so-called recreational drugs. Eating modifications, such as overeating or undereating, can also be used as inappropriate attempts to cope.

Hostility Versus Humor

Hostility, reflected through anger, irritability, childish reactions, or demonstration of temper, may reflect coping activity in some clients. A more positive expression of feelings that can reflect coping is humor. Humor is a commonly used coping activity (Weinberger, 1991). Many clients tell jokes or make light of serious situations when they are under stress.

Fatalism

Even fatalism can be used as a coping strategy. When using fatalism, clients say they will take a wait-and-see attitude, leave it in God's hands, or accept what has happened to them. Fatalism is usually accompanied by a sense that there is nothing that can be done about the problem.

Social Support

Social support by family, friends, and the community often can be a powerful aid in coping and can be extremely important to those in need of health care. By seeking support from others, people can gain information, physical help, and other forms of assistance. Both the type of help and the number of people willing to help can make a difference in the client's coping success.

Hospital rules and regulations often interfere with a client's ability to obtain the social support he or she needs. The interference with support can be especially acute within ethnic groups with large, close, and supportive families, such as in the Hispanic culture. Loss of social support can result when hospitalization occurs at a physical distance from the client's family, when elderly clients have outlived friends and relatives, or when the client has a socially stigmatizing illness, such as acquired immunodeficiency syndrome (AIDS). The inability to use a coping strategy on which one had previously depended, such as social support, can result in further stress.

Faith

Faith in God, a deity, or an ultimate meaning of life can be an effective aid to coping. For people who have a strong faith, the attitude of relinquishing control to God or believing in transcendence can be beneficial. Prayer, increased religious activity, and even a calm acceptance of God's will or an ultimate purpose are all forms of coping when they help reduce the perception of stress.

Event Rehearsal

If time allows, coping often begins before the stress event occurs, through event rehearsal. Event rehearsal involves mental or physical preparation in anticipation of an event or the practice of coping strategies before the event occurs. For example, clients who are to undergo elective surgery begin to plan their coping strategies before the actual surgery occurs. If time allows before a potentially stressful event, clients may mentally envision how they will react or handle the situation. Some authors have called this preparatory coping the "work of worrying" (Janis, 1985). However, that phrase implies that clients are concerned with only the negative aspects of an upcoming experience and ignores the fact that clients may focus on the positive aspects as well.

Event Review

After a stressful event, many people cope by reviewing the event. This review can be mental, verbal, or both. Event review probably helps people to cope by giving them the opportunity to understand what has happened to them. Often, there is no time during a stress event to process the incoming information. Review after an event occurs when there is time and energy available for processing. Nurses aid coping through review by encouraging clients to think or talk about their experiences.

People cope with the same problem in a variety of ways. Most nurses agree that coping in the hospital setting can be successfully accomplished through any one of a number of avenues. Common coping strategies are presented in Table 8–3.

TABLE 8-3

Common Coping Strategies	
Coping Strategy	**Examples**
Event rehearsal	• Mental and verbal preparation • Practice of coping strategies
Confrontation	• Aggressive information-seeking • Anger • Refusal of treatments
Distancing or denial	• Unwillingness or inability to talk about events • Going on as if nothing has happened
Self-control	• Stoicism • Showing no feelings
Social support	• Seeking out family, friends, or others in similar situations
Accepting responsibility	• Verbally placing responsibility for a situation on oneself
Faith	• Praying • Reading religious material • Seeking out clergy or religious guidance
Problem-solving	• Making plans • Verbally outlining what to do next
Positive reappraisal	• Speaking of how the situation has fostered growth
Event review	• Discussing situations or coping that has occurred

THEORIES ABOUT ADAPTATION

If a client has coped effectively, the stress or the emotional reaction to stress is eliminated or managed and a sense of equilibrium is restored. Restored equilibrium that results from coping is called adaptation. Some nurse theorists, such as Roy and Roberts (1981), have incorporated the concept of adaptation into their theory or model of nursing practice.

Adaptation is dependent on accurate appraisal of a stressful situation and effective coping. Adaptation can have many outcomes. The two results with the most significance to nursing are psychological and physical well-being.

Psychological Adaptation: Morale

People who cope adequately, it is hoped, will be satisfied with how they coped and the outcome reached. If a client believes that the correct decision was made with regard to health care issues, such as agreeing to hospitalization, choosing medical professionals, or handling pain or discomfort, the challenge of the stress has been met and coping is viewed as effective. The ability to see stress as a challenge to be overcome is important to the long-term maintenance of morale.

Morale is related to emotional equilibrium and the sense of well-being. In the past, many researchers considered well-being as the absence of depression or other signs of poor psychological health. More recently, the approach has changed: well-being is assessed through positive indicators, such as happiness and contentment. Healthy psychological adaptation is reflected in the client's sense of well-being.

Physical Adaptation: Somatic Health

Stress is consistently blamed for causing all illness and unhappiness. Diseases in which it can be determined that the mind influences the body's processes are called *psychophysiologic* (previously called psychosomatic). Stress is thought to be a major factor in psychophysiologic disease. Interestingly, the link between stress and illness is far from clear. Some evidence indicates that stress may suppress the effectiveness of the immune system and thus predispose a person to infection, cancer, and other diseases thought to be related to the immune system (see Table 8–1). Stress may also weaken the body so that any pathogens or toxic agents are more damaging than they would otherwise be. Other evidence indicates that stress may precipitate damage so that it occurs at a faster rate than normal, such as in cardiovascular disease.

At one time, it was hoped that a direct link could be found either between the stress event and illness or between personality type and illness. At that time, it was not uncommon to hear professionals speak of a colitis, ulcer, or arthritis personality. However, none of these theories has held up under study. No research has been able to show a strong relationship among incidence of illness, personality type, and stress.

The Concept of Hardiness

Research into the relationship between illness and personality characteristics is currently focused on hardiness, which is the ability to resist the effects of stress. The attribute of hardiness may be one reason why some people are negatively affected by exposure to stress and others are not. Hardiness is related to three personality characteristics:

■ Hardy people have a sense of *commitment* to work, a way of life, or ideals that provides them with a sense of satisfaction, motivation, and possibly achievement.
■ Hardy people look at life's occurrences as *challenges*, not threats. These people welcome change for the growth it promotes. They are optimistic and curious about life.
■ Hardy people have a sense of *control* over their lives. They do not feel helpless in the face of what happens to them. On the other hand, people who are low in measures of hardiness usually appear bored, are hopeless, and lack enthusiasm.

Commitment, challenge, and control may be three rea-

TABLE 8–4

Techniques for Increasing Hardiness

Personality Characteristic	Techniques
Commitment	• Capitalize on skills and interests to develop hobbies • Reduce time spent watching television • Develop a list outlining why one's work is important to the community • Recognize and acknowledge self-worth • Join a volunteer organization that provides services to help others • Join political, social, or religious organizations
Challenge	• Take a controlled physical risk, e.g., become involved in Outward Bound, take a glider flight or parachute jump, or undertake a new sport • Take a vacation that involves little or no planning • Take a course or attend a talk on a topic that questions one's own values • Vary daily activities and change routines
Control	• Set aside a period of time each week to do exactly what one wants • Volunteer for leadership positions in clubs and organizations • Become active in the political process; vote • Seek work situations in which control is increased • Recognize the enormous amount of control one can exercise over his or her own life

sons why differences exist in the ability to adapt to stress. Hardiness may actually help buffer the effects of stress. People who are hardy may be more resilient, or "tougher," in the face of life's ups and downs.

Because hardiness may be a personality characteristic, experts are unsure as to whether people can be taught to be hardy. However, attempts to increase hardiness may be beneficial. Table 8–4 shows a few examples of ways in which clients may increase commitment, challenge, and control in everyday life.

COLLABORATIVE MANAGEMENT

 Assessment

The first step in helping clients to deal with stress is to obtain an accurate assessment of the stress situation. The problem may be in the client's appraisal of the situation, in how the client is coping, or in the inherent stressfulness of the situation, which cannot be controlled or changed. The nurse should assess all aspects of the stress

response before determining which nursing interventions are appropriate.

➤ *Assessment of Stress*

The nurse assesses for physiologic signs that identify that the client is experiencing stress (Chart 8–1).

Physical Assessment: Clinical Manifestations

One of the most obvious physiologic indicators is increased heart rate. Although increased heart rate is a stress-related response, heart rate by itself has not proved to be a reliable indicator of the presence of stress. Among the reasons for this unpredictability is that heart rate

Chart 8–1

Nursing Care Highlight: Assessing for Common Signs of Stress

Physical Signs
• Sleep problems
• Headaches
• Shaking
• Inability to sit still
• Muscle tension
• Rapid speech, stuttering, or stammering
• Fatigue
• Increased heart rate
• Digestive troubles
• Increased perspiration
• Light-headedness
• Cold chills
• Hot flashes
• Palpitations
• Dry mouth
• Frequent urination
• Menstrual cycle changes
• Crying

Psychosocial Signs
• Resentment toward health care workers
• Anger, loss of temper
• Feelings of helplessness
• Resistance to treatments or tests
• Overuse of drugs, including prescription and over-the-counter drugs
• Withdrawal from friends and family
• Overuse of alcohol
• Excessive excitement
• Confusion and forgetfulness
• Nervousness
• Irritability
• Complaints of anxiety

varies with almost any stimulus, from movement to illness. Thus, heart rate is not specific enough to be a valid sign of stress. The correlation of stress and blood pressure has demonstrated the same problem.

A variety of physical complaints may also reflect stress in the client. Examples of stress-related complaints are headaches, neckaches, stomachaches, muscular cramping, and other signs of muscular tension. Some people perspire, some get pale, and others become flushed under stress. Many people experience alterations in their patterns of elimination, both bowel and urinary. Eating patterns may also reflect change, with some people eating more than usual and others eating less. Sleep patterns may be disrupted, with some clients experiencing insomnia and others wanting to sleep more than usual. The patterns of these changes are as different as the people involved.

Psychosocial Assessment

Nurses use many obvious psychosocial signs to assess stress behavior (see Chart 8–1). Many of the signs used to assess stress actually reflect coping activity. The more common signs attributed to stress include emotional excesses, such as agitation, anxiety, anger, and apathy. Other signs may include inappropriate or ineffectual coping behaviors, such as denial and blaming. Stress in people may be signaled by expressions of hopelessness, powerlessness, or loss of control; alterations in normal communication patterns, such as a change from extreme talkativeness to silence; and changes in thought processes. Even signs that are considered pathologic, such as manipulative behavior, depression, and withdrawal, may only reflect a person's reaction to tremendous stress.

Laboratory Assessment

Levels of epinephrine and norepinephrine are somewhat more predictive of stress than other laboratory values. Unlike steroid products, epinephrine and norepinephrine are released almost instantly in response to stress. Initial research has focused on athletes, astronauts, and others exposed to intense but transient stress-provoking episodes. Norepinephrine levels almost always rise when a person is subjected to a stressor, but epinephrine levels tend to stabilize after a brief period of elevation. Although these results are promising, they are only preliminary findings. In addition, it is not always possible to obtain blood for laboratory analysis, and this procedure is invasive.

► Assessment of Appraisal and Coping

The study of coping, including individual appraisal, is a new area of research, and many questions remain unanswered. Until further studies are available, nurses are best guided by the client in the perception of what is stressful and the best coping strategies to be used.

Assessment of Appraisal

The nurse first tries to determine what the client perceives as stressful. The nurse asks specific questions about which aspects of hospitalization or illness are stressful.

The assessment relates specifically to the appraisal process, with the nurse considering such factors as perceived ambiguity, predictability, and uncertainty of events. The nurse also asks specific questions about how much the client knows about diagnosis, diagnostic testing, and expected length of hospitalization.

The nurse next attempts to learn how stressful these items are perceived to be by the client. Stress is an individual matter, so it is the client's perception, or appraisal, that is important. One way of determining the level of stress is to ask the client to name the most stressful event possible and then compare the new stressor with that event.

After determining the client's appraisal of the event and the coping methods used, the nurse learns the successful coping strategies that the client has used in the past for similar problems.

Figure 8–3 depicts a guide for interviewing clients about stress and coping.

Assessment of Specific Coping Strategies

Nurses should remember that different individuals cope with the same problem in a variety of ways. If the chosen coping strategy is working, the nurse should support the client in that effort. If the coping strategy is not effective, the nurse works with the client to develop alternatives.

The nurse may note that clients are using event rehearsal if they discuss or talk about the upcoming event or if, when asked, say they have been thinking about the situation. If the event rehearsal is to be effective, clients need information about the stressor. Nurses may also make an assessment that clients are using event rehearsal when clients seek information. Many clients actively solicit information from health care providers, friends, or relatives.

Calling friends and family on the telephone, encouraging visitors, and socializing with others who are in the hospital may reflect the client's use of social support as a coping strategy. Talking with others about what has occurred may reflect the use of event review.

Developing a plan to eliminate or reduce the effect of the stressor can be another form of coping that is reflected in information-seeking behavior. When clients use planned problem-solving, they need accurate information so that the plans they make are based on reality.

If clients purposefully appear to keep their emotions or behaviors in check, they may be using self-control to aid their coping. Stoicism can reflect a personality type or even a culturally approved coping strategy. Other, more expressive clients may not keep their emotions and feelings in check and may be using confrontive coping strategies. The nurse may also assess anger, hostility, and argumentative behavior in the client as coping strategies.

Nurses may make an assessment of denial or distancing in clients who exhibit avoidance behavior, such as refusing to look at surgical scars or not learning self-care. Clients who do not talk about their conditions, do not prepare for upcoming events, or appear to go on as if nothing had happened to them may also be using denial. Some clients may even exhibit withdrawal behavior by

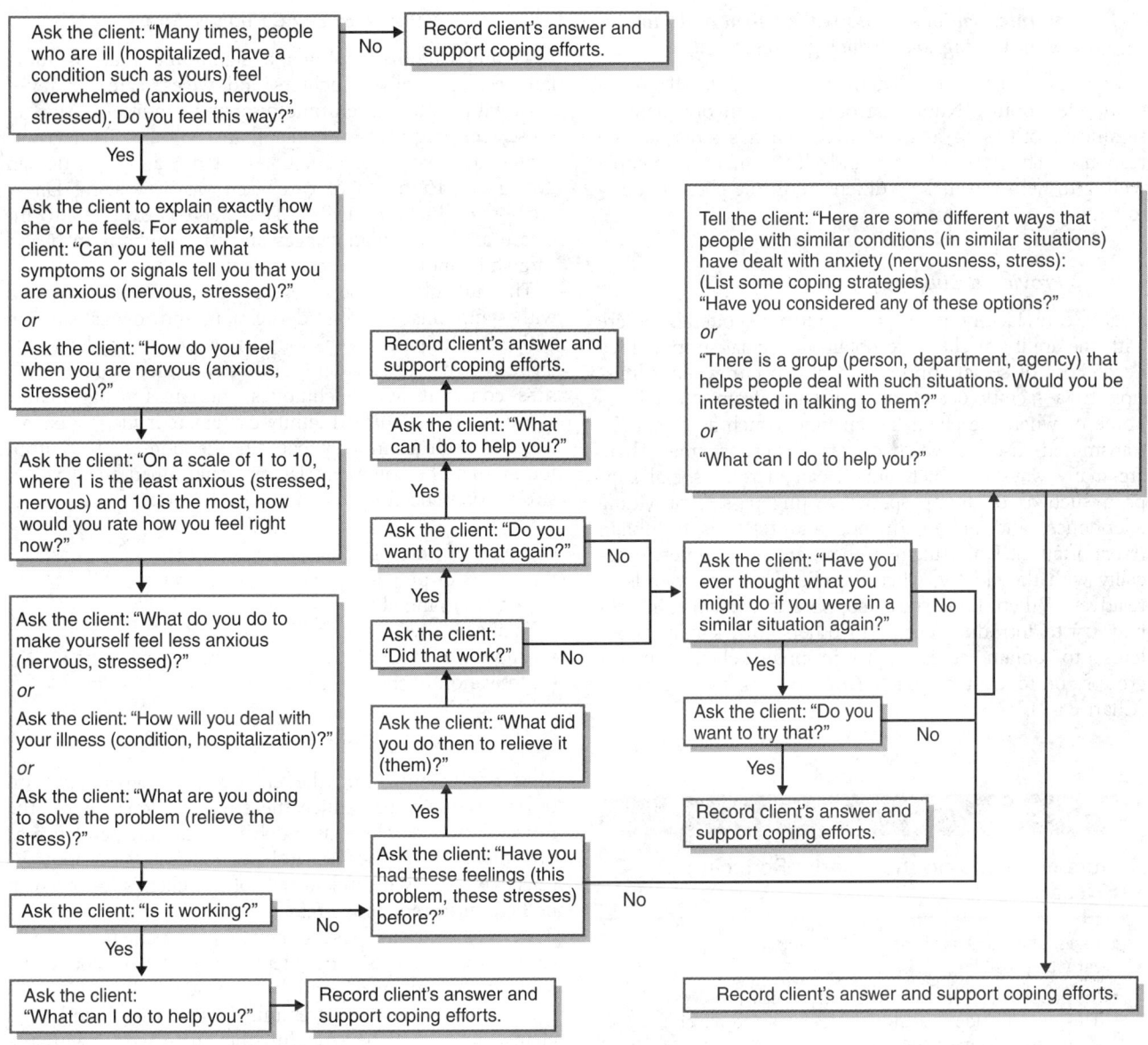

Figure 8–3. A guide for interviewing clients for stress and coping.

refusing to communicate or by communicating only minimally.

Clients who blame themselves for their illness or hospitalization may be using the coping strategy of self-blame. Clients who use faith as a coping strategy may request clergy visits, use religious articles, and engage in prayer, which are signs that the nurse can observe.

Interventions

After the nurse has assessed that there is a problem in the client's ability to appraise or to cope, many interventions are available. Because of the personal nature of stress, appraisal, and coping, the nurse must remember that there are no universal, standard nursing interventions.

➤ Interventions to Assist the Client in Appraisal

Nurses can help clients make more accurate appraisals through client education. Nurses assist clients to recognize and correct faulty appraisal, and they provide positive reinforcement of correct appraisal. Appraisal depends on accurate information. For example, nurses aid clients in appraisal by supplying information about the scheduling and the duration of events in an attempt to avoid ambiguity, confusion, and fear of the unknown.

Another important step in assisting clients with appraisal is exploring perceptions of stress and stressors to determine whether appraisals are accurate. The nurse encourages the client to verbalize perceptions and to help the nurse identify and correct faulty appraisal. If appraisals are inaccurate, the nurse intervenes to supply correct information and aids clients in changing their perception.

➤ *Interventions to Assist the Client and Family in Coping and Reducing Stress*

The social support provided by friends and family is essential to coping. Nurses encourage the involvement of significant others to assist with the client's stress-coping response. The type of help and the number of people willing to help can make a difference in the client's ability to cope.

Providing Support

Health care facility rules and regulations often interfere with the ability of clients to obtain the social support they need. Loss of social support can also occur when admission to a facility occurs at a distance from the client's home or when the client has an illness such as a sexually transmitted disease, which carries a social stigma. There are many ways in which nurses can increase social support, such as obtaining special visiting passes, providing telephones, and helping friends and relatives to obtain transportation. Unfortunately, there are many times, especially with the elderly, when the client has few friends or relatives. When little social support is available, nurses may try to introduce clients to others with similar problems, to obtain access to appropriate client support groups, or to contact pastoral or hospital social services (Chart 8–2).

Chart 8-2

Nursing Focus on the Elderly: Reducing Stress

- Assess the client's available social support systems as early as possible.
- Introduce the client to others with similar problems. This may include a change of roommates to match clients to help meet this need.
- Request spiritual support by contacting clergy, requesting religious articles, or saying a prayer, depending on the client's preference. Consider the client's cultural background.
- Take time to listen to the client's concerns.
- Collaborate with the social services department in identifying support systems for the client.
- Allow the client to be as independent as possible, even if it takes more time for a task, such as feeding, to be completed.
- To the extent possible, give the client an opportunity to make decisions about activities of daily living, hospital activities, and nursing interventions.
- Teach information about surgery, procedures, tests, and so forth at a slower pace than for a younger adult.
- Teach the importance of proper rest, sleep, exercise, and nutrition.
- Teach progressive muscle relaxation and guided imagery, if appropriate.

Assisting with Lay Caregiver Stress

Lay caregiving has become a significant issue as more families, especially daughters and wives, care for loved ones with acute and chronic disabling conditions. Most of those receiving care are older than 65 years. Twelve percent of the work force in the United States provides an average of 15 hours of care each week to aging family members (Hirshom, 1997). This trend is expected to increase as the population ages and the emphasis in health care shifts more toward cost containment.

The difficulty of the caregiver role has been associated with symptoms of stress, depression, and low satisfaction with life. Ruppert (1996) found that providing classes for lay caregivers helps them understand more about wellness, communication techniques, and stress management.

Smith (1994) studied family caregivers managing clients needing high-technology care in the home. The author found that the following factors determined the level of stress experienced by the family caregivers:

- Length of time providing care
- Amount of preparation for the caregiver
- Family coping ability
- Financial solvency of the family
- Amount of assistance from other family members
- Motivation of the caregiver

Providing Control

Most adults, including the elderly, find dependency on others stressful. To reduce the stress of dependency, the nurse allows the client as much physical independence as possible. When physical independence is not possible, sensitive care by a nurse aware of the client's feelings can be helpful in reducing stress.

In most client illnesses, health care personnel expect certain role changes. The client is expected to cooperate, focus on getting well, and be dependent. Each of these role changes can be stressful. If the client finds the change in role to be stressful, the nurse works with the client to develop a plan of care that incorporates maintenance of important role behaviors. Whenever possible, nurses should allow clients who desire it to have control over other activities of daily living, hospital activities, and nursing interventions. Control over such things as times of bathing, food choices, awake and sleep times, and scheduling of therapies and procedures can be very helpful in reducing stress and in maintaining self-esteem.

Providing Information

Adequate knowledge may also help clients gain control. Nursing research has shown the importance of client preparation for diagnostic tests and procedures (Johnson & Lauver, 1989). Among the content that should be included in client education is knowledge of the duration of events, expected behaviors, sensations involved, and sequencing of activities. Nurses should remember that even everyday experiences in the hospital or nursing home, such as the administration of intravenous therapy, can be extremely stressful to the client and the family.

Research Applications for Nursing

Communicating with Families Can Reduce Stress and Anxiety

Johnson, M. J., & Frank, D. I. (1995). Effectiveness of a telephone intervention in reducing anxiety of families of patients in an intensive care unit. Applied Nursing Research, 8, 42–43.

This study evaluated the results of a program designed to keep family members apprised of their loved one's status while in the intensive care unit. A total of 24 telephone calls were made to family members of the experimental group over a 48-hour period. The calls were brief, lasting less than 5 minutes. An additional 10 verbal contacts were made with this group. The anxiety scores of the experimental group decreased significantly more than those of the control group who did not receive the calls.

Critique. Although the sample was fairly small (20 families in each group), the study showed how a simple nursing intervention can help relieve the stress and anxiety of family members who are critically ill. This study supports the findings of other researchers who also had success with telephone programs.

Possible Nursing Implications. This study suggests that nurses need to take the time to communicate with families to minimize their anxiety. Some of the nurses who made calls in the study were reluctant to do so because they thought they were too time-consuming or not part of their role. Nurses in all health care settings should incorporate the family and significant others in their client care.

Not all clients and their families want to know about *all* aspects of care and hospitalization. For clients who want to know, it is vital that they receive detailed information about those areas in which lack of knowledge is perceived as stressful.

Families also experience anxiety and stress when they are not informed or an unpredictable event occurs. A study by Johnson and Frank (1995) showed that a telephone intervention helped reduce anxiety of families of clients in an intensive care unit (see the Research Applications for Nursing box).

A client's coping strategy of event rehearsal also depends on adequate and correct information about events. Many clients actively seek information from health care providers, friends, relatives, and even comparative strangers who have undergone similar experiences.

After a stress-provoking event, nurses can aid clients' coping through event review by encouraging clients to think or talk about their experiences. Nurses should allow clients to verbally review as much as they need to, even when the account is repetitive. The repetition of thoughts about a threatening event can facilitate coping.

Recognizing Client Feelings

When experiencing or responding to stress, clients can have a number of feelings. For example, if the client becomes hostile, nurses should not react personally. Instead, acknowledging the client's feelings of anger and aggression is often helpful. For example, the nurse might say, "I can understand why you're angry. I would be angry too, if that had happened to me." After anger is acknowledged, it often decreases or disappears. If the anger does not diminish, the nurse allows the client to explore his or her anger no matter how irrational it may seem. After the anger has been reduced, the nurse can explore the more logical reasons why the feelings arose.

Occasionally, people become so angry that they become a danger to themselves or others around them. If the client loses control over his or her emotions, the nurse should follow institutional guidelines governing such situations.

The nurse can often best facilitate coping by supporting the client's own coping strategies. For example, when clients use self-controlling mechanisms, they should be supported in those efforts rather than forced to share their feelings or to demonstrate their emotions if they are not comfortable in doing so.

► Interventions to Aid Family Coping

Families also experience many of the same stressors that the ill or hospitalized client does. Families under stress also use coping strategies, such as seeking social support, reviewing events, and venting hostility. Nurses can aid the family and significant others in appraisal of stress and coping just as they do for the client. The nurse can also refer them to social service agencies and other support services.

► Interventions to Reduce the Effects of Stress

When clients are facing illness, surgery, and other health-related events, they may experience a high level of stress that is not immediately reducible. The introduction of further stress can inhibit coping effectiveness. Nursing action that eliminates or reduces additional stress allows the client to concentrate his or her coping activities on the major stressor and not divert his or her energies to coping with annoyances.

Although many stressful aspects of illness or hospitalization can be reduced or eliminated, there are still many other aspects with which clients either cannot or will not cope. Some stressors cannot be eliminated or avoided. In such cases, effective nursing care may involve teaching the client techniques that may reduce the physical impact of stress on the body as well as provide a means of physical or emotional control to the client. Examples are biofeedback, progressive muscle relaxation (PMR), meditation, and guided imagery. These interventions are also considered complementary therapies (see Chapter 4). If these techniques are not effective, psychotherapy and/or medication, such as antianxiety drugs, may help.

Biofeedback

Biofeedback can be an effective treatment when obvious signs of stress, such as headaches, high blood pressure, muscle tension, and heart palpitations, occur frequently, are debilitating, or may be dangerous. Biofeedback works

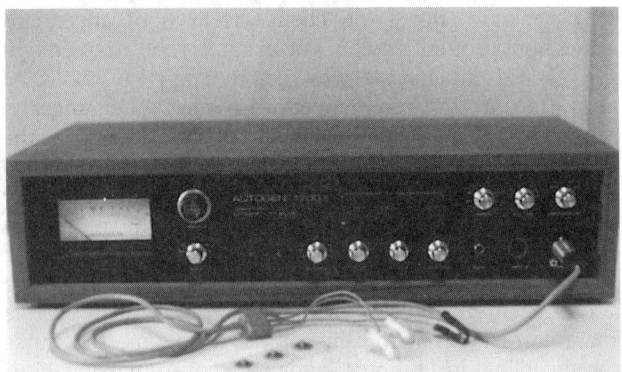

Figure 8-4. An example of a biofeedback system used to reduce stress. (Courtesy of Autogenic Systems, Inc., Newton, MA.)

Meditation

Meditation is a learned process through which a person attempts to quiet the mind. The methods used to quiet the mind involve consciously removing disturbing thoughts or filling the mind with only one thought, such as a *mantra* or prayer. By removing other thoughts, it is believed that stress can be reduced. Meditation is probably best learned through a mentor, although books and other audiovisual aids are available. If clients are inter-

by training the client to reverse the subtle changes that lead to a somatic, or physical, response. For instance, if a headache is the result of muscle tension in the forehead, the client can be trained to relax that tension before a headache results.

Biofeedback involves using electronic instrumentation to signal the user about selected somatic changes. The machinery is sensitive to minute changes within a body system. For example, if the biofeedback is directed toward sampling muscle activity, the machine detects small changes in the electrical activity of the muscles. If brain wave activity is the variable considered, the machine signals the type of brain waves that are occurring at a given moment. Cardiovascular and skin surface activity can also be monitored. After the physical clues are learned, the client can use them to gain control over and to reduce the undesired activity (Fig. 8-4).

Many hospitals and clinics have biofeedback equipment and trained personnel available. If not, referrals can usually be made to a local practitioner.

Progressive Muscle Relaxation

Stress commonly causes muscle tension, which results in many of the nagging physical symptoms of stress, such as headaches and neckaches. Control of muscle tension appears to help reduce the physical effects of such tension as well. PMR is one method used to reduce muscular tension.

PMR involves the tensing and then the relaxing of all the major muscle groups, usually in sequential steps. In PMR, the nurse guides the client through relaxation of each major body part, having the client first tighten and then relax each part. The following is a suggested sequence: feet, thighs, buttocks, stomach, chest, hands, forearms, shoulders, neck, and head. The nurse instructs the client in PMR until he or she can comfortably perform it alone without prompting. If time is a problem, the client can use a tape recorder and prerecorded PMR tape after completing the initial instruction (Chart 8-3). PMR is useful in nursing practice because it is easy to teach and can be used for a wide spectrum of clients. It is also inexpensive, unlike methods that use machinery, such as biofeedback.

Chart 8-3

Education Guide: Progressive Muscle Relaxation

- Take a minute and feel your body's different parts. Think about what portions of your body feel tense and which parts feel relaxed.

- We are going to do an exercise that will help you to relax and remove the tension from your body. I am going to talk you through this exercise, so just relax and follow my directions.

- I am going to ask you to tense one body part at a time. When you tense the body part, try to make the muscle as tight as possible. If you feel pain or a cramp when you tighten, reduce the tightness. This tightening is called tension.

- After you hold that muscle tightness for 5 to 10 seconds, I am going to ask you to let all the tightness out of that body part—to let it go limp. This is called relaxation.

- First, point your feet and curl your toes. Feel the tension in your feet. Hold that feeling until I tell you to relax.

- Relax—let your feet go limp. Feel the difference in going from tension to relaxation. Take a few moments to feel the relaxation.

- Now tighten the muscles in your lower legs. Feel the tension in your calves. Feel the tightness of your muscles. Hold that feeling until I say relax.

- Now relax your lower legs. Let them go limp. Feel the tightness leave and the feeling of relaxation take over.

- Now tighten the muscles of your neck by clenching your lower jaw. Feel the tightness of your muscles. Feel the tenseness as you clench your jaw.

- Relax your neck and jaw. Let the tightness go—feel the relaxation take over. Feel the difference between tension and relaxation.

- Close your eyes tightly and try to tighten all the other muscles in your face. Feel how tight your face feels.

- Now relax your face and let the tenseness flow out.

- Finally, I want you to let your whole body go limp—let it all relax. Remember those feelings of relaxation and let those feelings take over. Release any feelings of tension.

- Now, it is time to end this exercise. I want you to take your time as you slowly begin to move. When you are ready, you may resume your normal activities.

ested in learning meditative techniques, they should be referred to an appropriate source.

Guided Imagery

Similar to meditation, imagery also attempts to control the mind's thoughts. Guided imagery seeks to fill the mind with positive and pleasant mental pictures. Usually, imagery involves thinking about a peaceful scene or one in which there is total relaxation. Thinking processes are directed toward the promotion of relaxation rather than stress.

NURSING AND STRESS

Nurses as well as clients experience stress. Many nurses are affected by stress that exceeds their ability to cope. Nurses are exposed to tremendous numbers of stressors in their work each day, from exposure to death to sometimes unrealistic expectations of the work environment.

The effect of managed care in the 1990s and into the 21st century has been especially stressful for nurses in all health care settings, particularly hospitals. The decreasing census of many hospitals has led to layoffs of nurses and, in some cases, replacements of nurses with unlicensed assistive personnel. All health care agencies are attempting to contain costs in a number of ways. Nurses are very concerned that quality of care may be sacrificed in this cost containment era.

Many programs are available to aid the nurse in reducing stress, and there are also a variety of strategies that the nurse may use. In addition to the strategies outlined for clients, the following stress management techniques may be effective (Schultes, 1997):

- Learn assertiveness techniques to present feelings and thoughts in an honest, direct, and acceptable manner. Remember that hostile expression of anger and aggression usually inflame, rather than reduce, stress feelings.
- Acknowledge the positive aspects of work and do not dwell on the negatives. Happier people have been found to be less "realistic" in their assessments of situations, in that they focus on the funny and the positive aspects of life.
- Develop alternative plans for situations known to cause stress. For example, if transportation is a problem, arrange for a friend or coworker to serve as a back-up when trouble develops.
- Follow the same health care practices that nurses recommend to others. Get adequate sleep, eat a healthy diet, reduce caffeine consumption, get regular exercise, stop smoking, and use alcohol only in moderation, if at all.
- Use humor to cope with stress as well as to help clients cope and heal.

SELECTED BIBLIOGRAPHY

*Cannon, W. B. (1931). *The wisdom of the body.* New York: W. W. Norton.

Corley, M. C., Ferriter, J., Zeh, J., & Gifford, C. (1995). Physiological and psychological effects of back rubs. *Applied Nursing Research, 8,* 39–42.

*DeLongis, A., Coyne, J. C., Dakof, G., Folkman, S., & Lazarus, R. S. (1982). Relationship of daily hassles, uplifts and major life events to health status. *Health Psychology, 1,* 119–136.

Gio-Fitman, J. (1996). The role of psychological stress in rheumatoid arthritis. *MedSurg Nursing, 5*(6), 422–426.

Hirshom, E. (1997). Case study: Meeting the challenges of dementia management. *Continuing Care, 16*(2), 19–21.

*Holmes, T. H., & Rahe, R. H. (1967). The social readjustment rating scale. *Journal of Psychosomatic Research, 11,* 213–218.

Hunt, R. & Zurek, E. L. (1997). *Introduction to community based nursing.* Philadelphia: J. B. Lippincott.

*Janis, I. L. (1985). Coping patterns among patients with life-threatening diseases. *Issues in Mental Health Nursing, 7,* 461–476.

*Johnson, J. E., & Lauver, D. R. (1989). Alternative explanations of coping with stressful experiences associated with physical illness. *Advances in Nursing Science, 11,* 39–52.

Johnson, M. J., & Frank, D. I. (1995). Effectiveness of a telephone intervention in reducing anxiety of families of patients in an intensive care unit. *Applied Nursing Research, 8,* 42–43.

*Kobasa, S. C. (1979). Stressful life events, personality, and health: An inquiry into hardiness. *Journal of Personality and Social Psychology, 37,* 1–10.

*Lazarus, R. S., & Folkman, S. (1984). *Stress, appraisal and coping.* New York: Springer.

*Moos, R. H., & Tsu, V. D. (1977). The crisis of physical illness. In R. H. Moos (Ed.), *Coping with physical illness.* New York: Plenum.

*Pollock, S. E. (1989). The hardiness characteristic: A motivating factor in adaptation. *Advances in Nursing Science, 11,* 53–62.

*Pollock, S. E., Christian, B. J., & Sands, D. (1990). Response to chronic illness: Analysis of psychological and physiological adaptation. *Nursing Research, 39,* 300–304.

*Pollock, S. E., & Duffy, M. E. (1990). The health-related hardiness scale: Development and psychometric analysis. *Nursing Research, 39,* 218–222.

*Robinson, L. (1990). Stress and anxiety. *Nursing Clinics of North America, 25,* 935–943.

*Roy, C., & Roberts, S. (1981). *Theory construction in nursing: An adaptation model.* Englewood Cliffs, NJ: Prentice-Hall.

Ruppert, R. A. (1996). Caring for the lay caregiver. *American Journal of Nursing, 96*(3), 40–45.

Sarna, L., van Servellen, G., & Padilla, G. (1996). Comparison of emotional distress in men with acquired immunodeficiency syndrome and in men with cancer. *Applied Nursing Research, 9,* 209–212.

Schultes, L. S. (1997). Humor with hospice clients: You're putting me on. *Home Healthcare Nurse, 15*(8), 561–566.

*Selye, H. (1946). General adaptation syndrome and diseases of adaptation. *Journal of Clinical Endocrinology, 6,* 117–230.

Smith, C. (1994). A model of caregiving effectiveness for technologically dependent adults residing at home. *Advances in Nursing Science, 17*(2), 27–40.

*Weinberger, R. (1991). Teaching the elderly stress reduction. *Journal of Gerontological Nursing, 17*(10), 23–27.

SUGGESTED READINGS

Corley, M. C., Ferriter, J., Zeh, J., & Gifford, C. (1995). Physiological and psychological effects of back rubs. *Applied Nursing Research, 8,* 39–43.

    This nursing pilot study examined the physiologic and psychological effects of a back rub on elderly residents in a nursing home. Mood ratings improved in both the experimental group (those receiving back rubs) and the control group (those who rested), but the mood was significantly better in the experimental group. The study has implications for nursing practice because back rubs are often not provided for residents in long-term care.

Ruppert, R. A. (1996). Caring for the lay caregiver. *American Journal of Nursing, 96*(3), 40–45.

    This article discusses the effects of prolonged caregiving by family members in the home. The author shares her experience providing classes for caregivers to help them prepare for their caregiving experience as well as alert them to the need to take care of themselves.

PAIN

Pain is a protective mechanism for the body in that it occurs when tissues are being damaged (Guyton, 1996). The person in pain usually takes action to remove the pain or its cause, if possible. Indeed, pain is the number one symptom or complaint that causes people to seek health care. It alters or compromises the quality of life more than any other single health-related problem.

OVERVIEW

Everyone experiences pain at some time in life, but although this is likely a universal experience, it is also a complex and private one. Because it is such a personal experience, it is very difficult to describe or explain to others. Many factors make hard to understand and assess, including psychosocial, cultural, and developmental factors and the influence of gender, the environment, and the subjectivity of pain itself. The interpretation of pain, based solely on the person's actions or behaviors can be misleading, because the amount of pain and responses to it vary from person to person.

Definitions of Pain

Several attempts have been made to define pain in descriptive or measurable terms; however, no one definition is more accepted than another. Among the most popular definitions of pain are those of Sternbach (1968), Mc-

Caffery (1979), and the International Association on Pain (1979). Sternbach (p. 8) asserted that pain is "an abstract concept which refers to:

- A personal, private sensation of hurt
- A harmful stimulus which signals current or impending tissue damage
- A pattern of responses to protect the organism from harm"

This comprehensive definition serves to explain pain through a physiologic, psychological, and social approach.

McCaffery (1979) offered a more personal explanation of pain when she stated that pain "is whatever the experiencing person says it is and exists whenever he says it does" (p. 11). This understanding of pain requires that the client be seen as the authority on the pain and the only one who can define the experience.

Finally, the International Association on Pain (1979) described pain as an unpleasant sensory and emotional experience associated with actual or potential tissue damage.

Regardless of the definition, most people agree that pain has both sensory and behavioral components and is strongly influenced by various physiologic, psychological, and sociologic factors. A comprehensive understanding of pain requires a knowledge of the descriptive definitions, theories, and physiology of pain. The nurse can use this knowledge as a basis to develop an appreciation of the variety of clinical pain situations and skill in pain intervention. This understanding can also help the nurse develop a personal philosophy of pain management.

Theoretical Bases for Pain

Several theories have been proposed to explain the complex phenomenon of pain. Early theories emphasized the recognition of specific pathways of pain transmission. Later theories attempted to uncover the complexity of central processing of pain in specific areas of the brain. More recently, the concept of a pain-modulating network was introduced. This concept describes the various links and connections in the spinal cord and brain, specifically the medulla and the midbrain. The identification of chemical mediators involved in the pain response has helped in an understanding of pain transmission and perception.

Early Theories of Pain

The specificity theory was first proposed in the early 1800s and was accepted for almost 100 years as the most popular theoretical explanation for pain. This theory emphasized the highly specific structures and pathways responsible for pain transmission. Its premise was based on the existence of free nerve endings in the periphery of the body that were capable of accepting sensory input and transmitting it along highly specific nerve fibers. Although this theory set the stage for further research, its major biological orientation was not sufficient to account for the complexity of pain.

Later, in the early 1900s, an opposing pattern theory was developed. Goldscheider (cited in Melzack, 1973), the originator of this theory, identified two major pain fibers: a rapidly conducting fiber and a slowly conducting fiber. Both fibers synapse in the spinal cord and relay information to the brain. The concept of central summation was introduced: As pain fibers converge at the level of the spinal cord, the summation of impulses from these fibers ascends to various levels of the brain. The amount, intensity, and type of sensory input permit the brain to interpret the sensation.

Both the pattern theory and the specificity theory failed to explain the influences of psychological variables, such as anxiety and depression, on pain. Also, neither theory provided a reasonable explanation for failure of pain to resolve after pain pathways and spinal nerves were interrupted.

Gate Control Theory

The gate control theory was proposed to explain the observed relationship between pain and emotion. Melzack and Wall (1982), who first introduced this theory, concluded that pain is not just a physiologic response, but that psychological variables, such as behavioral and emotional responses, also influence the perception of pain.

According to the gate control theory, a gating mechanism occurs in the spinal cord. Pain impulses are transmitted from the periphery of the body by nerve fibers (A delta and C fibers). The impulses travel to the dorsal horns of the spinal cord, specifically to the area of the cord called the *substantia gelatinosa*. The cells of the substantia gelatinosa can inhibit or facilitate pain impulses that are transmitted to the trigger cells (T cells). When T-cell activity is inhibited, the gate is closed and impulses are less likely to be transmitted to the brain. When the gate is opened, pain impulses ascend to the brain (Fig. 9–1).

Similar gating mechanisms exist in the descending nerve fibers from the thalamus and cerebral cortex. These areas of the brain regulate a person's thoughts and emotions, including beliefs and values. When pain occurs, a person's thoughts and emotions can modify perceptual phenomena as they reach the level of conscious awareness.

The gate control theory has helped nurses and other

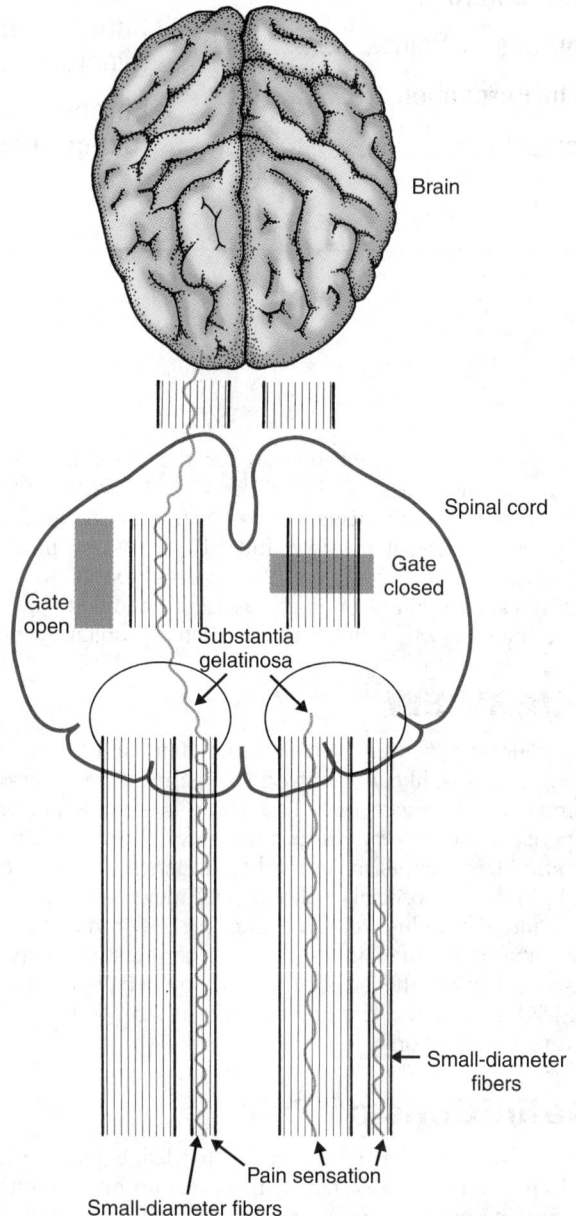

Figure 9–1. The gate control theory of pain.

health care professionals recognize the *holistic* nature of pain. As a result, many interventions, such as imagery and distraction (discussed later), are used to help relieve a client's pain.

Anatomic and Physiologic Bases for Pain

Pain Stimuli

Various types of noxious pain stimuli account for the perception of pain. A wide range of sensory input is capable of producing pain. In addition, tissue ischemia and muscle spasm cause pain. Free nerve endings, or receptors capable of responding to painful stimuli, are often referred to as nociceptors. Nociceptors are located in various body tissues and are activated by thermal, mechanical, and chemical stimuli. In addition to nociceptors, other receptors in the body respond to almost any type of intense stimulation, sometimes resulting in pain.

In most circumstances, painful stimuli cause actual tissue damage, which leads to the release of certain chemical substances, such as histamine, bradykinin, serotonin, norepinephrine, and certain acids that sensitize the nociceptors, including leukotrienes, prostaglandins, and substance P. These chemicals are believed to activate pain receptors. For example, the accumulation of lactic acids leads to the pain associated with ischemic tissue damage (Guyton, 1996). Muscle contraction or spasm can also produce ischemic-type pain. The muscle's oxygen demands are increased, but the blood supply is limited because of compressed blood vessels.

Pain Fibers and Pathways

Usually, painful stimuli originate in the periphery of the body. For the painful stimuli to be perceived, however, they must first be transmitted to the spinal cord and then to the central areas of the brain, as described by the gate control theory of pain (Fig. 9–1). In the periphery, two specific fibers can transmit stimuli: A delta fibers, which are found primarily in the skin and muscle, and C fibers, which are distributed in muscle, periosteum, and viscera. Both of these nerve fibers comprise the first-order neurons capable of accepting nociceptive stimuli.

A delta fibers are myelinated fibers that carry rapid, sharp, pricking, or piercing sensations. A person feeling these sensations can generally localize them readily to a fairly well-defined area. Because these fibers respond predominantly to mechanical stimuli, rather than to chemical or thermal stimuli, they are called mechanical nociceptors.

C fibers are unmyelinated or poorly myelinated fibers that conduct thermal, chemical, and strong mechanical impulses. Pain conduction from C fibers is more diffuse and dull, burning, or achy—quite different from the sensations of A delta fibers. In contrast to the intermittent nature of A delta sensations, C fibers usually produce constant pain.

Second-order neurons or pain pathways of the ascending pain tracts are found in the dorsal horn of the spinal cord and terminate in the thalamus. The spinothalamic tract is divided into two spinal tracts known as the lateral or neospinothalamic tract and the medial or paleospinothalamic tract. The neospinothalamic tract is responsible for sensory pain discrimination, as it transmits painful stimuli more directly to the sensory cortex where pain is eventually perceived and interpreted. The paleospinothalamic tract synapses in other parts of the brain, such as the limbic system (or emotional center) and the reticular formation (or sleep-wake center), subjecting the painful stimuli to emotional and behavioral influences.

Central Nervous System Processing

The central processing of pain occurs at three different levels of the brain: the thalamus, midbrain, and cortex. These areas of the brain cooperate to raise the awareness of pain, interpret the painful stimuli, and produce a response to the pain. The thalamus acts as the relay station for sensory input from the spinothalamic tract of the spinal cord. The midbrain signals the cortex to increase the awareness of the stimuli. The cortex seems to be involved in the discrimination of well-localized pain as well as in the interpretation of the pain experience.

Inhibitory and Facilitatory Mechanisms

Sensory input to the spinal cord may be influenced by chemical substances known as *neuroregulators*. These are classified as neurotransmitters or neuromodulators.

Neurotransmitters

Neurotransmitters are chemicals that exert inhibitory or excitatory activity at postsynaptic nerve cell membranes. Acetylcholine, norepinephrine, epinephrine, and dopamine are documented neurotransmitters.

Neuromodulators

Neuromodulators, also called endogenous opiates, are protein hormones found in the brain. They have been implicated in the modification of pain. These substances are composed of large amino acid peptides called *alpha-* and *beta-endorphins* and *enkephalins*. The speculation that these natural opiate-like substances were responsible for pain relief was confirmed when induced analgesic effects were reversed with naloxone (Narcan), an opioid antagonist.

Endorphins and enkephalins are similar to morphine-like substances, only more potent. They are believed to play a major role in the biological response to pain. The larger peptides (endorphins) exert more prolonged analgesic effects than do the enkephalins. Endorphins are produced by the anterior pituitary gland and the hypothalamus. The smaller peptides (enkephalins) tend to be more widespread throughout the brain and the dorsal horn of the spinal cord. Several types of endorphins and enkephalins have been identified. Each acts on highly specific opiate receptors in the central nervous system.

Opioid receptors are binding sites for not only endogenous opiates but also opioid analgesics that are taken to relieve pain also bind to these receptors. There are several types of opioid receptors: mu, kappa, delta, epsilon, and sigma. The mu receptors are found throughout the central nervous system, especially in the periaqueductal gray matter in the brain stem, the limbic system, and the dorsal horn. Morphine and morphine agonists bind to the mu receptors. Specific subtypes of the mu receptor are responsible for analgesia, bradycardia and sedation, and opioid agonist binding, which is associated with respiratory depression, euphoria, and physical dependence.

Various factors influence the production of neuromodulators. The activity of endorphins and enkephalins may be enhanced by prolonged strenuous activity (Fig. 9–2), transcutaneous electrical nerve stimulators (see later discussions about interventions for pain and chronic pain), and antidepressant therapy, which often increases serotonin levels in the body. Adequate amounts of serotonin, a neurotransmitter, have been shown to enhance analgesia through the activity of endorphins and enkephalins. Similarly, pain and stress are strong activators of the endogenous opiate system.

Sources of Pain

There are three major categories of pain sources: somatic, visceral, and neuropathic. Another arbitrary classification for the physiological sources of pain is based on pain that involves the activation of nociceptors and nonnociceptive pain or neuropathic pain. For a complete characterization of the physiological sources of pain, consult Table 9–1.

Somatic Pain

Somatic structures are the first source of pain. These structures are further classified as cutaneous and deep.

Cutaneous structures make up the superficial parts of the body, such as the skin and subcutaneous tissue. The cutaneous structures are well supplied with nerves; therefore, painful stimuli are well defined and localized.

Deep somatic structures include nerve receptors originating in bone, blood vessels, nerves, muscles, and other supporting tissues. Because these structures are poorly supplied with nerves, this pain is usually dull and poorly localized. Deep pain may produce an autonomic nervous system response, including nausea, pulse and blood pressure changes, and sweating.

Visceral Pain

The second source of pain is visceral and is defined as pain arising from body organs. The scarcity of nerve receptors in these structures produces poorly localized and diffuse pain. Visceral receptors are sensitive to stretching, inflammation, and ischemia, but they are not sensitive to cuts and extremes of temperature.

Visceral pain is well known for its ability to produce referred pain, which is a type of pain that a person perceives in an area other than the site of the stimuli. Referred pain occurs because visceral fibers synapse at the level of the spinal cord, close to fibers supplying certain subcutaneous tissue areas of the body. A common example of referred pain is pain in the right posterior shoulder that is related to gallbladder disease. The referred pain occurs because the subcutaneous tissue fibers of the scapula are close to the fibers of the gallbladder that are transmitting the painful stimuli. Other referred pain sites are illustrated in Figure 9–2.

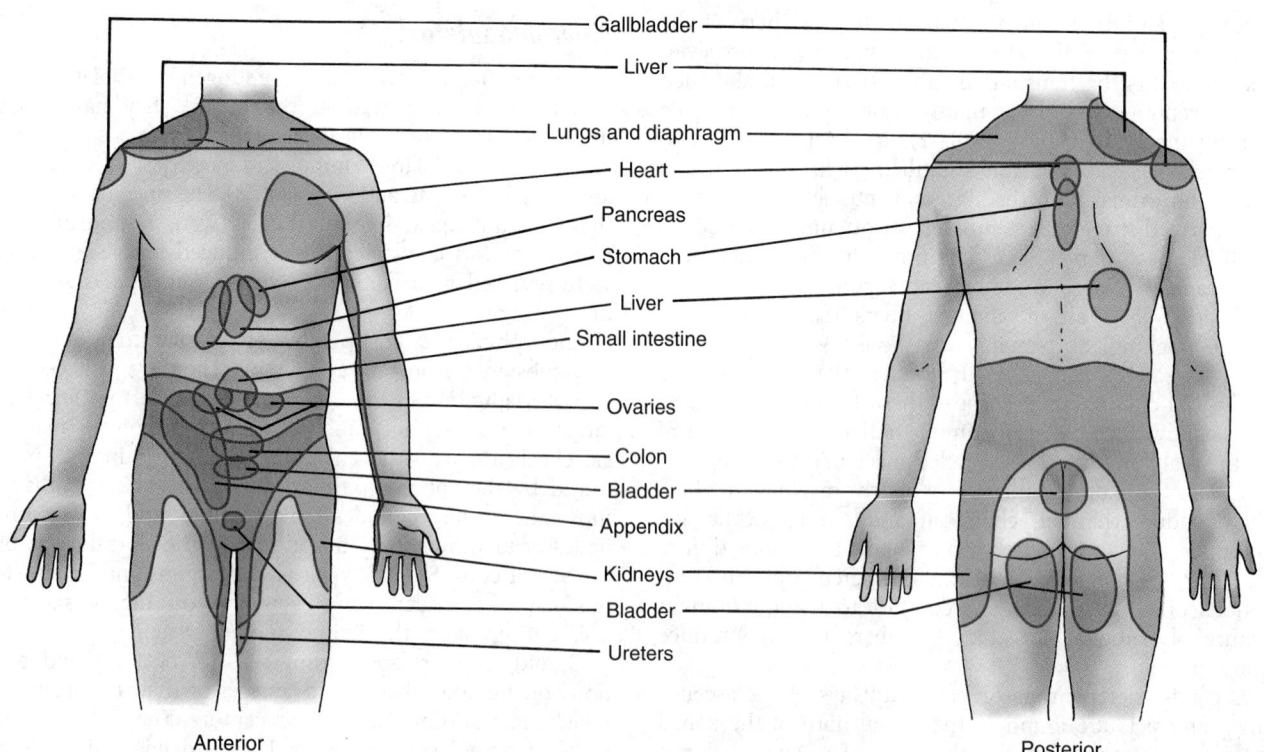

Figure 9–2. Anterior and posterior referred pain sites.

TABLE 9–1

Physiologic Sources of Pain					
Type of Pain	Physiologic Structures	Mechanism of Pain	Characteristics of Pain	Sources of Acute Postoperative Pain	Sources of Chronic Pain Syndromes
Somatic pain	Cutaneous: skin and subcutaneous tissues Deep somatic: bone, muscle, blood vessels, connective tissues	Activation of nociceptors	Well localized Constant and achy	Incisional pain, pain at insertion sites of tubes and drains, wound complications, orthopaedic procedures, skeletal muscle spasms	Bony metastases, osteo- and rheumatoid arthritis, low back pain, peripheral vascular disease
Visceral pain	Organs and the linings of the body cavities	Activation of nociceptors	Poorly localized Diffuse, deep, cramping or splitting	Chest tubes, abdominal tubes and drains, bladder distention or spasms, intestinal distention	Pancreatitis, liver metastases, colitis
Neuropathic pain	Nerve fibers, spinal cord, and central nervous system	Nonnociceptive Injury to the nervous system structures	Poorly localized Shooting, burning, fiery, shock-like, sharp, and painful numbness	Phantom limb pain, postmastectomy pain, and pain from nerve compression	Diabetic, human immunodeficiency virus, chemotherapy-induced neuropathies, postherpetic neuralgia, cancer-related nerve injury

Neuropathic Pain

The third major source of pain is neuropathic. Neuropathic pain is that caused by injury or destruction to peripheral nerves, pathways in the spinal cord, and neurons located in the brain. This injury results in disruptions in the transmission of afferent and efferent impulses in the periphery, spinal cord, and brain. Interruptions in the processing of painful stimuli give rise to peripheral and/or central perceptual phenomena, alterations in sensory modalities (touch, pressure, and temperature), and sometimes motor dysfunction. Central pain may be evident when the brain senses painful stimuli even though there may be no obvious or documented physiologic cause for the pain. Phantom limb pain, which may occur after the removal of an extremity or body part or severe damage to a major nerve plexus that innervates a particular extremity is one example of neuropathic pain.

Neuropathic pain represents a variety of complex painful mechanisms. This category of pain is receiving increased attention in the literature because it may not be as easily relieved by opioid analgesics as is somatic or visceral pain. Successful treatment of neuropathic pain usually requires a combination of pharmacologic approaches and sometimes pain-relieving procedures.

Pain Perception

The subjectivity of the pain experience limits our understanding of the perception and response to pain. This situation is further complicated by the knowledge that even when pain pathways are surgically interrupted, the perception of pain may persist. However, even though the perception of pain is difficult to measure, it can be characterized as the actual awareness of the painful feeling or sensation.

The pain threshold is the amount or degree of noxious stimuli that leads a person to first interpret a sensation as painful. More specifically, this term refers to the point at which a person feels pain and reports it as such.

Even though all pain is real, it sometimes persists without any detectable physical cause. Such pain may be highly influenced by emotional and social factors. In these situations, the lack of a physiologic or organic cause may lead health professionals, families, and clients to doubt the validity of the pain.

Pain tolerance refers to the ability of a person to endure the intensity of pain. Pain tolerance is usually characterized by an overt expression of behavior. Unlike pain perception and pain threshold, the ability to tolerate pain is more a function of psychological and social variables than of biological characteristics.

The nurse should be aware that many variables affect a person's perception of and response to pain. Demographic factors, such as age, gender, and sociocultural background, personality characteristics, and cognition, may influence the client's ability to process pain sensations and react to them.

Age

ELDERLY CONSIDERATIONS

Researchers agree that there are some variations in threshold associated with the chronologic age of the nervous system, but there are no clear trends (Zatzick & Dimsdale, 1990). Some researchers believe that the perceptual acuity of pain diminishes as a result of aging, although this finding has not been validated (Acute Pain Management Guideline Panel, 1992; Neeley, 1993). The perception of cutaneous pain may diminish because of age-related skin changes, but the perception of visceral pain may increase in older adults (Egbert, 1991).

Little attention has been paid to assessing pain in elderly people who are cognitively impaired and hospitalized, those residing at home, or residents of long-term care facilities (Harkins, 1996; Miller et al., 1996). Miller et al. (1996) examined various ways of assessing pain in elderly clients who were acutely confused.

Older adults generally receive less analgesia and tend to report pain less often than do younger adults (Neeley, 1993). These findings may be related to beliefs and concerns that the elderly have about pain and the reporting of pain. Many elderly people hold the following beliefs and concern about pain (Neeley, 1993):

- Pain is something that they must live with.
- Expressing pain is unacceptable or is a sign of weakness.
- Complaining of pain will label them as "bad" clients.
- Nurses are too busy to listen to complaints of pain.
- Pain signifies a serious illness or impending death.

Nurses should be aware of the beliefs that elderly clients hold to manage their pain. Nurses and other caregivers frequently undermedicate elderly clients and are sometimes reluctant to administer prescribed analgesics. Unfounded concerns about overmedication, addiction, and decreases in pain perception may contribute to undermedication (Champlin, 1992; Ferrell et al., 1992b; Greipp, 1992; Haviley et al., 1992).

Gender

Gender differences in types of pain and responses to it have been described by several researchers (Faucett, 1994; Vallerand, 1995). Physiologic, hormonal, and anatomic influences on pain are unclear, but it is apparent that some painful conditions are more common in either men or women (Ruda, 1993). Women suffer more frequently from migraine headaches, arthritis, and facial pain, whereas cluster headaches, back pain, and chest pain are more common among men (Faucett, 1994; Vallerand, 1995).

Gender effects on pain in clinical situations have been identified in some studies but not in others. Such studies must be interpreted with caution, as gender-oriented pain research is based largely on male responses. Women may be more likely to discuss their pain and distress and therefore are mistakenly labeled as less likely to deal effectively with their pain. Some investigators have demonstrated that men tolerate pain better than women do, whereas others have found no gender differences. It is widely believed that men exhibit greater stoicism than do women (Zatzick & Dimsdale, 1990). Research has shown that nurses expect men to be stoic but accept more emotional responses from women in pain (Walding, 1991).

Whatever gender differences do exist in the perception of and response to pain, nurses must acknowledge the effects of gender bias. Studies investigating the attitudes of caregivers toward the client in pain suggest that women are treated less aggressively, and their complaints are viewed with suspicion (Vallerand, 1995). In a recent study of physicians' pain management practices for clients with cancer, being female was an important predictor of inadequate analgesia (Cleeland et al., 1994).

TRANSCULTURAL CONSIDERATIONS

The American Nurses' Association emphasizes the need for nurses to appreciate the cultural diversity of their clients in all aspects of nursing practice. Weber (1996) contends that cultural sensitivity is critical to the understanding of factors that influence pain and expressions of pain. More importantly, the evolving integration of traditional ethnic heritage and modern American socialization gives rise to unique and highly individualized cultural expressions of pain. Yet, sociocultural groups are still sometimes categorized according to their ability to tolerate pain. This leads to unfair stereotypes and expectations of certain ethnic groups; for example, "Italian-Americans are very dramatic when they are in pain" or "Mexican-Americans have a low pain tolerance" (Calvillo & Flaskerud, 1991). A recent investigation of ethnic pain styles in clients experiencing myocardial infarction found few ethnographic correlates of pain dimensions (Neill, 1993), although higher mean pain scores and lower socioeconomic status were related. The dominant social class in the United States may still value less expressive responses to pain.

Many studies have shown a relationship between pain and a person's culture, but the study methods and results have not been consistent (Zatzick & Dimsdale, 1990). Descriptions of the study sample must be carefully evaluated for similar and dissimilar characteristics compared with patients in clinical practice. Findings from ethnic groups studied in other countries may not apply to culturally diverse populations living in America and socialized in the American culture. Also, studies that lack evidence of acceptable psychometric or measurement properties for the pain instruments must be interpreted cautiously. Finally, cross-cultural comparisons performed on pain measurement data substantially improve the ability to identify similarities and differences in the perceptions of and responses to pain across cultures.

Few nursing studies have examined the transcultural aspects of pain, yet nurses assess pain and make decisions regarding pain management for individuals in various ethnic groups. For example, many Mexican-American clients, especially women, moan or cry when they are uncomfortable. As a result, they are often identified by nurses as complainers who cannot tolerate pain (Calvillo & Flaskerud, 1991). Nurses who value the stoic model or "norm" for pain response interpret behaviors such as moaning and crying as an inability to tolerate pain and a request for intervention. In the Mexican culture, however, these behaviors might help the client relieve pain rather than communicate a need for intervention (Calvillo & Flaskerud, 1991).

Nurses must also consider language when dealing with people from various cultures. If English is not the person's first language within an English-speaking culture, the ability of the person to express pain may be limited, or expressions of pain may be misinterpreted. The nurse may need to rely on nonverbal communication, which can also be misinterpreted. Gaston-Johansson and colleagues (1990) examined the similarities in pain descriptions from four different cultural groups and found that people with diverse cultural and educational backgrounds may use similar words to describe the terms pain, hurt, and ache. Fortunately, some researchers have provided evidenced-based data to support the use of several standardized pain measures in clinical practice among culturally diverse groups diagnosed with cancer. Research on 536 persons with cancer of different ethnic backgrounds showed that evaluations of sensory pain using the McGill Pain Questionnaire were congruent across ethnic populations; however, descriptions of pain using affective terminology varied significantly (Greenwald, 1991). The multidimensional structure of the Brief Pain Inventory (BPI) has consistently demonstrated a high degree of reliability and validity when administered to samples from other countries (Cleeland & Ryan, 1994; Cleeland et al., 1996).

Personality Traits

According to the gate control theory of pain, a person's perception of pain and pain tolerance can be influenced by personality and other psychosocial factors. For example, people who are outgoing, or extroverts, may be more likely to express their pain than those who are quiet and shy.

Another personality factor that can influence pain perception and tolerance is anxiety. Many researchers have linked the presence of anxiety with pain. Other associated characteristics are feelings of powerlessness and the inability to cope with anxiety and pain. Nursing interventions to reduce anxiety and increase the ability to cope have also helped to relieve pain (Walding, 1991). However, the way in which pain is interpreted or appraised influences the coping strategies or methods selected by clients to deal with their pain (Arathuzik, 1991).

In addition to personality and other factors that cannot be changed, such as age and gender, other factors that are present at a given time may influence a person's experience of pain. Factors that tend to *decrease* the threshold for and tolerance of pain include discomfort, insomnia, fatigue, anxiety, fear, anger, sadness, depression, mental isolation, introversion, and past experience. Factors that tend to *increase* the threshold for and tolerance of pain include relief of symptoms, sleep, rest, sympathy, understanding, diversion, elevation of mood, analgesics, anxiolytic agents, and antidepressants. Because many of these factors can be altered, nursing interventions for pain often include minimizing factors that lower the pain threshold and tolerance and increasing or maximizing factors that increase the pain threshold and tolerance.

Research on Pain

Nurse-researchers have been concerned with the concept of pain, most often in relation to measuring the effects of nonpharmacologic interventions aimed at relieving pain. It is important for nurses to recognize the value of non-drug measures in alleviating pain and the associated distress. However, these techniques, when used for surgical pain and cancer-related pain, should compliment and not replace analgesic therapy.

In a classic study by Wells (1982), the effects of postoperative relaxation training were evaluated in a small sample of clients who had undergone cholecystectomy. Relaxation training reduced the psychological discomforts related to pain but demonstrated no measurable changes on any physiologic measures, such as blood pressure or pulse rate.

The overall effectiveness of relaxation techniques, including exercise, imagery, rhythmic breathing, and medication, has been evaluated by several investigators (Hyman et al., 1989). The result of their meta-analysis of published clinical studies indicated that relaxation techniques positively affect some clinical symptoms. Headaches were found to be consistently relieved through these techniques, whereas effects for chronic pain and anxiety were low to moderate and for acute pain were quite low.

In another evaluation of the effects of nursing intervention, Keller and Bzdek (1986) investigated the effects of therapeutic touch on tension headache pain. In this study, the McGill-Melzack Pain Questionnaire (Fig. 9–3) was used to demonstrate an average 70% pain reduction in the group who received touch intervention compared with the group who did not. Ferrel-Torry and Glick (1993) successfully used therapeutic massage as a nursing intervention to modify anxiety and the perception of cancer pain. Mulloney and Wells-Federman (1996) documented the powerful healing potential for therapeutic touch, including relief of pain, for selected clients. More recently, the benefits of progressive muscle relaxation and of therapeutic touch on pain and distress associated with degenerative arthritis were compared in older persons. Although both were effective, the greatest benefits for pain and distress were found with progressive muscle relaxation (Eckes Peck, 1997).

Music therapy as an intervention for pain has been shown to reduce postoperative pain and promote restorative sleep (Zimmerman et al., 1996). Benefits of music therapy have also been noted for clients experiencing cancer-related pain.

Pain Attitudes and Practices

Negative and mistaken beliefs about pain and its treatment currently prevail in the health care system. When such beliefs are perpetuated in clinical settings, it is difficult for health professionals to accept research-based information over traditional practices that are shaped by myths and misconceptions. Numerous studies have been conducted to help health professionals be more insightful and sensitive to these misconceptions that continue to obstruct views of pain and efforts to management it.

Attitudes of Nurses

Nurses' attitudes toward pain easily influence the way they perceive clients in pain and interact with them. Studies have suggested that practicing nurses perceive nu-

McGill-Melzack
PAIN QUESTIONNAIRE

Patient's name _____ Age _____
File No. _____ Date _____
Clinical category (e.g., cardiac, neurologic)
Diagnosis: _____
_____
_____
Analgesic (if already administered):
1. Type _____
2. Dosage _____
3. Time given in relation to this test _____
Patient's intelligence: circle number that represents best estimate.

   1 (low)   2   3   4   5 (high)

****

This questionnaire has been designed to tell us more about your pain. Four major questions we ask are
1. Where is your pain?
2. What does it feel like?
3. How does it change with time?
4. How strong is it?

It is important that you tell us how your pain feels now. Please follow the instructions at the beginning of each part.

_____
© R. Melzack, Oct. 1970

Part 1. Where Is Your Pain?

Please mark, on the drawings below, the areas where you feel pain. Put E if external, or I if internal, near the areas you mark. Put EI if both external and internal.

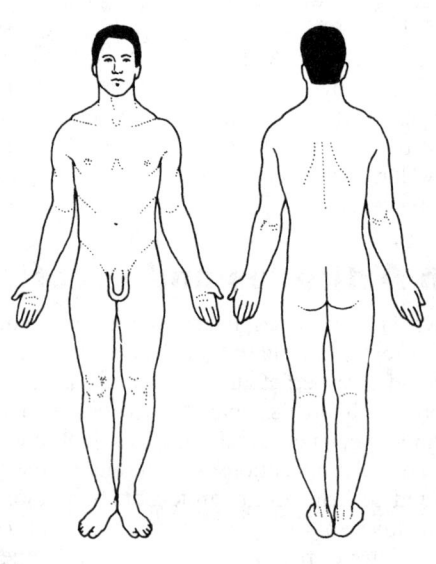

Part 2. What Does Your Pain Feel Like?

Some of the words below describe your *present* pain. Circle *ONLY* those words that best describe it. Leave out any category that is not suitable. Use only a single word in each appropriate category—the one that applies best.

1	6	11	16
Flickering	Tugging	Tiring	Annoying
Quivering	Pulling	Exhausting	Troublesome
Pulsing	Wrenching		Miserable
Throbbing	**7**	**12**	Intense
Beating	Hot	Sickening	Unbearable
Pounding	Burning	Suffocat-	
2	Scalding	ing	**17**
Jumping	Searing		Spreading
Flashing	**8**	**13**	Radiating
Shooting	Tingling	Fearful	Penetrating
3	Itchy	Frightful	Piercing
Pricking	Smarting	Terrifying	**18**
Boring	Stinging	**14**	Tight
Drilling	**9**	Punishing	Numb
Stabbing	Dull	Grueling	Drawing
Lancinating	Sore	Cruel	Squeezing
4	Hurting	Vicious	Tearing
Sharp	Aching	Killing	**19**
Cutting	Heavy	**15**	Cool
Lacerating	**10**	Wretched	Cold
5	Tender	Blinding	Freezing
Pinching	Taut		**20**
Pressing	Rasping		Nagging
Gnawing	Splitting		Nauseating
Cramping			Agonizing
Crushing			Dreadful
			Torturing

Part 3. How Does Your Pain Change With Time?

1. Which word or words would you use to describe the *pattern* of your pain?

1	2	3
Continuous	Rhythmic	Brief
Steady	Periodic	Momentary
Constant	Intermittent	Transient

2. What kind of things *relieve* your pain?

3. What kind of things *increase* your pain?

Part 4. How Strong Is Your Pain?

People agree that the following 5 words represent pain of increasing intensity. They are:

1	2	3	4	5
Mild	Discomforting	Distressing	Horrible	Excruciating

To answer each question below, write the number of the most appropriate word in the space beside the question.

1. Which word describes your pain right now? ____
2. Which word describes it at its worst? ____
3. Which word describes it when it is least? ____
4. Which word describes the worst toothache you ever had? ____
5. Which word describes the worst headache you ever had? ____
6. Which word describes the worst stomach ache you ever had? ____

Figure 9-3. The McGill-Melzack Pain Questionnaire. (From Melzack, R. [1975]. The McGill Pain Questionnaire: Major properties and scoring methods. *Pain, 1,* 272–281.)

merous barriers to effective pain management outcomes (Ferrell et al., 1992a; Fife et al., 1993; Wallace et al., 1995). Without an adequate knowledge of pain and principles of analgesic therapy, nurses may not be able to understand their clients' pain and confidently participate with physicians and other professionals in its treatment. Similarly, surveys of nursing faculty have shown that they too are ill prepared to care for clients in pain (Deikmann & Wassem, 1991; Ferrell et al., 1993)

Nurses who may have little personal experience with pain may not appreciate the magnitude of painful conditions associated with diseases and medical and surgical interventions. Nurses may expect that clients with chronic pain will react similarly to those with acute pain. They may assume that reactions to pain, including complaints about pain, will fall within a certain norm on the basis of their own cultural values. The more the response of a person with pain varies from these expected norms, the more likely it is that the attitude of the nurse toward the client will be biased, either positively or negatively.

Attitudes of Clients

Many client are reluctant to report pain, and when they do, they may underestimate its severity (Von Roenn et al., 1993). Clients may not complain of pain because they want to be a "good" client or they may not want to bother or distract their caregivers from other issues in their care. In clients with a history of cancer, pain can be an unwanted reminder of the disease and its progression.

Clients may also be reluctant to take pain medication, especially opioid analgesics, because of fear that they will become addicted or used to the medication (Ward & Gatwood, 1994). Compliance with medications can be affected by the complexity of the medication schedule or experience with untoward side effects, such as sedation or constipation.

Attitudes of Physicians

Undertreatment of pain, especially cancer pain, is a serious problem in the United States and elsewhere in the world. In 1983, the World Health Organization estimated that on any given day, 3.5 million people in the world experience cancer pain that could be relieved (Haviley et al., 1992).

Despite increased education about pain, many physicians underprescribe medication for clients in pain, especially opioids such as morphine. Some investigators have assessed several factors that account for this practice (Von Roenn et al., 1993).

First, cultural and societal attitudes exist about opioid use, especially in the United States. In some states, clients who use these drugs have to register with state regulatory agencies in a manner similar to that required of people enrolled in methadone programs. Requiring this procedure equates the client with a drug abuser. Some state regulations make it mandatory that triplicate prescriptions are used for schedule II controlled substances, which can deter physicians from prescribing some opioid analgesics.

Second, government regulatory agencies do not set practical guidelines for drug use in people with severe or chronic pain. A physician may be reprimanded by the medical board for prescribing what the board considers an inappropriate amount or type of pain medication.

Third, there is still a lack of knowledge about the effects of analgesics. Most of the studies on a person's response to drug therapy have been done with people who were not in pain. In many of these studies, subjects were volunteers who were former drug addicts imprisoned for drug abuse. The fear of respiratory depression that some physicians have is unnecessary because pain prevents or diminishes the respiratory effect of opioids (Haviley et al., 1992; Hill, 1990).

Types of Pain

There are several ways to classify types of pain. In 1986, the National Institutes of Health Consensus Conference on Pain categorized pain according to its cause. The participants at the conference identified three types of pain: acute, chronic malignant, and chronic nonmalignant. Acute pain results from acute injury, disease, or surgery. Chronic nonmalignant pain is associated with tissue injury that is not progressive or that has healed. Pain that is associated with cancer or another progressive disease is called chronic malignant pain. The nurse is usually concerned with two basic types of pain in practice: acute pain and chronic pain.

Acute Pain
Characteristics of Acute Pain

Acute pain is experienced by almost everyone at some time. Certain characteristics distinguish this type of pain from the more chronic, or long-term pain that is often associated with chronic illness. A major distinction between acute and chronic pain is the effect of pain on biological responses. Acute pain serves a biological purpose. It acts as a warning signal because it can activate the sympathetic nervous system. This stimulation causes the release of catecholamine neurotransmitters, such as epinephrine, which give rise to various physiologic responses. As a result, clients experiencing acute pain exhibit physiologic responses similar to those found in "fight-or-flight" reactions (see Chap. 8). These responses include increased heart rate, blood pressure, and respiratory rate; dilated pupils; and sweating. Behavioral signs of acute pain may include restlessness, an inability to concentrate, apprehension, and overall distress (Table 9–2).

Acute pain is usually temporary, of sudden onset, and easily localized. The client can frequently describe the pain, which may subside with or without treatment. Acute pain frequently results from sudden, accidental trauma, such as fractures, burns, and lacerations, or from surgery, ischemia, and acute inflammation. Acute pain is often the result of trauma involving superficial or cutaneous structures. This pain is confined to the affected area. As the painful area heals, the quality or sensation of the pain changes. Acute pain, although possibly severe, is limited over time and generally can be managed successfully. Both the caregiver and the client can see an end to the pain, which makes coping somewhat easier.

TABLE 9–2

Physiologic and Behavioral Responses to Acute and Chronic Pain		
Pain Type	Physiologic Response	Behavioral Response
Acute	• Increased blood pressure initially • Increased pulse rate • Increased respiratory rate • Dilated pupils • Perspiration	• Restlessness • Inability to concentrate • Apprehension • Distress
Chronic	• Normal blood pressure • Normal pulse rate • Normal respiratory rate • Normal pupils • Dry skin	• Immobility or physical inactivity • Withdrawal • Despair

Postoperative Pain

Pain accompanying surgery is one of the most common examples of acute pain, but it is poorly understood and not always well managed. It is conservatively estimated that 20% of all clients who undergo surgery experience mild pain, 20% to 40% experience moderate pain, and 40% to 70% experience severe pain (Bonica, 1983). According to some authorities, the alarmingly high number of clients who experience pain after surgery can be attributed to inadequate analgesia (Acute Pain Management Guideline Panel, 1992). As discussed earlier, others believe that inadequate pain control stems from societal attitudes and believe that people in pain should "grin and bear it." Still others identify the fear of addiction as a major factor in physician-prescribing practices such as administering less than optimal amounts of analgesics after surgery. Whatever the reason, some people undergoing surgery suffer needlessly.

Pain is an expected outcome of surgery. Not only is there a sensory component arising from the area of tissue destruction, there is also a major psychosocial component.

RELATIONSHIP TO TYPE OF SURGICAL APPROACH. According to several studies, the type and site of the operation are the most important predictors in determining the incidence, severity, and duration of postoperative pain. Similarly, the extent of the operation, the degree of tissue trauma, and the positioning of the client during surgery contribute to the overall incidence and severity of postoperative pain.

Intrathoracic and upper intra-abdominal surgical approaches are generally associated with more severe, steady wound pain, as well as pain on movement in the postoperative period. Conversely, many clients who undergo superficial surgery of the head and neck, chest wall, or limbs report minimal or no pain postoperatively. Muscle-splitting procedures are far more painful than muscle-stretching procedures. On the basis of this information, surgeons have modified their techniques over the years in an attempt to reduce or minimize the components of this type of pain.

INFLUENCE OF PSYCHOSOCIAL VARIABLES. A person's postoperative pain experience is not limited to the level of tissue trauma. Postoperative pain is also influenced by many psychosocial variables. Personal factors, such as age and sociocultural group, may be important determinants for predicting patterns of expressing and coping with postoperative pain.

Anxiety is perhaps the best-explored psychological determinant in predicting postoperative pain. A highly anxious client may appear to be more distressed and affected by pain. Numerous studies have been done in an attempt to correlate preoperative information with postoperative pain (Acute Pain Management Guideline Panel, 1992). Some nursing studies, such as that of Johnson et al. (1978), indicate that clients who receive preoperative procedural or sensory information (i.e., a description of the expected sensation, as well as techniques to enhance relaxation) seem to cope better with postoperative pain. In addition, these clients recover more quickly than clients given only factual information about the anticipated postoperative experience.

Highly anxious clients, however, may be given minimal procedural information, such as the location of the incision, the sequence of events before surgery (e.g., preoperative sedation and visits from perioperative personnel), and postoperative care regimens. For these clients, too much information can exacerbate fear and pain (Acute Pain Management Guideline Panel, 1992).

The nurse stresses to the client the importance of requesting analgesia when he or she perceives pain. The nurse should repeat these instructions at regular intervals if the client is anxious, because anxiety interferes with the ability to process information. The nurse also uses nonpharmacologic interventions, such as distraction and relaxation, to help the highly anxious client (see later).

Chronic Pain
Characteristics of Chronic Pain

Chronic pain is a major health problem. It has been estimated that in the United States alone, 25% of people, many of them older than 65 years, are affected with a chronic illness and chronic pain. In contrast to acute pain, chronic pain serves no biological purpose. After the pain's initial warning signal, the body must learn to adapt to the persistent pain impulses by blocking or adjusting to the activation of the sympathetic nervous system, which causes the fight-or-flight reaction in acute pain. Because of this adaptation, many of the obvious symptoms that are associated with physiologic responses to pain are absent or less obvious in the client with chronic pain.

Chronic pain is defined as pain that persists or recurs for indefinite periods, usually for more than 2 months.

Onset is gradual, and the character and quality of the pain change over time. Because chronic pain frequently involves deep somatic and visceral structures, it is usually diffuse, poorly localized, and often difficult to describe. If the underlying cause of the chronic pain cannot be treated medically, controlling the long-term effects of chronic pain may be a difficult clinical challenge.

Chronic pain is associated with a variety of health problems, such as cancer, connective tissue diseases, peripheral vascular diseases, and musculoskeletal disorders. It is also seen in post-traumatic problems, such as phantom limb pain and low back pain. The degree of chronic pain varies, depending on the type of problem and whether it is progressive, stable, or capable of resolution. Unless the disease process is arrested or reversed, the severity of chronic pain may worsen to the point that the client is physically and emotionally debilitated. Even when the physiologic pain stimuli are eliminated or tissue damage has resolved, the client's perception of pain may linger. This is sometimes called the "chronic pain syndrome." A client's response to chronic pain is influenced by his or her ability to cope, the availability of family support and social resources, and the severity of the physiologic and emotional consequences (see Table 9–2).

Because chronic pain persists for extended periods, it can interfere with activities of daily living and personal relationships. It can also result in emotional and financial burdens. Thus, the efforts of an interdisciplinary health care team are needed to manage the situation effectively. If pain is inadequately managed, it is an overwhelming, frustrating experience for both sufferer and caregiver. Although many of the characteristics of chronic pain are similar in different clients, the nurse should be aware that each chronic pain situation is unique and requires a highly specialized plan of care.

Chronic Nonmalignant Pain

Chronic nonmalignant pain may be caused by chronic diseases such as rheumatoid arthritis, lupus, sickle cell anemia, diabetic neuropathy, and peripheral vascular disease. It may also be related to painful conditions such as fibromyalgia, low back pain, chronic headaches, osteoporosis, and facial pain. Whenever possible, the source(s) of the chronic nonmalignant pain should be targeted and managed with nonopioid analgesics and nondrug measures. However, chronic opioid therapy has gained wide acceptance in selected populations when other therapies have failed to provide optimal pain relief.

In the past, physicians were reluctant to consider opioid therapy in clients who did not have cancer. Clients experiencing nonmalignant pain were traditionally managed with nonopioid analgesics or adjuvant drugs, and nondrug measures. However, today some clients with chronic nonmalignant pain are managed with long-term opioid therapy. This type of therapy is generally reserved for clients who have a documented physiologic source for the pain—more specifically, those with chronic diseases. Structured regimens using long-acting or extended-release opioids with occasional short-acting analgesics, if necessary, are preferred.

There is enough evidence to suggest that the benefits of alleviating pain and suffering with chronic opioid therapy far outweigh any risks. Several published reports in selected client populations have documented favorable clinical outcomes such as improved function, better quality of life, less psychological distress, and less dependence on the health care system when opioids have been used (Schofferman et al., 1993; Vallerand, 1991). Moreover, the risk of addiction remains exceedingly low. Even when chronic opioids are given to clients with nonmalignant pain having a known history of substance abuse, drug-seeking behavior is seldom a significant problem (Dunbar & Katz, 1996).

Only those clients who have demonstrated measurable benefits from opioids should be considered for long-term use of these medications for nonmalignant pain. Compassionate use of opioids may be considered for the elderly with debilitating pain (i.e., compression fractures of the spine) both at home and in extended care facilities. The nurse recognizes that the elderly may be more prone to side effects of opioids (i.e., sedation, constipation, mental status changes) and implements measures to reduce the risk of opioid-induced adverse effects.

Chronic Pain Syndrome

Clients sometimes have chronic pain associated with a physical problem. Eventually, the physiologic alterations resolve or become less detectable, and the etiology for the pain is unclear. Sometimes these painful conditions are referred to as idiopathic pain, pain of unknown etiology, or chronic pain syndrome. However, the perception or sensation of pain persists. The degree of pain appears to be out of proportion to the physical findings, yet the pain is real to the person experiencing it. Clients in this situation often subject themselves to a variety of medical tests and frequent hospitalization while searching for a cause for or explanation of their pain. So-called doctor shopping is common in this group of clients. Some clients invest an incredible amount of time and energy in the health care system in the hope of uncovering a solution for their pain. As a result, clients with chronic pain syndrome focus on what they cannot do rather than what they can to do. Clients often demonstrate learned helplessness, powerlessness, dependency, and sick role behaviors. They may experience loss of confidence, disuse of their bodies, risks of losing income, and difficulty in adapting to social and work situations. When pain persists for long periods, family members are often emotionally drained, frustrated, and in need of help in dealing with the client.

Interdisciplinary pain centers, like pain clinics or programs, are best equipped to handle the complex psychosocial pain issues associated with chronic pain syndromes. Published data show that comprehensive pain centers have demonstrated modest success in eliminating the need for prescription analgesics, reducing dependence on the health care system, and reintegrating clients into social and occupational networks (Flor et al., 1992). Behavioral and cognitive approaches, which focus on family-centered care, are useful strategies for these clients.

Chronic Malignant (Cancer-Related) Pain

Although many clients with advanced malignant disease experience severe pain, adequate pain control could be achieved for most of them. Even when the best pain management techniques are used, however, the complexity and progressive nature of this type of pain often limit the success of pain management efforts.

Cancer-related pain arises from a variety of mechanisms. For example, as a malignant tumor invades the bone, chemicals known as prostaglandins are released. These substances sensitize nerve receptors in the bone and increase their sensitivity to painful stimuli. In part, this explains the extreme degree of pain associated with bony metastases. Other causes of cancer-related pain include arterial ischemia, venous engorgement, nerve compression, infection, inflammation, necrosis, and ulcerations. In addition, the sources of these problems are usually in deep somatic and visceral structures. These types of painful sensations, coupled with the diffuse nature of the pain, hamper the client's ability to describe and localize cancer pain.

The psychological impact of cancer can be devastating, especially if clients must contend with unrelieved pain (see Research Applications for Nursing). Investigators have documented marked psychological distress among clients with higher pain intensities and poorer relief of pain. (Polomano, 1995; Zimmerman et al., 1996).

▶ Research Applications for Nursing

Psychological Variables and Their Effect on Cancer Pain

Zimmerman, L., Turner Story, K., Gaston-Johansson, F., & Rowles, J. (1996). Psychological variables and cancer pain. Cancer Nursing, 19(1), 44–53.

The purpose of this study was to determine whether cancer clients with pain had higher scores of depression, anxiety, somatization, and hostility than did cancer clients without pain. Thirty clients in each group were given the Brief Symptom Inventory (BSI), the McGill Pain Questionnaire (MPQ), and a visual analogue scale for pain. Clients with pain scored higher on all four subscales of the BSI, meaning that they were experiencing more depression, anxiety, somatization, and hostility. However, these differences were only significant for somatization and hostility. For all subjects, there were significant positive relationships between the scores on the MPQ and all four subscales. Higher MPQ scores, indicative of more pain, were associated with higher BSI subscale scores, which reflect poorer outcomes

Critique. This study was an attempt to further clarify the nature of affective, cognitive, and behavioral components of pain. The small convenience sample limits the ability to generalize these findings to other clients with cancer but points the way to further research.

Possible Implications for Nursing. The findings suggest a relationship between psychological status and dimensions of the pain experience. Nursing interventions for the client in pain should be directed at assessing and modifying both pain level and psychological status.

Most clients with advanced cancer have more than one location of and physiologic source of pain. Approximately one third of these clients experience a component of neuropathic pain or nerve injury pain (Polomano, 1995). Because the pharmacologic approaches may vary depending on whether clients have somatic, visceral, and/or neuropathic pain, it is important for the nurse to identify the cause or causes of the pain in each location. (For additional information on this type of pain, see Chapter 26 and consult Management of Cancer Pain Clinical Practice Guidelines, 1994.)

Collaborative Management

 Assessment

▶ History

The nurse asks the client about the pain experience, including the sequence of events (precipitating and relieving factors); the nature of adjustments, if any, in the client's life or in the family; and beliefs about the cause of the pain and what should be done about it (client's expectations). Personal characteristics, such as the client's age and culture, influence attitudes about reporting a pain history. Families and significant others are included in this information-gathering process.

Clients may report pain in the absence of any observable or documented physiologic changes in the body. The nurse keeps in mind that all pain is real and operates from the premise that pain is "whatever the person experiencing it says it is." The nurse respects the client's verbal and nonverbal expressions of pain without making judgments or inferences about the reality of the pain. If clients perceive that health professionals doubt the existence of their pain, mistrust and other negative feelings can arise and interfere with a therapeutic nurse-client relationship.

The nurse also assesses the length of time the client has experienced pain. Clients who experience acute pain may welcome an opportunity to discuss their pain with the nurse, because acute pain is a relatively short-term experience and is easily described by clients. However, clients with chronic pain can be frustrated when they are unable to adequately describe their vague, diffuse pain experience. Structured interviews using assessment aids, such as pain scales and descriptors, often help clients to express their pain.

ELDERLY CONSIDERATIONS

The elderly client's complaints of pain may be ignored by caregivers. Herr and Mobily (1991) found that some elderly clients in a residential center stopped expressing their discomfort because they were treated as "chronic complainers." Other elders stated that the response to their complaints was "What do you expect at your age?" Older adults do not typically have age-related pain.

Nurses should also consider that when they take a history from elderly clients, the clients may be anxious or temporarily disoriented as a result of pain or because they

Nursing Focus on the Elderly: The Elderly Client Experiencing Pain

When taking a client history

- Realize that the prevalence of pain is estimated to be double those younger than 60 years and well over 70% among elders in care facilities.
- Consider the elderly at risk for the undertreatment of pain, especially cancer pain, because of inappropriate beliefs about pain sensitivity, tolerance, and ability to use opioids.
- Recognize that cognitive impairment in the elderly may pose barriers to pain assessment, but the elderly with mild to moderate cognitive impairment may be able to accurately report pain at the moment or when prompted.
- Cognitively impaired elderly may require more frequent assessments of pain than clients who are not impaired.
- Use visual representations of pain meases rather than mental images of pain rating scales. Be sure that the client is wearing glasses and hearing aid(s), if needed and available.
- Alter a written pain scale to include large lettering, adequate space between lines, nonglossy paper, and color for increased visualization.
- Provide adequate lighting and privacy to avoid distracting background noise.

If the client cannot verbally communicate

- Assess for nonverbal indicators of pain, such as grimacing or crying.
- Observe for changes in the client's behavior, such as increased confusion or combativeness.
- Respond to complaints of pain promptly—they are typically not age-related complaints.
- Administer the prescribed amount of analgesics for postoperative pain in a timely manner. If pain is not relieved, evaluate the effectiveness of the analgesic regimen and immediately notify the physician.
- Use nondrug pain relief measures.

Data from the Acute Pain Management Guideline Panel. (1994). *Acute pain management: Operative or medical procedures and trauma. Clinical practice guideline.* AHCPR Pub. No. 92-0032. Rockville, MD: Agency for Health Care Policy and Research, Public Health Service, U.S. Department of Health and Human Services.

are in an unusual environment. The nurse observes for nonverbal indicators of pain, such as grimacing, and checks for changes in behavior. For example, if a client becomes restless, hostile, or combative, the nurse considers pain as a possible underlying reason. Too often a client who behaves in this manner is labeled with a diagnosis of dementia or other cognitive impairment or is categorized by the nursing staff as "difficult." Chart 9–1 highlights key points for assessing an elderly client in pain.

➤ Essential Data for a Complete Pain History

Information about a client's pain can be helpful in understanding the factors that are associated with the client's present pain or previous episodes of pain. If the client is

in pain when the nurse is taking the history, the nurse should keep the session reasonably short or continue at a later time. Data to obtain include

- *Precipitating factors.* Does the client associate any activities, ingestion of food, or other environmental factors with the onset of pain? What does the client think causes the present pain? Was the onset of pain sudden or insidious? Has the client done anything or taken anything to relieve the pain? What were the results of the intervention?
- *Aggravating factors.* What factors make the pain worse? What influence has this pain had on the client's activity? What changes in life activity have been affected (e.g., diet, job, sleep)?
- *Localization of pain.* Can the client localize the pain or describe where it travels or radiates?
- *Character and quality of pain.* What words does the client use to describe the pain, its character, quality, or intensity?
- *Duration of pain.* How long has the client experienced this pain?

➤ Physical Assessment/Clinical Manifestations

The overt or observable clinical manifestations of pain include physiologic responses, motor or body movements, and affective behaviors such as crying. Although physiologic changes occur in response to acute noxious stimuli, these changes are usually *not* reliable indicators of chronic pain. Acute pain, with its property of warning an individual about harm, elicits several physiologic signs and symptoms. These signs and symptoms are largely a function of sympathetic nervous system stimulation. Clients with acute pain often manifest pronounced changes in vital body functions, such as tachycardia and blood pressure changes. The blood pressure is usually elevated initially and is then decreased. In addition, clients with acute pain may become diaphoretic, restless, and apprehensive.

Physiologic changes in response to chronic pain are usually masked as the body attempts to compensate for and adapt to the noxious stimuli. The pain no longer serves as a necessary warning. Changes in vital signs related to chronic pain may be evident only when preexisting pain occurs or as new sites of painful stimuli arise.

Certain motor or body movements may be associated with acute or chronic pain. Some may be more exaggerated or obvious than others. Clients in pain may support or shield ("splint"), holding painful body parts while moving, or lie listlessly because they are afraid to move. The nurse assesses the functional status and degree of impairment in the client with pain.

Location of Pain

The nurse assesses the location of pain from two dimensions: the level of pain, either deep or superficial, and the position or location of pain. Most clients, whether they are experiencing acute or chronic pain, can usually describe the depth of pain perceived. However, the actual area or location of the pain may not be as easily identified.

The nurse asks the client whether the pain is superficial or deep. In general, clients who have pain involving superficial or cutaneous structures describe their pain as superficial and can often localize the pain to a specific area. These structures have an abundant nerve supply, which contributes to the ease and accuracy of the client localizing the pain. In contrast, clients who perceive pain from deeper somatic or visceral structures within the body may have difficulty localizing their pain (a result of the poor innervation of this area).

Pain may be described as belonging to one of four categories, related to its location:

- Localized pain—pain confined to the site of origin
- Projected pain—pain along a specific nerve or nerves
- Radiating pain—diffuse pain around the site of origin that is not well localized
- Referred pain—pain perceived in an area distant from the site of painful stimuli

A client who has difficulty specifying the exact location of pain can be asked to point to the painful areas on his or her own body or on another person. Sometimes having the client point to or shade in the painful areas on a diagram of the front and back of the human body is helpful (see Fig. 9-2). When clients cannot identify the painful areas and state that they just "hurt all over," the nurse encourages the client to focus on parts of the body that are not painful. The nurse asks the client to concentrate on different body parts, beginning with the hand and fingers of one extremity, while asking him or her to identify the presence or absence of pain. As the nurse focuses attention on selected areas of the body, the client is assisted in localizing painful areas. Often clients who state that they hurt everywhere begin to realize that some parts of the body are not painful.

Clients may present with more than one discrete painful site. In fact, about one half of clients with advanced cancer report having pain in more than one location. As painful areas are identified, the nurse helps the client to understand the origin of the pain. This understanding is particularly important for clients with cancer because every new pain often raises the suspicion of metastasis (spread of disease). The pain may be caused by other reasons, such as immobility or constipation.

Character and Quality of Pain

After asking the client to locate the pain, the nurse asks him or her to describe how the pain feels. Clients may use a word or group of words to convey the sensations or feelings of the pain. The nurse avoids suggesting descriptive words for the pain. Some clients who are frustrated and are having difficulty describing their pain may benefit from using the McGill-Melzack Pain Questionnaire (see Fig. 9-3). With this measurement tool, the nurse asks the client to circle descriptive terms in the appropriate categories to best describe the pain. This questionnaire may be too difficult for clients with poor reading or verbal skills. The Short-Form McGill Pain Questionnaire (SF-MPQ) provides a simpler way of describing the sensory and affective components of pain (Melzack, 1987) (see Fig. 9-5). Its use is of particular value in measuring

changes in sensations of the pain when adjuvant or non-opioid analgesics such as tricylcic antidepressants and anticonvulsants are tried.

Another useful strategy is to ask the client to describe the sensation by comparing it to a situation or event that may be comparable to the feeling of pain. For example, a man with excruciating diffuse abdominal pain from advanced cancer once said that his pain felt as if a soldier were walking around inside his abdomen, with no set path or destination, stepping on mines. For this man, pain was unpredictable and never-ending and produced "blowing-up" sensations.

Pattern of Pain

Pain is rarely the same at all times. It is perceived differently over time and is subjected to various precipitating and aggravating factors (see earlier discussion under History).

Intensity of Pain

Subjective measurements of pain intensity are more reliable and accurate than the overt or observable parameters of pain. Only the client can determine the amount or severity of pain experienced. Various visual analog scales, numeric rating scales (NRS), descriptive word scales, and other measures have been designed to help clients communicate the magnitude or severity of pain and to help nurses quantify the pain.

The nurse uses pain intensity scales to measure pain in the clinical setting and to assess and determine the effectiveness of relief-oriented interventions. The client is presented with an appropriate pain scale and asked to rate the amount of painful stimuli. Clients with more than one discrete painful site may wish to specify their pain levels by location. Clinicians have recently been encouraged to elicit self-report measures of pain that reflect not only present pain levels but also the average or general pain level and least and worst pain intensities.

When describing varied levels of pain, the client is asked to recall the pain over a specified time interval.

A variety of scales can be used to measure pain intensity, and some also assess the emotional aspects of pain. Verbal descriptive scales typically group words such as "none," "moderate," or "severe" and permit an intensity rating of pain. Visual analog scales (VAS) usually use a 10-cm line to represent a continuum of pain intensity and include verbal anchors that describe the intensity of the stimuli. Numeric rating scales (0-10) (NRS) are commonly employed in clinical practice because they are easily communicated and interpreted. Studies have shown strong correlations between the NRS and the VAS (Puntillo & Weiss, 1994). For examples of such pain intensity rating scales, see Figure 9-4.

Variations in the scales are important determinants for selecting the appropriate measurement tool. Clients with chronic, nagging, diffuse pain may have difficulty using broad numeric ranges such as the NRS. Some clients are better able to use word associations and prefer measurements that contain descriptive words or phrases rather than just numbers. The Faces Rating Scale is particularly useful for assessing pain in culturally diverse populations

PAIN INTENSITY SCALES

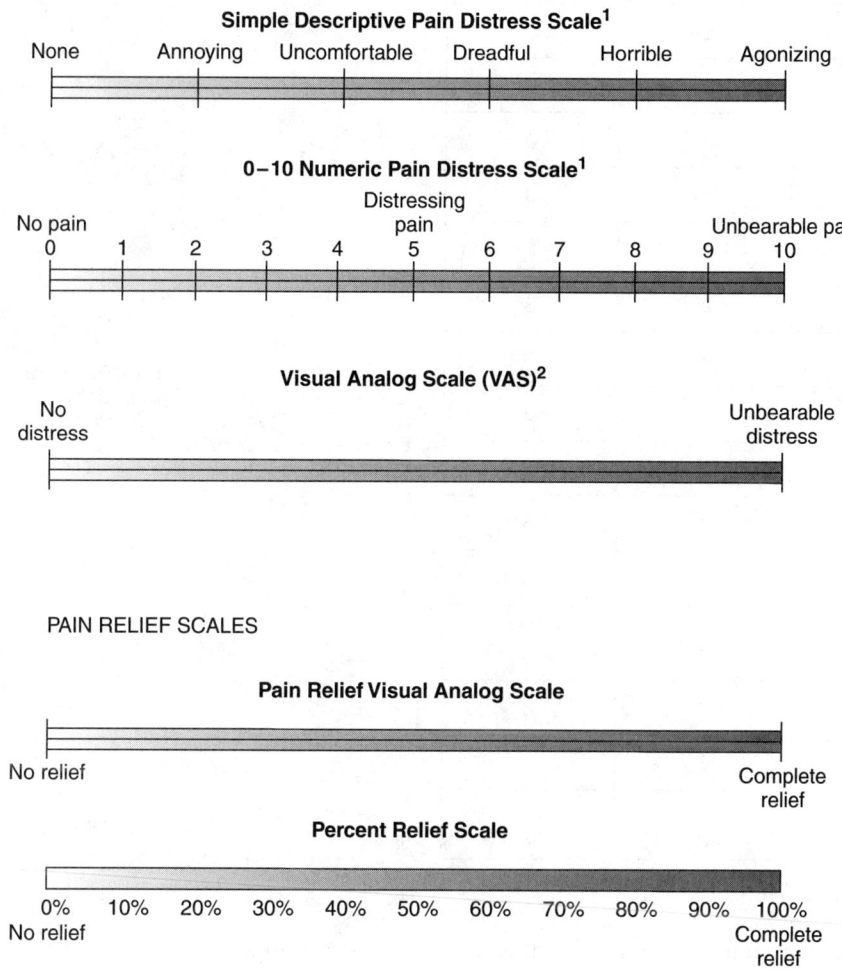

Figure 9–4. Pain rating scales and pain relief scales. (Simple Descriptive Pain Distress Scale, 0–10 Numeric Pain Distress Scale, and Visual Analog Scale redrawn from Acute Pain Management Guideline Panel. [1992]. *Acute pain management: Operative or medical procedures and trauma. Clinical practice guideline.* AHCPR Pub. No. 92-0032. Rockville, MD: Agency for Health Care Policy and Research, Public Health Service, U.S. Department of Health and Human Services; Pain Relief Visual Analog Scale redrawn from Fishman, B., Pasternak, S., Wallenstein, S. L., Houde, R. W., Holland, J. C., & Foley, K. M. [1987]. The Memorial Pain Assessment Card: A valid instrument for the evaluation of cancer pain. *Cancer, 60*[5], 1151–1158; Percent Relief Scale redrawn from the Brief Pain Inventory. Pain Research Group, Department of Neurology, University of Wisconsin-Madison.)

[1]If used as a graphic rating scale, a 10-cm baseline is recommended.

[2]A 10-cm baseline is recommended for VAS scales.

who encounter language barriers in expressing their pain.

Perception of Pain Relief

Pain relief is a dimension separate from pain intensity. Therefore, the amount of relief that is achieved from pain therapies, in addition to the amount or level of pain experienced, should be assessed. Valid measures of pain relief can be obtained by using relief scales. As with pain intensity measures, it is critical to provide a time frame for evaluating the pain therapy. Evaluation of pain relief can be accomplished with either a pain relief analogue scale or a percent rating scale (see Figure 9–4).

Issues in Pain Measurement

It is critical that reliable and valid measures be used to evaluate dimensions of pain. Nurses should avoid using self-report scales that have not been adequately tested in

clinical practice settings. Pain measures should be appropriate for the client's cognitive level and issues with pain.

ELDERLY CONSIDERATIONS

When using tools to measure pain in elderly clients, the nurse considers possible visual or hearing limitations. The client should wear glasses and one or two hearing aids, if appropriate. Increased lighting with nonglare bulbs may improve visual perception. The tools may be altered to include large lettering, adequate spacing between lines, and color on a white background (Herr & Mobily, 1991). Pasero and McCaffery (1994) provide additional strategies for assessing pain in the elderly.

➤ Psychosocial Assessment

Acute Pain

All pain holds significant meaning for the person experiencing it. For clients experiencing acute pain from sur-

Type	None	Mild	Moderate	Severe
Throbbing	0	1	2	3
Shooting	0	1	2	3
Stabbing	0	1	2	3
Sharp	0	1	2	3
Cramping	0	1	2	3
Gnawing	0	1	2	3
Hot-burning	0	1	2	3
Aching	0	1	2	3
Heavy	0	1	2	3
Tender	0	1	2	3
Splitting	0	1	2	3
Tiring/exhausting	0	1	2	3
Sickening	0	1	2	3
Fearful	0	1	2	3
Punishing/cruel	0	1	2	3

Figure 9–5. The Short-Form McGill Pain Questionnaire (Recreated from Melzack, R. [1987]. The Short-Form McGill Pain Questionnaire. *Pain, 30,* 191–197.)

gery, the pain may be interpreted as necessary and expected. The pain may be viewed with relief as a sign that some greater problem has been resolved or alleviated by the surgery. Knowledge that the duration of the pain is limited may allow the client to deal with unpleasant sensations without too much difficulty. In contrast, acute chest pain associated with angina may mark the beginning of a life of fear and uncertainty for the client.

Chronic Pain

Psychosocial factors that influence chronic pain vary. Some are similar to those found in the acute pain experience, such as anxiety or fear related to the meaning of the pain for each client. Because pain persists in the chronic situation or is perhaps only partially relieved, the client may feel powerless, angry, hostile, or desperate. The client with chronic pain is also vulnerable to labels such as "chronic complainer" or "fake." Because many of the behavioral manifestations of acute pain (e.g., sweating, writhing, increased blood pressure) are absent in the client with chronic pain, the caregiver might doubt the existence of the pain. In some chronic pain conditions (e.g., myofacial pain disorders), there may be an absence of objective physical findings that corroborate the report of pain. This may produce problems of depression, difficulties socializing, and conflicts with others. Clients may

need outside assistance to resolve their illness-specific controversies with others.

The status of family and other close relationships, along with the breadth of social resources available to the chronic pain client, must be assessed. The existence of pain-specific conflict with a spouse or significant other may affect or limit pain coping strategies (Faucett, 1994). Other people may react to chronic pain with depression, social withdrawal, and preoccupation with physical symptoms.

If the pain is chronic and associated with a progressive disease, such as cancer, rheumatoid arthritis, or peripheral vascular disease, the client may have worries and concerns about the consequences of the illness. Clients suffering from cancer-related pain may fear death or body mutilation. Some may think that they are being punished for some wrongdoing in life. Others may attach a religious or spiritual significance to lingering pain and may think that suffering on earth exemplifies the experience of pain so often associated with those in the Bible.

The nurse asks open-ended questions (e.g., "Tell me how your pain has affected your job or role as a mother") to allow the client to describe personal attitudes about pain and its influence on his or her life. This opportunity can help a client whose life has been changed by pain. However, some clients choose not to share private information or fears related to the meaning of their pain readily, and this decision should be respected by the nurse.

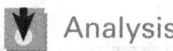 Analysis

> *Common Nursing Diagnoses and Collaborative Problems*

The actual diagnoses for a client with pain are divided into two main categories:

- Pain
- Chronic Pain

The etiologic factors are not included here because they vary, depending on the cause of the pain and each client's response.

> *Additional Nursing Diagnoses and Collaborative Problems*

In addition to the common nursing diagnoses, the client experiencing acute or chronic pain may have one or more of the following nursing diagnoses:

- Anxiety related to loss of control
- Fear related to pain
- Powerlessness related to illness-related regimen
- Altered Role Performance related to a change in health status and impaired coping
- Altered Sexuality Patterns related to illness and pain
- Impaired Physical Mobility related to pain and discomfort
- Activity Intolerance related to pain and/or depression
- Sleep Pattern Disturbance related to pain
- Self-Care Deficit (total or partial) related to pain
- Altered Health Maintenance related to a feeling of hopelessness

> *Pain*

 Planning and Implementation

Pharmacologic measures are the major means used to relieve acute pain. Nonpharmacologic measures, such as the use of a pillow for splinting an incision and complementary therapies, are also effective, but these measures are usually used in conjunction with drug therapy.

Drug Therapy. Clients who achieve adequate analgesia during the postoperative phase experience fewer complications and have shorter recovery periods than clients who have a significant degree of pain (Acute Pain Management Guideline Panel, 1992). Nurses must ensure that clients receive adequate interventions to manage their pain.

Nonopioid Analgesics. Many people underestimate the effectiveness of nonopioid analgesics, also referred to as peripheral-acting analgesics. Acetylsalicylic acid (ASA; aspirin, Ancasal♣), 650 mg, and acetaminophen (Datril, Tylenol, Ace-Tabs♣), 650 mg (which are nonopioids), produce pain relief comparable to that of codeine, 32 mg orally, and meperidine (Demerol), 50 mg orally, which are opioids, for mild pain. Aspirin has direct analgesic effects because it inhibits prostaglandin synthesis in the presence of inflammation.

Over-the-counter (OTC) medications are not given alone for the treatment of severe pain. They are usually administered in conjunction with opioid analgesics. Aspirin or aspirin-containing compounds must be used with caution after surgery because they can irritate the gastrointestinal tract and interfere with platelet aggregation. The nurse monitors the client carefully for bleeding and bruising.

Nonsteroidal anti-inflammatory drugs (NSAIDs) are also popular nonopioids that possess anti-inflammatory properties, largely by inhibiting prostaglandins. Ketoprofen (Orudis), also an NSAID, seems to block the synthesis of leukotrienes, which also sensitize the nociceptors. These drugs are particularly useful in the management of acute inflammation caused by tissue destruction. Parenteral ketorolac (Toradol) is one of the most popular NSAIDs prescribed by physicians for short-term use in cases of acute pain. Unlike other NSAIDs, this drug is available in both oral and parenteral form. Table 9–3 outlines the NSAIDs most commonly prescribed for acute pain.

The side effects of NSAIDs are similar to those of aspirin—gastric irritation and upset, renal toxicity and effects on coagulation. They can also cause sodium and water retention, which is of special concern in elderly clients, who can easily develop congestive heart failure from fluid retention. The elderly may also be more at risk for renal toxicity and should be monitored closely with renal function blood values. The nurse observes for and teaches the client and family to observe for these untoward effects of medication.

Opioid Analgesics. Opioid analgesics (also called opioids or narcotics) are central-acting analgesics that are the cornerstone of pharmacologic acute pain management (Acute Pain Management Guideline Panel, 1992). These drugs work by binding with opioid receptors, both within and outside of the central nervous system. For acute pain, they may be administered by the oral, rectal, intramuscular, intraspinal, intravenous, or subcutaneous route.

Classification of Opioids. Opioid analgesics are classified as full agonists, partial agonists, or mixed agonist-antagonists. "Full agonists produce a maximal response within the cells to which they bind; partial agonists produce a lesser response; and mixed agonist-antagonists activate one type of opioid receptor while simultaneously blocking another type" (Acute Pain Management Guideline Panel, 1992, p. 17).

The most important type of opioid receptor is the mu receptor. Commonly used opioids that bind with mu (mu opioids) are short-acting morphine (Roxanol, MSIR, Statex♣); controlled-released morphine (MS Contin, Oramorph); hydromorphone (Dilaudid); codeine; short-acting oxycodone (Roxicodone) and in combination with acetaminophen (Percocet, Roxicet, Tylox), controlled-released oxycodone (OxyContin), meperidine (Demerol), and fentanyl (Sublimaze). Clients receiving these agonists should not receive mixed agonist-antagonists, such as pentazocine (Talwin), nalbuphine (Nubain), butorphanol (Stadol), or tramadol (Ultram), or partial agonists like buprenorphine because they may negate the effect of the agonists. Table 9–4 lists common opioid agonists with dosing guidelines and additional information.

Meperidine (Demerol) used to be routinely prescribed by physicians after surgery because it was mistakenly

TABLE 9-3

Nonsteroidal Anti-Inflammatory Drugs for the Treatment of Acute Pain

Drug	Usual Adult Dose	Comments
Oral NSAIDs		
Acetaminophen	650–975 mg q 4 hr	Acetaminophen lacks the peripheral anti-inflammatory activity of other NSAIDs
Aspirin	650–975 mg q 4 hr	The standard against which other NSAIDs are compared. Inhibits platelet aggregation; may cause postoperative bleeding
Choline magnesium trisalicylate (Trilisate)	1000–1500 mg bid	May have minimal antiplatelet activity; also available as oral liquid
Diflunisal (Dolobid)	1000 mg initial dose followed by 500 mg q 12 hr	
Etodolac (Lodine)	200–400 mg q 6–8 hr	
Fenoprofen calcium (Nalfon)	200 mg q 4–6 hr	
Ibuprofen (Motrin, others)	400 mg q 4–6 hr	Available as several brand names and as generic; also available as oral suspension
Ketoprofen (Orudis)	25–75 mg q 6–8 hr	
Magnesium salicylate	650 mg q 4 hr	Many brands and generic forms available
Meclofenamate sodium (Meclomen)	50 mg q 4–6 hr	
Mefenamic acid (Ponstel)	250 mg q 6 hr	
Naproxen (Naprosyn)	500 mg initial dose followed by 250 mg q 6–8 hr	Also available as oral liquid
Naproxen sodium (Anaprox)	550 mg initial dose followed by 275 mg q 6–8 hr	
Salsalate (Disalcid, others)	500 mg q 4 hr	May have minimal antiplatelet activity
Sodium salicylate	325–650 mg q 3–4 hr	Available in generic form from several distributors
Parenteral NSAID		
Ketorolac	30 or 60 mg IM initial dose followed by 15 or 30 mg q 6 hr Oral dose following IM dosage: 10 mg q 6–8 hr	Intramuscular dose not to exceed 5 days

Acute Pain Management Guideline Panel. (1992). *Acute pain management: Operative or medical procedures and trauma. Clinical practice guideline* (pp. 110–111). AHCPR Pub. No. 92–0032. Rockville, MD: Agency for Health Care Policy and Research, Public Health Service, U.S. Department of Health and Human Services.

thought to possess certain advantages over morphine and other opioids. Often, an insufficient amount was prescribed, resulting in less than optimal pain control. Meperidine is only effective for 2.5 to 3.5 hours, and a dose of 75 mg is equivalent to only 5 to 7.5 mg of morphine.

ELDERLY CONSIDERATIONS

Elderly clients and those with renal disease should not take meperidine because of the prolonged half-life of its drug metabolite normeperidine (Acute Pain Management Guideline Panel, 1992). Normeperidine, an excitotoxin, accumulates with repeated dosing and can lead to life-threatening seizures. The drug is also contraindicated in elderly clients, as they may excrete the metabolite more slowly, making them more at risk for cerebral irritation, which leads to seizures, memory loss, hallucinations, paranoia, and depression (Hofland, 1992). Some

institutions have established guidelines to restrict the use of meperidine, monitor the duration of therapy, and offer alternative choices for the use of other opioids.

All mu opioids may cause urinary retention, constipation, sedation, respiratory depression, and nausea and vomiting. Urinary retention and respiratory depression are less common among opioid-dependent clients or those who take opioids for extended periods. Opioid-induced side effects generally correlate with the blood level of the medication. The nurse observes for these problems and reports their occurrence to the physician. The nurse remembers that pain and the stress and anxiety that accompany it are potent respiratory *stimulants* that may negate the respiratory depressive action of the drugs. The nurse also keeps in mind that the effect of all opioid analgesics may be potentiated in a client who is elderly, has reduced blood volume or renal disease, or has received anesthetic agents or other central nervous system depressants.

TABLE 9-4

Dosing Guidelines for Opioids in the Treatment of Acute Pain*†

Drug	Approximate Equianalgesic Oral Dose	Approximate Equianalgesic Parenteral Dose	Recommended Starting Dose (Adults More Than 50 kg Body Weight)		Recommended Starting Dose (Children and Adults Less Than 50 kg Body Weight)‡	
			Oral	Parenteral	Oral	Parenteral
Opioid Agonist						
Morphine§	30 mg q 3–4 hr (around-the-clock dosing) 60 mg q 3–4 hr (single dose or intermittent dosing)	10 mg q 3–4 hr	30 mg q 3–4 hr	10 mg q 3–4 hr	0.3 mg/kg q 3–4 hr	0.1 mg/kg q 3–4 hr
Codeine¶	130 mg q 3–4 hr	75 mg q 3–4 hr	60 mg q 3–4 hr	60 mg q 2 hr (intramuscular/subcutaneous)	1 mg/kg q 3–4 hr**	Not recommended
Hydromophone§ (Dilaudid)	7.5 mg q 3–4 hr	1.5 mg q 3–4 hr	6 mg q 3–4 hr	1.5 mg q 3–4 hr	0.06 mg/kg q 3–4 hr	0.015 mg/kg q 3–4 hr
Hydrocodone (in Lorcet, Lortab, Vicodin, others)	30 mg q 3–4 hr	Not available	10 mg q 3–4 hr	Not available	0.2 mg/kg q 3–4 hr**	Not available
Levorphanol (Levo-Dromoran)	4 mg q 6–8 hr	2 mg q 6–8 hr	4 mg q 6–8 hr	2 mg q 6–8 hr	0.04 mg/kg q 6–8 hr	0.02 mg/kg q 6–8 hr
Meperidine (Demerol)	300 mg q 2–3 hr	100 mg q 3 hr	Not recommended	100 mg q 3 hr	Not recommended	0.75 mg/kg q 2–3 hr
Methadone (Dolophine, others)	20 mg q 6–8 hr	10 mg q 6–8 hr	20 mg q 6–8 hr	10 mg q 6–8 hr	0.2 mg/kg q 6–8 hr	0.1 mg/kg q 6–8 hr
Oxycodone (Roxicodone, also in Percocet, Percodan, Tylox, others)	30 mg q 3–4 hr	Not available	10 mg q 3–4 hr	Not available	0.2 mg/kg q 3–4 hr**	Not available
Oxymorphone§ (Numorphan)	Not available	1 mg q 3–4 hr	Not available	1 mg q 3–4 hr	Not recommended**	Not recommended
Opioid Agonist-Antagonist and Partial Agonist						
Buprenorphine (Buprenex)	Not available	0.3–0.4 mg q 6–8 hr	Not available	0.4 mg q 6–8 hr	Not available	0.004 mg/kg q 6–8 hr
Butorphanol (Stadol)	Not available	2 mg q 3–4 hr	Not available	2 mg q 3–4 hr	Not available	Not recommended
Nalbuphine (Nubian)	Not available	10 mg q 3–4 hr	Not available	10 mg q 3–4 hr	Not available	0.1 mg/kg q 3–4 hr
Pentazocine (Talwin, others)	150 mg q 3–4 hr	60 mg q 3–4 hr	50 mg q 4–6 hr	Not recommended	Not recommended	Not recommended

*__Note:__ Published tables vary in the suggested doses that are equianalgesic to morphine. Clinical response is the criterion that must be applied for each client; titration to clinical response is necessary. Because there is not complete cross tolerance among these drugs, it is usually necessary to use a lower than equianalgesic dose when changing drugs and to retitrate to response.

†__Caution:__ Recommended doses do not apply to clients with renal or hepatic insufficiency or other conditions affecting drug metabolism and kinetics.

‡__Caution:__ Doses listed for clients with body weight less than 50 kg cannot be used as initial starting doses in babies less than 6 months of age. Consult the *Clinical Practice Guideline for Acute Pain Management: Operative or Medical Procedures and Trauma* section on management of pain in neonates for recommendations.

§For morphine, hydromorphone, and oxymorphone, rectal administration is an alternate route for clients unable to take oral medications, but equianalgesic doses may differ from oral and parenteral doses because of pharmacokinetic differences.

¶__Caution:__ Codeine doses above 65 mg often are not appropriate due to diminishing incremental analgesia with increasing doses but continually increasing constipation and other side effects.

**__Caution:__ Doses of aspirin and acetaminophen in combination opioid/NSAID preparations must also be adjusted to the client's body weight.

Acute Pain Management Guideline Panel. (1992). *Acute pain management: Operative or medical procedures and trauma. Clinical practice guideline* (pp. 112–113). AHCPR Pub. No. 92-0032. Rockville, MD: Agency for Health Care Policy and Research, Public Health Service, U.S. Department of Health and Human Services.

When respirations fall below 10, the nurse should rouse the client. If respirations do not increase, the health care provider typically orders naloxone (Narcan), an opioid antagonist, to reverse the respiratory depression. Naloxone can potentially reverse the effects of the opioid analgesic. Doses of more than 0.2 mgs generally reverse analgesia and precipitate acute physiologic withdrawal in clients who are opioid dependent. Smaller doses (< 0.2 mg) can be given and titrated slowly to reduce the respiratory depressant effects of opioid agonist drugs. Naloxone is always given with caution to clients who are physically dependent on opioids and only in life-threatening situations. In the hospital or nursing home setting, this drug is kept in an emergency drug box or cabinet on each unit for use as necessary.

Opioid Analgesic Regimens. Immediately after surgery or traumatic injury, the health care provider typically prescribes oral or parenteral opioid analgesics on a continuous time schedule or on an intermittent as needed (PRN) schedule. Round-the-clock dosing schedules should be used during the first 24 to 36 hours following surgery (Acute Pain Management Guideline Panel, 1992). Oral drugs are the most convenient and least expensive but should be prescribed in doses equianalgesic to parenteral ones.

When the health care provider orders an intermittent schedule, the client depends on the nurse to give the medication when requested. Not all clients will ask for medication. It is imperative for the nurse to offer the medication at the prescribed intervals and to anticipate the need for medication based on behavioral and nonverbal cues.

Use of Opioids for Substance Abusers. Acute pain management for clients who are known or suspected substance abusers is a difficult but increasingly common problem. Some hospitals have pain management teams that assist with this type of problem in managing a client's pain. The team members usually represent several disciplines, including, but not limited to, nurses, physicians, clinical pharmacists, and social workers.

Clients who are substance abusers often have traumatic injuries and other health problems that cause acute pain. Chart 9–2 lists some recommendations that the nurse can follow when planning and implementing pain management for a client who is a substance abuser. It is important for the nurse to recognize that substance abusers, typically those abusing opioids, are often tolerant to the pain-relieving effects of opioid analgesics and generally require increase doses. There is always the danger of abrupt physiologic withdrawal when recreational users of opioid agonists are given mixed agonist-antagonists and partial *agonists.*

Adjuvant Drugs for Acute Opioid Analgesia. A relatively common practice in the treatment of acute pain is the administration of adjuvant drugs—drugs that add to the action or effects of opioids. The ones most frequently used are hydroxyzine pamoate (Vistaril) and promethazine (Phenergan, Histanil✷). These drugs were once thought to potentiate the action of opioids, but evidence has shown that they enhance the sedating effects of the opioid and not the actual pain-relieving effects. They do help to relieve the anxiety and nausea that frequently follow general anesthesia and accompany acute pain. Some analgesic effects have been demonstrated with hydroxyzine alone in the treatment of postoperative pain. The nurse observes clients receiving promethazine or hydroxyzine in addition to opioid analgesics for the side effect of sedation.

Anxiolytic agents such as the benzodiazepines may be helpful in reducing the anxiety that accompanies acute pain. However, these agents do cause sedation and should be cautiously administered along with opioids.

Patient-Controlled Analgesia. Patient-controlled analgesia (PCA) is one way to combat the problem of inadequate analgesia in the management of acute and chronic pain. This method allows the client to control the dosage of opioid analgesia received. This approach to pain control can improve pain relief and increase client satisfaction. It can also decrease the amount of opioid consumption per day when compared with intermittent dosing methods.

Clients receiving medication on an as needed basis for postoperative pain must sense the pain, report it to the nurse, and wait until the nurse is aware of the client's need and has the time to administer the analgesic. Considerable time may pass in this sequence because the client may wait too long before asking for the medication. Alternatively, the nurse may not understand the need to respond promptly to the request, or the nurse may have other equally pressing responsibilities. Whatever the reasons, the client's pain may be more severe or out of control by the time the analgesic is received. More medication is then required to relieve the pain adequately.

However, clients who have ready access to an analgesic are more likely to medicate themselves before the pain becomes severe, and thus they may require a reduced

---

Chart 9–2

Nursing Care Highlight: Pain Management for the Substance Abuser

- Define the exact source(s) of pain and treat them; e.g., heat for muscle spasms, antibiotics for infection.
- Follow the principles of opioid use, such as not giving agonist-antagonists to clients receiving opioid agonists.
- Use nonopioid therapies, including medication, cutaneous stimulation techniques, and cognitive and behavioral strategies.
- Monitor the client for drug abuse while in the health care agency to ensure that drugs are not being stolen or hoarded.
- Set limits and negotiate with the client about drug choices and dosing.
- Provide clear instructions about drug use and dosing schedules.
- Consult with other members of the health care team, such as physicians, psychiatrists, psychologists, pharmacists, and social workers.

Data from the Acute Pain Management Guideline Panel. (1992). *Acute pain management: Operative or medical procedures and trauma. Clinical practice guideline.* AHCPR Pub. No. 92-0032. Rockville, MD: Agency for Health Care Policy and Research, Public Health Service, U.S. Department of Health and Human Services.

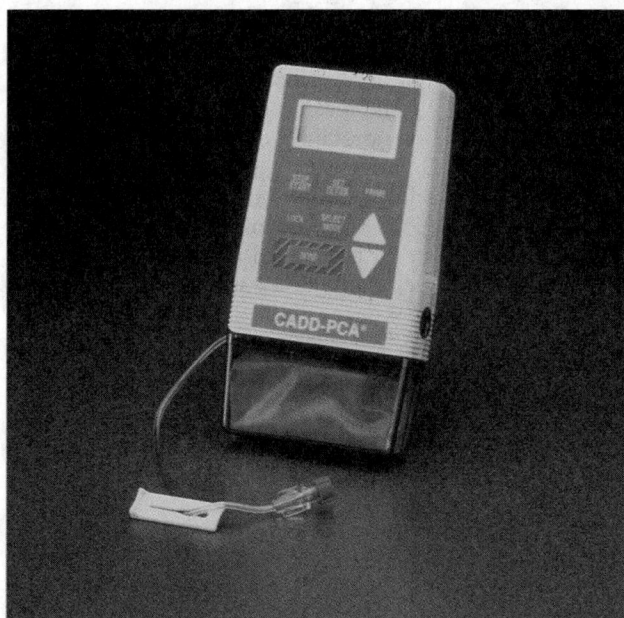

Figure 9–6. An ambulatory patient-controlled analgesia (PCA) infusion pump. (CADD-PCA is a registered trademark of Pharmacia Deltec.)

amount. Having control over when the drug can be administered also reduces the client's anxiety, which helps relieve pain.

Patient-controlled analgesia is achieved through the use of a PCA infusion pump (Fig. 9–6). Both stationary pole pumps for hospital use and ambulatory pumps for nursing home or home use are available. The infusion pump delivers the desired amount of medication through a conventional intravenous route for acute pain. The most commonly used drug for PCA is morphine. However, the use of PCA hydromorphone (Dilaudid) and fentanyl (Sublimaze) is gaining popularity. Meperidine (Demerol) is still reserved for short-term use, usually less than 48–72 hours, because its toxic metabolite, normeperidine, which is capable of inducing confusion and seizures, may accumulate in the blood.

Drug security to avoid overdosing is achieved through a locked syringe pump system or locked drug reservoir system. The device is programmed to deliver a certain amount of drug within a specific interval known as a lockout interval. The physician specifies the amount of the demand dose. Morphine doses typically range from 1 to 2 mg; hydromorphone, 0.15 to 0.4 mg; fentanyl, 12.5 to 25.0 μg; and meperidine, 10 to 15 mg. Doses may vary according to the client's degree of pain and tolerance for opioids. The lockout interval is usually 5 to 15 minutes.

The nurse programs the dosing parameters into the PCA delivery device. When the client presses the button or pendant (on ambulatory pumps), the appropriate bolus or demand dose is delivered. If the client attempts access to the drug before the designated time interval between doses has elapsed, no drug will be administered. With this technique, there is little chance of clients overmedicating themselves.

The PCA regimen may consist of a demand-dosing-only schedule or a continuous infusion or basal rate and demand dosing. With demand or self-administered dosing only, the client relies soley on a push of the pendant or bolus feature of the device to seek pain relief. Continuous or basal infusions of the opioid in addition to demand dosing provide more consistent analgesia and allow the client to sleep without fear of missing pain medication. The usual morphine dose prescribed by the health care provider for postoperative pain is 1 to 2 mg per hour; hydromorphone, 0.15 to 0.4 mg per hour; and fentanyl, 12.5 to 25.0 μg. A continuous infusion of meperidine is not recommended. When a continuous infusion is added to the regimen, clients may be at greater risk for opioid-induced side effects (i.e., nausea and vomiting, sedation, respiratory depression), especially if the hourly dose is too much for the client.

The nurse's role in caring for clients using PCA is to teach them how to use the device and to report side effects, such as dizziness, nausea and vomiting, and inability to void. As with all opioids, the nurse monitors the client's vital signs frequently—at least every 4 hours. In some cases, the nurse may need to anticipate the client's need for pain medication and administer doses of the drug if the client is unable to do so. For example, the client who is confused or cannot move may need the nurse to push the pump button to administer the drug. The physician specifies the PCA demand doses, or bolus amounts, along with the lockout interval.

Epidural Analgesia. *Epidural* analgesia, also known as peridural or extradural analgesia, refers to the instillation of a pain-blocking agent, usually an opioid analgesic alone or in combination with a local anesthetic into the epidural space (the space between the dura mater and the vertebral column). Epidural analgesia is far more popular for management of acute pain, such as postoperative pain. It has been used since the 1950s, but it has become more popular as newer and more innovative approaches to acute pain control are explored. Epidural analgesia is used with clients who are predisposed to respiratory complications, including those undergoing thoracic surgery, those with pre-existing respiratory disease, and those who are obese.

Morphine (preservative free) and fentanyl (Sublimaze) are the most commonly used opioids for epidural administration. A local anesthetic such as bupivacaine, which affects both sensory and motor nerves, may be given alone or in combination with an opioid. Low concentrations of local anesthetics are used to avoid significant sensory and motor deficits that can accompany epidural anesthesia. With the introduction of ropivacaine, a new local anesthetic that is selective for sensory nerves, the incidence of lower motor weakness is far less (Cederholm, 1997).

A temporary externalized epidural catheter is used for acute pain control. This device is not sutured to the skin and is easily dislodged. The nurse tapes the catheter in two places to anchor it properly. Some clinicians do not recommend transparent dressings, because the catheter may be dislodged when the dressing is removed. The catheter is generally placed in either the lumbar or thoracic region. Rarely is the catheter placed above the level of sixth thoracic vertebra, as the diaphragmatic muscle may be affected by the analgesia.

Complications of Epidural Analgesia. In caring for a client with epidural analgesia, the nurse helps to prevent associated complications, monitors the client for them, and implements prescribed medical therapies for managing side effects (Polomano et al., 1993). Complications that occur with epidural analgesia are directly related to catheter placement, catheter maintenance, and the type of analgesic used.

Pruritus (itching) and nausea and vomiting are common side effects of epidural opioids. Pruritus is treated with a small amount of naloxone (Narcan) first. Because epidural-induced pruritus does not appear to be mediated by histamine release, diphenhydramine (Benadryl, Allerdryl✦) may not be effective in relieving itching and may only work via its sedating effects. The physician usually prescribes an antiemetic for nausea and vomiting.

Infection results from failure to maintain aseptic technique during catheter placement, direct drug instillation, and infusion solution and tubing changes. Infection also results from failure to maintain aseptic conditions for indwelling catheters at the site of insertion or at the site of tube junctions. To prevent infections, the nurse ensures that all catheter line connections are secure and that an occlusive sterile dressing is maintained over the catheter site.

ELDERLY CONSIDERATIONS

The nurse also observes the elderly or restless client carefully for possible dislodgement of the catheter. The older client may become confused or disoriented as a result of surgery and try to pull out the temporary catheter. The catheter usually stays in place for about 48–72 hours, depending on the reason for the analgesia and the hospital policy.

Clients who receive epidural opioids are also at risk for respiratory depression resulting from high plasma and/or cerebrospinal fluid concentrations of the instilled drug. Clients receiving just epidural therapy with local anesthetic are not at risk for respiratory depression. Morphine, because of its potential for greater rostral or vertical spread up the spinal cord, is more likely to cause respiratory depression than fentanyl. When a larger distribution of analgesia is required, such as for the relief of pain from extensive abdominal wounds, morphine is preferred to fentanyl.

The nurse monitors respirations frequently and immediately reports to the physician respiratory rates below 10 per minute during and after the administration of epidural opioids. Opioid-induced respiratory depression usually occurs within the first few hours after the administration of fentanyl but may not be seen for 12 hours or more when morphine is given. This complication is managed by the administration of low doses (< 0.2 mg) of naloxone (Narcan), either intravenously or intramuscularly.

Urinary retention is another common problem associated with epidural analgesia, but it occurs no more frequently than postoperative urinary retention in clients not receiving epidural analgesia. Although the cause is not clear, this problem usually occurs during the first or second day of analgesia administration and may be treated with bethanecol chloride (Urecholine) or intermittent urinary catheterization. The incidence of this complication is less than 25% and is more likely to occur in men than in women (Wild & Coyne, 1992).

Lower motor weakness is more common when an epidural local anesthetic is used. Clients who get out of bed for the first time should be assisted by the nurse to determine the degree, if any, of leg weakness.

Intrapleural Opioid Analgesia. While not commonly used, local anesthetics may be administered via the intrapleural route to achieve pain control. This method is sometimes used postoperatively for clients who have had a videothoracoscopy and less frequently for open thoracotomy (chest surgery) (Polomano et al., 1993).

Placebos. The clinical use of placebos in non–research-based therapies has not been shown to have a sustained effect on pain relief. McCaffery's definition of a placebo is "any medical treatment (medication or procedure, including surgery) or nursing care that produces an effect in a patient because of its implicit or explicit or nursing care therapeutic intent and not because of its specific nature (physical or chemical properties)" (1979, p. 160). Placebos are substances or actions that produce an effect regardless of their intrinsic known value. When a client responds favorably to a placebo, it is known as the *placebo effect.*

Some clients who receive placebos report pain relief. Evidence has shown that these clients release endogenous opiates, such as endorphins, because of the power of suggestion, trust in the caregiver's interventions, or belief that something, regardless of what it is, will help the pain. A client's favorable response to a placebo does not mean that the pain was not real or was imaginary. Placebos should never be used to determine whether a client's pain is real. Even clients with documented physiologic causes for pain can respond favorably to placebos.

Placebos are sometimes used incorrectly and unethically. For example, placebos such as intramuscular saline may be administered and the client informed that the injection contains a pain medication. This practice deceives the client and perpetuates mistrust in caregivers and the health care system. Some health care providers are concerned that placebos may not be legal; therefore, they are not used in many settings.

Physical Measures. Physical measures may be used instead of or in addition to drug therapy for the relief of acute pain. Cutaneous stimulation strategies to relieve pain have been in use for many years. Various types of stimulation to the skin and subcutaneous tissue produce pain relief. Mobily et al. (1994) have identified areas of nursing practice that are critical to the successful implementation of cutaneous stimulation. Nurses play an important role in educating clients about these techniques. Methods of cutaneous stimulation include techniques such as

- Transcutaneous electrical nerve stimulation (TENS)
- Application of heat, cold, and pressure
- Therapeutic touch

- Massage
- Vibration

Whatever the method, several characteristics of cutaneous stimulation must be considered:

- The benefits of these techniques are highly unpredictable and may vary from application to application.
- Pain relief is generally sustained only as long as the stimulation continues.
- Multiple trials may be necessary to establish the desired effects.
- Stimulation itself may aggravate pre-existing pain or may produce new pain.

Despite these drawbacks to cutaneous stimulation, these methods are effective in the management of both acute and chronic pain. These techniques have physiologic as well as psychological effects on the client. The use of cutaneous stimulation techniques also gives clients an opportunity to participate actively in the management of their pain.

Transcutaneous Electrical Nerve Stimulation. Transcutaneous electrical nerve stimulation (TENS) involves the use of a battery-operated device capable of delivering small electrical currents to the skin and underlying tissues. The first-generation, or conventional, TENS unit is used most frequently. Electrodes connected to a small box are placed over the painful sites. The voltage or current is regulated by adjusting a dial to the point at which the client perceives a prickly, "pins and needles" sensation. The current is adjusted on the basis of the client's degree of pain relief and level of comfort.

The physician, nurse, or physical therapist (depending on the health care setting) assists the client in applying the electrodes either on the painful area or above or below it (Fig. 9–7). A conducting substance (usually a gel) is placed between the electrode and the client's skin.

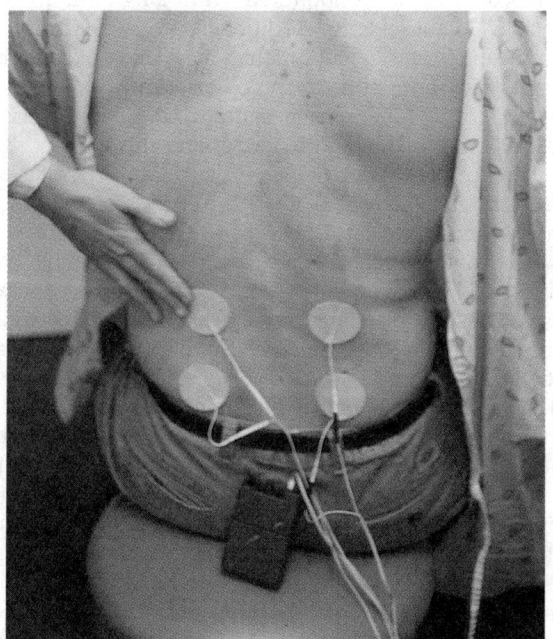

Figure 9–7. Application of a TENS unit.

The advantages of these units are that the client can wear the unit and achieve a level of pain relief while participating in activities of daily living. The unit is easy to use and can be worn for several hours. However, the skin at the site of the electrode placement may become irritated. To prevent this, the nurse teaches the client to rotate electrode sites.

In general, clients use TENS units for the management of both acute and chronic pain. This type of therapy is indicated for localized pain, such as postoperative or local chronic pain, particularly low back pain (Fishbain et al., (1996).

Other Cutaneous Techniques. Additional cutaneous stimulation techniques, such as the use of touch, pressure, massage, and vibration, as well as the application of heat and cold, stimulate the skin and somehow interrupt the pain pathway. These interventions are relatively easy for the client to learn and are fairly economical. Table 9–5 summarizes these techniques.

Cognitive and Behavioral Strategies. Cognitive and behavioral strategies to relieve pain, such as distraction, have also been popular for years, either as adjuncts to drug therapy or as alternative interventions. Theoretical explanations for the effectiveness of these measures reflect the premises of the gate control theory.

Distraction can be an effective method of acute pain relief. Simple measures such as holding a client's hand, taking the client for a walk, or encouraging deep breathing exercises can divert attention from the pain. Nurses often observe that clients request less pain medication when family members are present. After visiting hours are over, many clients request something for pain. Instead of viewing distraction as a therapeutic pain relief measure, some nurses may question the presence or severity of the pain if a client is easily distracted from it.

Distraction alters the perception of pain, but it does not influence the cause or peripheral mechanism of pain. It is a transient method of pain relief and is probably best used with other pain control measures.

Nurses can provide several methods of distraction. Visual distractors, such as pictures or television, can divert the client's attention to something pleasant or interesting. Auditory distractors, which include music or relaxation tapes, can have a calming effect. Changing the environment can remove unpleasant stressors or reminders that may enhance the client's pain. Physical distractions, such as deep breathing exercises, help the client concentrate on other physiologic sensations.

Distraction is used for

- Exacerbations of pain
- Painful procedures (e.g., dressing changes or invasive procedures)
- Interrupting the client's constant perception of pain

➤ *Chronic Pain*

 Planning and Implementation

The client is expected to experience a reduction in or relief of the pain, modification of the pain, or prevention of the recurrence or worsening of the pain.

TABLE 9–5

Cutaneous Stimulation Techniques Used to Interrupt the Pain Pathway		
Technique	**Method of Application**	**Comments**
Therapeutic touch or "laying on of hands"	• The hands of the caregiver are placed on or close to the client's body.	• The intent to help on the part of the caregiver may contribute to the success of this technique. This technique may extend the nurse-client relationship.
Pressure	• A hand or other object is placed firmly over or around the painful area.	• Pressure seems to relieve pain, decrease bleeding, and prevent swelling. Release of pressure is associated with increased blood flow and return of pain.
Massage	• The hands or fingers are moved slowly or briskly over a body part. A lubricant or other substance is sometimes used.	• Effects include muscle relaxation and sedation.
Vibration	• Electrical and battery-operated vibrators produce a massage effect.	• Vibration may decrease the intensity of the noxious (pain) stimuli.
Application of heat and cold	• Heat may be applied in a variety of ways, including short-wave diathermy, microwave diathermy, sonography, use of melted paraffin and Hubbard tank, use of hot water bottle or heating pad, use of heat cradle and lamp, application of moist pads or towels, use of hot tub or shower, or use of gel packs. • Cold may be applied in a dry or moist way, similar to heat applications. Ice chips, cold towels and packs, and chilled gel packs are commonly used.	• Both heat and cold may reduce muscle spasm and decrease pain. Cold probably slows the conduction velocity of nerves. Heat increases the tendency for bleeding and therefore should not be used after trauma. Heat may also increased edema and is not indicated if circulation is poor. Both heat and cold should be used cautiously if clients have impaired sensation or cannot communicate.

Data from McCaffery, M. (1979). *Nursing management of the patient with pain* (2nd ed., pp. 117–126). Philadelphia: J. B. Lippincott.

The goals for chronic pain management are accomplished by interrupting the relentless cycle of pain, anxiety, and sometimes depression. Nonsurgical methods of pain reduction are generally used before surgical techniques are tried. The client may eventually need a combination of nonsurgical and surgical measures.

Nonsurgical Management. A pharmacologic approach to the treatment of chronic pain is the most effective and reliable method of pain management. Other measures may be used in combination with drug therapy.

Drug Therapy. Although a number of drugs have been used in the management of chronic pain, the physician most commonly prescribes nonopioid and opioid analgesics.

Nonopioid Analgesics. Acetylsalicylic acid (aspirin, Ancasal✦), acetaminophen (Tylenol, Ace-Tabs✦), and nonsteroidal anti-inflammatory drugs (NSAIDs) such as ibuprofen (Motrin, Amersol✦) are effective in the management of mild chronic pain. They are also effective in combination with opioid analgesics. Aspirin and NSAIDs possess anti-inflammatory properties, in that they peripherally inhibit prostaglandins. This property makes them particularly useful in treating the inflammation associated with arthritis and cancer. The requirements for opioid analgesics in the client with chronic pain can be reduced by aspirin and NSAIDs. However, both aspirin and NSAIDs can cause gastric disturbances and can have an

effect on platelets, which results in a tendency toward bleeding. The nurse observes the client for gastric discomfort or vomiting and bleeding or bruising and reports these problems to the physician immediately. NSAIDs can cause renal toxicity; therefore, renal function blood tests should be routinely monitored with long-term therapy, especially in the elderly. Additionally, NSAIDs can cause sodium and water retention that may lead to congestive heart failure, more often in the older client.

Salicylates (choline magnesium trisalicylate [Trilisate]) also have anti-inflammatory effects, and this class of drugs has certain benefits. Compared with aspirin, salicylates cause less gastrointestinal upset and are less toxic to the kidneys and have little effect on platelet aggregation. These advantages make salicylates a more favorable alternative to NSAIDs in clients undergoing cancer therapy, those at risk for bleeding, and elderly clients who may be more susceptible to the renal effects of NSAIDs (see Table 9–6).

The health care provider also commonly prescribes acetaminophen for chronic pain. Acetaminophen exerts its analgesic action by blocking peripheral pain receptors, thus increasing the threshold of these receptors to painful stimuli. Reports of liver toxicity have been associated with higher doses of this drug (1000 mg) taken more frequently than every 4 hours for long-term use. Current recommendations restrict the total daily amount of acetaminophen to no more than 4000 mg or 4 g. Therefore, nurses must check all combination analgesic products for

TABLE 9–6

Nonopioid Analgesics for Chronic Pain		
Drug	**Usual Dose for Adults and Children ≥50 kg Body Weight**	**Usual Dose for Children* and Adults† ≤50 kg Body Weight**
Acetaminophen and Over-the-Counter NSAIDs		
Acetaminophen‡	650 mg q 4 h 975 mg q 6 h	10–15 mg/kg q 4 h 15–20 mg/kg q 4 h (rectal)
Aspirin§	650 mg q 4 h 975 mg q 6 h	10–15 mg/kg q 4 h 15–20 mg/kg q 4 h (rectal)
Ibuprofen (Motrin, others)	400–600 mg q 6 h	10 mg/kg q 6–8 h¶
Prescription NSAIDs		
Carprofen (Rimadyl)	100 mg tid	
Choline magnesium trisalicylate (Trilisate)**	1,000–1,500 mg tid	25 mg/kg tid
Choline salicylate (Arthropan)**	870 mg q 3–4 h	
Diflunisal (Dolobid)††	500 mg q 12 h	
Etodolac (Lodine)	200–400 mg q 6–8 h	
Fenoprofen calcium (Nalfon)	300–600 mg q 6 h	
Ketoprofen (Orudis)	25–60 mg q 6–8 h	
Ketorolac tromethamine (Toradol)‡‡	10 mg q 4–6 h to a maximum of 40 mg/day	
Magnesium salicylate (Doan's, Magan, Mobidin, others)	650 mg q 4 h	
Meclofenamate sodium (Meclomen)§§	50–100 mg q 6 h	
Mefenamic acid (Ponstel)	250 mg q 6 h	
Naproxen (Naprosyn)	250–275 mg q 6–8 h	5 mg/kg q 8 h
Naproxen sodium (Anaprox)	275 mg q 6–8 h	
Sodium salicylate (Generic)	325–650 mg q 3–4 h	
Parenteral NSAIDs		
Ketorolac tromethamine (Toradol)‡‡,¶¶	60 mg initially, then 30 mg q 6 h intramuscular dose not to exceed 5 days	

Management of Cancer Pain Guideline Panel. (1994). *Management of cancer pain: Clinical practice guidelines* (pp. 48 and 49). AHCPR Pub. No. 94-0592. Rockville, MD: Agency for Health Care Policy and Research, Public Health Service, U.S. Department of Health and Human Services.
*Only drugs that are FDA approved as an analgesic for use in children are included.
†Acetaminophen and NSAID dosage for adults weighing less than 50 kg should be adjusted for weight.
‡APAP lacks the peripheral anti-inflammatory and antiplatelet activities of the other NSAIDs.
§The standard against which other NSAIDs are compared. May inhibit platelet aggregation ≥1 week and may cause bleeding. Aspirin is contraindicated in children with fever or other viral disease because of its association with Reye's syndrome.
¶Not FDA approved for use in children as an over-the-counter drug; has FDA approval for use in children as a prescription drug for fever. However, clinicians have experience in prescribing ibuprofen for pain in children.
**May have minimal antiplatelet activity.
††Administration with antacids may decrease absorption.
‡‡For short-term use only.
§§Coombs-positive autoimmune hemolytic anemia has been associated with prolonged use.
¶¶Has the same GI toxicities as oral NSAIDs.
NOTE: Only the above NSAIDs have FDA approval for use as simple analgesics, but clinical experience has been gained with other drugs as well.

their acetaminophen content and caution the client regarding maximum dosing.

Capsaicin (Zostrix), an over-the-counter cream, can be applied to the skin in painful areas. Its pain-relieving qualities lie in its ability to deplete the painful site of substance P, a pain mediator. The preparation is marketed for painful arthritis, diabetic neuropathy, and other chronic pain conditions. For the first few applications, the cream produces noticeable pain as the release of substance P is intensified, but, this can be alleviated with the addition of a local anesthetic cream or ointment. Regular applications are recommended to sustain its pain-relieving properties.

Adjuvant Drugs. Other nonopioid drugs that are used to control the pain of certain neuralgias (pain along the distribution of nerves) or nerve injury pain include carbamazepine (Tegretol, Mazepine✦), phenytoin (Dilantin), and valproic acid (Depakene). The exact mechanism of action of these drugs is unknown, but it is believed that they inhibit or reduce the paroxysmal firing of nerve impulses. Both carbamazepine and phenytoin are associated with a wide variety of side effects (hematopoietic, hepatic, and pulmonary effects and central nervous system toxicity). Therefore, these drugs are used with extreme caution.

Tricyclic antidepressants, such as amitriptyline (Elavil), nortriptyline (Pamelor), imipramine (Tofranil), desipramine, and doxepin (Sinequan) may be beneficial in the treatment of chronic neuropathic pain. Both tricyclic antidepressants and other antidepressants like trazodone (Desyrel), fluoxitine (Prozac), paroxitine (Paxil), and sertraline (Zoloft) help treat the depression that can accompany chronic pain. They also stimulate the activity of endogenous opiates (endorphins and enkephalins) by increasing levels of serotonin, a neurotransmitter. Perhaps the greatest advantage of this group of drugs, particularly the tricyclic antidepressants, is the sedative effect, which can be helpful in promoting sleep when administered at bedtime.

In some cases, antianxiety agents help relax the client and thus help relieve pain. The physician selects the drugs that have the fewest side effects, because many of these drugs cause confusion, drowsiness, and hypotension. Examples of drugs that may be ordered include alprazolam (Xanax), clorazepate (Tranxene, Novoclopate✦), lorazepam (Ativan), and oxazepam (Serax, Zapex✦). Clonazepam (Klonopin), also used for anxiety, has been shown to be particularly helpful for certain types of nerve injury pain.

Oral local anesthetics such as mexilitine (Mexitil) act by suppressing aberrant electrical activity of both peripheral nerves and neurons in the CNS. They are useful for lancinating, electric shock-like pain, and continuous pains. Mexilitine is contraindicated for clients who have cardiac conduction defects or arrhythmias or are currently taking cardiac antiarrhythmic medications.

Opioid Analgesics. Opioid analgesics are drugs capable of relieving pain by binding to various opiate receptors located in the central nervous system (see the discussion under Nursing Interventions for Pain). For chronic pain, opioids are more commonly administered by the oral route; however, other acceptable routes include transdermal, rectal, sublingual, subcutaneous, intravenous, or intraspinal.

An equianalgesic guide (Table 9–7) can help determine the appropriate dose conversions when switching routes of a drug or from one drug to another. Equianalgesic refers to the dose and route of administration of one drug that produces approximately the same degree of analgesia as the given dose and route of another drug. Most commonly, 10 mg of morphine is the standard dose against which other opioids are measured. Equianalgesic opioid drug guides only provide the comparative analgesic potencies among these drugs. Dose modifications may be necessary according to each client's response to the drugs. When converting from one opioid to another in clients on higher than usual opioid amounts, the new opioid should be started at one half of the equianalgesic dose. This is because incomplete cross-tolerance between opioids may occur.

Considerations with Long-Term Use of Opioids. The side effects of opioid analgesics are discussed under Nursing Interventions for Pain. The long-term use of these agents is associated with some concerns.

Physical Dependency. Physical dependency is associated with the administration of opioids on a long-term basis. Physical dependency is *not* the same as addiction. However, it is sometimes confused with addiction. Nursing textbooks and resource materials often fail to make the appropriate distinctions (Ferrell et al., 1992a). Physical dependency is a physiologic adaptation of the body tissues that requires continued administration of the drug for normal tissue function. When a client who has become physically dependent on opioids abruptly ceases using them, so-called withdrawal symptoms result. These symptoms result from autonomic nervous system responses, which include nausea and vomiting, abdominal cramping, muscle twitching, profuse perspiration, delirium, and convulsions. When it is necessary to discontinue opioid analgesia for a client who is opioid dependent, a slow tapering, or weaning, of the drug dosage lessens or alleviates physical withdrawal symptoms.

Addiction. Addiction is a common fear of health professionals who administer or prescribe opioids and of clients who receive them. Addiction is a term used to describe persistent craving and abuse of a drug for recreational purposes. Addiction is a psychologic phenomenon, not a physical one. Physical dependence does occur in many people who become addicted; however, it does not define the problem of addiction. Although addiction rarely occurs in clients who use opioids for medicinal relief of pain, the fear of addiction is a major factor contributing to the inadequate prescription and administration of opioid analgesics.

Clients also worry about becoming addicted to analgesics (Champlin, 1992). They may be concerned about the possibility of drug withdrawal symptoms, which are often associated with the "street addict." The nurse clarifies the term addiction with clients while stressing the concept of physical dependency.

Drug Tolerance. The client may also experience drug tolerance from opioid analgesic therapy. Tolerance is

TABLE 9–7

Dose Equivalents for Opioid Analgesics in Opioid-Naive Adults*

Drug	Approximate Equianalgesic Dose		Usual Starting Dose for Moderate to Severe Pain	
	Oral	Parenteral	Oral	Parenteral
Opioid Agonist†				
Morphine‡	30 mg q 3–4 h (repeat around-the-clock dosing) 60 mg q 3–4 h (single dose or intermittent dosing)	10 mg q 3–4 h	30 mg q 3–4 h	10 mg q 3–4 h
Morphine, controlled-release†§ (MS Contin, Oramorph)	90–120 mg q 12 h	N/A	90–120 mg q 12 h	N/A
Hydromorphone§ (Dilaudid)	7.5 mg q 3–4 h	1.5 mg q 3–4 h	6 mg q 3–4 h	1.5 mg q 3–4 h
Levorphanol (Levo-Dromoran)	4 mg q 6–8 h	2 mg q 6–8 h	4 mg q 6–8 h	2 mg q 6–8 h
Meperidine (Demerol)	300 mg q 2–3 h	100 mg q 3 h	N/R	100 mg q 3 h
Methadone (Dolophine, other)	20 mg q 6–8 h	10 mg q 6–8 h	20 mg q 6–8 h	10 mg q 6–8 h
Oxymorphone‡ (Numorphan)	N/A	1 mg q 3–4 h	N/A	1 mg q 3–4 h
Combination Opioid/NSAID Preparations¶				
Codeine** (with aspirin or acetaminophen)	180-200 mg q 3–4 h	130 mg q 3–4 h	60 mg q 3–4 h	60 mg q 2 h (IM/SC)
Hydrocodone (in Lorcet, Lortab, Vicodin, others)	30 mg q 3–4 h	N/A	10 mg q 3–4 h	N/A
Oxycodone (Roxicodone, also in Percocet, Percodan, Tylox, others)	30 mg q 3–4 h	N/A	10 mg q 3–4 h	N/A

*Caution: Recommended doses do not apply for adult patients with body weight less than 50 kg. For recommended starting doses for children and adults <50 kg body weight, see Table 9–4.

†Caution: Recommended doses do not apply to patients with renal or hepatic insufficiency or other conditions affecting drug metabolism and kinetics.

‡Caution: For morphine, hydromorphone, and oxymorphone, rectal administration is an alternate route for patients unable to take oral medications. Equianalgesic doses may differ from oral and parenteral doses because of pharmokinetic differences.

§Transdermal fentanyl (Duragesic) is an alternative option. Transdermal fentanyl dosage is not calculated as equianalgesic to a single morphine dosage. See the package insert for dosing calculations. Doses above 25 μg/hr should not be used in opioid-naive patients.

¶Caution: Doses of aspirin and acetaminophen in combination opioid-NSAID preparations must also be adjusted to the patient's body weight. Aspirin is contraindicated in children in the presence of fever or other viral disease because of its association with Reye's syndrome.

**Caution: Codeine doses above 65 mg often are not appropriate because of diminishing incremental analgesia with increasing doses but increasing nausea, constipation, and other side effects.

NOTE: Published tables vary in the suggested doses that are equianalgesic to morphine. Clinical response is the criterion that must be applied for each patient; titration to clinical responses is necessary. Because there is not complete cross-tolerance among these drugs, it is usually necessary to use a lower-than-equianalgesic dose when changing drugs and to retitrate to response.

N/A = not available; N/R = not recommended.

Management of Cancer Pain Guideline Panel. (1994). *Management of cancer pain: Clinical practice guidelines* (pp. 52 and 53). AHCPR Pub. No. 94-0592. Rockville, MD: Agency for Health Care Policy and Research, Public Health Service, U.S. Department of Health and Human Services.

characterized by a gradual resistance of the body to the effects of an opioid, including its pain-relieving properties. When tolerance occurs, clients usually require more of the drug to achieve the same analgesic effects. Tolerance should be recognized, and appropriate analgesic plans should be designed to account for increased opioid requirements at times of acute exacerbations of chronic or procedural-related pain. Issues with sedation and analgesia for clients with cancer can be especially difficult (Polomano, et al., 1997).

Tolerance to opioid analgesics is particularly a problem in clients who are substance abusers (see Chart 9–2). Keep in mind that tolerance is measured not only by the analgesic effects but also by the body's ability to adjust to the adverse reactions.

Continuous Intravenous Opioid Analgesia. For chronic cancer pain management, hourly doses of continuous opioid infusions vary, depending on the severity of the pain and the client's tolerance to the opioid. If the hourly dose needs to be increased, the physician usually increases it no more than 10% to 20% of the hourly rate and no sooner than every 3 to 4 hours. It may be necessary for the nurse to monitor the client's vital signs frequently (at least every hour) until an adequate and safe level of drug is achieved.

Patient-controlled analgesia (PCA) can provide effective relief of chronic pain. Although the principles of how PCA works are the same for both and acute and chronic pain, dosing guidelines and methods of administration differ. PCA for chronic pain, typically cancer pain, can be administered either by intravenous or subcutaneous routes. The idea is to provide most of the analgesia in a continuous rate. The physician calculates demand doses based on the amount of continuous hourly opioid administration. Usually the PCA demand dose is a minimum of 33% of the basal or continuous rate, but sometimes it may be as high as 100% of the hourly rate. The lockout interval, unlike in PCA for acute pain, is usually longer, between 20 and 30 minutes. Longer lock-out intervals with higher demand doses keep the client from having to work hard at managing the pain.

Continuous Subcutaneous Opioid Analgesia. Continuous subcutaneous opioid analgesia is best for clients who have compromised venous access or for those whose central venous lines are being used for other fluids (Haviley et al., 1992). Subcutaneous infusion is accomplished through the use of a small (25- or 27-gauge) butterfly-type catheter or a special subcutaneous needle device placed under the skin into the subcutaneous tissue.

Typically, the subclavicular tissue underneath the clavicle or the abdomen is used. Placing the catheter in the extremities should be avoided, if possible, especially in terminally ill clients, because peripheral circulation may be impaired or edema may be present, possibly affecting absorption of the drug. The nurse applies an occlusive dressing over the site and rotates the site every 3 to 7 days, depending on the drug and the volume delivered. The physician usually orders no more than 3 to 6 mL per hour.

Morphine is the most common drug given by this route. Occasionally, hydromorphone (Dilaudid) is used; however, this drug is more irritating to the tissues, requiring more site changes. If the physician orders a PCA demand-dosing schedule in addition to the continuous infusion, the volume of the bolus dose does not usually exceed 1 mL. In addition, the lockout interval, or time between doses that the client may access more opioids, is usually no more frequent than 30 to 60 minutes. Clients receiving continuous narcotic infusions with a PCA feature may require dose adjustments in their continuous rates if more than 6 to 12 bolus doses per day are used.

The nurse observes for and reports complications of subcutaneous infusion, which include leakage of fluid around the insertion site, inadequate pain relief, and edema around the site (Haviley et al., 1992).

Neuraxial Delivery of Analgesia. Neuraxial drug delivery involves the epidural, subarachnoid or intrathecal, and intraventricular routes. Neuraxial administration is sometimes referred to as the intraspinal route. There are two major methods for administering intraspinal analgesia: epidural and intrathecal. Intraspinal therapy is particularly useful for intractable pain that is refractory to systemic opioids (Rauck, 1997) or patients who may not be able to tolerate the effects of systemic opioid analgesics.

Long-term epidural analgesia, also known as peridural or extradural analgesia, refers to the instillation of a pain-blocking agent, usually an opioid analgesic alone or in combination with a local anesthetic, into the epidural space (the space between the dura mater and the vertebral column) through an externalized catheter (Fig. 9–8), an implantable port, or an implantable drug delivery system. *Intrathecal* (subarachnoid) analgesia, in which a pain-blocking agent is introduced into the space between the arachnoid mater and pia mater of the spinal cord where cerebrospinal fluid is located, is the route of choice for long-term management (>3 months) of intractable pain.

Action of Intraspinal Analgesia. The goal of both types of intraspinal analgesia is to interrupt the conduction of pain at the point that the sensory fibers exit from the spinal cord. Morphine (preservative free) is the opioid of choice for long-term intraspinal administration; however, fentanyl (Sublimaze) and hydromorphone (Dilaudid) may also be used. The addition of a local anesthetic, such as bopivacaine or ropivacaine, may provide an opioid-sparing effect and is often considered for many intractable neuropathic pain syndromes. For intraspinal analgesia, lower concentrations of local anesthetics are used to minimize significant sensory and motor deficits that often accompany intraspinal anesthesia. Similar to opioids, tolerance may also develop to local anesthetics, necessitating increasing doses over time.

Long-Term Intraspinal Analgesia. Long-term intraspinal opioid administration may be used for the management of chronic, intractable (uncontrollable or unyielding) pain, usually from cancer. A permanent *epidural catheter* may be inserted. Several catheter devices are available for this purpose. The DuPen Silastic catheter (Davol) is the most commonly used *external* catheter. A portion of the catheter exits the skin, where drugs can be intermittently injected, or the catheter can be attached to an infusion device for continuous drug administration.

Implantable devices are also used. The epidural Port-A-Cath (SIMS Deltec, Inc.) is implanted under the skin, and the catheter portion is inserted into the epidural space. Like the DuPen catheter, this device can be injected with drugs intermittently or can be connected to an infusion device for continuous opioid delivery. Injectable ports have been shown to reduce the incidence of catheter dislodgement and early infection. (de Jong & Kansen, 1994). Systems that consist of either an externalized catheter or a drug delivery device are rarely used for intrathecal or subarachnoid drug administration. The SynchroMed pump (Medtronic, Inc.) is a totally implantable system that contains a drug reservoir, which is filled on a routine basis and is capable of continuously administering a certain volume of drug each day (Fig. 9–8).

Side effects of intraspinal opioids are more common in clients who have had little exposure to opioids in the past. Clients who receive intraspinal therapy are usually

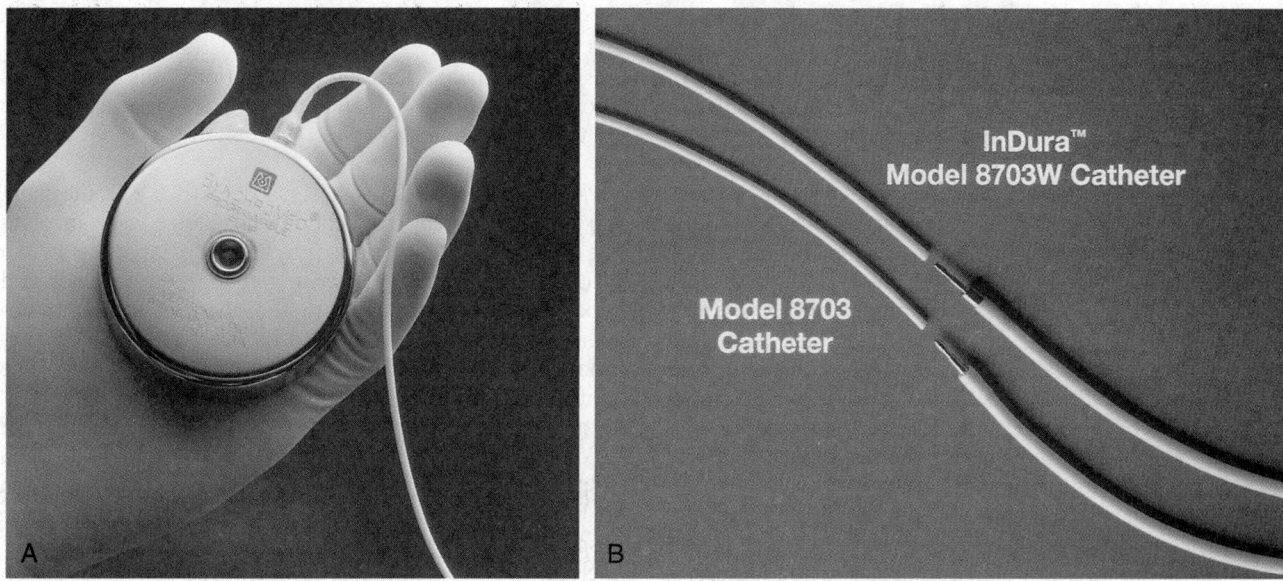

Figure 9–8. A SynchroMed implantable pump (*A*) and spinal catheters (*B*) for delivery of a precise volume of long-term intraspinal analgesia each day. (Courtesy of Medtronic, Inc., Columbia Heights, MN.)

more tolerant of the effects of opioids and may not require the rigorous monitoring needed for postoperative analgesia. Some male clients on long-term spinal opioids may complain of sexual dysfunction, decreased libido, and difficulty maintaining an erection, whereas female clients may experience amenorrhea (Paice et al., 1994). If sexual problems occur in male clients, testosterone injections seem to help improving sexual function.

Transdermal Opioid Administration. Transdermal opioid administration is now possible with the transdermal fentanyl system (Duragesic). Duragesic is available in patch dose strengths of 25 mcg/hr, 50 mcg/hr, 75 mcg/hr, and 100 mcg/hr. This system is used for clients who can take nothing by mouth, have difficulty taking pills, or cannot comply with their analgesic regimen. Duragesic is reserved for those with continuous and relatively stable pain. Because of the extended length of time needed to achieve steady state optimal serum concentrations of the opioid, the application of a Duragesic patch is supplemented with intermittent opioid administration of short-acting opioids. Intermittent "rescue" dosing should continue if the client has periods of episodic pain requiring an increased need for opioid analgesia. Duragesic should be used for clients with a known opioid requirement that is effective in relieving pain as it is difficult to titrate quickly to pain relief.

The system is applied by removing the adhesive backing and placing it on the skin of the client's chest, either front or back, preferably on an area without hair. If hair is present on the chest, the nurse clips it. Once the patch is applied, it delivers a specified amount of drug into the skin. The drug absorbs over 72 hours. The physician calculates the appropriate dosage from the client's previous opioid requirement; if the requirement is known, the lowest patch strength is used initially. Transdermal administration should be used cautiously when the requirement is *not* known.

The nurse teaches the client and family how to apply the patch and to report side effects, such as dizziness, sedation, nausea, or a decrease in respiratory rate, to the physician or nurse. The nurse also explains that when the patch is first applied, it may take up to 24 hours before pain relief is apparent. Supplemental analgesia with short-acting opioids is usually ordered until adequate blood levels of the transdermal drug are reached. The absorption of transdermal analgesics is affected by the client's body temperature. The nurse teaches the client and family that a fever of 102° F (38.9° C) or greater might accelerate absorption of the drug from the skin and increase side effects. Clients should be monitored closely for increased effects of the medication, such as sedation when fever is present. Once the system is removed, the client is monitored for about 24 hours, as the drug may still be released into the bloodstream from the site of application.

Complementary Therapies. Cognitive and behavioral strategies including imagery, relaxation, hypnosis, and biofeedback, are often effective in the relief of chronic pain. Analgesic therapy is an essential component of pain management, but cognitive and behavioral strategies may be effectively used in addition to and sometimes instead of drug therapy. A recent study provided support for the value of progressive muscle relaxation and guided imagery for the attenuation of cancer pain (Sloman, 1995). Subjects in this study reported a significant reduction in pain sensation, present pain intensity, overall pain severity, and the consumption of nonopioid analgesic medication. However, these interventions failed to reduce the affect or worry associated with pain, suggesting that knowledge of the potential threat to life that can accompany a cancer diagnosis was not relieved by these techniques.

Imagery. Imagery is a form of distraction in which the client is encouraged to visualize or think about some pleasant or desirable feeling, sensation, or event. Guided imagery takes place when a person, frequently a nurse, assists the client in sustaining a sequence of thoughts aimed at diverting the client's attention away from pain. Clients require intense concentration to visualize images. Clients who are extremely anxious, agitated, or unable to concentrate may benefit first from mild distraction.

Imagery is particularly useful with clients who experience chronic pain. Clients who practice this technique can mentally experience sights, sounds, smells, events, or other sensations vividly. First, the nurse assesses the client's level of concentration to determine if he or she can sustain a particular thought or thoughts for a desired time. The time interval for mental imagery can vary from 5 to 60 minutes. Behaviors that are helpful in assessing a client's capacity for imagery include the following:

- Reading and comprehending the newspaper
- Listening to music or other auditory stimuli
- Having the ability to follow and participate in sustained conversation
- Having an interest in environmental surroundings

When the client has demonstrated some ability to concentrate, the nurse assists the client in identifying a pleasant or favorable thought. The client is then encouraged to focus on this thought to divert attention away from painful stimuli. Audiotapes may help clients form and maintain images. The nurse, client, or family may wish to create such tapes for the client's use, or commercially available tapes may be used. An example of guided imagery instructions follows: "Imagine yourself on the beach on some deserted island. You can hear the sound of waves rushing onto the shore, the cry of sea gulls flying high above, and the rustling of trees as they are brushed gently by the wind. You can feel the warmth of the sun over your body and the cooling breeze."

Relaxation Techniques. Clients may use relaxation techniques to reduce anxiety, tension, and emotional stress, which may exacerbate pain. Techniques to help clients relax can be both physical and psychological. Physical techniques include

- The client receiving a body massage, back rub, or warm or hot bath
- Modifications in the client's environment to reduce distractions
- The client moving into a comfortable position.

Psychological techniques include

- The use of pleasant conversation
- The use of music
- The use of relaxation tapes

There are relaxation tapes that assist the client with progressive relaxation of the muscles. Relaxation exercises can be effectively coupled with guided imagery, distraction, and hypnosis. Chapter 8 describes relaxation techniques in detail.

Hypnosis. Hypnosis is defined as an altered state of consciousness in which a person enters a trance and loses an overall sense of reality. Although the person is in a trance, he or she has some sense of awareness and contact with reality and an understanding of what is actually happening. Hypnosis is used to treat a variety of pain syndromes, particularly chronic pain. It is used to help clients overcome the emotional consequences of pain and can promote a positive state of mind. Although nurses do not usually teach clients hypnosis, they are in a key position to help clarify misconceptions, instruct clients about relaxation and distraction, and encourage clients to practice self-hypnosis.

Biofeedback. Biofeedback is used to treat chronic pain, anxiety, and other stress conditions. Biofeedback involves the monitoring of various physiologic responses by an electric device capable of sensing changes in the body and reporting this information to the client. Certain physiologic signals are transmitted to the feedback unit by electrode sensors, which are placed on the client's skin. The biofeedback unit amplifies and transforms physiologic information into visual signals (usually meter readings or colored lights). Clients are first alerted to stress-related responses, such as increased muscle tension or elevation in blood pressure. Then they are taught to regulate these responses through a combination of techniques, which include deep breathing exercises, progressive relaxation exercises, distraction, and visual imagery.

Biofeedback units vary. Some measure muscle contraction via electromyography and brain activity via electroencephalography. Galvanic skin response and skin temperature, which can reflect changes in blood flow, heart rate, or blood pressure, are also measured. Whatever the technique, physiologic responses that tend to worsen or prolong the client's pain are voluntarily controlled.

The client who is interested in learning biofeedback techniques to control pain is usually trained by a skilled therapist. The client is taught to observe the feedback information, report sensations or feelings that become apparent, and practice stress-reducing or pain-reducing techniques. Clients may need several sessions before they can recognize and control these responses. The client eventually becomes aware of even the most subtle changes in body function that indicate the onset or worsening of pain and automatically responds without the help of the biofeedback unit.

Biofeedback training helps the client gain control over pain. Clients require training and self-discipline if biofeedback and all other cognitive therapy strategies are to be used effectively.

Invasive Pain Management Techniques for Chronic Pain. Invasive techniques are used to interrupt the pain pathways when pain is intractable or severely debilitating. Depending on the technique, some degree of nerve destruction and neurologic deficits is expected. When chronic or persistent pain can no longer be adequately controlled with drugs or other pain-reducing methods, various invasive techniques are used (Fig. 9–9).

Nerve Blocks. Nerve blocks can be used for both diagnostic and treatment purposes. These procedures are usually indicated for pain that is confined to a specific area or nerve distribution. The technique involves localizing a nerve root (or roots) and injecting either a local anesthetic for temporary relief or diagnostic evaluations or a chemical agent (e.g., phenol or alcohol) to achieve permanent neurolysis or destruction of the nerve(s). Nerve areas where temporary blocks or permanent destruction (neu-

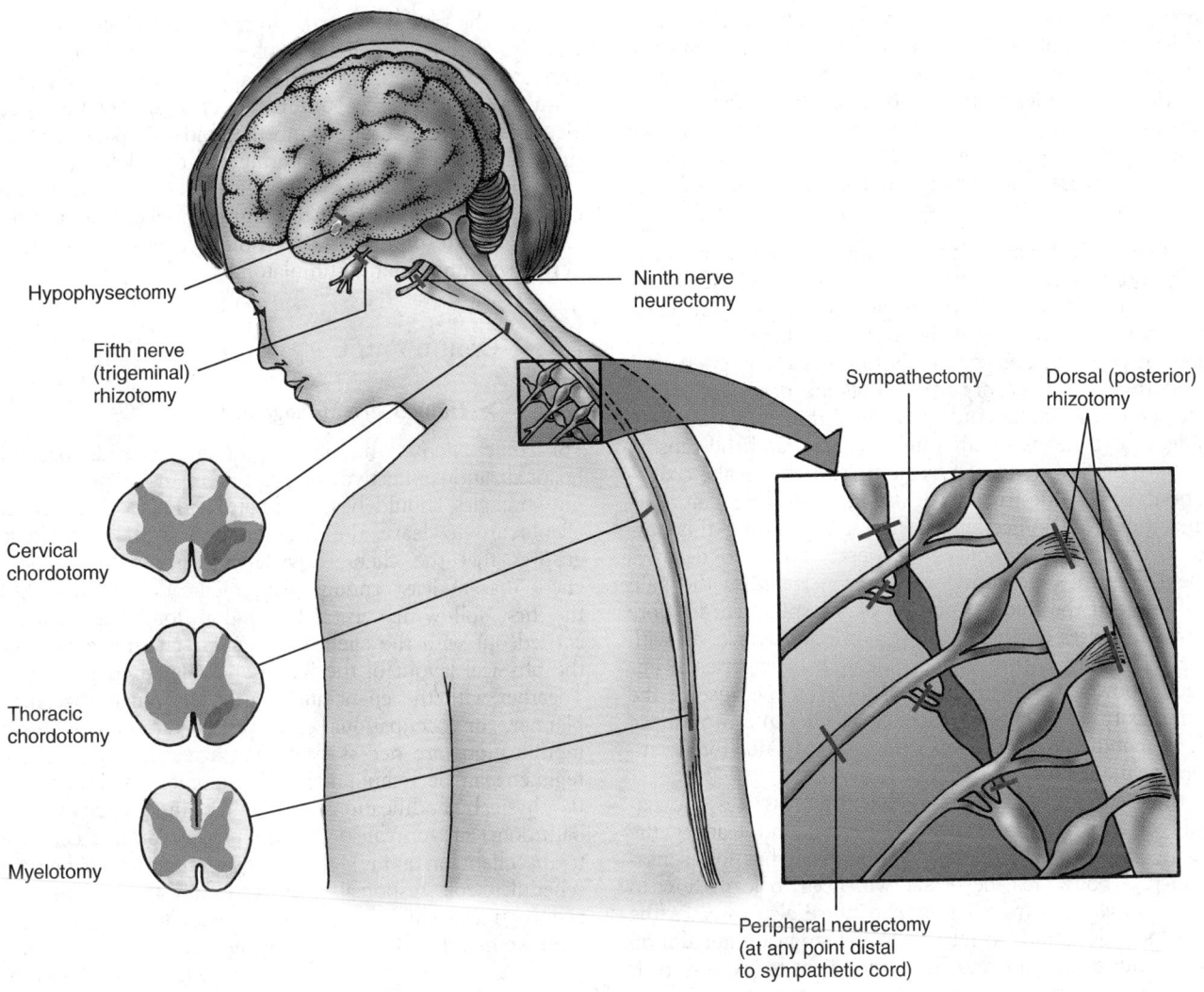

Figure 9–9. Surgical procedures designed to alleviate pain.

roablation) might be considered include intercostal nerves, celiac plexus, superior hypogastric block, or craniofacial nerves.

Complications associated with this technique vary. Injections into peripheral nerve root with local anesthetic or chemical agents generally lead to decreased sensation in the area, with no effect on motor function. Injections into the lumbosacral area of the spinal cord area with local anesthetic may cause transient motor and bowel and bladder dysfunction. However, neurolysis of lumbosacral nerves can damage motor nerve roots, resulting in lost or impaired bowel, bladder, or sexual function. This procedure is generally reserved for clients who have intractable cancer-related pain. Before permanent neurolysis is considered, a temporary nerve block may be given to determine the degree of relief if nerve impulses are disrupted. Although the intent of neurolysis is to permanently destroy nerve transmission, clients may only experience short-term pain relief because of nerve cell regeneration or the development of alternative pathways capable of transmitting pain. Although relatively new, permanent ablation of nerve roots can be done with thermal techniques

such as radiofrequency ablation, which uses heat, or cyroanalgesia, which involves cold.

Because a nerve block is an invasive procedure performed by anesthesiologists, neurosurgeons, surgeons, and neurologists, the physician is responsible for informing the client about the procedure, its risks, and alternative treatments. The nurse reinforces this information with the client and family.

Epidural steroids may also be used for pain; however, their use in certain pain conditions is controversial. Some investigators have looked at the evidence for use of epidural steroids in clients with low back pain (Koes et al., 1995). Their review of 12 randomized clinical trials found this treatment to be effective in only half of the published studies. They concluded that the benefits of epidural injection, if any, are of short duration.

Spinal Cord Stimulation. Spinal cord stimulator therapy offers a more invasive method of nerve stimulation. This technique involves the use of electrodes implanted under the skin into the area of nerve(s) responsible for the pain. At first, a trial of spinal cord stimulation is attempted through the use of temporary externalized electrodes, which are implanted and connected to an stimulator device. The amount of electrical current is adjusted to provide pain relief without additional discomfort. If successful, the client is taken to the operating room for placement of a permanent implantable stimulator. Forrest (1996) discusses the nursing implications associated with this technique.

Surgical Techniques. Some techniques aimed at surgically interrupting the transmission of pain include rhizotomy and cordotomy. With the new, improved pain management measures currently available, these procedures are not performed as commonly today (see Fig. 9–10).

In rhizotomy, sensory nerve roots are destroyed where they enter the spinal cord. In a *closed* rhizotomy, a percutaneous catheter is inserted into the area, and the sensory nerve roots are destroyed by neurolytic chemicals, coagulation, or cryodestruction (extreme cold). For an *open* rhizotomy, a laminectomy is necessary. During this surgery, the physician isolates the nerve roots and destroys them. With a cordotomy, the surgeon transects the pain pathways at the midline portion of the spinal cord before nerve impulses ascend to the spinothalamic tract. As with the other surgical procedures, clients may experience impaired bowel, bladder, or sexual function. Because of the complexity of the pain experience, the interruption of nerve conduction and pain pathways may not totally interrupt the client's sensation of pain.

After surgical intervention, the nurse assesses the nature of the neurologic deficits, if any, and teaches the client how to adapt to them. If the client has lost sensation in a body area, he or she will need to learn how to protect that area from harm. The nurse also assesses the client's expectations in relation to the surgical interruption of painful sensations and helps the client to express realistic expectations.

Stimulation Techniques. Acupuncture and dorsal column stimulation are means of achieving pain control through stimulating certain parts of the nervous system.

Acupuncture. The practice of acupuncture originated in China. According to ancient beliefs, the body is divided into 10 hypothetic sections by parasagittal lines, or meridians. Specific acupuncture points are located within these meridians. The acupuncturist inserts tiny needles into the skin and subcutaneous tissues at these points, and manual vibration or electrical stimulation is delivered. This technique is used to relieve pain and is thought to cure certain diseases.

Acupuncture is still widely acclaimed in China, but it is less popular in the West. Because the physiologic basis for this technique is unclear, many Western health professionals are skeptical about its usefulness. Nonetheless, acupuncture is practiced for anesthetic purposes during diagnostic procedures, during labor and delivery, during surgery, and for the treatment of pain. It is also used to help clients change behavior, for example, to stop smoking. More than 1000 acupuncture sites have been identified, and 14 "lines" exist as *meridians* (Fig. 9–10).

Dorsal Column Stimulation. Dorsal column stimulation is a temporary or permanent way of stimulating nerve

roots in the spinal cord to override the painful stimuli. Usually, good candidates for this procedure are those who derive some benefit from the application of transcutaneous electrical nerve stimulation (TENS). Percutaneous electrodes can be inserted into the epidural space in close proximity to nerve roots entering the dorsal horn of the spinal cord. The electrodes are then connected to an external device capable of delivering an electrical current. Clients who respond to this technique may go on to have permanent implantable stimulators.

 Continuing Care

> *Home Care Management*

For some clients, the pain experience extends beyond hospitalization. Effective analgesic regimens or pain-relieving strategies should be coordinated prior to discharge if clients are to leave the hospital with pain. The nurse ensures that the client, especially the opioid-dependent client, has at least enough pain medication to last until the first follow-up visit. Preparation for home care is carried out with the client and family. The nurse assesses the physical layout of the home and related environment. Together with the client and family, the nurse, discharge planner, or occupational therapist determines whether modifications are necessary so that a reasonably pain-free regimen can be maintained after the client is discharged. If physical modifications (e.g., installing a downstairs bathroom) are unrealistic (too expensive or unacceptable to the client or family), the caregiver suggests changes in schedules, role responsibilities, and daily routines to help avoid fatigue, which heightens the awareness of pain.

At home, clients may require referral for physical therapy, especially to continue treatment with cutaneous stimulation, TENS, or heat or cold techniques. Clients may need a psychiatric clinical nurse specialist or social worker to help them develop coping strategies or maintain adequate family dynamics. In the management of terminally ill clients, hospice referral (hospital based or within the community) can help maintain continuity of care. Clients with cancer may be at risk for developing uncontrolled pain that, if not managed at home, will result in hospitalization (Plaisance, 1997). Importantly, nurses knowledgeable about palliative care and end-of-life issues are better able to manage pain crises.

The growing number of home infusion therapy programs provides a wide variety of services to clients who require technology-supported pain care at home. Many of these services depend on insurance-carrier approval generally before analgesic options are considered and placement of technology is performed. Well-defined home agency practices and professional support at home are key if clients are required to leave the hospital with infusional pain therapy (Gorski & Grothman, 1996).

> *Health Teaching*

The nurse directs educational efforts toward involving clients and their families in continuing health care behaviors that will relieve pain and improve psychological well-being and overall functional status. The nurse teaches the

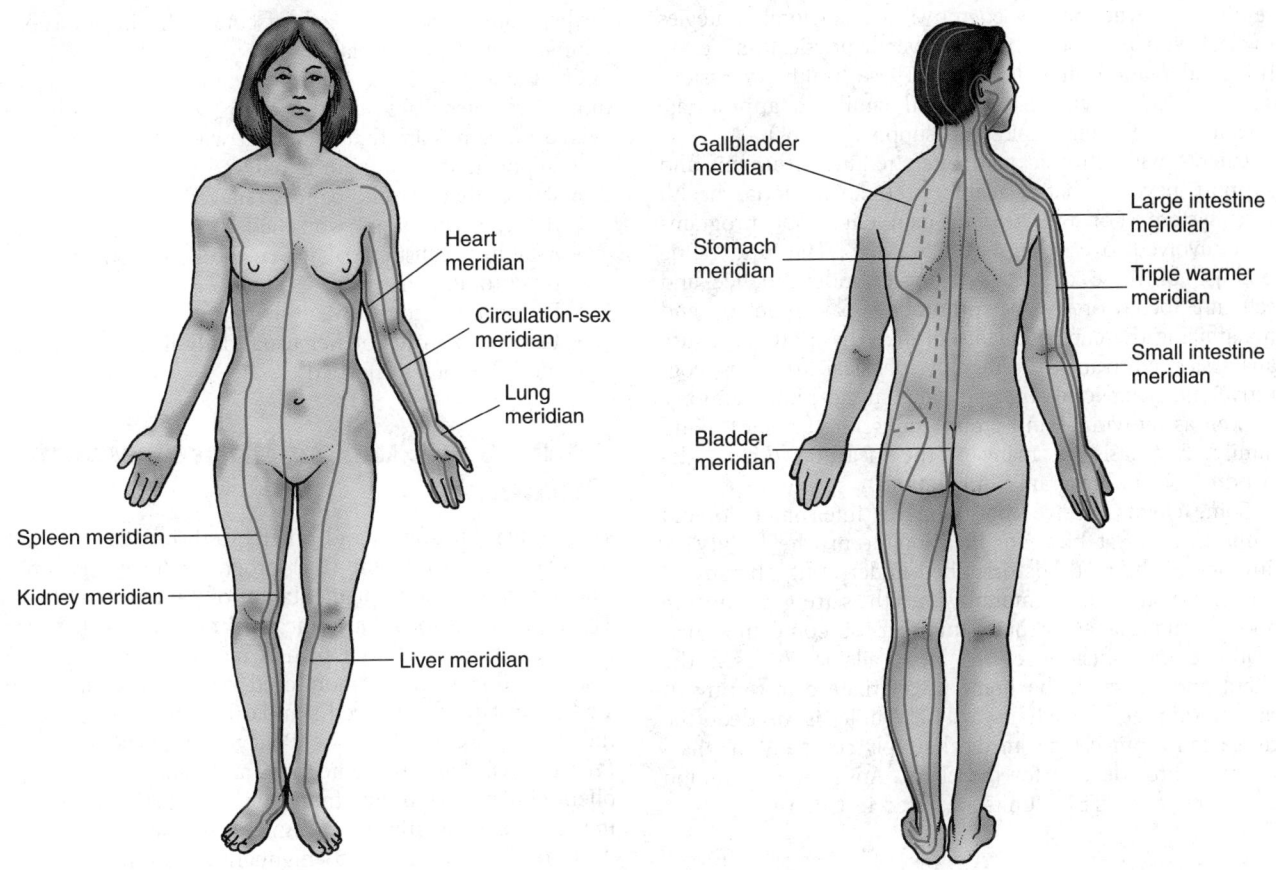

Figure 9–10. Acupuncture meridians.

client and family about analgesic regimens, the purpose and action of medications, their side effects or adverse reactions, and the importance of dosage intervals.

The nurse explains that ideally the analgesic regimen should not interfere with the client's sleep, rest, appetite, or level of physical mobility. If such interference occurs, the nurse encourages the family or significant other to consult with the physician or the visiting nurse.

In clients with pain from advanced cancer, all efforts should be directed toward maximizing pain relief and symptom control at home to eliminate unnecessary readmissions. This may mean that the physician prescribes a flexible analgesic schedule that allows the client to titrate analgesics based on the amount of pain. The nurse teaches the client and family how to safely increase the medication within the prescribed dosing guidelines.

The nurse evaluates family support systems to assist the client in adhering to and continuing the proposed medical and nursing plans. Family members are informed about and included in activities during and after hospitalization.

To achieve a reasonable level of expectation for the client, the nurse suggests ways to continue participation in household, social, sexual, and work-oriented activities after discharge. The nurse can help the client identify important activities and plan them around adequate rest schedules.

The client with chronic pain needs continued support

to cope with the anxiety, fear, and powerlessness that often accompany this type of pain. The nurse helps the client and family or significant others to identify coping strategies that have worked in the past. Outside support systems are also identified. Chapter 8 discusses stress and coping in detail.

➤ Health Care Resources

A home health nurse referral is made when it is anticipated that clients will require assistance or supervision with their pain relief regimen at home. This referral should include specific information from the hospital-based staff nurse about the client's overall physical condition, general level of sedation, weakness or fatigue, possible constipation or nutritional problems, and sleep patterns.

In addition to explaining the client's physical status to the home health nurse, the staff nurse also describes the client's levels of anxiety and depression and general expectations about pain status after discharge. The nurse describes family interactions and determines whether the client or family anticipates any altered role functions at home. The client's close relationships and available support network are important factors in providing ongoing support for effective pain intervention strategies.

Referrals to the clinical nurse pain specialist, social worker, or psychologist are appropriate ways to continue to provide emotional support to the client and family, reinforce instructions for cognitive or behavioral strategies to deal with pain, and evaluate overall physical and emotional adaptation after discharge. These health professionals can also direct the client and family to appropriate resources (e.g., pain clinics and support groups).

Clients with chronic pain often require treatment and support beyond that available in the traditional health care system. For this reason, pain clinics or programs have evolved over the past 25 years. The underlying premise of these clinics is to foster independence and self-care behaviors while promoting pain control and maximizing the client's quality of life. These programs use analgesics, adjuvant drug therapy, physical measures, cognitive and behavioral strategies, and surgical interventions, as well as individual and group counseling for clients and family. Emphasis on many of the measures differs, depending on the program's orientation.

Some clients receive continuous or intermittent opioid administration at home or in a long-term care facility by any one of the methods described under Drug Therapy. If the nurse in the community health setting is unsure about drug management, a number of companies that manufacture infusion set-ups are available to assist the client and nurse in the home or alternate care setting. If other equipment, such as a TENS unit, is needed, the nurse can arrange for a medical supply company or pharmacy to provide one for the client. Answers to common questions about TENS units are listed in Chart 9–3.

 Evaluation

Historically, inadequate attention has been given to evaluating the effects of pain interventions. Caregivers may not assess the degree of pain relief and intensity accurately or often enough. Furthermore, nurses may not establish pain relief goals that are consistent with the client and families' expectations. Because of this, the client is at risk for further pain, frustration, lack of control, feelings of abandonment, and social isolation.

On the basis of the identified nursing diagnoses, the nurse evaluates care for the client with pain. The expected outcomes are that the client will

- Report that acute pain is relieved or reduced.
- Report that chronic pain is relieved or reduced or that the pain is not worsened.
- Establish realistic goals given the limitations imposed by chronic pain.
- Perform activities of daily living.
- Participate in his or her usual daily lifestyle, with modifications as needed.

Pain as a Quality Improvement Outcome

Today, many hospitals and other health care facilities rely on quality improvement (QI) programs to evaluate pain care and direct the implementation of pain care strategies. These programs focus on critical pain outcomes that serve as indicators of how well pain is managed. Indicators are assessed, documented, monitored over time, and evaluated against predetermined standards. The introduction of the Agency for Health Care Policy and Research *Clinical Practice Guidelines* for acute pain and cancer pain (1992) offers clinicians a useful framework for designing quality improvement initiatives. The American Pain Society Quality Care Committee (1995) highlights five critical components of a QI program for pain. Programs should be based on the following tenets: 1) unrelieved pain should attract clinicians' attention; 2) information about analgesics should be accessible where orders are written; 3) clients should be assured of responsive analgesic care and urged to communicate pain; 4) policies and safeguards should be implemented for the use of technology-supported pain care; and 5) implementation of these measures should be assessed and coordinated.

Some investigators have used self-report measures of pain and assessments of analgesic therapy as a QI initiative to gauge the level of compliance with the Agency for Health Care Policy and Research Clinical Practice Guidelines for Acute Pain (1992) (Dietrick-Gallagher et al., 1994). Others have identified systems and caregivers' barriers to pain control through QI monitoring (Bookbinder et al., 1996).

Costs of Pain Care

When caring for clients with pain, the nurse appreciates the financial aspects of pain care, especially in the current climate of managed care. Kolassa (1994) identifies several factors associated with medication costs. First, costs differ depending on the location of administration. Parenteral drug therapy administered in a hospital setting may be more costly than at home. Second, the commercial success of the agent influences the price of a pharmaceutical product. Third, the type of manufacturer and history of drug development and testing influences the market price of a drug. Drug innovations like extended-release or controlled-release products may be more costly per tablet

---

Chart 9–3

Education Guide: TENS Units

- The cost of using your TENS unit should be comparable to that for a regimen of prescription drugs or surgery.
- Insurance usually covers the cost of buying or leasing a TENS unit.
- You can get a TENS unit only through the physician who prescribed it.
- Whether a TENS unit works for you will depend on your type of pain. These units have been used successfully on back pain, arm and leg pain, pain from neuralgia, arthritis pain, and other types of pain. A trial period under a physician's care is generally advised.
- TENS units are relatively simple to operate. You simply attach color-coded electrodes to your skin over the painful area. You then turn the unit on and, depending on your level of pain, you make day-to-day adjustments.

TABLE 9-8

Economics of Pain Care: Cost Analysis Framework

Costs associated with oral alternative route medications
Costs associated with parenteral/neuraxial administration
Unreimbursed charges of medication therapy
Costs of surgical interventions
Costs of specialized pain care
Costs of nondrug measures
Expenditures to justify costs
Reimbursement issues
Expenditures by various health care settings and home costs associated with preventing and treating complications of pain/pain therapy

Adapted from Agency for Health Care Policy and Research. (1994). *Clinical Practice Guidelines for Cancer Pain.* From: Ferrell, B. R., Griffith, H. (1994). Cost issues related to pain management: Report from the Cancer Pain Panel of the Agency for Health Care Policy and Research. *Journal of Pain and Symptom Management, 9*(4), 221–234.

than short-acting agents. However, the cost of the overall therapy (dose per day) may be similar or only slightly more. A cost-analysis framework for evaluating the economic implications for pain care is provided in Table 9–8).

Technology-supported pain care is always associated with increased costs, but the financial expenditures in selected populations may be worth it in terms of improved clinical outcomes. Epidural analgesia and patient-controlled analgesia in the immediate postoperative period have shown significant benefits in improving pain control and recovery, compared with intermittent nurse-administered analgesics. The use of technology in delivering analgesia may also be cost-efficient for certain clients with intractable chronic nonmalignant and cancer-related pain. Despite the inflated costs of extended-release or controlled-release preparations, clients report better compliance and achieve better pain control.

For long-term management of pain, the oral route is preferred. The nurse considers the cost of both opioid and nonopioid analgesics to ensure that the cost expenditures for drug therapy are within the client's financial budget. Knowledge of the client's prescription plan aids the nurse in assessing "out of pocket" expenses by the client. Certainly, the nurse must factor in any other health care expenditures for the client and/or family. Some pharmaceutical companies, usually manufacturers of opioid analgesics, supply indigent clients with free medication if they meet certain eligibility criteria.

Significant health care costs are associated with hospitalizations for pain control (Grant et al., 1995). The nurse recognizes the importance of aggressive pain care to facilitate discharge and prevent subsequent hospitalizations for pain.

SELECTED BIBLIOGRAPHY

*Acute Pain Management Guideline Panel. (1992). *Acute pain management: Operative or medical procedures and trauma. Clinical practice guideline.* AHCPR Pub. No. 92-0032. Rockville, MD: Agency for Health Care Policy and Research, Public Health Service, U.S. Department of Health and Human Services.

Allock, N. (1996). The use of different research methodologies to evaluate the effectiveness of programmes to improve the care of patients in postoperative pain. *Journal of Advanced Nursing, 23*(1), 32–38.

Altman, G. B., & Lee, C. A. (1996). Strontium-89 for treatment of painful bone metastasis from prostate cancer. *Oncology Nursing Forum, 23*(3), 523–527.

*American Pain Society. (1989). *Principles of analgesic use in the treatment of acute pain and chronic cancer pain: A concise guide to medical practice.* Washington, D.C.: American Pain Society.

American Pain Society Quality of Care Committee. (1995). Quality improvement guidelines for the treatment of acute pain and cancer pain. *Journal of American Medical Association, 274*(23), 1874–1880.

*Arathuzik, M. D. (1991). The appraisal of pain and coping in cancer clients. *Western Journal of Nursing Research, 13*(6), 714–731.

*Barker, E. (1987). Pain. *Journal of Neurosurgical Nursing, 19*, 233–234.

*Bonica, J. (1983). The importance of education and training in pain diagnosis and therapy. In R. Rizzi & M. Visentin (Eds.), *Pain therapy* (pp. 1–10). Amsterdam: Elsevier Biomedical.

Bookbinder, M., Coyle, N., Kiss M., Goldstein, M. L., Holritz, K., Thaler, H., Gianella, A., Derby, S., Brown, M., Racolin, A., Ho, M.-N., & Portenoy, R. K. (1996). Implementing national standards for cancer pain management: Program model and evaluation. *Journal of Pain & Symptom Management, 12*(6), 334–347.

*Burckhardt, C. S. (1990). Chronic pain. *Nursing Clinics of North America, 25*, 868–870.

*Burke, S. O., & Jerrett, M. (1989). Pain management across age groups. *Western Journal of Nursing Research, 11*, 164–178.

*Calvillo, E. R., & Flaskerud, J. H. (1991). Review of literature on culture and pain of adults with focus of Mexican-Americans. *Journal of Transcultural Nursing, 2*, 16–23.

*Calvillo, E. R., & Flaskerud, J. H. (1993). Evaluation of the pain response by Mexican-American and Anglo-American women and their nurses. *Journal of Advanced Nursing, 18*, 451–459.

*Carroll, K. C., & Magruder, C. C. (1993). The role of analgesics and sedatives in the management of pain and agitation during weaning from mechanical ventilation. *Critical Care Nursing Quarterly, 15*(4), 68–77.

Cederholm, I. (1997). Preliminary risk-benefit analysis of ropivacaine in labour and following surgery. *Drug Safety, 16*(6), 391–402.

*Champlin, L. (1992). Inadequate analgesia: Clients endure pain, fear addiction. *Geriatrics, 47*(8), 71–74.

*Clark, I. M. (1993). Management of postoperative pain. *Lancet, 341*, 27.

Clarke, E. B., French, B., Bilodeau, M. L., Capasso, V. C., & Empoliti, J. (1996). Pain management knowledge, attitudes and clinical practice: The impact of nurses' characteristics and education. *Journal of Pain & Symptom Management, 11*(1), 18–31.

Cleeland, C. S., Gonin, R., Hatfield, A. K., Edmonson, J. H., Blum, R. H., Stewart, J. A., & Pandya, K. J. (1994). Pain and pain treatment in outclients with metastatic cancer: The Eastern Cooperative Oncology Group's outpatient pain study. *The New England Journal of Medicine, 330*, 592–596.

Cleeland, C. S., & Ryan, K. M. (1994). Pain assessment: Global use of the Brief Pain Inventory. *Annals of the Academy of Medicine, Singapore, 23*(2), 129–138.

Cleeland, C. S., Nakamura, Y., Mendoza, T. R., Edwards, K. R., Douglas, J., & Serlin, R. C. (1996). Dimensions of the impact of cancer pain in a four-country sample: New information from multidimensional scaling. *Pain, 67*(2–3), 267–273.

Cobb, S. C. & Mindel, S. A. (1996). Creating a cost-effective pain management task force in a community hospital. *MEDSURG Nursing, 5*(6), 445–448.

*Deikmann, J. M., & Wassem, R. A. (1991). A survey of nursing students' knowledge of cancer pain control. *Cancer Nursing, 14*, 314–320.

deJong, P. C., & Kansen, P. J. (1994). A comparison of epidural catheters with or without subcutaneous injection ports for treatment of cancer pain. *Anesthesia and Analgesia, 78*(1), 94–100.

Dietrick-Gallagher, M., Polomano, R. C., & Carrick, L. (1994). Pain as a quality management initiative. *J Nurs Care Qual 9*(1), 30–42.

*Dobkin de Rios, M., & Achauer, B. M. (1991). Pain relief for the Hispanic burn patient using cultural metaphors. *Plastic and Reconstructive Surgery, 88*(1), 160–164.

*Donovan, M. W. (1990). Acute pain relief. *Nursing Clinics of North America, 25*, 851–861.

Dunbar, S. A., & Katz, N. P. (1996). Chronic opioid therapy for nonmalignant pain in clients with a history of substance abuse: Report of 20 cases. *Journal of Pain and Symptom Management, 11*(3), 163–171.

Eckes Peck, S. D. (1997). The effectiveness of therapeutic touch for decreasing pain in elders with degenerative arthritis. *Journal of Holistic Nursing, 15*(2), 176–198.

*Egbert, A. M. (1991). Help for the hurting elderly: Safe use of drugs to relieve pain. *Postgraduate Medicine, 89*(4), 217–228.

Faucett, J. A. (1994). Depression in painful chronic disorders: The role of pain and conflict about pain. *Journal of Pain and Symptom Management, 9*(8), 520–526.

*Ferrell, B. A., Ferrell, B. R., & Osterweil, D. (1990). Pain in the nursing home. *Journal of the American Geriatrics Society, 38*, 409–414.

Ferrell, B. R., & Griffith, H. (1994). Cost issues related to pain management: Report from the Cancer Pain Panel of the Agency for Health Care Policy and Research. *Journal of Pain and Symptom Management, 9*(4), 221–234.

*Ferrell, B. R., McCaffery, M., & Grant, M. (1991). Clinical decision making and pain. *Cancer Nursing, 14*, 289–297.

*Ferrell, B. R., McCaffery, M., & Rhiner, M. (1992a). Pain and education: An urgent need for change in nursing education. *Journal of Pain and Symptom Management, 7*(2), 117–124.

*Ferrell, B. R., McCaffery, M., & Ropchan, R. (1992b). Pain management as a clinical challenge for nursing administration. *Nursing Outlook, 40*, 263–268.

*Ferrell, B. R., McGuire, D. B., & Donovan, M. I. (1993). Knowledge and beliefs regarding pain in a sample of nursing faculty. *Journal of Professional Nursing, 9*(2), 79–88.

Ferrell, B., Whedon, M., & Rollins, B. (1995). Pain and quality assessment/improvement. *Journal of Nursing Care Quality, 9*(3), 69–85.

*Ferrell-Torry, A. T., & Glick, O. J. (1993). The use of therapeutic massage as a nursing intervention to modify anxiety and the perception of cancer pain. *Cancer Nursing, 16*, 93–101.

*Fife, B. L., Irick, N., & Painter, J. D. (1993). A comparative study of the attitudes of physicians and nurses toward the management of pain. *Journal of Pain and Symptom Management, 8*(3), 132–139.

Fishbain, D. A., Chabal, C., Abbott, A., Heine, L. W., & Cutler R. (1996). Transcutaneous electrical nerve stimulation (TENS) treatment outcome in long-term users. *Clinical Journal of Pain, 12*(3), 201–214.

*Flor, H., Fydrich, T., & Turk, D. C. (1992). Efficacy of multidisciplinary pain treatment centers: A meta analytic review. *Pain, 49*, 221–230.

Forrest, D. M. (1996). Spinal cord stimulator therapy. *Journal of Perianesthesia Nursing, 11*(5), 349–352.

*Gaston-Johansson, F., Albert, M., Fagan, E., & Zimmerman, L. (1990). Similarities in pain descriptions of four different ethnic-culture groups. *Journal of Pain and Symptom Management, 5*(2), 94–100.

Gorski, L. A., & Grothman L. (1996). Home infusion therapy. *Seminars in Oncology Nursing, 12*(3), 193–201.

Grant, M., Ferrell, B. R., Rivera, L. M., & Lee, J. (1995). Unscheduled readmissions for uncontrolled symptoms. *Nursing Clinics of North America, 30*(4), 673–682.

*Greenwald, H. P. (1991). Interethnic differences in pain perception. *Pain, 44*(2), 157–163.

*Greipp, M. (1992). Undermedication for pain: An ethical model. *Advances in Nursing Science, 15*(1), 44–53.

Guyton, A. C. (1996). *Textbook of medical physiology* (9th ed.) Philadelphia: W. B. Saunders.

Harkins, S. W. (1996). Geriatric pain. Pain perceptions in the old. *Clinics of Geriatric Medicine, 12*(3), 435–459.

*Haviley, C., et al. (1992). Pharmacological management of cancer pain: A guide for the health professional. *Cancer Nursing, 15*, 331–346.

Heiser, R. M., Chiles, K., Fudge, M., & Gray, S. E. (1997). The use of music during the immediate postoperative recovery period. *AORN Journal, 65*(4), 777–785.

*Herr, K. A., & Mobily, P. R. (1991). Complexities of pain assessment in the elderly. *Journal of Gerontological Nursing, 17*(4), 12–19.

*Herr, K. A., & Mobily, P. R. (1992). Interventions related to pain. *Nursing Clinics of North America, 27*, 347–370.

Hitchcook, L. S., Ferrell, B. R., & McCaffery, M. (1994). The experience of chronic nonmalignant pain. *Journal of Pain and Symptom Management, 9*(5), 312–318.

*Hofland, S. L. (1992). Elder beliefs: Blocks to pain management. *Journal of Gerontological Nursing, 18*(6), 19–40.

*Hyman, R. B., Feldman, H. R., Harris, R. B., et al. (1989). The effects of relaxation training on clinical symptoms: A meta-analysis. *Nursing Research, 38*(4), 216–220.

*International Association on Pain, Subcommittee of Taxonomy. (1979). Pain terms: A list with definitions and notes on usage. *Pain, 6*, 249.

*Jacox, A. K. (Ed.) (1977). *Pain: A source book for nurses and other health care professionals.* Boston: Little, Brown.

*Johnson, J., Rice, V., Fuller, S., et al. (1978). Sensory information, information in a coping strategy, and recovery from surgery. *Research in Nursing and Health, 1*, 4–17.

*Keeney, S. A. (1993). Nursing care of the postoperative patient receiving epidural analgesia. *MEDSURG Nursing, 2*(3), 191–196.

*Keller, E., & Bzdek, V. (1986). Effects of therapeutic touch on tension headache pain. *Nursing Research, 35*, 101–105.

Koes, B. W., Scholten, R. J., Mens, J. M., & Bouter, L. M. (1995). Efficacy of epidural steroid injections for low back pain and sciatica: A systematic review of randomized clinical trials. *Pain, 63*, 279–288.

Kolassa, E. M. (1994). Guidance for clinicians in discerning and comparing the price of pharmaceutical agents. *Journal of Pain and Symptom Management, 9*(4), 221–234.

*Kreiger, D. (1975). Therapeutic touch: The imprimatur of nursing. *American Journal of Nursing, 75*, 784–787.

Malek, C. J., & Olivieri, R. J. (1996). Pain management—Documenting the decision making process. *Nursing Case Management, 1*(2), 64–74.

Management of Cancer Pain Guideline Panel. (1994). *Management of cancer pain: Clinical practice guidelines.* AHCPR Pub. No. 94-0592. Rockville, MD: Agency for Health Care Policy and Research, Public Health Service, U.S. Department of Health and Human Services.

*McCaffery, M. (1979). *Nursing management of the patient with pain.* (2nd ed.) Philadelphia: J. B. Lippincott.

*McCaffery, M. (1980). Relieving pain with noninvasive techniques. *Nursing '80, 10*(12), 54–57.

*McCaffery, M. (1990). Pain management: Nurses lead the way to new priorities. *American Journal of Nursing, 90*, 45–50.

*McCaffery, M., & Beebe, A. (1989). *Pain: Clinical manual for nursing practice.* St. Louis: C. V. Mosby.

*McCaffery, M., Ferrell, B., O'Neil-Page E., Lester, M., & Ferrell, B. (1990). Nurses' knowledge of opioid analgesic drugs and psychological dependence. *Cancer Nursing, 13*(1), 21–27.

*McGuire, D. B. (1984). The measurement of clinical pain. *Nursing Research, 33*, 152–156.

McGuire, L. (1994). The nurse's role in pain relief. *MEDSURG Nursing, 3*(2), 94–107.

*Melzack, R. (1973). *The puzzle of pain.* New York: Basic Books.

*Melzack, R. (1975). The McGill Pain Questionnaire: Major properties and scoring methods. *Pain, 1*, 277–299.

*Melzack, R. (1983). The McGill Pain Questionnaire. In R. Melzack (Ed.), *Pain assessment and management* (pp. 41–47). New York: Raven Press.

*Melzack, R. (1987). The short form McGill Pain Questionnaire. *Pain, 30*, 191–197.

*Melzack, R., & Wall, P. D. (1982). *The challenge of pain.* New York: Basic Books.

Miller, J., Neelon, V., Dalton, J., Ng'andu, N., Bailey, D., Layman, E., & Hosfeld, A. (1996). The assessment of discomfort in elderly confused patients: A preliminary study. *Journal of Neuroscience Nursing, 28*(3), 175–182.

Mobily, P. R., Herr, K. A., & Nicholson, A. C. (1994). Validation of cutaneous stimulation interventions for pain management. *International Journal of Nursing Studies, 31*(6), 533–544.

Mulloney, S. S., & Wells-Federman, C. (1996). Therapeutic touch: A healing modality. *Journal of Cardiovascular Nursing, 10*(30), 27–82.

*National Institutes of Health. (1986). *The integrated approach to the management of pain: Consensus Development Conference statement.* Washington, D. C.: U.S. Government Printing Office.

*Neeley, M. A. (1993). Pain management in elderly clients. *MEDSURG Nursing Quarterly, 1*(4), 32–51.

*Neill, K. M. (1993). Ethnic pain styles in acute myocardial infarction. *Western Journal of Nursing Research, 15*(5), 531–547.

Paice, J. A., Penn, R. D., & Ryan, W. G. (1994). Altered sexual function and decreased testosterone in clients receiving intraspinal opioids. *Journal of Pain and Symptom Management, 9*, 126–131.

*Pasero, C. L. (1994). Pain control. *American Journal of Nursing, 94*(2), 22–23.

Pasero, C. L., & McCaffery, M. (1994). Avoiding opioid-induced respiratory depression. *American Journal of Nursing, 94*(4), 25–30.

Plaisance, L. (1997). Managing cancer pain crisis effectively in the home. *Home Health Nurse, 15*(6), 411–413.

Polomano, R. C. (1995). *The relationship of pain characteristics, type of cancer, and opioid consumption to quality of life, psychological distress and pain outcomes* [Unpublished doctoral dissertation]. University of Maryland, Baltimore, MD.

*Polomano, R. C., Blumenthal, N., Schiavonne-Gatto, P., & O'Brien, J. (1993). Recommendations for developing policies and procedures for the administration of continuous epidural narcotics/local anesthetics with or without patient controlled epidural analgesia. *MEDSURG Nursing, 2*(3), 195–196.

*Polomano, R. C., Blumenthal, N. P., & Riegler, F. X. (1993). Intrapleural analgesia for the management of postoperative pain. *MEDSURG Nursing, 2*(3), 185–190.

Polomano, R. C., Soulen, M., & McDaniel, C. (1997). Sedation and analgesia with interventional radiology for oncology patients. *Critical Care Nursing Clinics of North America, 9*(3), 335–353.

*Poniatowski, B. C. (1991). Continuous subcutaneous infusions for pain control. *Journal of Intravenous Nursing, 14,* 30–35.

Puntillo, K., & Weiss, S. J. (1994). Pain: Its mediators and associated morbidity in critically ill cardiovascular surgical clients. *Nursing Research, 43*(1), 31–36.

Rauck, R. L. (1997). Intraspinal therapy in the management of refractory cancer pain. *Techniques in Regional Anesthesia and Pain Management, 1*(1), 38–48.

*Ruda, M. A. (1993). Gender and pain. *Pain, 53,* 1–2.

Sloman, R. (1995). Relaxation and the relief of cancer pain. *Nursing Clinics of North America, 30*(4), 697–709.

*Sternbach, R. A. (1968). *Pain: A psychophysiological analysis.* New York: Academic Press.

*Stevens, K. (1990). Clients' perceptions of music during surgery. *Journal of Advanced Nursing, 15,* 1045–1051.

*Thomas, B. L. (1990). Pain management for the elderly: Alternative interventions (Part 1). *AORN Journal, 52,* 1268–1272.

*Vallerand, A. H., (1991). The use of narcotic analgesics in chronic nonmalignant pain. *Holistic Nursing Practice, 6*(1), 17–23.

Vallerand, A. H., (1994). Street addicts and clients with pain: Similarities and differences. *Clinical Nurse Specialist, 8*(1), 11–12.

Vallerand, A. H. (1995). Gender differences in pain. *Image: Journal of Nursing Scholarship, 27*(3), 235–237.

*Von Roenn, J. H., Cleeland, C. S., Gonin, R., Hatfield, A. K., & Pandya, K. J. (1993). Physician attitudes and practices in cancer pain management: A survey from the Eastern Cooperative Oncology Group. *Annals of Internal Medicine, 119,* 121–126.

*Walding, M. F. (1991). Pain, anxiety, and powerlessness. *Journal of Advanced Nursing, 16,* 388–397.

Wallace, K. G., Reed, B. A., Pasero, C., & Olsson, G. L. (1995). Staff nurses' perceptions of barriers to effective pain management. *Journal of Pain and Symptom Management, 10*(3), 205–213.

Ward, S., & Gatwood, J. (1994). Concerns about reporting pain and using analgesics. *Cancer Nursing, 17*(3), 200–206.

Weber, S. E. (1996). Cultural aspects of pain in childbearing women. *Journal of Obstetric, Gynecologic, & Neonatal Nursing, 25*(1), 67–72.

*Wells, N. (1982). The effect of relaxation on postoperative pain. *Nursing Research, 31,* 236–238.

*Wild, L., & Coyne, C. (1992). The basics and beyond: Epidural analgesia. *American Journal of Nursing, 92*(4), 26–34.

Wilke, D. J. (1995). Neural mechanisms of pain: A foundation for cancer pain assessment and management. In D. B. McGuire, C. H. Yarbro, & B. R. Ferrell (Eds.) *Cancer pain management* (2nd ed.; pp. 61–87). Boston: Jones and Bartlett Publishers.

Willens, J. S. (1994). Giving fentanyl for pain outside the OR. *American Journal of Nursing, 94*(2) 24–28.

*Zatzick, D. F., & Dimsdale, J. E. (1990). Cultural variations in response to painful stimuli. *Psychosomatic Medicine, 52,* 544–557.

Zimmerman, L., Nieveen, J., Barnason, S., & Schmaderer, M. (1996). The effects of music therapy on postoperative pain and sleep in coronary artery bypass graft (CABG) patients. *Scholarly Inquiry for Nursing Practice, 10*(2), 153–170.

Zimmerman L., Story, K. T., Gaston-Johansson, F., & Rowles, J. R. (1996). Psychological variables and cancer pain. *Cancer Nursing, 19*(1), 44–53.

SUGGESTED READINGS

Heiser, R. M., Chiles, K., Fudge, M., & Gray, S. E. (1997). The use of music during the immediate postoperative recovery period. *AORN Journal, 65*(4), 777–784.

This study examined the effect of music therapy on pain management in the post-anesthesia care unit (PACU). Two groups of clients were compared—one group listened to music during the last 30 minutes of their surgery and during the first hour in the PACU. No differences were found in pain management between the treatment group and the control group, but the clients who heard music stated that it helped them relax and functioned as a distractor.

Malek, C. J. & Olivieri, R. J. (1996). Pain management—Documenting the decision making process. *Nursing Case Management, 1*(2), 64–74.

The authors examined hospital nurses' clinical decisions regarding pain management and found that they did not adequately document pain assessments or pain relief and that they undertreated pain by not administering the amount of analgesia that was ordered. Additionally, there was minimal documentation of cognitive, behavioral, or physical interventions for pain.

BODY IMAGE

Self-concept is the sum of self-esteem, role performance, and body image (Fig. 10–1). Body image involves both conscious and unconscious information, perceptions, and feelings about one's body. Many illnesses, diseases, and disabilities affect a person's body image.

OVERVIEW

If someone's body image is definite and consistent with reality, the person is likely to feel satisfied with himself or herself. When illness or chronic disability is present, it is a challenge for someone to integrate the physical changes into his or her body image. Nurses, by diagnosing and treating responses to health problems in a holistic manner, are concerned about the total experience of body image development. Therefore, to assess client responses accurately, medical-surgical nurses must understand how illness can change the body image.

Definition of Body Image

Body image includes perceptions of shape, size, mass, function, structure, and significance of the physical, living body in relation to its parts. It also may include inanimate objects that are part of a person's daily contact with the body (e.g., make-up, jewelry, eyeglasses, clothing, wheelchair, crutches, or other appliances). Body image is a complex concept that is difficult to assess in nursing practice and is influenced by many factors.

Factors Affecting Body Image

Body image is influenced by several factors, including aging, culture, gender roles, and technology.

AGING. The Western World continues to place a major emphasis on the "ideal body," which represents youth, an ideal body weight, beauty, and agility. If a person does not fit this social image, as the middle-aged and older adult *may* not, he or she may receive negative messages about his or her value as a human being. Therefore, the normal aging process can influence body image.

CULTURE. The role of culture in the formation of body image can also be significant. People learn to judge themselves by how well they live up to the expectations and demands of their culture. The Western World places a high value on physical appearance and popularity with peers. If a person does not meet these expectations, the culture may perceive him or her less favorably. For example, the adult with anorexia nervosa or obesity may be the brunt of cruel jokes. Therefore, the negative attitudes of a person's culture can contribute to the creation of a poor body image.

GENDER ROLES. Gender roles play a major role in body image and the way in which it develops. The women's movement in the Western World has emphasized that although women and men are different, they

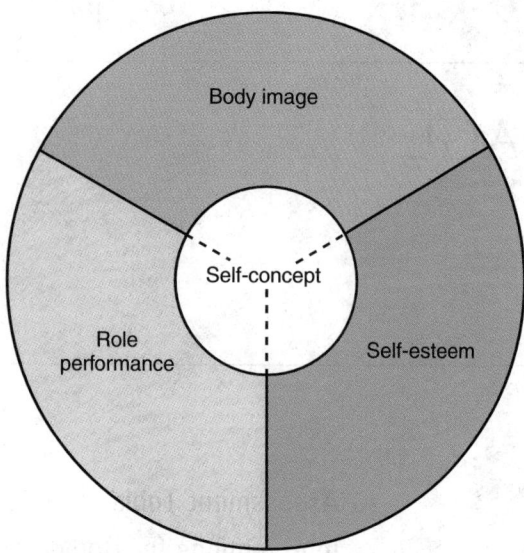

Figure 10–1. Relationship of self-concept to its components. Self-concept is the sum of self-esteem, role performance, and body image.

are of equal *value*. Nevertheless, boys and girls learn at an early age that society's expectations of them may differ greatly.

Body image and sexuality tend to go hand in hand. However, a positive body image does not necessarily predict positive feelings about sexuality or sexual satisfaction. (For more information on human sexuality, see Chapter 11.)

TECHNOLOGY. In the past decade, there have been many technological developments in health care. For example, joint replacements with artificial materials are now very common. Kidney and liver transplants are also common. Never before has so much replacement of human body parts been possible. However, these advances have an impact on body image, although this impact is not clearly understood.

The Life Cycle of Body Image

The body attempts to achieve consistency throughout the life cycle. A person's body image does readjust and adapt through interaction with significant others and the environment; that is, body image development is an ongoing process of learning and maturation through the cycle of life.

Most developmental theorists say that development of body image does not begin until after birth. The newborn is unable to distinguish clear boundaries between itself and the environment: Therefore, the newborn has no perceived body image. Table 10–1 summarizes body image development from infancy through adolescence. Body image development during adulthood is described here.

Young Adulthood (Ages 18–35 Years)

RELATIONSHIPS. Young adults are normally very concerned with developing intimate relationships with others.

Over time, body image becomes more stable and positive as a young adult develops these relationships. Without these relationships, the young adult experiences feelings of isolation. A healthy and realistic body image requires positive social reinforcement because people tend to become what others tell them they are. Unfortunately, stereotyping is common during this stage of development. For example, a young, overweight woman may be stereotyped as undisciplined and inactive when she may be just the opposite. This social reinforcement can strongly influence body image development.

PERSONAL CHARACTERISTICS. Body image develops and changes as the physical body changes. However, certain personal characteristics seem to be more crucial to body image than others. Sexual identification is central to body image, and any circumstance that alters or threatens this identification can affect it. For example, the woman who experiences a mastectomy (breast removal) may begin to question her sexuality and femininity and wonder "Am I still desirable and attractive?" "Am I still a woman?" "Who am I?"

WORK. The kind of work in which the young adult engages is another characteristic that influences body image. A person's identity may center on a career or occu-

TABLE 10–1

Development of Body Image from Infancy Through Adolescence	
Period of the Life Cycle	**Body Image Development Task**
Infancy (birth to age 1 year)	• Develops and uses touch • Perceives the differentiation between self and environment
Toddlerhood (age 1–3 years)	• Learns about body parts • Begins to trust feelings
Preschool (age 3–6 years)	• Develops a sexual identity • Begins to understand the concepts of normal and different, pretty and not pretty
Middle childhood (age 6–12 years)	• Recognizes differences in body types and structures • Focuses on physical appearance, peer relationships, and adherence to social group norms
Adolescence (age 12–18 years)	• Undergoes many internal and external physical changes • Makes comparisons with others and strives for the "perfect" body • Is confused by sexual feelings

pation, such as nurse, artist, farmer, or homemaker. Injury, illness, or change in career may require a total readjustment of body image. A musician who is no longer able to play an instrument because of amputation must readjust and adapt to the changes in his or her body. A painter who is affected by macular degeneration, which causes blindness, also faces the developmental task of body image readjustment.

Women usually have clearer and more accurate images of their bodies than men. Women tend to equate body more with self and are more aware of physical changes, especially around the face. Perhaps these images have related to the historical roles of woman as nurturer and mother, which are closely identified with the body. On the contrary, men have tended to be much less specific in how they view their bodies, perhaps because their roles have traditionally related more toward life accomplishments and attaining power and position in their careers than to their bodies.

Middle Adulthood (Ages 35–65 Years)

The body image of the middle-aged adult (the "middlescent") continues to develop as his or her interaction with the environment becomes more complex. During this period, the middlescent must readjust his or her body image to adapt to the psychological and physical changes of normal aging. This readjustment can be adaptive or maladaptive.

An example of *maladaptive* readjustment of body image is the middlescent who attempts to recapture or mimic youth by applying excessive cosmetics, wearing extremely youthful clothes, or adopting youthful hairstyles. If such an adult continues to perceive his or her physical appearance negatively, the negative body image may result in depression, irritability, and anxiety. The tendency to use maladaptive readjustment strategies depends on a person's personality and level of satisfaction with life up to middlescence.

An example of *adaptive* readjustment is the middle-aged adult who views the changes of this period as evidence of maturity, experience, and knowledge. Such an adult might participate in regular exercise programs, which may slow the normal physical aging process. The middle-aged adult who has successfully developed a realistic body image accepts the self and the body while realizing that acceptance from others cannot be expected unless self-acceptance is present.

Late Adulthood (Older Than 65 Years)

No matter when older adults begin to consider themselves as "elderly," they tend to undergo a marked change in body image. For example, sensory deficits resulting from normal aging are common in the older adult and may decrease the ability to enjoy hobbies, such as reading or listening to music. Decreased strength and increased fatigue may reduce the ability to remain a productive, active worker. These reduced abilities may lead to feelings of worthlessness and despair, which influence body image. Other events that can affect both body image and self-concept as a whole are retirement, loss of a spouse,

and loss of other close family members and friends (see Chap. 5).

Body Image Disturbance

Illness, whether chronic or acute, can change both external and internal body appearance and function. Changes in *external* body appearance and function can be devastating to body image. Chronic illness is usually more disabling than acute illness because it requires continuous body image reintegration as the disease process continues. For example, a client who has had a stroke is aware each day of the mobility or communication deficits that the illness has caused. As a result, the client continuously attempts to reintegrate not only the current body changes into the body image but also the ever-present fear of future immobility or communication losses that can result from further strokes.

Illness can also affect a person's *internal* function. For instance, a woman who has had a hysterectomy appears physically unchanged but has lost organs that contribute to her image as a woman. The medical-surgical nurse must be aware of these less obvious causes of body image disturbance.

The Theory of Readjustment to Body Image Disturbance

Body image readjustment is a lengthy process. Stages of this adaptation process include (1) psychological shock, (2) withdrawal, (3) acknowledgment, and (4) integration (Fig. 10–2).

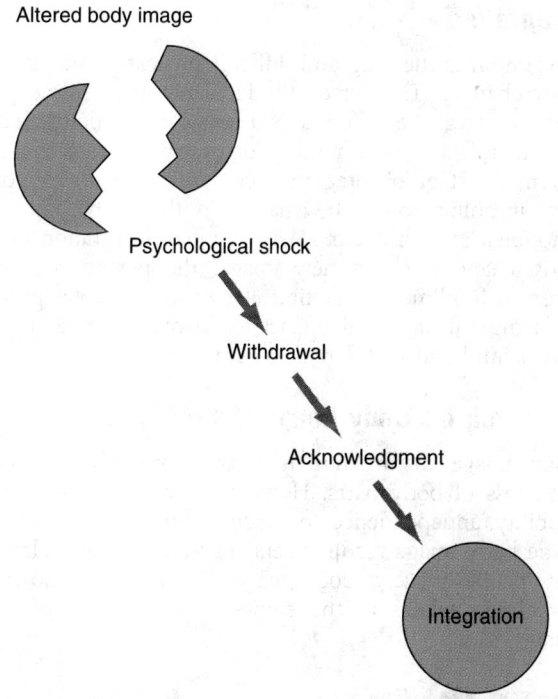

Figure 10–2. Readjustment to altered body image. Stages of the adaptation process include psychological shock, withdrawal, acknowledgment, and integration.

Psychological Shock

Psychological shock is often the initial emotional reaction to the impact of the life change that occurs when a person first becomes aware of a problem. This shock may occur at the time of an injury, illness, or developmental change, or it may occur later, when body changes are seen or experienced more acutely. Psychological shock is a defense mechanism that people use in reaction to anxiety. Denial and anger are common reactions during this stage.

Withdrawal

Withdrawal is the next stage of readjustment. Once the person becomes aware of an injury, illness, or developmental change and begins to think about the future, he or she may feel an overwhelming desire to run away from the reality of the situation. Because this is not physically possible, emotional retreat serves as a coping mechanism. This withdrawal provides an opportunity for the person to replenish physical and psychological energies used during the emotional shock phase. The person may become passive and dependent and lack motivation.

Acknowledgment

Acknowledgment occurs gradually, as the person recognizes the change in body image. Once the loss or change is acknowledged, the person can begin mourning (see Chapter 12 on grieving, death, and dying). The person may contemplate the meaning of the change and its implications for the future. This acknowledgment allows the person to view the body change itself and to begin reintegration of the body image.

Integration

Integration is the long and difficult process of adapting to body changes. The person thinks about future life experiences that will be different as a result of the body change and identifies ways to manage or deal with these changes. Often, the stage of integration can create for the person a new meaning about the change in the body part, and emotional growth occurs. As a result of integration of the body changes into a new image, the person regains a sense of fulfillment over time. However, the total process of change, from initial impact to adaptation, can be long and painful and is different for everyone.

Research on Body Image Disturbance

Body image disturbance is most commonly associated with loss of body parts. However, any type of loss (e.g., mobility, independence, or a body function) necessitates some body image readjustment. Research has not clarified how people perceive body image after a loss and how this perception relates to the emotional component of body image.

Loss of Mobility

People value the drive and ability to be mobile. Mobility is of such fundamental importance that healthy adults, even during resting periods, turn or change position frequently. Mobility enables people to exert control or influence over their environment. This control is threatened when mobility is restricted or lost (Hanna, 1996).

People view immobility, whether temporary or permanent, as a loss that can influence body image. This loss and the lifestyle changes that result can threaten the survival of the immobilized person. In this respect, body image in relation to immobility can have a considerable impact on nursing practice.

Pain

Pain can play a role in body image development. The impact of illness and pain on body image can be overwhelming. If severe pain continues, the painful body part can become isolated from the rest of the body to the point that it becomes alienated from the body image.

Cancer

Cancer often changes the way people feel about their personal appearance (Burt, 1995). Alopecia (hair loss) that occurs during the treatment of disease is one important factor. Cancer clients with alopecia have a lower self-image than cancer clients without alopecia. For these clients, alopecia is seen as a constant reminder of their disease. With or without hair loss, the experience of cancer can affect the body image.

Chronic Illness

Certain chronic illnesses can affect body image, whether or not pain is involved. For example, people with deforming arthritis, such as the rheumatoid type, are usually very self-conscious about their appearance. Some of these people refuse to socialize or be seen in public. The presence of chronic pain further affects the body image of these people.

Nicholas and Leuner (1992) studied people with another type of chronic illness—chronic obstructive pulmonary disease (COPD). They found that the body image of these people decreased as the disease became more severe.

Surgery

For any client, the anticipation of surgery can create anxiety, a fear of mutilation, and an unrealistic body image (see the Research Applications for Nursing box). Facial disfigurement resulting from surgical treatment of head and neck cancer, in particular, can cause severe body image disturbances. Likewise, the deformity that may result from burns or burn surgery can seriously affect a person's body image.

Another procedure that can cause body image disturbances is mastectomy. For most women, a mastectomy results in the loss of a body part that is viewed as essential for maintaining femininity, attractiveness, and self-esteem. This loss is based on the historical (or traditional) belief that the female breast is a symbol of femininity and maternity.

Research Applications for Nursing

Does Body Image Perception Change After Lumbar Laminectomy?

Neatherlin, J. S., & Brillhart, B. (1995). Body image in preoperative and postoperative lumbar laminectomy patients. Journal of Neuroscience Nursing, 27(1), 43–46.

This study was conducted to determine whether patients undergoing lumbar laminectomy had a change in body image perception between the preoperative and postoperative phases. Twenty-four middle-aged and elderly clients were assessed using the Body-Cathexis Scale. Scores on the tool were higher postoperatively, indicating that body image perception changed. In addition, the subjects rated a difference in energy level and sexual activity.

Critique. This was a comparative study using a small convenience sample. The researchers stated that a larger sample and more time are needed to see if the perceptions remain the same after surgery.

Possible Nursing Implications. Although nurses may not categorize a laminectomy as a deforming surgery that changes external appearance, this study shows that any type of surgery is a threat to body image. Therefore, nurses need to help all surgical clients cope with body image changes.

Body image disturbances are also common after the surgical creation of an ostomy (Giese & Terrell, 1996). These disturbances can result from the person's perception of the appearance of the stoma and from the reaction to the stoma by significant others. The person and significant others may equate the stoma with the genital region. Thus, exposure and direct handling of the stoma can be especially damaging to body image.

For body image to remain healthy, it must accurately incorporate the actual physical changes of surgery. That is, the person must accept the body as it has become. For example, the client with an ostomy must recognize that the stoma is probably lifesaving and that it serves the same purpose as the bowel tract and rectum. This recognition is realistic.

Amputation, Paralysis, and Deformity

For a person with a limb amputation or any type of paralysis, body image reintegration is required. In clients with an amputation, phantom limb pain, in which the limb is gone but pain continues, creates different body perceptions that necessitate body image reintegration.

Limb amputation, paralysis, and deformity can all limit mobility. For example, the client with a spinal cord injury also experiences serious changes in mobility. These changes in mobility can, in turn, affect body image.

Eating Disorders

Obesity, anorexia nervosa, and bulimia nervosa commonly reflect body image disturbances (Amara & Cerrato, 1996; Segal-Isaacson, 1996). People with these conditions have a tendency to overestimate their body size, both during and after weight loss. This overestimation results in a feeling of having lost no weight even after dieting has produced a significant weight loss. (Also see Chapters 63 and 64 for more information on body image and eating disorders.)

Collaborative Management

 Assessment

➤ History

The North American Nursing Diagnosis Association (NANDA) (1992) states that to justify a diagnosis of Body Image Disturbance, the client must have a verbal or nonverbal response to an actual or perceived change in body structure and/or function. To assess and understand a body image disturbance, the nurse collects data about how the client perceives and has adapted to a body change (Chart 10–1).

View of Self

The nurse begins the nursing assessment by obtaining data that identify the client's view of self. As the client shares information about body image, the nurse can better diagnose Body Image Disturbance and its cause. The nurse gathers data by inquiring about the client's recent physical body change. Is this perceived positively or negatively? What feelings does this change create? Are current feelings a change from feelings before this illness? Does the client describe herself or himself as hopeful or helpless?

Perception of Body Change

After assessing the client's view of self, the nurse identifies the body change as perceived by the client and his or her family or significant others. The nurse must assess both client and family perceptions because they may conflict and/or lend insight into further assessment and interven-

---

Chart 10–1

Nursing Care Highlight

Specific Factors to Consider When Taking a History of the Client with Body Image Disturbance

- What is the client's view of himself or herself? (e.g., "How would you describe your body to another person?")
- What is the client's or family's perceived body change?
- What is the client's developmental level?
- What are the client's or family's past successful coping strategies?
- What is the client's current occupation or work history?
- What was the client's past experience with pain?
- What is the client's environment?

tion. For example, do the client and family understand the actual physiologic surgical alteration? Is the body change perceived a certain way (e.g., lifesaving, positive, or negative)? What does this mean to them?

Developmental Level

When assessing body image disturbance, the nurse should take into account the client's developmental level. A young adult client may be functioning only as an adolescent. Therefore, the client's body image may not be developed to the level of an adult, and certain expectations will not be appropriate. The nurse assesses the developmental level of a client by evaluating responses of the client to questions and by noticing the way he or she is affected during an interview. Body language and maturity of responses are important clues to the developmental level of a client. For example, does the client give inconsistent verbal responses to questions? Does he or she have poor eye contact? Is the client unable to answer some questions because he or she does not understand?

Coping Strategies

To establish baseline data regarding coping behaviors, nurses should identify the client's and/or family's past successful coping strategies. The nurse can assess these strategies by asking
- "How have you dealt with hard times in your life in the past?"
- "What did you do in the past that helped you get through them?"
- "Have you been doing some of these same things this time?"
- "Do you think that these things might help you now?"

Chapter 8 discusses the assessment of coping in detail.

Occupation or Work History

The client's current occupation or work history can lend further insight into his or her self-image and body image. For example, is the client currently employed, laid off, fired, or retired? Does this work situation create any negative feelings or problems? Does the client anticipate return to work, or is he or she not currently working? Does the client feel useful?

Experience with Pain

Body image assessment must also include data about the client's past experience with pain. Has the client ever experienced pain before? Was this pain chronic or acute? Did this pain control the client's life? What caused the pain? How did the client deal with the pain? Were friends or family supportive about the pain? Did the pain change the client's life in any way? The nurse assesses the client's pain experience regardless of whether it is a past or current problem.

Environment

As well as assessing the client and family, the nurse also collects data about the client's immediate environment. The environment includes the immediate physical area at

home, social supports, and community. Does the client have easy access to follow-up care? Is the home environment conducive to self-care needs (e.g., one-level versus two-level home, steps into home, bathroom and bedroom locations)? Is the community supportive of this client's needs (e.g., presence of wheelchair ramps, easy transportation)? By collecting all of this information, the nurse can assess body image disturbances more accurately.

➤ Physical Assessment/Clinical Manifestations

The nurse completes a collection of data concerning body changes. NANDA identifies the following *objective* clinical manifestations, or defining characteristics, for assessment of Body Image Disturbance. Although these defining characteristics have not been clinically validated by research, they provide direction for nursing assessment. NANDA's definition and defining characteristics have not been revised or refined since 1986:
- Missing body part
- Actual change in structure or function
- Not looking at body part
- Not touching body part
- Hiding or overexposing body part (intentional or unintentional)
- Trauma to nonfunctioning body part
- Change in social involvement
- Change in ability to estimate spatial relationship of body to environment

➤ Psychosocial Assessment
Personalization of a Body Part

The North American Nursing Diagnosis Association (NANDA) has also identified as indicative of a body image disturbance client extension of the body boundary to incorporate environmental objects and personalization of the body part or loss by name. However, research has not established these characteristics as unhealthy behavior. For example, could it be that the client who envisions the body and wheelchair as one has successfully adapted to the new body image? Has the client who calls the colostomy "Sam" successfully incorporated this body change into a healthy image of the body? Future research may clarify these questions.

The client who depersonalizes the body part or loss by the use of impersonal pronouns (e.g., "it") may exhibit difficulty in adapting to the body change. The use of an impersonal pronoun to refer to a mastectomy, colostomy, or stump demonstrates one's inability to perceive the body change as part of the self. Such a reference keeps the body change impersonal and may facilitate denial of the change. By using denial, the client may demonstrate a refusal to verify the actual body change. This refusal then prolongs the grieving and coping process and can interrupt body image reintegration.

Coping and Support Systems

The nurse assesses the client's current coping behaviors and the client's attempts at body image adaptation to the change. Current coping behaviors can also be compared with past coping behaviors to assist the client with body

Subjective Interview
Points

____ 1. I will be undergoing a major change in my job status as a result of this experience.
____SA ____A ____U ____D ____SD
If so, what?
____Decrease in job status ____Job loss
____Change in job ____Other (specify)
_____

____ 2. I do not have someone available to help me or talk to.
____SA ____A ____U ____D ____SD
If someone is available, who?
____Spouse ____Parents
____Close friend ____Children
____Significant other ____Nurse
(relative)

____ 3. I think of myself differently as a result of this experience.
____SA ____A ____U ____D ____SD
If so, how?
____Negatively ____Other (specify)
____Increased physical _____
complaints

____ 4. My ability to move around by myself has changed as a result of this experience.
____SA ____A ____U ____D ____SD
If so, how?
____Less mobile ____Other (specify)
____No change _____

____ 5. I have definite feelings about specific parts of my body.
____SA ____A ____U ____D ____SD
If so, what?
____Hate ____Fear

____Disgust ____Other (specify)
_____

____ 6. I am more fearful now than before this experience.
____SA ____A ____U ____D ____SD
If so, why?
____Fear of falling ____Fear of pain
____Fear of recurrence ____Fear of inability
of problem to care for self
____Fear of others' ____Other (specify)
reactions _____

Objective Interview

7. Does the patient display any prominent body feature?
____Obesity ____Disfigurement
____Limb loss ____Other (specify)_____
____Paralysis

8. Does the patient exhibit evidence of or complain of pain?
____Facial expression
____Physical strain or fatigue
____Body language (immobile, purposeless, protective, rubbing)
____Sleep disturbances
____Other (specify)_____

9. Does the patient exhibit any major change in affect?
____Withdrawal ____Crying
____Hostility ____Other (specify)_____

10. Is there any equipment present?
____Foley's catheter ____Traction
____NG or other tubes ____Tracheotomy
____Walker or crutches ____Cardiac monitor
____Cast ____Side rails up
____Other (specify)_____

SA, strongly agree; A, agree; U, undecided; D, disagree; SD, strongly disagree, IV, intravenous; NG, nasogastric.

Figure 10–3. The Baird Body Image Assessment Tool. (Courtesy of Susan Baird Holmes.)

image changes. The client who has used anger to cope with past stressful life events may need to demonstrate anger in response to body changes. With the knowledge of these data, the nurse is better prepared to treat a body image disturbance. (Also see Chapter 8.)

Nurses also evaluate the client's current family role to gain an understanding about communication patterns, support systems, and family dynamics. The client's role in the family may be a significant part of the client's identity. If this image of self is interrupted by a body change, major problems with body image may occur. In addition, family members may be significantly influenced by the client's body change and inability to perform previous family roles.

The nurse assesses client and family support systems. The success or failure of a client and family to deal with physical body changes can depend greatly on the existence of support systems. Support systems may consist of specific people, groups, communities, financial plans, or assistive devices. The nurse initiates this assessment on first contact with the client. However, much of this data collection is ongoing. To develop an effective plan of care, the nurse should know the client and family support systems.

➤ Assessment Tools

Various written tools have been developed, primarily through the efforts of psychology researchers who study self-concept and body image. However, these tools are time-consuming for clients to complete and difficult to evaluate. To assist the nurse in identifying body image disturbances, a clinically useful nursing assessment tool is needed. The Baird Body Image Assessment Tool (BBIAT) attempts to clarify potential versus actual body image disturbances (Fig. 10–3). The client completes the subjective portion, answering each question with "strongly agree" (SA), "agree" (A), "undecided" (U), "disagree" (D), or "strongly disagree" (SD). The nurse asks clients to respond to questions 1 through 6. Points are then assigned to each answer as follows: SA = 5, A = 4, U = 3, D = 2, SD = 1. The total possible score for the subjective portion of the BBIAT is 30. Reliability and validity of this nursing tool have been established. A score of 23 to 30 points may indicate a serious need for nursing intervention; 19 to 22 points, a potential need that requires nursing intervention; and 18 or lower, no need for nursing intervention or the client has adapted to body changes.

The BBIAT is meant to be used only as a guide or tool to clarify for nurses, in daily practice, the assessment of body image alterations. The nurse uses the objective portion to identify other physical evidence that may have an impact on body image reintegration. No score is given for this portion. However, if so many objective variables exist that the nurse is unsure whether the client has a body image disturbance, this portion of the tool may help the nurse clarify the nursing diagnosis, etiology, or both. Further research and tool refinement are needed before one can draw any conclusions.

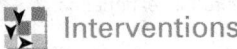 Interventions

Research has established the role of teaching in providing reassurance to clients who are about to undergo surgical body alterations. For example, preoperative teaching can decrease anxiety before and after surgery (see Chap. 20). Visits to clients by people who have had the same health problems have also been effective in assisting the client to adjust to the body image alteration.

If accepted by the client's culture, light touch to an extremity may be used by the nurse during discussion to help clients in re-establishing changed body boundaries. This practice can convey to the client a sense of being valued and that the physical body is still present. Talking to clients at equal eye level can be especially helpful in establishing an open, trusting relationship with those who may be feeling anxious or fearful.

The nurse encourages client verbalization and active thinking by providing for client participation in planning for the client's own needs. A client's sense of independence and responsibility is also enhanced by self-initiated activity. For example, a client with a spinal cord injury usually requires extra time for self-care. The nurse asks the client to suggest the best time for physical therapy appointments according to the client's need to have sufficient time to prepare for the appointment.

Nursing interventions for body image disturbance also focus on helping clients cope with alterations in body structure function.

➤ *Understanding the Grieving Process*

The nurse teaches the client and family or significant other the components of the healthy grieving process. Teaching begins by increasing client and family awareness of the various stages of grieving as well as understanding coping behaviors that are used in response to loss. For example, the client, family member, or significant other who responds with anger or denies the body change that has occurred may not be aware of his or her response. The nurse specifically helps the person to discuss feelings, recognize current behaviors, and possibly identify other therapeutic coping strategies. The nurse should also teach an understanding of healthy body image development throughout the life span. Clients and families should be better prepared to understand their fears and concerns and should be more effective in coping by developing an awareness about body image development.

➤ *Goal Setting*

Nursing interventions also focus on setting small, achievable goals; the nurse does this together with the client, family, or both. Goals are established during hospitalization to provide positive reinforcement about remaining strengths as well as effective coping strategies. For example, a client may be convinced that a burn site is noticeable, even under clothing, and may refuse to leave the hospital room. The nurse helps the client set a goal to dress in personal clothes of his or her choice and visit the gift shop in the hospital. The client meets the goal within 3 days and by the end of the week is in the visitors' lounge every afternoon, meeting new people and enjoying social interaction. Meeting the public for the first time after surgery can be threatening, and clients may become progressively desensitized to physical body changes. The nurse helps the client to be aware of his or her feelings about being stared at in public and to plan coping strategies to deal with these feelings.

Clients need to realize their remaining strengths and capabilities. In addition, the nurse can assist the client and/or family with identification of long-term effective coping mechanisms by validating realistic concerns and fears. For example, the amputee who in the past coped with life events by jogging every day needs assistance to identify and practice new coping behaviors. In addition, the nurse may arrange for another client who has experienced similar body changes and has successfully reintegrated these changes into a new body image to visit the client and to discuss concerns.

➤ *Family Support*

Family members and significant others need the same kind of assistance as the client in coping with body changes. Family members need support so that they in turn can be supportive to the client. The family must be able to deal with both any feelings about previous problems concerning the client and new feelings related to the kind and extent of body changes incurred by the client. For example, family members may feel guilty about a belief that their mother's leg might have been saved if they had gotten her to the doctor sooner. The nurse serves as the client's and family's most consistent health caregiver. This consistency establishes a caring rapport, which increases comfort in discussing these sensitive issues.

Providing empathy, *not* sympathy, can be the single most important intervention when treating body image disturbance. For example, an empathic supporting statement to a client might be, "This must be very difficult for you." A sympathetic statement to a client might be, "I'm so sorry for you." The nurse may convey sensitivity and empathy more clearly to the client and family by the use of a light touch to the arm or hand during these discussions. In addition, the nurse should sit at eye level with the client and family or significant others to facilitate even more open verbalization of concerns.

The nurse may also actively attempt to involve the family in the client's care during hospitalization, but only as they desire. This intervention may increase both the client's and family's sense of control over the situation and may decrease feelings of powerlessness. In addition, with this involvement in care, family members are impressed with the importance for the client to gradually increase responsibility for self-care and other activities. For example, teaching family members how to care for a stump at home after an amputation provides the client with positive reinforcement about the physical change and assists the family in recognizing that the client is still their loved one.

The client and family may need to restructure their relationships, depending on the extent and impact of the body change. The nurse can assist with this restructuring by serving as a buffer between client and family, if necessary. The nurse may also provide knowledge about community or hospital resources if family roles have changed as a result of the body alteration. For example, if the client is unable to maintain the family role as breadwinner, community resources may assist with financial needs. By helping the client and family share concerns or fears and solve problems together, the nurse can alleviate miscommunication problems and can enhance existing support systems.

SELECTED BIBLIOGRAPHY

Amara, A., & Cerrato, P. L. (1996). Eating disorders—Still a threat. *RN, 59*(6), 30–35.

*Baird, S. E. (1985). Development of a nursing assessment tool to diagnose altered body image in immobilized patients. *Orthopaedic Nursing, 4,* 47–54.

Beer, J. (1995). Body image of patients with ESRD and following renal transplantation. *British Journal of Nursing, 4*(10), 591–598.

Burt, K. (1995). The effects of cancer on body image and sexuality. *Nursing Times, 91*(7), 36–37.

Carpenter, J. S., & Brockopp, D. Y. (1994). Evaluation of self-esteem of women with cancer receiving chemotherapy. *Oncology Nursing Forum, 21*(4), 751–757.

Cowen, L., Clark, C., MacGillivary, C., Harper, R., & Wilson, L. (1995). Positive images of aging. *Elder Care, 7*(1), 14–15.

*Fischer, S. (1964). Sex differences in body perception. *Psychological Monographs,* 1–22.

Giese, L. A., & Terrell, L. (1996). Sexual health issues in inflammatory bowel disease. *Gastroenterology Nursing, 19*(1), 12–17.

Hanna, B. (1996). Sexuality, body image, and self-esteem: The future after trauma. *Journal of Trauma Nursing, 3*(1), 13–17, 19–20.

*Leonard, B. J. (1972). Body image changes in chronic illness. *Nursing Clinics of North America, 7,* 687–695.

Lisanti, P., & Verdisco, L. A. (1994). Perceived body space and self-esteem in adult females with chronic low back pain. *Orthopaedic Nursing, 13*(2), 55–63.

*Morris, C. A. (1985). Self-concept as altered by the diagnosis of cancer. *Nursing Clinics of North America, 20,* 611–630.

Neatherlin, J. S., & Brillhart, B. (1995). Body image in preoperative and postoperative lumbar laminectomy patients. *Journal of Neuroscience Nursing, 27*(1), 43–46.

*Nicholas, P. K., & Leuner, J. D. (1992). Relationship between body image and chronic obstructive pulmonary disease. *Applied Nursing Research, 5,* 83–84.

Paier, G. S. (1996). Specter of the crone: The experience of vertebral fracture. *Advances in Nursing Science, 18*(3), 27–36.

Price, B. (1994). The asthma experience: Altered body image and noncompliance. *Journal of Clinical Nursing, 3*(3), 139–145.

Segal-Isaacson, C. J. (1996). American attitudes toward body fatness. *Nurse Practitioner, 21*(3), 9–10, 12–13.

Walsh, B. A., Grunert, B. K., Telford, G. L., & Otterson, M. F. (1995). Multidisciplinary management of altered body image in the patient with an ostomy. *Journal of Wound, Ostomy, and Continence Nursing, 22*(5), 227–236.

SUGGESTED READINGS

Beer, J. (1995). Body image of patients with ESRD and following renal transplantation. *British Journal of Nursing, 4*(10), 591–598.

This study examines the need for nurses and other health care professionals to understand the social consequences and emotional aspects of clients living with a long-term illness, such as end stage renal disease (ESRD). Although the clients in the study accepted dialysis and other treatment options, they had difficulty adjusting to the disfiguring changes that occurred to their bodies.

Burt, K. (1995). The effects of cancer on body image. *Nursing Times, 91*(7), 36–37.

Nurses often dismiss the changes in body image experienced by clients who have cancer and cancer treatments. This article emphasizes the need for nurses to counsel clients and help them adjust to these changes.

Walsh, B. A., Grunert, B. K., Telford, G. L, & Otterson, M. F. (1995). Multidisciplinary management of altered body image in the patient with an ostomy. *Journal of Wound, Ostomy, and Continence Nursing, 22*(5), 227–236.

This article presents selected cases in which a multidisciplinary approach was successful in facilitating adaptation to an altered body image caused by an ostomy. The team included an enterostomal therapist, a nurse, and a psychologist. Clients with ostomies also have difficulty with personal acceptance, sexual concerns, and reduced self-care skills.

HUMAN SEXUALITY

A person's sexual health and well-being are created by the relationships among various factors. Sexual health can be described as a person's freedom from physical and psychological impairment that would compromise expression of one's sexuality. Sexual well-being includes the individual's awareness of open and positive attitudes toward one's body and sexual functioning, accurate knowledge about sexual anatomy and physiology, and acceptance of sexual arousal and responsibility for sexual behaviors.

OVERVIEW

Medical-surgical nurses are concerned with issues of sexual health and well-being. In providing nursing care, the nurse recognizes the importance of sexuality and encourages the growth and development of clients as sexual beings. The nurse also intervenes in a variety of situations to promote sexual health and to prevent sexual dysfunctions related to illness and injury throughout a client's life cycle.

Conceptual Model of Sexual Health and Well-Being

Throughout the life cycle, various factors determine an individual's optimal status of sexual health and well-be-

ing. Sexual health and well-being are holistic concepts that suggest the interrelationships among biological, psychological, social, and spiritual aspects of being human:

- Physical factors are associated with maturational changes in one's body; these include age, reproductive history, level of sexual functioning, past and present illnesses and injuries, the use of medications, and specific sexual behaviors.
- Psychological factors are associated with the mind; these include both emotional and cognitive processes. These factors include body image, self-esteem, gender identity, knowledge of sexuality, attitudes toward gender roles, beliefs about sexuality, and preference for sexual partners.
- Sociocultural factors include race, ethnicity, social status, marital status, family and social connectedness, occupation, and level of education.

External threats to the individual—in the form of physical illness, injury, or medical and surgical interventions—may lead to alterations in these factors and can reduce a person's level of sexual health and well-being. Similarly, threats to a person's psychological and sociocultural domains, such as family violence or changes in family composition, may result in changes that diminish sexual health and well-being.

To promote optimal sexual health in clients, the medical-surgical nurse assesses these factors and compares current findings with past patterns that clients have reported. The nurse evaluates the impact of external threats on these dimensions and provides nursing interventions that reduce or prevent the negative effects of the threats. The nurse also anticipates potential threats to optimal sexual health and well-being and provides guidance congruent with health-promoting goals.

Effect of Anatomy and Physiology on Sexual Health and Well-Being

The physical structure and function of the body affect a person's sexual health. Internal reproductive organs, such as the ovaries and uterus in a woman and the testes in a man, constitute one aspect of the anatomy that influences sexual health. In addition, external structures, such as the breasts and external genitalia, affect sexual health. A deformity, injury, disease, or surgical alteration of any of these internal or external structures poses a threat to one's sexual health. The endocrine system also maintains both structure and function of the reproductive organs.

Psychosexual Development

A person's psychosexual and physiologic development begin at the moment of conception and continue throughout young adulthood. Females are generally physically mature by the late teen years, whereas males may continue to develop mature secondary sexual characteristics into their early to late 20s. Overt sexual behaviors are observed in adults of all ages. Age, illness or injury, and life experiences have major impacts on an adult's sexuality. Attitudes and values are generally more firmly established in the adult than in the adolescent and influence overt sexual behavior. Although a man may reach his peak of sexual urgency in his 20s, a woman may not reach her peak until her 30s or 40s. This "mismatch" may lead to conflicts within marriage or other intimate heterosexual relationships.

Research on Human Sexuality

The history of research in human sexuality is fairly short. Before Alfred Kinsey's surveys of human sexual behavior in the 1930s, most research had addressed people with deviant or criminal behavior and little was known about average or typical sexual behavior. Kinsey trained interviewers who questioned more than 18,000 people in the United States about their sexual histories. Some of these findings led to new understandings about the sexual activities of women and of people with a homosexual orientation. In addition, the findings enabled the U.S. public to redefine the social code of acceptable sexual activities and to acknowledge more openly the reality of human sexual characteristics.

In the late 1950s and 1960s, the team of Masters and Johnson (1970) began to observe couples engaging in sexual activity and used various instruments to measure the responses of both men and women. In addition to using case studies and clinical and experimental research designs to increase the knowledge base of human sexual response and behavior, this team developed and tested interventions for use with couples who had recognizable sexual dysfunctions. The contributions of Masters and Johnson to the field of sexology as well as to the knowledge of the general public are well documented.

Sexual Response Cycle of the Adult

In the 1960s, Masters and Johnson described and measured in detail the sexual response cycle of both male and female adults. This cycle consists of four phases: excitement, plateau, orgasm, and resolution (Table 11–1). The underlying physiology of this cycle consists of vasocongestion and myotonia. *Vasocongestion* refers to blood trapped in tissues of the breast, vulva, and penis. This congestion results in erection of the nipples, clitoris, and penis. *Myotonia* refers to the tension of both voluntary and involuntary muscles that occurs during sexual excitement and orgasm. The differences in male and female sexual response cycles are illustrated in Figure 11–1. The problems of sexual dysfunction in adults are categorized according to the different phases of these cycles.

Sexual Preferences
Homosexuality

Sexual behavior and preference for partners may change over one's life span. Although most children and many adolescents engage in some types of overt homosexual activities as a normal part of sexual play, only a small percentage of adults identify themselves as homosexual. *Homosexuality* is defined as a person's attraction to one or more persons of the same sex. This preference is the most common of the sexual minorities.

Many stereotypic myths remain about homosexual (gay) men and lesbian women. Many such myths are based on homophobia, an irrational fear of homosexuality. However, the nurse who is equipped with an appropriate knowledge base and positive attitude toward human sexuality can help to dispel these myths and provide nursing care that includes attention to the person's sexual preference or orientation.

Although nursing care of homosexual clients does not differ from care of heterosexual ones and these groups have much in common, they also have some different concerns. For example, lesbians may experience the same concerns about gynecologic and breast problems as heterosexual women but may not have the same needs for contraception. Furthermore, lesbians are less likely to become pregnant than women who are sexually active with heterosexual partners. However, there is an increasing interest in parenting among homosexual couples, and artificial insemination followed by pregnancy is becoming more frequent in this population. Moreover, there is evi-

TABLE 11–1

The Adult Sexual Response Cycle

Phase	Male Response	Female Response
Excitement	• Skin flushing begins on the abdomen, then spreads to the neck and face. • The nipples become erect. • Myotonia of the legs and arms occurs. • Erection of the penis may subside and return. • The testes become elevated. • Pulse and blood pressure increase.	• Skin flushing begins on the abdomen and throat, then spreads to the breasts. • The nipples become erect, the veins distend, areolae darken, and the breasts enlarge by 25%. • Myotonia of the entire body occurs. • The clitoris becomes erect. • The vagina is lubricated. • Pulse and blood pressure increase.
Plateau	• Myotonia increases, with carpopedal spasms and facial grimaces. • The penis remains erect and darkens. • The testes continue to swell and elevate toward the perineum. • Pulse, respirations, and blood pressure increase.	• Myotonia increases, with carpopedal spasms, flared nostrils, and an arched back. • The clitoris retracts under its hood. • The vaginal barrel distends, and contractions begin. • Pulse, respirations, and blood pressure increase.
Orgasm	• The skin flush is maximal. • Myotonia of the entire body occurs, and the rectal sphincter contracts. • Semen is ejaculated through the penis. • Pulse and blood pressure increase. • The respiratory rate doubles.	• The skin flush is maximal. • Myotonia of the entire body occurs. • The clitoris remains retracted. • Pulse and blood pressure increase. • The respiratory rate doubles.
Resolution	• The skin flush disappears within 5 minutes in most men, followed by perspiration. • The muscles relax. • The nipples return to normal. • The penis returns to its normal size in two stages. • The testes return to their normal size and position. • Pulse, respirations, and blood pressure return to normal.	• The skin flush disappears and may be followed by perspiration. • The muscles relax. • The nipples and breasts return to their normal color and size. • The clitoris returns to its normal position within 10 seconds. • The vagina collapses and loses its dark color. • Pulse, respirations, and blood pressure return to normal.

dence that some pregnant teenagers are lesbians who want to be mothers.

Many lesbians approach the health care system cautiously because of widespread homophobia among health professionals. Because of the lesbian's fear and suspicions about the type of care that she may receive, she may pay incomplete attention to minor problems that have the potential to become serious.

Similarly, gay men may avoid the traditional health care system and thus may receive inadequate preventive or primary health care. Nonetheless, gay men have many of the same concerns about genitourinary problems as heterosexual men. However, because of the high incidence of anal intercourse among gay men, these clients seek treatment more frequently for injuries of the rectum and for gastrointestinal infections known as the "gay bowel syndrome." Gay men with this syndrome are infected and reinfected with microorganisms that cause one or more gastrointestinal infections. The incidence of sexually transmitted diseases (STDs) is also higher among gay men. At this time, gay men also represent the group with the highest incidence of acquired immunodeficiency syndrome (AIDS) (see Chap. 25).

Other Sexual Variations

The nurse should be familiar with other sexual variations, such as the following:

BISEXUALITY. *Bisexuality* refers to a person's preference for intimate relationships with members of either sex.

INTERSEXUALITY. *Intersexuality* refers to a person having been born with either ambiguous genitalia (i.e., it is not clearly apparent whether the baby is male or female) or with internal and external genitalia of both sexes (e.g., penis, scrotum, and uterus).

TRANSSEXUALITY. *Transsexuality* refers to a person being dissatisfied with his or her gender assignment and being convinced that he or she is trapped within the wrong body. Sex reassignment surgery for the man who has a strong urge to live as a woman includes orchiectomy (removal of the testes), penectomy (removal of the penis), and vaginoplasty (construction of a vagina). Hormone replacement treatment is also given. A woman who

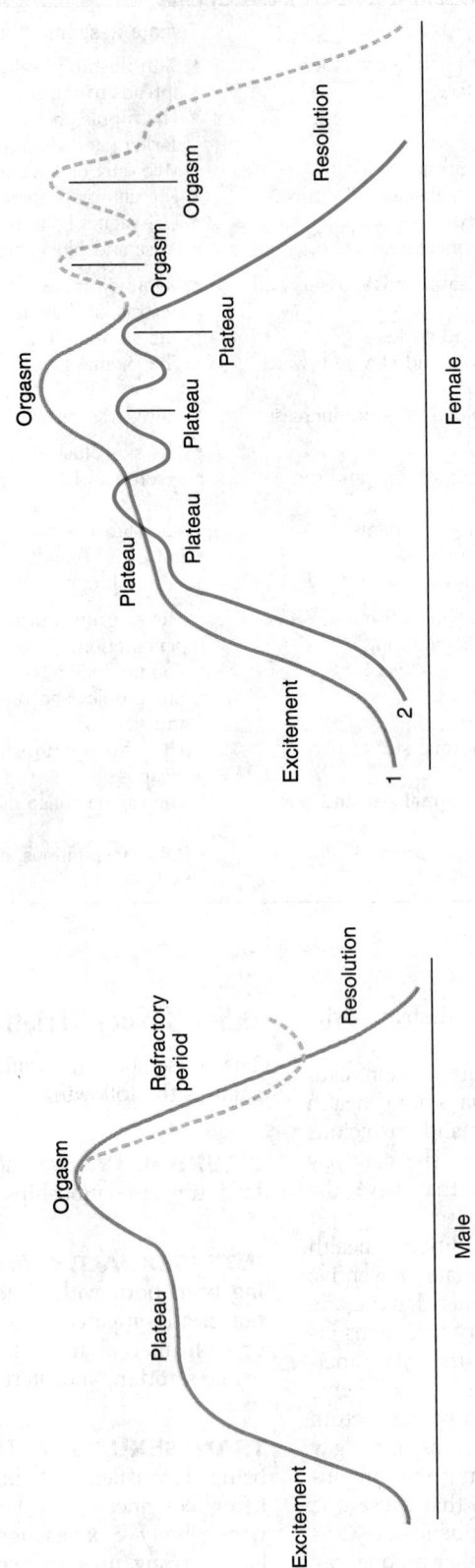

Figure 11–1. The male and female adult sexual response cycles. In the male sexual response cycle, a refractory period usually follows orgasm before another erection occurs. Women respond in various ways to sexual stimulation: Pattern 1 depicts single or multiple orgasms; pattern 2 shows some peaks but no orgasm.

is reassigned as a man undergoes hysterectomy (uterus removal), oophorectomy (ovary removal), and mastectomy (breast removal) along with hormone replacement therapy.

TRANSVESTISM. Also known as cross-dressing, *transvestism* refers to a person liking to wear clothes associated with the opposite sex for the sake of his or her sexual arousal. Transvestism is more common in men than in women. Unlike the transsexual, the transvestite does not have a conflict about his or her gender; some transvestites are married, and most engage in transvestism in private.

PEDOPHILIA. Pedophilia is a sexual preference for children. It is a psychiatric disorder (not discussed in this chapter).

Changes in Sexual Function Associated with Aging

Physical, social, and psychological changes affect sexual functioning throughout the life cycle. Chart 11–1 summarizes the major changes in the older adult. For more information on sexuality during each phase of adult development, see Chapter 5.

Effects of Illness on Sexuality

Many illnesses and injuries can have a negative effect on sexual health and well-being. In some cases, sexual dysfunctions may result that can be temporary or permanent (Table 11–2).

Chart 11–1

Nursing Focus on the Elderly

Changes Affecting Sexuality

Physical Changes
- In women, vaginal tissue gradually atrophies.
- Women become infertile; male fertility varies.
- Sexual arousal takes longer, and sperm count and the force of ejaculation in men decrease.

Social Changes
- Men and women experience increased losses in social networks.
- Men and women experience a heightened need for human contact and intimacy.
- Society views the elderly as asexual, having no sexual desires or needs.
- Health care providers often ignore the sexual needs and desires of the elderly.

Psychological Changes
- Men and women engage in life review and desire to be useful.
- The elderly may experience negative body image and lowered self-esteem.

Hospitalization

People often perceive the process of hospitalization as impersonal. Elements of sexual identity and behaviors associated with gender roles are frequently denied or seriously curtailed by the social milieu in most hospitals. Hospitals provide little privacy; in addition, symbols of sexual identity, such as certain clothing and jewelry, are usually removed. Behaviors that express sexual arousal and satisfaction are discouraged.

Acute Illness

When a person is hospitalized for acute illness or injury, sexual health may be impaired. Not only is the social climate not conducive to sexual expression for the reasons just identified, but a client's physical and psychological conditions may not be congruent with optimal sexual health and well-being. Acute medical conditions for which a client may be hospitalized can render the person physically unable to engage in sexual activity because of anxiety, fatigue, pain, malaise, or direct tissue damage or surgery that interferes with sexual arousal.

Specific acute disorders, such as sexually transmitted diseases (STDs), or complications associated with these disorders may affect the sexuality of the hospitalized person (see Chap. 80). Nurses should consider care that includes assessment of risk factors and sexual contacts when caring for the client with an acute condition requiring hospitalization. Because of the social stigma associated with the diagnosis of STDs, the hospitalized client may also suffer from guilt, embarrassment, and low self-esteem, which may impair his or her pursuit of behaviors that would lead to sexual health.

Specific acute bacterial or viral infections, such as pneumonia, hepatitis, gastroenteritis, and prostatitis, affect sexual health. In addition to the fatigue and malaise that are associated with these conditions, specific changes in body function may threaten an ill person's body image and self-esteem. These physical problems are closely related to psychological aspects of sexual well-being.

Chronic Illness

The sexual health of the client with a chronic illness or impairment may be threatened in various ways. For example, clients with hypertension, connective tissue disease, cancer, cardiovascular disease, diabetes, end-stage renal disease (ESRD), chronic respiratory disease, chronic liver disease, or spinal cord injury face limitations in sexual behavior patterns. These clients must deal with changes in body structure, function, or both in addition to psychological factors, such as uncertainty, fear, and depression. The client's body image is threatened, and tissue damage may disrupt the sexual response cycle or may render the client unable to engage in preferred sexual activities. (See also Chapter 10 on Body Image.)

HYPERTENSION. Adults who experience hypertension are at risk for problems in sexual functioning. Centrally acting adrenergic inhibitor drugs, such as methyldopa (Aldomet and Amodopa) and beta-adrenergic blockers such

TABLE 11–2

Effects of Illness on Adult Sexuality		
Illness	**Effects on Men**	**Effects on Women**
Arthritis	• Decreased libido • Low self-esteem • Altered body image • Depression, anxiety	• Dyspareunia • Low self-esteem • Altered body image • Depression, anxiety
Cancer	• Altered body image • Erectile dysfunction • Decreased libido • Depression, anxiety • Low self-esteem	• Altered body image • Dyspareunia • Decreased libido • Depression, anxiety • Low self-esteem
Cardiovascular disease	• Erectile dysfunction • Low self-esteem • Depression, anxiety	• Decreased libido • Low self-esteem • Depression, anxiety
Diabetes	• Erectile dysfunction • Retrograde ejaculation • Decreased fertility	• Decreased libido • Orgasmic dysfunction • Decreased fertility • Dyspareunia • Chronic vaginitis • Decreased vaginal lubrication
Hepatic disease	• Loss of libido • Sexual unresponsiveness • Erectile dysfunction	• Decreased libido • Orgasmic dysfunction • Amenorrhea
Hypertension	• Decreased libido • Erectile failure • Ejaculatory failure • Gynecomastia	• Decreased libido • Galactorrhea
Renal disease	• Low self-esteem • Altered body image • Loss of libido • Erectile dysfunction • Decreased fertility • Depression, fatigue	• Low self-esteem • Altered body image • Loss of libido • Orgasmic dysfunction • Decreased fertility • Depression, fatigue
Respiratory disease	• Low self-esteem • Decreased libido • Erectile dysfunction	• Low self-esteem • Decreased libido • Orgasmic dysfunction
Spinal cord injury	• Erectile dysfunction • Possible infertility • Retrograde ejaculation • Ejaculatory dysfunction • Orgasmic dysfunction • Low self-esteem • Impaired body image • Loss of libido	• Orgasmic dysfunction • Amenorrhea • Low self-esteem • Impaired body image • Loss of libido

as propranolol (Inderal, Novopranol✦), have been associated with decreased libido (sexual desire) in both men and women. In addition, men may experience erectile and ejaculatory failure, whereas women may experience galactorrhea (the presence of milk in the breasts) and an inability to have an orgasm. These adverse effects usually disappear within 2 weeks after medication is discontinued.

Clonidine hydrochloride (Catapres), another antihypertensive agent, may lead to urinary retention, impotence, and gynecomastia (breast enlargement in men), thus affecting the sexual response cycle. Calcium-channel–blocking drugs such as nifedipine (Procardia, Adalat) and amlodipine besylate (Norvasc) reportedly have fewer sexual side effects. Metoprolol tartrate (Lopressor) also contributes to impotence in men. The nurse should assess the effects of such drugs in both men and women so that the physician may consider changes in dosages or types of medication if needed.

CONNECTIVE TISSUE DISEASE. Clients with connective tissue diseases, such as rheumatoid arthritis and systemic lupus erythematosus, face a chronic disabling condition characterized by problems with mobility, pain, and weakness. Although research on the specific incidence of sexual dysfunction among people with arthritis is lacking, obvious physical barriers exist to the usual sexual activities of such clients. Limited joint movement, weakness, fatigue, pain, swelling, and stiffness of extremities make activities of daily living, including sexual activity, difficult.

In addition to the often deforming nature of some forms of arthritis, large dosages of corticosteroid drugs may alter an arthritic person's physical appearance, which can result in lowered self-esteem and altered body image. Depression and anxiety about the unrelenting course of arthritic conditions may interfere with interpersonal communication and result in decreased sexual desire. Dyspareunia (painful intercourse) may result from changes in secretory function of the vagina, as seen in clients with Sjögren's syndrome.

CANCER. Various types of cancer directly affect sexual functioning and body image. Cervical or uterine cancer that results in hysterectomy and breast cancer that results in mastectomy are among the obvious malignancies affecting both sexual functioning and body image in women. In men, testicular and prostatic cancer may result in radical surgery that alters both sexual functioning and body image.

Other primary malignant tumors also contribute to the decline of a person's sexual health. These include cancers of the gastrointestinal tract, urinary system, and larynx, often necessitating surgical diversion or radical neck dissection. In addition to the damaging effects of malignant growths and surgical procedures, radiation and chemotherapy affect the sexual response cycle, appearance, and self-esteem of a client with cancer. Clients may experience alopecia (loss of hair), fatigue, anorexia, malaise, decline in libido, and secondary ovarian or testicular failure as a result of these therapies.

CARDIOVASCULAR DISEASE. Cardiovascular disease affects a person's sexual health and well-being because sexual activity makes demands on the cardiopulmonary system. Cardiovascular disease also affects the client's self-concept, self-esteem, and role function. When a person is resuming sexual activity after a myocardial infarction, for example, the activity should be planned and implemented on an individual basis. The conditions under which sexual activity is pursued (e.g., relaxing versus anxiety-provoking conditions) and the amount of physical stress that the heart can handle must be considered. The severity of tissue damage and the effects of medications may limit the degree to which people with chronic cardiovascular disease can pursue sexual activity. With physical conditioning programs, regulation of drug therapy, and adequate teaching and support, a client may continue to resume previous patterns of sexual activity or develop new and satisfying ones (see Research Applications for Nursing).

DIABETES MELLITUS. Diabetes has long been associated with sexual problems. Secondary erectile dysfunction (impotence) in men is often associated with microvascular

▷ Research Applications for Nursing

Clients May Want to Talk About Sexual Functioning and Cardiovascular Disease

Quadagno, D., Nation, A. J., Johnson, D., Waitley, C., Waitley, N., Epstein, D., & Satterwhite, A. (1995). Cardiovascular disease and sexual functioning. Applied Nursing Research, 8(3), 143–146.

Researchers studied 29 married men (mean age = 56.1 years) and 8 married women (mean age = 59.2 years) who had experienced cardiovascular problems, including heart transplant, myocardial infarction, bypass surgery, and hypertension. A questionnaire was distributed to the subjects at their cardiologist's office and included questions about general health, sexual activity, and sexual concerns. The subjects were also asked if health care workers had discussed resuming sexual activity and had provided them with adequate information about resuming normal activities following their cardiovascular health problem.

The majority of men and women in the sample reported having received no information from their health care providers about resuming sexual activities. Older subjects were less likely to receive this information than younger subjects, and they were also less likely to resume previous levels of sexual activity. Health care providers were also less likely to discuss sexual activity with women than with men.

These findings indicate that health care providers continue to perpetuate the myth that elderly clients have less sexual desire or fewer sexual needs than younger clients. Similarly, they suggest that women with cardiovascular disease do not receive information about resuming sexual activity. Nurses could fill an important gap in providing preliminary information to these clients.

Critique. The results of this study are limited by the small sample size, self-reported data, and use of questionnaires rather than interviews. However, the topic is important to nurses who care for these clients.

Possible Nursing Implications. Any nurse caring for clients undergoing surgery or receiving medical treatment for cardiovascular disease should be aware of the importance of sexuality. The nurse can provide preliminary information about resuming sexual activity and should be available to answer questions and provide emotional support to these clients. Moreover, nurses can be client advocates and assist such clients in requesting information from their physicians.

---

changes and neuropathy and occurs in more than half of men who have diabetes. A small percentage of diabetic men may experience retrograde ejaculation (the ejaculate is released into the urinary bladder instead of through the urinary meatus). This difficulty and the presence of disease of long duration may contribute to problems with fertility in diabetic men. Comparable changes in women lead to decreased libido, orgasmic dysfunctions, and infertility. A decrease in vaginal lubrication and increased risk of infection contribute to chronic vaginitis in diabetic women. The incidence of sexual problems in people who have had diabetes for longer periods is increased.

END-STAGE RENAL DISEASE. The effects of end-stage renal disease (ESRD) are monumental. Every system in the body is affected by impairment of the metabolism and regulation of electrolytes. In addition to the physical limitations resulting from fatigue, pruritus (itching), anorexia, lethargy, and muscle cramping, the client with ESRD faces overwhelming psychosocial changes. The client's self-concept, body image, and self-esteem suffer as a result of the gradual deterioration of body functions and structures. Role functions and issues of dependency are altered if the client is forced to stop working or cannot manage usual responsibilities in the home and community. The financial burdens of lost income and expensive treatments add to the stressors for the person with chronic renal disease. As a result of these multiple factors, the person may experience depression, loss of libido, decreased frequency of sexual activity, impotence, and sterility. New patterns of sexual expression must be explored to promote sexual well-being.

CHRONIC RESPIRATORY DISEASE. A person with chronic respiratory disease may experience increased levels of fatigue with accompanying threats to self-esteem. For example, people with chronic airflow limitation often report difficulty in continuing sexual intercourse. A review of the adult sexual response cycle indicates that respiratory rates double during plateau and orgasmic phases, which makes coitus difficult for both men and women with respiratory disease. Clients may need to learn alternative methods and positions for satisfying sexual activity.

LIVER DYSFUNCTION. Chronic conditions affecting the liver and immune system frequently lead to impaired sexual health. Clients experiencing anorexia, fatigue, joint pain, nausea, fever, and jaundice associated with chronic hepatitis may become uninterested in sexually overt behavior. In addition, the client may experience complications such as erectile dysfunction or sexual unresponsiveness. Similarly, many clients with cirrhosis of the liver related to malnutrition, infection with parasites, or alcohol abuse experience a loss of libido and specific pathologic conditions, including gynecomastia and erectile dysfunction in men and amenorrhea in women.

SPINAL CORD INJURY. Clients with spinal cord injury experience various sexual dysfunctions as a result of altered physical functioning and psychosocial changes. The dysfunctions depend on the extent and location of the injury, and they differ for men and women. Men with injury to the cervical spinal cord usually continue to have reflexive erections of the penis. Men whose injury occurred at lower levels of the spine experience erectile dysfunction because the neural pathways from the spinal cord are damaged or destroyed.

Incomplete injury to the spinal cord permits some sensation and motor function of the genitalia; complete injury results in loss of libido in both men and women, loss of erection and ejaculation in men, and orgasmic dysfunction in women. Men in whom the lumbosacral cord has been completely cut are infertile because of retrograde ejaculation or damaged sperm. Women, however, may experience temporary amenorrhea, may retain fertility, and may be capable of a full-term pregnancy. Each person's injury must be addressed individually.

Psychosocial problems may contribute to a decline in sexual health for spine-injured clients because of the accompanying change in body image and decrease in self-esteem. However, many people with spinal cord injuries continue to have satisfying sexual activity when their physical, psychological, and social problems are addressed. Many resources are available to assist them in promoting satisfying sexual expression. Women with spinal cord disabilities are often overlooked by health care providers concerning their needs for specialized menstrual products, contraception, and pregnancy. Many have suffered from the oppressive attitudes and behaviors of others who fail to appreciate their struggle for reproductive freedom (Waxman, 1994). Nurses can be strong advocates for these women in helping to design feminine hygiene products and obtaining optimal sexual health care services.

Effects of Drug and Alcohol Abuse

Nurses should not overlook the possibility of drug abuse or alcoholism as a central factor when suspecting or validating sexual problems in men and women. As middle adulthood approaches, some people turn to alcohol or other drugs to ease their anxieties, including anxiety specifically related to diminished sexual functioning (Table 11–3). The primary effects of limited alcohol intake are often initially stimulating, and both men and women may experience release of inhibitions, relief of anxiety, and an increase in libido. However, as the amount or frequency of alcohol intake increases, clients experience several negative effects. In women, for example, the desire for sexual activity may gradually decrease until there is no interest. Women in the stages of late alcoholism also experience a gradual decrease in vaginal lubrication and sensitivity. It takes more time for such women to have an orgasm, and they experience fewer orgasms.

Men in the late stage of alcoholism experience decreased desire, often accompanied by an increase in aggression and, finally, a total loss of desire and profound aggression. A delay in penile erection leads to an inability to attain an erection even with maximum stimulation, and the man's orgasm may be tentative or may not occur under any circumstances. The man may also experience diminished pleasurable sensations associated with sexual arousal. Although erection is still possible, the resolution stage is prolonged, and the man experiences a loss of sexual satisfaction.

Alcohol and drug use have also been implicated in risky sexual behaviors among adolescents and young adults, sometimes leading to unplanned pregnancies, sexually transmitted diseases, and personal violence. The role of alcohol and drug abuse as a factor in family violence is beyond the scope of this chapter, but the nurse should be aware of the increased risk to young pregnant women and to both males and females who may be raped when a sexual partner is a substance abuser.

TABLE 11–3

Effects of Alcohol and Other Drugs on Sexual Functioning

Drug	Effects on Men	Effects on Women
Alcohol	• Decreased libido • Increased aggression, possibly leading to sexual abuse • Erectile dysfunction • Decreased fertility • Low sexual satisfaction	• Decreased libido • Increased passivity, possibly leading to sexual abuse from partner • Orgasmic dysfunction • Amenorrhea, sterility • Low sexual satisfaction
Antidepressants	• Erectile dysfunction • Delayed ejaculation	• Delayed orgasm
Antihypertensives	• Decreased libido • Erectile dysfunction • Ejaculatory dysfunction • Retrograde ejaculation	• Decreased libido • Anovulation, amenorrhea • Galactorrhea • Impaired orgasm
Cocaine and amphetamines	• Delayed orgasm • Delayed ejaculation	• Orgasmic dysfunction • Decreased libido
Opioids	• Decreased libido • Erectile dysfunction • Delayed ejaculation	• Decreased libido • Spontaneous abortion • Amenorrhea
Tranquilizers	• Retrograde ejaculation • Erectile dysfunction	• Galactorrhea • Amenorrhea, anovulation

TRANSCULTURAL CONSIDERATIONS

Many factors affect a person's sexual health and his or her willingness to discuss this very private part of life. Spanish-speaking clients and Native Americans tend to be hesitant to talk about sexually related matters. In some cases, people from these groups may talk more freely to a nurse or other health care professional of the same sex or from the same culture (Giger & Davidhizar, 1995).

Cultural or religious background can also influence one's willingness to discuss sexual matters. This background may permit certain practices and prohibit others. The teachings of the Roman Catholic Church, for instance, prohibit the use of artificial contraception.

The decision to circumcise a male is also culturally based. In the United States, for example, 80% to 90% of males are circumcised, although fewer boys today are being circumcised than 20 years ago. In other countries of the world, such as Canada, England, Sweden, and China, circumcision is thought to be unnecessary. Some religious groups, such as Jews and Muslims, include circumcision as part of their religious practice. Other groups, like Hispanics and Native Americans, do not traditionally practice male circumcision (Jarvis, 1996). There is scant scientific evidence that circumcision is necessary, although penile carcinoma occurs more frequently in men who are not circumcised.

Female circumcision is not traditionally performed in the United States. However, immigrants from central Africa and India may enter the formal health care system with complications directly related to this practice. Female circumcision varies from minor procedures such as removal of the prepuce of the clitoris to infibulation, which is complete excision of the clitoris, labia minora, and parts of the labia majora and partial closure of the vaginal opening. Most of these procedures are done as tribal rituals associated with coming of age and often are performed without sterile conditions and anesthetics. Incisions are rarely sutured: A small piece of wood or some other hard object may be inserted into the vagina to permit flow of menstrual blood, and often the girl's legs are bound together to facilitate healing. Some young women hemorrhage or suffer from urinary retention and infection. Others face delayed complications such as vaginal stenosis, chronic urinary tract infections, and chronic pelvic inflammatory disease (Walker & Morgan, 1995). The culturally sensitive nurse provides care without judging the morality of cultural customs that promote these practices.

Nurses' Comfort with Sexuality

Our increased knowledge and awareness of human sexuality throughout the life cycle have led to an increased demand for solutions to problems in sexual functioning. Nursing, as a major provider of health care services, has responded to this demand by developing strategies to prevent the development of sexual problems and to promote sexual health.

In addition to having an adequate knowledge base in human sexuality, the nurse should feel comfortable in addressing the sexual health needs of clients. To help clients achieve optimal sexual health and well-being, nurses should have an attitude of openness and willingness to approach the subject. Nurses must first be aware of their personal attitudes toward sexuality and their ability to promote the sexual health and well-being of others

TABLE 11–4

Values Clarification Exercise

Situation: Mary is a 26-year-old single woman hospitalized for a radical hysterectomy. She has a malignancy. Which of the following responses by nurses is most like your response to assessing, diagnosing, and intervening with regard to her actual and potential sexual problems?

Nurse A: "I hope she doesn't ask about having sexual relations or I'll just die of embarrassment!"

Nurse B: "I know how I'll handle any questions about sex. I'll just refer her to the head nurse. She can handle that stuff."

Nurse C: "It's OK if she asks about sex, but I'm not sure I know all the answers. I know I can listen and try to help her find answers if I don't know them."

Nurse D: "It's just fine if she asks about how this will affect her sexually. In fact, even if she doesn't bring it up, I will. I really believe it's an important aspect of her health."

Clarification of values in responses: If you answered that you feel most like one of the nurses above, check below to clarify what this means.

Nurse A: This nurse feels uncomfortable handling concerns about sexual health and needs to do more reading and talking about her feelings with other health professionals.

Nurse B: This nurse also feels uncomfortable and is willing to shirk responsibility, passing it on to one with more authority. Again, more learning and exploration of his or her attitudes are needed.

Nurse C: This nurse feels comfortable. Being able and willing to look for additional information is essential to helping the client.

Nurse D: This nurse also feels comfortable and is willing to take more responsibility for including sexual health in client care.

(Table 11–4). If inquiring about sexual functioning or behavior is embarrassing to the nurse, he or she must be willing to acknowledge this and refer the client to another nurse with more experience. This nurse should also attempt to learn more about human sexuality and its relationship to health and well-being.

Sexual Harassment

There has been an increased realization of and discussion about sexual harassment in the workplace and other settings. Because most nurses are women, it is possible that they will be harassed at some point while caring for their clients. Sexual harassment by a client can interfere with the nurse's ability to complete a sexual health assessment and effectively intervene for specific sexual problems.

In addition to the possibility of being sexually harassed by clients, the nurse may encounter harassment from other members of the health care team or the client's family members or visitors. Several court cases have determined that people should be protected from harassment and the offenders legally punished.

Collaborative Management

 Assessment

> *History*

In managing the sexual health of hospitalized clients, the nurse takes a brief sexual history that is integrated with the general health history. Nurses need to be sensitive to clients' willingness to discuss this private part of their lives. Factors such as the age of both the client and the nurse may affect the client's willingness to disclose such personal information. For example, elderly clients may be reluctant to discuss sexual health, especially if they were taught that sex should not be discussed openly. An equally embarrassing situation might be one in which a young female nurse interviews a young heterosexual male; both people may feel hesitant about discussing this topic.

Nurses address three areas in taking the sexual health history:

- Physical development and situational changes in sexual functioning
- Alterations in body image, gender identity, sex role, and self-esteem
- Sociocultural factors, such as ritualistic practices and beliefs

Here are some examples of questions that the nurse can ask while obtaining a history:

- "Have you ever experienced any injury or disease of the genitourinary system? Is there any history of sexually transmitted diseases?"
- "What was the pattern of development of secondary sexual characteristics (e.g., onset of menstruation)? Have there been any changes in these characteristics (e.g., hirsutism [excessive hair growth in females] or gynecomastia)? What changes do you attribute to your age?"
- "Have you ever experienced any unwanted or traumatic sexual events such as incest, rape, or sexual harassment?"
- "Have you noticed any changes in sexual functioning in the past related to the use of alcohol or other drugs?"
- "Have you experienced any changes in sexual functioning or desire for sexual activity since your current illness, injury, or surgery?"
- "Has this physical problem (illness, injury, or surgical treatment) changed the way you view your body or feel about yourself as a woman or man?"
- "As a result of this physical problem, have you noticed changes in your usual activities as a woman or man, or changes in your usual roles, such as those of wife or mother, or husband or father?"
- "What are some of your beliefs and practices about sexual behavior? Have any of these been affected by your current illness, injury, or surgery?"

Although some of these questions may be answered easily with "yes" or "no," the nurse should pose them in such a way as to invite the client to discuss his or her sexual identity, roles, or activity. The nurse should phrase questions in language that the client understands, according to his or her educational level and sociocultural background. Beginning each phrase with "Tell me how" may encourage further information. Taking a sexual history is one way to identify misinformation that should be corrected as part of the nursing intervention. Chart 11–2 summarizes the information contained in a brief sexual history and assessment.

Chart 11–2

Nursing Care Highlights

Brief Sexual History and Assessment Guide
History: Current Assessment
Physical

- Note development of secondary sexual characteristics (onset and pattern of menses in woman): Observe and palpate. Note changes over time.
- Note use of contraceptives; problems with fertility or pregnancy. Assess.
- Note current use and problems with contraception; issues of fertility or pregnancy.
- Note episodes of sexually transmitted diseases.
- Note recent changes in sexual activity level or pattern.
- Ask about past genitourinary disease, injury, or surgery.
- Note thickening or discharge from the breast or genitalia.
- Ask about past use of alcohol or other drugs.
- Note current drug use.
- Ask about past patterns of sexual function.
- Note changes in levels of sexual arousal or function.

Psychological

- Ask about past sexual dysfunction.
- Identify knowledge of sexual function.
- Ask about past problems with body image, gender role, or self-esteem.
- Note current values and current feelings about body parts and functions and self-esteem.
- Take history of incest, rape, or other unwanted sexual experiences.
- Identify recent unwanted sexual experiences.

Social

- Ask about cultural rituals, beliefs, and inhibitions (e.g., circumcision, menses, marriage).
- Note cultural expectations for sexual behavior.
- Note family composition and roles.
- Note changes in composition of family or peers.
- Ask about pattern of marital or sexual status and living arrangements.
- Note change in living arrangements or marital status.
- Ask about past sexual orientation and preference (e.g., homosexuality, bisexuality, heterosexuality, transsexuality).
- Identify current sexual preference and patterns of sexual activity.

➤ *Physical Assessment/Clinical Manifestations*

The nurse incorporates the sexual health assessment into a general physical assessment. Subjective data concerning body image may be gathered as the nurse palpates various parts of the body, moving from relatively neutral areas, such as the face and extremities, to the breasts and external genitalia. Nurses should always have concern for the client's dignity when assessing these more private areas. The nurse explains what is to be examined, in what manner, and for what reason. As in other physical assessments, the nurse pays attention to external appearance, palpation of internal structures, and any discharges (which may also need to be further assessed in the laboratory) as well as the client's subjective response to this examination.

While assessing the client's genitalia and breasts, the nurse may elicit additional information about sexual activity, knowledge, and attitudes. For example, when inspecting the external genitalia, the nurse might ask the client to describe his or her usual pattern of sexual activities and ask whether there is any discomfort or anxiety related to these behaviors.

Chapter 76 includes a detailed description of the physical assessment of genitalia and breasts. The clinical manifestations described in this chapter relate specifically to sexual functioning.

Dyspareunia

Dyspareunia (painful intercourse) in women may be related to several factors, such as

- An intact hymen
- Scarring from an episiotomy or infibulation
- Infections of the vagina or vulva, including venereal warts or other sexually transmitted diseases (STDs)
- Insufficient vaginal lubrication
- Irritation from chemical products, such as contraceptives, douches, and feminine deodorants

Pathologic conditions of the uterus, cervix, ovaries, and fallopian tubes may also result in dyspareunia. Such conditions should be ruled out through referral to a gynecologist or other physician. In a classic study by Gloeckner (1991), dyspareunia was the major complaint of women who had undergone a proctocolectomy (surgical removal of the colon and rectum). Dyspareunia may also be related to psychogenic factors, such as trauma from rape, incest, or other unwanted sexual experiences, or to previous experience with an inconsiderate partner.

In men, dyspareunia may be associated with inflammation or infection of the penis, prostate, urinary bladder, urethra, or testes. Men infrequently experience pain related to exposure to vaginal contraceptive creams or foams or lubricants on condoms or from irritation from the partner's intrauterine device (IUD). An increase in latex allergies must be considered as a possible cause of painful inflammatory responses in both men and women where condoms are routinely used.

Hypoactive Sexual Desire

Hypoactive sexual desire is a loss of interest in sexual activity or a decline in libido. In women it may be related to several factors, including

- Hormonal replacement therapy
- Use of oral contraceptives
- Eating disorders (e.g., anorexia nervosa or bulimia nervosa)
- Weight gain or loss
- Substance abuse
- Chronic illness (e.g., cancer or end-stage renal disease)

Psychosocial factors, such as abuse, marital or partner discord, family violence, depression, anxiety, fear, or other environmental stressors, may be major contributing factors.

In men, hypoactive sexual desire may be related to

- The use of antihypertensive drugs
- Substance abuse
- A chronic illness that affects energy levels

The psychosocial factors that affect men are the same as those affecting women.

Vaginismus

In a woman with vaginismus, the muscles of the outer third of the vaginal barrel contract powerfully and prevent insertion of a tampon or other object. This condition may be related to physical factors, such as sexual activity during the healing phase after childbirth, infections of the vagina and vulva, abnormalities of the hymen, and atrophy of the vagina. Other contributing factors include the person's lack of information, anxiety, and fear. Vaginismus is more likely to be related to psychogenic causes, including strong religious teachings, rape trauma, physical or psychosocial abuse, or homosexual experimentation about which the individual has conflicting feelings.

For an accurate assessment of vaginismus, the physician or nurse practitioner or nurse specialist must perform a direct pelvic examination.

Vaginitis

Vaginitis may be either acute or chronic. Because the vulva perspires more than other parts of the body, wearing restrictive clothing that is nonabsorbent places the woman at risk for irritation and infection. Strenuous exercising such as bike riding or horse-back riding in tight clothing can cause such irritation. Heterosexual intercourse without condoms changes the pH balance of the vagina, making it more alkaline and thus vulnerable to infection in the presence of other contributing factors. Other factors that contribute to vaginitis include stress, chemical irritants such as tampons containing deodorants and scented douches, and the use of antibiotics to treat other infections (Northouse, 1995).

Orgasmic Dysfunction

Orgasmic dysfunction is defined as the inability to achieve orgasm (primary dysfunction) or as the inability to achieve orgasm with intercourse or at an appropriate time during intercourse (secondary dysfunction). These dysfunctions are the most common sexual complaints of adult women. Orgasmic dysfunctions are related to physical factors, such as adhesions of the clitoris that interfere with stimulation, lack of strength in the pubococcygeal

muscles, and diminished contractions of the uterus. The nurse should refer women with these conditions to a nurse practitioner or physician for confirmation.

Other factors contributing to orgasmic dysfunction are psychogenic and may include

- Feelings of anxiety or guilt
- Lack of knowledge
- Poor communication skills
- Marital or partner discord/family violence

Fear of rejection and conscious withholding of orgasm may lead to secondary orgasmic dysfunctions. General expectations of the culture or society may also be contributing factors.

Erectile Dysfunction

Erectile dysfunction (impotence) is the inability of a man to attain or maintain an erection of the penis of sufficient firmness to permit penetration. This problem can be primary (the man has never been able to sustain an erection) or secondary (he has experienced at least one erection of sufficient firmness to permit penetration). The term *erectile dysfunction* is preferred to *impotence*.

Organic causes include spinal cord injury, diabetes mellitus, alcoholism, neurologic disease (such as multiple sclerosis), endocrine disorders, various infections or surgical procedures involving the genitourinary system, and specific drug use and abuse. Psychosocial factors contributing to erectile dysfunction include marital or partner discord, anxiety, depression, excessive weight gain or loss, insomnia, and fatigue.

Premature Ejaculatory Dysfunction

A man with a premature ejaculatory dysfunction ejaculates after penetration but sooner than either partner desires. Although there are no established norms for the timing of ejaculation during intercourse, this timing is important to the satisfaction of both partners involved in sexual activity. If the man is unable to exercise any voluntary control over the timing of this learned response, premature ejaculation may become a problem.

Organic causes are rare, if they exist at all; psychosocial factors contribute to the learning of this response. A man's feelings of anxiety, guilt, and fear, along with situations in which he may hurry toward a climax, may result in this type of dysfunction.

Retrograde Ejaculation

Retrograde ejaculation, or "dry orgasm," may sometimes be confused with ejaculatory incompetence because there is no external evidence of the ejaculate. Men experiencing retrograde ejaculation discharge semen in a reverse manner—into the urinary bladder rather than forward through the penis. This may result from prostatic surgery, diabetes, multiple sclerosis, structural defects of the urethra and bladder neck, or the use of tranquilizers. During orgasm, the bladder neck does not close and the semen is forced directly into it. The man experiences the sensation of orgasm but is infertile. In some cases, live sperm have been harvested from the urinary bladder and used for in vitro fertilization.

➤ *Psychosocial Assessment*

Once a sexual problem is identified or suspected, the nurse completes a more comprehensive and specific sexual health history. Although the general sexual history described earlier is an essential part of a nursing assessment, the nurse should obtain additional information about the psychological and social factors related to past and present sexual functioning when making a nursing diagnosis of sexual dysfunction. Subjective responses include the way in which the client perceives the problem as well as how he or she feels, thinks, and acts. The following questions may guide the nurse in making a more complete assessment of past and present factors related to sexual dysfunctions:

- How does the client describe the problem? What specific behaviors, thoughts, feelings, or attitudes are problematic?
- What is the client's perception of what caused the problem or what continues to contribute to the problem?
- What environmental or situational factors were present at the onset of the problem? Do these factors continue to interfere with sexual health and well-being?
- How has the problem changed over time? Has it become more severe or less severe? Does it occur in more than one setting?
- What has the client previously done to seek help from others, both professionals and peers? What forms of self-help has he or she tried? Have they been effective or ineffective and in what ways?
- What are the client's expectations and goals, both realistic and ideal, for therapeutic intervention and resolution of the problem?

In addition to this direct assessment of the client's sexual health, the nurse may notice problems of sexuality as a result of the client's "acting-out" behaviors. An example would be a client who exhibits inappropriate behaviors, such as exposing genitalia or overtly soliciting sexual favors from the nurse. The nurse should realize that such behavior may represent a coping mechanism on the part of the client, who may be overwhelmed by actual or potential threats to body image, gender identity, gender role, and sexual functioning. This pattern of behaviors may also indicate unresolved issues related to early sexual abuse or trauma.

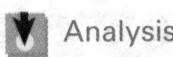 Analysis

➤ *Common Nursing Diagnoses and Collaborative Problems*

The major sexual problems addressed through the nursing process are sexual dysfunctions. Common problems related to sexual dysfunctions may affect either men or women or both and include

1. Sexual Dysfunction related to dyspareunia or hypoactive sexual desire
2. Sexual Dysfunction related to vaginismus or orgasmic dysfunction

3. Sexual Dysfunction related to erectile dysfunction, premature ejaculatory dysfunction, or retrograde ejaculation

➤ *Additional Nursing Diagnoses and Collaborative Problems*

In addition to the common nursing diagnoses, some clients may experience one or more of the following diagnoses:

- Ineffective Individual Coping related to loss of control over body part or body function
- Anxiety related to feelings of failure or loss of control
- Pain related to infectious process, inflammation, or muscle spasm
- Self Esteem Disturbance related to loss of function or physical appearance
- Body Image Disturbance related to change in physical appearance

 Planning and Implementation

➤ *Sexual Dysfunction Related to Dyspareunia or Hypoactive Sexual Desire*

Planning: Expected Outcomes

The outcomes, determined with the client, are that the client is expected to be free from pain or discomfort during sexual intercourse and resume interest in sexual activity.

Interventions

The nursing care for the man or woman who experiences dyspareunia depends in part on the cause of the problem.

Interventions for Dyspareunia in Women. Nursing interventions for the woman with dyspareunia depend on the contributing factors. When pain results from physical factors (e.g., an intact hymen, scarring from an episiotomy or infibulation, or pathologic conditions of the reproductive organs), the nurse refers the client to a gynecologist. Infections of the vagina or vulva also require medical diagnosis and treatment. If infection is present, the nurse administers prescribed antibiotics, provides increased fluid intake, and encourages the client to rest and avoid sexual activity. The nurse can use therapeutic communication and education to reduce further episodes of infection by listening with a nonjudgmental attitude and explaining about the risk of multiple partners, if this is a factor. The nurse also explains the risks associated with the client's usual sexual activities. For example, chronic irritations may result from foreign objects placed into the vagina without adequate lubrication, the use of chemical irritants, or wearing restrictive clothing.

When the major contributing factors include inadequate vaginal lubrication or irritation from excessive use of chemical contraceptives, douches, or feminine deodorants, clients need accurate information and specific suggestions for behavioral changes. The nurse reviews anatomy and physiology and emphasizes the ability of the vagina to clean itself. The nurse describes alternative methods of contraception and encourages the client to use unscented feminine products, including tampons or sanitary pads. Increasing vaginal lubrication through the use of over-the-counter water-soluble gels or a vaginal dilator may also be suggested.

Interventions for Dyspareunia in Men. When dyspareunia results from inflammation or infection of organs within the man's genitourinary system, the nurse administers prescribed antibiotics and encourages the client to drink fluids and to rest. The nurse encourages the man with acute inflammation or infection to avoid sexual intercourse with his partner until the acute condition is resolved. Alternative sexual activities that avoid intercourse are suggested and explored with both partners. Much literature is available to assist clients in trying alternative behaviors.

When the major contributing factor for dyspareunia in the man is exposure to vaginal contraceptive creams and foams or an intrauterine device (IUD) in the sexual partner, the nurse may suggest alternatives to both partners, such as mutual body massage and caressing until the infection clears.

Interventions for Hypoactive Sexual Desire. If hypoactive sexual desire in the woman is related to hormonal replacement therapy or oral contraceptive use, the nurse may present alternatives or refer the client to a gynecologist. For example, contraceptive foams, creams, or patches may be used in place of oral contraceptives. To increase the client's interest and sexual arousal, the nurse may suggest that the client use erotic reading or video materials or change the time and setting of usual sexual activities.

When drug or alcohol abuse or chronic illness is the major contributing factor in clients with hypoactive sexual desire, medical management of the underlying factor is required before other interventions can be tried. Certain hypothalamopituitary disorders result in loss of desire as well as problems with vaginal lubrication and orgasm (Hulter & Lundberg, 1994). If the prognosis for any of these conditions is poor, the outcome for the sexual problem is often poor. The nurse informs the client about the relationship between the underlying causes and the resulting sexual dysfunction.

Psychosocial factors that affect the development of hypoactive sexual desire are similar in both men and women. Marital or partner discord, depression, anxiety, and fear may be sufficiently severe to require the specialized education and experience of a nurse specialist or clinician with expertise in the area of psychology or psychiatry. Other psychiatric diagnoses such as depression may be associated with hypoactive sexual desire (American Psychiatric Association, 1994). Nursing interventions include therapeutic communication, encouraging the client to pursue intensive therapy with a qualified sex therapist, and referring the client to a competent professional. Often the process involves either the client or his or her sexual partner or partners or all of these people.

➤ Sexual Dysfunction Related to Vaginismus and Orgasmic Dysfunction

Planning: Expected Outcomes

The outcomes are that the client is expected to (1) relieve or prevent the involuntary spasms of the vagina and (2) experience an orgasm by any personally satisfying means.

Interventions

Interventions are often focused toward relieving the cause of the problem.

Interventions for Vaginismus. The nursing interventions for an actual problem of vaginismus aim to relieve the underlying contributing factors. The interventions for a potential problem of vaginismus are directed at educating the woman who is at risk for this response, thus preventing its occurrence.

If the major contributing factor is psychogenic, such as trauma from rape, conflicts surrounding homosexual experimentation, or strong religious teachings, the interventions are similar to those already discussed and range from giving permission to express anxiety and conflict to providing intensive therapy. If the major contributing factor is a physical one, such as sexual activity too soon after birth trauma, infection, abnormality of the hymen, or atrophy of the vagina, referral to a gynecologist may be indicated. Nursing interventions include encouraging the client to explore alternatives to vaginal intercourse during the healing process. The nurse also educates the woman and her sexual partner about the relationship between physical factors and involuntary muscular response.

Interventions for Orgasmic Dysfunction. When the major contributing factors in primary or secondary orgasmic dysfunction are psychogenic, the nurse provides opportunities for the client to talk about this situation. The nurse teaches the client about the relationship between stressors and the physical response of orgasm. The nurse also explains Kegel exercises, which strengthen the pubococcygeal muscles, and encourages general exercise to strengthen the pelvic musculature. Instructions for Kegel exercises are provided in Chart 11-3.

The client may need more intensive therapy, such as marriage counseling or in-depth counseling, for issues of anxiety and guilt. The nurse might refer the client to a nurse specialist or other professional in one or both of these specialties.

Chart 11-3

Education Guide

Kegel Exercises

1. Tighten the muscles as you would when stopping the flow of urine.
2. Hold for 2 to 3 seconds, then release.
3. Contract and relax these muscles 10 to 12 times and repeat this series several times daily.

If adhesions of the clitoris result in orgasmic dysfunction, the nurse refers the client to a physician for possible surgical intervention and provides encouragement that the condition may be corrected.

➤ *Sexual Dysfunction Related to Erectile Dysfunction, Premature Ejaculatory Dysfunction, or Retrograde Ejaculation*

Planning: Expected Outcomes

The outcomes are that the client is expected to (1) attain or maintain an erection, (2) delay ejaculation until he and his sexual partner are satisfied, and (3) accept the alteration of retrograde ejaculation and adjust to the resulting possibility of sterility.

Interventions

Interventions usually include treatment of the underlying cause of the problem(s).

Interventions for Erectile Dysfunction. For nursing interventions to influence the client's symptoms of erectile dysfunction, underlying diseases (e.g., diabetes mellitus, alcoholism, multiple sclerosis, endocrine disorders, and infections of the genitourinary system) must be under medical supervision. Appropriate nursing interventions include education; specific suggestions, such as the "sensate focus" technique; and alternatives for satisfying sexual activities. The sensate focus technique may also be used when the underlying factors are psychogenic. The nurse instructs the client and his partner in the following steps:

1. Mutual body touching and pleasuring without contact in the area of the genitalia
2. Genital stimulation, resulting in penile erection but not followed by intercourse
3. Orgasm and ejaculation through manual or oral stimulation (not vaginal penetration)
4. Vaginal penetration without orgasm or ejaculation (simple containment)
5. Vaginal penetration with orgasm and ejaculation
6. Dialogue between partners throughout steps

As with all sexual problems in which the major contributing factors are psychogenic, therapeutic communication and intensive therapy are indicated. The nurse makes the appropriate referrals, and the nurse specialist, psychotherapist, or psychiatrist provides therapy directed at alleviating underlying marital or partner discord, anxiety, or depression.

In the absence of underlying disease or obvious psychological factors, the use or abuse of various drugs may be the major etiologic factor in erectile dysfunction. The nurse explains the effects of such drugs as antihypertensives, barbiturates, sedatives, and amphetamines on the sexual response cycle. The nurse refers the client to a physician to evaluate the drug regimen so that an alternative drug, dosage, or therapy may be considered.

The client may also need referral to a urologist who treats men by self-injection of papaverine (Pavatine) and phentolamine (Regitine, Rogitine✝). These drugs are vasodilators that allow more blood to flow to the penis and facilitate erection. Many men have found these drugs to be successful. The nurse explains about possible side effects, including prolonged erection, bruising, and liver abnormalities. Another drug, prostaglandin E_1, has been found effective with intracavernosal self-injection (into the shaft of the penis) for use in elderly males (Godschalk et al., 1994).

Interventions for Premature Ejaculation. Nursing interventions for premature ejaculation include educating the client and sexual partner about the relationship between emotions and the sexual response cycle. The nurse may teach the client, partner, or both systematic relaxation exercises to alleviate anxiety as a major contributing factor. The nurse should be sure to include the client's sexual partner in the treatment, because the partner's communication of desires and expressions of distress may be instrumental in maintaining the dysfunction.

With appropriate preparation, the nurse may instruct the client and his partner in the "squeeze technique" for learning voluntary control for premature ejaculatory dysfunction. The man's partner can provide two types of squeezes.

In the traditional method, the partner places the thumb and first and second fingers just above and below the head of the penis and applies a squeezing pressure. In the basilar method, the thumb and fingers are placed at the base of the penis rather than at the head. Either position is held firmly for approximately 4 seconds, then released. The partner is instructed to always apply the pressure from the front to back of the shaft of the penis and never from side to side because this may result in tissue injury. The nurse should stress the importance of avoiding injury from the fingernails. The partner applies the squeeze shortly after erection occurs, and periodically thereafter, until both partners are ready for penetration to take place. Once the man has been aroused to the point of ejaculatory inevitability, this squeeze technique should not be used; instead, ejaculation should be allowed to continue.

Interventions for Retrograde Ejaculation. When the man's problem is retrograde ejaculation, the underlying cause is physiologic. Men who have diabetes, prostatic disease, multiple sclerosis, or abnormalities of the bladder and urethra must be referred to a urologist for further evaluation and medical or surgical intervention. With the exception of a physical abnormality, clients with diabetes, multiple sclerosis, or prostatic disease have an irreversible condition, and nursing interventions are thus directed at assisting them with coping skills. These men have an altered sensation from previous ejaculations and may be rendered sterile.

Education and counseling of the client and his sexual partner are important nursing interventions. The nurse reassures both partners that there are no harmful effects to the ejaculate being deposited in the bladder. Some clients who wish to have children are referred to an infertility clinic. It is possible for semen to be centrifuged from the urine and prepared for in vitro fertilization.

Continuing Care

When preparing clients to return home after hospitalization for illness, injury, or surgery, the nurse should anticipate plans for follow-up care and sexual counseling.

The nurse teaches the client and sexual partner, when appropriate, about the relationship of the illness, injury, or surgery to sexual functioning. For example, when clients have surgery or chemotherapy for cancer, they may experience temporary alterations in sexual desire. It is appropriate for the nurse to explain this situation and offer suggestions for less strenuous expressions of intimacy. Similarly, the nurse should counsel the client who has had a myocardial infarction about his or her anxiety related to resuming sexual intercourse.

The nurse teaches clients to report any adverse effects of medications on their sexual functioning. Nurses must be aware of how specific drugs affect sexual functioning and provide appropriate information to clients who will continue to receive these medications after discharge.

When clients are discharged to home health care, additional follow-up may be directed at the family caregiver. The caregiver who takes primary responsibility for care of a client in the absence of professional home health caregivers is often a spouse whose own health needs must also be considered.

Providing nursing care and being a sexual partner of the client may present conflicts for a spouse who accepts the role of family caregiver. Nurses should anticipate and prevent such conflict by discussing these roles with the family caregiver. The home health nurse can offer counseling or seek more expert assistance as the situation warrants.

 Evaluation

The expected outcomes are that the client
- Does not experience pain or discomfort associated with intercourse
- Describes restored levels of interest in sexual activity
- States that sexual activity is no longer accompanied by painful involuntary spasms of the vaginal wall
- Experiences orgasm as desired
- Reports satisfaction and enjoyment of orgasm
- Attains or maintains erections of the penis of sufficient firmness to permit vaginal penetration in at least 50% of attempts
- Learns voluntary control over the ejaculatory response

SELECTED BIBLIOGRAPHY

American Psychiatric Association. (1994). *Diagnostic and statistical manual of mental disorders (4th ed.).* Washington, D. C.: American Psychiatric Association.

*Cholewinski, J. T., & Burge, J. M. (1990). Sexual harassment of nursing students. *Image: Journal of Nursing Scholarship, 22,* 106–110.

Giger, J. N., & Davidhizar, R. E. (1995). *Transcultural nursing: Assessment and intervention* (2nd ed.). St. Louis: Mosby–Year Book.

Gloeckner, M. (1991). Perception of sexuality after ostomy surgery. *Journal of Enterostomal Therapy, 18*(1), 36–38.

Godschalk, M. F., Chen, J., Katz, P. G., & Mulligan, T. (1994). Prostaglandin E1 as treatment for erectile failure in elderly men. *Journal of the American Geriatric Society, 42,* 1263–1265.

Hulter, B., & Lundberg, P. O. (1994). Sexual function in women with hypothalamo-pituitary disorders. *Archives of Sexual Behavior, 23,* 171–183.

Jarvis, C. (1996). *Physical examination and health assessment* (2nd ed.). Philadelphia: W. B. Saunders.

Kendall, J. (1996). Human association as a factor influencing wellness in homosexual men with human immunodeficiency virus disease. *Applied Nursing Research, 9,* 195–203.

*Masters, W. M., Johnson, V. E., & Kolodny, R. C. (1985). *Human sexuality* (2nd ed.). Boston: Little, Brown.

Northouse, C. (1995). *Women's bodies, women's wisdom.* New York: Bantam Books.

Quadagno, D., Nation, A. J., Johnson, D., Waitley, C., Waitley, N., Epstein, D., & Satterwhite, A. (1995). Cardiovascular disease and sexual functioning. *Applied Nursing Research, 8*(3), 143–146.

*Roth, S., & Newman, E. (1991). The process of coping with sexual trauma. *Journal of Traumatic Stress, 4,* 279–297.

*Schiavi, R. C. (1992). Normal aging and the evaluation of sexual dysfunction. *Psychiatric Medicine, 10,* 217–225.

Skidmore-Roth, L. (1995). *Mosby's 1995 nursing drug reference.* St. Louis: Mosby.

Walker, L. R. & Morgan, M. C. (1995). Female circumcision: A report of four adolescents. *Journal of Adolescent Health, 17,* 128–132.

Waxman, B. F. (1994). Up against eugenics: Disabled women's challenge to receive reproductive health services. *Sexuality and Disability, 12,* 155–171.

SUGGESTED READINGS

Aloni, R., Schwartz, J., & Ring, H. (1994). Sexual function in post-stroke female patients. *Sexuality and Disability, 12,* 191–199.
   These researchers studied the sexual functioning in female patients 26 to 59 years of age who experienced strokes. They found their sexual functioning, including sexual desire, to be related to the severity of neurologic impairment. The article has good implications for nurses caring for young and middle-aged women with neurologic impairment.

Kendall, J. (1996). Human association as a factor influencing wellness in homosexual men with human immunodeficiency virus disease. *Applied Nursing Research, 9,* 195–203.
   This nursing study presents findings from in-depth interviews with 29 gay men with human immunodeficiency virus infection. The subjects stated that the need for intimacy and community were crucial to their well-being. The authors suggested that nurses should help clients connect and interact with others to enhance their wellness.

LOSS, DEATH, AND DYING

Loss, dying, and death are integral parts of living that accompany the developmental stages of late adulthood and are frequently associated with illness. Because nurses frequently face loss and death in their work, knowledge of responses to loss is essential in assisting clients and families to cope with these experiences.

LOSS
Overview

Loss is being deprived of or being without something valued that one once had. We begin life with loss, cast from the womb, and we experience losses throughout life. Although death may be considered the ultimate loss, it is not the only loss worthy of attention. There are various types of loss, each of which gives rise to grief reactions. Even minor losses give rise to grief, and insufficient attention to such losses could have a more profound impact on an individual in the long run than a loss through death.

Mitchell and Anderson (1983) have identified six major types of loss. The first is material loss, loss of a physical object to which one has important attachment. The second type is relationship loss, the ending of opportunities to relate to another human being. Although death is one example of this type of loss, any temporary or permanent separation of two human beings can be a relationship loss. Intrapsychic loss, the third type of loss, occurs when a person loses an emotionally important image of herself or himself. This experience often involves a vision or

dream of how things might have been; a change in one's perception of another; loss of emotions such as faith, hope, or courage; or emotions that occur on successful completion of a major task.

Functional loss, the fourth type of loss, involves the loss of a functional ability, as in the bodily decline of illness or aging. Role loss, the fifth type of loss, is loss of one's accustomed place in a social network. Role loss can occur through retirement or promotion, when one goes from being single to being married or vice versa, or when a person becomes a client.

Systemic loss, the sixth type of loss, occurs when one loses contact with certain interactional behaviors within a system. An employee leaving the workplace or a child leaving home affects the interactional behaviors within the workplace or the family.

Responses to Loss
Grief

Grieving is the psychologic, social, and physical reaction to the perception of significant loss. It is a natural response to loss and varies from one person to another, manifested as thoughts, feelings, and behaviors associated with often overwhelming distress or sorrow. Although a grief reaction can result from the loss of any precious element in a person's life, loss through death is used as the major example of grief for the remainder of this chapter.

Mourning is the process of doing the grief work. There

are numerous conceptualizations of mourning (or grieving), which use different labels to describe stages or phases. Conceptualizations differ in their focus or names. All were developed to describe reaction to loss, and all cover similar basic feelings. A major limitation of conceptualizations is that they describe only part of the grieving process.

Kübler-Ross's (1969) stages of coping with imminent death was one of the first conceptualizations to describe grieving after loss and included shock and disbelief, denial, anger, bargaining, depression, and acceptance.

SHOCK AND DISBELIEF. During this phase, the person has a desire to avoid the acknowledgment of loss because it is too overwhelming to deal with. Numbness and disbelief are prominent, and people are often confused, dazed, and unable to comprehend what has happened.

DENIAL. When a person is faced with an overwhelming loss, denial often buffers reality, allowing him or her to absorb the loss a little at a time. Denial is often therapeutic.

ANGER. At several times after news of an actual or anticipated loss, the client or family members feel and possibly express anger. Family members may be angry at the client or the deceased for leaving them and at God or fate for allowing the illness or death. Survivors of deceased people may be angry at family, friends, or caregivers for not saving the person's life. A person who is dying might ask, "Why me?"

BARGAINING. In this stage, people bargain with fate, physicians, the disease, or a deity for a short-term or long-term postponement of the loss. Characteristic responses are "I'll do anything as long as he lives . . ." and "Just let me live until my daughter gets married."

DEPRESSION. Crying and tearfulness are common during this stage. People lose interest in life and its meaning. Some isolate themselves socially, withdrawing from any conversation. Survivors may avoid discussions or activities, such as hobbies, that they had shared with the lost loved one. Many see life as a weighty burden and describe a lack of pleasure. They cannot believe that life will ever hold meaning and joy again. They may talk of suicide during the first year of bereavement and express a strong desire for reunion with the deceased.

The intensity of these negative feelings can be frightening. People who have had relatively stable or calm personalities may have a horror of losing emotional control. Their fears can be intensified by memory lapses and difficulty in concentrating. To gain control, they center on themselves, which can be interpreted as selfishness by themselves as well as by others.

Depression contributes to the bereaved's difficulty in concentrating and fuels excesses of anger, guilt, and extreme sadness. The bereaved may focus exclusively on the deceased and reject all offers of comfort.

ACCEPTANCE. The feelings and symptoms of grief do not simply stop completely one day. Sadness decreases only gradually, and a new life, based on the acceptance of a new reality, emerges slowly as time passes. With time, the bereaved may experience a new awareness of the precious gift each day brings.

Although Kübler-Ross and other theorists described grief in stages, it is now believed that these stages are not necessarily sequential, nor must each person go through each stage. More recent grief theorists describe reactions as opposed to stages, which include, but are not limited to, reactions described previously. These include guilt ("I should have done more;" or "It's my fault she died"), identification with the deceased (taking up one of his or her hobbies), "grief attacks" manifested as waves and pangs of emotional or physical pain, and visual or auditory hallucinations.

Manifestations of grief vary widely; people may take one step forward and two steps back, then half steps from side to side as they cycle through healing. Many people achieve healthy accommodation to a loss by doing the grief work or mourning rapidly, with very little disruption in their lives. Others' response may involve great life disruption.

Although estimates of a "normal" duration for grieving have been made, it is now believed that there is no fixed timetable by which a person passes through grieving. Normal grief is now viewed as a long-term process that may require long-term bereavement follow-up at critical points in the mourner's life. Because such a wide range of normal responses exist, nurses may need to consult with bereavement experts before labeling a reaction abnormal.

Rando (1993) identified six processes of mourning necessary for healthy accommodation to any loss:

- Recognizing the loss through acknowledgment and understanding
- Reacting to the separation by experiencing the pain and some form of expression of all the psychological reactions
- Realistically recollecting and reviewing the relationship with the lost object or person
- Relinquishing old attachments to the lost object or person and the old assumptive world
- Readjusting and adapting to the new world, developing a new relationship with the lost object or person, and adopting new ways of being in the new world (forming a new identity)
- Reinvesting in the new world

Complicated Mourning

Complicated mourning describes a state of compromise, distortion, or failure of one of the six processes of mourning (given a realistic amount of time since the loss). In all forms of complicated mourning, there are attempts to deny, repress, or avoid aspects of the loss and to hold onto and avoid relinquishing the loss. High-risk factors for complicated mourning are either associated with the specific loss (e.g., death) or are antecedent and subsequent variables (see Chart 12–1).

Chart 12–1

Nursing Care Highlight: High-Risk Factors for Complicated Mourning

Factors Associated with Death

• Sudden, unanticipated death (especially when traumatic, violent, mutilating, or random)
• Death from an overly lengthy illness
• Loss of a child
• Mourner's perception that the death was preventable

Antecedent and Subsequent Variables

• A premorbid relationship with deceased that was markedly angry, ambivalent, or dependent
• Prior or concurrent mourner liabilities of unaccommodated losses and/or stresses or mental health problems
• The mourner's perceived lack of social support

Collaborative Management

 Assessment

> *History*

In assessing a person who is grieving a death, the nurse obtains information on the relationship to and age of the deceased, cause of death and length of illness (if appropriate), length of preparation for the death, and degree of intimacy or intensity of the relationship. The nurse also obtains information on the bereaved person's age, education, employment, economic status, history of losses, history of depressions, personality or mental health problems, substance abuse, ethnic background, family structure, social support, coping strategies, and spiritual aspects (sense of meaning and purpose). Nurses must understand that the process of eliciting the material for a thorough assessment from the bereaved also can be a therapeutic encounter.

In all likelihood, the grieving client will not be able to supply all information in a business-like and straightforward manner. There will be pauses at certain questions for either the control or expression of feelings. Because it is difficult to predict which parts of the assessment will affect individual clients and in what ways, the nurse moves from topic to topic, not necessarily in order but guided by the client's response. The key is to keep the information flowing while comforting the person as much as possible.

> *Review of Loss*

Because most newly bereaved people have a need to repeat the circumstances of the terminal episode and the death, questions related to this need are asked at the beginning of the assessment. Often, by retelling the story to an empathic listener and possibly discharging tears, guilt, or anger, the client feels accepted and understood and does not react to the more factual and sensitive assessment items as intrusive or callous.

> *Physical Assessment/Clinical Manifestations*

Grief can cause physiologic distress in addition to emotional pain, which may lead to serious illness. Recent studies indicate that the physical health of caregivers often deteriorates while caring for a loved one, and caregivers often delay contact with health providers because they are preoccupied with their loved one's needs. The nurse should always assess survivors for any physical signs and symptoms of serious disease.

TRANSCULTURAL CONSIDERATIONS

 Most of the research on loss, grieving, and death has focused on Caucasian, English-speaking populations. The grieving responses of other cultural groups have not been widely studied, except in relation to religious origin. Table 12–1 lists specific beliefs and customs about death and dying of various religious groups.

 Analysis

> *Common Nursing Diagnoses and Collaborative Problems*

The nursing diagnoses given the highest priority when caring for a client reacting to potential death are

• Potential for Ineffective Individual Coping related to loss of significant other
• Anticipatory Grieving related to an actual or perceived loss

> *Additional Nursing Diagnoses and Collaborative Problems*

One or more of the following common diagnoses and collaborative problems may apply:

• Avoidance Coping related to support system deficit
• Compromised Family Coping related to knowledge deficit, emotional conflicts, role changes, or exhaustion of supportive capacity
• Disabling Family Coping related to unexpressed guilt, hostility, or anxiety of family member
• Spiritual Distress related to challenged belief and value system due to the loss
• Social Isolation related to others' intolerance to loss

Planning and Implementation

> *Potential for Ineffective Individual Coping*

Planning: Expected Outcomes. The client and family or significant others are expected to readjust, adapt, and be able to reinvest in the new world.

Interventions. Interventions are largely psychosocial and aim to provide sensitive support.

Offering Physical and Emotional Support. The nurse intervenes with those mourning a death by "being with" as opposed to "being there." "Being with" implies that the nurse is physically and psychologically with the grieving client, empathizing to provide emotional support. Listen-

TABLE 12–1

Major Religious Groups in the United States: Concepts and Practices Related to Death

Religious Group	Afterlife	Rituals	Handling of the Body After Death	"Extraordinary" Life-Prolonging Measures
Eastern Orthodoxy (including Greek and Russian Orthodoxy)	• Yes; the soul blends into the spiritual cosmos	• The client's arms are crossed after death, with the fingers set in the shape of a cross • Special prayers are said for those who have been baptized to bless the sick and dying • Last Rites must be delivered while the person is still conscious • Holy Communion is obligatory	• Autopsy and embalming are discouraged • Organ and body donation are discouraged • Cremation is discouraged	• Encouraged
Judaism	• The dead will be resurrected with the coming of the Messiah • A person lives on in the memories of his or her survivors • For Reform Jews, no concept of eternal punishment	• The dying and dead are never left unattended before burial because the soul should depart in the presence of people • The body is ritually washed, sometimes by members of a ritual burial society • Burial is in a wooden casket within 24 hours or as soon as possible after death • Five stages of mourning extend over a year • Funerals are very simple, with no flowers (flowers are a symbol of life)	• Orthodox Jews prohibit autopsy and allow no removal of body parts Conservative and Reform Jews permit autopsy For Orthodox Jews, no embalming is allowed • Beliefs about organ and body donation vary Orthodox Jews generally prohibit both but may agree, with rabbinical consent • Cremation is largely prohibited, but beliefs vary Reform Jews allow cremation but recommend burial of ashes in a Jewish cemetery	• Generally discouraged after irreversible brain damage is determined Orthodox Jews advocate life support without "heroic measures"

ing and somehow acknowledging the legitimacy of the client's pain are often more therapeutic than speaking. Physical support such as gentle touching, holding hands, and hugging are especially important during the first phases of grief. When necessary, nurses facilitate the expression of grief by giving the person mourning permission to express herself or himself. The nurse's manner and words show that the expression of grief is not only acceptable and expected but also healthy. Nurses can say something like "Just let the tears come. Don't hold back."

Being Realistic. The pain of loss cannot be, nor should it be, taken away no matter how committed the nurse may be to the client's comfort. The nurse avoids trite assurances such as "Things will be fine. Don't cry" or "Don't be upset. She wouldn't want it that way" or "In a year you will have forgotten." Such comments comfort the nurse—not the client. The nurse accepts whatever the griever says about the situation and remains present, ready to listen attentively and guide gently. In this way, nurses help the bereaved prepare for the necessary reminiscence and integration of the loss.

Avoiding Explanations of the Loss. The nurse should not try soon after the death to explain the loss in philosophical or religious terms. Statements such as "Everything happens for the best" or "God sends us only as much as we can bear" are not helpful when the bereaved person has yet to express feelings of anguish or anger. Telling someone too soon that they have other children to

TABLE 12–1

Major Religious Groups in the United States: Concepts and Practices Related to Death *Continued*				
Religious Group	Afterlife	Rituals	Handling of the Body After Death	"Extraordinary" Life-Prolonging Measures
Roman Catholicism	• The faithful go to Heaven, but those who reject God's grace go to Hell • The soul goes to Purgatory for a time and is released by prayers and Masses • Resurrection occurs at the second coming of Christ	• The family and priest choose prayers • Holy Communion and rites for anointing the sick are mandatory • Confession may be desired but is not mandatory; however, repentance is recommended	• Autopsy is permitted, but all body parts must be buried appropriately • Organ and body donation are unrestricted provided that the donor is not harmed • Cremation is not restricted	• Discouraged
Protestantism	• Varies; Episcopalians, Presbyterians, and Lutherans strongly believe in an afterlife, Quakers strongly do not	• Varies; anointing rites, confession, and communion may be available but are not mandatory • Healing services may be available, but there are no official sacraments • The client and family may have a large role in planning services and prayer; services range from traditional funerals to memorial services • Clergy may minister through prayer, scripture reading, and counseling	• Beliefs about autopsy, organ and body donation, and cremation vary by group from no restriction to individual choice to preferred	• Discouraged
Nonaffiliated	• Varies	• Spontaneous and individualized, possibly including reading of original or traditional prayers or songs such as Psalm 23 • Traditional secular funeral or memorial services are used	• Autopsy, organ and body donation, and cremation are by individual preference	• Individual preference

rely on or that there are other family members who need them does not diminish the intensity of the grief. In fact, doing so can create feelings of anger and resentment toward the nurse because it reflects an insensitivity to the acute initial pain.

"Being with" remains important as the weeks or months pass and the funeral crisis supports dissipate. The out-of-town relatives return home, and friends and local relatives resume their own lives. The nurse offers physical and emotional support by encouraging the bereaved to eat, drink, rest, and stay as physically active as possible. Exercise to tolerance levels is a wonderful psychic as well as physical energizer.

Referral to Bereavement Counselors. The nurse informs the family about bereavement counselors and groups for persons who have experienced the death of a loved one. This process can be especially effective if the nurse can help locate a group to meet the family's special needs. Many survivors experience uncomfortable feelings during the grief work, which they often don't discuss. They question their own mental stability and worry about what others will think of them. Seeing a counselor or being a part of a support group can help people discover that others have gone through a similar sequence and intensity of emotion, making them more likely to share their feelings and thus gain some comfort from others.

Chart 12–2

Education Guide: Common Physical Signs and Symptoms of Approaching Death

Coolness of Extremities

- Circulation to the extremities is decreased; the skin may become mottled or discolored
  - Cover the client with a blanket
  - Do not use an electric blanket, hot water bottle, electric heating pad, or hair dryer to warm the client

Increased Sleeping

- Metabolism is decreased
  - Spend time sitting quietly with the person
  - Do not force the person to stay awake
  - Talk to the person as you normally would, even if he or she does not respond

Fluid and Food Decrease

- Metabolic needs have decreased
  - Do not force the person to eat or drink
  - Offer ice chips or small sips of liquids frequently if the person is alert
  - Use glycerine swabs to keep the mouth moist and comfortable
  - Coat the lips with lip balm or petroleum jelly

Incontinence

- Perineal muscles relax
  - Keep the area clean and dry
  - If the person would be more comfortable, use urine catheters

Congestion and Gurgling

- The person is unable to cough up secretions effectively
  - Suctioning can be used to remove secretions, but this may cause the person discomfort
  - Medications can decrease the production of secretions

Breathing Pattern Change

- Slowed circulation to the brain may cause the breathing pattern to become irregular, with brief periods of no or shallow breathing
  - Elevate the person's head
  - Position the person on his or her side

Disorientation

- Decreased metabolism and slowed circulation to the brain may occur
  - Identify yourself whenever you communicate with the person
  - Speak softly, clearly, and truthfully

Restlessness

- Decreased metabolism and slowed circulation to the brain may occur
  - Play soothing music
  - Do not restrain the person
  - Massage the person's forehead
  - Reduce the number of people in the room

Adapted from the Hospice of North Central Florida, Inc.

➤ *Anticipatory Grieving*

Anticipatory grieving refers to accomplishing part of the grief work before the actual loss. Although dying clients experience anticipatory grieving, the term most often describes the process undergone by the families of clients with terminal illness. Anticipatory grieving can be beneficial if it helps people progress to a healthier state after the loss.

Planning: Expected Outcomes. The family or significant others should be able to accept the reality of the loss and share grief with others.

Interventions. Interventions aim to provide the family members of the dying client with appropriate information and emotional support.

Teaching About the Physical Signs of Death. Witnessing the death of a loved one is one of the most effective experiences in helping the family accept the reality of the loss. If death is anticipated, the nurse gives the client and family or significant others information about the signs of death, using nontechnical language. The nurse describes the physical signs in detail, realistic enough to be unmistakable, yet not so graphic as to alarm the listeners. Chart 12–2 describes common signs and symptoms of approaching death in lay terms. Such charts are often shared with family and friends anticipating a loved one's death.

Ensuring Palliative Care. When family and friends anticipate the death of a loved one, they may fear that the death will be characterized by pain and suffering. The nurse reassures families that clients will be monitored closely for any sign or symptom of distress and that appropriate medications will be administered as needed until pain is controlled. The nurse also reassures families that significant advances have been made in pain and symptom control. (See Interventions under Active Dying.)

 Evaluation

The nurse evaluates the care of the client and family anticipating or grieving loss on the basis of identified nursing diagnoses. Expected outcomes include that the client and family

- State acceptance and adaptation to the loss
- Share their grief with others

ACTIVE DYING
Overview
Death

Death is manifested as cessation of respiration and heartbeat caused by physiologic dysfunction, generally related to an illness or trauma that overwhelms the body's compensatory mechanisms. Direct causes of death include respiratory failure (PCO_2 accumulation and PO_2 deficit) and hypovolemic, septic, or cardiogenic shock, manifested as inadequate blood flow to meet the demands of vital organs. Inadequate blood flow to tissues deprives cells of their source of oxygen and biochemical exchange, the ultimate factor in their death. *Clinical death* refers to the short interval after cessation of heartbeat and cessation of breathing when no evidence of brain function is present. If this termination of function occurs suddenly, as in cardiac arrest or massive hemorrhage, a brief time remains before vital organs lose their viability, and cardiopulmonary resuscitation (CPR) may succeed. People with healthy organs are most likely to survive resuscitation. CPR is likely to be futile, and therefore inappropriate in resuscitating those with terminal disease. However, legal and ethical standards of care must be followed.

Most agencies require that CPR be initiated on clients when breathing or heartbeat ceases unless a doctor's order of "do not resuscitate" (DNR) is obtained. Because CPR is generally futile (and often inappropriate) in terminal illness, nurses need to address advance directives and DNR status with all clients who are actively dying.

Dying

Death is the termination of life. Dying is a process. Emotional responses of dying patients are similar to those described previously in responses to loss. Chart 12–3 lists some of the common emotional symptoms that the dying client may express. However, as death nears, clients

---

Chart 12–3

Education Guide: Common Emotional Signs of Approaching Death

Withdrawal

• The person is preparing to "let go" from surroundings and relationships.

Vision-like Experiences

• The person may talk to people you cannot see or hear and see objects and places not visible to you. These are not hallucinations or drug reactions.
  • Do not deny or argue with what the person claims
  • Affirm the experience

Letting Go

• The person may become agitated or continue to perform repetitive tasks. Often, this indicates that something is unresolved or preventing the person from letting go. As difficult as it may be to do or say, when loved ones are able to say such things as "It's okay to go. We'll be all right," the dying person takes on a more peaceful demeanor.

Saying Goodbye

• When the person is ready to die and you are ready to let go, saying "Goodbye" is important for you both. Touching, hugging, crying, and saying "I love you," "Thank you," "I'm sorry," or "I'll miss you so much" are all natural expressions of your sadness and loss. Verbalizing these sentiments can bring comfort to the dying person as well as to those left behind.

Adapted from the Hospice of North Central Florida, Inc.

Chart 12–4

Nursing Care Highlight: Contents of Symptom Relief Kit

• For unrelieved pain: Morphine solution, 20 mg/mL, 1–2 mL (PO/SL) q2–3h PRN
• For unrelieved dyspnea: Morphine solution, 20 mg/mL, 0.25–0.5 mL (PO/SL) q2h PRN
• For nausea or vomiting: Prochlorperazine, 25 mg suppository, 1 PR q8h PRN
• For unrelieved nausea, vomiting, restlessness: ABR* suppository, 1 PR q8h PRN
• For severe agitation and restlessness:
  • Determine if client is in pain; treat accordingly
  • Determine if client is constipated or having urinary retention; take appropriate action
  • If agitation persists and safety of client or caregiver is at risk, administer pentobarbitol suppository 1 PR, q4–6h PRN
• For loud, wet respirations or excessive secretions: Levsin/SL tablets, 1–2 PO or SL q4–6h PRN
• For unrelieved respiratory fluid accumulation: Furosemide (Lasix) 40–80 mg PO, SC, IM, or IV q2h PRN

Printed with permission from VNA Hospice, Optima Health Visiting Nurse Services, Manchester, NH.
  *Many hospice and palliative care organizations will use pharmacist-compounded suppositories for symptom relief. One such combination is ABR, which stands for Ativan, Benadryl, and Reglan (lorazepam, diphenhydramine, and metoclopramide).

---

may manifest fear, anxiety, and physical symptoms of distress, which require treatment and control. Although the majority of symptoms near death can be controlled, expert clinical judgment and knowledge of palliative care are often required. Even with optimal care, a certain percentage of clients have intractable symptoms that may require sedation until death. Providers on oncology units or in hospice services are often knowledgeable about palliative care. Chart 12–4 summarizes the contents of a symptom relief kit used by hospice nurses to provide immediate relief from uncomfortable or distressing symptoms. Palliative care nurses and physicians may be consulted if clients cannot be transferred to these services.

Hospice Services

Hospice care was developed in the United States in the 1970s in response to unmet needs of terminally ill clients. As both a philosophy and a system of care, hospice care seeks to facilitate quality of life and death with dignity for clients with terminal disease, using a multidisciplinary approach. Hospice programs are frequently affiliated with home care agencies, providing services to clients at home or in an extended care facility. Some communities also have hospice "houses," which admit clients in the terminal phase of their illness, allowing them to die there.

Not all hospices restrict their services to the terminally ill. Some hospice agencies divide their services into "supportive care" for clients with advanced disease not necessarily limited to a 6-month prognosis and "hospice" for clients with a documented prognosis of 6 months or less.

This facilitates the delivery of expert palliative care to clients whose exact prognosis might not be known, and/or when clients, families, and/or physicians referring clients are averse to the word "hospice." To many, *hospice* connotes only the negative aspects of death.

Collaborative Management

 Assessment

➤ History

The nurse obtains information on the client's diagnosis, past medical history, and recent state of health to identify possible risks for symptoms near death. For example, clients with lung cancer, cardiac failure, or chronic respiratory disease are at high risk for respiratory distress near death. Clients with pain syndromes may continue with the same pain intensity or have more or less pain as death nears.

➤ *Physical Assessment/Clinical Manifestations*

The nurse assesses for signs and symptoms of impending death. Most research on symptoms near death has been conducted on clients with cancer. These studies have identified anywhere from 14 to 44 symptoms during the active phase of dying (see Charts 12–2 and 12–3), including pain, dyspnea, delirium, nausea, and vomiting, as the most distressing symptoms occurring near death in clients with terminal cancer.

The nurse assesses vital signs, respiratory rate, breath sounds, cough, bowel sounds, abdominal distention, last bowel movement, and urine output to determine any possible or potential symptom of distress. All clients or family members are subjectively assessed for pain or discomfort. Any discomfort is rated by the client, using a visual or verbal analog scale if possible. Information on pain is also elicited with regard to its location, character, level of intensity in the past, reaction to medication, effect on activities, and effect on sleep. Frequency and amount of medications to treat and control pain are documented at least daily, along with client satisfaction and goals regarding pain control. Chapter 9 provides detailed information regarding types of pain and methods of control.

TRANSCULTURAL CONSIDERATIONS

Mainstream United States values affect how middle-class, upper-middle-class, and upper-class people in the United States deal with "dying." These groups believe that an answer or solution is always possible and that choices should always be available. This is probably why the dying process in this country is so frequently oriented to a "high-tech" hospital setting and why family demands for testing and treatment are common, even when clients themselves prefer a palliative approach.

Hispanic-Americans tend to see dying as a family affair: One primary caregiver, usually a wife or daughter, tends to take responsibility for the majority of care. For Southeast Asians, discussing dying brings bad luck, and hospitals and treatments are alien. Some Southeast Asians, especially if uneducated, are likely to avoid visiting terminally ill family members for fear of contracting the disease.

Various other values, religious beliefs, practices of healing (e.g., faith healing), and family structures can also affect dying in both positive challenging and negative ways. Nurses need to assess cultural beliefs of both clients and families to assess their potential effect on the process of dying and symptom control. (See Chapter 9 for transcultural pain considerations.)

Interventions

Interventions for the actively dying client are to prevent and control symptom distress until death.

Food and Fluids

Because of weakness and fatigue, clients should be restricted to bed during the active phase of dying, unless they express the desire to be up in a recliner. Because they are weak and fatigued, they commonly experience impaired swallowing. They may also lack desire to eat or drink. In either of these situations, caregivers should refrain from providing anything by mouth because of the risk of regurgitation and aspiration. Nurses need to reassure family that anorexia is frequently normal at the end of life. Families may have great difficulty accepting that their loved ones are not being fed and may request that intravenous fluids be initiated. With great sensitivity, nurses reinforce that cessation of food and liquids is thought to be a natural process and that hydration can actually increase discomfort in a person with multisystem slow-down. Discomfort from fluid replacement could lead to respiratory secretions (and distress), increased gastrointestinal secretions, nausea, vomiting, edema, and ascites.

With poor or no fluid intake, the client's mouth becomes uncomfortably dry. However, comfort can be provided by moistening the mouth and lips with applicators and saturated gauze and by applying emollient to the lips.

Nausea and vomiting can be controlled with a variety of antiemetic agents. Combinations of antiemetics often must be individualized for clients for maximal relief of nausea and vomiting (see Chart 12–4).

Pain Management

Pain is the symptom that dying clients fear the most; although not universal, pain is common. There are many possible causes for pain in dying clients. Diseases such as cancer often cause tumor pain due to infiltration of malignant cells into organs, nerves, and bones. Other causes of pain in dying clients include "disturbance" pain resulting from headaches, osteoarthritis, muscle spasms, and stiff joints caused by immobility.

Clients who have had their pain controlled by long-acting narcotics (e.g., clients with cancer or HIV) may or may not have an increase in pain near death. These clients must still continue scheduled doses of opioids to prevent any recurrence of pain. Increases in pain require immediate-relief analgesics (e.g., morphine sulfate immediate-release liquid) and possibly an increase in long-acting opioids. Long-acting opioids may be increased by an amount equal to the previous day's total opioid requirement as frequently as every 24 hours, with physician guidance. Clients who cannot safely swallow receive analgesics by rectum, sublingually, or by subcutaneous or intravenous infusion.

Nurses are often concerned that high doses of opioids may cause a client's death and are often reluctant to administer opioids, especially when death is near. Nurses should understand the importance of medicating clients when *any* symptoms of pain manifest, regardless of level of consciousness. According to the Agency for Health Care Policy and Research *Management of Cancer Pain Clinical Practice Guideline* (1994), "when death due to progressive cancer is imminent, a risk of earlier death counts little against the benefit of pain relief and a painless death" (p. 64). Nurses should be knowledgeable about equigesic doses and formulas to calculate bolus dosages for breakthrough pain (see Chap. 9).

Respiratory Distress

Accumulation of mucus in the large bronchi may cause loud, noisy respirations. This noise, known as the "death rattle," is very distressing to family members. The secretions can be reduced with sublingual administration of anticholinergic agents such as hyoscyamine (Levsin). If this is not effective, a diuretic such as furosemide (Lasix) may be tried. The client may be made more comfortable by a change of position onto his or her side with the head slightly elevated (supported on a pillow).

Dyspnea and/or labored respirations, which often require morphine, are common symptoms near death. The starting dose for treating dyspnea is 2.5 to 5.0 mg of oral morphine every 4 hours, which can be increased to 5 to 10 mg orally or subcutaneously every 2 hours (see Chart 12–4). Clients who are already receiving morphine for pain control usually require a 50% increase for relief of dyspnea. Other interventions to relieve dyspnea include opening a window, administering oxygen, and administering antianxiety drugs such as lorazepam (Ativan).

Anxiety and Agitation

The dying client may experience restlessness or agitation. When such symptoms are present, the client should be assessed for pain or urinary retention. If analgesia and catheterization do not relieve restlessness, sedation can be prescribed to promote a peaceful death. Once adequate sedation is achieved, sedatives should be continued around the clock to prevent further restlessness and terminal agitation.

Skin Changes

The client's skin may be damp with cold perspiration even though he or she complains of feeling overly warm. The nurse keeps the client dry by frequent sponging if a fever is present. Only a light covering is necessary.

As the peripheral circulation lessens, the client's hands, feet, ears, and nose become cold. The client's hands and feet may become mottled and cyanotic. If blood pressure has been monitored, the nurse will notice that it becomes lower and then disappears. The dying person's pulse may double in rate, weaken, gradually decrease, and stop. Meanwhile, respirations become shallow until they too stop. Death has taken place when respirations and heartbeat cease.

Sensory Perception

The family and health care professionals should be aware that the dying client's sense of hearing may remain intact even though it appears that he or she can perceive no other stimuli. Conversation in the room and near the client should be carried on as if the client were alert. Caregivers should be encouraged to talk softly to the client and to touch and gently stroke him or her. The dying person may not respond, but the family will feel better maintaining a normal interchange. This activity fosters a sense of active, reciprocal communication for everyone right up to the end. Soft music might also be played on a tape recorder.

Postmortem Care

The dying client may have such reduced physical activity that actual death can be difficult to ascertain. Chart 12–5 lists physical manifestations of death.

After a client's death, the nurse or the physician (depending on the state of death) pronounces death. He or she then completes a death certificate, which must accompany the body to the funeral home. The nurse or other member of the nursing staff prepares the body for immediate postmortem viewing. All tubes and linens are removed or cut according to agency policy, the eyes are closed, dentures are replaced, and the body is straightened. The nurse removes all pillows except for one supporting the head, kept in place to delay blood pooling and discoloration of the face. Pads are placed under the client's hips and around the perineum to absorb fecal material and fluid. Each health care agency has its own policies and procedures for postmortem care. Chart 12–6 lists typical postmortem nursing interventions.

Chart 12–5

Education Guide: Physical Manifestations of Death

- No breathing
- No heartbeat
- Release of bowel and bladder contents
- No response to name, environmental sounds, touch, or pain
- Eyelids slightly open
- Pupils enlarged and not constricting in response to light
- Eyes fixed on a certain spot
- No blinking in response to air moving over the eyes or to a light touch on the eye
- Jaw relaxed and mouth slightly open

Chart 12–6

Nursing Care Highlight: Postmortem Care

- Ensure that the nurse or physician has completed and signed the death certificate
- Ask the family or significant others if they wish to wash or help wash the client
- Remove or cut all tubes and lines according to health care agency policy
- Close the client's eyes
- Replace dentures or other dental appliances, if worn
- Straighten the client and lower the bed to a flat position
- Place a pillow under the client's head
- Wash the client as needed; comb and arrange the client's hair
- Place pads under the client's hips and around the perineum to absorb feces and urine
- Clean up the client's room or unit
- Allow the family or significant others to see the client in private and perform any religious or cultural customs they wish
- Notify the hospital chaplain or appropriate community religious leader if requested by the family or significant others
- Prepare the client for transfer to either a morgue or funeral home; wrap the client in a shroud and attach identification tags per agency policy (if the client is to be transferred to the morgue)

The family or significant others may then have privacy while they join the deceased in the room. They may perform religious or cultural customs, as described in Table 12–1. If the family wishes to see a member of the clergy, the nurse notifies the hospital chaplain or appropriate community religious leader.

After the family or significant others view the body, the nurse follows agency procedure for preparing the client for transfer to either the morgue or a funeral home. The necessary materials, such as a shroud and identification tags, are usually supplied in a packet.

Home Care

Most people who choose hospice care prefer the home to other caregiving environments during the final episodes of the illness. Although there are exceptions, being surrounded by familiar people and things and having ready access to friends and relatives and the freedom from institutional restriction often make the home setting more comfortable and give the client and family more control. Clients whose cases are being followed by home hospice agencies have access to nurses, social workers, spiritual and/or bereavement counselors, and volunteers to assist in dealing with multiple end-of-life issues. Multidisciplinary hospice team meetings are regularly scheduled to review client needs and solve problems.

Although home care is less costly than any sort of inpatient care, it generally requires that a friend or family member(s) take on the responsibility of providing most physical and emotional care. Some families may not be able to manage the physically and psychologically de-

manding schedule of 24-hour, 7-day-a-week care. Depending on insurance benefits, some families may be entitled to assistive personnel for personal client care in the home. Generally, health care aides are only allowed to assist in the home for 1 to 2 hours once a day, sometimes twice each day if clients are bedbound or incontinent. Families who require more assistance with personal (custodial) care are often referred to agencies that hire out private duty nursing assistants. However, the family must pay for these services, and many families cannot afford them. If families are exhausted from providing care, respite care of the client in a hospital or nursing home for a short time may be available to allow caregivers a few days of rest.

Some family members may have crippling anxiety about what to do when clients manifest symptoms such as pain, dyspnea, or difficulty breathing. Hospices generally provide 24-hour on-call services to facilitate client needs, and medications to control symptoms of distress should be readily available in the home. Because it is not always possible to predict the final phase of the terminal process, some hospices have arranged for pharmacies to supply clients (by prescription) with "symptom relief kits." These provide a limited amount of commonly used medications effective in treatment of symptoms near death. Chart 12–4 describes contents and directions for a "hospice symptom relief kit" to facilitate "safe passage" in the home.

End-of-Life Issues

Under some conditions, keeping someone alive through technological life support rather than actively and arbitrarily ending his or her life can provide time—time to try an experimental new therapy or perhaps for a remission. Unfortunately, an interval like this is not always "good" or "quality" time for peace and growth but is time fraught with pain, suffering, and confusion. The occurrence and fear of pain and suffering have stimulated movements that provide and support the controversial practice of euthanasia in our society.

Euthanasia, derived from a Greek word meaning "easy or pleasant death," implies that under some circumstances, death is preferable to life. *Active euthanasia* refers to an act of commission that directly and *intentionally* shortens a person's life. *Passive euthanasia* is an act of omission and usually refers to letting the person die by either withdrawing or withholding a treatment that might prolong life.

Although active euthanasia, or "mercy killing," is condemned by many professional organizations (e.g., the American Nurses' Association, the American Medical Association) and religious communities (e.g., the Catholic Church), the rights of clients or their surrogates to refuse or stop life-sustaining treatment (e.g., mechanical ventilation, tube feedings, antibiotics) are actually supported by these same communities. Advance directives (e.g., durable power of attorney for health care, living will) have allowed United States residents to make their wishes known about treatment at the end of life, helping surrogate decision-makers to make their own decisions when clients are unconscious or incompetent. The Patient Self-

▷ Research Applications for Nursing

Painful Deaths for Seriously Ill Hospitalized Patients Continue Despite a Physician Education Intervention

A controlled trial to improve care for seriously ill hospitalized patients. (1995). Journal of the American Medical Association, 274, 1591–1598.

The objectives of this two-phase study were to improve end-of-life decision-making and to reduce the frequency of mechanically supported, painful, prolonged dying in seriously ill hospitalized clients. The sample involved 9105 adults hospitalized with one or more of nine life-threatening diseases in one of five major teaching hospitals in the United States. Phase I, a 2-year prospective observational study, found that only 47% of physicians knew when their clients preferred to avoid cardiopulmonary resuscitation (CPR); 38% of clients who died spent at least 10 days in an intensive care unit; and family reports of moderate to severe pain occurred at least half the time in 50% of clients near death.

In phase II (intervention phase), physicians were provided with estimates of client 6-month survival (given their disease and condition), estimates of outcomes for CPR, and estimates on functional disability for clients at 2 months. This phase also included a specially trained nurse making multiple contacts with clients, families, physicians, and hospital staff to elicit preferences, improve understanding of outcomes, encourage attention to pain control, and facilitate advance directive planning and client-physician communication. Results of phase II were that clients experienced no improvement in client-physician communication, no improvement occurred in physicians' knowledge of client preferences not to be resuscitated, the number of days clients spent on mechanical ventilation or comatose in intensive care units did not decrease, and the level of pain reported by families of clients near death did not decrease.

Critique. This study was rigorous in its experimental design and large sample size. However, it does not explain why aggressive treatment was continued despite poor odds for recovery. For example, did clients change their minds? Did physicians simply ignore what clients and nurses communicated? Did they see the teaching hospital as one that assumes aggressive care, regardless of the odds? A qualitative component to the study might shed light on findings.

Possible Nursing Implications. The role of the nurse in discussing end-of-life issues in acute care may not be deemed appropriate by providers making treatment decisions. Despite this perception, nurses are generally guided by state nurse practice acts to obtain comprehensive assessment data on all clients, and nurses are often the best equipped to initiate discussions on end-of-life issues. Nurses working with clients with serious illnesses should identify and fulfill their educational needs regarding end-of-life issues and effectively communicate their knowledge and concerns to physicians, clients, and families when appropriate.

Determination Act (1990) requires that all clients admitted to health care agencies be asked if they have drafted advance directives. The Act's intent was to facilitate end-of-life treatment decisions prior to a crisis situation. Clients who have not drafted advance directives should be given information about the process and implications of having (or not having) these in place and should be assisted in drafting them.

Much confusion exists regarding euthanasia and treatment of dying clients. It is important that health care providers, clients, and families understand the distinctions of active and passive euthanasia and assisted suicide versus appropriate treatment of pain and symptoms of distress. Because nurses spend more time with clients than any other health provider, they should be competent in and committed to initiating discussions of end-of-life issues when appropriate. Recent research indicates that many hospitalized clients die undergoing aggressive treatment and pain, without regard for their wishes. Better communication between clients and health providers and more collaboration among physicians and nurses are needed if end-of-life decisions of clients in acute care are to be heeded (see Research Applications for Nursing).

SELECTED BIBLIOGRAPHY

*Amenta, M., & Bohnet, N. (1986). *Nursing care of the terminally ill.* Boston: Little, Brown.
*American Nurses' Association. (1987). *Standards and scope of hospice nursing practice.* Kansas City: American Nurses' Association.
Benzein, E., & Saveman, B. (1998). Nurses' perception of hope in patients with cancer: A palliative care perspective. *Cancer Nursing, 21*(1), 10–16.
Callanan, M. (1994). Farewell messages. *American Journal of Nursing, 94*(5), 19–20.
*Carmack, B. J. (1992). Balancing engagement/detachment in AIDS-related multiple losses. *Image: Journal of Nursing Scholarship, 24,* 9–14.
A controlled trial to improve care for seriously ill hospitalized patients. (1995). *Journal of the American Medical Association, 274,* 1591–1598.
*Cooley, M. E. (1992). Bereavement care: A role for nurses. *Cancer Nursing, 15*(2), 125–129.
Corless, I. B., Germino, B. B., & Pittman, M. (1994). *Dying, death, and bereavement: Theoretical perspectives and other ways of knowing.* Boston: Jones and Bartlett.
Dean, G. E. (1995). Symptom management for the dying patient. *Quality of Life—A Nursing Challenge 3*(3), 61–66.
Edwards, B. S. (1994). When the family can't let go. *American Journal of Nursing, 94*(1), 52–56.
*Farberow, N. L. (1992). Changes in grief and mental health of bereaved spouses of older suicides. *Journal of Gerontology, 47,* 357–366.
*Gardner, D. L. (1992). Presence. In G. M. Bulachek & J. C. McCloskey (Eds.), *Nursing interventions: Essential nursing treatments* (2nd ed., pp. 191–200). Philadelphia: W. B. Saunders.
Gavrin, J., & Chapman, C. R. (1995). Clinical management of dying patients. *Caring for patients at the end of life [Special Issue]. Western Journal of Medicine, 163,* 268–277.
Kazanowski, M. (1997). A commitment to palliative care—Could it impact assisted suicide? *Journal of Gerontological Nursing, 3*(3), 1–7.
Kemp, C. (1995). *Terminal illness.* Philadelphia: J. B. Lippincott.
*Kübler-Ross, E. (1969). *On death and dying.* New York: Macmillan.
*Lindemann, E. (1944). Symptomatology and management of acute grief. *American Journal of Psychiatry, 101,* 141–149.
*Lindley-Davis, B. (1991). Process of dying: Defining characteristics. *Cancer Nursing, 14,* 328–333.
Management of Cancer Pain Guideline Panel. (1994). *Management of cancer pain clinical practice guideline.* AHCPR Pub. No. 94-0592. Rockville, MD: Agency for Health Care Policy and Research.
Meares, C. (1994). Terminal dehydration: A review. *The American Journal of Hospice & Palliative Care, 11*(3), 10–14.
*Mitchell, K. R., & Anderson, H. (1983). *All our losses, all our griefs.* Philadelphia: Westminster Press.
*Nuland, S. B. (1993). *How we die.* New York: Vintage Books.
*Rando, T. A. (1984). *Grief, dying, and death.* Champaign, IL: Research Press.

*Rando, T. A. (1993). *Treatment of complicated mourning.* Champaign, IL: Research Press.

Sheehan, D. C., & Forman, W. B. (1996). *Hospice and palliative care.* Sudbury, MA: Jones and Bartlett.

*United States Congress. (1990). *Omnibus Budget Reconciliation Act of 1990* (pp. 101–508). Pub L Washington, D. C.: United States Congress.

SUGGESTED READINGS

Dean, G. E. (1995). Symptom management for the dying patient. *Quality of Life—A Nursing Challenge* 3(3), 61–66.

This article provides a concise, valuable description of common symptoms of distress in patients with cancer near death. Causes and interventions are discussed for pain, dyspnea, restlessness, agitation, problems with elimination, and fatigue.

Kazanowski, M. (1997). A commitment to palliative care—Could it impact assisted suicide? *Journal of Gerontological Nursing,* 3(3), 1–7.

This is one of several articles on end-of-life issues published in a special issue of the *Journal of Gerontological Nursing.* In support of palliative care, the author describes how this philosophy differs from the acute care model and suggests that more widespread knowledge about both the existence and goals of palliative care might make assisted suicide less appealing.

Meares, C. (1994). Terminal dehydration: A review. *The American Journal of Hospice & Palliative Care,* 11(3), 10–14.

This article is based on a review of the literature on terminal dehydration near death. The author describes the physiology, patient symptoms, ethical and legal issues, and physician and nurse perceptions of withholding fluid near death. The author points out that the vast majority of hospice nurses studied believe that aggressive nutritional support in a dying patient does more harm than good.

Chapter 13

REHABILITATION OF CLIENTS WITH CHRONIC AND DISABLING CONDITIONS

CHAPTER

HIGHLIGHTS

A chronic illness or condition is one that has existed for at least 3 months. A disabling condition is any physical or mental health problem that can cause disability. This text focuses on physical health problems; mental health problems are discussed in textbooks on mental health nursing.

Clients with chronic and disabling conditions often participate in rehabilitation programs to prevent disability, maintain functional ability, and restore as much function as possible. The nurse is a vital rehabilitation team member.

OVERVIEW

Chronic illness is a major health problem in the United States. Approximately 50% of the population have one or more chronic illnesses. About 35 million people, or one in seven, experience activity limitations because of their chronic health problems. Most of these individuals are in residential settings.

In the United States, the annual cost of chronic and disabling conditions is more than $200 billion in medical care and lost productivity. Disability occurs slightly more often in men than in women and in families with lower incomes (Institute of Medicine, 1991).

Stroke is the leading cause of disability, costing more than $30 billion each year in medical costs and loss of productivity (Collins, 1997). Coronary artery disease, cancer, chronic airflow limitation (CAL), and arthritis are other common chronic conditions that may result in varying degrees of disability. Most of these conditions occur in people older than 65 years.

Chronic and disabling conditions are not always diseases such as cancer; they may also result from accidents. Accidents are the leading cause of death among young adults and the third leading cause of death in people 45 to 54 years old. Today, increasing numbers of people survive accidents because of advances in medical technology. These survivors are often faced with chronic or disabling conditions, such as head and spinal cord injuries (SCIs). Therefore, the need for rehabilitation is on the rise. Such survivors may need months to years of follow-up health care after returning to the community.

CONCEPTS RELATED TO REHABILITATION

Rehabilitation is the process of learning to live with chronic and disabling conditions, often those resulting from trauma. The goal of rehabilitation is to return the client to the fullest possible physical, mental, social, vocational, and economic capacity. However, rehabilitation is not limited to the return of function in post-traumatic situations. It includes education and therapy for any chronic illness characterized by a change in a body system function or body structure. Rehabilitation programs related to respiratory, cardiac, musculoskeletal, and oncologic disorders are common examples that do not involve trauma.

In any discussion of rehabilitation, it is important to define and distinguish the terms *impairment, disability,* and *handicap.* These terms have been used interchangeably in some settings; however, for this chapter, the terms are defined according to the classic, but still widely used, *International Classification of Impairments, Disabilities and Handicaps* (World Health Organization, 1980).

Impairment

Impairment is an abnormality of a body structure or structures or an alteration in a body system function resulting from any cause; it represents a disturbance at the organ level. Impairments can be temporary or permanent and may or may not be associated with an active pathologic condition.

Disability

Disability is the consequence of an impairment and is usually described in terms of a client's altered functional ability; it represents disturbance at the personal level. A variety of diseases or traumas impair mobility and may result in a decreased ability to function.

Handicap

A handicap is the disadvantage experienced by a person as a result of impairments and disabilities; it represents disturbance at the societal level. This disadvantage is based on interactions that the client experiences with the environment. Handicaps are associated with negative values that a person or society ascribes to the person's situation or experience. Handicaps are both preventable and reversible, although impairments caused by pathologic changes in a body organ and the resulting disabilities are often unpreventable or irreversible.

REHABILITATION AS PART OF CONTINUING CARE

After a client's acute condition or injury has been stabilized in a hospital, the client may be discharged to continue the healing process, generally under the follow-up care of a nonhospital health care provider, such as a family physician. The nurse provides home care prepara-

tion, health teaching, psychosocial preparation, and information about various health care resources to help the client resume their usual roles in society.

Some health problems, however, require the intermediate step of rehabilitation, which can take place in a number of settings. Rehabilitation starts in the acute care hospital (sometimes called acute rehabilitation) and continues after discharge from the hospital. The nurse's coordination of care from acute care through continuing care is critical to the success of rehabilitation.

Settings for Rehabilitation

For continuing rehabilitation services, the most common settings are freestanding rehabilitation hospitals, rehabilitation units within hospitals, and skilled nursing home units to which the client is typically admitted for 1 to 4 weeks (Fig. 13–1). Outpatient (ambulatory) rehabilitation departments and home rehabilitation programs may be needed to continue less intensive rehabilitative services after discharge from one of the inpatient settings or as an alternative to inpatient rehabilitation.

Some hospitals and nursing homes have converted one or more inpatient units into subacute care units or transitional care units (TCUs). The client can then stay in the same health care system for both acute and continuing rehabilitative care.

After disabled clients become more confident and independent in the inpatient setting, they may choose to live at home or in a group home. These living centers are facilities in which clients live independently while together with other disabled adults. Each client or group of clients has a care provider, such as a personal care aide,

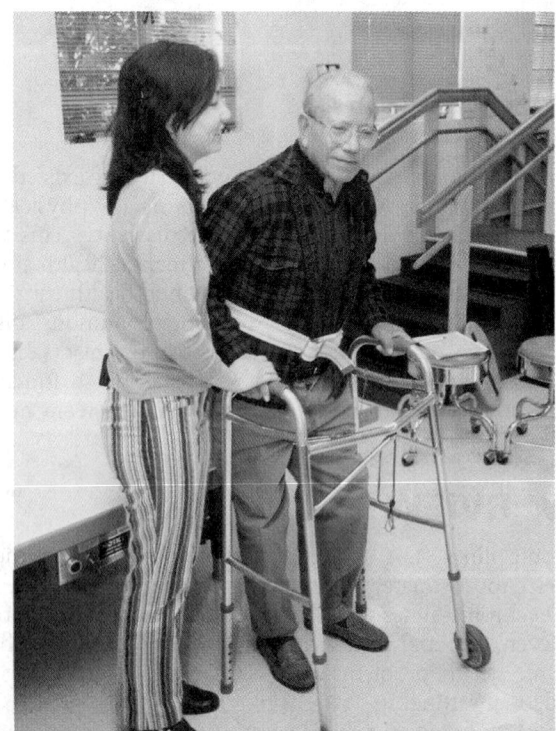

Figure 13–1. A physical therapist helping a client to ambulate.

to assist with the activities of daily living (ADLs) and decisions requiring accurate judgments. The clients may or may not be employed. The goal of these centers is to provide independent living arrangements outside an institution, especially for younger clients with head injury or spinal cord injury.

The Rehabilitation Team

Successful rehabilitation depends on the coordinated effort of a group of health care professionals—the interdisciplinary rehabilitation team—and the involvement of the client, family, and other support systems in planning and implementing care.

Goals of the Rehabilitation Team

The rehabilitation team has two basic goals: prevention of injury and restoration of function. The aim of prevention is to maintain the client's activity levels to avoid the deterioration of an unaffected organ or part and to eliminate possible hazards or factors that may contribute to further injury. Prevention is a continuous aspect of care for the chronically ill or disabled client. For example, meticulous skin care is necessary to prevent the formation of pressure ulcers. The other major goal of the rehabilitation team is restoration of as much function as possible to the injured or diseased body part or system to facilitate the client's independence.

Members of the Rehabilitation Team

The interdisciplinary health care team members in the rehabilitation setting include physicians, nurses, physical therapists, occupational therapists, speech-language pathologists, recreational therapists, cognitive therapists, aides, social workers, psychologists, vocational counselors, the clients themselves, and family members or significant others. Not all settings that offer rehabilitation services have all of these members on their team.

PHYSIATRISTS. The physician who specializes in rehabilitative medicine is called a physiatrist. Most inpatient rehabilitation settings, except for most freestanding skilled nursing facilities, employ physiatrists.

REHABILITATION NURSES. The rehabilitation nurse coordinates the efforts of the team members and is, therefore, usually designated as the clients' case manager. In clients undergoing rehabilitation, health problems are characterized by an altered functional ability and a diminished quality of life. The goal of rehabilitation nursing is to assist clients in restoring and maintaining optimal health. The rehabilitation nurse must be innovative and patient in helping clients regain independence.

THERAPISTS. Physical therapists (PTs) intervene to help the client achieve mobility (e.g., by facilitating ambulation and teaching the client to use a walker). They may also teach techniques for performing certain ADLs, such as transferring (e.g., moving into and out of bed), ambulating, and toileting.

Occupational therapists (OTs) work to develop the client's fine motor skills used for ADLs, such as those required for eating, maintaining hygiene, dressing, and driving. OTs may also teach the client skills related to coordination, such as hand movements (Fig. 13–2).

Speech-language pathologists (SLPs) evaluate and retrain clients with speech, language, or swallowing problems. Speech is roughly defined as the ability to say words, and language is the ability to understand and put words together in a meaningful way. Some clients, especially those with head injury or cerebrovascular accident (CVA, or stroke), have difficulty with both speech and language. Clients who have experienced CVAs also typically have dysphagia (difficulty with swallowing).

Recreational or activity therapists work to help clients continue or develop hobbies or interests. These therapists often coordinate their efforts with those of the OT.

Cognitive therapists, usually neuropsychologists, work primarily with clients with head injuries who have cognitive impairments. These therapists often use computers to assist with cognitive retraining.

Aides and health care assistants work in the nursing or therapy departments to assist in the care of clients. These rehabilitation team members are under the direct supervision of the nurse or therapist.

COUNSELORS. Various counselors are helpful in promoting community reintegration of the client and acceptance of the disability or chronic illness. Social workers help clients identify support services and resources, including financial assistance. They usually coordinate the clients' transfer to or discharge from the rehabilitation setting. Psychologists also counsel clients and families on their psychological problems and on strategies to cope with disability.

Vocational counselors assist the client with job placement, training, or further education. Work-related skills

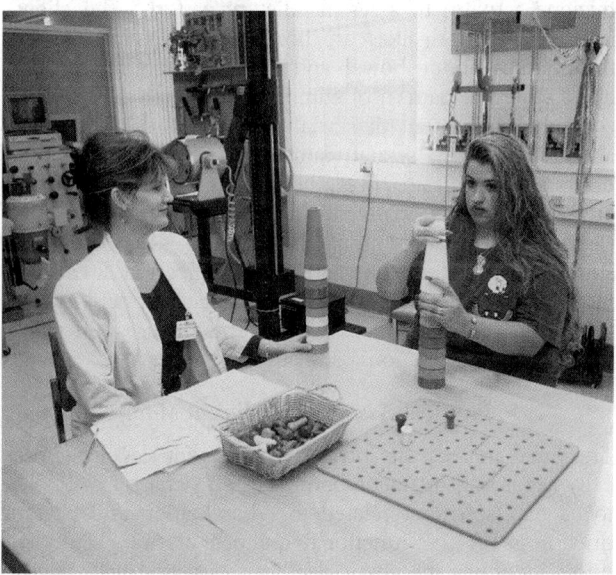

Figure 13–2. An occupational therapist working with a client.

are taught if the client needs to change careers because of the disability. If the client has not yet completed high school, educational tutors may help the client in the rehabilitation setting to complete the requirements for graduation.

Interdisciplinary team conferences for the exchange of ideas are held with the client, family members and significant others, and health care providers on a regular basis. Chart documentation is shared and read by all team members.

Collaborative Management

 Assessment

➤ History

As the case manager, the nurse collects the client's health history, including the history of the present condition, any current medications, and any treatment programs in progress.

General Background Data. The nurse obtains general background data about the client and family. These data include financial status, occupations, educational levels, cultural background, and home situation. In collaboration with the occupational therapist, the nurse addresses architectural features of the environment, such as the layout of the home. The nurse determines whether the physical layout at home, such as the presence of stairs or the width of doorways, will present a problem to the client. Data are gathered on the client's neighborhood, such as the location of shopping centers and available transportation. The nurse determines who will do the client's shopping, cooking, and housework. This information is essential for discharge planning.

Daily Schedule and Habits. The nurse also assesses the client's usual daily schedule and habits of everyday living. These include hygiene practices, eating, and elimination; sexual activity; and sleep. The nurse asks about the client's preferred method and time of bathing and hygiene activity. In assessing dietary patterns, the client's food likes and dislikes are noted. The nurse also elicits information about bowel and bladder function and the client's normal pattern of elimination.

In the assessment of sexuality patterns, the nurse asks about changes in sexual function since the onset of the disability (see Chap. 11). The client's current and previous sleep habits, patterns, usual number of hours of sleep, and use of hypnotics are also assessed. The nurse should ask whether the client feels well rested after sleep. Sleep patterns have a significant impact on activity patterns. Assessment of activity patterns focuses on work, exercise, and recreational activities.

➤ Physical Assessment/Clinical Manifestations

The nurse collects the physical assessment data systematically according to major body systems (Chart 13–1). The focus of assessment related to rehabilitation and chronic disease is on the functional abilities of the client. The nurse identifies the client's ability to use self-help devices during this portion of the assessment.

Cardiovascular System. An alteration in cardiac status may affect the client's cardiac output or cause activity intolerance. The nurse assesses the manifestations of decreased cardiac output, such as chest pain and fatigue, and determines when the client experiences these symptoms and what relieves them. The nurse seeks medical consultation before the client continues activities that provoke these symptoms. The physician may order a change in medications or may prescribe a prophylactic dose of nitroglycerin to be taken before the client resumes the activities. The nurse collaborates with the physician and appropriate therapists to determine whether activities can be modified to be accomplished without these symptoms.

For the client showing fatigue, the nurse and the client together plan methods of using the client's limited energy resources. For instance, the client could take frequent rest periods throughout the day, especially before undertaking activities. Major tasks could be performed in the morning because most people have the most energy at that time.

A great hindrance to rehabilitation for clients with cardiac disorders is fear. A client may have survived a life-threatening experience, such as a myocardial infarction, but now is so afraid of recurrence (and death) that he or she is unable, or unwilling, to resume any activity. The client with cardiac disorders experiencing fear usually benefits from participation in a structured cardiac rehabilitation program. The nurse discusses available programs with the client and the family (see Chapter 40 for a complete description of cardiac rehabilitation).

Respiratory System. The nurse asks the client whether he or she is experiencing shortness of breath during or after activity. It is important to determine the level of activity that the client can accomplish without experiencing shortness of breath. For example, can the client climb one flight of stairs without shortness of breath, or does shortness of breath occur after the client climbs only two steps?

The fear associated with any inability to breathe normally can render a person dependent in many facets of life. Some problems related to disorders of the respiratory system can be resolved or diminished, but some breathing difficulties must be endured (e.g., in emphysema).

Gastrointestinal System and Nutrition. The nurse assesses the client's oral intake and pattern of eating. The client is also assessed for the presence of anorexia, dysphagia, nausea, vomiting, or discomfort related to or interfering with oral intake. In collaboration with the physician and the dietitian, the nurse assesses the client's height; weight; hemoglobin; and hematocrit levels; and serum albumin, transferrin, and blood glucose concentrations (see Chapter 64 for complete nutritional assessment). Weight loss or gain is particularly significant and may be related to an associated disease or to the illness that caused disability.

Elimination habits vary from person to person; they are often related to daily job or activity schedules, dietary patterns, and family or cultural background. Elimination habits may be difficult to assess, because many nurses are hesitant to request—and many clients are afraid to volunteer—information pertaining to elimination. When assessing the client's elimination status, the nurse first asks

Nursing Care Highlight: Physical Assessment of Clients Undergoing Rehabilitation

Body System	Relevant Data
Cardiovascular system	• Chest pain • Fatigue • Fear of cardiac failure
Respiratory system	• Shortness of breath or dyspnea • Activity tolerance • Fear of inability to breathe
Gastrointestinal system and nutrition	• Oral intake, eating pattern • Anorexia, nausea, and vomiting • Dysphagia • Laboratory data (e.g., serum albumin level) • Weight loss or gain • Bowel elimination pattern or habits • Change in stool • Ability to get to toilet
Renal-urinary system	• Urinary pattern • Fluid intake • Urinary incontinence or retention • Urine culture or urinalysis
Neurologic system	• Motor function • Sensation • Cognitive abilities
Musculoskeletal system	• Functional ability • Range of motion • Endurance • Muscle strength
Integumentary system	• Risk of skin breakdown • Presence of skin lesions

what the usual elimination patterns were for that person before the injury or the illness.

The nurse is attuned to any changes in the client's bowel routine or the consistency of the stool. If the client is noticing any change in elimination pattern, the nurse tries to determine whether this alteration can be attributed to a change in diet, activity pattern, or use of medications that could cause increased or decreased motility of the gastrointestinal tract. Bowel habits are evaluated on the basis of what is normal for that person.

The nurse also determines whether the client can manage bowel functions independently. Independence in bowel elimination requires cognition, manual dexterity, sensation, muscle control, and mobility. If the client requires help, the nurse determines whether there is someone available at home to provide the assistance. The client's (and family's) ability to cope with any dependency in bowel elimination must be assessed as well.

Renal/Urinary System. When assessing the client's urinary system, the nurse determines the client's baseline urinary patterns, asking about the number of times the client usually voids and whether the client routinely awakens during the night to empty the bladder or has uninterrupted sleep. The client's fluid intake patterns and volume are recorded, including the type of fluids ingested and the timing of fluid consumption throughout the day.

The nurse determines whether the client has experienced any problems with urinary incontinence or retention in the past. Laboratory reports, especially the results of urine culture and urinalysis, are also monitored.

Neurologic System. In rehabilitation, the neurologic assessment identifies the functional aspects of motor ability, sensation, and cognition. The nurse assesses the client's pre-existing problems, general physical condition, and communication abilities.

Motor Ability. The movement of an extremity is compared with the function of the opposite extremity to identify paresis (weakness) or paralysis (absence of movement).

Sensation. The identification of sensory-perceptual alterations is important in assessing the client's risk for injury. The nurse assesses the client's response to light touch, hot or cold temperature, and position change in each extremity and on the trunk. Levels of decreased sensation are identified. For a perceptual assessment, the nurse evaluates the client's ability to receive and understand what is heard and seen and the ability to express appropriate motor and verbal responses. During this portion of the assessment, the nurse can also begin assessing short- and long-term memory.

Cognitive Abilities. The nurse also assesses the client's cognitive abilities, especially if there is a head injury or stroke. Several tools are available to evaluate cognition. One of the most common is the Mini-Mental State Examination, which is described in detail in Chapter 44.

Musculoskeletal System. As is the case for other body systems, the rehabilitation nursing assessment of the musculoskeletal system focuses on function. The nurse assesses the client's musculoskeletal status, response to the impairment, and demands of the home, work, or school environment. The nurse determines the client's endurance level and measures both active and passive range of motion (ROM) of joints. The nurse reviews the results of manual muscle testing by physical therapy, which identifies the client's ROM and resistance against gravity. In this procedure, the therapist determines the degree of muscle strength present in each body segment. The grading system usually ranges from 0 (no evidence of muscle contractility) to 5 (normal muscle contractility) (see Chap. 52).

Integumentary System. In assessing a client's integumentary system, the nurse identifies actual or potential interruptions in the integrity of the skin.

Risk for Skin Breakdown. To maintain healthy skin, the body must have adequate food, water, and oxygen intake; intact waste removal mechanisms; sensation; and functional mobility. Changes in any of these variables can lead to rapid and extensive skin breakdown. If the client cannot protect or maintain the skin, the nurse must be able to assess and plan for the client's needs. The nurse monitors the client to determine the risk of skin breakdown before it occurs.

Some rehabilitation settings use special skin assessment tools to identify clients at risk for skin breakdown. For example, the classic Braden Scale for Predicting Pressure Sore Risk (see Chap. 70) assesses six areas: sensory perception, skin moisture, activity level, nutritional status, and potential for friction and shear.

Several other skin risk assessment tools are available. Some tools also include additional indicators of nutritional status, such as the serum albumin or transferrin level. When either of these levels is low, the client is at high risk for pressure sores. Some tools include incontinence and altered mental state as risk factors. Regardless of which tool is used, Braden and Bergstrom (1992) recommended the following schedule for skin assessment:

- For clients in critical care units: during every nursing shift when the client is unstable and at least daily when the client is stable
- For clients in medical-surgical units: every other day when the client's condition is stable and when the condition changes significantly (e.g., after surgery)
- For clients in nursing homes or rehabilitation units: weekly for 1 month and then monthly after the first month unless there is a significant change in the client's condition

Actual Skin Breakdown. If a pressure ulcer or other change in skin integrity develops, the nurse accurately assesses the problem and its possible causes. The nurse inspects the client's skin every 2 hours, or more often if needed, until the client has learned to inspect his or her own skin several times a day. The nurse documents the depth and diameter of the open skin area in centimeters or inches, depending on the facility's policy. The area around the open lesion must also be assessed to determine the presence of cellulitis or other tissue damage. Chapter 70 includes a widely used classification system for staging skin breakdown. The nurse also assesses the client's understanding of the cause and treatment of skin breakdown as well as his or her ability to inspect the skin and participate in maintaining skin integrity.

In many health care agencies, a skin assessment and documentation tool, or "skin sheet," is used to keep track of each area of skin breakdown. A baseline assessment is conducted on admission to the agency, and the form is updated periodically, depending on the agency's policy and the nurse's judgment. In some long-term care or rehabilitation settings, photographs of the client's skin are taken at various intervals with the client's permission to document the skin's condition.

➤ Functional Assessment

Functional ability refers to the client's ability to perform activities of daily living (ADLs), such as bathing, dressing, feeding, and ambulating, and instrumental activities of daily living (IADLs), such as using the telephone, shopping, preparing food, and housekeeping. Functional assessment tools are used to assess a person's abilities (Research Applications for Nursing). Rehabilitation nurses, physiatrists, or therapists complete one or more of these assessment tools on the basis of the client's abilities and the policy of the health care setting. Some of the commonly used tools are briefly described next. For further information, consult corresponding references in this chapter.

PULSES Profile. One of the earliest tools used was the PULSES profile. It was developed in 1957 and adapted in 1975 to evaluate and classify functional capacity in the chronically ill and aging client population. The six categories included for evaluation are
- Physical condition (basic health status)
- Upper limb function (self-care)
- Lower limb function (mobility)
- Sensory components (sight, communication)
- Excretory function
- Support factors

Scoring uses four numeric grades for each category; scores increase as functional ability is diminished. The maximum score is 24. High scores indicate greater levels of dependency for the client. The adapted form of the PULSES profile has been a useful tool in many rehabilitation programs. It indicates the level of independence in life-functioning skills necessary for a person to make adaptations to community living.

Katz Index of Activities of Daily Living. One of the best known and most widely used instruments was developed during the 1950s from observations of clients with

▶ Research Applications for Nursing

Do Spinal Cord–Injured (SCI) Clients Retain Their Self-Care Skills Learned in Acute Rehabilitation?

Boss, B. J., Pecanty, L., McFarland, S. M., & Sasser, L. (1995). Self-care competence among persons with spinal cord injury. SCI Nursing, 12(2), 48–53.

This study examined the self-care competence of 48 clients with SCI from two Veterans Affairs Medical Centers and a state university–affiliated rehabilitation program to determine the retention of cognitive and functional skills after discharge from these programs. The data collection tool was the Self-Care Assessment Tool, which measures eight functional areas, such as bathing and grooming, skin management, and bladder management. The score of the study participants was high, indicating that they retained both the cognitive information and functional skills that had been emphasized in their rehabilitation programs.

Critique. Although the sample was fairly small and purposefully selected, this study was an attempt to examine outcomes over an extended period of time. As the health care industry continues to move toward managed care, measurement of both quality and cost outcomes is critical.

Possible Nursing Implications. Additional studies to determine the long-term effect of nursing and interdisciplinary interventions are needed. Activities that promote self-care enable clients to be independent and maintain their highest level of wellness.

Level of Rehabilitation Scale. The Level of Rehabilitation Scale (LORS), developed by Carey and Posavec (1978), provides a general assessment of the client's functioning for program evaluation rather than clinical assessment. The LORS provides an overview through measurement of function regarding ADLs, cognition, home activities, activities outside the home, and social interactions. The LORS was then expanded to include 11 items related to activities of daily living, mobility, and communication (Posavec & Carey, 1982). These items receive a score of 0–4, determined through the use of a coding manual ascribing numeric values to behavioral terms.

Functional Independence Measure. Assessment tools have also been designed for use on a national level; thus, uniform outcome data can be obtained from numerous rehabilitation programs. An example of this kind of system—a uniform data system—is the Functional Independence Measure (FIM), developed by Granger and Gresham (1984). The FIM, as a basic indicator of the severity of a disability, attempts to quantify what the person actually does, whatever the diagnosis or impairment. It does not measure what a person should do or how the person would perform under a different set of circumstances. To eliminate the bias of a particular discipline, the assessment may be done by trained clinicians; the entire assessment may be done by one person, or certain categories may be performed by representatives of various disciplines.

Categories for assessment are self-care, sphincter control, mobility and locomotion, communication, and cognition. Scoring is done with numbers using predetermined criteria for measurement. The evaluation is performed when the client is admitted to and discharged from a rehabilitation institution and at a specified follow-up time. The FIM assessment system has also been adapted for use in other health care settings, including acute care and home care.

▶ Psychosocial Assessment

The nurse must understand the theories of body image and self-esteem to assess the client's psychosocial needs adequately. These concepts serve as a basis for understanding psychological responses to chronic illness and resulting disability. The client's self-esteem and body image are assessed through the client's verbal indicators and descriptions of self-care. Body image can also be assessed by tools such as the Baird Body Image Assessment Tool (BBIAT) (see Chap. 10).

The nurse assesses the client's use of defense mechanisms and manifestations of anxiety, such as those noted in facial expressions and communication patterns. To assess the client's response to loss, the nurse asks the client to describe feelings concerning the loss of a body part or function. The nurse also notes any stress-related physical problems. The client may experience symptoms of depression, such as fatigue, a change in appetite, or feelings of powerlessness.

The nurse assesses the availability of support systems for the client. The major support system is typically the family or significant others. The family interactions and coping patterns are assessed.

fractured hips. The Katz Index of Activities of Daily Living addresses six functional tasks: bathing, dressing, toileting, achieving transfers, level of continence, and feeding (Katz et al., 1963). Each of the six areas is scored as either "dependent" or "independent" on the basis of the client's need for help in performing the task (Table 13–1). The overall functional status is then assigned a grade from A (independent in feeding, being continent, transferring, toileting, dressing, and bathing) through G (dependent in all six functions) from total scores.

The Katz Index has been used for clients with many types of chronic illnesses. It is a valuable tool for evaluating care and developing data about the course of an illness over time.

Barthel Index. The Barthel Index was designed to measure functional levels and mobility in the physically impaired client. This tool consists of 10 variables according to which the clients are scored by their degree of independence in performance. Categories include feeding, bathing, and mobility. The scoring system consists of two descriptive areas: doing an activity with help and performing an activity independently. Scores range from 0, indicating total dependence, to 100, indicating complete independence. The Barthel Index was intended for use in both immediate and long-term care rehabilitation programs.

TABLE 13-1

Katz Index of Activities of Daily Living

Independence means without supervision, direction, or active personal assistance, except as specifically noted below. This is based on actual status and not ability. A patient who refuses to perform a function is considered as not performing the function, even though he or she is deemed able.

Bathing (sponge, shower, or tub)

Independent: assistance only in bathing a single part (back or disabled extremity) or bathes self completely

Dependent: Assistance in bathing more than one part of body; assistance in getting in or out of tub; does not bathe self

Dressing

Independent; gets clothes from closets and drawers; puts on clothes, outer garments, braces; manages fasteners; act of tying shoes is excluded.
Dependent: does not dress self or remains partly undressed

Going to Toilet

Independent: gets to toilet; gets on and off toilet; arranges clothes, cleans organs of excretion (may manage own bedpan used at night only and may or may not be using mechanical supports)
Dependent: uses bedpan or commode or receives assistance in getting to and using toilet

Transfer

Independent: moves in and out of bed and in and out of chair independently (may or may not be using mechanical supports)
Dependent: assistance in moving in or out of bed and/or chair; does not perform one or more transfers

Continence

Independent: urination and defecation entirely self-controlled
Dependent: partial or total incontinence in urination or defecation; partial or total control by enemas, catheters, or regulated use of urinals and/or bedpans

Feeding

Independent: gets food from plate or its equivalent into mouth (precutting of meat and preparation of food, as buttering bread, are excluded from evaluation)

Dependent: assistance in act of feeding (see above); does not eat at all or parenteral feeding

Evaluation Form

Name _____ Date of Evaluation _____

For each area of functioning listed below, circle description that applies (the word "assistance" means supervision, direction, or personal assistance).

Bathing—either sponge bath, tub bath, or shower

Receives no assistance (gets in and out of tub by self if tub is usual means of bathing)	Receives assistance in bathing only one part of body (such as back or a leg)	Receives assistance in bathing more than one part of body (or does not bathe self)

Dressing—gets clothes from closets and drawers; puts on clothes, including underclothes, outer garments; manages fasteners (including braces, if worn)

Gets clothes and gets completely dressed without assistance	Gets clothes and gets dressed without assistance except for tying shoes	Receives assistance in getting clothes or in getting dressed or stays partly or completely undressed

Toileting—going to the "toilet room" for bowel and urine elimination; cleaning self after elimination and arranging clothes

Goes to "toilet room," cleans self, and arranges clothes without assistance (may use object for support such as cane, walker, or wheelchair and may manage night bedpan or commode, emptying same in morning)	Receives assistance in going to "toilet room" or in cleansing self or in arranging clothes after elimination or in use of night bedpan or commode	Does not go to room termed "toilet" for the elimination process

Transfer

Moves in and out of bed and in and out of chair without assistance (may use object for support such as cane or walker)	Moves in or out of bed or chair with assistance	Does not get out of bed

Continence

Controls urination and bowel movement completely by self	Has occasional "accidents"	Supervision helps keep urine or bowel control; catheter is used or is incontinent

Feeding

Feeds self without assistance	Feeds self except for getting assistance in cutting meat or buttering bread	Receives assistance in feeding or is fed partly or completely by tubes or intravenous fluids

From Katz, S., et al. (1963). Studies of illness in the aged. The index of ADL: A standardized measure of biological and psychosocial function. *Journal of the American Medical Association, 185,* 914–919. Copyright 1963, American Medical Association.

➤ *Vocational Assessment*

The rehabilitation nurse assists the client in maximizing functional status, allowing the client to resume many usual activities. The nurse should be aware of appropriate resources for each client in compiling a vocational data base for the client. In collaboration with vocational counselors, the nurse helps the client find meaningful training, education, or employment after discharge from the rehabilitation setting. The nurse gathers data on the client's educational and employment history, including previous jobs held. The nurse also obtains employers' attitudes toward the disabled client and information on the client's performance on the job, such as absenteeism and work record.

The nurse informs clients who are United States residents about the 1991 Americans with Disabilities Act passed by Congress to prevent employer discrimination against disabled people. Within reason, the employer must offer assistance to the disabled to allow them to perform the job. For example, if a client has a severe hearing loss, the employer may need to hire an interpreter for sign language so that the client can work.

The nurse also notes the cognitive and physical demands of the jobs held and ascertains whether the client can return to the former job or whether retraining in another field will be needed. The physical demands of jobs range from light in sedentary occupations (0–10 pounds frequently lifted) to heavy (more than 100 pounds frequently lifted). The nurse must also consider other aspects of the job, such as strength, mobility, or senses required in the job (e.g., hearing).

Job analysis also involves assessing the work environment of the client's former job. The nurse works with the vocational counselor to determine whether the environment is conducive to the client's return. Union contracts must also be considered, and any job modifications must be noted. If the injured worker requires vocational rehabilitation, the nurse refers the client to vocational rehabilitation personnel and assists the client to work with the counselors on evaluating present skills and learning new skills for employment. The nurse may also help with job placement in the community.

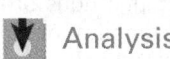 Analysis

➤ *Common Nursing Diagnoses and Collaborative Problems*

Regardless of the client's age or specific disability, the following nursing diagnoses are commonly applicable to the client with chronic illness or disability:

1. Impaired Physical Mobility related to neuromuscular impairment, sensory-perceptual impairment, pain, activity intolerance, fatigue, or the effects of trauma or surgery
2. Self-Care Deficit (total or partial) related to effects of trauma or chronic illness, muscular weakness, pain, immobility, or perceptual or cognitive impairment
3. Risk for Impaired Skin Integrity related to altered sensation or immobility

4. Altered Urinary Elimination related to sensorimotor impairment or immobility
5. Constipation related to neuromuscular or musculoskeletal impairment or immobility
6. Ineffective Individual Coping related to the effects of chronic illness, the loss of control over a body part or a body function, or major changes in lifestyle
7. Body Image Disturbance related to a change in body structure or function

➤ *Additional Nursing Diagnoses and Collaborative Problems*

Additional nursing diagnoses may apply, depending on the client's specific disability. For example, a client with rheumatoid arthritis also experiences chronic pain. The client with a spinal cord injury may also have sexual dysfunction.

 Planning and Implementation

➤ *Impaired Physical Mobility*

Planning: Expected Outcomes. The primary outcomes are that the client is expected to achieve the maximal physical mobility possible with the least restriction of activity and not experience complications resulting from immobility.

Interventions. Most problems requiring rehabilitation relate to impaired physical mobility. Clients with neurologic disease or injury, amputations, arthritis, severe burns, and cardiopulmonary disease experience some degree of impaired mobility. Physical and occupational therapists are the key rehabilitation team members who help clients meet mobility goals. Clients often spend several hours every day working in the physical therapy department to regain function and skills.

ELDERLY CONSIDERATIONS

Older clients may not be able to tolerate extensive therapy work-outs and may need shorter sessions to prevent extreme fatigue or physical complications. The nurse reinforces the physical therapist's instructions and must be aware of the client's progress and abilities.

Transfer Techniques. Clients with decreased mobility may require assistance with transfers, for example, from a bed to a chair, a commode, or a wheelchair. Because the degree of assistance required varies with the client and the specific disability, the nurse carefully assesses the client's mobility status before attempting a transfer. The physical or occupational therapist usually specifies how a particular client is to be transferred. For example, a quadriplegic client may use a sliding board for transfer. The client with an above-knee amputation may need a wheelchair with removable arms. In any case, the nurse always plans the transfer technique before initiating it. The desired outcome is that the client will eventually be able to transfer independently and safely.

Basic techniques for the nurse to use for assisting in the transfer of the client from a bed to a chair or a wheelchair, and vice versa, are identified in Chart 13–2. These techniques are also taught to the family member or other caregiver who will be caring for the client at home.

Alternative Transfer Techniques. Some clients cannot bear weight. For example, a client with a spinal cord injury resulting in quadriplegia either uses a sliding board (which requires balance skills) or, with the nurse or therapist, uses a "bear hug" technique. The sitting client places his or her arms around the nurse's neck while the nurse lifts the client from the bed to the chair, or vice versa. Another person assists with the transfer by stabilizing the wheelchair and holding onto the client's waist. Most physical therapists recommend that the client wear pants or a gait belt so that the assistant can hold on to the belt during the transfer.

Potential Problems with Transfers. Before any client transfer, the nurse carefully observes the client for potential problems. Orthostatic, or postural, hypotension is a common problem for the client in rehabilitation. If the client moves from a lying to a sitting or standing position too quickly, the client's blood pressure drops and he or she becomes dizzy or faints as a result. This complication contributes to falls, which are common in any client with

impaired mobility. The problem is worsened when the client, especially if elderly, is taking antihypertensive medications. The nurse helps the client change positions slowly with frequent rest periods to allow the blood pressure to stabilize. The nurse may take the client's blood pressure with the client in lying, sitting, and standing positions to examine the differences. More than a 20-mmHg drop in systolic pressure or a 10-mmHg drop in diastolic pressure between positions indicates orthostatic hypotension. The nurse notifies the physician about this change.

Another potential problem for the client who requires transfers is weight gain. Because the client undergoing rehabilitation has impaired mobility, he or she tends to gain weight. Excessive weight hinders transfers both for the nurse or the therapist who is assisting and for the client, who is learning to transfer independently. The client is usually weighed every week to check for weight gain or loss.

Gait Training. The physical therapist works with clients for gait training if they are able to ambulate. While regaining the ability to ambulate, clients may need to use canes or walkers (Fig. 13–3). When working with clients who are using such assistive devices, also known as ambulatory aids, the physical therapist ensures that the client has a level surface on which to walk. The nurse reinforces the physical therapist's instructions and encourages the client to practice. The goal is for the client to walk independently with or without an assistive device. Elderly clients typically use a walker for a broader base of support. Younger clients or clients with minimal impairment often progress to the use of a hemi-cane or straight cane. Chart 13–3 outlines how to use assistive devices for ambulation.

Some clients never regain the ability to walk because of their impairment, such as multiple sclerosis and spinal cord injury. These clients may become wheelchair dependent and need to learn wheelchair mobility skills. With the help of physical and occupational therapy, most clients can learn to move anywhere they want in the wheelchair.

Prevention of Complications. During the rehabilitation phase, clients are vulnerable to complications of immobility. Table 13–2 lists common complications and major strategies that the nurse can use to help prevent each complication. Implementing range-of-motion (ROM) routines, adhering to schedules for turning and repositioning, and maintaining skin care are constant components of rehabilitation nursing care to prevent the complications of immobility. The key is to increase the client's mobility.

One way to increase mobility, even with clients who are bedridden, is through ROM exercises. ROM techniques are beneficial for any client with decreased mobility (Table 13–3). Although basic ROM techniques are presented in basic nursing textbooks, a few key principles are pertinent for rehabilitation nursing care:

- The human body contains more joints than simply the knees, the hips, the elbows, and the shoulders. For ROM techniques to be effective in preventing musculoskeletal contractures, the client must exercise

---

Chart 13–2

Nursing Care Highlight: Transfer Techniques

Bed to Wheelchair or Chair

1. Place the chair at an angle to the bed on the client's strong side.
2. Lock the wheelchair brakes or secure the chair position.
3. Assist the client to stand and move his or her strong hand to the armrest.
4. Keep the client's body weight forward and pivot.
5. When the client's legs touch the chair edge, assist the client in sitting.

Wheelchair or Chair to Bed

1. Place the chair with the client's strong side next to the bed.
2. Lock the wheelchair brakes or secure.
3. Assist the client to stand and move the client's strong hand to the armrest.
4. Keep the client's body weight forward and pivot.
5. When the client's legs touch the bed edge, assist the client in sitting and then reclining.

Use of a Sliding Board

1. Place the chair or wheelchair as close to the bed as possible.
2. Remove the armrest from the chair or (if removable) wheelchair.
3. Powder the sliding board.
4. Place the sliding board under the client's buttocks.
5. Instruct the client to reach toward the client's side.
6. Assist the client in sliding gently to the bed.

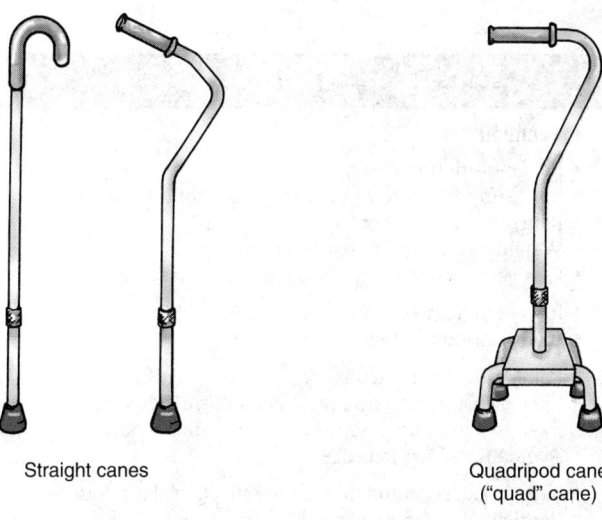

Straight canes
Quadripod cane ("quad" cane)

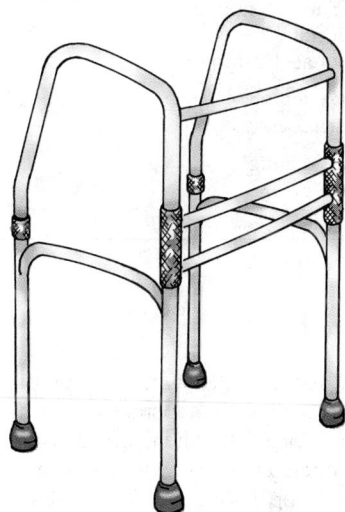

Standard walker

Figure 13–3. Assistive devices for ambulation. Assistive devices vary in the amount of support they provide. A straight cane provides less support than a quadripod cane or walker.

all joints, including each joint of the fingers, hands, toes, and so forth.
■ In performing ROM activities, the nurse or client completes full-range movement of each joint five times or more and completes the entire process at least three times daily.
■ The nurse does not move joints beyond points at which the client expresses pain or the nurse perceives stiffness or difficulty.

Clients with decreased mobility who are able to follow directions are taught by the nurse and the physical therapist to perform active or active-assisted ROM exercises.

► Self-Care Deficit

Planning: Expected Outcomes. The primary outcome is that the client is expected to become independent in

ADLs to the extent possible based on the client's disability.

Interventions. Activities of daily living, or self-care activities, include eating, bathing, dressing, grooming, and toileting. The nurse encourages clients to perform as much self-care as possible. The nurse and occupational therapist collaborate to identify ways in which self-care activities can be modified so that the client can perform them independently. For example, the occupational therapist teaches a hemiplegic client to put a shirt on by placing the affected arm in the sleeve first and putting the unaffected arm in the appropriate sleeve next. The nurse reinforces this dressing technique and encourages the client to practice.

Use of Assistive-Adaptive Devices. A variety of assistive-adaptive devices are available for clients with chronic illness and disability. An assistive-adaptive device, or self-care support device, is any item that enables the client to perform all or part of an activity independently. Table 13–4 identifies common devices and describes their use.

Many department stores carry clothing and assistive-adaptive devices designed for clients with disabilities. The occupational therapist works with the client to determine specific needs with regard to such equipment. In addition, the nurse and the occupational therapist help the client look for creative and inexpensive alternatives to meeting needs. For example, barbecue tongs may be used as "reachers" for pulling up pants or obtaining items on

---

Chart 13–3

Nursing Care Highlight: Gait Training Techniques

Walker Assisted

1. Apply a gait belt around the client's waist.
2. Assist the client to a standing position.
3. Assist the client in placing both hands on the walker.
4. Ensure that the client is well balanced.
5. Assist the client repeatedly to perform the following sequence:
   a. Lift the walker.
   b. Move the walker 2 ft forward and set it down on all legs.
   c. While resting on the walker, take small steps.
   d. Check balance.

Cane Assisted

1. Apply a gait belt around the client's waist.
2. Assist the client to a standing position.
3. Assist the client in placing his or her strong hand on the cane.
4. Ensure that the client is well balanced.
5. Assist the client repeatedly to perform the following sequence:
   a. Move the cane forward.
   b. Move the weaker leg one step forward.
   c. Move the stronger leg one step forward.
   d. Check balance.

TABLE 13–2

Prevention of Some Common Hazards of Immobility

Body System	Complication	Prevention
Musculoskeletal	• Contractures • Foot drop • Osteoporosis • Susceptibility to fractures • Muscular atrophy	• Range-of-motion exercises • Foot support while in bed, range-of-motion activities • Range-of-motion exercises • Weight-bearing exercises • Passive or active range-of-motion exercises
Gastrointestinal	• Constipation	• Increased activity level • Increased fluid intake
Cardiovascular	• Decreased cardiac output • Increased venous stasis • Thrombus formation • Embolism	• Range-of-motion exercises • Exercise, support hose, or antiembolism stockings • Exercise, support hose, or antiembolism stockings • Avoidance of leg massage
Neurologic	• Disorientation • Postural hypotension	• Sleep-wake schedule in accord with light-dark pattern • Reorientation (to person, place, and time) • Control of sensory stimulation • Avoidance of sudden position changes
Renal/urinary	• Calculi	• Decreased dietary calcium level • Increased fluid intake • Maintenance of acidic urine
Respiratory	• Pneumonia	• Frequent repositioning • Respiratory exercises
Integumentary	• Pressure ulcers	• Frequent repositioning • Pressure relief devices • Skin care

TABLE 13–3

Types of Range-of-Motion Exercises

Type	Description	Indications
Passive	• Exercises are performed by the nurse for the client.	• The client is too weak to participate actively.
Active	• Exercises are performed by the client.	• The client is able to complete range-of-motion movements.
Assisted, or active assisted	• Exercises are performed by the client but are guided by the nurse or the therapist.	• The client is weak and needs assistance.
Resistive	• The actions of the client are in opposition to those performed by the nurse or the therapist.	• The client has full range of motion, and an increase in strength is desired.

high shelves. A foam curler with the plastic insert removed may be placed over a pencil or eating utensil to make a built-up device. The client might use an extended shoe horn to operate light switches from wheelchair height. Hook-and-loop fasteners (Velcro) sewn on clothes can prevent the frustrations caused by buttons and zippers.

Energy Conservation. Nurses work with occupational therapists to assess the client's self-care abilities and to determine possible ways of conserving energy. Fatigue is commonly associated with chronic and disabling conditions. The nurse and the therapist develop strategies for energy conservation after evaluating the client's self-care routines. Preparation for ADLs can be helpful in reducing the client's effort and energy expenditure (e.g., the client gathers all needed equipment before starting grooming routines). The nurse can teach the client with high energy levels in the morning to schedule energy-intensive activities in the morning rather than later in the day or evening. Spacing activities is also helpful for saving energy. Additionally, allowing time to rest before and after eating and toileting decreases the strain on the client's energy level.

► Risk for Impaired Skin Integrity

Planning: Expected Outcomes. The primary outcome is that the client is expected to have intact skin.

TABLE 13–4

Uses of Assistive-Adaptive Devices

Device	Use
Buttonhook	• Threaded through the buttonhole to enable clients with weak finger mobility to button shirts. • Alternative uses include serving as a pencil holder or a cigarette holder.
Extended shoe horn	• Assists in the application of shoes for clients with decreased mobility. • Alternative uses include turning light switches off or on while the client is in a wheelchair.
Plate guard	• Applied to a plate to assist clients with weak hand and arm mobility to feed themselves.
Gel pad	• Placed under a plate or a glass to prevent dishes from slipping and moving. • Alternative uses include placement under bathing and grooming items to prevent their moving.
Foam build-ups	• Applied to eating utensils to assist clients with weak handgrasps to feed themselves. • Alternative uses include the application to pens and pencils to assist with writing or over a buttonhook to assist with grasping the device.
Hook and loop fastener (Velcro) straps	• Applied to utensils, a buttonhook, or a pencil to slip over the hand and provide a method of stabilizing the device when the client's handgrasp is weak.
Long-handled reacher	• Assists in obtaining items located on high shelves or at ground level for clients who are not able to change positions easily.

Interventions. An enormous variety of topical and mechanical remedies have been used to prevent and treat pressure ulcers, with varying success. Pressure reduction is a nursing intervention that may be achieved when the nurse temporarily repositions the client or alters the physical properties of the mattress surface, such as adding a mattress overlay.

Turning and Repositioning. The best intervention to prevent skin impairment is frequent position changes in combination with adequate skin care and sufficient nutritional intake. In general, the nurse turns and repositions the client every 2 hours; however, this may not be sufficient for people who are frail and have thin skin, especially elderly people (Chart 13–4). Therefore, the nurse assesses the client's skin condition each time the client is

turned and repositioned to determine the best turning schedule. For example, if the client has been sleeping for 2 hours and the nurse decides to postpone turning for 1 hour, reddened areas over the client's bony prominences may be present. If such reddened areas do not fade within 30 minutes after pressure relief or do not blanch, they may be classified as pre-ulcer areas, or stage I pressure areas (see Chap. 70). Some clients need to be turned and repositioned every hour to prevent the development of pressure sores; others may tolerate 2–3 hours between turnings.

For clients who sit for prolonged periods in a wheelchair, the nurse repositions them at least every 1–2 hours. Clients who are able are taught to perform "wheelchair pushups" by using their arms to lift their buttocks off the wheelchair seat for 10 seconds or longer every hour, or more often if needed. The physical therapist helps clients strengthen arm muscles in preparation for teaching wheelchair pushups.

Skin Care. Adequate skin care is an essential component of prevention. The nurse performs or assists clients in completing skin care each time they are turned, repositioned, or bathed. Skin care includes cleaning soiled areas, followed by careful drying and application of body lotion. For clients who are incontinent, topical barrier creams or ointments can help to protect the skin from moisture, which facilitates skin breakdown. If pre-ulcer (reddened) areas are noted, the nurse does not rub these areas because this causes more extensive damage to the already fragile capillary system. Instead, the nurse carefully observes the pre-ulcer areas for further breakdown and relieves pressure on the areas as much as possible. Bed pillows are often good pressure-relieving devices (see Chapter 70 for a complete discussion of skin care interventions).

Chart 13–4

Nursing Focus on the Elderly: Special Considerations in Rehabilitation

• When getting the client out of bed, move the client or instruct the client to move or sit up slowly to prevent orthostatic hypotension. This problem is most common in elderly clients who take antihypertensive medications.
• Turn the client more often than every 2 hours even if it is just a minor position change. Skin becomes thinner and more fragile with age.
• Determine whether the client had any problem with urinary patterns before the illness or rehabilitation. A client with a previous problem may not have a successful bladder training program.
• Be aware that intestinal motility decreases with age, which leads to constipation.
• Assess the client's support system of family and significant others. Many elderly clients have no spouse or close friends who would usually serve as a support network.

Nutrition. Clients need sufficient nutrition both to repair wounds and to prevent pressure ulcers. The nurse collaborates with the dietitian to assess the client's food selection and ensure that it contains adequate protein and carbohydrates. Both the nurse and the dietitian closely monitor the client's weight and serum albumin and transferrin levels. If either of these indexes decreases significantly, the client may be given high-protein, high-carbohydrate food supplements, such as milkshakes, or commercial preparations, such as Ensure Plus (also see Chap. 64).

Mechanical Devices. Pressure-relieving devices include waterbeds, foam (egg crate) or gel mattresses or pads, air mattresses, alternating-pressure mattresses, low air loss overlays or beds, and air-fluidized beds. Mattress overlays, such as foam, air, and gel types, are controversial because their effectiveness has not been proven. The nurse and the client usually decide the type of device. The use of any mechanical device (except air-fluidized beds) does not eliminate the need for turning and repositioning.

Specialty beds are categorized as either "low air loss" or "air fluidized." Air-fluidized therapy (e.g., Clinitron or FluidAir bed) provides the most effective pressure relief. The client is maintained in a nearly pressure-free environment (Fig. 13–4). These beds are generally not used for the prevention of skin breakdown, because most insurers will not reimburse the agency for the use of the bed. Special beds are, therefore, usually reserved for severe skin problems that have not healed with use of a conventional bed or other mechanical device. If optimal nutrition and healing conditions are maintained, skin breakdowns that have occurred should heal with continued use of air-fluidized therapy. The primary disadvantage is its expense, which may exceed several hundred dollars for each day of use. The cost of air-fluidized therapy may be reimbursed by some health insurance providers, such as Medicare.

➤ *Altered Urinary Elimination*

Planning: Expected Outcomes. The primary outcomes are that the client is expected to achieve a personally acceptable form of urinary elimination and be free from urinary complications, such as infection.

Interventions. Neurologic disabilities may interfere with successful bladder control in a client undergoing rehabilitation. These disabilities result in three basic functional types of neurogenic bladder: reflex (spastic) bladder, flaccid bladder, and uninhibited bladder.

A reflex or spastic (upper motor neuron) bladder causes incontinence characterized by sudden gushing voids. However, the bladder does not usually empty completely. A reflex bladder is also sometimes referred to as a "spastic" bladder. Neurologic problems affecting the upper motor neuron typically occur with high-level or mid-level spinal cord injuries, above the 12th thoracic vertebra (T-12). These injuries result in a failure of impulse transmission from the lower spinal cord areas to the cortex of the brain. When the bladder fills and transmits impulses to the spinal cord, the client is not conscious of the filling sensation. However, because there is no injury at the lower spinal cord level and the voiding reflex arc is intact, the efferent (motor) impulse is relayed and the bladder contracts.

A flaccid (lower motor neuron) bladder results in urinary retention and overflow (dribbling). Injuries that cause damage to the lower motor neuron at the spinal cord level of S2–4 (e.g., multiple sclerosis and spinal cord injury below T-12) may directly interfere with the reflex arc or may result in inappropriate interpretation of the impulses to the brain. The bladder fills, and afferent (sensory) impulses conduct the message via the spinal cord to the cortical region of the brain. Because of the injury, however, the impulse is not interpreted correctly by the cortical bladder center in the brain, and there is a failure to respond with a message for the bladder to contract.

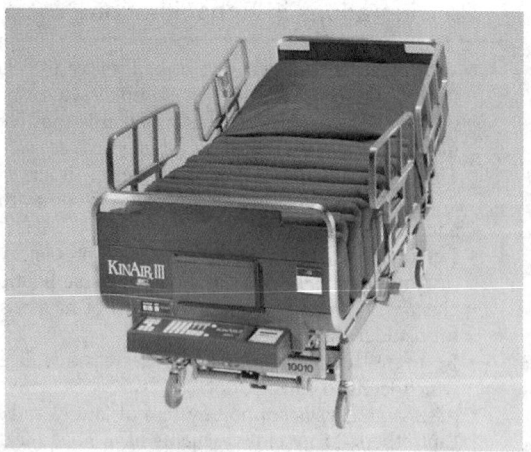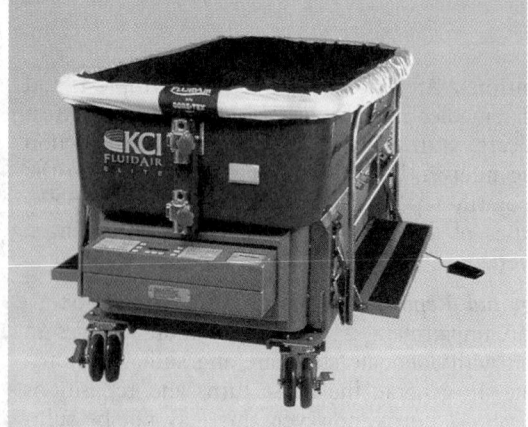

Figure 13–4. Pressure relief devices. *Left,* KinAirIII beds provide controlled air suspension to redistribute body weight away from bony prominences. *Right,* FluidAir Elite beds use airflow and bead fluidization. Both of these beds are covered with GORE-TEX fabric, which resists tearing. This fabric is also waterproof and acts as a barrier against bacteria. (Courtesy of Kinetic Concepts, Inc., San Antonio, TX.)

An uninhibited bladder may occur when the client has a neurologic problem that affects the cortical bladder center of the brain (frontal lobe), such as stroke or brain injury. When the bladder needs to empty, the client has little sensorimotor control and cannot wait until he or she is on the commode or bedpan before voiding. Therefore, the client is incontinent, but the bladder may not completely empty.

Bladder Training. The nurse can teach three techniques to assist the client in "repatterning" voiding, or bladder training:

- Facilitating, or triggering, techniques
- Intermittent catheterization
- Consistent scheduling of toileting routines

These techniques may not be as effective in a client with physiologic changes associated with aging.

Facilitating or Triggering Techniques. The nurse uses facilitating (triggering) techniques to stimulate voiding (Table 13–5). If there is an upper motor neuron problem, and the reflex arc is intact (reflex bladder pattern), any stimulus that sends the message to the spinal cord level S2–4 that the bladder might be full can initiate the voiding response. Such techniques include stroking the medial aspect of the thigh, pinching the area above the groin, pulling pubic hair, massaging the penoscrotal area, pinching the posterior aspect of the glans penis, and providing digital anal stimulation.

When the client has a lower motor neuron problem, the voiding reflex arc is not intact (flaccid bladder pattern) and additional stimulation may be needed to initiate voiding. Two techniques used to facilitate voiding are the Valsalva maneuver and Credé's maneuver. In teaching the client the Valsalva maneuver, the nurse instructs the client to hold his or her breath and bear down as if trying to defecate. The nurse assists the client in performing Credé's maneuver by placing the client's hand in a cupped position directly over the bladder area and instructing the client to push inward and downward as if massaging the bladder to empty.

Intermittent Catheterization. This is a method of bladder training frequently used for disorders involving a flaccid bladder, generally caused by a lower motor neuron problem. In assisting the client with intermittent catheterization, the nurse inserts a urinary catheter every 2–3 hours initially. Insertion is done after the client has attempted voiding and has used the Valsalva and Credé's maneuvers. If less than 150 mL of residual urine is obtained, the nurse increases the interval between catheterizations. The interval may be to 3–4 hours, according to the physician's order or health care agency protocol. The interval may be gradually increased to 4–6 hours, but the client should not go beyond 8 hours between catheterizations. The exception occurs when the residual urine volume is less than 150 mL each time with an adequate intake of fluids. If the client will be performing intermittent self-catheterization at home after discharge from the rehabilitation facility, the nurse instructs the client about clean (not sterile) technique.

Intermittent catheterizations may also be done to determine residual urine volumes for the client with a reflex (upper motor neuron) or uninhibited bladder. The client with this types of neurogenic bladder can void but often does not empty the bladder completely. The nurse catheterizes the client within 10 minutes after the client voids to determine the residual amount of urine in the bladder. For most clients, the desired amount is less than 100 mL of residual urine.

Toileting Schedule. Consistent toileting routines may be the best way of re-establishing voiding continence when the client displays an uninhibited bladder pattern (associated with brain damage or head injury). The nurse assesses the client's previous voiding pattern and determines the client's daily routine. At a minimum, the nurse assists the client with voiding in the morning after rising, before and after meals, before and after physical activity, and at bedtime. The nurse considers the client's bladder capacity, which may range from 100 to 500 mL, as well as the client's mobility limitations and clothing that may be restrictive. Bladder capacity is determined by measuring the client's urine output. The nurse ensures that the client is aware of nearby bathrooms at all times or has a call system to contact the nurse for assistance.

TABLE 13–5

Management of Altered Urinary Elimination

Functional Type	Neurologic Disability	Clinical Manifestations	Re-establishing Voiding Patterns
Reflex (spastic)	• Upper motor neuron spinal cord injury above T-12	• Urinary frequency, incontinence	• Triggering or facilitating techniques • Medications
Flaccid	• Lower motor neuron spinal cord injury below T-12 (affects S2–4 reflex arc)	• Urinary retention, overflow	• Valsalva and Credé maneuvers • Medications
Uninhibited	• Brain damage from injury or stroke	• Frequency, urgency, incontinence, voiding in small amounts	• Intermittent catheterization • Consistent toileting schedule • Regulation of fluid intake

Drug Therapy. Medications that may be used for urinary elimination problems include cholinergics (to promote bladder emptying), antispasmodics (to prevent incontinence), and skeletal muscle relaxants (to decrease spasticity, which promotes self-care) (Chart 13–5). Medications are not usually prescribed by the physician in the initial management of bladder problems but may be used to assist a bladder training program. The nurse reports the client's progress in bladder training to the health care provider so that he or she can make the best decision regarding drug therapy. In general, anticholinergics, antispasmodics, and skeletal muscle relaxants help to promote continence in clients with a reflex (upper motor neuron) bladder. Cholinergics, such as bethanechol chloride (Urecholine), may decrease urinary retention problems in the client with a flaccid bladder. This drug type may also facilitate complete bladder emptying in a client with a large residual volume, such as in reflex bladder problems. The client with an uninhibited bladder does not routinely require medications for bladder training programs unless urinary function is affected by additional pathologic changes.

Chart 13–5

Drug Therapy for Clients in Bladder-Training Programs

Drug	Usual Dosage	Nursing Interventions	Rationale
Cholinergics			
Bethanechol chloride (Urecholine)	• 10–50 mg bid-qid PO	• Give 1 hr before or 2 hr after meals. • Instruct clients to change positions slowly. • Give 1 hr before toileting or triggering or facilitating measure.	• This agent may cause nausea and vomiting. • Orthostatic hypotension is a possible side effect. • The drug is effective when using other measures for bladder training.
Antispasmodics			
Oxybutynin chloride (Ditropan)	• 5 mg bid or tid PO	• Instruct the client to avoid driving. • Instruct the client to avoid hot environmental temperatures. • Assess the client for urinary retention.	• Vertigo, drowsiness, and blurred vision may occur. • Sweating is suppressed. • Retention may be a side effect of the drug.
Flavoxate hydrochloride (Urispas)	• 100–200 mg tid or qid PO	• Instruct the client to avoid driving. • Instruct the client to avoid hot environmental temperatures. • Assess the client for urinary retention.	• Drowsiness, mental confusion, and blurred vision may occur. • Sweating is suppressed. • Retention may be a side effect of the drug.
Skeletal Muscle Relaxants			
Dantrolene (Dantrium)	• 25 mg once daily PO initially; increase to 25 mg bid–qid, then by 25-mg increments up to 100 mg	• Instruct the client to avoid driving. • Instruct the client to avoid prolonged sun exposure.	• Fatigue, dizziness, and muscular weakness are side effects. • Photosensitivity may occur.
Baclofen (Lioresal)	• 5 mg tid PO; may increase by 5 mg daily until desired effect attained to maximum of 80 mg	• Instruct the client to avoid alcohol. • Instruct the client to avoid driving.	• Alcohol potentiates the drug's effects. • Drowsiness and dizziness may occur.

Fluid Intake. The nurse instructs the client to maintain an adequate intake of fluids, at least 2000–2500 mL/day. The nurse encourages the client to drink fluids that promote an acidic urine, including large amounts of cranberry juice, prune juice, bouillion, tomato juice, and water. Fluids that promote an alkaline urine are discouraged, including citrus juices, excessive amounts of milk and milk products, and carbonated beverages. An acidic urine minimizes risks of urinary tract infection and calculus (stone) formation, although this belief is controversial. Some microorganisms, such as *Escherichia coli*, grow best in acidic environments.

In addition, the nurse discourages high-calorie fluids for overweight clients. Disabled clients have more difficulty with mobility and self-care if weight is not controlled.

ELDERLY CONSIDERATIONS

The nurse may decrease fluid intake to prevent complications in clients with congestive heart disease or renal problems, especially elderly clients. Some clients, especially those with flaccid bladder patterns, decrease fluid intake after 6 or 7 PM to avoid the need for catheterization during the night.

Prevention of Complications. The client with altered urinary elimination is at risk for skin breakdown from incontinence, urinary tract infection from urinary retention, and urinary calculi from urinary retention and stasis. The nurse keeps the client clean and dry and provides skin care as described under Risk for Impaired Skin Integrity earlier in this chapter. (See Chapter 73 for preventive measures for urinary tract infection and calculi.)

➤ Constipation

Planning: Expected Outcomes. The primary outcomes are that the client is expected to achieve a personally acceptable form of bowel elimination and be free from bowel elimination complications, such as impaction or diarrhea.

Interventions. Neurologic problems often affect the client's bowel pattern by causing a reflex (spastic) bowel, a flaccid bowel, or an uninhibited bowel.

Upper motor neuron diseases and injuries, such as a high-level or midlevel spinal cord injury, may result in a reflex (spastic) bowel pattern, with defecation occurring suddenly and without warning. With a reflex pattern, any facilitating or triggering mechanism may lead to defecation if the lower colon contains stool. Examples of facilitating or triggering techniques include providing anal stimulation (by inserting a finger, using either a finger cot or rubber glove and lubrication, to the first joint), gently pinching the anus, and pulling pubic hair. Digital stimulation should not be used for clients with cardiac disease because of the risk of inducing a vagal response (a rapid decrease in heart rate).

Lower motor neuron diseases and injuries interfere with transmission of the nervous impulse across the reflex arc and may result in a flaccid bowel pattern, with defecation occurring infrequently and in small amounts. The use of facilitating and triggering mechanisms in combination with a toileting schedule, suppository use, and disimpaction yields the best results. Clients may be able to self-administer the suppository or disimpact if necessary.

Neurologic injuries affecting the brain may cause an uninhibited bowel pattern, with frequent defecation, urgency, and complaints of hard stool. Clients may manage uninhibited bowel patterns through a consistent toileting schedule, a high-fiber diet, and the use of stool softeners.

Bowel Training. An overview of management techniques for bowel dysfunction is presented in Table 13–6. In many cases, clients are not able to regain control over their bowel function in the manner previously possible. The nurse assists clients in designing a bowel elimination program that accommodates the disability.

The nurse works with clients to schedule bowel elimi-

TABLE 13–6

Management of Bowel Dysfunction

Functional Type	Neurologic Disability	Dysfunction	Re-establishing Defecation Patterns
Reflex (spastic)	• Upper motor neuron spinal cord injury above T-12	• Defecation without warning	• Triggering mechanisms • Facilitation techniques • High-fiber diet • Suppository use • Consistent toileting schedule
Flaccid	• Lower motor neuron spinal cord injury below T-12 (affects S2–4 reflex arc)	• Infrequent, small stools	• Triggering or facilitating techniques • High-fiber diet • Suppository use • Consistent toileting schedule • Manual disimpaction
Uninhibited	• Brain damage from injury or stroke	• Frequent, urgency, and constipation	• Consistent toileting schedule • High-fiber diet • Stood softener use

nation as close to their previous routine as possible. For example, a client who had stools at noon every other day before the illness or injury should have the bowel program scheduled in the same way. An exception is the client who prefers another time that best fits into his or her daily routine. If the client is employed during the day, a time-consuming bowel elimination program in the morning may not be reasonable. The client may prefer to change the bowel protocol until the evening, when there is more time.

Drug Therapy. Bowel training programs for clients with neurologic problems are often designed to include the combination of suppository use and a consistent toileting schedule. Although medications should not be a first choice when a bowel training program is being formulated, the nurse routinely considers the need for a suppository if clients do not re-establish defecation habits through consistent scheduling of toileting, dietary modification, anal stimulation, and disimpaction.

The most common agents prescribed by physicians as suppositories in bowel training programs are bisacodyl (Dulcolax) and glycerin. Suppositories must be placed against the bowel wall to stimulate the sacral reflex arc and promote rectal emptying. Both agents are equivalent in effect; results occur in 15–30 minutes. The suppository is administered by the nurse when the client expects to defecate. For example, if a client had a previous bowel habit of defecating every other day after breakfast, the suppository is administered every other day after breakfast. Ordinarily, administering the suppository every second or third day is effective in re-establishing defecation patterns. Depending on each client's need, other medications, such as laxatives, may be indicated for bowel training programs.

Nutrition. Bowel elimination is directly related to the type and quality of food and fluid ingested. A high-fiber diet is a mainstay of most bowel training programs and includes whole-grain foods, bran, and fresh and dried fruits. Increasing dietary fiber is effective in facilitating defecation only if the client reduces fat intake.

Prevention of Complications. Common complications of any bowel training program are constipation, diarrhea, and flatulence. The nurse assesses clients for these complications and modifies the bowel training program accordingly, in collaboration with the physician and the dietitian.

➤ Ineffective Individual Coping

Planning: Expected Outcomes. The major outcome is that the client is expected to learn to cope with the chronic illness or disability and participate in the rehabilitation program.

Interventions. The client with a disability often has a poor self-concept because of changes in body image from structural or functional changes. The use of an assistive device, such as a wheelchair, also differentiates the client from most other people, and the client may not want to accept the need for the device. The nurse encourages the client to discuss feelings and asks questions to elicit specific information that can help in assessing the client's acceptance of and coping with the disability.

A disability also affects a person's role in society. For instance, a young medical student may fall from a ladder and become a paraplegic, and plans for a career as a surgeon are altered. A middle-aged farmer may be burned severely when his tractor catches on fire. He can no longer care for his farm, and his wife takes over during his rehabilitation process. An elderly woman who cares for her grandchildren is crippled with rheumatoid arthritis and can no longer provide child care. Disability requires role changes and always involves losses in the lives of those affected.

In addition to role changes, relationships with people change. Socializing with friends and family may be a strain when a person feels "different." Intimate relationships are affected because sexual dysfunction may result from disability. The nurse should be sensitive to these issues and should not avoid discussing them.

The nurse assesses coping strategies and support systems that the client has used in the past so that they can be used during rehabilitation if needed. The nurse asks the client what strategies have been used in the past to cope successfully with life crises, if any. Spiritual and religious beliefs are important for some people and should not be overlooked as the nurse helps the client identify sources of support.

➤ Continuing Care

The nurse begins discharge planning at or before client admission. If the client is being transferred from a hospital to a rehabilitation unit or facility, the nurse orients the client to the change in routine and emphasizes the importance of self-care. When the client is admitted to the rehabilitation unit or facility, the nurse assesses the client's current living situation at home. The nurse determines, with the client and family members or significant others, the adequacy of the client's current situation and potential needs after discharge to the home. The client with chronic illness and disability may require home care, assistance with ADLs, nursing care, or physical or occupational therapy after discharge. The nurse case manager assesses these needs and plans with the client, family or significant other, social worker, physical or vocational therapist, and physician for the best ways to meet identified needs.

Other health care professionals may be necessary to meet the unique needs of special populations. For example, brain-injured clients benefit from life planning, a process that examines and plans to meet the lifelong needs of clients. Case managers specializing in life planning are often part of the interdisciplinary rehabilitation team.

➤ Home Care Management

Before the client returns home, the nurse assesses the client's readiness for discharge from the rehabilitation facility. The client's home may be assessed in multiple ways.

Predischarge Assessment. The case manager or occupational therapist may visit the home before discharge to assess the home's layout and accessibility. These professionals may be employed by the health care agency or third-party payer, such as a health maintenance organization (see Chapter 3 for a discussion of third-party payers). For example, because of the stress of hospitalization, a client with a fractured hip who is ambulating well with a walker may neglect to explain to the nurse that the home has three steps at the entrance and that the bathroom is accessible by stairway only. The client may not consider it important to mention to the nurse that throw rugs, which do not provide a completely level surface on which to use a cane, are scattered throughout the apartment.

During a predischarge visit to the home, the case manager assesses the accessibility of the home in general and of the bathrooms, bedrooms, and kitchen. If the client will be wheelchair dependent after discharge from the facility, ramps are needed to replace steps, and doorways should be checked for adequate width. Usually, a doorway width of 36–38 inches (slightly less than 1 m) is sufficient for a standard-sized wheelchair. Any room that the client needs to use is checked. The bedroom should have sufficient space for the client to maneuver transfers to and from the wheelchair and the bed.

Space requirements vary, depending on the client's need to use a wheelchair, a walker, or a cane. In the bathroom, grab bars may need to be installed before the client comes home. Bathtub benches can provide support for the client who has difficulty with mobility and, when used in combination with a hand-held showerhead, can provide easily accessible bathing facilities. Assessment of the kitchen may or may not be critical, depending on whether the client has help with cooking and preparing meals. If the client will be responsible for cooking after discharge from the hospital or facility, the kitchen is assessed for wheelchair or walker accessibility, appliance accessibility, and the need for adaptive equipment.

Leave-of-Absence Visit. A second method of assessing the client's home is through a brief home visit, also called a leave-of-absence (LOA) visit, by the client before discharge. The nurse prepares the client by explaining the need for the trial home visit and by assessing the client's comfort level with this idea. The client who has been hospitalized for a lengthy period may feel intense anxiety about returning home. The nurse may allay such anxieties with careful preparation. Before the visit, the nurse meets with the client and family members or significant others to set goals for the visit and to identify specific tasks that the client should attempt during the time at home. After the client has been home, the nurse interviews the client to determine the success of the visit and to assess additional education or training needs before final discharge.

Going home may not be an option for all clients. Some clients may not have a support network of family members or significant others. For example, many elderly clients have no spouse or close friends living nearby. Children may reside at a distance, which can make home care difficult. If there is no caregiver available, the family must decide whether care can be provided in the home by an outside resource or whether the client needs to be admitted to a 24-hour supervised health care setting, such as a nursing home. Rehabilitation services are available in most long-term care settings (skilled nursing facilities) at least 5 days a week.

➤ Health Teaching

Education of the client and the family is the cornerstone of nursing care. The nurse assesses every component of the client's care to determine how the client can be taught to perform activities of daily living (ADLs) independently. The nurse assesses the client's learning potential and cognitive capacity. As care is provided, the nurse explains the procedure and its rationale. The client is encouraged to perform or direct the technique independently to verify understanding. The nurse gives written material explaining the steps in the procedure to the client and family members to reinforce learning and to provide support with the technique after discharge. However, before giving the client written material, the nurse assesses the reading level of the material and determines whether it is appropriate for the client's reading ability and language skills.

Any chronic illness or disability necessitates changes in a client's lifestyle and body image. The nurse assists the client in dealing with such changes by encouraging the client to verbalize feelings and emotions. The nurse also helps the client focus on existing capabilities instead of disabilities.

The client may fail to relate psychologically to the disability during hospitalization. For example, the client may display anger or frustration in attempting to perform self-care routines before discharge from the rehabilitation facility. The nurse encourages the client to be open about such feelings and to talk about ways to prevent worries from becoming realities after discharge.

The leave-of-absence home visit assists the client and family members or significant others in psychosocial preparation for discharge. It allows the client to experience the home situation while being able to return to the hospital environment after a few hours. Often the client finds that fears were not realized during the home visit, but frequently find new problems in the home that must be addressed before discharge. The nurse reviews this information with the client in preparation for discharge to the home.

➤ Health Care Resources

Various health care resources, such as physical therapy, home care nursing, and vocational counseling, are available to the client with chronic illness and disability after discharge to the home. The nurse assesses the client's need for additional care and support throughout the client's hospitalization and works with the case manager and physician in arranging for home services.

 Evaluation

On the basis of the identified nursing diagnoses and collaborative problems, the client and the nurse evaluate the rehabilitation interventions for the client with a disabling or chronic condition. Expected outcomes may include that the client will

- Ambulate independently, with or without assistive devices, or be independent in wheelchair mobility skills
- Perform ADLs independently with or without assistive-adaptive devices
- Have intact skin
- Demonstrate effective urinary elimination through an individualized bladder training program
- Demonstrate effective bowel elimination through an individualized bowel training program
- State acceptance of the disability and use coping strategies effectively

SELECTED BIBLIOGRAPHY

Badley, E. M. (1995). The impact of disabling arthritis. *Arthritis Care Research, 8*(4), 221–228.

Boss, B. J., Pecanty, L., McFarland, S. M., & Sasser, L. (1995). Self-care competence among persons with spinal cord injury. *SCI Nursing, 12*(2), 48–53.

*Boynton De Sepulveda, L. I., & Chang, B. (1994). Effective coping with stroke disability in a community setting: The development of a causal model. *Journal of Neuroscience Nursing, 26*(4), 193–203.

*Braden, B. J., & Bergstrom, N. (1992). Pressure reduction. In G. M. Bulachek & J. C. McCloskey (Eds.), *Nursing interventions: Essential nursing treatments* (2nd ed., pp. 94–108). Philadelphia: W. B. Saunders.

*Carey, R. G., & Posavec, E. J. (1978). Program evaluation of a physical medicine and rehabilitation unit: A new approach. *Archives of Physical Medicine and Rehabilitation, 59*, 330–337.

Collins, R. C. (1997). *Neurology.* Philadelphia: W. B. Saunders.

Donohoe, K. M., Wineman, N. M., & O'Brien, R. A. (1996). Are alternative long-term-care programs needed for adults with chronic progressive disability? *Journal of Neuroscience Nursing, 28*(6), 373–380.

Edwards, P. A. (1996). Health promotion through fitness for adolescents and young adults following spinal cord injury. *SCI Nursing, 13*(3), 69–73.

Evans, R. W. (1997). The role of the neuropsychologist in life care planning for brain-injured populations. *The Journal of Care Management, 3*(5), 46–47, 49.

Galindo-Ciocon, D., Ciocon, J. O., & Galindo, D. (1995). Functional impairment among elderly women with osteoporotic vertebral fractures. *Rehabilitation Nursing, 20*(2), 79–83.

*Granger, C. V., & Gresham, G. E. (1984). *Functional assessment in rehabilitation medicine.* Baltimore: Williams & Wilkins.

*Granger, C. V., Hamilton, B. B., Lenacre, J. M., Heinemann, A. W., & Wright, B. D. (1993). Performance profiles of the Functional Independence Measure. *Journal of Physical Medicine and Rehabilitation, 72*, 84–89.

Hamilton, L., & Lyon, P. S. (1995). A nursing-driven program to preserve and restore functional ability in hospitalized elderly patients. *Journal of Nursing Administration, 25*(4), 30–37.

*Hellman, E. A., & Williams, M. A. (1994). Outpatient cardiac rehabilitation in elderly patients. *Heart and Lung, 23*(6), 506–512.

Hickey, J. V. (1996). *The clinical practice of neurological and neurosurgical nursing* (4th ed.). Philadelphia: J. B. Lippincott.

Huntt, D. C., & Growick, B. S. (1997). Managed care for people with disabilities. *Journal of Rehabilitation*, July/August/September, 10–14.

Ignatavicius, D. D. (1998). *Introduction to long term care nursing.* Philadelphia: F. A. Davis.

*Institute of Medicine. (1991). *Disability in America.* Washington, DC: National Academy Press.

*Katz, S., et al. (1963). Studies of illness in the aged. The index of ADL: A standardized measure of biological and psychosocial function. *Journal of the American Medical Association, 185*, 914–919.

*Mason, M., & Bell, J. (1994). Functional outcomes of rehabilitation in the frail elderly: A two-year retrospective review. *Perspectives, 18*(2), 7–9.

*Miller, J. M. (1991). *Coping with chronic illness: Overcoming powerlessness* (2nd ed.). Philadelphia: F. A. Davis.

Neal, L. J. (1995). The rehabilitation nurse in the home care setting: Treating chronic wounds as a disability. *Rehabilitation Nursing, 20*(5), 261–264.

*Posavec, E. J., & Carey, R. G. (1982). Using a level of function scale (LORS-II) to evaluate the success of inpatient rehabilitation programs. *Rehabilitation Nursing, 7*(6), 17–19.

*Redeker, N. S., Mason, D. J., Wykpisz, E., Glica, B., & Miner, C. (1994). First postoperative week activity patterns and recovery in women after coronary artery bypass surgery. *Nursing Research, 43*(3), 168–173.

Somervill, B. A. (1997). Transitional and subacute care. *Case Review, 3*(3), 61–63.

Wojner, A. W. (1996). Optimizing ischemic stroke outcomes: An interdisciplinary approach to rehabilitation in acute care. *Critical Care Nursing Quarterly, 19*(2), 47–61.

*World Health Organization. (1980). *International classification of impairments, disabilities and handicaps.* Geneva: Author.

SUGGESTED READINGS

Hamilton, L., & Lyon, P. S. (1994). A nursing-driven program to preserve and restore functional ability in hospitalized elderly patients. *Journal of Nursing Administration, 25*(4), 30–37.

In this article, the authors discuss the hazards of hospitalization for the elderly and the successful implementation of a six-bed unit for geriatric assessment and rehabilitation in a community hospital. Although interdisciplinary in focus, the entire program was managed and evaluated by the nursing staff.

Hellman, E. A., & Williams, M. A. (1994). Outpatient cardiac rehabilitation in elderly patients. *Heart and Lung, 23*(6), 506–512.

The authors review available data regarding exercise training in elderly clients with heart disease. Both female and male clients improve in functional capacity and reduced myocardial work as a benefit of exercise. A quiz for continuing education contact hours follows this article.

Neal, L. J. (1995). The rehabilitation nurse in the home setting: Treating chronic wounds as a disability. *Rehabilitation Nursing, 20*(5), 261–264.

Rehabilitation nurses, along with other home care nurses, treat clients with chronic wounds, including a focus on lifestyle modification. Rehabilitation nurses also treat clients with other disabilities who are at risk for developing wounds and instruct them in wound prevention.

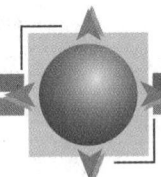

Management of Clients

with Fluid, Electrolyte,

and Acid-Base Imbalances

FLUID AND ELECTROLYTE BALANCE

Every body system is affected by the fluids in and around the tissues and cells. For proper physiologic function, body fluids must be regulated carefully. This regulation ensures adequate distribution, total volume, and concentrations of various substances, especially electrolytes, dissolved in body water. Excesses and deficiencies of body water or electrolytes can cause organ dysfunction that may lead to death. Therefore, all nurses must understand the processes involved in fluid and electrolyte balance to assess accurately each client's total health status.

ANATOMY AND PHYSIOLOGY REVIEW
Physical and Biological Influences on Fluid and Electrolyte Balance

Many physical and biological processes control the normal balance of body fluids and electrolytes. These processes work together to regulate homeostasis (equilibrium) so that even when the external environment undergoes dramatic changes, the body's internal environment remains stable.

Being familiar with the terminology related to solutions is necessary to understand the processes involved in fluid and electrolyte balance (Table 14–1). Body fluids are composed of water and particles dissolved or suspended in water. *Solvent* is the water portion of body fluids. *Solutes* are the particles dissolved in the water. Solutes vary in type and concentration from one body fluid compartment to another. Proper body function is highly dependent on maintaining the correct balance of fluid and specific electrolytes within each body fluid compartment.

Important processes involved in fluid and electrolyte balance include filtration, diffusion, osmosis, and active transport. Capillary dynamics also affect fluid and electrolyte balance. All of these processes or events influence the movement of fluids and particles across biological membranes.

Filtration
Definition

Filtration is the movement of fluid through a biological membrane because of hydrostatic pressure differences on both sides of the membrane. Because filtration depends on hydrostatic pressure, knowledge about the factors influencing hydrostatic pressure is necessary.

All fluid has weight. The overall weight of the fluid is related to the amount of fluid present in the confined space. Water molecules in a confined space constantly

TABLE 14–1

Terminology Associated with Fluid and Electrolyte Balance

Term	Definition
Active transport	• Assisted movement of a substance through a permeable membrane between two fluid compartments against a concentration, electrical, or pressure gradient; requires the expenditure of chemical energy
Adenosine triphosphate (ATP)	• A substance that is generated by the metabolism of glucose or fat within cells and that releases chemical energy for physiologic function when a high-energy phosphate bond ($\sim$P) is broken
Aldosterone	• A hormone secreted by the adrenal cortex that stimulates the renal reabsorption of sodium and water and the renal excretion of potassium
Anion	• A molecule (electrolyte) that carries an overall negative charge when dissolved in water
Antidiuretic hormone (ADH)	• A hormone secreted from the posterior pituitary gland that increases the renal reabsorption of pure water and decreases urinary output
Atrial natriuretic peptide (ANP)	• A hormone secreted by cardiac atrial cells that increases renal excretion of sodium and water
Brownian motion	• Inherent molecular motion
Capillary (plasma) hydro-static pressure	• The force generated by fluid within a capillary that tends to move fluid out from the capillary and into the interstital space
Capillary (plasma) osmotic pressure	• The force generated by the concentration of plasma solutes (osmotic and oncotic pressures) that tends to retain fluid within the capillary or move fluid from the interstitial space into the capillary
Cation	• A molecule (electrolyte) that carries an overall positive charge when dissolved in water
Cofactor	• A substance required to enhance the activity of an enzyme or a physiologic reaction
Colloidal oncotic pressure	• The osmotic pressure exerted by the concentration of colloids (proteins) within a solution
Diffusion	• Unimpeded movement of a substance through a permeable membrane between two fluid compartments down a concentration gradient; does not require the expenditure of chemical energy
Disequilibrium	• A state in which two fluid compartments are unequal in at least one characteristic
Electrolytes	• Substances that carry an electrical charge when dissolved in water
Electroneutrality	• A state in which a body fluid has an equal number of cations and anions, so that the fluid does not express an electrical charge
Equilibrium	• A state in which two fluid compartments are equal in one or more characteristics
Extracellular fluid (ECF)	• Body fluid present outside of cells; includes plasma, interstitial fluid, and transcellular fluid
Facilitated diffusion	• Assisted movement of a substance through a permeable membrane between two fluid compartments down a concentration gradient; does not require the expenditure of chemical energy
Filtration	• The movement of fluid through a biologic membrane as a result of hydrostatic pressure differences on the two sides of the membrane
Gradient	• A graded difference in some characteristic between two fluid compartments
Hydrostatic pressure	• The force of pressure exerted by static water in a confined space—"water-pushing" pressure

press outward against the confining boundaries. *Hydrostatic pressure* is the force water molecules exert against the confining walls of the space. This pressure is caused by the weight of fluid against the walls. Hydrostatic pressure may be thought of as "water-pushing" pressure, because it is a major force in moving water outward from a confined space through a membrane (Fig. 14–1).

Physiologic Activity

Water is the largest component of any body fluid. The amount of water in any body fluid compartment is a main factor in determining the hydrostatic pressure of that compartment. The proportion of water present in a fluid is inversely related to the *viscosity* (thickness) of that fluid. Viscosity is a property of fluid relating to its density, specific gravity, and surface tension. Blood, a viscous fluid (one that is thicker than water), is confined within the blood vessels of the vascular system. Blood has hydrostatic pressure because of its weight and volume and also because of cardiac contraction causing the ejection of blood into the arterial circulation.

Whenever a permeable (porous) membrane separates two fluid compartments, the hydrostatic pressures of the two compartments can be compared. If hydrostatic pressure is the same in both fluid compartments, then a state

TABLE 14–1

Terminology Associated with Fluid and Electrolyte Balance *Continued*

Term	Definition
Hypertonic (hyperosmotic)	• Any solution with a solute concentration (osmolarity) greater than that of normal body fluids (>310 mOsm/L)
Hypotonic (hyposmotic)	• Any solution with a solute concentration (osmolarity) less than that of normal body fluids (<270 mOsm/L)
Impermeable membrane	• A membrane separating two fluid compartments that does not permit the movement of one or more substances through the membrane (by diffusion) from one compartment to the other
Insensible fluid loss	• Unregulated fluid losses from the skin, the gastrointestinal tract, wounds, and the pulmonary epithelium
Interstitial fluid	• Fluid present in tissues between cells
Intracellular fluid (ICF)	• Fluid found inside cells
Isotonic (isosmotic)	• Any solution with a solute concentration equal to the osmolarity of normal body fluids or normal saline (0.9% NaCl), ~300 mOsm/L
Obligatory urinary output	• The minimal amount of urinary output necessary to ensure the excretion of metabolic wastes (~400 mL/day)
Osmolality	• The concentration of solute within a solution as measured by the amount of solute osmoles per kilogram of solvent
Osmolarity	• The concentration of solute within a solution as measured by the amount of solute osmoles per liter of solution
Osmoreceptor	• Specialized sensory nerve cells in the thalamus or the hypothalamus that are sensitive to changes in the osmolarity of extracellular fluid
Osmosis	• Diffusion of water only through a selectively permeable membrane from an area of lower osmotic pressure to an area of greater osmotic pressure
Osmotic pressure	• The pressure exerted by a solution that contains a relatively high concentration of solute; this pressure draws water from areas or compartments with lower concentrations of solute into the areas or compartments with higher concentrations of solute—"water-pulling" pressure
Permeable membrane	• A membrane separating two fluid compartments that permits movement of one or more substances through the membrane (by diffusion) from one compartment to the other
Solubility	• The degree to which any given solute completely dissolves (dissociates) in water
Solute	• The solid particles dissolved in a solution
Solvent	• The fluid (water) portion of a solution
Tissue hydrostatic pressure (THP)	• The force generated by fluid within the interstitial spaces that tends to move fluid into the capillary from the interstitial space
Tissue osmotic pressure (TOP)	• The force generated by the concentration of interstitial fluid solutes that tend to retain fluid in the interstitial space or move fluid from the capillary into the interstitial space
Transcellular fluid	• Extracellular fluid confined to a specific area or region of the body (cerebrospinal fluid, pericardial fluid, visceral fluid, aqueous humor, peritoneal fluid, and pleural fluid)
Viscosity	• Gumminess or thickness of the molecules in a solution, causing friction within that solution

of *equilibrium* exists for hydrostatic pressure. If the hydrostatic pressure is not the same in both compartments, then a state of *disequilibrium* exists. This means that the two compartments have a *gradient*, or graded difference, of hydrostatic pressure: One compartment has a higher hydrostatic pressure than the other. Because the human body is a dynamic system and constantly seeks equilibrium, a gradient across a membrane causes forces to rearrange the distribution of substances on both sides of the membrane until an equilibrium is reached (Fig. 14–2).

In most instances, substances move or are rearranged in the direction from the greater amount of pressure or concentration to the lesser amount. Thus, when a hydrostatic pressure gradient exists between two fluid compartments, fluid from the compartment with the higher hydrostatic pressure moves (filters) through the membrane into the fluid compartment with the lower hydrostatic pressure. This filtration continues only as long as the hydrostatic pressure gradient exists. When enough fluid leaves the compartment that initially had the higher pressure and enters the compartment that initially had the lower pressure to make the hydrostatic pressure in both compartments equal, an equilibrium is reached.

When the two compartments are in equilibrium for hydrostatic pressure, a gradient no longer exists between them. Although water molecules may be exchanged

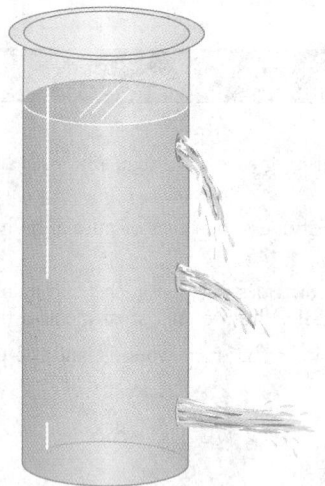

Figure 14–1. Hydrostatic pressure. The pressure water molecules exert against the sides of the container is highest where the weight of the water is greatest. (From Nave, C., & Nave, B. [1985]. Hydrostatic pressure. In *Physics for the health sciences* [3rd ed.]. Philadelphia: W. B. Saunders.)

evenly back and forth between two compartments in equilibrium, no net filtration of fluid occurs. In equilibrium, neither compartment gains or loses water molecules, and the hydrostatic pressure in both compartments remains the same.

Clinical Function and Significance

Blood pressure is a hydrostatic filtering force measured in millimeters of mercury (mmHg). It moves whole blood from the heart to tissue areas where filtration can occur. Filtration is important for the exchange of water, nutri-

ents, and waste products when blood arrives at the tissue capillaries. One factor that determines whether fluid leaves the vascular system and enters the tissue spaces (interstitial fluid) is the difference between the hydrostatic pressure of the fluid in the capillaries and that of the fluid in the interstitial tissue spaces.

The lining of capillaries is only one cell layer thick. Therefore, the wall holding blood in the capillaries is thin. In addition, large spaces, or *pores,* between the cells in the capillary membrane (Fig. 14–3) help water filter freely through capillary membranes in either direction if a hydrostatic pressure gradient is present. This concept is discussed later in this chapter under the heading Capillary Dynamics.

Edema (tissue swelling) can develop as a result of changes in normal hydrostatic pressure gradients, such as in clients with right-sided congestive heart failure. In this clinical situation, the volume of blood in the right side of the heart increases greatly because the right ventricle is too weak to efficiently pump blood into the pulmonary vascular system. As blood volume accumulates, blood backs up into the venous system, and the venous hydrostatic pressure rises. The increased venous pressure causes capillary hydrostatic pressure to increase until it is higher than the hydrostatic pressure in the interstitial spaces. Excess filtration of fluid from the capillaries into the interstitial tissue spaces then occurs, resulting in the formation of visible edema.

Diffusion
Definition

Diffusion is the free movement of particles across a permeable membrane down a *concentration gradient,* that is,

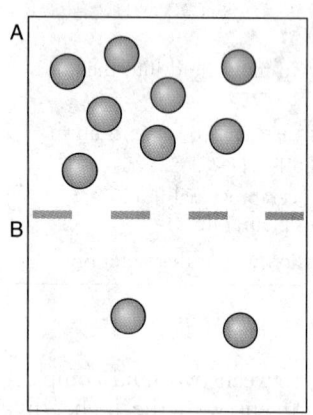

Compartment A has more water molecules and greater hydrostatic pressure than does compartment B.

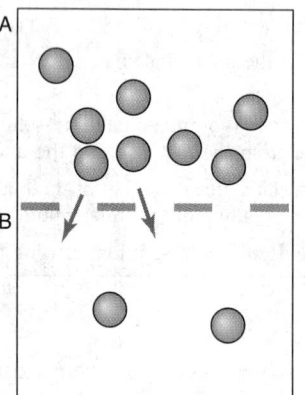

Water molecules move down the hydrostatic pressure gradient from compartment A through the permeable membrane into compartment B, which has a lower hydrostatic pressure.

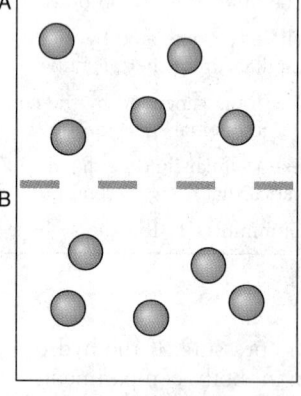

Enough water molecules have moved down the hydrostatic pressure gradient from compartment A into compartment B that both sides now have the same amount of water and the same amount of hydrostatic pressure. An equilibrium of hydrostatic pressure now exists between the two compartments, and no further *net* movement of water will occur.

Figure 14–2. The process of filtration. (© M. Linda Workman, 1992. All rights reserved.)

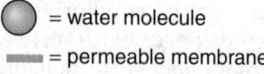

● = water molecule

▬▬ = permeable membrane

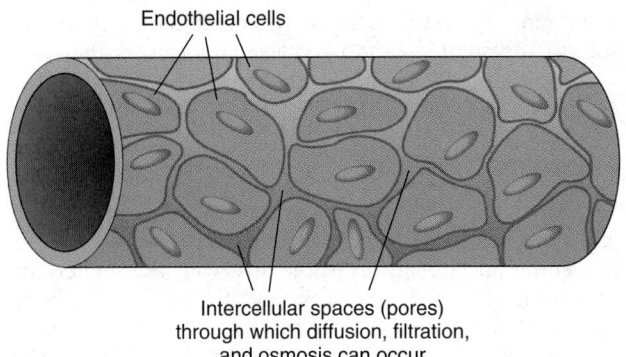

Endothelial cells

Intercellular spaces (pores)
through which diffusion, filtration,
and osmosis can occur

Figure 14–3. The basic structure of a capillary.

from an area of higher concentration to an area of lower concentration. Diffusion controls the movement of particles in solution across various body membranes.

Physiologic Activity

Diffusion of particles into and out of cells and fluid compartments occurs via *brownian motion,* the kinetic energy of molecular motion. Brownian motion is the vibration of individual molecules caused by electrons orbiting at the core of a molecule. It produces totally random movement of molecules. This random movement causes molecules to move and collide with each other within a confined space. The collisions usually cause a temporary increase in the speed of the movement after the molecules hit.

As a result of these collisions, molecules in a solution spread out evenly through whatever space is available. They move from an area of higher concentration of atoms and molecules to an area of lower concentration, until an equality of concentrations is achieved in all areas. The number of collisions is related to the concentration of molecules in a confined space. Spaces with many molecules have more collisions and faster molecular motion than spaces with fewer molecules.

A concentration gradient exists when two areas have different concentrations of the same type of molecules. Brownian motion of the molecules causes them to move down the concentration gradient. As a result of the brownian motion, any membrane that separates two areas is struck repeatedly by molecules. When the molecule strikes a pore in the membrane that is large enough for it to pass through, diffusion occurs (Fig. 14–4). The likelihood of any single molecule colliding with the membrane and going through a pore is much greater on the side of the membrane with a higher molecule concentration.

The speed of diffusion is directly related to the degree of concentration difference between the two sides of the membrane. The degree of concentration difference is usually referred to as the steepness of the gradient: The larger the concentration difference between the two sides, the steeper the gradient. Diffusion occurs more rapidly when the concentration gradient is steeper (just as a ball rolls downhill more rapidly when the hill is steep than when the hill is nearly flat). The greater the difference in concentration, the more rapidly diffusion occurs from the

area of higher concentration to the area of lower concentration.

Diffusion of solute particles continues through the membrane as long as a concentration gradient exists between the two sides of the membrane. When the concentration of solute is the same on both sides of the membrane, an equilibrium exists and an equal exchange—not a net movement—of solute continues.

Clinical Function and Significance

Diffusion is important in the transport of gases and in the movement of most electrolytes, atoms, and molecules through biological membranes. Unlike capillary membranes, which permit diffusion of most small-sized substances down a concentration gradient, cell membranes are *selective.* That is, they permit movement of some substances and inhibit movement of other substances. Some molecules cannot move across a cell membrane, even when a steep "downhill" gradient exists, because the membrane is impermeable (not porous) to that molecule. Thus, the concentration gradient is maintained across the membrane.

This impermeability, along with special transport mechanisms, accounts for differences in concentrations of specific substances from one fluid compartment to another. For example, under normal conditions the extracellular fluid (ECF) contains almost ten times more sodium ions than the fluid inside the cell, the intracellular fluid (ICF). The relative impermeability of the cell membrane to sodium and a special "sodium pump" that moves any extra sodium out of the cell "uphill" against its concentration gradient and back into the extracellular fluid account for this extreme concentration difference.

In some instances, diffusion cannot occur without assistance, even down steep concentration gradients, because of membrane selectivity. A clinical example is the fact that even though the concentration of glucose is much higher in the ECF than it is in the intracellular

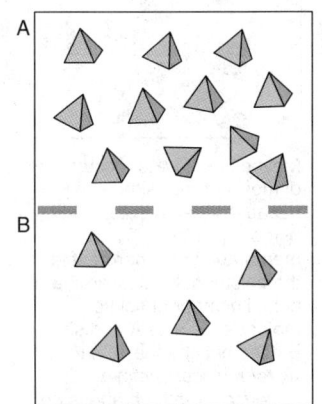

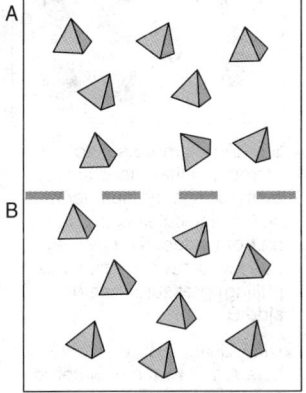

The concentration of solute is greater on side A than on side B, with a permeable membrane separating the two compartments.

Solute molecules have diffused from side A through the membrane into side B until an equilibrium of solute exists and the concentration of solute is the same on both sides.

Figure 14–4. Diffusion of a solute.

fluid (ICF), creating a steep gradient for glucose, glucose cannot cross most cell membranes without the assistance of insulin. When insulin is present in the ECF, it binds to insulin receptor sites on cell membranes. When insulin binds to the cell membranes, the membranes become much more permeable to glucose.

Glucose can then cross the cellular membrane down its concentration gradient until either an equilibrium of glucose concentration is created or insulin binding decreases. Diffusion across a cell membrane requiring the assistance of a transport system or membrane-altering system, such as insulin, is called *facilitated diffusion* or *facilitated transport*. Because this type of transport occurs down a concentration gradient and requires no energy expenditure by the cell, it is considered a form of diffusion.

Osmosis

Definition

Osmosis is the process by which only the water molecules (solvent) move through a selectively permeable membrane. A membrane must separate two fluid compartments for osmosis to occur. At least one of these fluid compartments must contain a solute that cannot move through the membrane. (The membrane is therefore impermeable to this solute.) A concentration gradient of this solute must also exist. If the membrane were permeable to this solute, then the solute would diffuse through the membrane down its concentration gradient until the concentrations of solute were equal on both sides of the membrane. However, because the membrane is impermeable to the solute, these particles cannot cross the membrane (although water molecules can).

Physiologic Activity

For the fluid compartments to have equal concentrations of solute, the water molecules must move down their concentration gradient from the side with the higher concentration of water molecules (and thus a lower concentration of solute molecules) to the side with the lower concentration of water molecules (and thus a higher concentration of solute molecules). This movement continues until both compartments contain the same proportions of solute to solvent. The less concentrated fluid contains proportionately fewer solute molecules and more water molecules than the more concentrated fluid. Water therefore moves by osmosis down its concentration gradient from the area of more dilute solute to the area of more concentrated solute until a new equilibrium is achieved (Fig. 14–5).

At this point, the concentrations of solute in the fluid compartments (the proportion of solute to solvent) on both sides of the membrane are equal, even though the total numbers of solute and volume of water may be different. This equilibrium is achieved by the movement of water molecules rather than the movement of solute molecules.

Factors that determine whether and how rapidly osmosis occurs include

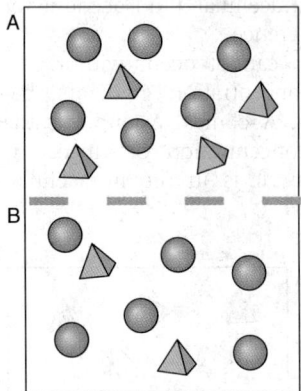
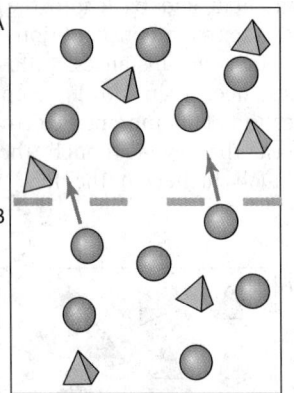
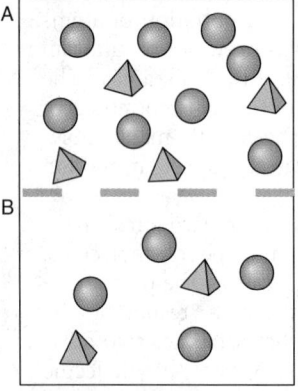

Side A has more solute molecules than does side B, even though the number of water molecules is the same on both sides. Thus, side A has a greater osmotic (water pulling) pressure than does side B.

DISEQUILIBRIUM
side A 1.5:1 ratio of water to solute
side B   3:1 ratio of water to solute

Movement of water occurs by osmosis toward side A because it has greater osmotic pressure. The membrane is *not* permeable to the solute molecules, so the actual number of solute molecules is side A and side B does not change. *Only the water molecules move because the membrane is not permeable to the solute molecules.*

Enough water molecules have moved from side B into side A that the actual concentration of solute is now the same on both sides, with a ratio of water to solute of 2:1. An equilibrium of osmotic pressure now exists between the two compartments, and no further *net* movement of water molecules or solute molecules will occur.

EQUILIBRIUM
side A 2:1 ratio of water to solute
side B 2:1 ratio of water to solute

● = water molecule

━━━ = permeable membrane

△ = solute molecule

Figure 14–5. The process of osmosis.

- The overall concentration of osmotically active particles (solute) in solution
- The solubility of the solute (how easily the solute dissolves in water)
- The amount of membrane available for osmosis

Concentration of Solute. The concentration of particles in human body fluids is expressed in milliequivalents per liter (mEq/L), millimoles per liter (mmol/L), and milliosmoles per liter (mOsm/L). Osmoles and milliosmoles are used to express the total concentration of solute particles (including electrolytes) contained within a solution. The number of milliosmoles present in body fluids can be expressed as either osmolarity or osmolality.

Osmolarity is defined as the number of milliosmoles in a *liter* of solution; *osmolality* is defined as the number of milliosmoles in a *kilogram* of solution. The normal osmolarity value for plasma and other body fluids ranges from 270 to 300 mOsm/L (Guyton & Hall, 1996).

The body functions best when the osmolarity of the fluids in all compartments is about 300 mOsm/L. Many mechanisms function to maintain solute concentration homeostasis. When all body fluids have this solute concentration, the osmotic pressures (water-pulling) of the various fluid compartments are essentially equal and no *net* water movement occurs. In such a situation, the body fluids are said to be *isosmotic* to each other. Another term with essentially the same meaning is *isotonic* (sometimes called *normotonic*). Examples of specific intravenous solutions with overall concentrations of specific substances equaling 270 to 300 mOsm/L include 0.9% sodium chloride in water and the complex formula of Ringer's lactate in water (Trissel, 1994). Because these substances are isotonic, or isosmotic, to plasma, their addition to plasma does not change plasma osmolarity or plasma osmotic pressure.

Fluids with osmolarities (solute concentrations) greater than 300 mOsm/L are said to be hyperosmotic, or hypertonic, compared with isosmotic fluids. Hyperosmotic fluids have a greater osmotic pressure than do isosmotic fluids and tend to pull water from the isosmotic fluid compartment into the hyperosmotic fluid compartment until an osmotic balance is achieved.

Fluids with osmolarities of less than 270 mOsm/L are said to be hypo-osmotic, or hypotonic, compared with isosmotic fluids. Hyposmolar fluids have a lower or smaller osmotic pressure than isosmotic fluids. As a result, water tends to be pulled from the hypo-osmotic fluid compartment into the isosmotic fluid compartment until an osmotic balance is achieved (Metheny, 1996).

Solubility of Solute. *Solubility* refers to the degree to which a solute dissolves or dissociates completely in water. Solubility is directly related to osmotic pressure: The greater the solubility of the solutes in a fluid, the higher the osmotic pressure of that fluid.

Amount of Available Membrane. The greater the amount of membrane available for osmosis, the faster the rate of osmosis. More membrane increases the chances that water molecules will strike the membrane at a point where penetration is possible.

Clinical Function and Significance

The process of osmosis acts with the process of filtration in capillary fluid dynamics to regulate both extracellular and intracellular fluid volumes. The thirst mechanism is an excellent example of the importance of osmosis in maintaining homeostasis. Thirst results from activation of cells in the hypothalamus of the brain that respond to changes in extracellular fluid (ECF) osmolarity. These cells are so sensitive to changes in ECF osmolarity that they are called *osmoreceptors*. When a person loses body fluids, especially water, such as through excessive sweating during prolonged heavy exercise, the ECF volume is decreased and the osmolarity is increased (hypertonic conditions exist). The cells in the thirst center shrink as water moves from the cells into the hypertonic ECF. Shrinking of these cells stimulates a person's awareness of thirst and increases the urge to drink. The person will usually drink enough fluid to replace that lost through sweating and restore the ECF osmolarity to its normal value. After the ECF volume and osmolarity return to normal levels, the osmoreceptors return to their normal size and no longer send stimulatory messages.

Active Transport
Definition

A cell must expend energy to move a substance across the cell membrane against a concentration gradient (uphill). Such movement is called *active transport,* because the cell must make active efforts for the net movement to occur. Because of its energy demands and uphill movement, active transport is sometimes called "pumping," and the mechanisms are known as membrane pumps.

Physiologic Activity

Active transport systems, or pumps, are usually located in the cell membrane and act as "gatekeepers" to maintain special environments inside cells. Some active transport pumps can carry more than one substance across the membrane at the same time. In these instances, the pump usually moves one substance into a cell and a different substance out of the cell at the same time. This process is called *cotransport*. Both transports are uphill against individual concentration gradients and require energy. The sodium-potassium pump is an example of such a double active transport system.

Sodium tends to diffuse slightly down its concentration gradient into the intracellular fluid (ICF) because it has such a high extracellular fluid (ECF) concentration compared with its ICF concentration. Similarly, because potassium has such a high concentration inside the cells compared with its concentration in ECF, it tends to diffuse slightly down its concentration gradient into the ECF. The action of the sodium-potassium pump moves the extra sodium out of the cell, while returning the lost potassium back into the cell. The sodium-potassium pump requires cellular energy expenditure.

The cellular energy for this process usually comes from breaking a high-energy bond ($\sim P$) when a phosphate group is split off from an adenosine triphosphate (ATP) molecule. Functioning of active transport pumps depends on the presence of adequate cellular ATP.

Clinical Function and Significance

Cells use active transport to control the intracellular concentration of many substances and to regulate cell volume. All cells function best when their internal environments are maintained separately from the changes occurring in the extracellular fluid (ECF) environment.

A clinical example of the results of active transport failure is the series of events following hypoxia (decreased oxygen supply in the body). Without adequate oxygen, ATP cannot be produced in sufficient amounts. Without ATP, the sodium-potassium pump cannot remove the extra sodium ions that have diffused from the ECF into the cell. The increased sodium concentration inside the cell increases the osmolarity and the osmotic pressure of the fluid inside the cell. Water moves into the cell in response to the increased osmotic pressure, which causes the cell to swell and perhaps to lyse (break open) and die if oxygen is not provided.

Table 14–2 summarizes the membrane processes involved in fluid and electrolyte balance.

Capillary Dynamics

The circulatory system distributes nutrients and removes wastes at the tissue level. The most important blood vessels for nutrient–waste exchange are the thin-walled, porous capillaries. Nutrient distribution and waste removal depend on capillary fluid movement.

Fluid movement at the capillary level is dynamic not only because it is continuous but also because relative homeostasis of vascular and interstitial fluid volumes

must be maintained. Opposing processes must occur for nutrients to move into tissue spaces, for wastes to move into circulation, and for the fluid volumes of both the vascular and tissue spaces to be maintained. In these processes, some fluid with nutrients must leave the capillary and enter the interstitial (tissue space) fluid compartment for a short period, which temporarily expands the interstitial fluid volume. The nutrients in the interstitial fluid are then taken up by the cells through various membrane transport processes. Water may be exchanged between the intracellular compartment and the interstitial compartment, but under normal circumstances, no net change in water volume occurs. Metabolic wastes created in the cells are moved into the interstitial fluid. Any extra fluid in the interstitial space, together with the waste products excreted from cells, must be returned via the capillary to the systemic circulation. Without a way to return the fluid originally lost into the interstitial compartment back to the blood, the vascular volume would become depleted to the point of circulatory failure and the interstitial fluid compartment would greatly expand.

Capillary Forces Influencing Fluid Movement

Forces at the capillary level permit capillary fluid loss to be followed by a return of fluid to the capillary so that a near-equilibrium of fluid distribution is maintained at the capillary-tissue level. These forces, known as *Starling's forces*, are outlined in Figure 14–6. The near equilibrium is based on the fact that forces tending to move fluid out from the capillary at the arterial end are nearly equal to the forces tending to move fluid from the interstitial compartment back into the capillary at the venous end.

Blood flowing from the arterial end of the capillary to the venous end is controlled by

TABLE 14–2

Summary of Membrane-Fluid Actions		
Action	**Definition**	**Specific Characteristics**
Filtration	• The movement of fluid through a biologic membrane as a result of hydrostatic pressure differences on both sides of the membrane	• Does not require energy • Is limited to solvent and low–molecular-weight solute • Usually occurs from capillaries to the interstitial fluid • Depends on hydrostatic pressure differences • Occurs more rapidly with steep gradients
Diffusion	• Free movement of substances across a permeable membrane down a concentration gradient	• Does not require energy • Is not pressure-dependent • Moves solute as well as solvent down their individual gradients • Occurs more rapidly with steep gradients • Is directly related in speed to the amount of membrane available • Occurs in both directions across capillary and cell membranes • Is responsible for maintaining tissue nutrition
Osmosis	• The process by which only the *solvent* diffuses through a selectively permeable membrane	• Does not require energy • Involves movement of water only • Depends on hydrostatic and osmotic pressures • Occurs more rapidly with steep gradients
Active transport	• The movement of a substance across a selectively permeable membrane against a concentration, electrical, or pressure gradient	• Requires energy • Requires a transport system (pump) • Helps maintain a special intracellular environment

Capillary blood normally flows from the arterial to the venous end:

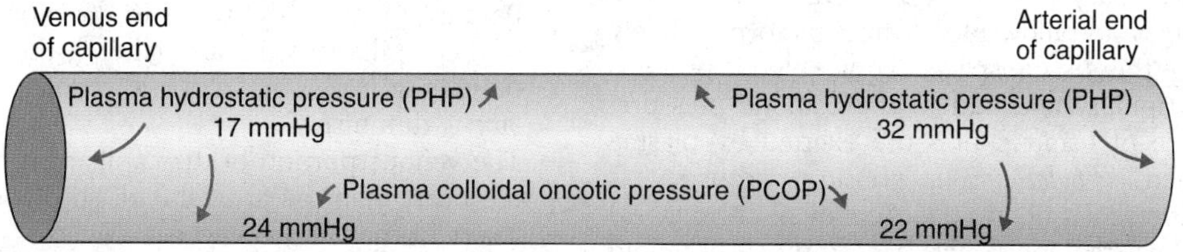

Venous end
of capillary

Arterial end
of capillary

Plasma hydrostatic pressure (PHP) ↗
17 mmHg

Plasma hydrostatic pressure (PHP)
32 mmHg

Plasma colloidal oncotic pressure (PCOP)↘
24 mmHg

22 mmHg

Tissue hydrostatic pressure (THP) 8 mmHg
Tissue osmotic pressure (TOP) 6 mmHg

Tissue hydrostatic pressure (THP) 4 mmHg
Tissue osmotic pressure (TOP) 10 mmHg

At the arterial end, the forces that tend to move fluid from the capillary into the tissue space are
Plasma hydrostatic pressure 32 mmHg
+
Tissue osmotic pressure 10 mmHg
_____
Total forces moving fluid out = 42 mmHg
At the arterial end, the forces that tend to move fluid from the tissue spaces into the capillary are
Tissue hydrostatic pressure 4 mmHg
+
Plasma colloidal oncotic pressure 22 mmHg
_____
Total forces moving fluid in = 26 mmHg
The total forces tending to move fluid out at the arterial end are 16 mmHg higher than the total forces tending to move fluid in at the arterial end (42 − 26 = 16). Thus, at the arterial end, fluid leaks out of the capillary into the tissue (interstitial) spaces.
At the venous end of the same capillary, the forces that tend to move fluid from the capillary into the tissue space are
Plasma hydrostatic pressure 17 mmHg
+
Tissue osmotic pressure 6 mmHg
_____
Total forces moving fluid out = 23 mmHg
At the venous end of the capillary, the forces that tend to move fluid from the tissue spaces back into the capillary are
Tissue hydrostatic pressure 8 mmHg
+
Plasma colloidal oncotic pressure 24 mmHg
_____
Total forces moving fluid in = 32 mmHg
The total forces tending to move fluid out at the venous end are 9 mmHg lower than the total forces tending to move fluid into the capillary at the venous end (32 − 23 = 9). Thus, at the venous end, fluid moves from the tissue spaces back into the capillary.
Because the pressures tending to move fluid out of the capillary at the arterial end (16 mmHg) are greater than the pressures that tend to move fluid back into the capillary at the venous end (9 mmHg), more fluid is lost from the capillary than is returned to it. Lymph drainage eventually returns this extra lost fluid to systemic circulation.

Figure 14–6. Capillary dynamics.

- Hydrostatic pressure of blood
- Dynamic ejection of blood from the left ventricle of the heart
- Patency or openness of the capillaries

The blood entering the arterial end of the capillary has a blood pressure, or a capillary (plasma) hydrostatic pressure (PHP), of about 32 mmHg. The capillary membrane is thin and permeable. The usual tissue hydrostatic pressure is low. These factors create a natural tendency for filtration from the blood outward into the tissue spaces. The fluid portion of the blood, along with most of the smaller substances dissolved in the blood, filters through the capillary membrane into the tissue spaces. Through this process, nutrients and other essential substances can reach the cells.

If net filtration, as a result of plasma hydrostatic pres-

sure, were the only force or factor involved at this level, blood volume would be progressively lost from the vascular space and would appear in the tissues. Fortunately, other mechanisms that favor the reabsorption of tissue fluid into the capillaries are also part of capillary dynamics. These mechanisms are plasma osmotic pressure and tissue hydrostatic pressure.

Osmosis (of water) through the capillary membrane (in either direction) occurs in response to differences in the concentrations of osmotically active substances in the capillary blood and in the tissue fluid. Tissue osmotic pressure (TOP) tends to draw fluid out of the capillary. Plasma osmotic pressure (POP) in the capillary tends to keep fluid in the capillary and to draw fluid from the interstitial space into the capillary. Under normal conditions, capillary plasma osmotic pressure is greater than tissue osmotic pressure because of the higher concentration of proteins in the blood compared with the protein concentration in the interstitial fluid.

Because the capillary membrane is highly impermeable to proteins, it does not allow blood proteins to pass freely through it into the tissue space. Thus, blood proteins remain in the capillary and add to the osmotic pressure. The specific type of osmotic pressure exerted by plasma proteins is called *colloidal oncotic pressure* because it is caused by the presence of proteins (colloidal substances) rather than dissociated ions such as sodium (crystalloid substances). The average colloidal oncotic pressure in capillary blood is about 22 mmHg.

Blood pressure (hydrostatic pressure) is greater than colloidal oncotic pressure at the arterial end of the capillary. Capillary hydrostatic pressure favors the filtration of fluid from the capillary into the tissue spaces, and colloidal oncotic pressure favors the reabsorption of fluid from the interstitial space into the capillary. The difference between these two capillary pressures at the arterial end of the capillary indicates a greater filtering force outward than a reabsorbing force inward.

Tissue Forces Influencing Fluid Movement

Tissue forces also influence the movement of solutions at the capillary level. These forces are tissue hydrostatic pressure (THP) and tissue osmotic pressure (TOP). Usually, both are relatively small forces. However, in some diseases, these forces increase greatly and significantly alter capillary dynamics.

To determine the direction of fluid movement in any one area of the capillary, the forces that move fluid out of the capillary are compared with the forces that move fluid into the capillary. Two forces at the arterial end that move fluid out of the capillary are the plasma hydrostatic pressure (PHP) (normally about 32 mmHg) and the tissue osmotic pressure (TOP) (normally about 10 mmHg). The pressures at the arterial end that return fluid to the capillary are the plasma colloidal oncotic pressure (normally about 22 mmHg) and the tissue hydrostatic pressure (THP) (normally about 4 mmHg). Because the outward filtration force is 16 mmHg higher than the inward reabsorbing force, the overall result at the arterial end of the capillary is the outward filtration of fluid and small solute particles into the tissue spaces.

Plasma hydrostatic pressure (PHP) decreases along the length of the capillary as blood flows through it. As filtration proceeds along the capillary, water is lost from the capillary, and the PHP gradually decreases. Therefore, the pressures that create the outward filtration force (from the capillary into the interstitial fluid) decrease, while the pressures that create the inward reabsorption force (from the interstitial fluid into the capillary) remain the same. Eventually, the outward filtration pressures and the inward reabsorption pressures become equal.

Clinical Function and Significance

Finally, at the venous end of the capillary, the inward reabsorption forces exceed the outward filtration forces. The venous end of the capillary has a much lower hydro-

static pressure than does the arterial end. This decreased hydrostatic pressure has two causes:

■ Because much of the water in the blood was filtered out of the capillary at the arterial end, the volume of water remaining in the blood at the venous end of the capillary is diminished.
■ The venous portion of the capillary is farther away from the heart than the arterial end, so blood pressure is lower in the venous end.

The hydrostatic pressure in the venous end of the capillary is low, and the interstitial fluid (tissue) hydrostatic pressure is high (because water moved from the arterial end of the capillary into the interstitial space). The colloidal osmotic pressure at the venous end of the capillary exceeds that at the arterial end because water was lost, increasing the concentration of proteins. The tissue osmotic pressure at the venous end of the capillary is lower than at the arterial end of the capillary because the water lost from the capillary has diluted the solute concentration of the tissue fluid. As a result, forces favoring the return of water from the tissues into the capillary are greater than the forces favoring filtration, and some water returns from the interstitial space back into the capillary at the venous end.

Lymph

Usually, not all the fluid that leaves the capillary at the arterial end and enters the interstitial space is returned to the capillary at the venous end. A small amount remains in the tissues. If this situation were not balanced by another mechanism to return the fluid to the systemic circulation, the circulating volume would become depleted and the interstitial areas would constantly be edematous. Instead, this extra fluid leaking out from the capillaries is returned to systemic circulation as *lymph*.

Lymph fluid is similar to blood plasma (from which it is formed) but contains far less protein. It is returned to systemic circulation by components of the auxiliary venous system known as lymph vessels, or *lymphatics*. Lymphatics begin as small, thin-walled, vein-like vessels that merge to form larger lymphatic vessels. Two large groups of lymphatic vessels connect the entire lymph system with the general circulatory system. The left thoracic lymph duct drains lymph from the abdomen, the gastrointestinal tract, the pelvis, the lower extremities, the left side of the thorax, the left arm, and the left side of the head and neck into the left subclavian vein at the point where it joins the left internal jugular vein (Fig. 14–7). Lymph from the right arm, the right side of the thorax, and right side of the head and neck drains into the right subclavian vein through three lymph ducts. Lymph nodes are situated along the lymphatic paths and act as lymph fluid filters.

Lymphatics carry lymph fluid in one direction— toward the heart. Lymph flow is slower than blood flow because lymph has no pump and no direct connection between the arterial blood circulation and the lymphatic system. The physical mechanisms that enhance lymph flow are skeletal muscle contractions, intrathoracic pres-

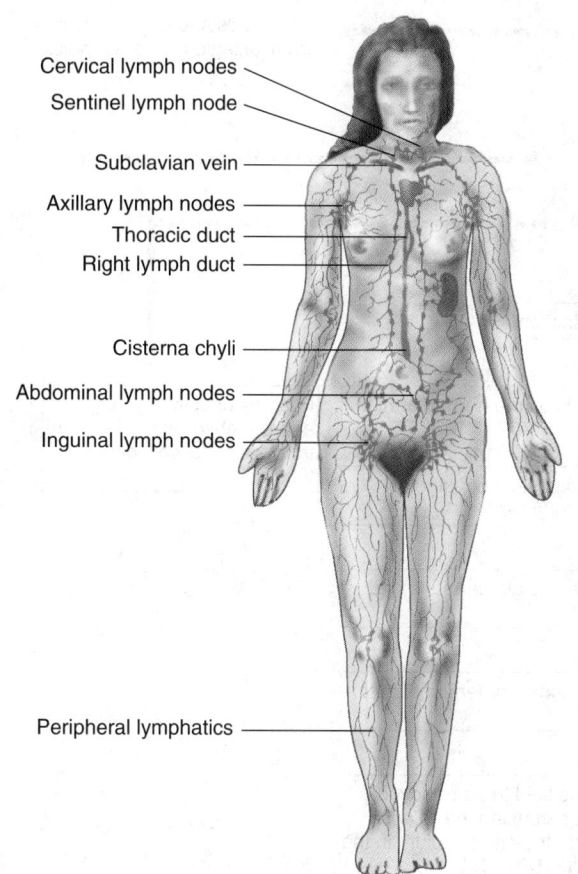

Cervical lymph nodes

Sentinel lymph node

Subclavian vein

Axillary lymph nodes

Thoracic duct

Right lymph duct

Cisterna chyli

Abdominal lymph nodes

Inguinal lymph nodes

Peripheral lymphatics

Figure 14–7. Patterns of lymph drainage. (From Lymph drainage. In Guyton, A., & Hall, J. [1996]. *Textbook of medical physiology* [9th ed., p. 194]. Philadelphia: W. B. Saunders.)

sure changes that occur during pulmonary ventilation, and an intrinsic peristalsis-like motion in lymph vessels.

Hormonal Influences on Fluid and Electrolyte Balance

Many endocrine mechanisms assist in the regulation of fluid and electrolyte balance. Three hormones that help control these critical balances are aldosterone, antidiuretic hormone (ADH), and atrial natriuretic peptide (ANP).

Aldosterone

Aldosterone is a *mineralocorticoid* (a naturally occurring steroid) secreted by the adrenal cortex. Aldosterone secretion is stimulated by either a decreased sodium level in the extracellular fluid (ECF) or an increased sodium level in urine. Aldosterone, angiotensinogen, and angiotensin secretion and function are outlined in Figure 14–8. Aldosterone directly influences sodium balance by preventing sodium loss. Because sodium in body fluids exerts osmotic (water-pulling) pressure, water attempts to follow sodium in physiologically proportionate amounts (Guyton

& Hall, 1996). As a result of this sodium-water relationship, aldosterone secretion also indirectly regulates water balance.

In the kidney, blood is supplied to the glomerulus of nephrons via the afferent arteriole. Specialized cells (juxtaglomerular cells) inside the afferent arteriole near the glomerulus are sensitive to changes in serum concentrations of sodium. This area of the afferent arteriole comes into direct contact with a specialized area of the distal convoluted tubule (the macula densa). Together, the juxtaglomerular cells and the macula densa form a functional group called the *juxtaglomerular complex*. When this complex senses that actual serum sodium concentrations are lower than normal or that the total blood volume is low, the macula densa stimulates juxtaglomerular cells to secrete renin.

Renin acts enzymatically on an inactive plasma protein called *angiotensinogen*, converting it to angiotensin I. Angiotensin I is immediately further degraded by an enzyme called angiotensin-converting enzyme into angiotensin II. Angiotensin II causes massive vasoconstriction of many blood vessels and stimulates increased secretion of aldosterone from the adrenal cortex.

Aldosterone acts on the distal convoluted tubules of the nephrons. When serum osmolarity is too low, aldosterone secretion stimulates these areas to reabsorb sodium (in exchange for potassium) from the filtrate (urine) back into systemic circulation, thus increasing serum osmolarity. Aldosterone secretion increases when blood osmolarity or serum sodium levels are low, and its presence is normally required to prevent excessive renal excretion of sodium. Aldosterone secretion also helps prevent serum potassium levels from becoming too high. Secretion of aldosterone is inhibited when serum sodium level or blood osmolarity is greater than normal.

Antidiuretic Hormone

Antidiuretic hormone (ADH), also known as *vasopressin*, is synthesized in specific areas of the brain and stored in the posterior pituitary gland. The release of ADH from the posterior pituitary gland is controlled by the hypothalamus in response to changes in blood osmolarity. The hypothalamus contains specialized cells, known as osmoreceptors, that are sensitive to changes in blood osmolarity. Increased blood osmolarity, especially an increase in plasma sodium concentration, results in slight shrinkage of these cells and triggers the hypothalamus to stimulate the posterior pituitary to release ADH.

Antidiuretic hormone acts directly on the renal tubules and collecting ducts, making them more permeable to water. As a result, more water is reabsorbed by these tubules and returned to the systemic circulation, causing the blood to have decreased osmolarity by becoming more dilute. When the blood osmolarity decreases, especially when the plasma sodium concentration is below normal, the osmoreceptors swell slightly and inhibit the release of ADH. Then, less water is reabsorbed and more is lost from the body in the urine. As a result, the amount of water in the extracellular fluid (ECF) decreases, bringing osmolarity to normal.

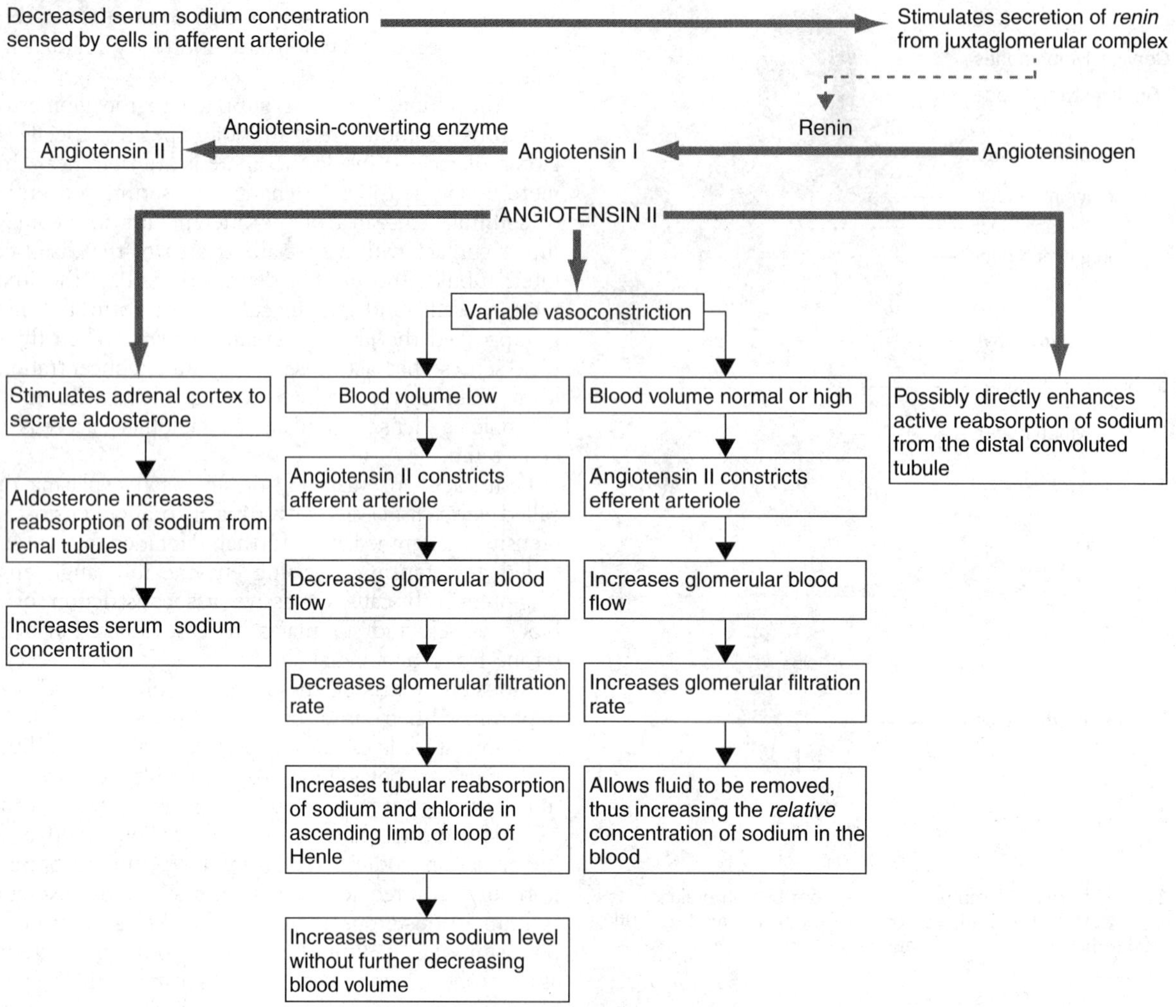

Decreased serum sodium concentration sensed by cells in afferent arteriole → Stimulates secretion of *renin* from juxtaglomerular complex

Angiotensin II ← Angiotensin-converting enzyme ← Angiotensin I ← Renin ← Angiotensinogen

ANGIOTENSIN II

Variable vasoconstriction

Stimulates adrenal cortex to secrete aldosterone

Aldosterone increases reabsorption of sodium from renal tubules

Increases serum sodium concentration

Blood volume low

Angiotensin II constricts afferent arteriole

Decreases glomerular blood flow

Decreases glomerular filtration rate

Increases tubular reabsorption of sodium and chloride in ascending limb of loop of Henle

Increases serum sodium level without further decreasing blood volume

Blood volume normal or high

Angiotensin II constricts efferent arteriole

Increases glomerular blood flow

Increases glomerular filtration rate

Allows fluid to be removed, thus increasing the *relative* concentration of sodium in the blood

Possibly directly enhances active reabsorption of sodium from the distal convoluted tubule

Figure 14–8. The role of aldosterone, angiotensinogen, angiotensin I, and angiotensin II in the renal regulation of water and sodium.

Atrial Natriuretic Peptide

Atrial natriuretic peptide (ANP) is secreted by special cells lining the atria of the heart in response to increased blood volume and blood pressure. ANP binds to receptor sites in the collecting ducts of the nephrons, creating effects opposite to those of aldosterone. Tubular reabsorption of sodium is inhibited at the same time that glomerular filtration is increased (Briggs et al., 1996). The outcome is increased output of urine with a high sodium content, which results in decreased circulating blood volume and decreased blood osmolarity.

Body Fluids

Fluids constitute approximately 55% to 60% of total adult body weight and consist of the extracellular fluid (ECF) and intracellular fluid (ICF). The ECF compartment is approximately 15 L (40%) of total body water and includes interstitial fluid, blood plasma, lymph, bone and connective tissue water, and the fluid within special spaces (called transcellular fluid), such as cerebrospinal fluid, synovial fluid, peritoneal fluid, and pleural fluid. ICF composes the remaining 25 L (60%) of total body water. Figure 14–9 shows the normal distribution of total body water.

A person's age, gender, and lean mass to body fat ratio influence the amounts and distribution of body fluids. An elderly adult has less body water than a younger adult. Because fat cells contain practically no water compared with other cells, an obese person has less water than a lean person of the same body weight.

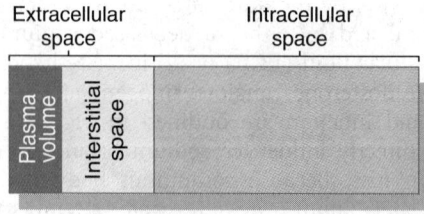

Figure 14–9. Normal distribution of total body water.

WOMEN'S HEALTH CONSIDERATIONS

w A woman of any age usually has less total body water than does a man of similar stature of the same age. This difference is because men have greater muscle mass than women, and women have a higher percentage of fat body weight. Differences in muscle mass and percentage of fat body weight are partly due to the influence of sex hormones. This difference in fat to lean body weight may be responsible for some differences seen in women's and men's responses to drugs.

Body fluids are solvents and transport substances. They allow the nutrition of cells and transport biological molecules (such as hormones) important to the regulation of normal physiologic functions. Most physiologic processes occur only in a liquid environment. Body fluids are constantly renewed, purified, and replaced as fluid balance is maintained through intake and output. The total amount of water within each fluid compartment is stable, but water movement occurs continually among all compartments. Water in any compartment is not static but rather is exchanged constantly while maintaining a volume equilibrium. Table 14–3 summarizes key points regarding fluid and electrolyte balance.

Sources of Fluid Intake

Fluid intake is regulated through the thirst drive. Fluids enter the body primarily as liquids (Table 14–4). Because solid foods contain up to 85% water, some fluid also enters the body in ingested solid foods. In addition, water

TABLE 14–3

Summary of Key Points Regarding Fluid and Electrolyte Balance

- All plasma electrolyte values must remain within a narrow range for proper physiologic functioning
- The plasma is the entrance and exit site for all fluids and electrolytes
- The primary organs or tissues of fluid and electrolyte regulation are the hypothalamus, the kidney, the adrenal glands, the posterior pituitary gland, the thyroid gland, and the parathyroid glands
- The total number of positive charges within a solution must be balanced by an equal number of negative charges to maintain electroneutrality
- Although the specific types and concentrations of substances (solute) dissolved in body fluid vary from one fluid compartment to another, the total concentration of all solutes is the same in all fluid compartments (270–300 mOsm/L)
- Whenever possible, the body's regulatory mechanisms attempt to create or maintain an osmolar equilibrium in all body fluid compartments
- A fluid compartment that is hyposmolar (hypotonic) to normal body fluids will expel water from the compartment
- A fluid compartment that is hyperosmolar (hypertonic) to normal body fluids will draw water into it

TABLE 14–4

Routes of Fluid Ingestion and Excretion

Intake	Output
Measurable	
Oral fluids	Urine
Parenteral fluids	Emesis†
Enemas*	Feces†
Irrigation fluids*	Drainage from body cavities
Not Measurable	
Solid foods	Perspiration
Metabolism	Vaporization through the lungs

* Measured by subtracting the amount returned from the amount instilled.
† Measurement accurate only when these substances are excreted in liquid form.

is a byproduct of cellular metabolism. This byproduct is called the water of oxidation. Approximately 10% (300 mL) of daily water requirements is met by the water of oxidation. A rising plasma osmolarity or a decreasing plasma volume stimulates the sensation of thirst. Other sensory input to the hypothalamus, such as dryness of the oral mucosa or sensorimotor input from higher brain areas, can trigger the thirst drive. An adult consumes an average of 1500 mL of fluid per day and obtains an additional 800 mL of fluid from ingested foods.

Routes of Fluid Loss

The body has several routes by which excessive water and waste products are removed (Table 14–4). Of all the water loss pathways, the renal route is the most important and most sensitive. Fluid loss via the renal route is closely regulated and is adjustable. The volume of urine excreted daily varies, depending on the amount of fluid intake and the body's need to conserve fluids.

The minimum amount of urine per day needed to dissolve and excrete the toxic waste products of metabolism ranges from 400 to 600 mL. This minimal volume is called the *obligatory urinary output*. If the 24-hour urine volume falls below the obligatory output amount, metabolic wastes are retained and can cause lethal electrolyte imbalances, acidosis, and toxic build-up of nitrogen. This urine is maximally concentrated, with a specific gravity (weight of the liquid compared with weight of pure water) of 1.032 or higher, and an osmolarity of at least 1200 mOsm/L.

Urine can also become maximally dilute, with a specific gravity of 1.005 and an osmolarity of 200 mOsm/L. This dilution can result from a large fluid intake and is reflected in a large volume of urine output. The concentrating and diluting capacity of the renal tubules is a response to changes in the osmolarity of the extracellular fluid (ECF), the volumes and pressures of the ECF compartments, and variation in the secretion of aldosterone, antidiuretic hormone (ADH), and atrial natriuretic peptide (ANP).

Other normal water loss occurs through the skin, the lungs, and the gastrointestinal tract. Additional water losses can occur via salivation, drainage from fistulas and drains, and gastrointestinal suction.

Water loss from the skin, lungs, and stool, termed *insensible water loss,* can be significant. In a healthy adult, insensible water loss is about 15 to 20 mL/kg per day. Insensible water loss can increase dramatically in hypermetabolic states such as thyroid crisis, trauma, burns, states of extreme stress, and fever. For every degree Celsius of increase in body temperature, insensible water loss increases by 10%. When atmospheric conditions are hot and dry, insensible water loss also increases. Examples of clients at risk for increased insensible water loss include those undergoing mechanical ventilation and those with rapid respirations (tachypnea). Insensible water loss (not including sweat) is pure water and does not contain electrolytes. Therefore, excessive amounts of insensible water loss result in a more hypertonic extracellular fluid (ECF) of a smaller volume. If this loss is not balanced by intake, the hypertonic ECF and accompanying dehydration can lead to *hypernatremia* (elevated serum sodium level).

Loss by sweating is variable and can reach a maximal rate of about 2 L/hour. Sweat, although it contains electrolytes, is slightly hypotonic to plasma. The amount of sweating is regulated by the autonomic nervous system, body temperature, and the skin blood flow.

Water loss through stool is normally minimal. However, in severe diarrhea or excessive fistula drainage, this loss can increase significantly. Clients with ulcerative colitis can have diarrheal fluid loss of several liters per day. Diarrheal fluid contains water, potassium, sodium, bicarbonate, and chloride. Thus, with diarrhea, hypotonic fluid containing some electrolytes is lost.

Electrolytes

Electrolytes, or ions, are substances in body fluids that carry an electrical charge. *Cations* are positively charged ions; *anions* are negatively charged ions. The body fluids are electrochemically neutral: positive ions are balanced by negative ions. However, the composition and distribution of ions differ in the extracellular fluid (ECF) and the intracellular fluid (ICF) (Fig. 14–10).

Most electrolytes have different concentrations in the ICF and in the ECF. This concentration difference helps maintain membrane excitability and transmit impulses. The electrolyte concentration ranges in these fluid compartments are extremely narrow. Thus, even small changes in these concentrations can result in major pathologic alterations.

Table 14–5 lists the major body fluid electrolytes together with their normal serum concentrations and primary functions. Most electrolytes enter the body in the form of ingested food.

Electrolyte homeostasis is controlled by balancing the dietary intake of electrolytes with the renal excretion or reabsorption of electrolytes. For example, plasma potassium concentration is maintained between 3.5 and 5.1 mmol/L. Potassium in common foods could in theory dramatically increase the ECF potassium concentration and lead to major pathologic consequences. However, the renal excretion of potassium keeps pace with potassium intake and prevents major changes in the plasma potassium concentration.

Sodium

Sodium (Na^+) is the major cation in the extracellular fluid (ECF) and is the main factor responsible for maintaining ECF osmolarity. The activity of the sodium-potassium pump keeps the sodium concentration of the intracellular fluid (ICF) low (about 14 mmol/L) while maintaining high sodium concentrations in the plasma and other ECFs. Preserving this difference in sodium concentration is vital for these normal physiologic functions:

- Initiation of skeletal muscle contraction
- Initiation of cardiac contractility
- Transmission of neuronal impulses
- Maintenance of ECF osmolarity
- Maintenance of ECF volume
- Maintenance of the renal urine-concentrating system

The concentration of sodium in the ECF determines whether water is retained, excreted, or moved from one body compartment to another.

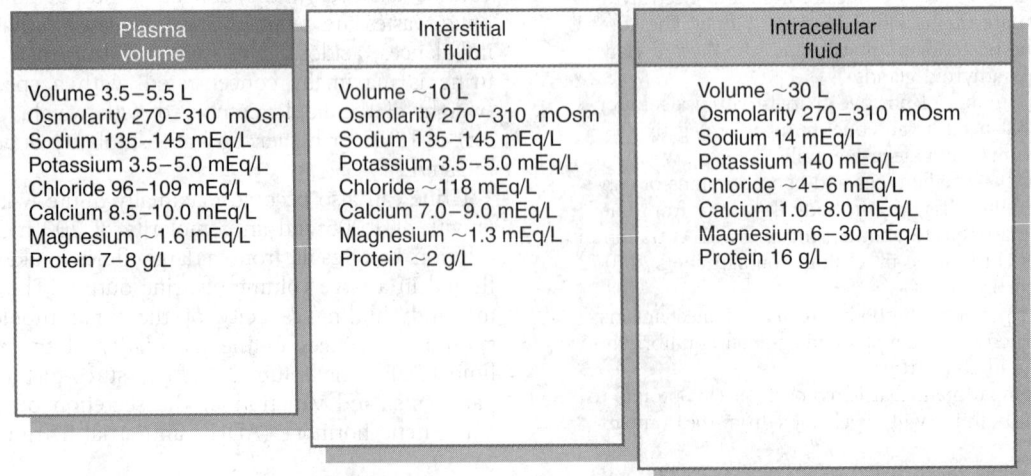

Plasma volume	Interstitial fluid	Intracellular fluid
Volume 3.5–5.5 L	Volume ~10 L	Volume ~30 L
Osmolarity 270–310 mOsm	Osmolarity 270–310 mOsm	Osmolarity 270–310 mOsm
Sodium 135–145 mEq/L	Sodium 135–145 mEq/L	Sodium 14 mEq/L
Potassium 3.5–5.0 mEq/L	Potassium 3.5–5.0 mEq/L	Potassium 140 mEq/L
Chloride 96–109 mEq/L	Chloride ~118 mEq/L	Chloride ~4–6 mEq/L
Calcium 8.5–10.0 mEq/L	Calcium 7.0–9.0 mEq/L	Calcium 1.0–8.0 mEq/L
Magnesium ~1.6 mEq/L	Magnesium ~1.3 mEq/L	Magnesium 6–30 mEq/L
Protein 7–8 g/L	Protein ~2 g/L	Protein 16 g/L

Figure 14–10. The composition of various body fluids.

TABLE 14–5

Major Serum Electrolyte Concentrations and Functions

Electrolyte	Reference Range	International Recommended Units	Functions
Sodium (Na$^+$)	136–145 mEq/L	136–145 mmol/L	• Maintenance of plasma and interstitial osmolarity • Generation and transmission of action potentials • Maintenance of acid-base balance • Maintenance of electroneutrality
Potassium (K$^+$)	3.5–5.1 mEq/L	3.5–5.1 mmol/L	• Regulation of intracellular osmolarity • Maintenance of electrical membrane excitability • Maintenance of plasma acid-base balance
Calcium (Ca^{2+})	8.6–10.0 mg/dL	2.15–2.5 mmol/L	• Cofactor in blood clotting cascade • Excitable membrane stabilizer • Adds strength/density to bones and teeth • Essential element in cardiac, skeletal, and smooth muscle contraction
Chloride (Cl$^-$)	98–107 mEq/L	98–107 mmol/L	• Maintenance of plasma acid-base balance • Maintenance of plasma electroneutrality • Formation of hydrochloric acid
Magnesium (Mg^{2+})	1.6–2.6 mg/dL	0.66–1.07 mmol/L	• Excitable membrane stabilizer • Essential element in cardiac, skeletal, and smooth muscle contraction • Cofactor in blood clotting cascade • Cofactor in carbohydrate metabolism • Cofactor in DNA and protein synthesis
Phosphorus (Pi)	2.7–4.5 mg/dL	0.87–1.45 mmol/L	• Activation of B-complex vitamins • Formation of adenosine triphosphate and other high-energy substances • Cofactor in carbohydrate, protein, and lipid metabolism

Data from Tietz, N. (Ed.) (1995). *Clinical guide to laboratory tests* (3rd ed.). Philadelphia: W. B. Saunders.

The concentration of sodium, a cation, within a body fluid must be matched by an equal concentration of anions to maintain electrical balance. Each cation in the ECF must be balanced by an anion so that the fluid does not carry either an overall positive or an overall negative charge. When such a balance is maintained, a state of *electroneutrality* exists in that fluid. Changes in the plasma sodium concentration profoundly affect the fluid volume and the distribution of other electrolytes.

The normal concentration of plasma sodium ranges between 136 and 145 mEq/L or mmol/L (see Table 14–5). Sodium enters the body from ingestion of many foods and fluids (Table 14–6). The average dietary intake of sodium is about 6 to 12 g/day. Sodium is also stored in interstitial fluid areas deep within the renal tissues and can be released to ECF as needed. Despite great variations in sodium intake, serum sodium concentration usually remains within the normal range. Plasma sodium balance is regulated by the kidney under the influences of aldosterone, antidiuretic hormone (ADH), and atrial natriuretic peptide (ANP).

Low serum sodium levels inhibit ADH and ANP secretion while stimulating aldosterone secretion. These actions together increase serum sodium concentration by increas-

TABLE 14–6

Common Food Sources of Sodium*

Food Source	Amount (mg)
Table salt (1 tsp)	2000
Cheddar cheese (1 oz)	176
Cottage cheese (4 oz)	457
American cheese (1 oz)	439
Whole milk (8 oz)	120
Skim milk (8 oz)	126
Butter (1 tsp)	123
White bread (1 slice)	123
Whole-wheat bread (1 slice)	159
Soy sauce (1 tbsp)	1029
Ketchup (1 tbsp)	156
Mustard (1 tbsp)	188
Beef, lean (4 oz)	60
Pork, lean, fresh (4 oz)	60
Pork, cured (4 oz)	850
Chicken, light meat (4 oz)	70
Chicken, dark meat (4 oz)	70

Data from Pennington, J. (1994). *Bowe's and Church's food values of portions commonly used* (16th ed.). Philadelphia: J. B. Lippincott.

* U. S. Department of Agriculture recommended daily allowance for adults: 1100–3300 mg.

ing renal reabsorption of sodium and enhancing renal loss of water.

High serum sodium levels inhibit aldosterone secretion and directly stimulate ADH and ANP secretion. Together, these hormones cause an increase in the renal excretion of sodium and the renal reabsorption of water.

Potassium

In contrast to sodium, potassium (K^+) is the major cation of the intracellular fluid (ICF). The normal plasma concentration of potassium ranges from 3.5 to 5.1 mEq/L or mmol/L (see Table 14–5). The normal ICF concentration of potassium is about 140 mEq/L (mmol/L). Because of its high concentration inside cells, potassium exerts some control over intracellular osmolarity and volume. Maintaining this large difference in potassium concentration between ICF and the extracellular fluid (ECF) is critical for enabling excitable tissues to generate action potentials and to transmit impulses. Intracellular and extracellular functions of potassium include

- Regulation of protein synthesis
- Regulation of glucose use and storage
- Maintenance of action potentials in excitable membranes

Because ECF potassium levels are so low, any alteration in concentration is poorly tolerated by the body and profoundly affects physiologic activities. For example, a decrease in plasma potassium of only 1 mEq/L (from 4 mEq/L to 3 mEq/L) represents a significant difference (25%) in total ECF potassium concentration, whereas a decrease in plasma sodium of 1 mEq/L (from 140 mEq/L to 139 mEq/L) represents a much smaller change (less than 1%) in total ECF sodium concentration.

Potassium drifts out of cells down its concentration gradient into the ECF. In addition, almost all foods contain potassium (Table 14–7). Potassium intake averages about 2 to 20 g/day. Despite heavy potassium ingestion and the drifting of potassium from cellular storage sites into the ECF, the healthy body keeps plasma potassium levels within the narrow range of normal values required for physiologic function.

The primary controller of ECF potassium concentration is the sodium-potassium pump within the membranes of all body cells. The pump removes three sodium ions from the fluid inside the cell for every two potassium ions that it returns to the cell. In this way, the concentration differences for both ions are maintained.

Some potassium regulation also occurs through renal function. The kidney is the excretory route for ridding the body of ECF potassium (80% of potassium removed from the body occurs via the kidney). Unlike sodium, no hormone has been identified that directly controls renal reabsorption of potassium, and thus, the kidney does not conserve potassium directly.

Calcium

Calcium (Ca^{2+}) is a mineral whose presence and functions are closely related to those of phosphorus and magnesium. Calcium is a *divalent cation* (an ion expressing

TABLE 14–7

Common Food Sources of Potassium*

Food Source	Amount (mg)
Corn flakes (1¼ c)	26
Cooked oatmeal (¾ c)	99
Egg (1 large)	66
Codfish, raw (4 oz)	400
Salmon, pink, raw (3½ oz)	306
Tuna fish (4 oz)	375
Apple, raw with skin (1 medium)	159
Banana (1 medium)	451
Cantaloupe (1 c pieces)	494
Grapefruit (½ medium)	175
Orange (1 medium)	250
Raisins (½ c)	700
Strawberries, raw (1 c)	247
Watermelon (1 c pieces)	186
White bread (1 slice)	27
Whole-wheat bread (1 slice)	44
Beef (4 oz)	480
Beef liver (3½ oz)	281
Pork, fresh (4 oz)	525
Pork, cured (4 oz)	325
Chicken (4 oz)	225
Veal cutlet (3½ oz)	448
Whole milk (8 oz)	370
Skim milk (8 oz)	406
Avocado (1 medium)	1097
Carrot (1 large)	341
Corn (4-inch ear)	196
Cauliflower (1 c pieces)	295
Celery (1 stalk)	170
Green beans (1 c)	189
Mushrooms (10 small)	410
Onion (1 medium)	157
Peas (¾ c)	316
Potato, white (1 medium)	407
Spinach, raw (3½ oz)	470
Tomato (1 medium)	366

Data from Pennington, J. (1994). *Bowe's and Church's food values of portions commonly used* (16th ed.). Philadelphia: J. B. Lippincott.
* U. S. Department of Agriculture recommended daily allowance for adults: 1875–5625 mg.

two positive charges) that exists in the body in two forms: bound and ionized (unbound or free).

Bound calcium is usually connected to specific serum proteins, especially albumin. Ionized calcium is present in blood and other extracellular fluids (ECFs) as free calcium. Free calcium is physiologically active and must be maintained within a narrow range in the ECF. The body functions best when plasma calcium concentrations are maintained between 8.6 and 10.0 mg/dL, or 2.15 and 2.5 mmol/L. Because the intracellular fluid (ICF) concentration of calcium is low, calcium has a steep gradient between ECF and ICF. Calcium functions in many ways and in many specialized body systems, including

- Biochemical cofactor (a substance required to enhance the activity of enzymes or reactions)
- Skeletal muscle contraction
- Cardiac contractility

TABLE 14-8

Common Food Sources of Calcium*	
Food Source	**Amount (mg)**
Cheddar cheese (1 oz)	204
Cottage cheese (4 oz)	68
American cheese (1 oz)	174
Whole milk (8 oz)	288
Skim milk (8 oz)	302
Yogurt, low-fat (1 c)	415
Broccoli, raw (½ c)	75
Carrot (1 large)	37
Collard greens, raw (3 oz)	200
Green beans (1 c)	62
Rhubarb (1 c)	266
Spinach, raw (3½ oz)	93
Tofu (3 oz)	100

Data from Pennington, J. (1994). *Bowe's and Church's food values of portions commonly used* (16th ed.). Philadelphia: J. B. Lippincott.
* U. S. Department of Agriculture recommended daily allowance for adults: 800–1200 mg.

- Regulation of neural impulse transmission
- Blood clotting
- Bone strength and density

Calcium enters the body by dietary intake and subsequent absorption through the intestinal tract (Table 14–8). Absorption of dietary calcium requires the active form of vitamin D. Calcium is stored in the bones. When both plasma calcium levels and stored calcium levels are adequate, intestinal absorption of dietary calcium is inhibited and urinary excretion of excess calcium increases. When more plasma calcium is needed, parathyroid hormone (PTH, or parathormone) is secreted and released from the parathyroid glands (Table 14–9). PTH causes ECF calcium levels to increase through the following processes:

- Release of free calcium from bone storage sites directly into the ECF (*resorption*)

- Stimulation of vitamin D activation, thus increasing intestinal absorption of dietary calcium
- Inhibition of renal excretion of calcium and stimulation of renal tubular reabsorption of calcium

When excess calcium is present in plasma, secretion of PTH is inhibited and secretion of thyrocalcitonin (TCT), a hormone secreted by the thyroid gland, is increased. TCT causes the plasma calcium level to decrease through the following processes:

- Inhibition of bone resorption of calcium
- Inhibition of activation of vitamin D; decreased gastrointestinal uptake of calcium
- Increased renal excretion of calcium in the urine

Phosphorus

Phosphorus (P) is present in the body in both inorganic and organic forms. Normal plasma levels of phosphorus range from 2.7 to 4.5 mg/dL, or 0.87 to 1.45 mmol/L. The majority of phosphorus (80%) can be found in the bones. Phosphorus is the major anion in the intracellular fluid (ICF), and its concentration inside cells is much higher than that in extracellular fluid (ECF). Phosphorus is vital to the following intracellular activities:

- Activation of B-complex vitamins
- Formation and activation of high-energy substances, including adenosine triphosphate (ATP)
- Cell division
- Carbohydrate metabolism
- Protein metabolism
- Lipid (fat) metabolism

Extracellular fluid phosphorus functions include acid-base buffering and calcium homeostasis. Phosphorus is present in a variety of foods, such as nuts, legumes, dairy products, red meat, organ meat, bran, and whole grains (Table 14–10). The average diet is high in phosphorus (1–2 g/day).

Phosphorus balance and calcium balance are intertwined. Normally, plasma concentrations of calcium and

TABLE 14-9

Hormonal Regulation of Calcium	
Hormone	**Action**
Parathyroid Hormone (PTH)	
Secreted in response to low or low-normal serum calcium levels Secretion results in a rise in serum calcium concentration	• Increases bone resorption of calcium (leaching of stored calcium) • Increases the absorption of ingested calcium from the gastrointestinal tract into extracellular fluid • Increases renal reabsorption of calcium at the proximal convoluted tubule
Thyrocalcitonin (TCT)	
Secreted by the thyroid gland in response to high or high-normal serum calcium levels Secretion results in a reduction of the serum calcium concentration	• Increases bone uptake of calcium • Inhibits the absorption of calcium from the gastrointestinal tract so that ingested calcium is excreted from the body in feces • Inhibits renal reabsorption of calcium at the proximal convoluted tubule so that more calcium is excreted in the urine

TABLE 14–10

Common Food Sources of Phosphorus*	
Food Source	**Amount (mg)**
Rolled oats, cooked (¾ c)	133
Egg (1 large)	90
Codfish (3 oz)	175
Tuna fish, white, canned (6½ oz)	405
Raisins (½ c)	75
White bread (1 slice)	26
Whole-wheat bread (1 slice)	23
Cheddar cheese (1 oz)	145
American cheese (1 oz)	211
Whole milk (8 oz)	228
Skim milk (8 oz)	247
Yogurt, low-fat (8 oz)	326
Beef (4 oz)	215
Beef liver (4 oz)	375
Pork, fresh (4 oz)	325
Chicken (4 oz)	200
Almonds (1 oz)	141
Peanuts (1 oz)	110

Data from Pennington, J. (1994). *Bowe's and Church's food values of portions commonly used* (16th ed.). Philadelphia: J. B. Lippincott.
* U. S. Department of Agriculture recommended daily allowance for adults: 800 mg.

phosphorus exist in a reciprocal relationship, in that the product of the plasma concentrations remains constant. Therefore, a change in the concentration of phosphorus results in an equal and opposite change in the concentration of calcium (and vice versa).

The regulation of ECF phosphorus occurs through the activity of parathyroid hormone (PTH). Increased PTH secretion results in a net loss of phosphorus. Reduced PTH levels enhance renal reabsorption of phosphorus, resulting in increased ECF phosphorus concentrations.

Magnesium

Magnesium (Mg^{2+}) is another mineral that forms a cation when dissolved in water. The adult human body has an average of 25 g of magnesium, most of which (60%) is stored in bones and cartilage. Little magnesium is present in the extracellular fluid (ECF), and more than 25% of that is bound to albumin. Plasma levels of ionized magnesium range from 1.6 to 2.6 mg/dL, or 0.66 to 1.07 mmol/L. Much more magnesium is present in the intracellular fluid (ICF), and it has more functions inside the cells than in the plasma. Magnesium is critical for the following intracellular reactions or activities:

- Muscle contraction
- Carbohydrate metabolism
- Activation and use of adenosine triphosphate (ATP)
- Activation of many B-complex vitamins
- DNA synthesis
- Protein synthesis

Extracellular magnesium regulates blood coagulation and skeletal muscle contractility.

Magnesium is abundant in many foods, such as nuts, vegetables, fish, and whole grains (Table 14–11). The daily magnesium requirement for adults is about 300 mg.

Although magnesium is similar to calcium in many respects and its presence in plasma must be maintained within a narrow range of normal values, little is known about its regulation. Magnesium is absorbed from the intestinal tract at the same point as for calcium. The absorption of phosphorus inhibits magnesium absorption. Parathyroid hormone (PTH) stimulates the release of magnesium from bone in much the same way that it stimulates the release of calcium.

Chloride

Chloride (Cl^-) is the major anion of the extracellular fluid (ECF). It works with sodium in maintaining ECF osmotic pressure. Chloride is important in the formation of hydrochloric acid in the stomach. The normal plasma concentration of chloride ranges from 98 to 107 mEq/L, or 98 to 107 mmol/L.

Only a small quantity of chloride is present inside the cells because negatively charged particles on the cell membrane repel chloride and prevent it from crossing the cell membranes. However, extracellular chloride can enter cells when it is exchanged for another anion that is leaving the cell. This situation, a *chloride shift*, results in decreased plasma chloride concentration but no net body loss of chloride. Bicarbonate (HCO_3^-) is the anion most commonly exchanged for chloride. Chloride enters the body through dietary intake. Because chloride, with sodium, potassium, and many other minerals, is a part of a

TABLE 14–11

Common Food Sources of Magnesium*	
Food Source	**Amount (mg)**
Rolled oats, cooked (¾ c)	42
Tuna fish, white, canned (6½ oz)	59
Raisins (½ c)	25
Beef (4 oz)	24
Pork (4 oz)	30
Chicken (4 oz)	26
Whole milk (8 oz)	33
Skim milk (8 oz)	28
Yogurt, low-fat (8 oz)	40
Peanut butter (1 tbsp)	22
Avocado (1 medium)	70
Broccoli (1 stalk)	24
Cauliflower (1 c pieces)	24
Peas (¾ c)	35
Potato (1 medium)	34
Spinach, raw (3½ oz)	88

Data from Pennington, J. (1994). *Bowe's and Church's food values of portions commonly used* (16th ed.). Philadelphia: J. B. Lippincott.
* U. S. Department of Agriculture recommended daily allowance for adults: 300–350 mg.

Chart 14–1

Nursing Focus on the Elderly: Impact of Age-Related Changes on Fluid and Electrolyte Balance

System	Change	Result
Integumentary	• Loss of elasticity • Decreased turgor • Decreased oil production	• An unreliable indicator of fluid status • Dry, easily damaged skin
Renal	• Decreased glomerular filtration • Decreased concentrating capacity	• Poor excretion of waste products • Increased water loss
Muscular	• Decreased muscle mass	• Decreased total body water • Greater risk of dehydration
Neurologic	• Diminished thirst reflex	• Decreased fluid intake, increasing risk of dehydration
Endocrine	• Adrenal atrophy	• Poor regulation of sodium and potassium, predisposing the client to hyponatremia and hyperkalemia

salt, most diets contain enough chloride to meet the body's normal needs.

Fluid and Electrolyte Changes Associated with Aging

Only 45% to 50% of the body weight of elderly people is water, compared with 55% to 60% in younger adults. This decrease represents a net loss of muscle mass and a reduced ratio of lean body weight to total body weight. The decrease in total body water places elderly people at greater risk for water-deficit states. Multiple symptoms point to fluid volume deficit in the elderly person.

Skin *turgor* (the normal resiliency of a pinched fold of skin) is not always an accurate assessment of extracellular fluid (ECF) volume deficit in the elderly person because the natural aging process is associated with decreased

turgor (Chart 14–1). Furthermore, the elderly person may have a diminished thirst sensation and decreased renal function, both of which contribute to risk of fluid volume deficit and make assessment more difficult. Accurate documentation of intake and output and accurate weight measurement are extremely important when nurses work with elderly clients because these measurements reflect hydration status more accurately than does skin turgor.

The normal concentration of serum electrolytes also changes with the aging process. Chart 14–2 lists the normal electrolyte values for people older than 60 years.

Electrolyte balance may be more difficult to maintain in older people. Small changes in the concentrations of potassium and calcium in particular may produce unexpectedly profound results. Although plasma and intracellular fluid (ICF) electrolyte ranges may remain normal, the balance is fragile and more easily disturbed in an elderly

---

Chart 14–2

Nursing Focus on the Elderly: Normal Plasma Electrolyte Values for People Older than 60 Years

Electrolyte	Reference Range	International Recommended Units
Calcium (Ca^{2+}) > 90 years	8.8–10.2 mg/dL 8.2–9.6 mg/dL	2.2–2.55 mmol/L 2.05–2.40 mmol/L
Chloride (Cl^-) > 90 years	98–107 mEq/L 98–111 mEq/L	98–107 mmol/L 98–111 mmol/L
Magnesium (Mg^{2+}) > 90 years	1.6–2.4 mg/dL 1.7–2.3 mg/dL	0.66–0.99 mmol/L 0.70–0.95 mmol/L
Phosphorus (Pi)	2.3–3.7 mg/dL (male) 2.8–4.1 mg/dL (female)	0.74–1.20 mmol/L 0.90–1.32 mmol/L
Potassium (K^+)	3.5–4.5 mEq/L (male) 3.4–4.4 mEq/L (female)	3.5–4.5 mmol/L 3.4–4.4 mmol/L
Sodium (Na^+) > 90 years	136–145 mEq/L 132–146 mEq/L	136–145 mmol/L 132–146 mmol/L

Data compiled from: Tietz, N. (Ed.) (1995). *Clinical guide to laboratory tests* (3rd ed.). Philadelphia: W. B. Saunders.

person. Part of this fragility is related to decreased regulatory functions that occur with aging. Age-related renal changes include decreased renal blood flow, decreased glomerular filtration rate, and decreased numbers of functional nephrons. Renal and membrane changes associated with hypertension may also be present in the elderly person.

 Assessment of Fluid and Electrolyte Balance

➤ History

A client's nutritional history can often reveal an underlying pathophysiologic process influencing fluid and electrolyte balance. The nurse directly elicits this information because the client may not understand the connection between dietary intake and the onset of fluid and electrolyte imbalances.

Guidelines for obtaining a thorough fluid and electrolyte history do not differ from those for assessing any other system; however, the information collected is more quantitative. For example, intake and output volumes are often extremely important, as are serial daily weights. The nurse may need to guide clients in accurately reporting the amount of fluid ingested and changes in voiding patterns. The nurse also assesses the types of fluids and foods ingested to determine osmolarity as well as amount. In addition, many clients do not consider solid food to contain liquid. Solid foods such as ice cream, gelatin, and ices are liquids at body temperature, and the nurse includes them when calculating fluid intake.

Output fluids include not only losses through urine but also those through significant diaphoresis and diarrhea and insensible loss during fevers. The nurse asks specific questions about prescribed and over-the-counter medications that the client has taken and ascertains the dosage, the length of time taken, and the client's compliance with the medication regimen. A client taking diuretics can have an imbalance of fluid, potassium, sodium, or hydrogen ions if additional threats to water balance, such as vomiting or excessive sweating, also occur.

Elderly people frequently use laxatives, which can disturb fluid and electrolyte balance. Misuse and overuse of these drugs can lead to serious imbalances.

Other pertinent areas of the client history include body weight changes, thirst or excessive drinking, exposure to environmental heat, and the presence of other preexisting disorders such as renal or endocrine diseases (e.g., Cushing's disease, Addison's disease, diabetes mellitus, and diabetes insipidus). The nurse makes a general assessment of the client's level of consciousness and mental status, because changes in mental status may further support findings of imbalance. In such cases, the nurse may need to verify with family members the accuracy of historical data.

➤ Physical Assessment

Hydration is the normal state of fluid balance. A normally hydrated adult is alert, has moist eyes and mucous mem-

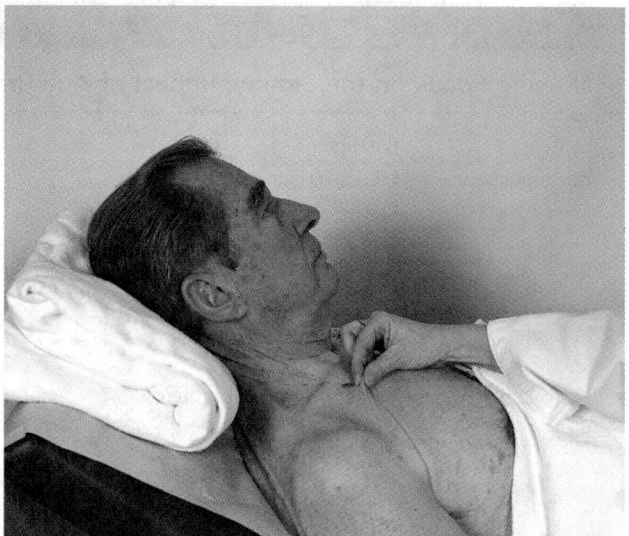
Figure 14–11. Examining the skin turgor of an elderly client.

branes, has a urinary output appropriate for the amount of fluid ingested (with a urine specific gravity of approximately 1.015), and has an adequate state of skin hydration as assessed by skin turgor.

The nurse assesses skin turgor by pinching a fold of skin. This pinched fold should return immediately to its original shape after release. Decreased turgor, a sign of dehydration, is present when the fold remains in a pinched shape after being released and rebounds slowly (*tenting*) (Fig. 14–11). The nurse can best assess skin turgor in body areas that contain little adipose tissue, such as over the sternum or on the back of the hand. An elderly person may have poor skin turgor because of the loss of tissue elasticity related to the aging process; thus, a true state of hydration may be more difficult to assess in an older adult than in a younger adult. The test areas for assessing turgor in the elderly are over the sternum and on the forehead.

Skin hydration assessment also includes an examination for dryness. The mucous membranes and the conjunctiva are normally moist. An assessment of fluid balance always includes an examination of the eyes, the nose, and oral mucous membranes. A dry, sticky, "cottony" mouth; the absence of tearing; the presence of weight loss; and decreased urinary output all indicate an actual fluid volume deficit.

A major criterion used in assessing fluid and electrolyte status is accurate measurement of fluid intake and output. Accurate assessment of actual fluid intake and output is the nurse's responsibility, and volumetric measuring devices must be used.

Behavioral and neurologic assessments are included in fluid assessment because changes in fluid balance can result in alteration of neurologic function. In hypertonic states, neuronal cell shrinkage may induce serious nervous system excitability and hyperactivity, and convulsions may occur. Another variable to assess is the degree of thirst. Thirst may be difficult to gauge in a confused elderly client.

The nurse approximates insensible water loss (e.g., sweat) in every client. Special situations also require an assessment of fluid loss from other routes, including

- Fluid losses from wounds
- Gastric or intestinal drainage
- Blood loss from hemorrhage
- Drainage of body secretions, such as bile and pancreatic juices, through surgical fistulas

Electrolytes control the activity of excitable membranes, and electrolyte imbalances are associated with altered function of these membranes. Electrolyte assessment includes a complete neuromuscular assessment of muscle tone and strength, movement, coordination, and tremors. Assessment of other systems, including cardiac (heart rate, the strength of contractions, and the presence of dysrhythmias) and gastrointestinal (peristalsis) systems, may indicate alterations of excitable membrane function.

Part of the nurse's assessment focuses on changes from previous findings (including mental status, physical examination data, and laboratory data). Fluid and electrolyte imbalances can occur quickly; therefore, the nurse must be familiar with the client's baseline assessment data to detect any changes.

➤ Psychosocial Assessment

Psychosocial assessment related to fluid and electrolyte status includes both psychologic and cultural factors that might influence balance. Depressed clients may refuse fluids or forget to drink adequate fluids. Clients with bulimia or anorexia nervosa (eating disorders) may use laxatives to excess or may induce vomiting, resulting in fluid and electrolyte imbalances. The nurse also assesses social practices. For example, excessive alcohol or drug use may lead to fluid or electrolyte imbalance.

➤ Diagnostic Assessment

Laboratory results are crucial in identifying specific fluid and electrolyte imbalances or disorders that alter fluid and electrolyte status. Normal serum electrolyte values are presented in Table 14–5, and normal values for people older than 60 years appear in Chart 14–2. Other laboratory values helpful in assessing fluid and electrolyte status include blood urea nitrogen level, glucose concentration, creatinine level, pH, bicarbonate level, osmolarity, hemoglobin, and hematocrit.

The urine test results may be helpful in assessing fluid status (Table 14–12). If a laboratory report is not avail-

TABLE 14–12

Normal Urine Electrolyte Values

Electrolyte/Characteristics	Normal Value*	Significance of Abnormal Value†
Calcium	2.5–7.5 mmol/day	Increased: Malignancy, thyrotoxicosis, hyperparathyroidism, osteoporosis, vitamin D intoxication Decreased: Hypoparathyroidism, rickets, kidney disease, hypothyroidism
Chloride	100–250 mEq/day 110–250 mmol/day	Increased: Increased salt intake, drug-induced diuresis, adrenocortical insufficiency Decreased: Reduced salt intake, water retention, vomiting, cerebral edema, adrenocortical hyperfunction
Magnesium	3.0–5.0 mmol/day	Increased: Alcohol intake, diuretics, corticosteroid therapy, cisplatin therapy Decreased: Dietary insufficiency
Phosphorus	12.9–42.0 mmol/day	Increased: Hyperparathyroidism, renal tubular damage, immobility, nonrenal acidosis Decreased: Hypoparathyroidism
Potassium	25–125 mmol/day (varies with diet)	Increased: Early starvation, hyperaldosteronism, metabolic acidosis Decreased: Addison's disease, renal disease
Sodium	40–220 mEq/day 40–220 mmol/day	Increased: Increased dietary intake, adrenal failure, diuretic therapy Decreased: Low sodium intake, sodium and water retention, adrenocortical hyperfunction, excessive diaphoresis, diarrhea
Osmolarity (osmolality)	300–900 mOsm/kg water	Increased: Dehydration, SIADH Decreased: Diabetes insipidus, primary polydipsia
Specific gravity	1.015–1.025	Increased: Dehydration, SIADH, diabetes mellitus, toxemia of pregnancy Decreased: Chronic renal insufficiency, diabetes insipidus, lithium toxicity, early renal disease

* Based on 24-hour total volume urine sample.
† Common conditions associated with abnormal values.
Data from Tietz, N. (Ed.) (1995). *Clinical guide to laboratory tests* (3rd ed.). Philadelphia: W. B. Saunders.

able, the nurse can perform various tests using a dipstick to help determine fluid and electrolyte status, including detecting substances that should not be present in the urine, such as glucose, acetone, protein, and blood. Urine measurements such as pH and specific gravity also can be determined in this way.

SELECTED BIBLIOGRAPHY

Bove, L. (1996). Restoring electrolyte balance: Sodium & chloride. *RN*, *59*(1), 25–29.

Bove, L. (1996). Restoring electrolyte balance: Calcium & phosphorus. *RN*, *59*(3), 47–52.

Braxmeyer, D., & Keyes, J. (1996). The pathophysiology of potassium balance. *Critical Care Nurse*, *16*(5), 59–71.

Briggs, J., Singh, I., Sawaya, B., & Schnermann, J. (1996). Disorders of salt balance. In J. Kokko and R. Tannen (Eds.), *Fluid and electrolytes* (3rd ed., pp 3–62). Philadelphia: W. B. Saunders.

Ferrin, M. (1996). Restoring electrolyte balance: Magnesium. *RN*, *59*(5), 31–35.

Frizzell, J. (1998). Avoiding lab test pitfalls. *American Journal of Nursing*, *98*(2), 34–38.

Guyton, A., & Hall, J. (1996). *Textbook of medical physiology* (9th ed.). Philadelphia: W. B. Saunders.

Kokko, J., & Tannen, R. (1996). *Fluids and electrolytes* (3rd ed.). Philadelphia: W. B. Saunders.

Metheny, N. (1996). *Fluid and electrolyte balance: Nursing considerations* (3rd ed). Philadelphia: Lippincott-Raven.

Norris, M. K. (1994). Checking chloride levels. *Nursing94*, *24*(3), 76.

O'Donnell, M. (1995). Assessing fluid and electrolyte balance needs in elders. *American Journal of Nursing*, *95*(1), 41–46.

Pennington, J. (1994). *Bowe's and Church's food values of portions commonly used* (16th ed.). Philadelphia: J. B. Lippincott.

Terry, J. (1994). The major electrolytes: Sodium, potassium, and chloride. *Journal of Intravenous Nursing*, *17*(5), 240–247.

Tietz, N. W. (ed.) (1995). *Clinical guide to laboratory tests* (3rd ed.). Philadelphia: W. B. Saunders.

Toto, K. (1994). Regulation of plasma osmolality. *Critical Care Nursing Clinics of North America*, *6*(4), 661–674.

Toto, K., & Yucha, C. (1994). Magnesium: Homeostasis, imbalances, and therapeutic uses. *Critical Care Nursing Clinics of North America*, *6*(4), 767–783.

Trissel, L. (1994). *Handbook on injectable drugs* (8th ed.). Bethesda, MD: American Society of Hospital Pharmacists.

Yu-Yahiro, J. (1994). Electrolytes and their relationship to normal and abnormal muscle function. *Orthopaedic Nursing*, *13*(5), 38–40.

SUGGESTED READINGS

O'Donnell, M. (1995). Assessing fluid and electrolyte balance needs in elders. *American Journal of Nursing*, *95*(1), 41–46.

This excellent article provides realistic cues to assist nurses in the differentiation between age-related skin changes and manifestations of actual fluid imbalances in the elderly. A case presentation approach is used to identify common signs and symptoms of fluid or electrolyte imbalances. Self-assessment questions are included at the end of the article.

Terry, J. (1994). The major electrolytes: Sodium, potassium, and chloride. *Journal of Intravenous Nursing*, *17*(5), 240–247.

This article describes the sources, activities, and regulation of three common electrolytes. The information is presented in a user-friendly and practical format, highlighted with nursing considerations.

Toto, K. (1994). Regulation of plasma osmolality. *Critical Care Nursing Clinics of North America*, *6*(4), 661–674.

A thorough explanation of the physiology of water balance is provided. The author describes the interaction of the thirst reflex and antidiuretic hormone in maintaining normal plasma osmolarity. Clinical examples and graphic artwork help the reader visualize the physiologic applications.

Chapter 15

INTERVENTIONS FOR CLIENTS WITH FLUID IMBALANCE

A proper balance of all body fluids is required for normal physiologic functioning. All clients are at risk for some degree of fluid imbalance because many health problems can disrupt fluid intake or output. This chapter focuses only on the problems surrounding fluid imbalances, although most fluid imbalances are accompanied by electrolyte imbalances.

Dehydration

Overview

In dehydration, the body's fluid intake is not sufficient to meet the body's fluid needs, resulting in a fluid volume deficit. Three basic types of dehydration are possible (Fig. 15–1):

- *Isotonic dehydration*, in which water and dissolved electrolytes are lost in equal proportions
- *Hypertonic dehydration*, in which water loss exceeds electrolyte loss
- *Hypotonic dehydration*, in which electrolyte loss exceeds water loss

Dehydration is a clinical state rather than a disease and can be caused by many factors. Dehydration may be an actual decrease in total body water caused by either inadequate fluid intake or excessive fluid loss. Dehydration also can occur without an actual decrease in total body water, such as when water shifts from the plasma into the interstitial space.

Pathophysiology

Isotonic Dehydration

Isotonic dehydration, or hypovolemia, is the most common type of dehydration. Problems associated with isotonic dehydration result from a reduction in plasma volume. Isotonic dehydration involves loss of isotonic fluids from the extracellular fluid (ECF) compartment (both the plasma and the interstitial space). Because isotonic fluid is lost, plasma osmolarity remains normal. This type of dehydration does not result in a shift of fluids between compartments; thus the intracellular fluid (ICF) volume remains normal. Isotonic dehydration results in decreased circulating blood volume and inadequate tissue perfusion. Compensatory mechanisms attempt to maintain adequate tissue perfusion to vital organs in spite of decreased vascular volume (Fig. 15–2).

Hypertonic Dehydration

Hypertonic dehydration is the second most common type of fluid volume deficit. The problems associated with hypertonic dehydration result from alterations in the concentrations of specific plasma electrolytes.

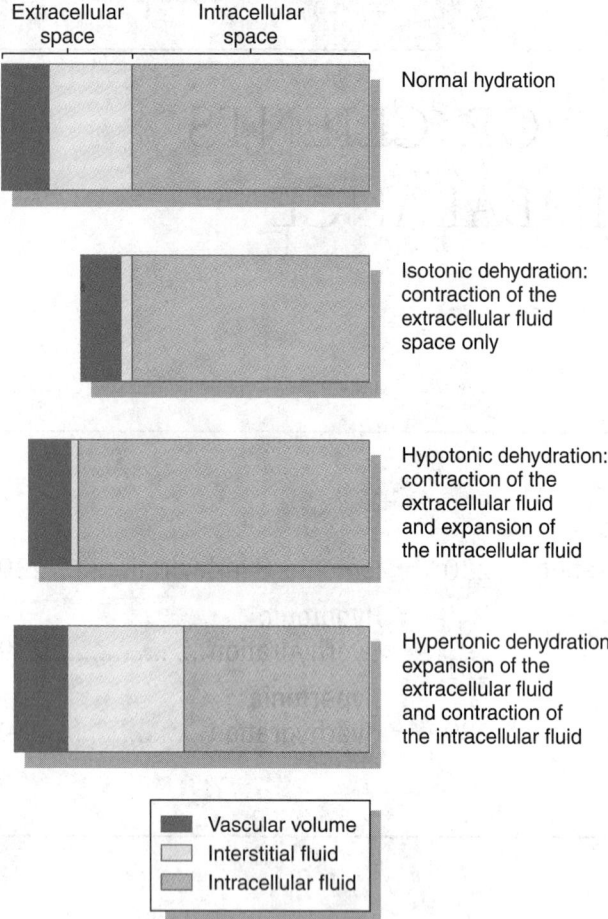

Hypertonic dehydration occurs when water loss from the ECF exceeds electrolyte loss. This water loss increases the osmolarity of the remaining plasma, making it hypertonic or hyperosmolar compared with normal ECF. The hyperosmolar plasma has an increased osmotic pressure that causes fluid to move from the ICF into the plasma and interstitial fluid spaces. This fluid shift results in cellular dehydration and shrinkage. The fluid shift also causes the plasma volume to approach (or perhaps exceed) normal levels. Thus, the compensatory mechanisms and signs and symptoms of hypovolemic shock are not present. However, excitable membrane activity and cardiac contractility are affected by altered plasma levels of potassium and calcium. Compensatory mechanisms for hypertonic dehydration occur in response to the increased ECF osmolarity (Fig. 15–3).

Hypotonic Dehydration

Hypotonic dehydration is the least common type of dehydration. The problems associated with hypotonic dehydration result from fluid shifts between compartments, causing a decrease in plasma volume.

Hypotonic dehydration involves the excessive loss of sodium and potassium from the ECF. This loss results in decreased osmolarity of the remaining ECF, making it hypotonic compared with normal ECF. The decreased ECF osmolarity lowers the osmotic pressure of plasma and interstitial fluids to below that of the fluid inside the cells (the ICF). As a result of this difference in osmotic pressure, water moves from the plasma and interstitial spaces into the cells, creating a plasma volume deficit and causing the cells to swell.

Intracellular swelling causes widespread problems and symptoms. Because brain cells are more sensitive to cellular fluid changes than the cells of other tissues, neurologic dysfunction usually accompanies hypotonic dehydration. Hypotonic fluid also dilutes the normal electrolyte concentrations and causes sodium and potassium imbalances.

Etiology
Isotonic Dehydration

Isotonic dehydration has many causes (Table 15–1). These include inadequate intake of fluids and solutes, fluid shifts between compartments, and excessive losses of isotonic body fluids.

Hypertonic Dehydration

Hypertonic dehydration results from the loss of any body fluid that is hypotonic (low osmolarity, or decreased concentration of solute particles compared with isotonic body fluid). Common causes of hypertonic dehydration are conditions that increase insensible fluid loss. Such conditions include excessive perspiration, hyperventilation, ketoacidosis, prolonged fevers, diarrhea, early-stage renal failure, diabetes insipidus, and ketoacidosis in the diuretic phase (see Table 15–1).

Hypotonic Dehydration

Hypotonic dehydration is usually associated with chronic illness. Chronic renal failure, in which the kidneys waste sodium, leads to hypotonic dehydration. Chronic malnutrition and excessive ingestion of hypotonic fluids also cause hypotonic dehydration.

Incidence/Prevalence

Although the actual incidence of dehydration is not known, virtually every ill client is at risk. Elderly clients are at high risk because they have less total body water than younger adults. Conditions contributing to inadequate fluid intake in the elderly include diminished thirst sensation and possible difficulty with ambulation or other motor skills necessary for ingesting fluids. Nursing home residents older than 85 years appear to be at greatest risk for dehydration (see Research Applications for Nursing, p. 232).

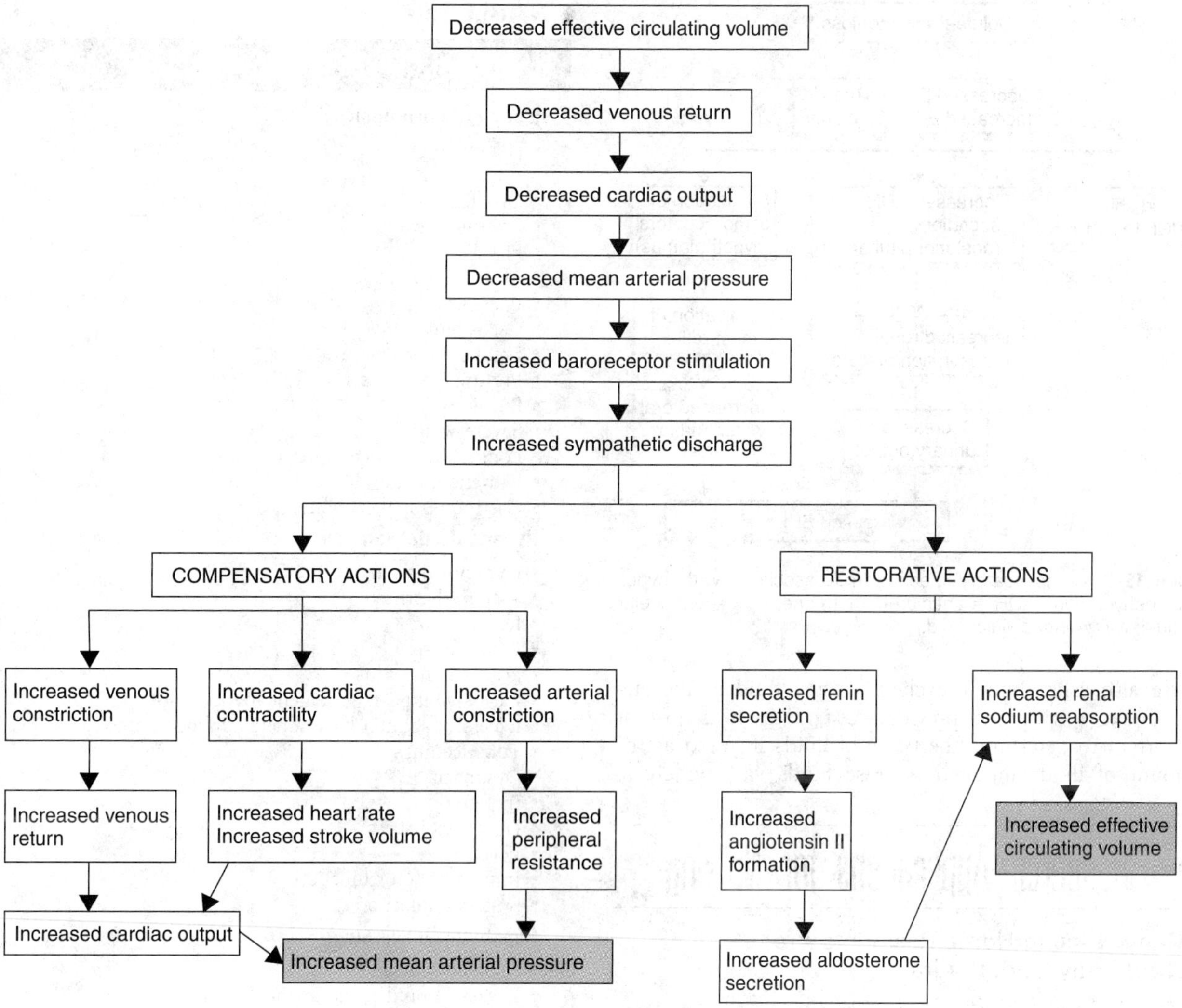

Decreased effective circulating volume

↓

Decreased venous return

↓

Decreased cardiac output

↓

Decreased mean arterial pressure

↓

Increased baroreceptor stimulation

↓

Increased sympathetic discharge

COMPENSATORY ACTIONS

Increased venous constriction → Increased venous return → Increased cardiac output

Increased cardiac contractility → Increased heart rate / Increased stroke volume → Increased mean arterial pressure

Increased arterial constriction → Increased peripheral resistance → Increased mean arterial pressure

RESTORATIVE ACTIONS

Increased renin secretion → Increased angiotensin II formation → Increased aldosterone secretion → Increased renal sodium reabsorption → Increased effective circulating volume

Figure 15–2. Compensatory mechanisms associated with isotonic dehydration.

Collaborative Management

 ## Assessment

➤ History

The nurse collects data on risk factors and factors causing dehydration (Table 15–2).

Age. This is an important consideration because dehydration in the elderly develops in response to relatively small fluid losses. In addition, elderly people are more likely to have chronic illnesses or to be taking medications that can lead to fluid and electrolyte imbalances (Anderson, 1996; O'Donnell, 1995).

Height and Weight. Measuring height and weight is important for calculating approximate fluid needs. If this information is not known or if the client is confused, the nurse obtains these measurements directly. Because weight and liquid measurements are related, changes in daily weights are good indicators of fluid losses or excesses. One liter of water weighs approximately 1 kg (2.2 pounds). Therefore, a weight change of 1 pound corresponds to a fluid volume change of about 500 mL.

Other Changes. The nurse questions the client about changes in the tightness of clothing, rings, and shoes. A sudden decrease in tightness may indicate dehydration; an increase may reflect a fluid shift to the interstitial space. Other relevant findings include the sensation of palpitations or lightheadedness on moving from a lying or a sitting position to a standing position (caused by orthostatic, or postural, hypotension).

The nurse further asks about any abnormal or excessive fluid losses, such as perspiration, diarrhea, bleeding, vomiting, urination, salivation, and wound drainage. Other important history information includes chronic illnesses, recent acute illnesses, recent surgery, and medications.

The nurse asks specific questions about urine output, including the frequency and amount of voidings. The

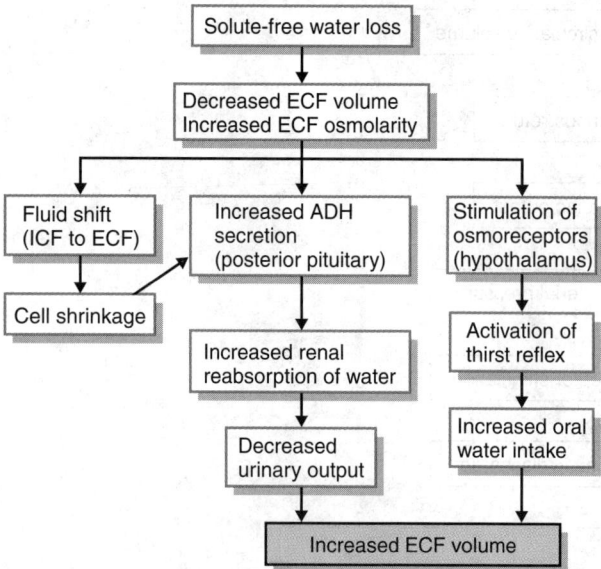

Figure 15–3. Compensatory mechanisms associated with hypertonic dehydration. (ADH = antidiuretic hormone; ECF = extracellular fluid; ICF = intracellular fluid.)

nurse also asks about the client's usual fluid intake and the intake during the previous 24 hours. It is just as important to determine the types of fluids ingested as the amount of fluids ingested because fluids vary widely in

▷ Research Applications for Nursing

Many Nursing Home Residents Are Chronically Underhydrated

Colling, J., Owen, T., & McCreedy, M. (1994). Urine volumes and voiding patterns among incontinent nursing home residents. Geriatric Nursing, 15(4), 188–192.

This prospective, descriptive clinical study observed 24-hour voiding patterns for 88 elderly nursing home residents a total of 14 times each over a 9-month period. Clients were mostly female and older than 85 years. Most clients had physical or mental impairments that limited their ability to obtain oral liquids independently. Oral intake was accurately measured. Liquid output was measured volumetrically when available and by weight when clients were incontinent.

Clients rarely exceeded a 1500-mL output for 24 hours, and more than 33% averaged less than 1000 mL total output for 24 hours. The two major findings of this study were that most clients were underhydrated and most experienced higher output at night.

Critique. The study was well designed. The conclusions were supported by the data obtained. The study could have been strengthened by the inclusion of additional objective data indicative of hydration status, however.

Possible Nursing Implications. Cognitively and physically impaired elders are dependent on caregivers to provide adequate oral hydration. Little attempt is made in nursing homes to assess accurately each resident's intake and output patterns, however. Implementing an action plan of regularly scheduling oral hydration breaks or offerings in a manner similar to medication administration could improve the hydration status of impaired elders.

TABLE 15–1

Common Causes of Dehydration

Isotonic Dehydration
- Hemorrhage
- Vomiting
- Diarrhea
- Profuse salivation
- Fistulas
- Abscesses
- Ileostomy
- Cecostomy
- Frequent enemas
- Profuse diaphoresis
- Burns
- Severe wounds
- Long-term NPO (nothing by mouth)
- Diuretic therapy
- Gastrointestinal suction

Hypertonic Dehydration
- Hyperventilation
- Watery diarrhea
- Renal failure
- Ketoacidosis
- Diabetes insipidus
- Excessive fluid replacement (hypertonic)
- Excessive sodium bicarbonate administration
- Tube feedings
- Dysphagia
- Impaired thirst
- Unconsciousness
- Fever
- Impaired motor function
- Systemic infection

Hypotonic Dehydration
- Chronic illness
- Excessive fluid replacement (hypotonic)
- Renal failure
- Chronic or severe malnutrition

osmolarity. The nurse also asks whether the client has recently engaged in strenuous physical activity and, if so, whether the activity took place in hot or dry environmental conditions.

TABLE 15–2

Risk Factors for Dehydration

Illnesses	Other Situations
• Vomiting	• Extremes of age: elderly, infants
• Diarrhea	
• Burns	• Unconsciousness
• Large draining wounds	• Motor limitations
• Liver dysfunction	**Therapies**
• Diabetes mellitus	
• Diabetes insipidus	• Surgery
• Renal disease	• Diuretics
• Hemorrhage	• Nothing by mouth
• Major venous obstruction	• Excessive hypertonic enemas
• Prolonged febrile state	• Nasogastric suction

> *Physical Assessment/Clinical Manifestations*

The clinical manifestations of dehydration depend on which fluid compartments lose fluid, although all body systems are affected to some degree (Chart 15–1). The most obvious and life-threatening clinical manifestations are seen when dehydration causes a decrease in the plasma volume.

Cardiovascular Manifestations. Cardiovascular changes are the most reliable indicators of changes in plasma volume. The heart rate increases with plasma volume deficits. Peripheral pulses are weaker, difficult to find, and easily blocked with light pressure. If interstitial edema accompanies the dehydration, the peripheral pulses may not be palpable. Blood pressure also decreases, as does the pulse pressure, with a greater decrease in the systolic blood pressure. Hypotension is more profound with the

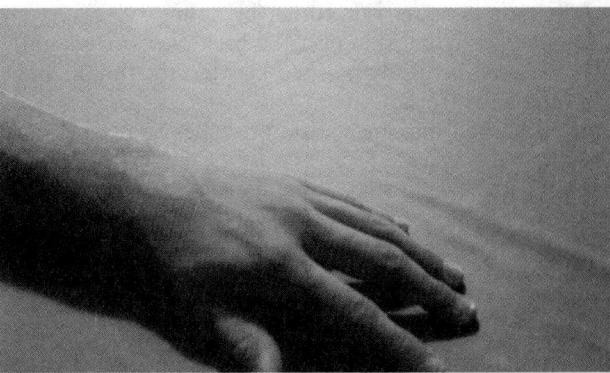

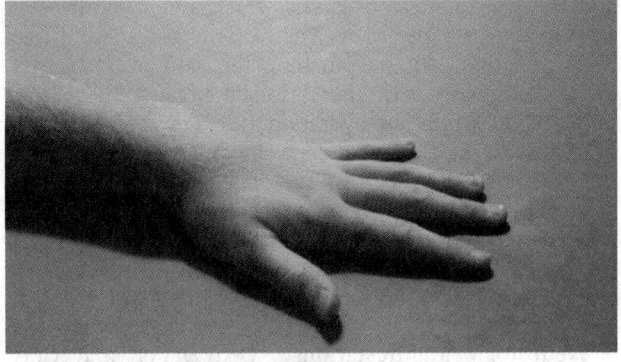

Figure 15–4. Hand veins full and bulging in the dependent position (*top*). Hand veins collapsed (*bottom*).

Chart 15–1

Key Features of Dehydration

Manifestations of Dehydration in General*

Cardiovascular

- Increased pulse rate
- Thready pulse quality
- Decreased blood pressure
- Postural hypotension
- Flat neck and hand veins in dependent positions
- Diminished peripheral pulses

Respiratory

- Increased respiratory rate
- Increased depth of respirations

Neuromuscular

- Decreased central nervous system activity (lethargy to coma)
- Fever

Renal

- Decreased urinary output
- Increased specific gravity

Integumentary

- Skin dry and scaly
- Turgor poor, tenting present
- Mouth dry and fissured, paste-like coating present

Gastrointestinal

- Decreased motility
- Diminished bowel sounds
- Constipation
- Thirst

Manifestations of Hypotonic Dehydration

- Skeletal muscle weakness

Manifestations of Hypertonic Dehydration

- Hyperactive deep tendon reflexes
- Increased sensation of thirst
- Pitting edema

*These manifestations are most severe with hypotonic dehydration.

---

client in the standing position than in the sitting or the lying position. Because the blood pressure with the client standing may be much lower than in other positions, blood pressure is measured first with the client lying down, then sitting, and finally standing.

Another cardiovascular indicator of hydration status is the degree of neck and hand vein filling. Normally, hand veins fill and become engorged when the hands are lower than the level of the heart. As the hands are raised above the level of the heart, the veins flatten or collapse (Fig. 15–4). Neck veins are normally distended when a client is in the supine position. These veins flatten when the client moves to a sitting position. When dehydration involves a plasma volume deficit, neck and hand veins are flat, even when not raised above the level of the heart. These cardiovascular changes are not seen in hypertonic dehydration.

Respiratory Manifestations. Respiratory rate increases directly with the degree of fluid loss from plasma volume. When acidosis accompanies dehydration, respirations become deep and rapid. This type of respiratory pattern is called *Kussmaul breathing.*

Integumentary Manifestations. Integumentary changes may be useful indicators of hydration. The nurse assesses for changes in the skin and mucous membranes that may indicate dehydration, including skin color, moisture, skin turgor, and edema. In elderly clients, this information is less reliable because of poor skin turgor resulting from the loss of elastic tissue and the loss of tissue fluids with aging.

The nurse assesses skin turgor by noting
- How easily the skin over the back of the hand and arm can be gently pinched between the thumb and the forefinger to form a "tent"
- How soon the pinched skin resumes its normal position after release
- Whether depressions (pits) remain in the skin after a finger is pressed firmly but gently (over the shin, over the sternum, and over the sacrum)
- How deep the depression is (in millimeters)
- How long the depression remains

In generalized dehydration, skin turgor is poor, with the tenting remaining for minutes after pinching the skin, and no skin depressions occur with gentle pressure. The skin appears dry and scaly. The nurse assesses skin turgor in an elderly client by pinching the skin over the sternum, the forehead, or the abdomen because these areas more reliably indicate hydration (see Fig. 14–11). As a person ages, the skin loses elasticity and tents on extremities even if the person is well hydrated.

In dehydration, oral mucous membranes are not moist. They may be covered with a thick, sticky, paste-like coating and may have cracks and fissures. The surface of the tongue may have deep furrows.

Neurologic Manifestations. Dehydration may cause changes in body temperature and mental status. The client with dehydration typically has a low-grade fever. A client with a temperature exceeding 39° C (102° F) for longer than 6 hours is especially at risk. Elderly clients who normally have a body temperature range of 35.4° to 36.6° C (96°–98° F) are at greater risk for dehydration during episodes of fever. Mental status changes are also common with dehydration. Chart 15–2 outlines how to assess mental status quickly.

Renal Manifestations. The volume and the composition of urine output indicate the hydration status of the renal system. The nurse closely monitors urine output, comparing total output to total fluid intake and daily weight. Accurate intake and output measurement is a major nursing responsibility. Urine output below 500 mL/day for any client without renal disease is cause for concern. A client with fluid imbalance is weighed each day at the same time and on the same scale. When possible, the client should be wearing the same amount and type of clothing for each weigh-in. Usually, metabolic tissue loss (even in starvation) accounts for only about 1/2 pound of weight loss per day. Any weight loss in excess of this amount is considered fluid loss.

▶ *Psychosocial Assessment*

The nurse observes the client for behavioral changes that accompany dehydration. Initially, a dehydrated client may have a flat affect and may seem unconcerned or indifferent about the state of health and possible treatment regimens. As dehydration worsens, the client's psychosocial activities reflect abnormal functioning of the central nervous system. The client may become apprehensive, rest-

---

Chart 15–2

Nursing Care Highlight: Brief Check of Mental Status

- Is the client awake?
- If the client is not awake, what type of stimulation is needed to waken the client?
  - Calling the client's name in a normal voice volume
  - Calling the client's name in a louder voice volume
  - Touching the client's arm or face while calling name
  - Gently tapping or shaking an arm
  - Vigorously shaking a hand or arm
  - Applying a painful stimulus
- If the client is awake, ask questions that require more than a "yes" or "no" response to establish orientation to time and place.
- Avoid the use of nonsense questions (such as "Do helicopters eat their young?").
- Ask questions that are reasonable and likely to be known by the client, such as "When is your birthday?" Avoid questions such as "Who was vice president under Truman?"
- Is it necessary to repeat questions to obtain a response?
- Does the response answer the question asked?
- Does the client have difficulty with word choices in forming responses?
- Is the client irritated or upset by the questions?
- Can the client concentrate on a question long enough to provide an appropriate response or is the attention span short?
- Can the client count by threes?
- Can the client count backward from 100 by threes?
- Does the client know the names of immediate family members?
- Does the client know who the questioner is (not necessarily the questioner's name but that person's role in the client's care such as nurse, doctor, chaplain, therapist)?
- Does the client know his or her immediate location (e.g., home, hospital, clinic)?
- Does the client know the year?

---

less, lethargic, and confused. These behavioral changes are more obvious in hypertonic and hypotonic dehydration because of intracellular fluid (ICF) shifts in brain cells, resulting in shrinkage or swelling of the cells. If the conditions causing the dehydration continue, circulation to cerebral tissues becomes so impaired that delirium and coma can occur.

▶ *Laboratory Assessment*

No single laboratory test result confirms or rules out dehydration. Instead, a diagnosis of dehydration must be based on laboratory findings along with presenting signs and symptoms. Such laboratory findings depend on the type of dehydration present (Chart 15–3). Isotonic and hypotonic dehydration states with accompanying plasma volume deficits are manifested as hemoconcentration, with elevated levels of hemoglobin and increased hematocrit, and as increased serum osmolarity, with increased levels of glucose, protein, blood urea nitrogen (BUN), and

---

Chart 15–3

Laboratory Profile: Dehydration

Values*	Isotonic Dehydration	Hypotonic Dehydration	Hypertonic Dehydration
Blood Values			
BUN	• Normal or increased	• Increased	• Increased
Creatinine	• Normal or increased	• Increased	• Increased
Sodium	• Normal	• <120 mEq/L (mmol)	• >150 mEq/L (mmol)
Osmolality	• Normal	• Decreased	• Increased
Hematocrit	• Increased	• Increased	• Normal or decreased
Hemoglobin	• Increased	• Increased	• Normal or decreased
WBCs	• Increased	• Increased	• Normal or decreased
Protein	• Increased	• Increased	• Increased
Urine Values			
Specific gravity	• >1.010	• <1.010	• >1.030
Osmolality	• Increased	• Increased	• Increased
Volume	• Decreased	• Decreased	• Decreased

*All values reflect dehydration states alone and not the underlying pathologic changes or disease states contributing to the dehydration.
BUN = blood urea nitrogen; WBC = white blood cell.

---

various electrolytes. Hemoconcentration is not evident when dehydration results from hemorrhage, because loss of all blood and plasma products occurs.

Specific urine laboratory values can help to determine dehydration if the client does not have renal dysfunction. Usually, the urine of clients with dehydration is highly concentrated, with a specific gravity exceeding 1.030. Volume is decreased, and osmolarity is greatly increased. Usually, the color is dark amber, and a strong odor is evident.

 Analysis

➤ Common Nursing Diagnoses and Collaborative Problems

The priority nursing diagnoses to consider when caring for a client with dehydration are as follows:

1. Fluid Volume Deficit related to excessive fluid loss or inadequate fluid intake
2. Decreased Cardiac Output related to insufficient plasma volume
3. Altered Oral Mucous Membranes related to inadequate oral secretions

The primary collaborative problem is Potential for Dysrhythmias.

➤ Additional Nursing Diagnoses and Collaborative Problems

In addition to the common nursing diagnoses and collaborative problems, one or more of the following may apply:

■ Constipation related to decreased body fluids
■ High Risk for Injury (fall) related to orthostatic (postural) hypotension
■ Knowledge Deficit related to medication regimen and preventive measures
■ High Risk for Impaired Skin Integrity related to deficiencies of interstitial fluid and inadequate tissue perfusion
■ Ineffective Airway Clearance related to thick, tenacious secretions
■ Potential for Hypovolemic Shock
■ Potential for Electrolyte Imbalances

 Planning and Implementation

➤ Fluid Volume Deficit

Planning: Expected Outcomes. The expected outcome is that the client will have normal body fluid levels.

Interventions. Management of dehydration aims to prevent further fluid losses and increase fluid compartment volumes to normal ranges. Diet therapy, oral rehydration therapy, and drug therapy are the methods of choice.

Diet Therapy. Mild to moderate dehydration may be successfully treated with oral fluid replacement if the client is alert enough to swallow and can tolerate oral fluids. The nurse or assistive personnel encourages and measures all fluid intake. The specific type of fluid needed for replacement varies with the type of dehydration.

The client's compliance in ingesting oral replacement fluids can be enhanced by using fluids the client enjoys at temperatures with which the client is comfortable and by carefully timing the intake schedule. Dividing the total amount of fluids needed by nursing shifts helps to meet fluid needs more evenly with less danger of overhydration. The nurse or assistive personnel offers the conscious

TABLE 15–3

Commercial Solutions for Oral Rehydration Therapy

Brand Name	Na+ (mEq/L)	K+ (mEq/L)	Cl- (mEq/L)	Citrate (mEq/L)	Sugar or Starch	Calories (kcal/L)
Ricelyte (Mead-Johnson)	50	25	45	34	Rice syrup (30 g)	126
Resol (Wyeth-Ayerst)	50	20	50	34	Dextrose (20 g)	84
Rehydralyte (Ross Labs)	75	20	65	30	Dextrose (25 g)	100
Pedialyte (Ross Labs)	45	20	35	30	Dextrose (25 g)	100
Gastrolyte (Rorer)	60	20	60	10	Dextrose (17.8 g)	75
Rapolyte (Richmond)	90	20	80	30	Dextrose (20 g)	84
Lytren (Mead-Johnson)	50	25	45	30	Dextrose (20 g)	84
Naturalyte (United Beverages)	45	20	35	48	Dextrose (25 g)	100
Oralyte (Rugby)	45	20	25	48	Dextrose (25 g)	100

Data from United States Pharmacopeial Convention, Inc. (1998). USPDI Vol I, *Drug information for the health care professional.* Rockville, MD: United States Pharmacopeial Convention. Printed by Rand McNally, Taunton MA.

client small volumes of fluids every hour to increase compliance.

Oral Rehydration Therapy. Oral rehydration therapy (ORT) is the most cost-effective way to replace fluids and treat the client with diarrhea. Specifically formulated solutions containing glucose and electrolytes cause water to be absorbed even in the presence of diarrhea and vomiting. Fluid losses from diarrhea are usually 2 to 3 L/day and should be replaced liter for liter, especially in elderly clients. A typical physician's order might be "Resol 1 L every 8 hours." Table 15–3 lists commercially available ORT solutions.

Drug Therapy. Drug therapy for dehydration is directed at restoring fluid balance and controlling the conditions causing dehydration. Whenever possible, fluids are replaced by the oral route. When dehydration is severe or life-threatening, intravenous (IV) fluid replacement may be necessary. Calculation of the volume of replacement fluids needed is based on both the client's weight loss and presenting symptoms. The rate of fluid replacement depends on the client's degree of dehydration and the presence of pre-existing cardiac, pulmonary, or renal problems.

The type of fluid ordered by the physician varies with the type of dehydration and the client's cardiovascular status. The desired outcomes of therapy are appropriate fluid replacement and normal volumes in all body fluid compartments. Usually, the client receives IV infusions of water with whatever solutes (especially electrolytes) are determined necessary on the basis of laboratory values. Table 15–4 lists the osmolarity, caloric content, and tonicity of common IV fluids. Generally, isotonic dehydra-

tion is treated with isotonic fluid solutions; hypertonic dehydration, with hypotonic fluid solutions; and hypotonic dehydration, with hypertonic fluid solutions.

Drug therapy includes the use of medications to correct the underlying cause of the dehydration. Antidiarrheal medications are ordered when excessive diarrhea causes dehydration. Antimicrobial therapy may be used in clients with bacterial diarrhea. Antiemetics to control vomiting may be necessary when excessive vomiting produces dehydration. Antipyretics to reduce body temperature are helpful when fever contributes to dehydration.

► Decreased Cardiac Output

Planning: Expected Outcomes. The expected outcomes are that the client should
- Have cardiac output restored to normal levels
- Maintain adequate oxygenation to vital organs

Interventions. Interventions aim to increase circulating fluid volume, support compensatory mechanisms, and prevent ischemic complications mainly through drug therapy and oxygen therapy.

Drug Therapy. Drug therapy to increase body fluid volume and prevent excessive fluid loss is the same as that for the client with fluid volume deficit. Drugs to increase venous return or improve cardiac contractility are used only when a co-existing cardiac problem is present.

Oxygen Therapy. Oxygen can be delivered by mask, hood, nasal cannula, nasopharyngeal tube, endotracheal tube, or tracheostomy tube. Usually, masks and nasal cannulas are used to administer oxygen to clients with dehydration. The nurse administers water-nebulized oxy-

TABLE 15-4

Characteristics of Common Intravenous Therapy Solutions

Solution	Osmolarity (mOsm/L)	pH	Calories* (kcal)	Tonicity
0.9% saline	308	5	0	Isotonic
0.45% saline	154	5	0	Hypotonic
5% dextrose in water (D_5W)	272	3.5–6.5	170	Isotonic†
10% dextrose in water ($D_{10}W$)	500	3.5–6.5	340	Hypertonic†
5% dextrose in 0.9% saline	560	3.5–6.5	170	Hypertonic†
5% dextrose in 0.45% saline	406	4	170	Hypertonic†
5% dextrose in 0.225% saline	321	4	170	Isotonic†
Ringer's lactate	273	6.5	9	Isotonic
5% dextrose in Ringer's lactate	525	4.0–6.5	179	Hypertonic†

Data from Trissel, L. (1994). *Handbook on injectable drugs* (8th ed.). Bethesda, MD: American Society of Hospital Pharmacists.
*Calories are calculated on the basis of a volume of 1000 mL.
†*Solution tonicity at the time of administration.* Within a short time after administration, the dextrose is metabolized, and the tonicity of the infused solution decreases in proportion to the osmolarity or tonicity of the nondextrose components (electrolytes) within the water.

gen to the client at the rate or amount specified by the physician's order.

Monitoring. Monitoring vital signs and level of consciousness is an important responsibility of nurses caring for dehydrated clients. The nurse or assistive personnel monitors the client's pulse, blood pressure, pulse pressure, central venous pressure, respiratory rate, skin and mucous membrane color, and urinary output at least every hour until the fluid imbalance is resolved.

➤ Altered Oral Mucous Membranes

Planning: Expected Outcomes. The expected outcomes are that the client should experience less discomfort and remain free of complications.

Interventions. Interventions include drug therapy, fluid replacement, good oral hygiene, and the early diagnosis and prevention of complications. Diet therapy may also be used to resolve the dehydration.

Drug Therapy. Drug therapy to increase body fluid volume and prevent excessive fluid loss is the same as that discussed earlier for fluid volume deficit. Commercial preparations of artificial saliva can reduce the sensation of mouth dryness. The nurse avoids using such agents in an unconscious client, however, to prevent aspiration.

Oral Hygiene. Nursing actions to promote oral hygiene can increase the client's comfort. The nurse keeps the client's lips clean and moistens them with a petrolatum-based lubricant. The thick, sticky coating on the oral cavity during episodes of dehydration can be reduced with frequent oral hygiene measures.

Mouth care includes gentle tooth brushing several times a day and rinsing hourly. The nurse teaches the client to avoid commercial mouthwashes that contain alcohol and glycerin-containing washes and swabs, because these products dry the oral mucosa further and may cause increased discomfort by stinging or burning open fissures in the mucosa. Rinsing the mouth with dilute solutions of hydrogen peroxide two or three times per day is a good form of oral hygiene; however, when used more frequently, this treatment increases oral dryness. Tap water and normal saline rinses can be used safely as often as the client wishes.

Prevention of Complications. A dry mouth contributes to the development of sores and fissures in the mucosa, providing a portal of entry for many pathogens. The thick, sticky coating also is an excellent breeding ground for microorganisms. A major complication of mouth dryness is a wide variety of oral infections. Chart 15-4 summarizes nursing interventions for mouth care.

Chart 15-4

Nursing Care Highlight: Mouth Care for Clients with Dehydration

- Examine the client's mouth (including under the roof, on the tongue, and between the teeth and cheek) every 4 hours.
- Document the location, size, and character of fissures, blisters, sores, or drainage.
- Obtain an order to culture sores or drainage.
- Brush the client's teeth and tongue with a soft-bristled brush or sponges every 8 hours.
- Rinse the client's mouth with a 50:50 solution of ½ peroxide and ½ normal saline every 12 hours.
- Avoid the use of alcohol or glycerin-based mouthwashes.
- Assist the conscious client to swish and spit room-temperature tap water or normal saline PRN.
- Apply petrolatum jelly to the client's lips after each episode of mouth care and PRN.
- Assist the client in using artificial saliva.
- Assist the client in menu choices to avoid spicy or hard foods.
- Offer complete mouth care before and after every meal.

PRN = as necessary.

➤ Potential for Dysrhythmias

Planning: Expected Outcomes. The expected outcome is that the client will maintain his or her normal cardiac rhythm.

Interventions. Interventions are aimed at correcting the dehydration and recognizing dysrhythmias so appropriate drug therapy can be initiated.

Drug Therapy. Drug therapy to increase body fluid volume and prevent excessive fluid loss is the same as that discussed earlier for fluid volume deficit.

Elevated potassium or calcium level can cause life-threatening dysrhythmias. Drug therapy to reduce these electrolytes may be ordered. If potassium levels are elevated, a combination of 20 units of regular insulin in 100 mL of 20% dextrose may be administered to promote movement of potassium into the ICF. Drugs such as etidronate (Didronel) and plicamycin (Mithracin) may be administered to reduce an elevated serum calcium level.

Monitoring. The nurse monitors the client for signs and symptoms of cardiac dysrhythmias every 15 minutes until the client is fully rehydrated. The rate, rhythm, and quality of the apical pulse are assessed and compared with the client's baseline measurements. The nurse further assesses the client for fatigue, chest discomfort or pain, and shortness of breath. Hand grasps and deep tendon reflexes are assessed, and changes from baseline are noted.

Clients at risk for dysrhythmias are monitored using electrocardiography (ECG). The pattern may show tall T waves or a shortened ST segment. Any change from the client's baseline ECG is reported to the physician immediately.

 Continuing Care

No extensive home care preparations are necessary for clients with mild dehydration or for those with dehydration of sudden onset. The imbalance is corrected before discharge from the facility and, with minimal precautions, is unlikely to recur. Clients who are most likely to be discharged before the imbalance is completely corrected and who are susceptible to recurrent episodes are those with chronic pathologic conditions, such as renal insufficiency, diabetes, malignancy, adrenal insufficiency, and specific endocrine disorders. These clients often require long-term diet and drug therapy.

➤ Health Teaching

Education is important in the prevention and early detection of dehydration. The teaching plan for any client at risk for dehydration includes diet, drug regimens, and the signs and symptoms of dehydration.

➤ Home Care Management

The nurse, occupational therapist, or social worker evaluates the client's home environment with regard to precipitating factors for dehydration. Particular attention is paid to environmental temperature and humidification. Kitchen

and bathroom access are assessed, and suggestions for modifications made as necessary.

Home adjustments may be necessary for elderly clients or clients whose dehydration is caused by chronic illness. One contributing factor to dehydration in the elderly is the fear of incontinence. Clients may limit fluid intake to reduce their need to go to the bathroom. This tactic is used frequently among elderly women who do not have a toilet available on the same floor where they spend most of their time. A portable toilet on the living floor can remedy this situation if home remodeling is not an option.

The nurse instructs the family to keep appropriate fluids for the client in places that the client can access. Container modifications, such as opening zip-top cans and covering them with foil, can be made to ensure the client can easily open container lids. Sipper containers not only provide easy access but also are unbreakable and reduce spillage.

The nurse performs a focused assessment (Chart 15–5)

Chart 15–5

Focused Assessment for Home Care Clients at Risk for Dehydration

- Assess cardiovascular status.
  - Vital signs, including apical pulse, pulse pressure, presence or absence of orthostatic hypotension, and quality and rhythm of peripheral pulses
  - Presence or absence of peripheral edema
  - Hand vein filling in the dependent position
  - Neck vein filling in the recumbent and sitting positions
  - Weight gain or loss
- Assess cognition and mental status.
  - Level of consciousness
  - Orientation to time, place, and person
  - Can the client accurately read a seven-word sentence containing no words greater than three syllables?
- Assess condition of skin and mucous membranes.
  - Presence or absence of skin tenting over the sternum or the forehead
  - Moistness of skin, most reliable on chest and back
  - Presence or absence of coating on tongue or teeth
  - Can the client spit?
- Assess neuromuscular status.
  - Reactivity of patellar and biceps reflexes
  - Oral temperature
  - Handgrip strength
  - Steadiness of gait
- Assess renal system.
  - Observe urine specimen for color, odor, cloudiness, and amount
- Ask about the following:
  - 24-hour fluid intake and output
  - 24-hour diet recall
  - 24-hour activity recall
  - Over-the-counter and prescribed medications the client has taken
- Assess client's understanding of illness and compliance with treatment.
  - Signs and symptoms to report to health care provider
  - Medication plan (correct timing and dose)

and a mental status check at every home visit to a client at risk for dehydration. Medication regimens, signs and symptoms of dehydration, and health care resources are reviewed with the client and family.

➤ Health Care Resources

A client with severe chronic health problems may be discharged to a nursing home or extended-care facility on a permanent or a temporary basis. The hospital nurse uses the transfer chart to communicate all important information about the client's individual needs and special care problems. The nurse refers the client discharged to home to specific resources available for client education and family support. Two examples of such support agencies are the American Diabetes Association and the Kidney Foundation.

A home care nurse may be needed to assess the client's hydration status and adherence to drug and diet therapies. If the client lives alone, a daily visit by a home health aide to assist with activities of daily living and reinforce an oral intake plan may be helpful.

 Evaluation

On the basis of the identified nursing diagnoses, the nurse evaluates the care of clients with dehydration. Outcomes include that the client is expected to
- Ingest at least 1500 mL of hypotonic fluids each day
- Maintain a fluid output that is approximately equal to the fluid intake
- State that oral mucosal discomfort is relieved
- Experience no oral mucosal complication

Overhydration

Overview

Overhydration, also referred to as fluid overload, is an excess of body fluid. It is not an actual disease but rather a clinical manifestation of a physiologic problem in which fluid intake or retention exceeds the body's fluid needs. Overhydration may be characterized as either an actual excess of total body fluid or a relative fluid excess in one or more fluid compartments. The three basic types of fluid volume excess are isotonic overhydration, hypotonic overhydration, and hypertonic overhydration (Figure 15–5).

Pathophysiology

Most problems associated with overhydration are related to fluid volume excess in the vascular space or to dilution of specific electrolytes and blood components. Clinical manifestations vary with the type and degree of overhydration (Chart 15–6).

Isotonic Overhydration

Isotonic overhydration is also called *hypervolemia* because its associated problems result from excessive fluid in the

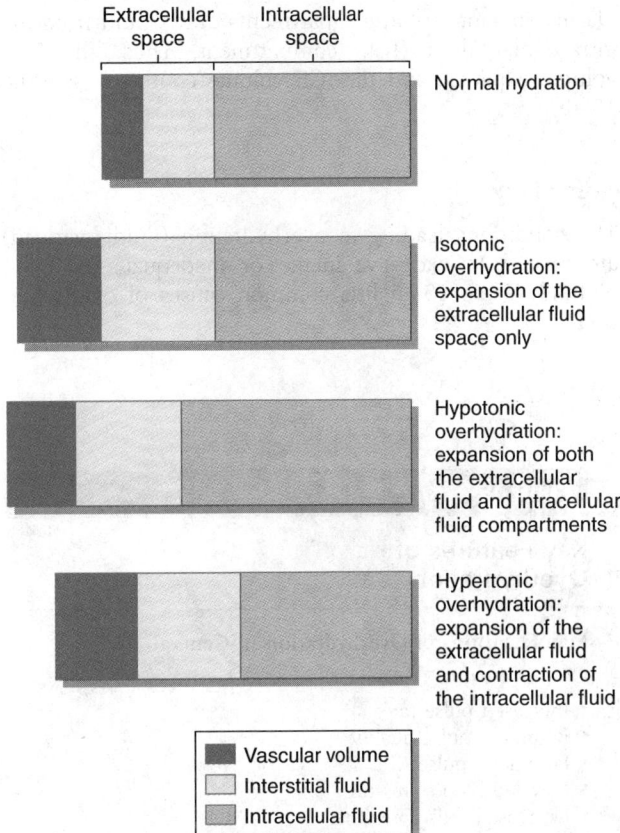

Figure 15–5. Three types of overhydration. (© 1992 M. Linda Workman. All rights reserved.)

extracellular fluid (ECF) compartment. In isotonic overhydration, isotonic fluids are ingested or retained, so that osmolarity remains normal. Only the ECF compartment is expanded, and fluid does not shift between the extracellular and intracellular compartments. The effects of severe isotonic overhydration are circulatory overload and the formation of interstitial edema. Figure 15–6 outlines the compensatory mechanisms associated with mild to moderate isotonic overhydration. When isotonic overhydration is severe or when it occurs in a person with poor cardiac status, overhydration results in congestive heart failure and pulmonary edema.

Hypotonic Overhydration

In hypotonic overhydration (water intoxication), the excess fluid is hypotonic to normal body fluids. Thus, the osmolarity of the ECF decreases, and hydrostatic pressure increases. The excessive fluid moves into the intracellular space because of the decreased vascular osmotic pressure, and all body fluid compartments expand (see Figure 15–5). Because the excessive fluid is hypotonic, electrolyte imbalances resulting from dilution accompany hypotonic overhydration.

Hypertonic Overhydration

Hypertonic overhydration is rare and is caused by an excessive sodium intake. The hyperosmolarity of the plasma and interstitial compartments draws fluid from the intracellular fluid (ICF) compartment. Thus, the ECF volume expands, and the ICF volume contracts (see Fig. 15–5).

Etiology

The conditions leading to overhydration (fluid overload) are related to excessive intake or inadequate excretion of fluid. Table 15–5 lists common causes of overhydration.

Chart 15–6

Key Features of Overhydration

Manifestations of Overhydration in General

Cardiovascular

- Increased pulse rate
- Bounding pulse quality
- Peripheral pulses full
- Elevated blood pressure
- Decreased pulse pressure
- Elevated central venous pressure
- Distended neck and hand veins
- Engorged venous varicosities

Respiratory

- Respiratory rate increased
- Shallow respirations
- Dyspnea increases with exertion or in the supine position
- Moist crackles present on auscultation

Integumentary

- Pitting edema in dependent areas
- Skin pale and cool to touch

Neuromuscular

- Altered level of consciousness
- Headache
- Visual disturbances
- Skeletal muscle weakness
- Paresthesias

Gastrointestinal

- Increased motility

Manifestations of Isotonic Overhydration

- Liver enlargement
- Ascites formation

Manifestations of Hypotonic Overhydration

- Polyuria
- Diarrhea
- Nonpitting edema
- Cardiac dysrhythmias associated with electrolyte dilution
- Projectile vomiting

TABLE 15–5

Common Causes of Overhydration

Isotonic Overhydration

- Poorly controlled intravenous therapy
- Renal failure
- Long-term corticosteroid therapy

Hypotonic Overhydration

- Early renal failure
- Congestive heart failure
- Syndrome of inappropriate antidiuretic hormone
- Poorly controlled intravenous therapy
- Replacement of isotonic fluid loss with hypotonic fluids
- Psychogenic polydipsia
- Irrigation of wounds and body cavities with hypotonic fluids

Hypertonic Overhydration

- Excessive sodium ingestion
- Rapid infusion of hypertonic saline
- Excessive sodium bicarbonate therapy

Collaborative Management

 Assessment

Clinical manifestations of overhydration vary with the specific type, the fluid compartments involved, and the degree of overhydration. Clients with isotonic overhydration or hypertonic overhydration have signs and symptoms associated with circulatory overload. Clients with hypotonic overhydration have problems associated with ICF increase and electrolyte dilution. Chart 15–6 summarizes the common clinical manifestations of overhydration.

A diagnosis of overhydration is based on physical assessment findings together with the results of several laboratory tests. In isotonic overhydration, serum electrolyte values are normal, but decreased hemoglobin, hematocrit, and serum protein levels may result from *hemodilution* (excessive water in the vascular compartment). Elevated levels of most electrolytes, along with increased BUN and creatinine levels, are associated with overhydration caused by renal failure. Hypotonic overhydration is accompanied by decreased complete blood count and decreased protein and electrolyte levels.

Interventions

Interventions for clients with fluid volume excess aim to restore normal fluid balance, provide supportive care until the imbalance is resolved, and prevent future fluid overload. Drug and diet therapies form the basis of intervention.

➤ *Drug Therapy*

The physician may order diuretics for clients with overhydration if renal failure is not the cause. Diuretics work on

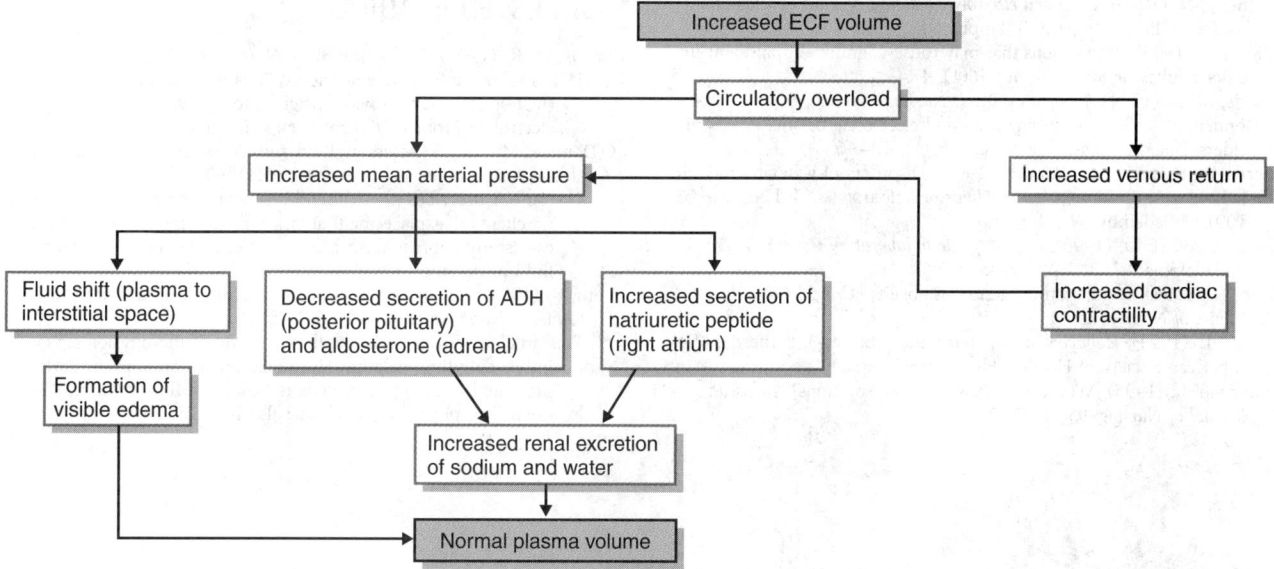

Figure 15–6. Compensatory mechanisms associated with hypervolemia. (ADH = antidiuretic hormone; ECF = extracellular fluid.)

the kidneys to increase the excretion of water or sodium from the body. Osmotic diuretics, such as mannitol, are typically prescribed first to prevent severe electrolyte imbalances. Osmotic diuretics primarily cause renal excretion of water rather than excretion of sodium or potassium. If osmotic diuretics are not effective, the physician may prescribe high-ceiling (loop) diuretics, such as furosemide (Lasix, Furoside*).

The nurse monitors the client for response to medication, especially weight loss and increased urine output. The nurse also observes the client for signs and symptoms of electrolyte imbalance and assesses laboratory findings every 8 hours.

➤ Diet Therapy

For the client with mild or chronic overhydration, long-term diet therapy may be valuable in controlling fluid volume through restrictions of both fluid and sodium intake. The client's serum sodium concentration should be considered whenever overhydration is present.

➤ Monitoring

Intake and Output. The nurse or assistive personnel accurately measures fluid intake and output and explains the reason for any fluid restriction. In addition to regulating the total amount of fluid ingested in a 24-hour period, the nurse carefully schedules fluid offerings throughout the 24 hours. Urine also is monitored for color, character, and specific gravity.

If the client is receiving IV therapy, the nurse administers the exact amount ordered by the physician and monitors the client for increased fluid overload.

Weight. Fluid retention may not be visible. However, a sudden weight gain indicates fluid retention. The nurse weighs the client at the same time every day (before breakfast) using the same scale. Whenever possible, the client wears the same type of clothing for each weigh-in.

 CASE STUDY for the Client with Dehydration

■ You are making a home visit to an 86-year-old woman who underwent hip replacement 2 months ago. She lives alone. When the client answers the door, you find that she is confused. She says she is thirsty and that "it hurts when I piddle." You find a half-empty pan of soup on the stove and evidence of vomiting in the bathroom. Her vital signs are as follows: blood pressure, 102/80 mm Hg; pulse, 102 (thready); respirations, 32; and oral temperature, 38.6° C (101° F).

Q U E S T I O N S :
1. What additional assessment techniques would you perform?
2. How would you assess hydration status?
3. What other data would you gather?
4. What are your action priorities?

SELECTED BIBLIOGRAPHY

Anderson, S. (1996). Fluid and electrolyte disorders in the elderly. In J. Kokko & R. Tannen (Eds.), *Fluids and electrolytes* (3rd ed., pp. 831–839). Philadelphia: W. B. Saunders.
Colling, J., Owen, T., & McCreedy, M. (1994). Urine volumes and voiding patterns among incontinent nursing home residents. *Geriatric Nursing, 15*(4), 188–192.
Frizzell, J. (1998). Avoiding lab test pitfalls. *American Journal of Nursing, 98*(2), 34–38.
Guyton, A., & Hall, J. (1996). *Textbook of medical physiology* (9th ed.). Philadelphia: W. B. Saunders.
Halperin, M., & Goldstein, M. (1994), *Fluid, electrolyte and acid-base physiology: A problem-based approach* (2nd ed). Philadelphia: W. B. Saunders.
Kokko, J., & Tannen, R. (1996). *Fluids and electrolytes* (3rd ed.). Philadelphia: W. B. Saunders.
Kuhn, M. (1996). Laboratory analysis. *Critical Care Nurse, 16*(5), 74–76.

Metheny, N. (1996). *Fluid and electrolyte balance: Nursing considerations* (3rd ed.). Philadelphia: J. B. Lippincott.

Miller, C. (1995). Medications that may cause cognitive impairment in older adults. *Geriatric Nursing, 16*(1), 47.

Norris, M. K. (1994). Evaluating BUN. *Nursing94, 24*(5), 80.

O'Donnell, M. (1995). Assessing fluid and electrolyte balance needs in elders. *American Journal of Nursing, 95*(1), 40–46.

Sterns, R., Spital, A., & Clark, E. (1996). Disorders of water balance. In J. Kokko & R. Tannen (eds.), *Fluids and electrolytes* (3rd ed., pp. 63–109). Philadelphia: W. B. Saunders.

Tietz, N. W. (Ed.). (1995). *Clinical guide to laboratory tests* (3rd ed.). Philadelphia: W. B. Saunders.

Toto, K. (1994). Regulation of plasma osmolality. *Critical Care Nursing Clinics of North America, 6*(4), 661–674.

Trissel, L. (1994). *Handbook on injectable drugs* (8th ed.). Bethesda, MD: American Society of Hospital Pharmacists.

Vonfrolio, L. (1995). Would you hang these IV solutions? *American Journal of Nursing, 95*(4), 37–39.

SUGGESTED READINGS

Norris, M. K. (1994). Evaluating BUN. *Nursing94, 24*(5), 80.

This brief but informative article explains how blood urea nitrogen (BUN) values can provide insight into the type of fluid and electrolyte problem a client is experiencing.

O'Donnell, M. (1995). Assessing fluid and electrolyte balance needs in elders. *American Journal of Nursing, 95*(1), 40–46.

The author describes physical and behavioral characteristics of geriatric clients that place them at risk for fluid imbalances using a case study approach. An assessment checklist for elders with fluid or nutritional deficits is included.

Toto, K. (1994). Regulation of plasma osmolality. *Critical Care Nursing Clinics of North America, 6*(4), 661–674.

This article provides an in-depth discussion of the physiologic factors influencing fluid balance. Hormonal regulation is particularly well presented. Although the focus is mainly on fluid balance, some electrolyte physiology (sodium) also is presented.

Chapter 16

INTERVENTIONS FOR CLIENTS WITH ELECTROLYTE IMBALANCES

Mild electrolyte imbalances occur frequently in healthy people as a result of variation in fluid intake and output. Such imbalances are of short duration and do not require interventions from health care professionals. Severe electrolyte imbalances, however, are life-threatening and can occur in any setting. Elderly clients and clients taking medications that alter fluid and electrolyte status are at greater risk for electrolyte imbalances.

POTASSIUM IMBALANCES

Hypokalemia

Overview

Because 98% of total body potassium (K^+) is intracellular, minor changes in extracellular potassium levels cause major changes in cell membrane excitability as well as in other cellular processes. Hypokalemia is indicated by a serum potassium level below 3.5 mEq/L (mmol/L). A relatively common electrolyte imbalance, hypokalemia is potentially life-threatening because every body system can be affected.

Pathophysiology

Decreased serum potassium level increases the difference in potassium concentration between the fluid inside the cells, or intracellular fluid (ICF), and the extracellular fluid (ECF). This increased difference reduces the excit-ability of cells. Consequently, the cell membranes of all excitable tissues, such as nerve and muscle, are less re-sponsive to normal stimuli.

The severity of problems caused by hypokalemia is directly related to how rapidly the serum potassium level decreases. When extracellular potassium loss is gradual, cells adjust and intracellular potassium decreases in pro-portion to the ECF potassium level. In this situation, the potassium concentration difference between the two fluid compartments remains unchanged, and symptoms of hy-pokalemia may not appear until the potassium loss is extreme. Rapid changes in extracellular potassium levels (representing a more rapid loss of potassium) cannot be compensated for quickly, and result in dramatic changes in body function.

Etiology

Hypokalemia may result either from actual total body potassium loss or from movement of potassium from the ECF to the ICF, causing a relative decrease in extracellu-lar potassium level. Table 16–1 summarizes the common causes of hypokalemia.

Actual potassium depletion occurs when potassium loss is excessive or when potassium intake is not sufficient to match normal potassium loss. Relative hypokalemia oc-curs when total body potassium levels are normal but the potassium distribution between fluid compartments is ab-normal. Conditions that increase the cellular uptake of

TABLE 16–1

Common Causes of Hypokalemia

Actual Potassium Deficits

Excessive Potassium Loss

- Inappropriate or excessive use of drugs
  - Diuretics
  - Digitalis
  - Corticosteroids
- Increased secretion of aldosterone
  - Cushing's syndrome
- Diarrhea
- Vomiting
- Wound drainage (especially gastrointestinal)
- Prolonged nasogastric suction
- Heat-induced excessive diaphoresis
- Renal disease impairing reabsorption of potassium

Inadequate Potassium Intake

- Nothing by mouth

Relative Potassium Deficits

Movement of Potassium from Extracellular Fluid to Intracellular Fluid

- Alkalosis
- Hyperinsulinism
- Hyperalimentation
- Total parenteral nutrition

Dilution of Serum Potassium

- Water intoxication
- Intravenous therapy with potassium-poor solutions

potassium, leading to hypokalemia, include metabolic alkalosis and insulin administration.

Incidence/Prevalence

Exact statistics about the incidence of hypokalemia are not available. This imbalance occurs frequently in both hospitalized clients and in those receiving ambulatory care. Hypokalemia may be associated with any illness (Braxmeyer & Keyes, 1996). Elderly clients are especially at high risk for hypokalemia resulting from chronic illness or prescribed medications.

Collaborative Management

 Assessment

➤ History

The nurse collects data from clients at risk as well as those with actual hypokalemia.

Age. This is an important consideration because renal capacity to concentrate urine decreases with aging, increasing potassium loss. Moreover, elderly clients are more likely to use medications that promote potassium loss.

Medication Use. The nurse questions the client about medication use, especially diuretics and corticosteroids. These drugs increase potassium loss through the kidneys.

One of the most common causes of hypokalemia is the use and misuse of diuretics. In clients taking digitalis preparations such as digoxin (Lanoxin, Novodigoxin✦), hypokalemia increases the sensitivity of the myocardium to the drug and may result in digitalis toxicity, even when the dosage is within the therapeutic range.

The nurse questions whether the client takes a prescribed potassium supplement, such as potassium chloride (KCl). The client may not be taking the potassium chloride as prescribed because of its unpleasant taste.

Other Factors. Any acute or chronic disease state may lead to hypokalemia. The nurse asks about recent illnesses and medical or surgical interventions. A thorough diet history, including a typical day's food and beverage intake, helps the nurse identify clients at risk for hypokalemia.

➤ Physical Assessment/Clinical Manifestations

Clinical manifestations of hypokalemia are associated with altered function of many systems (Chart 16–1).

Chart 16–1

Key Features of Hypokalemia

Cardiovascular

- Variable pulse rate, more often rapid
- Pulse quality thready and weak
- Peripheral pulses difficult to palpate
- Orthostatic (postural) hypotension
- Electrocardiographic abnormalities
  - ST depression
  - Inverted T wave
  - Prominent U wave
  - Heart block

Respiratory

- Shallow, ineffective respirations resulting from profound weakness of the skeletal muscles of respiration
- Diminished breath sounds

Neuromuscular

- Anxiety, lethargy, confusion, coma
- Loss of tactile discrimination
- General skeletal muscle weakness
- Deep tendon hyporeflexia
- Eventual flaccid paralysis

Gastrointestinal

- Decreased motility
- Hypoactive to absent bowel sounds
- Nausea
- Vomiting
- Abdominal distention
- Paralytic ileus
- Constipation

Renal

- Decreased ability to concentrate urine
- Polyuria
- Decreased specific gravity

Musculoskeletal Manifestations. Skeletal muscles become weak in response to hypokalemia, and a stronger stimulus is needed to begin muscle contraction. A client may be so weak as to be unable to stand. Handgrasps are weak, and hyporeflexia (a decreased response to deep tendon reflex stimulation) may be noted. Severe hypokalemia can lead to flaccid paralysis. The nurse assesses the degree of muscle weakness and determines the client's ability to perform activities of daily living (ADLs).

Respiratory Manifestations. The respiratory system can be profoundly affected by hypokalemia through depression of the nerves and muscles needed for breathing. Weakness of the skeletal muscles of respiration results in shallow respirations. The nurse assesses breath sounds, ease of respiratory effort, color of nail beds and mucous membranes, and rate and depth of respiration. The nurse assesses the client's respiratory status at least every 2 hours, because respiratory insufficiency frequently accompanies hypokalemia and is a major cause of death (Tannen, 1996).

Cardiovascular Manifestations. Cardiovascular changes often accompany hypokalemia. The nurse assesses the cardiovascular system by first palpating peripheral pulses. In the client with hypokalemia, the pulse is usually thready and weak. Palpation is difficult, and the pulse is easily blocked with light pressure. The pulse rate ranges from excessively slow to excessively rapid, depending on whether a dysrhythmia (irregular heartbeat) is present. The nurse measures blood pressure with the client in lying, sitting, and standing positions, because orthostatic (postural) hypotension accompanies hypokalemia.

Neurologic Manifestations. Neurologic manifestations of hypokalemia include changes in mental status. The client may experience short-term irritability and anxiety followed by lethargy progressing to confusion and coma as hypokalemia worsens. Severe hypokalemia affects sensory nerves by decreasing sensory awareness. For example, the client may not be able to identify mild sensations of pain, touch, heat, and cold.

Gastrointestinal Manifestations. Hypokalemia results in decreased smooth muscle contractility within the gastrointestinal system, leading to decreased peristalsis. The affected client has hypoactive bowel sounds and may experience nausea, vomiting, constipation, and abdominal distention. The nurse assesses distention by measuring abdominal girth. The nurse also assesses bowel sounds in all four abdominal quadrants to determine the extent of decreased peristalsis. Severe hypokalemia can cause paralytic ileus (the absence of peristalsis).

➤ *Psychosocial Assessment*

Because hypokalemia is seldom a long-term problem, any associated behavioral changes usually occur within a short period. Information about the client's behavior may need to be obtained from close family members or friends, depending on the client's condition.

The nurse collects data about the onset and duration of behavioral changes as well as their association with any other physical signs and symptoms. These data are impor-

tant and need to be as accurate as possible. The client may be lethargic and unable to perform simple problem-solving tasks that require concentration, such as counting backward from 100 by threes. As hypokalemia progresses, the client may become increasingly confused, in particular being disoriented to time and place. In severe hypokalemia, coma may develop.

➤ *Laboratory Assessment*

Hypokalemia is confirmed by a serum potassium value below 3.5 mEq/L (mmol/L). However, this value does not indicate whether a true potassium deficit exists or whether a shift of potassium from the blood to the intracellular fluid (ICF) has occurred.

➤ *Other Diagnostic Assessment*

The physician usually orders a baseline electrocardiogram (ECG) followed by continuous cardiac monitoring for a client with severe hypokalemia. Hypokalemia causes electrical conduction abnormalities, including ST-segment depression, flat or inverted T waves, and increased U waves. Dysrhythmias can result in death, particularly in elderly clients taking digitalis.

 Analysis

➤ *Common Nursing Diagnoses and Collaborative Problems*

The priority nursing diagnoses for clients with hypokalemia are as follows:
1. High Risk for Injury related to skeletal muscle weakness
2. Constipation related to smooth muscle atony.

The primary collaborative problem is High Risk for Ineffective Breathing Pattern Related to Neuromuscular Impairment.

➤ *Additional Nursing Diagnoses and Collaborative Problems*

In addition to the common nursing diagnoses and collaborative problems, clients with hypokalemia may have one or more of the following:
- Impaired Mobility related to skeletal muscle weakness
- Total Self-Care Deficit related to skeletal muscle weakness
- Decreased Cardiac Output related to dysrhythmia.

 Planning and Implementation

➤ *High Risk for Injury*

Planning: Expected Outcomes. The client is expected to avoid injury and show a return to a normal serum potassium level.

Interventions. These aim to prevent potassium loss, increase serum potassium levels, and provide a safe environment for the client. Drug and diet therapies help restore normal serum potassium levels.

Drug Therapy. Potassium supplements (oral or intravenous [IV]) are commonly given for the treatment and prevention of hypokalemia.

Potassium Supplements. Most potassium supplements (replacements) consist of potassium chloride. The amount and the route of potassium replacement depend on the degree of potassium loss. A client with a serum potassium level of 3 mEq/L needs 100 to 200 mEq of potassium supplement, for example, and one with a serum potassium level of 2.0 mEq/L needs 500 to 600 mEq (Tannen, 1996).

Potassium is given IV for severe hypokalemia. A dilution of no more than 1 mEq/10 mL of solution is recommended. The maximum recommended infusion rate is 5 to 10 mEq/hour, *never to exceed 20 mEq/hour under any circumstances.* Elderly clients may not be able to handle this rate. Because rapid infusion of potassium can cause cardiac arrest, the nurse never gives potassium by IV push.

Potassium is a severe tissue irritant and is never administered as an intramuscular or subcutaneous injection. Tissues damaged by potassium can become necrotic and slough, leading to loss of function and requiring reconstructive surgery. IV potassium solutions irritate veins and can cause phlebitis. The nurse checks the physician's orders carefully to ensure that the client receives the correct amount of potassium. The nurse assesses the IV site every 2 hours and asks the client whether he or she feels burning or pain at the site. The IV solution is stopped immediately if infiltration occurs.

Oral potassium preparations may be administered as liquids or solids. Potassium chloride has a strong, unpleasant taste that is difficult to mask. Because potassium chloride can cause nausea and vomiting, it should not be taken on an empty stomach.

Potassium-Sparing Diuretics. Diuretics that increase renal excretion of potassium commonly cause hypokalemia. These classes of diuretics include high-ceiling, or loop, diuretics, such as furosemide (Lasix, Furoside✦), bumetanide (Bumex), and ethacrynic acid (Edecrin), and the thiazide diuretics, such as chlorothiazide (Diuril), hydrochlorothiazide (Esidrix, Nefrol✦), and quinethazone (Hydromox, Aquamox✦). Thus, these drugs are avoided in clients with actual hypokalemia and in those who are susceptible to hypokalemia. For a client with hypokalemia who requires diuretic therapy, a potassium-sparing diuretic may be appropriate. Potassium-sparing diuretics cause diuresis without increasing potassium excretion. Diuretics with this action include spironolactone (Aldactone, Novospiroton✦), triamterene (Dyrenium), and amiloride (Midamor).

Diet Therapy. The nurse consults with the dietitian in teaching the client how to increase dietary potassium intake. Eating food naturally rich in potassium helps restore normal potassium levels and prevent further loss. Table 14–7 lists foods with a high potassium content.

Safety Measures. For a client experiencing muscle weakness, the nurse uses safety measures and eliminates hazards. The nurse or assistive personnel assists the client with ambulation. Obstacles or slippery areas are removed from the ambulation path, and the client wears nonslip footgear. When ambulating with assistance, the client wears a gait belt around the waist.

➤ Constipation

Planning: Expected Outcomes. The client's normal bowel elimination pattern is expected to be restored.

Interventions. These aim to restore normal serum potassium levels and induce gastric motility. Specific interventions include drug and diet therapies to restore serum potassium levels to normal values (discussed earlier under drug and diet therapies for High Risk for Injury) and stimulate intestinal peristalsis as well as interventions designed to prevent constipation.

Drug Therapy. Laxatives that add bulk or fiber may be used to stimulate peristalsis. Other drugs that enhance gastric emptying and stimulate gastrointestinal motility, such as metoclopramide (Reglan, Maxeran✦), are used to treat constipation associated with hypokalemia.

Diet Therapy. The nurse provides high-fiber foods and plenty of liquids for the client who is not on fluid restrictions. To ensure client cooperation, the nurse prepares a list of foods that contain high concentrations of fiber and asks the client to select favorite items from that list.

Comfort Measures. The nurse or assistive personnel can help the client maintain normal bowel elimination patterns in several ways. When the client is using the toilet or bedpan, privacy is provided. The door is closed, privacy curtains are drawn, and visitors are asked to step out of the room. Physical activity and exercise promote gastric motility. The client is encouraged to ambulate whenever his or her condition permits. A bedridden client benefits from frequent position changes and mild bed exercises.

➤ Ineffective Breathing Pattern

Planning: Expected Outcomes. The client is expected to have a breathing pattern adequate to maintain gas exchange.

Interventions. The nurse monitors the client's rate and depth of respiration at least once per hour, noting particularly increased rate and decreased depth. The effectiveness of respiratory muscles can also be determined by assessing the client's ability to cough. The nurse also examines the client's face, oral mucosa, and nail beds for pallor or cyanosis. The nurse evaluates arterial blood gas values for *hypoxemia* (decreased blood oxygen concentration) and *hypercapnia* (increased arterial carbon dioxide concentration). (Chapters 29 and 30 discuss respiratory assessment and interventions in more detail.)

➤ Continuing Care

No extensive home care preparations are necessary for clients with mild hypokalemia and those with sudden-onset hypokalemia. The imbalance is corrected before discharge and, with minimal precautions, is unlikely to recur. Clients who are most likely to be discharged before the imbalance is completely corrected and who are susceptible to recurrent episodes of imbalance have chronic pathologic conditions or diseases. These clients often require long-term diet and drug therapy.

➤ Health Teaching

The nurse instructs the at-risk client (especially one receiving diuretics or corticosteroids) regarding the proper use of medications, the signs and symptoms of hypokalemia, when to seek medical help, and foods rich in potassium. The nurse also teaches the client to assess the rate, rhythm, and quality of peripheral pulses at least once each day and whenever any signs or symptoms of hypokalemia are present. The nurse discusses with a chronically ill client how potassium is lost from the body so that the client can act to reduce potassium loss before actual deficits occur. The nurse reinforces how often the client should have serum potassium levels assessed.

➤ Home Care Management

When hypokalemia is resolved and the underlying cause is controlled, home care management techniques are individualized to the client's baseline physical and mental functioning. The home environment is assessed for the client's ability to perform ADLs safely.

A client with a chronic condition that increases his or her risk for hypokalemia and other electrolyte imbalances may not be able to live alone. The nurse assesses the ability and willingness of family members to share in the client's care. The nurse also determines whether and what type of home care assistance may be needed.

A home health aide may be needed to assist with hygiene and ensure a safe environment. Weekly visits by a nurse may also be needed to assess changes and ensure compliance with the medication regimen. At every home visit to a client at risk for hypokalemia, the nurse performs a focused assessment (Chart 16–2). Medication regimens, signs and symptoms of hypokalemia, and health care resources are reviewed with the client and family.

➤ Health Care Resources

Because hypokalemia is a manifestation of other health problems rather than a distinct disease, needed health care resources vary with the client's underlying health problem. For the client with chronic health problems that increase the risk for hypokalemia, appropriate health care resources include the physician, home care nurse, pharmacist, and nutritionist or dietitian. When special equipment needs or financial problems interfere with the client's ability to obtain necessary food or medications, the nurse contacts the social services department of the facil-

---

Chart 16–2

Focused Assessment for Home Care Clients at Risk for Hypokalemia

- Assess respiratory status.
  - Rate, depth, rhythm of respiration
  - Color of lips, tongue, nail beds
  - Can the client complete a sentence without taking a breath?
- Assess cardiovascular status.
  - Vital signs, including apical pulse, pulse pressure, presence or absence of orthostatic hypotension, and quality and rhythm of peripheral pulses
  - Presence or absence of peripheral edema
  - Hand vein filling in the dependent position
  - Neck vein filling in the recumbent and sitting positions
  - Weight gain or loss
- Assess cognition and mental status.
  - Level of consciousness
  - Orientation to time, place, and person
  - Can the client accurately read a seven-word sentence containing no words greater than three syllables?
- Assess condition of skin and mucous membranes.
  - Presence or absence of skin tenting over the sternum or the forehead
  - Moistness of skin, most reliable on chest and back
  - Presence or absence of coating on tongue or teeth
  - Can the client spit?
- Assess neuromuscular status.
  - Reactivity of patellar and biceps reflexes
  - Oral temperature
  - Handgrip strength
  - Steadiness of gait
- Assess renal system.
  - Observe urine specimen for color, odor, cloudiness, and amount
- Ask about the following:
  - 24-hour fluid intake and output
  - 24-hour diet recall
  - 24-hour activity recall
  - What over-the-counter and prescribed medications has the client taken?
  - Has the client experienced any dizziness or lightheadedness?
  - Does the client have a headache (what time of day, associated with what activities)?
  - Muscle twitches, cramps, pain, or spasms
- Assess client's understanding of illness and compliance with treatment.
  - Signs and symptoms to report to health care provider
  - Medication plan (correct timing and dose)

---

ity. The client with chronic health problems frequently requires assistance with self-care. If no one is available to perform these functions, home care nursing may be necessary or the client may have to be placed in an extended-care facility. Specific organizations related to the chronic disease or organ problem causing the hypokalemia may be helpful. Such organizations include the Kidney Foundation and the American Diabetes Association.

 Evaluation

On the basis of the identified nursing diagnoses and collaborative problems, the nurse evaluates the care of the client with hypokalemia. The client is expected to

- Return to and maintain a normal serum potassium level (between 3.5 and 5.1 mEq/L)
- Comply with drug and diet therapies as prescribed
- State the early signs and symptoms of hypokalemia
- Avoid injury
- Have normal bowel elimination patterns
- Maintain adequate gas exchange
- Maintain regular cardiac rate and rhythm

Hyperkalemia

Overview

Hyperkalemia occurs when the serum potassium level exceeds 5.1 mEq/L (mmol/L). Because the range of normal serum potassium values is narrow, even slight increases above normal values can have serious adverse effects on the physiologic function of excitable tissues, especially the myocardium.

Pathophysiology

An elevated serum potassium level produces a decreased potassium concentration difference between the intracellular fluid (ICF) and the extracellular fluid (ECF). This decreased difference increases cell excitability, so excitable tissues respond to less intense stimuli and may even discharge spontaneously.

Hyperkalemia alters the function of all excitable membranes to some degree. The myocardium is the excitable membrane most sensitive to serum potassium increases; thus, the more serious complications of hyperkalemia are associated with altered cardiac function.

Pathologic changes associated with hyperkalemia are directly related to how rapidly ECF potassium levels increase. Sudden increases in serum potassium levels cause profound functional changes at potassium levels between 6 and 7 mEq/L. When serum potassium levels increase slowly, problems with excitable membrane function may not be obvious until potassium levels reach 8 mEq/L.

Etiology

Hyperkalemia may result from an actual increase in the amount of total body potassium. It also may result from abnormal movement of potassium from the cells to the ECF. Table 16–2 summarizes common causes of hyperkalemia.

Hyperkalemia is rare in persons with normally functioning kidneys. Most cases of hyperkalemia occur in hospitalized clients and those undergoing medical treatment. Clients at greatest risk for hyperkalemia are the chronically ill, debilitated, and elderly.

TABLE 16–2

Common Causes of Hyperkalemia

Actual Potassium Excesses

Excessive Potassium Intake

- Overingestion of potassium-containing foods or medications
  - Salt substitutes
  - Potassium chloride
- Rapid infusion of potassium-containing intravenous solution
- Bolus intravenous potassium injections

Decreased Potassium Excretion

- Adrenal insufficiency (Addison's disease, adrenalectomy)
- Renal failure
- Potassium-sparing diuretics

Relative Potassium Excesses

Movement of Potassium from Intracellular Fluid to Extracellular Fluid

- Tissue damage
- Acidosis
- Hyperuricemia
- Hypercatabolism

Collaborative Management

 Assessment

➤ History

The client's age is an important factor because renal function decreases with aging. The nurse asks about chronic illnesses, particularly renal disease and diabetes mellitus, and recent medical or surgical interventions. The client is questioned about urine output, including the frequency and amount of voidings. The nurse also inquires about medication use, particularly potassium-sparing diuretics. The nurse obtains a diet history to pinpoint possible causative factors, such as the intake of potassium-rich foods. The client is specifically asked about the use of salt substitutes, many of which contain potassium salts.

The nurse collects data pointing to symptoms related to hyperkalemia. The client is asked whether he or she has experienced palpitations, skipped heartbeats, or other cardiac irregularities as well as muscle twitching, weakness in leg muscles, and unusual tingling or numbness in the hands, feet, or face. The nurse inquires about recent changes in bowel habits, especially diarrhea, colic, and explosive bowel movements.

➤ Physical Assessment/Clinical Manifestations

The clinical manifestations of hyperkalemia are summarized in Chart 16–3.

Cardiovascular Manifestations. Cardiovascular changes are the most severe results of hyperkalemia and are the most common cause of death in clients with hyperkalemia (Tannen, 1996). The nurse, therefore, carefully assesses the cardiac status of all clients with hyperkalemia through careful observation and cardiac monitoring. Conduction changes indicating hyperkalemia include gradual worsening of bradycardia; heart block; tall, peaked T waves; prolonged PR intervals; flattened or absent P waves; and widened QRS complexes (Fig. 16–1).

As serum potassium levels rise, impulse conduction through the cardiac Purkinje system slows and may be blocked at the atrioventricular (AV) node. The heart muscle dilates and becomes flaccid. As electrical conduction is blocked at the AV node, ectopic beats (beats generated outside the normal conduction system in the ventricles) may appear. Complete heart block, ventricular standstill, and ventricular fibrillation are major life-threatening complications of severe hyperkalemia.

Besides noting specific ECG changes, the nurse also assesses cardiac status through peripheral pulse and blood pressure measurements. The client with hyperkalemia usually has a slow, weak pulse and low blood pressure.

Neuromuscular Manifestations. The neuromuscular response to hyperkalemia has two phases. In the early stages of hyperkalemia, skeletal muscles twitch, and the client may be aware of unusual nerve sensations, such as tingling and burning, followed by numbness in the hands and feet and around the mouth. As hyperkalemia progresses, muscle twitching changes to weakness followed

by flaccid paralysis. The weakness ascends from distal to proximal areas and initially affects the muscles of the arms and the legs. Trunk, head, and respiratory muscles are not affected until serum potassium levels reach lethal levels.

Gastrointestinal Manifestations. The smooth muscle of the gastrointestinal tract responds to hyperkalemia by increasing peristalsis. The nurse assesses the gastrointestinal system by listening to bowel sounds and observing stools. The client may experience diarrhea and spastic colonic activity. Bowel sounds are hyperactive, with frequent audible rushes and gurgles. Bowel movements may be frequent, watery, and explosive.

➤ Laboratory Assessment

A serum potassium value exceeding 5.1 mEq/L confirms hyperkalemia. If hyperkalemia results from dehydration, levels of other serum electrolytes, hematocrit, and hemoglobin may be elevated. Hyperkalemia associated with renal failure is usually accompanied by elevated serum creatinine and blood urea nitrogen levels, decreased blood pH, and normal or low hematocrit and hemoglobin levels.

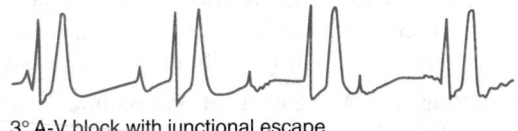

3° A-V block with junctional escape

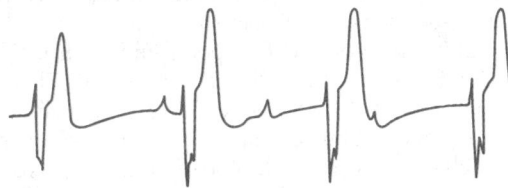

3° A-V block with ventricular escape

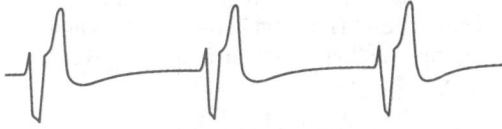

Idioventricular without atrial activity

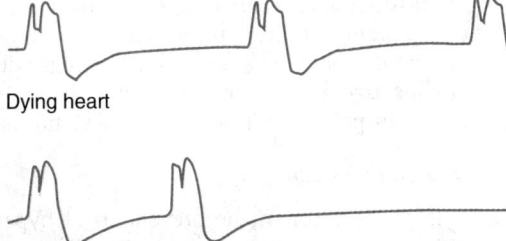

Dying heart

Asystole

Figure 16–1. Electrocardiographic (ECG) changes associated with hyperkalemia. (Modified with permission from John M. Clochesy.)

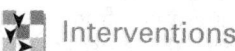 Interventions

Although identifying the causes of hyperkalemia is important, interventions are aimed at immediately reducing the serum potassium level. Drug therapy is useful for restoring normal potassium balance.

➤ Drug Therapy

The aims of drug therapy are to prevent further increases in serum potassium level by eliminating potassium administration, enhancing potassium excretion, and promoting the movement of potassium from the extracellular fluid (ECF) into the cells.

Eliminating Potassium Administration. When hyperkalemia occurs, the nurse stops infusions of potassium-containing IV solutions, but keeps the IV catheter open. Oral potassium supplements are withheld, and a potassium-restricted diet is ordered.

Increasing Potassium Excretion. If renal function is not impaired, the physician orders administration of potassium-excreting diuretics, such as furosemide (Mendyka, 1992). For a client with renal problems, drug therapy to increase potassium excretion includes cation exchange resins that promote gastrointestinal sodium absorption and potassium excretion, such as sodium polystyrene sulfonate (Kayexalate). Sodium polystyrene sulfonate may take many hours to reduce potassium levels, however. If potassium levels are dangerously high, additional measures, such as dialysis and ultrafiltration, are necessary.

Promoting the Movement of Potassium. Potassium movement from the ECF into the cells is enhanced by the presence of insulin. Insulin increases the activity of the membrane-bound sodium-potassium pump (see Chapter 14), resulting in movement of potassium from the blood and other ECFs into the cell (Tannen, 1996). The physician may order IV fluids that contain substantial amounts of glucose and insulin to help decrease the serum potassium levels (usually 100 mL of 10% to 20% glucose with 10 to 20 units of regular insulin). These IV solutions are hypertonic and are administered through a central venous catheter or in a vein with a high blood flow to avoid local vein inflammation. The nurse observes the client for signs and symptoms of hypokalemia and hypoglycemia during this therapy.

➤ Cardiac Monitoring

Prevention of lethal dysrhythmias depends not only on reducing potassium levels but also on recognizing early signs and symptoms of the adverse response of cardiac muscle. The nurse compares recent ECG tracings with the client's baseline tracings or with tracings obtained when the client's serum potassium level was close to normal.

➤ Health Teaching

Education is a key factor in the prevention of hyperkalemia and in the early detection of its life-threatening complications. The teaching plan for the client at risk for hyperkalemia includes diet, medications, and recognition of the signs and symptoms of hyperkalemia. Diet educa-

---

Chart 16–4

Education Guide: Dietary Management of Hyperkalemia

You Should Avoid	You May Eat
• Organ meats	• Eggs
• Fish	• Breads
• Fresh fruits	• Cereals
• Dried fruits	• Butter
• Beef	• Sugar
• Chicken	
• Pork	
• Milk	
• Vegetables	

---

tion includes knowledge of foods to avoid (those high in potassium) and permissible foods containing little potassium (Chart 16–4). The nurse instructs the client to examine medication and food package labels to determine the potassium content and to avoid salt substitutes, because these preparations usually contain potassium.

SODIUM IMBALANCES

Hyponatremia

Overview

Hyponatremia is a serum sodium (Na^+) level below 135 mEq/L (mmol/L). Because sodium is the major cation of the blood and interstitial fluid and is primarily used for maintaining the osmolarity of these fluids, sodium imbalances are usually associated with fluid volume imbalances.

Pathophysiology

The pathophysiologic changes underlying hyponatremia involve two mechanisms. The first mechanism is a change in cell excitability or activity. As the concentration of sodium in the blood and other extracellular fluid decreases, the sodium concentration gradient between the extracellular fluid (ECF) and the intracellular fluid (ICF) also decreases. Less sodium is available to move across the excitable membrane, causing delayed and slower membrane depolarization. The second mechanism is the movement of water from the ECF space into the ICF space. Cells swell and their functions are impaired.

Etiology

Various conditions can lead to hyponatremia by causing either an actual or a relative decrease in sodium content (Table 16–3). Hyponatremia can represent a loss of total body sodium, movement of sodium from the blood to other fluid spaces, or dilution of serum sodium as a result of excessive water in the plasma.

WOMEN'S HEALTH CONSIDERATIONS

 Hyponatremia as a complication during early postoperative recovery has a relatively high occurrence

TABLE 16-3

Common Causes of Hyponatremia

Actual Sodium Deficits

Increased Sodium Excretion

- Excessive diaphoresis
- Diuretics (high-ceiling diuretics)
- Wound drainage (especially gastrointestinal)
- Decreased secretion of aldosterone
- Hyperlipidemia
- Renal disease (scarred distal convoluted tubule)

Inadequate Sodium Intake

- Nothing by mouth
- Low-salt diet

Relative Sodium Deficits

Dilution of Serum Sodium

- Excessive ingestion of hypotonic fluids
- Psychogenic polydipsia
- Freshwater drowning
- Renal failure (nephrotic syndrome)
- Irrigation with hypotonic fluids
- Syndrome of inappropriate antidiuretic hormone secretion
- Hyperglycemia
- Congestive heart failure

in the United States, ranging from 1% to 5%. Although this complication occurs as often among men as women, more women develop brain damage and die from coma or seizure activity. The accompanying Research Applications for Nursing feature suggests a physiologic basis for this gender difference in response to hyponatremia.

Collaborative Management

 Assessment

The clinical manifestations of hyponatremia are associated with its effects on excitable cellular activity. The cells especially affected are involved in cerebral, neuromuscular, and gastric smooth muscle functions (Chart 16–5).

➤ *Cerebral Manifestations*

Changes in cerebral function are the most obvious signs and symptoms of hyponatremia. Because these changes may be seen as either depressed activity or excessive activity (and sometimes both), establishing the client's usual cerebral function and behavioral patterns is essential to detecting changes associated with hyponatremia. Behavioral changes result from cerebral edema and increased intracranial pressure. The nurse closely observes and documents the client's behavior. The nurse assesses the client's current mental status, starting with the level of consciousness, in the same manner described under neurologic manifestations of dehydration (p. 000).

➤ *Neuromuscular Manifestations*

The nurse assesses the client's neuromuscular status during each nursing shift for changes from baseline values. The neuromuscular response to hyponatremia is generalized muscle weakness. Muscle tone and deep tendon reflex responses diminish.

Muscle weakness associated with hyponatremia occurs bilaterally and is worse in the extremities. The nurse assesses deep tendon reflexes by lightly tapping the patellar (knee) tendons and Achilles (heel) tendons with a reflex hammer and documenting the degree of reflex movement. The technique for assessing motor strength and reflexes is described in depth in Chapter 43.

➤ Research Applications for Nursing

Men and Women Differ in Their Ability to Recover from Postoperative Hyponatremia

Ayus, J. C., & Arieff, A. (1996). Brain damage and postoperative hyponatremia: The role of gender. Neurology, 46(2), 323–328.

This article is a meta-analysis of the incidence and treatment of postoperative hyponatremia in the United States from 1935 to 1990. This analysis determined that postoperative hyponatremia occurred at a minimum frequency of 1% in 25 million inpatient surgical procedures. Hyponatremia induces cerebral encephalopathy with neuronal swelling and hypoxia. The incidence of postoperative hyponatremia is nearly equal among men and women; however, more women than men suffer severe complications of encephalopathy, permanent brain damage, or death.

The investigators explored an animal model for gender differences in hyponatremic encephalopathy. In female rats, the hypoxic effects of hyponatremia were compounded by estrogen and vasopressin interacting to decrease cerebral perfusion. Male rats, without the interactive effect of estrogen on vasopressin activity, did not experience cerebral hypoxia.

The investigators found that the hyponatremia in both male and female animal models could be reversed with the administration of intravenous (IV) hypertonic saline. The literature review confirmed that patients who were treated with hypertonic saline, water restriction, and loop diuretics had better outcomes than those who received standard isotonic or hypotonic fluid therapy.

Critique. This study blended prospective experimental bench research with retrospective clinical research in an attempt to explain a life-threatening phenomenon. Although the results are not absolute, the findings are compelling enough to call into question the practice of supporting postoperative clients with IV hypotonic fluids.

Possible Nursing Implications. Increasing the IV fluid rate in clients whose urine output is below 20 mL/hour is common in postoperative recovery. When the client is a woman aged 18 to 55 years, and the urine output remains decreased for 2 consecutive hours with no other indications of hemorrhage or hypovolemia, the nurse should consider the possibility of surgically induced hyponatremia before aggressively administering IV fluids. Serum electrolytes showing a dilutional pattern (decreased sodium, potassium, chloride, hematocrit, and hemoglobin) can alert the nurse to the possibility of hyponatremia leading to encephalopathy.

> ## Chart 16–5
>
> ## Key Features of Hyponatremia
>
> **Cardiovascular***
> - Normovolemic
>   - Rapid pulse rate
>   - Normal blood pressure
> - Hypovolemic
>   - Rapid pulse rate
>   - Pulse quality thready and weak
>   - Hypotensive
>   - Central venous pressure normal or low
>   - Flat neck veins
> - Hypervolemic
>   - Rapid, bounding pulse
>   - Central venous pressure normal or elevated
>   - Blood pressure normal or elevated
>
> **Respiratory**
> - Late manifestations related to skeletal muscle weakness
>   - Shallow, ineffective respiratory movements
> - Hypervolemia
> - Pulmonary edema
>   - Rapid, shallow respiration
>   - Moist rales
>
> **Neuromuscular**
> - Generalized skeletal muscle weakness
> - Diminished deep tendon reflexes
>
> **Cerebral**
> - Personality changes
> - Headache
>
> **Renal**
> - Increased urinary output
> - Decreased specific gravity
>
> **Gastrointestinal**
> - Increased motility
> - Nausea
> - Hyperactive bowel sounds
> - Diarrhea

*Symptoms vary with changes in vascular volume.

➤ Gastrointestinal Manifestations

The smooth muscle of the gastrointestinal system responds to decreased serum sodium levels with increased gastrointestinal motility, causing nausea, diarrhea, and abdominal cramping. The nurse assesses the gastrointestinal system by listening to bowel sounds and observing stools. Bowel sounds are hyperactive, with frequent rushes and gurgles, especially over the splenic flexure and in the lower left quadrant. Bowel movements are frequent, watery, and explosive. Peristaltic movements may be palpated through the abdominal wall and may even be visible on the abdominal surface.

➤ Cardiovascular Manifestations

Hyponatremia has little direct effect on cardiac muscle contractility; however, alterations in cardiac output are associated with hyponatremia. When hyponatremia is accompanied by changes in the plasma volume, these fluid changes alter cardiac function. Generally, cardiac responses to hyponatremia with accompanying hypovolemia (decreased plasma volume) are manifested as a rapid, weak, thready pulse. Peripheral pulses are difficult to palpate and are easily blocked with light pressure. Neck veins are flat with the client in the upright position and possibly also in the supine position. Blood pressure, especially diastolic pressure, is decreased. The client may have severe hypotension when moving from a lying or sitting position to a standing position. The central venous pressure is low.

When hyponatremia is accompanied by plasma hypervolemia (increased plasma volume), cardiac manifestations include a rapid, full pulse. Blood pressure is normal or elevated. Central venous pressure is normal or elevated depending on how well the left ventricle handles the extra fluid. Peripheral pulses are full and difficult to block; however, if edema is present, peripheral pulses may not be palpable.

 Interventions

Interventions aim to restore serum sodium levels to normal values and prevent further decreases in serum sodium levels. Primary treatment modalities are drug therapy and diet therapy.

➤ Drug Therapy

Drug therapy attempts to restore the serum sodium level to normal. Drug therapy regimens vary depending on whether fluid imbalance accompanies hyponatremia.

When hyponatremia occurs with a fluid deficit (hypovolemia), the physician orders IV saline infusions to restore both sodium content and fluid volume. The nurse monitors the infusion rate and the client's response. The infusions are delivered through a controller or a pump to prevent accidental alterations in infusion rate.

When hyponatremia is accompanied by fluid excess, drug therapy includes administration of diuretics that primarily promote the excretion of water rather than sodium. These drugs are osmotic diuretics, such as mannitol (Osmitrol♣). The nurse assesses the client hourly for signs of excessive losses of fluids and potassium and dramatic increases in sodium levels.

Drug therapy for hyponatremia as a result of inappropriate or excessive secretion of antidiuretic hormone (ADH) includes agents that antagonize ADH, such as lithium and demeclocycline (Declomycin).

➤ Diet Therapy

Diet therapy can help restore normal sodium balance in mild hyponatremia. Table 14–6 lists the sodium content of common foods. The nurse collaborates with the dietitian in teaching the client about which foods to increase in the diet. Therapy consists of increasing oral sodium intake and restricting oral fluid intake to some degree. When overhydration with oral hypotonic fluids is the underlying cause of the hyponatremia or when renal fluid excretion is impaired, fluid restriction may be a long-term regimen. The nurse or assistive personnel measures fluid intake and output. The nurse also verbally reinforces the purpose of the fluid restriction.

Hypernatremia

Overview

Hypernatremia is a serum sodium level exceeding 145 mEq/L. Increased serum sodium level can be caused by or can cause changes in fluid volumes. Table 16–4 lists common causes of hypernatremia.

As the extracellular sodium level rises, a larger sodium concentration difference occurs between the extracellular fluid (ECF) and the intracellular fluid (ICF). More sodium is available to move rapidly across cell membranes. With mild hypernatremia, almost all excitable tissues are excited more easily, a condition called *irritability*. This irritability causes excitable tissues to overrespond to stimuli. As the extracellular sodium concentration increases, however, the osmolarity of the ECF also increases. This situation causes water to move from the cells into the ECF as a compensatory action to dilute the hyperosmolar ECF. When hypernatremia persists or worsens, the compensatory action causes severe intracellular dehydration, and excitable tissues may no longer be able to respond to stimuli.

Collaborative Management

 Assessment

The clinical manifestations of hypernatremia vary with the degree of imbalance and whether a fluid imbalance is also present. Rapid increases in serum sodium level generally produce more obvious and severe symptoms. Gradual in-

TABLE 16–4

Common Causes of Hypernatremia

Actual Sodium Excesses

Decreased Sodium Excretion

- Hyperaldosteronism
- Renal failure
- Corticosteroids
- Cushing's syndrome

Increased Sodium Intake

- Excessive oral sodium ingestion
- Excessive administration of sodium-containing intravenous fluids

Relative Sodium Excesses

Decreased Water Intake

- Nothing by mouth

Increased Water Loss

- Increased rate of metabolism
- Fever
- Hyperventilation
- Infection
- Excessive diaphoresis
- Watery diarrhea
- Dehydration

Chart 16–6

Key Features of Hypernatremia

Cardiovascular

- Decreased myocardial contractility
- Diminished cardiac output
- Heart rate and blood pressure respond to vascular volume

Respiratory

- Problems associated with pulmonary edema when hypernatremia is accompanied by hypervolemia

Central Nervous System*

- Hypernatremia and normovolemia or hypovolemia
  - Increased neural activity
  - Agitation, confusion, seizures
- Hypernatremia and hypervolemia
  - Decreased neural activity
  - Lethargy, stupor, coma

Neuromuscular

- Mild or early hypernatremia
  - Spontaneous muscle twitches
  - Irregular contractions
- Severe or late hypernatremia
  - Skeletal muscle weakness
  - Deep tendon reflexes diminished or absent

Renal

- Decreased urinary output
- Increased specific gravity

Integumentary

- Dry, flaky skin
- Presence or absence of edema related to accompanying fluid volume changes

*Upper neural function changes are related to volume changes as well as sodium increases.

---

creases in serum sodium levels may produce no observable physical changes, however, even when sodium levels increase to well above normal ranges. Clinical manifestations of hypernatremia are primarily associated with changes in cell membrane activity, especially among excitable tissues involved in cerebral, neuromuscular, and cardiac functions (Chart 16–6).

➤ *Central Nervous System Manifestations*

Altered cerebral function is the most common manifestation of hypernatremia. The nurse assesses the client's mental status in terms of attention span, recall of recent events, and ability to perform cognitive functions. In hypernatremia with normal or decreased fluid volumes, the client may have a short attention span and be agitated or confused about the sequence of recent events. If serum sodium concentration continues to increase, the client may become manic or experience convulsions. When hypernatremia is accompanied by an extracellular volume overload, the client may exhibit lethargy, drowsiness, stupor, and even coma.

➤ Neuromuscular Manifestations

Skeletal muscles respond differently to various degrees of hypernatremia. Mild hypernatremia causes muscle twitching and irregular muscle contractions. As hypernatremia worsens, the ability of skeletal muscle and nerves to respond to a stimulus diminishes. Muscles become progressively weaker and demonstrate rigid paralysis. Deep tendon reflexes are diminished or absent. The nurse assesses neuromuscular status by observing for twitching in muscle groups. The nurse also assesses muscle strength by having the client perform handgrip and arm flexion against resistance. Muscle weakness associated with hypernatremia occurs bilaterally and has no specific progressive pattern. The nurse assesses peripheral nerve response by lightly tapping the patellar (knee) tendons and Achilles (heel) tendons with a reflex hammer and measuring the degree of movement. (For an in-depth description of nursing assessment of mental status, deep tendon reflexes, and muscle strength, see Chapter 43.)

➤ Cardiovascular Manifestations

Increased serum sodium level prevents movement of calcium into the myocardium, thus decreasing the ability of the myocardium to contract. The nurse assesses cardiovascular status by taking blood pressure and measuring the rate and quality of apical and peripheral pulses. Pulse rate and blood pressure may be normal, above normal, or below normal during hypernatremic episodes, depending on the fluid volume and the speed with which the imbalance occurs.

In clients with hypernatremia and hypovolemia, the pulse rate is increased. Peripheral pulses may be difficult to palpate and are easily blocked with light pressure. The client is hypotensive, with severe orthostatic (postural) hypotension, and pulse pressure is greatly diminished.

Clients with hypernatremia and hypervolemia have slow to normal bounding pulses. Peripheral pulses are full and difficult to block. Neck veins are distended, even with the client in the upright position. Blood pressure, especially diastolic, is increased.

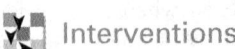 Interventions

Interventions aim to prevent further increases in serum sodium levels and decrease elevated serum sodium levels. Drug administration and diet therapy play important roles in restoring normal sodium balance. Other interventions used when hypernatremia becomes life-threatening include hemodialysis, peritoneal dialysis, and blood ultrafiltration.

➤ Drug Therapy

When hypernatremia is caused by fluid loss, drug therapy focuses on restoring fluid balance. The physician orders IV infusions of glucose and water (e.g., 5% dextrose in water). When hypernatremia is caused by fluid and sodium losses, it may be necessary to replace the fluid with IV administration of isotonic sodium chloride (NaCl) solutions. When hypernatremia is caused by inadequate renal excretion of sodium, drug therapy with diuretics pro-

moting sodium loss, such as furosemide (Lasix, Furoside✦), bumetanide (Bumex), and ethacrynic acid (Edecrin), is ordered. The nurse assesses the client hourly for symptoms indicating excessive loss of fluids, sodium, or potassium.

➤ Diet Therapy

Dietary sodium restriction is useful in preventing hypernatremia. Often fluids must be restricted as well. The nurse collaborates with the dietitian in helping the client understand how to determine the sodium content of foods, beverages, and medications and the importance of complying with the diet.

CALCIUM IMBALANCES

Hypocalcemia

Overview

Hypocalcemia is a total serum calcium (Ca^{2+}) level below 8.6 mg/dL or 2.15 mmol/L. Calcium is stored in bone, and only a small fraction of the total body calcium is present in ECF. Because the normal serum level of calcium is so low, small changes in serum calcium levels have major effects on body function.

Pathophysiology

Calcium ions decrease excitable membrane permeability to sodium ions, preventing spontaneous depolarization. Calcium is considered a membrane stabilizer, regulating depolarization and the generation of action potentials. Low serum calcium levels increase the permeability of excitable membranes to sodium, so that depolarization occurs more easily and at inappropriate times.

Excitable tissues vary in their sensitivity to low serum calcium levels. Peripheral nerves, skeletal muscles, cardiac muscle, and the smooth muscle of the gastrointestinal system demonstrate the most obvious responses to decreased serum calcium levels. The severity of the manifestations associated with hypocalcemia depends on the degree of the calcium imbalance.

Hypocalcemia can also cause pathologic effects on bone. Bone is the primary storage site for calcium and can release calcium into the bloodstream when needed. Excessive calcium loss from bone can cause bone to weaken its supporting structure. Chronic hypocalcemia leads to progressive osteoporosis, resulting in bones that are less dense and more susceptible to fracture or deformity. (See Chapter 53 for a discussion of osteoporosis.)

Etiology

Hypocalcemia can result from various chronic and acute pathologic states as well as specific medical or surgical treatments. Table 16–5 lists common causes of hypocalcemia.

Actual calcium loss (a reduction in total body calcium) occurs in response to conditions that either inhibit calcium absorption from the gastrointestinal tract or increase the loss of calcium from the body.

TABLE 16–5

Common Causes of Hypocalcemia

Actual Calcium Deficits

Inhibition of Calcium Absorption from the Gastrointestinal Tract

- Inadequate oral intake of calcium
- Lactose intolerance
- Malabsorption syndromes
  - Celiac sprue
  - Crohn's disease
- Inadequate intake of vitamin D
- End-stage renal disease

Increased Calcium Excretion

- Renal failure—polyuric phase
- Diarrhea
- Steatorrhea
- Wound drainage (especially gastrointestinal)

Relative Calcium Deficits

Conditions That Decrease the Ionized Fraction of Calcium

- Hyperproteinemia
- Alkalosis
- Calcium chelators or binders
  - Citrate
  - Mithramycin
  - Penicillamine
  - Sodium cellulose phosphate (Calcibind)
  - Aredia
- Acute pancreatitis
- Hyperphosphatemia
- Immobility

Endocrine Disturbances

- Removal or destruction of parathyroid glands
  - Thyroidectomy
  - Radiation to thyroid
  - Strangulation
  - Neck injuries

Relative calcium loss causes the total body calcium concentration to remain normal while serum calcium levels are too low. This type of hypocalcemia occurs in response to conditions that either decrease the free, or ionized (unbound), calcium in the body or decrease parathyroid gland function.

TRANSCULTURAL CONSIDERATIONS

Many African-American clients have a lactose intolerance related to a genetic deficiency of the enzyme lactase. These clients cannot use the nutrients present in milk, and they experience cramping, diarrhea, and abdominal pain after ingesting dairy products. Dairy products, especially milk, are a common and rich source of both calcium and vitamin D. Clients with lactose intolerance may, therefore, experience difficulty obtaining enough calcium and vitamin D from other sources to maintain normal calcium levels in the blood and bones.

WOMEN'S HEALTH CONSIDERATIONS

Postmenopausal women are susceptible to hypocalcemia. This occurrence appears to be related to reduced weight-bearing activities and a decrease in sex hormone (estrogen) levels. Osteoporosis occurs when weight-bearing activity decreases or is limited. Because women generally are smaller framed than men, the female skeleton does not experience as much weight-bearing as the male skeleton. In addition, as they age, many women decrease weight-bearing activities, such as running and walking. Also, the estrogen secretion that protects against osteoporosis diminishes. All of these factors increase the risk of hypocalcemia in women, particularly the elderly.

Hypocalcemia and the Elderly

Elderly people are at risk for most electrolyte imbalances. Major organs and body systems undergo changes with aging. For example, an older adult has a smaller fluid volume per body weight than a younger adult, so that any variation in fluid volumes or electrolyte levels leads to imbalances more quickly. The elderly client is also more likely to be taking prescription or over-the-counter medications that affect fluid or electrolyte balance. Some elderly clients have dietary calcium or vitamin D deficits because of economic conditions or general problems with obtaining, preparing, or eating food.

Collaborative Management

 Assessment

The most critical factor in assessing for the risk of actual or potential hypocalcemia is the diet history. The nurse questions clients regarding the intake of calcium-containing foods (see Table 14–8). The nurse also identifies whether the client uses a calcium supplement on a regular basis.

One indicator of hypocalcemia is a report of frequent, painful muscle spasms (charley horses) in the calf or foot during periods of inactivity or sleep. Other information that can alert the nurse to a possible risk of hypocalcemia is a history of recent orthopedic surgery or bone healing. Disorders and treatments related to endocrine disturbances are significant for hypocalcemia. History of thyroid surgery, therapeutic radiation to the upper middle chest and neck area, or a recent anterior neck injury predisposes the client to hypocalcemia.

The most common clinical manifestations of hypocalcemia are related to overstimulation of nerves and muscles (see Chart 16–7).

➤ Neuromuscular Manifestations

Although all nerves and muscles are affected by hypocalcemia to some degree, the client usually notices symptoms first in the limbs, with distal to proximal movement from the hands and feet. At first, paresthesias may be noted, with sensations of tingling alternating with sensations of numbness. If hypocalcemia continues or worsens, these sensations may progress to actual muscle twitching or painful cramps and spasms. Paresthesias may also af-

---

Chart 16–7

Key Features of Hypocalcemia

Cardiovascular

- Decreased heart rate
- Decreased myocardial contractility
- Diminished peripheral pulses
- Hypotension
- Electrocardiographic abnormalities
  - Prolonged ST interval
  - Prolonged QT interval

Respiratory

- Not directly affected
- Respiratory failure or arrest can result from decreased respiratory movement because of muscle tetany or seizure activity

Neuromuscular*

- Anxiety, irritability, psychosis
- Paresthesias followed by numbness
- Irritable skeletal muscles—twitches, cramps, tetany, seizures
- Hyperactive deep tendon reflexes
- Positive Trousseau's sign
- Positive Chvostek's sign

Gastrointestinal

- Increased gastric motility
- Hyperactive bowel sounds
- Abdominal cramping
- Diarrhea

---

*The neuromuscular system is most profoundly affected by hypocalcemia.

fect the lips, nose, and ears. These symptoms signal the approach of serious neuromuscular overstimulation and tetany.

The nurse assesses for hypocalcemia by testing for Trousseau's and Chvostek's signs. To test for Trousseau's sign, the nurse places a blood pressure cuff around the upper arm, inflating the cuff to greater than the client's systolic pressure and keeping it inflated for 1 to 4 minutes. Under these hypoxic conditions, a positive Trousseau's sign occurs if the hand and fingers go into spasm in palmar flexion (Fig. 16–2). To test for Chvostek's sign, the nurse taps on the face just below and anterior to the ear (over the facial nerve) to trigger facial twitching of one side of the mouth, nose, and cheek (Fig. 16–3).

➤ Cardiovascular Manifestations

The heart rate may be slower or slightly faster than normal, but myocardial contractility is weaker, resulting in a diminished pulse quality. Severe hypocalcemia causes profound hypotension and ECG changes, including a prolonged ST interval leading to a prolonged QT interval.

➤ Gastrointestinal Manifestations

Overstimulation associated with hypocalcemia increases peristaltic activity. The nurse auscultates the abdomen for

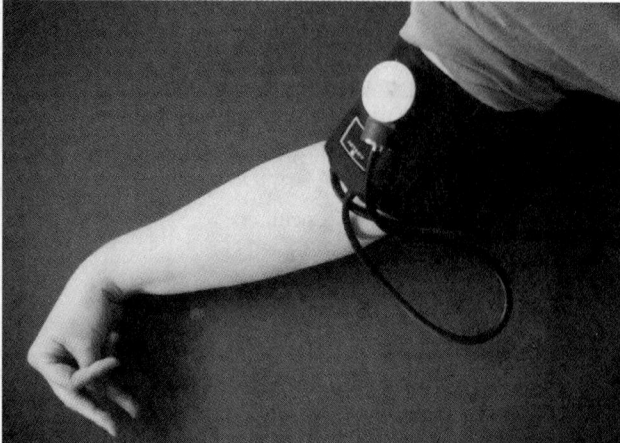

Figure 16–2. Palmar flexion—positive Trousseau's sign in hypocalcemia.

hyperactive bowel sounds. The client may report painful abdominal cramping and diarrhea.

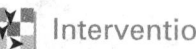 **Interventions**

Interventions aim to prevent further decreases in serum calcium levels, restore normal serum calcium levels, and prevent complications. Appropriate interventions may include drug therapy, diet therapy, reduction of environmental stimuli, and injury prevention.

➤ Drug Therapy

Drug therapy for hypocalcemia consists of direct calcium supplements or replacements, drugs that enhance absorption of calcium, and drugs that decrease nerve and muscle responsiveness to overstimulation. Chart 16–8 lists different drug types used to manage hypocalcemia.

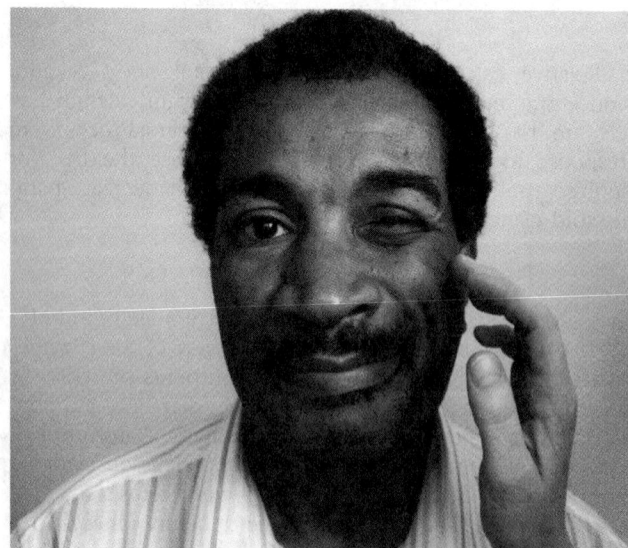

Figure 16–3. Facial muscle response—positive Chvostek's sign in hypocalcemia.

Chart 16–8

Drug Therapy for Hypocalcemia

Drug	Precautions
Oral Calcium Supplements	
Calcium carbonate	Dose must be increased in elderly clients because of decreased intestinal absorption.
Calcium citrate	Use with thiazide diuretics can increase the risk for hypercalcemia.
Calcium gluconate	Use with phenytoin decreases the bioavailability of both drugs; phenytoin should not be
Calcium lactate	given within 3 hours of calcium administration.
Intravenous Calcium	
Calcium acetate	All must be administered slowly, not to exceed 27 g/min.
Calcium chloride	Clients should be monitored for electrocardiographic changes during administration.
Calcium gluconate	Observe client for infiltration; calcium is a severe tissue irritant/vesicant.
	Potential for hypercalcemia and hypomagnesemia.
	Injection should be warmed to body temperature before administration.
Agents That Increase Calcium Absorption	
Aluminum hydroxide	Reduces serum phosphorus levels, causing the countereffect of increasing calcium levels; potential for hypophosphatemia. Signs and symptoms include bradycardia, decreased deep tendon reflexes, shortness of breath, confusion.
Vitamin D	Increases the intestinal absorption of calcium; potential for hypercalcemia.
Alfacalcidol	This is a fat-soluble vitamin and is stored to some degree; risk for vitamin D toxicity
Calcifediol	resulting in renal failure and/or cardiac failure.
Calcitriol	
Dihydrotachysterol	
Agents That Reduce Nerve and Skeletal Muscle Excitability	
Magnesium sulfate	Tissue irritant; the preferred route of administration is intravenous.
	Potential for hypermagnesemia; signs and symptoms of toxicity include bradycardia, flushing, headache, nausea, vomiting, shortness of breath, hypotension.
Methocarbamol	These agents act at the level of the central nervous system to decrease skeletal muscle
Robaxin	activity.
Carbacot	All have some sedative effect.
Metaxalone	All have some risk for psychological dependency and abuse.
Skelaxin	
Orphenadrine	
Banflex	
Flexoject	
Myolin	
Diazepam	
Valium	
Rival	
Epam✚	
Carisoprodol	
Soma	
Vanadom	

➤ Diet Therapy

A high-calcium diet is indicated for clients with mild hypocalcemia and for those with chronic conditions that cause them to be at continuous risk for hypocalcemia. The nurse consults with the dietitian to assist the client in selecting calcium-rich foods. Common sources of calcium are listed in Table 14–8.

➤ Reduction of Environmental Stimuli

The excitable membranes of both the nervous and the skeletal systems are overstimulated in hypocalcemia. The

nurse, therefore, provides an environment that reduces extraneous stimulation of these systems.

➤ Prevention of Injury

The nurse places the client on seizure precautions, which include padding the side rails of the bed and keeping emergency equipment, such as oxygen and suction, at the bedside. An emergency cart equipped with emergency drugs and an endotracheal tray is positioned just outside the client's room.

The client with long-standing calcium loss may have brittle, fragile bones that fracture at only slight provocation and cause little pain. When lifting or moving a client with fragile bones, the nurse and assistive personnel use a lift sheet rather than pull or grasp the client directly. The nurse also observes the client for any unusual surface projections or depressions over bony areas as well as for normal range of joint motion.

Hypercalcemia

Overview

Hypercalcemia occurs when the total serum calcium level exceeds 10 mg/dL or 2.5 mmol/L. Because the normal range for serum calcium is extremely narrow, even small increases can have severe effects on body function. Although the effects of hypercalcemia are most noticeable in body systems that depend on cell excitability, all body systems are affected to some degree.

Pathophysiology

Hypercalcemia indicates either that the amount of serum calcium is so great that the normal calcium-regulating mechanisms are overburdened or that at least one calcium-regulating mechanism is not functioning properly. Because extracellular calcium ions function as stabilizers of excitable cell membranes, hypercalcemia causes excitable tissues to be less sensitive to normal stimuli and require a stronger stimulus to function. Excitable tissues that demonstrate obvious and serious immediate responses to hypercalcemia are cardiac muscle tissue, nerve tissue, skeletal muscle, and gastrointestinal smooth muscle.

Calcium is also a critical cofactor for many of the enzymes involved in the blood-clotting process. Hypercalcemia usually results in faster clotting times. This condition may cause clots to form at inappropriate times and places. Excessive clotting related to hypercalcemia is more likely in vessels or organs in which blood flow is slow or blocked.

Etiology

Underlying causes of hypercalcemia include increased absorption of calcium, decreased excretion of calcium, and increased bone resorption of calcium (Table 16–6).

Collaborative Management

 Assessment

Clinical manifestations of hypercalcemia are related to both the severity of the imbalance and how quickly the imbalance occurred. The client with mild excess of serum calcium level that occurred rapidly usually experiences more severe signs and symptoms than the client whose hypercalcemic state is severe but developed slowly. The clinical manifestations of hypercalcemia are primarily associated with alterations of excitable membrane activity (Chart 16–9). Thus, the body systems most affected by hypercalcemia include the cardiovascular, neuromuscular, gastrointestinal, and renal–urinary systems.

TABLE 16–6

Common Causes of Hypercalcemia

Actual Calcium Excesses

Increased Calcium Absorption

- Excessive oral intake of calcium
- Excessive oral intake of vitamin D

Decreased Calcium Excretion

- Renal failure
- Use of thiazide diuretics

Relative Calcium Excesses

Increased Bone Resorption of Calcium

- Hyperparathyroidism
- Malignancy
  - Direct invasion (cancers of breast, lung, prostate, and osteoclastic bone and multiple myeloma)
  - Indirect resorption (liver cancer, small cell lung cancer, and cancer of the adrenal gland)
- Hyperthyroidism
- Immobility
- Use of glucocorticoids

Hemoconcentration

- Dehydration
- Use of lithium
- Adrenal insufficiency

➤ Cardiovascular Manifestations

The most serious and life-threatening clinical manifestations of hypercalcemia involve alterations in cardiac function. Mild hypercalcemia initially causes increased heart rate and blood pressure. Severe or prolonged hypercalcemia affects electrical conduction.

The nurse assesses cardiac status by measuring pulse and blood pressure and observing for indications of inadequate tissue perfusion such as cyanosis and pallor. The nurse also observes ECG tracings for indications of dysrhythmias, especially a shortened QT interval.

Although hypercalcemia does not directly cause formation of blood clots, increased calcium levels produce clot formation more easily whenever abnormal conditions are present. Thus, the client with hypercalcemia may be at an increased risk for clot formation in locations where blood vessel or tissue damage have occurred and in vessels or organs in which blood flow is blocked. Blood clotting is more likely in the lower legs, the pelvic region, areas where blood flow is blocked by internal or external constrictions, and regions where internal blood vessel obstruction occurs.

The nurse assesses each client at risk for hypercalcemia for indications of slowed or impaired blood flow. Calf circumferences are measured with a soft tape measure and recorded. The nurse asks the client to alternately dorsiflex and plantar flex the ankles and state whether calf pain occurs in either position. The nurse assesses the lower legs for temperature, color, and capillary refill to determine the adequacy of blood flow to and from the area.

Chart 16-9

Key Features of Hypercalcemia

Cardiovascular
- Increased heart rate (early phase)
- Increased blood pressure
- Bounding, full peripheral pulses
- Electrocardiographic abnormalities
  - Shortened ST segment
  - Widened T wave
- Potentiation of digitalis-associated toxicities
- Decreased clotting time
- Late phase
  - Bradycardia
  - Cardiac arrest, sinus arrest

Respiratory
- Ineffective respiratory movement related to profound skeletal muscle weakness

Neuromuscular
- Disorientation, lethargy, coma
- Profound muscle weakness
- Diminished or absent deep tendon reflexes

Renal
- Increased urinary output
- Dehydration
- Formation of renal calculi

Gastrointestinal
- Decreased motility
- Hypoactive bowel sounds
- Anorexia, nausea
- Abdominal distention
- Constipation

➤ Neuromuscular Manifestations

The neuromuscular manifestations of hypercalcemia include severe muscle weakness without accompanying paresthesia and greatly diminished deep tendon reflexes. Central nervous system manifestations include altered level of consciousness ranging from disorientation and lethargy to coma.

➤ Gastrointestinal Manifestations

Decreased peristalsis is an early manifestation of hypercalcemia. The nurse assesses the gastrointestinal tract by auscultating for bowel sounds in all four abdominal quadrants. Bowel sounds are hypoactive or absent. The abdomen increases in size because intestinal contents remain in the gastrointestinal tract instead of being propelled to the outside. The nurse assesses abdominal size by measuring abdominal girth with a soft tape measure in a line circling the abdomen at the level of the umbilicus. The client may report constipation, anorexia, nausea, vomiting, and abdominal pain.

➤ Renal Manifestations

Hypercalcemia causes increased urinary output and leads to serious dehydration. Chronic hypercalcemia results in the formation of renal calculi (stones) in the kidney tubular system, because the excessive calcium precipitates out of solution in a solid form. The nurse or assistive personnel measures intake and output, assesses voided urine for blood or cloudiness, and strains the urine for the presence of renal calculi.

Interventions

Interventions for hypercalcemia aim to prevent further increases in serum calcium levels and decrease excessive serum calcium levels through drug therapy and dialysis.

➤ Drug Therapy

Drug therapy for the treatment of hypercalcemia restores normal calcium balance by preventing additional calcium administration and promoting calcium excretion. IV infusions of solutions containing calcium are stopped. In addition, administration of oral drugs containing calcium or vitamin D, such as calcium-based antacids, is discontinued.

Fluid volume replacement alone can help restore normal serum calcium levels. The physician usually orders IV normal saline (isotonic sodium chloride) because it does not contain calcium.

Thiazide diuretic administration is discontinued for clients with hypercalcemia. Diuretics that enhance the excretion of calcium such as furosemide (Lasix, Furoside♣) are prescribed instead.

Agents that act as calcium chelators (calcium binders) can be useful in lowering serum calcium levels. Such drugs include plicamycin (Mithracin) and penicillamine (Cuprimine, Pendramine♣).

Other drugs that may be useful in treating hypercalcemia include agents that inhibit calcium resorption from bone, such as phosphorus, calcitonin (Calcimar), bisphosphonates (etidronate), and prostaglandin synthesis inhibitors (aspirin, nonsteroidal anti-inflammatory drugs).

➤ Dialysis

In severe hypercalcemia that causes life-threatening cardiac problems, drug therapy may not reduce serum calcium levels quickly enough to prevent death. Dialysis (either hemodialysis or peritoneal dialysis) or blood ultrafiltration may be necessary.

➤ Cardiac Monitoring

Clients with hypercalcemia usually undergo continuous cardiac monitoring to identify possible dysrhythmias and decreased cardiac output. The nurse compares recently obtained ECG tracings with the client's baseline tracings or those obtained when the client's serum calcium level was normal. The nurse observes the ECG for changes in the T waves and the QT interval as well as changes in rate and rhythm.

PHOSPHORUS IMBALANCES

Hypophosphatemia

Overview

Hypophosphatemia is a serum phosphorus level below 2.7 mg/dL. Even though the serum concentration of phosphorus has a narrow range of normal values (2.7–4.5 mg/dL), body functions are not significantly impaired as a result of rapid, wide changes in serum phosphorus levels. Alterations in function are more obvious when hypophosphatemia is chronic.

Pathophysiology

Most of the pathophysiologic effects of hypophosphatemia are related to decreased energy metabolism and altered levels of other electrolytes and body fluids. Because of the reciprocal relationship between phosphorus and calcium, decreases in serum phosphorus levels are accompanied by increases in serum calcium levels.

Etiology

Three main processes underlie decreased serum phosphorus levels: decreased absorption of phosphorus, increased excretion of phosphorus, and intracellular phosphorus shift (Table 16–7).

Collaborative Management

 Assessment

Clinical manifestations of hypophosphatemia occur when the decrease in serum phosphorus levels is severe or pro-

---

TABLE 16–7

Common Causes of Phosphorus Imbalance

Hypophosphatemia

Insufficient Phosphorus Intake
- Malnutrition
- Starvation
- Use of aluminum hydroxide–based antacids
- Use of magnesium-based antacids

Increased Phosphorus Excretion
- Hyperparathyroidism
- Hypocalcemia
- Renal failure
- Malignancy

Intracellular Shift
- Hyperglycemia
- Hyperalimentation
- Respiratory alkalosis

Hyperphosphatemia
- Decreased renal excretion resulting from renal insufficiency
- Tumor lysis syndrome
- Increased intake of phosphorus
- Hypoparathyroidism

Chart 16–10

Key Features of Hypophosphatemia

Cardiovascular
- Decreased contractility
- Cardiomyopathy (reversible)

Respiratory
- Shallow respirations

Musculoskeletal
- Weakness
- Rhabdomyolysis
- Decreased deep tendon reflexes

Central Nervous
- Irritability
- Confusion
- Seizures

Hematologic
- Increased bleeding
- Decreased platelet aggregation
- Immunosuppression

---

longed. Acute manifestations of hypophosphatemia are related to the decreased availability of high-energy compounds (such as adenosine triphosphate [ATP]) necessary to perform normal cellular metabolic functions. These clinical manifestations include alterations in cardiac, musculoskeletal, hematologic, and central nervous system functions (Chart 16–10).

➤ *Cardiovascular Manifestations*

The cardiac manifestations of hypophosphatemia include decreased stroke volume and decreased cardiac output. Peripheral pulses are slow, difficult to find, and easy to block. Myocardial depression is caused by low intracellular energy stores. Without sufficient quantities of energy in myocardial cells, contractions are weak and ineffective. Prolonged hypophosphatemia can lead to progressive, but reversible, myocardial damage.

➤ *Musculoskeletal Manifestations*

The mechanism of hypophosphatemia that weakens cardiac muscles also appears to be responsible for weakening skeletal muscles. The weakness is generalized, and paresthesias usually are not present. When the skeletal muscle weakness becomes profound, respiratory movements are ineffective, which can lead to respiratory failure. The nurse assesses for muscle strength and observes respiratory ability.

The clinical manifestations of chronic hypophosphatemia are most evident in the skeletal system. Bone density is decreased, possibly causing fractures and alterations in bone shape. These changes result from the calcium resorption that often accompanies hypophosphatemia. The nurse assesses the client for unusual lumps, projections, or depressions over bony areas indicating fracture of demineralized bone.

➤ *Central Nervous System Manifestations*

Central nervous system manifestations are not apparent until hypophosphatemia is severe. These first appear as increased irritability and may progress to seizure activity followed by coma.

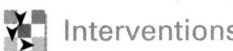 ## Interventions

➤ *Drug Therapy*

Administration of drugs that contribute to the development of hypophosphatemia, such as antacids, osmotic diuretics, and calcium supplements, is discontinued. Generally, oral replacement of phosphorus along with a vitamin D supplement is sufficient to correct hypophosphatemia. IV phosphorus administration is initiated only when serum phosphorus levels fall below 1 mg/dL and the client has serious clinical manifestations. IV phosphorus is administered slowly because problems associated with hyperphosphatemia are equally serious.

➤ *Diet Therapy*

Diet therapy for hypophosphatemia consists primarily of increasing the intake of phosphorus-rich foods while decreasing the intake of calcium-rich foods (Chart 16–11).

Hyperphosphatemia

Overview

Hyperphosphatemia occurs when the serum phosphorus level exceeds 4.5 mg/dL. Elevated serum phosphorus levels above normal are tolerated well by most body systems.

The health problems associated with hyperphosphatemia center on the hypocalcemia that results when serum phosphorus levels increase. These problems include increased sensitivity of excitable membranes to the extent that they may depolarize spontaneously and inappropriately.

Underlying causes of increased serum phosphorus levels include renal insufficiency, some cancer treatments,

increased phosphorus intake, and hypoparathyroidism. Table 16–7 lists specific common causes of hyperphosphatemia.

Collaborative Management

Hyperphosphatemia produces few direct problems with body function. However, hypocalcemia is usually present as well because the calcium and phosphorus ions exist in the blood in a balanced reciprocal relationship: when one increases, the other decreases. The accompanying hypocalcemia dramatically alters the physiologic functioning of many body systems and has the potential for causing serious and life-threatening side effects. Thus, the management of hyperphosphatemia entails the management of hypocalcemia.

MAGNESIUM IMBALANCES

Hypomagnesemia

Overview

Hypomagnesemia occurs when the serum magnesium (Mg^{2+}) level decreases below 1.6 mg/dL. Because most conditions resulting in hypomagnesemia are related either to decreased magnesium intake or to increased magnesium loss, measurable hypomagnesemia reflects a decrease in total body magnesium concentration.

The direct pathophysiologic effects of hypomagnesemia are related to alterations in the function of excitable membranes and accompanying imbalances of serum calcium and potassium. These problems include increased sensitivity of excitable membranes, especially nerve cell membranes, to the extent that they may depolarize spontaneously and inappropriately.

Hypomagnesemia results from either decreased absorption of dietary magnesium or increased renal excretion of magnesium. Table 16–8 lists specific causes of hypomagnesemia.

Collaborative Management

 ## Assessment

Most clinical manifestations of hypomagnesemia result from alterations in the activity of excitable cell membranes. The most common manifestations are seen in the neuromuscular, central nervous, and gastrointestinal systems (Chart 16–12).

➤ *Neuromuscular Manifestations*

The neuromuscular manifestations of hypomagnesemia result from increased nerve impulse transmission at some synaptic areas. Normally, magnesium inhibits the release of the neurotransmitter acetylcholine from the presynaptic cell. Decreased magnesium levels allow greater release of acetylcholine, which increases the transmission of impulses from nerve to nerve or from nerve to skeletal muscle. The client with hypomagnesemia has hyperactive deep tendon reflexes (+4) accompanied by painful paresthesia (numbness and tingling) and tetanic muscle contractions. Positive Chvostek's and Trousseau's signs may

---

Chart 16–11

Education Guide: Dietary Management of Hypophosphatemia

You Should Avoid	You May Eat
• Milk	• Fish
• Cheese	• Beef
• Yogurt	• Chicken
• Collard greens	• Pork
• Rhubarb	• Organ meats
	• Nuts
	• Whole-grain breads and cereals

TABLE 16–8

Common Causes of Magnesium Imbalance

Hypomagnesemia

Insufficient Magnesium Intake

- Malnutrition
- Starvation
- Diarrhea
- Steatorrhea
- Celiac disease
- Crohn's disease

Increased Magnesium Excretion

- Drugs (diuretics, aminoglycoside antibiotics, cisplatin, amphotericin B, cyclosporine)
- Citrate (blood products)
- Ethanol ingestion

Intracellular Movement of Magnesium

- Hyperglycemia
- Insulin administration
- Sepsis
- Alkalosis

Hypermagnesemia

- Increased magnesium intake
  - Magnesium-containing antacids and laxatives
  - Intravenous magnesium replacement
- Decreased renal excretion of magnesium resulting from renal insufficiency

be present because hypomagnesemia may be accompanied by hypocalcemia (see prior discussion of these assessment signs under Hypocalcemia). Skeletal muscle weakness may be present if intracellular magnesium levels are also decreased in an attempt to restore normal magnesium balance. As hypomagnesemia progresses, the client may experience tetany and seizures.

► Central Nervous System Manifestations

The central nervous system manifestations of hypomagnesemia are related to a general increase in the transmission of nerve impulses. Increased central nervous system irritability may manifest as psychological depression, psychosis, and confusion.

► Gastrointestinal Manifestations

Gastrointestinal manifestations are associated with decreased contractility of intestinal smooth muscle. Clients have decreased gastric motility with anorexia, nausea, and abdominal distention. If the hypomagnesemia is severe, a paralytic ileus may occur.

 Interventions

Interventions for hypomagnesemia aim to correct the electrolyte imbalance and manage the specific condition that caused the hypomagnesemia. In addition, because hypocalcemia frequently accompanies hypomagnesemia, some

interventions also aim to restore normal serum calcium levels.

► Drug Therapy

The administration of drugs that contribute to the development of hypomagnesemia, such as high-ceiling (loop) diuretics, osmotic diuretics, aminoglycosides, and drugs containing phosphorus, is discontinued. Magnesium is replaced IV in the form of magnesium sulfate ($MgSO_4$) when hypomagnesemia is severe. The IV route is used because $MgSO_4$ causes pain and tissue damage when injected intramuscularly. Oral preparations of magnesium frequently cause diarrhea and increase magnesium loss. If hypocalcemia is also present, the physician prescribes drug therapy to increase serum calcium concentration.

► Diet Therapy

Diet therapy for hypomagnesemia consists of increasing the intake of foods that contain high concentrations of magnesium (see Table 14–11).

Chart 16–12

Key Features of Hypomagnesemia

Cardiovascular

- Electrocardiographic changes
  - Tall T waves
  - Depressed ST segments
- Dysrhythmias
  - Ectopic beats
  - Ventricular tachycardia
  - Ventricular fibrillation
- Hypertension

Gastrointestinal

- Decreased motility
- Anorexia
- Nausea
- Abdominal distention
- Decreased bowel sounds

Respiratory

- Shallow respirations

Neuromuscular

- Fasciculations
- Twitches
- Paresthesias
- Positive Trousseau's sign
- Positive Chvostek's sign
- Hyperreflexia
- Tetany
- Seizures

Central Nervous

- Irritability
- Confusion
- Psychosis

Hypermagnesemia

Overview

Hypermagnesemia occurs when the serum magnesium level exceeds 2.6 mg/dL. Magnesium is a membrane stabilizer. When excesses of magnesium occur, excitable membranes require a stronger-than-normal stimulus to respond and thus are less sensitive or less excitable. If hypermagnesemia is severe, excitable membranes may not respond to any stimulus.

Hypermagnesemia results from increased intake of magnesium coupled with decreased renal excretion of magnesium. Table 16–8 lists specific causes of hypermagnesemia.

Collaborative Management

 Assessment

Most clinical manifestations of hypermagnesemia occur as a result of alterations in the activity of excitable cell membranes. Usually, manifestations are not apparent until serum magnesium levels exceed 4 mg/dL. The most common manifestations are seen in the cardiac, central nervous, and neuromuscular systems.

➤ *Cardiovascular Manifestations*

Cardiac manifestations of hypermagnesemia are related to bradycardia, peripheral vasodilation, and hypotension. These become more severe as serum magnesium concentration increases. ECG changes include a prolonged PR interval with a widened QRS complex. Bradycardia can be severe; cardiac arrest is possible during diastole of the cardiac cycle. Hypotension with a wide pulse pressure is also severe; the diastolic pressure is much lower than normal. Clients with severe hypermagnesemia are in grave danger of cardiac arrest.

➤ *Central Nervous System Manifestations*

Central nervous system manifestations of hypermagnesemia are related to depressed transmission of nerve impulses at specific synaptic points. Clients may be drowsy to the point of lethargy. Coma may occur if the hypermagnesemia is prolonged or becomes severe.

➤ *Neuromuscular Manifestations*

Neuromuscular manifestations of hypermagnesemia are related to decreased transmission of impulses from nerves to skeletal muscles. Deep tendon reflexes are greatly diminished or even absent. Voluntary skeletal muscle contractions become progressively weaker and finally stop.

➤ *Respiratory Manifestations*

Hypermagnesemia has no direct effect on the organs of respiration. However, when the skeletal muscles of respiration are involved, respiratory insufficiency may occur, leading to respiratory failure and death from anoxia.

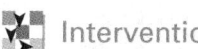 Interventions

Interventions for hypermagnesemia aim to reduce the serum magnesium level and correct the underlying pathologic change that initiated or contributed to the development of hypermagnesemia.

➤ *Drug Therapy*

All oral and parenteral administration of magnesium is discontinued. When renal failure is not a contributing factor, administration of magnesium-free IV fluids can assist in reducing serum magnesium levels. Administration of high-ceiling (loop) diuretics such as furosemide (Lasix, Furoside✦) can further reduce serum magnesium levels. When cardiac manifestations are severe, administration of calcium may reverse the cardiac effects of hypermagnesemia.

➤ *Diet Therapy*

Diet therapy is most effective in preventing hypermagnesemia when other chronic pathologic conditions predispose the client to the development of excess serum magnesium levels. Dietary restrictions involve limiting the ingestion of meat, nuts, legumes, fish, vegetables, and whole-grain cereal products.

 CASE STUDY for the Client with Hypokalemia

■ An 89-year-old woman is one of your nursing home residents. She has a history of myocardial infarction, congestive heart failure, and adult-onset diabetes mellitus. Her medication orders include Lasix, 80 mg qd, Digoxin, 0.125 mg qd, potassium chloride, 40 mEq qd, and Orinase, 500 mg.

Today the resident seems confused when you bring her morning medications. She says she feels "sick to her stomach" and does not want breakfast. The nursing assistant reports that the client's pulse is weak and slightly irregular at 62 bpm and her blood pressure is 102/68 mm Hg.

QUESTIONS:

1. When taking a history from this resident, what important questions should you ask?
2. What additional physical assessment techniques would you perform?
3. During respiratory assessment, you find that the client's respirations are rapid and shallow. Breath sounds are present in both lungs with no crackles or wheezes audible on auscultation. Given these assessment findings, what should you do first?

SELECTED BIBLIOGRAPHY

Anderson, S. (1996). Fluid and electrolyte disorders in the elderly. In J. Kokko & R. Tannen (Eds.), *Fluids and electrolytes* (3rd ed., pp. 831–839). Philadelphia: W. B. Saunders.

Ayus, J. C., & Arieff, A. (1996). Brain damage and postoperative hypo-natremia: The role of gender. *Neurology, 46*(2), 323–328.

Bove, L. (1996). Restoring electrolyte balance: Calcium and phosphorus. *RN, 59*(3), 47–52.

Bove, L. (1996). Restoring electrolyte balance: Sodium & chloride. *RN, 59*(1), 25–29.

Braxmeyer, D., & Keyes, J. (1996). The pathophysiology of potassium balance. *Critical Care Nurse, 16*(5), 59–71.

Bryce, J. (1994). S.I.A.D.H. *Nursing94, 24*(4), 33.

*Chenevey, B. (1987). Overview of fluids and electrolytes. *Nursing Clinics of North America, 22*(4), 749.

Dennis, V. (1996). Phosphate disorders. In J. Kokko & R. Tannen (Eds.), *Fluids and electrolytes* (3rd ed., pp. 359–390). Philadelphia: W. B. Saunders.

Ellis, S. (1995). Severe hyponatremia: Complications and treatment. *Quarterly Journal of Medicine, 88*(12), 905–909.

Fenves, A., Thomas, S., & Knochel, J. (1996). Beer potomania: Two cases and review of the literature. *Clinical Nephrology, 45*(1), 61–64.

Ferrin, M. (1996). Restoring electrolyte balance: Magnesium. *RN, 59*(5), 31–34.

Guyton, A., & Hall, J. (1996). *Textbook of medical physiology* (9th ed.). Philadelphia: W. B. Saunders.

Halperin, M., & Goldstein, M. (1994), *Fluid, electrolyte and acid-base physiology: A problem-based approach* (2nd ed.). Philadelphia: W. B. Saunders.

Held, J. (1995). Correcting fluid and electrolyte imbalances. *Nursing95, 25*(4), 71.

Kaplan, R. (1994). Hypercalcemia of malignancy. *Oncology Nursing Forum, 21*(6), 1039–1046.

Kokko, J., & Tannen, R. (1996). *Fluids and electrolytes* (3rd ed.). Philadelphia: W. B. Saunders.

Kuhn, M. (1996). Laboratory analysis. *Critical Care Nurse, 16*(5), 74–76.

Kumar, R. (1996). Calcium disorders. In J. Kokko & R. Tannen (Eds.), *Fluids and electrolytes* (3rd ed., pp. 391–419). Philadelphia: W. B. Saunders.

McConnell, E. (1994). What's wrong with this patient? *Nursing94, 24*(5), 92–93.

McConnell, E. (1995). What's wrong with this patient? *Nursing95, 24*(4), 73–74.

*Mendyka, B. (1992). Fluid and electrolyte disorders caused by diuretic therapy. *AACN Clinical Issues in Critical Care Nursing, 3*(3), 672–680.

Metheny, N. (1996). *Fluid and electrolyte balance: Nursing considerations* (3rd ed.). Philadelphia: J. B. Lippincott.

Miller, C. (1995). Medications that may cause cognitive impairment in older adults. *Geriatric Nursing, 16*(1), 47.

Norris, M. K. (1994). Checking chloride levels. *Nursing94, 24*(3), 76.

O'Donnell, M. (1995). Assessing fluid and electrolyte balance needs in elders. *American Journal of Nursing, 95*(1), 40–46.

Rude, R. (1996). Magnesium disorders. In J. Kokko & R. Tannen (Eds.), *Fluids and electrolytes* (3rd ed., pp. 421–445). Philadelphia: W. B. Saunders.

Sica, D. (1994). Renal disease, electrolyte abnormalities, and acid-base imbalance in the elderly. *Clinics in Geriatric Medicine, 10*(1), 197–211.

Tannen, R. (1996). Potassium disorders. In J. Kokko & R. Tannen (Eds.), *Fluids and electrolytes* (3rd ed., pp. 111–199). Philadelphia: W. B. Saunders.

Tietz, N. W. (Ed.). (1995). *Clinical guide to laboratory tests* (3rd ed.). Philadelphia: W. B. Saunders.

Toto, K., & Yucha, C. (1994). Magnesium: Homeostasis, imbalances, and therapeutic uses. *Critical Care Nursing Clinics of North America, 6*(4), 767–783.

Trissel, L. (1994). *Handbook on injectable drugs* (8th ed.). Bethesda, MD: American Society of Hospital Pharmacists.

Vonfrolio, L. (1995). Would you hang these IV solutions? *American Journal of Nursing, 95*(4), 37–39.

Yucha, C., & Toto, K. (1994). Calcium and phosphorus derangements. *Critical Care Nursing Clinics of North America, 6*(4), 747–766.

Zelingher, J., Putterman, C., Ilan, Y., Dann, E., Zveibil, F., Shvil, Y., & Galun, E. (1996). Case series: Hyponatremia associated with moderate exercise. *American Journal of the Medical Sciences, 311*(2), 86–91.

SUGGESTED READINGS

Braxmeyer, D., & Keyes, J. (1996). The pathophysiology of potassium balance. *Critical Care Nurse, 16*(5), 59–71.
This outstanding article presents potassium physiology, deficits, and excesses in a comprehensive, yet user-friendly manner. The article is enhanced by flow charts, clear discussions of nursing actions and implications, and associated self-assessment questions.

Mendyka, B. (1992). Fluid and electrolyte disorders caused by diuretic therapy. *AACN Clinical Issues in Critical Care Nursing, 3*(3), 672–680.
This article presents in text and tables the mechanisms of action and electrolyte effects of the major diuretic categories. Normal nephron function is reviewed. Nursing care considerations for specific electrolyte disturbances are summarized.

O'Donnell, M. (1995). Assessing fluid and electrolyte balance needs in elders. *American Journal of Nursing, 95*(1), 40–46.
The author describes physical and behavioral characteristics of geriatric clients that place them at risk for electrolyte imbalances, using a case study approach. An assessment checklist for elders with nutritional deficits is included.

INFUSION THERAPY

The term "infusion therapy" refers to a wide variety of techniques and procedures health care professionals utilize to deliver parenteral medications and fluids to their clients. The delivery of these medications and fluids may be into clients' vascular systems, such as in intravenous therapy or arterial therapy. Some clients require administration of fluids and medications into their tissue (subcutaneous therapy) or into their epidural or intrathecal spaces as in central nervous system therapies. Infusion of fluids or medications into a client's body cavity is intraperitoneal therapy; into a client's bones is intraosseous therapy.

INTRODUCTION TO INFUSION THERAPY

Approximately 90% of hospitalized clients receive some type of infusion therapy. Health care providers prescribe infusion therapy for their clients for a variety of reasons or therapeutic goals, including maintenance, replacement, treatment, diagnosis, monitoring, palliation, or a combination of these.

Not long ago, most clients received their infusion therapies as inpatients in acute care facilities. With the advent of computerized ambulatory and implantable infusion control devices, as well as long-term infusion access devices, clients now receive infusion therapy in virtually any setting—from their homes to long-term care facilities.

Some agencies have specialized teams that focus on all of the procedures associated with infusion therapy. These infusion or intravenous (IV) teams develop infusion policies and procedures, initiate peripheral intravenous and peripherally inserted central catheters, administer parenteral fluids and medications, administer parenteral nutrition and blood products, maintain infusion devices, provide input to agency purchasing departments regarding infusion devices and equipment, monitor infusion-related complications, provide consultation to health care providers and clients regarding device selection and placement, and engage in quality improvement activities.

The continued use of IV teams in health care settings is a controversial issue. In this time of "downsizing," "rightsizing," and "re-engineering," many agencies have disbanded their IV teams, leaving these responsibilities to nurse generalists or unlicensed technicians. The Veteran's Affairs Medical Center in Pittsburgh, Pennsylvania, however, founded its IV team in 1992. As a result of its IV team, the hospital reported a decrease in IV-related bacteremia to 1.5 per 1000 patient discharges from 4.6 per 1000 client discharges on the medical-surgical units of its 330-bed acute care facility. In the critical care areas, where house staff and general staff nurses continued to care for IV lines, there was no change in the rate of IV-related bacteremia. The study demonstrated a significant decrease in morbidity and mortality in the medical surgical clients at this institution, and the authors estimate that the IV team saved $124,906 during the year, considering the decrease in the treatment of bacteremias (Miller et al., 1996).

The Intravenous Nurses Society (INS), the professional nursing organization for infusion therapy nurses, publishes standards of care that provide the basis for the practice of infusion nursing. Its affiliate organization, the Intravenous Nurses Certification Corporation (INCC), offers a written certifying examination. Nurses who successfully complete this examination may use the initials "CRNI," which stand for "certified registered nurse infusion." The INS is currently the only organization offering certification in infusion therapy. Many agencies offer basic and advanced instruction in infusion therapy.

INFUSION SYSTEMS

Nurses administering infusion therapies need to understand the way in which infusion systems work. This knowledge ensures that the nurse can optimize a particular system's advantages while minimizing any potential complications.

Containers

Infusion containers are generally made of glass or plastic. Each of these systems has advantages as well as disadvantages (Table 17–1).

Glass infusion systems are of two types—the separate airway design and the integral airway system. The separate airway design has a plastic tube or "straw" attached to the inside of the thick, hard cork-type stopper. This tube extends almost the entire length of the bottle to above the fluid level of a full bottle. Unfiltered air enters through the straw and exerts pressure on the surface of the fluid, allowing the fluid to pass through the administration set. The integral airway design glass system is also an "open" system. In this system, air enters through a

side port filter on the administration set. This type of set is often referred to as "vented" tubing.

Plastic containers may be soft and totally collapsible or semirigid. Both of these systems are considered "closed" systems as they do not rely on outside air to allow the fluid to infuse. Instead, atmospheric pressure pushes against the flexible sides of the container, allowing the fluid to flow by gravity. For this reason, plastic containers use "nonvented" or "unvented" tubing.

The totally collapsible variety of plastic containers is usually made of PVC (polyvinyl chloride). Some PVC materials cause container-medication compatibility problems with nitroglycerin, insulin, and fat emulsions. Nitroglycerin and insulin adhere to the walls of the PVC container, making it impossible to know exactly how much medication the client is receiving. Fat emulsions leach the plasticizer diethylhexylphthalate (DEHP), a component of some PVC containers, thereby unintentionally making this substance part of the client's infusion.

Although they are plastic, semirigid containers do not have the same compatibility problems associated with containers made of PVC. This container, as its name indicates, is less flexible than totally collapsible plastic containers.

Administration Sets

The administration set is the connection between the client's access device and the solution container. Numerous administration sets are available in many different configurations. The type and purpose of the infusion assists in determining the type of administration set the nurse should choose. Many sets are generic, meaning that they are appropriate for most infusions. Some sets are specialty sets to be used for specific types of infusions; still other sets are dedicated, meaning that they must be used with a specific manufacturer's infusion control device. Nurses

TABLE 17–1

Advantages and Disadvantages of Infusion Containers		
Container Type	**Advantages**	**Disadvantages**
Glass	Able to withstand trauma and varying pressures during sterilization process	Difficult to see small cracks, which alter the integrity of the system
	Clarity allows the nurse to inspect the container for any particulate matter	Rigid sides make storage and disposal bulky
	Rigid sides allow nurse to accurately determine the container's volume	Requires a source of air to allow fluid to drip, thereby making it an "open" system
	Glass is an inert product and will not react with solutions or medications	
Plastic	Not likely to break when dropped or bumped	Not clear, making it difficult to visualize particulate matter
	Some designs may be stored on top of one another for ease	May be pierced by needle when making additions to the bag
	Because they collapse when empty, disposal is easier and less bulky than glass	Difficult to accurately measure volumes because sides collapse as the bag empties
	Able to withstand freezing and thawing	Compatibility problems with some medications
	Can be manufactured to hold any volume and still be manageable for most nurses	

From Booker, M. F., & Ignatavicius, D. D. (1996). *Infusion therapy: Techniques and medications.* Philadelphia: W. B. Saunders.

can usually find information on the packaging that describes the proper use of the administration set inside. Table 17–2 and Charts 17–1 and 17–2 describe some of the standard and miscellaneous components of administration sets and the factors determining their use.

Filters remove particulate matter suspended in the infusion solution while allowing the fluid to pass through to the client. The nurse may see filters of two types: membrane filters and depth filters. Either of these filters may be "in-line" (an integral part of the administration set) or "add-on" (a filter set that is separate and must be added to the administration set).

A membrane filter has tiny pores or holes sized to prevent the passage of particles into the filter. These pores capture any particles that may be in the solution and trap them on the surface of the filter. One problem associated with membrane filters is that they are prone to "loading," a phenomenon that occurs when the filter's surface is completely coated with particulate matter, rendering it inoperable and therefore of no value. It is for this reason that membrane filters are best suited as final filters rather than the primary or singular filtering mechanism.

A depth filter has a maze-like configuration. Any particles suspended in the fluid pass through the surface and become trapped in the multitude of passages as they travel through the labyrinth. Additionally, depth filters also have adsorption properties that cause any particles to adhere to the filter material itself. The size of the particle does not influence the adsorption of the filter material.

Both membrane and depth filters are rated by the size

Chart 17–1
Nursing Care Highlight: Piggybacking an Intermittent Medication

1. Verify the order from the health care provider.
2. Check the compatibility between the medication and the large-volume parenteral (LVP) and its additives.
3. Spike the medication mini-bag with the secondary set.
4. Prime the secondary set, close the roller clamp, and hang the mini-bag on the other arm of the intravenous (IV) pole.
5. Place the hanger that comes with the secondary set on the IV pole with the LVP.
6. Cleanse the lowest "Y-site" injection port on the LVP administration set.
7. Attach the secondary set to the "Y-site."
8. Lower the level of the LVP by hanging it from the hanger. Do not adjust the LVP roller clamp. (The rate will decrease and then stop when the secondary set is opened.)
9. Open the roller clamp on the secondary set and regulate the flow to the desired rate.
10. When the intermittent infusion completes, the LVP will automatically begin again. Hang the LVP from the IV pole and adjust the roller clamp to deliver the prescribed rate.

Chart 17–2
Nursing Care Highlight: How to Use a Burette

1. To fill the burette, close the main clamp below the burette.
2. Open the clamp between the solution container and the burette, allowing the fluid to flow into the burette.
3. When the burette contains the amount of fluid desired, close the clamp between the solution container and the burette.
4. If using the burette for administration of intermittent medications, add the prescribed medication now and gently swirl the burette.
5. Regulate the rate of the infusion from the burette with the lower clamp.

---

of the smallest particles they hold back. A 0.22-micron filter retains any particles 0.22 micron and larger. These particles may be particulate matter or organisms such as *Escherichia coli* and *Pseudomonas.*

Needleless Systems

In July 1992, the Occupational Safety and Health Administration published its guidelines entitled *Occupational Exposure to Bloodborne Pathogens, Final Rule.* This document requires health care organizations to initiate engineering controls "that isolate or remove the bloodborne pathogen hazard from the workplace." Currently, there are a number of products available and more entering the market every day designed to minimize health care workers' exposure to contaminated needles. Some of these products include devices that use blunt metal cannulae or needles recessed into a plastic housing; others use a blunt plastic cannula, and still others include valves. It is estimated that needleless systems can eliminate up to 80% of the traditional metal needles used in a hospital setting (Beason et al., 1993). Figure 17–1 displays some of the common needleless systems currently available.

Infusion Regulation Devices

The ability to regulate the rate and volume of infusions is critical to the safe and accurate administration of medications and fluids to clients. Nurses have a choice of numerous devices designed to regulate infusions. Most are classified as either controllers or pumps and require either AC (alternating current) or a battery as a power source.

Nurses and clients who use infusion pumps and controllers reap the benefits of some of the latest computer technology. Infusion regulation devices can save nursing time and prevent runaway infusions, as well as reduce the incidence of infiltration and keep infusion access devices patent. However, the nurse must remember that the use of these devices does not decrease the practitioner's responsibility to carefully monitor the client's infusion site and the infusion rate.

Not every regulation device is appropriate for every

TABLE 17–2

Components of Administration Sets

Component	Description or Characteristics	Purpose or Function
Standard Components		
Spike	Hard plastic tube with a sharp point; plastic cover or sheath over spike must be removed before use	Sharp point penetrates the solution container; sheath maintains sterility of spike
Shield	Hard plastic disk below the spike	Prevents the nurse's hands from slipping onto the spike when inserting it into the fluid container
Drip chamber	Plastic tube between the shield and the tubing; the bottom of the spike extends into this chamber	Used to prime the administration set and to verify continued flow
Bottom of spike	Plastic or metal piece that extends into the drip chamber	Size controls the volume of fluid in each drop; may be macrodrip or mini- or microdrip. Volume of a macrodrip varies among manufacturer from 10 to 20 drops/mL (gtt/mL); micro- or minidrip is 60 gtt/mL
Tubing	May be of varying lengths and diameters	Connects the drip chamber to the connector device
Clamps	May be screw clamp or roller clamp	Controls the rate of fluid flow through the administration
Flashball	A piece of latex with small circles on the surface that highlight areas reinforced with self-sealing material	Connects the tubing to the connector; reinforced areas used for needle access to infusion to administer intravenous push medications
Connectors	At the end of the tubing, may be slip tip, luer lock, or slip luer	Connects the administration set to the client's access device
Y-site	Set may have one or more; may be called injection site or side-arm; hard plastic tube; upper end has either a self-sealing injection port or a valve; the bottom of the Y-site is an integral part of the administration set tubing	Used for piggybacking intermittent medications into the client's primary infusion (Chart 17–1)
Miscellaneous Components		
On-off clamps	May be slide or clip; not appropriate for regulating rate of flow	Used to open or close the administration set to flow
Burettes	Reservoir that is either incorporated into the administration set or an add-on device; the reservoir holds between 100 and 150 mL of fluid; the burette is calibrated on the side to assist with accurate measurement; at the top or bottom of the burette is a rubber cap that looks like the end of a "Y site"; through this self-sealing cap, the nurse can add any medications or additives ordered for the client	The burette is useful for mixing intravenous medications for administration or for controlling the amount of fluid available for administration, a critical consideration in the care of the young child or the elderly client (Chart 17–2)
Back-check valves	When present, a back-check valve is built into the administration set; the device is a hard plastic one-way valve	Back-check valves allow fluid to travel away from the solution container but prevent fluid from flowing upstream toward the container
Passive flow control devices	Usually an add-on device that looks like an extension set with a dial	Regulates the rate of infusion in mL/hr; all other clamps are left open, and the passive flow control device regulates the administrations at the prescribed rate

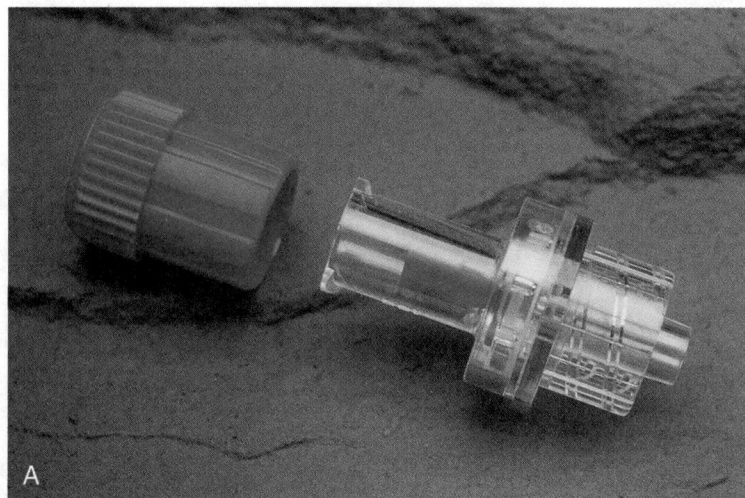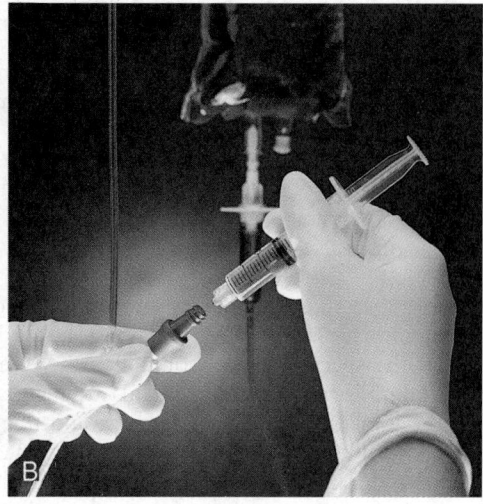

Figure 17–1. Needleless infusion systems. *A*, Burron Safesite IV System valve and "deadhead." *B*, Clave system in use. (*A*, courtesy of B. Braun Medical, Inc., Bethlehem, PA; *B*, courtesy of ICU Medical, Inc., San Clemente, CA.)

situation. It is important for the nurse to consider the purpose of the infusion, the drug or solution, the client, the client care setting, and the type of access device the client has before deciding on a particular type of infusion regulation device.

A controller is a stationary (pole-mounted) electronic device that can be classified as either nonvolumetric or volumetric. Nonvolumetric controllers rely completely on gravity for flow. A drop sensor attached to the drip chamber of the administration set regulates flow. Volumetric controllers also count drops and electronically convert the drops to mL/hr. Because controllers rely on counting drops, which may and do vary in size and therefore volume, controllers are not as accurate as pumps.

Pumps may be either stationary (pole mounted or tabletop), ambulatory (portable), or implantable (surgically implanted into the client). As their name indicates, these devices actually pump medications or solutions under pressure. Stationary pumps may be nonvolumetric or volumetric. Nonvolumetric pumps count drops and, as with controllers, are inherently inaccurate because of the variation in drop size. Three types of volumetric pumps are available: syringe, cassette, and peristaltic.

Syringe pumps use a mechanism that continuously closes the plunger at a selected mL/h rate. The use of syringe pumps is limited for small-volume continuous infusions or for administration of intermittent medications such as antiinfectives. Syringe pumps are generally not appropriate for use in the continuous administration of larger volumes, as they require very frequent syringe changes.

Cassette pumps use special sets (dedicated sets) that include a pumping chamber of exact volume. This volume is displaced by means of either a piston or a diaphragm at the selected mL/hr rate. Cassette pumps usually require special techniques to prime the administration set but are appropriate for use when delivering large volume infusions.

Peristaltic pumps are also appropriate for large-volume infusions. They control the rate of the infusion by squeezing the tubing with finger-like projections intermittently walking across the administration set tubing.

Ambulatory pumps are generally used for home care clients and allow clients to return to their usual activities while receiving infusion therapy.

Implantable pumps usually include a catheter as part of the pump. The physician places the catheter in a vessel feeding the "target organ," or structure. Implantable pumps also have a chamber that holds the medication and at least one self-sealing septum that the clinician uses to access the medication chamber for (re)filling and emptying the medication chamber. Implantable pumps are placed in the client's trunk via a laparotomy. Usual implant sites are the lower abdomen, the subclavicular area, and the subscapular area. Common uses for these pumps include regional chemotherapy and continuous intraspinal pain management.

TYPES OF INFUSION THERAPY
Intravenous Therapy

Intravenous (IV) therapy involves infusing medications and/or solutions into a client's veins through a venous access device (VAD). The tip placement of the IV cannula determines whether the therapy is considered peripheral or central venous therapy. In peripheral venous therapy the tip of the cannula remains in the client's peripheral veins. Central venous therapy involves placing the tip of the cannula or catheter into the client's superior vena cava (SVC).

Peripheral Intravenous Therapy
Description

Peripheral IV therapy is the most common *method* of gaining access to the client's venous system. Nurses competent in venipuncture insert the needle or flexible cannula percutaneously (through the skin) into a client's veins. Under most circumstances, the peripheral veins offer the quickest and easiest approach to establishing a route for administering IV solutions and medications. These solutions and medications may be administered for therapeutic or diagnostic purposes. Replacement of fluid, electrolyte, and nutrient losses; administration of anti-infectives; blood and blood product transfusions; and medication administration can be accomplished via the peripheral venous system. Enhancing agents for diagnostic imaging may also be administered via the peripheral veins.

An order from a health care provider is necessary before the nurse initiates IV therapy. The order usually includes the specific type of solution to be given; the rate of the administration written in mL/hr, mg/hr, μg/hr, or u/hr; the total volume of the infusion; and the number of hours for infusion. If the health care provider orders medication for IV administration, the dose, volume, solution or diluent, rate, and frequency of administration are usually included in the order. In many agencies, the infusion pharmacist determines the solution and volume for the medication admixture.

When determining which site to use to initiate the client's peripheral intravenous therapy, the nurse considers the client's age, history, and diagnosis; the type and duration of the prescribed therapy; and, whenever possible, the client's preference. Chart 17–3 lists some criteria for the placement of peripheral venous access devices.

The veins considered the most appropriate for most peripheral IV therapy are in the upper extremities and include the metacarpal, basilic, cephalic, and median veins, as well as their branches (Fig. 17–2). Veins that are resilient, long, and straight are the best choices for cannula placement. Veins that are hard, knotty, or sclerotic are difficult to encannulate and are likely to infiltrate. For short-term therapy, it is recommended that the

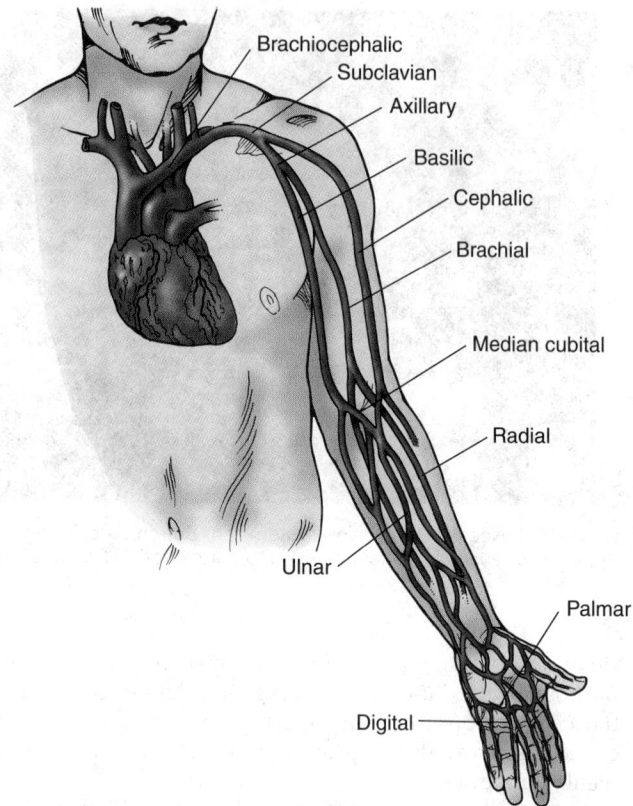

Figure 17–2. The superficial veins of the arm.

nurse place the initial IV catheter in the most distal site of the client's arm and use more proximal sites for subsequent IV cannula insertions.

The product to be infused requires the nurse's consideration when determining which vein and which type of peripheral access device to use. The administration of an isotonic solution, such as D5W, does not require any specific precautions related to the size of the vein or type of catheter the nurse uses for the infusion. However, the administration of medications or solutions that are viscous or those with a high osmolality or a high or low pH can be harsh and cause vein irritation. Medications or solutions with these properties require that the nurse consider the use of a larger vein to increase hemodilution and thereby decrease the potential for complications. Additionally, a midline or midclavicular catheter provides more reliable and longer-term access for solutions that are potentially irritating to veins.

Intravenous administrations that are of short duration, such as a one-time dose of an IV push medication that does not have vein-irritating properties, may be given into most veins. An infusion of a medication or solution with vein-irritating properties requires a larger vessel to reduce the probability of complications.

Devices

The nurse considers the age and condition of the client; the size, location, and condition of the available veins;

Chart 17–3

Nursing Care Highlight: Criteria for Placement of Peripheral Venous Access Devices

- Obtain a health care provider's order for placing a peripheral intravenous (IV) cannula.
- For adults, place a peripheral IV catheter only in the upper extremities.
- Use the client's nondominant hand when possible.
- Do not use the arm on the side where the client has a mastectomy, a lymph node dissection, an arteriovenous shunt or fistula, or venous revision.
- Use the most distal area of the client's arm above the wrist for the initial insertion and work your way up the client's arm to more proximal sites for subsequent insertions.
- Avoid placing a peripheral IV catheter over a joint.
- Avoid placing a peripheral IV cannula in a vein that is bruised, has puncture wounds from other venipunctures, is streaked, is hard, has a palpable cord, or is tender to touch.

and the type and duration of the infusion. The shortest, smallest-gauge device that accommodates the vein, type of infusion, and duration of therapy is the nurse's best choice when selecting an IV catheter.

Intravenous access devices may be categorized in a variety of ways. For the purpose of this discussion, peripheral IV catheters are categorized by dwell time (the amount of time the catheter may stay in the vein before being replaced)—either short-term dwell or long-term dwell.

SHORT-TERM DWELL CATHETERS. Winged metal sets and most over-the-needle catheters are short-term dwell catheters. Most short-term dwell peripheral catheters have a dwell time of 48–72 hours (Pearson et al., 1996).

A metal winged IV set is commonly known as a butterfly. Many practitioners consider these catheters easy to insert, but they may contribute to practitioner needlesticks. The practitioner holds the wings between the thumb and forefinger to insert the device. After insertion, the wings lie flat against the client's skin.

The standard over-the-needle catheter is between ¾ and 3 inches long and ranges in gauge size from 14 G to 26 G. The over-the-needle catheter consists of a needle inside a polyethylene or plastic catheter. The practitioner removes the needle after making the venipuncture, and the plastic catheter remains inside the vessel. Some manufacturers make over-the-needle winged sets. The nurse inserts these catheters in the same manner as a metal-winged set. However, after the insertion, the needle-stylet is removed, leaving only the catheter in the vessel.

LONG-TERM DWELL CATHETERS. Longer dwell time peripheral catheters, such as the midline or midclavicular catheters, are usually through-the-needle catheters. Through-the-needle catheters have either a break-away needle or a plastic peel-away sheath to encase the needle after the catheter is advanced through it. Some controversy exists over the amount of time these longer-dwell catheters may stay in place. Some believe that the midline and mid-clavicular catheters may remain in place for as long as the client exhibits no complications, or until the client no longer requires venous access (Pearson et al., 1996). In a position paper, the Intravenous Nurses Society (INS) recommends that maximum dwell time for midline catheters be limited to 2–4 weeks and to 2–3 months dwell time for midclavicular catheters (INS, 1997). Blood specimens may be drawn from indwelling peripheral catheters (see Research Applications for Nursing).

A midline catheter is a through-the-needle catheter that the nurse usually inserts at the antecubital fossa into the basilic, cephalic, or median cubital veins. The tip of the midline rests in the vein about 6–8 inches above the insertion site.

A mid-clavicular catheter is a through-the-needle catheter that is longer than the midline catheter. The tip of the mid-clavicular catheter usually rests at the mid-clavicular line. This area is the approximate junction of the axillary and subclavian veins.

▷ Research Applications for Nursing

What Is the Proper Discard Volume When Drawing Blood Through an Indwelling Catheter?

Yucha, C. B., & DeAngelo, E. (1996). The minimum discard volume. Journal of Intravenous Nursing, 19(3), 141–146.

Nurses frequently use indwelling central venous catheters for acquiring venous blood samples from their clients in both inpatient and outpatient settings. Most protocols involve withdrawing some blood to clear the catheter dead space and to remove the impact of the catheter's flushing solution on the test results. How does the nurse know how much blood should be withdrawn before acquiring the test sample? Does the appropriate amount vary with the test to be completed? The type of flush? Or the type of catheter?

Yucha and DeAngelo conducted a study to quantify the minimum amount of blood to be discarded from an indwelling peripheral intravenous catheter to obtain an accurate hematocrit reading. Using a study sample of nine subjects, repeat blood sampling was used to develop a mathematical model (Michaelis-Menton curve) describing the mixing of the flush solution and blood. This model was used to estimate the hematocrit when different volumes of blood are discarded. The differences between the computed hematocrit and true hematocrit were determined for each subject. When 1.5 mL (three times the deadspace volume) is discarded, the 95% confidence interval is within 0.6% of the true hematocrit.

Critique. This study was performed on nine young, healthy subjects with peripheral intravenous catheters. Only hematocrit readings were quantified in this study. For these reasons, the conclusions cannot be generalized to include other types of catheters, other types of laboratory determinations, ill clients, or those in other age groups. Further studies are therefore indicated.

Possible Nursing Implications. The nurse's ability to know the amount of discard required to ensure accurate laboratory testing has direct implications on client care and treatment, as well as on costs. Spurious laboratory results can cause the client to receive inappropriate doses of medication or unnecessary treatments. Having to repeat laboratory tests to get accurate results places the client at risk and adds to the cost of client care.

ELDERLY CONSIDERATIONS

Elderly clients receiving intravenous (IV) therapy have special needs. The normal aging process presents changes in the skin and vessels that require the nurse's attention.

The elderly person's skin may be described as loose, thin, and transparent. As people age, they lose subcutaneous fat, the dermis thins, and the density and amount of collagen lessen. Elastin fibers just below the dermis become more abundant but less effectively organized. The fine elastin fibers in the dermis disappear. All of these changes account for the decreased elasticity found in the elderly client's skin.

The elderly client's veins appear tortuous and large because of inadequate venous pressure. The veins are likely to roll, as there is little connective tissue to hold them, and the veins themselves become more fragile. These changes may require the nurse to alter the IV insertion technique in the elderly. Chart 17–4 outlines special considerations for the elderly client receiving peripheral IV therapy.

Central Intravenous Therapy

Description

Central venous therapy involves the placement of a flexible catheter into one of the client's central veins. The tip of the catheter is situated in the superior vena cava. Drugs, fluids, nutrients, enhancing agents, and blood and blood products may be infused through a central IV line. At times a central venous catheter (CVC) is placed be-cause the client's peripheral venous access is inadequate for the duration or type of IV therapy required. In some clients, a CVC allows the nurse to measure and monitor central venous pressure (CVP). In other cases, a CVC is inserted to ensure venous access when IV therapy is prescribed.

There are a number of criteria to consider when determining the type of CVC a client will have. The type and duration of therapy, the setting in which the client is to receive the therapy, and the client's lifestyle, activity, and personal preference all play a role in determining the type of catheter the client will receive.

Each of the devices discussed here, with the exception of the peripherally inserted central catheter (PICC), requires a physician to insert the catheter.

Devices

Nontunneled catheters may be placed at the client's bedside. The physician places the catheter percutaneously (through the skin) in a manner similar to a through-the-needle peripheral IV catheter. The site of placement may be into the client's chest or neck veins (usually the subclavian, or internal or external jugular veins). The catheters are made of polyurethane or silastic and may be single lumen or multiple lumen. The chest and neck vein sites are generally used for short-term therapy for clients who will remain as inpatients in a facility or who are outpatients. After placement and before it is used for infusions, the catheter's placement is checked by x-ray.

The PICC is another type of nontunneled catheter (Fig. 17–3). The PICC is currently the only type of central venous catheter that falls within the realm of nursing practice. Boards of nursing in every state now recognize the specially trained nurse's ability to safely and efficiently access the client's central venous system with a PICC. Many agencies and regulating boards agree that before a nurse be considered "PICC competent," he or she must complete a minimum of 8 hours of didactic (classroom) training and perform at least three successful PICC placements under the guidance of a preceptor or clinical trainer.

The PICC is appropriate for any setting and for administration of any IV therapy. As with other direct insertion catheters, PICCs are available in single or multiple lumen and require an x-ray to verify placement before use. According to the INS's position paper, a PICC that is functioning well may remain in place for up to 12 months (INS, 1997).

Tunneled CVCs include the Broviac, Hickman, Leonard, and Groshong catheters. These catheters, named for their developers, are made from silicone or polyurethane. Some of the differences among these catheters have to do with their inside diameters or gauge of lumen and the catheter tips. Before the nurse uses these catheters, the physician will confirm the placement of the catheter tip by radiography.

The Broviac catheter is usually a smaller-bore catheter than the Hickman, Leonard, or Groshong. Like the Hickman and Leonard, the Broviac is an open-ended catheter, meaning that it has a tip that is open, similar to that of peripheral venous catheters. The external portions of the

---

Chart 17–4

Focus on the Elderly: Special Considerations for the Elderly Client Receiving Peripheral Intravenous Therapy

- If the client's veins appear large and tortuous, do not use a tourniquet. Having the client hold the arm in a dependent position may fill the veins sufficiently for venipuncture.
- Do not use hand veins for starting an IV line. These veins are too small and limit the elderly client's ability to perform activities of daily living.
- Use the smallest-gauge intravenous (IV) catheter possible, preferably 21 G or smaller. (Most 24-G catheters allow the delivery of 100 mL/h.)
- Do not use a traditional tourniquet. A blood pressure cuff is easier on the elderly client's skin.
- Take time to find the most suitable vein.
- Use strict aseptic technique, because the elderly client is typically immunocompromised.
- Do not slap the arm to visualize the client's veins.
- Use a decreased angle for insertion—usually between 5 and 15 degrees.
- Set the flow rate of IV medications, especially antibiotics, to no more than 100 mL/h; for clients with congestive heart failure or renal failure set the rate at 50 mL/h.
- Use a protective skin preparation before applying a transparent dressing over the IV insertion site; dry gauze pads may be best for clients with tissue-thin skin.
- Cover the IV dressing with flexible netting. If netting is unavailable, use minimal tape or an elastic bandage to secure the dressing and protect the site; keep the insertion site visible at all times.
- Do not use circumferential restraints on the extremity with the IV catheter.
- Do not use the client's lower extremities for IV insertion, because the circulation may be impaired in the client's legs and feet.
- Assess the client's mental status at least every 4 hours.
- Use pumps, controllers, or burettes to control infusion volume and rate.

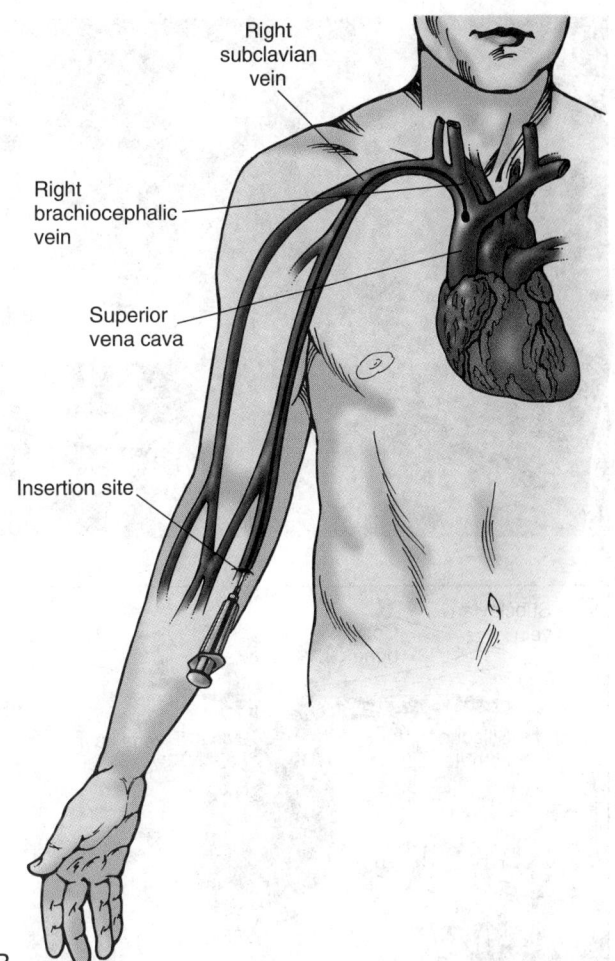

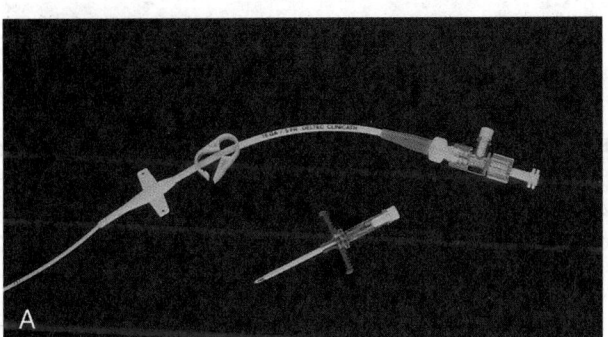

Figure 17–3. *A,* A ClinicCath peripherally inserted central venous catheter (courtesy of SIMS Deltec, Inc., St Paul, MN). *B,* Usual placement.

Hickman and Broviac catheters have a reinforced area on each lumen. When the catheter is not being used for infusions, the lumens are clamped at the reinforced area to avoid air embolism.

The Groshong catheter is a closed-end catheter. Toward the tip of the Groshong catheter on the side there is a slit-valve that opens out and allows fluid to infuse if there is positive pressure in the catheter and opens in and allows blood to be aspirated if there is negative pressure in the catheter. When the pressure in the catheter is neutral, the valve is closed. The Groshong catheter is not supplied with clamps, and the manufacturer's instructions state that the catheter should not be clamped to maintain the integrity of the valve. The Groshong tip is available on PICC catheters as well as tunneled catheters.

The rest of the features of the Broviac, Hickman, and Groshong catheters are similar in design. Each of these catheters is available in single, double, triple, and quadruple lumen. The catheters are usually 42–90 cm in length until the physician trims them during insertion. Each has a cuff positioned inside the subcutaneous tunnel. This cuff is designed to rest just inside the tunnel, under the skin. Fibrous tissue develops around it after insertion to

secure the catheter in place and produce a physical barrier to the migration of organisms up the tunnel into the client's bloodstream.

Implanted ports consist of a portal body, a central septum, a reservoir, and a catheter (Fig. 17–4). The port is surgically placed in a subcutaneous pocket in the client's trunk. The surgeon threads the catheter into the central vascular system and positions the tip in the superior vena cava. The catheter is attached to the portal body. The distal tip of the catheter is either open end or closed end. The septum is made of self-sealing silicone, located in either the center or on the side of the portal body. The nurse uses a noncoring device to access the system by piercing the skin over the portal body and puncturing the septum.

Complications of Intravenous Therapy

Vigilant nursing care is the key to decreasing the incidence of complications associated with all infusion therapy. A major nursing responsibility when caring for clients receiving infusion therapies is prevention, assessment, and management of complications. Table 17–3 de-

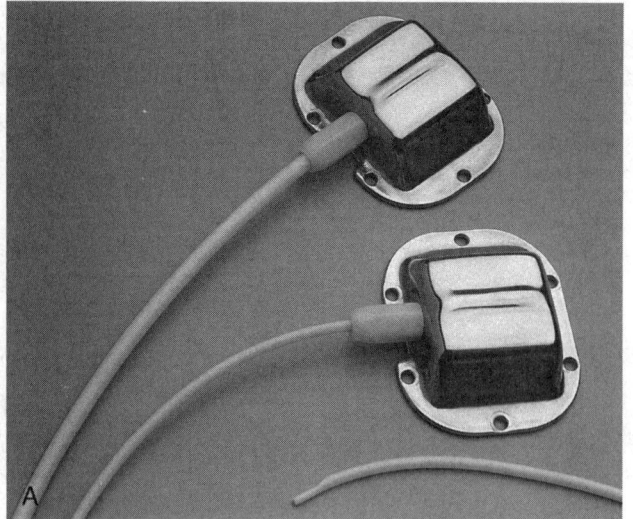

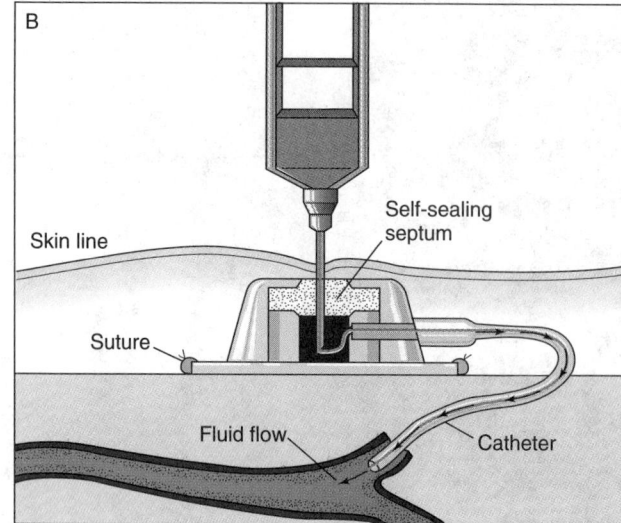

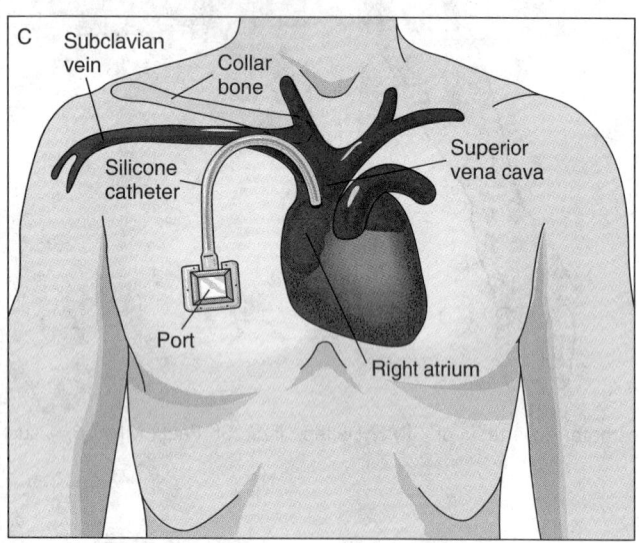

Figure 17–4. *A,* A dual-access implantable port for venous access. *B,* A needle puncture through the skin into the port allows drugs, fluids, and blood to be administered. *C,* For systemic drug and fluid delivery, the catheter is placed in the subclavian vein. (*A,* courtesy of Harbor Medical Devices, Inc., Boston, MA. *B* and *C,* redrawn from Winters, B. [1984]. Implantable vascular access devices. *Oncology Nursing Forum, 11*[6], 25–30.)

scribes local and systemic complications of peripheral intravenous (IV) therapy.

Arterial Therapy
Description

The use of a client's arteries for infusion therapy is usually to provide the client with intra-arterial chemotherapy (IAC). Chemotherapy administered arterially allows the administration of a high concentration of drug to the tumor site before it is diluted in the circulatory system or metabolized in the liver or kidneys. A high drug concentration at the tumor site optimizes tumor site cell kill while minimizing systemic side effects. This action is important to clients who are receiving chemotherapy because frequently debilitating systemic side effects may lead to discontinuation of some therapeutic regimens or alteration of others. Additionally, enough drug is available systematically to treat undetected micrometastases.

The physician is responsible for initiating the arterial catheter because the catheter placement is usually a surgical procedure or completed as an interventional radiologic procedure. The nurse's responsibility is the monitoring and maintenance of IAC.

The artery selected for encannulation (placement of a catheter) is specific to the diseased organ or structure to be treated. The physician usually prescribes IAC to treat a client's localized inoperable tumor in the liver, head, neck, or bones. Liver tumors are usually treated through the hepatic artery or branches of the celiac artery. The nurse may see the external carotid artery used in the treatment of head and neck tumors and the internal carotid artery used for the treatment of brain tumors.

Generally, the length of the therapy regimen and number of treatments determine which type of catheter the client will have. If the client is going to have intermittently scheduled therapy for a limited number of times, the physician will likely place a nonpermanent catheter using a radiologic procedure in the x-ray department. If the client is prescribed continuous therapy over a period of weeks or months, the physician will likely elect to place a permanent arterial catheter and a surgically implanted port. In either case, the physician places the catheter in a main artery that feeds the target organ or structure.

Devices

Catheters placed under radiography are usually made of polymer or Teflon. The catheters inserted surgically are usually ports. These ports are similar to those discussed in the central venous therapy section of this chapter, but the lumen of the catheter is generally smaller.

Whether the physician is placing the catheter surgically or radiologically, the catheter is threaded into the main artery feeding the tumor site. Some clients may have several vessels supplying the tumor site or the target vessel cannot be infused without infusing other adjacent vessels. When this occurs, the physician may elect to occlude these other vessels by injecting Gelfoam or metal coils through the catheter. Embolizing the arteries in this way may cause the tumor to shrink without the chemotherapy. The body absorbs the Gelfoam within a few days, re-establishing circulation. Metal coils provide permanent vascular occlusion. Until the client's body establishes collateral circulation, the client may complain of general malaise and pain in the area occluded.

Complications

Catheter displacement is the most common problem associated with temporary arterial catheters. Clients whose catheters become displaced may exhibit dyspepsia, excessive nausea and vomiting or diarrhea, gastric pain from peptic ulcers, or abdominal pain from pancreatitis. Treatment may include discontinuation of the chemotherapy infusion temporarily until the client can be treated with antiemetics and antacids.

A subintimal tear is the separation of the intima and media of the arterial wall, resulting from manipulation during placement. The client may complain of pain near the target organ during the infusion. Subintimal tears can delay therapy for weeks until the tear heals.

Arterial occlusion may occur with either a temporary radiologically placed catheter or a surgically placed catheter. The physician may order heparin in the chemotherapy infusion or have the client take 650 mg of aspirin twice daily to avoid catheter occlusion. Even with this prophylactic therapy, the nurse may observe transient or permanent loss or decrease in the client's pulse distal to the insertion site. The nurse must report these symptoms immediately. If the physician diagnoses the client with an embolism, the physician will either remove the catheter or use the fibrolytic agent urokinase (Abbokinase) in an attempt to lyse the clot.

Intraperitoneal Therapy
Description

Intraperitoneal (IP) therapy is the administration of therapeutic agents (cytotoxic drugs and biological response modifiers [BRMs]) into the peritoneal cavity. Intraperitoneal therapy is usually prescribed for the treatment of tumors that are confined to the peritoneal cavity. Carcinomas of the ovaries and fallopian tubes generally meet this criterion.

Devices

There are three categories of IP catheters generally available: temporary indwelling catheters, semipermanent indwelling external catheters, and implantable IP ports. The initiation of an IP catheter is a physician responsibility, but the administration and monitoring of the therapeutic agent is generally a nursing responsibility.

Administration of the IP therapy includes three phases: the instillation phase, the dwell phase, and the drain phase. The peritoneal cavity generally acts as a tumor refuge, separated from the bloodstream by a cellular enclosure similar to the blood-brain barrier. This enclosure protects IP tumors from systemically infused chemotherapeutic agents. IP therapy, like intraarterial therapy allows for the administration of antineoplastic agents directly to the tumor sites. This enhances the drug's penetration and cell kill while restricting systemic effects.

Temporary indwelling catheters include the temporary peritoneal dialysis catheter, paracentesis catheters, and a 16- or 18-gauge over-the-needle IV catheter. Semipermanent indwelling external catheters include the Tenckhoff catheter, the Gore-tex catheter, and the column-disk catheter. IP implanted ports are similar to intravenous and arterial ports, but the portal body and the catheter diameter are larger.

Temporary indwelling catheters may be inserted and removed at the bedside. Clients receiving a temporary indwelling catheter benefit from having a new catheter inserted at the time of each therapy. Complications such as the development of fibrous sheaths and infection do not plague these clients.

Semipermanent indwelling external catheters and IP implanted ports are inserted in the operating room. Both of these catheters are appropriate for longer-term therapy.

Complications

Exit site infection, indicated by redness, tenderness, and warmth of the tissue around the catheter, is more often seen in clients who have Tenckhoff catheters. Frequent dressing changes to the exit site using sterile technique can help prevent this complication.

Microbial peritonitis is the inflammation of the peritoneal membranes from the invasion of microorganisms. The client may experience a fever and complain of abdominal pain. There may be abdominal rigidity and rebound tenderness. This condition is preventable with strict aseptic technique in the handling of all equipment and infusion supplies. Treatment includes antimicrobial therapy either intravenously or intraperitoneally.

Chemical peritonitis is the irritation of the peritoneal membranes by the chemotherapeutic agent. The client may complain of symptoms similar to those experienced with microbial peritonitis. If severe, chemical peritonitis may delay further treatment.

Occlusion is the inability to administer fluids into the

TABLE 17–3

Complications of Peripheral Intravenous Therapy

Complication	Definition	Cause	Signs and Symptoms	Treatment	Prevention
Local Complications					
Infiltration	Infusion or seepage of intravenous (IV) solution or medication into the extravascular tissue	Access device either partially or completely dislodges from the vein	IV rate slows down; increasing edema above IV insertion site; client may complain of burning and tightness at IV site	If recent, ice may prevent any further seepage into the surrounding tissue; if older, warm moist compresses will assist with reabsorption of the fluid	Stabilize the IV catheter well, use the smallest catheter than will accomplish the infusion, avoid placement over area of flexion; monitor site frequently
Phlebitis	Inflammation of the vein	May be mechanical due to insertion technique or not stabilizing catheter well; may be chemical due to the pH or osmolality of the solution or medication	Client may complain of pain at IV site; nurse may observe that vein appears red and inflamed along the length; client may spike temperature; vein may become hard and cord-like	Remove the catheter; warm compresses to relieve pain; adjustment of infusion solution or admixture to prevent further injury	Change short-term IV catheter every 72 hours; when infusing medications or solutions with high osmolality, choose large veins; anchor catheters well to avoid movement in vein
Hematoma	Leaking of blood into the surrounding tissue	May be caused by piercing the back of the vein during insertion of the catheter; client may have faulty coagulation ability or be on anticoagulants	Discolored area of bruising around IV site; client may complain of pain; area may be swollen	Remove IV device and apply pressure; see treatment for infiltration	Carefully advance catheter, staying parallel with the client's skin; select the smallest catheter that will accomplish the task
Local infection	Bacterial contamination at the IV site	Break in aseptic technique during insertion or the handling of sterile equipment	Site appears red, swollen, and warm; client may complain of tenderness at the site; may observe purulent or malodorous exudate	Remove IV catheter and allow site to bleed for a few seconds and use 2 × 2 to express discharge; send catheter tip for culture; clean site with antibacterial solution and cover with dry sterile dressing; physician to evaluate for septic phlebitis and need for surgical intervention	Use careful technique when inserting IV; change site every 72 hours
Catheter embolism	A shaving or piece of catheter breaks off and floats freely in the vessel	May occur if needle of an over-the-needle catheter is reinserted into the catheter or if the catheter of a through-the-needle catheter is inadvertently pulled back through the catheter	Client will experience a decrease in blood pressure and complain of pain along the vein; pulse becomes weak, rapid, and thready, and the nurse may note cyanosis of the nail beds and circumorally; client may lapse into unconsciousness	Discontinue the catheter and apply a tourniquet high on the limb of the catheter site; inspect the catheter for any rough edges; an x-ray is taken to determine the presence of any catheter piece; surgical intervention may be necessary	When inserting over-the-needle catheters, never reinsert the needle into the catheter; avoid pulling a through-the-needle catheter back through the needle during insertion

Systemic Complications

Bloodstream infection	Pathogenic organisms enter the client's circulation	Early symptoms include fever, chills, headache, and general malaise; if left untreated, the client may experience severe infection, which may lead to vascular collapse and death	Same as for local infection above
Circulatory overload	The disruption of fluid homeostasis with excess fluid in the circulatory system	Client may complain of shortness of breath and cough; client's blood pressure is elevated, and there is puffiness around the eyes and edema in dependent areas; the client's neck veins may be engorged, and the nurse may hear moist breath sounds	Slow the IV rate and notify the physician; raise the client to an upright position; monitor vital signs and administer oxygen as ordered; administer diuretics as ordered
Speed shock	A systemic reaction to the rapid infusion of a substance unfamiliar to the client's circulatory system	Rapid infusion of drugs or bolus infusion, which causes the drug to reach toxic levels quickly	Immediately discontinue the drug infusion and hang D5W to keep the vein open; monitor the client's vital signs carefully and notify the physician for further treatment orders
Speed shock (cont.)		Client may complain of lightheadedness or dizziness and chest tightness; the nurse may note that the client has a flushed face and an irregular pulse; without intervention, the client may lose consciousness and go into shock and cardiac arrest	The nurse is aware of the appropriate infusion rate of medications and adheres to them; use of infusion control devices assists in prevention of speed shock
Allergic reaction	A local or general response to an allergen	May be the response to tape, cleansing agent, drug, solution, or IV device	
Allergic reaction (cont.)		The client having a local reaction may exhibit a wheal, redness, or itching at the IV site; in the case of a general reaction, the client may complain of itching, running nose, and tearing; the nurse may note bronchospasm, wheezing, and a truncal rash; without treatment, the client may experience anaphylaxis	
Bloodstream infection (cont.)	Result of poor aseptic technique or contaminated infusion or if the catheter site is not changed regularly		Change the entire infusion system from solution to IV device; notify physician, obtain cultures, and administer antibiotics as ordered; if the infusate is the suspected cause, send a specimen to the laboratory for evaluation

Monitor intake and output carefully and notify the physician as soon as an imbalance is noticed between the client's intake and output

peritoneum or withdraw fluid from the peritoneum. Occlusion is caused by formation of fibrous sheaths or fibrin clots or plugs inside the catheter or around the tip or by compartmentalization of fluid due to adhesions or twisting, kinking, or displacement of the catheter. Management may include the infusion of a lysing agent such as urokinase. If the catheter is an indwelling external catheter, the physician may attempt to dislodge the clot by using a push-pull method with a syringe and 0.9% normal satire solution (NSS). Sometimes, the physician may insert a sterile stylet through an external catheter to dislodge the catheter.

Subcutaneous Therapy

Description

Subcutaneous (SC) therapy involves the insertion of a small-gauge needle into the client's subcutaneous space and the continuous administration of isotonic fluids or medications at a slow rate—usually 1 mL/min. Continuous subcutaneous infusion (CSQI) has been used as an alternative to intravenous therapy for maintenance, treatment, and palliation.

Devices

The nurse implements CSQI by cleansing any area on the client's body that has sufficient SC tissue. The nurse primes the attached tubing and, gently pinching an area of approximately 2 inches, inserts a small-gauge needle. Appropriate needle choices for CSQI include a 25- to 27-gauge butterfly needle or a Sub-Q-Set (Baxter). If using a butterfly needle, the nurse inserts the device at a 35- to 45-degree angle. The Sub-Q-Set is inserted at a 90-degree angle. After anchoring the needle, the nurse covers the site with a transparent dressing.

Clients who benefit from CSQI are those who

- Are unable to take oral medications (e.g., have dysphagia, gastrointestinal obstruction, or malabsorption)
- Have intractable nausea and vomiting
- Require parenteral medication but have poor venous access
- Require subcutaneous injections for longer than 48 hours
- Have a need for prolonged use of parenteral medication
- Need a continuous level of medication to control pain
- Cannot cope with the expense of intravenous therapy
- Are confused or depressed

Complications

Insertion site irritation, evidenced by erythema, heat, or swelling, is a local complication of CSQI. Rotation of the SC site approximately every 5–7 days usually helps prevent this problem.

Central Nervous System Therapy

Central nervous system therapy involves the infusion of medications into the epidural space or intrathecally.

Epidural Therapy

In epidural therapy, the physician or specially trained nurse administers medication into the epidural space of the spinal column. Located between the wall of the vertebral canal and the dura mater, the epidural space consists of fat, connective tissue, and blood vessels that protect the spinal cord. The most common uses of epidural therapy are to relieve postoperative or chronic pain and the pain associated with labor and delivery. The physician, usually an anesthesiologist or neurosurgeon, initiates epidural therapy. There are four different categories of catheters used for epidural therapy. The choice of one over the other depends on the purpose and duration of therapy. Table 17–4 describes each type and lists their indications.

Opioids administered epidurally slowly diffuse across the dura mater to the dorsal horn of the spinal cord and lock onto receptors and block pain impulses from ascending to the brain. The client receives pain relief from the level of the injection caudally (toward the toes). Local anesthetics administered epidurally work on the sensory nerve roots in the epidural space to block pain impulses. After the physician administers the first dose of medication, depending on state law, the type of medication, and facility policies, nurses trained in epidural therapy administer subsequent doses. In all cases, it is a nursing responsibility to monitor the client receiving epidural therapy for any signs of complications.

Complications associated with epidural therapy are usually caused by the medications administered. Table 17–5 outlines medication-related complications seen in the administration of epidural opiates and local anesthetics.

Intrathecal Therapy

Intrathecal therapy provides a means of administering chemotherapy, pain medication, or antibiotics directly into the ventricular cerebral spinal fluid (CSF) of clients who suffer from CSF malignancies or metastases, chronic cancer pain, or CSF infections. Some medications used to treat CSF neoplasms, such as methotrexate and cytarabine, cannot be administered intravenously because they cannot cross the blood-brain barrier. Others must be administered in very large doses to cross this natural protective mechanism. Large doses of chemotherapy may not be possible due to the severe systemic side effects associated with them. Administration of medications via the intrathecal route eliminates this problem, as the medication is administered directly into the CSF.

The Ommaya reservoir is the catheter commonly used for intrathecal therapy. A neurosurgeon is usually responsible for the placement of the catheter in the operating room under strict asepsis. The Ommaya reservoir consists of two pieces: a mushroom-shaped self-sealing dome made of silicone and a catheter that attaches to the dome. The tip of the catheter is placed in one of the lateral ventricles. The reservoir is attached and placed beneath a flap in the client's scalp. Some models of the reservoir have a side outlet tube that can be used as a shunt to remove excess CSF in the client with increased intracra-

TABLE 17–4

Catheters Used for Epidural Therapy

Type of Device	Description	Indications
Percutaneous catheter	Flexible nylon catheter threaded through a spinal needle into the epidural space. The external end has a standard female Luer-Lok hub, which accepts an intermittent injection cap.	Temporary pain relief post-operatively or during labor and delivery. For pain control in clients with end-stage cancer or a temporary measure to determine if the chronic pain client will receive relief with epidural therapy.
Subcutaneous tunneled catheter	A Silastic catheter tunneled from the point where it exits the spine to a point on the client's trunk, usually on the side just above the waist. Like a tunneled central venous catheter, the catheter has a Dacron cuff that prevents the migration of micro-organisms along the catheter into the epidural space.	A more permanent catheter indicated for clients in whom epidural therapy has proved to be effective and who have a life expectancy of weeks to months.
Totally implantable reservoir or port	Appears identical to a venous or arterial port. The surgeon places the portal body over a bony prominence, such as the spine itself, or one of the client's lower ribs.	Indicated for clients who respond to epidural therapy and have a life expectancy of months to years. Another indication is the client who is confused and repeatedly pulls out his or her subcutaneous tunneled catheter.
Totally implantable infusion pump	Consists of a catheter whose tip sits in the epidural space at the appropriate level. The catheter is tunneled subcutaneously and attached to the pump, which is usually implanted in a pocket in the abdominal region of chest wall. As described earlier, the medication is in the pump's reservoir.	The most expensive method of administering epidural therapy. Indicated for clients who will require therapy for a long period (chronic pain) and who have a life expectancy of months to years.

nial pressure. The physician or, in some cases, the chemotherapy nurse administers the medication by inserting a needle through the client's skin into the Ommaya dome. After removing the amount of CSF equal to the volume of the medication to be administered, the physician slowly injects the medication. The physician removes the needle and pumps the dome of the reservoir to release the medication into the catheter for delivery to the

TABLE 17–5

Medication-Related Complications of Epidural Therapy

System	Epidural Opiates	Epidural Local Anesthetics
Cardiovascular	No postural hypotension Minor changes in heart rate	Postural hypotension Decrease in heart rate
Respiratory	If occurs, may be early at 1–2 hours due to systemic absorption or late after dose at 6–24 hours due to migration to brain	Usually unimpaired
Central nervous system	Sedation may be marked Convulsions absent	Sedation absent to mild Convulsions possible due to rapid vascular absorption Sensory losses Motor weakness
Genitourinary	Urinary retention	Urinary retention
Integumentary	Pruritis	Pruritis rarely occurs
Gastrointestinal	Nausea and vomiting	Nausea and vomiting rarely occurs

From Booker, M. F., & Ignatavicius, D. D. (1996). *Infusion therapy: Techniques and medications.* Philadelphia: W. B. Saunders.

CSF. The nurse is responsible for monitoring the client for any complications.

Complications of Central Nervous System Therapy

Infection in the client receiving either epidural or intrathecal therapy is the result of a lack of asepsis when handling the medication or during the administration. There may be local evidence of infection, such as redness or swelling at the catheter exit site or over the Ommaya reservoir. The client may also exhibit neurological and systemic signs of infection, such as headache, stiff neck, or temperature higher than 101° F (38.3° C). The nurse may observe cloudy CSF, indicating a proliferation of white blood cells in clients undergoing intrathecal therapy.

Misplacement or migration of the catheter may occur at the time of placement, or the catheter can move or become kinked after placement. In clients with epidural catheters, when the nurse aspirates to check placement, he or she may observe clear free-flowing fluid (CSF), indicating that the catheter has migrated into the subarachnoid space, or the nurse may withdraw blood, indicating that the catheter has migrated into a blood vessel. An inadvertent administration of local anesthetics directly into the subarachnoid space may lead to high or total spinal block and convulsions or cardiovascular depression. Clients who mistakenly receive local anesthetics intravenously may experience toxic reactions with convulsions. In the client receiving intrathecal therapy via an Ommaya reservoir, the physician may observe no or very slow filling when "pumping" the dome. The client may exhibit new neurologic symptoms if the catheter has migrated.

Intraosseous Therapy

Description

Intraosseous (IO) therapy is a previously used and re-emerging method of gaining access to a client's vascular system. Primarily utilized in critically injured clients with vascular collapse, IO therapy is the topic of a number of research studies that confirm that it is a viable option for other clients requiring infusion therapy as well. In some states, prehospital providers such as emergency medical technicians (EMTs) and paramedics, as well as trained clinicians in trauma centers and emergency departments, initiate IO therapy.

Intraosseous therapy allows access to the rich vascular network located in the client's long bones. This vascular network is more prominent in children younger than 6 years. Victims of trauma, burns, cardiac arrest, and other life-threatening conditions benefit from IO therapy, because frequently clinicians are unable to access these clients' vascular systems using traditional methods such as intravenous therapy. Research indicates that absorption rates of large volume peripheral infusions (LVPs) and medications administered via the IO route are similar to those achieved with peripheral or central venous administration.

Devices

Theoretically, any needle may be used to provide IO therapy and access the medullary space. However, there are criteria that make some needles superior to others for IO therapy. A needle that has a removable stylet that screws into the cannula to keep the needle from retracting during insertion, a short shaft to eliminate accidental dislodgment after placement, an adjustable guard to stabilize the needle at skin level, and graduations along the needle to guide the practitioner during the insertion are features that make a needle well suited for IO therapy.

Complications

Improper needle placement is the most common complication of IO therapy. An accumulation of fluid under the skin at either the insertion site or on the other side of the limb indicates that the needle is either not far enough in to penetrate the bone marrow or is too far into the limb and has protruded through the other side of the shaft.

Needle obstruction occurs when the puncture has been accomplished but there has been delay in flushing. This delay may cause the needle to become clotted with bone marrow.

Osteomyelitis is a very serious complication of IO therapy. This infection in the bone tissue is unusual, but when it occurs it is generally due to leaving the cannula in place too long or the client having had a source of infection prior to the needle's insertion.

Embolus is a complication of any orthopedic procedure, and IO therapy is no exception. Embolus occurs when a bone fragment or fat enters the peripheral circulation. The client exhibits classic symptoms of respiratory distress, tachycardia, hypertension, tachypnea, fever, and petechiae. Laboratory data indicate an increased sedimentation rate and decreased red blood cell and platelet counts.

Compartment syndrome is a condition in which increased tissue pressure in a confined anatomic space causes decreased blood flow to the area. The decreased circulation to the area leads to hypoxia and pain in the area. This is very rare in IO therapy, but the nurse should monitor the site of the IO therapy carefully and alert the physician promptly should the client exhibit any signs of decreased circulation to the limb, such as coolness, swelling, mottling, and discoloration. Without improvement in perfusion to the limb, the client may require amputation of the limb.

SELECTED BIBLIOGRAPHY

*Beason, R., Bourguignon, J., Fowle, D., et al. (1993). Evaluation of a needle-free intravenous access system. *Journal of Intravenous Nursing,* 15(1), 11–15.

Booker, M. F., & Ignatavicius, D. D. (1996). *Infusion therapy: Techniques and medications.* Philadelphia; W. B. Saunders.

Clemence, M. A., Walker, D., & Farr, B. M. (1995). Central venous catheter practices: Results of a survey. *American Journal of Infection Control,* 23(1), 5–12.

Hunt, M. L., & Rapp, R. P. (1996). Intravenous medication errors. *Journal of Intravenous Nursing,* 19(3S), S9–S15.

Intravenous Nurses Society. (1997) Position paper: Midline and midclavicular catheters. *Journal of Intravenous Nursing,* 20(4), 175–178.

Intravenous Nurses Society. (1997). Position paper: Peripherally inserted central catheters. *Journal of Intravenous Nursing, 20*(4), 172–174.

Miller, J. M., Goetz, A., et al. (1996). Reduction in nosocomial intravenous device-related bacteremias after institution of an intravenous therapy team. *Journal of Intravenous Nursing, 19*(2), 103–106.

Pearson, M. L., et al. (1996). Guideline for prevention of intravascular-device–related infections. *Infection Control and Hospital Epidemiology, 17*(7), 438–473.

Treston-Aurand, J., Olmsted, R. N., et al. (1997). Impact of dressing materials on central venous catheter infection rates. *Journal of Intravenous Nursing, 20*(4), 201–206.

SUGGESTED READINGS

Clemence, M. A., Walker, D., & Farr, B. M. (1995). Central venous catheter practices: Results of a survey. *American Journal of Infection Control, 23*(1), 5–12.

This article describes the significant diversity among health care agencies in the care of central venous catheters. Certain protocols, still in use, that have been linked to an increase in bloodstream infections are presented, as well as suggestions for further research.

Treston-Aurand, J., Olmsted, R. N., et al. (1997). Impact of dressing materials on central venous catheter infection rates. *Journal of Intravenous Nursing, 20*(4), 201–206.

In the mid-1980s, many health care organizations changed their central venous catheter dressing regimens from gauze to transparent semipermeable polyurethane dressings. However, some studies have linked these dressings with microbial growth under the dressing and, consequently, an increase in catheter-related infections (CRIs). This article discusses the positive impact that the use of a highly permeable transparent dressing had on CRIs in one facility.

Hunt, M. L., & Rapp, R. P. (1996). Intravenous medication errors. *Journal of Intravenous Nursing, 19*(3S), S9–S15.

This article provides a brief history of modern hospital pharmacy practices, as well as a thorough discussion of the factors related to intravenous medication errors and strategies for physicians, pharmacists, and nurses to avoid them.

ACID-BASE BALANCE

Acids and bases regulate the body's hydrogen ion (H^+) production and elimination. Body fluid pH is a measure of its hydrogen ion concentrations. Even small changes in the hydrogen ion concentration, or *pH,* of body fluids can cause major problems in bodily function. Body fluid pH has the narrowest range of normal and the tightest control mechanisms of all electrolytes. Acids and bases perform the processes that release or bind hydrogen ions.

The normal hydrogen ion concentration of blood and other body fluids is quite low (< 0.0001 mEq/L) compared with the body fluid concentrations of other electrolytes (see Chapters 14 and 16). Because it is so low, hydrogen ion concentration is measured in pH units, calculated as the negative logarithm of the concentration in milliequivalents per liter (Fig. 18–1). Normal pH ranges from 7.35 to 7.45 for arterial blood and from 7.32 to 7.42 for venous blood.

Because pH is calculated in negative logarithm units, the value of pH is inversely related to the concentration of hydrogen ions. In other words, the lower the pH value of a fluid, the higher is the concentration of hydrogen ions in that fluid. In the 14-point pH scale, *a change of 1 pH unit actually represents a 10-fold change in hydrogen ion concentration.* Therefore, even a pH unit change of one tenth (e.g., a change from 7.4 to 7.3) represents a large increase in the hydrogen ion concentration of a given

solution. Table 18–1 lists terms used to describe acid-base balance.

Changes in pH interfere with many normal physiologic functions, including

- Altering the shape or position of hormones and enzymes to the extent that they can no longer perform their designated functions
- Changing the distribution of other electrolytes, causing fluid and electrolyte imbalances
- Altering the responses of excitable membranes, so that the heart, nerves, skeletal muscles, and gastrointestinal tract are either less or more active than normal
- Decreasing the uptake, activity, and distribution of many hormones and drugs, possibly reducing their effectiveness

Fortunately, the body has many well-regulated mechanisms to ensure minimal changes in hydrogen ion concentration. Table 18–2 lists the key concepts of acid-base balance.

ACID-BASE BALANCE

As discussed in Chapters 14 and 16, body fluids are electrically neutral even though they contain ions with an overall positive charge (cations or protons) and ions with

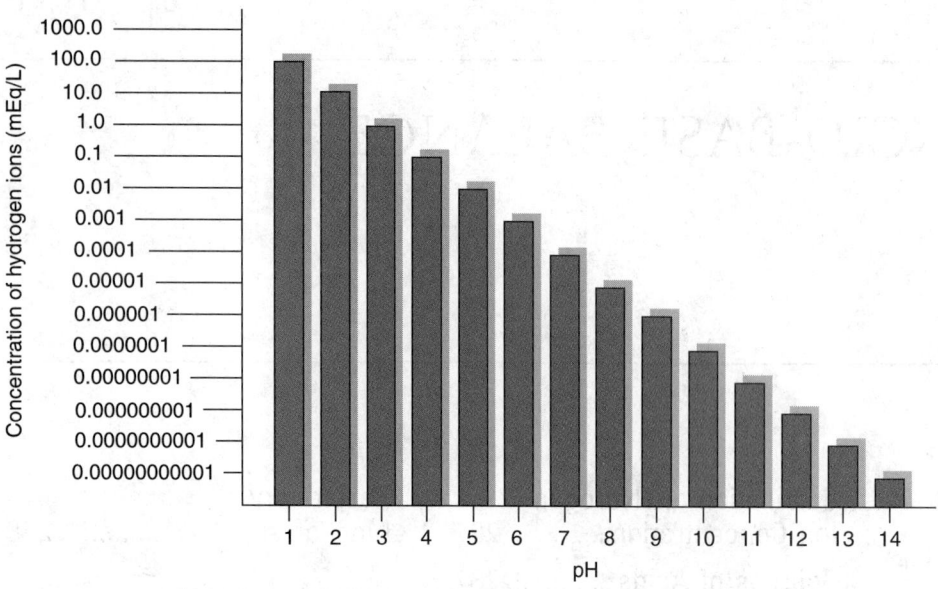

Figure 18–1. Relationship between pH and concentration of hydrogen ions.

an overall negative charge (anions). When fluids contain an equal number of positive and negative charges, the electrical charge remains neutral. The system maintains a body fluid pH between 7.35 and 7.45 in a similar manner; however, this value is not strictly neutral (7.0 is neutral) but rather is slightly alkaline. Normal body fluid pH remains at a near-neutral value when the acid components and base components are in relative balance, thus limiting the total number of free hydrogen ions. That is, acid-base balance occurs by matching the rate of hydrogen ion production with the activity of mechanisms for hydrogen ion removal and uptake.

Acid-Base Chemistry

Acids

Acids are substances that donate, or release, a hydrogen ion when the substance is dissolved in water (H_2O). An

TABLE 18–1

Pertinent Acid-Base Balance Terminology

Term	Definition
Acid	• Any substance releasing a hydrogen ion when dissolved in water
Anaerobic metabolism	• Cellular metabolism occurring without the presence of oxygen
Base	• Any substance binding a hydrogen ion when dissolved in water
Buffer	• A substance capable of binding a hydrogen ion from body fluids (acting as a base) or releasing a hydrogen ion into body fluids (acting as an acid)
Chemoreceptors	• Special cells in the respiratory center of the brain sensitive to changes in the carbon dioxide concentration of extracellular fluid
pH	• The concentration of hydrogen ions in a solution, calculated as the negative logarithm of the milliequivalent concentration per liter

TABLE 18–2

Key Concepts of Acid-Base Balance

- The normal pH of the body's extracellular fluids (including blood) is 7.35–7.45.
- The pH in the body can be described as the relationship of bicarbonate to carbonic acid, or a 20:1 ratio.
- Carbon dioxide is the most changeable component of carbonic acid.
- The concentration of carbon dioxide is directly related to the concentration of hydrogen ions.
- An acid gives up hydrogen ions in solution; a base binds hydrogen ions in solution.
- Acids are formed in the body as a result of metabolism and incomplete oxidation of glucose and fats.
- Acid-base balance is regulated by chemical, respiratory, and renal mechanisms.
- Chemical buffers are the immediate way that acid-base imbalances are corrected.
- The lungs control the amount of carbon dioxide that is retained or exhaled.
- The kidneys regulate the amount of hydrogen and bicarbonate ions that are retained or excreted by the body.
- Compensation is the process in which the body uses its three regulatory mechanisms to correct for changes in the pH of body fluids.

acid in solution thus increases the concentration of free hydrogen ions in that solution. The strength of an acid is determined by how easily it releases a hydrogen ion in solution. A strong acid, such as hydrochloric acid (HCl), dissociates (separates) completely in water and readily releases all its hydrogen ions:

$$HCl + H_2O \longrightarrow H^+ + Cl^- + H_2O$$

hydrochloric acid   water   hydrogen ion   chloride ion   water

A weak acid does not completely dissociate in water; it releases only some of its total hydrogen ions. In the following example, each molecule of acetic acid (CH_3COOH), a weak acid, contains a total of four hydrogen molecules. When acetic acid combines with water, it releases only one of its four hydrogen molecules. The other three hydrogen molecules remain bound to the acetic acid molecule:

$$CH_3COOH + H_2O \longrightarrow H^+ + CH_3COO^- + H_2O$$

Bases

A base is a substance that binds free hydrogen ions in solution. Thus, bases are hydrogen acceptors: they reduce the concentration of free hydrogen ions in solution. Strong bases bind hydrogen ions easily. Some may bind more than one hydrogen ion to one base molecule. Examples of strong bases include sodium hydroxide (NaOH) and ammonia (NH_3); weak bases include aluminum hydroxide ($Al(OH)_3$) and bicarbonate (HCO_3^-).

Weak bases bind hydrogen ions less readily. Although bicarbonate is a relatively weak base, bicarbonate ions in the body are crucial in preventing major disturbances in body fluid pH.

Buffers

Buffers are substances that either release a hydrogen ion into a fluid or bind a hydrogen ion from a fluid. Most substances, when dissolved in water, react by either releasing a hydrogen ion (an acidic substance) or binding a free hydrogen ion (a basic substance). Buffers dissolved in water can react in two ways: either as an acid, releasing a hydrogen ion, or as a base, binding a hydrogen ion.

How a buffer reacts when dissolved in water or other fluid depends on the existing acid-base balance of that fluid. Buffers always try to bring the fluid as close as possible to a normal body fluid pH of 7.35 to 7.45. Thus, if the fluid is basic (with few free hydrogen ions), the buffer will release hydrogen ions into the fluid (Fig. 18–2). If the fluid is acidic (with many free hydrogen ions), the buffer will act as a base, binding some hydrogen ions. In a sense, buffers are hydrogen ion "sponges," soaking up hydrogen ions when too many are present in a fluid and squeezing out hydrogen ions when too few are present in a fluid. Because of this flexibility, buffers are important regulators of body fluid pH or hydrogen ion concentration (acid-base balance).

Solutions with a pH of 7.0 are considered neutral; they contain a set concentration of hydrogen ions whose number and strength of acid and base components are in equilibrium. Figure 18–3 is an artificial yet concrete representation of the concept of neutral pH. This repre-

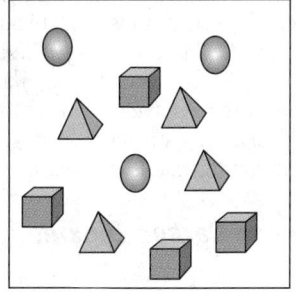

Fluid pH 7.38 (normal). The number and strength of acid components are equal to the number and strength of base components. Hydrogen ion concentration is limited and constant.

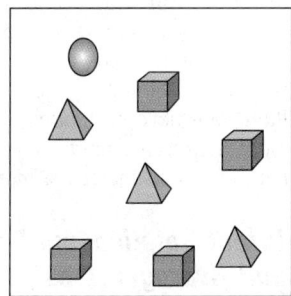

Fluid pH 7.51 (alkaline). The number and strength of base components are greater than the number and strength of acid components. Hydrogen ion concentration is below normal.

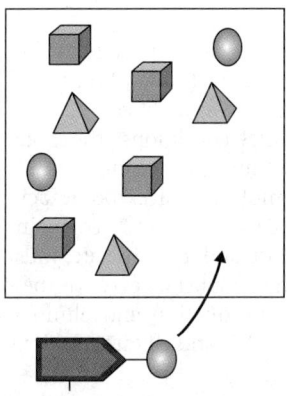

Buffer is added to the alkaline fluid.

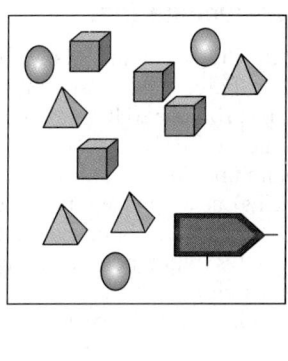

The buffer acts as an acid, releasing a hydrogen ion.

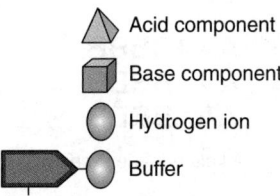

△ Acid component

▢ Base component

◯ Hydrogen ion

⬠ Buffer

Figure 18–2. Action of buffer in solution. (© 1992 by M. Linda Workman. All rights reserved.)

AAABBB   AAAABBB   AAABB
AAABBB   AAAABBB   AAABB
AAABBB   AAAABBB   AAABB

Neutral   Acidic (acid excess)   Acidic (base deficit)

Figure 18–3. Concept of acidic versus normal pH. (A = acid; B = base.)

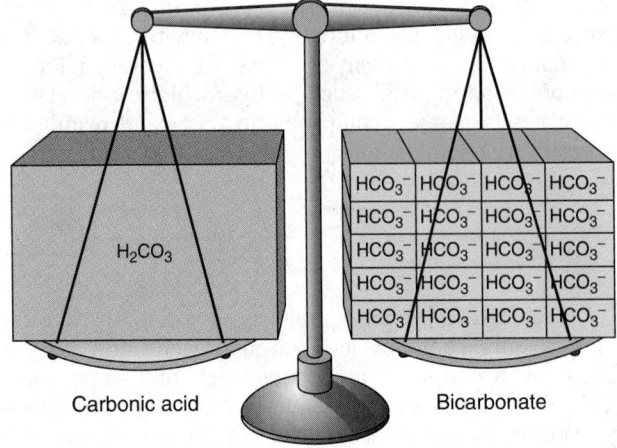

Figure 18–5. Normal ratio of carbonic acid to bicarbonate is 1:20.

sentation indicates that the strength as well as the amount of all acid components is equal to the strength as well as the amount of all the base components in a given solution. Although this is never the actual case in human physiology, in acid-base homeostasis, the relative amounts and strengths of acids and bases are approximately equal, so the overall hydrogen ion concentration remains constant.

Solutions with a pH from 1.0 to 6.99 contain an excessive amount or strength (or both) of the acid components compared with the amount or strength (or both) of the base components. Such solutions are considered *acidic* (see Fig. 18–3). This results in more hydrogen ions being released than bound, greatly increasing the number of free hydrogen ions.

Solutions with a pH ranging from 7.01 to 14.0 have an excessive amount or strength (or both) of the base components compared with the amount or strength (or both) of the acid components. These solutions are considered *basic*. This results in more hydrogen ions being bound than released, causing a deficit in the number of free hydrogen ions (Fig. 18–4).

Body Fluid Chemistry

Bicarbonate Ions

Body fluids contain many different acidic substances and a few bases. The most common base in human body fluid is bicarbonate (HCO_3^-); the most common acid is carbonic acid (H_2CO_3). Under normal conditions, the body maintains these substances within extracellular fluids (ECFs) at a constant ratio of 1 molecule of carbonic acid to 20 free bicarbonate ions (1:20) (Fig. 18–5). To maintain this ratio, both carbonic acid and bicarbonate must be carefully controlled. Both these substances and their constant ratio are related to the production and elimination of both carbon dioxide (CO_2) and hydrogen ions (H^+).

A key concept that aids understanding acid-base balance is the *carbonic anhydrase equation* (shown next). This equation, driven by the enzyme carbonic anhydrase, demonstrates how hydrogen ion concentration and carbon dioxide concentration are directly related to one another, so that an increase in one causes a corresponding increase in the other:

$$CO_2 + H_2O \longleftrightarrow H_2CO_3 \longleftrightarrow H^+ + HCO_3^-$$
$$\text{carbon dioxide} \quad \text{water} \quad \text{carbonic acid} \quad \text{hydrogen ion} \quad \text{bicarbonate ion}$$

Carbon dioxide is a gas that, when combined with water, forms carbonic acid. Carbon dioxide thus is a changeable part of carbonic acid. Because carbonic acid is not stable and the body needs to maintain a 1:20 ratio of carbonic acid to bicarbonate, as soon as carbonic acid is formed from water and carbon dioxide, it immediately dissociates (separates) into free hydrogen ions and bicarbonate ions. *Therefore, the carbon dioxide content of a fluid is directly related to the hydrogen ion concentration of that fluid. Whenever conditions cause carbon dioxide to increase, more hydrogen ions are created. Likewise, whenever hydrogen ion production increases, more carbon dioxide is produced.*

Direct Relationship Between Carbon Dioxide and Hydrogen Ions

When excess carbon dioxide is produced, the concentration of carbon dioxide increases and the carbonic anhydrase equation shifts to the right, demonstrating an increase in the hydrogen ion concentration (and a decrease in pH):

$$CO_2 + H_2O \Longrightarrow H_2CO_3 \Longrightarrow H^+ + HCO_3^-$$

When very little carbon dioxide is produced, no hydrogen ions are generated by the carbonic anhydrase equation.

When excess hydrogen ions are produced or brought into the body, the carbonic anhydrase equation shifts to the left, demonstrating the creation of more carbon dioxide:

AAABBB   AAABBBB   AABBB
AAABBB   AAABBBB   AABBB
AAABBB   AAABBBB   AABBB

Neutral   Alkaline (base excess)   Alkaline (acid deficit)

Figure 18–4. Concept of alkaline versus normal pH. (A = acid; B = base.)

$$CO_2 + H_2O \longleftrightarrow H_2CO_3 \longleftrightarrow H^+ + HCO_3^-$$

When the body fluids are low on hydrogen ions, no extra carbon dioxide is produced.

Calculation of Hydrogen Ion Concentration

The pH is a calculated measurement of hydrogen ion concentration in body fluids, because the actual number or percentage of hydrogen ions in these fluids is not easily measured. The pH calculations are derived from the Henderson-Hasselbalch equation, a mathematical formula that expresses the interrelatedness of three factors: the concentration of free hydrogen ions, the concentration of bases, and the concentration of acids in a solution. When other influences (such as temperature and pressure) remain constant, if two of the three factors are known, then the third factor can be calculated.

$$pH = 6.1 + \log \frac{[HCO_3^-]}{[H_2CO_3 + CO_2]}$$

Because the ratio of carbonic acid and bicarbonate concentration in ECF is 1:20 under normal physiologic conditions, the major factor in the equation that tends to change is the carbon dioxide concentration. Whenever the carbon dioxide concentration changes, pH changes correspondingly.

In the Henderson-Hasselbalch formula, carbon dioxide concentration is on the bottom of the equation, making it inversely related to pH while it is directly related to the hydrogen ion concentration. Thus, when the carbon dioxide concentration of a solution increases, the pH drops, indicating an increase in the hydrogen ion concentration. Conversely, when the carbon dioxide concentration of a solution decreases, the pH rises, indicating a decrease in the hydrogen ion concentration.

An increase in the bicarbonate concentration causes the hydrogen ion concentration to decrease and the pH to increase, or become more alkaline (basic). Conversely, an increase in the carbon dioxide concentration causes the hydrogen ion concentration to increase and the pH to decrease, or become more acidic. In either case, the normal 1:20 ratio is changed and the pH of the blood is also changed.

Because the kidneys control bicarbonate concentration and the lungs control carbon dioxide concentration in the body, pH can also be described as the function of the kidneys divided by the function of the lungs, or

$$pH = \frac{Kidneys\ (bicarbonate)}{Lungs\ (carbon\ dioxide)}$$

Sources of Acids

Acids are formed in the body as byproducts of normal metabolism. Common sources of hydrogen ions are carbon dioxide production, metabolism of proteins and fats, anaerobic metabolism of glucose or fats, and destruction of cells.

Production of Carbon Dioxide

Carbon dioxide is a byproduct of glucose breakdown and many other metabolic reactions. (The complete breakdown of 1 molecule of glucose results in the formation of 36 molecules of adenosine triphosphate, 6 molecules of water, and 6 molecules of carbon dioxide.) Because of the relationship between carbon dioxide and hydrogen ions through the carbonic anhydrase equation, any increase in carbon dioxide concentration in body fluids always leads to the formation of increased amounts of hydrogen ions in those fluids, with a resulting decrease in pH.

Carbon dioxide is exhaled by the lungs during breathing. Therefore, one determinant of blood pH is how much carbon dioxide is produced by body cells during metabolism versus how rapidly carbon dioxide is removed by respiration.

Metabolism of Fats and Proteins

The catabolism (breakdown) of food for energy results in the formation of *fixed acids*. Protein catabolism creates sulfuric acid. Fat catabolism creates fatty acids.

Anaerobic Metabolism of Glucose and Fats

Incomplete oxidation—as occurs whenever cells continue to metabolize substances under anaerobic, or no oxygen, conditions—of glucose leads to the formation of lactic acid. Incomplete breakdown of fatty acids, either because excessive amounts of fatty acids are being metabolized or because insufficient oxygen is present during any fatty acid breakdown, results in the formation of ketoacids (Guyton & Hall, 1996).

Destruction of Cells

Whenever cells are damaged or destroyed, plasma membranes are broken and intracellular contents are released. Some cell structures contain acids that are released into the extracellular fluid (ECF) when this occurs.

Sources of Bicarbonate Ions

Bicarbonate is the principal buffer of the ECF. Sources of bicarbonate in the ECF include the breakdown of carbonic acid, gastrointestinal absorption of ingested bicarbonate, pancreatic synthesis and secretion of bicarbonate, movement of intracellular bicarbonate into the ECF, and renal reabsorption of filtered bicarbonate. Once bicarbonate is in the ECF, it is maintained at a concentration 20 times greater than that of carbonic acid.

Homeostasis

As long as body cells are capable of metabolism, the production of various acids, carbon dioxide, and hydrogen ions is a normal and continuous process. Despite this production, homeostasis of body fluids in terms of hydrogen ion, bicarbonate, oxygen, and carbon dioxide concentrations is maintained under normal physiologic conditions. Chart 18–1 lists normal values for these substances

---

Chart 18–1

Laboratory Profile: Acid-Base Assessment

	Normal Range for Adults		
Test	Arterial	Venous	Significance of Abnormal Findings
pH >90 years	7.35–7.45 7.25–7.45	7.32–7.43	Increased: metabolic alkalosis, loss of gastric fluids, decreased potassium intake, diuretic therapy, fever, salicylate toxicity Decreased: metabolic or respiratory acidosis, ketosis, renal failure, starvation, diarrhea, hyperthyroidism
PaO_2 (mm Hg) >90 years	83–108 >50		Increased: increased ventilation, oxygen therapy, exercise Decreased: respiratory depression, high altitude, carbon monoxide poisoning, decreased cardiac output
$PaCO_2$ (mm Hg)	35–48	41–55	Increased: respiratory acidosis, emphysema, pneumonia, cardiac failure, respiratory depression Decreased: respiratory alkalosis, excessive ventilation, diarrhea
Bicarbonate (mEq/L or mmol/L)	22–26	24–29	Increased: bicarbonate therapy, metabolic alkalosis Decreased: metabolic acidosis, diarrhea, pancreatitis
Lactate (mg/dL)	<11.3	8.1–15.3	Increased: hypoxia, exercise, insulin infusion, alcoholism, pregnancy Decreased: fluid overload

PaO_2 = partial pressure of arterial oxygen; $PaCO_2$ = partial pressure of arterial carbon dioxide.

---

in arterial and venous blood. This homeostasis depends on three factors:

- Hydrogen ion production must be consistent and not excessive.
- Carbon dioxide loss from the body through breathing must occur at a rate that keeps pace with hydrogen ion production.
- The ratio between carbonic acid and bicarbonate must be maintained at 1:20.

Acid-Base Regulatory Mechanisms

To maintain the hydrogen ion concentration (pH) of the extracellular fluid (ECF) within the narrow ranges of normal, the body has three well-regulated mechanisms for acid-base balance: chemical, respiratory, and renal (Table 18–3).

Chemical Mechanisms

Buffers are the first line of defense against changes in hydrogen ion concentration. Because they are constantly present in body fluids, buffers can take immediate action to reduce or raise the hydrogen ion concentration to normal. By acting as hydrogen ion "sponges," buffers can bind hydrogen ions when the concentration is too high or release hydrogen ions when the concentration is too low. Fluid buffers are composed of chemicals or proteins.

CHEMICAL BUFFERS. Chemical buffers are paired mixtures, usually consisting of a weak base and the conjugated salt of an acid. The two most common chemical buffer systems are bicarbonate buffers (which are active in both the ECF and intracellular fluid [ICF]) and phosphate buffers (which are active in the ICF).

PROTEIN BUFFERS. Proteins are the largest source of buffers. Proteins in body fluids can either bind or release hydrogen ions as needed. Both intracellular and extracellular proteins serve as buffers.

The major intracellular protein buffer is hemoglobin. Hemoglobin buffers hydrogen ions directly, and also buffers whole acids formed during the synthesis and transport of carbon dioxide. When the hydrogen ion concentration of the blood increases, some of the excess hydrogen ions cross the plasma membrane of red blood cells and bind to the large numbers of hemoglobin molecules in each red blood cell.

Extracellular buffering proteins include albumins and globulins. These proteins buffer both carbonic acid and the fixed acids present in the ECF as a result of catabolism.

Respiratory Mechanisms

When chemical buffers alone cannot prevent changes in body fluid pH, the respiratory system is the second line of defense against changes. Breathing controls hydrogen ion concentration by regulating the carbon dioxide concentration in arterial blood. Carbon dioxide is converted into hydrogen ions through the carbonic anhydrase reaction; therefore, the carbon dioxide concentration is directly related to the hydrogen ion concentration. Breathing is a major mechanism for ridding the body of

TABLE 18-3

Acid-Base Regulatory Mechanisms

Chemical Mechanisms

Protein buffers
  Extracellular
    Albumin
    Globulins
  Intracellular
    Hemoglobin
Chemical buffers
  Extracellular
    Bicarbonate
  Intracellular
    Phosphate
    Bicarbonate

- Very rapid
- Provide immediate response to changing conditions
- Can handle relatively small fluctuations in hydrogen ion production and elimination encountered under normal metabolic and health conditions

Respiratory Mechanisms

Increased hydrogen ions
Increased carbon dioxide
  Stimulates central respiratory neurons, leading to increased rate and depth of breathing, causing more carbon dioxide to be lost and decreasing the hydrogen ion concentration
Decreased hydrogen ions
Decreased carbon dioxide
  Inhibition of central respiratory neurons, leading to decreased rate and depth of breathing, causing normally produced carbon dioxide to be retained, increasing the hydrogen ion concentration

- Primarily assist buffering systems when the fluctuation of hydrogen ion concentration is acute

Renal Mechanisms

Mechanisms to decrease pH
  Increased renal excretion of bicarbonate
  Increased renal reabsorption of hydrogen ions
Mechanisms to increase pH
  Decreased renal excretion of bicarbonate
  Decreased renal reabsorption of hydrogen ions

- The most powerful regulator of acid-base balance
- Respond to large or chronic fluctuations in hydrogen ion production or elimination

---

is exhaled during breathing and is lost from the body. Because the partial pressure (concentration) of carbon dioxide in atmospheric air is nearly zero, carbon dioxide usually continues to be exhaled at an appropriate rate even when breathing is impaired to some degree.

HYPERVENTILATION. Respiratory regulation of acid-base balance is under the control of the nervous system (Fig. 18–6). Special chemoreceptors in the areas of the brain that directly regulate the rate and depth of respiration are sensitive to changes in the carbon dioxide concentration in the cerebral extracellular fluid (ECF). As the carbon dioxide concentration begins to rise in cerebral blood and tissues, these central chemoreceptors stimulate the neurons that control the rate and depth of respiration. Under this stimulation, both the rate and the depth of respiration increase, so that more carbon dioxide is exhaled ("blown off") from the alveoli and the carbon dioxide concentration of the ECF decreases. When the arterial carbon dioxide concentration returns to normal, the rate and depth of respiration return to levels normal for the individual.

HYPOVENTILATION. If the ECF hydrogen ion concentration is too low, then the carbon dioxide concentration is also too low. Central chemoreceptors sense these low carbon dioxide levels and inhibit stimulation of neurons in the respiratory control centers. As a result of this lack of stimulation, the rate and depth of respiration dramatically diminish, so that less carbon dioxide is lost through the lungs and more carbon dioxide is retained in arterial blood. This retention, coupled with the normal carbon dioxide–generating metabolic reactions, results in a rapid return of the arterial carbon dioxide concentration (and hydrogen ion concentration) to normal levels. When these levels are normal, the rate and depth of respiration also return to basal levels.

The respiratory system's response in regulating acid-base balance is rapid. Changes in the rate and depth of respiration occur within minutes after changes in the hydrogen ion concentration or carbon dioxide concentration of the ECF occur.

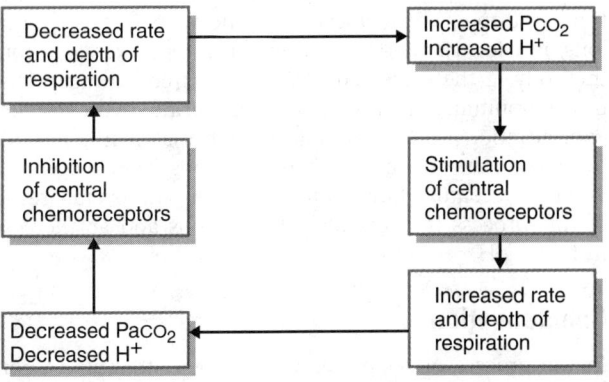

Figure 18–6. Neural regulation of respiration and hydrogen ion concentration. (PaCO$_2$ = partial pressure of arterial carbon dioxide; H$^+$ = hydrogen ion.)

carbon dioxide, which is created as a byproduct of metabolism.

The carbon dioxide concentration in venous blood increases during normal metabolism. This carbon dioxide is transported to the capillaries of the lungs. Because the partial pressure (concentration) of carbon dioxide is far higher in capillary blood than in the atmospheric air in the alveoli, carbon dioxide diffuses freely from the blood into the alveolar air. Once in the alveoli, carbon dioxide

Renal Mechanisms

The kidneys are the third line of defense against fluctuations in body fluid pH. Renal mechanisms are the most powerful mechanism for regulating acid-base balance, but take longer to start than the chemical and respiratory mechanisms. When changes in body fluid pH are persistent, renal mechanisms that increase excretion and reabsorption rates of acids or bases (depending on the direction of the pH changes) begin to operate (Fig. 18–7). These mechanisms include renal tubular movement of bicarbonate, formation of acids, and formation of ammonium.

TUBULAR MOVEMENT OF BICARBONATE. This first renal mechanism occurs in the kidney tubules in two ways: (1) renal movement of bicarbonate produced elsewhere in the body and (2) renal movement of bicarbonate produced in the kidneys. Much of the bicarbonate made in other body areas is absorbed into the blood and filtered from the blood into early urine in the nephron. When blood hydrogen ion levels are high, this filtered bicarbonate is reabsorbed from the tubules back into systemic circulation, where it can help buffer excess hydrogen ions. When blood hydrogen ion levels are low, the filtered bicarbonate remains in the urine and is excreted. When a hydrogen ion excess is evident, the kidney tubules can respond by making additional bicarbonate that will be reabsorbed.

FORMATION OF ACIDS. The second renal mechanism occurs through the phosphate-buffering mechanism inside the cells of the kidney tubules. When the newly created bicarbonate made in the tubule cells is reabsorbed into systemic circulation along with the sodium, the urine has an excess of anions, including phosphate (HPO_4^{2-}). This negatively charged environment draws hydrogen ions into the urine. Once the hydrogen ion is in the urine, it combines with the phosphate ion, forming an acid, H_2PO_4, which is then excreted from the body in the urine.

FORMATION OF AMMONIUM. In the third renal mechanism, ammonium (NH_4^+) is formed from ammonia, which is a byproduct of normal amino acid catabolism (Guyton & Hall, 1996). Ammonia is excreted into the tubular urine, where it can combine with free hydrogen ions and form ammonium. Afterward, it is excreted from the body in the urine. This trapping of free hydrogen ions in ammonium prevents the tubular urine hydrogen ion concentration from becoming so high that it inhibits diffusion or transport of free hydrogen ions from blood and other extracellular fluids into the urine. The overall result of this process is a loss of hydrogen ions and an increase in blood pH.

Compensation

In the process of *compensation*, the body attempts to correct for changes in body fluid (blood) pH. A pH below 6.9 or above 7.8 is usually fatal. The normal pH range for human extracellular fluids is 7.35 to 7.45.

Renal Compensation

A healthy renal system can correct or compensate for changes in pH when the respiratory system is either overwhelmed or is actually a cause of the imbalance. For example, in a person with chronic airflow limitation (CAL), the respiratory system cannot exchange gases adequately. Carbon dioxide is thus retained, and the pH of the extracellular fluid (ECF) falls, or becomes more acidic. To counteract this process, the renal system increases its excretion of hydrogen ions and increases the reabsorption of bicarbonate back into the body. As a result, the pH of body fluids remains either within or closer to the normal range. When these back-up mechanisms are completely effective, respiratory problems are fully compensated and the pH of the blood returns to normal, even though the concentration of other substances (such as oxygen and bicarbonate) may be abnormal.

Sometimes, however, the respiratory factors contributing to the acid-base imbalance are so severe that renal actions can only partially compensate, and thus the pH is not normal. Even partial compensation is critically important to acid-base balance because it prevents the imbalance from becoming severe (and possibly life-threatening).

Respiratory Compensation

The respiratory system can compensate for acid-base imbalances of a metabolic origin. For example, when prolonged running causes excess build-up of lactic acid, hydrogen ion concentration in the ECF increases and the pH drops. To bring the pH back to normal, the healthy respiratory system is stimulated by the increased carbon dioxide concentration to increase both the rate and depth of respiration. These respiratory efforts cause the blood to lose carbon dioxide with each exhalation, so ECF levels of carbon dioxide and hydrogen ions gradually decrease. When the respiratory system can fully compensate, the pH returns to normal.

Both the renal and respiratory systems can compensate for acid-base imbalances but are not equal in their compensatory actions and reactions. The respiratory system is much more sensitive to acid-base changes and can begin compensation efforts within seconds to minutes after a change in pH. These efforts are limited and can be overwhelmed easily, however. The renal compensatory mechanisms are much more powerful and result in dramatic changes in ECF composition. However, these more powerful mechanisms are not fully stimulated until the acid-base imbalance has been sustained for a period ranging from several hours to several days.

AGE-RELATED CHANGES IN ACID-BASE BALANCE

The elderly are more susceptible to pH disturbances than younger people because their normal physiologic mechanisms are less able to respond to minor fluctuations in hydrogen ion production or elimination. In addition, an elderly person may be taking medications that alter the activity of normal pH-compensating mechanisms (Chart 18–2).

1. TUBULAR MOVEMENT OF BICARBONATE

METHOD A: Movement of Pre-existing Bicarbonate   **METHOD B:** Movement of New Bicarbonate

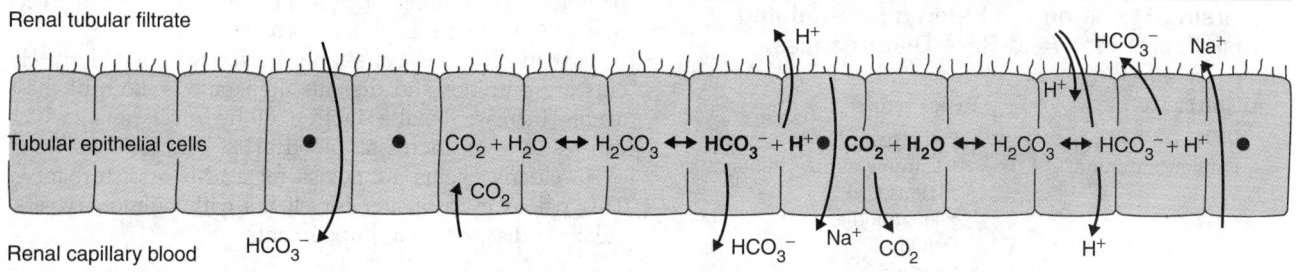

Bicarbonate filtered at the glomerulus into the filtrate ("early urine") is reabsorbed across the renal tubular epithelium into the renal capillaries and returned to the systemic circulation. This movement of bicarbonate into the systemic circulation increases blood pH (makes blood less acidic).

If Blood CO_2 Levels Are High
Carbon dioxide enters the tubular epithelium, shifting the carbonic anhydrase equation to the right to form bicarbonate and hydrogen ions. Bicarbonate moves into the renal capillaries. Hydrogen moves into the tubular filtrate in exchange for sodium. The loss of hydrogen ions from blood increases its pH (makes it less acidic).

To prevent excess hydrogen in the renal tubular filtrate, hydrogen ions must combine with other substances. The second and third renal mechanisms of acid-base balance now come into play.

If Blood CO_2 Levels Are Low
Hydrogen ions from the tubular filtrate are reabsorbed into the renal capillaries in exchange for sodium. This flow of hydrogen may be direct, or it may shift the carbonic anhydrase equation to the left so that carbon dioxide is reabsorbed into the systemic circulation and bicarbonate moves into the renal tubular filtrate. Retention of acids and excretion of bases reduce blood pH (makes blood more acidic).

2. FORMATION OF TITRATABLE ACIDS

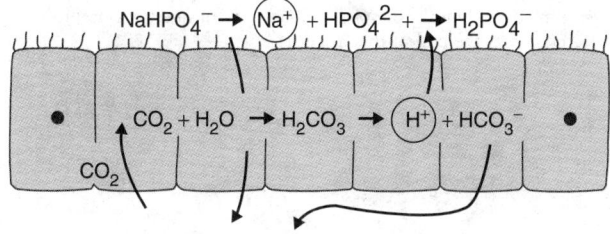

After the newly generated bicarbonate and the cation sodium are passed into the systemic circulation, the renal tubular filtrate has an excess of anions, including phoshate. The cation hydrogen is attracted to the negatively charged environment of the renal tubular filtrate. There, hydrogen binds with phosphate to form the titratable acid H_2PO_4, which is excreted in urine.

3. FORMATION OF AMMONIUM

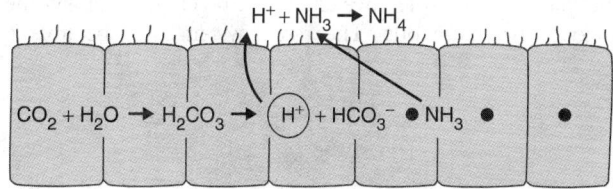

Ammonia produced by amino acid (glutamine) catabolism is excreted into the renal tubular filtrate. There, ammonia combines with hydrogen cations to form ammonium, which is excreted in urine.

Figure 18–7. Renal mechanisms of acid-base balance. (CO_2 = carbon dioxide.)

Chart 18-2

Nursing Focus on the Elderly: Age-Related Risk Factors for Acid-Base Disturbances

Disturbance	Risk Factors

• Increased hydrogen ion concentration	• Pulmonary diseases
	  • Chronic airflow limitation (CAL)
	  • Pneumonia
	• Dehydration
	• Infection
	• Renal disease
	• Vascular disease
	  • Atherosclerosis
	  • Arteriosclerosis
	  • Angiitis

• Decreased hydrogen ion concentration	• Overhydration
	• Congestive heart failure
	• Drugs
	  • Diuretics (loop and thiazide)
	  • Digitalis preparations
	  • Insulin
	  • Antibiotics
	  • Chemotherapeutic agents

The effectiveness of gas exchange during breathing is also reduced as a person ages. There is less alveolar membrane for gas exchange in older people, and many also have some degree of blood vessel thickening, which further impairs gas diffusion through capillaries. These conditions can cause carbon dioxide retention, increasing the concentration of hydrogen ions.

Because renal function diminishes with age, elderly people are less able to excrete hydrogen ions or synthesize bicarbonate ions. The renal system may be able to handle ordinary changes resulting from normal metabolism, but it cannot compensate adequately when other pathologic conditions (such as pneumonia, fever, or infection) interfere with acid-base balance.

Two medications commonly prescribed for elderly clients are diuretics and digitalis preparations. Both of these agents increase renal excretion of hydrogen ions, which can result in an increased blood pH.

All elderly clients are at risk for acid-base disturbances. This risk is even greater for clients with pulmonary, vascular, cardiac, or renal impairments.

SELECTED BIBLIOGRAPHY

Cornock, M. (1996). Making sense of arterial blood gases and their interpretation. *Nursing Times, 92*(6), 30–31.

Guyton, A., & Hall, J. (1996). *Textbook of medical physiology* (9th ed.). Philadelphia: W. B. Saunders.

Halperin, M., & Goldstein, M. (1994), *Fluid, electrolyte and acid-base physiology: A problem-based approach* (2nd ed.). Philadelphia: W. B. Saunders.

Kuhn, M. (1996). Laboratory analysis. *Critical Care Nurse, 16*(5), 74–76.

Mays, D. (1995). Turn ABGs into child's play. *RN, 58*(1), 36–40.

Metheny, N. (1996). *Fluid and electrolyte balance: Nursing considerations* (3rd ed.). Philadelphia: J. B. Lippincott.

O'Donnell, J. (1995). Can you prevent respiratory depression? *Nursing95, 25*(4), 32JJ.

Tasota, F., & Wesmiller, S. (1994). Assessing A.B.G.s: Maintaining the delicate balance. *Nursing94, 24*(5), 34–46.

Tietz, N. W. (Ed.). (1995). *Clinical guide to laboratory tests* (3rd ed.). Philadelphia: W. B. Saunders.

SUGGESTED READINGS

Mays, D. (1995). Turn ABGs into child's play. *RN, 58*(1), 36-40.
  The author uses a game approach to describe a simple method of determining the pH status for an individual client. Practice opportunity is provided through the use of several case presentations.

Tasota, F., & Wesmiller, S. (1994). Assessing A.B.G.s: Maintaining the delicate balance. *Nursing94, 24*(5), 34–46.
  This well-written article describes the interaction among oxygenation, ventilation and acid-base balance. Several case studies are presented as clinical examples. Self-assessment questions are included at the end of the article.

Chapter 19

INTERVENTIONS FOR CLIENTS WITH ACID-BASE IMBALANCE

Acid-base balance, or hydrogen ion concentration as measured by pH, is the most carefully regulated body parameter. The normal pH range of body fluids is 7.35 to 7.45. Changes in the pH of blood indicate either problems with the body's acid-base regulatory mechanisms or exposure of the body to dangerous conditions. Severe impairment of normal physiology accompanies acid-base imbalances and can be life-threatening. Table 19–1 lists key points associated with acid-base imbalance.

ACIDOSIS

Overview

In acidosis, the acid-base balance of the blood and other extracellular fluid (ECF) is disturbed. Acidosis is characterized by an excess of hydrogen ions (H^+), or an arterial blood pH below 7.35. The concentration or strength, or both, of acid components is greater than normal compared with the concentration or strength of the base components.

Acidosis is not a disease but rather a condition caused by a disease or pathologic process. Acidosis can be caused by metabolic problems, respiratory problems, or both.

Pathophysiology

Acidosis can result from an actual or relative increase in the concentration or strength of acid components. In an actual acid excess, acidosis results from processes that cause either an overproduction of acids (and release of hydrogen ions) or an underelimination of normally produced acids (retention of hydrogen ions).

In *relative* acidosis, the actual amount or strength of acid components does not increase. Instead, the concentration or strength (or both) of the base components decreases (to create a *base deficit*), which makes the fluid relatively more acidic than basic. A relative acid-excess acidosis (or *actual base deficit*) results from processes that cause either an overelimination (usually in the form of bicarbonate ions [HCO_3^-]) or an underproduction of base components (Fig. 19–1).

Regardless of its origin, acidosis causes major changes in physiologic function. Its primary pathologic effects are related to the fact that hydrogen ions are cations (positively charged electrolytes). An increase in hydrogen ion concentration creates imbalances of other electrolytes, especially potassium, the principal cation in intracellular fluid, which then disrupts functions of excitable membranes, such as nerve and cardiac tissue. Many of the early signs and symptoms associated with acidosis thus appear in the neuromuscular, cardiac, respiratory, and central nervous systems (Metheny, 1996). Even slight increases in hydrogen ion concentration cause many body hormones and enzymes, as well as medications, to become inactive and may lead to death.

TABLE 19–1

Key Points Related to Acid-Base Imbalances

- Acidemia is defined as an increase in the hydrogen ion concentration (pH) of the blood, and is reflected by an arterial blood pH below 7.35.
- Acidemia can result from an actual acid excess or a relative base deficit.
- Metabolic acidosis usually results from a lack of bicarbonate or an excess acid production in the body.
- Respiratory acidosis results from retention of carbon dioxide in the body, causing increased carbonic acid production.
- Manifestations of acidemia are related to fluid and electrolyte imbalances that accompany acid-base imbalance, such as hyperkalemia.
- Chronic respiratory acidosis is common in the medical-surgical setting as a result of chronic obstructive pulmonary disease, such as emphysema.
- Alkalemia is defined as a decrease in the hydrogen ion concentration of the blood, reflected by an arterial blood pH above 7.45.
- Alkalemia can result from an actual base excess or an acid deficit.
- Metabolic alkalosis most often occurs when body acids are lost, such as in prolonged vomiting or nasogastric suctioning.
- Respiratory alkalosis most often occurs when hyperventilation causes excessive carbon dioxide loss.
- Dehydration and hypokalemia are associated with metabolic alkalosis, and account for most of the clinical manifestations seen in this acid-base imbalance.
- The goal of management for any type of acid-base imbalance is to restore fluid, electrolyte, and acid-base balance to normal or near normal.

Etiology

Acidosis can be caused by metabolic disturbances, respiratory disturbances, or combined metabolic and respiratory disturbances. The causes of metabolic and respiratory acidosis are summarized in Table 19–2.

Metabolic Acidosis

Four processes can result in metabolic acidosis: overproduction of hydrogen ions, underelimination of hydrogen ions, underproduction of bicarbonate ions, and overelimination of bicarbonate ions.

OVERPRODUCTION OF HYDROGEN IONS. Three metabolic processes that can increase body fluid hydrogen

AAABBB	AAAABBB	AAABB
AAABBB	AAAABBB	AAABB
AAABBB	AAAABBB	AAABB
Acid-base balance	Actual acidosis (acid excess)	Relative acidosis (base deficit)

Figure 19–1. Concepts of actual and relative acidosis. (A = acid; B = base.)

TABLE 19–2

Common Causes of Acidosis

Pathology	Condition
Metabolic Acidosis	

Overproduction of Hydrogen Ions	• Excessive oxidation of fatty acids
	  • Diabetic ketoacidosis
	  • Starvation
	 • Hypermetabolism
	  • Heavy exercise
	  • Seizure activity
	  • Fever
	  • Hypoxia, ischemia
	 • Excessive ingestion of acids
	  • Ethanol intoxication
	  • Methanol ingestion
	  • Salicylate intoxication

Underelimination of Hydrogen Ions	• Renal failure
Underproduction of Bicarbonate	• Renal failure • Pancreatitis • Liver failure • Dehydration
Overelimination of Bicarbonate	• Diarrhea • Buffering of organic acids
Respiratory Acidosis	

Underelimination of Hydrogen Ions	• Respiratory depression
	  • Anesthetics
	  • Drugs (especially opioids)
	  • Poisons
	  • Electrolyte imbalance
	  • Trauma
	    Cerebral edema
	    Spinal cord injuries
	  • Neuritic diseases
	    Guillain-Barré
	    Polio
	    Myasthenia gravis
	 • Inadequate chest expansion
	  • Skeletal deformities
	  • Muscle weakness
	  • Nonpulmonary restriction
	    Obesity
	    Fluid
	    Tumor
	 • Airway obstruction
	  • Asthma
	  • Cancer
	  • Bronchiolitis
	 • Alveolar-capillary block
	  • Thrombus or embolus
	  • Vascular occlusive disease
	  • Pneumonia
	  • Pulmonary edema
	  • Tuberculosis
	  • Cystic fibrosis
	  • Atelectasis
	  • Adult respiratory distress syndrome (ARDS)
	  • Emphysema
	  • Cancer

ion concentration are excessive breakdown of fatty acids, hypermetabolism (anaerobic lactic acidosis), and excessive ingestion of acidic substances.

Excessive Breakdown of Fatty Acids. Excessive breakdown of fatty acids is usually a result of diabetic ketoacidosis or starvation. When glucose is not readily available for metabolic fuel, the body metabolizes fats (lipids) instead. The metabolites from fatty acid breakdown form strong acids called *ketoacids*, which release large amounts of hydrogen ions.

Hypermetabolism (Anaerobic Lactic Acidosis). When cells are forced to use glucose without adequate oxygen (anaerobic metabolism), glucose is incompletely metabolized and forms lactic acid. Lactic acid molecules leave the cell, enter the extracellular fluid (ECF), and release hydrogen ions, causing acidosis. Anaerobic metabolism that results in lactic acidosis occurs whenever the body has insufficient oxygen. Some conditions leading to lactic acidosis include strenuous exercise, seizure activity, fever, and presence of tissue hypoxia.

Excessive Intake of Acidic Substances. Excessive ingestion of acidic substances floods the body directly with hydrogen ions. Some of the most common substances that cause acidosis when ingested in excess include ethyl (for drinking) alcohol, methyl alcohol (a poison), and acetylsalicylic acid (aspirin).

UNDERELIMINATION OF HYDROGEN IONS. The major routes for hydrogen ion elimination are respiratory (via the lungs) and renal (via the kidneys). Renal failure causes acidosis when the renal tubules cannot secrete hydrogen ions into the urine. As a result, too many hydrogen ions are retained.

UNDERPRODUCTION OF BICARBONATE IONS. As discussed in Chapter 18, bicarbonate is the most common base in the fluid outside the cells and is responsible for buffering carbonic acid (H_2CO_3). When body fluid levels of bicarbonate are too low, a base-deficit state exists. Base-deficit acidosis occurs when hydrogen ion production and elimination are normal, but too few molecules of bicarbonate ions are present to balance the hydrogen ions. Such base deficits occur when bicarbonate ions are not produced at the normal rate. Because bicarbonate is made in the kidney tubules and in the pancreas, renal failure and diminished hepatic or pancreatic function can result in a base-deficit acidosis (Guyton & Hall, 1996).

OVERELIMINATION OF BICARBONATE IONS. Base-deficit acidosis can also occur when hydrogen ion production and elimination are normal but too many bicarbonate ions have been eliminated (overelimination). The most common example of overelimination is diarrhea.

Respiratory Acidosis

Respiratory acidosis results from an impairment in any area of respiratory function, causing an inadequate exchange of oxygen (O_2) and carbon dioxide (CO_2). This impairment causes carbon dioxide retention. Because any increase in carbon dioxide concentration causes a corresponding increase in hydrogen ion concentration, carbon dioxide retention leads to acidosis, as demonstrated in the carbonic anhydrase equation:

$$CO_2 + H_2O \longleftrightarrow H_2CO_3 \longleftrightarrow H^+ + HCO_3^-$$

An excess of carbon dioxide forces the equation to the right, first increasing the production of carbonic acid. The carbonic acid then rapidly dissociates (separates) into hydrogen ions and bicarbonate ions. This increase in the free hydrogen ion concentration of the blood is acidosis.

Unlike metabolic acidosis, respiratory acidosis results from only one primary mechanism: retention of carbon dioxide, causing an underelimination of hydrogen ions. Virtually all causes of respiratory acidosis result in an acid-excess acidosis. Four types of respiratory problems can cause respiratory acidosis: respiratory depression, inadequate chest expansion, airway obstruction, and interference with alveolar-capillary diffusion.

RESPIRATORY DEPRESSION. Respiratory depression involves a change in the function of brain stem neurons stimulating inhalation and exhalation. The overall result is a reduced rate and depth of respiration, causing inadequate gas exchange and a retention of carbon dioxide. Respiratory depression may be chemical or physical in origin.

Chemical Depression. Chemical depression of respiratory neurons in the brain can result from the action of anesthetic agents, drugs (especially opioids), and poisons that cross the blood-brain barrier. Specific electrolyte imbalances (see Chapter 16 for hyponatremia, hypercalcemia, and hyperkalemia) also slow or inhibit respiratory neurons.

Physical Depression. Physical depression of respiratory neurons can occur in response to many conditions. Respiratory neurons can be damaged or destroyed by trauma or when problems in other areas of the brain cause an increase in intracranial pressure. Such an increase causes edema of brain tissues, which then presses into the respiratory centers located in the brain stem. Conditions causing cerebral edema with resultant respiratory depression include brain tumors, cerebral aneurysm, cerebrovascular accidents, overhydration, and hyponatremia.

INADEQUATE CHEST EXPANSION. Any condition that restricts or limits chest expansion can result in inadequate gas exchange. Inadequate chest expansion can result from skeletal trauma or deformities, respiratory muscle weakness, or non–respiratory-associated movement restrictions.

Skeletal Problems. Respiratory movement of the chest wall will be restricted if broken or malformed bones distort the shape of the chest. Broken ribs restrict chest movement because they cannot provide the rigid structure needed for thoracic pressure changes (as in flail chest).

Pain from broken ribs may also cause voluntary restriction of chest movement.

Respiratory Muscle Weakness. Conditions causing respiratory muscle weakness that can make chest expansion inadequate include electrolyte imbalances (especially hyperkalemia and hyponatremia), fatigue, muscular dystrophy, rhabdomyosarcoma, and inflammatory myositis.

Nonrespiratory Conditions. Nonrespiratory conditions also can restrict the chest movement necessary for full lung expansion. Causes of restricted chest movement include body cast enclosure of the thoracic cavity, tight scar tissue formation around the chest, severe obesity, abdominal masses, ascites, and hemothorax (blood in the thoracic cavity).

AIRWAY OBSTRUCTION. Prevention of air movement in and out of the lungs through airway obstruction can lead to ineffective gas exchange, carbon dioxide retention, and acidosis. The upper airway can be obstructed externally by restrictive clothing, neck edema, and regional lymph node enlargement. Internal obstruction of the upper airway can be caused by aspiration of foreign objects, constriction of bronchial smooth muscles, and edema. Internal obstruction of the lower airways is caused by constriction of smooth muscle, edema, and excessive mucus, which occurs in asthma, bronchiolitis, and emphysema.

INTERFERENCE WITH ALVEOLAR-CAPILLARY DIFFUSION. Most pulmonary gas exchanges occur by diffusion where the alveolar membrane and the capillary membranes meet. Any condition that prevents or slows this diffusion process can cause retention of carbon dioxide and acidosis. Conditions or disease that can prevent alveolar-capillary diffusion include pneumonia, pulmonary edema, aspiration of fluids, pneumonitis, tuberculosis, emphysema, adult respiratory distress syndrome, chest trauma, pulmonary emboli, and pulmonary edema.

Combined Metabolic and Respiratory Acidosis

Metabolic and respiratory acidosis can occur simultaneously. Uncorrected acute respiratory acidosis always leads to anaerobic (lacking molecular oxygen) metabolism and lactic acidosis (Metheny, 1996). The resulting acidosis is more profound than that caused by either metabolic acidosis or respiratory acidosis alone. Cardiac arrest is an example of a condition leading to combined metabolic and respiratory acidosis. Another example is the development of severe diarrhea in a client with chronic obstructive lung disease.

Incidence/Prevalence

Because acidosis is a manifestation of many pathologic conditions rather than a separate disease state, its actual incidence is not known. Mild metabolic acidosis resulting from lactic acidosis is common even among healthy people, however. Normal respiratory compensation usually prevents this acidosis from becoming severe or prolonged, and no intervention is necessary. Clients at particular risk

---

Chart 19–1

Nursing Focus on the Elderly: The Elderly Client Experiencing Acid-Base Imbalance

When Taking a Client's History

- Assess risk factors for acid-base imbalance, including medications, chronic health problems (especially renal disease, pulmonary disease), and acute health problems.
- Take the history when the client is awake and more familiar with surroundings.
- Ask the client to list all prescribed and over-the-counter medications (especially diuretics and antacids). If the client cannot recall this information or seems confused, ask the significant other to bring medications from home to show the nurse.
- Ask the client to recall what liquids she or he has taken in the past 24 hours and whether the client has urinated as much as usual.

When Assessing the Client

- Compare the client's mental status with what the family, significant other, or health record states is the client's baseline.
- Observe the rate and depth of respiration.
  - Can the client complete a sentence without stopping to take a breath?
  - Examine the color of the client's nail beds and mucous membranes.
- Obtain a specimen of urine and observe for color and character. Test for specific gravity and pH.
- Examine skin turgor for dehydration. Attempt to pinch the skin up to form a tent over the sternum and on the forehead. If a tent forms, record how long it remains.
- Measure the rate and quality of the pulse.

Observe the client's clinical responses and laboratory values carefully while the acid-base imbalance is being corrected.
Administer intravenous therapy by pump or controller.

---

for acidosis are those with conditions that impair any aspect of respiratory function to any degree, as in the elderly (see Chart 19–1).

Collaborative Management

 Assessment

➤ *History*

When obtaining a history from any client, the nurse collects data related to risk factors as well as causative factors related to the development of acidosis, specifically age, nutrition, and presenting symptoms.

Age. The elderly are more vulnerable to conditions that may cause an acid-base imbalance. Such conditions include impairments of cardiac, renal, and pulmonary functions. In addition, elderly persons are more likely to be taking prescribed or over-the-counter medications that interfere with acid-base, fluid, and electrolyte balance, especially diuretics, aspirin, and products containing alcohol. The nurse asks about specific risk factors, such as any type of respiratory problem, renal failure, diabetes mellitus, diarrhea, pancreatitis, and fever.

Nutrition. The nurse obtains a detailed diet history to determine total caloric intake as well as approximate proportions of carbohydrates, fats, and proteins ingested. The nurse specifically asks the client whether he or she has fasted or followed a strict diet during the preceding week.

Symptoms. Because the client's central nervous system is frequently depressed in acidosis, the nurse may question a close family member or the client's significant other. The nurse asks the client whether he or she has experienced headaches, behavior changes, increased drowsiness, reduced alertness, reduced attention span, lethargy, anorexia, abdominal distention, nausea or vomiting, muscle weakness, or increased fatigue. Having the client relate activities of the previous 24 hours may disclose additional information about activity intolerance, changes in behavior, and unexplained fatigue.

> ### ➤ *Physical Assessment/Clinical Manifestations*

The key clinical manifestations of acidosis are similar whether the cause is metabolic or respiratory (Chart 19–2). Clinical manifestations are associated primarily with changes in activity of excitable membranes involved in cerebral, neuromuscular, and gastric smooth muscle functions.

Central Nervous System Manifestations. Depression of central nervous system function is common in acidosis

---

Chart 19–2

Key Features of Acidosis

Central Nervous System Manifestations
- Depressed activity (lethargy, confusion, stupor, and coma)

Neuromuscular Manifestations
- Hyporeflexia
- Skeletal muscle weakness
- Flaccid paralysis

Cardiovascular Manifestations
- Delayed electrical conduction
  - Bradycardia to block
  - Tall T waves
  - Widened QRS complex
  - Prolonged PR interval
- Hypotension
- Thready peripheral pulses

Respiratory Manifestations
- Kussmaul respirations (in metabolic acidosis with respiratory compensation)
- Variable respirations (generally ineffective in respiratory acidosis)

Integumentary Manifestations
- Warm, flushed, dry skin in metabolic acidosis
- Pale to cyanotic and dry skin in respiratory acidosis

---

and may be manifested as lethargy that progresses to confusion, especially in elderly clients. As acidosis worsens or if it is accompanied by hyperkalemia, the client may become stuporous and unresponsive. The nurse assesses the client's level of consciousness (see Chap. 43).

Neuromuscular Manifestations. An increase in serum hydrogen ion concentration, along with any accompanying hyperkalemia, causes a decrease in muscle tone and deep tendon reflexes. The nurse assesses muscle strength by having the client

- Squeeze the nurse's hand
- Attempt to keep arms flexed while the nurse pulls downward on the lower arms
- Push both feet against a flat surface while the nurse applies resistance

Muscle weakness associated with acidosis is bilateral and can progress to flaccid paralysis. Respiratory efforts are reduced when skeletal muscles become weak.

Cardiovascular Manifestations. Early cardiac manifestations of acidosis include increased heart rate and cardiac output. As acidosis worsens or if it is accompanied by hyperkalemia, electrical conduction through the myocardium is reduced and the heart rate decreases. The nurse monitors for clinical as well as electrocardiographic changes. Peripheral pulses may be hard to find and are easily blocked with light pressure. The client may experience hypotension as a result of vasodilation.

Respiratory Manifestations. The nurse assesses the client's respiratory system by observing the rate, depth, and ease of respirations. Pulse oximetry is performed to determine the effectiveness of oxygen delivery to peripheral tissues. Some agencies are using protective shields for pulse oximetry sensors, reducing costs by allowing the sensors to be reused. This manipulation of the sensor does not appear to alter its accuracy (see Research Applications for Nursing).

Metabolic Causes. If acidosis is metabolic in origin, the rate and depth of respiration increase in proportion to the increase in the hydrogen ion concentration. Respirations are deep, rapid, and not under voluntary control. This pattern is called *Kussmaul respiration.*

Respiratory Causes. If acidosis is respiratory in origin, the effectiveness of respiratory efforts is greatly reduced. Respirations are usually shallow and quite rapid.

Integumentary Manifestations. Respiration is unimpaired and respiratory rate increased in metabolic acidosis. The increased gas exchange, coupled with a vasodilation, makes the client's skin and mucous membranes warm, dry, and pink. Because respirations are ineffective in respiratory acidosis, skin and mucous membranes are pale to cyanotic.

> ### ➤ *Psychosocial Assessment*

It is vital that the nurse complete a psychosocial assessment, because behavioral changes resulting from central nervous system effects may be the first observable clinical manifestations of acidosis. The nurse observes and docu-

⊳ Research Applications for Nursing

Save Money on Pulse Oximetry Without Sacrificing Accuracy

Russell, G., & Graybeal, J. (1995). Accuracy of laminated disposable pulse-oximetry sensors. Respiratory Care, 40(7), 728–733.

The purpose of this study was to determine whether pulse-oximetry sensors protected with a disposable, plastic-laminated shield were as sensitive and accurate at measuring oxygen saturation (SPO_2) as unshielded sensors. Pulse-oximeter accuracy reported by the manufacturers is ±2 percentage points for values in the 70 to 100% range and ±3 percentage points for values below 70%. Five healthy adult male volunteers had arterial blood gases measured at the same time pulse oximetry was measured using both shielded and unshielded sensors. All subjects were subjected to hypoxemic episodes by exposure to a hypoxic gas mixture of 8 to 10% oxygen in balance with helium. A total of 20 hypoxemic episodes were measured. Desaturation was measured every 10 seconds during each hypoxemic episode for a total of 907 pulse oximetry pairs. For SPO_2 measurements above 70% saturation, both the shielded and unshielded sensors were within the manufacturer's reported accuracy. Response times to reductions in SPO_2 were also unaffected. Both shielded and unshielded sensors were less consistently accurate below 70% saturation.

Critique. The study was well controlled and answered the question with a high degree of confidence. These studies were performed over a relatively short period of time, however (each hypoxemic episode lasted only 10 minutes). No data are available to determine whether lamination affects sensor accuracy with multiple uses over a longer period (such as 24 hours).

Possible Nursing Implications. It may be possible to reuse disposable sensors labeled "single use only" without sacrificing accuracy. Cross-contamination is a danger in reusing any equipment, however. Until such reuse has been demonstrated to not increase the risk for cross-contamination and infection, use should be limited to high-volume areas with immunocompetent clients only.

ments the client's presenting behavior by description (objectively) rather than by interpretation (subjectively). For example, the nurse may state that "the client is unable to recognize close family members" rather than "the client is confused" or "the client spit out the oral medication" rather than "the client is uncooperative." The nurse questions family members and significant others further to determine whether the client's presenting behavior and mental status are typical.

⊳ *Laboratory Assessment*

Arterial blood pH is the laboratory value used to confirm acidosis. When arterial blood pH is less than 7.35, acidosis is present. This test alone does not indicate the underlying pathologic condition or the origin of the acidosis, however. Because the clinical manifestations of metabolic acidosis and respiratory acidosis are similar but their effective treatments are different, it is critical that the nurse obtain and interpret additional laboratory data, such as arterial blood gas (ABG) values and measurements of certain serum electrolytes (Chart 19–3).

Metabolic Acidosis. Pure metabolic acidosis is indicated by a low pH, a low bicarbonate level, a normal partial pressure of arterial carbon dioxide ($PaCO_2$), and an elevated serum potassium level.

pH. The pH is low because buffering and respiratory compensation are not adequate to maintain the hydrogen ion concentration at a normal level.

Bicarbonate. Decreased bicarbonate level, coupled with the normal carbon dioxide level, indicates metabolic acidosis. The bicarbonate level is below normal for any one (or all) of the following reasons:
- Bicarbonate has been lost from the body, creating actual base-deficit acidosis.
- Bicarbonate has not been produced in sufficient quantities, creating actual base-deficit acidosis.
- Bicarbonate may be bound to other substances during the buffering of organic acid–stimulated acidosis.

Carbon Dioxide and Oxygen. The carbon dioxide level is normal or even slightly decreased because gas

---

Chart 19–3

Laboratory Profile: Acid-Base Imbalances

Imbalance	Laboratory Value Changes						
	pH	HCO_3^-	PaO_2	$PaCO_2$	K^+	Ca^{2+}	Cl^-
• Metabolic acidosis	↓	↓	Ø	Ø	↑	Ø	↑
• Respiratory acidosis	↓	↑	↓	↑	↑	Ø	↑↓
• Combined acidosis	↓	↑	↓	↑	↑	Ø	↑↓
• Metabolic alkalosis	↑	↑	Ø	↑	↓	↓	↓
• Respiratory alkalosis	↑	↓	Ø	↓	↓	↓	↑
• Combined alkalosis	↑	↑	Ø	↓	↓	↓	↓

↑ = above normal; ↓ = below normal; Ø = normal; HCO_3^- = bicarbonate ions; PaO_2 = partial pressure of arterial oxygen; $PaCO_2$ = partial pressure of arterial carbon dioxide; K^+ = potassium ions; Ca^{2+} = calcium ions; Cl^- = chloride ions.

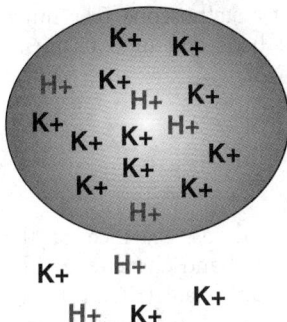

Under normal conditions, the intracellular potassium content is much greater than that of the extracellular fluid. The concentration of hydrogen ions is low in both compartments.

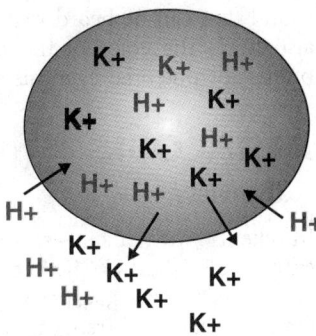

In acidemia, the extracellular hydrogen ion content increases, and the hydrogen ions move into the intracellular fluid. To keep the intracellular fluid electrically neutral, an equal number of potassium ions leave the cell, creating a relative hyperkalemia.

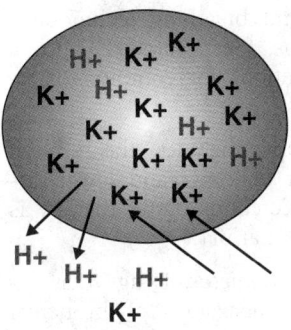

In alkalemia, more hydrogen ions are present in the intracellular fluid than in the extracellular fluid. Hydrogen ions move from the intracellular fluid into the extracellular fluid. To keep the intracellular fluid electrically neutral, potassium ions move from the extracellular fluid into the intracellular fluid, creating a relative hyperkalemia.

Figure 19–2. Movement of potassium in response to changes in the extracellular fluid hydrogen ion concentration. (© 1992 M. Linda Workman. All rights reserved.)

exchange is adequate and carbon dioxide retention is not a factor. The oxygen level is normal because gas exchange is adequate.

Potassium. The serum potassium level is frequently elevated in metabolic acidosis as a result of the body's attempt to maintain electroneutrality during buffering. In some cases, prolonged elevation of potassium in the blood may contribute to the development of metabolic acidosis.

Figure 19–2 demonstrates movement of potassium ions associated with changes in serum pH. As the hydrogen ion concentration of the blood increases, some of the excess hydrogen ions enter cells (especially red blood cells), the site of intracellular buffering mechanisms. The movement of hydrogen ions into the cells creates an intracellular excess of positive ions. To prevent intracellular charge imbalances, an equal number of potassium ions then move from the cells into the blood. This increases the extracellular potassium concentration, causing hyperkalemia.

Respiratory Acidosis. Low pH, elevated $PaCO_2$, and decreased partial pressure of arterial oxygen (PaO_2) indicate respiratory acidosis. Changes in bicarbonate and serum potassium levels vary with the duration of the acidosis and the degree of renal compensation (see Chap. 18).

pH. The increase in the ECF hydrogen ion concentration lowers pH. If the renal system partially compensates for this acidosis, then pH is low but not as abnormal as could be expected, considering the degree of derangement apparent in the retention of carbon dioxide.

Bicarbonate. Rapid onset of respiratory acidosis is characterized by a normal bicarbonate level. When respiratory acidosis persists for 24 hours or longer, renal compensation for the acidosis results in increased generation and reabsorption of bicarbonate. An elevated bicarbonate

level, coupled with increased $PaCO_2$, indicates chronic respiratory acidosis.

Carbon Dioxide and Oxygen. $PaCO_2$ is elevated and PaO_2 is decreased because the cause of this acid-base disturbance is impaired gas exchange. The impairment causes carbon dioxide retention, and the client cannot inhale adequate amounts of oxygen.

Potassium. Serum potassium levels are elevated in acute respiratory acidosis. Serum potassium levels are normal or low in chronic respiratory acidosis when renal compensation is present.

Interventions

Interventions for acidosis focus on correcting the underlying problem and supporting aerobic metabolism. To ensure appropriate interventions, the specific type of acidosis must first be identified.

➤ *Metabolic Acidosis*

Interventions for metabolic acidosis include hydration therapy and specific drugs or treatments to control or eliminate the condition causing the acidosis. For example, if the acidosis is a result of diabetic ketoacidosis, insulin is given to correct the hyperglycemia and production of ketone bodies. If the acidosis is a result of prolonged diarrhea, rehydration and antidiarrheal drugs are administered. Bicarbonate is administered only if serum bicarbonate levels are low.

➤ *Respiratory Acidosis*

Interventions for respiratory acidosis aim at maintaining a patent airway and enhancing gas exchange. Such interventions can include drug therapy, oxygen therapy, pulmonary hygiene (positioning and breathing techniques), and prevention of complications. (See Chapter 32 for a complete discussion of interventions for common disorders causing respiratory acidosis.)

Drug Therapy. Drug therapy includes the use of agents to increase the diameter of upper and lower airways and to thin pulmonary secretions. Drug therapy is not aimed directly at altering arterial pH.

Drugs to Increase Airway Diameter. Drugs that increase airway diameter induce relaxation of bronchial smooth muscle. Many of these agents are adrenergic agonists, sympathomimetic agents, antimuscarinic drugs, and methylxanthines. These drugs include albuterol (Novo-Salmol♣, Proventil, Ventolin), ephedrine, fenoterol (Berotec), isoproterenol (Isuprel), metaproterenol (Alupent), pirbuterol (Maxair), terbutaline (Brethine, Bricanyl), ipratropium (Atrovent), atropine, aminophylline (Phyllocontin, Truphylline), and theophylline (Bronkodyl, Theo-Dur♣).

Clients may take agents that increase bronchodilation by reducing inflammation of bronchial luminal tissues. These agents are primarily cortisol (steroid) based, such as beclomethasone (Vanceril, Beclovent), dexamethasone (Decadron Respihaler, Dexasone♣), flunisolide (AeroBid, Bronalide♣), and triamcinolone (Azmacort).

Drugs to Thin Bronchial Secretions. Some drugs can break up mucus when thick, tenacious pulmonary secretions contribute to airway obstruction. These agents are classified as mucolytic; an example is acetylcysteine (Mucomyst, Mucosil). (For a discussion of drugs used for clients with chronic obstructive pulmonary disease or chronic airflow limitation [CAL], see Chapter 32.)

Oxygen Therapy. Oxygen therapy can help promote gas exchange for clients with respiratory acidosis. However, the nurse must use caution when administering oxygen to clients with CAL and carbon dioxide retention, as evidenced by a high $PaCO_2$ level in arterial blood. The only respiratory trigger for these clients is a decreased arterial oxygen level. Administration of too much oxygen to these clients decreases their respiratory efforts and increases carbon dioxide retention.

Pulmonary Hygiene. To promote effective gas exchange, the nurse considers client positioning, techniques to enhance excretion of pulmonary secretions, and specific breathing techniques to change airway resistance and maintain inflated alveoli. The nurse helps clients assume a Fowler's or semi-Fowler's position to help increase lung expansion. Increasing clients' fluid intake also may reduce the thickness of pulmonary secretions and assist in their excretion.

Prevention of Complications. Monitoring clients' respiratory status is critical in preventing pulmonary complications. At least every 2 hours, the nurse assesses the respiratory status of clients experiencing chronic respiratory acidosis. In addition to assessing the rate and depth of respiration, the nurse auscultates breath sounds. The nurse notes the ease with which air moves in and out of the lungs, including any muscle retractions, use of accessory muscles, and whether respiratory effort produces a

sound that can be heard without a stethoscope. The nurse also notes the color of the nail beds and mucous membranes for potential cyanosis.

ALKALOSIS

Overview

In clients with alkalosis, the acid-base balance of the extracellular fluid (ECF) is disturbed and characterized by an excess of bases, especially bicarbonate (HCO_3^-). The concentration or strength, or both, of the base components is greater than normal compared with the concentration or strength of acid components. Alkalosis is defined as a decrease in the hydrogen ion concentration of the blood, reflected by an arterial blood pH above 7.45. Like acidosis, alkalosis is not a disease but rather a manifestation of a disease or pathologic process. Alkalosis can be caused by metabolic problems, respiratory problems, or both.

Pathophysiology

Alkalosis can result from an actual or relative increase in the concentration or strength, or both, of base components. In an actual base excess, alkalosis is the result of processes that cause either an overproduction of base components or an underelimination of normally produced base components (usually bicarbonate).

In *relative* alkalosis, the actual amount or strength of base components does not increase. Instead, the concentration or strength (or both) of the acid components decreases (creating an *acid deficit*), which makes the fluid relatively more basic than acidic. A relative base-excess alkalosis (or *actual acid deficit*) results from processes that cause either an overelimination or an underproduction of acid components (Fig. 19–3).

Alkalosis can cause serious and life-threatening disturbances in metabolism and in pulmonary respiration. Because alkalosis is the manifestation of another abnormal process (or processes), treatment is most effective when directed at the underlying abnormal processes. Treatment that is effective for metabolic alkalosis is different from treatment that is effective for respiratory alkalosis. Therefore, one must be able to distinguish between metabolic and respiratory alkalosis to prevent and manage this condition.

Whether its origin is metabolic, respiratory, or both, alkalosis greatly affects specific physiologic functions. Its pathologic effects are related to the accompanying electrolyte imbalances that occur in response to decreased blood cation concentration. The most common manifestations of

AAABBB	AAABBBB	AABBB
AAABBB	AAABBBB	AABBB
AAABBB	AAABBBB	AABBB
Acid-base balance	Actual alkalosis (base excess)	Relative alkalosis (acid deficit)

Figure 19–3. Concepts of actual and relative alkalosis. (A = acid; B = base.)

alkalosis are associated with increased stimulation of the central nervous, neuromuscular, and cardiovascular systems.

Etiology

Alkalosis can be caused by metabolic disturbances, respiratory disturbances, or combined metabolic and respiratory disturbances. The causes of alkalosis are listed in Table 19–3.

Metabolic Alkalosis

Most conditions that result in metabolic alkalosis create the acid-base disturbance through either of two mechanisms: an actual increase of base components or an actual decrease of acid components.

INCREASE IN BASE COMPONENTS. Increases in base components (base excesses) occur as a result of oral or parenteral ingestion of bicarbonates, carbonates, acetates, citrates, and lactates. Excessive use of oral antacids

TABLE 19–3

Common Causes of Alkalosis	
Pathology	**Condition**
Metabolic Alkalosis	

Increase of base components	• Oral ingestion of bases
	  • Antacids
	  • Milk-alkali syndrome
	• Parenteral base administration
	  • Blood transfusion
	  • Sodium bicarbonate
	  • Total parenteral nutrition

Decrease of acid components	• Prolonged vomiting • Nasogastric suctioning • Cushing's syndrome (hypercortisolism) • Hyperaldosteronism • Thiazide diuretics
Respiratory Alkalosis	

Excessive loss of carbon dioxide	• Hyperventilation
	  • Fear
	  • Anxiety
	  • Mechanical ventilation
	  • Central nervous system stimulation
	    • Salicylates
	    • Catecholamines
	    • Progesterone
	• Hypoxemia
	  • Asphyxiation
	  • High altitudes
	  • Shock
	  • Early-stage pulmonary problems
	    • Pneumonia
	    • Asthma
	    • Pulmonary emboli

containing sodium bicarbonate or calcium carbonate can also cause a metabolic alkalosis. Other base excesses can occur as a result of medical treatments, such as citrate excesses during rapid or massive blood transfusions, acetate and lactate excesses during hyperalimentation, and intravenous sodium bicarbonate administration to correct lactic acidosis or ketoacidosis.

DECREASE IN ACID COMPONENTS. Decreases in acid components (acid deficit) can occur in response to disease processes or medical treatment. Contributing conditions include prolonged vomiting, Cushing's syndrome (hypercortisolism), and hyperaldosteronism. Medical treatments that promote acid loss and can cause metabolic alkalosis include the use of thiazide diuretics and prolonged nasogastric suctioning.

Respiratory Alkalosis

The primary mechanism responsible for respiratory alkalosis is the excessive loss of carbon dioxide through hyperventilation (rapid respirations). Clients may hyperventilate in response to anxiety, fear, or improper settings on mechanical ventilators. Hyperventilation can also result from direct stimulation of central respiratory centers. Conditions that directly stimulate these centers include fever, respiratory compensation for metabolic acidosis, central nervous system lesions, and certain drugs (e.g., salicylates, catecholamines, and progesterone).

Collaborative Management

 Assessment

➤ *Physical Assessment/Clinical Manifestations*

Clinical manifestations of alkalosis are consistent whether metabolic or respiratory in origin. Many symptoms are the result of the hypocalcemia (low calcium levels) and hypokalemia (low potassium levels) that usually accompany alkalosis. These key manifestations are associated with changes in central nervous system, neuromuscular, and cardiovascular functions (Chart 19–4).

Central Nervous System Manifestations. Overexcitement of the central and peripheral nervous systems is the major cause of symptoms associated with alkalosis. Clients experience lightheadedness, agitation, confusion, and hyperreflexia, which may progress to seizure activity. Paresthesias may be present as tingling or numbness around the mouth and in the toes. Other reliable indicators of alkalosis with accompanying hypocalcemia are positive Chvostek's and Trousseau's signs (see Chap. 16).

Neuromuscular Manifestations. Alkalosis with hypocalcemia or hypokalemia increases nervous system activity. This nerve stimulation, in turn, causes nonvoluntary skeletal muscle contractions manifested as cramps, twitches, and charley horses. Deep tendon reflexes are hyperactive. *Tetany* (continuous spasms) of isolated muscle groups also may be present. Tetany is painful and indicates a rapidly worsening condition.

Although skeletal muscles may contract as a result of

Chart 19–4

Key Features of Alkalosis

Central Nervous System Manifestations
- Increased activity
- Anxiety, irritability, tetany, seizures
- Positive Chvostek's sign
- Positive Trousseau's sign
- Paresthesias

Neuromuscular Manifestations
- Hyperreflexia
- Muscle cramping and twitching
- Skeletal muscle weakness

Cardiovascular Manifestations
- Increased heart rate
- Normal or low blood pressure
- Increased digitalis toxicity

Respiratory Manifestations
- Increased rate and depth of ventilation in respiratory alkalosis
- Decreased respiratory effort associated with skeletal muscle weakness in metabolic alkalosis

nerve overstimulation, the skeletal muscles themselves become weaker because of the alkalosis and hypokalemia. Handgrip strength diminishes, and the client may be unable to walk or support his or her own weight. Respiratory efforts also become less effective as the skeletal muscles of respiration weaken.

Cardiovascular Manifestations. Alkalosis causes increased irritability of the myocardium, especially when accompanied by hypokalemia. The heart rate increases, and the pulse is thready. When hypovolemia (decreased blood volume) is also present, the client may experience profound hypotension. Alkalosis also increases myocardial sensitivity to digitalis derivatives, resulting in increased risk for digitalis toxicity.

Respiratory Manifestations. Alterations in the rate and depth of respiration are the underlying causes of respiratory alkalosis. Tidal volume (the volume of air inhaled and exhaled with each breath) is nearly normal, but minute respiratory volume (the total volume of air inhaled and exhaled in 1 minute) rises in proportion to the increase in respiratory rate. The increase in minute respiratory volume may result from other physiologic changes or from anxiety.

➤ Laboratory Assessment

As in acidosis, arterial blood pH confirms alkalosis. When arterial blood pH is above 7.45, alkalosis is present. This test alone does not identify the underlying pathologic condition or the origin of the alkalosis, however. Because the clinical manifestations of metabolic alkalosis are similar to those of respiratory alkalosis, it is critical that the nurse obtain additional laboratory data, especially arterial

blood gas (ABG) values and specific serum electrolytes levels (see Chart 19–3).

Metabolic Alkalosis. Metabolic alkalosis is indicated by
- High pH (> 7.45)
- Elevated bicarbonate level (> 28 mEq/L)
- Normal PaO_2
- Rising $PaCO_2$
- Decreased serum potassium levels
- Decreased serum calcium levels

The pH is high because buffering and respiratory compensation are not adequate to maintain the hydrogen ion concentration at a normal level.

The increased bicarbonate level, coupled with a rising $PaCO_2$, is the hallmark of metabolic alkalosis. The rising $PaCO_2$ compensates for the decreased hydrogen ion concentration. The serum potassium level decreases as the body attempts to maintain electroneutrality (see Fig. 19–2). As the pH increases, calcium binding increases and the serum calcium concentration decreases, creating an accompanying state of hypocalcemia. Most of the serious clinical manifestations of alkalosis are attributed to this accompanying hypocalcemia.

Respiratory Alkalosis. Arterial blood data that demonstrate respiratory alkalosis are
- High pH
- Low bicarbonate level
- Low $PaCO_2$
- Low serum potassium level
- Low serum calcium level

The pH is high because buffering and renal compensation cannot maintain the hydrogen ion concentration at a normal level.

The classic respiratory alkalosis profile is a reduced bicarbonate level (not usually < 15 mEq/L) coupled with a very low $PaCO_2$. The carbon dioxide level is so low because it is being exhaled through hyperventilation more rapidly than it is being produced. The bicarbonate level is reduced in response to the pH increase. Various blood and intracellular buffers generate hydrogen ions, which immediately combine with the serum bicarbonate ions and form carbonic acid, thus reducing the serum concentration of bicarbonate.

As in metabolic alkalosis, the serum potassium level is reduced as the body attempts to maintain electroneutrality. Again, as the pH increases, calcium binding increases and the concentration of serum calcium decreases, resulting in hypocalcemia.

 Interventions

Interventions aim to prevent further losses of hydrogen, potassium, calcium, and chloride ions and to restore fluid balance.

Drug therapy is the intervention of choice for alkalosis. Drugs are prescribed to resolve the underlying causes of alkalosis and to restore normal fluid, electrolyte, and acid-base balance. For example, the client with metabolic alkalosis caused by diuretic therapy receives fluid and electrolyte replacement and is then re-evaluated by the physician for the need to resume a diuretic. The physician may prescribe a potassium-sparing diuretic to prevent potassium loss. The physician orders antiemetic medications to halt vomiting in the client experiencing emesis. Fluids and electrolytes are replaced orally or parenterally. The nurse carefully monitors the client's progress and titrates fluid and electrolyte therapy. Serum electrolyte values are monitored daily until they return to normal or near normal.

SELECTED BIBLIOGRAPHY

Ahern, J. (1995). A guide to blood gases. *Nursing Standard, 10*(49), 50–52.

Anderson, S. (1996). Fluid and electrolyte disorders in the elderly. In J. Kokko & R. Tannen (Eds.), *Fluids and electrolytes* (3rd ed., pp. 831–839). Philadelphia: W. B. Saunders.

Cornock, M. (1996). Making sense of arterial blood gases and their interpretation. *Nursing Times, 92*(6), 30–31.

Guyton, A. C., & Hall, J. (1996). *Textbook of medical physiology* (9th ed.). Philadelphia: W. B. Saunders.

Halperin, M., & Goldstein, M. (1994), *Fluid, electrolyte and acid-base physiology: A problem-based approach* (2nd ed.). Philadelphia: W. B. Saunders.

Kelly, M. (1996). Acute respiratory failure. *American Journal of Nursing, 96*(12), 46.

Kokko, J., & Tannen, R. (1996). *Fluids and electrolytes* (3rd ed.). Philadelphia: W. B. Saunders.

Mays, D. (1995). Turn ABGs into child's play. *RN, 58*(1), 36–40.

Metheny, N. (1996). *Fluid and electrolyte balance: Nursing considerations* (3rd ed.). Philadelphia: J. B. Lippincott.

Molony, D., Schiess, M., & Dosekum, A. (1996). Respiratory acid-base disorders. In J. Kokko & R. Tannen (Eds.), *Fluids and electrolytes* (3rd ed., pp. 267–342). Philadelphia: W. B. Saunders.

O'Donnell, J. (1995). Can you prevent respiratory depression? *Nursing95, 25*(4), 32JJ.

Russell, G., & Graybeal, J. (1995). Accuracy of laminated disposable pulse-oximetry sensors. *Respiratory Care, 40*(7), 728–733.

Schwartz-Goldstein, B., Malik, A., Sarwar, A., & Brandstetter, R. (1996). Lactic acidosis associated with a deceptively normal anion gap. *Heart & Lung, 25*(1), 79–80.

Sica, D. (1994). Renal disease, electrolyte abnormalities, and acid-base imbalance in the elderly. *Clinics in Geriatric Medicine, 10*(1), 197–211.

Tasota, F., & Wesmiller, S. (1994). Assessing A.B.G.s: Maintaining the delicate balance. *Nursing94, 24*(5), 34–46.

Tietz, N. W. (Ed.). (1995). *Clinical guide to laboratory tests* (3rd ed.). Philadelphia: W. B. Saunders.

Toto, R., & Alpern, R. (1996). Metabolic acid-base disorders. In J. Kokko & R. Tannen (Eds.), *Fluids and electrolytes* (3rd ed., pp. 201–266). Philadelphia: W. B. Saunders.

White, V. (1997). Hyperkalemia. *American Journal of Nursing, 97*(6), 35.

SUGGESTED READINGS

Kelly, M. (1996). Acute respiratory failure. *American Journal of Nursing, 96*(12), 46.

This brief but informative article uses a case presentation approach to help readers identify the key indicators of acute respiratory failure. The pathophysiology is explained in understandable terms, and the reader directed toward appropriate interventions.

O'Donnell, J. (1995). Can you prevent respiratory depression? *Nursing95, 25*(4), 32JJ.

This brief article can assist the nurse in preventing respiratory depression when administering opioids and benzodiazepines, two classes of agents commonly implicated in causing respiratory depression among clients in acute care settings. Assessment and intervention tips are presented in a logical, easy-to-remember format.

Sica, D. (1994). Renal disease, electrolyte abnormalities, and acid-base imbalance in the elderly. *Clinics in Geriatric Medicine, 10*(1), 197–211.

This comprehensive article includes a detailed section on acid-base abnormalities commonly seen among elderly clients. Although written for a medical audience, the article is clear and concise and outlines realistic therapy and medical interventions.

UNIT 4

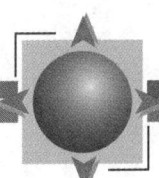

Management of

Perioperative Clients

Chapter 20

INTERVENTIONS FOR PREOPERATIVE CLIENTS

CHAPTER

HIGHLIGHTS

With cost reduction as a driving force over the past decade, new or re-engineered policies and procedures have changed the way a surgical client is handled by the health care community. Outpatient surgical services have expanded, more clients are being admitted as inpatients *after* a procedure (rather than before), and the length of hospital stay after a procedure has been shortened. Perioperative, or surgical, nursing focuses on client care before (preoperative), during (intraoperative), and after (postoperative) surgery, regardless of setting.

Overview

The preoperative period begins when the client is scheduled for surgery and ends at the time of transfer to the surgical suite. The nurse acts as an educator, an advocate, and a promoter of health. Perioperative nursing places special emphasis on safety.

After a thorough assessment, the nurse develops an individualized teaching care plan to help the client and family through the surgical experience. Preoperative care mainly consists of education to reduce anxiety and postoperative complications and to promote cooperation in postoperative procedures. In preoperative teaching, the nurse uses adult teaching and learning principles and

validates and clarifies information that the physician has provided.

Categories and Purposes of Surgery

The nurse understands the terminology for surgical procedures to provide the client and family members with comprehensive information. Procedures are usually categorized according to

- The reason for the surgery
- The urgency of the procedure
- The degree of risk
- The anatomic location
- The extent of surgery required

The primary purposes, or reasons, for surgery can be divided into five general subcategories: diagnostic, curative, restorative, palliative, and cosmetic. Palliative surgery makes the client more comfortable, and cosmetic surgery reconstructs the skin and underlying structures. The urgency of the procedure can be divided into three subcategories: elective, urgent, and emergent. The degree of risk is classified as minor or major. Classification by location

TABLE 20–1

Selected Categories of Surgical Procedures		
Category	**Description**	**Condition or Surgical Procedure**
Reasons for Surgery		
Diagnostic	• Performed to determine the origin and cause of a disorder or the cell type for cancer	• Breast biopsy • Exploratory laparotomy
Curative	• Performed to resolve a health problem by repairing or removing the cause	• Cholelithiasis • Mastectomy • Hysterectomy
Restorative	• Performed to improve a client's functional ability	• Total knee replacement • Finger reimplantation
Palliative	• Performed to relieve symptoms of a disease process, but does not cure	• Colostomy • Nerve root resection • Tumor debulking • Ileostomy
Cosmetic	• Performed primarily to alter or enhance personal appearance	• Liposuction • Revision of scars • Rhinoplasty • Blepharoplasty
Urgency of Surgery		
Elective	• Planned for correction of a nonacute problem	• Cataract removal • Hernia repair • Hemorrhoidectomy • Total joint replacement
Urgent	• Requires prompt intervention; or may be life-threatening if treatment delayed more than 24–48 hr	• Intestinal obstruction • Bladder obstruction • Kidney or ureteral stones • Bone fracture • Eye injury • Acute cholecystitis
Emergent	• Requires immediate intervention because of life-threatening consequences	• Gunshot or stab wound • Severe bleeding • Abdominal aortic aneurysm • Compound fracture • Appendectomy
Degree of Risk of Surgery		
Minor	• Procedure without significant risk, often done with local anesthesia	• Incision and drainage (I&D) • Implantation of a venous access device (VAD) • Muscle biopsy
Major	• Procedure of greater risk, usually longer and more extensive than a minor procedure	• Mitral valve replacement • Pancreas transplant • Lymph node dissection
Extent of Surgery		
Simple	• Only the most overtly affected areas involved in the surgery	• Simple/partial mastectomy
Radical	• Extensive surgery beyond the area obviously involved; is directed at finding a root cause	• Radical prostatectomy • Radical hysterectomy

is based on the area of the body on which surgery occurs: for example, abdominal surgery, intracranial surgery, and heart surgery. The extent can be simple, modified, or radical. Table 20–1 explains the categories and gives examples of surgical procedures.

Surgical Settings

The term *inpatient* refers to a client who is admitted to a hospital. The client may be admitted the day before or the day of surgery (often termed same-day admission

[SDA]) or may already be an inpatient when the need for surgical intervention is identified. In contrast, the term *outpatient* refers to a client who goes to the surgical area the day of the surgery and returns home on the same day (i.e., same-day surgery [SDS]). Hospital-based ambulatory surgical centers, freestanding surgical centers, physicians' offices, and ambulatory care centers are becoming increasingly more common.

One of the many advantages of outpatient surgery is that clients are not separated from the comfort and security of their home and family. With continuous improvements in surgical techniques and anesthesia, more procedures are being safely performed on an outpatient basis. However, changes in the surgical experience present particular challenges for the client without an adequate or available support system. An elderly spouse may be unable to assist in the preoperative and postoperative care of the client. A client who is primarily responsible for others may be unable to perform his or her usual tasks within the family. Clients may try to continue their family role but jeopardize their own health by doing so. As a result, the client's stress, fears, and anxieties about the surgical experience and about returning home immediately after surgery may be increased.

Collaborative Management

 Assessment

➤ *History*

Collection of data about the client before surgery begins in various settings (e.g., the surgeon's office, the preadmission or admission office, the inpatient unit, and over the telephone). The nurse provides privacy to increase the client's comfort with the interview process. Anesthesia and surgery are both physical and emotional stressors for the client. The nurse collects the following data:

- Age
- Tobacco, alcohol, and illicit substance use, including marijuana
- Current medications
- Medical history
- Prior surgical procedures and experiences
- Prior experience with anesthesia
- Autologous or directed blood donations
- Allergies
- General health
- Family history
- Type of surgery planned
- Knowledge and understanding about events during the perioperative period
- Support system adequacy and availability

When taking a history, the nurse screens the preoperative client for risks that may contribute to complications during the perioperative period. Some conditions that could either increase the surgical risk or increase the possibility of postoperative complications are outlined in Table 20–2.

Age. Elderly clients are at increased risk. The normal aging process decreases immune system functioning and delays wound healing. Frequency of chronic illness increases in elderly clients. See Chart 20-1 for other physiologic changes in elderly clients.

Medication and Substance Use. The use of tobacco products increases the risk of pulmonary complications because of changes they cause to the lungs and thoracic cavity. Excessive alcohol and illicit substance use can alter the effects of anesthesia and response to pain medication. Withdrawal of alcohol in preparation for surgery may precipitate delirium tremens. Prescription and over-the-

TABLE 20–2

Selected Factors That Increase Surgical Risk or Increase the Risk of Postoperative Complications

Age
- Older than 65 yr

Medications
- Antihypertensives
- Tricyclic antidepressants
- Anticoagulants — *COUMADIN · ASPIRIN*
- Nonsteroidal anti-inflammatory drugs (NSAIDs)

Medical History
- Decreased immunity
- Diabetes
- Pulmonary disease
- Cardiac disease
- Hemodynamic instability
- Multisystem disease
- Coagulation defect or disorder
- Anemia
- Dehydration
- Infection
- Hypertension
- Hypotension
- Any chronic disease

Prior Surgical Experiences
- Less-than-optimal emotional reaction
- Anesthesia reactions or complications
- Postoperative complications

Health History
- Malnutrition or obesity
- Medication, tobacco, alcohol, or illicit substance use or abuse
- Altered coping ability

Family History
- Malignant hyperthermia
- Cancer
- Bleeding disorder

Type of Surgical Procedure Planned
- Neck, oral, or facial procedures (airway complications)
- Chest or high abdominal procedures (pulmonary complications)
- Abdominal surgery (paralytic ileus, deep vein thrombosis)

Chart 20-1

Nursing Focus on the Elderly

Changes of Aging as Surgical Risk Factors

Physiologic Change	Nursing Interventions	Rationale
Cardiovascular system Decreased cardiac output Increased blood pressure Decreased peripheral circulation	• Determine normal activity levels and note when the client tires. • Monitor vital signs, peripheral pulses, and capillary refill.	• Knowing limits helps prevent fatigue. • Having baseline data helps detect deviations.
Respiratory system Reduced vital capacity Loss of lung elasticity Decreased oxygenation of blood	• Teach coughing and deep breathing exercises. • Monitor respirations and breathing effort.	• Pulmonary exercises help prevent pulmonary complications. • Having baseline data helps detect deviations.
Renal/urinary system Decreased blood flow to kidneys Reduced ability to excrete waste products Decline in glomerular filtration rate Nocturia common	• Monitor intake and output. • Assess overall hydration. • Monitor electrolyte status. K^+ Na^+ • Assist frequently with toileting needs, especially at night.	• Ongoing assessment helps detect fluid and electrolyte imbalances and decreased renal function. • Frequent toileting helps prevent incontinence and falls.
Neurologic system Sensory deficits Slower reaction time Decreased ability to adjust to changes in the surroundings	• Orient the client to the surroundings. • Allow extra time for teaching the client. • Provide for the client's safety.	• An individualized preoperative teaching plan is developed on the basis of the client's orientation and any neurologic deficits. • Safety measures help prevent falls and injury.
Musculoskeletal system Increased incidence of deformities related to osteoporosis or arthritis	• Assess the client's mobility. • Teach turning and positioning. • Encourage ambulation. • Place on fall precautions, if indicated.	• Interventions help prevent complications of immobility. • Safety measures help prevent injury.

---

counter medications may also affect how the client reacts to the perioperative experience. The potential effects of specific medications are noted in Table 20-3.

Medical History. The nurse asks the client about his or her medical history. The presence of certain chronic illnesses increases perioperative risks and is considered when planning care. For example, a client with systemic lupus erythematosus may need additional medication to offset the physical and emotional stress of the surgery. A diabetic client may need a more extensive preoperative bowel preparation because of decreased gastrointestinal motility. An infection may need to be treated before surgery.

Prior Cardiac History. The nurse obtains a history of cardiac disease because complications from anesthesia could occur in clients with cardiac problems. Cardiac disorders that increase risks associated with surgery include coronary artery disease, angina pectoris, myocardial infarction (MI) within 6 months before surgery, congestive heart failure, hypertension, and dysrhythmias. These disorders impair the client's ability to withstand and re-

spond to both anesthesia and the hemodynamic changes during surgery. The risk of intraoperative MI is also higher in clients with pre-existing heart problems.

Pulmonary History. Adults with chronic respiratory problems, elderly people, and smokers are at risk for pulmonary complications because of physiologic pulmonary changes. Increased rigidity of the thoracic cavity and loss of lung elasticity reduce the efficiency of anesthesia excretion. Smoking increases the level of circulating carboxyhemoglobin (carbon monoxide in the oxygen-binding sites of the hemoglobin molecule), which in turn decreases oxygen delivery to organs. Concurrently, mucociliary transport decreases, which leads to increased secretions and predisposes the client to infection (pneumonia) and atelectasis (collapse of alveoli). Atelectasis prevents the exchange of oxygen and carbon dioxide and causes intolerance of anesthesia. Chronic conditions such as asthma, emphysema, and chronic bronchitis also reduce the elasticity of the lungs, which causes an ineffective exchange of carbon dioxide and oxygen. As a result, clients with these conditions have decreased oxygen diffusion and decreased oxygenation of the tissues.

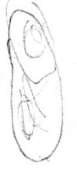

TABLE 20–3

Effects of Routine Medications Taken Preoperatively

Drug	Implications for the Perioperative Experience	Nursing Interventions	Rationale
Antiarrhythmics Quinidine gluconate (Quinate✦, Quinaglute Dura-Tabs) Procainamide hydrochloride (Pronestyl, Procan-SR)	• Antiarrhythmic medications affect the client's tolerance of anesthesia and potentiate anesthetics that are neuromuscular blockers. • Antiarrhythmics depress cardiac function by decreasing cardiac output and slowing the pulse rate. • Antiarrhythmics may cause peripheral vasodilation.	• Communicate the use and type of antiarrhythmics to the anesthesia personnel. • Monitor vital signs. • Obtain a baseline electrocardiogram, as ordered. • Assess the client's peripheral circulation.	• Cardiac complications during surgery can be life-threatening. • Ongoing monitoring helps to detect deviations and potential complications.
Antihypertensives Methyldopa (Aldomet, Novomedopa✦) Captopril (Capoten) Clonidine hydrochloride (Catapres)	• Antihypertensive agents alter the client's response to muscle relaxants and opioid analgesics by inhibiting synthesis and storage of norepinephrine. • Antihypertensives may cause a hypotensive crisis intraoperatively and postoperatively.	• Monitor blood pressure and pulse frequently. • Assess for hypotension during transfer and turning.	• Ongoing monitoring helps to detect deviations and potential complications. • Hypotensive crisis can occur and may be prevented through timely assessments.
Corticosteroids Dexamethasone (Decadron, Dexasone✦) Hydrocortisone sodium (Solu-Cortef) Prednisone (Deltasone, Winpred✦)	• Surgery increases the demand for corticosteroids in the client with no adrenal function. • Steroids delay wound healing because of blockage of collagen formation. • Steroids increase the serum glucose level and block fibroblast formation. • Steroids increase the risk of hemorrhage. • Steroids mask the signs and symptoms of infection.	• Continue steroid therapy during surgery. • Monitor vital signs. • Assess for signs of hyperglycemia. • Assess for subtle signs of infection and bleeding. • Monitor wound healing, support the incision area with binders, and splint the wound when the client is turning, coughing, and deep breathing.	• Continuation of steroid therapy avoids problems associated with abrupt withdrawal. • Ongoing monitoring helps to detect deviations and potential complications. • It is important to detect early signs and symptoms of infection. • Specific wound and incision care helps to prevent complications.
Anticoagulants Warfarin sodium (Coumadin, Warfilone sodium✦) Heparin sodium (Lipo-Hepin, Hepalean✦) Aspirin (acetylsalicylic acid, Ancasal✦, Astin✦, Coryphen✦)	• Anticoagulant therapy increases the risk of hemorrhage intraoperatively and postoperatively.	• Monitor coagulation studies (APTT, PT). • Monitor for signs of bleeding. • Gradually discontinue anticoagulants 24–48 hr before surgery, as ordered. • Have an antidote (protamine sulfate for heparin and vitamin K [Mephyton] for warfarin sodium) available to reverse the effects of the anticoagulant.	• Coagulation studies help detect bleeding disorders. • Anticoagulant administration is discontinued to avoid hemorrhage. • An antidote needs to be available to prevent complications of bleeding in an emergency situation.

Previous Surgery and Anesthesia. The number and type of previous surgeries and previous surgical experiences affect the preoperative client's readiness for surgery. Previous perioperative complications may contribute to the client's fears and concerns about the scheduled surgery. The nurse asks about the client's experience with anesthetic agents and all allergies. These data provide the nurse with information about tolerance of and possible fears about the use of anesthesia. The client's sensitivity or allergy to certain substances alerts the nurse to a possi-

TABLE 20–3

Effects of Routine Medications Taken Preoperatively *Continued*			
Drug	**Implications for the Perioperative Experience**	**Nursing Interventions**	**Rationale**
Antiseizure Medications			
Phenobarbital (Luminal✦, Gardenal✦)	• Seizure activity can cause injury to the surgical wound. • Antiseizure medications alter the metabolism of anesthetic agents.	• Maintain use of the drug. • Inform the anesthesiologist or anesthetist to allow for adjustment of the dosage of the anesthetic. • Assess for seizure activity. • Pad the side rails of the bed. • Place suction equipment at the bedside.	• Antiseizure medications prevent seizures. • Safety measures prevent injury.
Glaucoma Medications			
Demecarium bromide (Humorsol) Echothiophate (Phospholine iodide) Pilocarpine hydrochloride (Isopto-Carpine, Pilocar, Miocarpine✦) Timolol maleate (Timoptic)	• Glaucoma medications have cumulative systemic effects and can cause respiratory and cardiovascular collapse, especially during surgery.	• Consult the physician about stopping Humorsol at least 2 weeks before surgery. • Monitor respiratory status and cardiac output. • Assess for increased intraocular pressure.	• Collaboration with the physician helps prevent complications. • Ongoing monitoring helps to detect complications.
Antidiabetic Agent			
Insulin	• Insulin needs decrease preoperatively when the client is on NPO status. • Postoperative insulin demands increase because of IV administration of dextrose. • Insulin levels may fluctuate during healing because of dietary and activity restrictions and the physical stress of surgery.	• Monitor serum glucose levels. • Administer antibiotics and other intermittent medications in normal saline instead of dextrose when possible, as ordered, or as per facility policy.	• Monitoring will detect an increased or a decreased need for insulin. • The use of normal saline prevents complications.

ble reaction to anesthetic agents or to substances that are used for preoperative skin preparation. For example, povidone-iodine used for skin preparation contains some of the same components found in shellfish. The family medical history and problems with anesthetics may indicate possible intraoperative needs and reactions to anesthesia, such as malignant hyperthermia.

Autologous or Directed Blood Donations. Clients may donate their own blood (autologous donations) in the few weeks immediately before the scheduled surgery date. If clients then need blood because of their surgery, an autologous blood transfusion can be given. This practice eliminates the possibility of transfusion reactions and the transmission of disease.

Clients may be candidates for autologous blood donations up to 5 weeks preoperatively if they are afebrile, have a hemoglobin level greater than 11 g/dL (110 g/L), and have a physician's recommendation. The physician usually orders supplemental iron beginning before the first donation. Autologous donations can be made as fre-

quently as every 3 days if the other criteria can be met. Usually, a total of 2 to 4 units is donated. The last donation cannot be less than 72 hours before surgery.

A special tag is affixed to the transfusion bag when an autologous blood donation has been made. The blood donor center gives the client a matching tag that he or she brings to the surgical area preoperatively. This procedure helps to ensure that the client receives only his or her own blood. If the client does not use the blood, the blood goes to the blood bank to be used as would any other unit of donated blood.

Clients may wish to have family and friends donate blood exclusively for their use, if needed. This practice of *directed* blood donation is possible only if the blood types are compatible and the donor's blood is acceptable. Clients may fear disease transmission from unknown blood and feel more comfortable knowing who gave the blood. Some blood collection centers and other health care personnel are discouraging the practice, stating that it gives the client a false sense of security. As with autologous blood donations, a special tag is affixed to the blood. This tag notes the names of the client and the donor and has the client's signature.

The nurse asks whether autologous or directed blood donations have been made and documents this information in the chart. It may be important to know the specific blood collection center and whether the blood has arrived before the client goes into surgery.

Planning for Bloodless Surgery. Growth in bloodless surgery programs is helping to provide another alternative for clients with religious or medical contrandications to blood transfusions. These programs reduce or eliminate the need for transfusion during and after surgery. Some techniques employed include limiting preoperative blood samples (the number of samples as well as the volume of blood drawn per sample) and stimulating the client's own red cell production with epoetin alfa (EPO) before, during, and after surgery. The physician may prescribe supplemental iron, folic acid, vitamin B_{12}, and vitamin C preoperatively to further stimulate erythropoiesis. Special equipment and techniques used during the surgical procedure allows less blood loss than usually expected. The nurse assesses, monitors, teaches, and supports the client during the bloodless surgery process (Vernon & Pfeifer, 1997).

Discharge Planning. The nurse also assesses the client's home environment, self-care capabilities, and support systems. The nurse anticipates the client's postoperative needs during the preoperative period. All clients should have discharge planning. Elderly people and dependent adults may need referrals for transportation to and from the physician's office. They may need a home care nurse to monitor their postoperative recovery and to provide instruction on wound care. All clients with inadequate support systems may need follow-up care at home.

➤ Physical Assessment/Clinical Manifestations

The preoperative client may be of any age, with a health status that varies from well to debilitated. The nurse performs a complete preoperative physical assessment to obtain baseline data. During physical assessment, the nurse also identifies current health problems, potential complications related to the administration of anesthesia, and potential postoperative complications.

When beginning the assessment, the nurse obtains a complete set of vital signs. The nurse may need to obtain vital signs several times for accurate baseline values. Abnormal vital signs may cause the postponement of surgery until the underlying problem is treated and the client's condition is stable. The nurse also assesses for anxiety, which could increase the client's blood pressure, pulse, and respiratory rate, and documents this in the client's chart as part of the overall assessment.

Throughout the physical assessment, the nurse focuses on problem areas identified from the client's history and on all body systems affected directly or indirectly by the surgical procedure. The elderly (Chart 20–2; see also Chapter 6) or chronically ill client is at increased risk for intraoperative and postoperative complications. Perioperative morbidity and mortality are higher in elderly and

chronically ill clients owing to their preoperative physical condition.

The nurse reports any abnormalities found on physical assessment to the physician and anesthesiology personnel. In this manner, the nurse functions as a proactive client advocate and is exercising his or her legal responsibility.

Cardiovascular System. Alterations in cardiac status are responsible for as many as 30% of perioperative deaths. The nurse evaluates the client for hypertension, which is common, often undiagnosed, and can affect surgery. Cardiovascular assessment also includes auscultation of heart sounds for rate, regularity, and abnormalities. The nurse evaluates the client's extremities for temperature, color, peripheral pulses, capillary refill, and edema. Any physical alterations, such as absent peripheral pulses and pitting edema, or cardiac symptoms, such as chest pain, shortness of breath, and dyspnea, are reported to the physician for further assessment and evaluation. (Chapter 35 further discusses cardiovascular assessment.)

Respiratory System. In assessing the client's respiratory status, the nurse considers the client's age and history of smoking and the presence of chronic illness. The nurse observes the client's posture; respiratory rate, rhythm, and depth; overall respiratory effort; and lung expansion. Clubbing of the fingertips (swelling at the base of the nailbeds caused by a chronic lack of oxygen) or any cyanosis is noted. The nurse auscultates the lungs to determine the quality and presence of any adventitious (crackles, wheezes, rubs) or abnormal breath sounds. (More information is found in Chapter 29.)

Renal/Urinary System. Renal and urinary function affects the filtration and eventual excretion of waste products. If renal and urinary function is not optimal, fluid and electrolyte balance can be altered, especially in the elderly client. The nurse asks the client about the presence or absence of symptoms such as urinary frequency, dysuria (painful urination), nocturia (awakening during nighttime sleep because of a need to void), difficulty

---

Chart 20–2

Nursing Focus on the Elderly

Specific Considerations When Planning Care for the Elderly Preoperative Client

- Greater incidence of chronic illness
- Greater incidence of malnutrition
- More allergies
- Increased incidence of impaired self-care abilities
- Inadequate support systems
- Decreased ability to withstand the stress of surgery and anesthesia
- Increased risk of postoperative cardiopulmonary complications
- Risk of a change in mental status when admitted (related to unfamiliar surroundings, change in routine, medications administered, and so forth)
- Increased risk of a fall and resultant injury

starting urine flow, and oliguria (scant amount of urine). The nurse also asks about the appearance and odor of the urine. Equally important is an assessment of the client's usual fluid intake and degree of continence. If the client is suspected of having underlying renal or urinary problems, the nurse consults with the physician about further client work-up. (Chapter 72 further discusses renal/urinary assessment.)

Abnormal renal function can decrease the excretion rate of preoperative medications and anesthetic agents. As a result, the drug's effectiveness may be altered. Scopolamine (Buscospan✢), morphine, meperidine (Demerol), and barbiturates frequently cause confusion, disorientation, apprehension, and restlessness when administered to clients with decreased renal function.

Neurologic System. The nurse assesses the client's overall mental status, including level of consciousness, orientation, and ability to follow commands, before planning preoperative teaching and postoperative care. A deficit in any of these areas affects the type of care required during the perioperative experience. The nurse determines the client's baseline neurologic status to be able to identify changes that may occur later. The nurse also assesses for any motor or sensory deficits. (See Chapter 43 for complete nervous system assessment.)

The usual neurologic status of a mentally impaired or elderly client may be difficult to assess. The client who has been independent and oriented while in the home environment may become disoriented in an unfamiliar hospital setting. Family members and significant others can often provide information about what the client was like at home.

Often, as part of the neurologic assessment, the nurse assesses the client's risk of falling, especially for elderly clients. Factors such as mental status, muscle strength, steadiness of gait, and sense of independence are evaluated to determine the client's risk. The client's ability to ambulate and his or her steadiness of gait are noted preoperatively as baseline data.

Musculoskeletal System. Deformities of the musculoskeletal system may interfere with intraoperative and postoperative positioning of the client. For example, clients with arthritis may be able to assume conventional intraoperative positions but then have unnecessary discomfort postoperatively from prolonged immobilization of joints. Other anatomic characteristics, such as the shape and length of the client's neck and the shape of the thoracic cavity, may interfere with respiratory and cardiac function and positioning during surgery.

The nurse asks about a history of joint replacements. During surgery, the nurse ensures that electrocautery pads, which could cause an electrical burn, are not placed near the area of the prosthesis.

Nutritional Status. Malnutrition and obesity can increase surgical risks. Surgery usually increases the body's metabolic rate and consequently depletes potassium, ascorbic acid, and B vitamins, all of which are needed for wound healing and fibrin formation. In malnourished clients, hypoproteinemia retards postoperative recovery.

Negative nitrogen balance may result from depleted protein stores. This situation increases the risk of perioperative morbidity and mortality from delayed wound healing, possible dehiscence or evisceration (see Chap. 22), fluid volume deficit, and sepsis.

Some elderly clients are susceptible to nutritional imbalances because of chronic illness, diuretic or laxative use, poor dietary planning or habits, anorexia, lack of motivation, and financial limitations. Clinical indications of alterations in the fluid and nutritional status of the client preoperatively include brittle nails, muscle wasting, dry or flaky skin, hair alterations (e.g., dull, sparse, dry), decreased skin turgor, orthostatic (postural) hypotension, decreased serum albumin levels, and abnormal serum electrolyte values.

The obese client is often malnourished because of poor eating habits and an imbalanced diet and has an increased chance of poor or incomplete wound healing because of excessive adipose tissue. Fatty tissue lacks nutrients, is not as vascular, and has little collagen, and nutrients, vascularity, and collagen are important for wound healing. Obesity causes increased stress on the heart and reduces the available lung volumes, which can affect the client's intraoperative experience and postoperative recovery.

➤ Psychosocial Assessment

The nurse performs a psychosocial assessment and preparation of the client to determine the client's level of anxiety, coping ability, and support systems; provide information; and offer support.

A client scheduled for surgery experiences some preoperative anxiety and fear. The extent and type of these reactions vary for each client according to the kind of surgery, the perceived effects of the surgery and its potential outcome, and the client's basic personality. Surgery may be seen as a threat to the client's biological integrity, body image, self-esteem, self-concept, or lifestyle. Clients may fear death, pain, helplessness, decreased socioeconomic status, a diagnosis of life-threatening conditions, possible disabling or crippling effects, and the unknown.

The client's anxiety and fear affect his or her ability to learn, cope, and cooperate with preoperative teaching and perioperative procedures. Anxiety and fear may also influence the amount and type of anesthesia needed and may retard postoperative recovery. The nurse is aware of potential fears and anxieties when interviewing the client and planning preoperative teaching.

The nurse assesses coping mechanisms used by the client under similar situations or in the past when the client had been confronted with a stressful situation. The nurse asks open-ended questions pertaining to the client's feelings about the entire perioperative experience. The nurse assesses factors that influence coping, including age, previous surgical and sick-role experiences, emotional and physical signs of fear, anxiety, and discomfort. Signs of fear and anxiety include anger, crying, restlessness, diaphoresis (sweating, usually profusely), increased pulse rate, palpitations, sleeplessness, diarrhea, and urinary frequency. (For more information on stress and coping, see Chapter 8.)

➤ Laboratory Assessment

Preoperative laboratory tests provide baseline data about the client's health and help predict potential complications. The client scheduled for surgery in a surgical center or admitted to the hospital on the morning of or day before surgery may have preadmission testing performed 48 hours to 21 days before the scheduled surgery, depending on the facility's policy. The results of prior tests are usually valid unless there has been a change in the client's condition that warrants repeated testing. Depending on the test or tests needed, the hospitalized client has testing done under similar time guidelines.

The choice of routine preoperative laboratory tests varies among facilities and depends on the client's age and medical history and type of anesthesia planned. The most common tests are

- Urinalysis
- Blood type and cross-match
- Complete blood count or hemoglobin level and hematocrit
- Coagulation studies (prothrombin time [PT], activated partial thromboplastin time [APTT], and platelet count)
- Electrolyte levels
- Serum creatinine

Depending on a female client's age, a pregnancy test may also be ordered.

A preoperative urinalysis is performed to assess for the presence of protein, glucose, blood, and bacteria, all of which are abnormal constituents of the urine. If renal disease is suspected or the client is elderly, the physician may order other tests to determine the type and degree of disease present.

The nurse reports electrolyte imbalances or other abnormal results to the surgeon before surgery. Hypokalemia (decreased serum potassium level) increases the risk of digitalis toxicity (if the client is receiving a digitalis preparation), slows recovery from anesthesia, and increases cardiac irritability. Hyperkalemia (increased serum potassium level) increases the risk of cardiac dysrhythmias, especially with the use of anesthesia. Both hypokalemia and hyperkalemia should be treated before the surgery.

The physician may order other studies, depending on the client's medical history. For example, baseline arterial blood gas (ABG) values are assessed before surgery for clients with chronic pulmonary problems. Chart 20-3 presents abnormal laboratory findings and their possible causes.

➤ Radiographic Assessment

A chest radiograph, when ordered by the physician or anesthesiologist, is commonly obtained to determine size and contour of the heart, lungs, and major vessels and to determine the presence of any infiltrates that could indicate pneumonia or tuberculosis. A chest radiograph also provides baseline data in the event of postoperative complications. Abnormal radiograph results alert the physician to potential cardiac or pulmonary complications. The presence of congestive heart failure, cardiomyopathy, pneumonia, or infiltrates may cause cancellation or delay of elective surgery. For emergency surgery, radiograph results assist the anesthesiologist in the selection of anesthesia. In many facilities, chest radiograph results are valid when done within 6 months before surgery, provided that there has not been a change in the client's condition.

Other radiographic studies are based on individual client need, medical history, and nature of the surgical procedure. For example, a client with back pain may have computed tomography (CT) or magnetic resonance imaging (MRI) done before a laminectomy to identify the exact location of the abnormality.

➤ Other Diagnostic Assessment

An electrocardiogram (ECG) may routinely be required for all clients older than a specific age who are to have general anesthesia. The age varies among facilities but is often 40–45 years. An ECG may also be ordered for clients with a history of cardiac disease or those at risk for cardiovascular complications. An ECG provides baseline information on new or pre-existing cardiac conditions, such as an old anterior wall myocardial infarction. A client with a known cardiac condition may require a preoperative consultation with a cardiologist. Prophylactic medication, such as nitroglycerin and antibiotics, may be needed during the perioperative period to reduce or prevent stress on the cardiovascular system. Abnormal or potentially life-threatening ECG results may cause the cancellation of surgery until the client's cardiac status is stable.

A focused assessment of the preoperative client is shown in Chart 20–4.

 Analysis

➤ Common Nursing Diagnoses

Two nursing diagnoses are common to the preoperative client:

1. Knowledge Deficit related to a lack of education and lack of exposure to the specific perioperative experience
2. Anxiety related to the threat of a change in health status or fear of the unknown

➤ Additional Nursing Diagnoses

In addition to the common diagnoses, other nursing diagnoses may apply:

- Sleep Pattern Disturbance related to internal sensory alterations (e.g., illness and anxiety)
- Ineffective Individual Coping related to the impending surgery
- Anticipatory Grieving related to the effects of surgery
- Body Image Disturbance related to anticipated changes in the body's appearance or function
- Ineffective Family Coping: Compromised related to temporary family disorganization and role changes
- Powerlessness related to the health care environment, loss of independence, and loss of control of one's body
- Altered Family Processes related to situational crisis

Chart 20–3

Laboratory Profile

Perioperative Assessment

		Significance of Abnormal Findings	
Test	**Normal Range for Adults**	**Increased in**	**Decreased in**
Potassium (K^+) level	• 3.5–4.5 mEq/L, or 3.5–4.5 mmol/L	• Dehydration • Renal failure • Acidosis • Cellular/tissue damage • Hemolysis of the specimen	• NPO states when K^+ replacement is inadequate • Excessive use of non–K^+-sparing diuretics • Vomiting • Malnutrition • Diarrhea • Alkalosis
Sodium (Na^+)	• Up to 90 yo: 136–145 mEq/L, or 136–145 mmol/L • >90 yo: 132–146 mEq/L, or 132–146 mmol/L	• Cardiac or renal failure • Hypertension • Excessive amounts of IV fluids containing normal saline • Edema • Dehydration (hemoconcentration)	• Nasogastric drainage • Vomiting or diarrhea • Excessive use of laxatives or diuretics • Excessive amounts of IV fluids containing water • Syndrome of inappropriate antidiuretic hormone secretion (SIADH)
Chloride (Cl^-)	• Up to 90 yo: 98–107 mEq/L, or 98–107 mmol/L • >90 yo: 98–111 m Eq/L, or 98–111 mmol/L	• Respiratory alkalosis • Dehydration • Renal failure • Excessive amounts of IV fluids containing sodium chloride (NaCl)	• Excessive nasogastric drainage • Vomiting • Excessive use of diuretics • Diarrhea
Carbon dioxide (CO_2)	• Up to 60 yo: 23–29 mEq/L, or 23–29 mmol/L • 60–90 yo: 23–31 mEq/L, or 23–31 mmol/L • >90 yo: 20–29 mEq/L, or 20–29 mmol/L	• Chronic pulmonary disease • Intestinal obstruction • Vomiting or nasogastric suctioning • Metabolic alkalosis	• Hyperventilation • Diabetic ketoacidosis • Diarrhea • Lactic acidosis • Renal failure • Salicylate toxicity
Glucose (fasting)	• Up to 60 yo: 74–106 mg/dL, or 4.1–5.9 mmol/L • 60–90 yo: 82–115 mg/dL, or 4.6–6.4 mmol/L • >90 yo: 75–121 mg/dL, or 4.2–6.7 mmol/L	• Hyperglycemia • Excess amounts of IV fluids containing glucose • Stress • Steroid use • Pancreatic or hepatic disease	• Hypoglycemia • Excess insulin

Creatinine	• Females:
	  • Up to 60 yo: 0.6–1.1 mg/dL, or 53–97 μmol/L
	  • 60–90 yo: 0.6–1.2 mg/dL, or 53–106 μmol/L
	  • >90 yo: 0.6–1.3 mg/dL, or 53–115 μmol/L
	• Males:
	  • Up to 60 yo: 0.9–1.3 mg/dL, or 80–115 μmol/L
	  • 60–90 yo: 0.8–1.3 mg/dL, or 71–115 μmol/L
	  • >90 yo: 1.0–1.7 mg/dL, or 88–150 μmol/L
		• Renal damage with destruction of large number of nephrons
		• Renal insufficiency
		• Acute renal failure
		• Chronic renal failure
		• End-stage renal disease (ESRD)
			• Atrophy of muscle tissue

Continued

CHART 20–3. Laboratory Profile   Continued

Perioperative Assessment

Test	Normal Range for Adults	Significance of Abnormal Findings	
		Increased in	**Decreased in**
Blood urea nitrogen (BUN)	• Up to 60 yo: 6–20 mg/dL, or 2.1–7.1 mmol/L • 60–90 yo: 8–23 mg/dL, or 2.9–8.2 mmol/L • >90 yo: 10–31 mg/dL, or 3.6–11.1 mmol/L	• Dehydration • Renal failure • Excessive protein in diet • Liver failure	• Overhydration • Malnutrition
Prothrombin time (Pro Time, PT)	• 11–15 sec, 85%–100%, or 1–1.1 client/control ratio	• Coagulation defect (bleeding disorder) • Liver disease • Anticoagulant therapy (aspirin, warfarin)	• Coagulation (clotting) disorder such as thrombophlebitis or pulmonary embolus • Extensive cancer
Partial thromboplastin time, activated (APTT)	• Less than 35 sec	• Coagulation defect (bleeding disorder) • Anticoagulant therapy (heparin) • Liver disease	• Coagulation (clotting) disorder such as thrombophlebitis or pulmonary embolus • Extensive cancer
White blood cell (WBC) count (leukocyte count)	• Total: 4.5–11.0 × 10³ cells/μL, or 7.4 IRU • African Americans: 3.6–10.2 × 10³ cells/μL	• Infection • Inflammation • Stress • Tissue necrosis	• Immune disorder • Immunosuppressant therapy

Hemoglobin, total	• Females:
	  • 18–44 yo: 11.7–15.5 g/dL, or 117–155 g/L
	  • 45–64 yo: 11.7–16.0 g/dL, or 117–160 g/L
	  • 65–74 yo: 11.7–16.1 g/dL, or 117–161 g/L
	• Males:
	  • 18–44 yo: 13.2–17.3 g/dL, or 132–173 g/L
	  • 45–64 yo: 13.1–17.2 g/dL, or 131–172 g/L
	  • 65–74 yo: 12.6–17.4 g/dL, or 126–174 g/L
		• Dehydration
		• Polycythemia
		• Chronic pulmonary disease
		• Congestive heart failure
			• Blood loss
			• Anemia
			• Renal failure

Hematocrit	• Females:
	  • 18–44 yo: 35%–45%
	  • 45–74 yo: 35%–47%
	• Males:
	  • 18–44 yo: 39%–49%
	  • 45–64 yo: 39%–50%
	  • 65–74 yo: 37%–51%
		• Dehydration
		• Polycythemia
		• High altitude
			• Blood loss
			• Anemia
			• Renal failure

IRU = international recommended unit; yo = years of age; NPO = nothing by mouth.

 Planning and Implementation

➤ *Knowledge Deficit*

Planning: Expected Outcomes. Two outcomes are that the client will

- Verbalize and comply with preoperative procedures
- Demonstrate techniques to prevent postoperative complications

Interventions. Because the perioperative experience is foreign to many people, the nurse focuses on preoperative education of the client and family members. Preoperative teaching typically begins in the surgeon's office for planned or elective surgery. Pamphlets and written instructions may be given and sent to the client as well. More teaching may occur when the client has preadmission testing. Some facilities conduct preoperative classes for groups of clients who are having the same or similar

Focused Assessment of the Preoperative Client

As part of the cardiopulmonary assessment, take and record vital signs; report the following:

- Hypotension or hypertension
- Heart rate of less than 60 or more than 120 beats/min
- Irregular heart rate
- Chest pain
- Shortness of breath or dyspnea
- Tachypnea
- Pulse oximetry reading of <94%

Assess for and report any signs or symptoms of infection, including

- Fever
- Purulent sputum
- Dysuria or cloudy, foul-smelling urine
- Any red, swollen, draining intravenous or wound site
- Increased white blood cell count

Assess for and report signs or symptoms that could contraindicate surgery, including

- Increased Pro Time or activated partial thromboplastin time
- Hypokalemia or hyperkalemia
- Client report of possible pregnancy or positive pregnancy test

Assess for and report other clinical conditions that may need to be evaluated by a physician or advanced nurse practitioner before proceeding with the surgical plans, including

- Change in mental status
- Vomiting
- Rash
- Recent administration of an anticoagulant medication

surgical procedures. A tour of the operating suite and the postanesthesia care unit (PACU) may be included.

Information about informed consent, dietary restrictions, preoperative preparation (bowel and skin preparations), and postoperative exercises and procedures promotes the client's participation in health care. A sample preoperative educational checklist is shown in Table 20–4. Because education of the client takes place in a variety of settings, coordination of client teaching efforts is particularly challenging. The nurse who cares for the client immediately before surgery (same-day, ambulatory surgery outpatient or inpatient hospital unit) assesses the client's knowledge and provides additional information as needed.

Ensuring Informed Consent. Surgery of any type involves invasion of the body and requires informed consent from the client or legal guardian (Fig. 20–1). Consent implies that one has been provided with information necessary to understand the following:

- The nature of and reason for surgery
- All available options and the risks associated with each option
- The risks of the surgical procedure and its potential outcomes
- The risks associated with the administration of anesthesia

Signed permission helps protect the client from any unwanted procedures and the physician and the facility from lawsuit claims related to unauthorized surgery or uninformed clients.

The physician is usually responsible for having the consent form signed before preoperative sedation is given and before surgery is performed. The nurse is not responsible for providing detailed information about the surgical procedure. Rather, the nurse clarifies facts that have been presented by the physician and dispels myths that the client and family may have about the perioperative experience. The nurse ensures that the consent form is signed and serves as a witness to the signature, not to the fact that the client is informed. The surgeon is contacted and requested to see the client for clarification of information if the nurse believes that the client has not been adequately informed. The nurse documents this action in the client's chart.

Clients who cannot write may sign with an **X**, which must be witnessed by two people. In an emergency, telephone or telegram authorization is acceptable and should be followed with written consent as soon as possible. The number of witnesses (usually two) and the type of documentation vary according to the facility's policy. In a life-threatening situation in which every effort has been made to contact the person with medical power of attorney, consent is desired but not essential. In lieu of written or oral consent, written consultation by at least two physicians who are not associated with the case may be requested by the physician. This formal consultation legally supports the decision for surgery until the appropriate person can sign a consent form. If the client is not capable of giving consent and has no family, the court can appoint a legal guardian to represent the client's best interests.

TABLE 20–4

Preoperative Teaching Checklist

Consider the following items when planning individualized preoperative teaching for clients and families:

  Fears and anxieties
  Surgical procedure
  Preoperative routines (e.g., NPO, enemas, blood samples, showering)
  Invasive procedures (e.g., lines, catheters)
  Coughing, turning, deep breathing
  Incentive spirometer
    How to use
    How to tell when used correctly
  Lower extremity exercises
  Stockings and pneumatic compression devices
  Early ambulation
  Splinting
  Pain management

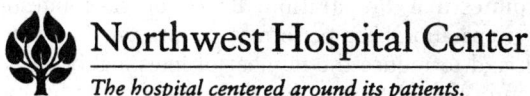

Northwest Hospital Center
The hospital centered around its patients.

**REQUEST AND AUTHORIZATION FOR
MEDICAL AND/OR SURGICAL TREATMENT,
BLOOD PRODUCTS ADMINISTRATION**

1. I hereby request and authorize Dr._____ and/or his/her associates and whomever they may designate as their assistants, to administer such treatment as is necessary and to perform the following operation_____
    _____
    and such additional operations or procedures as are considered necessary on the basis of conditions that may be revealed during the course of said operation or treatment.

2. The reasons why the above named surgery and/or treatment is considered necessary, its advantages, probability of success, possible complications, and risks, as well as possible alternative modes of treatment were explained to me by
    Dr._____.

3. I request and authorize the administration of such anesthetics and/or other medications as are necessary.

4. Final disposition of any tissues or parts surgically removed is to be handled in accordance with the customary practices of the hospital.

5. I am aware that the practice of medicine and surgery is not an exact science and I acknowledge that no guarantees have been made to me concerning the results of the operation or procedure.

6. I hereby acknowledge that I have read and fully understand the above request and authorization for medical and/or surgical treatment.

7. I consent to the admittance of permitted observers, the use of closed-circuit television, taking of photographs (including motion pictures), and the preparation of drawings and similar illustrative material, and I also consent to the use of such photographs and other material for scientific purposes, provided my identity is not revealed by the pictures or by the descriptive text accompanying them.

8. I consent to release of my social security number in accordance with the Safe Medical Device Act.

_____   _____   _____
Date   Time   Signature of Patient or Patient Surrogate

_____   _____
Witness   Signature of Physician

CONSENT TO BLOOD/BLOOD PRODUCTS TRANSFUSION

After discussing the risks, benefits and alternatives to transfusion of blood (donor/autologous) (circle one or both) or blood products with my physician or his designee, I consent to the administration of these products.

_____   _____   _____
Date   Time   Signature of Patient or Patient Surrogate

_____   _____
Witness   Signature of Physician

703/1019-3-R-8/97   (40-1331)

Figure 20–1. A surgical consent form. (Courtesy of Northwest Hospital Center, Randallstown, MD.)

A blind client is capable of signing his or her own consent form, which usually needs to be witnessed by two people. Clients who speak a language other than the general language in the agency require a translator and a second witness. Some facilities have consent forms written in more than one language.

Some surgical procedures require a special permit in addition to the standard consent. National and local governing bodies and the individual surgical facility determine which procedures require a separate permit. Intraocular lens implants, sterilization, and experimental procedures are examples of procedures for which the extra form is usually required. Separate consents for anesthesia and the administration of blood products may be required as well.

Implementing Dietary Restrictions. Regardless of the type of surgery and anesthesia planned, the client is restricted to nothing by mouth (NPO) for 6 to 8 hours before surgery. *NPO* means no eating of food, drinking (including water), or smoking (nicotine stimulates gastric secretions). It is common practice to begin NPO status for all preoperative clients at midnight on the night before surgery. This extra precaution ensures that the stomach contains a limited volume of gastric secretions, which helps decrease the possibility of aspiration. Outpatients and clients who are scheduled for admission to the hospital on the same day that surgery is performed must receive written and oral instructions about remaining NPO after midnight. The nurse emphasizes the importance of compliance; failure to comply can result in cancellation of surgery or an increased risk of intraoperative or postoperative aspiration.

Administering Regularly Scheduled Medications. On the day of surgery, the client's usual medication schedule may need to be altered. The nurse consults the client's medical physician for instructions about administration of medications, such as those used for diabetes mellitus, cardiac disease, and glaucoma, as well as regularly scheduled anticonvulsants, antihypertensives, anticoagulants, antidepressants, and corticosteroids. The physician may order some medications to be stopped until after surgery. The physician may order other medications to be administered by the intravenous (IV) route to maintain the client's blood level of the medication. Medications for cardiac disease and hypertension are commonly allowed with a sip of water if taken at least 2 hours before surgery. Some antihypertensive or antidepressant medications may be withheld on the day of surgery because of a possible adverse affect on the blood pressure intraoperatively.

The diabetic client who is taking insulin may be given a reduced dose of intermediate- or long-acting insulin on the basis of the serum glucose level, or the client may be given regular (fast-acting) insulin subcutaneously in divided doses on the day of surgery. An alternative method of diabetes management is an IV infusion of 5% dextrose in water given with the insulin to prevent hypoglycemia intraoperatively. Because of numerous treatment approaches to diabetes, the nurse clarifies medication and IV orders with the physician. (More information about the surgical client with diabetes is found in Chapter 68.)

Gastrointestinal Preparation. Bowel or gastrointestinal (GI) preparations are performed to prevent injury to the colon and to reduce the number of intestinal bacteria. Evacuation of the GI tract is done when a client is having major abdominal, pelvic, perineal, or perianal surgery. The surgeon's preference and type of surgical procedure determine the type of bowel preparation. Table 20–5 shows typical GI preparation regimens for common surgical procedures and complications of the regimens. An enema ordered to be given until return flow is clear is a physically stressful procedure for anyone but especially for the elderly client. Repeated enemas can cause electrolyte imbalance (especially potassium depletion), fluid volume deficit, vagal stimulation, and postural (orthostatic) hypotension. Enemas also cause severe anorectal discomfort in clients with hemorrhoids. To prevent complications, some physicians prescribe potent laxatives (e.g., polyethylene glycol–electrolyte solution [GoLYTELY]) instead of enemas, especially for elderly clients. Bowel preparation procedures can be exhausting, and the nurse takes safety precautions to prevent client falls.

Skin Preparation. The skin preparation may be embarrassing or uncomfortable for the client, especially if the surgical site is in a sensitive or generally private area. The nurse provides a warm, comfortable, and private environment for the client during the procedure.

The skin is the body's first line of defense against infection. A break in this protective mechanism increases the risk of infection, especially for elderly clients. Preoperative skin preparation is the initial step in the prevention of wound infection. One or two days before the scheduled surgery, the surgeon may require the client to shower using an antiseptic solution such as povidone-iodine (Betadine) or hexachlorophene. The physician may want the client to be especially attentive to cleaning around the proposed surgical site. If the patient is hospitalized before surgery, the showering and cleaning is often repeated the night before surgery or in the morning before the client is transferred to the surgical suite. This cleaning reduces contamination of and the number of microorganisms on the surgical field. After the final cleaning procedure, especially for an orthopedic surgery, the area may be covered with sterile towels or drapes to prevent contamination.

A controversial step in preoperative skin preparation after the cleaning or showering is the shave. Many health care practitioners believe that the shaving procedure itself is a possible source of contamination of the surgical area and traumatizes the skin around the area where the incision will be made. Those factors believed to predispose the client to wound contamination include bacteria found in hair follicles, disruption of the normal protective mechanisms of the skin, and nicks in the skin (e.g., from shaving). Shaving of hair creates the potential for infection. Clipping of the hair with electrical surgical clippers is becoming increasingly popular to decrease the complications associated with traditional razors. In the United States, the Centers for Disease Control and Prevention recommend that if shaving is necessary, the hair should be removed using disposable sterile supplies and aseptic principles *immediately* before the start of the surgical pro-

TABLE 20–5

Complications of Common Bowel Preparations for the Surgical Client

Surgical Site	Preparation	Complications
Stomach, duodenum, and proximal jejunum	• Oral laxative (e.g., castor oil preparation or bisacodyl [Dulcolax, Laxit✦]) • Clear liquid diet the evening before surgery • NPO after midnight	• Abdominal cramping • Dehydration • Electrolyte imbalance • Fatigue
Small intestine	• Oral laxative (e.g., magnesium citrate) • Clear liquid diet the evening before surgery • Multiple-position enema the evening before surgery • NPO after midnight	• Abdominal cramping • Dehydration • Electrolyte imbalance • Fatigue
Large intestine to rectum	• Multiple or combination of oral laxatives 12–24 hr before surgery • Multiple-position tap water or antibiotic (neomycin) enemas (three times or until the return flow is clear) the evening and morning before surgery • Oral antibiotics to sterilize the bowel (e.g., neomycin and erythromycin) 24 hr before surgery • Clear liquid diet the day before surgery • NPO after midnight	• Abdominal cramping • Fatigue and weakness • Fluid excess or deficit • Potassium or sodium deficit • Decreased cardiac output from vagal stimulation • Irritation of bowel and rectal mucosa from enemas

cedure. Thus, shave preparations are performed in the treatment room, the holding area of the operating suite, or the operating room. Figure 20–2 shows areas shaved for various surgical procedures. Shaving of hair, especially from the head or genital area, can be emotionally upsetting to the client, and regrowth of this hair can be uncomfortable.

Preparing the Client for Tubes, Drains, and Intravenous Access. The nurse prepares the client for possible insertion of tubes, drains, and IV access devices. Preparation reduces the client's postoperative anxiety and fear. The nurse is careful not to scare the client while providing information about the purpose of each tube.

Tubes. The client may require an indwelling urinary catheter (Foley) before, during, or after surgery to keep the bladder empty and to enable monitoring of renal function. The client having major abdominal or genitourinary surgery usually has a Foley catheter.

A nasogastric tube may be inserted before emergency surgery or major abdominal surgery for decompressing or emptying the stomach and the upper bowel. However, it is more often inserted after the induction of anesthesia, when insertion is less disturbing to the client and is easier to perform.

Drains. Drains are frequently inserted during surgery to promote the evacuation of fluid from the surgical site. Some drains are under the dressing, whereas others are visible and require emptying. Drains come in various shapes and sizes (see Chapter 22). The nurse informs the client that drains are often used routinely and that generally they are not painful. The nurse further discusses with

clients the reasons why they should not kink or pull on the drain.

Intravenous Access. An IV access (line) is placed by the nurse or anesthesia personnel for all clients receiving general anesthesia and some clients receiving other types of anesthesia. An access is needed to administer medication and fluids before, during, and after surgery. Clients who are dehydrated or who are at risk for dehydration, such as elderly clients, may receive fluids before surgery. Elderly clients are more susceptible to dehydration because their fluid reserves are lower than those of young or middle-aged adults. Careful monitoring is required for the elderly and for clients with cardiac disease receiving IV fluids. (See Chapter 17 for more information on IV therapy.)

The IV access is usually placed in the arm or the posterior aspect of the hand using a large, short catheter (e.g., 18 gauge, 1 inch). This type of catheter provides the least resistance to fluid or blood infusion, especially in an emergency when rapid infusions may be necessary. Depending on the individual client's needs and the facility's policies and practices, the IV can be placed before surgery when the client is in the hospital room, in the holding or admission area of the surgical suite, or in the operating room.

Teaching About Postoperative Procedures and Exercises. The nurse instructs the client and family members about postoperative exercises and procedures, e.g., checking dressings and obtaining vital signs frequently (see the Client Care Plan). Preoperative teaching reduces the client's apprehension and fear, increases the client's cooperation and participation in postoperative care, and decreases

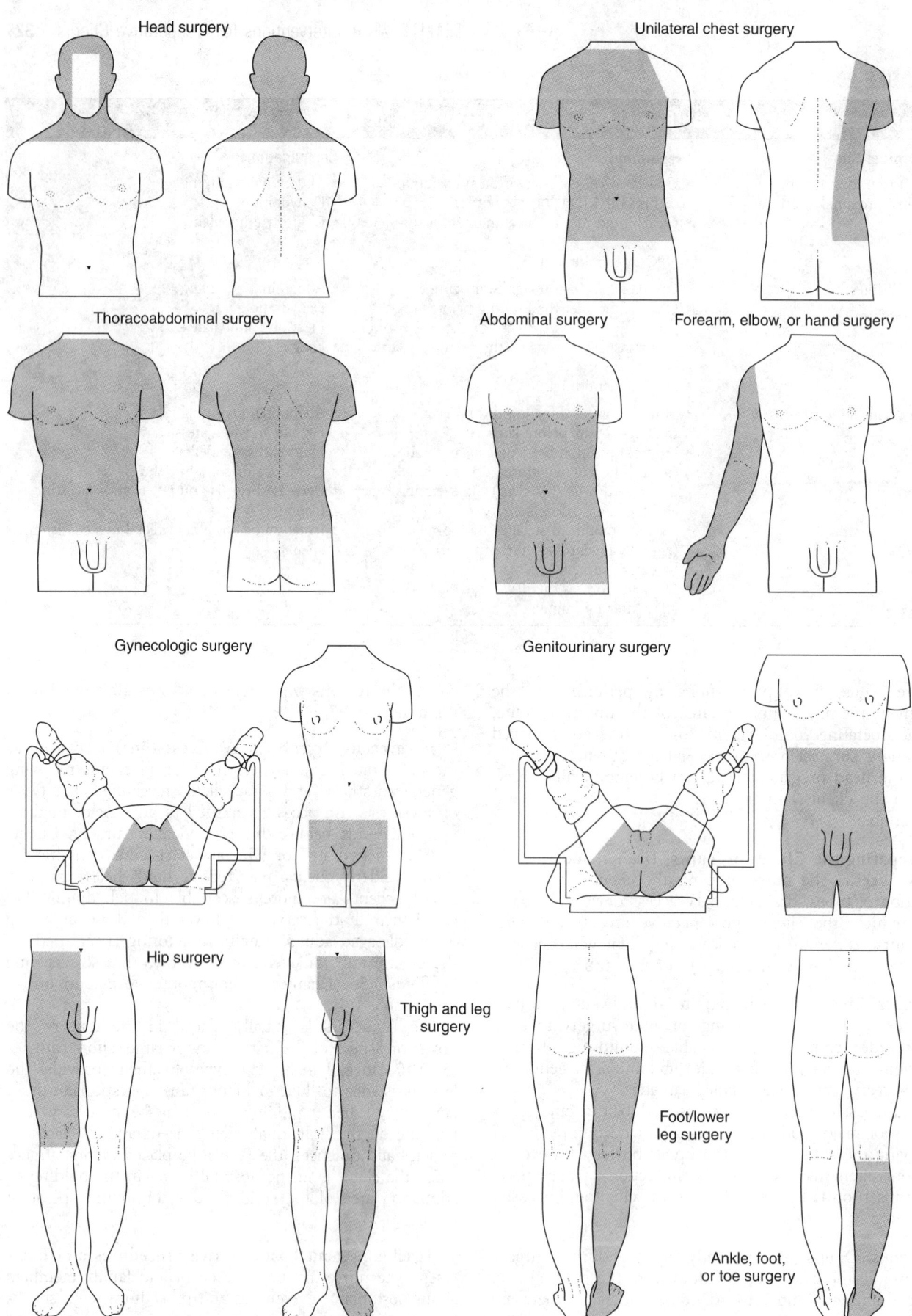

Head surgery

Unilateral chest surgery

Thoracoabdominal surgery

Abdominal surgery

Forearm, elbow, or hand surgery

Gynecologic surgery

Genitourinary surgery

Hip surgery

Thigh and leg
surgery

Foot/lower
leg surgery

Ankle, foot,
or toe surgery

Figure 20–2. Skin preparation of common surgical sites. Shaded areas indicate areas of hair removal.

Client Care Plan

The Preoperative Client

Nursing Diagnosis No. 1: Knowledge Deficit related to lack of exposure to the specific perioperative experience

Expected Outcomes	Nursing Interventions	Rationale
The client will Verbalize an understanding of the perioperative routine.	■ Assess the client's current level of knowledge and provide information about the perioperative routine, as necessary.	■ By assessing the client's knowledge base, the nurse is able to individualize the preoperative teaching.
State reasons for and expected frequency of the postoperative exercises.	■ Discuss with the client and significant others the reasons for the postoperative exercises. ■ Discuss and demonstrate correct breathing and leg exercises.	■ Clients are more likely to comply when they understand the reasons for the activities. ■ Significant others are able to reinforce instructions and encourage the client postoperatively.
Demonstrate correct use of an incentive spirometer (IS). State the goals to achieve with the IS.	■ Encourage the client to practice the exercises. ■ Supplement instructions with written materials, videos, and so on, as available.	■ Repetition helps the learning process. ■ Reinforcement of instructions in more than one format facilitates learning.
Demonstrate splinting of the anticipated surgical area.	■ Discuss and demonstrate the technique for splinting.	■ Client demonstration preoperatively will make it easier to perform postoperatively.

Nursing Diagnosis No. 2. Anxiety related to the threat of a change in health status or fear of the unknown

Expected Outcomes	Nursing Interventions	Rationale
The client will Verbalize the reasons for anxieties or fears, if possible.	■ Assess the client's level of anxiety. ■ Encourage the client to verbalize concerns and fears. ■ Review perioperative events and routines.	■ By assessing the client's anxiety level, support systems, and coping mechanisms, the nurse is able to individualize the plan for anxiety reduction. ■ Familiarity with the usual perioperative events decreases the unknown, which is often a source of anxiety.
Demonstrate relaxation breathing exercises. Identify available diversional activities. Use successful coping mechanisms.	■ Teach relaxation breathing. ■ Provide distractions such as music and television. ■ Assess the client's support systems and coping mechanisms. ■ Incorporate the client's methods of reducing stress, as indicated.	■ Focused thoughts and distractions help to decrease anxiety. ■ Focused thoughts and distractions help to decrease anxiety. ■ When the client is able to continue familiar activities and actions, anxiety is reduced.
State that anxiety is reduced or manageable.	■ Encourage the client to identify which specific interventions reduce anxiety.	■ When client is aware of successful interventions, outcomes can be met in a more timely fashion.

the incidence and severity of postoperative complications. However, when the client's fear or anxiety level is high, the nurse explores the client's attitudes and feelings before discussing procedures (Cipperley et al., 1995). Discussion, demonstration, and return demonstration and practice by the client aid in the ability to perform various breathing (Chart 20–5) and leg (Chart 20–6) exercises during postoperative recovery. The nurse emphasizes the need to begin exercises early in the recovery phase and to continue them, with five to ten repetitions each, every 1 to 2 hours after surgery for at least the first 48 hours. The nurse also explains that the client may need to be awakened for these activities.

Breathing Exercises. In deep, or diaphragmatic, breathing, the diaphragm flattens during inspiration, enlarging the upper abdominal cavity. During expiration, the abdominal muscles and diaphragm contract, which completely expands the lungs. After the nurse demonstrates and explains the technique, the client is encouraged to practice the five steps of deep breathing.

For clients with chronic pulmonary disease or limited upper chest expansion, as seen in elderly clients because of the aging process, expansion breathing exercises are useful. For the client having thoracic surgery, expansion breathing exercises strengthen accessory muscles and should be initiated preoperatively. Expansion breathing may be used postoperatively during chest physiotherapy (percussion, vibration, and postural drainage) to assist with loosening secretions and maintaining an adequate air exchange.

Incentive Spirometry. Incentive spirometry is another way to encourage the client to take deep breaths. Its purpose is to promote complete lung expansion and to prevent respiratory complications. Various types of incentive spirometers are available; some examples are shown in Figure 20–3. With all types, the client must be able to seal his or her lips tightly around the mouthpiece, inhale spontaneously, and hold his or her breath for 3 to 5 seconds to achieve effective lung expansion. Goals (e.g., attaining specific volumes) can be set according to the client's ability and the type of incentive spirometer. Visualization by seeing a light move up a column or a bellows expanding often reinforces and motivates the client to continue performance.

Coughing and Splinting. Coughing may be performed in conjunction with deep breathing every 1 to 2 hours postoperatively. The purposes of coughing are to promote expectoration of secretions, keep the lungs clear, allow full aeration, and prevent pneumonia and atelectasis. Coughing may be uncomfortable for the client, but when performed correctly, it should not harm the surgical area. Splinting (e.g., holding) the incision area provides support, promotes a feeling of security, and reduces pain during coughing. The proper technique for splinting the incision site and coughing was described in Chart 20–5. A folded bath blanket is helpful to use as a splint.

Some practitioners think that coughing exercises should no longer be encouraged routinely. Their belief is that coughing has the potential to harm the surgical wound and that it would be better to emphasize other, safer

---

Chart 20–5

Education Guide: Perioperative Respiratory Care

Deep (diaphragmatic) breathing

1. Sit upright on the edge of the bed or in a chair, being sure that your feet are placed firmly on the floor or a stool. [After surgery, deep breathing is done with the client in Fowler's position or in semi-Fowler's position.]
2. Take a gentle breath through your mouth.
3. Breathe out gently and completely.
4. Then take a deep breath through your nose and mouth, and hold this breath to the count of five.
5. Exhale through your nose and mouth.

Expansion breathing

1. Find a comfortable upright position, with your knees slightly bent. [Bending the knees decreases tension on the abdominal muscles and decreases respiratory resistance and discomfort.]
2. Place your hands on each side of your lower rib cage, just above your waist.
3. Take a deep breath through your nose, using your shoulder muscles to expand your lower rib cage outward during inhalation.
4. Exhale, concentrating first on moving your chest, then on moving your lower ribs inward, while gently squeezing the rib cage and forcing air out of the base of your lungs.

Splinting of the surgical incision

1. Unless coughing is contraindicated, place a pillow, towel, or folded blanket over your surgical incision and hold the item firmly in place.
2. Take three slow, deep breaths to stimulate your cough reflex.
3. Inhale through your nose, then exhale through your mouth.
4. On your third deep breath, cough to clear secretions from your lungs while firmly holding the pillow, towel, or folded blanket against your incision.

---

measures for pulmonary hygiene, such as the deep breathing and incentive spirometer exercises. When routine coughing exercises are contraindicated for a client, such as after a hernia repair, the physician usually writes a "do not cough" order.

Leg Procedures and Exercises. Antiembolism stockings (TED stockings or Jobst hose), elastic (Ace) wraps, or pneumatic compression devices (e.g., "sequentials" and "boots") may be used perioperatively in combination with leg exercises and early ambulation to promote venous return. Venous stasis can lead to deep vein (venous) thrombosis (DVT) or a pulmonary embolus (PE) if the blood clot breaks off and travels to the lungs. Interventions depend on the client's risk factors. Clients at greater risk for deep vein thrombosis

- Are obese
- Are older than 40 years of age
- Have a concurrent cancer diagnosis

Chart 20–6

Education Guide: Postoperative Leg Exercises

Exercise No. 1

1. Lie in bed with the head of your bed elevated to about 45 degrees. [Using semi-Fowler's position during postoperative leg exercises improves peripheral circulation, prevents thrombus formation, and strengthens muscles.]
2. Beginning with your right leg, bend your knee, raise your foot off the bed, and hold this position for a few seconds.
3. Extend your leg by unbending your knee, and lower the leg to the bed.
4. Repeat this sequence four more times with your right leg, then perform this same exercise five times with your left leg.

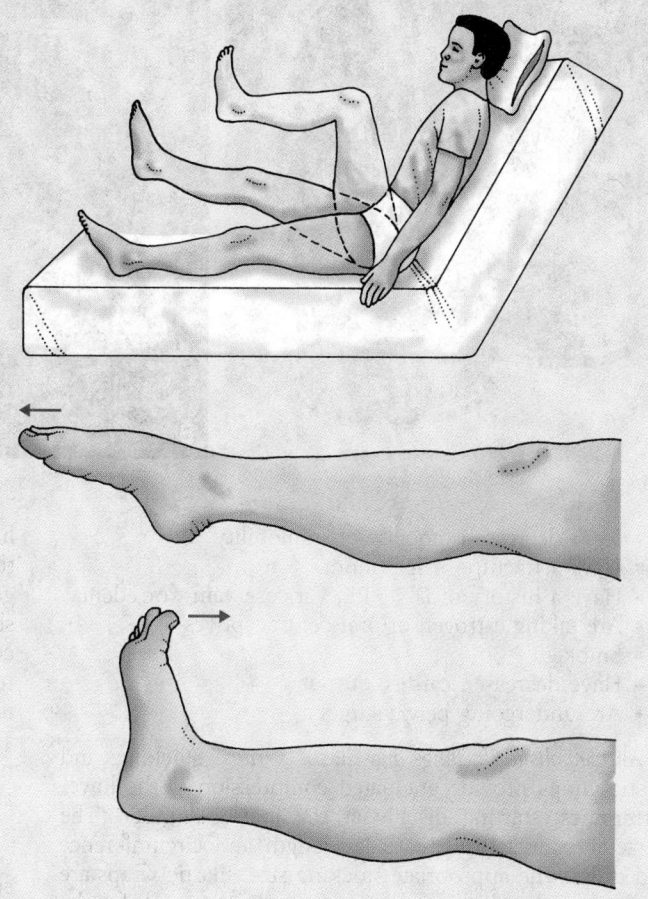

Exercise No. 2

1. Beginning with your right leg, point your toes toward the bottom of the bed.
2. With the same leg, point your toes up toward your face.
3. Repeat this exercise several times with your right leg, then perform this same exercise with your left leg.

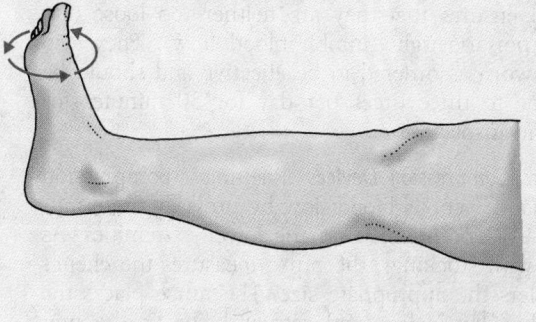

Exercise No. 3

1. Beginning with your right leg, make circles with your ankles, first to the left, then to the right.
2. Repeat this exercise several times with your right leg, then perform this same exercise with your left leg.

Exercise No. 4

1. Beginning with your right leg, bend your knee and *push* the ball of your foot into the bed or floor until you feel your calf and thigh muscles contracting.
2. Repeat this exercise several times with your right leg, then perform this same exercise with your left leg.

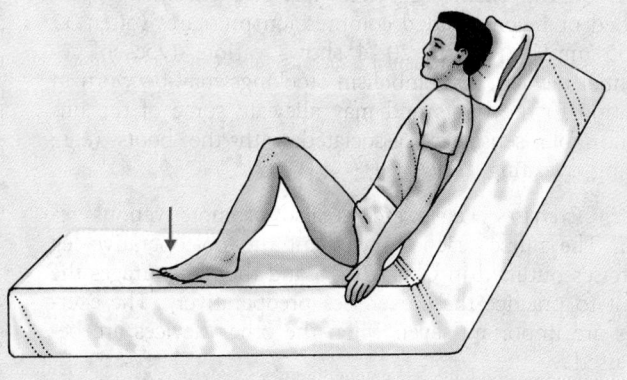

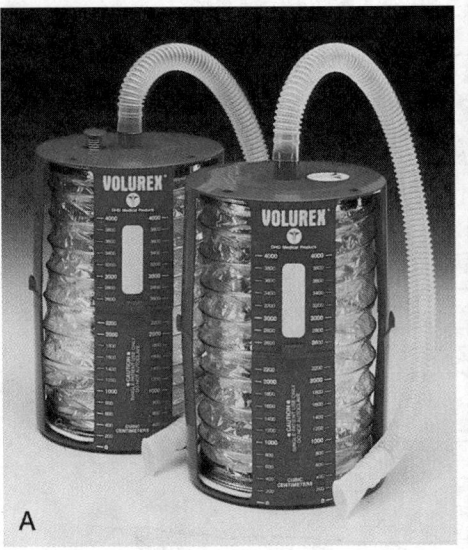 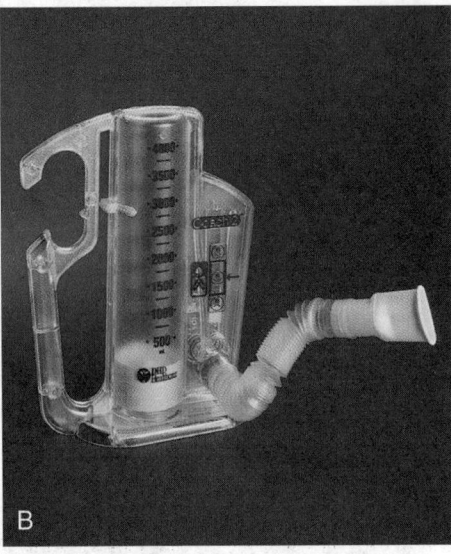

Figure 20–3. Examples of volume incentive spirometers for lung expansion. *A.* A volume displacement incentive spirometer. *B,* A volumetric incentive spirometer. (Courtesy of DHD Healthcare, Canastota, NY.)

- Have decreased mobility or immobility
- Have a fracture or leg trauma
- Have a history of DVT, PE, varicose veins, or edema
- Are taking estrogen or oral contraceptives
- Smoke
- Have decreased cardiac output
- Are undergoing pelvic surgery

Antiembolism Stockings and Elastic Wraps. Stockings and elastic wraps provide graduated compression of the lower extremities, starting distally at the foot and ankle. The nurse measures the client's leg length and circumference and orders the appropriate stocking size. Elastic wraps are used when the client's leg is too large or too small for the stockings. The nurse assists the client in applying the devices and ensures that they are neither too loose (are ineffective) nor too tight (inhibit blood flow). They also need to be worn as ordered to be effective and should be removed one to three times per day for 30 minutes for skin care and inspection.

Pneumatic Compression Devices. Pneumatic compression devices enhance venous blood flow by providing intermittent periods of compression on the lower extremities. As is the case with stockings, the nurse measures the client's leg and orders the appropriate size. The nurse places the boots on the client's legs and sets and checks the prescribed or recommended compression pressures (often 35 to 55 mmHg). Figure 20–4 shows various types of sequential devices. Antiembolism stockings may be worn in addition to the boots and may alleviate some of the uncomfortable sensations associated with the boots (e.g., itching, sweating, heat).

Leg Exercises. Leg exercises also promote venous return. The nurse teaches the client the postoperative leg exercises outlined in Chart 20–6 and then encourages the client to practice these exercises preoperatively. The exercises are important, even when the other devices are being used.

Early Ambulation. Mobility soon after surgery (early ambulation) stimulates gastrointestinal motility, enhances

lung expansion, mobilizes secretions, promotes venous return, prevents rigidity of joints, and relieves pressure. In general, the nurse instructs the client that he or she should turn at least every 2 hours after surgery while confined to bed. To aid clients, the nurse teaches them how to use the bed side rails safely for turning and how to protect the surgical wound (splinting) when turning. The nurse assures clients that assistance will be given as needed to alleviate any anxiety they may have about this activity.

For certain surgeries, such as some brain, spinal, and orthopedic surgeries, the physician may order turning restrictions. The nurse discusses with the physician other interventions to prevent complications associated with immobility in clients with turning restrictions. The nurse informs the client of anticipated turning restrictions during preoperative teaching.

Many clients are allowed and encouraged to get out of bed the day of or the day after surgery. The nurse assists the client into a chair or with ambulation the evening after the surgery or the next day, depending on the type and time of surgery and the physician's preference. If a client must remain in bed, he or she must turn, deep breathe, and perform leg exercises at least every 2 hours to prevent the complications of postoperative immobility.

Range-of-Motion Exercises. Passive or active range-of-motion (ROM) exercises help prevent joint rigidity and muscle contracture. The client should do these exercises three to five times each, three to four times a day while bedridden. The nurse instructs the client in these procedures and informs the client that he or she will receive assistance as needed postoperatively. (Guidelines for ROM exercises are found in Chapter 24.)

➤ *Anxiety*

Planning: Expected Outcomes. The outcomes are that the client will

- Verbalize decreased or manageable preoperative anxiety
- Demonstrate evidence of relaxation when at rest

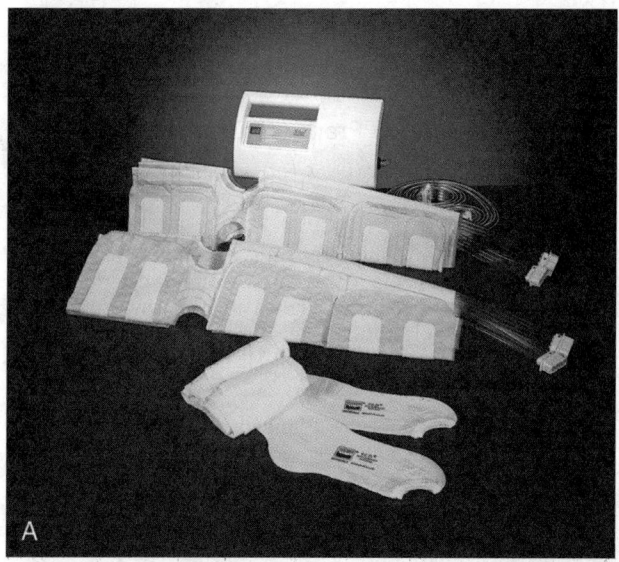

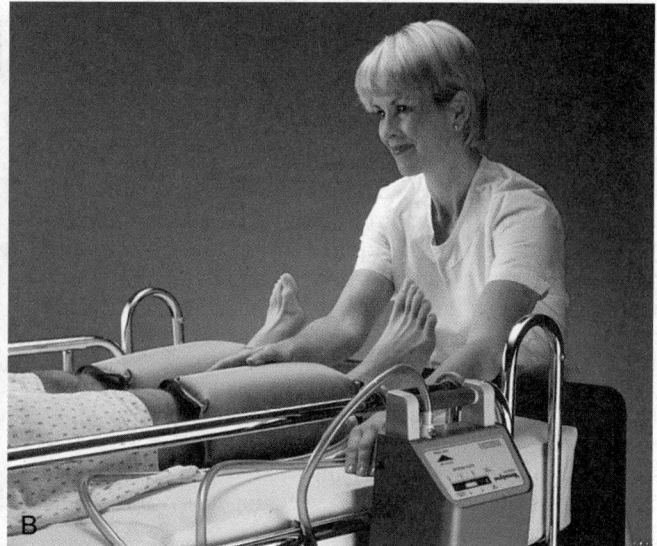

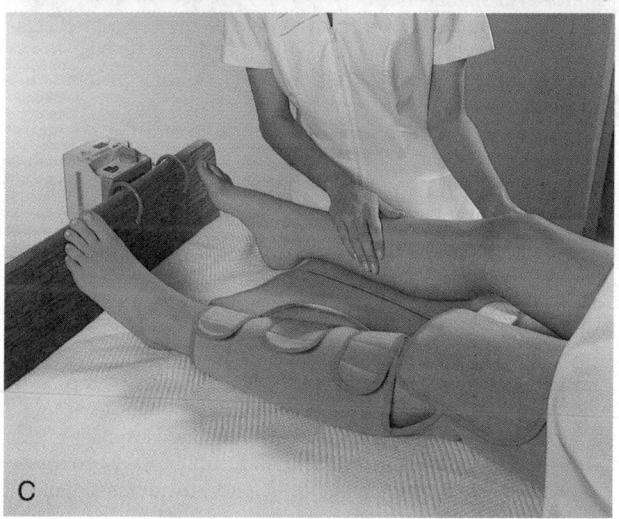

Figure 20–4. Examples of external pneumatic compression devices used to promote venous return and prevent deep vein thrombosis (DVT). *A.* Kendall SCD machine, sleeves, and TED stockings (Courtesy of Kendall Healthcare Company). *B,* Venodyne pneumatic compression system (Courtesy of Venodyne, Inc.). *C,* Flowtron DVT calf garments (Courtesy of Huntleigh Healthcare).

Interventions. Preoperative anxiety frequently causes the client to exhibit physical symptoms such as restlessness and sleeplessness. The surgical client perceives the perioperative experience as a threat to biopsychosocial integrity. The nurse first assesses the client's level of anxiety, as discussed earlier in this chapter. Interventions such as teaching and communicating with the client preoperatively, enabling the client to utilize previously successful coping mechanisms, and administering antianxiety agents help to reduce the anxiety and subsequent complications. The nurse incorporates appropriate and available support systems into the plan of care.

Preoperative Teaching. The nurse assesses the client's knowledge about the perioperative experience that he or she has acquired from prior surgical experiences and procedures and from other sources (see Knowledge Deficit earlier in this chapter). The nurse provides factual information about the surgery and the perioperative experience

to promote the client's understanding. The nurse allows ample time for the client's questions. The nurse responds to the client's questions appropriately and accurately and refers unanswered questions to the proper person. During the discussion between the client and the nurse, the nurse continually assesses the client's responses and anxiety level. The nurse must be careful not to provide information that might increase anxiety. Clients have ranked psychosocial support as the most important component during preoperative teaching. The informed, educated client is better able to anticipate events and maintain self-control and is thus less anxious.

Encouraging Communication. Stating feelings, fears, and concerns is an appropriate way to reduce anxiety. The nurse develops a trusting relationship with the client so he or she can express feelings freely without fear of ridicule or judgment. The nurse keeps the client informed, clarifies information, answers questions, and allays some of the client's apprehensions about surgery.

Promoting Rest. The stress and anxiety of impending surgery frequently interfere with the client's ability to sleep and rest the night before surgery. The preoperative experience is physically and emotionally stressful. To assist the client in relaxing, the nurse determines what the client usually does to relax and fall asleep. If permitted and able, the client is encouraged to continue these methods of relaxation. A back rub is a relaxing and therapeutic measure and can be performed by a nurse or family member. The physician may prescribe a sedative or short-acting hypnotic to ensure that the client is well rested for surgery.

Using Distraction. The nurse may plan distraction as an intervention for anxiety. Especially in the 24 hours immediately before surgery, listening to music (see Research Applications For Nursing) or comedy audiotapes may decrease anxiety, as may watching television, reading, or visiting with family members.

Teaching Family and Significant Others. The nurse assesses the readiness and desire of the family or significant others to take an active part in the client's care. The involved family provides support for the client and helps reduce anxiety. A positive sign of family interest is members' initiation of questions about the perioperative experience. After family readiness is determined, the nurse keeps family members informed and encourages their involvement in all aspects of preoperative education with the client. The nurse emphasizes the important role of the family preoperatively but guides discussions and practice sessions so that family members do not dominate the sessions. Family members can encourage and help the client practice postoperative exercises.

The nurse informs the family of the time for surgery, if known, and of any schedule changes. If the client is an outpatient, he or she and the family need clear directions regarding any specific night-before procedures, what time and where to report, and what to bring with them. The family is encouraged to stay with the client preoperatively for support.

Most families are anxious about the surgery planned for their loved one. To reduce their anxiety, the nurse explains the intraoperative and postoperative routine to them. The nurse explains that after the client leaves the hospital room or admission area, there is usually a 30- to 60-minute preparation period in the operating area (holding room, treatment area, and so on) before the surgery actually begins. After surgery, the client is taken to the postanesthesia care unit (PACU) for 1 to 2 hours before returning to the hospital room or discharge area. The nurse instructs the family about the best place to wait for the client or surgeon according to the facility's policy and the physician's preference. Many hospitals and surgical centers have designated surgical waiting areas so families can wait in comfortable surroundings and be easily located when the procedure is completed.

➤ *Preoperative Chart Review*

The nurse reviews the client's chart to ensure all documentation, preoperative procedures, and orders are completed. The nurse checks the surgical informed consent

---

➤ Research Applications for Nursing

Music May Reduce Preoperative Anxiety

Augustin, P., & Haines, A. A. (1996). Effect of music on ambulatory surgery patients' preoperative anxiety. AORN Journal, 63(4), 750, 753–758.

In this study, 42 ambulatory surgical clients were assigned to either an experimental or a control group to determine the effect music had on reducing preoperative anxiety. Vital signs and client self-reports of anxiety, using the State-Trait Anxiety Inventory, were measured. All clients received preoperative instruction.

Critique. This sample was limited to 42 ambulatory patients. Anxiety is generally believed to have an effect on heart and respiratory rates and blood pressure. In this study, heart rates were found to be significantly lower in the experimental group, but the effect on blood pressure and respiratory rate approached significance only.

Further studies are needed to validate the physical effects of anxiety and to describe the physical effects related to different causes of anxiety. Additionally, studies on interventions that could reduce preoperative anxiety should be expanded to include the same-day admission and the hospitalized client. The study of music effects on clients awaiting consultation, diagnostic tests, or other, nonsurgical procedures could also be studied.

Possible Nursing Implications. Health care professionals caring for clients before ambulatory surgery may need to start interventions aimed at reducing preoperative anxiety earlier than in the immediate preoperative period. Ambulatory surgical suites may need to consider having a variety of music for clients to choose from while awaiting surgery and will need an adequate number of listening devices to accommodate their usual number of cases per day. Hospitals could assess their physical environment and their inpatient routines to determine how they might be able to provide music intervention to their preoperative clients.

---

form and, if indicated, any other special consent forms to see that they are signed, dated, and contain the witnesses' signatures. Allergies should be noted according to facility policy. Accurate documentation of height and weight is important for proper dosage calculation of the anesthetic agents. The results of all laboratory, radiographic, and diagnostic tests should be on the chart; any abnormal results are documented and reported to the physician and the anesthesiologist or anesthetist. If the client was an autologous blood donor or had directed blood donations made, those special slips must be included in the chart. The nurse records a current set of vital signs (within 1–2 hours of the scheduled surgery time) and documents any significant physical or psychosocial observations. The nurse reports special needs and concerns of the client to the surgical team. For example, the nurse advises the surgical team whether the client is a member of Jehovah's Witnesses and does not accept blood products or whether the client is hard of hearing and does not have his or her hearing aid. This information assists the surgical team in providing continuity of care while the client is in the surgical area.

➤ *Preoperative Client Preparation*

Facilities generally require that the client remove most clothing and wear a hospital gown into the operating room. Underwear may be permitted for surgery above the waist; socks may be worn, except for foot or leg surgery. If ordered by the surgeon, antiembolism stockings are applied preoperatively.

The client's valuables, including jewelry, money, and clothes, are locked in a safe place, according to the facility's policy. The nurse tapes in place rings that cannot be removed. Religious emblems may be pinned or fastened securely to the client's gown; in some facilities, paper emblems are available from a religious leader.

The client wears an identification band that clearly gives first and last names and hospital number. A bracelet designating that a blood sample for type and crossmatch has been drawn may be worn, depending on the facility's policy.

Dentures, including partial dental plates, are removed and placed in a labeled denture cup. The removal of dentures is a safety measure to prevent aspiration and obstruction of the airway. If a client has any capped teeth, the nurse documents this finding on the preoperative checklist.

All prosthetic devices, such as artificial eyes and limbs, are removed and safely stored, as are contact lenses, wigs, and toupees. The nurse checks for hairpins and clips, which, if not removed, can conduct electrical current used during surgery and cause scalp burns.

Some facilities allow hearing aids in the surgical suite to facilitate communication before and after surgery. If the client is sent to surgery with a hearing aid, the nurse communicates this to the surgical nurse to prevent accidental loss of or damage to the aid. Some facilities allow dentures, wigs, glasses, and so on to be worn by the client into the operating suite to prevent embarrassment to the client. These items can then be removed when absolutely necessary.

The removal of fingernail polish or artificial nails is controversial. Polish is flammable, and artificial nails may affect the accuracy of pulse oximetry readings. In some facilities, at least one artificial nail must be removed for this reason.

After the client is prepared for surgery and the operating suite is ready to receive the client, the nurse asks the client to empty his or her bladder to prevent incontinence or overdistention and to provide a starting point for intake and output measurement. An overly full bladder may hinder access to the surgical site. The nurse answers any final questions the client has, offers reassurance as needed, and administers any ordered preoperative medication.

➤ *Preoperative Medications*

Preoperative medication may be ordered for clients, regardless of the type of planned anesthesia. Various preoperative medications reduce anxiety, promote relaxation, reduce pharyngeal secretions, prevent laryngospasm, inhibit gastric secretions, and decrease the amount of anesthetic required for the induction and maintenance of anesthesia. The selection of medication is based on the client's age, physical and psychological condition, medical history, and height and weight; the medications that the client takes routinely; the results of preoperative tests; and the type and extensiveness of the surgical procedure. If more than one pharmacologic response is required, combination therapy is usually ordered. A typical combination consists of a sedative or tranquilizer, an opioid analgesic, and an anticholinergic agent.

The preoperative medication is often ordered when the client is "on call" to the surgical suite. After the nurse positively identifies the client (using the arm band) and makes sure the operative permit is signed, he or she administers the correct medication. Then the nurse raises the side rails, places the call system within easy reach of the client while reminding him or her not to try to get out of bed, and places the bed in a low position. The nurse tells the client that he or she may become drowsy and have a dry mouth owing to the medication.

An increasingly common practice is for the premedication to be given *after* the client is transferred to the operating area. This practice permits the operating and anesthesia personnel to make more accurate assessments and have last-minute discussions with a client not yet affected by medication. In addition, after the client is in the operating area, medications can be given via the IV route. The oral (PO) or intramuscular (IM) route is less desirable because of unpredictable absorption rates.

➤ *Client Transfer to the Surgical Suite*

In the immediate preoperative preparation, the nurse reviews and updates the client's chart, reinforces preoperative teaching, ensures that the client is appropriately dressed for surgery, and administers preoperative medication, if ordered. The nurse uses a preoperative checklist to assist in the smooth, efficient transfer of the client to the surgical suite (Fig. 20–5). The client, along with the signed consent form, the completed preoperative checklist, the chart, and the addressograph plate, is transported to the surgical suite.

Most clients in the hospital setting are transferred to the surgical suite on a stretcher with the side rails up. In special circumstances (e.g., clients requiring traction, those having orthopedic surgery, and those who should be moved as little as possible immediately after surgery), the client is transferred in his or her hospital bed. Other factors that influence the nurse's decision to transfer the client in a bed are the client's age, size, and physical condition.

▲ Evaluation

The nurse evaluates the care of the preoperative client according to the identified nursing diagnoses. The outcomes for the client in the preoperative phase of the perioperative experience include that the client

- States that he or she understands informed consent as it applies to surgery
- Complies with the nothing by mouth requirement before surgery

NORTHWEST HOSPITAL CENTER
PRE-OPERATIVE CHECKLIST

Date of Surgery_____

Addressograph Plate

ALLERGIES

CLINICAL DATA:	YES	NO	COMMENTS
Authorization for Surgical Treatment Completed			
Height & Weight Charted			
History and Physical			
Chest X-Ray			
EKG Report			
Urine Report			
Blood Sugar Within Range of (75-250mg%)			
Hematocrit Within Range of (27-55%)			
Potassium Within Range of (3.2-5.5mEq/L)			
Results Out of Range Reported to Dept. of Anesthesia			
Anesthesiologist	Time:		By:
PATIENT PREPARATION:	**YES**	**NO**	**COMMENTS**
Jewelry Removed			
Hair Piece, Wig, Hairpin, Barrettes, Beads, Rubberbands Removed			
Loose Teeth or Caps Noted			
Dentures Removed			
Artificial Eye, Contact Lenses, Glasses Removed			
Any Prosthetic Appliance Removed			
Voided or Catheterized - I&O Sheet on Chart			
Identification Bracelet in Place			
Parenteral Fluids Patent & Infusing at cc/hr			
B/P, T.P.R. Charted			
Premedication Given As Ordered			
Side Rails Up-Pt. Care Data & Care Plan on Chart			
Is Patient on Isolation - If Yes, What Type			
COMMUNICATION ASSESSMENT:	**Normal**	**Abnormal**	**COMMENTS**
Vision			
Hearing			
Mental			
Speech			
Other			
Patient's Preferred Name:			
Limb For Burial ☐ Yes ☐ No Funeral Home:			

R.N. Completing Checklist

Figure 20–5. A preoperative checklist. (Courtesy of Northwest Hospital Center, Randallstown, MD.)

- Verbalizes an understanding of and the reason for a bowel preparation, if applicable
- States the purpose of the skin preparation
- Verbalizes an understanding of how tubes, drains, and IV lines and catheters may be used during and after surgery
- Demonstrates postoperative exercises: turning, deep breathing, splinting, coughing, and performing specific leg exercises
- Demonstrates the use of an incentive spirometer
- States that preoperative anxiety is lessened after preoperative teaching

CASE STUDY For the Preoperative Client

■ Mrs. James, a 68-year-old diabetic woman, is scheduled for a left below-the-knee amputation. You get a report from the off-going nurse who tells you that her preoperative checklist is completed. Three hours later, the operating room calls for Mrs. James. You have her void, take and record a set of vital signs, note that no premedication is ordered, and send her to the operating suite. Five minutes later, an angry holding room nurse calls you and says, "You sent this patient to the operating suite without a signed consent, without an armband, and with her wedding ring on!"

QUESTIONS:

1. How should you respond to the holding room nurse?
2. The holding room nurse continues to be quite angry for this situation, causing delays within the operating room and blames you personally— even threatens to report you to your supervisor. On what should your response focus?
3. How could you prevent this situation from reoccurring?

SELECTED BIBLIOGRAPHY

Augustin, P., & Haines, A. A. (1996). Effect of music on ambulatory surgery patients' preoperative anxiety. *AORN Journal, 63*(4), 750, 753–758.

Balcom, C. (1994). The new code of ethics: Implications for perioperative nurses. *Canadian Operating Room Nursing Journal, 12*(1), 6–8.

Blake, G. J. (1994). Administering prophylactic antibiotics before surgery: Consult this chart for the regime your patient will need. *Nursing94, 24*(12), 18.

Brick, J. (1996). OR nursing law. Informed consent and perioperative nursing. *AORN Journal, 63*(1), 258, 261.

Bright, L. D. (1994). How to protect your patient from DVT. *American Journal of Nursing, 94*(12), 28–32.

Brumfield, V. C., Kee, C. D., & Johnson, J. Y. (1997). Preoperative patient teaching in ambulatory surgery settings. *AORN Journal, 64*(6), 941, 943–946, 948, 951–952.

Burden, N. (1994). Patient and family education in the ambulatory surgery setting. *Seminars in Perioperative Nursing, 3*(3), 145–151.

*Caldwell, L. M. (1991). The influence of preference for information on preoperative stress and coping in surgical outpatients. *Applied Nursing Research 4*(4), 177–183.

Chalfin, D. B., et al. (1994). Preoperative evaluation and postoperative care of the elderly patient undergoing major surgery. *Clinics in Geriatric Medicine, 10*(1), 51–70.

Chapman, A. (1996). Current theory and practice: a study of preoperative fasting. *Nursing Standard, 10*(18), 33–36.

Chiarella, M. (1995). The consent form: Perils and possibilities. *Australian Confederation of Operating Room Nurses Journal, 8*(4), 21–22.

Chiarella, M. (1996). The consent form: Perils and possibilities—part 2. *Australian Confederation of Operating Room Nurses Journal, 9*(1), 29–30.

Cipperley, J. A., Butcher, L. A., & Hayes, J. E. (1995). Research utilization: The development of a preoperative teaching protocol. *MED-SURG Nursing, 4*(3), 199–206.

Cirina, C. L. (1994). Effects of sedative music on patient preoperative anxiety. *Today's OR Nurse, 16*(3), 15–18.

DeFazio-Quinn, D. M. (1997). Ambulatory surgery. *Nursing Clinics of North America, 32*(2), 375–488.

*Dellasega, C., & Burgunder, C. (1991). Perioperative nursing care for the elderly surgical patient. *Today's OR Nurse, 13*(6), 12–17, 30–31.

Diabetic patients require special care in same-day surgery. (1994). *Same-Day Surgery, 18*(3), 33–36.

*Drago, S. S. (1992). Banking on your own blood. *American Journal of Nursing, 92*(3), 61–64.

Droogan, J., et al. (1996). Pre-operative patient instruction: Is it effective? *Nursing Standard, 10*(35), 32–33.

Etchason, J., Petz, L., Keeler, E., et al. (1995). The cost effectiveness of preoperative autologous blood donations. *New England Journal of Medicine, 332*(11), 719–724.

Evans, M. M., et al. (1994). Music: A diversionary therapy. *Today's OR Nurse, 16*(4), 17–22.

*Friedman, S. B., Fitzpatrick, S., & Badere, B. (1992). The effects of television viewing on preoperative anxiety. *Journal of Post Anesthesia Nursing, 7*(4), 243–250.

*Gaberson, K. B. (1991). The effect of humorous and musical distraction on preoperative anxiety. *AORN Journal, 62*(5), 784–788+.

Giordano, B. P. (1996). Clinical exemplars demonstrate perioperative nurses' courage and commitment to quality patient care. *AORN Journal, 63*(1), 15, 18.

Giordano, B. P. (1996). Ensuring the readability of patient education materials is one way to demonstrate perioperative nurses' value. *AORN Journal, 63*(4), 699–700.

Green, D. (1995). Patient assessment for surgery. *British Journal of Theatre Nursing, 5*(1), 10–12.

Groves, H. (1994). Preoperative patient fasting regimes. *British Journal of Theatre Nursing, 4*(2), 14–16.

Hnatiuk, O. W., Dillard, I. A., & Torrington, K. G. (1995). Adherence to established guidelines for preoperative pulmonary function testing. *Chest, 107*(5), 1294–1297.

*Johnson, G. M., & Bowman, R. J. (1992). Autologous blood transfusion: Current trends, nursing implications. *AORN Journal, 56*(2), 281–285, 288–293, 296–298.

*Kapp, M. B. (1990). Informed, assisted, delegated consent for elderly patients. *AORN Journal, 52*(4), 857–862.

*Keene, A. (1991). Perioperative assessment and nursing implications for the elderly. *Plastic Surgical Nursing, 11*(4), 143–150, 163–167.

Kendrick, J. M., & Powers, P. H. (1994). Perioperative care of the pregnant surgical patient. *AORN Journal, 60*(2), 203–219.

*Leckrone, L. (1991). Preparing your patient for surgery. *Nursing91, 21*(7), 46–49.

*Leske, J. S. (1992). Practice-based perioperative research. *AORN Journal, 55*(2), 581–590.

*Litwak, K. (1991). What you need to know about administering preoperative medications. *Nursing91, 21*(8), 44–47.

Marshall, W. J. (1994). Perioperative nutritional support. *Care of the Critically Ill, 10*(4), 163–167.

Martin, D. (1996). Pre-operative visits to reduce patient anxiety: A study. *Nursing Standard, 10*(23), 33–38.

McGaughey, J., et al. (1994). Understanding the pre-operative information needs of patients and their relatives in intensive care units. *Intensive & Critical Care Nursing, 10*(3), 186–194.

Meckes, P. F. (1995). Geriatric surgery. In M. H. Meeker & J. C. Rothrock (Eds.), *Alexander's care of the patient in surgery* (10th ed., pp. 1195–1209). St. Louis: Mosby–Year Book.

Meeker, M. H., & Rothrock, J. C. (Eds.). (1995). *Alexander's care of the patient in surgery* (10th ed.). St. Louis: Mosby–Year Book.

*Moore, L. W., et al. (1993). Communicating effectively with elderly surgical patients. *AORN Journal, 58*(2), 345, 347, 349–350+.

Moran, S., et al. (1995). Quality indicators for patient information in short-stay units. *Nursing Times, 91*(4), 37–40.

Moss, V. A. (1994). Assessing learning abilities, readiness for education. *Seminars in Perioperative Nursing, 3*(3), 113–120.

Nash, C. A., & Jensen, P. L. (1994). When your surgical patient has hypertension. *American Journal of Nursing, 94*(12), 39–45.

Null, S. L. (1994). Preadmission testing: A coordinator can be the answer. *AORN Journal, 59*(5), 1051–1056, 1059–1060.

Oberle, K., Allen, M., & Lynkowski, P. (1994). Follow-up of same day surgery patients. *AORN Journal, 59*(5), 1016–1025.

*Oetker-Black, S. L., Hart, F., Hoffman, J., et al. (1992). Preoperative self-efficacy and postoperative behaviors. *Applied Nursing Research, 5*(3), 134–139.

*Persson, A. V., Davis, R. J., & Villavicencio, J. L. (1991). Deep vein thrombosis and pulmonary embolism. *Surgical Clinics of North America, 71*(6), 1195–1209.

*Peterson, K. J. (1992). Nursing management of autologous blood transfusion. *Journal of Intravenous Nursing, 15*(3), 128–134.

Planchock, N. Y., et al. (1994). Preoperative assessment and teaching: Physiological and psychological preparation. *Seminars in Perioperative Nursing, 3*(2), 61–69.

Proposed recommended practices for surgical skin preparation (1996). *AORN Journal, 63*(1), 221–224, 227.

Redmond, C. (1994). Postoperative instructions: Is your timing right? . . . postoperative instructions should be given prior to the day of surgery. *Breathline, 14*(3), 1, 8.

Salzbach, R. (1995). Presurgical testing improves patient care. *AORN Journal, 61*(1), 210–212, 215–216, 218.

Schwartz-Barcott, D., et al. (1994). Client-nurse interaction: Testing for its impact in preoperative instruction. *International Journal of Nursing Studies, 31*(1), 23–35.

SDS program streamlines pre-admit assessment . . . same-day surgery program (1995). *Same-Day Surgery, 19*(2), 18–20.

*Shea, S. I. (1992). Our patients face recovery with confidence. *RN, 55*(6), 17–18, 20.

Small, S. P. (1996). Preoperative hair removal: A case report with implications for nursing. *Journal of Clinical Nursing, 5*(2), 79–84.

Stewart, B. (1994). Teaching culturally diverse populations. *Seminars in Perioperative Nursing, 3*(3), 160–167.

Sutherland, R. (1994). Is this the way forward? . . . the role of the nurse in day surgery. *British Journal of Theatre Nursing, 4*(1), 12–13.

Swan, B. A. (1994). A collaborative ambulatory preoperative evaluation model: Implementation, implications, evaluation. *AORN Journal, 59*(2), 430–437.

Take a close look at pre-op visits: How much is too much? (1995). *Same-Day Surgery, 19*(2), 13–17.

Thomas, D. R., & Ritchie, C. (1995). Preoperative assessment of older adults. *Journal of the American Geriatrics Society, 43*(7), 811–821.

Tietz, N. W. (1995). *Clinical guide to laboratory tests* (3rd ed.). Philadelphia: W. B. Saunders.

Toy, P. T. C., & Kerr, K. (1996). Preoperative autologous blood donation. *AACN Clinical Issues: Advanced Practice in Acute and Critical Care, 7*(2), 221–228.

Vernon, S., & Pfeifer, G. M. (1997). Are you ready for bloodless surgery? *American Journal of Nursing, 97*(9), 40–47.

Watson, D. S., & Sangermano, C. A. (1995). Ambulatory surgery. In M. H. Meeker & J. C. Rothrock (Eds.), *Alexander's care of the patient in surgery* (10th ed., pp. 1125–1144). St. Louis: Mosby–Year Book.

Webb, R. A. (1995). Preoperative visiting from the perspective of the theatre nurse. *British Journal of Theatre Nursing, 4*(16), 919–925.

West, B. J. M., et al. (1995). Day surgery: Cheap option or challenge to care? *British Journal of Theatre Nursing, 5*(1), 5–8.

When the fast track isn't the best track (1995). *Same-Day Surgery, 19*(9), 104–105.

*Which presurgical tests are worthwhile? (1992). *Emergency Medicine, 24*(14), 88–90.

Wicker, P. (1995). Pre-operative visiting—making it work. *British Journal of Theatre Nursing, 5*(7), 16–19.

Young, R., et al. (1994). Effect of preadmission brochures on surgical patients' behavioral outcomes. *AORN Journal, 60*(2), 232–236, 239–241.

SUGGESTED READINGS

Brick, J. (1996). OR nursing law. Informed consent and perioperative nursing. *AORN Journal, 63*(1), 258, 261.

This two-page article gives a brief but informative review of battery and negligence as may arise from lack of consent. Specific examples involving nurses are included. Consent terminology, such as implied consent and informed consent, is explained.

Bright, L. D. (1994). How to protect your patient from DVT. *American Journal of Nursing, 94*(12), 28–32.

This easy-to-read article first identifies risk factors for deep vein thrombosis and then discusses interventions for the low-, medium-, and high-risk patient. The article reviews the physiologic principles of graduated compression stockings, how to apply them, and what complications to assess for. In discussing pneumatic compression devices, the authors differentiate the intermittent from the sequential device and provide much nursing detail, including cost factors.

Cipperley, J. A., Butcher, L. A., & Hayes, J. E. (1995). Research utilization: The development of a preoperative teaching protocol. *MEDSURG Nursing, 4*(3), 199–206.

These authors wanted to develop a preoperative teaching tool that would enhance patient outcomes; e.g., reduced pain, complications and length of stay. First they describe findings from their literature search, which focused on preoperative instruction in two main areas: educational content and instructional methods. Then a protocol was developed, which includes content in the procedural, behavioral, and sensory domains. The authors explain that after the nurse assesses the client's level of fear and anxiety, a pathway is decided on for teaching. Both the protocol and a surgical teaching flow sheet are reprinted in the article.

INTERVENTIONS FOR INTRAOPERATIVE CLIENTS

As the client enters the surgical suite, the intraoperative phase of the perioperative experience begins. This is an anxious time for the client, as he or she enters into unfamiliar experiences involving unknown outcomes. Nursing care during the intraoperative period addresses all of the client's physical needs, as well as his or her comfort, safety, dignity, and psychological status. Specific procedures and policies may differ among agencies, but similarities are evident and reflect the standards and recommended practices for perioperative nursing, as published by the Association of Operating Room Nurses.

OVERVIEW
Members of the Surgical Team

The surgical team consists of the surgeon, one or more surgical assistants, the anesthesiologist and/or nurse anesthetist, and operating room nurses.

Operating room nurses include the holding area nurse, circulating nurse, scrub nurse, and any specialty nurses. The number of assistants, circulating nurses, and scrub nurses depends on the complexity and projected length of the surgical procedure. For some minor diagnostic or outpatient procedures, only a scrub nurse or a circulating nurse may be required in addition to the surgeon.

Surgeon and Surgical Assistant

The surgeon is a physician who assumes responsibility for the surgical procedure and any surgical judgments about the client. The surgical assistant might be another surgeon (or physician, such as a resident or intern) or a physician's assistant, nurse, or surgical technologist. Under the direction of the surgeon, the assistant may hold retractors, suction the wound (to allow visualization of the operative site), cut tissue, suture, and dress wounds. Regulating agencies determine who may qualify to be a surgical assistant and usually delineate the functions of the surgical assistant.

Anesthesiologist and Nurse Anesthetist

The anesthesiologist is a physician who specializes in the administration of anesthetic agents. A certified registered

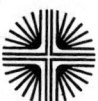

Our Lady of Lourdes Medical Center
1600 Haddon Avenue Camden, N.J. 08103

PRE-OPERATIVE RECORD

PRE-OPERATIVE

Patient Name _____ Surgeon _____ Date _____

Procedure _____

Arrival _____ **ID** ☐ Verbal ☐ Nameband **Pt Verbalizes** ☐ Procedure Site ☐ Surgeon **NPO** Since _____

Allergies: ☐ NDA ☐ Latex ☐ Other _____ ☐ Drugs _____

Lab Data: ☐ CBC   Reports: Consents: Blood Products - # of units
    ☐ Urinalysis   ☐ EKG   ☐ Surgical   In OR _____
    ☐ Chemistry   ☐ Chest   ☐ Blood   Blood Bank _____   ☐ Autologus _____
    ☐ Coag Studies   ☐ H & P   ☐ Anesthesia   ☐ Type and Screen _____ ☐ Directed _____
    _____ ☐ Pregnancy Test   ☐ Other   ☐ Type and Cross _____ ☐ Homologus _____

Equipment: ☐ IV's ☐ Foley ☐ Ventilator ☐ Cardiac Monitor ☐ IABP ☐ Other _____
Prosthesis: ☐ None ☐ Opthalmic ☐ Otic ☐ Dental ☐ Jewelry   Disposition of Prosthesis _____
Orientation: ☐ Awake ☐ Oriented ☐ Sedated ☐ Confused ☐ Agitated ☐ Crying

Implants / Other Comments:_____

_____ RN SIGNATURE _____

INTRA OPERATIVE

Identification: ☐ Verbal ☐ Nameband   Scrub Nurse: ☐ Sees Permits ☐ Aware of Allergies

Skin Condition: ☐ Intact ☐ Presence of Lesions - Type / Location _____

Skin Prep: ☐ Betadine ☐ Hibiclens ☐ Other _____

Position: ☐ Supine ☐ Prone ☐ Lithotomy ☐ Lateral ☐ Jackknife ☐ Fracture Table
    ☐ Other _____ Positioned by _____

Equipment Codes: **Supports:**
= - Safety Strap applied by _____ ☐ Kidney Rest _____
X - Grounding Pad applied by _____ ☐ Stirrups _____
T - Tourniquet applied by _____ ☐ Arms @ Side _____
Δ - Pressure Pads applied by _____ ☐ Arms on Armboard _____
S - Sandbag applied by _____ ☐ Action Pads _____
R - Roll applied by _____ ☐ Black Leg Positioner _____
A - Action Donut applied by _____ ☐ Bean Bag _____
Z - Zoll Defib Pad applied by _____

Tourniquet Unit # _____ mm/Hg _____ Inflated _____ Deflated _____

Warming Blanket Unit # _____ Temp _____ On _____ Off _____

Electrocautery Unit # _____ Coag @ _____ Cut @ _____

Pad # _____ Exp. Date _____ ESU Pad Skin Site _____

Defibrillator # _____ Time / Joules _____

BiPolar Unit # _____ Setting _____ Other Equipment _____

Comments _____

_____ RN SIGNATURE _____

FORM #PO1 (REV. 4/96)

Figure 21–1. A perioperative nursing record with areas for charting preoperatively upon the client's arrival in the operating room (OR) suite and upon initial preparation intraoperatively. (Courtesy of Our Lady of Lourdes Medical Center, Camden, NJ.)

nurse anesthetist (CRNA) is a specially trained registered nurse with additional credentials who administers anesthetics under the supervision of an anesthesiologist, surgeon, dentist, or podiatrist. The anesthesiologist or CRNA administers anesthetic drugs to induce and maintain anesthesia and administers other medications as indicated to support the client's physical status during surgery.

The anesthesiologist or nurse anesthetist usually monitors the client intraoperatively by measuring, assessing, and monitoring the following:

- The level of anesthesia (i.e., by using a peripheral nerve stimulator)
- Cardiopulmonary function (via electrocardiographic [ECG] monitoring, pulse oximetry, end-tidal CO_2 monitoring, arterial blood gases, and hemodynamic monitoring via arterial lines and/or pulmonary artery catheters)
- Vital signs
- Intake and output

Depending on the client's needs, anesthesia personnel administer intravenous (IV) fluids, including blood and blood components, to maintain the client's physiologic homeostasis.

(See Units 3, 6, and 7 for further discussion on fluid balance and acid-base balance; oxygenation; and cardiac monitoring, assessment, and function.)

Operating Room Nurses

Operating room (OR) nurses assume several roles within the operating suite, depending on their education, experience, skill, and job responsibilities.

HOLDING AREA NURSE. Some operating suites feature a presurgical holding area adjacent to the main ORs. The client waits in this area until the OR is ready. The holding room nurse manages the client's care while the client is in this area. This nurse greets the client on arrival, reviews the chart and preoperative checklist, and ensures the operative consent forms are signed. The nurse assesses the client's physical and emotional status, lends emotional support, answers questions, and provides additional education as needed. The nurse initiates documentation on a perioperative nursing record (Fig. 21–1).

The holding area can be very busy, with many staff members performing a number of preoperative procedures (e.g., establishing IV lines or inserting nasogastric tubes). The holding area nurse maintains an atmosphere conducive to the client's overall well-being and intervenes on behalf of the client to maintain comfort, privacy, and confidentiality.

CIRCULATING NURSE. The circulating nurse (who must be a registered nurse) coordinates, oversees, and participates in the client's nursing care while the client is in the OR. The circulating nurse's actions are vital to the smooth flow of events before, during, and after the operation. The circulator sets up the OR, ensures that necessary supplies and equipment are readily available, and checks that all equipment is safe and functional before the surgery. The circulating nurse makes the operating bed (formerly called the OR table) with gel pads (to prevent pressure sores) and heating pads (to prevent hypothermia) under the sheets as indicated.

If there is no holding room nurse, the circulator assumes the responsibilities of that nursing role as well. Even when there is a holding room nurse, the circulator also greets the client and reviews findings with the holding area nurse because the circulator is responsible for continuity of client care.

Once the client is ready to move into the OR, the circulating nurse assists the OR team in transferring the client onto the operating bed. The nurse then positions the client, protecting bony prominences with extra padding as indicated while comforting and reassuring the client. The circulating nurse also assists the anesthesiologist or CRNA with the induction of anesthesia and then may "prep" (scrub) the surgical site before the client is draped with sterile drapes.

Throughout the surgery, the circulating nurse

- Monitors traffic in the room
- Assesses the amount of urine and blood loss
- Reports findings to the surgeon and anesthesia personnel
- Ensures that the surgical team maintains sterile technique and a sterile field
- Documents care, events, interventions and findings

Depending on facility policy, the circulating nurse may obtain and record medications, blood, and blood components. (This may partially be a function of anesthesia personnel.) Before the surgical procedure is over, the circulating nurse completes documentation (Fig. 21–2; see also Fig. 21–1). The nurse notes drains or catheters in place, length of surgery, and a count of all sponges, "sharps" (needles, blades), and instruments. The nurse notifies the postanesthesia care unit (PACU) of the client's estimated time of arrival and any special needs of the client.

SCRUB NURSE AND SURGICAL TECHNOLOGIST. The scrub nurse sets up the sterile field (Fig. 21–3), assists with draping the client, and hands sterile supplies and instruments to the surgeon and the assistant. Knowledge of anatomy and physiology and familiarity with the surgical procedure allow the scrub nurse to anticipate which instruments and types of sutures the surgeon will need; the nurse's ability to anticipate these needs reduces the duration of anesthesia for the client. Throughout the surgical procedure, the scrub nurse (with the circulating nurse) maintains an accurate account of sponges, sharps, and instruments and the amounts of irrigation fluid used.

The scrub role may be performed by a specially trained person who is not a nurse. Such people are called operating room technicians (ORTs) or surgical technologists. (The term *CST* may be used for those who are certified surgical technologists.)

SPECIALTY NURSES. The specialty coordinator nurse is educated in a particular type of surgery (e.g., orthopedic, cardiac, ophthalmologic) and is responsible for intraoperative nursing care specific to clients needing that type of surgery. The specialty coordinator nurse also cares for and maintains equipment and instruments used in the specialty and maintains needed supplies. During surgery, the specialty nurse may function as the scrub or circulating nurse.

If the facility has laser technology, nurses specially trained in the use, care, and maintenance of the laser should be on hand. Such a nurse may be called a laser specialty nurse or a laser nurse coordinator. *Laser* is an

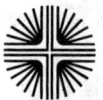

Our Lady of Lourdes Medical Center
1600 Haddon Avenue Camden, N.J. 08103

INTRA-OPERATIVE RECORD

Patient Name _____ Date _____ Suite _____

☐ Scheduled ☐ Emergency ☐ Add On   In Room _____ Began _____ End _____ Out_____

Surgeon _____ Assistant _____

Anesthesia _____ Perfusion/Other _____

Type of Anesthesia: ☐ General   ☐ Spinal   ☐ Epidural   ☐ Regional Block   ☐ Local ASB   ☐ Local

Scrub _____ Circulator _____

Relief _____ Relief _____

Preoperative Diagnosis _____
_____

Postoperative Diagnosis _____
_____

Procedure _____
_____
_____

Clamp/Bypass on _____ off_____   EBL _____

Specimens: Cultures ☐ **Aerobic** ☐ **Anerobic** _____   Implant Log# _____
_____   **Irrigation:** _____
_____   Wound Classification:
_____   Pre-Op   I   II   III   IV
_____   Post-Op   I   II   III   IV
                                                          ASA Classification   I   II   III   IV

Medication Dispensed to OR Table (Include time, drug, amt used, site/route should be prepared by and given by)
_____
_____
_____
_____
_____
_____
_____

Counts: ☐ Correct _____ ☐ Incorrect _____ Comments: _____
_____

Intra operative X-ray   ☐ Yes   ☐ No   Type _____

Drains / Packing: ☐ None ☐ Foley   Inserted by _____ ☐ Immediate urine output
☐ Jackson Pratt / Davol _____ ☐ Hemovac_____ ☐ Penrose _____ ☐ Packing _____ Other _____
☐ Chest Tubes # and size _____ ☐ Pleuravac ☐ Auto transfusion pleuravac

Post Op Skin Condition:_____

ESU Pad Skin Site _____ Dressing Site _____

Receiving Unit ☐ PACU ☐ CVU ☐ ICU / CCU ☐ SDS ☐ Nursing Unit _____ Report given to _____

RN Signature _____ Surgeon Signature _____

FORM #PO2 (REV. 7/96)   White - Original Copy   Yellow - O.R. Copy   Pink - Surgeon Copy   Goldenrod - Pharmacy Copy

Figure 21–2. An interdisciplinary intra-operative record. Names of all personnel involved are listed, and both the circulating nurse's and surgeon's signatures are required for completion. (Courtesy of Our Lady of Lourdes Medical Center, Camden, NJ.)

acronym for light amplification by the stimulated emission of radiation. A laser emits a high-powered beam of light that cuts tissue more cleanly than scalpel blades do. This process produces intense heat for rapid coagulation of blood vessels or tissue and can turn tissue (such as a tumor) into vapor. It is essential for all personnel to observe safety measures (e.g., eye shields, door signs) during laser procedures.

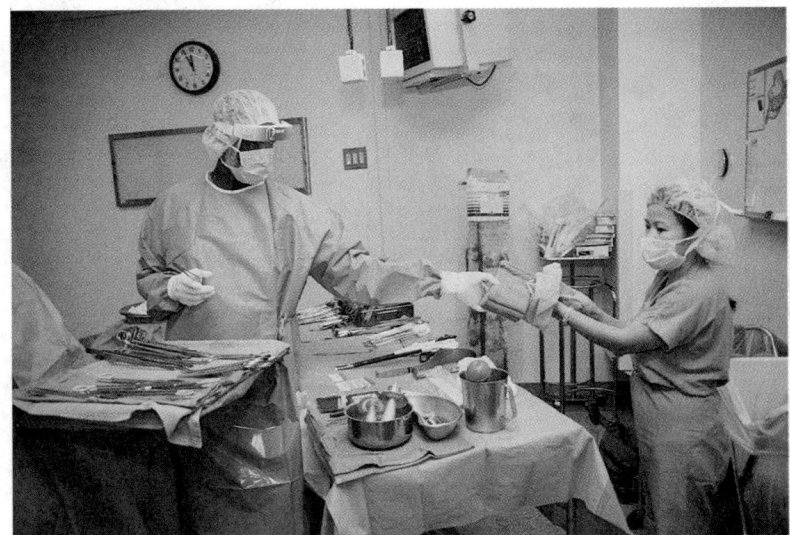

Figure 21–3. Setting up the sterile table.

Preparation of the Surgical Suite and Team Safety

During the intraoperative phase, safety of the client is a primary concern of all members of the surgical team. The operating room (OR) layout is designed to prevent infection by limiting the source of contaminants. The staff uses safety straps for the client and securely locks the operating bed in place. Heating pads are used to prevent hypothermia, and interventions are instituted to prevent skin breakdown.

The nurse ensures electrical safety through proper placement of grounding pads and use of electrical equipment that meets safety standards. All equipment that might be used during surgery must be appropriately cleaned and sterilized and in proper working condition. The nurse ensures a correct count of surgical instruments and sponges before, during, and after surgery.

Fire prevention is of utmost concern to OR personnel, as is prevention of complications associated with the use of hazardous and potentially toxic substances. A cool room temperature and low humidity are optimal, and staff and clients must be protected against thermal or chemical burns caused by fire or spills. The nurse is aware of appropriate emergency measures to take in the event of a fire or spill.

Layout

The surgical suite should be located out of the mainstream of the hospital or facility and adjacent to the postanesthesia unit (PACU) and support services (e.g., blood bank, pathology and laboratory departments). Traffic flow should be such that contamination from outside the suite is minimal. Within the suite, clean and contaminated areas must be separate. Traffic flow is controlled by designating areas as unrestricted, semirestricted, and restricted.

The size of a surgical suite depends on the size and surgical capabilities of the facility. The average suite contains staff changing rooms (staff locker rooms) and staff lounges, an admission (or preoperative holding) area, a scrub area (for staff), a number of ORs, designated cabinets for sterile supplies, separate utility rooms for clean and soiled equipment, and a clean linen room.

Figure 21–4 shows a typical OR. The exact number of tables and specialized equipment used in the room is based on the needs of each client. A reliable communication system provides the vital link between the OR and the main desk of the surgical unit or suite. The system should include an intercom and the capability to differentiate between routine and emergency calls.

Health and Hygiene of the Surgical Team

Everyone has a large number of potentially pathogenic bacteria on the skin and hair and in the respiratory tract. Because these pathogens can be transmitted to the client, special health requirements and dress are required. Health standards require that all members of the surgical team and other support personnel in the surgical suite be free from communicable diseases. Anyone who has an open wound, cold, or other infection should not participate in surgery.

Good personal hygiene aids in the control of infection, as does frequent and appropriate hand washing. Shedding of microorganisms and skin debris is greatest immediately after showering, so surgical staff should bathe a few hours before changing into OR attire. Jewelry, which can carry multiple microorganisms, should be minimal.

In preparing for surgery, all personnel must wash their hands between procedures and more frequently when indicated. Specimens from the hands of surgical personnel may be obtained for culture periodically to maintain an awareness of the potential for nosocomial (hospital-acquired) infections and to identify the source of pathogenic invasion. Further interventions or cultures are necessary if quality reports (e.g., through the Quality Improvement Program or Quality Reviews) indicate a problem. The average time between routine cultures is 3 to 6 months. Surgical attire and the surgical scrub are additional interventions that help to prevent contaminations.

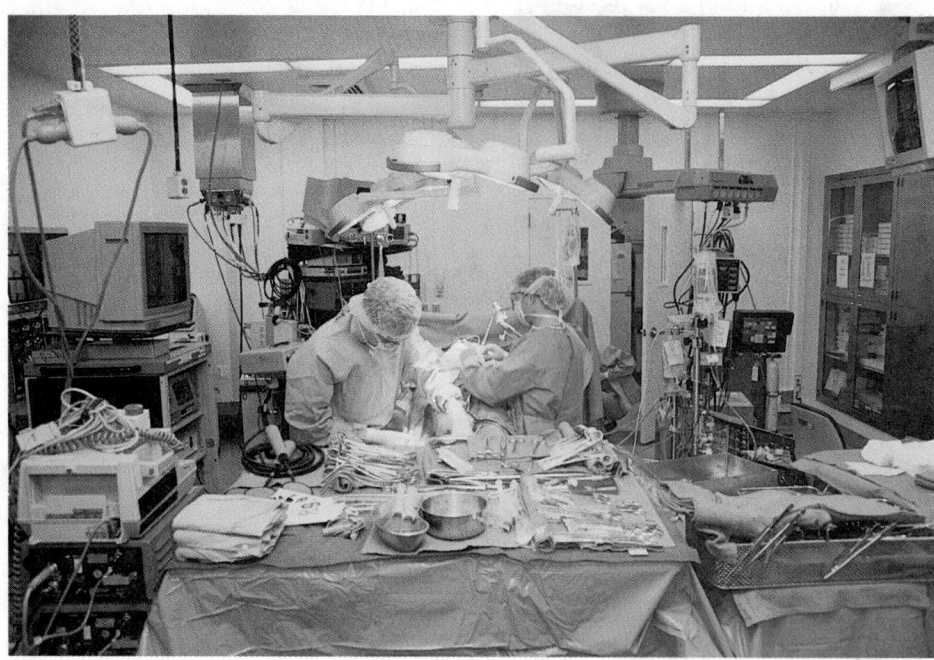

A

Figure 21–4. *A,* A typical operating room. *B,* A typical anesthesia station with an anesthesia machine.

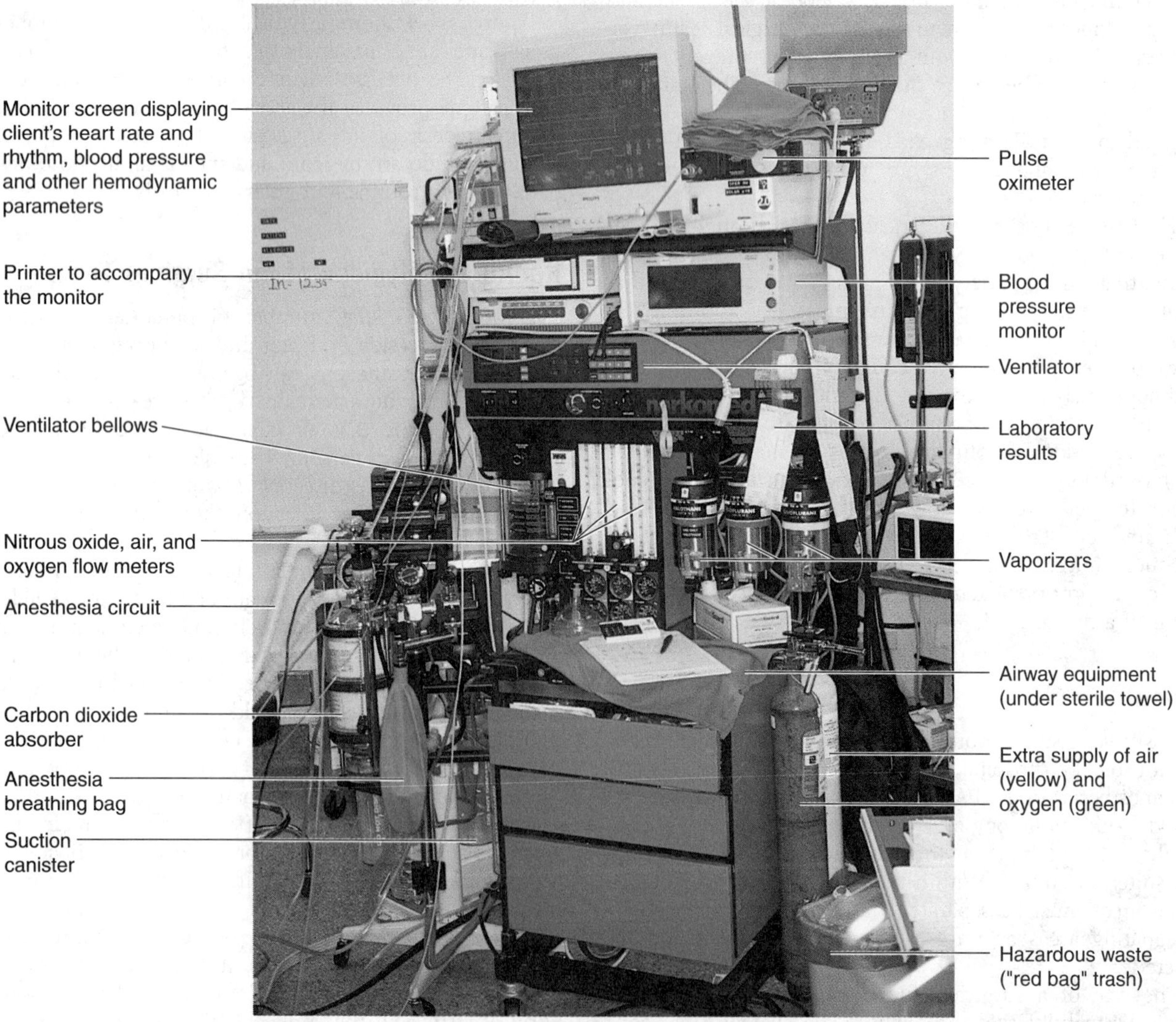

Monitor screen displaying client's heart rate and rhythm, blood pressure and other hemodynamic parameters

Printer to accompany the monitor

Ventilator bellows

Nitrous oxide, air, and oxygen flow meters

Anesthesia circuit

Carbon dioxide absorber

Anesthesia breathing bag

Suction canister

Pulse oximeter

Blood pressure monitor

Ventilator

Laboratory results

Vaporizers

Airway equipment (under sterile towel)

Extra supply of air (yellow) and oxygen (green)

Hazardous waste ("red bag" trash)

B

Surgical Attire

All members of the surgical team and all OR personnel must wear scrub attire. Scrub attire is clean, not sterile. It is worn to decrease contamination from microorganisms. As one enters the operating *suite,* the basic attire consists of a shirt and pants, a cap or hood (Fig. 21–5), and shoe coverings. Staff change into clean surgical attire in the operating suite locker rooms, not at home. All members of the surgical team must cover their hair.

In addition to basic attire, anyone who enters an OR must wear a mask. Members of the surgical team who are scrubbed to be at the bedside of the client during the surgical procedure must also be in a sterile gown, with sterile gloves and eye protectors (Fig. 21–6). Members of the surgical team in the OR who are *not* scrubbed (e.g., anesthesiologist and circulating nurse) usually wear cover scrub jackets to prevent shedding of organisms from bare arms.

Surgical Scrub

The surgeon, all assistants, and the scrub nurse perform the surgical scrub after putting on a mask and before putting on the sterile gown and gloves (Fig. 21–7). The scrub does not make the hands and forearms sterile; however, when it is effectively carried out, it reduces the number of microorganisms.

A disposable scrub brush or sponge, impregnated with an antimicrobial solution, and a nail cleaner are used. As with hand washing, the effectiveness of the scrub depends on the application of friction from the fingertips to the elbow. The surgical scrub usually continues for 3 to 5 minutes (see Research Applications for Nursing), followed by a rinse. During the rinse, surgical personnel position their hands and arms in such a way that water runs off, rather than up or down, their arms. After scrubbing,

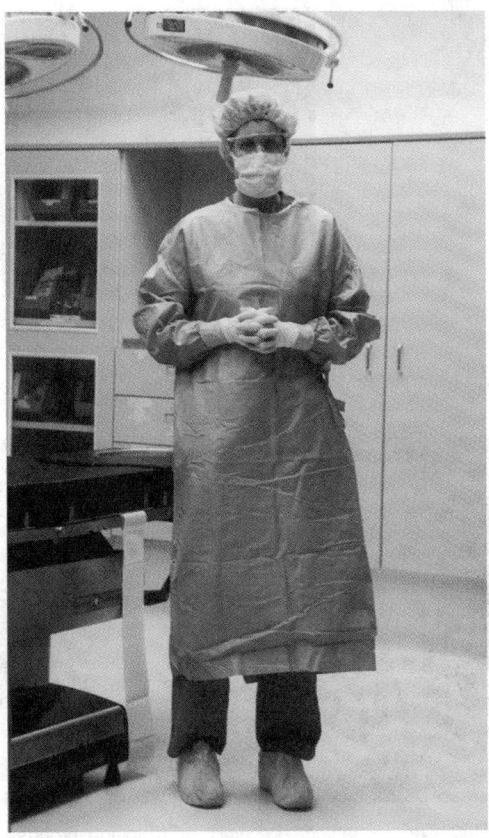

Figure 21–6. Typical attire for all scrubbed personnel. Note complete hair covering, eye shields, mask, sterile gloves over the sleeves of the sterile gown, and shoe coverings. Note that when not in use, the hands are typically folded in front of the body, never below the waist.

personnel enter the OR with their hands held higher than the elbows and thoroughly dry their hands and forearms with a sterile towel. After drying, the scrubbed staff member is assisted into a sterile gown ("gowning") and puts on sterile gloves ("gloving").

Gowns, gloves, and materials used at the operative field must be sterile and are changed between surgical procedures. The areas of the surgical gown considered sterile are the front of the gown from 2 inches below the neck to the waist area, and the elbow to wrist area. Only when they are properly scrubbed and attired should members of the surgical team handle sterile drapes and other equipment.

Anesthesia

The word *anesthesia* comes from the Greek word *anesthesis,* meaning "negative sensation." Administration of anesthesia is an exact and sophisticated science requiring the skill of a licensed anesthesiologist or a certified registered nurse anesthetist (CRNA).

Anesthesia is an artificially induced state of partial or total loss of sensation, occurring with or without loss of consciousness. The purpose of anesthesia is to block the transmission of nerve impulses, suppress reflexes, promote muscular relaxation, and, in some cases, achieve a

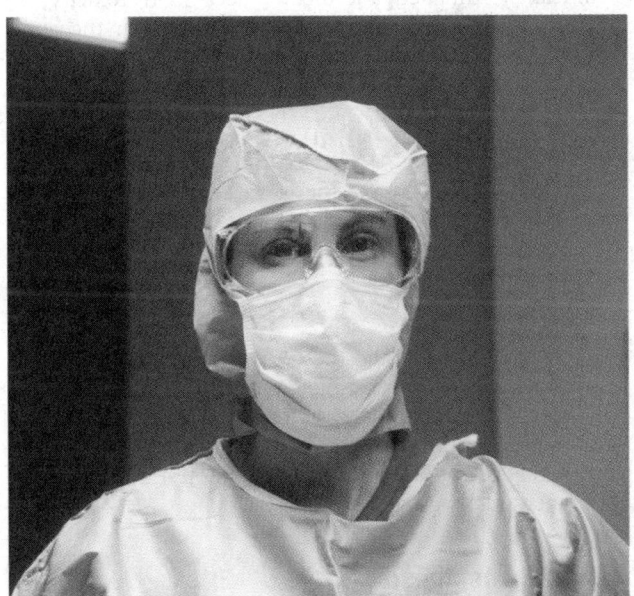

Figure 21–5. An example of a hood-type hair covering that adequately covers facial and scalp hair.

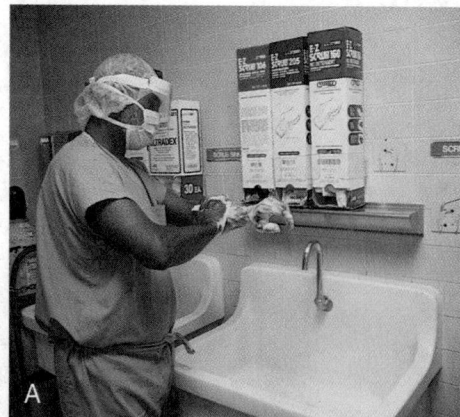
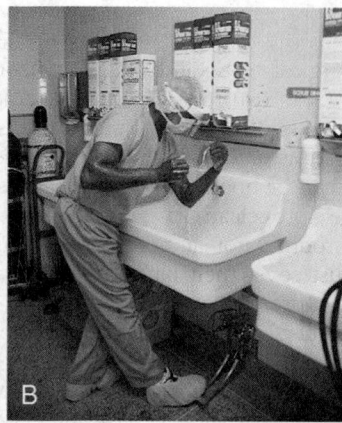
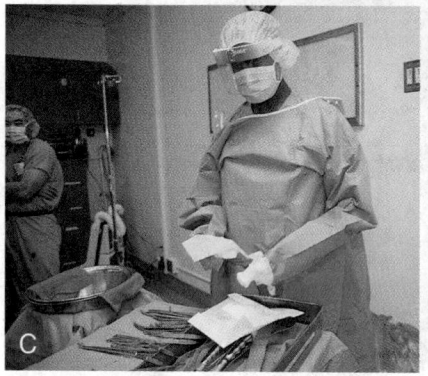
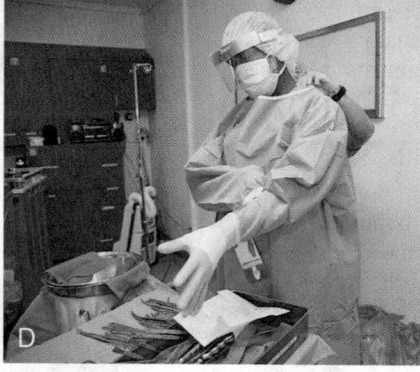
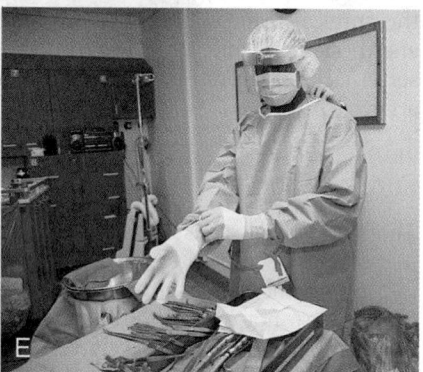

Figure 21–7. The scrubbing, gowning, and gloving process. *A*, The surgical scrub. *B*, Rinsing. Note the water falling off the hands and arms. Also note the foot-operated handle that controls the water flow. (After scrubbing and rinsing, the scrub nurse dries his hands and arms with a sterile towel inside the operating room, then is assisted into a sterile gown.) *C*, The scrub nurse prepares sterile gloves. Note that the scrub nurse's hands are *inside* the sleeve of the gown and that he is touching the sterile gloves only with the sterile sleeve. *D*, The scrub nurse puts on his first sterile glove while the sterile gown is being tied in the back. Note again that his hand never emerges from under the sterile sleeve. *E*, The scrub nurse puts on his second sterile glove.

controlled level of unconsciousness. Anesthesia personnel use a separate anesthesia record for documentation (Fig. 21–8).

The choice of anesthesia is determined primarily by the anesthesiologist or CRNA after consultation with the surgeon and consideration of specific client-related factors. The nurse or client or both communicate the client's preference and fears related to a particular type of anesthesia to the anesthesiologist or CRNA. Specific problems noted in the client's history or preoperative physical examination are major factors in the selection and dosage of anesthesia. Selection is also influenced by the following factors:

- Type and duration of the procedure
- Area of body being operated on
- Whether the procedure is an emergency
- How long it has been since the client ate
- The client position indicated for the surgical procedure

The administration of anesthesia begins with the selection and administration of preoperative medication, if any (see Chap. 20).

The nurse should know the pharmacologic characteristics of commonly used agents and their effects on the client during and after surgery. Anesthesia produces multiple systemic effects, which can affect the client's care

and can compound other coexisting problems. For example, most anesthetics are metabolized by the liver and excreted by the kidneys. Hepatic or renal dysfunction can significantly enhance anesthetic effects and toxicity. In addition, drug interactions may occur between the anesthetic agents and other medications the client has been receiving.

The state of anesthesia may be produced in a number of ways (Table 21–1):

- General or balanced anesthesia
- Local or regional anesthesia
- Hypnosis or hypnoanesthesia
- Cryothermia
- Acupuncture

Hypnosis or hypnoanesthesia (which induces a passive trance-like state), cryothermia (use of cold—for example, with ice—to lower the surface temperature of the surgical site), and acupuncture are not commonly used in the United States or Canada. However, interest in the use of these methods is growing.

General Anesthesia

General anesthesia is a reversible state in which the client loses consciousness as a result of the inhibition of neuro-

Research Applications for Nursing

A 2-Minute Scrub May Be as Effective as a 3-Minute Scrub

Wheelock, S. M., & Lookinland, S. (1997). Effect of surgical hand scrub time on subsequent bacterial growth. AORN Journal, 65(6), 1087–1090, 1092, 1094–1098.

The researchers note that the effectiveness of the surgical hand scrub, which is supposed to reduce surgical wound infections, has not been confirmed by study. They review the history of handwashing and gloving during surgery and note that today, scrub times vary facility to facility from 2 to 10 minutes. They cite studies that have shown a 5-minute scrub to be as effective as a 10-minute scrub and report on a study that concluded that 3 minutes was an effective scrub time.

In this study, 25 surgical nurses and technologists performed either a 2- or 3-minute scrub. Then, using a cross-over sampling scheme after a minimum of 7 days in between, the same subject scrubbed a second time for the alternate amount of time. After the scrub, the subject wore sterile gloves and went about his or her regular duties, but without contact with patients or any of the sterile fields. After 1 hour, samples of the subject's glove juice were taken.

On average, the bacteria count after the 2-minute scrub was higher than that after the 3-minute scrub. In 11 instances, however, the 2-minute scrub performed better than the 3-minute scrub. Both the 2- and 3-minute scrubs resulted in bacteria counts of less than 0.5 log, which is the threshold for practical and clinical significance. This finding suggests that 2-minute scrubs are as effective as 3-minute scrubs. The incidence of glove perforation was 4%.

Critique. Not all subjects in the study used the same surgical scrub agent, although one of the three most popular agents was used in all cases.

Possible Nursing Implications. If surgical scrub times can be reduced without untoward effects, the operating staff will have more time to devote to other aspects of patient care, increasing the cost-effectiveness of their care. Cost savings would be achieved from using less water. Further, because of a possible decrease in hand irritations, staff may not lose as much time from work.

nal impulses in the brain. This state is achieved by the administration of a single agent or a combination of chemical agents. The anesthetic agents used induce depression of the central nervous system (CNS), a depression characterized by analgesia (pain relief or pain suppression), amnesia (memory loss of the surgery), and unconsciousness, with loss of muscle tone and reflexes. The client is unconscious, unaware, and anesthetized. Some indications for general anesthesia include surgery of the head, neck, and upper torso; extensive abdominal surgery; and situations in which clients are unable to cooperate.

STAGES OF GENERAL ANESTHESIA. Four stages of general anesthesia are classically described. Table 21–2 presents the client's physiologic responses and nursing interventions for each stage.

The speed of *emergence*, or recovery from the anesthesia, depends on the type of anesthetic agent, the length of time the client is anesthetized, and whether a reversal agent for the neuromuscular blocking agent has been administered. Although not as common as they once were (because of advances made in the pharmacology of anesthesia), retching, vomiting, and restlessness may occur during emergence; the nurse has suction equipment available to prevent aspiration. During recovery, shivering, rigidity, and slight cyanosis are not uncommon; these phenomena may reflect a temporary disturbance in the body's temperature control. The nurse provides the client with warm blankets, radiant light, and oxygen to decrease the undesirable effects of emergence.

ADMINISTRATION OF GENERAL ANESTHESIA. The two methods of administering general anesthesia are inhalation and intravenous (IV) injection.

Inhalation. Inhalation is the most controllable method of administering general anesthesia because intake and elimination of the anesthetic are accomplished primarily by respiration. The lungs act as a passageway for entrance and exit of the anesthetic agent. The client inhales the anesthetic vapor of a volatile liquid or the anesthetic gas via mask; the anesthetic then passes across the alveolar membrane to the general circulation. It is transported, via the bloodstream, to the various tissues, where it is metabolized.

To improve ventilation and control the anesthesia, respiration may be assisted or controlled. With *assisted* respiration, an endotracheal (ET) tube is inserted. It is then connected to a reservoir (breathing) bag of the anesthesia machine (see Fig. 21–4). The anesthesiologist overrides, or "assists," the client's own respiratory effort to initiate the respiratory cycle by manually compressing the reservoir bag.

Controlled respiration can be accomplished with the use of a mechanical device (such as a mechanical ventilator) that automatically and rhythmically inflates the lungs with intermittent positive pressure; the client is not required to participate. Controlled ventilation is initiated after the anesthesiologist has produced apnea either through hyperventilation or by administering respiratory depressant or neuromuscular blocker drugs.

The anesthesiologist or CRNA inserts the ET tube, with the assistance of the circulating nurse. A laryngoscope is used to visualize the vocal cords, and the tube is placed in the trachea (Fig. 21–9). With the ET tube safely in place, the client has an open airway (through the tube) and an avenue for the safe administration of the inhaled anesthetic and oxygen.

Inhalation anesthetic agents are divided into two categories: gases and volatile agents. Table 21–3 lists the advantages, disadvantages, and related nursing implications of various inhalation anesthetic agents.

GASEOUS AGENTS. In the past, gaseous agents included ether and cyclopropane gas. *Nitrous oxide* (N_2O) is now the most commonly used gaseous anesthetic agent and is usually administered with oxygen. It is a colorless, odor-

OUR LADY OF LOURDES MEDICAL CENTER
CAMDEN, NEW JERSEY

ANESTHESIA RECORD

DATE	ANESTHESIA RECORD NUMBER
CONSENT	PHYS. STATUS 1 2 3 4 E1 E2 E3 E4 5
PREMEDICATION (DRUG, DOSE, TIME, EFFECT)	

NAME
ADDRESS
ROOM
MEDICAL RECORDS NUMBER
SEX
AGE
BUSINESS DATA PLATE

15 30 45 15 30 45 15 30 45 15 30 45 15 30

AGENTS: N_2O, O_2

FLUIDS

B.P. V Λ
PULSE •
START ANES X
START OP ⊙
END ANES ⊗
TEMP Δ
SUCTION S
REC. ROOM R

°C: 38, 36, 34, 32, 30

240, 220, 200, 180, 160, 140, 120, 100, 80, 60, 40, 20, 10

RESP. O: SPON., ASST., CONT., VENT.

SYMBOLS

PREOPERATIVE DIAGNOSIS

AGENTS	TECHNIQUES	DOSAGE
A.		
B.		
C.		
D.		
E.		
F.		
G.		

REMARKS (INDUCTION, MAINTENANCE, EMERGENCE)

FLUID SUMMARY	RECOVERY (OR)
DEXTROSE - H_2O	REFLEX IN OR YES______NO ___
RING - LAC	CONSC. IN OR YES ______NO ___
SALINE	NAUSEA ______EMESIS ______
PLASMA	HYPOTENSION
BLOOD	
OTHER	
BLO. LOSS, HOW MEASURED	

POST OPERATIVE DIAGNOSIS

OPERATION

SURGEON | ANESTHETIST

1. OP NP OT NT (D - B)
2. CUFF-PACK TUBE SIZE______
3. TECHNICAL DIFFICULTY
4. MACHINE
   VAPORIZER
   MONITOR

OLLH FORM F20 (12/81)

Figure 21–8. An anesthesia record. (Courtesy of Our Lady of Lourdes Medical Center, Camden, NJ.)

TABLE 21–1

Advantages and Disadvantages of Various Types of Anesthesia

Type	Advantages	Disadvantages
General		
Inhalation	• Most controllable method • Induction and reversal accomplished with pulmonary ventilation • Few side effects	• Must be used in combination with other agents for painful or prolonged procedures • Limited muscle relaxant effects • Postoperative nausea and shivering common • Explosive
Intravenous	• Rapid and pleasant induction • Low incidence of postoperative nausea and vomiting • Requires little equipment	• Must be metabolized and excreted from the body for complete reversal • Contraindicated in presence of hepatic or renal disease • Increased cardiac and respiratory depression • Retained by fat cells
Balanced	• Minimal disturbance to physiologic function • Minimal side effects • Can be used with elderly and high-risk clients	• Drug interactions can occur • Pharmacological effects on the body may be unpredictable
Regional or Local	• Gag and cough reflexes stay intact • Allows participation and cooperation by the client • Less disruption of physical and emotional body functions • Decreased chance of sensitivity to the agent • Decreased intraoperative stress	• Difficult to administer to an uncooperative or upset client • No way to control agent after administration • Absorbs rapidly into the blood and causes cardiac depression (hypotension) or overdose • Increased nervous system stimulation (overdose) • Not practical for extensive procedures because of the amount of drug that would be required to maintain anesthesia

less, nonirritating gas and provides analgesia equivalent to 10 mg of morphine sulfate.

VOLATILE AGENTS. Liquids vaporized for inhalation are considered volatile agents. Oxygen acts as a carrier, flowing over or bubbling through the liquid in the vaporizer system on the anesthesia machine. All volatile agents can produce postoperative shivering in the client because of an effect on the hypothalamus. Awakening is usually rapid, within 15 to 20 minutes.

Halothane (Fluothane). Halothane is a halogenated hydrocarbon that depresses the cardiovascular system. The intraoperative use of epinephrine to control bleeding may exacerbate or precipitate a dysrhythmia when halothane is used. Clients can have memory impairment for up to 24 hours later.

Enflurane (Ethrane). Enflurane is an inhalation anesthetic agent that reduces the client's ventilations and decreases blood pressure as the depth of anesthesia increases.

Isoflurane (Forane). Isoflurane is another halogenated compound and appears to be a preferred inhalation agent.

Desflurane (Suprane). Desflurane produces a rapid induction of anesthesia but can cause coughing and excitation during the process. The rapid elimination of desflurane produces awakening in 8 to 10 minutes. Cardiopulmonary depressant effects and malignant hyperthermia are the most common adverse effects.

Sevoflurane (Sevoflurane). Sevoflurane is like desflurane, except less coughing and laryngospasm occur with sevoflurane. Adverse effects are similar to those associated with desflurane.

Intravenous (IV) Injection. Intravenous anesthetic agents are injected, usually via a peripheral IV line, into the circulation. A pleasant, rapid, and smooth dissipation of the agent occurs. The drug is diluted by the blood, but it travels in high concentration to the organs of high

TABLE 21-2

The Four Stages of General Anesthesia and Related Nursing Interventions

Stage	Description	Nursing Interventions	Rationale
Stage 1 (Analgesia and Sedation, Relaxation)	• Begins with induction and ends with loss of consciousness. • Client feels drowsy and dizzy, has a reduced sensation to pain, and is amnesic. • Hearing is exaggerated.	• Close operating room doors, dim the lights, and control traffic in the operating room. • Position client securely with safety belts. • Keep discussions about the client to a minimum.	• Avoiding external stimuli in the environment promotes relaxation. • Using safety measures in stage 1 prepares for stage 2. • Being sensitive to the client maintains his or her dignity.
Stage 2 (Excitement, Delirium)	• Begins with loss of consciousness and ends with relaxation, regular breathing, and loss of the eyelid reflex. • Client may have irregular breathing, increased muscle tone, and involuntary movement of the extremities during this stage. • Laryngospasm or vomiting may occur. • Client is susceptible to external stimuli.	• Avoid auditory and physical stimuli. • Protect the extremities. • Assist the anesthesiologist or CRNA with suctioning as needed. • Stay with client.	• Sensory stimuli can contribute to the client's response. • Safety measures help to prevent injury. • Staying with the client is emotionally supportive.
Stage 3 (Operative Anesthesia, Surgical Anesthesia)	• Begins with generalized muscle relaxation and ends with loss of reflexes and depression of vital functions. • The jaw is relaxed, and there is quiet, regular breathing. • The client cannot hear. • Sensations are lost (i.e., to pain).	• Assist the anesthesiologist or CRNA with intubation. • Place client into operative position. • Prep (scrub) the client's skin over the operative site as directed.	• Providing assistance helps promote smooth intubation and prevent injury. • Performing procedures as soon as possible promotes time management to minimize total anesthesia time for the client.
Stage 4 (Danger)	• Begins with depression of vital functions and ends with respiratory failure, cardiac arrest, and possible death. • Respiratory muscles are paralyzed, apnea occurs. • Pupils fixed and dilated.	• Prepare for and assist in treatment of cardiac and/or pulmonary arrest. • Document occurrence in the client's chart.	• Teamwork and preparedness help decrease injuries and complications, and promote the possibility of a desired outcome for the client.

blood flow (brain, liver, and kidneys). The reversal and removal of the agent from circulation are not possible with IV injection, and the recovery from the agent is directly related to the client's metabolism. Table 21-4 lists advantages, disadvantages, and related nursing implications of various intravenous anesthetic agents.

BARBITURATES. Barbiturates are often used for IV induction of anesthesia. These drugs act directly on the central nervous system, producing a reaction ranging from mild sedation to unconsciousness. The principal barbiturate used is thiopental sodium (Pentothal), which can also be used for rectal induction. Intravenously, it acts rapidly, resulting in unconsciousness in 30 seconds. Because thiopental is a potent respiratory and cardiovascular system depressant, the client's vital signs must be monitored continuously during administration.

KETAMINE (KETALAR). Ketamine is a dissociative anesthetic agent (one that promotes a feeling of dissociation from the environment). It acts by selectively interrupting various pathways in the brain. Rapid onset of a trance-like, analgesic state occurs. It is commonly used for diagnostic and short surgical procedures or to supplement weaker agents, such as nitrous oxide.

During the client's recovery from ketamine, emergence reactions are expected. The OR nurse reports the use of the drug to the postanesthesia nurse so that safety precautions can be implemented. If the client is combative or restless, the nurse pads the side rails of the bed to prevent injury. The nurse minimizes external stimuli until the client awakens naturally. For severe reactions during the recovery phase, small doses of diazepam (Valium, Vivol♣, Novodipam♣) may be given as needed. The medical-surgical nurse continues interventions until the effects of the drug have worn off.

PROPOFOL (DIPRIVAN). Propofol is in a newer classification of IV anesthetic agents, the alkylphenols. Its short action makes it desirable as an anesthetic agent. Hypnosis occurs

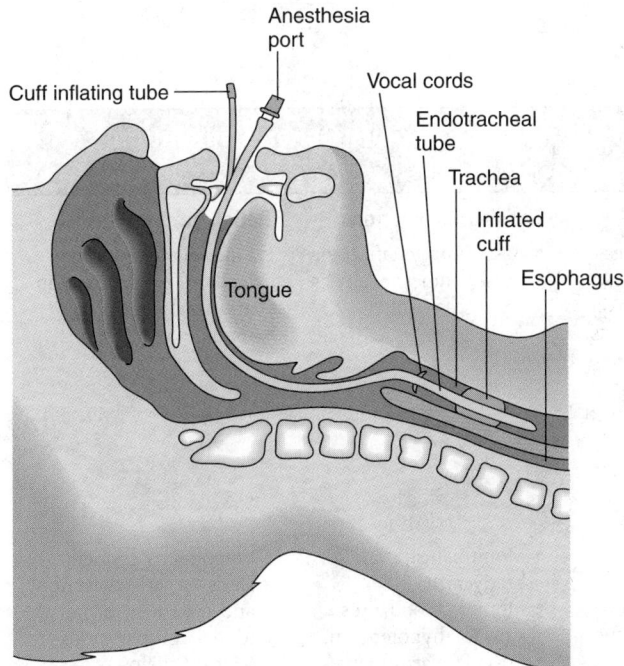

Figure 21–9. An oral endotracheal tube in position. The cuff of the tube was placed just below the vocal cords, then inflated to seal off the airway.

in less than 1 minute from the time of injection, and because the drug is so rapidly metabolized, it does not accumulate during maintenance of the anesthesia. The client becomes responsive quickly after the infusion is ended (within 8 minutes). Propofol is also used to supplement nitrous oxide during short procedures and is used as a hypnotic agent with regional anesthesia.

ADJUNCTS TO THE GENERAL ANESTHESIA AGENTS.
Other drugs, such as hypnotics, opioid analgesics, and neuromuscular blocking agents, may be used as part of the anesthesia regimen.

Hypnotics. The benzodiazepines may be used for various effects. Common drugs in this classification include midazolam (Versed), lorazepam (Ativan, Novolorazem✤), and diazepam (Valium, Vivol✤, Novodipam✤). All have hypnotic, sedative, antianxiety, muscle relaxant, and amnesic effects. Generally, lower doses are ordered for preoperative sedation. Each may be used as part of an IV conscious sedation regimen for diagnostic or endoscopic procedures. Higher doses of midazolam may be used to induce general anesthesia. The benzodiazepines may also be used intraoperatively in conjunction with regional or local anesthesia. Adverse reactions include respiratory depression, apnea, and oversedation.

Opioid Analgesics. Common opioid analgesics used to supplement inhalation anesthesia include morphine sulfate (Statex✤), meperidine hydrochloride (Demerol), fentanyl citrate (Sublimaze), and sufentanil (Sufenta). The

use of opioids during surgery contributes to postoperative analgesia. All opioid analgesics decrease alveolar ventilation and are respiratory depressants. The nurse monitors respirations and maintains an open airway. Reduced dosages are prescribed for the elderly, the client with a circulatory problem (such as heart failure), and the debilitated client.

Fentanyl and sufentanil provide analgesia in lower doses, but at higher doses, they can be used as the anesthetic agent. Fentanyl has a potency 75 to 125 times greater than that of morphine (Omoigui, 1995). Sufentanil has five to seven times the analgesic potency of fentanyl (Omoigui, 1995) and produces a more rapid onset of central nervous system effects than does fentanyl. It is often used in open heart surgery when the sternum must be opened. The nurse monitors the client who has received sufentanil for bradycardia and decreased cardiac output.

Neuromuscular Blocking Agents. The neuromuscular blockers are used to relax the jaw and vocal cords immediately after induction so the anesthesiologist or certified registered nurse anesthetist (CRNA) can pass the endotracheal tube. These drugs are also used throughout the surgical procedure to provide continued overall muscle relaxation. Neuromuscular blocking agents act on the striated muscles of the body by interfering with impulse transmission at the neuromuscular junction. The drugs are administered intravenously in small amounts and may cause circulatory alterations and decreased respirations or apnea from muscle paralysis. The nurse ensures the client's safety by securing the client on the operating bed with safety straps and assists the anesthesiologist or CRNA with intubation. Throughout the surgery, the anesthesiologist or CRNA checks the effectiveness of the blocker agent by using a peripheral nerve stimulator. There are two types of neuromuscular blocking agents: non-depolarizing and depolarizing.

NON-DEPOLARIZING BLOCKER AGENTS. The non-depolarizing blockers block acetylcholine at the neuromuscular junction. Only skeletal muscles are blocked, and the drug is easily reversed with an antidote of neostigmine and atropine. Examples of non-depolarizing blockers include pancuronium (Pavulon), atracurium (Tracrium), vecuronium (Norcuron), doxacurium (Nuromax), tubocurarine (Tubarine✤), and mivacurium (Mivacron). Pancuronium has has a relatively long effect (45–60 minutes) compared with vecuronium (25–30 minutes) or mivacurium (6–16 minutes). The longer the effect of the drug, the longer it takes for the client to recover.

DEPOLARIZING BLOCKER AGENTS. The depolarizing blocker agents, also called "noncompetitive" blockers, depolarize the motor end plate at the neuromuscular junction. In the process, potassium is forced out of the muscle cells and into general circulation, which can cause hyperkalemia. Clients often experience transient intraoperative muscle twitching, which can result in generalized muscle aches after awakening. There is no specific antidote. Other side effects include increased salivation, which puts the client

TABLE 21-3

Advantages, Disadvantages, and Related Nursing Implications of Various General Inhalation Anesthetic Agents

Agent	Advantages	Disadvantages	Nursing Implications	Rationale
Nitrous oxide (N₂O)	• Rapid induction and recovery • Useful for short procedures • When used with other agents, reduces the required concentration of the other agents • Minimal cardiovascular and respiratory depression	• Relatively weak anesthetic agent • May produce hypoxia if the concentration is high • Needs addition of other agents for longer procedures	• Assess oxygenation via pulse oximetry, physical assessment.	• Ongoing assessment leads to early detection and treatment of potential complications.
Halothane (Fluothane)	• Rapid and smooth induction • Low incidence of postoperative nausea and vomiting • Less irritating to the respiratory tract than other inhalation agents • Sweet smell makes it easy to use in children • Tolerated well by children	• Shivering common postoperatively • Malignant hyperthermia is possible in susceptible clients. • Metabolized by the liver • Hypotension and bradycardia may occur. • Can sensitize the myocardium to dysrhythmias	• Monitor heart rate for bradycardia. • Monitor blood pressure for hypotension. • Provide warm blankets, radiant heat.	• Ongoing assessment leads to early detection and treatment of potential complications. • Warmth helps promote client comfort and decrease shivering.
Enflurane (Ethrane)	• Rapid induction and recovery • Does not alter heart rate or rhythm	• Respiratory depression and hypotension may occur. • Malignant hyperthermia is possible in susceptible clients. • Lowers seizure threshold	• Monitor respiratory rate and depth for hypoventilation. • Assess oxygenation via pulse oximetry, physical assessment. • Monitor blood pressure for hypotension.	• Ongoing assessment leads to early detection and treatment of potential complications.
Isoflurane (Forane)	• Rapid induction and recovery • Has some muscle relaxant properties • Stimulates heart, which helps keep a stable heart rate • Is not significantly metabolized; no renal or hepatic damage	• Respiratory depression may occur. • Malignant hyperthermia is possible in susceptible clients.	• Monitor respiratory rate and depth for hypoventilation.	• Ongoing assessment leads to early detection and treatment of potential complications.
Desflurane (Suprane)	• Rapid induction, recovery and awakening	• May cause coughing and excitement during induction. • Deep levels of anesthesia may increase heart rate and blood pressure. • Malignant hyperthermia is possible in susceptible clients. • May cause changes in mental function.	• Monitor heart rate and blood pressure. • Caution client and family that client should not drive or operate hazardous machinery until mental status has returned to preoperative baseline.	• Ongoing assessment leads to early detection and treatment of potential complications. • Specific instructions will help prevent other injuries or accidents.

TABLE 21-4

Advantages, Disadvantages, and Related Nursing Implications of Various General Intravenous Anesthetic Agents				
Agent	**Advantages**	**Disadvantages**	**Nursing Implications**	**Rationale**
Barbiturates				
Thiopental sodium (Pentothal), methohexital sodium (Brevital), thiamylal sodium (Surital)	• Rapid, pleasant induction and recovery • Acts directly on the central nervous system • Short-acting • Low incidence of postoperative nausea and vomiting	• Strong respiratory and cardiovascular depressant effect • No antagonist medication available • Mild to severe local tissue reaction with extravasation • Poor analgesic, muscle relaxant effects	• Monitor respiratory rate and depth for hypoventilation. • Monitor heart rate for bradycardia. • Monitor blood pressure for hypotension. • Assess IV site.	• Ongoing assessment leads to early detection and treatment of potential complications.
Nonbarbiturates				
Ketamine hydrochloride (Ketalar)	• Rapid induction • Short-acting • Can be given IM or IV • No respiratory depression or loss of muscle tone (protects the airway) • Protective reflexes remain intact • Stimulates the cardiovascular system • Can use for clients with respiratory or cardiac disorders • Good amnesic effect • Postop emergence reactions generally last only 24 hr	• Emergence reactions are common: hallucinations, irrational behaviors, distorted images, unpleasant dreams, restlessness • Increased heart rate • Increased blood pressure • Increased cardiac output • Poor muscle relaxant effect • Nausea, vomiting, and aspiration can occur	• Minimize external stimuli: noise, light, touch, movement. • Speak in a calm, soothing voice. • Reassure client and family that emergence reactions are common and temporary. • Have suction equipment near. • Monitor blood pressure for hypertension. • Monitor heart rate for tachycardia.	• Stimuli increase the severity of the emergence reaction. • Quiet promotes comfort, decreases anxiety. • Reassurance decreases anxiety. • Suction may be needed in the event of vomiting to prevent aspiration. • Ongoing assessment leads to early detection and treatment of potential complications.
Propofol (Diprivan)	• Short-acting • Rapidly metabolized • Client becomes responsive quickly postoperatively • Minimal postoperative nausea, vomiting, or sedation	• Allergic skin reactions have occurred • Client becomes aware of postoperative pain and discomfort sooner than with other anesthetics	• Be prepared to administer analgesic medications as ordered early in the postoperative period. • Plan for nonpharmacologic pain interventions (see Chapter 9).	• Awareness of pain very early in the postoperative period can be frightening. • Pain can increase blood pressure and increase anxiety.
Opioids (as adjunct)				
Fentanyl (Sublimaze)	• Excellent postoperative analgesia • Long-acting analgesia	• Significant respiratory depression can occur several hours after administration • Cardiovascular depression can occur	• Monitor respiratory rate and depth for hypoventilation. • Monitor blood pressure for hypotension. • Have atropine, naloxone (Narcan), vasopressors, and resuscitative equipment nearby.	• Ongoing assessment leads to early detection and treatment of potential complications. • Having necessary supplies and equipment available provides for prompt response to an emergency.

at risk for aspiration, and increased intraocular pressure, which may be contraindicated with glaucoma. An example of a depolarizing blocker is succinylcholine (Anectine).

BALANCED ANESTHESIA. Balanced anesthesia is widely used. It provides a safe and controlled anesthetic experience, especially for elderly and high-risk clients. A combination of agents is used to provide hypnosis, amnesia, analgesia, muscle relaxation, and relaxation of reflexes with minimal disturbance of the client's physiologic function. An example of balanced anesthesia is the use of a barbiturate (such as thiopental) administered intravenously for induction, nitrous oxide for amnesia, morphine for analgesia, and a muscle relaxant (such as pancuronium) to provide additional relaxation of the muscles.

A second example of balanced anesthesia is the use of 70% nitrous oxide for induction and maintenance (to prevent awareness throughout the procedure and to prevent recall afterward), 30% oxygen to maintain the client's oxygenation saturation greater than 90%, along with an opioid and a muscle relaxant. Many combinations are possible, and selection reflects assessment of the individual client and the specific surgical procedure.

COMPLICATIONS FROM GENERAL ANESTHESIA OR ANESTHESIA MANAGEMENT. Complications can range from minor and annoying to the most severe—death.

Malignant Hyperthermia. Malignant hyperthermia (MH) is an acute, life-threatening complication of general anesthesia. The client with a genetic predisposition for MH is at risk for this complication from certain MH-triggering general anesthetic agents, including halothane, enflurane, isoflurane, desflurane, sevoflurane, and succinylcholine. Stressors, such as severe fatigue, strenuous exercise, muscle injury, and emotional stress, may also trigger this crisis. A biochemical reaction occurs as a result of a defect in the muscle cell membrane, causing a rise in the circulating calcium level, an increase in metabolic rate, hyperkalemia, and metabolic and respiratory acidosis.

Signs of malignant hypothermia include tachycardia or other dysrhythmia; muscle rigidity, especially of the jaw (masseter muscle rigidity) and upper chest; hypotension; tachypnea; and skin mottling, cyanosis, and myoglobinuria (cola-colored urine). The first indication is an unexpected rise in the end-tidal CO_2 level with a decrease in oxygen saturation (Dunn, 1997). The second indication may be unexplained sinus tachycardia. Extremely elevated temperature, perhaps as high as 44° C (111.2° F), is a late sign of MH. Treatment and survival of the client depend on early diagnosis and cooperation of the entire surgical team.

Once a client or family history of MH is known, close family members can undergo a muscle biopsy to determine whether they are at risk. In the case of a known history or predetermination, the client can be treated preoperatively, intraoperatively, and postoperatively with dantrolene to prevent this complication. Chart 21–1 summarizes the nursing care of the client with malignant hyperthermia.

Overdose. An anesthesia overdose can occur if the client's pharmacokinetics do not react or respond as expected. Drugs (e.g., antihypertensive medications) also alter the pharmacokinetics, and drug interactions can occur between the anesthetic agents and other regularly administered medications. Accurate, accessible information about the client, such as height, weight, and history, is

---

Chart 21–1

Nursing Care Highlight: Malignant Hyperthermia

The Susceptible Client

- Assess client and family history preoperatively for signs and symptoms of malignant hyperthermia (MH) or of muscular dystrophy.
- Counsel client regarding quadriceps femoris muscle biopsy to determine his or her predisposition to MH.
- Assist client in finding a muscle biopsy testing center.
- Provide information about MH and the MH Association of the United States (MHAUS).
- Reassure the client that surgery can still be performed safely.

The Client in Malignant Hyperthermia Crisis

- Call for help!
- Assist the physician and anesthesiologist and/or certified registered nurse anesthetist with the immediate discontinuation of surgery.
- Hyperventilate with 100% oxygen (15–20 L/min).
- Call the malignant hyperthermia hotline at 800-644-9737.
- Reconstitute dantrolene (Dantrium) with sterile *distilled* water.
- Give 2.5–10.0 mg/kg of dantrolene (Dantrium) intravenously as ordered.
- With increasing body temperature, or if temperature is greater than 40° C (104° F), cool the client with external ice packs, iced intravenous (IV) saline; iced lavages of the rectum, stomach, and wound; and hypothermia blankets for over and under the client as ordered. Discontinue cooling when the client's body temperature is less than 38° C (100.4° F).
- Collect urine and blood specimens as ordered.
- Have sodium bicarbonate, mannitol (Osmitrol✦), procainamide (Pronestyl), hydrocortisone (Solu-Cortef), furosemide (Lasix, Furoside✦), regular insulin, 50% dextrose, 10% calcium chloride, 2% lidocaine, and heparin (Hepalean✦) available to treat acidosis, hyperkalemia, dysrhythmias and DIC, and to maintain urinary output.
- Assist with monitoring urinary output (insert Foley catheter), serum potassium and calcium levels, ABGs, clotting studies, and cardiac rhythms as indicated.
- Document the event, detailing times, interventions, and client response. Submit an adverse metabolic reaction to anesthesia report to the North American Malignant Hyperthermia Registry at 717-531-6936.

ABGs = arterial blood gases; DIC = disseminated intravascular coagulation.

---

vital in determining anesthetic type and dosage. Intraoperative death, however, is more often related to the client's premorbid condition, rather than overdosage of anesthetics.

Unrecognized Hypoventilation. The respiratory system is most frequently involved when the client experiences a damaging event related to anesthesia. Failure to ventilate can lead to cardiac arrest, central nervous system

TABLE 21–5

Advantages, Disadvantages, and Related Nursing Implications of Local or Regional Anesthetic Agents				
Agent	Advantages	Disadvantages	Nursing Implications	Rationale
Procaine (Novocain) Tetracaine (Pontocaine) Lidocaine (Xylocaine) Mepivacaine (Carbocaine, Polocaine) Bupivacaine (Marcaine, Sensorcaine)	• Easily administered • Rapid onset (4–17 min) • Can be administered topically or by injection • Excellent muscle relaxant effects • Protective reflexes (cough, gag) remain intact • Client does not lose consciousness • Many are available with epinephrine added	• Absorbs into the bloodstream • Can cause cardiac depression and dysrhythmias with absorption • Difficult to control dosage • Drug interactions with monoamine oxidase (MAO) inhibitors can cause hypertension • Tremors, twitching shivering, respiratory arrest can occur with absorption	• Assess for return of movement and sensation in the area anesthetized. • Monitor blood pressure and pulse. • Assess administration site for pallor, drainage. • Protect area anesthetized until full sensation has returned.	• Movement returns first, then sense of touch, pain, warmth, and cold, in that order. • Ongoing assessment leads to early detection and treatment of potential complications. • Protection prevents injury to the area. • Duration of the anesthetic is 3–6 hr.

damage (e.g., permanent brain damage), and death. Monitoring standards include the use of an end-tidal carbon dioxide monitor to confirm carbon dioxide in the client's expired gas and a breathing system disconnect monitor to detect any break in the breathing circuit equipment.

Complications Related to Specific Anesthetic Agents. Specific complications were discussed earlier in the chapter. The elderly or debilitated client may be more susceptible to complications of anesthesia because of an intolerance to the agent, decreased metabolism, or general physical condition. (For preoperative risk factors, see Chapter 20.)

Complications of Intubation. Many complications can occur from intubation; for example, broken or injured teeth and caps, swollen lip, or vocal cord trauma. Intubation may be difficult because of the individual client's anatomy or disease process (e.g., small oral cavity, tight mandibular joint, tumor). Improper extension of the client's neck during intubation may cause injury. The surgeon should be in the operating room (OR) in case an emergency arises (e.g., a tracheostomy is needed) when the endotracheal tube is placed. Placement of the endotracheal tube causes some degree of irritation and edema of the trachea and accounts for the client's sore throat postoperatively.

Local or Regional Anesthesia

Local or regional anesthesia temporarily interrupts the transmission of sensory nerve impulses from a specific area or region. Motor function may or may not be affected, and the client does not lose consciousness. Thus, the client is able to follow instructions throughout the procedure. Because the gag and cough reflexes remain intact, there is little risk of aspiration or other respiratory complications. Local or regional anesthesia is typically supplemented with sedatives, opioid analgesics, and/or hypnotics.

The OR nurse provides the client with information, directions, and emotional support before, during, and after the procedure. Table 21–5 describes various anesthetic agents and related nursing interventions.

LOCAL ANESTHESIA. Techniques used to administer local anesthesia include topical anesthesia and local infiltration. Sometimes when the term *local* is used, it means *any* form of anesthesia that is not general anesthesia. The client could be receiving regional anesthesia, but local anesthetic agents are used.

Topical Anesthesia. Topical anesthesia refers to an anesthetic applied *directly* to the surface of the area to be anesthetized. Often the anesthetic is in the form of an ointment or spray. This method is often used for respiratory intubation or for diagnostic procedures, such as laryngoscopy, bronchoscopy, or cystoscopy. The onset of action is 1 minute, and the duration is 20 to 30 minutes. Collapse or depression of the cardiovascular system may occur after the topical anesthetic is applied to the respiratory tract.

Local Infiltration. Local infiltration is the injection of an anesthetic agent intracutaneously and subcutaneously *into* the tissue surrounding an incision, wound, or lesion. The anesthetic blocks peripheral nerve stimulation at its origin. Local infiltration is commonly used during the suturing of superficial lacerations.

REGIONAL ANESTHESIA. Regional anesthesia—a type of local anesthesia—may be used as follows:

■ When general anesthesia is contraindicated because of the presence of medical problems (e.g., dysrhythmias and respiratory disease)

- When the client has experienced previous adverse reactions to general anesthetic agents
- When the client has a preference and a choice is possible

If the client has eaten and the surgery is an emergency, it may be possible to perform the procedure with the client under regional anesthesia (depending on the procedure) to decrease the risks associated with gastric contents (e.g., aspiration). Types of regional anesthesia include field block, nerve block, spinal, and epidural.

Field Block. A field block is produced by a series of injections *around* the operative field. Injecting around a specific nerve or group of nerves depresses the entire sensory nervous system of a localized area. This type of blocking is used for thoracic procedures, herniorrhaphy (hernia repair), dental procedures, and plastic surgery.

Nerve Block. A nerve block is achieved by injection of the local anesthestic agent *into or around* a nerve or nerves supplying the involved area. Nerve blocks interrupt sensory, motor, or sympathetic transmission. They are used surgically to prevent pain during a procedure, diagnostically to identify the cause of pain, and therapeutically to relieve chronic pain and increase circulation in some vascular diseases.

Figure 21–10 shows common nerve block sites. Lidocaine (Xylocaine) or bupivacaine (Marcaine) is frequently the agent used. A nerve block takes effect within minutes after the injection, and the anesthesia lasts longer than is achieved with local infiltration. Epinephrine added to the anesthetic agent potentiates the drug, causing a prolonged effect. Seizures, cardiac depression, dysrhythmias, and/or respiratory depression may occur if the nerve-blocking agent is injected into the bloodstream. The nurse observes for signs of systemic absorption, sensitivity, or overdose.

Spinal Anesthesia. Spinal anesthesia—intrathecal block —is achieved by injection of the anesthetic agent into the subarachnoid space (Fig. 21–11). The drug acts on the nerves as they emerge from the spinal cord and before they leave the spinal canal through the intervertebral foramen, thereby inhibiting conduction in the autonomic, sensory, and motor systems. The drug is rapidly absorbed into the nerve fibers and produces analgesia with relaxation, which is effective for lower abdominal and pelvic surgical procedures.

Epidural Anesthesia. The anesthetic is injected into the epidural space so that the protective coverings of the spinal cord (dura mater and arachnoid mater) are never entered. Because the anesthetic can diffuse or float up the vertebral column, the client can achieve anesthetic effects as high as the T-4 level; however, potential respiratory complications may make injection at this high a level undesirable.

Epidural anesthesia is used for anorectal, vaginal, and perineal procedures, as well as for hip and lower extremity operations, such as total hip or knee replacements. Two important advantages are associated with this type of anesthesia:

- Decreased cardiopulmonary complications—particularly important for the elderly client
- Ability to retain the epidural catheter for postoperative analgesic administration (see Chap. 9)

COMPLICATIONS OF LOCAL OR REGIONAL ANESTHESIA. Major intraoperative complications are usually attributable to client sensitization to the anesthetic agent (anaphylaxis), incorrect administration technique, systemic absorption, and overdosage. The nurse observes for signs of a systemic toxic reaction, which is manifested by central nervous system (CNS) stimulation followed by CNS

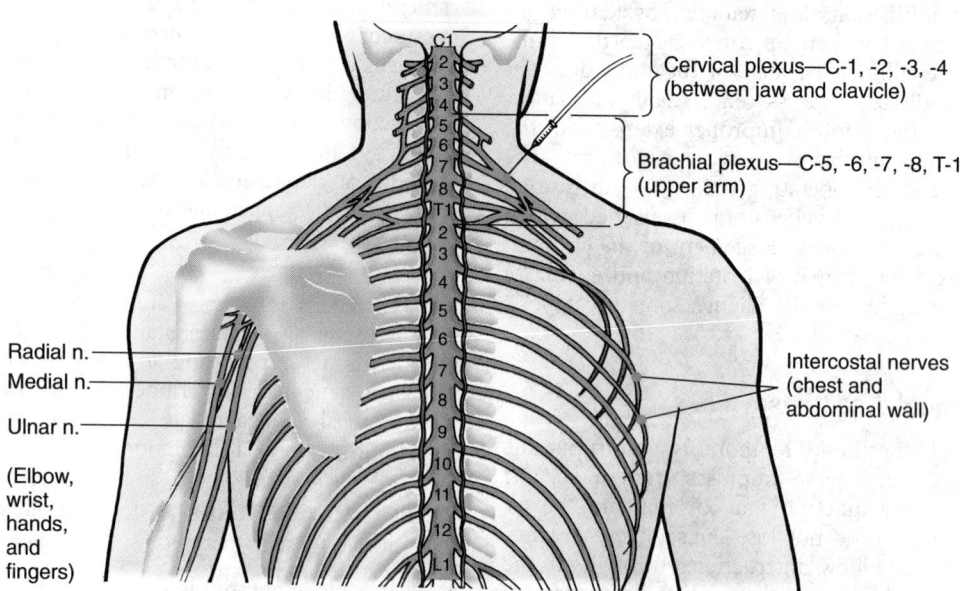

Figure 21–10. Nerve block sites.

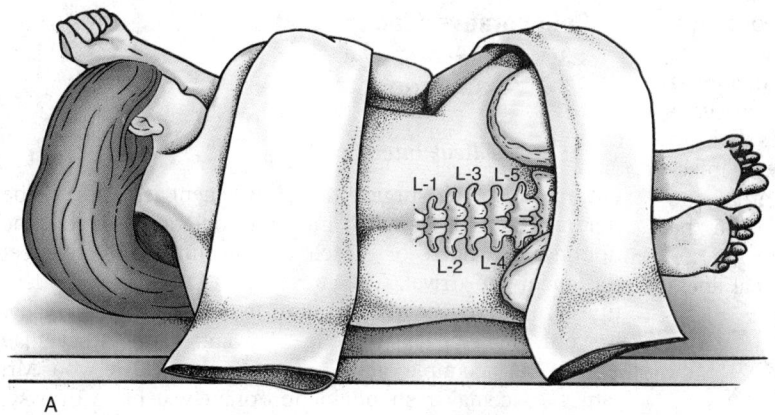

A

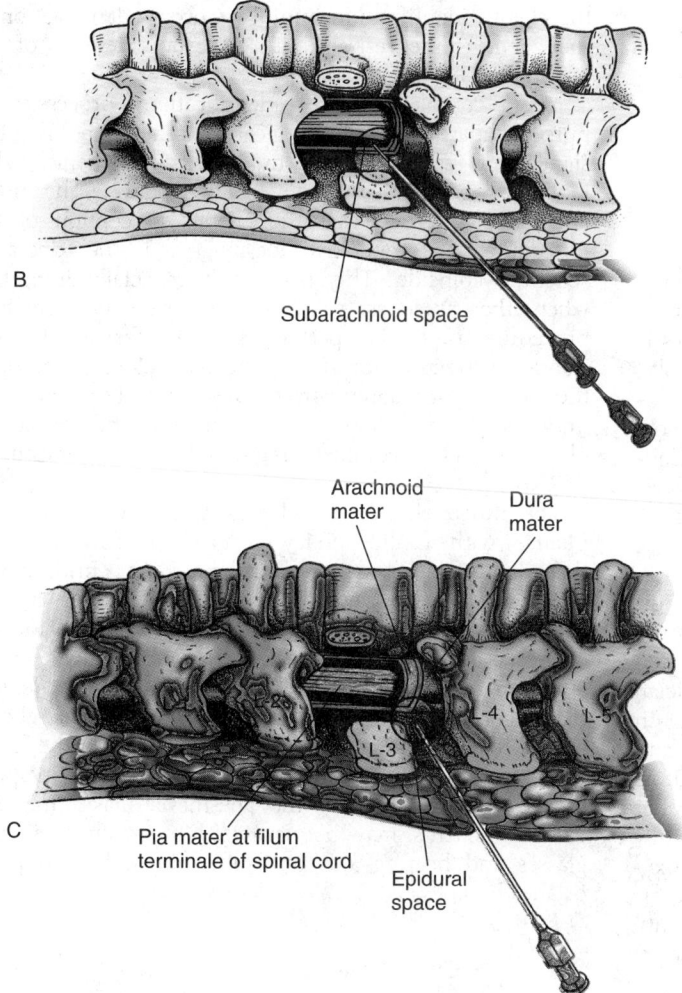

B
Subarachnoid space

Arachnoid mater   Dura mater

L-4   L-5
L-3

C
Pia mater at filum
terminale of spinal cord
Epidural space

Figure 21–11. Administration of spinal and epidural anesthesia. *A,* Spinal or epidural anesthesia is administered by inserting a spinal needle between the second and third or the third and fourth lumbar vertebrae (L2–3 or L3–4). The client is placed in the flexed lateral (fetal) position (shown here) or seated on the edge of the operating bed with the back arched and the chin tucked to the chest. *B,* Spinal anesthesia (viewed from the side). A large needle is inserted to the surface of the dura mater, and a second, smaller needle is passed through the first to penetrate the dura mater and arachnoid mater. An anesthetic is injected, sometimes through an indwelling catheter, directly into the cerebrospinal fluid in the subarachnoid space. *C,* Epidural anesthesia (viewed from the side). The needle is inserted to the surface of the dura mater, and the anesthetic is injected, usually through an indwelling catheter, into the epidural space.

and cardiovascular depression. The nurse assesses for such initial behaviors as restlessness; excitement; incoherent speech; headache; blurred vision; metallic taste; nausea; vomiting; tremors; seizures; and increased pulse, respirations, and blood pressure. Nursing interventions include establishing and maintaining an open airway, administering oxygen, and notifying the surgeon. It is usu-

ally necessary to administer a fast-acting and short-acting barbiturate. If the client's toxic reaction remains untreated, unconsciousness, hypotension, apnea, cardiac arrest, and death may result.

A cardiac arrest may rarely occur as a complication of spinal anesthesia, possibly related to unknown autonomic nervous system effects. Epinephrine may prevent the arrest when administered to the client who develops sudden, unexplained bradycardia (Biddle, 1994).

Localized complications include edema and inflammation initially, with possible abscess, necrosis, and/or gangrene later. Inflammation and abscess usually result from a break in sterile technique occurring at the time of injection of the anesthetic agent. Necrosis and gangrene are rare but may occur as a result of vasoconstriction in the area of the injection.

The nurse's role in the administration of regional anesthesia consists of

- Assisting the anesthesiologist or certified registered nurse anesthetist (CRNA)
- Observing for breaks in sterile technique
- Providing physical and emotional support for the client
- Staying with the client
- Providing the client a chance to verbalize feelings
- Offering information, encouragement, and reassurance
- Positioning the client comfortably and safely

Conscious Sedation

Conscious sedation, usually administered by direct intravenous (IV) injection ("IV push"), is given to dull or reduce the intensity of pain or awareness of pain during a procedure without loss of defensive reflexes. Usually a combination of opioid analgesics and sedative-hypnotics is used (Berkowitz, 1997). Diazepam (Valium, Vivol✦, Novodipam✦), midazolam (Versed), meperidine (Demerol), fentanyl (Sublimaze), alfentanil (Alfenta), and morphine sulfate are the most commonly used drugs. Conscious sedation is typically used for procedures such as endoscopy, cardiac catheterization, closed fracture reduction, percutaneous transluminal cardiac angiography (PTCA), cardioversion, and other special procedures.

The physician determines whether the client is a candidate for IV conscious sedation and often administers the first dosages. In most states, a credentialed registered nurse may administer conscious sedation under physician supervision. Credentialing involves advanced training in IV medication administration, airway management, and advanced cardic life support (ACLS). The nurse monitors the client during and after the procedure for his or her response to drug administration. The nurse carefully monitors the client's airway, level of consciousness, oxygen saturation via pulse oximetry, electrocardiographic (ECG) status, and vital signs every 15 to 30 minutes until the client is fully awake, alert, and oriented and when vital signs have returned to preprocedural levels.

Clients receiving IV conscious sedation may be discharged to go home with a responsible adult. If the client returns to the general medical-surgical nursing unit, the unit staff nurses continue to monitor the client. The client is expected to be sleepy but arousable for several hours after the procedure. The nurse usually does not permit oral intake until 30 minutes after the client has received medication or, in other cases, according to physician order. When fluids are permitted, the nurse makes sure that the client is awake and positioned to avoid aspiration.

Collaborative Management

 Assessment

► Client Interview

On arrival in the surgical suite, the client is taken to the holding area or directly into the operating suite. The holding area nurse or the circulating nurse or both greet the client on arrival. The nurse verifies the client's identity with his or her identification bracelet and asks, "What is your name?" This practice prevents errors that may occur. For example, if a client is asked, "Are you Mr. James?" He may respond inappropriately if he is drowsy, anxious, or sedated. The nurse always validates the identification obtained using the chart, the client's name, and the client's identification number. Correct identification of the client is the responsibility of every member of the health care team.

After completing the identification process, the nurse validates that the surgical consent form has been signed and witnessed. The nurse asks the client, "What kind of operation are you having today?" The nurse checks to ascertain that the client's perception of the procedure, the operative permit, and the operative schedule coincide. This practice is especially important when the nurse is validating the side on which a procedure is to be performed (e.g., for amputation, cataract extraction, or hernia repair). Before proceeding, the nurse thoroughly investigates *any* discrepancy in information and notifies the surgeon and anesthesiologist and/or certified registered nurse anesthetist (CRNA).

The nurse checks the client's attire to ensure compliance with facility policy. The nurse checks to see that dentures and dental prostheses (e.g., bridges and retainers), jewelry, eyeglasses, contact lenses, hearing aids, wigs, and other prostheses are removed for the client's safety during surgery. The nurse pays special attention to the removal of dentures, because the denture plate could become loose and obstruct the client's airway during surgery. Occasionally, the anesthesiology team may request that the dentures be left in place to ensure a snug fit of the anesthesia mask. In some facilities, clients may be permitted to retain their eyeglasses and hearing aids until after the induction phase of anesthesia.

► Chart Review

The circulating nurse and anesthesia personnel review the client's chart in the holding area (or in the operating room if there is no holding area). The chart provides information needed to identify potential and actual needs of the client during the intraoperative period and allows the circulating nurse to assess and plan for the client's needs during and after surgery. The client's chart is a primary source of information on the type and location of the planned surgical procedure. A check of the chart ensures that all required data are present before the procedure is begun.

Allergies and Previous Reactions to Anesthesia or Transfusions

In reviewing the chart, the nurse asks the client about allergies and previous reactions to anesthesia or blood transfusions. Allergies or sensitivity to iodine products or shellfish may indicate the potential for a reaction to the antimicrobial agents used to clean the surgical area. The nurse clearly indicates the allergies on the chart and notifies the operating room (OR) team. The client's previous experience with anesthesia helps the nurse and anesthesiologist or CRNA plan and anticipate the client's needs. For example, if a client is restless or agitated as a reaction to anesthesia, the nurse can have padding for the stretcher side rails and protective restraints available. The use of blood and blood products during surgery may be influenced by the client's history, religious beliefs or preferences, and type of transfusion reaction in the past.

Autologous Blood Transfusion

Increasingly, autologous blood transfusion (reinfusing the client's own blood) is being used for surgery. This method of blood transfusion eliminates the risk of acquiring blood-borne infections, such as hepatitis B and human immunodeficiency virus (HIV), from another person. Chapter 20 discusses autologous blood transfusion in more detail, and Chart 21–2 outlines key points of intraoperative autologous blood transfusion.

Laboratory and Diagnostic Test Results

The OR nurse reviews preoperative laboratory and diagnostic test results. The nurse assesses most recent laboratory results to inform the surgical team about the client's medical condition and to alert them to potential intraoperative and postoperative interventions. The most recent results are usually obtained within 24 to 28 hours before surgery for hospitalized clients and within 2 weeks for ambulatory surgery clients. The nurse reports all abnormalities to the surgeon and anesthesiologist or CRNA. Laboratory values significantly greater than or less than the normal range are potentially life-threatening for any client, but especially for the client undergoing surgery (see Chap. 20). For example, if the hemoglobin concentration is less than 10 g/dL, the client's oxygen transport capacity is lessened; this condition affects the amount and type of anesthesia used and the potential impact of blood loss during surgery.

Medical History and Physical Examination Findings

The OR nurse checks that the client's medical history and examination findings, including usual pulse and blood pressure, are recorded. This information provides the circulating nurse, surgeon, anesthesiologist and/or CRNA, and postanesthesia care unit (PACU) nurse with baseline data to assess the client's reaction to the surgical procedure and anesthesia. Medications the client has routinely taken preoperatively may affect the client's reaction to surgery and wound healing. For example, aspirin has an anticoagulant effect and can cause increased clotting time and danger of hemorrhage.

Knowing the client's medical history and age (Chart 21–3) allows the nurse to take special precautions and plan appropriate interventions for the care and safety of high-risk clients. The nurse carefully monitors elderly clients and those with cardiac disease for potential fluid overload, which can be life-threatening.

After completing the chart review, the nurse may insert an intravenous catheter and perform a surgical shave. The circulating nurse provides additional emotional support and explains procedures to the client. The client is never left unattended. If the client is in the holding area, he or she is transferred to the OR after the preoperative routine is completed.

Chart 21–2

Nursing Care Highlight: Intraoperative Autologous Blood Salvage and Transfusion

- Be aware of the cell-processing method to be used.
- Make sure that collection containers are labeled for the client.
- Assist with sterile set-up as necessary.
- Assist with processing and reinfusing procedures as needed.
- Document the transfusion process.
- Monitor the client's vital signs during the transfusion procedure.

Chart 21–3

Nursing Focus on the Elderly: Intraoperative Nursing Interventions

- Allow clients to retain eyeglasses and hearing aids until anesthesia has been administered.
- Use a small pillow under the client's head if his or her head and neck are normally bent slightly forward.
- Lift clients into position to prevent shearing forces on fragile skin.
- Position arthritic and artificial joints carefully to prevent postoperative pain and discomfort from strain on those joints.
- Pad bony prominences to prevent pressure sores.
- Provide extra padding for those clients with decreased peripheral circulation.
- Use head caps to prevent heat loss through the scalp.
- Place stockinette on extremities to conserve body heat.
- Warm prepping solutions and intravenous and irrigation fluids as indicated.
- Follow strict aseptic technique.
- Carefully monitor intake and output, including blood loss.

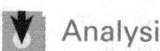 Analysis

> ### Common Nursing Diagnoses and Collaborative Problems

Common nursing diagnoses for intraoperative clients include

1. Risk for Perioperative Positioning Injury related to immobilization and effects of anesthesia
2. Impaired Skin Integrity and Impaired Tissue Integrity related to the surgical incision

A common collaborative problem for the intraoperative client is Potential for Hypoventilation.

> ### Additional Nursing Diagnoses and Collaborative Problems

Additional nursing diagnoses and collaborative problems may apply to intraoperative clients:

- Risk for Infection related to break in skin integrity, i.e., incision, invasive lines
- Risk for Injury related to fire and electrical hazards within the operating environment
- Risk for Disuse Syndrome related to decreased level of consciousness or to immobilization
- Hypothermia related to evaporation from skin and exposed tissue in a cool environment, body heat loss, alteration in the hypothalamus from anesthetic agents, inadequate body covering, or aging
- Ineffective Thermoregulation related to sedation, fluctuating environmental temperature, medications, or age extremes
- Fear related to threat of death, actual or perceived, or to anticipation of events posing a threat to self-esteem
- Anxiety related to loss of control or threat of death
- Fluid Volume Deficit related to decreased intake, evaporative fluid loss through the skin and exposed tissue, or blood loss
- Potential for Peripheral Nerve Damage related to intraoperative positioning

 Planning and Implementation

> ### Risk for Perioperative Positioning Injury

Planning: Expected Outcomes. The primary goal is for the client to be free of injury.

Interventions. Interventions are directed toward preventing injury resulting from intraoperative positioning.

Because of preoperative medication, anesthetic agents, and the narrowness of the bed, the client's normal defense mechanisms cannot guard against nerve or joint damage and muscle stretch and strain. Proper positioning, therefore, is important. The circulating nurse pads the operating bed with foam and/or silicone gel pads, properly places the grounding pads, coordinates the transfer of the client to the operating bed, and helps the client obtain a comfortable position. The circulating nurse assesses

the skin, especially of the elderly, for bruising or injury, placing extra padding as indicated.

The client is usually in a dorsal recumbent (supine) position after transfer to the operating bed. Anesthesia may be administered with the client supine, and the client may be repositioned for surgery. When general anesthesia is used, the nurse repositions the client after he or she is in stage 3 (see Table 21–2).

The circulating nurse coordinates repositioning of the client for surgery and modifies the position according to the client's safety and special needs. Factors influencing the *timing* of repositioning include

- The surgical site
- The age and size of client
- Anesthetic administration technique
- Pain experienced by the conscious client on movement

Factors influencing the actual *position* include

- The specific procedure being performed
- The surgeon's request
- The client's age, size, and weight
- Any respiratory, skeletal, or neuromuscular limitations, such as rheumatoid arthritis, joint replacements, or emphysema

Table 21–6 presents possible complications related to prolonged surgical immobility and preventive nursing actions.

The dorsal recumbent, prone, lithotomy, and lateral positions are frequently used for surgery. Figure 21–12 illustrates common surgical positions and the use of protective padding. When general anesthesia is used, the nurse positions the client slowly to prevent vasogenic hypotension. The nurse ensures proper positioning by assessing for

- Physiologic alignment
- Minimal interference with circulation and respiration
- Protection of skeletal and neuromuscular structures
- Optimal exposure of the operative site and intravenous line
- Adequate access to the client for the anesthesiologist or CRNA
- The client's comfort and safety
- Preservation of the client's dignity

The nurse must be aware of potential complications related to specific positions and modifies care as indicated. For example, clients in lithotomy position may develop leg swelling, pain in the legs or back, and diminished sensation or pulses. The nurse ensures proper padding and position changes at regular intervals. Throughout the intraoperative period, the nurse assists in preventing obstruction of circulatory, respiratory, or neurologic systems caused by tight straps, improperly placed pads and pillows, or position of the bed.

> ### Impaired Skin Integrity and Impaired Tissue Integrity

Planning: Expected Outcomes. The primary goal is that the client will experience minimal skin and tissue impairment and contamination as a result of surgery.

TABLE 21-6

Interventions to Prevent Neuromuscular Complications Related to Intraoperative Positioning

Anatomic Area	Complications	Interventions
Brachial plexus	• Paralysis • Loss of sensation in the arm and shoulder	• Pad the elbow. • Avoid excessive abduction. • Secure the arm firmly on an arm board, positioned at shoulder level.
Radial nerve	• Wrist drop	• Support the wrist with padding. • Do not overtighten wrist straps.
Medial or ulnar nerves	• Hand deformities	• Place a safety strap above or below area.
Peroneal nerve	• Foot drop	• Place pillow or padding under knees. • Support lower extremities. • Do not overtighten leg straps.
Tibial nerve	• Loss of sensation on the plantar surface of the foot	• Place a safety strap above the ankle. • Do not place equipment on lower extremities.
Joints	• Stiffness • Pain • Inflammation	• Place pillow or foam padding under bony prominences. • Maintain good body alignment. • Slightly flex joints and support with pillows, trochanter rolls, or pads.

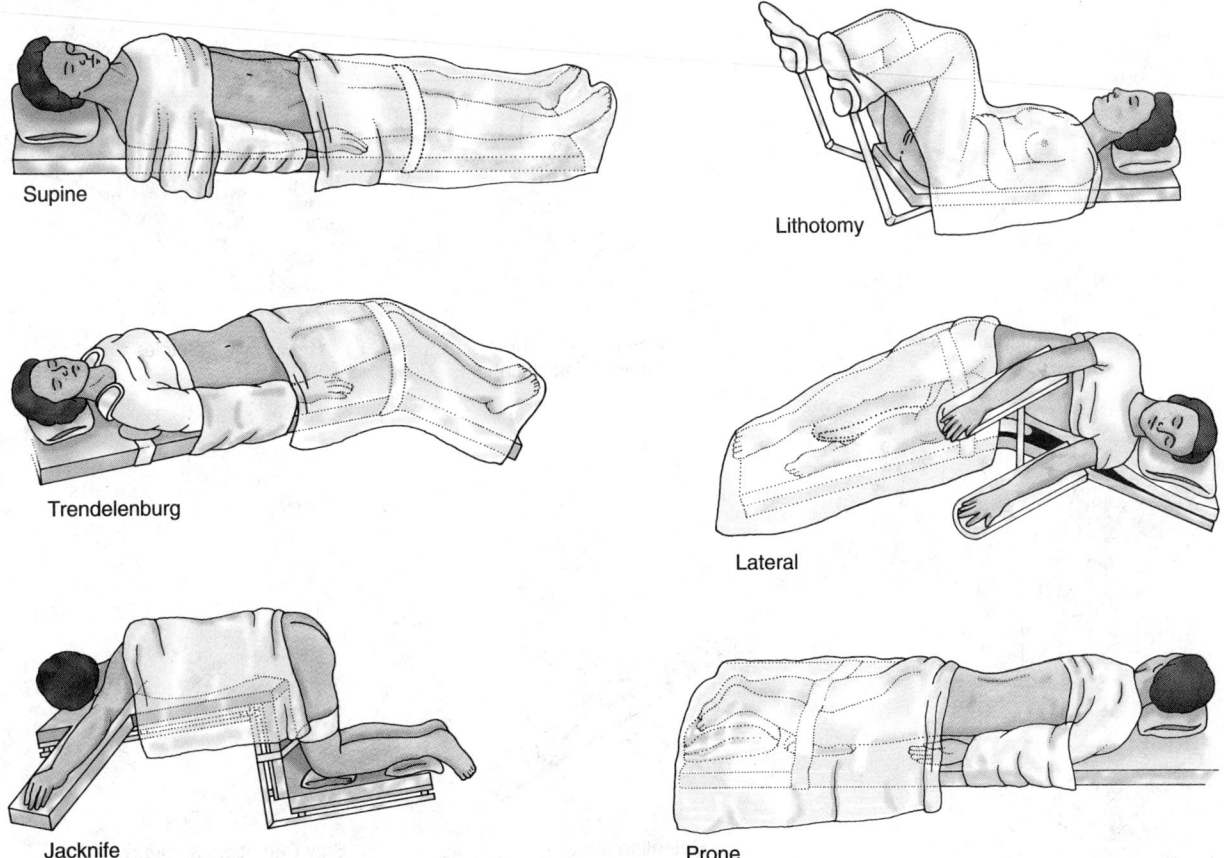

Supine

Lithotomy

Trendelenburg

Lateral

Jacknife

Prone

Figure 21–12. Common surgical positions.

Interventions. Surgery is an invasive procedure that places the client at risk for complications related to the surgical wound (such as incisional tears and lacerations), bacterial contamination, and loss of body fluids from the wound during and after surgery. Sterile surgical technique and the use of protective drapes, skin closures, and dressings help to minimize complications and promote wound healing.

Plastic Adhesive Drapes. If a sterile plastic adhesive drape is used, the scrub nurse helps the surgical assistant apply the drape after the surgical site has been cleaned and dried. The plastic drape is applied directly to the client's skin to prevent shifting and exposure of skin edges. The surgeon makes the incision through the plastic drape. The cut edge remains adherent to the skin and keeps the surgical incision sealed from the migration of bacteria into the wound. The scrub nurse and surgical assistant *gently* remove the drape after closure of the surgical incision. The nurse pays special attention to the elderly and to clients with fragile skin to prevent skin tearing when the adhesive drape is removed.

Skin Closures. Skin and tissue closures, such as sutures and staples, are used for several reasons:

- To approximate wound edges until wound healing is complete
- To occlude the lumen of blood vessels, preventing hemorrhage and loss of body fluids
- To prevent wound contamination

The quality of the approximated tissue and the type of closure material are two factors that determine the strength and integrity of the closure. The wound is usually closed in layers to maintain tissue integrity and promote healing with minimal scarring. The surgeon selects the method and type of closures to be used on the basis of the surgical site, the tissue involved, the size and depth of the surgical wound, and the age and medical history of the client. A combination of sutures and clips is commonly used for closure of internal layers of the wound. Staples, stay and retention sutures, and skin closure tapes (Steri-Strips) are used for closure of superficial wounds of the epidermis. Figure 21–13 illustrates commonly used wound closures.

A suture consists of one or more strands of material and is designated by its size, or gauge. The size designation sequence, from largest diameter to smallest, is 5, 4, 3, 2, 1, 0, 2-0, 3-0, 4-0, and so forth, to 11-0. Size 5 may be used to close the deep layers of an abdominal wound; 11-0 is the smallest-diameter suture and is used in plastic surgery and ophthalmology. Other characteristics of the suture material, such as type (nylon, silk, Vicryl), color (e.g., green, blue, black, white, violet), and structure (twisted, braided), are often listed on the package.

Suture material can be absorbable or nonabsorbable. *Absorbable* sutures are digested over time by body enzymes. These sutures first lose strength and then gradually disappear from the tissue. Catgut suture, such as "plain gut" and "chromic gut," was a common type of

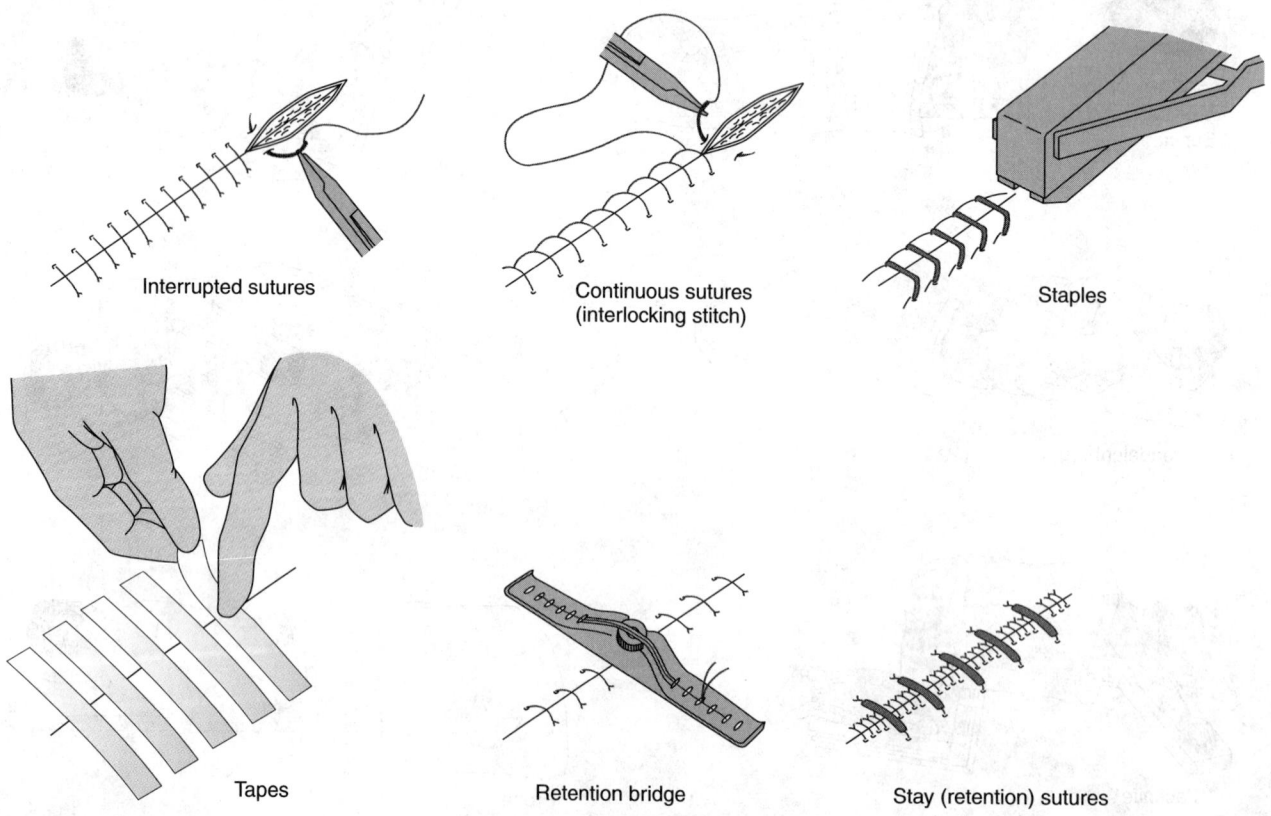

Interrupted sutures

Continuous sutures
(interlocking stitch)

Staples

Tapes

Retention bridge

Stay (retention) sutures

Figure 21–13. Common skin closures.

absorbable suture material that is still in use today, although not as frequently as it once was. Other absorbable sutures are made of synthetics and are labeled as such on the package. The client's physical status, the presence of inflammation, and the type of suture used all influence the rate of absorption, which is usually up to about 2 weeks.

Nonabsorbable sutures are not affected by body enzymes. Nonabsorbable sutures become encapsulated in the tissue during the healing process and remain embedded in the tissue unless they are removed. These sutures are made of silk, cotton, steel, nylon, polyester, or other synthetic material. Nonabsorbable sutures are used for vascular anastomosis, "wiring" the sternum together after open heart surgery, and closing external wounds. The surgeon may use a double or interlocking stitch to increase the integrity of the closure. Retention and stay sutures (see Fig. 21–13) may be used in addition to standard suture material for high-risk clients (those having major abdominal surgery, obese clients, diabetic clients, and clients taking steroids, which inhibit wound healing).

After the incision is closed, the physician may inject a local anesthetic or instill an antibiotic into the wound. A gauze or spray dressing may be applied to protect it from contamination. A variety of dressings may also be used to absorb drainage and provide support to the incision. A pressure dressing may be applied to prevent or stop a vascular area from bleeding postoperatively. One or more drains (see Chap. 22) may be inserted to prevent the accumulation of secretions within tissues around the surgical area. These secretions, if not drained, impede healing and serve as a medium for bacterial growth, which could result in wound infection.

After the dressing is secure, the nurse coordinates the surgical team in repositioning and transferring the client as indicated. A roller board or a lift sheet is used to transfer the client safely from the operating bed to a stretcher or bed. The circulating nurse and anesthesiologist or certified registered nurse anesthetist (CRNA) accompany the client to the postanesthesia care unit (PACU) and give a report of the client's intraoperative experience to the PACU nurse (see Chap. 22).

➤ *Potential for Hypoventilation*

Planning: Expected Outcomes. The primary goal is for the client to be free of damaging events related to hypoventilation.

Interventions. Interventions are directed toward preventing injury resulting from anesthesia (see earlier). The nurse, physician, and anesthesiologist or CRNA monitor the client according to official standards. These standards, which have been adopted by both the American Society of Anesthesiologists and the American Association of Nurse Anesthetists, include continuous monitoring of ventilation, circulation, and cardiac rhythms; blood pressure and heart rate recordings every 5 minutes; and the continuous presence of an anesthesiology practitioner during the case (Biddle, 1994).

 Evaluation

On the basis of identified nursing diagnoses, collaborative problems, and desired outcomes, the nurse evaluates the care of the intraoperative client and ensures that the client

- Is safely anesthetized without complications
- Does not experience any injury related to intraoperative positioning or equipment
- Is free of skin or tissue contamination during surgery
- Is free of skin tears, bruises, redness, abrasion, or maceration over pressure points and elsewhere

 CASE STUDY for the Intraoperative Client

■ You are an operating room nurse having lunch in the hospital cafeteria with one of your friends who works in the open-heart surgery unit. He says to you, "Boy, we seem to get a lot of patients out of the OR with skin breakdown on the back of their heads." On further discussion, he tells you that most often the breakdown is black eschar.

QUESTIONS:

1. Is it possible that these patients developed the skin breakdown while in the operating suite? Why or why not?
2. What should you do with the information your friend passed on to you and why?
3. How could this situation have been prevented?

SELECTED BIBLIOGRAPHY

Atkinson, L. J. (1996). *Berry & Kohn's operating room technique* (8th ed.). St. Louis: Mosby–Year Book.

Ball, K. A. (1995). *Lasers: The perioperative challenge* (2nd ed.). St. Louis: C. V. Mosby.

*Ball, K. A. (1990). The basics of laser technology. *Nursing Clinics of North America, 25*(3), 619–634.

Ballantyne, G. H., Leahy, P. F., & Modlin, I. M. (1994). *Laparoscopic surgery*. Philadelphia: W. B. Saunders Co.

Beck, C. F. (1994). Malignant hyperthermia: Are you prepared? *AORN Journal, 59*(2), 367, 370–372, 374–378+.

Berkowitz, C. M. (1997). Conscious sedation: A primer. *RN. 60*(2), 32–36.

Biddle, C. (1994). AANA journal course: Update for nurse anesthetists—outcome measures in anesthesiology: Are we going in the right direction? *American Association of Nurse Anesthetists Journal, 62*(2), 117–124.

Boike, L., et al. (1995). Development of an outpatient perioperative care record. *Journal of Post Anesthesia Nursing, 10*(3), 140–150.

Brown, K. A. (1997). Malignant hyperthermia. *American Journal of Nursing, 97*(10), 33.

*Bruton-Maree, N. (1990). Anesthesia and the aging population. *CRNA, 1*(1), 25–31.

*Burden, N. (1988). Post-anesthesia: While the patient is unconscious. *RN, 51*(4), 34–44.

Clinch, C. (1996). Pressure area care in one operating theatre. *British Journal Theatre Nursing, 6*(3), 25–27.

Corey-Plett, P. (1994). Fluid replacement therapy and perioperative management. *Canadian Operating Room Nursing Journal, 12*(4), 18–21.

*Cruz, L. D. (1991). A history of the RN first assistant. *AORN Journal,* 53(6), 1536–1537.

Curry, M. (1994). Perioperative nursing care of the elderly patient: A case study. *ACORN Journal,* 7(2), 23–26.

*Davidhizar, R. (1992). When patients die in the operating room. *Today's OR Nurse,* 14(1), 4.

*Davidson, J. E. (1991). Neuromuscular blockade. *Focus on Critical Care—AACN,* 18(6), 512–520.

*Dellasega, C., & Burgunder, C. (1991). Perioperative nursing care of the elderly surgical patient. *Today's OR Nurse,* 13(6), 12–17.

Dougherty, J. (1996). Same-day surgery: The nurse's role. *Orthopedic Nursing,* 15(4), 15–18.

Dunn, D. (1997). Malignant hyperthermia. *AORN Journal,* 65(4), 728–762.

*Entrup, M. H. (1991). Perioperative complications of anesthesia. *Surgical Clinics of North America,* 71(6), 1151–1173.

Fawcett, D. L., et al. (1996). A pilot study appraising the climate for perioperative research. *AORN Journal,* 63(1), 205–208.

*Fiesta, J. (1992). Anesthesia-related liability. *Nursing Management,* 23(10), 28–30.

Fogg, D. M. (1996). Clinical issues. Length of sterile drapes; counts; alcohol skin preps; food and drink in ORs; houseplants in OR lounges. *AORN Journal,* 63(1), 262–264, 267.

*Gallagher, M. T., & Kahn, C. (1990). Lasers: Scalpels of light. *RN,* 53(5), 46–53.

Gerber, D. E., et al. (1995). Death in the operating room and postanesthesia care unit: Helping nurses to cope. *Journal of Post Anesthesia Nursing,* 10(2), 84–88.

Gillette, V. A. (1996). Applying nursing theory to perioperative nursing practice. *AORN Journal,* 64(2), 261–264, 267–268, 270.

Golanowski, M. (1995). Do not resuscitate: Informed consent in the operating room and postanesthesia care unit. *Journal of Post Anesthesia Nursing,* 10(1), 9–11.

Green, S. (1996). Positioning the patient for surgery. *British Journal Theatre Nursing,* 6(5), 35–38.

Gruendemann, B. J., & Fernsebner, B. (1995). *Comprehensive perioperative nursing.* Sudbury, MA: Jones & Bartlett.

Haney, P. E., Raymond, B. A., Hernandez, J. M., et al. (1996). Tuberculosis makes a comeback. *AORN Journal,* 63(4), 705, 707, 709, 713–715.

Hankela, S., et al. (1996). Intraoperative nursing care as experienced by surgical patients. *AORN Journal,* 63(2), 435–442.

Hussar, D. A. (1997). New drugs (ropivacaine HCl). *Nursing97,* 27(6), 38.

*Hussar, D. A. (1992). New drugs (mivacurium chloride). *Nursing92,* 22(12), 61.

*Jackson, M. F. (1989). Implications of surgery in very elderly patients. *AORN Journal,* 50(4), 859–869.

*Jarpe, M. B. (1992). Nursing care of patients receiving long-term infusion of neuromuscular blocking agents. *Critical Care Nurse,* 12(7), 58–63.

*Johnson, G. M., & Bowman, R. J. (1992). Autologous blood transfusion. *AORN Journal,* 56(2), 282–298.

Jonasen, A. M. (1994). Therapeutic touch: A holistic approach to perioperative nursing. *Today's OR Nurse,* 16(1), 7–12, 50–51.

*Keene, A. (1991). Perioperative assessment and nursing implications for the elderly. *Plastic Surgical Nursing,* 11(4), 143–167.

Keffer, M. J. & Keffer, H. L. (1994). The do-not-resuscitate order: Moral responsibilities of the perioperative nurse. *AORN Journal,* 59(3), 641–650.

Kobs, A. (1997). Conscious sedation: Questions about the anesthesia continuum. *Nursing Management,* 28(4), 14, 17.

Leske, J. S. (1995). Effects of intraoperative progress reports on anxiety levels of surgical patients' family members. *Applied Nursing Research,* 8(4), 169–173.

Leske, J. S. (1996). Intraoperative progress reports decrease family members' anxiety. *AORN Journal,* 64(3), 424–436.

Ley, S. J. (1996). Intraoperative and postoperative blood salvage. *AACN Clinical Issues in Advanced Practice of Acute Critical Care,* 7(2), 238–248.

McCraine, J. (1994). Fire safety in the operating room. *Today's OR Nurse,* 16(1), 33–37.

McEwen, D. R. (1996). Intraoperative positioning of surgical patients. *AORN Journal,* 63(6), 1059–1063, 1066–1075, 1077–1082, 1084–1085.

Meckes, P. F. (1995). Geriatric surgery. In M. H. Meeker & J. Rothrock (Eds.), *Alexander's care of the patient in surgery* (10th ed., pp. 1195–1209). St. Louis: Mosby–Year Book.

Meeker, M. H., & Rothrock, J. (1995). *Alexander's care of the patient in surgery* (10th ed.). St. Louis: Mosby–Year Book.

Miller, R. D. (1994). *Anesthesia* (Vols. 1 & 2, 4th ed.). New York: Churchill Livingstone.

*Moore, J. L., & Rice, E. L. (1992). Malignant hyperthermia. *American Family Physician,* 45(5), 2245–2251.

Moss, M. T. (1995). Perioperative nursing in the managed care era. Collaborative relationships in the operating room part II—hospitals and nurses: Strategies of partnership. *Nursing Economics,* 13(5), 310, 313.

*Murphy, E. K. (1991). Liability for injury resulting from poor patient positioning. *AORN Journal,* 53(6), 1361–1365.

Null, S., et al. (1995). Development of a perioperative nursing diagnoses flow sheet. *AORN Journal,* 61(3), 547–550.

Nussbaum, W., et al. (1994). Perioperative challenges in the care of the Jehovah's Witness: A case report. *American Association of Nurse Anesthetists Journal,* 62(2), 160–164.

Omoigui, S. (1995). *The anesthesia drugs handbook* (2nd ed.). St. Louis: Mosby–Year Book.

Ouellette, R. G. (1994). Perioperative hypothermia. *Current Reviews For Nurse Anesthetists,* 16(22), 195–200.

Palmerini, J. (1996). Practical innovations. Developing a comprehensive perioperative nursing documentation form. *AORN Journal,* 63(1), 239–242, 245–247.

Patient outcomes: Standards of perioperative care (1997). *AORN Journal,* 65(2), 408–416.

Paulson, D. S. (1994). Comparative evaluation of five surgical hand scrub preparations. *AORN Journal,* 60(2), 249, 251–256.

Pearlman, R. C., et al. (1994). Intraoperative neural monitoring: An introduction for perioperative nurses . . . to determine whether nerve impulses are being conducted at normal levels. *AORN Journal,* 60(4), 648, 650–651.

*Pereira, L. J., Lee, S. M., & Wade, K. J. (1990). The effect of surgical handwashing routines on the microbial counts of operating room nurses. *American Journal of Infection Control,* 18(6), 354–364.

*Peterson, K. J. (1992). Nursing management of autologous blood transfusion. *Journal of Intravenous Nursing,* 15(3), 128–134.

*Polis, S. L. (1992). Competency-based laser education: Its implementation in the OR. *AORN Journal,* 55(2), 567–572.

Position statement: AORN position statement on perioperative care of patients with do-not-resuscitate (DNR) orders (1995). *AORN Journal,* 61(6), 954–955.

Position statement: AORN recommended education standards for RN first assistant programs (1995). *AORN Journal,* 61(3), 476–478.

Prior, L. (1996). Caring for patients from ethnic minority groups. *British Journal Theatre Nursing,* 6(3), 28–30.

*Proposed recommended practices—disinfection (1991). *AORN Journal,* 54(1), 75–80.

Proposed recommended practices for establishing and maintaining a sterile field (1996). *AORN Journal,* 63(1), 211, 213–218.

Proposed recommended practices for sterilization in the practice setting (1994). *AORN Journal,* 60(1), 109–110, 112–117, 119–120.

Proposed recommended practices for surgical attire (1994). *AORN Journal,* 60(1), 282, 284–286, 289–290+.

Proposed recommended practices for surgical hand scrubs (1994). *AORN Journal,* 60(2), 270, 273–274, 276, 279.

Proposed recommended practices for surgical skin preparation (1996). *AORN Journal,* 63(1), 221–224, 227–228.

Pursell, S. (1996). The role of the OR nurse in relation to HIV. *ACORN Journal,* 9(1), 23–24, 26–28.

*Ratner, L. E., & Smith, G. W. (1993). Intraoperative fluid management. *Surgical Clinics of North America,* 73(2), 229–241.

*Recommended practices: Aseptic technique (1991). *AORN Journal,* 54(4), 819–824.

Recommended practices: Documentation of perioperative nursing care (1996). *AORN Journal,* 63(6), 1145, 1148.

Recommended practices: Environmental cleaning for the surgical practice setting (1996). *AORN Journal,* 64(4), 611–615.

Recommended practices for the care and cleaning of surgical instruments and powered equipment (1997). *AORN Journal,* 65(1), 124–128.

Recommended practices for managing the patient receiving conscious sedation/analgesia (1997). *AORN Journal,* 65(1), 129–134.

*Recommended practices: Laser safety in the practice setting (1993). *AORN Journal, 58*(5), 1027–1031.

Recommended practices: Positioning the patient in the perioperative practice setting (1996). *AORN Journal, 64*(2), 278, 281–284.

Recommended practices: Safe care through identification of potential hazards in the surgical environment (1996). *AORN Journal, 63*(4), 802–806.

Recommended practices: Sponge, sharp, and instrument counts (1996). *AORN Journal, 64*(4), 616, 618–622.

Recommended practices: Traffic patterns in the perioperative practice setting (1996). *AORN Journal, 63*(3), 655–656, 658.

*Recommended practices: Universal precautions in the perioperative practice setting (1993). *AORN Journal, 57*(2), 554–558.

Recommended practices: Use and selection of barrier materials for surgical gowns and drapes (1996). *AORN Journal, 63*(3), 650, 653–654.

*Reeder, J. M. (1993). Do-not-resuscitate orders in the operating room. *AORN Journal, 57*(4), 947–951.

*Revised AORN official statement on RN first assistants (1993). *AORN Journal, 57*(1), 47–51.

Ringler, J. D. (1995). The use of diazepam and ketamine for IV conscious sedation in outpatient surgery settings. *AORN Journal, 62*(4), 638–645.

Roth, R. A. (1995). *Perioperative nursing core curriculum: Achieving competency in clinical practice.* Philadelphia: W. B. Saunders.

Rothrock, J. C. (1996). *Perioperative nursing care planning* (2nd ed.). St. Louis: Mosby–Year Book.

*Rowell, C. C. (1990). The nosocomial wound infection report: Its impact in the OR. *Today's OR Nurse, 12*(10), 21–23, 50–51.

*Rivelli, D. (1993). Local and regional anesthesia: Nursing implications. *Nursing Clinics of North America, 28*(3), 547–572.

*Scott, S. M., Mayhew, P. A., & Harris, E. A. (1992). Pressure ulcer development in the operating room: Nursing implications. *AORN Journal, 56*(2), 242–250.

*Smalley, P. J. (1992). Laser nursing—a perioperative challenge. *Canadian Operating Room Nursing Journal, 10*(1), 18–22+.

Smith, C. J. (1994). Preparing nurses to monitor patients receiving local anesthesia: Using the decision-making process. *AORN Journal, 59*(5), 1033, 1036–1041.

*Smith, K. A. (1990). Positioning principles: An anatomical review. *AORN Journal, 52*(6), 1196, 1198, 1200–1202+.

Somerson, S. J., et al. (1995). Insights into conscious sedation. *American Journal of Nursing, 95*(6), 26–33.

Standards and recommended practices for perioperative nursing (1996). Denver, CO: Association of Operating Room Nurses.

Standards: Perioperative nursing care. The function of the nurse as first assistant (1995). *Canadian Operating Room Nursing Journal, 13*(2), 25–28.

Stein, R. H. (1995). The perioperative nurse's role in anesthesia management. *AORN Journal, 62*(5), 794–795, 797–797, 801+.

*Stephens, G. (1992). Technology and its effect on OR nursing. *Canadian Operating Room Nursing Journal, 10*(1), 6–7.

*Takes, K. L. (1992). Cost-effective practice: Do OR nurses care? *Nursing Management, 23*(4), 96Q–R, V–X.

*Tappen, R. M. (1991). Alzheimer's disease: Communication techniques to facilitate perioperative care. *AORN Journal, 54*(6), 1279–1286.

Tappen, R. M., et al. (1996). Inadvertent hypothermia in elderly surgical patients. *AORN Journal, 63*(3), 639–644.

*Thomas, S. D. (1989). Malignant hyperthermia. *Critical Care Nurse, 3*(6), 58–69.

Thompson, J. (1996). AORN's multisite clinical study of bloodborne exposures in OR personnel. *AORN Journal, 63*(2), 428–430, 433.

*Treat, M. R., Oz, Mehmet C., & Bass, L. S. (1992). New technologies and future applications of surgical lasers: The right tool for the right job. *Surgical Clinics of North America, 72*(3), 705–742.

Walsh, J. (1994). AANA journal course: Update for nurse anesthetists—patient positioning. *American Association of Nurse Anesthetists Journal, 62*(3), 289–298.

*Walsh, J. (1993). Postop effects of OR positioning. *RN, 56*(2), 50–57.

*Watson, D. S. (1991). Safe nursing practices involving the patient receiving local anesthesia. *AORN Journal, 53*(4), 1055, 1058–1059.

Watson, D. S., & Sangermano, C. A. (1995). Ambulatory surgery. In M. H. Meeker & J. Rothrock (Eds.), *Alexander's care of the patient in surgery* (10th ed., pp. 1125–1144). St. Louis: Mosby–Year Book.

Wheelock, S. M., & Lookinland, S. (1997). Effect of surgical hand scrub time on subsequent bacterial growth. *AORN Journal, 65*(6), 1087–1090, 1092, 1094–1098.

Williams, M. (1996). The expanding role of the nurse in laparoscopic surgery. *British Journal Theatre Nursing, 6*(4), 34–35.

Wilson, L. (1995). Continuous quality improvement: A staff nurse perspective. *Canadian Operating Room Nursing Journal, 13*(1), 29–33.

Winter, M. J. (1994). Music reduces stress and anxiety of patients in the surgical holding area. *Journal of Post Anesthesia Nursing, 9*(6), 340–343.

Woodin, L. M. (1996). Resting easy. How to care for patients receiving I.V. conscious sedation. *Nursing96, 26*(6), 33–41.

Wound closure manual (1994). Somerville, NJ: Ethicon. (Pub. No. EPB010).

Wynd, C. A., et al. (1994). Bacterial carriage on the fingernails of OR nurses. *AORN Journal, 60*(5), 796, 799–805.

*Young, M. A., Meyers, M., McCulloch, L. D., et al. (1992). Latex allergy: A guideline for perioperative nurses. *AORN Journal, 56*(3), 485–497.

SUGGESTED READINGS

Dunn, D. (1997). Malignant hyperthermia. *AORN Journal, 65*(4), 728–762.

This very comprehensive and current article on malignant hyperthermia discusses pathophysiology, incidence, triggering agents, signs and symptoms, crisis management, testing for susceptibility, preparedness for an episode of malignant hyperthermia, and future research considerations. Numerous tables and charts help the reader comprehend the topic. A case study, numerous references, and a continuing education test are included.

McEwen, D. R. (1996). Intraoperative positioning of surgical patients. *AORN Journal, 63*(6), 1059–1063, 1066–1075, 1077–1082, 1084–1085.

The positioning injuries of pressure ulcers (occiput), alopecia, nerve injuries, and respiratory and cardiovascular compromise are discussed in this article. An extensive table outlining upper and lower extremity neuropathies associated with intraoperative positioning and how to correctly position to prevent these injuries is included. Risk factors, positioning considerations, and positioning devices are all addressed. Positioning devices needed to prevent specific injuries in the supine, prone, lateral, sitting, and lithotomy positions are detailed. The article concludes with a 38-item reference list and a 40-question CEU test.

Woodin, L. M. (1996). Resting easy. How to care for patients receiving I.V. conscious sedation. *Nursing96, 26*(6), 33–41.

This comprehensive article on intravenous conscious sedation follows an outpatient having an esophageal gastric dilation and biopsy. General indications for conscious sedation, as well as specific preprocedural nursing assessments, are included. The opioids and benzodiazepines and their antagonists and monitoring related to these medications are discussed in detail. Appropriate emergency responses to potential complications are addressed. A 13-item CEU test is included.

INTERVENTIONS FOR POSTOPERATIVE CLIENTS

The postoperative period begins with completion of the surgical procedure. Ambulatory surgery clients who had local anesthesia may be able to be discharged home. Clients who received conscious sedation will move to a quiet area where they can be observed and monitored until discharge criteria are met. Other clients move from the operating room (OR) to another area for specialized nursing care (often a postanesthesia care unit [PACU]), until their condition stabilizes. The postoperative period continues after the client's condition is stabilized and after the client is discharged from the ambulatory surgery facility or hospital. The actual time spent away from home after surgery varies according to the client's age, physical health, self-care ability, support systems, type and length of surgical procedure, anesthesia, complications (if any), and community resources.

Overview

The postanesthesia care unit is usually located close to the operating department. The unit is usually a large and open room to provide maximal visibility of clients, appropriate ventilation and lighting, and easy access to supplies and emergency equipment. The client area in the unit is often divided into individual cubicles. Curtains or screens for privacy are available but are usually closed only during bedside procedures. Each cubicle is stocked with equipment and supplies commonly used by the nurse to monitor and care for the client, such as oxygen, suction equipment, cardiac monitors, airway equipment, and emergency medications.

After the surgical procedure is completed, the circulating nurse and the anesthesiologist or nurse anesthetist (certified registered nurse anesthetist, or CRNA) accompany the client to the PACU. In some situations, such as when the client is in critical condition, he or she may go directly from the operating department to the intensive (critical) care unit. On arrival, anesthesiology personnel and the circulating nurse give the postanesthesia nurse a verbal report (Table 22–1).

The postanesthesia nurse is skilled in the care of clients of all ages with multiple medical and surgical problems immediately after surgery. This nurse has in-depth knowledge of anesthetic agents, analgesics, pain management, and surgical procedures; is skilled in physical and psychosocial assessment; and can make quick decisions if emergencies or complications occur. The postanesthesia nurse monitors the client closely and consults with the anesthesiology personnel and the surgeons as needed.

TABLE 22–1

Report Guidelines on Arrival in the Postanesthesia Care Unit

Anesthesiology personnel explain the following:
- Type and extent of the surgical procedure
- Type of anesthesia
- Client's tolerance of anesthesia and the surgical procedure
- Client's allergies
- Pathologic condition
- Status of vital signs
- Type and amount of intravenous fluids and medications administered
- Estimated blood loss (EBL)
- Any intraoperative complications, such as a traumatic intubation

The circulating nurse adds information related to
- Client's primary language spoken and any sensory impairments
- Client's anxiety level before receiving anesthesia
- Special requests that were verbalized by the client preoperatively
- Client's preoperative and intraoperative respiratory function and dysfunction
- Pertinent medical history
- Location and type of incisions, dressings, catheters, tubes, drains, or packing
- Intake and output, including current intravenous fluid administration and estimated blood loss
- Joint or limb immobility while in the operating room, especially in the elderly client
- Other intraoperative positioning that may be relevant in the postoperative phase
- Any other important intraoperative occurrences

Collaborative Management

 Assessment

➤ History

The postanesthesia nurse uses the information from the surgical team's report in planning care for the client. After receiving the report and assessing the client, the PACU nurse reviews the chart for information about the client's history and his or her presurgical physical and emotional status. In ideal situations, the postanesthesia nurse reviews pertinent information before the client arrives in the unit. If the client is remaining as an inpatient, the nurse on the medical-surgical unit later incorporates all of the surgical and postanesthesia information into the client's postoperative plan of care. Chapter 20 identifies clinical situations that put a client at risk for the following postoperative complications:

- Allergic reactions
- Hypothermia
- Hyperthermia
- Hypertension
- Hypotension

- Hypovolemic shock
- Renal failure
- Electrolyte imbalances
- Dysrhythmias
- Congestive heart failure
- Paralytic ileus
- Acute urinary retention
- Deep venous thrombosis
- Pulmonary embolism
- Atelectasis or pneumonia
- Laryngeal edema
- Ventilator dependence
- Gastrointestinal (GI) bleeding
- Disseminated intravascular coagulation (DIC)
- Anemia
- Wound evisceration

➤ Physical Assessment/Clinical Manifestations

The postanesthesia nurse assesses the client and compiles data on a PACU record form (Fig. 22–1). Assessment data include the client's temperature, pulse, respiration, and blood pressure. The nurse examines the surgical area for bleeding. The postanesthesia nurse initiates assessments, and the intensive care or medical-surgical nurse continues assessments when the client is discharged to the inpatient unit. The frequency of vital signs measurement is based on the facility's policy and the surgeon's orders. Vital signs are often recorded every 15 minutes for four times, every 30 minutes for four times, every 2 hours for four times, and then every 4 hours for 24 to 48 hours if the client's condition is stable. Thereafter, vital signs are assessed according to the facility's policy, the client's condition, and the nurse's judgment.

The health care team determines the client's readiness for discharge from the postanesthesia area by noting a postanesthesia recovery score on the postanesthesia recovery scale of at least 10 (see Figure 22–1). In addition, the facility may have specific criteria for discharge (e.g., stable vital signs, normothermia, no overt bleeding, and return of gag, cough, and swallow reflexes). After the nurse determines that all criteria have been met, the client is discharged by the anesthesiologist to the hospital unit or to home. When an anesthesiologist has not been involved, such as may be the case with local anesthesia or conscious sedation, the surgeon or nurse discharges the client once the discharge criteria have been met.

Physical assessment continues from the PACU to the intensive care or medical-surgical nursing unit. If the client is to be discharged from the PACU to the home, physical assessment is continued by home care nurses or by the client or family members themselves after adequate instruction.

Respiratory System

Airway Assessment. When the client is admitted to PACU, the nurse immediately assesses for a patent airway and adequate respiratory exchange. An artificial airway, such as an endotracheal (ET) tube, a nasal trumpet, or an oral airway, may be in place. If the client is receiving supplemental oxygen, the nurse notes the type of delivery device and the concentration or liter flow of the oxygen.

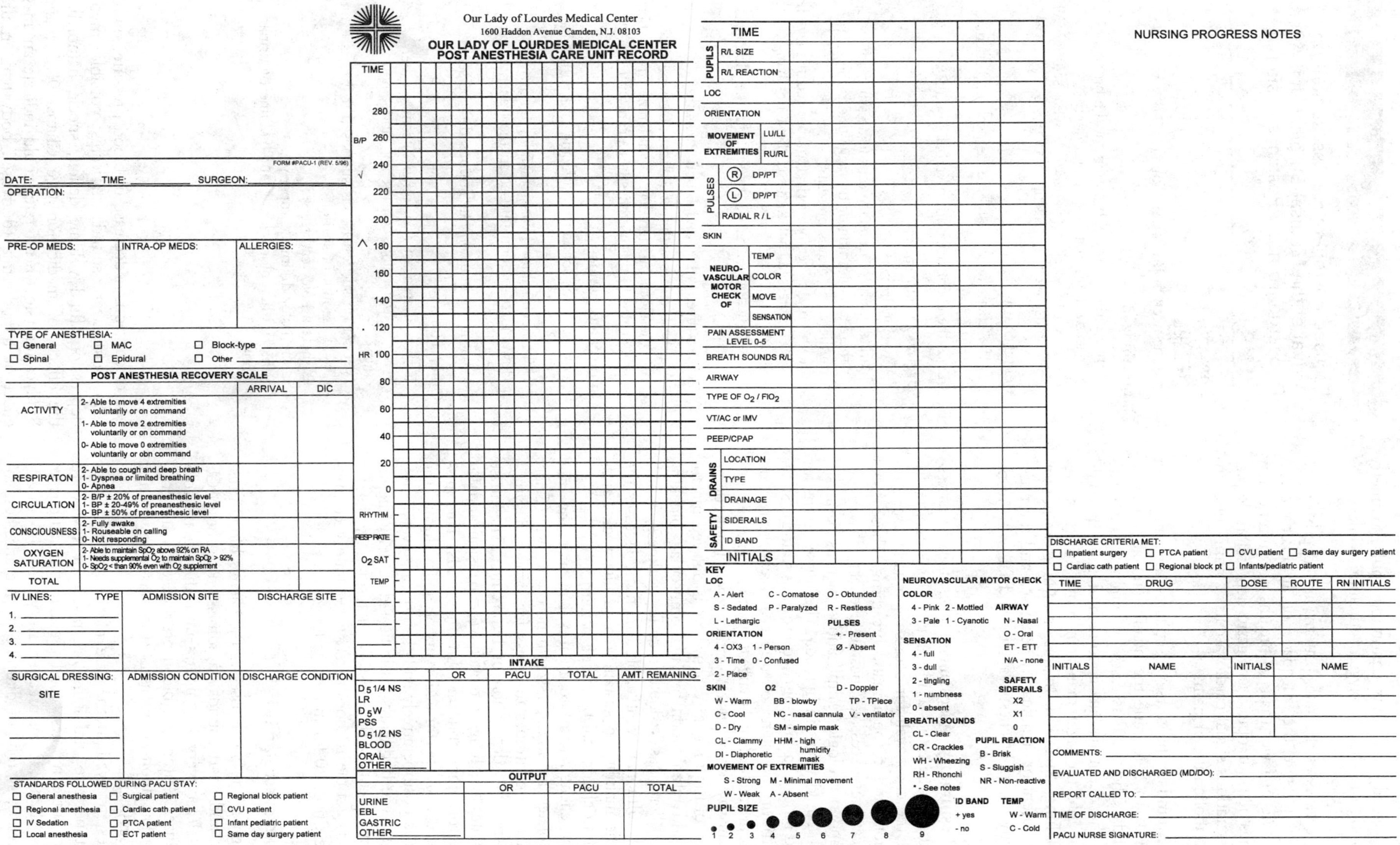

Our Lady of Lourdes Medical Center
1600 Haddon Avenue Camden, N.J. 08103

OUR LADY OF LOURDES MEDICAL CENTER
POST ANESTHESIA CARE UNIT RECORD

FORM #PACU-1 (REV. 5/96)

DATE: ________ TIME: ________ SURGEON: ________
OPERATION:

PRE-OP MEDS:	INTRA-OP MEDS:	ALLERGIES:

TYPE OF ANESTHESIA:
☐ General ☐ MAC ☐ Block-type ________
☐ Spinal ☐ Epidural ☐ Other ________

POST ANESTHESIA RECOVERY SCALE		ARRIVAL	DIC
ACTIVITY	2- Able to move 4 extremities voluntarily or on command 1- Able to move 2 extremities voluntarily or on command 0- Able to move 0 extremities voluntarily or obn command		
RESPIRATON	2- Able to cough and deep breath 1- Dyspnea or limited breathing 0- Apnea		
CIRCULATION	2- B/P ± 20% of preanesthesic level 1- BP ± 20-49% of preanesthesic level 0- BP ± 50% of preanesthesic level		
CONSCIOUSNESS	2- Fully awake 1- Rouseable on calling 0- Not responding		
OXYGEN SATURATION	2- Able to maintain SpO_2 above 92% on RA 1- Needs supplemental O_2 to maintain SpO_2 > 92% 0- SpO_2 < than 90% even with O_2 supplement		
TOTAL			

IV LINES:	TYPE	ADMISSION SITE	DISCHARGE SITE
1.			
2.			
3.			
4.			

SURGICAL DRESSING:	ADMISSION CONDITION	DISCHARGE CONDITION
SITE		

STANDARDS FOLLOWED DURING PACU STAY:
☐ General anesthesia ☐ Surgical patient ☐ Regional block patient
☐ Regional anesthesia ☐ Cardiac cath patient ☐ CVU patient
☐ IV Sedation ☐ PTCA patient ☐ Infant pediatric patient
☐ Local anesthesia ☐ ECT patient ☐ Same day surgery patient

TIME
B/P 280 260 240 220 200 180 160 140 120 HR 100 80 60 40 20 0
RHYTHM
RESP RATE
O_2 SAT
TEMP

INTAKE	OR	PACU	TOTAL	AMT. REMANING
D_5 1/4 NS				
LR				
D_5W				
PSS				
D_5 1/2 NS				
BLOOD				
ORAL				
OTHER____				

OUTPUT	OR	PACU	TOTAL
URINE			
EBL			
GASTRIC			
OTHER____			

TIME						
PUPILS R/L SIZE						
PUPILS R/L REACTION						
LOC						
ORIENTATION						
MOVEMENT OF EXTREMITIES LU/LL						
MOVEMENT OF EXTREMITIES RU/RL						
PULSES Ⓡ DP/PT						
PULSES Ⓛ DP/PT						
PULSES RADIAL R / L						
SKIN						
NEURO-VASCULAR MOTOR CHECK OF TEMP						
COLOR						
MOVE						
SENSATION						
PAIN ASSESSMENT LEVEL 0-5						
BREATH SOUNDS R/L						
AIRWAY						
TYPE OF O_2 / FIO_2						
VT/AC or IMV						
PEEP/CPAP						
DRAINS LOCATION						
DRAINS TYPE						
DRAINS DRAINAGE						
SAFETY SIDERAILS						
SAFETY ID BAND						
INITIALS						

KEY
LOC: A - Alert, C - Comatose, O - Obtunded, S - Sedated, P - Paralyzed, R - Restless, L - Lethargic
ORIENTATION: 4 - OX3, 1 - Person, 3 - Time, 0 - Confused, 2 - Place
PULSES: + - Present, Ø - Absent
SKIN: W - Warm, C - Cool, D - Dry, CL - Clammy, DI - Diaphoretic
O2: BB - blowby, NC - nasal cannula, SM - simple mask, HHM - high humidity mask, D - Doppler, TP - TPiece, V - ventilator
MOVEMENT OF EXTREMITIES: S - Strong, M - Minimal movement, W - Weak, A - Absent
PUPIL SIZE: 1 2 3 4 5 6 7 8 9

NEUROVASCULAR MOTOR CHECK
COLOR: 4 - Pink, 2 - Mottled, 3 - Pale, 1 - Cyanotic
SENSATION: 4 - full, 3 - dull, 2 - tingling, 1 - numbness, 0 - absent
BREATH SOUNDS: CL - Clear, CR - Crackles, WH - Wheezing, RH - Rhonchi, * - See notes
AIRWAY: N - Nasal, O - Oral, ET - ETT, N/A - none
SAFETY SIDERAILS: X2, X1, 0
PUPIL REACTION: B - Brisk, S - Sluggish, NR - Non-reactive
ID BAND: + yes, - no
TEMP: W - Warm, C - Cold

NURSING PROGRESS NOTES

DISCHARGE CRITERIA MET:
☐ Inpatient surgery ☐ PTCA patient ☐ CVU patient ☐ Same day surgery patient
☐ Cardiac cath patient ☐ Regional block pt ☐ Infants/pediatric patient

TIME	DRUG	DOSE	ROUTE	RN INITIALS

INITIALS	NAME	INITIALS	NAME

COMMENTS: ________
EVALUATED AND DISCHARGED (MD/DO): ________
REPORT CALLED TO: ________
TIME OF DISCHARGE: ________
PACU NURSE SIGNATURE: ________

Figure 22–1. Example of a postanesthesia care unit record. (Courtesy of Our Lady of Lourdes Medical Center, Camden, NJ.)

The nurse usually maintains continuous pulse oximetry for monitoring the client's oxygen saturation while in the PACU.

The nurse assesses the rate, pattern, and depth of respirations to measure the adequacy of air exchange. A respiratory rate of fewer than 10 breaths per minute may indicate anesthetic or opioid analgesic depression. Rapid, shallow respirations signal cardiovascular compromise, increased metabolic rate, or pain.

Breath Sounds. The nurse auscultates the lungs over all lung fields to determine the quality and adequacy of breath sounds. The nurse assesses for symmetry of breath sounds. If the client has an endotracheal tube, it could move down into the right mainstem bronchus, thus preventing left lung expansion. In this case, lung sounds on the left are absent or significantly decreased and the nurse observes only the right chest wall rise and fall with respirations.

Other Respiratory Assessments. Respiratory assessment by the postanesthesia nurse includes ongoing inspection of the chest wall for accessory muscle use, sternal retraction, and diaphragmatic breathing. These signs could indicate an excessive anesthetic effect, airway obstruction, and neurologic complications such as paralysis, all of which could result in hypoxia. The nurse listens for snoring and stridor (a high-pitched crowing sound). Snoring and stridor are signs of upper airway obstruction resulting from tracheal or laryngeal spasm or edema, mucus in the airway, or occlusion of the airway from edema or relaxation of the tongue. When there is delayed metabolism of and elimination of neuromuscular blocking agents, the client has residual muscle weakness, which could affect pulmonary ventilation. The nurse assesses the client for the inability to sustain a head lift, weak handgrasps, and an abdominal breathing pattern.

When the client returns to an inpatient unit, the unit nurse completes an initial assessment on arrival (Chart 22–1) and then continues to assess for signs and symptoms of respiratory depression or hypoxemia. The nurse also auscultates the lungs for effective expansion and for adventitious or other abnormal breath sounds. This auscultation is usually performed every 4 hours during the first 24 hours postoperatively and then during every nursing shift, or more frequently, as indicated. Elderly clients, smokers, and clients with a history of respiratory disease are more susceptible to postoperative respiratory complications (see Chap. 20 for more details).

Cardiovascular System

Vital Signs. The nurse assesses the client's blood pressure, pulse, and heart sounds on admission to the PACU and then at least every 15 minutes until the client's condition stabilizes. Automated blood pressure cuffs and continuous cardiac monitoring assist the nurse in making frequent assessments.

All nurses involved in the care of the surgical client review postoperative vital signs for upward or downward trends. The nurse reports blood pressure fluctuations of more or less than 25% of preoperative values (15- to 20-point difference, systolic or diastolic) to the anesthesiologist or surgeon. A decrease in blood pressure, pulse pressure, and heart sounds indicates possible myocardial depression, fluid volume deficit, shock, hemorrhage, or the effects of medication (see Chaps. 9, 15, and 39). Bradycardia (slow heart rate) could indicate an anesthesia effect or hypothermia (decreased body temperature). El-

---

Chart 22–1

Focused Postoperative Assessment on Arrival at the Medical-Surgical Unit After Discharge from the Postanesthesia Care Unit

Airway

Is it patent?
Is the neck in proper alignment?

Breathing

What is the quality and pattern of the breathing?
What is the respiratory rate and depth?
Is the client receiving oxygen? At what setting? What is the pulse oximetry result?

Mental Status

Is the client awake, able to be aroused, oriented, and aware?
Does the client respond to verbal stimuli?

Surgical Incision Site

How is it dressed?
Mark amount of drainage on the dressing immediately.
Is there any bleeding or drainage under the client?
Are there any drains present?
Are the drains set properly (compressed if they should be compressed, not kinked, client not lying on them, etc.)?
How much drainage is present in the drainage container?

Temperature, Pulse, and Blood Pressure

Are these values within the client's baseline range?
Are these values significantly different than when the client was in the postanesthesia care unit (PACU)?

Intravenous Fluids

What type of solution is infusing and with what additives?
How much solution was remaining on arrival?
How much solution infused in the transport time from PACU?
What is the infusion rate supposed to be set at? Is it?

Other Tubes

Is there a nasogastric or other intestinal tube?
What is the color, consistency, and amount of drainage?
Is it set on suction if it is supposed to be? Is it on the right amount of suction?
Is there a Foley catheter?
Is the Foley draining properly?
What is the color, clarity, and volume of urinary output?

derly clients are especially predisposed to hypothermia because of aging changes in the hypothalamus (the temperature regulation center), loss of subcutaneous tissue, and coolness of the operating suite. An increased pulse rate could indicate hemorrhage, shock, or pain.

Cardiac Monitoring. Cardiac monitoring is routinely maintained until the client is discharged from the PACU. For clients at risk for dysrhythmias, monitoring may continue on either specialized telemetry units or on general medical-surgical units. In assessing the vital signs of a client who is not undergoing continuous monitoring, the nurse determines the rate, rhythm, and quality of the client's apical pulse compared with those of a peripheral pulse such as the radial pulse. A pulse deficit (a difference between the apical and peripheral pulses) could indicate a dysrhythmia.

Peripheral Vascular Assessment. Anesthesia and positioning during surgery (e.g., the lithotomy position for genitourinary procedures) may compromise the client's peripheral circulation. The nurse assesses the client's peripheral circulation by comparing distal pulses bilaterally for the presence and quality of pulsation, noting the color and temperature of extremities, evaluating sensation, and determining the speed of capillary refill. Palpable dorsalis pedis pulses indicate adequate circulation and tissue perfusion of the distal lower extremities.

As part of the ongoing assessment, the nurse assesses the lower extremities for redness, pain, warmth, swelling, and the presence of Homan's sign, any of which could indicate the presence of deep venous thrombosis (DVT), a life-threatening condition. Assessment of the lower extremities may be performed once during a nursing shift, once daily, or once per visit, depending on the risk of complications and the facility's or agency's policy. (Chapters 20, 38, and 54 have further information on deep venous thrombosis.)

Neurologic System

General Cerebral Functioning. Regardless of the type of surgical procedure, the postanesthesia nurse assesses cerebral function and the level of consciousness or awareness of all clients who have received general anesthesia (Table 22–2) or any type of sedation. To assess the client's level of consciousness, the nurse observes for lethargy, restlessness, or irritability and tests coherence and orientation. The nurse determines awareness by observing responses to calling the client's name, touching the client, and giving simple commands such as "Open your eyes" and "Take a deep breath." Eye opening in response to a command indicates wakefulness or arousability but not necessarily awareness. The nurse determines the degree of orientation to person, place, and time by asking the conscious client to answer simple questions, such as "What is your name?" (person), "Where are you?" (place), and "What day is it?" (time).

For an elderly client, a rapid return to his or her prior level of orientation may not be realistic. The preoperative, intraoperative, and postoperative medications and anesthetic agents often affect the elderly client's reorientation ability (see Chaps. 20 and 21).

TABLE 22–2

Immediate Postoperative Neurologic Assessment: Return to Preoperative Level

Order of Return to Consciousness After General Anesthesia

1. Muscular irritability
2. Restlessness and delirium
3. Recognition of pain
4. Ability to reason and control behavior

Order of Return of Motor and Sensory Functioning After Local or Regional Anesthesia

1. Sense of touch
2. Sense of pain
3. Sense of warmth
4. Sense of cold
5. Ability to move

The nurse compares the client's preoperative baseline neurologic status with the postoperative assessment findings. Clients with altered cerebral functioning preoperatively as a result of a pre-existing condition continue to have that alteration postoperatively. After the client has returned to a satisfactory consciousness level (and all other criteria have been met), he or she is discharged from the PACU. Assessment of the client's level of consciousness continues every 4 to 8 hours or as indicated by the client's condition and the facility's policy.

Motor/Sensory Assessment. For all clients receiving general and regional anesthesia, motor and sensory function is assessed. General anesthesia renders clients unconscious and depresses voluntary motor function; regional anesthesia alters the motor and sensory function of only part of the body. (See Chapter 21 for more information on anesthesia.) Motor and sensory assessment is especially important after the client has had epidural or spinal anesthesia. The postanesthesia nurse evaluates motor function by instructing the client to move each extremity. The client who had epidural or spinal anesthesia remains in the PACU until sensory function (feeling) and voluntary motor movement of the lower extremities have returned (see Table 22–2). In addition, the nurse assesses the strength of each limb and compares the results bilaterally.

The postanesthesia nurse also tests for the return of sympathetic nervous system tone by gradually elevating the client's head and monitoring for hypotension. This evaluation begins after the client's sensation has returned to at least the spinal dermatome level of T-10. (See Chapter 43 for further neurologic assessment.) After the client is transferred to the nursing unit, the medical-surgical nurse continues neurologic assessment as indicated.

Fluid and Electrolyte Balance

Fasting before and during surgery, the loss of fluid during the procedure, and the type and amount of blood or IV fluid administered affect the client's postoperative fluid and electrolyte balance. Either fluid volume deficit or fluid volume overload may occur after surgery. Sodium, potassium, chloride, and calcium imbalances also may result, as may alterations in other electrolyte levels. Complications of fluid and electrolyte imbalances occur more often in elderly or debilitated clients and in clients with medical problems such as diabetes mellitus, Crohn's disease (especially after major intestinal surgery), and heart failure.

Intake and Output. Intraoperative intake and output measurement is part of the operative record and part of the circulating nurse's report to the postanesthesia nurse. The postanesthesia nurse records any intake or output, including intravenous (IV) fluid intake, vomitus, urine, and nasogastric (NG) tube drainage. When he or she gives report, the medical-surgical nurse needs to know the total intake and output from both the OR and the PACU to assess fluid balance accurately and to complete the 24-hour intake and output record.

Hydration Assessment. The medical-surgical nurse continues to assess the client's hydration. The nurse inspects the color and moist appearance of mucous membranes; the turgor, texture, and "tenting" of the skin (test over the sternum or forehead of an elderly client); the amount of drainage on dressings; and the presence of axillary sweat, which indicates adequate hydration. The nurse measures total output (e.g., NG tube drainage, urinary output, and wound drainage) and compares it with total intake to identify a possible fluid imbalance. The nurse considers insensible fluid loss when reviewing total output. The nurse continues to assess the client's intake and output while the client is at risk for fluid imbalances. Some facilities have policies that require intake and output to be measured if the client receives IV fluids or has a catheter, drains, or an NG tube.

Intravenous Fluids. The nurse administers and closely monitors IV fluids to promote fluid and electrolyte balance. Standard isotonic solutions such as lactated Ringer's (LR) and 5% dextrose with lactated Ringer's (D5/LR) are used for IV fluid replacement and maintenance in the PACU. After the client returns to the medical-surgical unit, the type and rate of administration of IV solutions are based on the individual client's need. A typical IV solution for the client when admitted to the nursing unit is 5% dextrose with 0.45% normal saline (D5/½ NSS). (See Chapters 15 and 17 for further discussion of IV fluid administration, electrolyte balance, and assessment of hydration.)

Acid-Base Balance

Acid-base balance may be affected by preoperative, intraoperative, and postoperative respiratory status, intraoperative metabolic changes, and losses of acids or bases in drainage. For example, NG tube drainage or vomitus represents a loss of hydrochloric acid. The nurse assesses acid-base status mostly through arterial blood gas measurement and other laboratory values. (See Chapter 19 for more detailed information on acid-base imbalances.)

Renal/Urinary System

Voluntary control of urinary function may return immediately after surgery or may not return for 6 to 8 hours or longer after inhalation, IV, and epidural or spinal anesthe-

sia. The effects of preoperative medications and anesthetic agents and manipulation during surgery, in combination or alone, can cause urinary retention. The nurse assesses for this complication by inspection, palpation, and percussion of the client's lower abdomen for bladder distention. Assessment may be difficult to perform when the client has had lower abdominal surgery. Urinary retention is common in the early postoperative period and requires appropriate intervention, often one or more intermittent (straight) catheterizations to empty the bladder.

When the client has an indwelling urinary (Foley) catheter, the nurse assesses the urine for color, clarity, and amount. If the client is voiding, the nurse also assesses the urinary frequency, associated amount per void, and any symptoms. Urinary output should correlate with total input for a 24-hour period, but other sources of output need to be considered. The nurse reports a urinary output of less than 30 mL/hour (240 mL/8-hour nursing shift) to the physician. Decreased urinary output may indicate hypovolemia or renal complications. (Refer to Chapter 72 for complete information on the assessment of renal/urinary function, including the interpretation of specific gravity, electrolyte values, and osmolality of urine.)

Gastrointestinal System

Nausea and Vomiting. One of the most common postoperative reactions is nausea and vomiting. Approximately 30% of clients receiving general anesthesia have some form of gastrointestinal upset within the first 24 hours after surgery. Clients with a history of motion sickness are more likely to develop postoperative nausea and vomiting. Obese individuals may be at risk because many anesthetics are retained by fat cells and, therefore, have a lingering effect. Abdominal surgery and the use of opioid analgesics reduce intestinal peristalsis after surgery. These situations predispose the client to nausea and vomiting for longer than the first 24 hours after surgery.

Postoperative nausea and vomiting can cause stress and irritation of abdominal and gastrointestinal (GI) wounds, increase intracranial pressure in clients who had head and neck surgery, elevate intraocular pressure in clients who had eye surgery, and increase the risk of aspiration and aspiration pneumonia. The nurse assesses for nausea and vomiting continuously. Often a client experiences nausea as the head of the bed is raised in the early postoperative period. This symptom may occur with or without associated dizziness. The nurse has the client in side-lying position before raising his or her head slowly.

Gastrointestinal Peristalsis. The nurse in the postanesthesia care unit and later on the medical-surgical unit assesses for the return of peristaltic function. Peristalsis may be delayed because of the length of time under anesthesia, the amount of bowel handling intraoperatively, and opioid analgesic use.

Assessment. The nurse auscultates for bowel sounds in all four abdominal quadrants and at the umbilicus. If the client is undergoing nasogastric (NG) suctioning, the suction must be turned off before auscultation of the abdomen. Otherwise, the nurse could mistake the sound of the suction for bowel sounds. In addition, the nurse asks the client whether flatus has been passed. Both bowel sounds and flatus passage indicate peristalsis, but abdominal cramping denotes trapped, nonmoving gas and not peristalsis.

Complications. Decreased peristalsis can occur in clients with paralytic ileus. The intestine wall is distended and there is no movement of the intestinal wall (aperistalsis). The nurse assesses for the clinical manifestations of paralytic ileus. These include few or absent bowel sounds, distended abdomen, diffuse abdominal discomfort (as a result of the distention), vomiting, lack of flatus, and no passage of stool.

The client may also experience constipation postoperatively owing to anesthesia, analgesia (especially codeine [Paveral✦] and other opioid analgesics), decreased activity, and decreased oral intake. The nurse assesses the client's abdomen by inspection, palpation, percussion, and auscultation and records the client's elimination pattern to determine whether interventions are needed. Increased dietary fiber intake, the administration of mild laxatives or bulk-forming agents, or the use of enemas may be necessary.

Nasogastric Tube Drainage. An NG tube may be inserted intraoperatively to decompress and drain the stomach, to promote gastrointestinal rest, to allow the lower gastrointestinal tract to heal, and to provide an enteral feeding route. It may also be used to monitor the occurrence of bleeding and prevent intestinal obstruction. The Levin tube and the Salem sump tube are the two most common tubes used. The Salem tube is a double-lumen tube with an air vent to keep the tube from adhering to the gastric mucosa. This feature allows easy drainage of the stomach and prevents gastric mucosal damage. The Levin tube is a single-lumen tube with no air vent. To promote drainage, varying degrees of suction (high, medium, or low) are applied to the nasogastric tube. Suction is either continuous (recommended for the Salem tube) or intermittent on the basis of the surgeon's preference and the tube type.

Assessment. The nurse records the color, consistency, and amount of the drained material every 8 hours (Table 22–3). In some instances, the results of an occult blood test (Gastroccult) may also be recorded. Normal NG drainage fluid is greenish-yellow; red drainage fluid indicates active bleeding, and brown liquid or coffee-ground drainage indicates the possibility of old bleeding.

Complications. The nurse assesses the client for possible complications related to NG tube use, including fluid and electrolyte imbalances, aspiration, and nares discomfort. To prevent aspiration, the nurse checks the tube placement every 4 to 8 hours and before the instillation of irrigation solution into the tube (see Chapter 58 for information on tube placement and care). After gastric surgery, the tube should not be manipulated or irrigated without an order from the physician. Fluid and electrolyte imbalances can result from NG drainage and tube irrigation with water instead of saline. Imbalances include fluid volume deficit (see Chap. 15), hypokalemia and hyponatremia (see Chap. 16), hypochloremia, and metabolic alkalosis (see Chap. 19).

TABLE 22–3

Calculating Nasogastric Tube Drainage

Formula

drainage in collection device − amount of irrigant = true (actual) amount of drainage

Example

A client's drainage container was marked at 150 mL at 7 AM. At 3 PM, there was 525 mL in the container. During the nursing shift, the nurse instilled 30 mL of saline as an irrigant into the tube four times, as ordered by the physician.

525 mL − 150 mL = 375 mL of drainage

30 mL × 4 = 120 mL of irrigant

375 mL − 120 mL = 255 mL of actual drainage

Integumentary System

The clean surgical wound heals itself at skin level in approximately 2 weeks in the absence of trauma, connective tissue disease, malnutrition, and the use of some medications such as steroids. Smokers, elderly clients, obese clients, and those with diseases that decrease immunity have delayed wound healing. Complete healing of underlying tissue and return to presurgical integrity may take 6 months to 2 years. The physical condition and age of the client, size and location of the wound, and stress on the surgical wound also affect the length of time for wound healing. Because of rich blood supply, wounds of the face and head heal more quickly than abdominal and leg wounds.

Normal Wound Healing. During the first few days of normal wound healing, the incised tissue regains blood supply and begins to bind together. Fibrin from the clotting process and a thin layer of epithelial cells seal the incision. After 1 to 4 days, epithelial cells continue to grow along the fibrin while growing strands of collagen begin to fill in the gaps in the wound (Strimike et al., 1997). This process continues for 2 to 3 weeks when the wound appears to be healed; however, healing is not complete for up to 2 years until the scar is strengthened. (See Chapter 70 for discussion of wound healing and wound infection.)

When the client is an inpatient, the surgeon usually removes the original postoperative dressing the first or second postoperative day. The nurse assesses the incision on a regular basis, usually every 8 hours, for redness, increased warmth, swelling, tenderness or pain, and the type and amount of drainage. Some drainage is normal during the first few days, changing from sanguineous (bloody) to serosanguineous to serous (serum-like or yellow). Serosanguineous drainage continuing beyond the fifth postoperative day should alert the nurse to the possibility of dehiscence, and the surgeon should be notified. Slight crusting on the incision line is normal, as is a pink color to the line itself owing to inflammation from the surgical procedure. Slight swelling under the sutures or staples is also normal. Redness or swelling of or around the incision line, excessive tenderness or pain on palpation, and purulent or odorous drainage could indicate wound infection and is reported to the surgeon.

Ineffective Wound Healing. Ineffective wound healing may be caused by wound infection, distention from edema or paralytic ileus, stress at the surgical site, and pre-existing conditions that cause delayed wound healing. Wound *dehiscence* is a partial or complete separation of the outer layers of the wound, sometimes described as a "splitting open of the wound". *Evisceration* is the total separation of the layers and extrusion of internal organs or viscera (usually abdominal) through the open wound (Fig. 22–2). Both of these alterations in wound healing are more often seen between the 5th and 10th postoperative days and occur more frequently in obese clients or others predisposed to delayed wound healing. Wound dehiscence or evisceration may be preceded by excessive coughing, not splinting the surgical site, vomiting, or straining. The client may state, "Something gave way" or "I feel as if I just split open."

Dressings and Drains. All dressings, including casts and elastic (Ace) bandages, are assessed for bleeding or other drainage on admission to the PACU and then frequently until the client is discharged to home or transferred to the inpatient unit. The medical-surgical nurse assesses the client's dressing each time vital signs are taken. When inspecting the dressing, the nurse checks for drainage and notes the amount, color, consistency, and odor of the drainage fluid. The nurse also checks underneath the client, because drainage (often blood from hemorrhage) may leak from the side of the dressing and yet

not appear on the dressing itself. The dressing should not restrict circulation or sensation.

To confine or contain drainage, the surgeon inserts a drain into or close to the wound if more than a minimal amount of drainage is expected. A Penrose drain (a single-lumen, soft latex tube) is a gravity-type drain under the dressing. The nurse assesses closed-suction drains such as Hemovac, VacuDrain, and Jackson-Pratt drains to ensure maintenance of compression and thus suction. The surgeon may place a T tube after abdominal cholecystectomy to drain bile. Figure 22–3 shows commonly used drains.

The nurse assesses all drains for patency when the client is admitted to the PACU and every time vital signs are taken during the postoperative period. The nurse monitors the amount, color, and consistency of the drainage while the client is in the PACU and at least every 8 hours after the client is transferred to the medical-surgical nursing unit. For example, large amounts of sanguineous drainage may indicate internal bleeding.

Discomfort/Pain Assessment

The surgical client almost always reports pain. Postoperative pain is related to the surgical wound, tissue manipulation, presence of drains, and intraoperative positioning. In assessing the client's discomfort or pain and need for medication, the nurse considers the type, extent, and length of the surgical procedure. The nurse assesses for physical and emotional signs of pain such as increased pulse and blood pressure, increased respiratory rate or hyperventilation, diaphoresis (profuse perspiration), restlessness, increased confusion (in the elderly), wincing, moaning, and crying. When possible, the nurse asks the client to quantify or rate the discomfort or pain before and after medication is given (e.g., on a scale of 1 to 10, with 1 being least intense and 10 being extreme pain). In addition, the nurse observes for a return of the client's normal (baseline) physical behaviors. (See Chapter 9 for further discussion of pain assessment.)

Discomfort or pain assessment is initiated by the postanesthesia nurse. After the client is transferred from the PACU, the medical-surgical nurse continues to assess the client's comfort level. Postoperative pain generally reaches its peak on the second postoperative day, when the client is more awake and the anesthetics and analgesics given intraoperatively have been metabolized and excreted.

► Psychosocial Assessment

As the nurse completes the physical aspects of postoperative assessment, the psychological, social, and cultural characteristics of the client are considered. This assessment may be delayed or difficult to perform in the PACU when the client is drowsy or incoherent. The nurse considers the client's age and medical history, surgical procedure, and impact of the procedure on the client's recovery, body image, roles, and lifestyle.

Physical signs indicating anxiety include restlessness; increased pulse, blood pressure, and respiratory rate; and crying. The client may be anxious and ask questions about the results or findings of the surgical procedure.

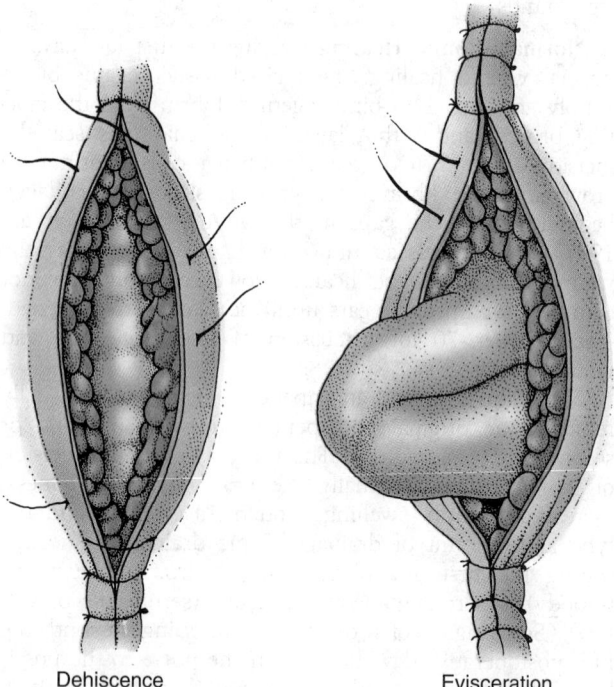

Dehiscence   Evisceration

Figure 22–2. Complications of wound healing.

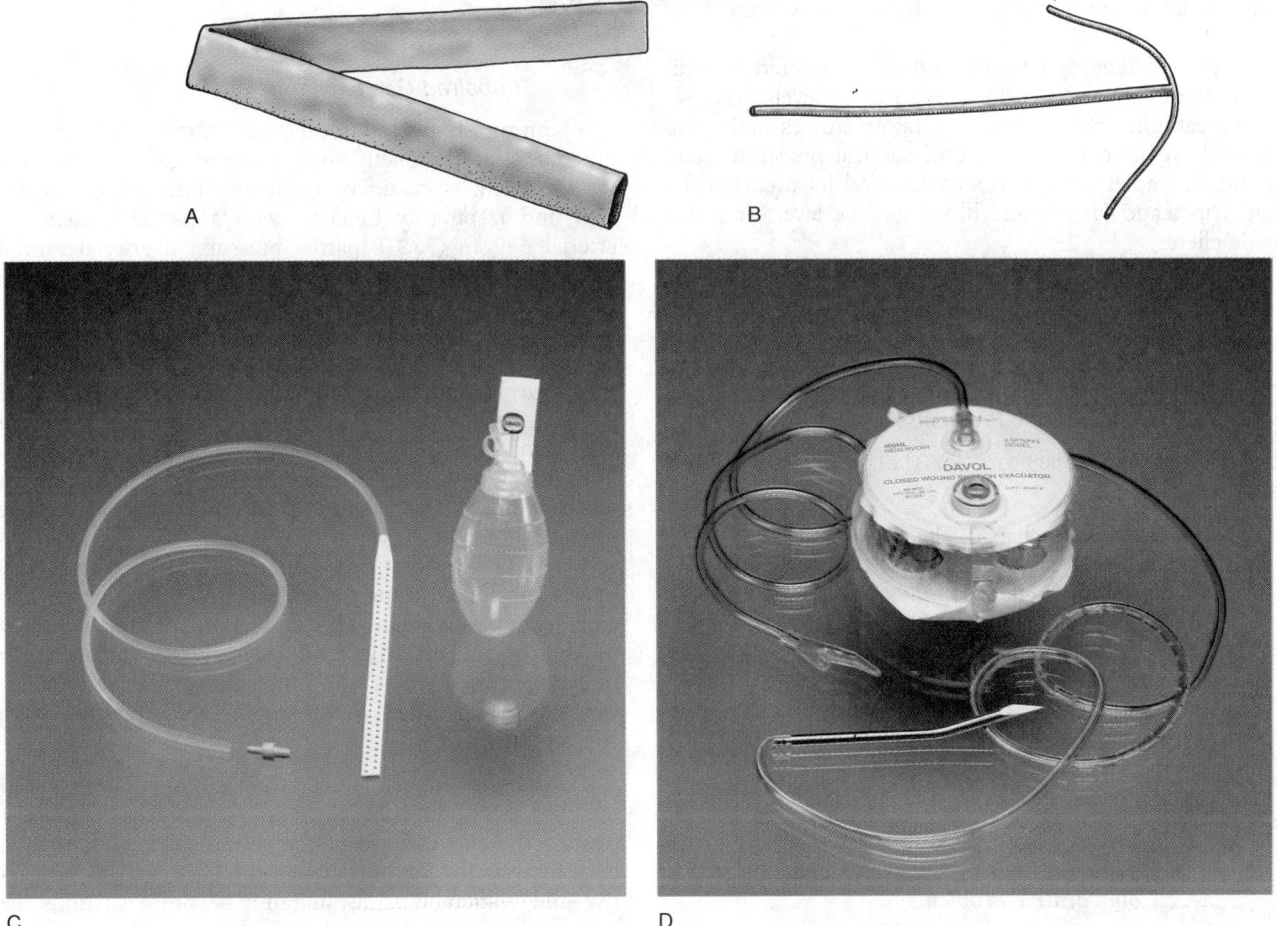

Figure 22–3. Types of surgical drains. Gravity drains, such as the Penrose *(A)* and the T tube *(B)* drain directly through a tube from the surgical area. In closed wound drainage systems, such as the Jackson-Pratt *(C)* and Hemovac *(D)*, drainage collects in a collecting vessel by means of compression and reexpansion of the system. *(C* and *D,* courtesy of C. R. Bard, Inc., Covington, GA.)

The nurse reassures the client that the surgeon will speak with him or her after the client is fully awake. If the surgeon has already spoken with the client, the nurse reinforces what was said. (Chapter 8 has further information on stress.)

After the client returns to the medical-surgical unit, the medical-surgical nurse continues the psychosocial assessment of the client and assesses significant others as well.

➤ *Laboratory Assessment*

Postoperative laboratory tests are performed to monitor the client for complications. Tests are based on the surgical procedure and the client's medical history and postoperative clinical manifestations. Common postoperative serum tests include analysis of electrolytes and a complete blood count (see Chart 20–3). A change in laboratory test results (e.g., electrolyte levels, hematocrit, and hemoglobin levels) commonly occurs during the first 24 to 48 hours postoperatively because of blood and fluid loss and the body's reaction to the surgical process. Fluid loss without significant blood loss may result in hemoconcentrated laboratory values (decreased fluid in the blood with resultant increased concentration). The laboratory test re-

sult is reported as increased, but actually represents a concentrated normal value.

A subtle early indication of infection is an increase in the band cells (immature neutrophils) in the white cell differential count. This increase is termed a *shift to the left.* The source of infection may be the respiratory system, urinary tract, wound, or IV site. The nurse obtains appropriate specimens for culture and sensitivity testing and monitors the culture results reported from the microbiology laboratory at 24, 48, and 72 hours. The nurse notifies the physician of positive culture results. (See Chapter 28 for more information on infection.)

Arterial blood gas (ABG) determinations may be indicated for clients with a history of respiratory or cardiac disease, those undergoing prolonged mechanical ventilation postoperatively, and those having had surgery involving the thoracic cavity. The nurse interprets ABG results and notifies the surgeon of any deviation from the expected norm for that client (acid-base imbalance or hypoxemia). The anion gap can be calculated from serum electrolyte values or recorded by the chemistry laboratory. An increase in the anion gap alerts the nurse to the possibility of metabolic acidosis. (For more discussion on arterial blood gases and acidosis, see Chapters 18 and 19.)

Urine and renal laboratory studies are ordered as indicated (e.g., urinalysis, urinary electrolyte levels, and serum creatinine levels). Other laboratory studies performed depend on the diagnosis, type of surgical procedure, and so on. Examples are serum amylase level for a client who had pancreatic surgery and blood glucose level for a diabetic client.

 Analysis

> ### Common Nursing Diagnoses and Collaborative Problems

Common nursing diagnoses for the postoperative client are

1. Impaired Gas Exchange related to the residual effects of anesthesia, pain, the use of opioid analgesics, and immobility
2. Impaired Skin Integrity related to surgical wounds, inflammatory processes, drains and drainage, and tubes
3. Pain related to the surgical incision and positioning during surgery

A common collaborative problem for the postoperative client is potential for hypoxemia.

> ### Additional Nursing Diagnoses and Collaborative Problems

Depending on the type and extent of surgery, the family structure, and so on, there may be additional nursing diagnoses or collaborative problems for the postoperative client (see the discussion of surgical management in other chapters as appropriate), such as

■ Risk for Aspiration related to decreased mobility, anesthesia, and opioid analgesic use
■ Ineffective Airway Clearance related to ineffective or absent cough
■ Fluid Volume Deficit related to decreased oral intake and abnormal fluid loss
■ Potential for Hypovolemic Shock
■ Potential for Deep Venous Thrombosis and Pulmonary Embolism
■ Constipation related to decreased mobility, anesthesia, and opioid analgesic use
■ Risk for Infection related to surgery and invasive lines, catheters, and tubes
■ Urinary Retention related to anesthesia, surgical procedures, and decreased mobility
■ Sleep Pattern Disturbance related to the use of medications and hospitalization
■ Self-Care Deficit related to surgical procedures and decreased mobility
■ Body Image Disturbance related to surgical procedures, loss of a body part or function, and pain
■ Altered Family Processes related to the impact of surgery and illness on the family system
■ Altered Sexuality Patterns related to surgery, pain, and hospitalization

 Planning and Implementation

Impaired Gas Exchange

Planning: Expected Outcomes. The major expected outcomes for the client with impaired gas exchange are for the client to attain or maintain optimal lung expansion and respiratory function with a partial pressure of arterial oxygen (PaO_2), partial pressure of arterial carbon dioxide ($PaCO_2$), and oxygen saturation values within baseline range.

Interventions

Airway Maintenance. After assessing the airway, the postanesthesia nurse may need to insert an oral airway if the client does not already have one. The oral airway pulls the tongue forward and holds it down to prevent obstruction. If the client has clenched teeth, a large tongue, or upper airway obstruction, the nurse could insert a nasal airway (nasal trumpet) to keep the airway open. The nurse keeps the manual resuscitation bag and emergency equipment for intubation or tracheostomy nearby. For clients whose only airway is a tracheostomy or laryngectomy stoma, the nurse alerts other staff members by posting signs in the room, notes on the chart, and so forth.

Positioning. Immediate care by the nurse in the PACU includes positioning the client in a side-lying position or turning the client's head to the side to prevent aspiration of secretions (or vomitus) while the client is still unreactive and vulnerable to aspiration. The nurse suctions the mouth, nose, and throat to keep the airway clear of mucus or vomitus as necessary.

The postanesthesia nurse keeps the client's head flat to prevent hypotension and possible shock, unless this position is contraindicated by the client's condition or surgical procedure. (For example, after intracranial surgery, the head of the bed or stretcher is elevated to promote respiratory function and prevent postoperative cerebral edema.) The nurse administers oxygen via face tent, nasal cannula, or mask to facilitate the excretion of inhalation anesthetic agents, to increase arterial oxygen levels, and to raise the level of consciousness. After the client is fully reactive and stable, the postanesthesia nurse raises the head of the bed to promote respiratory function.

Breathing Exercises. After the client regains the gag and cough reflex and meets the agency's criteria for extubation (if intubated), the airway or endotracheal (ET) tube is removed. Examples of extubation criteria are the client's ability to raise and hold the head up and evidence of thoracic breathing. The nurse encourages the client to cough (with the incision splinted) and deep breathe to expand the lungs, promote gas exchange, and hasten the elimination of inhalation anesthetic agents. Chart 20–5 reviews the teaching of postoperative breathing exercises and splinting of the surgical wound area to the client. As soon as the client is awake enough to follow commands, and throughout the postoperative period, the nurse encourages the client to cough, use the incentive spirometer, and take deep breaths. The client who is unable to expectorate mucus or sputum voluntarily may require oral or nasal suctioning. Meticulous mouth care is important after the removal of secretions.

Mobilization. The client is out of bed and ambulating as soon as possible to help mobilize secretions and promote lung expansion. Even for the hospitalized client with extensive surgery, the goal may be to get the client out of bed the same day as or the first day after surgery. If this is not possible, given the individual client's situation, the nurse turns the client at least every 2 hours (side to side) and ensures that the client performs his or her respiratory exercises and leg exercises (see Chart 20–6). Early ambulation minimizes the risk of pulmonary complications, including a pulmonary embolism, which could arise from impaired venous circulation in the legs. The client may report pain and resist getting up, but the nurse stresses the importance of activity to prevent postoperative complications. When indicated, the nurse offers pain medication 30 to 45 minutes before the client gets out of bed.

Impaired Skin Integrity

Planning: Expected Outcomes. The expected outcome for the client with impaired skin integrity is for the client to have incision healing without postoperative wound complications.

Interventions. Nursing assessment of the surgical area postoperatively is critical (see the discussion of integumentary system assessment earlier in this chapter). Although most wound complications can be treated without additional surgical intervention, emergency surgical procedures may be necessary.

Nonsurgical Management. Postoperative nonsurgical wound care usually includes changing and care of the dressing, assessment of the wound for signs of infection, and care of drains, including emptying, measuring, and documenting characteristics of the drainage. The nurse emphasizes to the client the importance of early deep-breathing exercises (see Chap. 20) to prevent respiratory complications that could cause forceful coughing. The nurse encourages hip flexion when the client is in the supine position to reduce tension on a chest or abdominal wound. The nurse also reminds the client always to splint the incision when coughing. The nurse promotes an atmosphere conducive to wound healing and protective of the skin in general, especially for the elderly client (Chart 22–2).

Dressings. The surgeon usually performs the first dressing change to assess the wound, remove any packing, and advance (pull partially out) or remove drains as indicated. Before the first dressing change, the nurse reinforces the dressing if it becomes wet from drainage. The nurse documents the reinforcement as well as the color, type, amount, and odor of drainage fluid and time of observation in the client's chart. The nurse assesses the surgical area frequently and reports any unexpected findings to the surgeon.

After removal of the surgical dressing, the surgeon may wish to leave the suture or staple line open to the air, which allows easy assessment of the wound and early

---

Chart 22–2

Nursing Focus on the Elderly: Postoperative Skin Care

- Improve perfusion to the wound to promote wound healing:
  - Keep the client adequately hydrated to maintain cardiac output.
  - Keep the airway patent and provide adequate oxygenation.
  - Keep the client's oxygen saturation on pulse oximetry at greater than 93%.
- Conserve the client's energy:
  - Allow the client to sleep in darkened, quiet room.
  - Administer medication to combat pain and sleeplessness, as ordered.
  - Provide rest periods throughout the day.
  - Control the client's room temperature.
  - Assist in activities of daily living.
- Place the client on a safety program to prevent falls, if indicated.
- Maintain strict aseptic technique in caring for breaks in the integument (intravenous or other catheters, indwelling urethral catheter, wound).
- Maintain the client's psychosocial health:
  - Prevent unnecessary stressors.
  - Allow the client liberal visitation of supportive others.
  - Enable the client to use individual successful coping mechanisms.
  - Keep the client well groomed and bathed.
- Protect fragile skin:
  - Minimize the use of tape on the skin.
  - Use hypoallergenic tape or Montgomery straps.
  - Change dressings as soon as they become wet.
  - Lift the client during transfer or repositioning.

Data from Jones, P. L., & Millman, A. (1990). Wound healing and the aged patient. *Nursing Clinics of North America, 25*(1), 263–277.

---

detection of poor approximation, drainage, swelling, or redness. Some surgeons believe that air-drying promotes healing. A draining wound, however, is always covered with a dressing.

Dressing changes are generally ordered by the surgeon, but the facility or unit may have standards or policies that dictate specific protocols for postoperative dressing changes and incision care. An unchanged wet or damp dressing becomes a source of infection. The nurse performs dressing changes under aseptic conditions until the sutures or staples are removed.

Dressings vary depending on the surgical procedure and the surgeon's preference. The standard postoperative dressing for a large incision consists of gauze or nonadherent pads covered with a larger absorbent pad held in place by tape or by Montgomery straps (Fig. 22–4). In other cases, the incision may be covered with a transparent plastic surgical dressing (such as Op-Site) or a spray in the operating room. This type of dressing stays intact for 3 to 6 days and allows visualization (observation) of the wound while preventing contamination and eliminating the need for dressing changes.

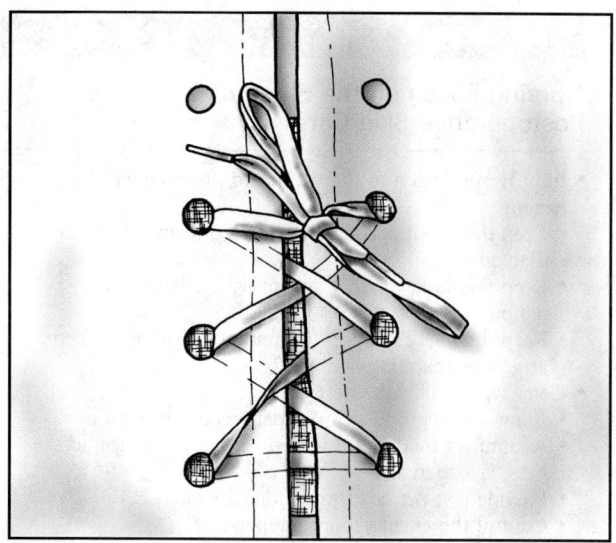

Figure 22–4. Montgomery straps may be used when frequent dressing changes are anticipated. They help to prevent skin irritation from frequent tape removal.

Wound or suture line care generally consists of changing gauze dressings at least once during a nursing shift or daily and may include cleaning the area with sterile saline or some other solution. The hospital's policy, the unit's standards, and the surgeon's preference determine what solution, if any, is used on the wound and also the frequency of the dressing changes. For extensive dressing changes or drain removal, the nurse offers the client an ordered analgesic before the procedure.

Skin sutures or staples are usually removed 6 to 8 days postoperatively, and the incision is secured with Steri-Strips. Either the surgeon or the nurse removes the sutures or staples, depending on the agency's policy. Before removing sutures, the nurse notes the condition and healing stage of the wound. If the wound does not appear to be healing well, the nurse notifies the surgeon before proceeding with suture removal.

Drains. Drains (see Figure 22–3) may be inserted into the wound or through a separate small incision (known as a stab wound) close to the operative site during surgery. The drain provides an exit through which air and fluids, such as blood and bile, can be evacuated. Drains also help prevent deep infections and abscess formation within the wound during healing.

The Penrose drain is a superficial device placed into the external aspect of the incision and that drains directly onto the client's dressing and perisurgical area (the skin around the incision). The nurse changes a damp or soiled dressing by carefully cleaning under and around the Penrose drain. The nurse then pads the area distal to the drain with absorbent pads to prevent skin irritation and contamination of the surgical wound. Whether sutured in place or not, the drain can easily be dislodged or accidentally pulled out during a dressing change. As the wound heals, the surgeon shortens (advances) the drain by pulling it out and removing the excess external portion until drainage stops.

Jackson-Pratt and Hemovac drains are two commonly used self-contained drainage systems by which the wound drains directly through a tube via gravity, suction, or vacuum. These drains are commonly sutured in place with a pursestring suture that seals the area when the drain is removed. The nurse empties the reservoir of the drain and records the amount and color of drainage during every nursing shift or more frequently if ordered by the surgeon. After emptying and compressing the reservoir, the nurse secures the drain to the client's gown or pajamas (never to the sheet or mattress) to prevent pulling and stress on the surgical wound.

Drug Therapy. Wound infection is a major postoperative complication. It usually results from contamination during surgery, preoperative infection, debilitation, or immunosuppression. A client at risk for wound infection may receive prophylactic antibiotic therapy with a broad-spectrum antibiotic or one that is effective in fighting organisms common to the specific surgical site. These antibiotics are usually continued for 24 to 72 hours postoperatively to ensure that adequate antibiotic levels are reached in this critical time period. The first dose may be administered IV before or during the surgery.

Wounds that become infected and open (without intact sutures) are usually treated with specific dressing changes and prolonged systemic antibiotic administration. Depending on physician order, the nurse irrigates the wound (e.g., with sterile saline, hydrogen peroxide, povidone-iodine, or acetic acid), loosely packs it with solution-soaked gauze (e.g., with neomycin, gentamicin, iodoform, povidone-iodine, saline, or acetic acid), and covers the wound with dry, sterile dressings. This procedure (wet-to-dry dressings) may be ordered one to three times daily. The packing promotes healing from within the wound and debridement (removal) of the infected tissue as the wound heals.

Surgical Management

Management of Dehiscence. If dehiscence (wound opening) occurs, the nurse applies a sterile nonadherent (such as Telfa) or saline dressing to the wound and notifies the surgeon. A wound that becomes infected dehisces by itself, or it may be opened by the surgeon through an incision and drainage (I&D) procedure. In either case, the wound is left open rather than resutured and is treated as described previously.

Management of Evisceration. An evisceration (a wound opening with the protrusion of internal organs or viscera) is considered a surgical emergency. One nurse tends to the client while another nurse immediately notifies the surgeon. Chart 22–3 outlines emergency care. The nurse provides emotional support by explaining what happened and reassuring the client that the emergency can, and will, be handled by competent, capable individuals.

The surgeon may order an NG tube to decompress the stomach and relieve some of the pressure internally or to remove the stomach's contents if the client has been eating and general anesthesia is planned. The nurse prepares the client for surgery (see Chap. 20) to close the wound. Regional or local anesthesia may be used, depending on the location of the wound and the surgeon's or the anes-

Chart 22–3

Nursing Care Highlight: Surgical Wound Evisceration

1. Call for help! Instruct the person who responds to notify the surgeon immediately and to bring any needed supplies into the client's room.
2. Stay with the client.
3. Cover the wound with a nonadherent dressing premoistened with warmed sterile normal saline. Note: The supplies needed for this emergency should be in the client's room, especially if the client is at high risk.
4. If premoistened dressings are not available, moisten sterile gauze or sterile towels in a sterile irrigation tray with sterile saline, then cover the wound.
5. If saline is not immediately available, cover the wound with gauze, and then moisten with sterile saline using a sterile irrigation tray as soon as someone brings saline.
6. Do not attempt to reinsert the protruding organ or viscera.
7. While covering the wound, note the client's response and assess for signs and symptoms of shock.
8. Place the client in a supine position with the hips and knees bent.
9. Take and document vital signs. Note: If the person who answered the call for help is back in the room before this, instruct that individual to take vital signs while you focus on covering the wound and repositioning the client.
10. Provide support and reassurance to the client.
11. Continue assessing the client, including vital signs assessment, every 5 to 10 min, until the surgeon arrives.
12. Keep dressings continuously moist by adding warmed sterile saline to the dressing as often as necessary. Do not let the dressing become dry.
13. When the surgeon arrives, report your findings and your interventions. Then follow the surgeon's directions.
14. Document the incident, the activity the client was engaged in at the time of the incident, your actions, and your assessments.

thesiologist's preference. Postoperative nausea and vomiting, which place undue stress on the already fragile incision, are minimized when regional or local anesthesia is used. To increase the incision's integrity, stay or retention sutures of wire or nylon are used over the standard suture or staple line (see Figure 21–13).

Pain

Planning: Expected Outcomes. The expected outcome for the client with pain is for the client to attain or maintain optimal comfort levels throughout the postoperative phase. This outcome entails the alleviation or reduction of pain or discomfort associated with the surgical wound and positioning during surgery.

Interventions. Postoperative pain management usually includes drug therapy and other methods such as positioning, massage, relaxation techniques, and diversion. Often the client achieves greater benefit from a combination of approaches. The nurse assesses the client's comfort level and the effectiveness of the therapies. (Chapter 9 provides a comprehensive discussion of pain assessment and management for the postoperative client.) The client who has optimal pain control is better able to cooperate with the therapies and exercises designed to prevent postoperative complications and to promote the postoperative rehabilitation process.

Drug Therapy. The use of opioids or other analgesics for the management of pain may mask or increase the amount and severity of symptoms of an anesthesia reaction. Therefore, these drugs must be administered with caution, especially in the PACU when the client's condition is not stabilized. Pain medication, when administered in the PACU, is usually given IV in small doses. After the nurse administers medication for pain, the client remains in the PACU for a defined period (often 30–45 minutes). The postanesthesia nurse assesses for hypotension, respiratory depression, and other side effects. Approximately 5 to 10 minutes after an IV injection, the nurse assesses the effectiveness of the medication (i.e., on a rating scale) in relieving the client's pain.

Opioid analgesics are routinely given during the first 24 to 48 hours after surgery to control acute pain. Around-the-clock administration is generally more effective than medicating on client demand because more constant blood levels can be obtained. Drugs commonly used include meperidine hydrochloride (Demerol), morphine sulfate (Statex♣), hydromorphone hydrochloride (Dilaudid), ketorolac (Toradol), codeine sulfate, butorphanol tartrate (Stadol), and oxycodone hydrochloride with aspirin (Percodan), or oxycodone hydrochloride with acetaminophen (Tylox, Percocet). The nurse assesses the type, location, and intensity of the pain before and after the administration of medication (see also Discomfort/Pain Assessment earlier in this chapter). The nurse monitors the client's vital signs closely, especially for hypotension and hypoventilation, after the administration of opioid analgesics. Chart 22–4 contains further information on various analgesics used during the postoperative period.

Patient-controlled analgesia (PCA) via IV or internal pump (the catheter is sutured into or proximal to the surgical area) and epidural analgesia are becoming more common to achieve better pain control. In PCA, the client adjusts the rate or dosage of infusion of an opioid analgesic on the basis of the pain level and physical response to the drug. This method allows more consistent pain relief and more control by the client. The maximal dose per hour is "locked in" to the pump so the client cannot accidentally overdose. Drugs commonly used by the PCA method include morphine, meperidine, and hydromorphone.

Epidural analgesia can be administered intermittently by the anesthesiologist or via continuous drip with or without PCA through an epidural catheter left in place after epidural anesthesia. Drugs commonly given by epidural catheter include the opioids fentanyl citrate (Subli-

Chart 22–4

Drug Therapy for Management of Postoperative Pain

Drug	Usual Dosage	Nursing Interventions	Rationale
Meperidine hydrochloride (Demerol)	• 50–150 mg q3–4h PO or IM • 12.5–25 mg IV • Maximum 6–8 doses	• Monitor blood pressure. • Move and ambulate the client slowly. • Monitor pulse rate. • Assess for decreased GI motility or GI upset.	• Common side effects include decreased blood pressure, orthostatic (postural) hypotension, and bradycardia. • Constipation, nausea, and vomiting can occur.
Morphine sulfate (Epimorph✤, Statex✤)	• 2–15 mg IM or IV incrementally • 10–30 mg q4h PO • Maximum 6 doses	• Monitor respiratory status. • Monitor blood pressure. • Assess for GI motility and urinary output.	• Respiratory depression can be severe and need medical intervention. • Hypotension, constipation, and urinary retention can occur.
Hydromorphone hydrochloride (Dilaudid)	• 1–4 mg q3–4h IV or IM • 2–4 mg q3–4h PO	• Monitor respirations. • Monitor blood pressure. • Monitor for food intolerance. • Monitor fluid and electrolyte balance. • Assess GI motility.	• Respiratory depression, hypotension, anorexia, nausea, vomiting, and constipation can occur.
Codeine sulfate, codeine phosphate (Paveral✤)	• 15–60 mg q4h IM or PO • Maximum 6 doses	• Monitor respiratory status. • Monitor for food intolerance. • Monitor fluid and electrolyte balance. • Assess GI motility.	• Respiratory depression, nausea, and vomiting can occur. • Constipation is common; prophylactic interventions may be indicated.
Butorphanol tartrate (Stadol)	• 1–4 mg q3–4h IM • 0.5–2 mg IV • Maximum 6–8 doses	• Monitor neurologic status and changes in level of consciousness. • Monitor respiratory status.	• Butorphanol can cause increased intracranial pressure and respiratory depression.
Oxycodone hydrochloride and aspirin (Percodan, Endocan✤, Oxycodan✤)	• 1–2 tablets (5–10 mg) q3–4h PO • Maximum 80 mg	• Assess GI tolerance of medication. • Assess for GI bleeding. • Monitor GI motility. • Monitor coagulation respiratory studies (PT, APTT). • Monitor respiratory status.	• The aspirin component can irritate the stomach and could cause GI bleeding. • Bleeding times and other coagulation study results may be increased because of the aspirin component. • Respiratory depression and constipation can be caused by the oxycodone component.
Oxycodone hydrochloride and acetaminophen (Tylox, Percocet, Endocet✤, Oxycocet✤)	• 1–2 tablets q3–4h PO • Maximum 12 tablets	• Monitor blood pressure and respiratory status. • Assess for GI motility.	• Respiratory depression, hypotension, and constipation can occur.

Continued

Chart 22–4. Drug Therapy for Management of Postoperative Pain   Continued

Drug	Usual Dosage	Nursing Interventions	Rationale
Ketorolac tromethamine (Toradol)	• 15–60 mg IM or IV q6h • Maximum 120 mg • 5 day administration maximum	• Monitor for GI bleeding. • Monitor for renal effects, especially in the elderly.	• GI bleeding, ulceration, and perforation can occur. • Decreased urinary output, increased serum creatinine, hematuria, and proteinuria can occur. • Ketorolac is cleared more slowly in the elderly. • The elderly are more sensitive to the renal effects of NSAIDs.
Ibuprofen (Motrin, Amersol✦, Novoprofen✦)	• 300–800 mg q4–6h PO • Maximum 2400 mg daily	• Monitor upper GI tolerance of medication. • Give with food or milk. • Monitor coagulation studies (PT, APTT). • Assess for signs of bleeding or delayed clotting.	• Food or milk helps decrease irritation of the stomach. • Bleeding times and other coagulation study results may be increased. • Monitoring leads to early detection of complications.

PT = prothrombin time; PTT = partial thromboplastin time; NSAID = nonsteroidal antiinflammatory drug; GI = gastrointestinal; PO = orally; IM = intramuscularly; IV = intravenously.

maze) and preservative-free morphine (Duramorph), and the local anesthetic bupivacaine (Marcaine).

The nurse uses care not to overmedicate or undermedicate the client, especially the elderly client. In assessing for overmedication, the nurse monitors the client's vital signs, especially blood pressure and respiratory rate, and level of consciousness. Complications from the use of opioid analgesics include respiratory depression, hypotension, nausea, vomiting, and constipation. An opioid antagonist such as naloxone hydrochloride (Narcan) may be administered to reverse the acute effects of opioid depression. Because of the short effect of the opioid antagonist, the nurse monitors the blood pressure and respirations closely (i.e., every 15–30 minutes) until the full effect of the opioid analgesic has passed. The nurse may need to give more doses of the opioid antagonist during this time. See Chart 22–5 for more information on the opioid antagonists. In addition, the client has breakthrough pain after the opioid antagonist is administered, so the nurse initiates other interventions to promote comfort.

The nurse assesses for undermedication by questioning the client about the effects of the medication and observing for nonverbal cues that indicate pain (e.g., restlessness, increased confusion, "picking" at bedcovers, and aggressive behaviors). The nurse offers pain medication after checking for hypotension and respiratory depression.

As the client's recovery progresses, the nurse administers pain medications in reduced doses and frequency. The medications are changed from injectable or PCA to oral as soon as the client can tolerate oral administration. Nonopioid analgesics, such as acetaminophen (Tylenol, Atasol✦), and nonsteroidal antiinflammatory drugs

(NSAIDs), such as ibuprofen (Motrin, Novoprofen✦, Amersol✦) and ketorolac (Toradol), are used during convalescence or can be given with an opioid analgesic as an adjunct. Antianxiety drugs, such as hydroxyzine (Vistaril, Novohydroxyzin✦), may be given in combination with an opioid analgesic. This combination decreases pain-related anxiety, alleviates muscle tension that could contribute to the client's pain or discomfort, and controls nausea.

Other Methods of Pain Control. The nurse provides comfort measures that may lower the amount of pain medication needed. These measures reduce anxiety and allow the client to relax and rest.

Positioning. In positioning the client, the nurse considers the client's position during surgery, the location of the surgical incision and drains, and medical problems such as arthritis and chronic pulmonary disease. The nurse assists the client in achieving a position of comfort, while enabling the client to maintain optimal function. The client's extremities are supported with pillows. No pillows are placed under the client's knees, and the knee gatch of the bed is not raised because this position could restrict circulation and increase the risk of thrombophlebitis. The nurse turns or helps the client turn at least every 2 hours while the client is bedridden to prevent pulmonary and other complications sometimes caused by immobility.

On the basis of the surgeon's orders and the nurse's assessment of the client's tolerance, the nurse encourages the client progressively to increase activity. Activity decreases stiffness, promotes lung expansion, and promotes

---

Chart 22–5

Drug Therapy for Management of Opioid Overdose

Drug	Usual Dosage	Nursing Interventions	Rationales
Naloxone hydrochloride (Narcan)	• 0.1–2 mg IV, SC, and IM; repeat every 2–3 minutes PRN on the basis of the client's response up to 10 mg	• Maintain an open airway. • Administer oxygen as ordered. • Have suction available. • Closely monitor vital signs and pulse oximetry readings until the client responds. • Do not leave the client unattended until he or she is fully responsive. • Observe for significant reversal of analgesia. • Continue to monitor the client for effects of the naloxone for at least 1 hour.	• A patent airway maximizes respiratory effort. • Oxygen helps to prevent hypoxemia. • Vomiting can occur with administration of naloxone; suction prevents aspiration. • The threat of hypoxemia and respiratory depression or arrest is a concern until the naloxone becomes effective. • Staying with the client promotes safety. • With reversal of the narcotic's respiratory-depressive effects, analgesic effects will also be reversed. • Continued monitoring leads to early detection of hypertension, hypotension, tachycardia, and dysrhythmias, which can be effects of naloxone.

venous circulation. When the client is initially allowed out of bed, the nurse assists him or her to the side of the bed and into a chair. The client splints the surgical wound for support and comfort during the transfer.

Massage. The nurse uses gentle massage of stiff joints or a sore back to decrease postoperative discomfort. The nurse positions the client in a side-lying position and applies lotion with smooth, gentle strokes to increase blood flow to the area and promote general relaxation. The legs, especially the calves, are not massaged because of the increased risk of loosening a thrombus and causing a pulmonary embolus, which can be life threatening.

Other Interventions. Relaxation and diversion are also used to control acute episodes of pain, such as during painful procedures such as dressing changes and injections. Chapters 8 and 9 discuss how the nurse instructs and guides the client through these pain control methods. Music and noise reduction have been shown to decrease awareness of discomfort. Chart 22–6 lists examples of other interventions that may help to reduce pain and promote comfort.

Potential for Hypoxemia

Planning: Expected Outcomes. The expected outcome for the client with hypoxemia is for the client to attain or maintain preoperative baseline PaO_2 values.

Interventions. The key to preventing hypoxemia is to follow the interventions appropriate to the nursing diagnoses of impaired gas exchange (discussed earlier), ineffective airway clearance, and ineffective breathing pattern. Postoperatively, the nurse and physician monitor the client's arterial blood gas and pulse oximetry results. A client who received conscious sedation with midazolam (Versed) or lorazepam (Ativan, Nu-Loraz✲) may be overly sedated or have cardiopulmonary depression sufficient to require reversal with flumazenil (Romazicon) (Chart 22–7). Postoperative hypothermia and its associated shivering causes increased oxygen demands and can contribute to hypoxemia. Various rewarming methods are used in PACUs, although prevention may be more important (see Research Applications for Nursing). The highest incidence of postoperative hypoxemia, however, is on the second postoperative day. Those clients who have a low normal PaO_2, such as those with underlying pulmonary disease or the elderly, are at higher risk for hypoxemia.

The physician treats the potential for hypoxemia with oxygen administration. Depending on the surgeon's preference and established guidelines, the physician may continue oxygen administration until after the second postoperative day. When hypoxemia occurs despite preventive care, the physician orders treatment to manage the cause of the hypoxemia and prescribes oxygen therapy, respiratory treatments, and mechanical ventilation as indicated.

% of arterial 0₂

Chart 22-6

Nursing Care Highlight: Examples of Nonpharmacologic Interventions to Reduce Postoperative Pain and Promote Comfort

- Control or remove noxious stimuli.
- Cushion and elevate painful areas; avoid tension or pressure on those areas.
- Provide adequate rest to increase pain tolerance.
- Encourage the client's participation in diversional activities.
- Instruct the client in relaxation techniques; use audiotapes and breathing exercises.
- Provide opportunities for meditation.
- Help the client to stimulate sensory nerve endings near the painful areas to inhibit ascending pain impulses.
- Use ice to reduce and prevent swelling, as indicated.
- Find a general position of comfort for the client.
- Help the client to stimulate the area contralateral (opposite) to the painful area.

 Continuing Care

Many clients are discharged after a brief hospital stay or directly from the PACU to home. Because of the shortened length of hospitalization, discharge planning, teaching, and referral begin preoperatively and continue postoperatively.

➤ *Health Teaching*

The teaching plan for the postoperative client and appropriate others includes
- Prevention of infection
- Care and assessment of the surgical wound
- Diet therapy
- Pain management
- Drug therapy
- Progressive increase in activity

If dressing changes are needed, the client and family members are instructed on the importance of proper hand washing to prevent infection. The nurse thoroughly explains and demonstrates wound care to the client and family. The client or a family member performs a return demonstration of that care. During teaching sessions, the nurse evaluates learning and promotes compliance after discharge. At the same time, the nurse teaches signs and symptoms of complications such as wound infection. The nurse also discusses with the client and family members appropriate measures to take if complications occur.

A diet high in protein, calories, and vitamin C promotes wound healing. A dietary consultation before the client is discharged helps him or her to select a balanced diet to promote healing. Supplemental vitamin C, iron, and multivitamins are often prescribed after surgery to aid in wound healing and in the formation of red blood cells. Often these supplements are prescribed for 10 to 14 days postoperatively. The nurse instructs the client with prior dietary restrictions about the importance of following the prescribed diet during convalescence. The elderly or debilitated client is encouraged to continue using dietary supplements, if ordered, between meals until the wound is completely healed and energy level restored.

Chart 22-7

Drug Therapy for Management of Benzodiazepine Overdose

Drug	Usual Dosage	Nursing Interventions	Rationales
Flumazenil (Romazicon)	• 0.2–1 mg IV at rate of 0.2 mg/min; repeat every 2–3 minutes PRN up to 3 mg in any 1 hour	• Maintain an open airway. • Administer oxygen as ordered. • Have suction available. • Closely monitor the client's level of sedation, vital signs and pulse oximetry readings until the client responds. • Do not leave the client unattended until fully responsive. • Observe for significant reversal of sedation. • Observe for up to 2 hours for re-sedation and respiratory depression.	• A patent airway maximizes respiratory effort. • Oxygen helps to prevent hypoxemia. • Vomiting can occur with administration of flumazenil; suction prevents aspiration. • Hypoventilation may not be fully reversed with flumazenil; sedation, amnesia, and psychomotor effects of the benzodiazepines should be reversed. • Seizures have occurred with reversal. • With reversal of the benzodiazepine's sedative and amnesia effect, the client will become more aware of pain/discomfort. • The duration of action of the benzodiazepines is longer than that of flumazenil.

▷ Research Applications for Nursing

Hypothermia Still a Problem in Postanesthesia Care Units

Hershey, J., Valenciano, C., & Bookbinder, M. (1997). Comparison of three rewarming methods in a postanesthesia care unit. AORN Journal, 65(3), 597–601.

These researchers noted how frequently clients enter the postanesthesia care unit (PACU) with temperatures less than 36° C (98.6° F). With hypothermia comes shivering, a finding that they and other researchers have concluded is a normal homeostatic response, because the temperatures of clients who shiver will return to normal more quickly than those who do not shiver. They report, however, that shivering increases oxygen demands by as much as 400%, which puts the elderly and those with cardiac conditions at risk.

The nurses studied three rewarming approaches common in PACUs. All clients received two warmed thermal blankets, but each of the study groups also received either a hospital bedspread; a reflective blanket and a bedspread; or a reflective blanket, a bedspread, and a reflective head covering. There were 48 clients in each study group. There were no significant differences among the three nursing interventions and duration of hypothermia.

Critique. All clients in the study were women between the ages of 20 and 60 years; all were having diagnostic laparotomy procedures. These factors may limit the interpretation of the findings.

Possible Nursing Implications. Warming interventions may need to be initiated earlier in the surgical client's experience to prevent hypothermia. For example, nurses can place head coverings on in the holding area, and circulating nurses can be sure to cover any exposed skin of the client while in the operating room. Irrigation and intravenous fluids could be warmed before use in the operating room. Further research is needed to determine whether interventions can be identified that will be effective in either preventing hypothermia in surgical clients or reducing the effects of hypothermia.

The nurse instructs the client about taking pain medication, with special attention to the proper dosage and frequency of administration. The nurse instructs the client to notify the surgeon if the medication does not control the pain or if the pain suddenly increases. If antibiotics or other medications are prescribed, the client is instructed to finish the entire prescription as ordered by the surgeon.

Surgery places physical and emotional stress on the body, and time and rest are required for healing. The nurse instructs the client to increase activity level slowly, balance rest with activity (e.g., plan rest periods), and avoid straining the surgical wound or the surrounding area. Depending on the type of surgery and the client's occupation and usual activities, the surgeon decides when the client may climb stairs, return to work, drive, and resume other usual activities such as sexual intercourse. The amount of weight a client may safely lift after dis-

charge from the facility needs to be specifically defined by the surgeon (i.e., in pounds or kilograms, as appropriate) and interpreted and reinforced as necessary by the nurse (grocery bags, laundry baskets, children, books, and so on).

The nurse also instructs the client in the use of proper body mechanics. A client whose work involves a moderate amount of physical labor may be allowed back to work 6 weeks after nonlaser abdominal surgery. The client may be eager to return to work or to other activities and may not follow activity restrictions. The nurse emphasizes the importance of compliance to prevent complications or disability. It is imperative that the client receive written discharge instructions for reinforcement at home. A visiting nurse may be necessary for follow-up.

▶ Home Care Management

If the client is discharged directly home, the nurse reviews data to help assess the home environment for safety, cleanliness, and availability of caregivers. The nurse uses the data base that was completed when the client was admitted to the hospital or the ambulatory surgical unit to ascertain the client's needs. For example, if the client is unable or not allowed to climb stairs and lives in a two-story house with only one bathroom, the nurse advises the client to rent a bedside commode. The social worker or discharge planner, in collaboration with the nurse, helps the client identify needs related to postoperative care, including meal preparation, dressing changes, and personal hygiene. A referral to a home care nursing agency may be indicated.

The client is usually apprehensive about postoperative complications, pain, and changes in the usual activity level; thus, the nurse must allay fears. The more extensive the surgical procedure is, the more fearful the client is of assuming self-care. The nurse supports the client and family members as they make discharge plans. The client whose surgical procedure has left visible scars may require more emotional support from his or her family for acceptance. (See Chapter 10 for further discussion of body image.) The client may express anger about the surgical outcome or temporary or permanent role changes and concern about financial matters and work. The surgical outcome may not have met the client's expectations, and further interventions may be necessary to assist the client in resolving his or her feelings. Referrals are made for additional counseling as indicated.

▶ Health Care Resources

After returning home, the client may need equipment and assistance with dressing changes, activities of daily living (ADL), and meal preparation. Referral to a home care agency is made and may be paid for by third-party insurance payers, including Medicare, if the client is homebound and requires skilled care. The home care nurse provides skilled nursing assessments, dressing supplies, education in self-care, and referrals for services as needed by the client. Such referrals include Meals on Wheels, support groups, and homemaker services (e.g., for housecleaning and food shopping).

Evaluation

On the basis of the identified nursing diagnoses, collaborative problems, and desired outcomes, the nurse evaluates the care of the postoperative client. The outcomes include that the client

- Maintains a patent airway
- Maintains adequate lung expansion and respiratory function as evidenced by clear breath sounds
- Has stable vital signs
- Returns to baseline arterial blood gas values
- Returns to preoperative mental state
- Has complete wound healing without complications
- States that postoperative pain is reduced or alleviated by interventions

---

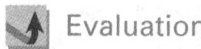 **CASE STUDY for the Postoperative Client**

■ You are a nurse working on a medical-surgical unit. Midway through your shift you are notified that a postoperative client was just placed in one of your rooms. You had not received any notice that you were receiving *any* patient in that room, nor did you get any report.

QUESTIONS:

1. What do you do first?
2. What do you say to the client?
3. What action should you take regarding not being notified of the admission and not receiving a report?

SELECTED BIBLIOGRAPHY

Acute pain management in adults: Operative procedures (AHCPR Pub. No. 92–0019). (1992). Rockville, MD: Agency for Health Care Policy and Research, U.S. Department of Health and Human Services.

*Aker, J. (1994). Immediate care in the postoperative period. *Current Review of Post Anesthesia Care Nurses, 16*(17), 147–154, 156.

Atsberger, D. B. (1995). Relaxation therapy: Its potential as an intervention for acute postoperative pain. *Journal of Post Anesthesia Nursing, 19*(1), 2–8.

Bach, D. M. (1995). Implementation of the Agency for Health Care Policy and Research postoperative pain management guideline. *Nursing Clinics of North America, 30*(3), 515–527.

Black, J. M. (1996). Surgical options in wound healing. *Critical Care Nursing Clinics of North America, 8*(2), 169–182.

Blinkhorne, K. (1995). Prepared for a smooth recovery?...Post-operative nausea and vomiting. *Nursing Times, 91*(28), 42–47.

Boike, L., et al. (1995). Development of an outpatient perioperative care record. *Journal of Post Anesthesia Nursing, 10*(3), 140–150.

*Bowman, A. M. (1992). The relationship of anxiety to development of postoperative delirium. *Journal of Gerontological Nursing, 18*(1), 24–30.

*Brockopp, D. Y., Warden, S., Colclough, G., et al. (1994). Postoperative pain: Getting a grip on the facts. *Nursing94, 24*(6), 49–50.

Brooks-Brunn, J. A. (1995). Consult stat. What accounts for pulmonary problems in these cases? *RN, 58*(11), 66.

Brooks-Brunn, J. A. (1995). Postoperative atelectasis and pneumonia: Risk factors. *American Journal of Critical Care, 4*(5), 340–351.

Brooks-Brunn, J. A. (1995). Postoperative atelectasis and pneumonia. *Heart Lung, 24*(2), 94–115.

Burden, N. (1995). Ambulatory approach. A case study: Identification

and treatment of narcotic depression in the ambulatory surgical patient. *Journal of Post Anesthesia Nursing, 10*(2), 94–99.

*Chalfin, D. B., et al. (1994). Preoperative evaluation and postoperative care of the elderly patient undergoing major surgery. *Clinics in Geriatric Medicine, 10*(1), 51–70.

*Dean, B. E. (1994). Overcoming sedation...Your postoperative patient refuses to take analgesics. *Nursing94, 24*(12), 28.

Dennison, R. D. (1997). Nurses' guide to common postoperative complications. *Nursing97, 27* (11), 56–57.

Dickinson, G. M., et al. (1995). Antimicrobial prophylaxis of infection. *Infectious Disease Clinics of North America, 9*(3), 783–804.

*Ehrlichman, R. J., Seckel, B. R., Bryan, D. J., & Moschella, C. J. (1991). Common complications of wound healing. *Surgical Clinics of North America, 71*(6), 1323–1351.

*Elmquist, L. (1992). Decision making for extubation of the post-anesthesia patient. *Critical Care Nursing Quarterly, 15*(1), 82–86.

Ferrara-Love, R., Sekeres, L., & Bircher, N. G. (1996). Nonpharmacologic treatment of postoperative nausea. *Journal of Perianesthesia Nursing, 11*(6), 378–383.

Ferrell, B. R. (1995). Controlling pain in the elderly. *Nursing95, 25*(7), 73.

Gerber, D. E., et al. (1995). Death in the operating room and postanesthesia care unit: Helping nurses to cope. *Journal of Post Anesthesia Nursing, 10*(2), 84–88.

Good, M. (1995a). A comparison of the effects of jaw relaxation and music on postoperative pain. *Nursing Research, 44*(1), 52–57.

Good, M. (1995b). Complementary modalities/part 2: Relaxation techniques for surgical patients. *American Journal of Nursing, 95*(5), 38–43.

Gordon, D. B., et al. (1995). Correcting patient misconceptions about pain. *American Journal of Nursing, 95*(7), 43–45.

*Heffline, M. S. (1992). Managing PACU emergencies. *Journal of Post Anesthesia Nursing, 7*(3), 215.

Hershey, J., Valenciano, C., & Bookbinder, M. (1997). Comparison of three rewarming methods in a postanesthesia care unit. *AORN Journal, 65*(3), 597–601.

*Hinojosa, R. J. (1992). Nursing interventions to prevent or relieve postoperative nausea and vomiting. *Journal of Post Anesthesia Nursing, 7*(1), 3–14.

Hinojosa, R. J. (1995). Postoperative nausea and vomiting: How nurses can help. *Plastic Surgery Nursing, 15*(2), 85–88, 98–100.

Holden, U. (1995). Dementia in acute units: Confusion. *Nursing Standards, 9*(17), 37–39.

Hunt, K. (1995). Perceptions of patient's pain: A study assessing nurses' attitudes. *Nursing Standards, 10*(4), 32–35.

*Hypoxemia on the general care floor. (1992). Newport Beach, CA: Communicore.

Jackson, A. (1995). Acupressure for post-operative nausea. *Nursing Times, 91*(26), 58.

*Jones, P. L., & Millman, A. (1990). Wound healing and the aged patient. *Nursing Clinics of North America, 25*(1), 263–277.

Kaempfe, G., & Goralski, V. J. (1996). Monitoring postop patients. *RN, 59*(7), 30–35.

*Kane, A. M., et al. (1994). Improving the postoperative care of acutely-confused older adults. *MedSurg Nursing, 3*(6), 453–458.

*Kearns, P. C. (1986). Exercises to ease pain after abdominal surgery. *RN, 49*(7), 45–48.

Komara, J. J., et al. (1995). The impact of a postoperative oxygen therapy protocol on use of pulse oximetry and oxygen therapy. *Respiratory Care, 40*(11), 1125–1129.

*Lawler, M. (1991). Preventing postop complications: Managing other complications. *Nursing91, 21*(11), 33, 40–48.

*Litwak, K. (1991). Managing postanesthesia emergencies. *Nursing91, 21*(9), 49–51.

*Litwak-Saleh, K. (1993). The elderly patient in the post anesthesia care unit. *The Nursing Clinics of North America, 28*(3), 507–518.

Lusis, S. A. (1996). The challenges of nursing elderly surgical patients. *AORN Journal, 64*(6), 954–955, 957–962.

Maklebust, J., & Palleschi, M. (1996). Promoting surgical wound healing. *Nursing96, 26*(6), 24c–24h.

Marley, R. A., et al. (1996). Patient discharge from the ambulatory setting. *Journal of Post Anesthesia Nursing, 11*(1), 39–49.

*Marshall, M. (1993). Postoperative confusion: Helping your patient emerge from the shadows. *Nursing93, 23*(1), 44–47.

*McConnell, E. A. (1990). Determining the cause of post-operative fever. *Nursing90, 20*(8), 82–83.

*McConnell, E. A. (1991). Preventing postop complications: Minimizing respiratory problems. *Nursing91, 21*(11), 33–39.

*McConnell, E. A. (1992a). Assessing postoperative chills and tremors. *Nursing92, 22*(4), 110–114.

*McConnell, E. A. (1992b). Assessing wound drainage. *Nursing92, 22*(7), 66.

*McConnell, E. A. (1992c). Diagnosing postoperative fatigue. *Nursing92, 22*(3), 70–74.

McConnell, E. A. (1995). What's wrong with this patient? When your patient's urine output decreases. *Nursing95, 25*(4), 73–74.

*Metzler, D. J., & Fromm, C. G. (1993). Laying out a care plan for the elderly postoperative patient. *Nursing93, 23*(4), 67–74.

Minnick, A., Roberts, M. J., Young, W. B. et al. (1995). An analysis of posthospitalization telephone survey data. *Nursing Research, 44*(6), 371–375.

Modderman, G. R. (1995). Barriers to pain management in elderly surgical patients. *AORN Journal, 61*(6), 1073–1075.

Morris, J. (1995). Monitoring post-operative effects in day-surgery patients. *Nursing Times, 91*(10), 32–34.

*Nash, C. A., & Jensen, P. L. (1994). When your surgical patient has hypertension. *American Journal of Nursing, 94*(12), 38–45.

*Neal, J. M. (1992). Management of postdural puncture headache. *Anesthesiology Clinics of North America, 10*(1), 163–178.

O'Donnell, M. E. (1995). Assessing fluid and electrolyte balance in elders. *American Journal of Nursing, 95*(11), 40–46.

O'Rourke, K. (1995). Epidural analgesia: Postoperative pain management. *CACCN, 6*(4), 12–15.

Ouellette, S. M. (1995). Postoperative myocardial ischemia: Etiology, recognition and management. *Current Review of Nurse Anesthetists, 18*(5), 38–44.

Paice, J., Mahon, S. M., & Faut-Callahan, M. (1995). Pain control in hospitalized postsurgical patients. *MedSurg Nursing, 4*(5), 367–372.

Pasero, C. L. (1996). Managing postoperative pain in the elderly. *American Journal of Nursing, 96*(10), 38–46.

*Pasero, C. L., & McCaffery, M. (1994). Avoiding opioid-induced respiratory depression. *American Journal of Nursing, 94*(4), 24–31.

*Peden, L. (1992). Helping postop patients to sleep. *RN, 55*(4), 24–26.

*Pediani, R. (1994). Recent developments in the control of surgical wound pain. *Journal of Wound Care, 3*(8), 394–396.

Rowbotham, D. (1995). Recognizing risk factors...Post-operative nausea and vomiting. *Nursing Times, 91*(28), 44–46.

*Rowland, M. A. (1990). Myths—and facts—about postop discomfort. *American Journal of Nursing, 90*(5), 60–64.

Schumacher, S. B. (1995). Monitoring vital signs to identify postoperative complications. *MedSurg Nursing, 4*(2), 142–145.

Sherman, D. W. (1997). Developing quality assurance programs in ambulatory surgery. *Nursing Management, 28*(9), 44–48.

Springhouse Corp. (1996). Controlling pain. Avoiding the I.M. route for analgesic administration. *Nursing96, 26*(1), 67.

Strimike, C. L., Wojcik, J. M., & Stark, B. A. (1997). Incision care that really cuts it. *RN, 60*(7), 22–26.

Swan, B. A. (1996). Assessing symptom distress in ambulatory surgery patients. *MedSurg Nursing, 5*(5), 348–354.

*Thomas, J. A., & McIntosh, J. M. (1994). Are incentive spirometry, intermittent positive pressure breathing, and deep breathing exercises effective in the prevention of postoperative pulmonary complication after upper abdominal surgery? A systematic overview and meta-analysis. *Physical Therapy, 74*(1), 3–16.

*Treloar, D. M. (1984). When a surgical wound bursts. *RN, 47*(6), 20–30, 78.

Wall, M. P. (1995). Dimensions of clinical practice. Postoperative respiratory complications. *Perspectives in Respiratory Nursing, 6*(4), 1, 3–4.

Weant, C. A. (1995). Soundwaves. What floor nurses want to hear from you. *Journal of Post Anesthesia Nursing, 10*(2), 100–101.

*Whitman, G. R. (1991). Hypertension and hypothermia in the acute postoperative period. *Critical Care Nursing Clinics of North America, 3*(4), 661–673.

*Wild, L., & Coyne, C. (1992). The basics and beyond: Epidural analgesia. *American Journal of Nursing, 92*(4), 26–35.

Wilkinson, R. (1996). A non-pharmacological approach to pain relief. *Professional Nurse, 11*(4), 222–224.

*Willens, J. S. (1994). Giving fentanyl for pain outside the OR. *American Journal of Nursing, 94*(2), 24–28.

Winslow, E. H., et al. (1995). Research for practice. Well-timed antibiotics prevent postop infection. *American Journal of Nursing, 95*(3), 60.

Wren, K. R., et al. (1996). Postsurgical urinary retention. *Urological Nursing, 16*(2), 45–49.

Zalon, M. L. (1997). Pain in frail, elderly women after surgery. *Image: Journal of Nursing Scholarship, 29*(1), 21–26.

SUGGESTED READINGS

Pasero, C. L. (1996). Managing postoperative pain in the elderly. *American Journal of Nursing, 96*(10), 38–46.

This article first addresses reasons why traditional pain management in the elderly may be less than optimal. The authors then introduce, define, and describe the multimodal approach to pain management, balanced analgesia, and preemptive analgesia, all of which have been found to be beneficial in the elderly. Specific interventions for managing pain in the elderly and for administering pain medication to the elderly are covered as are details related to different classifications of analgesic medication. Tips on minimizing adverse effects and situations to avoid are discussed. The article concludes with a section on planning for discharge. A continuing education test is included.

Strimike, C. L., Wojcik, J. M., & Stark, B. A. (1997). Incision care that really cuts it. *RN, 60*(7), 22–26.

The article begins with a physiologic description of the various stages of incisional healing. The authors then identify and discuss risk factors for wound complications. The remainder of the article addresses two factors to facilitate wound healing. The first is to perform wound care appropriate to the type of wound, and guidelines are included in the article. The second factor is adequate nutrition; an explanation of various nutrients and their role in wound healing is included in chart form.

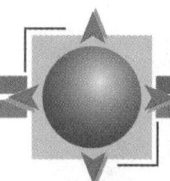

Problems of Protection:

Management of Clients

with Problems of the

Immune System

Chapter 23

CONCEPTS OF INFLAMMATION AND THE IMMUNE RESPONSE

Humans are susceptible to diseases caused by the invasion of microorganisms. Two major defenses, inflammation and immunity, protect the immunocompetent person against diseases and other problems when the body is invaded by microorganisms. These defenses also help the body to recover after injury or tissue damage. Therefore, inflammation and immunity have critical roles in maintaining health and preventing disease. Many diseases, injuries, and medical therapies alter immune function to some degree. These alterations in immune function may be temporary or permanent, but they always endanger the health of the client. Nurses need to understand the processes involved in inflammation and immunity to protect clients and minimize complications.

BASIC CONCEPTS OF INFLAMMATION AND IMMUNITY

Immunity encompasses a variety of functions that protect people against the effects accompanying injury or invasion of the body. People interact with many other living organisms in the environment. The size of these organisms varies from large (other humans and animals) to microscopic (bacteria, viruses, molds, spores, pollens, protozoa, and cells from other people or animals). As long as microorganisms do not enter the body's internal environment, they pose no threat to health. The body has some defenses to prevent microorganisms from gaining access to the internal environment. However, these defenses are not perfect, and invasion of the body's internal environment by microorganisms occurs often. Invasion occurs much more frequently than does an actual disease or illness because of proper immune functioning.

Purpose

The purpose of the immune system is to neutralize, eliminate, or destroy microorganisms that invade the internal environment. To accomplish this purpose without harming the body, immune system cells use defensive actions only against non-self proteins and cells. Therefore, immune system cells can differentiate between the body's own healthy self cells and other non-self proteins and cells.

Self Versus Non-Self

Non-self proteins and cells include infected or debilitated body cells, self cells that have become cancerous, and all invading cells and microorganisms. This ability to recognize self versus non-self, which is necessary to prevent healthy body cells from being destroyed along with the invaders, is called *self-tolerance*. The immune system cells are the only body cells capable of recognizing self from non-self. The process of self-tolerance is possible because of the different kinds of proteins present on cell membranes.

All organisms are made up of cells. Each cell is surrounded by a plasma membrane (Fig. 23–1). With any cell, many different proteins protrude through the plasma membrane. For example, in liver cells, many different proteins are present on the cell surface (protruding through the membrane). The amino acid sequence of each protein type differs from that of all other protein types. Some of these proteins are found on the liver cells of all animals (including humans) that have livers because these protein types are specific to the liver and actually serve as a marker for liver tissues. Other protein types are found only on the liver cells of humans, because these protein types are specific markers for humans. Still other protein types are found only on the liver cells of humans with a specific blood type. In addition, each person's liver cells have surface protein types that are specific to that individual. These proteins are unique to the person and would be identical only to the proteins of an identical twin. These unique proteins, found on the surface of all body cells of that individual, serve as a "universal product code" or a "cellular fingerprint" for that person (Workman et al., 1993). The proteins that make up the universal product code for one person are recognized as "foreign" by the immune system of another person. Because the cell-surface proteins would be recognized as foreign by another person's immune system, they are antigens, proteins capable of stimulating an immune response.

This unique universal product code for each person is composed of the human leukocyte antigens (HLAs). "Leukocyte" antigen is actually an incorrect term, because these antigens are also present on the surfaces of nearly all body cells, not just on leukocytes. HLAs are a normal part of the person and act as antigens only if they enter another person's body. These antigens specify the tissue type of a person. Other names for these personal cellular fingerprints are human transplantation antigens, human histocompatibility antigens, and class I antigens.

Humans have about 40 major HLAs (known as *histocompatibility antigens*) that are determined by a series of genes collectively called the major histocompatibility complex (MHC). However, the exact number of minor HLAs that any person has is not known. The specific antigens that any person has (of a large number of possible antigens) are genetically determined by which MHC genes were inherited from his or her parents.

This universal product code (HLA) is a key feature for recognition and self-tolerance. The immune system cells constantly come into contact with other body cells and with any invader that happens to enter the body's internal environment. At each encounter, the immune system cells compare the surface protein universal product codes (HLAs) to determine whether or not the encountered cell

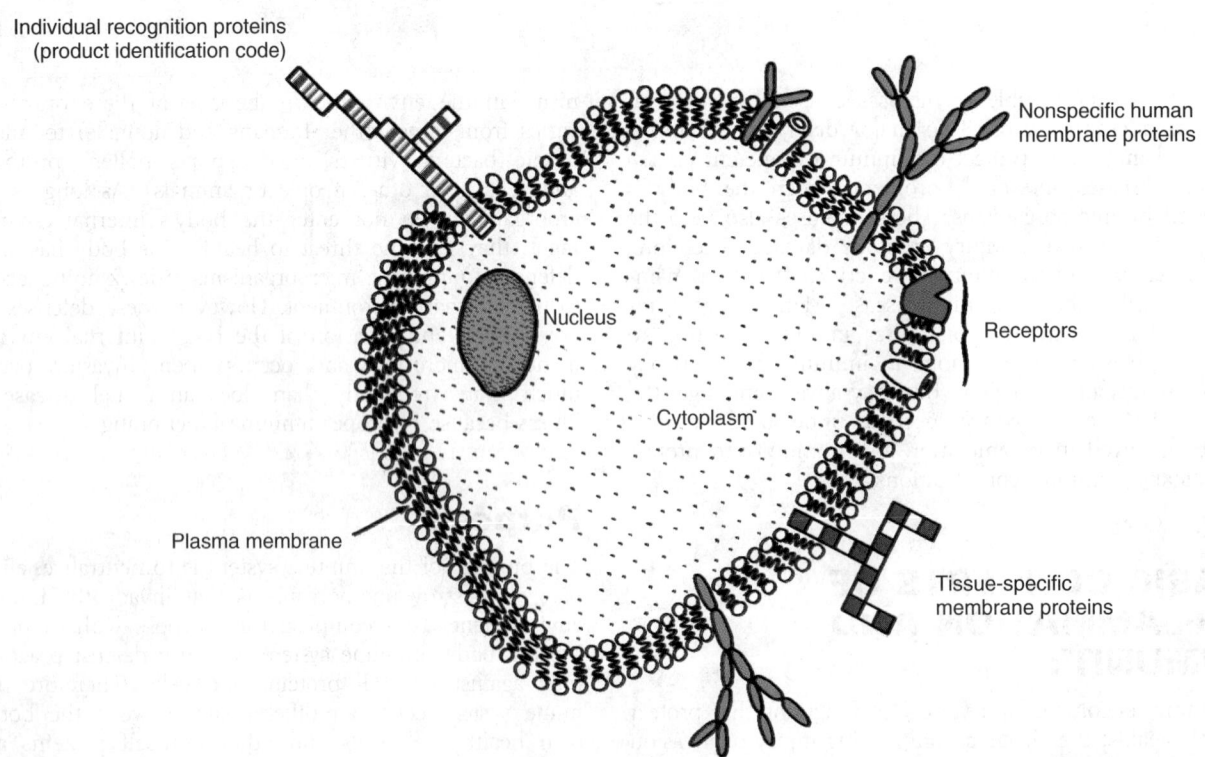

Figure 23–1. Properties of human cell membranes.

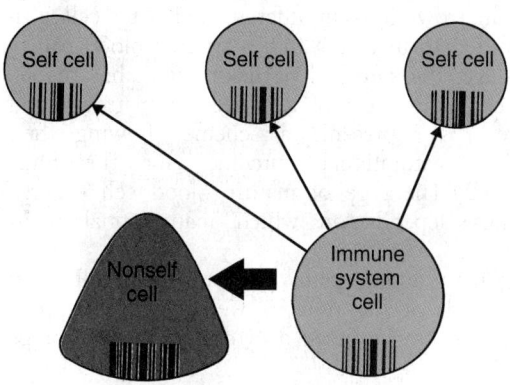

Figure 23–2. Determination of self versus non-self cells.

cell's universal product code (HLA) does not perfectly match the HLA of the immune system cell, the encountered cell is considered non-self or foreign. The immune system cell takes actions to neutralize, destroy, or eliminate the foreign invader.

Immune function changes during a person's life, according to nutritional status, environmental conditions, medications, the presence of disease, and age. Immune function is most efficient when people are in their 20s and 30s and slowly declines with increasing age. The elderly have decreased immune function, causing greater susceptibility to a variety of pathologic conditions (Chart 23–1).

belongs in the body's internal environment (Fig. 23–2). If the encountered cell's universal product code (HLA) perfectly matches the HLA of the immune system cell, the encountered cell is considered self and is not further molested by the immune system cell. If the encountered

Organization of the Immune System

The immune system does not reside in any one organ or area of the body. The cells of the immune system originate in the bone marrow. Some of these cells mature in

---

Chart 23–1

Nursing Focus on the Elderly: Changes in Immune Function Related to Aging

Immune Component	Functional Change	Nursing Implications
Inflammation	• Probable defect in neutrophil function	• Neutrophil counts may be normal, but activity is reduced or impaired.
	• Leukocytosis does not occur during episodes of acute infection	• Clients may have an infection but not show standard changes in white blood cell counts.
	• Elderly persons may not have a fever during inflammatory or infectious episodes	• Not only is there potential loss of protection through inflammation, but minor infections may be overlooked until the client becomes severely infected or septic.
Antibody-mediated immunity	• The total number of colony-forming B lymphocytes and the ability of these cells to mature into antibody-secreting cells are diminished	• The elderly are less able to make new antibodies in response to the presence of new antigens. Thus, the elderly should receive immunizations, such as "flu shots" and the pneumococcal vaccination.
	• There is a decline in natural antibodies, decreased response to antigens, and reduction in the amount of time the antibody response is maintained	• Elderly people may not have sufficient antibodies present to provide protection when they are re-exposed to microorganisms against which they have already generated antibodies. Thus, elderly clients need to avoid people with viral infections and to receive "booster" shots for old vaccinations and immunizations.
Cell-mediated immunity	• Thymic activity decreases with aging, and the number of circulating T lymphocytes decreases	• Skin tests for tuberculosis may be falsely negative. • Elderly clients are more at risk for bacterial and fungal infections, especially on the skin and mucous membranes, in the respiratory tract, and in the genitourinary tract.

the bone marrow; others leave the bone marrow and mature in different specific body sites. After maturation, most immune system cells are released into the blood, where they circulate to most areas of the body and exert specific effects.

The bone marrow is the source of all blood cells, including immune system cells. The bone marrow produces an immature, undifferentiated cell called a stem cell (Abbas et al., 1997). This immature stem cell is also described as pluripotent, multipotent, totipotent, and even omnipotent. These adjectives describe the potential future of the stem cell. When the stem cell is first created in the

bone marrow, it is undifferentiated. The cell is not yet committed to maturing into a specific blood cell type. At this stage, the stem cell is flexible and has the potential to become any one of a variety of mature blood cells. Figure 23–3 presents a scheme showing the major possible maturational outcomes for the pluripotent stem cell. The type of mature blood cell the stem cell becomes depends on which maturational pathway it follows.

The maturational pathway of any stem cell depends on body needs at the time as well as on the presence of specific hormones (termed cytokines, factors, or poietins)

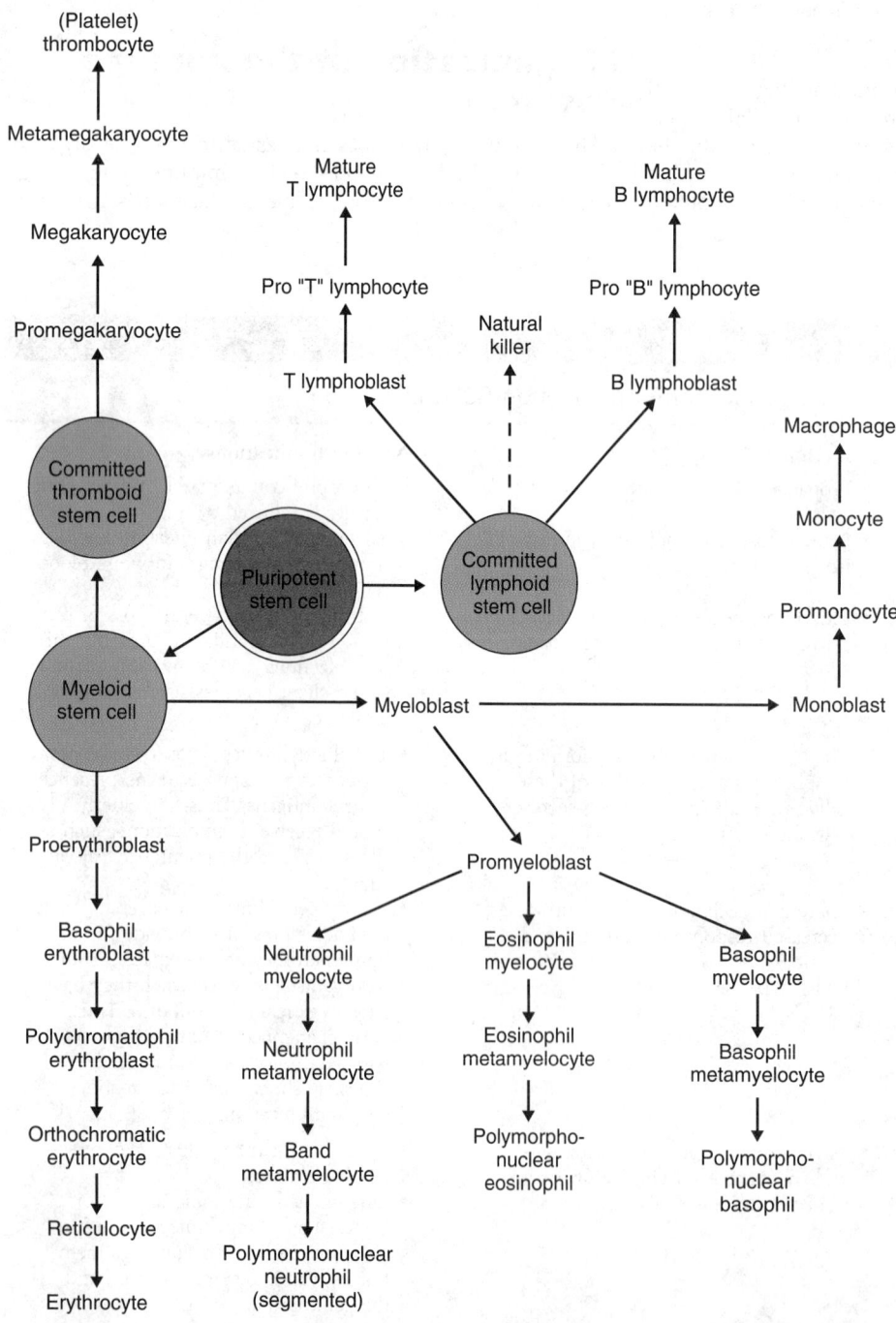

Figure 23–3. Stem cell differentiation and maturation.

TABLE 23-1

Immune Functions of Specific Leukocytes

Variable	Leukocyte	Function
Inflammation	Neutrophil	• Nonspecific ingestion and phagocytosis of microorganisms and foreign protein
	Macrophage	• Nonspecific recognition of foreign proteins and microorganisms; ingestion and phagocytosis
	Monocyte	• Destruction of bacteria and cellular debris; matures into macrophage
	Eosinophil	• Weak phagocytic action; releases vasoactive amines during allergic reactions
	Basophil	• Releases histamine and heparin in areas of tissue damage
Antibody-mediated immunity	B lymphocyte	• Becomes sensitized to foreign cells and proteins
	Plasma cell	• Secretes immunoglobulins in response to the presence of a specific antigen
	Memory cell	• Remains sensitized to a specific antigen and can secrete increased amounts of immunoglobulins specific to the antigen
Cell-mediated immunity	T lymphocyte helper–inducer T cell	• Enhances immune activity through secretion of various factors, cytokines, and lymphokines
	Cytotoxic–cytolytic T cell	• Selectively attacks and destroys non-self cells, including virally infected cells, grafts, and transplanted organs
	Natural killer cell	• Nonselectively attacks non-self cells, especially body cells that have undergone mutation and become malignant; also attacks grafts and transplanted organs

that direct commitment and induce maturation. For example, erythropoietin is made in the kidney. When immature stem cells are exposed to erythropoietin, the immature stem cells commit to the erythrocyte maturational pathway and become mature red blood cells.

White blood cells (leukocytes) are cells that protect the body from the effects of invasion by foreign microorganisms. These cells are the immune system cells. Table 23–1 summarizes the functions of different immune system cells. The leukocytes can provide protection through a variety of defensive actions (Abbas et al., 1997). These actions include

- Recognition of self versus non-self
- Phagocytic destruction of foreign invaders, cellular debris, and unhealthy or abnormal self cells
- Lytic destruction of foreign invaders and unhealthy self cells
- Production of antibodies directed against invaders
- Activation of complement
- Production of hormones that stimulate increased formation of leukocytes in bone marrow
- Production of hormones that increase specific leukocyte growth and activity

The three processes necessary for immunity and the cells involved in these responses can be categorized as inflammation, antibody-mediated immunity (AMI) (humoral immunity), and cell-mediated immunity (CMI).

These three processes represent different defensive actions (Fig. 23–4). Full immunity, or immunocompetence, requires the function and interaction of all three processes.

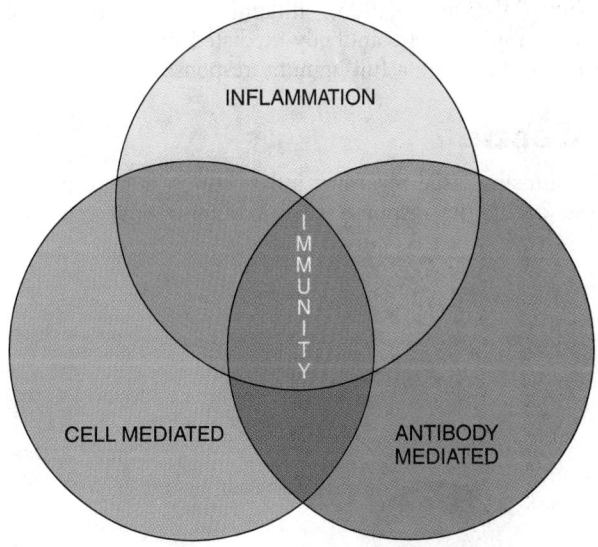

Figure 23–4. The three divisions of immunity. Each division (inflammation, antibody-mediated immunity, and cell-mediated immunity) has an important independent function. In addition, the function of each division of immunity is profoundly influenced by the other two divisions. Most important, optimal function of all three divisions is necessary for complete immunity.

INFLAMMATION

Inflammation provides immediate protection against the effects of tissue injury and invading foreign proteins. The ability to produce an inflammatory response is critical to health and well-being. Inflammation differs from AMI and CMI in two important ways:

1. Inflammatory responses provide immediate but short-term protection against the effects of injury or foreign invaders rather than sustained, long-term immunity on repeated exposure to the same foreign invaders.
2. Inflammation is a nonspecific body defense to invasion or injury.

Inflammation is nonspecific because the same tissue responses occur with any type of injury or invasion, regardless of the location on the body or the specific initiating agent. Therefore, the inflammatory processes stimulated by a scald burn to the hand are the same as the inflammatory processes stimulated by excessive acid in the stomach or the presence of bacteria in the middle ear. How widespread the symptoms of inflammation are in the body depends on the intensity, severity, duration, and extent of exposure to the initiating injury or invasion. For example, a splinter in the finger triggers an inflammatory response only at the splinter site, whereas a burn injuring 60% of the skin surface results in an inflammatory response involving the entire body.

Purpose

Inflammatory responses result in tissue actions that cause visible and uncomfortable symptoms. Despite the discomfort, these inflammatory actions are important in ridding the body of harmful microorganisms. However, if the inflammatory response is excessive, tissue damage may result (Workman, 1995). Inflammatory responses also help stimulate both antibody-mediated and cell-mediated actions to activate a full immune response.

Infection

A confusing issue regarding inflammation is that this process occurs in response to tissue injury as well as to invasion by microorganisms or other foreign proteins. Infection is usually accompanied by inflammation; however, inflammation can occur without invasion by microorganisms. For example, inflammatory responses not associated with infection occur with sprain injuries to joints, myocardial infarction, sterile surgical incisions, thrombophlebitis, and blister formation caused by temperature extremes. Examples of inflammatory responses associated with noninfectious invasion by foreign proteins include allergic rhinitis, contact dermatitis, and other immediate-type allergic reactions. Inflammatory responses associated with invasion by disease-causing microorganisms include otitis media, appendicitis, bacterial peritonitis, viral hepatitis, and bacterial myocarditis, among others. Thus, inflammation does not always mean that an infection is present.

Cell Types Involved in Inflammation

The leukocytes associated with inflammatory responses are neutrophils, macrophages, eosinophils, and basophils. Neutrophils and macrophages participate in phagocytosis, destroying and eliminating foreign invaders. Basophils and eosinophils act on blood vessels to cause tissue-level responses.

Neutrophils
Description and Origin

Mature neutrophils usually compose between 55% and 70% of the total white blood cell count. Neutrophils arise from the stem cells and complete the maturation process in the bone marrow (Fig. 23–5). They belong to the class of leukocytes known as granulocytes because of the large number of granules present inside each cell. Other names for neutrophils are based on their physical characteristics and degree of maturation. Mature neutrophils are also called segmented neutrophils ("segs") or polymorphonuclear cells ("polys") because of their segmented nucleus. Less mature neutrophils are called band neutrophils ("bands" or "stabs") because of their nuclear appearance.

Usually, maturation from the undifferentiated stem cell

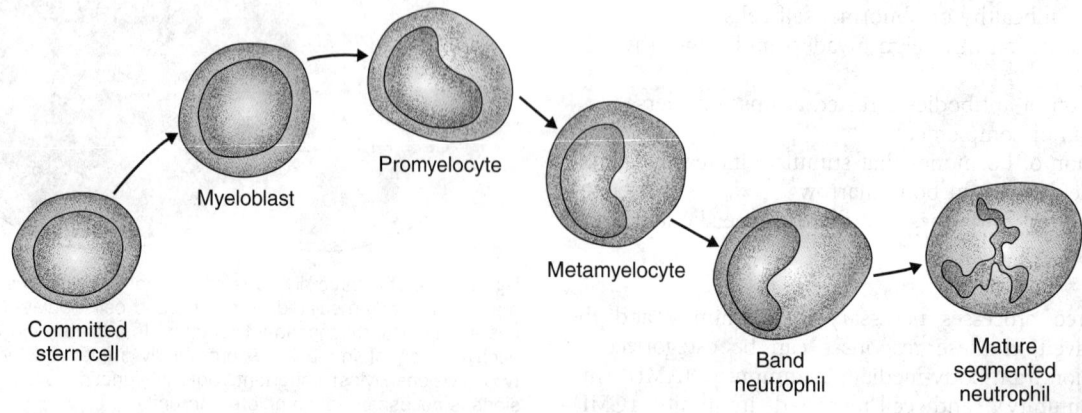

Committed stem cell — Myeloblast — Promyelocyte — Metamyelocyte — Band neutrophil — Mature segmented neutrophil

Figure 23–5. Neutrophil maturation.

to the functional segmented neutrophil requires 12 to 14 days. This time can be shortened by certain conditions that stimulate the body to produce specific cytokines such as granulocyte-macrophage colony–stimulating factor and granulocyte colony–stimulating factor. The purpose and action of cytokines are described later in this chapter under Cytokines.

In the immunocompetent, healthy person, more than 100 billion fresh, mature neutrophils are released from the bone marrow into the systemic circulation daily (Abbas et al., 1997). This massive production of neutrophils is necessary because the life span of a circulating neutrophil is extremely short, averaging only about 12 to 18 hours.

Function

Although the neutrophils are the largest group of circulating leukocytes, each individual cell is small. This army of powerful small cells provides the first internal line of defense, via phagocytosis, against foreign invaders (especially bacteria) in blood and extracellular fluid. It is the granules inside the neutrophils that cause the phagocytic destruction of foreign invaders. The mature neutrophil is filled with large numbers of granules containing various enzymes that can degrade different parts of foreign invaders.

Neutrophils have a small energy supply and no way of replenishing either that energy supply or the enzymes used in degradation. Thus, each neutrophil can participate in only one episode of phagocytic destruction before supplies are exhausted.

The mature, segmented neutrophil is the only neutrophil stage capable of effective phagocytosis. Because this cell type is responsible for continuous, instant, nonspecific protection against microorganisms, the percentage and actual number of circulating white blood cells that are mature neutrophils reliably measure a client's susceptibility to infection: the higher the numbers, the greater is the resistance to infection. This measurement is the *absolute neutrophil count* (sometimes called the absolute granulocyte count or total granulocyte count).

The differential of a normal white blood cell count indicates that most of the neutrophils released into the blood from the bone marrow are segmented neutrophils; only a small percentage are composed of band neutrophils (Fig. 23–6). The less mature neutrophil forms should not be present in the blood. Some conditions cause the major population of neutrophils in the blood to change from mostly segmented neutrophils to less mature forms. This situation is termed a *left shift* because the segmented neutrophil, which is seen at the far right of the neutrophil maturational pathway (see Fig. 23–5), no longer represents the greatest number of circulating neutrophils. Instead, the major population is made up of one of the cell types found farther left on the neutrophil maturational pathway.

A left shift is a clinical sign indicating that the client's bone marrow cannot produce enough mature neutrophils to keep pace with the continuing presence of microorganisms and is releasing immature neutrophils into the blood. Unfortunately, most of these immature neutrophils

Differential	%	/mm³
Total WBC	100	10,000
segs	62	6200
bands	5	500
monos	3	300
lymphs	28	2800
eosin	1.5	150
baso	0.5	50

Figure 23–6. Example of a laboratory slip showing the differential of a normal white blood cell (WBC) count.

are of no benefit to the client, because they are not capable of phagocytosis.

Macrophages
Description and Origin

Macrophages arise from the committed myeloid stem cell in the bone marrow and form the mononuclear phagocyte system. This cell first begins to differentiate into a monocyte and is released into the blood at this stage. Until they mature, monocytes have only limited activity. Most monocytes move into various tissues, where they complete the maturation process into macrophages. Some macrophages become "fixed" in position within the tissues, whereas others remain mobile in the tissue's interstitial fluid. Macrophages in various tissues have slightly different appearances and different names. Table 23–2 lists the names of the different tissue macrophages. Figure 23–7 shows the distribution of tissue macrophages throughout the body. The liver and spleen contain the greatest concentration of these cells.

Tissue macrophages have relatively long life spans, lasting from months to years. Macrophages are the largest of all the leukocytes and have granules containing many lytic enzymes.

TABLE 23–2

Tissue Macrophages

Tissue	Macrophage
Lung	• Alveolar macrophage
Connective tissue	• Histiocyte
Brain	• Microglial cell
Liver	• Kupffer cell
Peritoneum	• Peritoneal macrophage
Bone	• Osteoclast
Joints	• Synovial type A cell
Kidney	• Mesangial cell

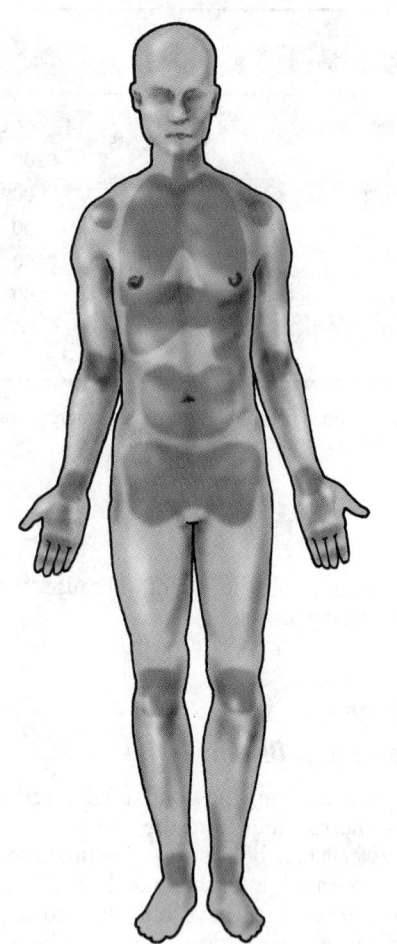

Figure 23–7. Areas of highest concentration of tissue macrophages.

Function

Macrophages play more than one role in protecting against invasion and tissue injury. These cells are important in immediate inflammatory responses and can also stimulate the longer lasting immune responses associated with antibody-mediated immunity (AMI) and cell-mediated immunity (CMI). Specific macrophage functions include phagocytosis, repair of injured tissues, antigen processing, and secretion of cytokines that help control the immune system.

The inflammation-associated macrophage function is phagocytosis. Macrophages are efficient at distinguishing between self and non-self and are especially effective at trapping invading cells. Unlike neutrophils, macrophages are able to regenerate the energy supplies and enzymes needed to degrade foreign protein. Therefore, each macrophage can participate in many phagocytic events during its life span.

Basophils
Description and Origin

The rarest leukocytes, basophils, arise from myeloid stem cells and are released from the bone marrow after a short maturation period. Basophils cause the obvious signs and symptoms accompanying inflammation.

Function

Basophilic granules contain many vasoactive chemicals that act on blood vessels, including heparin, histamine, serotonin, kinins, and leukotrienes. When released into the blood, most of these chemicals act on smooth muscle and blood vessel walls. Heparin inhibits coagulation of blood and other protein-containing extracellular fluids. Histamine constricts the smooth muscles of the respiratory system and small veins. Constriction of respiratory smooth muscle narrows the lumen of airways and restricts breathing. Constriction of venular smooth muscle inhibits blood flow through small veins and decreases venous return. This effect causes blood to collect in capillaries and small arterioles. Kinins cause vasodilation of arterioles and, together with serotonin, increased capillary permeability. These actions permit the plasma portion of the blood to leak into the interstitial space. This chemical-induced process is called *vascular leak syndrome*.

Eosinophils
Description and Origin

Eosinophils arise from the myeloid line and contain more vasoactive chemicals. Usually only 1% to 2% of the total white blood cell count is composed of eosinophils.

Function

Eosinophils are not efficient phagocytes, although they can act against infestations of parasitic larvae. Eosinophil granules contain many substances with vastly different actions. Some of these substances are vasoactive chemicals that produce inflammatory reactions when released. In addition, certain enzymes from eosinophils degrade vasoactive chemicals and in this way may control or modulate the extent of inflammatory reactions.

Phagocytosis

The key mechanism for the successful outcome of inflammation is *phagocytosis*, or the destruction of non-self cells. Phagocytosis is the process by which leukocytes engulf invaders and destroy them by enzymatic degradation. Phagocytosis rids the body of debris after tissue injury and destroys foreign invaders. Of all the leukocytes, neutrophils and macrophages perform phagocytosis most efficiently. Phagocytosis occurs in a predictable manner and involves the seven steps depicted in Figure 23–8.

Exposure and Invasion

Leukocytes that engage in phagocytosis and stimulate inflammation are present in the blood and most other extracellular fluids. For phagocytosis to be initiated, these leukocytes must first be exposed to debris from damaged tissues or foreign proteins (antigens). Therefore, the initiating event for phagocytosis is injury or invasion.

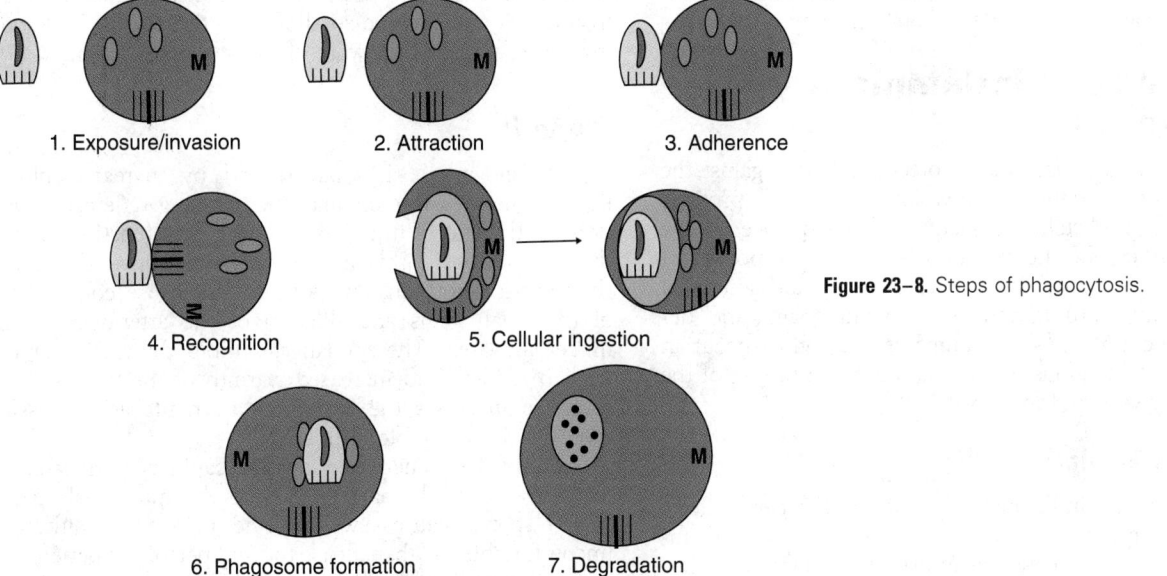

1. Exposure/invasion   2. Attraction   3. Adherence

4. Recognition   5. Cellular ingestion

Figure 23–8. Steps of phagocytosis.

6. Phagosome formation   7. Degradation

Attraction

Phagocytosis is effective only when the phagocytic cell comes into direct contact with the target (antigen, invader, or foreign protein). Special chemical substances can act as chemical magnets that attract neutrophils and macrophages. These substances are called chemotaxins, or leukotaxins. Damaged tissues and blood vessels secrete chemotaxins. In addition, substances that combine with surface components of invading foreign proteins serve as chemotaxins. This combining (and attracting) mechanism is described next.

Adherence

Because phagocytosis requires direct contact of the phagocyte with its intended target, the phagocytic cell must first bind to the surface of the target. A special process called *opsonization* helps provide direct contact of the phagocyte with its target.

Opsonization

The word *opsonin* is derived from the Greek and literally means "to cover food with a sauce in preparation for eating." In biological processes, opsonins coat a target cell (antigen or foreign protein); this changes the target cell's surface charge and makes it easier for phagocytic cells to stick to it. Many substances can act as opsonins. Some of these substances are particles from dead neutrophils, antibodies, and activated (fixated) complement components.

Complement Activation and Fixation

One mechanism of opsonization and phagocytic adherence to target cells is complement activation and fixation. Twenty different inactive protein components of the complement system are present in the blood. These components are made by the liver. With proper stimulation, individual complement proteins become activated and to-

gether cause dramatic actions as a result of fixation (adherence) to specific tissues. Complement fixation must occur quickly, but consequences can be devastating if its effects are exerted at the wrong time or in the wrong place. Therefore, the complement system works as a cascade reaction (chain reaction), with many sites of activation and control.

Recognition

When the phagocytic cell sticks to the surface of the target cell, recognition of non-self occurs. The body's phagocytic cells examine the universal product codes (HLAs) of whatever they encounter. Recognition of non-self is enhanced by opsonins on the surface of the target cell. Phagocytic cells proceed with phagocytosis only if the target cell is recognized either as foreign or as debris from damaged self cells.

Cellular Ingestion

Because phagocytic destruction is an intracellular process, the target cell or foreign protein must be brought inside the phagocytic cell. The phagocytic cell changes its shape and bends its membrane around to enclose (engulf) the target cell. Once the target is enclosed in the phagocytic cells, a vacuole is formed.

Phagosome Formation

When the phagocyte's granules are inside the vacuole, the structure is called a *phagosome* (or phagolysosome). These granules break open and release enzymes into the fluid of the phagosome and destroy the ingested target.

Degradation

The enzymes within the phagosome exert their specific effects on different parts of the ingested target. The target is broken down into smaller pieces until only minute particles remain to be removed from the body as debris.

Sequence of Inflammatory Responses

Inflammatory responses that protect the body against the effects of tissue injury or invasion by foreign proteins occur in a predictable sequence. The sequence is the same regardless of the initiating stimulus. Responses at the tissue level cause the five cardinal manifestations of inflammation: warmth, redness, swelling, pain, and decreased function. These inflammatory responses occur in three distinct functional stages, although the timing of the stages may overlap (Table 23–3).

Stage I (Vascular)

In stage I of the inflammatory response, the early effects involve changes at the blood vessel level. When inflammation results from tissue injury, this stage has two phases.

Phase I

The first phase is an immediate, short-term constriction of arterioles and venules as a direct result of physical trauma

to vascular smooth muscle. This phase lasts only seconds to minutes and may be so short that the person undergoing the response is unaware of the vasoconstriction.

Phase II

The second phase is characterized by increased blood flow to the area (hyperemia) and swelling (edema formation) at the site of injury or invasion. Injured tissues and the leukocytes in this area secrete vasoactive chemicals (histamine, serotonin, and kinins) that cause constriction of the small veins and dilation of the arterioles in the immediate area. These changes in blood vessel dilation lead to redness and increased warmth of the tissues. This response increases the supply of nutrients at the tissue level by increasing blood flow.

Some of these chemicals increase capillary permeability, allowing blood plasma to leak into the interstitial space. This response causes swelling and pain. Pain, although uncomfortable, is beneficial to the person experiencing inflammation. Pain increases the person's awareness that a problem exists and encourages action to avoid further injury or inflammation. Edema formation at the site of injury or invasion is also a helpful event. This swelling protects the area from further injury by creating a cushion of fluid. The extra fluid can dilute the concentration

TABLE 23–3

Stages of Inflammation

Stage	Onset	Cells Involved	Actions
Stage I: vascular	• Minutes after injury or invasion	• Tissue macrophages	• Limited phagocytosis of invading microorganisms or cell debris from injured tissues • Secretion of vasoactive amines (histamine, bradykinin, serotonin) to dilate blood vessels and increase capillary leak; this action results in redness, warmth, swelling, and pain at the site but also increases blood flow to the area; more nutrients are available to the tissues; plasma proteins moved into the tissues clot and "wall off" microorganisms, limiting their spread • Secretion of chemotaxins to draw more leukocytes into the area to sustain the inflammatory response • Secretion of cytokines to increase bone marrow production of granulocytes

Stage II: cellular exudate	• Hours after injury or invasion	• Granular myeloid cells
		  • Neutrophils
		  • Basophils
		  • Eosinophils
			• Increased phagocytosis
			• Secretion of slow-acting vasoactive amines to ensure a sustained inflammatory response
			• Secretion of substances to increase the rate of neutrophil maturation and macrophage maturation

Stage III: tissue repair and replacement	• Begins at initial injury and continues until new tissues are formed and mature or are functional	• Neutrophils • Macrophages	• Stimulation of mitotically active cells to divide; stimulation of fibroblasts in blood vessels to grow and release collagen to form scaffold on which to build scar tissue

of any toxins or microorganisms that have entered the area. The duration of these responses depends on the severity of the initiating event.

The major leukocyte involved in stage I of the inflammatory response is the tissue macrophage. The response of tissue macrophages is immediate, because they are already in place at the site of injury or invasion. However, this response is limited, because the number of such macrophages is so small. In addition to functioning in phagocytosis, the tissue macrophages secrete several cytokines to enhance the inflammatory response. One cytokine is colony-stimulating factor, which stimulates the bone marrow to reduce the time of leukocyte production from 14 days to a matter of hours. Tissue macrophages also secrete substances that increase the release of neutrophils from the bone marrow and attract them to the site of injury or invasion, which leads to the next stage of inflammation.

Stage II (Cellular Exudate)

Stage II of inflammation is characterized by neutrophilia (increased number of circulating neutrophils), secretion of many factors into the interstitial fluid, and formation of exudate.

The most active leukocyte in this stage is the neutrophil. Under the influence of chemotactic agents and cytokines, the neutrophil count can increase up to five times within 12 hours after the onset of inflammation. At the site of inflammation, neutrophils attack and destroy foreign materials and remove dead tissue through phagocytosis.

During acute inflammatory responses, the healthy person can produce enough mature neutrophils to keep pace with the effects of injury or invasion and to prevent the invaders from multiplying. At the same time, the leukocytes secrete cytokines, which increase reproduction of tissue macrophages and bone marrow production of monocytes. Although this reaction begins slowly, its effects are long lasting.

When infectious processes stimulating inflammation are longer or chronic, the bone marrow cannot produce and release enough mature neutrophils into the blood to keep pace with the ability of microorganisms to multiply. In this situation, the bone marrow begins to release only immature neutrophils. Such a reduction in the number of functional phagocytic neutrophils limits the effectiveness of the inflammatory response and increases the susceptibility to microbial infections.

Stage III (Tissue Repair and Replacement)

Although stage III is completed last, it begins at the time of injury and is critical to the ultimate function of the inflamed area.

Some of the leukocytes involved in inflammation start the replacement and repair of lost or damaged tissues by inducing the remaining healthy tissue to divide. In tissues that are nondividing, leukocytes stimulate new blood vessel growth and scar tissue formation. Because scar tissue does not behave like normal tissue, functional loss occurs where damaged tissues are replaced with scar tissue. The extent of the functional loss is determined by the percentage of tissue replaced by scar tissue.

Inflammation alone cannot confer immunity; however, the interaction of inflammatory cells with lymphocytes helps provide long-lasting immunity against re-exposure to the same microorganisms. Long-lasting immune actions are those generated by antibody-mediated immunity (AMI) and cell-mediated immunity (CMI).

ANTIBODY-MEDIATED IMMUNITY

Antibody-mediated immunity (AMI), also known as humoral immunity, involves antigen-antibody actions to neutralize, eliminate, or destroy foreign proteins. Antibodies for these actions are produced by populations of B lymphocytes.

Purpose

The primary functions of B lymphocytes are to become sensitized to a specific foreign protein (antigen) and to synthesize an antibody directed specifically against that protein. The antibody (rather than the actual B lymphocyte) then participates in one of several actions to neutralize, eliminate, or destroy that antigen.

Cell Types Involved in Antibody-Mediated Immunity

The leukocytes with the most direct role in AMI are the B lymphocytes. Macrophages and T lymphocytes (discussed later under Cell-Mediated Immunity) cooperate with B lymphocytes to start and complete antigen–antibody actions. Therefore, for optimal AMI, the entire immune system must function adequately.

B lymphocytes start life as pluripotent stem cells in the bone marrow, the primary lymphoid tissue. The pluripotent stem cells destined to become B lymphocytes commit early to the lymphocyte maturational pathway (see Fig. 23–3). At the point of commitment, these stem cells are no longer pluripotent but are limited to differentiation into lymphocytes. The committed lymphocyte stem cells are released from the bone marrow into the blood. They then migrate into various secondary lymphoid tissues, where maturation is completed.

In humans, the secondary lymphoid tissues for B lymphocyte maturation are the spleen, germinal centers of lymph nodes, tonsils, and Peyer's patches of the intestinal tract.

Antigen-Antibody Interactions

The body learns to make enough of any specific antibody to provide long-lasting immunity against specific microorganisms or toxins. Seven steps in a series of special interactions are required for the production of a unique and specific antibody directed against a unique and specific antigen whenever the person is exposed to that antigen: exposure and invasion, antigen recognition, lymphocyte sensitization, antibody production and release, antigen-antibody binding, antibody-binding reactions, and sustained immunity—memory (Fig. 23–9).

Exposure and Invasion

Antigen—antibody interactions occur in the body's internal environment. For the body to make an antibody that can exert its effects on a specific antigen, the antigen must first enter the body. Not all exposures result in the stimulation of antibody production, even when exposure includes penetration. Invasion by the antigen must occur in such large numbers that some of the antigen either evades detection by the normal nonspecific defenses or overwhelms the ability of the inflammatory response to neutralize, eliminate, or destroy the invader.

Take, for example, a person who has never contracted or even been exposed to the childhood viral disease chickenpox. This person baby-sits for three children who show chickenpox lesions within the next 10 hours. These children, in the pre-eruption stage, shed many millions of live chickenpox virus particles via the droplets from the upper respiratory tract. Because small children are often unconcerned about the finer points of infection control, they drink out of the baby-sitter's soft drink can, kiss the sitter directly (and wetly) on the lips, and sneeze and cough directly into the sitter's face. After spending 5 hours with the children at close range, the baby-sitter has been overwhelmingly invaded by the chickenpox virus (varicella zoster) and will become sick with this disease within 14 to 21 days. While the virus is incubating and the disease is developing, the sitter's leukocytes are partic-

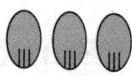

1. Invasion of the body by new antigens in sufficient numbers to stimulate an immune response.

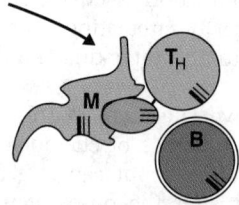

2. Interaction of macrophage (M) and T helper (T$_H$) cell in the processing and presenting of the antigen to the unsensitized "virgin" B lymphocyte (B).

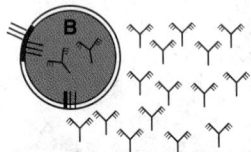

7. On reexposure to the same antigen, the sensitized lymphocytes and their progeny produce large quantities of the antibody specific to the antigen. In addition, new "virgin" B lymphocytes become sensitized to the antigen and also begin antibody production.

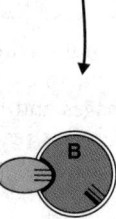

3. Sensitization of the virgin B lymphocyte to the new antigen.

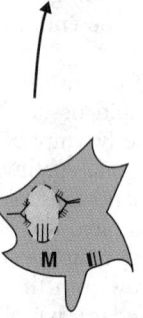

6. Antibody binding causes cellular events and attracts other leukocytes to the complex. The interaction of other leukocytes along with the cellular events results in the neutralization, destruction, or elimination of the antigen.

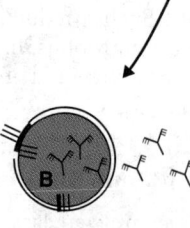

4. Antibody production by the B lymphocyte. These antibodies are directed specifically against the initiating antigen. The antibodies are released from the B lymphocyte and float freely in the blood and some other fluids.

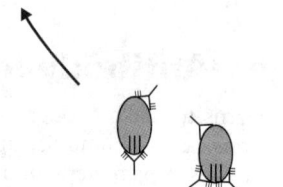

5. Antibodies bind to the antigen, forming an immune complex.

Figure 23–9. Sequence of events stimulating antibody-mediated immunity.

ipating in the next steps in the series of antibody-antigen interactions to prevent the development of chickenpox more than once.

Antigen Recognition

To begin to make antibodies against an antigen, the "virgin" or previously unsensitized B lymphocyte must first recognize the antigen as non-self. B lymphocytes cannot carry out this important function alone; they require the assistance of macrophages and helper/inducer T cells.

This cooperative effort is initiated by the macrophages. After the membrane of the antigen has been altered somewhat by opsonization (previously discussed under Adherence), the macrophage recognizes the invading foreign protein (antigen) as non-self and physically attaches itself to the antigen. This particular macrophage attachment to the antigen does not result in phagocytosis or in immediate destruction of the antigen. Instead, the macrophage brings the attached antigen in contact with a helper/inducer T cell. At this time, the helper/inducer T cell and the macrophage process the antigen in such a way as to expose the antigen's recognition sites (universal product code). After processing the antigen, the helper/inducer T cell brings the antigen into contact with the B lymphocyte

so that the B lymphocyte can recognize the antigen as non-self.

Lymphocyte Sensitization

Once the B lymphocyte recognizes the antigen as non-self, the B lymphocyte becomes sensitized to this antigen. An individual virgin B lymphocyte can undergo sensitization only once. Therefore, each B lymphocyte can be sensitized to only one antigen.

As a result of sensitization, this B lymphocyte can respond to any substance that carries the same antigens (codes) as the original antigen. Once it is sensitized to a specific antigen, the B lymphocyte always remains sensitized to that specific antigen. In addition, all daughter cells of that sensitized B lymphocyte are sensitized to that same specific antigen.

Immediately after it is sensitized, the B lymphocyte (or B blast) divides and forms two different types of lymphocytes, each one remaining sensitized to that specific antigen (Fig. 23–10). One new cell becomes a *plasma cell* and immediately starts to produce antibody directed specifically against the antigen that originally sensitized the B lymphocyte. The other new cell becomes a *memory cell*. The plasma cell functions immediately and has a short life span. The memory cell remains sensitized but functionally

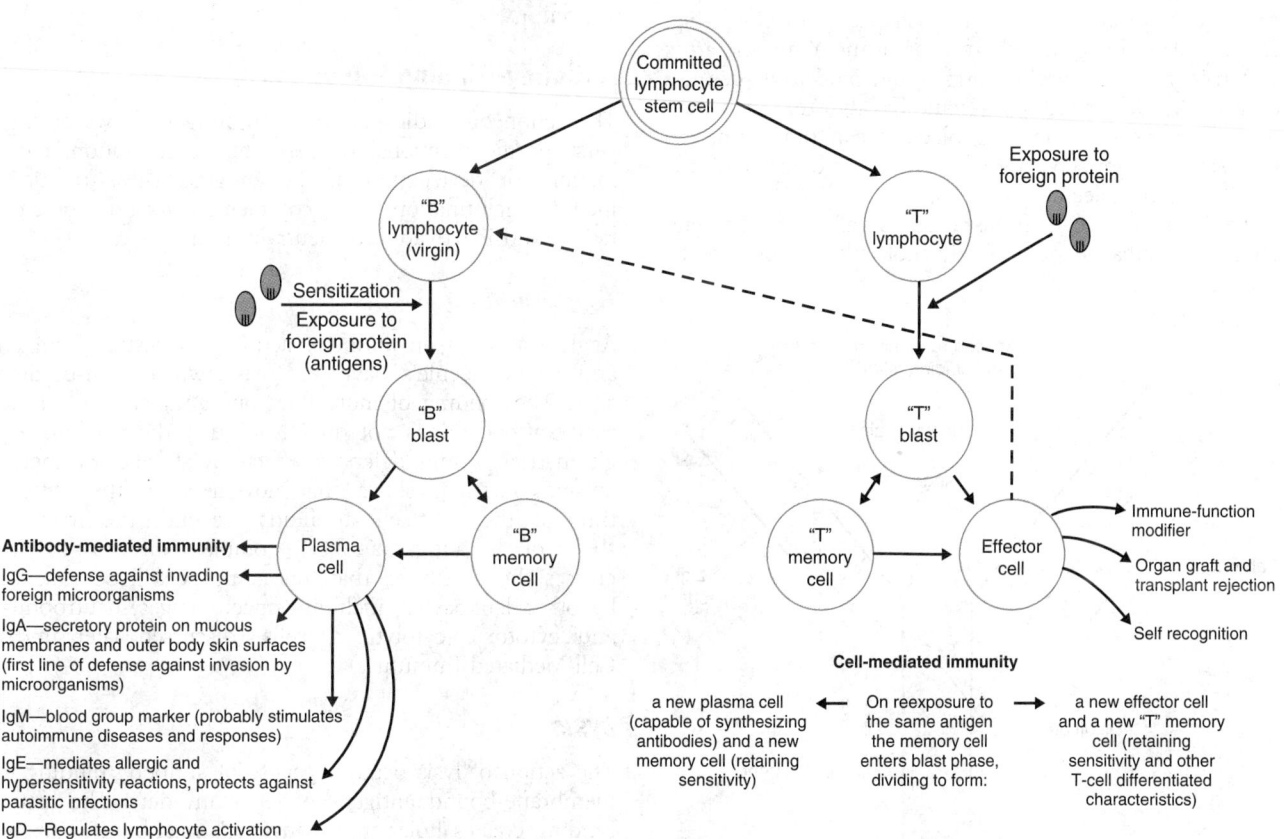

Figure 23–10. Differentiated functions of lymphocytes.

dormant until the next exposure to the same antigen (discussed later under Sustained Immunity–Memory).

Antibody Production and Release

Antibodies are produced by the plasma cell. When fully stimulated, each plasma cell can produce as much as 300 molecules of antibody per second. Each plasma cell produces antibody specific only to the antigen that originally sensitized the parent B lymphocyte. For example, in the case of the baby-sitter who was exposed to and invaded by chickenpox virus, the plasma cells derived from the B lymphocytes sensitized to the chickenpox virus can produce only antichickenpox antibodies. The exact antibody type (e.g., immunoglobulin G [IgG] or immunoglobulin M [IgM]) that the plasma cell can produce may vary, but the specificity of that antibody remains forever directed against chickenpox virus.

Antibody molecules produced by the plasma cells are secreted into the blood and other extracellular fluids as free antibody. Individual molecules of free antibody remain in the blood 3 to 30 days. Because the antibody circulates in body fluids (or body "humors") and is separate from the B lymphocytes, the immunity provided is sometimes called *humoral immunity*. Circulating antibodies can be transferred from one person to another to provide the receiving person with immediate immunity of short duration.

Antigen-Antibody Binding

An antibody is basically a **Y**-shaped molecule (Fig. 23–11). The tips of the short arms of the **Y** are the areas that recognize the specific antigen and bind to it. Because each individual antibody molecule has two tips (Fab fragments, or arms), antibody molecules can bind either to two separate antigen molecules or to two areas of the same antigen molecule.

The stem of the **Y** forms what is called the Fc fragment. This area of the antibody molecule can bind to Fc

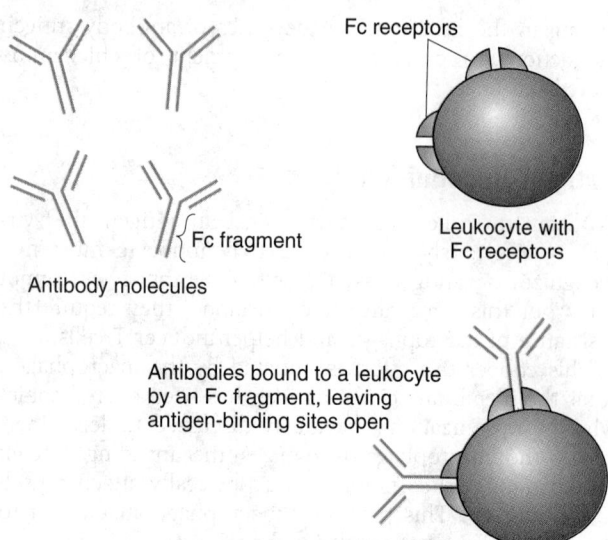

Figure 23–12. Antibody Fc receptors on leukocytes.

receptor sites on leukocytes, so that the leukocyte then has not only its own mechanisms of attacking antigens but also the added power of having antibodies on its surface that stick to antigens (Fig. 23–12).

The actual binding of antibody to antigen is not usually lethal to the antigen. Instead, the physical binding of the antibody to the antigen initiates other actions that result in the neutralization, elimination, or destruction of the antigen.

Antibody-Binding Reactions

The action of binding antibody to antigen allows or triggers specific reactions to cause the neutralization, elimination, or destruction of the antigen. These reactions include agglutination, lysis, complement fixation, precipitation, and inactivation or neutralization.

Agglutination

Agglutination is an antibody action that results from an antibody molecule's having at least two antigen-binding sites. The binding of more than one antigen molecule to each antibody does not directly destroy the antigen. Agglutination permits defensive effects by at least two mechanisms. First, it slows the movement of the antigen through the extracellular fluids. Second, the irregular shape of the antigen-antibody complex (Fig. 23–13) increases the likelihood that this complex will be attacked by other leukocytes, including macrophages, neutrophils, and cytotoxic–cytolytic T cells (discussed later under Cell-Mediated Immunity).

Lysis

The action of lysis occurs because of antibody binding to membrane-bound antigens of some invaders. The actual binding creates holes in the invader's membrane, causing lethal changes in its intracellular environment. This response usually requires that complement be involved in the antigen-antibody action. Bacteria and viruses are the

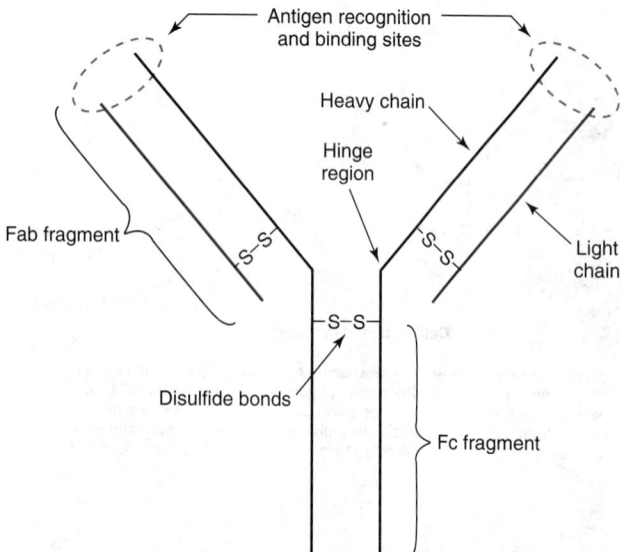

Figure 23–11. Basic antibody structure.

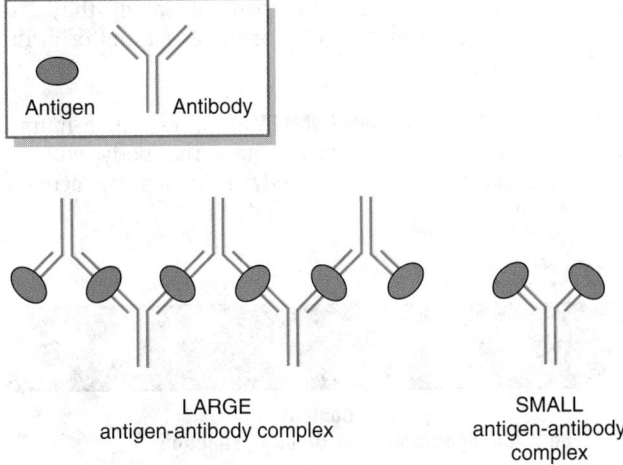

Figure 23-13. Antibody–antigen complexes.

non-self cells most susceptible to damage through lysis caused by the binding of antibody to membrane-surface antigens.

Complement Fixation

Specific classes of antibodies can cause the neutralization, elimination, or destruction of non-self antigen through activation of the complement cascade and complement fixation. (The mechanism by which complement assists in immunity was discussed earlier under Adherence.)

The two classes of antibody commonly associated with stimulating the complement system are IgG and IgM. Binding of antibody from either of these classes to an appropriate antigen provides a binding site for the first component of complement (C1q). Once C1q is activated, other components of the complement system are activated in a cascade.

Precipitation

Precipitation is similar to agglutination. However, in precipitation, antibody molecules bind so much antigen that large, insoluble antigen-antibody complexes are formed. These complexes cannot stay in suspension in the blood. Instead, they form a large, stationary precipitate, which can be acted on and removed by other nonspecific leukocytes.

Inactivation-Neutralization

Inactivation-neutralization is unique in that it does not result in the immediate destruction of the antigen. Usually, a relatively small area of the antigen is actually responsible for exerting harmful effects. The remainder of the antigen is not harmful to the host. Binding of antibody can interfere with the function of the active site by covering it up or changing its shape. Either mechanism inhibits the activity of the antigen and renders it harmless without destroying or eliminating it.

Sustained Immunity–Memory

The sustained immunity–memory function of AMI provides humans with long-lasting immunity to a specific antigen. Sustained immunity is provided by the action of the B-lymphocyte memory cells generated during the lymphocyte sensitization stage. These memory cells remain sensitized to the specific antigen to which they were originally exposed. On re-exposure to the same antigen, the memory cells are stimulated into rapid response. First, the cells divide and form new sensitized blast cells and new sensitized plasma cells. The blast cells continue to divide to generate even more sensitized plasma cells. The sensitized plasma cells begin to rapidly make and secrete large amounts of the antibody specific for the sensitizing antigen.

This ability of the sensitized memory cells to initiate events on re-exposure to the antigen that originally sensitized the B lymphocyte allows a rapid and widespread immune (*anamnestic*) response to the antigen. This response usually eliminates the invading antigen completely so that the person does not become ill. Because of this process, most people do not become ill with chickenpox or other viral diseases more than once, even though they are exposed many times to the causative organism. Without the process or action of memory, people would remain susceptible to specific diseases on subsequent exposure to the antigen, and no sustained immunity would be generated.

General Antibody Classification

All antibodies are referred to as immunoglobulins and gamma globulins. These names are based on the structure, location, and function of antibodies. A globulin is a type of protein structure that is globular rather than straight. Because antibodies are composed of this type of protein, they are globulins. The name immunoglobulin is appropriate for antibodies because they are globular proteins that assist in immune function. Antibodies are called gamma globulins because, during the process of electrophoresis, different groups of proteins in blood plasma separate out at different times, depending on how they move in response to electrical charge (Fig. 23–14). The protein groups are named according to when they emerge. The first group to emerge are the plasma albumins, which make up a large group. Three smaller groups emerge at specific times after the albumins. The fourth group, or protein fraction (gamma fraction), contains all five different types of antibody proteins. The five antibody types are classified by differences in antibody structure, molecular weight, and patterns of association (Table 23–4).

Acquiring Antibody-Mediated Immunity

Two broad categories of immunity are innate immunity and acquired immunity.

SEPARATION OF PLASMA PROTEINS BY ELECTROPHORESIS

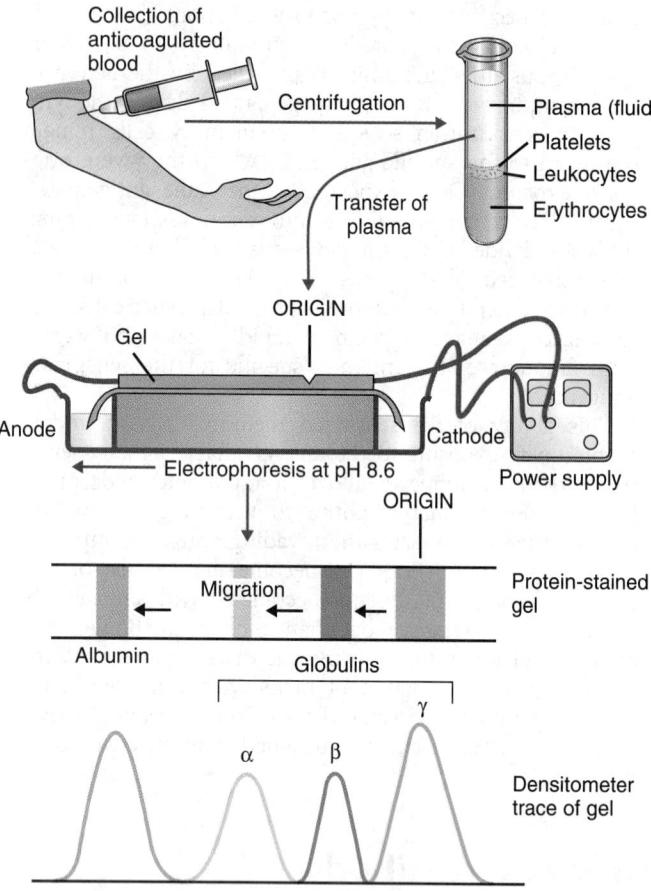

Figure 23–14. Electrophoresis of plasma proteins, including gamma globulin.

Innate Immunity

Innate immunity is a genetically determined characteristic of an individual, group, or species. A person either has or does not have innate immunity. For example, humans have many innate immunities to viruses and other microorganisms that cause specific diseases in animals. As a result, humans are not susceptible to such diseases as mange, distemper, hog cholera, or any of a variety of animal afflictions. This type of immunity cannot be developed or transferred from one person to another and is not an adaptive response to exposure or invasion by foreign proteins.

Acquired Immunity

Acquired immunity is the immunity that every person's body makes (or can receive) as an adaptive response to invasion by foreign proteins. AMI is an acquired immunity. Acquired immunity occurs either naturally or artificially and can be either active or passive.

Active Immunity

Active immunity occurs when antigens enter the body and the body responds by making specific antibodies against the antigen. This type of immunity is active be-

cause the body takes an active part in making the antibodies. Active immunity can occur under natural or artificial conditions.

NATURAL ACTIVE IMMUNITY. Natural active immunity occurs when an antigen enters the body without human assistance, and the body responds by actively

TABLE 23–4

Classification and Characterization of Antibodies

Type	Configuration	Content in Blood	Function
IgA	• Dimer	• <15%	• "Secretory"; present in body secretions, such as tears, mucus, saliva • Inhibits bacteria and viruses from adhering to skin and mucous membranes, making penetration into the internal environment more difficult
IgD	• Monomer	• <1%	• Modification of IgM activity
IgE	• Monomer	• <1%	• Degranulation of basophils and mast cells during inflammatory responses • Assists in clearance of parasites and prevention of pulmonary infections • Mediates many types of allergic reactions
IgG	• Monomer	• 75%	• Activates complement • Neutralizes toxins • Enhances phagocytosis • Provides significant sustained immunity against viral and bacterial infections
IgM	• Pentomer	• 10%	• Activates complement • Clears antigens through precipitation • Possibly mediates autoimmune reactions • Mediates ABO incompatibility reactions in blood transfusions

Ig = immunoglobulin.

making antibodies against that antigen (e.g., chickenpox virus). Most of the time, the first invasion of the body by the antigen results in manifestations of disease. However, processes occurring in the body at the same time confer immunity to that antigen, so that the person will not become ill after a second exposure to the same antigen. This type of immunity is the most effective and the longest lasting.

ARTIFICIAL ACTIVE IMMUNITY. Artificial active immunity is a type of protection developed against serious illnesses for which total avoidance is most desirable. Examples of diseases for which artificially acquired active immunity can be obtained include tetanus, diphtheria, measles, smallpox, mumps, and rubella. Small amounts of specific antigens are deliberately placed (as a vaccination) in the body, so that the body responds by actively making antibodies against the antigen. Because antigens used for this procedure have been specially processed to make them less likely to proliferate within the body, this exposure does not in itself cause the disease. Artificial active immunity lasts many years, although repeated but smaller doses of the original antigen are required as a "booster" for maintaining complete protection against the antigen.

Passive Immunity

Passive immunity occurs when antibodies against a specific antigen are in a person's body but were not created there. Rather, these antibodies are made in the body of one person or animal and then transferred to the body of another person. Because these antibodies are foreign to the individual, the body recognizes the antibodies as non-self and takes steps to eliminate them relatively quickly. For this reason, passive immunity can provide only immediate, short-term protection against a specific antigen.

Natural passive immunity occurs when antibodies are passed from the mother to the fetus via the placenta or to the infant through colostrum and breast milk.

Artificial passive immunity involves deliberately injecting one person with antibodies that were produced in another person or animal. This type of immunity is used when a person is exposed to a serious disease or illness for which he or she has little or no known actively acquired immunity. Instead, the injected antibodies are expected to inactivate the antigen. This type of immunity provides only temporary protection lasting for days to a few weeks. Some of the conditions or diseases for which artificial passive immunity may be used include exposure to rabies, tetanus, and poisonous snake bites.

Antibody-mediated immunity works with the inflammatory responses in providing protection against infection. However, AMI can provide the most effective, long-lasting immunity only when its actions are combined with the processes of cell-mediated immunity.

CELL-MEDIATED IMMUNITY

Cell-mediated immunity (CMI), or cellular immunity, involves many leukocyte actions, reactions, and interactions ranging from simple to complex. This type of immunity is provided by committed lymphocyte stem cells that mature in the secondary lymphoid tissues of the thymus and pericortical areas of lymph nodes. Certain CMI responses influence and regulate the activities of AMI and inflammation by producing and releasing cytokines. Therefore, for total immunocompetence, CMI must function optimally.

Cell Types Involved in Cell-Mediated Immunity

The leukocytes playing the most important roles in CMI include several specific T-lymphocyte subsets along with a special population of cells known as natural killer (NK) cells. T lymphocytes further differentiate into a variety of subsets, each of which has a specific function.

One way of identifying different T-lymphocyte subsets is to determine the presence or absence of certain "marker proteins" (antigens) on the cell membrane's surface. More than 50 different T-lymphocyte proteins have been identified on the cell membrane, and 11 of these (named T1 through T11) are commonly used in clinical situations to identify various immune system components. Antibodies have been made against each of these 11 proteins so that each T-lymphocyte subset can be identified by how the T lymphocyte reacts to the commercial antibodies. Most T lymphocytes have more than one antigen on their cell membranes. For example, all mature T lymphocytes contain T1, T3, T10, and T11 proteins. Certain subsets of T lymphocytes also contain other specific T-lymphocyte membrane antigens.

The names used to identify specific T-lymphocyte subsets include the specific membrane antigen and the overall functional activities of the cells in a subset. The three T-lymphocyte subsets critically important for the development and continuation of CMI are helper/inducer T cells, suppressor T cells, and cytotoxic–cytolytic T cells.

Helper/Inducer T Cells
Description

The cell membranes of these T cells contain the T4 protein. Usually, these cells are called T4+ cells or T_H cells. A newer name for helper/inducer T cells is CD4+ (cluster of differentiation 4). Several companies have made antibodies to the T4 cell membrane protein. These antibodies include OKT4 and Leu-3; thus, the helper/inducer T cells may also be referred to as cells that are OKT4 positive or Leu-3 positive.

Function

Helper/inducer T cells act efficiently in the recognition of self versus non-self. These important cells indirectly participate in CMI by stimulating the activity of many other leukocytes. In response to the recognition of non-self (antigen), helper/inducer T cells secrete lymphokines that can regulate the activity of other leukocytes.

In general, the lymphokines secreted by the helper/inducer T cells have overall stimulating effects on immune function. These lymphokines increase bone marrow production of stem cells and speed up the maturation of cells of myeloid and lymphoid origin. In effect, the helper/inducer T cells act as organizers in "calling to arms" various squads of leukocytes involved in inflammatory, antibody, and cellular defensive actions to destroy, eliminate, or neutralize antigens.

Suppressor T Cells
Description

The cell membranes of suppressor T cells contain the T8 lymphocyte antigen, and these cells are commonly called T8 cells, or T_S cells. Suppressor T cells participate in the regulation of CMI.

Function

Suppressor T cells prevent continuous overreaction or hypersensitivity reactions to exposure to non-self cells or proteins. This function is important in preventing the formation of autoantibodies directed against normal, healthy self cells, the basis for many autoimmune diseases.

The suppressor T cells secrete cytokines that have an overall inhibitory action on most and perhaps all cells of the immune system. These cytokines inhibit both the proliferation of immune system cells and the activation of immune system cells.

In general, suppressor T cells directly oppose the activity of helper/inducer T cells. Therefore, for optimal function of CMI, a balance between helper/inducer T-cell activity and suppressor T-cell activity must be maintained. This balance is usually provided when the helper/inducer T cells outnumber the suppressor T cells by a ratio of 2:1. When this ratio increases, overreactions can be expected, some of which are tissue-damaging as well as unpleasant. When the helper–suppressor ratio decreases, immune function is suppressed profoundly, and the body is much more vulnerable to invasion by non-self cells and infections of all types.

Cytotoxic–Cytolytic T Cells
Description

Cytotoxic–cytolytic T cells are also called T_C cells. Because they have the T8 protein present on their surfaces, they are a subset of suppressor cells. Cytotoxic–cytolytic T cells function in CMI by lysing (destroying) cells that contain a processed antigen–MHC complex. This activity is most effective against self cells infected by parasitic organisms, such as viruses or protozoa.

Function

Parasite-infected self cells have both self MHC proteins (universal product code) and the parasite's antigens on the cell surface. This allows the person's immune system cells to recognize the infected self cell as abnormal, and the cytotoxic–cytolytic T cell can bind to it.

The binding of the cytotoxic–cytolytic T cell to the infected cell's antigen–MHC complex stimulates activities that result in the death of the infected cell. The cyto-

toxic–cytolytic T cell bores a hole in the membrane of the infected cell and delivers a "lethal hit" of enzymes to the infected cell, causing it to lyse and die. Once the lethal hit has been administered to the infected cell, the cytotoxic–cytolytic T cell releases the dying infected cell and can attack and destroy other infected cells that carry the same antigen–MHC complex.

Natural Killer Cells
Description

Natural killer cells are extremely important in providing CMI. The actual site of differentiation and maturation of NK cells is unknown. Although this cell population has some T-cell characteristics, it is not considered a true T-cell subset (Abbas et al., 1997).

Function

NK cells direct cytotoxic–cytolytic effects on target non-self cells. Unlike cytotoxic–cytolytic T cells, NK cells can exert these cytotoxic effects without first undergoing a period of sensitization to non-self cell membrane antigens. Moreover, NK cells do not need to share any of the MHC proteins in common with the non-self cell to initiate defensive actions against the non-self cell. The defensive actions of NK cells appear to be totally unrelated to either antigen sensitivity or the interactions of other leukocytes. NK cells conduct "seek and destroy" missions in the body to eliminate invaders and unhealthy self cells.

NK cells are most effective in destroying unhealthy or abnormal self cells. The non-self cells most susceptible to defensive actions of NK cells are self cells that are virally infected and cancer cells.

Cytokines

The inducing and regulatory aspects of CMI are controlled through the selected production and activity of cytokines. Cytokines are small protein hormones produced by the various leukocytes. Cytokines made by the mononuclear phagocytes (macrophages, neutrophils, eosinophils, and monocytes) are termed *monokines*; cytokines produced by T lymphocytes are *lymphokines*.

Cytokine activity is similar to the action of any other kind of hormone: one cell produces and secretes a cytokine, which in turn exerts its effects on other cells of the immune system. The cells responding to the cytokine may be located close to or remote from the cytokine-secreting cell. The cells that change their activity in response to the cytokine are known as "responder" cells. For a responder cell to respond to the presence of a cytokine, the membrane of the responder cell must have a specific receptor for the cytokine to bind to and initiate changes in the responder cell's activity (Fig. 23–15).

Cytokines regulate a variety of inflammatory and immune responses. Most cytokines are produced as needed, and they are not stored to any great extent. The actions of some cytokines are pleiotropic in that the effects are widespread within the immune system, setting into motion various immunomodulating actions. Other cytokines have specific actions limited to only one type of cell.

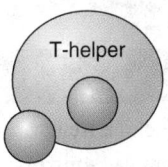

T-helper cell making and releasing a cytokine
(MAF—macrophage activating factor)

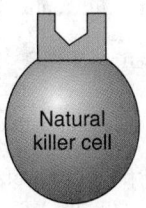

Leukocyte with one type
of surface receptor

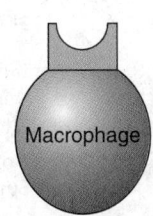

Leukocyte with a surface receptor
specific for the cytokine released
by the T-helper cell

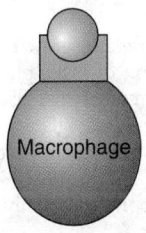

Cytokine binding to a cytokine-specific
receptor on the leukocyte (macrophage)

Figure 23–15. Cytokine receptors on leukocytes.

Table 23–5 summarizes the origins and activities of the currently known cytokines.

Protection Provided by Cell-Mediated Immunity

Cell-mediated immunity helps provide protection to the body through its highly developed ability to differentiate self from non-self. The non-self cells most easily recognized by CMI are those self cells infected by organisms that live within host cells and cancer cells. CMI provides a surveillance system for ridding the body of self cells that might potentially harm the body. CMI is important in preventing the development of cancer and metastasis after exposure to carcinogens.

Transplantation Rejection

Natural killer cells and cytotoxic–cytolytic T cells also destroy cells from other people or animals. Although this action is generally helpful, it is also responsible for rejection of grafts and transplanted organs. Because the solid organ transplanted into the host is seldom a perfectly identical match of universal product codes (HLAs) between the donated organ and the recipient host, the client's immune system cells recognize a newly transplanted organ as non-self. Without intervention, the host's im-

mune system initiates standard inflammatory and immunologic actions to destroy, eliminate, or neutralize these non-self cells. This activity causes rejection of the transplanted organ. Graft rejection is the result of a complex series of responses that change over time and involve different components of the immune system. Graft rejection can be hyperacute, acute, or chronic.

Hyperacute Rejection

Hyperacute graft rejection begins immediately on transplantation and is an antibody-mediated response. Antigen-antibody complexes form within the blood vessels of the transplanted organ. The host's blood has pre-existing antibodies to one or more of the antigens (including blood group antigens) present in the donated organ. The antigen–antibody complexes adhere to the lining of blood vessels and stimulate complement activation. The activated-fixated complement in the blood vessel linings initiates the blood clotting cascade; microcoagulation occurs throughout the organ vasculature. Widespread coagulation and occlusion lead to ischemic necrosis, inflammation with phagocytosis of the necrotic blood vessels, and release of lytic enzymes into the transplanted organ. These enzymes cause massive cellular destruction and graft loss.

Hyperacute rejection occurs primarily in transplanted kidneys. People at greatest risk for hyperacute rejection are

1. Those who have received donated organs of an ABO blood type different from their own
2. Those who have received multiple blood transfusions at any time in life before transplantation
3. Those who have a history of multiple pregnancies
4. Those who have received a previous transplant

The manifestations of hyperacute rejection become apparent within minutes of attachment of the donated organ to the host's blood supply. *The process cannot be stopped once it has started, and the rejected organ must be removed as soon as hyperacute rejection is diagnosed.*

Acute Rejection

Acute graft rejection occurs within 1 week to 3 months after transplantation. Two mechanisms are responsible. The first mechanism is antibody-mediated and results in vasculitis within the transplanted organ. This reaction differs from that of hyperacute rejection in that blood vessel necrosis (rather than thrombotic occlusion) leads to the organ's destruction.

The second mechanism is cellular. Host cytotoxic–cytolytic T cells and NK cells enter the transplanted organ through the blood, infiltrate the organ cells (rather than the blood vessel cells), and cause lysis of the organ cells.

Diagnosis of acute rejection is made by laboratory tests indicating impaired function of the specific organ, along with biopsy of the grafted organ. Manifestations of acute rejection vary with each client and with the specific organ transplanted. For example, when acute rejection occurs in a transplanted kidney, the client usually experiences some tenderness in the kidney area and may experience other general symptoms of inflammation.

TABLE 23–5

Summary of Cytokine Activity

Cytokine	Cellular Origin	Inducing Event	Cytokine Action
IL-1	Macrophages Monocytes Natural killer cells	Contact with gram-negative bacterial products Contact with CD4+ cell Presence of TNF	Stimulates increased production of prostaglandins Induces fever Increases proliferation of CD4+ cells Stimulates growth and differentiation of B lymphocytes Induces further secretion of IL-1 and IL-6
IL-2	Helper T cells (CD4+ T cells) CD8+ T cells	T-cell activation by antigens	Increases growth and differentiation of T lymphocytes Stimulates increased production of IL-2 from activated lymphocytes Enhances NK activity and activity of tumor-infiltrating lymphocytes
IL-3 (multilineage colony-stimulating factor)	Helper T cells (CD4+ T cells)	Infection or antigen invasion	Pluripotent (pleiotropic) stimulation of bone marrow stem cells
IL-4 (B-cell stimulatory factor)	Helper T cells (CD4+ T cells) Activated mast cells	Presence of anti-Ig antibody	Stimulates growth and differentiation of B lymphocytes Stimulates increased production of IgG and IgE Induces further secretion of IL-4, IL-5, and IL-6 Suppresses inflammation
IL-5 (B-cell growth factor)	Helper T cells (CD4+ T cells) Activated mast cells	Helminth infection Pulmonary infection	Stimulates growth and differentiation of eosinophils Stimulates increased production of IgA and IgE
IL-6	Activated T cells Fibroblasts Vascular endothelial cells Macrophages Monocytes	Infection or inflammation Presence of IL-1 TNF	Stimulates liver to produce fibrinogen, macroglobulin, protein C Stimulates growth of activated B lymphocytes Increases production of bone marrow stem cells
IL-7 (B-cell growth factor)	Bone marrow stromal cells	Presence of antigens	Stimulates growth and differentiation of committed B-lymphocyte stem cells Stimulates T-cell production of IL-2
IL-8 (monocyte chemotactic factor)	Activated T cells Macrophages Platelets Fibroblasts Endothelial cells	Infection or inflammation	Chemotactic factor for neutrophils, basophils, and eosinophils Stimulates neutrophil activation
IL-9	Helper T cells (CD4+ T cells)	Infection or inflammation	Stimulates mast cell growth Induces IL-4 production Stimulates lymphocyte activation
IL-10	Mature lymphocytes Macrophages Monocytes	Infection or inflammation	Enhances activity of cytotoxic–cytolytic T cells Suppresses inflammatory response
IL-11	Bone marrow stromal cells	Viral infection or inflammation	Enhances B-lymphocyte activity Stimulates platelet proliferation and maturation
IL-12	Macrophages Activated B cells	Infection or inflammation	Induces production of interferon Enhances NK activity and activity cytotoxic–cytolytic T cells Induces production of IL-2 and IL-4

TABLE 23–5

Summary of Cytokine Activity *Continued*

Cytokine	Cellular Origin	Inducing Event	Cytokine Action
IL-13	Activated T cells (CD4+ T cells and CD8+ T cells)	Infection	Induces B-lymphocyte proliferation Increases platelet and erythrocyte production Increases IL-6 production Decreases neutrophil activity
IL-14	Activated T cells	Infection, plasma cell malignancies	Induces B-lymphocyte proliferation Decreases Ig secretion Enhances B-cell differentiation
INF-α	Macrophages	Viral infection	Decreases viral proliferation
INF-β	Fibroblasts	Viral infection	Decreases viral proliferation
INF-γ	Helper T cells (CD4+ T cells) Suppressor T cells (CD8+ T cells) NK cells	Viral infection	Decreases viral proliferation Activates macrophages Induces differentiation of committed lymphoid stem cells Activates neutrophils Activates NK cells
TNF	Activated macrophages Activated mast cells Activated NK cells Activated T cells	Infection or inflammation (especially infection with gram-negative microorganisms)	Increases leukocyte adhesion Induces fever Stimulates production of CSF Induces cytolysis of virally infected cells Induces secretion of IL-1 and IL-6
GM-CSF	Activated T cells Macrophages Fibroblasts Vascular endothelial cells	Infection or inflammation	Increases growth and differentiation of committed myeloid stem cells Slightly activates macrophages
M-CSF	Fibroblasts Vascular endothelial cells	Infection or inflammation	Increases growth and differentiation of committed monocyte-macrophage progenitor cells
G-CSF	Macrophages Vascular endothelial cells Fibroblasts	Infection or inflammation	Increases proliferation and maturation of neutrophils

IL = interleukin; TNF = tumor necrosis factor; NK = natural killer; Ig = immunoglobulin; INF = interferon; G = granulocyte; M = macrophage; CSF = colony-stimulating factor.

An episode of acute rejection after solid organ transplantation does not automatically mean that the client will lose the transplant. Pharmacologic manipulation of host immune responses at this time may limit the damage to the organ and allow the graft to be maintained.

Chronic Rejection

The origin of chronic rejection is not clear, but it resembles the aftermath of chronic inflammation and scarring. Functional tissue of the transplanted organ is replaced with fibrotic, scar-like tissue. Because this fibrotic tissue does not resemble the organ tissue in either structure or function, the ability of the transplanted organ to perform differentiated tasks diminishes in proportion to the percentage of normal tissue replaced by fibrotic tissue. This type of reaction is long-standing and occurs continuously

as a response to chronic ischemia caused by blood vessel injury.

Although good control over host immune function can delay the manifestations of this type of rejection, the process probably occurs to some degree with all solid organ transplants. Because the fibrotic changes are permanent, there is no cure for chronic graft rejection. When the fibrosis increases to the extent that it significantly interferes with the functional capacity of the transplanted organ, the only recourse is retransplantation.

Treatment of Transplant Rejection

Rejection of transplanted solid organs involves all three components of immunity, although cell-mediated immune responses are most significant in the rejection process.

Maintenance Therapy

Three pharmacologic agents are generally used for routine immunosuppressive therapy after solid organ transplantation. These agents are azathioprine (Imuran); cyclosporine (Sandimmune); and one of the corticosteroids, such as prednisone (Apo-Prednisone✦, Deltasone) or prednisolone (Delta-Cortef). Drug dosage is adjusted for the immune response of each client. Treatment with these agents increases the client's risk for bacterial and fungal infections.

Rescue Therapy

Certain agents are used not to maintain the graft within the host but rather to reduce the host's immunologic responses during rejection episodes, especially acute rejection. These agents may be used in addition to or in place of any of the maintenance drugs in the host's post-transplantation treatment regimen.

Antilymphocyte Globulin

Antilymphocyte globulin (ALG) is an antibody (or group of antibodies) generated in an animal after the animal has been exposed to human lymphocytes. The globulin can be made more specific by exposing the animal to human T cells instead of mixed lymphocytes. When these antihuman lymphocyte antibodies are administered to humans, the antibodies selectively attack and clear lymphocytes from the blood, extracellular fluids, and tissues into which they have infiltrated (such as the transplanted organ). This agent is given only for a short time to combat the acute rejection episode.

Most clients receiving ALG have some associated immunologic response, ranging from low-grade fever and malaise to serum sickness and anaphylaxis. The response usually increases in intensity on repeated exposure to ALG.

OKT3

OKT3 is an antibody directed specifically against the human T-cell cell-surface antigen CD3. OKT3 is generated with a murine (mouse) model rather than an equine (horse) model. Because the agent is generated in mice, the humans receiving it rapidly develop antimouse antibodies. These antimouse antibodies attack the OKT3 and prevent its anti-T-cell activities. Thus, OKT3 is most effective against rejection during the first episode for which it is used. Its utility in combating graft rejection decreases with each subsequent use.

FK 506

FK 506 is used in maintenance therapy and rescue therapy, primarily after liver transplantation. It is similar in chemical composition to erythromycin and specifically suppresses T-cell actions, including synthesis of interleukin-2 (IL-2). These effects are achieved through various mechanisms. In the presence of FK 506, receptor sites for IL-2 are inhibited on helper/inducer T cells and cyto-

toxic–cytolytic T cells. Without continuous stimulation by IL-2, these lymphocytes are slow to reproduce and do not perform their usual functions. In addition, FK 506 is able to prevent activation of immature or unsensitized cytotoxic–cytolytic T cells. Because cytotoxic–cytolytic T cells are primarily responsible for immunologic destruction of transplanted cells and tissues, and because helper/inducer T cells boost the activity of cytotoxic–cytolytic T cells, selective suppression of the activity of these two cell populations allows the transplanted organ to remain free from immunologic destruction, yet does not result in so profound an immunosuppressive state as to put the host at great risk for infection.

SELECTED BIBLIOGRAPHY

Abbas, A., Lichtman, A., & Pober, J. (1997). *Cellular and molecular immunology* (3rd ed.). Philadelphia: W. B. Saunders.
Beck, G., & Habicht, G. (1996). Immunity and the invertebrates. *Scientific American, 275*(5), 60–66.
DeLaPena, L., Tomaszewski, J., Bernato, D. L., Kryk, J., Molenda, J., & Gantz, S. (1996). Programmed instruction: Biotherapy module IV. Interleukins. *Cancer Nursing, 19*(1), 60–74.
DeLaPena, L., Woolery-Antill, M., Tomaszewski, J., Gantz, S., Bernato, D. L., DiLorenzo, K., Molenda, J., & Kryk, J. (1996). Programmed instruction: Biotherapy module V. Hematopoietic growth factors. *Cancer Nursing, 19*(2), 135–150.
Ford, R., Tomayo, A., Martin, B., Niu, K., Claypool, K., Cabaniilas, F., & Ambrus, J. (1995). Identification of B-cell growth factors (interleukin-14; high molecular weight–B-cell growth factors) in effusion fluids from patients with aggressive B-cell lymphomas. *Blood, 86*(1), 283–293.
Gantz, S., Tomaszewski, J., DeLaPena, L., Molenda, J., Bernato, D. L., & Kryk, J. (1995). Programmed instruction: Biotherapy module III. Interferons. *Cancer Nursing, 18*(6), 479–494.
Guyton, A. C., & Hall, J. (1996). *Textbook of medical physiology* (9th ed.). Philadelphia: W. B. Saunders.
Krenitsky, J. (1996). Nutrition and the immune system. *AACN Clinical Issues: Advanced Practice in Acute and Critical Care, 7*(3), 359–369.
Lai, Y., Heslan, J., Poppema, S., Elliot, J., & Mosmann, T. (1996). Continuous administration of IL-13 to mice induces extramedullary hemopoiesis and monocytosis. *Journal of Immunology, 156*(9), 3166–3173.
Post-White, J. (1996). The immune system. *Seminars in Oncology Nursing, 12*(2), 89–96.
Roitt, I. (1994). *Essential immunology* (8th ed.). London: Blackwell Scientific.
Secor, V. (1994). The inflammatory/immune response in critical illness. *Critical Care Clinics of North America, 6*(2), 251–262.
Workman, M. L. (1995). Essential concepts of inflammation and immunity. *Critical Care Clinics of North America, 7*(4), 601–615.
*Workman, M. L., Ellerhorst-Ryan, J., & Koertge, V. (1993). *Nursing care of the immunocompromised patient*. Philadelphia: W. B. Saunders.
Workman, M. L. (1998). The lymphoid system and its role in immunocompetence. *Seminars in Oncology Nursing* (In press).

SUGGESTED READINGS

Secor, V. (1994). The inflammatory/immune response in critical illness. *Critical Care Clinics of North America, 6*(2), 251–262.
  The physiology of inflammatory and immune responses is presented, with mechanisms clearly depicted in line drawings. The article also discusses sepsis and systemic inflammatory response syndrome.
Workman, M. L. (1995). Essential concepts of inflammation and immunity. *Critical Care Clinics of North America, 7*(4), 601–615.
  This article reviews the normal immune and inflammatory responses. Clinical situations leading to altered immune function are presented. Traditional and new treatment modalities also are discussed.

Chapter 24

INTERVENTIONS FOR CLIENTS WITH CONNECTIVE TISSUE DISEASE

A *rheumatic disease* is any disease or condition involving the musculoskeletal system. Connective tissue disease (CTD) is the major focus of *rheumatology,* the study of rheumatic disease. In this text, CTDs are discussed separately from other musculoskeletal conditions because most CTDs are classified as probably autoimmune.

More than 37 million people in the United States, or 1 in 7, have one or more of over 100 CTDs. The primary clinical manifestation of many of these diseases is *arthritis,* the inflammation of one or more joints. Some CTDs present with additional localized clinical manifestations, whereas others are systemic. Management of clients with CTDs requires an interdisciplinary approach, including medicine, surgery, nursing, and physical and occupational therapy.

DEGENERATIVE JOINT DISEASE (OSTEOARTHRITIS)

Overview

Several terms describe degenerative joint disease (DJD), the most common connective tissue disease. *Osteoarthritis* (OA) and *osteoarthrosis* are used interchangeably with DJD; however, this condition is not a primary inflammatory disease, and thus osteoarthritis may not be the best term.

Pathophysiology

Degenerative joint disease is characterized by the progressive deterioration of and loss of articular cartilage in peripheral and axial joints. It is caused by prolonged or excessive use of these joints. Weight-bearing joints (hips and knees), the vertebral column, and hands are primarily affected because they are used most often and bear the stress of body weight. Therefore, DJD is also known as the "wear and tear disease." Most clients have the primary (idiopathic) form of the disease, but secondary DJD can result from other musculoskeletal conditions or from trauma.

In the affected joints, the normal bluish, translucent cartilage becomes soft, opaque, and yellow. Fissures, pitting, and ulcerations develop, and the cartilage thins. As cartilage and bone beneath the cartilage begin to erode, the joint space narrows and osteophyte (bone spur) formation occurs (Fig. 24–1). Inflammatory enzymes enhance tissue deterioration as a result of the alteration in cartilage metabolism. As a result, the repair process is unable to overcome the rapid process of degeneration.

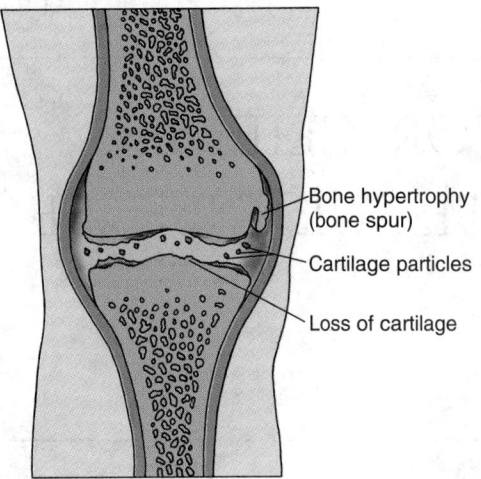

Bone hypertrophy (bone spur)

Cartilage particles

Loss of cartilage

Figure 24–1. Joint changes in degenerative joint disease.

Bone cysts and secondary synovitis are common in advanced disease. Eventually, subluxation and joint deformities cause marked immobility, pain, and muscle spasm.

Etiology

Although the causative mechanisms of primary DJD at the cellular level have not been well identified, the risk factors for DJD are known. Age is the strongest risk factor, but research does not support that aging alone is the cause of DJD (Mankin & Brandt, 1997). Joints that are used most often are typically affected. Obesity also contributes to the likelihood of degeneration, particularly in the hips and knees, the weight-bearing joints. Overuse or abuse of certain joints causes chronic pain and degeneration. Joint hyperextensibility, as seen in gymnasts, also predisposes the person to DJD. Certain heavy manual occupations, such as carpet installation, construction, and farming, cause increased mechanical stress to joints. The risk of hip and knee DJD is significantly increased in former athletes.

Congenital anomalies, trauma, and joint sepsis can result in secondary DJD. Certain metabolic diseases (such as diabetes mellitus and Paget's disease) and blood disorders (such as hemophilia) can also cause joint degeneration. Inflammatory joint diseases, such as rheumatoid arthritis, can also lead to secondary DJD.

Incidence/Prevalence

More than 20 million people in the United States have symptomatic DJD, but probably more than 40 million have degenerative joint changes that can be seen on x-ray examinations. Generalized disease is seen more often in women than in men.

ELDERLY CONSIDERATIONS

Prevalence increases with age; almost everyone older than 60 years has some degree of symptomatic joint degeneration. DJD of the hands is especially common in

the elderly, affecting more than 70% of those older than 70 years (Solomon, 1997).

TRANSCULTURAL CONSIDERATIONS

 Native Americans are affected more often than non–Native American groups, but the reason is unknown (Giger & Davidhizar, 1995).

Collaborative Management

◆ Assessment

➤ History

At the initial interview, the nurse collects information from the client that is specifically related to DJD. Because this disease is observed more often in older women, age and sex are important factors for the nursing history. The nurse asks about the client's occupation, nature of work, history of trauma, and current or previous involvement in sports. Even if the client appears to be within the ideal range for body weight, the nurse asks the client about a possible history of obesity. The nurse should also note a family history of "arthritis" because many CTDs seem to have familial tendencies.

Finally, the nurse determines whether the client has a current or previous medical condition that may cause joint manifestations. As with all musculoskeletal disorders, the nurse asks questions about the course of the disease.

➤ Physical Assessment/Clinical Manifestations

In the early stage of the disease, the clinical manifestations of degenerative joint disease (DJD) may appear similar to those of rheumatoid arthritis (RA). As the disease progresses, the distinction between DJD and RA becomes more evident. Table 24–1 differentiates the major characteristics of both diseases and their treatments.

Joint Pain. The major complaint of the client with DJD is typically nagging joint pain, which early in the course of the disease diminishes after rest and intensifies after activity. Later the pain occurs with slight motion or even when the person is at rest. Because cartilage has no nerve supply, the pain is probably due to joint and soft-tissue involvement and to spasms of surrounding muscles. During examination of the joints, the nurse can often elicit pain or tenderness by palpation or by putting the joint through range of motion. Crepitus, a continuous grating sensation, may be felt or heard as the joint is put through range of motion. One or more joints are affected. The client may also complain of joint stiffness that usually lasts less than 30 minutes after a period of inactivity.

Joint Changes. On inspection, the nurse notes that the joint is frequently enlarged because of bony hypertrophy; rarely does a joint appear to be hot and inflamed. The presence of inflammation in clients with DJD usually indicates a secondary synovitis. Approximately 50% of clients with hand involvement display the characteristic Heberden's nodes (at the distal interphalangeal joints) and

TABLE 24-1

Differential Features of Rheumatoid Arthritis and Degenerative Disease

Characteristic	Rheumatoid Arthritis	Degenerative Joint Disease
Typical onset	• At 35–45 yr	• At >60 yr
Sex affected	• Female (3:1)	• Female (2:1)
Risk factors or cause	• Probably autoimmune • Emotional stress	• Aging • Obesity • Trauma • Occupation
Disease process	• Inflammatory	• Degenerative
Disease pattern	• Bilateral, symmetric, multiple joints • Usually affects upper extremities first • Distal interphalangeal joints of hands spared • Systemic	• May be unilateral, single joint • Affects weight-bearing joints and hands, spine • Metacarpophalangeal joints spared • Nonsystemic
Laboratory findings	• Elevated rheumatoid factor, antinuclear antibody, ESR	• Normal or slightly elevated ESR
Drug therapy	• Salicylates • NSAIDs • Methotrexate • Gold or penicillamine • Corticosteroids • Other immunosuppressive agents • Other analgesics	• NSAIDs • Acetaminophen • Other analgesics

ESR = erythrocyte sedimentation rate; NSAIDs = nonsteroidal antiinflammatory drugs.

Bouchard's nodes (at the proximal interphalangeal joints). Although DJD is not a bilateral, symmetric disease, these large bony nodes appear in that pattern, especially in women. The nodes may be painful and red, but some clients do not experience discomfort from their presence. The nodes have a familial tendency and are usually a cosmetic concern to clients. The nodes feel hard when the nurse palpates them; clients may complain of tenderness on palpation.

Other Clinical Manifestations. Joint effusions are common when the knees are involved. When trying to differentiate the presence of fluid from subcutaneous tissue, the nurse is able to move fluid from the infrapatellar notch (the area directly below the knee) into the suprapatellar notch (the area directly above the knee). Subcutaneous tissue cannot be relocated.

The nurse also observes skeletal muscle atrophy from disuse. The vicious pain cycle of the disease discourages movement of painful joints, which then results in contractures, muscle atrophy, and further pain. Loss of function may result, depending on which joints are involved, Hip pain may cause the client to limp and restrict walking distance.

Degenerative joint disease can frequently affect the spine, especially the lumbar region at the L3-4 level or the cervical region at C4-6. Compression of spinal nerve roots may occur as a result of vertebral facet bone spurs. The client typically complains of radiating pain, stiffness, and muscle spasms in one or both extremities. Spinal and vertebral arteries may also become compressed.

In addition to performing a musculoskeletal assessment, the nurse performs a functional assessment of the client with DJD to determine mobility and ability to perform activities of daily living (ADLs). Severe pain and deformity interfere with ambulation and self-care. (Chapter 13 describes ADLs and functional assessment in depth.)

➤ Psychosocial Assessment

Degenerative joint disease is a chronic condition that may cause permanent changes in the client's lifestyle. A person's inability to care for oneself in advanced disease prevents socialization and results in role changes and other losses. Therefore, the client may exhibit a variety of behaviors indicative of the grieving process, such as anger and depression.

The client may experience a role change in the family, workplace, or both. The nurse asks the client about his or her roles before the disease developed to identify changes that have been or need to be made. The nurse and client mutually determine problem areas and adjustment in lifestyle that may still be needed as a result of the disease.

In addition to role change, joint deformities and bony nodules often cause an alteration in body image and self-esteem. The nurse observes the client's response to body changes. Does the client ignore them or seem overly occupied with them? How does the client refer to the changes—with anger, degradation, or humor? These clues help the nurse assess the client's acceptance of body alterations.

➤ Laboratory Assessment

There are no significant laboratory tests for DJD. The erythrocyte sedimentation rate (ESR) may be slightly elevated when secondary synovitis occurs.

➤ *Radiographic Assessment*

Routine x-rays are useful in determining structural joint changes. Specialized views are obtained when the disease cannot be visualized on standard x-ray but is suspected. A computed tomography (CT) scan may be used to determine vertebral involvement.

➤ *Other Diagnostic Assessment*

The health care provider may order magnetic resonance imaging (MRI) studies of the vertebral column to detect degenerative bony changes in the spine. A bone scan using technetium (Tc) 99m can often show early DJD years before typical x-ray changes appear.

 Analysis

➤ *Common Nursing Diagnoses and Collaborative Problems*

The priority for nursing diagnoses when the nurse is caring for a client with degenerative joint disease (DJD) is
1. Chronic Pain related to muscle spasm and/or inflammation
2. Impaired Physical Mobility related to pain and muscle atrophy

➤ *Additional Nursing Diagnoses and Collaborative Problems*

In addition to the common diagnoses, the client may have secondary problems caused by the pain and immobility common in DJD. These include
- Activity Intolerance related to pain and fatigue
- Self-Care Deficit (partial) related to pain, fatigue, and immobility
- Body Image Disturbance related to effects of loss of body function

 Planning and Implementation

Chronic Pain

Planning: Expected Outcomes. The major concern of the client with DJD is pain control. Therefore, the desired outcome is that the client is expected to experience a reduction in chronic pain.

Interventions. Pain control may be accomplished by drug and nondrug measures at home. If these measures become ineffective, surgery may be performed to reduce pain.

Nonsurgical Management. Management of chronic joint pain is difficult for both the client and the health care professional. A combination of modalities is often used, including medication, diet, physical therapy, and rest. Chapter 9 elaborates on methods of pain control for chronic pain.

Drug Therapy. The purpose of drug therapy is to reduce pain, relieve muscle spasm, and reduce secondary inflammation if present. The drug class of choice is usually nonsteroidal anti-inflammatory drugs (NSAIDs) (Chart 24–1). Acetaminophen (Tylenol, Atasol✢) may also be used. For temporary relief of pain in a single joint, the physician may inject the joint with a corticosteroid, such as cortisone, or a newer drug, Hyalgan (sodium hyaluronate). Muscle relaxants, such as cyclobenzaprine HCl (Flexeril), are sometimes given for severe muscle spasms, especially those occurring in the back. Potent analgesics are not usually appropriate for the client with DJD because of the chronic nature of the pain.

Rest. Several types of rest are used to treat clients with DJD:
- Local rest involves the immobilization of a joint with a splint or brace. If a joint becomes acutely inflamed, the joint is rested until inflammation subsides. The nurse or physician consults the occupational therapist (OT), who fits the client for the appropriate device and explains its use.
- Systemic rest refers to the immobilization of the entire body, such as a nap. The nurse teaches the client about the importance of sleeping about 10 hours and, if possible, resting an additional 1–2 hours each day.
- *Psychological* rest is equally important because it allows relief from daily stresses that can enhance pain.

Chapter 8 describes methods for relaxation and strategies for coping that the nurse can use to teach clients.

Positioning. Joints should be placed in their functional position, which may not be the position of comfort. When the client is in a supine position (recumbent), the nurse or assistive nursing personnel places a small pillow under the client's head or neck but avoids the use of other pillows. The client may quickly experience flexion contractures from the use of large pillows under the knees or head. If needed, the client's legs may be elevated 8–12 inches (20.3–30.5 cm) to reduce back discomfort. Lying prone twice a day is recommended if the client can tolerate that position. The nurse also reminds the client to use proper posture when standing and sitting to reduce undue strain on the vertebral column.

Heat. The client with DJD generally uses heat instead of cold to reduce pain. Cold application is usually reserved for acutely inflamed joints. The nurse suggests hot showers and baths, hot packs or compresses, and moist heating pads. Regardless of treatment, the nurse teaches the client to check that the heat source is not too heavy or so hot as to cause burns. A temperature just above the body's temperature is adequate to promote comfort.

A physical therapist may provide special heat treatments, such as paraffin dips, diathermy (use of electrical current), and ultrasonography (use of sound waves). Usually a 15- to 20-minute heat application is sufficient to temporarily reduce pain, spasm, and stiffness.

Diet Therapy. There is no "arthritis diet," as has been proposed by the media and uninformed authors. In collaboration with the dietitian, the nurse explains which foods are high in protein and vitamin C to promote tissue healing. In addition, the nurse encourages obese clients to lose weight to lessen stress on weight-bearing joints. Less weight reduces pain and slows the disease process in

Chart 24–1

Drug Therapy for Connective Tissue Disease

Drug	Usual Dosage	Nursing Interventions	Rationale
Salicylates (e.g., aspirin, buffered aspirin) (Ecotrin, Ascriptin, Ancasal✤)	12–18 tablets/d (4–6 g) are given in divided doses to achieve therapeutic effect.	• Give with meals or snacks. • Instruct client to observe for tinnitus, bleeding, or bruising (especially seen in elderly clients). Teach client to use soft-bristled toothbrush.	• Aspirin products can cause gastrointestinal problems, including bleeding and ulcers, because of increased stomach acid production. Drugs can damage eighth cranial nerve and prevent platelet aggregation, which causes clotting. • Gums may bleed easily because of decreased clotting.
NSAIDs, e.g., naproxen (Naprosyn, Apo-Naproxen✤), sulindac (Clinoril), indomethacin (Indocin, Apo-Indomethacin✤), ibuprofen (Motrin, Advil, Amersol✤), mefenamic acid (Ponstel, Ponstan✤), phenylbutazone (Butazolidin, Novobutazone✤), piroxicam (Feldene, Apo-Piroxicam✤), diclofenac sodium (Voltaren), flurbiprofen (Ansaid)	Dose varies depending on which drug is used. Piroxicam and naproxen are given in fewer doses because of longer half-life. Indomethacin and phenylbutazone are not as commonly used because of tendencies to cause peptic ulcer and CNS changes.	• Same as for salicylates above. • In addition, observe for fluid retention, increased blood pressure, and changes in renal function. • Monitor electrolyte and complete blood count values. • Observe for CNS changes, e.g., dizziness or confusion. • If a client is taking aspirin and an NSAID or is taking two NSAIDs, observe carefully for side effects or toxic effects.	• Same as for salicylates above. • Most NSAIDs cause sodium retention, which can lead to edema, hypertension, renal damage, and/or congestive heart failure. Drugs should be used with caution in elderly population. • Most NSAIDs cause increased sodium levels and can cause bone marrow suppression. • Most NSAIDs can cause CNS effects especially in the elderly. • Drugs are often used in combination, especially in clients with rheumatoid arthritis. Additive effects can cause serious complications.
Gold Auranofin (Ridaura)	Dose is 3 mg bid PO.	• Observe for and instruct client to report gastrointestinal problems, such as diarrhea, nausea/vomiting, abdominal cramping.	• This side effect causes discomfort and can lead to electrolyte imbalance.
Gold sodium thiomalate (water-based gold) (Myochrysine)	After a 10-mg test dose, 25 mg and then 50 mg is given every week until monthly maintenance of 50 mg IM is reached.	• Observe for rash or other skin change and for mouth ulceration (stomatitis).	• Drug may be discontinued for a short period, then restarted.

Continued

Chart 24–1. Drug Therapy for Connective Tissue Disease Continued

Drug	Usual Dosage	Nursing Interventions	Rationale
Aurothioglucose (oil-based gold) (Solganal)	Same as for gold sodium thiomalate. If total of 1000 mg is used and no clinical change is seen, gold is discontinued.	• Instruct client to expect metallic taste in mouth; teach importance of proper mouth care. • Monitor urine for protein and serum for CBC. If CBC is markedly decreased or if proteinuria is present, discontinue drug. • Give *deep* IM, preferably by Z-track technique. • After IM administration, observe for nitroid crisis, a form of anaphylactic reaction.	• Proper, frequent mouth care reduces risk of stomatitis and metallic taste. • These changes indicate serious toxic effects, and drug needs to be discontinued. • Drug is locally irritating to soft tissue. • Flushing, dyspnea, and anxiety may occur shortly after drug administration.
Hydroxychloroquine sulfate (Plaquenil)	200 mg PO each day is given.	• Instruct client to have frequent (every 3–6 mo) ophthalmologic examination.	• Drug can cause retinal damage.
Penicillamine (Cuprimine)	125–250 mg PO each day is used (may be given in two divided doses).	• Same as for IM gold, except no nitroid crisis occurs.	• Same as for IM gold.
Immunosuppressive agents, e.g., azathioprine (Imuran), cyclophosphamide (Cytoxan, Procytox✦), methotrexate (Mexate)	Dose varies depending on disease activity and route of drug administration.	• Observe for side effects and toxic effects, including, but not limited to, nausea/vomiting, bone marrow suppression, and alopecia. • Instruct client to avoid crowds and people with infections such as influenza.	• Side effects and toxic effects of these drugs can be devastating. Drugs are reserved for severe forms of CTDs in which organ involvement is potentially life threatening. • Bone marrow suppression or immune suppression increases risk of infection.
Prednisone (Deltasone, Apo-Prednisone✦)	Dose is 10–150 mg PO each day. For maintenance, attempt to give dose every other day (to allow client's adrenal glands to function).	• Observe for cushiongoid changes, e.g., moon-face, buffalo hump, striae, acne, thin skin, bruising, fluid retention, and increased blood pressure. • Monitor electrolyte and glucose levels. • Observe for long-term effects of chronic steroid therapy, such as osteoporosis, cataracts, hypertension, diabetes, and impaired healing. • Instruct client to avoid crowds and individuals with infections such as influenza.	• These changes are expected and tend to be dose related. Changes diminish as dose decreases. • Chronic steroid therapy can cause sodium or fluid retention, potassium depletion, and elevated glucose level. • These complications may need to be treated with other drugs or modalities. • Drug suppresses immune system (lymphocytes) and increases risk of infection or decreased healing.

NSAIDs = nonsteroidal anti-inflammatory drugs; CNS = central nervous system; CBC = complete blood count; CTDs = connective tissue diseases.

affected joints. If needed, the nurse collaborates with the dietitian to provide more in-depth client teaching about nutrition and meal planning.

Other Pain Relief Measures. Additional measures may be used for pain reduction. A transcutaneous electrical nerve stimulator (TENS) may be particularly helpful for vertebral involvement. The health care provider collaborates with the nurse and physical therapist to determine whether the client might benefit from this pain management modality. The client must be able to control the TENS unit for pain relief.

Complementary Therapies. Clients may also use acupuncture, hypnosis, music therapy, and imagery for pain relief (see Chaps. 4 and 9).

Surgical Management. When all other measures are inadequate to provide pain control for clients with DJD, surgery may be indicated. The most common surgical procedure performed for these clients is the total joint replacement (TJR). An osteotomy may be done to correct joint deformity instead, but this procedure is rare owing to the success rate of TJR.

Any synovial joint of the body can be replaced with a prosthetic system consisting of at least two parts, one for each joint surface. A TJR is the major type of arthroplasty (surgical creation of a joint) that is performed.

Indications. Total joint replacement is a procedure of last resort for pain management; it is used when all other methods of pain relief have been unsuccessful. Hips and knees are most commonly replaced, but replacements of finger and wrist joints, elbows, shoulders, and toe joints and ankles have become more popular in the past 20 years.

Although TJRs are performed most often for clients with degenerative joint disease (DJD), other conditions causing joint damage may also require surgery. These disorders include rheumatoid arthritis (RA), congenital anomalies, trauma, and avascular necrosis—bony necrosis secondary to lack of blood flow, usually from trauma or chronic steroid therapy.

Contraindications. The primary contraindications for TJR are infection anywhere in the body, advanced osteoporosis, and severe inflammation. An infection from a source in the body or from the joint being replaced can result in an infected TJR and subsequent prosthetic failure. If a client has a urinary tract infection, for example, the physician treats the infection before surgery. Advanced osteoporosis can cause bone shattering during replacement when the prosthetic device is inserted. Acute joint inflammation is treated before surgery because the mechanical stress of the procedure may promote further inflammation and prosthetic failure.

As a group, TJRs are quite successful. Many clients who have lived with chronic, unbearable pain for years and who could not function independently at home or in the workplace no longer experience pain in the diseased joint. The pain relief and psychological benefit may outweigh the perioperative risks, but the surgeon and client must make that decision. When the client is of advanced age, this decision may become an ethical issue in addition to a physical risk–versus–benefit decision.

Total Hip Replacement (THR). The most commonly replaced joint is the hip. Clients of any age have the surgery, but the procedure is done most often for clients older than 60. The special needs and normal physiologic changes of elderly clients often complicate the perioperative period and may result in additional postoperative complications. (See Chapters 20–22 for routine perioperative care and the special considerations needed for care of the elderly client.)

Preoperative Care. Some insurance companies assign TJR candidates to their case managers (CMs). During the assessment process, the CM determines whether the client will have support and caregiving services postoperatively. If none are available, the client's surgery is not approved until arrangements can be made for care in a nursing home or alternative placement.

As with any surgical procedure, preoperative care begins with assessment of the client's level of understanding about the impending replacement. The physician explains the procedure and postoperative care expectations during the office visit, but this explanation may have occurred weeks or months before the surgery was scheduled. Elderly clients, in particular, may forget some of the information or may not know what questions to ask. Many orthopedic surgeons employ nurses in the office who can follow up and address any of the client's special concerns. A clinical pathway outlining expectations during prehospitalization, hospitalization, and posthospitalization phases of care can be reviewed with the client and family.

In addition, nurse educators or orthopedic nurses may lead formal classes in the hospital several weeks before surgery to answer questions and clarify information. During class, the client is shown the prosthesis or a picture of the device and receives written instructions or teaching booklets to reinforce the information.

In some hospitals or orthopedic office practices, the physical therapist can meet the surgical candidate before surgery to explain ambulation and postoperative exercises.

Clients are admitted on the morning of surgery and do not come to the orthopedic, surgical, or medical-surgical unit until after surgery.

Operative Procedure. Before the start of the procedure, the operating room may be specially cleaned to reduce the risk of infection. Laminar airflow surgical suites and body exhaust systems ("spacesuits") may also be used. The surgery is usually scheduled early in the morning, if possible, and movement into and out of the room is kept to a minimum. The client is given a dose of intravenous antibiotics, usually a cephalosporin, such as cefazolin (Ancef), at least 1 hour before the initial surgical incision is made. Vancomycin (Vancocin) or clindamycin (Cleocin) may be used for clients allergic to cephalosporins.

The anesthesiologist or nurse anesthetist places the client under general or epidural anesthesia. Epidural induction reduces blood loss and the incidence of deep venous thrombosis. Intraoperative blood loss with hypotensive epidural anesthesia is usually less than 300 mL, which decreases the need for postoperative blood transfusions (Ranawat et al., 1997).

The 8- to 10-inch (20.3–24.5 cm) incision is usually longitudinal on the anterolateral thigh. A posterior incision may be used instead to preserve muscle, depending on surgeon preference.

If the prosthesis is cemented, polymethyl methacrylate (an acrylic fixating substance) is used. During the surgical procedure, the operative area is irrigated with a cool solution. To help prevent infection, the surgeon may mix an antibiotic with the cement or may use antibiotic-impregnated beads to plant deep into the wound. The surgeon also inserts one or two wound drains to remove exudate from the tissues that might serve as a medium for pathogenic growth and cause wound infection.

A major advance in joint replacement surgery is the increased use of noncemented prostheses, especially for hip replacements. Although polymethyl methacrylate is an excellent initial fixator, it has a finite life span and deteriorates over time, which causes loosening of the implant and pain. The average life span of a cemented hip is 10 years. When a prosthesis eventually loosens and causes pain, it is replaced; this procedure is called a *revision arthroplasty*. To prevent repeated replacements, several devices that do not require a fixating substance have been designed.

The most common mechanism that is used to avoid polymethyl methacrylate is a porous metal coating on the shaft of the femoral component and the back of the acetabular cap. By using a tight fit, known as a "press fit," the surgeon places the implant (prosthesis) snugly against the client's bone tissue. Most of the prostheses used today are custom designed by computers to match the size of the prosthesis with the size of the client's own joint. Figure 24–2 illustrates a typical noncemented hip replacement system.

New bone tissue grows between the pores of the prosthesis and "grafts" to the device within 6–12 weeks. The older the client, the longer the bone grafting may take. This bony ingrowth serves as the fixating mechanism and, ideally, lasts a lifetime. However, the earliest noncemented total joint systems, which were inserted in the 1970s and 1980s, have needed revisions, primarily because of undersizing of the prosthesis. As a result, the device loosens and is replaced with a new noncemented

TABLE 24–2

Nursing Interventions to Prevent Complications of Total Joint Replacement Surgery

Complication	Prevention/Intervention
Dislocation	• Position correctly. • For hip, keep legs slightly abducted. • For hip, prevent hip flexion beyond 90 degrees. • Assess for pain, rotation, and/or extremity shortening. • Keep client in bed. • Report immediately to physician.
Infection	• Use aseptic technique for wound care and emptying of drains. • Wash hands thoroughly when caring for client. • Culture drainage fluid. • Monitor temperature. • Report excessive inflammation and/or drainage to physician.
Deep venous thrombosis/pulmonary embolism	• Have client wear elastic stockings and/or sequential compression stockings. • Teach leg exercises to client. • Encourage fluid intake. • Observe for signs of thrombosis (redness, swelling, or pain). • Observe client for changes in mental status. • Keep client in bed. • Do not massage legs. • Do not use knee gatch on bed.
Hypotension, bleeding, or infection	• Take vital signs at least every 4 hr. • Observe client for bleeding. • Report excessively low blood pressure or bleeding to physician.

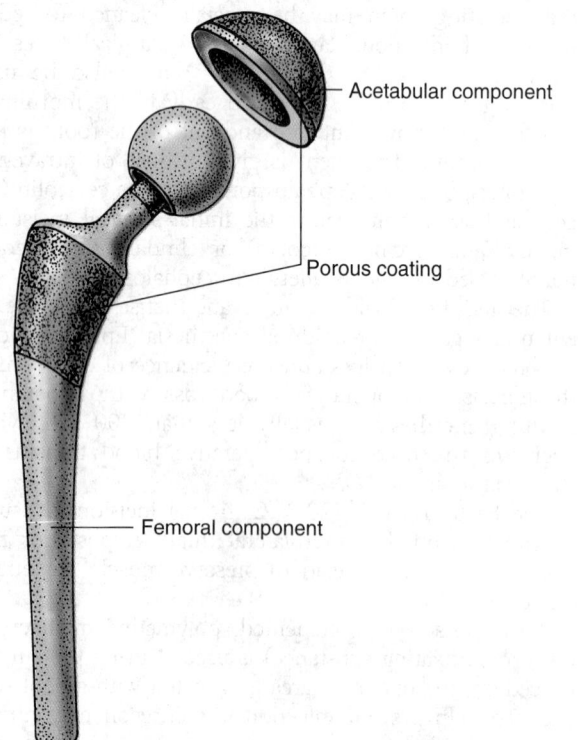

Figure 24–2. Noncemented, porous-coated hip replacement system.

Acetabular component

Porous coating

Femoral component

device. Freeze-dried bone grafts (*allografts*) are used to fill in bony defects that result from removing the old prosthesis. During the healing process, the essentially dead bone revascularizes and grafts with the client's own bone. Clients older than 75 and those who do not have sufficient bone mass are often not candidates for the noncemented hip.

Postoperative Care. In addition to providing the routine postoperative care discussed in Chapter 22, the nurse assesses for and assists in the prevention of postoperative complications that could occur after a joint replacement. Table 24–2 summarizes common postoperative complications of total hip replacement surgery, including nursing measures for prevention, assessment, and intervention.

Chart 24-2 highlights special concerns for the care of the elderly in the postoperative period.

Prevention of Dislocation. A common complication of total hip replacement is subluxation (partial dislocation) or total dislocation. Therefore, correct positioning is maintained at all times. When the client returns from the postanesthesia care unit (PACU), the nurse places the client in a supine position with the head slightly elevated. The nurse may place a trapezoid-shaped abduction pillow, wedge, sling, or splint, with or without straps, between the client's legs to prevent adduction beyond the body's midline. In some hospitals, this device is no longer used because it is uncomfortable for the client and not necessary in most cases. Abduction devices are usually reserved for clients who are very restless or who are unable to follow instructions, especially the elderly. One or two regular bed pillows are used instead for most clients.

The nurse may place and support the affected leg in neutral rotation by using a device such as the cradle boot. The cradle boot not only prevents rotation but also elevates the leg to the desired functional position and keeps the client's heel off the bed linen to prevent heel tissue breakdown. Keeping the heels off the bed is particularly important for the elderly client who is at high risk for pressure sores.

The nurse turns the client toward either side as long as the abduction or other pillow is in place. Some surgeons only allow turning directly onto one side or the other. This policy varies, depending on the surgeon's preference and the policy of the hospital unit.

The nurse observes the client for possible signs of hip dislocation, which include increased hip pain, shortening of the affected leg, and leg rotation. If any of these clinical manifestations occurs, the nurse keeps the client in bed and notifies the surgeon immediately. The surgeon manipulates and relocates the affected hip after the client receives analgesia or is anesthetized. The hip is then immobilized by an abduction splint or other device until healing occurs, usually in about 6 weeks.

Prevention of Infection. Another common potential complication of hip replacement is infection. As soon as the client's bowel sounds return and the client is voiding in sufficient quantity, the nurse discontinues intravenous therapy unless otherwise contraindicated.

The nurse also monitors the surgical incision and vital signs carefully: every 4 hours for the first several days and every 8 hours thereafter. The nurse observes for signs of infection, such as elevated temperature and excessive or foul-smelling drainage from the incision. An elderly client may not have a fever with infection but may experience an altered mental state instead. The nurse obtains a sample of the drainage for culture and sensitivity to determine the offending organisms and the antibiotics that may be needed for treatment.

An infection that occurs within 1 year of surgery is referred to as an early infection. It is most often due to contamination during surgery. In addition to antibiotics, laminar airflow operating rooms, body exhaust systems, ultraviolet light, and double gloving help reduce the incidence of infection. If an early infection occurs, the surgeon usually prescribes IV antibiotic therapy. Late infection can occur anywhere after 1 year postoperatively. If the late infection does not resolve with treatment, the surgeon may replace the prosthesis.

The clinical manifestations of infection are variable. The erythrocyte sedimentation rate (ESR) is elevated, and the client typically complains of incisional pain, swelling, erythema, and wound drainage.

Assessment of Bleeding and Prevention of Anemia. The nurse observes the surgical hip dressing for bleeding or other type of drainage at least every 4 hours or when vital signs are taken. The nurse empties and measures the fluid in the drain every shift. The nurse also observes and records the characteristics of the drainage, which is typically bloody. The total amount of drainage is usually less than 50 mL every 8 hours. If the client has received a plasma expander (such as dextran), this amount may be increased. The surgeon removes the drains and operative dressing 48–72 hours postoperatively. Care must be taken to prevent tape burns when the surgical dressing is removed, especially in an elderly client.

The surgeon also orders periodic hemoglobin and hematocrit assessments to determine whether the client is anemic and requires blood transfusions. Although some clients receive several units of blood during surgery, the hematocrit and hemoglobin may fall below the normal level so that additional blood is needed 2 or 3 days postoperatively. The client's blood pressure may be lower than usual because of blood loss during surgery or the use of cement, which tends to dilate blood vessels and cause hypotension.

Because total joint replacements (TJRs) are elective procedures, autologous blood transfusions are common. The

Chart 24-2

Nursing Focus on the Elderly: Total Hip Replacement

- Use an abduction pillow or splint to prevent adduction after surgery if the client is very restless or has an altered mental state.
- Keep the client's heels off the bed to prevent pressure sores.
- Do not rely on fever as a sign of infection; elderly clients often have infection without fever. Decreasing mental status typically occurs when the client has an infection.
- When assisting the client out of bed, move the client slowly to prevent orthostatic (postural) hypotension.
- Encourage the client to deep breathe and cough, and use the incentive spirometer every 2 hours to prevent atelectasis and pneumonia.
- As soon as permitted, get the client out of bed to prevent complications of immobility.
- Anticipate the client's need for pain medication, especially if the client is unable to verbalize the need for pain control.
- Expect a temporary change in mental state immediately after surgery as a result of the anesthesia and unfamiliar sensory stimuli. Reorient the client frequently.

client donates blood before surgery to be used as needed during and after surgery. This predeposit autologous blood donation is a cost-effective blood replacement alternative in clients with elective surgeries.

Another method for blood replacement is intraoperative or postoperative blood salvage. Intraoperatively, the shed blood is collected via aspiration from the surgical site. Using a cell saver, about 50% of the red blood cells are saved for reinfusion. This procedure is used most commonly for bilateral joint replacements or for revision surgeries. Postoperatively, blood can be replaced by collecting shed blood via suction into a reservoir, filtering the blood, and then reinfusing it. The American Association of Blood Banks recommends that the blood be reinfused within 6 hours of collection (Maher et al., 1994).

Assessment for Neurovascular Compromise. As with other bone surgery, frequent neurovascular assessments, which are performed at the same time as vital signs are checked, are necessary to monitor for possible compromise in circulation to the distal extremity.

Management of Incisional Pain. Although hip replacement is performed to relieve joint pain, the client experiences pain related to the surgical procedure. Many clients state that they have pain after surgery but that it is a different type and less excruciating than the pain before surgery. Pain control may be achieved by epidural analgesia, patient-controlled analgesia (PCA), intramuscular opioid analgesia, or a combination of techniques. (Chapter 9 contains a chart of commonly used opioid analgesics and related nursing interventions.)

The nurse anticipates the elderly client's need for pain medication if he or she cannot verbalize the need. Many elderly clients experience several days of increased disorientation or delirium as a result of surgery and anesthesia.

Regardless of the pain management method used, most clients do not require parenteral analgesia after the first two days. Oral opioids, such as oxycodone (Supeudol✦) or oxycodone plus acetaminophen (Percocet, Tylox), are then commonly prescribed until the client's pain can be controlled by NSAIDs, such as ibuprofen (Motrin, Apo-Ibuprofen✦).

Progression of Activity. The client with a total hip replacement is usually allowed to get out of bed the day after surgery, and physical therapy is initiated. Activities that are permitted differ among surgeons and hospitals, but prolonged bed rest can cause numerous complications, such as atelectasis and pneumonia, especially in the elderly. When getting the client out of bed, the nurse stands on the same side of the bed as the client's affected leg. After achieving a sitting position, the client stands on the unaffected leg and pivots to the chair with assistance. To prevent hip dislocation (Fig. 24–3), the nurse at all times ensures that the client does not flex the hips beyond 90 degrees. Raised toilet seats, straight-back chairs, and reclining wheelchairs help prevent hyperflexion.

The surgeon, the type of prosthesis, and the surgical approach all determine the resumption of weight-bearing on the affected leg. A client with a cemented implant is usually allowed partial weight-bearing (PWB) or full weight-bearing (FWB) to tolerance immediately. A client with an uncemented prosthesis cannot tolerate FWB until bony ingrowth occurs. PWB typically is only permitted for the first 6 weeks or until there is x-ray evidence of bony ingrowth.

The physical therapist (PT) teaches the client how to follow these weight-bearing restrictions and helps the client progress to full-weight-bearing (FWB) status, if possible. Most clients generally use a walker, although young clients may use crutches. Clients are usually advanced to a single cane or crutch if they can walk without a severe limp 1 month after surgery. When the limp disappears, they no longer need an ambulatory assistive device and are permitted to sit in normal-height chairs, use regular toilets, and drive a car.

Prevention of Thromboembolitic Complications. The risk of developing deep venous thrombosis postoperatively is high. Fatal pulmonary embolism syndrome occurs in 0.5% to 2% of cases (Ranawat et al., 1997). Elderly clients are especially at increased risk for thrombi because of age and compromised circulation before surgery. Obese clients and those with a history of deep venous thrombi are also at high risk for thrombi. In clients with total hip replacement, thrombi usually develop in the thigh; these thrombi become life-threatening emboli more readily than calf and other thrombi. For this reason, thigh-high stockings, elastic bandages, and sequential compression devices (SCDs) are used during the hospital stay (see Chap. 20).

Anticoagulants, such as aspirin (Ecotrin or buffered aspirin), warfarin (Coumadin, Warfilone✦), or subcutaneous low-molecular-weight (LMW) heparin (Lovenox), are prescribed in maintenance doses. Warfarin is the most commonly used anticoagulant. If the client takes warfarin, the dosage is adjusted to maintain an international normalized ratio (INR) of 2.0.

The PT teaches leg exercises, which are begun in the immediate postoperative period and continue until the client is fully ambulatory. These exercises include plantar flexion and dorsiflexion (heel pumping), circumduction (circles) of the feet, gluteal and quadriceps muscle setting, and straight-leg raises (SLRs). The client performs gluteal exercises by pushing the heels into the bed. The client achieves quadriceps-setting exercises ("quad sets") by straightening the legs and pushing the back of the knees into the bed. In addition to preventing clots, these exercises improve muscle tone, which aids in restoration of function of the extremity.

Promotion of Self-Care. The hospital's occupational therapy department often supplies assistive-adaptive devices to help with activities of daily living (ADLs). Particularly important for clients are devices designed for reaching to prevent them from bending or stooping and flexing at the hips more than 90 degrees. Extended handles on shoehorns and dressing sticks are particularly useful for helping clients achieve independence in ADLs.

Clients typically stay in the hospital for 3–5 days, but elderly clients or those experiencing postoperative complications may stay longer. Discharge may be to the home, a rehabilitation unit, transitional care unit (subacute unit), or a long-term care facility for rehabilitation or custodial care. The nurse provides written instructions for posthospital care and reviews them with clients and their family

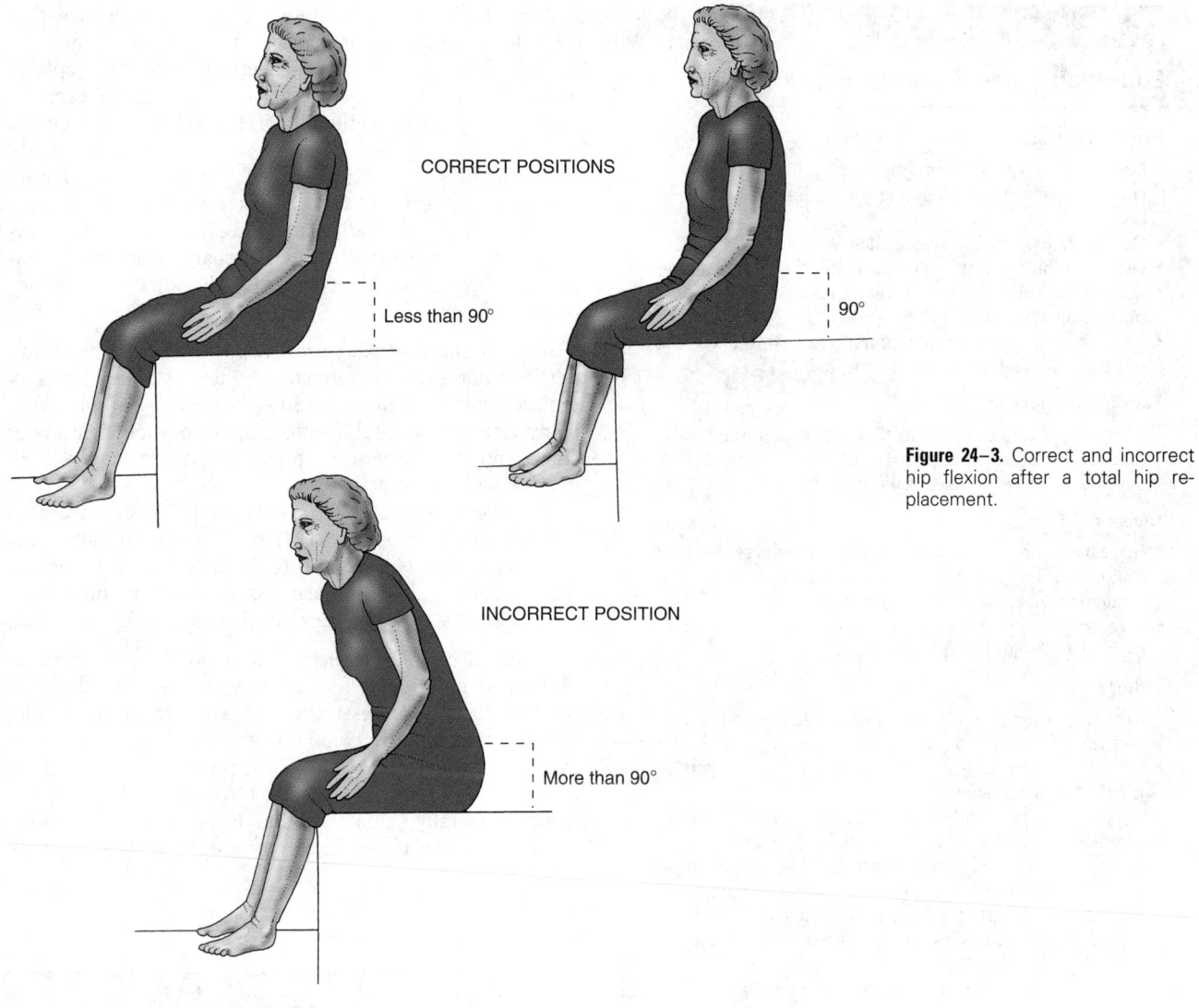

CORRECT POSITIONS

Less than 90°

90°

INCORRECT POSITION

More than 90°

Figure 24–3. Correct and incorrect hip flexion after a total hip replacement.

members (Chart 24–3). If the client is transferred to a facility, a copy of the posthospital instructions is sent with the client to the facility.

Total Knee Replacement (TKR). After total hip replacement, the second most common total joint replacement (TJR) procedure is for the knee. Before 1980, attempts at knee replacement were not successful, and most of the prostheses inserted before then have been removed. The knee is not a simple, hinged joint; it is a condylar joint that rotates slightly when flexed and extended. As seen in Figure 24–4, the typical total knee prosthesis is a three-part system: a femoral component, a tibial plate, and a patellar button. For some clients, only one surface is replaced.

Preoperative Care. Only severe symptoms and disability justify TKR in clients with DJD. TKRs are avoided in people younger than 60 years (Windsor & Insall, 1997). The preoperative care for clients undergoing a TKR is similar to that for total hip replacement. The major difference is the teaching, which depends on the postoperative protocol used by the orthopedic surgeon. After surgery,

clients may not be allowed to bend the operative knee for several days until a large, bulky pressure dressing is removed. Most surgeons have abandoned this traditional approach for the continuous passive motion (CPM) machine (see later in this chapter).

Operative Procedure. As with the hip, the knee can be replaced with the client under general or epidural anesthesia. The surgeon typically makes a central longitudinal incision, approximately 8–10 inches (20.3–25.4 cm) long. Osteotomies of the femoral and tibial condyles and of the posterior patella are performed; the surfaces are prepared for the prostheses. Noncemented implants, once popular in the 1980s, are used less for the knee than they are for the hip. The surgeon inserts one or two surgical drains and applies a pressure dressing to prevent bleeding.

Postoperative Care. Postoperative nursing care of the client with a total knee replacement is similar to that for the client with a total hip replacement, but maintaining abduction is not necessary. The surgeon usually orders a

Education Guide: Total Hip Replacement

Hip Precautions

- Do not sit or stand for prolonged periods.
- Do not cross your legs beyond the midline of your body.
- Do not bend your hips more than 90 degrees.
- Use an ambulatory aid, such as a walker, when walking.
- Use assistive-adaptive devices for dressing, such as for putting on shoes and socks.
- You can resume sexual intercourse as usual, but use the hip precautions learned in the hospital.

Pain Management

- Report increased hip pain to the physician immediately.
- Take oral analgesics, as prescribed, only as needed.
- Do not overexert yourself; take frequent rests.

Incisional Care

- Inspect your hip incision every day for redness, heat, or drainage; if any of these are present, call your physician immediately.
- Cleanse your hip incision with a mild soap and water every day; be sure to dry it thoroughly.

Other Care

- Continue walking and performing the leg exercises as you learned in the hospital.
- Report pain, redness, or swelling in your legs to your physician immediately.
- Report chest pain and/or shortness of breath to your physician immediately.
- If you are taking an anticoagulant for 4–6 weeks, follow the precautions learned in the hospital to prevent bleeding: avoid using a straight razor, avoid injuries, report bleeding or excessive bruising to your physician immediately.

Because dislocation is a rare problem for a client with a total knee replacement, special positioning is not required. Other complications affecting total hip replacement clients may affect these clients as well. Preventive measures described earlier for THRs are used for clients with TKRs.

On discharge from the hospital, the client should walk independently with a cane or walker and have 90 degrees of flexion in the operative knee. Use of a stationary bicycle can help gain flexion. After discharge from the hospital, the client should not hyperflex the knee or kneel for prolonged periods.

Total Shoulder Replacement. Replacement of the shoulder has not been performed as often as other types of replacement techniques. Because the joint is complex with many articulations, subluxation, or dislocation, is a major complication. A Neer-type prosthesis is commonly used, with or without cement.

The client's operative arm is typically placed in a continuous passive motion (CPM) machine shortly after surgery (see Chart 24–4). During the first few postoperative days, frequent neurovascular assessments are important. The hospital stay is shorter than that for a THR or a TKR.

Total Elbow Replacement. The elbow replacement is performed most often for clients with rheumatoid arthritis. It is usually successful in increasing range of motion, but infection is fairly common because of extensive tissue cutting during surgery. The Mayo prosthesis is commonly inserted, and the CPM device is often used postoperatively. Generally, elbow motion is allowed as tolerated. Physical therapy is not usually necessary for postoperative

CPM machine, which is can be applied in the postanesthesia care unit (PACU) or not used until 1–2 days after surgery (Fig. 24–5). The CPM keeps the prosthetic knee in motion and prevents scar tissue formation, which could impede mobility of the knee and exacerbate postoperative pain.

The surgeon, physical therapist, or technician presets the CPM machine for the appropriate range of motion and cycles per minute. A typical initial setting is 20–30 degrees range of motion at 2 cycles/minute, but this setting varies according to surgeon preference. The machine is generally used for 8–12 hours/day, and the range of motion is increased gradually. The current trend is intermittent use for several hours at a time. Each day the nurse notes the client's response to the use of the device.

Some machines do not allow the leg to achieve full extension, thus promoting flexion contractures; however, one solution is for the client to use the CPM machine during the day and sleep in a knee immobilizer at night to achieve the desired extension. Chart 24–4 outlines the nurse's responsibility when caring for a client using the CPM machine.

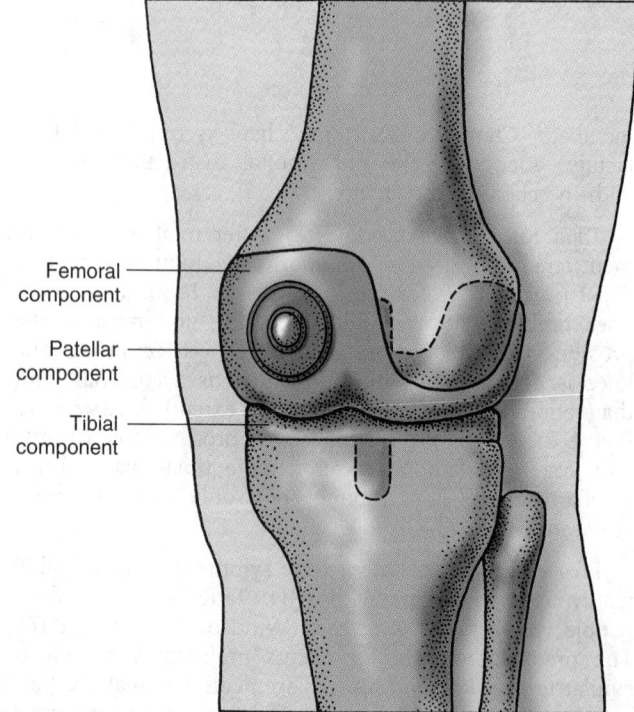

Femoral component
Patellar component
Tibial component

Figure 24–4. Typical three-part condylar knee replacement system.

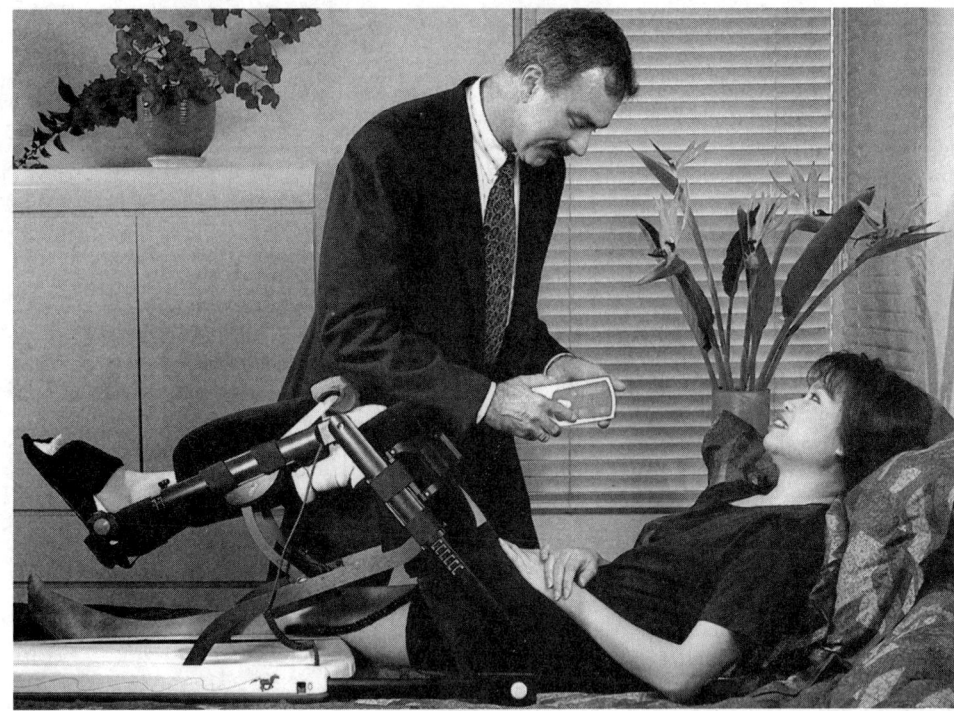

Figure 24–5. A continuous passive motion machine in use. (Courtesy of Orthologic, Tempe, AZ.)

clients with a total elbow replacement. Generalized swelling usually resolves in 3–6 months.

Finger and Wrist Replacements. Any joint of the hand can be replaced, often for clients with rheumatoid arthritis. The flexible, silicone prostheses are implanted without the use of polymethyl methacrylate because no weight-bearing is required for the prostheses.

Postoperatively, a bulky dressing is used temporarily and then replaced by a dynamic splint, brace, or cast or by a very small CPM machine. Edema formation is controlled if the client elevates the arm as much as possible. The rehabilitation program for finger arthroplasties may

last for weeks, until normal function and strength return. These procedures are typically performed in specialized hand centers.

Any bone of the wrist can be replaced, including the heads of the radius and ulna. The postoperative pressure dressing is removed in 2–3 days, and a splint or short arm cast is applied. The client usually regains full function within 6–12 weeks, but lifting may be restricted for a longer period. Occupational therapists are usually involved with upper extremity rehabilitation.

Ankle and Toe Replacements. Because the ankles support approximately 25% of the body's weight, developing an implant that is both small and strong enough to withstand the weight of the body has been difficult. When the ankle is replaced, usually an arthrodesis, or bone fusion, is performed for added stability. Replacing the ankle is not a common procedure.

The metatarsal implants are made of silicone and cannot bear excessive weight. Typically, the client has one or more osteotomies and fusions, which are immobilized by wires and a cast while healing occurs. Chapter 53 discusses foot osteotomies and their associated nursing care.

Impaired Physical Mobility

Planning: Expected Outcomes. The primary outcome for the client with DJD is that the client is expected to function independently in performing activities of daily living (ADLs) and ambulation.

Interventions. Management of the client with DJD is an interdisciplinary effort. The nurse collaborates with the physical and occupational therapists to meet the goal of independent function. The major interventions include therapeutic exercise and promotion of ADLs and ambula-

---

Chart 24–4

Nursing Care Highlight: The Client Using a Continuous Passive Motion (CPM) Machine

- Ensure that the machine is well padded with sheepskin or other similar material.
- Check the cycle and range-of-motion settings at least once per shift (every 8 hours).
- Ensure that the joint being moved is properly positioned on the machine.
- If the client is confused, place the controls to the machine out of the client's reach.
- Assess the client's response to the machine.
- Turn off the machine while the client is having a meal in bed.
- When the machine is not in use, do not store it on the floor.

tion through teaching about health and use of assistive-adaptive devices.

Exercise. Two types of exercise are recommended for the client with DJD: recreational and therapeutic. Recreational exercise includes hobbies and sports, with no planned purpose other than relaxation. Therapeutic exercise includes carefully planned activities that are designed to improve muscle strength and tone and joint ROM. Therapeutic exercise can also reduce pain and improve the client's psychological health.

Certain recreational activities may also be therapeutic, such as doing the breast stroke during swimming to enhance chest and arm muscles. Aerobic exercises, such as walking, biking, swimming, and aerobic dance, are recommended. Usually the physical therapist prescribes exercises for the client with DJD, but the nurse reinforces their techniques and principles. The ideal time for exercise is immediately after the application of heat. To prevent further joint damage, clients should rigorously follow the instructions for exercise outlined in Chart 24–5.

Use of Assistive-Adaptive Devices. The physical therapist evaluates the client's need for ambulatory aids, such as canes, walkers, or platform crutches. Although many clients do not like to use these aids or may forget how to use them, these aids help prevent further joint deterioration and pain. An occupational therapist evaluates the client's ability to perform ADLs and can provide ideas and devices for assistance.

 Continuing Care

The client with degenerative joint disease (DJD) is not usually hospitalized for the disease itself but for surgical management. However, the client may be admitted for

---

Chart 24–5

Education Guide: Exercises for Clients with Degenerative Joint Disease or Rheumatoid Arthritis

- Follow the exercise instructions that have been specifically prescribed for you. There are no universal exercises; your exercises have been specifically tailored to your own needs.
- Do your exercises on both "good" and "bad" days. Consistency is important.
- Respect pain. If pain increases as you exercise, stop and report this to your physician.
- Use active rather than active-assist or passive exercise whenever possible.
- Reduce the number of repetitions when the inflammation is severe and you have more pain.
- Do not substitute your normal activities or household tasks for the prescribed exercises.
- Avoid resistive exercises when your joints are severely inflamed.

Chart 24–6

Education Guide: Instructions for Joint Protection

- Use large joints instead of small ones; for example, place your purse strap over your shoulder instead of grasping the purse with your hand.
- Do not turn a doorknob clockwise. Turn it counterclockwise to avoid twisting your arm and promoting ulnar deviation.
- Use two hands instead of one to hold objects.
- Sit in a chair with a high, straight back.
- When getting out of bed, do not push off with your fingers; use the entire palm of both hands.
- Do not bend at your waist; bend your knees instead, while keeping your back straight.
- Use long-handled devices, such as a hairbrush with an extended handle.
- Use assistive-adaptive devices, such as Velcro closures and built-up utensil handles, to protect your joints.
- Do not use pillows in bed, except a small one under your head.
- Avoid twisting or wringing your hands.

---

another medical or surgical reason. The nurse considers the problems that are present as a result of arthritis before the client is discharged home.

➤ *Home Care Management*

If weight-bearing joints are markedly involved, the client may have difficulty going up or down stairs. Making arrangements to live on one floor with accessibility to all rooms is often the best solution. A home care nurse, physical therapist, or occupational therapist assesses the need for structural alterations to the home to accommodate ambulatory aids and to enable the client to perform activities. For example, a kitchen counter may need to be lowered or a seat and hand rails to be installed in the shower. If the client has a total hip replacement, an elevated toilet seat is necessary for several weeks postoperatively to prevent excessive hip flexion.

➤ *Health Teaching*

Learning how to protect the joint is the most important feature of client education. Preventing further damage to joints slows the progression of DJD and minimizes pain. The nurse explains general rules of joint protection and cites examples, as in Chart 24–6.

As with other diseases in which drugs and diet therapy are used, the nurse teaches the drug protocol, side effects, and toxic effects to the client and family. The nurse also emphasizes the importance of reducing weight and eating a well-balanced diet to promote tissue healing.

Many clients with "arthritis" become frustrated and desperate about the course of the disease and treatment, and they look for a cure. Unfortunately, there is no cure for these joint diseases, even though tabloids, books, and the media frequently cite "curative" remedies. People spend billions of dollars each year on quackery, including liniments, special diets, and copper bracelets. More hazardous substances, such as snake venom and industrial cleaners, are also advertised as remedies. The nurse instructs the client to always check with The Arthritis Foundation about new "cures." For example, if a client believes that wearing a copper bracelet or eating more foods with a high vitamin C content is helpful, the nurse may encourage the continuation of the practice as long as it is not harmful. If there is a potential for harm, the nurse instructs the client to avoid the modality and provides the rationale for doing so.

With most types of CTD, clients must live with a chronic, unpredictable, and painful disorder. Their roles, self-esteem, and body image may be affected by these diseases. Body image is often not as devastating in DJD as in the inflammatory arthritic diseases, such as rheumatoid arthritis. The psychosocial component is discussed in more detail under Rheumatoid Arthritis.

► Health Care Resources

The client who has undergone surgery is most likely to need help from community resources. After a joint replacement, the client needs extensive assistance with mobility. The client may be discharged to home, a long-term care facility, a subacute unit (transitional care unit), or a rehabilitation unit. The nurse collaborates with the social worker, discharge planner, case manager, and physician to find the best placement for each client. If the client is discharged to home, home care nurses visit for the first 2–3 weeks, depending on the client's concurrent systemic diseases. A nursing assistant may visit the home to help with hygiene-related needs; a physical therapist may work with the client on ambulatory and mobility skills. In addition, a client who has had a total hip or knee replacement should not be discharged to home alone. A family member or significant other must be in the home at all times for at least the first 4–6 weeks, when the client needs the most assistance.

The nurse provides written instructions about the care that is required, regardless of whether the client goes home or to another inpatient facility. For continuity of care, communication with the new care provider is ideal. Arrangements are made so that the client can return to the same acute care hospital if needed.

The Arthritis Foundation is an important community resource for all clients with CTD. This organization provides information to laypeople and health professionals and refers clients and their families to other resources as needed. Local support groups can help clients and their families cope with these diseases.

 Evaluation

The nurse evaluates the care provided by determining whether the client
- States that chronic pain is reduced as a result of interdisciplinary interventions

- Ambulates without personal assistance (although a mechanical aid such as a walker may be used)
- Is independent in ADLs (may use assistive-adaptive devices)

RHEUMATOID ARTHRITIS

Overview

Rheumatoid arthritis (RA) is the second most commonly occurring connective tissue disease but is the most destructive to joints. It is a chronic, progressive, systemic inflammatory process that affects primarily synovial joints.

The onset of RA is characterized by synovitis, or inflammation of the synovial tissue in joints. Inflammatory mediators, such as cytokines, chemokines, and proteases, attract and activate neutrophils and other cells (see Chapter 23 for a complete discussion of the inflammatory response). The synovium thickens and becomes hyperemic, fluid accumulates in the joint space, and a pannus forms. The pannus is vascular granulation tissue, composed of inflammatory cells, that erodes articular cartilage and eventually destroys bone. As a result, fibrous adhesions, bony ankylosis, and calcifications occur; bone loses density and secondary osteoporosis occurs.

If the disease is diagnosed early, permanent joint changes may be avoided. Early, aggressive treatment to suppress synovitis may cause a remission; about 25% of clients experience a remission, which may last as long as 20 years. Some clients also experience spontaneous remissions and exacerbations without treatment.

Rheumatoid arthritis is a systemic disease; that is, areas of the body—in addition to synovial joints—can be affected. Inflammatory responses similar to those occurring in synovial tissue may be seen in any organ or body system in which connective tissue is prevalent. If blood vessel involvement (*vasculitis*) occurs, the organ that is supplied by that vessel can be affected. The result is malfunction and eventual failure of the organ or system. These pathologic changes occur late in the disease process and cause life-threatening problems.

The etiology of RA remains a mystery, but research suggests a combination of environmental and genetic factors. The most popular theory to date—the immune complex hypothesis—states that unusual antibodies of the immunoglobulin (Ig) G or IgM type (rheumatoid factor) develop against IgG antigenic determinants to form complexes that lodge in synovium and other connective tissues. Local and systemic inflammatory responses result. RA has been found to be strongly associated with the human leukocyte antigen (HLA) DRw4. Other antigens have been identified but are observed less frequently. (See Chapter 23 on inflammation and the immune response.)

Although RA is probably an autoimmune disease, the origin of rheumatoid factor is unclear. A genetic predisposition for RA is most likely because the disease affects people with a family history of RA two to three times more often than the rest of the population.

Some researchers suspect that female reproductive hormones influence the development of RA because it affects women more often than men. Others suspect that a virus, such as Epstein-Barr virus, may trigger the autoimmune process. Physical and emotional stresses have been linked to exacerbations of the disorder and may be contributing factors in its development.

WOMEN'S HEALTH CONSIDERATIONS

 Rheumatoid arthritis affects 1% of the world's population, women three times more often than men. Women who are taking or who have taken oral contraceptives are less likely to have RA. The onset of the disease is typically between ages 35 and 45 years, but it can occur at any age.

There are no significant differences among geographic locations, despite the common lay belief that warmer, drier climates can be beneficial to people with RA. The incidence of RA in China is somewhat lower than elsewhere in the world (about 0.3%) and substantially higher among the Pima Indians in North America (about 5%) (Harris, 1997).

TRANSCULTURAL CONSIDERATIONS

With the exception of Native Americans, there are no major differences among races or ethnic groups. Studies of several northern Native American groups revealed RA prevalence rates that were three to seven times higher that those in non–Native American groups (Giger & Davidhizar, 1995).

Collaborative Management

Assessment

The onset of RA may be acute and severe or slow and insidious; clients may have vague complaints lasting for several months before diagnosis. The manifestations of RA can be categorized as early or late disease and as articular or extra-articular (Chart 24–7).

➤ Physical Assessment/Clinical Manifestations

Early Disease Manifestations. The client with RA typically complains of fatigue, generalized weakness, anorexia, and a weight loss of about 2 or 3 pounds (1 kg) early in the disease process. Persistent low-grade fever may accompany these complaints because RA is an inflammatory disease. In clients with early disease, the nurse notes that the upper extremity joints are involved initially, typically the proximal interphalangeal (PIP) and metacarpophalangeal (MCP) joints of the hands. These joints may be slightly reddened, warm, stiff, swollen, and tender or painful, particularly on palpation. The typical pattern of joint involvement in RA is bilateral and symmetric (e.g., both wrists), and the number of joints involved usually increases as the disease progresses.

ELDERLY CONSIDERATIONS

Rheumatoid arthritis developing in the elderly affects men more often than women. The client typically complains of stiffness; swelling of the hands, wrists, and forearms; and limb girdle pain (Harris, 1997).

Chart 24–7

Focused Assessment of the Client with Rheumatoid Arthritis

Early Manifestations
Joint

- Inflammation

Systemic

- Low-grade fever
- Fatigue
- Weakness
- Anorexia
- Paresthesias

Late Manifestations
Joint

- Deformities (e.g., swan neck or ulnar deviation)
- Moderate to severe pain and morning stiffness

Systemic

- Osteoporosis
- Severe fatigue
- Anemia
- Weight loss
- Subcutaneous nodules
- Peripheral neuropathy
- Vasculitis
- Pericarditis
- Fibrotic lung disease
- Sjögren's syndrome
- Renal disease

Late Disease Manifestations. As the disease worsens, the joints become progressively inflamed and quite painful. The client complains of morning stiffness (also called the gel phenomenon), which lasts between 30 minutes and several hours after awakening. On palpation, the nurse notes that the joints feel soft because of synovitis and effusions. The fingers often appear spindle like. The nurse may observe muscle atrophy, which can result from disuse secondary to joint pain, and a decreased range of motion in affected joints.

Eventually, most or all synovial joints are affected. In severe disease, the temporomandibular joint (TMJ) may be involved, but this involvement is infrequent. When the TMJ is affected, the client typically complains of pain when chewing or opening the mouth.

When the spinal column is involved, the cervical joints are most likely to be affected. The nurse palpates the posterior cervical spine to elicit pain or tenderness. Cervical disease may result in subluxation, especially the first and second vertebrae. This is a life-threatening complication because branches of the phrenic nerve that supply the diaphragm can be compressed and respiratory function may be subsequently compromised. The client is also in danger of becoming quadriparetic or quadriplegic.

Joint Manifestations. Joint deformity occurs as a late, articular manifestation, and secondary osteoporosis can cause bone fractures. The nurse observes common defor-

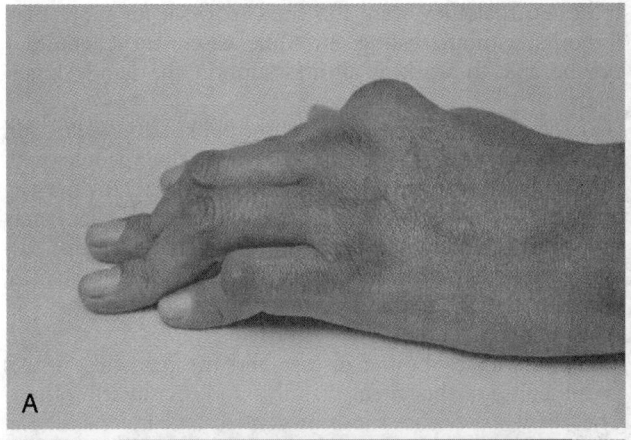

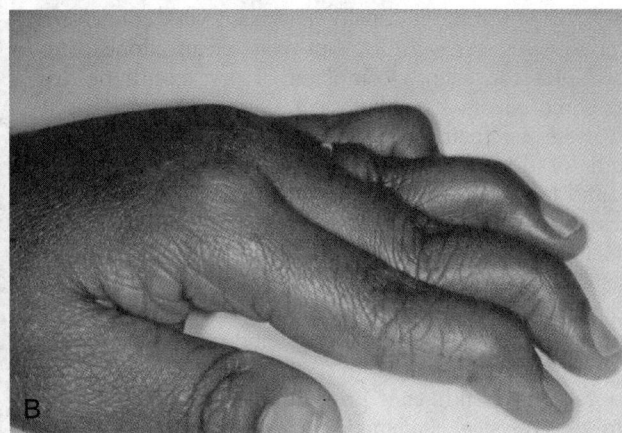

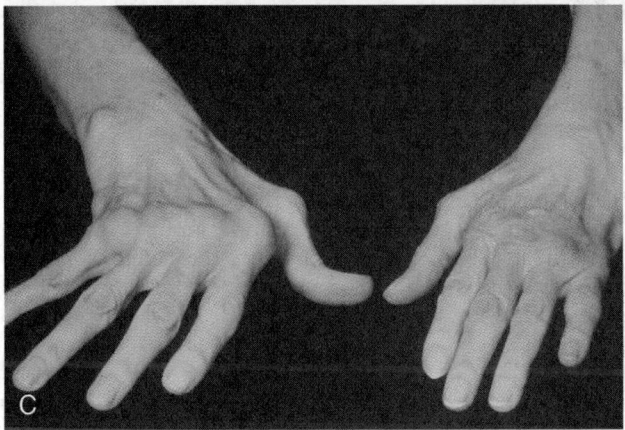

Figure 24-6. Common joint deformities seen in rheumatoid arthritis. *A,* Boutonniére, or buttonhole. *B,* Swan neck. *C,* Ulnar deviation (on left). (From the Arthritis Teaching Slide Collection, copyright 1980. Used by permission of the Arthritis Foundation.)

mities, especially in the hands and feet (Fig. 24-6). Extensive wrist involvement can result in carpal tunnel syndrome (see Chapter 54 for assessment and management).

The nurse palpates the tissues around the joints to elicit pain or tenderness associated with other rheumatoid complications. For example, Baker's cysts (enlarged popliteal bursae) may occur and cause tissue compression and pain. Tendon rupture is also common, particularly rupture of the Achilles tendon.

Systemic Manifestations. Numerous extra-articular clinical manifestations are associated with advanced disease. Consequently, the nurse assesses other body systems to ascertain systemic involvement. Moderate to severe weight loss, fever, and extreme fatigue are common in late disease exacerbations, often called "flares." Approximately 25% of clients have the characteristic round, movable, nontender subcutaneous nodules, which most often appear on the ulnar surface of the arm. These nodules disappear and reappear at any time and are associated with severe, destructive disease. They occasionally open and become infected, but otherwise they do not usually cause a problem.

Inflammation of the blood vessels results in vasculitis, particularly of small to medium-sized vessels. When arterial involvement (RA) occurs, major organs and body systems become ischemic and malfunction. Ischemic skin lesions appear in groups as small, brownish spots, most commonly around the nail bed (periungual lesions). The nurse and health care provider monitor the number of lesions and note their location each day. An increased number of lesions indicates increased vasculitis; a decreased number indicates decreased vasculitis. The nurse also carefully assesses any larger lesions that appear on the lower extremities; they often lead to ulcerations, which heal slowly as a result of decreased circulation. Peripheral neuropathy associated with decreased circulation can cause foot drop and paresthesias (burning and tingling sensations), most often in the elderly.

Respiratory complications manifest as pleurisy, pneumonitis, diffuse interstitial fibrosis, and pulmonary hypertension. Cardiac complications include pericarditis and myocarditis. The nurse also assesses for ocular involvement, which typically manifests as iritis and scleritis. If either of these complications is present, the nurse notes that the sclera of one or both eyes is reddened and the pupils have an irregular shape.

Associated Syndromes. Several syndromes are seen in clients with advanced RA. The most common is Sjögren's syndrome, which includes a triad of
- Dry eyes (keratoconjunctivitis sicca [KCS], or the sicca syndrome)
- Dry mouth (xerostomia)
- Dry vagina (in some cases)

In Sjögren's syndrome, immune complexes and inflammatory cells are thought to obstruct secretory glands and ducts. The syndrome is usually associated with connective tissue diseases such as RA but may occur alone. The nurse notes the client's complaint of dry mouth or dry eyes. Some clients state that their eyes feel "gritty," as if sand were in their eyes. The nurse also inspects the mouth for dry, sticky membranes and the eyes for redness and lack of tearing.

Less commonly observed is Felty's syndrome, which is characterized by RA, hepatosplenomegaly (enlarged liver and spleen), and leukopenia.

Caplan's syndrome is characterized by the presence of rheumatoid nodules in the lungs and pneumoconiosis, which is noted primarily in coal miners and asbestos workers. The health care provider diagnoses these syndromes by physical examination and diagnostic testing.

➤ *Psychosocial Assessment*

Rheumatoid arthritis can be a crippling disease. After 10–15 years of having the disease, fewer than 50% of clients are totally independent in ADLs. These physical limitations result in role changes in the family and society. For example, the person may not be able to cook for the family or be an active sexual partner. In addition, extreme fatigue often causes clients to desire an early bedtime and may result in a reluctance to socialize. In a classic nursing study by Crosby (1991), 52% of 101 people with RA indicated that they were too tired to work for more than 4 hours without resting. In some cases, the client may not be able to work at all and support the family financially.

Body changes may also cause poor self-esteem and body image. Because many societies value people with physically fit, attractive bodies, the client with RA may be embarrassed to be seen in public places. The client may grieve, may experience depression, and may attempt suicide. The client may experience a feeling of helplessness, accompanied by a loss of control over a disease that can "consume" the body.

Living with a chronic disease and the pain that results is difficult for the client, family, and significant others. The client experiences loss of control and independence. Chronic suffering affects quality of life (Dildy, 1996). The nurse assesses the client's emotional and mental status in relation to the disease and its problems and evaluates the client's support systems and resources.

➤ *Laboratory Assessment*

Laboratory tests help to support a diagnosis of rheumatoid arthritis, but no single test or group of tests can confirm it. Chart 24–8 summarizes the common laboratory tests that the health care provider uses for diagnosis of connective tissue disease.

Chart 24–8

Laboratory Profile: Connective Tissue Disease

Test	Normal Range for Adults	Significance of Abnormal Findings
Rheumatoid factor		
Rose-Waaler	• Negative	• Elevations of either titer (increase in number at right of colon) indicative of possible CTD
		• Increased Rose's titer indicative of RA (seropositive); not a sensitive test
Latex agglutination	• <1:16	• Latex titer not as specific to one disease, but quite sensitive test
ANA (total)	• Negative (if positive, types of ANA identified, e.g., anti-DNA, anti-DNP, anti-RNA, to indicate what part of cells involved)	• Elevations common in SLE, PSS, RA, and other inflammatory CTDs (5% of healthy adults have positive ANA results)
Serum complement (C' or CH$_{50}$)	• Varies greatly among laboratories	• Decreased value indicative of active autoimmune disease such as SLE
LE preparation	• Negative	• A type of ANA (anti-DNP); not reliable because negative result does not rule out SLE; can be used as screening test
SPEP		
Albumin	• 3.5–5.0 g/dL	• Increased levels of gamma globulins indicative of CTD (inflammatory type)
Globulin		
Alpha$_1$ globulin	• 0.1–0.3 g/dL	• Increased level of alpha globulins possible in RA
Alpha$_2$ globulin	• 0.6–1.0 g/dL	
Beta globulin	• 0.7–1.1 g/dL	
Gamma globulin	• 0.8–1.6 g/dL	
HLA testing (HLA-B27)	• None	• Presence of HLA-B27 indicative of Reiter's syndrome or ankylosing spondylitis

ANA = antinuclear antibody; CTD = connective tissue disease; DNP = dinitrophenol; SLE = systemic lupus erythematosus; PSS = progressive systemic sclerosis; LE = lupus erythematosus; SPEP = serum protein electrophoresis; RA = rheumatoid arthritis; HLA = human leukocyte antigen; ESR = erythrocyte sedimentation rate.

Rheumatoid Factor. The test for rheumatoid factor (RF) measures the presence of unusual antibodies of the IgG and IgM type that develop in a number of connective tissue diseases. Two methods may be used to ascertain the degree to which these antibodies are present in the body: Rose-Waaler and latex agglutination. In both procedures, values are reported as titers.

The Rose-Waaler test is more specific for a diagnosis of RA than the latex but is not as sensitive. A client with a positive Rose-Waaler result probably has RA and is seropositive; a client with a negative test result may or may not have the disease and is seronegative. About 60% of RA clients are seropositive and have a positive titer.

The latex agglutination test is sensitive but is not as specific for RA. Its normal value is less than 1:16 (Tietz, 1995). Generally, the higher the titer, the more active is the disease process.

Antinuclear Antibody Titer. The antinuclear antibody (ANA) test measures the titer of unusual antibodies that destroy the nuclei of cells and cause tissue death. When the fluorescent method is used, the test is sometimes referred to as FANA. If this test result is positive (a value higher than 1:8), various subtypes of this antibody are identified and measured. As with the RF, the higher the titer, the more active is the disease process. ANA is often negative until later in the disease process.

Erythrocyte Sedimentation Rate. The "sed rate," as the ESR is sometimes called, can confirm inflammation or infection anywhere in the body. It is particularly useful in connective tissue disease because the value directly correlates with the degree of inflammation and, later, with the severity of the disease.

Because several laboratory procedures are used to measure ESR, normal values vary; women have higher normal values than men. Generally, a value of 30–40 mm/hour indicates mild inflammation; 40–70 mm/hour, moderate inflammation; and 70–150 mm/hour, severe inflammation.

The ESR is also used to monitor a client's response to anti-inflammatory drug therapy. The value should decrease if the drug dosage is effective.

Serum Complement. In an attempt to destroy the immune complexes, complement (C') attaches to the complex. If a large amount of complement is used in this lytic process, the concentration of free-floating complement in the blood diminishes. Normal values vary considerably, depending on the laboratory technique used. An abnormal finding is indicated by a decrease in serum complement and is seen primarily in clients with vasculitis.

Serum Protein Electrophoresis. In serum protein electrophoresis, the protein fractions of the plasma are measured using electrical current to separate them. In acute inflammation, the level of alpha globulin is raised, but in chronic inflammatory conditions such as RA, the level of gamma globulin is increased because of the increase in immunoglobulins.

Immunoglobulins. The serum immunoglobulins can be separated into subtypes. In chronic inflammation, IgG is needed to combine with RF. Thus, in RA the IgG value is typically elevated.

Other Laboratory Tests. The presence of most chronic diseases usually causes mild to moderate anemia, which contributes to the client's fatigue. Therefore, the client's complete blood count (CBC) is monitored for a low hemoglobin, hematocrit, and red blood cell (RBC) count. An increase in white blood cell (WBC) count is consistent with an inflammatory response. A decrease in the WBC count may indicate Felty's syndrome. Thrombocytosis (increased platelets) is common in clients with RA. Additional laboratory tests may be performed, depending on the body systems and organs that may be affected by the disease. For example, if heart involvement is suspected, the health care provider may order cardiac enzymes.

➤ *Radiographic Assessment*

The standard x-ray is used to visualize the joint changes and deformities that are typical of RA. The computed tomography (CT) scan may help to determine the presence and degree of cervical spine involvement.

➤ *Other Diagnostic Assessment*

An *arthrocentesis* is a diagnostic procedure that may be used for clients with joint involvement. It may be done at the bedside or in a physician's office or clinic. After administering a local anesthetic, the physician inserts a large-gauge needle into the joint, usually the knee, to aspirate a sample of synovial fluid, which may also relieve pressure. The fluid is analyzed by use of tests described in Chart 24–8. After the procedure, the nurse monitors the insertion site for bleeding or leakage of synovial fluid. If either of these problems occur, the nurse notifies the physician.

A bone scan or joint scan can also assess the extent of joint involvement. Magnetic resonance imaging (MRI) may be performed to assess spinal column disease.

Because RA can affect multiple body systems, tests to diagnose specific systemic manifestations are performed as necessary. For example, electromyography helps to confirm peripheral neuropathy. Pulmonary function tests help to determine the presence of lung involvement.

 Interventions

As in other types of arthritis, the health care team manages pain by using a combination of drug and nondrug measures. When these measures are no longer effective, surgery may be indicated. The accompanying Client Care Plan highlights the most important nursing interventions for the client with RA.

Nonsurgical Management. Although numerous pain relief modalities are available, the client with RA often needs a variety of medications to relieve pain or slow the progression of the disease.

Drug Therapy. Medications that are prescribed for clients with RA have analgesic, antipyretic, and/or anti-inflammatory actions.

Client Care Plan

The Client with Rheumatoid Arthritis

Nursing Diagnosis No. 1: Chronic Pain related to joint inflammation

Expected Outcomes	Nursing Interventions	Rationale
The client will experience a reduction in joint pain.	■ Give prescribed drugs, as ordered, on time.	■ Giving drugs on time ensures a consistent blood level (e.g., salicylates).
	■ Give analgesic drugs as needed, if ordered, and periods of rest, especially after periods of increased activity (e.g., physical therapy).	■ Supplemental analgesics may be needed to control chronic pain; rest is necessary to prevent overuse of joints and help decreased inflammation.
	■ Provide a warm shower, tub bath, and/or hot compresses after periods of decreased activity or rest.	■ Heat application increases blood flow to the joints to decrease pain and increase joint mobility.
	■ Provide nonpharmacologic pain relief measures, such as imagery, massage, and music therapy. (Determine which of these measures are effective for each client.)	■ Independent nursing interventions help reduce pain and decrease the amount of analgesics needed for pain relief.
	■ Evaluate the effectiveness of all pain relief interventions and document/communicate the outcome to the physician and other involved health care team members. (Also see Chapter 9 for additional interventions and pain assessment tools.)	■ Evaluation of the effectiveness of pain relief interventions helps the health care team plan care for the client. Changes may be necessary if the plan is not effective in meeting the expected outcome.

Nursing Diagnosis No. 2: Impaired Physical Mobility related to fatigue, inflammation, and pain

Expected Outcomes	Nursing Interventions	Rationale
The client will ambulate independently, with or without ambulatory aids.	■ Reinforce the importance of and techniques for therapeutic joint and muscle exercises as taught by the physical therapist.	■ Therapeutic joint and muscle exercises increase joint mobility, decrease pain, and increase muscle strength.
	■ Teach the importance of recreational exercises, such as walking and swimming.	■ Walking and swimming increase muscle tone and enhance psychological well-being.
	■ Reinforce the importance of and techniques for use of ambulatory aids, such as a cane or walker; allow rest periods during ambulation.	■ Ambulatory aids help reduce stress on affected joints and, therefore, reduce pain and inflammation.
	■ Emphasize the client's abilities and strengths in mobility skills.	■ Focusing on the client's abilities rather than deficits builds the client's self-esteem and confidence.

Client Care Plan

Nursing Diagnosis No. 3: Self-Care Deficit (Partial) related to fatigue, pain, stiffness, and joint deformity

Expected Outcomes	Nursing Interventions	Rationale
The client will independently perform activities of daily living (ADLs) with or without the use of assistive-adaptive devices.	■ In collaboration with the occupational therapist, assess the client's abilities in ADLs.	■ The nurse allows the client to perform all ADLs independently. If the client needs assistance, the nurse plans ways to promote independence in these areas.
	■ Set up the client's try, if needed, by opening packages and cartons and cutting food; assess the need for assistive-adaptive devices.	■ The client may be able to self-feed if the tray is set up and/or if assistive devices, such as plate guard, are obtained.
	■ For dressing activities, assess the need for long-handled assistive-adaptive devices and other mechanical aids.	■ The client may be able to dress independently if assistive-adaptive devices are available.
	■ Encourage the client to use large muscle groups and joints instead of smaller ones, if possible.	■ Using larger joints helps prevent stress and pain in small joints (joint protection).
	■ Emphasize the client's abilities in performing ADLs.	■ Focusing on the client's abilities builds self-esteem and confidence.
	■ Teach the client to allow rest periods during ADLs.	■ Rest reduces fatigue that contributes to a decreased ability to perform ADLs.
	■ Assess the client's pain level, and intervene appropriately (see Nursing Diagnosis No. 1).	■ Pain and stiffness contribute to a decreased ability to perform ADLs.

Salicylates. A common drug of choice is salicylates, a type of nonsteroidal anti-inflammatory drugs (NSAIDs), although the selection of drugs varies by health care provider and geographic area. As seen in Chart 24–1, any one of several agents may be used. Large doses of aspirin (ASA, Ancasal✱) may be prescribed unless gastrointestinal distress (nausea, vomiting, or ulcers) occurs or the client has a history of one or more of these symptoms.

The initial dosage of aspirin is typically 12 to 18 tablets each day in divided doses (usually four times a day) until a therapeutic serum salicylate level of 20 to 25 mg/100 mL (25 mg/dL) is achieved, usually in 3 to 6 weeks. The health care provider regulates the dosage so that side effects are minimized and the serum level is less than 30 mg/100 mL. A level higher that this often results in signs of toxicity, such as tinnitus. The nurse asks the client whether he or she has experienced this symptom. If so, the health care provider usually reduces the daily dosage of the drug. Once the client's pain and other clinical manifestations are alleviated or reduced, the dosage can be adjusted to a maintenance level, which usually falls between 15 and 20 mg/100 mL (not > 1.45 mmol/L).

Nonsteroidal Anti-Inflammatory Drugs. These are often the drug of choice for inflammatory arthritis. The choice of which drug to administer depends on the client's needs and the physician's preference. To minimize gastrointestinal problems, the NSAID may be given with misoprostol (Cytotec), 100 to 200 μg/day. If after 6 weeks or so there is no clinical change, the health care provider may discontinue the NSAID, and another NSAID may be tried instead. This process may be repeated until the appropriate drug is found to be effective for that client.

ELDERLY CONSIDERATIONS

Adverse effects of NSAIDs include gastrointestinal distress and central nervous system changes, especially in the elderly. Many of these agents also cause retention of sodium and water, which poses a life-threatening risk to clients with hypertension, renal disease, or congestive heart failure. Elderly clients are especially vulnerable to these problems. The nurse carefully monitors these clients and reports problems as early as possible to the health care provider.

Gold Salts. When pain and inflammation are not reduced by NSAIDs, gold therapy may be added to the drug regimen as a second-line drug. Unlike the former drugs, gold can induce disease remission as well as reduce pain and inflammation. The most commonly used parenteral preparation is gold sodium thiomalate (Myochrysine). After a small test dose of 10 mg intramuscularly to detect an allergy to the drug, weekly gold injections are given. The dosage increases from 25–50 mg/week until improvement is evident or until a cumulative total of 1000 mg is administered.

If the client responds to gold without having toxic effects, such as rash, blood dyscrasias, or renal involvement, the injections are slowly tapered to every 2 weeks, then every 3 weeks, and then once a month. Before each drug administration, the client's urine is tested for protein level and a complete blood count is taken. If remission does not occur after a total of 1000 mg has been given, the drug is usually discontinued.

Because intramuscular administration of gold preparations is painful, auranofin (Ridaura), an oral gold product, is used more commonly. The client must take this drug daily to achieve a therapeutic serum level. Its major side effect is gastrointestinal symptoms, especially diarrhea, nausea, and vomiting. The nurse teaches the client to report any gastrointestinal problems to the health care provider.

Other Remittive Agents. Other remittive agents may be prescribed, such as the antimalarial drug hydroxychloroquine (Plaquenil) and penicillamine (Cuprimine). These drugs are not used as often as gold in rheumatoid disease because they produce numerous side effects and toxic effects and are often not as effective. The health care provider recommends that clients receiving hydroxychloroquine have an eye examination every 3–6 months to detect changes in vision, because retinal toxicity may occur. Retinal toxicity results in decreased visual acuity. If this complication occurs, the physician discontinues the drug. The side and toxic effects of penicillamine are similar to those of gold.

Cytotoxic Drugs. Methotrexate (MTX) in a low once-a-week dosage, has become the mainstay of therapy for advancing and sustaining RA because it is inexpensive, less toxic than other cytotoxic drugs, and effective. Because any cytotoxic drug can cause *Pneumocystis carinii* pneumonia, some rheumatologists advocate giving pentamidine to clients receiving MTX (Harris, 1997).

The nurse observes for the side and toxic effects of MTX, which include mouth sores, acute dyspnea from pneumonitis, chronic liver inflammation, and bone marrow suppression.

Other cytotoxic agents that may be used are azathioprine (Imuran) and cyclophosphamide (Cytoxan, Procytox✤). In addition to these adverse drug effects, lymphoma and bone marrow suppression may occur with

azathioprine administration. Cyclophosphamide (Cytoxan, Procytox✤) is sometimes given to control RA vasculitis; however, this drug may cause leukemia or other types of malignancy.

Chronic Steroid Therapy. For clients who do not experience relief of symptoms from the commonly administered medications, steroids, usually prednisone (Deltasone, Winpred✤, Apo-Prednisone✤), are given for their anti-inflammatory and immunosuppressive effects. Prednisone may also be used short term as bridge therapy when NSAIDs are insufficient and other second-line drugs (remittive agents) have not yet had an effect.

Unfortunately, chronic steroid therapy can result in devastating complications, such as diabetes mellitus, infection, fluid and electrolyte imbalances, hypertension, osteoporosis, and glaucoma. As shown in Chart 24–1, some drug effects are dose related, whereas others are not. The nurse observes the client for complications associated with chronic steroid therapy and reports them to the health care provider. For example, if the client's blood pressure becomes elevated or significant laboratory values change, the nurse notifies the physician.

Analgesic Drugs. Other analgesic drugs may be prescribed to supplement the anti-inflammatory drugs that are specific for RA. Some analgesics include acetaminophen (Tylenol, Exdol✤), propoxyphene (Darvon, Novopropoxyn✤), and propoxyphene napsylate (Darvocet-N). Propoxyphene and its associated products can cause headache, dizziness, and drowsiness. Over a long period, in clients with decreased metabolic rates, this slow-excreting drug may accumulate in the body and may cause death. The nurse teaches the client about the side and toxic effects of these drugs and advises the client to report any unusual symptom or complaint to the physician.

Rest, Positioning, Ice, and Heat. Adequate rest, proper positioning, and ice and heat application are important in pain management (see Chronic Pain in the discussion of degenerative joint disease). If acute inflammation is present, the physical therapist (PT) or assistive nursing personnel applies ice to the "hot" joints for pain relief until the inflammation lessens. The ice pack should not be too heavy.

To relieve morning stiffness or the pain of late-stage disease, the nurse recommends a hot shower for the client rather than a sponge bath or a tub bath. It is often difficult for the client with RA to get into and out of the bathtub, although special hydraulic lifts and tub chairs may be available. Hot packs applied directly to involved joints are also beneficial. Most physical therapy departments have hydrocollators that keep hot packs ready any time they are needed (Fig. 24–7).

Complementary Therapies. As in any client with arthritis, other nonpharmacologic pain relief techniques are available. For example, some clients may achieve relief with transcutaneous electrical nerve stimulation (TENS), hypnosis, acupuncture, imagery, or music therapy. Stress management is also becoming more popular as a pain relief intervention. Chapters 8 and 9 describe these interventions in detail.

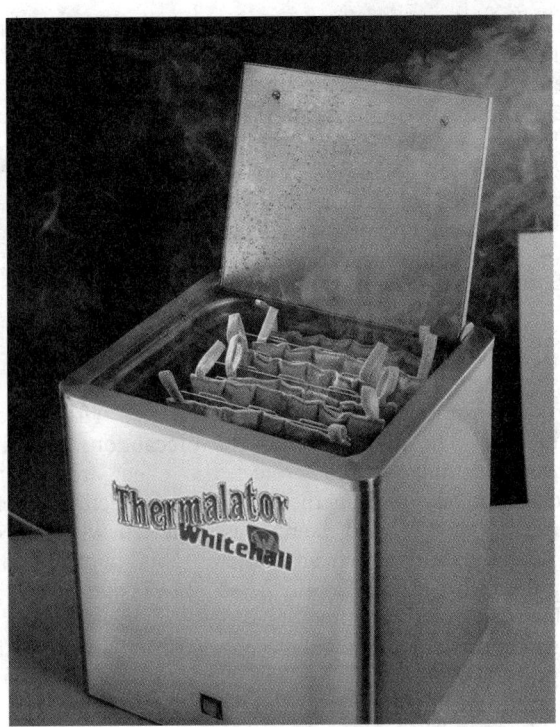

Figure 24–7. Heating units used for keeping hot packs warm. (Courtesy of Whitehall Manufacturing, City of Industry, CA.)

Experimental Therapies. In addition to the drug regimens described earlier, two techniques—pulse therapy and plasmapheresis—are being tried and evaluated to treat severe RA. In pulse therapy, the client receives rapid infusions of high-dose steroids or chemotherapeutic agents, usually over a period of several days. Plasmapheresis is a procedure in which the client's plasma is treated to remove the antibodies that are causing the disease. Sometimes called a plasma exchange, this procedure may be combined with pulse therapy for clients with severe life-threatening disease.

Promotion of Self-Care. Although the physical appearance of a client with severe RA may lead the nurse to believe that independence in ADLs is not possible, the client can use a number of alternative methods to perform these activities. The nurse should not automatically perform activities for the client; clients with RA do not want to be dependent. For example, hand deformities frequently prevent a client from opening packages of food, such as a box of crackers. The client may prefer to use his or her teeth to open the crackers rather than depend on someone else.

In the hospital or long-term care facility, a client may not eat because of the barriers of heavy plate covers, milk in cartons, small packages of condiments, and heavy containers. Styrofoam or paper cups may bend and collapse as the client attempts to hold them. A china or heavy plastic cup with handles may be easier to manipulate. The nurse and client collaborate with the dietitian to allow the client access to food and total independence in eating activity.

When fine motor activities (such as squeezing a tube of toothpaste) become impossible, larger joints or body surfaces can substitute for smaller ones. In this case, the nurse teaches the client to use the palm of the hand to press the paste onto the brush. Devices such as long-handled brushes can allow clients to brush their hair; dressing sticks can facilitate putting on pants. These examples illustrate the need for the nurse to assess the problem area, suggest alternative methods, and refer the client to an occupational or physical therapist for special assistive and adaptive devices if necessary.

Management of Fatigue. Nursing interventions depend, in part, on identifying the factors contributing to fatigue. For example, in a classic nursing study, Crosby (1991) found that increases in pain, sleep disturbance, and weakness were positively associated with increased fatigue. Anemia may also be a contributing factor and may be treated with iron (if an iron deficiency anemia is present), folic acid, or vitamin supplements, prescribed by the health care provider. Chronic normochromic or chronic hypochromic anemia frequently occurs in most chronic, systemic diseases. The nurse also assesses for drug-related blood loss, such as that caused by salicylate therapy or other NSAIDs, by checking the stool for gross or occult blood. Elderly Caucasian women are the most likely clients to experience gastrointestinal bleeding from these medications.

When a client's fatigue results from muscle atrophy, the physician prescribes an aggressive physical therapy program to strengthen muscles and to prevent further atrophy. Clients experience increased fatigue when pain prevents them from getting adequate rest and sleep. Measures to facilitate sleep include promoting a quiet environment, giving warm beverages, and administering hypnotics or relaxants as prescribed, if necessary. Pain relief measures have been discussed.

In addition to identifying and managing specific reasons for fatigue, the nurse assesses the client's daily activities and teaches principles of energy conservation, including

- Pacing activities
- Allowing rest periods
- Setting priorities
- Obtaining assistance when needed

Chart 24–9 lists specific suggestions for conserving the client's energy and thus increasing activity tolerance.

Enhancement of Body Image. A client's body image may be affected by the disease process and drug therapy as well. Steroids, for instance, can cause a moon-faced appearance, acne, striae, "buffalo humps," and weight gain. The nurse determines the client's perception of these changes and the impact of family and significant others' reactions to them. The most important intervention for the nurse is communicating acceptance of the client. When a trusting relationship is established, the nurse encourages the client to express his or her feelings.

Another way to improve body image while the client is in the hospital or nursing home is the use of personal items. The client's use of a hospital gown reinforces the sick role. The nurse encourages clients to wear their own

---

Chart 24–9

Education Guide: Energy Conservation for the Client with Arthritis

- Balance activity with rest. Take one or two naps each day.
- Pace yourself; do not plan too much for one day.
- Set priorities. Determine which activities are most important, and do them first.
- Delegate responsibility and tasks to your family and friends.
- Plan ahead to prevent last-minute rushing and stress.
- Learn your own activity tolerance and do not exceed it.

---

clothes, to brush their hair, and to use make-up if desired. The nurse assists in making the client as presentable as possible. The use of colored bows for hair, nail polish, and perfume may improve the female client's image and self-concept. Chapter 10 identifies additional strategies for care of a client with an altered body image.

As a reaction to body image disturbance and the presence of a chronic, painful disease, clients may display behaviors indicative of loss. They may use coping strategies ranging from denial or fear to anger or depression. In an attempt to regain control over the effects of the disease process, clients may appear to be manipulative and demanding and may sometimes be referred to as having an "arthritis personality." This personality, which has negative connotations, is a myth. Clients are trying to cope with the effects of their illness and should be treated with patience and understanding. The nurse continually assesses and accepts these behaviors but remains realistic in discussing goals to improve self-esteem. Clients' strengths are emphasized, and previously successful coping strategies are identified.

Nurses need to assess and intervene appropriately for clients who experience pain and suffering. A qualitative nursing study by Dildy (1996) found that clients with RA benefit from nurses who are empathetic, gentle, caring, and cheerful. Additionally, clients want nurses to decrease their suffering and provide comfort (Research Applications for Nursing).

 Continuing Care

Clients with RA are usually managed at home but may be institutionalized in a long-term care setting if they become restricted to bed or a wheelchair. Some clients may be discharged to a rehabilitation facility for several weeks to aid in developing strategies, techniques, and skills for independent living at home.

➤ Home Care Management

The amount of home care preparation depends on the severity of the disease. Structural changes may be necessary if there are deficits in ADLs or mobility. Doors must

be wide enough to accommodate a wheelchair or a walker if one is used. Ramps are needed to prevent the client in a wheelchair from being homebound. If the client cannot negotiate stairs, the client must have access to facilities for all ADLs on one floor.

To promote continued homemaking functions, structural changes of countertops and appliances may be needed. The client may also require hand rails and elevated chairs and toilet seats, which facilitate transfers (Fig. 24–8).

➤ Health Teaching

Health teaching is the most important nursing intervention for promoting the client's compliance with a treatment plan. The nurse should take precautions regarding myths and quackery to protect the client from harm. Information about drug therapy, joint protection, energy conservation, rest, and exercise is reviewed with the client, family, and significant others. This information is summarized in Charts 24–1, 24–5, 24–7, and 24–9.

The client with rheumatoid disease often complains of being on an "emotional roller coaster" from coping with a chronic illness every day of life. Control over one's life is an important human need. The client with an unpredictable chronic disease may lose this control, which lowers self-esteem. Health providers must allow the client to make decisions about care. Families and significant others must also include the client in decision making. Although the client's behavior may be perceived as demanding or manipulative, the client's self-esteem cannot be improved

---

▷ Research Applications for Nursing

Nurses Can Have an Impact on Client Suffering

Dildy, S. P. (1996). Suffering in people with rheumatoid arthritis. Applied Nursing Research, 9, 177–183.

This qualitative study attempted to describe the concept of suffering in clients with rheumatoid arthritis (RA). Fourteen people with RA were interviewed; all were Caucasian and well educated. Some clients were in remission, whereas others had active disease. The clients described the changes in their lives as a result of RA and the impact of their suffering. They also shared anecdotes regarding their experiences with nurses and other health care professionals. The general feeling was that nurses need to show empathy, be caring and gentle, and provide comfort, including the administration of medications as needed.

Critique. The study sample was small, and the group was homogeneous. However, the advantage of the interview technique for a qualitative study may outweigh this limitation. An enormous amount of information was collected and analyzed, which provides insight into the life of people with RA.

Possible Nursing Implications. The implications identified by the study were that nurses and other health care professionals need to be more empathetic when caring for clients with RA. Providing comfort is also a major nursing intervention, including touch, receptivity, and gentleness.

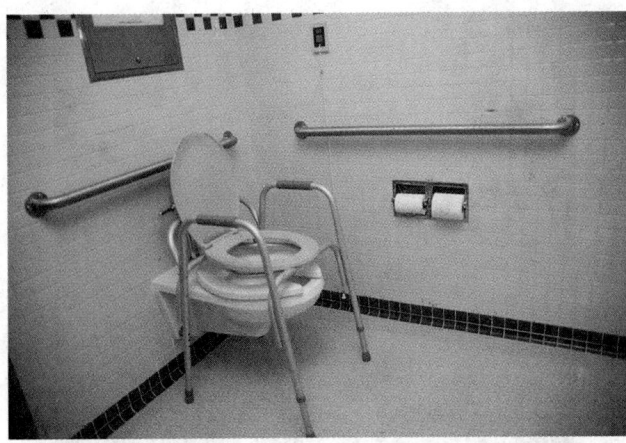

Figure 24–8. Handrails and an elevated toilet seat make transfers easier for the client.

without this important aspect of interpersonal relationships.

Increased dependency also affects the client's sense of control and self-esteem. Some clients ignore their health needs and portray a tough image for others by insisting that they need no assistance. The nurse emphasizes to the client and family that asking for help may be the best decision at times to prevent further joint damage and disease progression.

Social and work roles are dramatically affected by RA. The client may find new friends among others who have the same problem to be a support system to cope with these changes. Becoming an active member of and volunteering for The Arthritis Foundation can help the client to meet social and work needs. Loss of income from being unable to be gainfully employed can also be a major source of stress. The client may qualify for disability benefits through the federal Social Security program. If possible, the client can learn new skills for a less stressful career.

In addition to the interventions just described for self-esteem disturbance, the nurse may need to refer the client to a counselor or to a religious or spiritual leader for emotional support and guidance during times of crisis. The nurse should identify and recommend other support systems within the family and community when necessary.

➤ Health Care Resources

The need for health care resources for the client with RA is similar to that for the client with degenerative joint disease. A home health nurse or aide, physical therapist, or occupational therapist may be indicated. In collaboration with the discharge planner, the nurse in the hospital or nursing home identifies these resources and makes sure that they are available before the client is discharged.

 Evaluation

The nurse evaluates the care provided for the client with RA. The desired outcomes are that the client

- States that pain and stiffness are reduced after intervention
- Ambulates without personal assistance (may use an ambulatory aid such as a walker)
- Is independent in all ADLs (may use assistive-adaptive devices)
- States that fatigue is decreased
- Participates in daily activities at his or her own pace
- Demonstrates a positive self-esteem as evidenced by participation in daily activities and decision making

LUPUS ERYTHEMATOSUS

Overview

The word lupus is the Latin term for "wolf." In the mid-19th century, the facial rash that was seen in clients with the disease was thought to look like bites caused by a wolf. The rash was usually red, and thus the term *erythematosus*, a Latin word meaning reddened, was added to describe the disease.

There are two main classifications of lupus: discoid lupus erythematosus (DLE) and systemic lupus erythematosus (SLE). A small percentage of clients with lupus have the DLE type, which affects only the skin.

The systemic disorder is a chronic, progressive, inflammatory connective tissue disorder that can cause major body organs and systems to fail. It is characterized by spontaneous remissions and exacerbations, and the onset may be acute or insidious. The condition is potentially fatal, although the survival rate has dramatically improved over the past 20 years. Today more than 85% of clients with systemic lupus are alive 5 years after diagnosis (Hahn, 1997). Improvements in determining the cause, diagnosis, and treatment of lupus account for the prolonged survival of these clients.

Lupus is thought to be an autoimmune process; that is, abnormal antibodies are produced that react with the client's tissues. These antinuclear antibodies (ANAs) primarily affect the deoxyribonucleic acid (DNA) within the cell nuclei. As a result, immune complexes form in the serum and organ tissues, which causes inflammation and damage. The complexes invade organs directly or cause vasculitis (vessel inflammation), which deprives the organs of arterial blood and oxygen.

Many clients with SLE have some degree of kidney involvement, the leading cause of death. Other causes of death from SLE are cardiac and central nervous system involvement.

In kidney disease, renal biopsies show progressive changes within the glomeruli:

- In minimal lupus nephritis, the glomeruli are slightly irregular; immunoglobulins and complement are seen by electron microscopy.
- Focal, or mild, lupus nephritis is characterized by further glomerular changes, and immune complex deposits are common. In this type of lupus, the client begins to show clinical signs of renal impairment.
- In diffuse, severe proliferative nephritis, more than 50% of the glomeruli are affected, and the client is in renal failure.

Lupus affects women between the ages of 15 and 40 years at a rate 8–10 times more often than men. The onset of the disease is most often during the childbearing years, but it has been reported in young children and the elderly.

TRANSCULTURAL CONSIDERATIONS

 Although incidence and prevalence data vary, about 1 in 700 women between the ages of 15 and 64 years have the disease; 1 in 250 African-American women of this age group are affected.

Collaborative Management

 Assessment

It is impossible to describe a typical textbook picture of a client with lupus because of the extreme variability of symptoms among affected clients. When the disease is in remission, the client may appear healthy with no activity limitations. When the disease flares, the client may be so ill that admission to a critical care unit is required. Chart 24–10 highlights the clinical manifestations that occur in clients with systemic lupus.

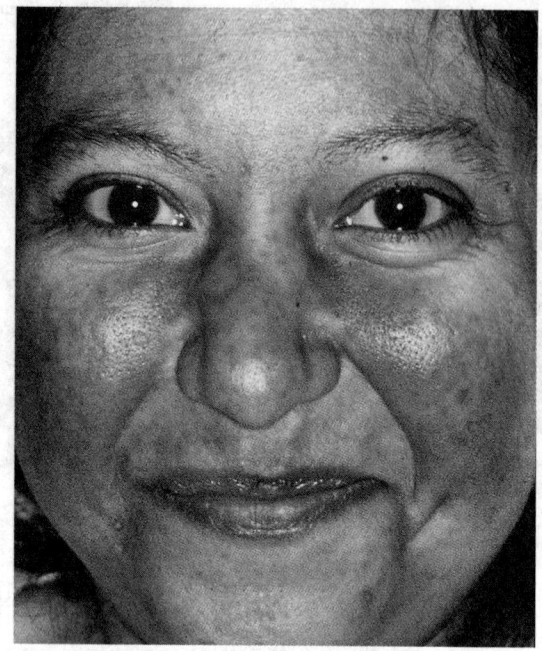

Figure 24–9. The characteristic "butterfly" rash of SLE.

Chart 24–10

Key Features of Systemic Lupus Erythematosus (SLE) and Progressive Systemic Sclerosis (PSS)

SLE	PSS
Skin Manifestations	
• Inflamed, red rash	• Inflamed
• Discoid lesions	• Fibrotic
	• Sclerotic
	• Edematous
Renal Manifestations	
• Nephritis	• Renal failure
Cardiovascular Manifestations	
• Pericarditis	• Myocardial fibrosis
• Raynaud's phenomenon	• Raynaud's phenomenon
Pulmonary Manifestations	
• Pleural effusions	• Interstitial fibrosis
Neurologic Manifestations	
• CNS lupus	• Not common
Gastrointestinal Manifestations	
• Abdominal pain	• Esophagitis
	• Ulcers
Musculoskeletal Manifestations	
• Joint inflammation	• Joint inflammation
• Myositis	• Myositis
Other Manifestations	
• Fever	• Fever
• Fatigue	• Fatigue
• Anorexia	• Anorexia
• Vasculitis	• Vasculitis

CNS = central nervous system.

➤ *Physical Assessment/Clinical Manifestations*

Skin Involvement. The major and usually only manifestation of discoid lupus is a dry, scaly, raised rash appearing on the face ("butterfly" rash) or upper body or individual round lesions, sometimes referred to as discoid (coin-like) lesions (Fig. 24–9). The nurse observes all skin changes and monitors changes daily while the client is in an acute care setting.

Musculoskeletal Changes. In addition to skin changes, articular involvement occurs in most clients with systemic lupus erythematosus (SLE). The initial joint changes are similar to those seen in rheumatoid arthritis (RA), but severe deformities are not common. Avascular necrosis (bone necrosis from lack of oxygen) is often seen in clients with SLE who have been treated for at least 5 years, usually with steroids. Chronic steroid therapy may cause constriction of small blood vessels supplying the joint causing the tissue to die. The hip is most commonly affected, and the client complains of pain and decreased mobility as a result.

The nurse observes for muscle atrophy, which can result from disuse or from skeletal muscle invasion by the immune complexes (myositis). Myalgia (muscle pain) may also occur. The nurse inspects and palpates major muscles, especially those in the extremities.

Systemic Manifestations. Because SLE is an inflammatory condition, fever is a common finding. The presence of fever is the classic sign of a flare, or exacerbation. Various degrees of generalized weakness, fatigue, anorexia, and weight loss occur. These signs may be the only evidence of impending disease, which makes diagnosis by the health care provider difficult. Consequently, some clients have a diagnosis of "probable SLE."

Any or all body systems may be affected by SLE. Because lupus nephritis is the leading cause of death, the nurse carefully assesses for signs of renal involvement (e.g., changes in urinary output, proteinuria, hematuria, and fluid retention). About 50% of clients with systemic lupus have some type of nephritis.

Pleural effusions are found in almost half of clients with SLE, but this complication is usually not life threatening. Pulmonary restrictive or obstructive changes may not result in overt clinical signs. However, progressive involvement can lead to dyspnea and arterial blood gas abnormalities. The nurse performs a complete respiratory assessment to determine any abnormalities in respiratory pattern or breath sounds.

Pericarditis is the most common cardiovascular manifestation and causes tachycardia, chest pain, and myocardial ischemia. The nurse monitors the client's vital signs at least every 4 hours while the client is in the hospital and reports chest pain immediately to the physician.

Raynaud's phenomenon is noted in 15% of clients with lupus. On exposure to cold or extreme stress, the client complains of the characteristic red, white, and blue color changes and severe pain in the digits caused by arteriolar vasospasm. The nurse may not observe these episodes but should ask clients whether color changes occur when their hands or feet are exposed to cold or when these clients are extremely stressed.

Neurologic manifestations are varied. Central nervous system effects include psychoses, paresis, seizures, migraine headaches, and cranial nerve palsies. Peripheral neuropathies are also common. The nurse performs a neurologic assessment as described in Chapter 43.

The nurse also monitors for reports of abdominal pain. Recurrent abdominal pain occurs frequently, but its cause may not be identified. Mesenteric arteritis, pancreatitis from arteritis of the pancreatic artery, and colonic ulcers can cause abdominal pain in the client with lupus. The nurse may note liver enlargement on assessment of the abdomen, but jaundice is rare. More than 50% of clients have lymph enlargement, and 10% have splenomegaly. The nurse palpates lymph nodes and documents findings.

➤ Psychosocial Assessment

The psychosocial results from lupus can be devastating. In either discoid or systemic disease, the rash can be disfiguring and embarrassing to the client. Young adult women who never had a blemish are confronted with a rash that cannot be completely covered with make-up. If chronic steroid therapy is used, side effects such as acne, striae, fat pads, and weight gain intensify the problem of an already altered body image.

Chronic fatigue and generalized weakness may prevent the client from being as active as in the past. The client may avoid social gatherings and may withdraw from family activities. The unpredictability and chronicity of SLE can cause fear and anxiety. Fear may heighten if the client knows another person with the disease, particularly if the other person has more advanced, severe disease. The myth that lupus is always a fatal condition is still common.

The nurse assesses the client's feelings about the illness to identify areas that require intervention. The nurse should assess the person's usual coping mechanisms and support systems before developing a plan of care.

(For additional information about psychosocial assessment of clients with chronic illness, see Rheumatoid Arthritis in this chapter.)

➤ Laboratory Assessment

Because discoid lupus is not a systemic condition, the only test that is significant is a skin biopsy. The physician gently scrapes skin cells from the rash for microscopic evaluation. The characteristic lupus cell and a number of inflammatory cells confirm the diagnosis.

The immunologic-based laboratory tests that are used to diagnose systemic lupus are the same as those performed for rheumatoid arthritis (RA): rheumatoid factor, antinuclear antibody, erythrocyte sedimentation rate, serum protein electrophoresis, serum complement, and immunoglobulins. The lupus cell preparation (LE cell prep) may also be performed, but this assay is a poor indicator of disease; rather, the test is best used for screening. (See the corresponding section under Rheumatoid Arthritis as well as Chart 24–8.)

In addition to immunologic testing, several tests are performed to evaluate possible involvement of major organs and body systems. A complete blood count (CBC) commonly shows pancytopenia (a decrease of all cell types), probably caused by direct attack of the blood cells or bone marrow by immune complexes. Serum electrolyte levels, renal function, cardiac and liver enzymes, and clotting factors are also routinely assessed to determine other body system functioning.

Interventions

The health care provider often prescribes potent drugs that are used topically and systemically. In addition, the client takes precautions to prevent further skin impairment and exacerbations (flare-ups) of the disease. Many of the skin lesions do not disappear, even with treatment, but they usually fade when the disease is in remission.

Drug Therapy. In discoid lupus, the client's major concern is the rash or discoid lesions. Clients with systemic lupus may also have concern about skin changes. Topical cortisone preparations help reduce inflammation and promote fading of the skin lesions. In addition, the health care provider may prescribe the antimalarial hydroxychloroquine (Plaquenil) for some clients to decrease the inflammatory response, but other systemic medications are usually not used (see Chart 24–1).

For clients with systemic lupus, the aim of management is to treat the disease aggressively until remission. In addition to medications for skin lesions, the health care provider often prescribes chronic steroid therapy to treat the systemic disease process. For clients with renal or central nervous system lupus, the health care provider may also order immunosuppressive agents, which are sometimes used for clients with rheumatoid arthritis (see Chart 24–1). Although clinical manifestations improve during remission, maintenance doses of these drugs are usually continued to prevent further exacerbations of disease. The nurse observes for side and toxic effects of these medications and reports their occurrence to the physician.

Skin Protection. Clients with lupus should avoid prolonged exposure to sunlight and other forms of ultraviolet lighting, including certain types of fluorescent light. The nurse instructs clients that, when outdoors, they may need to wear long sleeves and a large-brimmed hat. They should use sun-blocking agents with an SPF (sun protection factor) of 30 or higher on exposed skin surfaces.

In addition, the nurse teaches the client to clean the skin with mild soap (such as Ivory) and to avoid harsh, perfumed substances. The client rinses and dries the skin well and applies lotion. Excess powder and other drying substances are avoided. The client carefully selects cosmetics and should include moisturizers and sun protectors. The nurse may refer the client to a medical cosmetologist who specializes in applying make-up for clients with skin lesions of all types.

The client's hair should receive special attention because alopecia (hair loss) is common. The nurse recommends mild protein shampoos and avoidance of harsh treatments, such as permanents or frostings, until the hair regrows during remission.

 Continuing Care

Continuing care for the client with lupus is similar to that for rheumatoid arthritis. The client is generally managed at home but may need repeated hospitalizations during exacerbations of disease. Usually, however, the client does not need rehabilitation or a long-term care facility, because severe joint deformity and prolonged immobility are not common.

Two major differences exist between SLE and rheumatoid arthritis in terms of education of the client and family or significant others. First, the nurse teaches the client with SLE how to protect the skin (Chart 24–11).

Chart 24–11

Education Guide: Skin Protection and Care for Clients with Lupus Erythematosus

- Cleanse your skin with a mild soap like Ivory.
- Dry your skin thoroughly by patting rather than rubbing.
- Apply lotion liberally to dry skin areas.
- Avoid powder and other drying agents, such as rubbing alcohol.
- Use cosmetics that contain moisturizers.
- Avoid direct sunlight and any other type of ultraviolet lighting (including tanning beds).
- Wear a large-brimmed hat, long sleeves, and long pants when in the sun.
- Use a sun-blocking agent with a sun protection factor (SPF) of at least 30.
- Inspect your skin daily for open areas and rashes.

Second, body temperature is monitored carefully in SLE. Fever is the major sign of an exacerbation, during which the client can become seriously ill. The nurse teaches the client to report any other unusual or new clinical manifestation to the health care provider immediately.

Many clients become frustrated that family members, significant others, and the laypeople do not have a good understanding of lupus. When lupus is in complete remission, the client appears to be healthy. However, an exacerbation can necessitate rapid admission to a critical care unit. This unpredictability disrupts the client's life and can cause fear and anxiety. The nurse helps the client identify coping strategies and support systems that can help the client function in the community.

Although The Arthritis Foundation is a general resource for all clients with connective tissue disease, the Lupus Foundation is a national organization, with chapters in every state, that provides information and assistance for clients with lupus. Local support groups and services are offered without charge to the client.

PROGRESSIVE SYSTEMIC SCLEROSIS

Overview

Progressive systemic sclerosis (PSS), one of a family of diseases, is often referred to as systemic scleroderma. "Scleroderma" means hardening of the skin, which is only one clinical manifestation of PSS. As the name implies, PSS is a systemic disease. It is less common than systemic lupus erythematosus (SLE) but is associated with a higher mortality rate. Chart 24–10 shows a comparison of the clinical manifestations of these two diseases.

Progressive systemic sclerosis is a chronic connective tissue disease that is characterized by inflammation, fibrosis, and sclerosis of the skin and vital organs. The inflammatory process is so similar to that of lupus that clients are often diagnosed as having probable SLE until the disease progresses. The inflamed tissue undergoes fibrotic and then sclerotic changes. The most obvious tissue affected is the skin, but renal involvement is the leading cause of death. Unfortunately, clients with PSS do not respond well to steroids and immunosuppressants that are used for lupus, and the mortality rate is, therefore, higher.

The prognosis seems to be worse when the client presents with a group of manifestations that occur at the same time, the CREST syndrome:

- **C**alcinosis (calcium deposits)
- **R**aynaud's phenomenon
- **E**sophageal dysmotility
- **S**clerodactyly (scleroderma of the digits)
- **T**elangiectasia (spider-like hemangiomas)

The disease tends to progress rapidly, but spontaneous remissions and exacerbations can occur.

Little is known about the cause of PSS, but autoimmunity is suspected. The occurrence of more than one case per family is uncommon, although other connective tissue diseases may be noted in the family history.

Progressive systemic sclerosis has been described in

people of all races and in all geographic areas. Women are affected three to four times more often than men. The onset of the disease is usually between the ages of 30 and 50 years. The incidence is higher in coal miners, who have a high incidence of silicosis, which may be a predisposing or contributing factor to PSS.

Collaborative Management

 ## Assessment

➤ Physical Assessment/Clinical Manifestations

Arthralgia (joint pain) and stiffness are common manifestations that the nurse can elicit during the musculoskeletal examination. The acute inflammation that occurs in people with rheumatoid arthritis (RA) is not common, and deformities are rare.

Findings on inspection of the skin depend on the stage of the scleroderma. Typically, there is a painless, symmetric, pitting edema of the hands and fingers, which may progress to include the entire upper and lower extremities and face. In this edematous phase, the fingers are described as sausage like. The skin is taut, shiny, and free from wrinkles. If diffuse scleroderma occurs, swelling is replaced by tightening, hardening, and thickening of skin tissue; this phase is sometimes called the *indurative phase* (Fig. 24–10). The skin loses its elasticity, and range of motion is markedly decreased; ulcerations may occur. Joint contractures may develop, and the client may be unable to perform ADLs independently.

Major organ damage is likely to develop in clients with diffuse scleroderma, specifically affecting

- The gastrointestinal tract
- The cardiovascular system
- The pulmonary system
- The renal system

Gastrointestinal tract involvement, particularly of the esophagus, is common. The esophagus loses its motility, and dysphagia and esophageal reflux result. A small, slid-

ing hiatal hernia may be present, and swallowing may be difficult. Reflux of gastric contents can cause esophagitis and subsequent ulceration, particularly in the lower two thirds of the esophagus. Intestinal changes are similar to those of the esophagus. Peristalsis is diminished, which causes clinical manifestations similar to a partial bowel obstruction; malabsorption is a frequent complication.

In addition to assessing problems of the digestive tract, the nurse observes for cardiovascular manifestations. Raynaud's phenomenon occurs in various degrees in most clients with progressive systemic sclerosis. On exposure to cold or emotional stress, the small arterioles in the digits of both hands and feet rapidly constrict, which causes decreased blood flow. In severe cases, the client experiences digit necrosis, excruciating pain, and autoamputation of distal digits (the tips of digits fall off spontaneously). (See Chapter 38 for a complete discussion of this disorder.) The nurse notes vasculitic lesions, often around the nail beds (periungual lesions), in many clients. Myocardial fibrosis, another common problem, is evidenced by electrocardiographic (ECG) changes, cardiac dysrhythmias, and chest pain.

Lung involvement in the client with PSS may go undetected until autopsy. Fibrosis of the alveoli and interstitial tissues is present in almost all clients with the disease, but clinical manifestations may not be present.

Renal involvement is an important aspect of the overall disease process and frequently causes malignant hypertension and death. The nurse assesses for signs of impending organ failure, such as changes in urinary output.

➤ Laboratory Assessment

The laboratory findings in a client with PSS are similar to those in a client with systemic lupus. Clinical findings and the client's response to drug therapy help the health care provider differentiate the two diseases. Additional tests ordered for the client depend on which organs seem to be affected. Upper and lower gastrointestinal series are commonly performed because of the frequency of gastrointestinal clinical manifestations.

 ## Interventions

The aim of medical management of PSS is to force the disease into remission and thus slow disease progression. The health care provider uses drug therapy primarily for this purpose, but it is often unsuccessful. Systemic steroids and immunosuppressants are used in large doses and often in combination.

Local skin protective measures can help to maintain the client's skin integrity. The nurse teaches the client to use mild soap and lotions and gentle cleaning techniques. The skin should be inspected daily for further changes or open lesions. Skin ulcers are treated according to their type and location.

In addition to drug therapy to control the overall disease process, specific measures can provide comfort. The client with PSS not only experiences chronic joint pain but also has severe, acute pain during episodes of Raynaud's phenomenon. A bed cradle and footboard keep

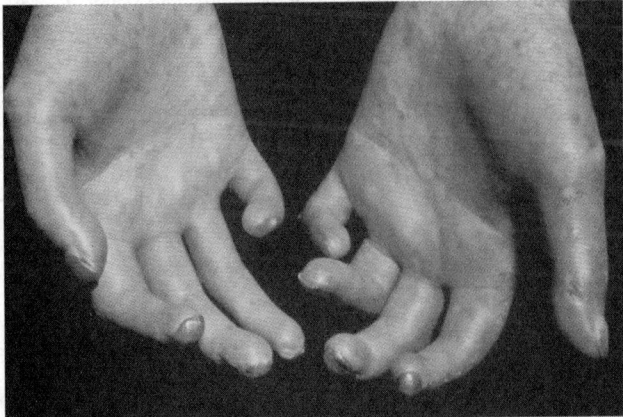

Figure 24–10. Late-stage skin changes seen in clients with progressive systemic sclerosis. (From the Arthritis Teaching Slide Collection, copyright 1980. Used by permission of the Arthritis Foundation.)

> ### Chart 24–12
>
> ### Nursing Care Highlight: The Client with Progressive Systemic Sclerosis and Esophagitis
>
> - Keep the client's head elevated at least 60 degrees during meals and for at least 1 hour after each meal.
> - Provide small, frequent meals rather than three large meals each day.
> - Give the client small amounts of food for each bite, and explain the importance of chewing each bite carefully before swallowing.
> - Provide semisoft foods, such as mashed potatoes and pudding or custard; liquids are most likely to cause choking.
> - Collaborate with the dietitian about the client's diet.
> - Teach the client to avoid foods that increase gastric secretion, for instance, caffeine, pepper, and other spices.
> - Give antacids if the physician prescribes them.

bed covers away from the skin in severe cases. The nurse adjusts the room temperature to prevent chilling, which can precipitate digit vasospasm. The client who can tolerate touching of the affected areas can wear gloves and socks to increase warmth. Because cigarette smoking and extreme emotional stress can also cause recurrence of symptoms, the client should try to avoid or minimize these factors as much as possible.

The client with esophageal involvement may need small, frequent meals rather than the traditional three meals daily. The client should minimize the intake of foods and liquids that stimulate gastric secretion (e.g., spicy foods, caffeine, and alcohol). The nurse instructs the client to keep his or her head elevated for 1–2 hours after meals. The client may need to be in this position continuously. Histamine antagonists and antacids help to reduce and neutralize gastric acid. To help the client avoid choking, the nurse collaborates with the dietitian for dietary changes (Chart 24–12).

Nursing care for the client with joint pain and decreased mobility is very similar to that for the client with rheumatoid arthritis (see Rheumatoid Arthritis earlier).

 Continuing Care

Continuing care for the client with PSS is similar to that for the client with lupus. The client is treated at home but may need frequent hospitalizations if major organ involvement occurs during exacerbations.

GOUT

Overview

Gout, or gouty arthritis, is a systemic disease in which urate crystals deposit in joints and other body tissues, causing inflammation. The cause and treatment of gout have been firmly established. The classic case of well-

advanced disease is seldom seen today unless the client does not comply with the therapeutic regimen. There are two major types of gout: primary and secondary.

Primary gout is the most common type and results from one of several inborn errors of purine metabolism. An end-product of purine metabolism is uric acid, which is usually excreted by the kidneys. In primary gout, uric acid production exceeds the excretion capability of the kidneys, and sodium urate is deposited in synovium and other tissues, which results in inflammation. Primary gout is inherited as an X-linked trait; males are affected through female carriers. About 25% of clients have a family history of gout. Primary gout affects middle-aged and older men (85–90% of clients with gout) and postmenopausal women. The peak time of onset is during a person's 30s and 40s.

Secondary gout involves hyperuricemia (excessive uric acid in the blood) that is caused by another disease. Secondary gout affects people of all ages. Renal insufficiency, diuretic therapy, and certain chemotherapeutic agents decrease the normal excretion of waste products, including uric acid. Disorders such as multiple myeloma and certain carcinomas bring about increased uric acid production because of greater turnover of cellular nucleic acids. Treatment involves management of the underlying disorder.

There are four phases of the primary disease process: asymptomatic hyperuricemic, acute, intercritical (intercurrent), and chronic. The client is usually unaware of the asymptomatic hyperuricemic phase unless he or she has had a serum uric acid level determination. The client's serum level is elevated, but no overt signs of the disease are present.

The first "attack" of gouty arthritis begins the acute phase. The client experiences excruciating pain and inflammation in one or more small joints, usually the metatarsophalangeal joint of the great toe. Of all clients with gout, 75% have inflammation of this joint (podagra) as the initial manifestation.

Months or perhaps years can pass before additional attacks occur; this is the intercritical, or intercurrent, phase of the disease. The client is asymptomatic, and no abnormalities are found on examination of the joints.

After repeated episodes of acute gout, deposits of urate crystals develop under the person's skin and within major organs, particularly in the renal system. The client is then classified as having chronic tophaceous gout. Urate kidney stone formation is more common than renal insufficiency in chronic gout.

Collaborative Management

 Assessment

The historical data that the nurse collects include age, sex, and a family history of gout. Gout affects men, particularly those who have relatives with gout. A complete medical history is needed to determine whether gout has been caused by another problem. In women, especially, there is a tendency to overuse diuretics, which can lead to secondary gout.

Acute Gout. Overt manifestations are present in the acute and chronic phases of gout. The nurse encounters a client with acute gout most often because chronic gout is not common today in the United States. Joint inflammation is the most frequent finding and is usually so painful that the client seeks medical care. The nurse uses inspection skills only; the inflamed area is usually too painful and swollen to be touched or moved.

Chronic Gout. When the client has chronic gout, the nurse inspects the skin for tophi, or deposits of sodium urate crystals (Fig. 24–11). Common sites for tophi are the ear, arms, and fingers near joints. The tophi are hard on palpation and are irregular in shape. When the skin over the tophi is irritated, it may break open, and a yellow, gritty substance is discharged. Infection may result. Although tophi may occur anywhere, they commonly appear on the outer ear.

Other manifestations of chronic gout include signs of renal calculi (stones) or renal dysfunction. Stones develop in about 20% of clients with gout. In some cases, urate kidney stones occur before the arthritis is present.

The health care provider orders determinations of serum uric acid levels to validate hyperuricemia. Because the serum uric acid level can be altered by food intake, serial measurements are usually taken. A consistent level of more than 8 mg/100 mL is generally considered abnormal. Urinary uric acid levels are also measured; an overproduction of uric acid is confirmed by an excretion of more than 600 mg per 24 hours after a 5-day restriction of purine intake.

The health care provider may order renal function tests, such as blood urea nitrogen (BUN) and serum creatinine level, to monitor possible kidney involvement. A definitive diagnostic test for the disease is synovial fluid aspiration (arthrocentesis) to detect the needle-like crystals that are characteristic of the disorder (see Other Diagnostic Assessment under Rheumatoid Arthritis.)

 Interventions

Gout is one of the easiest diseases for the health care provider to diagnose and treat in its early phases. If the client receives treatment and complies with drug therapy, the client should experience no further symptoms and no change in body image or lifestyle. The client with gout is usually treated on an outpatient basis.

Drug Therapy. Drug therapy is the primary component of management for clients with gout. In acute gouty "attacks," the inflammation subsides spontaneously within 3–5 days, but most clients cannot tolerate the pain for that long. The drugs used in acute gout are different from those used in chronic gout. The physician typically prescribes a combination of colchicine (Colsalide, Novocolchicine✤) and a nonsteroidal anti-inflammatory drug, such as indomethacin (Indocin, Novomethacin✤) or ibuprofen (Motrin, Amersol✤), for acute gout. The client takes these medications until the inflammation subsides, usually for 4–7 days, or until severe diarrhea occurs (a side effect of colchicine).

For clients with chronic gout, the health care provider prescribes drugs to promote uric acid excretion or to reduce its production on a continuous, maintenance basis. Allopurinol (Zyloprim) is the drug of choice. As a xanthine oxidase inhibitor, it prevents the conversion of xanthine to uric acid. Probenecid (Benemid, Benuryl✤) is also effective as a uricosuric drug in gout (it promotes excretion of excess uric acid). Combination drugs, such as ColBenemid, that contain probenecid and colchicine are also available. The health care provider and nurse monitor serum uric acid levels to determine the effectiveness of these medications.

Diet Therapy. Whether to recommend special dietary restrictions for clients with gout is controversial. Some physicians advocate a strict low-purine diet, advising the clients to avoid such foods as organ meats, shellfish, and oily fish with bones, such as sardines. Some health care providers and dietitians believe that limiting protein foods, especially red and organ meats, is sufficient. Still others do not believe that diet restrictions affect treatment. It is well known, however, that excessive alcohol intake and fad "starvation" diets can cause a gouty attack. The nurse helps clients determine which foods may precipitate a gout attack.

In addition to food and beverage restrictions, clients with gout should avoid all forms of aspirin and diuretics because they may precipitate an attack. Likewise, excessive physical or emotional stress can exacerbate the dis-

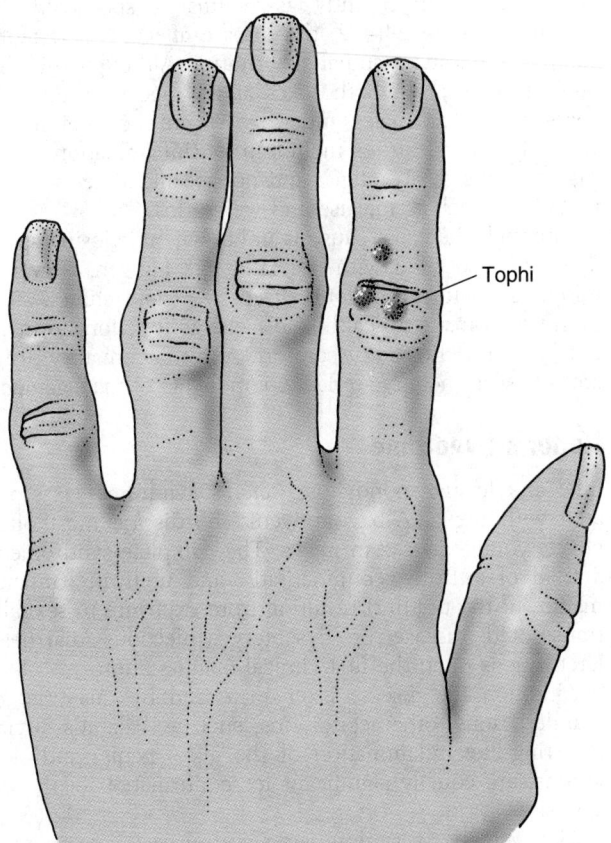

Figure 24–11. Typical appearance of tophi, which may occur in chronic gout, on an index finger.

ease. The nurse may need to teach stress management techniques (see Chap. 8).

Having the client drink more fluids is one of the best measures to prevent urinary stone formation. Such a measure helps to dilute the urine and prevent sediment formation. Uric acid is less likely to form urinary stones in urine that has a high pH because it is more soluble in that environment. The client's urinary pH can be increased by intake of alkaline ash foods, such as citrus fruits and juices, and milk and certain dairy products. However, the value of adhering to a strict diet that is rich in these foods is questionable.

The client with a diagnosis of gout is seldom hospitalized unless renal complications develop. If the client follows the prescribed interventions, chronic tophaceous gout should not develop.

OTHER CONNECTIVE TISSUE DISEASES

The care of clients with connective tissue diseases (CTDs) is often similar regardless of the specific diagnosis. This section describes other fairly common diseases that are classified as CTDs.

Polymyositis/Dermatomyositis

Polymyositis is a diffuse, inflammatory disease of striated muscle that causes symmetric weakness and atrophy. When a rash accompanies polymyositis, the disease is called *dermatomyositis*. Both diseases vary in their mode of onset and progression and are characterized by spontaneous remissions and exacerbations. Women are affected twice as often as men, and 30- to 60-year-olds are most susceptible to either disease.

In addition to proximal muscle and possible skin involvement, clients typically have polyarthritis, polyarthralgia (pain around multiple joints), and Raynaud's phenomenon (see Chap. 38). Clients with dermatomyositis have the characteristic heliotrope (lilac) rash and periorbital edema. Malignant neoplasms occur more frequently in these clients than in the rest of the population; as many as 30% of clients older than 55 have internal malignancies. Many clients have difficulty in swallowing or talking because of severe muscle weakness.

Clients are treated with high-dose steroids, immunosuppressive agents, and supportive care, with particular attention to nutrition.

Systemic Necrotizing Vasculitis

Necrotizing vasculitis is a term for a group of diseases whose primary manifestation is arteritis (inflammation of arterial walls), which causes ischemia in tissues usually supplied by the involved vessels.

Polyarteritis nodosa affects middle-aged men and involves every body system. Treatment is similar to that for clients with systemic lupus, but the prognosis is not as promising. Renal disorders and cardiac involvement are the most frequent causes of death.

Hypersensitivity vasculitis is the most common form of

vasculitis and primarily causes skin lesions as an allergic response to drugs, infections, or tumors.

Takayasu's arteritis, or the aortic arch syndrome, is also called the "pulseless" disease. Women in their 20s, particularly those of Japanese descent, are affected most often. Cerebral ischemia is manifested by visual changes, syncope, and vertigo.

The drug of choice for most types of vasculitis is chronic steroid therapy.

Polymyalgia Rheumatica

Polymyalgia rheumatica (PMR) is a clinical syndrome characterized by stiffness, weakness, and aching of the proximal musculature (i.e., the shoulder and pelvic girdles). Systemic manifestations, such as fever, arthralgias (pain around joints), and weight loss, occur in the majority of cases. The disease commonly occurs in women older than 50 years and typically responds to steroid therapy in 3–5 days.

Giant cell (temporal) arteritis is frequently associated with PMR. The branches of the aorta are vasculitic, which causes headaches and changes in vision. This disorder is easy to miss because most clients with PMR are elderly women who complain of declining vision (also an age-related change). Corticosteroids are highly effective in controlling giant cell arteritis.

Ankylosing Spondylitis

Ankylosing spondylitis is also known as Marie-Strümpell disease and, more recently, as rheumatoid spondylitis. As shown in Figure 24–12, the disease affects the vertebral column and causes spinal deformities. Although this disorder is present in both sexes at any age in adulthood, young Caucasian males under age 40 are most commonly affected. Other features include iritis (inflammation of the iris), arthritis or arthralgia, and nonspecific systemic manifestations, such as malaise and weight loss.

Although the exact cause is unknown, ankylosing spondylitis is associated with the HLA-B27 antigen. Compromised respiratory function caused by a rigid chest wall is the major threat to health. Most clients function normally but live with chronic discomfort. Anti-inflammatory drugs and physical therapy are key components of management.

Reiter's Syndrome

Like ankylosing spondylitis, Reiter's syndrome is associated with the HLA-B27 antigen. The disease most often affects young Caucasian males. The complete syndrome is a triad of arthritis, conjunctivitis, and urethritis (inflammation of the urethra) resulting from exposure to sexually transmitted disease or dysentery (infectious diarrhea). Urethritis is often the first clinical manifestation.

Although the disease is characterized by this triad of manifestations, other conditions, such as balanitis circinata (ring-like inflammation of the glans penis) and skin lesions, are equally significant for confirmation of the diagnosis.

Management is symptomatic and may be complex if there is organ involvement. Nonsteroidal anti-inflammatory drugs and physical therapy are generally prescribed.

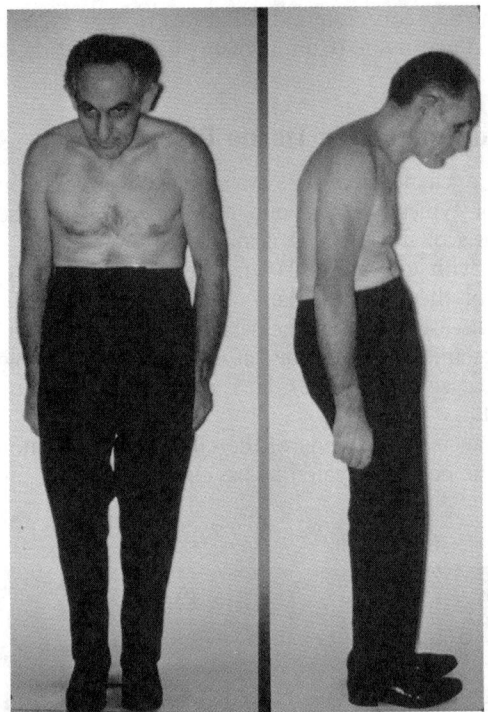

Figure 24–12. Spinal deformity and posture that are often seen in clients with advanced spondylitis. (From the Arthritis Teaching Slide Collection, copyright 1980. Used by permission of the Arthritis Foundation.)

Sjögren's Syndrome

In clients with Sjögren's syndrome, inflammatory cells and immune complexes obstruct secretory ducts and glands. As a result, the client has dry eyes (sicca syndrome), dry mouth (xerostomia), and dry vagina. In severe cases, swelling of the parotid and lacrimal areas and systemic manifestations, such as fever and fatigue, occur. Of clients with the syndrome, 50% have an associated disease, such as rheumatoid arthritis (RA).

Local management includes meticulous mouth, eye, and perineal care and the use of artificial tears and saliva. Systemic steroids may also be administered. Without treatment, the client can lose vision, and oral ulcerations, dental caries, and difficulty in swallowing or talking may ensue.

Infectious Arthritis

Any infectious agent can invade the joint space and cause inflammation and tissue destruction. Certain pathogens, such as *Staphylococcus aureus,* destroy tissue rapidly; others, especially viruses, do not cause irreversible damage. The cornerstone of management is local or systemic antibiotic therapy.

Lyme Disease

Lyme disease has been added to the list of connective tissue diseases (CTDs). Unlike many CTDs, however, the cause has been identified. The infected deer tick (*Ixodes*

dammini) transmits a bacterium (a spirochete) that causes a circular rash, malaise, fever, headache, and muscle or joint aches.

If Lyme disease is not diagnosed and treated, later complications, such as arthritis, enlarged lymph nodes, and neurologic and cardiac problems, can result. Prompt treatment with antibiotics, such as tetracycline, is usually effective. A new vaccine to prevent Lyme disease, Lymrex, is being tested for use in humans. Chart 24–13 lists ways to avoid Lyme disease.

Pseudogout

Pseudogout is a disease that mimics the clinical manifestations of gout. The crystals that deposit in joints, however, are calcium pyrophosphate, not sodium urate. Most often, these crystals migrate to cartilage, but they can also deposit in tendons, ligaments, and synovium.

The client most susceptible to pseudogout is an elderly male who is hospitalized. Although the cause is not certain, the incidence is highest in men who have metastatic cancer or endocrine imbalances, such as hypothyroidism. Nonsteroidal anti-inflammatory drugs usually control the manifestations of the disease.

Disease-Associated Arthritis

A number of diseases can cause secondary arthritis. Tuberculosis, Crohn's disease, ulcerative colitis, hemophilia, psoriasis, and sickle cell anemia are typical examples. To manage joint involvement, the primary disease is treated. For example, when a client with Crohn's disease has a remission, joint manifestations also subside. Conditions in which joint involvement can occur are presented in Table 24–3.

Chart 24–13

Health Promotion Guide: Prevention and Early Detection of Lyme Disease

- Avoid heavily wooded areas or areas with thick underbrush.
- Walk in the center of the trail.
- Avoid dark clothing. Lighter-colored clothing makes spotting ticks easier.
- Use an insect repellent on your skin and clothes in an area where ticks are likely to be found.
- Wear long-sleeved tops and long pants.
- Wear closed shoes and a hat or cap.
- Bathe immediately after being in an infested area, and inspect your body for ticks (about the size of a pinhead), paying special attention to your arms, legs, and hairline.
- Gently remove with tweezers or fingers any tick that you find. Dispose of the tick by flushing it down the toilet (burning a tick could spread infection).
- Wait 4 to 6 weeks after being bitten by a tick before being tested for Lyme disease (testing before this time is not reliable).
- Report symptoms, such as a rash or influenza-like illness, to your physician.

TABLE 24–3

Common Disorders Associated with Arthritis
• Crohn's disease
• Ulcerative colitis
• Tuberculosis
• Hemophilia
• Whipple's disease
• Intestinal bypass surgery
• Hyperparathyroidism
• Hyperthyroidism
• Diabetes mellitus
• Sickle cell anemia crisis
• Psoriasis
• Infection

Fibromyalgia

The term *fibromyalgia*, also called fibrositis, describes a syndrome characterized by trunk, extremity, and facial pain and tenderness without other objective findings. The primary manifestations are pain, muscle stiffness and spasm, sensory changes, and exhaustion, which may be attributable to severe sleep disturbances. Tender areas, known as trigger points, typically can be palpated to elicit pain in a predictable, reproducible pattern. Physical therapy, nonsteroidal anti-inflammatory drugs, and muscle relaxants usually provide temporary relief.

In most clients, fibrositis is the result of deep sleep deprivation. Clients may need hypnotics and other sleep-inducing methods to overcome this sleep disturbance. Antidepressive agents, such as amitriptyline (Elavil, Apo-Amitriptyline✦) or nortriptyline (Pamelor), may promote sleep and reduce muscle spasm. These drugs should be used with caution in the elderly because they can cause confusion and orthostatic hypotension. Trazodone (Desyrel) is the preferred drug for this population. The nurse observes the client for side effects and monitors for postural blood pressure changes.

Secondary fibrosis syndromes can accompany any connective tissue disease, particularly lupus and rheumatoid disease, and may not necessarily be related to sleep patterns.

Local Inflammatory Disorders

Two of the most common inflammatory conditions are localized to specific connective tissues: bursitis and tendinitis. Both problems are caused by repetitive motion and overuse related to aging, sports, or work injuries. Bursitis is an irritation of subcutaneous tissues and inflammation of the underlying bursae. Tendinitis is inflammation of one or more tendon sheaths.

Tight shoes often irritate the heel and cause bursitis. Diseases, such as rheumatoid arthritis (RA) and gout, and aerobic exercise can lead to bursitis and tendinitis.

The conservative management for both inflammatory conditions includes rest, ice, and nonsteroidal anti-inflammatory agents to relieve pain. More aggressive treatment may include corticosteroid injections or surgery to remove the inflamed tissue (Cunningham, 1994).

Mixed Connective Tissue Disease

When a client presents with clinical manifestations that are not typical of any one connective tissue disease, a diagnosis of mixed CTD is made. Approximately 10% of clients with CTDs are classified as having mixed disease. Some of these are overlap syndromes, in which two or more diseases occur at the same time. Common examples are systemic lupus erythematosus (SLE) plus progressive systemic sclerosis (PSS) and rheumatoid arthritis (RA) plus SLE.

Management depends of the clinical manifestations, but often the client is treated as having SLE.

CASE STUDY for the Client with Systemic Lupus Erythematosus

■ Susan, a 32-year-old Caucasian female, presents at her physician's office where you are a nurse with complaints of a facial rash. On further questioning, you find that she has been more fatigued than usual and has an achy left ankle. Her infant son is 4 months old, and she has just stopped bleeding from her traumatic vaginal delivery (the baby weighed 10 pounds, and she was in labor for 18 hours).

QUESTIONS:

1. When taking a complete history, what other questions should you ask Susan at this time?
2. If Susan has systemic lupus erythematosus (SLE), what other clinical manifestations might she have?
3. What risk factors does she have for SLE?
4. What laboratory tests will the physician most likely order?

SELECTED BIBLIOGRAPHY

Arcury, T. A., Bernard, S. L., Jordan, J. M., & Cook, H. L. (1996). Gender and ethnic differences in alternative and conventional arthritis remedy use among community-dwelling rural adults with arthritis. *Arthritis Care Research, 9*(5), 384–390.

*Crosby, L. (1991). Factors which contribute to fatigue associated with rheumatoid arthritis. *Journal of Advanced Nursing, 16*, 974–981.

Crutchfield, J., Zimmerman, L., Nieveen, J., et al. (1996). Preoperative and postoperative pain in total knee replacement patients. *Orthopaedic Nursing, 15*(2), 65–72.

Cunningham, M. (1996). Becoming familiar with fibromyalgia. *Orthopaedic Nursing, 15*(2), 33–38.

*Cunningham, M. E. (1994). Bursitis and tendinitis. *Orthopaedic Nursing, 13*(5), 13–16, 70.

Dildy, S. P. (1996). Suffering in people with rheumatoid arthritis. *Applied Nursing Research, 9*, 177–183.

Failla, S., Kuper, B. C., Nick, T. G., & Lee, F. A. (1996). Adjustment of women with lupus erythematosus. *Applied Nursing Research, 9*(2), 87–92.

Giger, J. N., & Davidhizar, R. E. (1995). *Transcultural nursing: Assessment and intervention* (2nd ed.). St. Louis, MO: Mosby Year Book.

Gio-Fitman, J. (1996). The role of psychological stress in rheumatoid arthritis. *MedSurg Nursing, 5*, 422–426.

Hahn, B. H. (1997). Management of systemic lupus erythematosus. In W. N. Kelley, S. Ruddy, E. D. Harris, & C. B. Sledge (Eds.), *Textbook of rheumatology* (5th ed., pp. 1040–1056). Philadelphia: W. B. Saunders.

Harris, E. D. (1997). Treatment of rheumatoid arthritis. In W. N. Kelley, S. Ruddy, E. D. Harris, & C. B. Sledge (Eds.), *Textbook of rheumatology* (5th ed., pp. 933–950). Philadelphia: W. B. Saunders.

*Maher, A. B., Salmond, S. W., & Pellino, T. A. (1994). *Orthopedic nursing*. Philadelphia: W. B. Saunders.

Mankin, H. J., & Brandt, K. D. (1997). Pathogenesis of osteo-arthritis. In W. N. Kelley, S. Ruddy, E. D. Harris, & C. B. Sledge (Eds.), *Textbook of rheumatology* (5th ed., pp. 1369–1382). Philadelphia: W. B. Saunders.

McGrath, A. (1997). Clinical snapshot: Raynaud's syndrome. *American Journal of Nursing, 97*(1), 34–35.

Ranawat, C. S., Miyasaka, K. C., Umlas, M. E., & Rodriguez, J. A. (1997). The hip. In W. N. Kelley, S. Ruddy, E. D. Harris, & C. B. Sledge (Eds.), *Textbook of rheumatology* (5th ed., pp. 1723–1738). Philadelphia: W. B. Saunders.

Schumacher, H. R., Jr. (1988). *Primer on the rheumatic diseases.* Atlanta: The Arthritis Foundation.

Solomon, L. (1997). Clinical features of osteoarthritis. In W. N. Kelley, S. Ruddy, E. D. Harris, & C. B. Sledge (Eds.), *Textbook of rheumatology* (5th ed., pp. 1383–1393). Philadelphia: W. B. Saunders.

Tietz, N. W. (1995). *Clinical guide to laboratory tests* (3rd ed.). Philadelphia: W. B. Saunders.

*Wetherbee, L. L. (1994). Caring for the client with rheumatoid arthritis. *Home Healthcare Nurse, 12*(1), 13–18.

Windsor, R. E. M., & Insall, J. N. (1997). The knee. In W. N. Kelley, S. Ruddy, E. D. Harris, & C. B. Sledge (Eds.), *Textbook of rheumatology* (5th ed., pp. 1739–1758). Philadelphia: W. B. Saunders.

Ulak, L. J. (1995). Special considerations for SLE patients. *MedSurg Nursing, 4*(2), 146–148.

SUGGESTED READINGS

Crutchfield, J., Zimmerman, L., Nieveen, J., et al. (1996). Preoperative and postoperative pain in total knee replacement patients. *Orthopaedic Nursing, 15*(2), 65–72.

The authors report the findings of their descriptive study, which compared pain levels in clients before and after total knee replacement. Participants in the study reported less pain after the surgery (on days 1 and 3) than before the surgery. The researchers also found that different words were used to describe the nature of acute and chronic pain.

*Cunningham, M. E. (1994). Bursitis and tendinitis. *Orthopaedic Nursing, 13*(5), 13–16, 70.

This article presents a thorough discussion of the pathophysiology, etiology, clinical manifestations, and treatment of two common local inflammatory conditions: bursitis and tendinitis. Nursing care of clients with these conditions is also described.

Gio-Fitman, J. (1996). The role of psychological stress in rheumatoid arthritis. *MedSurg Nursing, 5*, 422–426.

The author explores the relationship of rheumatoid arthritis (RA) and stress in this article. Studies that show a correlation between stress and RA are summarized. Nursing interventions that can help clients cope with their stress are also discussed.

Chapter 25

INTERVENTIONS FOR CLIENTS WITH HIV AND OTHER IMMUNOLOGIC DISORDERS

The purpose of immune function is to protect the body from disease and stimulate repair when tissue damage occurs. Problems of the immune system can result in inadequate function, excessive function, or inappropriate function. Clients who have inadequate immune function are at increased risk for infection and cancer. Clients who have excessive or inappropriate immune function are at increased risk for tissue damage. For some clients, malfunction of the immune system is the cause of disease; for others, it is the result. All clients with immunologic disorders are at high risk for development of other problems. Therefore, coordination of care through case management, which provides comprehensive, interdisciplinary care, can optimize client health outcomes.

IMMUNODEFICIENCIES

A deficient response of the immune system that is due to a missing or damaged immune component is an *immuno-deficiency*. The immunodeficient person cannot defend adequately against potentially harmful substances that an immunocompetent person can. An immunodeficient person's immune system cannot recognize or eliminate antigens normally, and the person is, therefore, susceptible to infection, malignancy, and other disease.

A *primary* or *congenital* immunodeficiency is one in which the immune malfunction is present from birth. An *acquired* or *secondary* immunodeficiency is one that occurs in a person who has a normally functioning immune system at birth but later becomes immunodeficient as a consequence of disease, injury, exposure to toxins, medical therapy, or unknown cause. These people are referred to as *immunocompromised* because their immune systems have been compromised, resulting in an impaired ability to neutralize, destroy, or eliminate antigens (see Chap. 23).

The immunodeficient client manifests clinical symptoms that vary in severity and occur in multiple body systems. For many immunodeficiencies, the cause is unknown or uncontrollable, the pathophysiology is not well understood, and effective treatment may not be available. The complications, not the actual immune defect, can be treated. Most immunodeficiencies are chronic conditions, and periods of wellness are interspersed with clinical problems.

Regardless of the cause, the immunodeficient person constantly faces the possibility that the next infection might be fatal. Normal environmental exposures to people, objects, and microorganisms may pose significant danger. The nurse is instrumental in teaching the immunodeficient person how to avoid infection and the signs and symptoms of infection. The nurse assesses the client for subtle changes related to early infection and treats the client quickly according to physician's orders. Supporting the client and family is an essential part of nursing care.

Acquired (Secondary) Immunodeficiencies

Acquired Immunodeficiency Syndrome

Overview

Acquired immunodeficiency syndrome (AIDS) is the late stage of a continuum of symptoms that result from infection with the human immunodeficiency virus (HIV). AIDS is not the same as HIV infection, and not everyone infected with HIV has AIDS. Persons with AIDS are profoundly immunosuppressed and usually have lived with HIV for several years before AIDS develops. The nurse provides education, physical care, and psychological support for the person living with AIDS.

AIDS is a serious, debilitating, and eventually fatal disease. To date, 84% of those with AIDS have been between the ages of 25 and 49 years (Table 25–1). To be diagnosed as having AIDS, a person must be infected with HIV and have a clinical disease that indicates cellular

TABLE 25–1

AIDS Cases Among Adults and Adolescents in the United States June 1, 1981–June 1997	
Age (years)	**No. Cases**
13–19	2,953
20–24	22,070
25–29	85,211
30–34	140,559
35–39	136,814
40–44	98,393
45–49	55,302
50–54	29,148
55–59	16,399
60–64	9,214
65+	8,113
Total	604,176 (374,656 deaths)

Data from the Centers for Disease Control and Prevention.
HIV/AIDS Surveillance Report, Mid-year 1997 Edition, *9*(1). Atlanta: Author.

▷ Research Applications for Nursing

AIDS Fears and Concerns Among Registered Nurses

Wang, J. F. (1997). Attitudes, concerns, and fear of acquired immune deficiency syndrome among registered nurses in the United States. Holistic Nursing Practice, 11(2), 36–49.

The purpose of this descriptive, correlational study was to explore the attitudes of registered nurses from different educational levels, work settings, and ages with regard to people with AIDS (PWAs). The study used a questionnaire that incorporated the Fear of AIDS (FOA) Scale II along with other questions related to demographics, working conditions, and HIV transmission knowledge. Participants (anonymous volunteers) were 376 registered nurses employed in a variety of settings within one mid-Atlantic state.

The results of this study indicate that, even though the health care profession does not carry a greater risk than the rest of the U.S. population for contracting AIDS, many registered nurses perceive the risk to be high and the stigma great. Not only do many of these nurses fear AIDS, but they have negative attitudes toward gays and IV drug abusers. Younger participants and those more involved with direct patient care likely to have blood contact had greater fear and more negative attitudes.

Critique. The study design was appropriate for the purpose. Reliability and validity data for the instruments used were not presented. The study could have been strengthened by obtaining information about the participants' knowledge level of HIV–AIDS, use of Standard Precautions, and personal experience with people who are HIV-positive.

Implications for Nursing. The study points out that, more than a decade after the cause and transmission paths of AIDS have been elucidated, registered nurses continue to harbor unjustified fear of AIDS and of people with AIDS. Accurate information regarding HIV–AIDS transmission should be integrated into all basic nursing education and agency orientation programs. Yearly updates in the workplace are advisable as are sensitivity training sessions to assist nurses in providing safe, compassionate, individualized nursing care to all clients.

immunodeficiency or CD4+ T-lymphocyte (T4) count below 200/mm³ or a CD4+ T-lymphocyte total percentage below 14.

The care of the person with AIDS can evoke complex personal issues for nurses. Nurses must acknowledge their own fear of acquiring HIV and any negative attitudes regarding possible client lifestyles contributing to HIV infection, such as intravenous (IV) drug use or homosexual behaviors (see Research Applications for Nursing). Knowledge and practice of appropriate infection control techniques can reduce nurses' fears about becoming infected. To provide competent, compassionate nursing care to the person with AIDS, nurses must suspend judgment.

Pathophysiology

The Centers for Disease Control and Prevention (CDC) classification scheme for HIV infection is based on clinical

TABLE 25–2

Centers for Disease Control and Prevention (CDC) Classification System for HIV Infection and AIDS Case Definition

Clinical Categories	Criteria	CD4+ T-Cell Categories
A1	Asymptomatic, acute (primary HIV or persistent generalized) Lymphadenopathy	≥ 500/μL
A2	Same as A1	200–400/μL
A3	Same as A1	< 200/μL*
B1	Symptomatic, not category A or C	≥ 500/μL
B2	Same as B1	200–400/μL
B3	Same as B1	< 200/μL*
C1	AIDS indicator conditions†	≥ 500/μL
C2	Same as C1	200–400/μL
C3	Same as C1	< 200/μL*

From U.S. Department of Health and Human Services, 1992.
* AIDS indicator T-cell count.
† Candidiasis (bronchi, trachea, lungs, or esophagus)
  Cervical cancer, invasive
  Coccidioidomycosis (disseminated or extrapulmonary)
  Cryptosporidiosis (chronic intestinal)
  Cytomegalovirus disease (other than liver, spleen, or nodes)
  Cytomegalovirus retinitis (with vision loss)
  Encephalopathy (HIV-related)
  Herpes simplex (chronic, or bronchitis, pneumonitis, or esophagitis)
  Histoplasmosis (disseminated or extrapulmonary)
  Isosporiasis (chronic intestinal)
  Kaposi's sarcoma
  Lymphoma (Burkitt's, immunoblastic, or primary brain)
  Mycobacterium avium-intracellulare complex or *M. kansasii* (disseminated or extrapulmonary)
  Mycobacterium tuberculosis
  Mycobacterium
  Pneumocystis carinii pneumonia
  Pneumonia, recurrent
  Progressive multifocal leukoencephalopathy
  Salmonella septicemia
  Toxoplasmosis (brain)
  Wasting syndrome resulting from HIV

conditions associated with HIV infection and three ranges of CD4+ T-lymphocyte counts (Table 25–2). The classification begins with acute infection and spans a continuum that culminates with AIDS. The person with HIV can transmit the virus to others at all stages of disease.

Acute infection (CDC group I) can occur within 1 to 8 weeks after infection with HIV and is characterized by a flu-like syndrome that resolves completely. The next stage is asymptomatic infection (CDC group II), in which the infected person has no signs or symptoms. The first symptomatic stage occurs with the appearance of persistent generalized lymphadenopathy (lymph node enlargement lasting more than 3 months) (CDC group III).

The next stage includes constitutional disease, which can include persistent fever or diarrhea (more than 1 month) or involuntary loss of more than 10% of body weight (CDC group IV-A). Neurologic disease, including dementia, neuropathy, and myelopathy, is an indicator for

CDC group IV-B classification. CDC groups IV-C and IV-D include a CD4 T-lymphocyte (see Chap. 23) count below 200/mm³ and such clinical conditions as opportunistic infections (infection by organisms that take advantage of a defective immune system), recurrent pneumonia, invasive cervical cancer, pulmonary tuberculosis, and other cancers.

The time from initial HIV infection to development of AIDS ranges from 18 months to more than 10 years. The range depends how HIV was acquired and a variety of personal factors. For people who have been transfused with HIV-contaminated blood, for instance, AIDS develops more quickly; for those who become HIV-positive as a result of a single sexual encounter, there is a longer latency period before the condition progresses to AIDS. Other personal factors that may influence progression to AIDS include frequency of re-exposures to HIV, presence of other sexually transmitted diseases (STDs), nutritional status, pregnancy, and stress.

Etiology

AIDS is caused by the profound suppression of immune responses resulting from infection with HIV. Two subtypes of the virus have been identified: type 1 (HIV-1) and type 2 (HIV-2). Type 1 is the form most frequently isolated from infected persons in the Western Hemisphere, Europe, and Asia. Type 2 is endemic to West Africa. Although they differ in viral surface molecules, both subtypes can cause AIDS.

HIV belongs to a special class of viruses known as *retroviruses,* which differ from other viruses in their efficiency of cellular infection. Retroviruses have only ribonucleic acid (RNA) as their genetic material. The most important difference between retroviruses and other viruses is a special complex of enzymes within the retrovirus called *reverse transcriptase* (RT). This enzyme complex increases the efficiency of viral replication once the retrovirus enters a human cell.

Once a retrovirus gains entry into the body and infects a human cell, the RT enzymes force the human cell's deoxyribonucleic acid (DNA) synthesis machinery to use the viral RNA as a pattern and make a piece of human DNA complementary to the viral RNA. This new piece of DNA is then incorporated successfully into the person's cellular DNA, where it acts as a template for viral production. HIV then spreads quickly throughout the lymphoid system, sequestering in macrophages and in the germinal centers of lymph nodes (Volberding, 1994). Throughout the course of infection, HIV is actively replicated by infected T lymphocytes, synthesizing up to 2 billion viral particles daily (Fig. 25–1). After many rounds of replication, these viral particles exhaust the immune system.

The HIV retrovirus attaches to, infects, and ultimately destroys immune system cells with a CD4 surface receptor. These cells include T4 lymphocytes (CD4+ cells) and macrophages. The T4 lymphocyte, also called the helper or inducer lymphocyte, regulates the activity of all immune system cells (see Chap. 23). When infected by HIV, the T4 cell does not function normally, causing general malfunction of the whole immune system. The results of HIV infection are

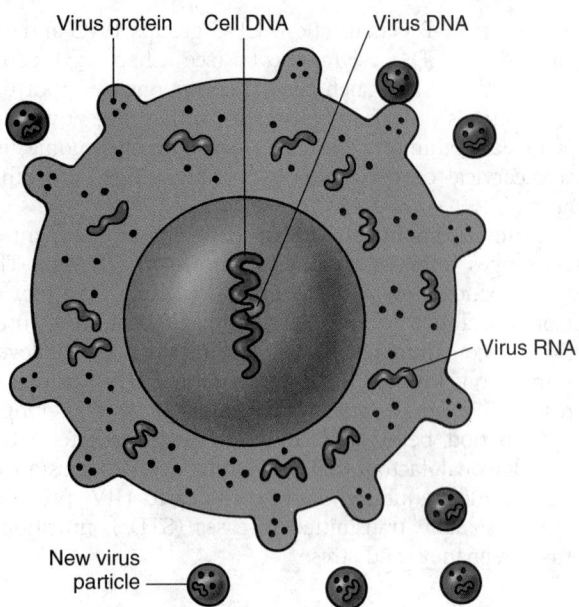

Figure 25–1. A T lymphocyte infected with human immunodeficiency virus. The virus can be seen budding from the infected T cell.

- Lymphocytopenia with selective T4 cell depletion
- Abnormal T-cell function
- Increased production of incomplete and nonfunctional antibodies
- Abnormally functioning macrophages

As a result of these immune dysfunctions, the client with HIV is susceptible to opportunistic infections and cancer. Macrophages infected by HIV are not destroyed by infection; they act as a reservoir for the virus.

Incidence/Prevalence

The incidence of AIDS in the United States has grown exponentially from the early 1980s. In 1981, 291 new cases of AIDS were reported; in 1995, 74,180 new cases were reported. From June 1981 through June 1997, there have been 604,176 reported cases and 374,656 AIDS-related deaths in the United States (Centers for Disease Control and Prevention, 1997). The Public Health Service (PHS) estimates that 1 million persons in the United States are infected with HIV. This includes those living with AIDS, those who have tested positive for HIV, and those who are positive but have not been tested.

Epidemiologic and demographic data have shown that most people with AIDS in the United States are (1) men who have had sex with other men (47%) or (2) persons of both sexes who have used IV drugs (22%) (Table 25–3). The fastest growing infected groups are women and minorities, with a disproportionate number of cases reported in racial and ethnic minority groups. Approximately 52% of all AIDS cases in North America have occurred in African-Americans and Hispanics, who constitute only 18.5% of the population. Between 1985 and 1995, the demographics of the disease changed dramatically. The rates for women increased 8.2%, and the inci-

dence of AIDS in minority groups increased 41.7% (Table 25–4).

AIDS is a disease with high mortality. The overall fatality rate is about 65% for adults (Centers for Disease Control and Prevention, 1997), and to date there have been no reports of a cure. Currently, there are 31 persons with AIDS identified as *nonprogressors,* individuals infected with HIV for at least 10 years who remain asymptomatic and have maintained CD4+ T-lymphocyte counts within a normal range. Researchers are studying nonprogressors to determine whether they resist disease because of differences in viral factors, such as infection with a weak HIV strain, or because they have an unusually strong immune response (Barnes, 1995).

TRANSCULTURAL CONSIDERATIONS

AIDS has been reported in 162 countries and in each of the United States (World Health Organization [WHO], 1991). In 1991, a total of 418,403 cases were reported worldwide (WHO, 1991), but reporting of AIDS cases to the WHO is generally incomplete. The pattern of HIV infection and manifestations of AIDS differ in countries such as West Africa, where HIV-2 is the predominant viral strain.

The main difference in HIV-2 infection is that it occurs primarily in the heterosexual population, with equal numbers of men and women infected. The modes of transmission are the same as those of HIV-1. The large number of infected females results in a high rate of perinatal transmission and large numbers of HIV-infected children.

WOMEN'S HEALTH CONSIDERATIONS

Women comprise the fastest growing group with HIV infection and AIDS (CDC, 1996). Women with HIV appear to have a poorer outcome with shorter survival than men. This outcome may be the result of late

TABLE 25–3

AIDS Cases Among Adults and Adolescents in the United States by Exposure Category: June 1, 1981–June 30, 1997

Category	No. Cases	%
Men who have sex with men	298,699	49
Injecting drug users (female and male heterosexual)	154,664	26
Men who have sex with men and inject drugs	38,923	6
Hemophilia	4,567	1
Heterosexual contact	54,571	9
Recipients of blood transfusion, blood components, or tissue	8,075	2
Other and unidentified risk	44,677	7
Total	604,176	100

Data from the Centers for Disease Control and Prevention.
HIV/AIDS Surveillance Report, Mid-year 1997 Edition, Vol. 9, No. 1. Atlanta: Author.

TABLE 25–4

Distribution of Adult/Adolescent AIDS Cases in the United States by Race and Ethnic Group, June 1, 1981–June 30, 1997	
Category	**No. Cases**
Caucasian, not Hispanic	277,672
African-American, not Hispanic	212,394
Hispanic	107,419
Asian/Pacific Islander	4,329
Native American	1,651
Unknown	711
Total	604,176

Data from the Centers for Disease Control and Prevention, 1997.

diagnosis and social and economic factors that reduce access to medical care rather than any viral pathology.

Gynecologic symptoms, particularly persistent or recurrent vaginal candidiasis, may be the first signs of HIV in women (Sabo & Carwein, 1994). Additional symptoms include genital herpes, pelvic inflammatory disease, and cervical neoplasia.

Most women with HIV are of childbearing age. The effect of pregnancy on the course of HIV infection is not known. There is conflicting evidence that it may or may not speed up the progression of disease.

ELDERLY CONSIDERATIONS

 Infection with HIV can occur at any age. The nurse or assistive nursing personnel should assess the elderly client for risk behaviors, including a sexual and drug use history. Decline in immune function may increase susceptibility to HIV infection in this population. In the older woman, changes in vaginal tissue as a result of aging may increase susceptibility to sexually transmitted HIV infection (Whipple & Scura, 1996).

Collaborative Management

Assessment

Continuous, careful, comprehensive assessment of the client with AIDS is crucial, because he or she may have signs and symptoms related to disease in multiple organ systems. Subtle changes must be assessed so infections and other clinical problems can be found early and treated effectively.

➤ History

Information relevant to HIV and AIDS from the general history includes age, gender, occupation, and residence. The nurse thoroughly assesses the current complaint or current illness, including its nature, when it started, severity of symptoms, associated problems, and any interventions to date. The nurse questions the client about when AIDS was diagnosed and what clinical symptoms led to that diagnosis. The client is asked to give a chronology of infections and clinical problems since the diagnosis. The nurse assesses health history, including whether the client received a blood transfusion between 1978 and 1985.

The client also is questioned about sexual practices, history of STDs, and history of major infectious diseases, including tuberculosis and hepatitis. If the client is a hemophiliac, the nurse asks about treatment with clotting factors. The client is asked about past or present drug use, including needle exposure and sharing. The nurse assesses the client's level of knowledge regarding the diagnosis, symptom management, diagnostic tests, treatments, community resources, and modes of transmission of the virus. The nurse also assesses the client's understanding of, familiarity with, and use of safer sex practices.

➤ Physical Assessment/Clinical Manifestations

The nurse or assistive personnel looks for many possible signs and symptoms. These include shortness of breath or cough, fever, night sweats, fatigue, nausea and vomiting, weight loss, lymphadenopathy, diarrhea, visual changes, headache, memory loss, confusion, seizures, personality changes, dry skin, rashes, skin lesions, pain, and discomfort (Chart 25–1).

Opportunistic Infections. Opportunistic infections occur because of the profound immune suppression of the person with AIDS (see Chart 25–1). They may result from primary infection or reactivation of a latent infection. Opportunistic infections account for most of the clinical manifestations observed in AIDS, and can be protozoan, fungal, bacterial, or viral. The nurse may note more than one infection in a client with AIDS.

Protozoal Infections. Pneumocystis carinii pneumonia (PCP) is the most common opportunistic infection in persons with HIV; its incidence ranges from 75% to 80% (Henry & Holzemer, 1992). The nurse notes dyspnea on exertion, tachypnea, a persistent dry cough, and fever. The client with PCP complains of fatigue and weight loss. On auscultation of the lungs, the nurse notes crackles.

Toxoplasmosis encephalitis, caused by *Toxoplasma gondii*, is acquired through contact with contaminated cat feces or ingesting infected, undercooked meat. The client may experience subtle changes in mental status, neurologic deficits, headaches, and fever. Other symptoms include difficulties with speech, gait, and vision, seizures, lethargy, and confusion. The nurse performs a comprehensive baseline mental status examination and monitors the client to detect subtle changes.

Cryptosporidiosis is a gastroenteritis caused by *Cryptosporidium*. In AIDS, this illness ranges from a mild diarrhea to a cholera-like syndrome with wasting and electrolyte imbalance. The nurse notes voluminous diarrhea, with a volume loss of up to 15 to 20 L/day.

Fungal Infections. Candida albicans is part of the natural flora of the gastrointestinal tract. In the person with AIDS, candidiasis occurs because the regulatory mechanisms of the immune system can no longer control fungal overgrowth. *Candida* stomatitis or esophagitis is a frequent finding in AIDS; clients complain of food tasting "funny,"

Chart 25-1

Key Features of AIDS

Immunologic Manifestations

- Low white blood cell counts:
  - T_4:T_8 ratio < 2
  - T_4 count < 200/mm³
- Hypergammaglobulinemia
- Opportunistic infections
- Lymphadenopathy
- Fatigue

Integumentary Manifestations

- Dry skin
- Poor wound healing
- Skin lesions
- Night sweats

Respiratory Manifestations

- Cough
- Shortness of breath

Gastrointestinal Manifestations

- Diarrhea
- Weight loss
- Nausea and vomiting

Central Nervous System Manifestations

- Confusion
- Dementia
- Headache
- Fever
- Visual changes
- Memory loss
- Personality changes
- Pain
- Seizures

Opportunistic Infections

- Protozoal Infections
  - *Pneumocystis carinii* pneumonia
  - Toxoplasmosis
  - Cryptosporidiosis
  - Isosporiasis
  - Microsporidiosis
  - Strongyloidiasis
  - Giardiasis
- Fungal Infections
  - Candidiasis
  - Cryptococcosis
  - Histoplasmosis
  - Coccidioidomycosis
- Bacterial Infections
  - *Mycobacterium avium-intracellulare* complex infection
  - Tuberculosis
  - Nocardiosis
- Viral Infections
  - Cytomegalovirus infection
  - Herpes simplex virus infection
  - Varicella-zoster virus infection

Malignancies

- Kaposi's sarcoma
- Non-Hodgkin's lymphoma
- Hodgkin's lymphoma
- Invasive cervical carcinoma

---

mouth pain, difficulty in swallowing, and retrosternal pain (pain behind the ribs). On examination of the mouth and the back of the throat, the nurse sees the characteristic "cottage cheese"–like, yellow-white plaques and inflammation. Esophagitis is diagnosed by endoscopic biopsy and culture. Women with AIDS may have vaginal candidiasis, characterized by severe pruritus (itching), perineal irritation, and a thick, white vaginal discharge.

Cryptococcosis is a severe, debilitating meningitis and occasionally a disseminated disease in AIDS. It is caused by *Cryptococcus neoformans*. Clinical manifestations of meningitis include fever, headache, blurred vision, nausea and vomiting, nuchal rigidity (stiff neck), mild confusion, and other mental status changes. The client sometimes experiences seizures and other focal neurologic abnormalities, or may present with mild symptoms and complain only of malaise and fever with or without headaches.

Histoplasmosis, caused by *Histoplasma capsulatum,* begins as a respiratory infection and progresses to disseminated infection in the person with AIDS. The nurse may note dyspnea, fever, cough, and weight loss. The client's spleen, liver, and lymph nodes may be enlarged.

Bacterial Infections. *Mycobacterium avium-intracellulare* complex (MAC) is the most common bacterial infection associated with AIDS. This complex is caused by *Mycobacterium intracellulare* or *Mycobacterium avium,* which infects the respiratory or gastrointestinal tract. MAC is a disseminated infection. Positive cultures may be obtained from lymph nodes, bone marrow, and blood. Clinical manifestations include fever, debility, weight loss, malaise, and sometimes lymphadenopathy or organ disease.

Tuberculosis, caused by *Mycobacterium tuberculosis,* occurs in 2% to 10% of persons with AIDS. People with HIV are at increased risk for active tuberculosis. More than 50% of all clients who have AIDS and tuberculosis have extrapulmonary disease sites, including the central nervous system, bones, liver, spleen, skin, and gastrointestinal tract. The client's systemic symptoms include fever, chills, night sweats, weight loss, and anorexia; pulmonary involvement causes cough, dyspnea, and chest pain. Symptoms of extrapulmonary infection vary with the site. The person with tuberculosis and a CD4+ count below 200/mm³ may not have a positive purified protein derivative (PPD) skin test because of an inability to mount an immune response to the antigen, a condition known as *anergy*. Other diagnostic measures should include chest x-ray film, acid-fast sputum smear, and sputum culture.

The nurse giving aerosol treatments such as pentamidine isethionate prophylaxis that induce coughing to clients with AIDS should be screened with a PPD skin test every 6 months.

Recurrent pneumonia from bacterial infections occurs frequently among immunocompromised clients. Under the 1993 revised CDC classification system for AIDS, two or more episodes of pneumonia in a 12-month period was added as an AIDS case definition. Symptoms include chest pain, productive cough, fever, and dyspnea.

Viral Infections. Cytomegalovirus (CMV) can infect multiple sites in people with AIDS, including the eye (CMV retinitis), respiratory and gastrointestinal tracts, and central nervous system. CMV infection can also result in many nonspecific symptoms associated with AIDS, such as fever, malaise, weight loss, fatigue, and lymphadenopathy. CMV retinitis causes visual impairment ranging from slight to total bilateral blindness.

Cytomegalovirus infection also causes colitis, with diarrhea, abdominal bloating and discomfort, and weight loss. In addition, CMV can cause encephalitis, pneumonitis, adrenalitis, hepatitis, and disseminated infection.

Herpes simplex virus (HSV) infections in people with AIDS occur in the perirectal, oral, and genital areas. Clients describe numbness or tingling at the site of infection up to 24 hours before vesicle formation. Vesicular lesions are painful, with chronic ulcerative lesions after vesicle rupture. The nurse notes fever, pain, bleeding, and lymph node enlargement in the affected area. Systemic symptoms include headache, myalgia, and malaise.

Varicella-zoster virus (VZV) infection usually does not represent a new infection for people with AIDS. This virus, present in nerve ganglia of many people, causes chickenpox. When these people are immunocompromised, VZV leave the nerve ganglia, enter body fluids and other tissue areas, causing *shingles*. Symptoms begin with pain and burning along dermatome nerve tracts. Large fluid-filled vesicles form and eventually crust over. Systemic symptoms include headache and low-grade fever.

Malignancies. The altered immunocompetence of AIDS increases the risk for cancer in this group. Cancers associated with AIDS include Kaposi's sarcoma (KS), Hodgkin's lymphoma, and non-Hodgkin's lymphoma.

Kaposi's Sarcoma. This is the most common malignancy associated with AIDS, occurring in 1% to 21% of clients with AIDS. Hemophiliacs with HIV have the lowest incidence of KS, and men infected through homosexual contact the highest.

Kaposi's sarcoma presents as small, purplish-brown, palpable discrete lesions that are usually not painful or pruritic; they can occur anywhere on the body. Most clients with KS present with mucocutaneous (skin or mucous membrane) lesions. In some, extracutaneous lesions develop, especially in the lymph nodes, gastrointestinal tract, or lungs. The nurse assesses KS lesions for number, size, and location and monitors their progression. KS is diagnosed by biopsy and histologic examination of the lesion.

Malignant Lymphomas. Malignant lymphomas associated with AIDS are primarily non-Hodgkin's B-cell lymphomas. Systemic symptoms include weight loss, fever, and night sweats. (See Chapter 42 on clinical course and care relevant to malignant lymphomas.)

Other Clinical Manifestations. All body systems are affected to some degree in AIDS; however, manifestations most consistently appear as changes in cognitive function, weight, and the skin.

AIDS Dementia Complex. HIV-associated dementia complex, or AIDS dementia complex (ADC), refers to the signs and symptoms of central nervous system involvement. ADC occurs in up to 70% of persons with AIDS. It is probably the result of direct infection of cells within the central nervous system by HIV. ADC is characterized by three components: cognitive, motor, and behavioral impairments (Chart 25-2). Symptoms range from subclinical to severe dementia.

Other neurologic complications may be due to HIV infection or drug side effects, including peripheral neuropathies and myopathies. Symptoms of peripheral neuropathies include paresthesias and burning sensations, pain, and gait changes. Myopathies are accompanied by leg weakness, ataxia, and muscle pain.

Wasting Syndrome. AIDS wasting syndrome is not due to any single factor. It may be the result of altered metabolism from malignancy or opportunistic infection. Diarrhea, malabsorption, anorexia, and oral and esophageal lesions can all contribute to persistent and sometimes

---

Chart 25-2

Key Features of AIDS Dementia Complex

Cognitive Impairment
- Slowed thinking
- Slowed reaction time to external stimuli
- Loss of concentration while thinking or speaking
- Memory loss
- Forgetfulness
- Wandering attention

Motor Impairment
- Loss of coordination
- Loss of balance
- Increased minor accidents such as tripping, bumping into things, or dropping things
- Slowed motor performance
- Leg weakness

Behavioral Impairment
- Apathy
- Withdrawal
  or
- Irritability
- Hyperactivity

extreme weight loss, and the client may appear quite emaciated.

Integumentary Changes. Many clients complain of dry, itchy, irritated skin and diffuse rashes of seborrheic dermatitis. The nurse may also observe folliculitis, eczema, or psoriasis; petechiae or bleeding gums may present as a result of a low platelet count.

➤ *Psychosocial Assessment*

Psychosocial data collection for a client with AIDS is extremely important. The nurse asks about the client's social support system, including family, significant others, and friends. To protect the client's confidentiality, the nurse assesses who in this support system is aware of the client's diagnosis so that the nurse does not inadvertently mention it. Some clients, because of real or threatened discrimination, are quite selective about whom they tell. Health care providers should respect the client's choices as much as possible without compromising care. The nurse can offer resources to help the client with disclosure to sexual partners or significant others.

The client may be closest to a lover or a friend who is not legally recognized as next of kin. The nurse obtains the name and telephone number of that person and learns whether a durable power of attorney document has been executed.

The nurse elicits information about the client's activities of daily living as well as any changes that may have occurred since diagnosis. The nurse assesses the client's employment status and occupation, social activities and hobbies, living arrangements, and financial resources, including health insurance.

To plan care and monitor changes, the nurse assesses the client's anxiety level, mood, and cognitive ability. The nurse also asks the client about any experiences with discrimination and how they were handled. After the nurse assesses the client's level of self-esteem and changes in body image, together the nurse and client identify the client's strengths and coping strategies. The nurse gathers information about any suicidal ideation, depression, or other psychological problems. The nurse also obtains information about the client's involvement with support groups or other community resources.

➤ *Laboratory Assessment*

Lymphocyte Counts. A lymphocyte count is generally performed as part of a complete blood count (CBC) with differential (see Chap. 23). The normal white blood cell count (WBC) is between 4500 and 11,000 cells/mm^3, with a differential of approximately 30% to 40% lymphocytes (an absolute number of 1500–4500). Clients with AIDS are often leukopenic, with a WBC count of less than 3500 cells/mm^3 and usually lymphopenic (less than 1500 cells/mm^3).

T4-T8 Ratio. The percentage and number of T4 and T8 cells are an important part of an immune profile. People with HIV infection usually have a lower than normal number of T4 cells. Some clients with AIDS have fewer than 100 cells/mm^3 (normal: between 800 and 1200 cells/mm^3), whereas the number of T8 cells is usually normal. The normal ratio of T4 to T8 cells is approximately 2:1. In AIDS, because of a low number of T4 cells, this ratio is low. Low T4 cell counts and a low T4–T8 ratio are associated with increased clinical manifestations of disease.

Antibody Tests. Antibody tests measure the client's response to the presence of the virus (the antigen) rather than to the virus itself. HIV antibody can be measured by enzyme-linked immunosorbent assay (ELISA) and Western blot analysis. After infection with the virus, it usually takes from 3 weeks to 3 months for a person to test positive for HIV antibodies. However, in some infected people, it can take up to 36 months for antibodies to be detectable (Imagawa et al., 1989). False-negative results (incorrectly indicating the absence of HIV infection) have been reported: early in the infection, in people with cancer, and in people on long-term immunosuppressive therapies.

Enzyme-Linked Immunosorbent Assay. The client's serum is mixed with HIV grown in culture. If the client has antibodies to HIV, they will bind to the HIV antigens and can be detected (a positive test). Two considerations in HIV antibody testing are sensitivity and specificity. False-positive test results (incorrectly indicating HIV infection) occur in approximately 0.1% of those tested with the ELISA. False-positive results (McMahon, 1988) have been reported in multiparous or pregnant women, intravenous drug users, people with a history of malaria, clients with lymphomas, and those with reactivity to the HLA-DR4 leukocyte antigen.

Western Blot. If the results of an ELISA are positive, they are confirmed by Western blot analysis. This test is not as widely available as ELISA because of its cost and complexity. The Western blot analysis is a more specific test to detect serum antibodies to four specific major HIV antigens. A positive Western blot is based on the presence of antibodies to two of the major HIV antigens.

The result is considered indeterminate if two of the major antibodies are not detected but other antibodies to HIV are. The person should then be retested. In people whose tests are positive, conversion from an indeterminate to a positive Western blot usually occurs within 6 months. If a person has a positive test result for HIV antibodies, it does not mean that he or she has AIDS, only that he or she has been infected with the virus.

Viral Culture. Virus culture techniques also can determine the presence of HIV. One method involves placing the infected client's blood cells in a culture medium and measuring the amount of reverse transcriptase (RT) activity over a 28-day period. The more RT present, the more actively the virus is thought to be replicating.

Viral Load Testing. Viral load testing (also called viral burden testing) measures the presence of HIV viral genetic material (RNA) or another actual viral protein in the client's blood rather than the body's response to the presence of the virus. These test types are quantitative and more directly indicate the level of viral burden or viral load. Such tests are very useful in monitoring disease progression or treatment effectiveness.

p24 Antigen Assay. The p24 antigen assay quantifies the amount of p24 (HIV viral core protein) in the client's serum. Antibodies to p24 are mixed with the serum and can detect even low levels of viral antigen present in serum. However, the assay is not as sensitive as antibody tests or assays of viral genetic material. Because this test is less expensive than measure of viral RNA, it is most frequently used to chart a client's disease progression rather than make an initial diagnosis.

Quantitative RNA Assays. Currently, three quantitative assays are available in some areas for viral load testing: RT-polymerase chain reaction (RT-PCR), branched DNA method (bDNA), and the nucleic acid sequence-based assay (NASBA). All three assays use gene amplification processes to determine the amount of HIV RNA present in a client's serum, and all have a specificity of 100% (Coste et al., 1996). Even if only a few infected cells are present in a serum sample, minute amounts of the HIV RNA are amplified by these methods in sufficient quantities to be detected. Such tests are useful in the clinical management of disease and in diagnosing HIV infection in people who have no other indication of infection. Limitations of viral load testing include cost and local availability of the gene amplification assays.

Other Laboratory Tests. Other laboratory tests establish and monitor the overall condition of the client and detect or diagnose any infections or secondary clinical processes. Standard tests include blood chemistries, CBC with differential and platelets, prothrombin time and partial thromboplastin time, serologic test for syphilis (STS), hepatitis B surface antigen, and immunoglobulin levels. Tests to evaluate further the immune profile of a client include skin testing for delayed hypersensitivity and bone marrow aspiration with biopsy and cultures.

➤ *Other Diagnostic Assessment*

On the basis of the clinical symptoms with which the client presents, other diagnostic tests are chosen, including stool for ova and parasites; biopsies of skin, lymph nodes, lungs, liver, gastrointestinal tract, or brain; chest x-ray film; gallium scans; bronchoscopy, endoscopy, or colonoscopy; liver and spleen scans; computed tomography scans; pulmonary function tests; and arterial blood gas analysis.

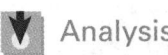 Analysis

➤ *Common Nursing Diagnoses and Collaborative Problems*

The most common nursing diagnoses relevant to the client with AIDS are

1. Impaired Gas Exchange related to anemia, respiratory infection or malignancy (PCP, CMV pneumonitis, pulmonary KS, and/or *Mycobacteria* infection), anemia, fatigue, or pain

2. Altered Nutrition: Less than Body Requirements related to high metabolic need, nausea/vomiting, diarrhea, difficulty chewing or swallowing, anorexia
3. Diarrhea related to infection, food intolerance, medications
4. Impaired Skin Integrity related to KS, infection, altered nutritional state, incontinence, immobility, hyperthermia, malignancy
5. Risk for Infection related to immune deficiency
6. Altered Thought Processes related to ADC, central nervous system infection, or malignancy
7. Self-Esteem Disturbance related to changes in body image changes, decreased self-esteem, and helplessness
8. Social Isolation related to stigma, virus transmissibility, infection control practices, and fear

The primary collaborative problem is Potential for Infection.

➤ *Additional Nursing Diagnoses and Collaborative Problems*

Clients with AIDS also may present with one or more of the following additional diagnoses:

- Activity Intolerance related to fatigue, discomfort, central nervous system defect, weakness, or anemia
- Risk for Injury related to central nervous system deficit, mental status changes, depression, and thrombocytopenia
- Pain related to neuropathy, myelopathy, malignancy, or infection
- Sensory/Perceptual Alterations (Visual) related to CMV retinitis and blindness
- Sleep Pattern Disturbance related to pain, discomfort, anxiety, or depression
- Ineffective Individual Coping related to the diagnosis of AIDS
- Ineffective Family/Significant Other Coping related to the diagnosis of AIDS
- Anticipatory Grieving related to potential loss of role and function and impending death

 Planning and Implementation

➤ *Impaired Gas Exchange*

Planning: Expected Outcomes. The client is expected to

- Maintain adequate oxygenation and perfusion
- Experience minimal dyspnea and discomfort

Interventions. As outlined in the clinical pathway, the nurse, respiratory therapist, or assistive personnel provides interventions, including drug therapy, respiratory support and maintenance, comfort, and rest.

Drug Therapy. Appropriate drug therapy is initiated after identification of an infectious or neoplastic cause for respiratory difficulty (Chart 25–3). One of the two treatments of choice for PCP is trimethoprim-sulfamethoxazole (Apo-sulfatrim♣, Bactrim, Protrin♣, Septra), given IV or orally, depending on the severity of infection. A high percentage of clients with AIDS experience adverse reac-

Chart 25–3

Drug Therapy for AIDS-Related Opportunistic Infections and Malignancies

Drug	Indication	Usual Dosage	Nursing Interventions	Rationale
Trimethoprim (TMP) and sulfamethoxazole (SMX) (Apo-sulfatrim✶, Bactrim, Protrin✶, Septra)	• *Pneumocystis carinii* pneumonia	• PO 160 mg TMP and 800 mg SMX every 12 hours	• Monitor I&O • Encourage fluids • Monitor CBC, urinalysis, bilirubin, creatinine, alkaline phosphatase. • Assess for sore throat, pallor, purpura, jaundice, weakness.	• I&O are monitored because TMP-SMX is nephrotoxic. • These values are monitored because TMP-SMX suppresses the immune system. • These signs are assessed for because TMP-SMX is hepatotoxic.
Pentamidine isethionate (Lomidine✶, Pentam)	• *P. carinii* pneumonia	• IM or IV 4 mg/kg once daily for 14–21 days	• Monitor blood pressure, heart rate, and rhythm. • Administer with client lying down. • Monitor for hypoglycemia. • Administer IV over 1 hour. • Monitor liver function, CBC.	• BP and heart rate are monitored because pentamidine causes hypotension when administered rapidly. • Monitoring is necessary because pentamidine causes severe hypoglycemia that may be fatal. • Liver function and CBC are monitored because pentamidine is hepatotoxic and immunosuppressive.
Pentamidine isethionate (Pentam, Pentarcarinate)	• *P. carinii* pneumonia	• Inhalant 300 mg every 4 weeks via nebulizer	• See above.	• See above.
Pyrimethamine (with sulfadiazine) (Daraprim)	• Toxoplasmosis	• PO 50–75 mg/day for 1–3 weeks, then 25 mg/day for 4–5 weeks	• Administer with food or milk. • Monitor CBC and platelets.	• Pyrimethamine irritates the GI tract. • The CBC and platelets are monitored because pyrimethamine suppresses bone marrow activity.
Sulfadiazine	• Toxoplasmosis • Nocardiasis	• PO 500–2000 mg daily every 6 hours for 3–4 weeks	• Monitor urine output, CBC. • Encourage fluids. • Advise client to avoid sun. • Assess for sore throat, pallor, purpura, jaundice, weakness.	• Urine output and the CBC are monitored because sulfadiazine causes renal toxicity. • Fluids are necessary because sulfadiazine suppresses bone marrow activity. • Clients should avoid the sun because sulfadiazine increases photosensitivity.
Dapsone (Avlosulfon✶, DDS)	• Toxoplasmosis	• PO 50–100 mg daily	• Monitor CBC. • Assess for fever, sore throat, purpura, jaundice.	• The CBC is monitored because dapsone suppresses bone marrow activity.

Continued

CHART 25–3. Drug Therapy for AIDS-Related Opportunistic Infections and Malignancies   Continued

Drug	Indicaton	Usual Dosage	Nursing Interventions	Rationale
Metronidazole (Flagyl, Novonidazol♣)	• Cryptosporidiosis • Giardiasis	• PO 7.5 mg/kg every 6 hours, IV 15 mg/kg initial dose, then 7.5 mg/kg every 6 hours	• Administer with food or milk. • Teach client to avoid alcohol during treatment. • Assess for dry mouth, dizziness, fungal infection.	• Food or milk is recommended because metronidazole irritates the GI tract. • Alcohol causes formation of acetaldehyde and headache, nausea, vomiting, and diarrhea.
Ketoconazole (Nizoral)	• Candidiasis • Coccidioidomycosis • Histoplasmosis	• PO 200–400 mg/day, single dose	• Administer with food or milk. • Avoid antacids for 2 hours. • Teach client to avoid sun and alcohol during treatment. • Monitor hepatic function.	• Ketoconazole irritates the GI tract. • Gastric acid is needed to activate drug. • Ketoconazole increases photosensitivity. • Hepatic function is monitored because ketoconazole is hepatotoxic.
Fluconazole (Diflucan)	• Candidiasis • Cryptococcal meningitis	• PO, IV 200–400 mg initially, then 100–200 mg daily for 2–4 weeks	• Monitor hepatic function. • Assess for abdominal pain, fever, diarrhea.	• Hepatic function is monitored because fluconazole is hepatotoxic.
Rifampin (Rifadin, Rofact♣)	• *Mycobacterium avium* complex • Tuberculosis	• PO 10 mg/kg/day	• Assess breath sounds, sputum. • Monitor hepatic function, CBC. • May turn body secretions orange.	• Assessment of breath sounds and sputum determines treatment effectiveness. • Rifampin is hepatotoxic.
Ethambutol (Myambutol, Etibi♣)	• *Mycobacterium avium-intracellulare* complex • Tuberculosis	• PO 25–30 mg/kg 2–3 times a week	• Assess vision changes. • Assess hepatic and renal function, CBC, urinalysis.	• Vision changes are assessed because ethambutol causes retrobulbar neuritis and decreased visual acuity (reversible). • This assessment is necessary because ethambutol increases uric acid concentrations. • Ethambutol suppresses bone marrow activity.
Amphotericin B (Fungizone)	• Candidiasis • Other fungal infections	• IV 0.3–1 mg/kg/day, maximum 50 mg/day	• Assess renal function. • Assess infusion site. • Assess CBC.	• Renal function is assessed because amphotericin B is nephrotoxic. • Amphotericin B causes thrombophlebitis. • The CBC is checked because amphotericin B suppresses bone marrow activity. • Amphotericin B is *very* toxic.

Continued

CHART 25–3. Drug Therapy for AIDS-Related Opportunistic Infections and Malignancies Continued

Drug	Indicaton	Usual Dosage	Nursing Interventions	Rationale
Ciprofloxacin (Cipro)	• *Mycobacterium avium-intracellulare complex* • Urinary tract infections	• PO 250–750 mg every 12 hours, IV 200–400 mg every 12 hours	• Monitor I&O. • Encourage fluids. • Administer on empty stomach (1 hour before or 2 hours after meals) if tolerated. • Teach client to avoid sun. • Assess for dizziness, fungal infection. • Infuse over 1 hour.	• An empty stomach is recommended for best absorption. • Clients should avoid the sun because ciprofloxacin increases photosensitivity.
Clofazimine (Lamprene)	• *Mycobacterium avium-intracellulare complex*	• PO 50–300 mg every day	• Assess vision changes, dizziness, drowsiness. • Instruct client to avoid sun. • Use lotions for dry skin. • Monitor hepatic and renal function.	• Vision changes and dizziness are assessed because clofazimine increases sedation. • Clofazimine increases photosensitivity (especially of eyes). • Clients should use lotions because clofazimine causes dry, scaly skin.
Pyrazinamide (Tebrazid❦)	• Tuberculosis	• PO 20–30 mg/kg/day	• Monitor hepatic function, uric acid. • Assess temperature every 4 hours.	• Pyrazinamide is hepatotoxic and increases uric acid concentration. • The client's temperature is assessed because pyrazinamide stimulates fever.
Isoniazid (Laniazid, Isotamine)	• Tuberculosis	• PO, IM 5–10 mg/kg/day or 15 mg/kg 2–3 times a week	• Administer on empty stomach. • Monitor hepatic function. • Assess for vision changes. • Instruct client to avoid alcohol and tyramine-containing foods.	• Taking isoniazid on an empty stomach enhances absorption. • Isoniazid is hepatotoxic. • Vision changes are assessed because isoniazid is neurotoxic. • Isoniazid is an MAO inhibitor.
Ganciclovir (Cytovene)	• Cytomegalovirus retinitis • PO 1000 mg every 8 hr	• IV 5 mg/kg every 12 hours for 14–21 days	• Monitor neutrophil and platelet count. • Infuse over 1 hour. • Give with food.	• Neutrophil and platelet counts are monitored because ganciclovir suppresses bone marrow activity.
Acyclovir (Zovirax)	• Herpes simplex • Herpes zoster • Varicella zoster	• PO 200–800 mg 5 times a day, IV 5–10 mg/kg every 8 hours for 7–10 days	• Monitor renal function. • Encourage fluids. • Rotate infusion site.	• Acyclovir is nephrotoxic. • Various infusion sites are used because acyclovir is a blood vessel irritant.

Continued

CHART 25–3. Drug Therapy for AIDS-Related Opportunistic Infections and Malignancies Continued

Drug	Indication	Usual Dosage	Nursing Interventions	Rationale
Zidovudine (Retrovir)	• HIV seropositivity	• PO 100–200 mg every 4 hours	• Must be administered around the clock. • Assess for dizziness. • Monitor CBC, hepatic and renal function.	• Zidovudine is given around the clock for maximum antiviral effect. • Dizziness is assessed because zidovudine crosses the blood-brain barrier. • Zidovudine suppresses bone marrow activity. • Zidovudine is hepatotoxic. • Zidovudine is nephrotoxic.
Didanosine (Videx)	• HIV seropositivity	• PO 125–300 mg every 12 hours	• Administer on empty stomach. • Instruct client to chew tablet or crush. • Monitor for dizziness, neuropathy, pancreatitis.	• Taking didanosine on an empty stomach enhances absorption. • Didanosine crosses the blood-brain barrier.
Zalcitabine (ddC)	• HIV seropositivity	• PO 0.75 mg every 8 hours (with AZT)	• Monitor liver function. • Given with AZT.	• This can cause serious liver damage. • Combination of ddC and AZT acts synergistically.
Lamivudine (Epivir, 3TC✤)	• HIV seropositivity • Prophylaxis—occupational exposure	• PO 150 mg tid	• Teach client to avoid fatty foods.	• This can cause severe pancreatitis.
Stavudine (d4T, Zerit)	• HIV seropositivity	• PO 40 mg bid	• Observe client's gait. Ask about paresthesia.	• This can cause severe peripheral neuropathy.
Ritonavir (Norvir)	• HIV seropositivity	• PO 600 mg bid	• Administer 1 hour before or 2 hours after meals. • Monitor triglyceride levels.	• Ritonavir is absorbed best in fasting state. • This can increase triglyceride levels.
Saquinavir (Invirase)	• HIV seropositivity	• PO 600 mg every 8 hours	• Administer with meals. • Warn client to avoid sun exposure.	• Saquinavir is absorbed best with a high-calorie, high-fat meal. • Saquinavir increases photosensitivity.
Interferon-alpha$_{2b}$	• Kaposi's sarcoma	• IM, SC 30 million IU/m² three times weekly	• Monitor vital signs, cardiac status. • Assess for bleeding, low-grade fever, malaise, muscle aches, headache, chills, infection, nausea.	• Vital signs and cardiac status are monitored because interferon-alpha$_{2b}$ poses a danger of hyperviscosity. • Interferon-alpha$_{2b}$ causes malaise and flu-like symptoms.

AIDS = acquired immunodeficiency syndrome; I&O = input and output; HIV = human immunodeficiency virus; CBC = complete blood count; MAO = monoamine oxidase; GI = gastrointestinal.

tions to this medication, including nausea, vomiting, hyponatremia, rashes, fever, leukopenia, thrombocytopenia, and hepatitis.

The second drug of choice is pentamidine isethionate (Lomidine✤, Pentam), usually given IV or intramuscularly (IM). Aerosolized pentamidine isethionate is used prophylactically in those with T4 counts below 200 and in those who have already had PCP.

Respiratory Support and Maintenance. The client also needs appropriate care to maintain respiratory function and avoid complications. The nurse, respiratory therapist, or assistive personnel assesses the client's respiratory rate, rhythm, and depth, breath sounds, and vital signs and monitors for cyanosis at least every 8 hours. The nurse applies and maintains oxygen therapy and room humidification, as ordered. In addition, the nurse monitors mechanical ventilation, performs suctioning and chest physical therapy as needed, and evaluates blood gas results.

Comfort. The nurse or assistive nursing personnel assesses the client's comfort. The client with respiratory difficulties often is more comfortable with the head of the bed elevated. The nurse helps the client pace activities to minimize shortness of breath and exhaustion. The nurse provides the patient with psychological support during periods of respiratory distress.

Rest and Activity. The nurse consults with the client to pace client activities to conserve energy. The nurse guides the client in active and passive range of motion (ROM) exercises, scheduling them and activities such as bathing so the client is not fatigued at mealtime.

➤ Altered Nutrition: Less Than Body Requirements

Many clients with AIDS have difficulty maintaining their weight and nutritional status. This problem may be associated with fatigue, anorexia, nausea and vomiting, difficult or painful swallowing, diarrhea, or wasting syndrome.

Planning: Expected Outcomes. The client is expected to maintain optimum weight through adequate nutrition and hydration.

Interventions. Because there are multiple factors for alterations in nutrition in AIDS, diagnostic procedures are undertaken to determine the cause. Once the cause is determined, appropriate therapy is initiated. For example, in the client who has candidal esophagitis, nutrition is affected because of the client's difficulty in swallowing.

Drug Therapy. Therapy can include ketoconazole (Nizoral) or fluconazole (Diflucan) orally, or IV amphotericin B (Fungizone). The nurse administers the medication as ordered and monitors the client for side effects such as nausea and vomiting, which further compromise nutritional status. The nurse provides mouth care and ice chips, and keeps unpleasant odors out of the client's environment. Antiemetics are used as ordered.

Diet Therapy. The nurse monitors the client's weight, intake and output, and calorie count. The nurse assesses the client's food preferences and any dietary cultural or religious practices. The nurse also instructs the client in a high-calorie, high-protein, low-microbial, nutritionally sound diet (see Chap. 42). In collaboration with the dietitian, the nurse provides an appropriate diet for the client, including small, frequent meals (better tolerated than large meals). Supplemental vitamins and fluids are indicated in some cases. For the client who cannot achieve adequate nutrition through food, tube feedings or total parenteral nutrition may be needed.

Mouth Care. For clients susceptible to oral ulceration or infection, the nurse or nursing staff member provides meticulous mouth care. Rinses of sodium bicarbonate with normal saline every 2 hours or several times a day are helpful. The client is given a soft toothbrush and advised to drink plenty of fluids. For oral pain that interferes with the client's ability to eat, analgesics or viscous lidocaine may be necessary.

➤ Diarrhea

Clients with AIDS frequently suffer from diarrhea. Sometimes an infectious cause (e.g., *Giardia* or *Amoeba*) can be determined and treated, or the cause is determined but no effective therapy is available, as in cryptosporidiosis or CMV colitis. In some cases, clients with AIDS have diarrhea and no infectious cause can be identified.

Planning: Expected Outcomes. The client is expected to

- Experience decreased diarrhea
- Maintain fluid, electrolyte, and nutritional status
- Minimize incontinence

Interventions. For most clients with AIDS and diarrhea, symptomatic management is all that is available. Antidiarrheals, such as diphenoxylate hydrochloride (Diarsed✚, Lomotil), given on a regular schedule, provide the client some degree of relief. In collaboration with the dietitian, the nurse offers dietary counseling and appropriate foods. Recommended dietary changes include less roughage; less fatty, spicy, and sweet foods; and no alcohol or caffeine. Some clients experience symptomatic relief if they eliminate dairy products from the diet or eat smaller amounts of food more often and drink plenty of fluids, especially between meals.

The nurse or assistive personnel provides the client a bedside commode or a bedpan if needed. Some clients cannot reach the bathroom in time because of immobility or anal sphincter weakness, others because of the urgency to defecate. The nurse provides privacy, support, and understanding.

➤ Impaired Skin Integrity

The most common skin lesion in AIDS is Kaposi's sarcoma (KS). Cutaneous involvement may be localized or disseminated. Large lesions can cause pain and restrict movement or ambulation. They can impede circulation, causing open, weeping, painful lesions. Another cause of impaired skin integrity is HSV infection.

Planning: Expected Outcomes. The client is expected to

- Experience healing of any existing lesions
- Avoid increased skin breakdown or secondary infection

Interventions. KS can be treated locally with radiotherapy, intralesional chemotherapy, or cryotherapy. KS responds to local radiation therapy but only transiently. Systemic therapy is used in clients with rapidly progressive disease or with significant involvement of the gastrointestinal tract, lungs, or other organs. These therapies include chemotherapy (single agent or combination), interferon-alpha, and interferon-alpha–zidovudine combinations.

Treatment of painful KS lesions includes the use of analgesics and comfort measures. Open, weeping KS lesions must be kept clean and dressed to minimize the risk of secondary infection. Many clients with cutaneous KS are concerned about their appearance and the risk of being identified as HIV-positive. Make-up (if open lesions are not present), long-sleeved shirts, and hats may help the client maintain a normal appearance.

For the client with an HSV abscess, the nurse provides meticulous skin care. The nurse or assistive personnel cleans the abscess regularly with a diluted solution of povidone-iodine (Betadine) and leaves it to air-dry or exposes it to a heat lamp. This infection can be painful and necessitates analgesics, assistance with position, and other comfort measures. Modified Burow's solution (Domeboro) soaks help to promote healing for some clients. HSV infection is treated with acyclovir (Zovirax) given IV, orally, or, in some cases, topically, depending on the severity of the infection.

➤ Risk for Infection

The client with AIDS is susceptible to opportunistic infections because of immunodeficiency secondary to HIV infection.

Planning: Expected Outcomes. The client is expected to remain free of opportunistic diseases.

Interventions. Several strategies can help the client minimize the chances of acquiring an infection. Some strategies are investigational, including drug therapy and immune function enhancement.

Drug Therapy. Chart 25–3 lists treatments for opportunistic infections and neoplasms. Several experimental medications have demonstrated antiretroviral effects in vitro and in animal studies. New regimens, called "cocktails," consisting of combinations of antiretroviral agents and protease inhibitors, are showing good results in reducing viral load and improving T4 lymphocyte counts.

Nucleoside Analogs. Zidovudine, or AZT (Retrovir), is an antiviral medication given orally or IV; the usual dose is 200 mg orally every 4 hours. Side effects include a potentially severe macrocytic anemia that often necessitates regular transfusions, mild headache, nausea, abdominal pain, diarrhea, and, less commonly, changes in WBC count or liver function tests. Didanosine, or ddI (Videx), is an antiviral used for persons who are unable to tolerate zidovudine or who have had continued loss of immune function despite AZT therapy. Two potential side effects are pancreatitis and peripheral neuropathy. Zalcitabine (ddC) is used in combination with AZT for those whose CD4+ count drops below 300 despite AZT treatment. Stavudine (d4T, Zerit) is used for those with CD4+ counts below 300 who are unable to tolerate AZT or ddI or for whom these drugs are ineffective. Lamivudine (3TC✦, Epivir) is used prophylactically after occupational exposure to HIV. It also is used in combination with either AZT or a

protease inhibitor for treatment of AIDS. The most common side effect for zalcitabine, stavudine, and lamivudine is peripheral neuropathy.

Protease Inhibitors. The newest drugs against HIV are the protease inhibitors, which block the HIV protease enzyme, preventing viral replication and release of viral particles. In recent studies, ritonavir (Norvir) reduced the viral load, slowed disease progression, and reduced the death rate in persons with AIDS. Potential side effects include diarrhea, nausea, vomiting, fatigue, and tingling around the mouth. Clinical benefits of other protease inhibitors, including indinavir (Crixivan) and saquinavir (Invirase), are under investigation. All three current protease inhibitors have fewer side effects than the nucleoside analogs but have shown rapid resistance (Bechtel-Boenning, 1996). Additionally, the protease inhibitors are extremely expensive; costs average more than $15,000 per client per year (McKinnon, 1996).

Immune Enhancement. Research is also being conducted to evaluate modalities that may enhance or reconstitute the immune system of clients who are made immunodeficient by HIV infection. Some of these methods include bone marrow transplantation, lymphocyte transfusion, and administration of lymphokines, particularly interleukin-2, and other biologic response modifiers (Ungvarsky, 1997).

Complementary Therapies. Complementary therapies to increase immune function are frequently used by people with HIV/AIDS (see Research Applications for Nursing). Such therapies include vitamins, shark cartilage, and botanical products available at health food stores. The clinical usefulness of these products has yet to be established through well-controlled clinical trials.

Health Promotion. HIV can remain latent inside a cell for long periods and cause active infection when the cell is stimulated. The specific signals for the cell to become activated are not known, but concurrent viral or parasitic infections are suspected. The nurse teaches the client to avoid exposure to infection.

➤ Altered Thought Processes

Neurologic changes and alterations in thought processes are major areas of concern for clients with AIDS. These changes may be due to psychological stressors accompanying the disease or to organic disorders caused by opportunistic infections, cancer, or HIV encephalitis.

Planning: Expected Outcomes. The client is expected to

- Demonstrate improved mental status
- Sustain no injury

Interventions. Clients with AIDS suffer from enormous loss and psychological stress, which complicate the assessment of any changes in behavior or affect. The nurse or assistive personnel establishes baseline neurologic and mental status by using neurologic assessment tools (see Chap. 43) to compare any changes. Subtle changes in memory, ability to concentrate, affect, and behavior are evaluated. Differential diagnosis is important

► Research Applications for Nursing

People with HIV Use Alternative Therapies

Nokes, K. M., Kendrew, J., & Longo, M. (1995). Alternative/complementary therapies used by persons with HIV disease. Journal of the Association of Nurses in AIDS Care, 6(4), 19–24.

The purpose of this descriptive study was to determine the types and frequency of use of alternative or complementary therapies by persons with HIV. The investigators developed an instrument that consisted of 55 alternative therapies based on a review of the literature and interviews with persons with HIV and experts in alternative therapies. Participants were asked to identify their familiarity with each therapy and how often they used it, if at all. A convenience sample of 145 persons with HIV, recruited from both inpatient and outpatient settings in two major cities, participated in the study. Participants were primarily young, Caucasian men whose HIV-related risk behavior was either male-to-male sex or bisexual sex. Each of the identified therapies on the questionnaire was used by at least one respondent. The five most frequently used alternative therapies were vitamins, relaxation, humor, spirituality, and meditation.

Critique. Content validity for the instrument was established through the literature, the input of content experts, and the population of interest. Reliability was established in this sample, with a Cronbach's alpha of .74. The use of a convenience sample and the demographics of the participants limit the generalizability of findings.

Possible Nursing Implications. Nurses caring for persons with HIV should include questions about alternative or complementary therapies in their assessments. They should also be familiar with the types of alternative therapies and understand each. This is necessary to teach the client about potential interactions between standard treatments and alternative therapies and to incorporate appropriate alternative therapies into the client's plan of care.

to determine whether the cause of the neurologic changes is treatable.

Orientation. The nurse reorients the confused client to person, time, and place as needed, reminding the client of the nurse's identity and explaining what is to be done at any given time. Using calendars, clocks, and radios and putting the bed close to a window also may help keep the client oriented. The nurse gives simple directions; uses short, uncomplicated sentences; explains activities in simple language; and involves the client in planning the daily schedule. Relatives or significant others are asked to bring in familiar items from home, and all items in the client's environment are arranged in the same location as at home.

Drug Therapy. Chart 25–3 lists agents appropriate for different conditions contributing to altered thought processes in the person with AIDS.

Safety Measures. Attention to safety is crucial to the well-being of the neurologically impaired client with AIDS. The client may not be aware of activities or surroundings, and may need assistance with bathing, dressing, eating, ambulating, and other activities of daily living. The environment, whether a hospital room, long-term care facility, or home, is made safe and comfortable. Some clients are prone to seizures. The nurse or assistive nursing personnel institutes seizure precautions, including using padded side rails and having an airway available. Anticonvulsants may be added to the client's medications.

The nurse assesses the client with neurologic disease for signs and symptoms of increased intracranial pressure. The nurse immediately reports any changes in level of consciousness, vital signs, pupil size or reactivity, or limb strength to the physician for appropriate intervention. Some clients are given corticosteroids to reduce intracranial pressure.

Support. The nurse and assistive personnel work closely with the family and significant others of the neurologically impaired client. There is great trauma in seeing a loved one unable to care for him- or herself or demonstrating unusual or child-like behavior. The nurse answers questions honestly and sensitively and teaches the family and significant others how to reorient the client. They are encouraged to continue to provide the client with news of family happenings or current events. The nurse, in collaboration with the social worker, identifies community resources for the client and family.

► Self-Esteem Disturbance

The client with AIDS is susceptible to changes in self-esteem and self-concept. Contributing to this are real and often dramatic changes in appearance that alter the person's body image. Many clients also experience abrupt, significant changes in their relationships with others and in day-to-day activities, including a job or other productive activities. All changes can disrupt the client's self-concept.

Planning: Expected Outcomes. The client is expected to
- Identify positive aspects of him- or herself
- Accept him- or herself

Interventions. The nurse and other members of the health care team provide a climate of acceptance for clients with AIDS by promoting a trusting relationship and helping clients express feelings and identify positive aspects of themselves. The nurse allows for client privacy but does not avoid or isolate the client. The nurse encourages the client's self-care, independence, control, and decision making, helping the client formulate short-term, attainable goals and offering encouragement and praise when achieved.

Complementary therapy in the form of guided imagery is used by many clients to increase their sense of control and enhance self-esteem. Imagery can focus on helping clients cope with distressing side effects or painful procedures. Other uses of imagery include picturing battle scenes in which the virus is killed by immune system cells.

► Social Isolation

Many clients with AIDS face discrimination, rejection, and isolation. Friends or health care workers sometimes avoid or refuse to have anything to do with these clients. Misunderstanding and fear lead to misuse of proper infection control procedures, and clients are inappropriately isolated.

Planning: Expected Outcomes. The client is expected to

- Identify behaviors that cause social isolation
- Demonstrate behaviors that reduce social isolation

Interventions. Interventions for social isolation focus on promoting interactions and on education to reduce fear of AIDS transmission.

Promotion of Interaction. The nurse does not isolate the client but establishes a therapeutic nurse–client relationship. The nurse shows understanding and concern while helping the client find ways to minimize feelings of rejection and isolation. The nurse reduces barriers to social contact for the client. Client social support resources are assessed. Family and significant others are taught about HIV transmission and use of Standard Precautions to reduce anxiety and increase contact with the client (see Chap. 28).

The nurse encourages the client to verbalize feelings about self, coping skills, and sense of ability to control the situation. The nurse helps the client identify support systems, including those already in place and those that need to be arranged.

Education. The most important aspect for prevention of HIV transmission is education. All people, regardless of age, sex, ethnicity, or sexual orientation, are susceptible to HIV infection. Because of the mode of viral transmission and the fragile nature of the virus, AIDS is a preventable disease.

HIV has been isolated from multiple body secretions and tissues, including blood, semen, vaginal secretions, breast milk, amniotic fluid, urine, feces, saliva, tears, cerebrospinal fluid, lymph nodes, cervical cells, Langerhans' cells, corneal tissue, and brain tissue. HIV is primarily transmitted in three ways:

- Sexual: genital, anal, or oral sexual contact with exposure of mucous membranes to infected semen or vaginal secretions
- Parenteral: sharing needles contaminated with infected blood or receiving contaminated blood products
- Perinatal: from the placenta, from contact with maternal blood and body fluids during birth, or from breast milk from an infected mother to child

HIV infection is not transmitted by casual contact in the home, school, or workplace. Studies of persons sharing household utensils, towels and linens, and toilet facilities in crowded households showed no evidence of HIV transmission (Friedland et al., 1990). Transmission by insect vectors is "highly improbable" (Gershon et al., 1990).

Sexual Transmission. Abstinence and mutually monogamous sex with a noninfected partner are the only absolutely safe methods of preventing HIV infection through sexual contact. However, this may not be feasible for personal, cultural, and economic factors.

Safer sex practices are those that reduce the risk of

| **Chart 25–4** |

Health Promotion Guide: Condom Use to Prevent Sexually Transmitted Diseases

- Use latex condoms rather than natural membrane condoms.
- Store condoms in a cool, dry place.
- Do not use condoms that were in damaged packages or those that show signs of age, such as those that are brittle, sticky, or discolored.
- Handle condoms carefully to avoid puncturing them.
- Put a condom on before making any genital contact. Hold the tip of the condom and unroll it onto the erect penis, making sure that no air is trapped in the tip. Leave space at the tip to collect semen.
- Use adequate lubrication. Use water-based lubricants only. Petroleum or oil-based lubricants such as petroleum jelly, cooking oil, shortening, and lotions can damage the condom.
- Using a spermicide-lubricated condom or additional spermicide can provide additional protection against sexually transmitted diseases.
- Replace a broken condom immediately. If ejaculation occurs after the condom breaks, there may be some protection in the immediate use of a spermicide.
- After ejaculation, the condom must remain on until the penis is withdrawn. While the penis is still erect, hold the condom against the base of the penis while withdrawing.
- Never reuse condoms.

From Centers for Disease Control. (1988). Condoms for prevention of sexually transmitted diseases. *Morbidity and Mortality Weekly Report, 37*(9), 133–137.

---

nonintact skin or mucous membranes coming in contact with potentially infected body fluids and blood (Chart 25–4). Such practices include using

- A latex condom and spermicide containing nonoxynol 9 for genital and anal intercourse
- A condom or latex barrier (dental dam) over the genitals or anus during oral-genital or oral-anal sexual contact
- Latex gloves for finger or hand contact with the vagina or rectum

Parenteral Transmission. Preventive practices to reduce parenteral transmission among IV drug users include the use of proper cleaning of "works" (needles, syringes, and other drug paraphernalia). Clients are instructed to clean a used needle and syringe by first filling and flushing with clear water. Next, the syringe should be filled with ordinary household bleach. The bleach-filled syringe should be shaken for 30 to 60 seconds. Drug users are advised to carry a small container with this solution whenever sharing needles. Some communities have a needle exchange program, in which needles and syringes are used only once and exchanged for clean ones.

The risk of AIDS transmission through blood and blood products has been reduced to a national average of 0.02%. Several measures have been implemented to protect the nation's blood supply. All donated blood in

North America is screened for the HIV antibody, and blood that reacts positively is discarded. However, current tests detect the antibody, not the virus itself. Because of time lag in antibody production (seroconversion) after exposure to HIV, infected blood can test negative for HIV antibodies. False-negative results also can occur. The small but real possibility of HIV transmission through blood and blood products has resulted in more stringent indications for transfusion and an increase in autologous transfusion.

Perinatal Transmission. The risk of perinatal transmission in pregnant clients with AIDS has been reported at 14% to 45% for each pregnancy. Studies have shown that pregnant women who received zidovudine had an 8.3% perinatal transmission rate compared with 25.5% in women who received a placebo (National Institute of Allergy and Infectious Disease, 1994). HIV transmission is thought to occur transplacentally in utero, intrapartally during exposure to blood and vaginal secretions during birth, or postpartally through breast milk. Women of childbearing age with HIV infection should be fully informed of the risks of perinatal transmission.

Transmission and Health Care Workers. Needlestick injuries are the primary means of HIV infection for health care workers. In addition, health care workers can be infected through exposure of nonintact skin and mucous membranes to blood and body fluids. Because there is a time lag between the time of infection with HIV and the pro-

---

Chart 25-5

Health Promotion Guide: CDC Recommendations for Human Immunodeficiency Virus (HIV) Testing

You should be tested for AIDS if you fall within one or more of the following groups:

- People with sexually transmitted disease
- Intravenous drug abusers
- People who consider themselves at risk
- Women of childbearing age with identifiable risks, including
  - Having used IV drugs
  - Having engaged in prostitution
  - Having had sexual partners who were infected or at risk
  - Having had contact with men from countries with high HIV prevalence
  - Having received a transfusion between 1978 and 1985
- People planning to get married
- People undergoing medical evaluation or treatment for signs and symptoms that may be HIV-related
- People admitted to hospitals
- People in correctional institutions such as jails and prisons
- Prostitutes and their customers

Modified from Centers for Disease Control. (1987). Public Health Service guidelines for counseling and antibody testing to prevent HIV infection and AIDS. *Morbidity and Mortality Weekly Report, 36*(31), 509–515.

TABLE 25-5

Recommendations for Preventing Human Immunodeficiency Virus by Health Care Workers

- Workers should adhere to Standard Precautions.
- Workers with exudative lesions or weeping dermatitis should not perform direct patient care or handle patient care equipment and devices used in invasive procedures.
- Workers must follow guidelines for disinfection and sterilization of reusable equipment used in invasive procedures.
- Workers infected with HIV are not restricted from practice of non-exposure–prone procedures, provided that they comply with Standard Precautions and sterilization/disinfection recommendations.
- Workers should identify exposure-prone procedures by institutions where they are performed.
- Workers who perform exposure-prone procedures should know their HIV antibody status.
- Workers who are infected with HIV should seek advice from an expert review panel before performing exposure-prone procedures to determine under what circumstances they may continue to practice these procedures. These circumstances would include notification of prospective clients of HIV positivity.

Adapted from Centers for Disease Control. (1991b). Recommendations for preventing transmission of human immunodeficiency virus and hepatitis B virus to patients during exposure-prone invasive procedures. *Morbidity and Mortality Weekly Report, 40*(RR-8), 1–9.

---

duction of serum antibodies (seroconversion), infected people can test negative for HIV and yet still transmit the virus. Therefore, the best prevention for health care providers is the scrupulous and consistent application of Standard Precautions for all clients as recommended by the Centers for Disease Control and Prevention (CDC) (see Chap. 28).

Reports of possible HIV transmission by a dentist during invasive dental procedures have alarmed the public about HIV transmission by health care workers. It is recommended that HIV-infected health care workers wear gloves when in contact with clients' nonintact skin or mucous membranes. Infected workers with weeping dermatitis or exudative lesions should not perform direct care activities. The CDC (1991) also has issued recommendations for preventing HIV transmission by health care workers during exposure-prone invasive procedures. These include any procedure in which there is a risk of percutaneous injury to the health care worker and the worker's blood is likely to make contact with the patient's body cavity, subcutaneous tissues, or mucous membranes. These recommendations aim to reduce the risk of HIV transmission to clients (Table 25-5).

Testing. Testing plays a role in prevention, because those who test positive can be educated and encouraged to modify their behaviors to prevent transmission to others. The CDC has issued recommendations describing who should be advised to seek HIV antibody testing (Chart 25-5). Pre- and post-test counseling must be performed

Chart 25–6

Education Guide: Recommendations for HIV-Positive People

- Seek regular medical evaluation and follow-up.
- Either avoid sexual activity or inform your prospective partner of your antibody test results and protect him or her from contact with your body fluids during sex. "Body fluids" include blood, semen, urine, feces, saliva, and women's genital secretions. Use a condom and avoid practices that may injure body tissues (e.g., anal intercourse). Avoid oral-genital contact and open-mouthed, intimate kissing.
- Inform your present and previous sex partners, and any persons with whom needles may have been shared, of their potential exposure to HIV and encourage them to seek counseling and antibody testing from their physicians or at appropriate health clinics.
- Don't share toothbrushes, razors, or other items that could become contaminated with blood.
- If you use drugs, enroll in a drug treatment program. Needles and other drug equipment must never be shared.
- Do not donate blood, plasma, body organs, other body tissue, or sperm.
- Clean blood or other body fluid spills on household or other surfaces with freshly diluted household bleach: 1 part bleach to 10 parts water. (Do not use bleach on wounds.)
- Inform your physician, dentist, and eye doctor of your positive HIV status so that proper precautions can be taken to protect you and others.
- Women with a positive antibody test should avoid pregnancy until more is known about the risks of transmitting HIV from mother to infant.

by appropriately trained personnel. Counseling helps the client make an informed decision about testing and provides an opportunity to teach the client risk-reduction behaviors. Post-test counseling is needed to interpret the results, discuss risk reduction, and provide psychological support and health promotion information for the client with a positive test result.

Recommendations for people who have had positive test results for antibody to HIV are presented in Chart 25–6. People who test positive should also be counseled on how to inform sexual partners and those with whom they have shared needles.

➤ Continuing Care

The usual course of illness is one of intermittent acute infections interspersed with periods of relative wellness over months or years and, ultimately, a chronic, progressive debilitation. Because of the fluctuating nature of HIV infection, the client often spends long periods at home between hospital admissions or clinic visits. In some instances, especially as the illness becomes more severe, the client may need referral to a long-term care facility, home health care agency, or hospice.

The nurse, in collaboration with the social worker, di-

etitian, and other available resources, works with clients to plan what will be needed and how they will manage at home with self-care and activities of daily living.

➤ Health Teaching

Educating the client, family, and significant others is a high priority, especially when preparing the client for discharge. The nurse instructs the client about modes of transmission and preventive behaviors (safer sex guidelines; not sharing toothbrushes, razors, and other potentially blood-contaminated articles). Caregivers also need instruction about infection control precautions to prevent transmission while caring for the client in the home (Chart 25–7), nursing techniques to use in the home, and coping and support strategies.

Chart 25–7

Education Guide: Infection Control for Home Care of the Person with AIDS

Direct Care
- Follow Standard Precautions and good handwashing techniques.
- Do not share razors or toothbrushes.

Housekeeping
- Wipe up feces, vomitus, sputum, urine, or blood or other body fluids and the area with soap and water. Dispose of solid wastes and solutions used for cleaning by flushing them down the toilet. Disinfect the area by wiping with a 1:10 solution of household bleach (1 part bleach to 10 parts water). Wear gloves during cleaning.
- Soak rags, mops, and sponges used for cleaning in a 1:10 bleach solution for 5 minutes to disinfect them.
- Wash dishes and eating utensils in hot water and dishwashing soap or detergent.
- Clean bathroom surfaces with regular household cleaners, then disinfect them with a 1:10 solution of household bleach.

Laundry
- Rinse clothes, towels, or bedclothes if they become soiled with feces, vomitus, sputum, urine, or blood. Then dispose of the soiled water by flushing it down the toilet. Launder these clothes with hot water and detergent with one cup of bleach added per load of laundry.
- Keep soiled clothes in a plastic bag.

Waste Disposal
- Dispose of needles and other "sharps" in a labeled puncture-proof container such as a coffee can with a lid, using Standard Precautions to avoid needlestick injuries. Decontaminate full containers by adding a 1:10 bleach solution. Then seal the container with tape and place it in a paper bag. Dispose of the container in the regular trash.
- Remove solid waste from contaminated trash such as paper towels or tissues, dressings, disposable incontinence pads, and disposable gloves, then flush the waste down the toilet. Place these items in tied plastic bags and dispose of them in the regular trash.

The nurse teaches the client, family, and significant others how to protect the client from infection, how to identify signs and symptoms of potential infections, and what to do if these appear. The nurse instructs the client about the importance of self-care strategies, such as good hygiene, balanced rest and exercise, skin care, mouth care, and safe administration of any ordered medications (including potential side effects). Dietary teaching stresses

- Good nutrition
- Avoidance of raw or rare fish, fowl, or meat
- Thorough washing of fruits and vegetables
- Proper food handling
- Refrigeration practices

The nurse also teaches the client about preventing infections by avoiding large crowds, especially in enclosed areas, not traveling to countries with poor sanitation, and not cleaning pet litter boxes.

➤ *Home Care Management*

If the client is discharged to home, the nurse carefully assesses the client's status, ability to function, and actual or potential needs for care. Some clients do not need home care but do need to maintain a link with the physician or primary care providers. Home care can range from assistance with activities of daily living for clients with weakness, debility, or limited function to around-the-clock nursing care, medications, and nutritional support for severely or terminally ill clients. The nurse assesses available resources, including family members and significant others willing and able to be caregivers. The nurse helps to make arrangements for outside caregivers or respite care, if needed. Clients may need referrals or help in planning housing, finances, insurance, legal services, funeral arrangements, and spiritual counseling.

Home health aids may be involved in daily or weekly care of the client with AIDS in the home. Usually a home care nurse makes routine visits for assessment purposes, especially as the client becomes increasingly debilitated. Chart 25–8 lists assessment areas for the client with AIDS at home.

➤ *Psychosocial Preparation*

Clients with AIDS are often concerned about the possible social stigma and rejection that they may experience. The nurse is aware that this fear is realistic, and helps the client to identify ways to avoid problems as well as coping strategies for difficult situations.

Family and significant others are supported in efforts to help the client and provide protection from discrimination.

The nurse encourages clients to continue as many usual activities as possible. Except when clients are too ill or too weak, they can continue to work and participate in most social activities. Because of potential stigma and discrimination, clients are supported in their selection of friends and relatives with whom to discuss the diagnosis. Sexual partners and care providers should be informed; beyond that, it is up to the client. Some clients experience severe depression or anxiety about the future. Almost all feel the burden of having a fatal disease widely

---

Chart 25–8

Focused Assessment for the Home Care Client with AIDS

Assess cardiovascular and respiratory status:

- Vital signs
- Presence of acute chest pain or dyspnea
- Presence of cough
- Presence of fever
- Activity tolerance

Assess nutritional status:

- Food intake
- Weight loss or gain
- General condition of skin
- Financial resources

Assess neurologic status:

- Cognitive changes
- Motor changes
- Sensory disturbances

Assess gastrointestinal status:

- Mouth and oropharynx
- Presence of dysphagia
- Presence of abdominal pain
- Presence of nausea, vomiting, diarrhea

Assess psychological status:

- Presence of anxiety
- Presence of depression

Assess activity and rest:

- Activities of daily living
- Mobility and ambulation
- Fatigue
- Sleep pattern
- Presence of pain

Assess home environment:

- Safety hazards
- Structural barriers affecting functional ability

Assess client's and caregiver's compliance and understanding of illness and treatment, including

- Signs and symptoms to report to nurse
- Medication schedule and side or toxic effects

Assess client's and caregiver's coping skills

---

considered unacceptable, and feel compelled to maintain some secrecy about the illness. Referrals to community resources, mental health professionals, and support groups can help the client verbalize fears and frustrations and cope with the illness.

➤ *Health Care Resources*

In many cities, community organizations have been set up to assist persons with AIDS. Often composed of volunteers, they offer excellent services to the community. The types and number of services vary by agency and city, but many include HIV testing and counseling, clinic services, buddy systems, support groups, respite care, education and outreach, referral services, and even housing. Clients may also need referrals to other local resources, such as home care agencies, companies that provide home IV therapy, community mental health agencies, Meals on Wheels, and others.

 Evaluation

The overall goals for care of clients with AIDS are to maintain the maximum possible level of function for as long as possible, minimize infections, and maintain quality of life and dignity during the course of progressive illness. On the basis of the identified nursing diagnoses, the nurse evaluates care for the client with AIDS. Expected outcomes include that the client should be able to

- Demonstrate adequate respiratory function
- Attain adequate weight, nutritional, and fluid status
- Maintain skin integrity
- Not develop opportunistic infections
- Remain oriented and/or in a safe environment
- Maintain self-esteem
- Maintain a support system and involvement with others
- Comply with the appropriate and available therapy

Nutrition-Related Deficiencies

Adequate and balanced nutrition is necessary for the proper functioning of the immune system. For example, lymphocytes are highly active metabolic cells that constantly shed surface components (such as immunoglobulin and marker antigens) and need nutrients to resynthesize these components. Immunodeficiency related to nutrition is an acquired abnormality and results from multiple factors—biologic, political, economic, and cultural. Acquired immunodeficiencies from inadequate or inappropriate nutrition are potentially preventable and treatable.

Malnutrition is a major cause of global immunodeficiency, seen with the greatest frequency in developing countries, in the urban and rural poor of developed countries, and in the chronically ill. Hospitalized adult medical-surgical clients also are at high risk for malnutrition. Four points should be kept in mind:

- Anorexia associated with chronic disease, acute infection, or treatment often leads to reduced oral intake.
- Absorption, assimilation, or utilization of nutrients is sometimes impaired because of gastrointestinal diseases or absorption problems.
- Host defense mechanisms mobilized in infection result in increased demand for nutrients, met at the expense of the body's stores.
- Hospitalized clients often receive a semistarvation regimen with many hours of nothing by mouth because of procedures that will be performed or because of IV fluid administration lacking essential nutrients.

Malnutrition can impair any or all aspects of the immune system; the degree of impairment is related to the severity of the malnutrition. An excess of nutrients, especially fats and certain carbohydrates, can also have a detrimental effect on immune function. Nutritional problems are almost never simple but a complex of deficiency or excess of one or multiple nutrients.

Protein-Calorie Malnutrition

Overview

Protein-calorie malnutrition (PCM) affects all aspects of the immune system. The greatest impairment is noted in cell-mediated immunity, with a decreased number of T lymphocytes, reduced delayed hypersensitivity, and thymic changes. The result is *anergy* (no cutaneous delayed hypersensitivity response to common antigens) and an increased incidence of infection. The incidence of PCM is unknown, but estimates range from 25% to 50% of hospitalized adult medical-surgical clients. PCM causes a deficiency in energy and protein synthesis, requiring that other body stores (if available) be used.

The usual manifestations of PCM in adults include

- Leanness and cachexia
- Decreased effort tolerance
- Lethargy
- Intolerance to cold
- Ankle edema
- Dry, flaking skin and various types of dermatitis
- Poor wound healing
- A higher than usual incidence of postoperative infection

Collaborative Management

The management strategy for clients with PCM is to treat the precipitating event and supply protein and calories, sometimes with nutrient supplements. In clients with severe PCM, any infection is first treated and fluid and electrolyte imbalances corrected. Then a gradual but steady repletion of protein and energy is undertaken. Often this refeeding begins parenterally, because a severely malnourished gut undergoes atrophy of the mucosa and depletion of gastric enzymes, resulting in an inability to tolerate food. Replenishment of protein and calories is accompanied by vitamin supplementation as appropriate, nutrition education, psychosocial stimulation, and a progressive increase in physical activity.

Protein-calorie malnutrition is easier to prevent than to treat. The nurse is aware of hospitalized clients at risk for PCM. To reduce this risk, the nurse

- Measures height and weight when the client is admitted to the agency, reweighing at least weekly
- Monitors the client's ability to eat the ordered diet and the amounts eaten
- Obtains dietary consultation when needed
- Evaluates whether nutrients consumed are sufficient to meet basal and stress-related energy needs
- Avoids prolonged use of standard IV fluids that provide less than 200 calories/L
- Assesses and monitors laboratory values for serum albumin, prealbumin, and leukocyte counts
- Schedules tests and procedures so that the client spends minimal time fasting

Obesity

Overview

The incidence and severity of infectious disease increase among obese people. Impaired cell-mediated immunity and decreased intracellular killing by neutrophils are associated with obesity, making obese people more susceptible to infection. Excess dietary fats have a generalized suppressive action on all aspects of immune function. In addition, the obese client may have a co-existing PCM.

Often the obese client is not recognized as malnourished because of the excessive weight. For these clients, nutritional status must be assessed by laboratory measurements and diet history.

Collaborative Management

Although more research is needed regarding the interaction between obesity and specific immune functions, appropriate nutrition is an important factor in maintaining and improving host immunologic defenses. The nurse, in consultation with the physician and dietitian, provides a diet that has sufficient calories and protein but is low in fat.

Because the obese client is somewhat immunodeficient, the nurse protects the client by maintaining a safe environment. Good hand washing is practiced before all contact with the client. All invasive procedures are conducted using strict aseptic technique. The nurse assesses the client every shift for signs and symptoms of local or systemic infection and notifies the physician of any suspected infection.

Therapy-Induced Immunodeficiencies

Overview

Some secondary immunodeficiencies may be related to other conditions that cause the loss of immunoglobulins or destruction of lymphocytes (T and B cells). The most common cause of secondary immunodeficiency is iatrogenesis, drugs, and other treatment modalities used for various diseases. Sometimes this is a desired effect, as in organ transplantation or the treatment of certain autoimmune disorders. At other times, immunosuppression is an undesirable, complicating side effect of therapy that is used for another intent, such as cancer chemotherapy, and may even necessitate altering the therapeutic regimen. Various therapies cause different types and degrees of immunosuppression. The challenge is deriving maximal therapeutic effect without leaving the client overly immunosuppressed and, therefore, susceptible to potentially serious complications.

Drug-Induced Immunodeficiencies

Several classes of drugs have powerful and significant immunosuppressive effects. Some induce general immunosuppression; others are more specific and target one part of the immune system more than another.

Cytotoxic Drugs

Cytotoxic drugs are usually not selective but interfere with all rapidly proliferating cells. White blood cells, including immunocompetent lymphocytes and phagocytes, rapidly proliferate and are, therefore, susceptible to this type of destruction (see Chaps. 23 and 27). The result is a decrease in the number of lymphocytes and phagocytic cells. Cytotoxic agents also interfere with the ability of lymphocytes to synthesize and release products such as lymphokines and antibodies, thereby causing a general immunosuppression. Most cytotoxic drugs are used to treat cancer (see Chap. 27) and autoimmune disorders.

Corticosteroids

Corticosteroids are adrenocortical hormones used to treat many immunologically mediated diseases, neoplasms, and several neurologic and endocrine disorders. Corticosteroids have both anti-inflammatory and immunosuppressive effects. They inhibit inflammation by stabilizing the vascular membrane and decreasing permeability, thereby blocking the migration and mobilization of neutrophils and monocytes. Corticosteroids disrupt the synthesis of arachidonic acid, the main precursor for a variety of vasoactive amines.

Corticosteroids sequester T cells in the bone marrow, reducing the number of circulating T cells and resulting in lymphopenia and suppressed cell-mediated immunity.

Corticosteroids appear to interfere with immunoglobulin G (IgG) synthesis and immunoglobulin binding to antigen. These drugs have many physiologic and immunologic effects, which can alter disease activity, and numerous side effects, including

- Central nervous system changes, such as euphoria, insomnia, or psychosis
- Cardiovascular changes, such as hypertension and edema
- Gastrointestinal tract effects, such as gastric irritation, ulcers, and increased appetite (with weight gain)
- Other changes, such as cataracts, hyperglycemia and glucose intolerance, muscle weakness, osteoporosis, delayed wound healing, redistribution of body fat

Cyclosporine

Cyclosporine (Sandimmune) is a specific immunosuppressant that selectively suppresses the helper subset of T lymphocytes by blocking proliferation and development (see Chap. 23). Cyclosporine has been used primarily to prevent organ transplant rejection and graft-versus-host disease (see Chaps. 42 and 75). The drug is undergoing clinical trials for use in other disorders, such as uveitis, rheumatoid arthritis, and other autoimmune diseases.

Radiation-Induced Immunodeficiency

Radiation is cytotoxic to proliferating and resting cells. Because most lymphocytes are sensitive to radiation, exposure can induce profound lymphopenia in lymphoid organs and in the circulation, causing general immunosuppression. Whether or not immunodeficiency occurs after radiation therapy depends on the location and dose of radiation. Exposure to the iliac and femur in adults can cause generalized immunosuppression because these medullary areas are the primary blood cell–producing sites. Total nodal irradiation is used in certain diseases, such as Hodgkin's disease, to induce immunosuppression, causing lymphopenia and decreased T-cell function.

Collaborative Management

Management of the client with treatment-induced immunodeficiency aims to improve immune function and protect the client from infection. The most severe immunosuppression occurs while the client is receiving the immunosuppressive drugs or during radiation treatment. The severity and duration of the immunosuppression are related directly to the dosage of specific drugs. Although this impairment is usually temporary, with good recovery of immune and inflammatory responses evident within weeks or months of therapy completion, the seriousness of the potential infection complications makes this problem a major treatment concern. The infectious processes most commonly observed during this period include those of fungal origin, yeast, some residual viral breakthrough, and a wide variety of bacteria.

The nurse works closely with the client and other health care professionals to provide safe care to clients at risk for infection. Chart 27–6 lists specific nursing care actions to prevent infection among clients with drug-induced immunosuppression. Good hand washing by the all health care professionals and unlicensed assistive personnel before contact with the client is the cornerstone for prevention of infection. Health care professionals must practice asepsis (prevention of contact with microorganisms) when any invasive technique or procedure must be done.

In some instances, drug-induced immunosuppression can be managed medically by the administration of biologic response modifiers (BRMs) to stimulate bone marrow production of immune system cells. Although not appropriate for all types of disorders, this supportive treatment can reduce the client's risk for infection during drug therapy. However, BRMs are expensive and not consistently covered by insurance. Further discussion of this treatment is presented in Chapters 27 and 42.

Many clients remain at home during periods of immunosuppression. The nurse teaches the client and family precautions to take to reduce the client's chances of developing an infection (see Chart 27–7).

For clients receiving chronic therapy with immunosuppressive drugs, drug dosages are regulated according to the client's responses. The aim is to give the lowest dose that will achieve the desired effect.

Congenital (Primary) Immunodeficiencies

Congenital, or primary, immunodeficiencies are disorders in which the immunodeficient person is born with a defect in the development or function of one or more of the

TABLE 25–6

Congenital Immunodeficiencies

Antibody-Mediated Immunodeficiencies
- X-linked agammaglobulinemia (Bruton's)
- Acquired hypogammaglobulinemia (common variable immunodeficiency)
- Selective IgA deficiency

Cell-Mediated Immunodeficiencies
- Congenital thymic aplasia (DiGeorge syndrome)
- Chronic mucocutaneous candidiasis

Combined Immunodeficiencies
- Severe combined immunodeficiencies
- Wiskott-Aldrich syndrome
- Immunodeficiency with ataxia-telangiectasia
- Nezelof syndrome

immune components. As a result, the immune response does not adequately protect the client from infection, cancer, or other disease. Fortunately, most congenital immunodeficiencies are rare.

Some congenital immunodeficiencies are inherited as an X-linked trait (such as Bruton's disease or Wiskott-Aldrich syndrome), and some are autosomal-recessive (such as immunodeficiency with ataxia-telangiectasia). For many congenital immunodeficiencies, however, the genetic defect and inheritance pattern have not been clearly identified. Examples of congenital immunodeficiencies are listed in Table 25–6.

Congenital immunodeficiencies are classified according to the type of immune function that is impaired: antibody-mediated, cell-mediated, and combined. Because cell-mediated and combined immunodeficiencies are so severe that the affected person usually does not survive infancy or childhood, only antibody-mediated immunodeficiencies (seen in adults) are discussed in this chapter.

Bruton's Agammaglobulinemia

Overview

A prototypic congenital antibody-mediated immunodeficiency is Bruton's or X-linked agammaglobulinemia. Boys born with this disease present at about 6 months of age, after the loss of maternal antibodies, with recurrent sinusitis, pneumonia, otitis, furunculosis, meningitis, and septicemia with extracellular pyogenic organisms, such as *Pneumococcus, Streptococcus,* and *Haemophilus.* Laboratory evaluation of the client with Bruton's agammaglobulinemia reveals an absence of circulating immunoglobulin.

Collaborative Management

Except for clients with poliomyelitis, chronic echovirus infection, or a lymphoreticular malignancy, the overall prognosis is fairly good if antibody replacement is begun early. IV or IM immune serum globulin is regularly given to these clients, usually about 100 to 400 mg/kg every 3 to 4 weeks (Chart 25–9). The dosage and schedule are

---

Chart 25–9

Nursing Care Highlight: Administration of Intravenous Immune Serum Globulin

Indications	Dosage	Interventions	Rationale

B cell or humoral immunodeficiencies
  Bruton's hypogammaglobulinemia
  Common variable immunodeficiency
  Combined immunodeficiencies: severe combined immunodeficiencies
Pediatric AIDS
	• Gamimune, 100–200 mg/kg or 2–4 mL/kg, IV once monthly
	or
	• Sandoglobulin, 0.2–0.3 g/kg, IV once monthly
	• Gammagard 200–400 mg/kg, IV once monthly
	• Iveegam 200–800 mg/kg, IV once monthly
		• Observe client closely and monitor vital signs during infusion and for 30–60 minutes thereafter.
		
		• Slow the rate of infusion or stop it temporarily if side effects occur.
			• Monitoring detects signs of anaphylaxis and routine side effects. Side effects occur in 10% of clients and include skeletal pain, back pain, nausea, chills, headache, chest tightness, and abdominal cramps.
			
			• Side effects appear to be related to the rate of infusion.

---

individualized. Intermittent courses of antibiotics are used for specific infections. Long-term prophylactic antibiotic therapy may also be used. Despite therapy, severe sinopulmonary disease later develops in some clients.

Common Variable Immunodeficiency

Overview

Common variable immunodeficiency, or acquired hypogammaglobulinemia, is characterized by recurrent bacterial infections similar to those seen in clients with Bruton's disease. The client has low levels of circulating immunoglobulins of all classes.

Acquired hypogammaglobulinemia differs from Bruton's disease in that it usually first appears later (in adolescence or young adulthood), occurs almost equally in males and females, and is associated with a less severe susceptibility to infection. Frequent complications include giardiasis (intestinal infection with the protozoon *Giardia lamblia*), bronchiectasis, gastric carcinoma, lymphoreticular malignancy, and cholelithiasis (gallbladder stones).

Collaborative Management

Treatment is similar to that for Bruton's disease. Regular administration of IV or IM immune serum globulin and regular or intermittent use of antibiotics protect the affected person against infection.

Selective Immunoglobulin A Deficiency

Overview

Selective immunoglobulin A (IgA) deficiency is the most common congenital immunodeficiency, occurring in 1 per 600 to 800 individuals (Cotran et al., 1994). The client may be asymptomatic or have chronic recurrent respiratory tract infections, atopic diseases, or collagen-vascular diseases. Usually, clients with selective IgA deficiency have a normal life span. Because IgA is the major immunoglobulin in secretions, bacterial infections are seen primarily in the respiratory, gastrointestinal, and urogenital tracts. Some adults with IgA deficiency also have a malabsorption syndrome.

Collaborative Management

Therapy for selective IgA deficiency is limited to appropriate and vigorous treatment of infections. Unlike other immunoglobulin deficiencies, selective IgA deficiency should never be treated with exogenous immune globulin for two reasons. First, exogenous immune globulin contains very little IgA. Second, because clients with selective IgA deficiency make normal amounts of all other classes of immunoglobulins, they are at high risk for severe allergic reactions to exogenous immune globulin. If malabsorption syndrome accompanies the selective IgA deficiency, the client will need nutritional supplementation (such as total parenteral nutrition).

HYPERSENSITIVITIES

Hypersensitivity is a state of altered reactivity in which a previously sensitized immune system reacts excessively or inappropriately, with resultant tissue damage and pathology. The primary function of the immune system is to protect the host from harm. However, the same protective mechanisms, if prolonged or excessive, have a deleterious effect and may produce tissue damage (Workman, 1995).

Immune mechanisms resulting in tissue damage to the host are classified into five basic types of hypersensitivity (Table 25–7) (Roitt, 1994):

- Type I: rapid hypersensitivity (anaphylactic) reactions
- Type II: (cytotoxic) reactions
- Type III: (immune complex–mediated) reactions
- Type IV: (delayed) hypersensitivity reactions
- Type V: (stimulatory) reactions

Clinical manifestations may be the consequence of one or any combination of these mechanisms of tissue injury.

TABLE 25-7

Mechanisms and Examples of Types of Hypersensitivities	
Mechanism	**Clinical Examples**
Type I: Immediate	
Reaction of IgE antibody on mast cells with antigen, which results in release of mediators	• Hay fever • Allergic asthma • Anaphylaxis
Type II: Cytotoxic	
Reaction of IgG with host cell membrane or antigen adsorbed by host cell membrane	• Autoimmune hemolytic anemia • Goodpasture's syndrome • Myasthenia gravis
Type III: Immune Complex–Mediated	
Formation of immune complex of antigen and antibody, which deposits in walls of blood vessels and results in complement release and inflammation	• Serum sickness • Vasculitis • Systemic lupus erythematosus • Rheumatoid arthritis
Type IV: Delayed	
Reaction of sensitized T cells with antigen and release of lymphokines, which activate macrophages and induce inflammation	• Poison ivy • Graft rejection • Tuberculosis • Sarcoidosis
Type V: Stimulated	
Reaction of autoantibodies with normal cell-surface receptors, stimulating a continual overreaction of the target cell	• Graves' disease • B-cell gammopathies

Type I: Rapid Hypersensitivity Reactions

Type I, or rapid, hypersensitivity occurs when IgE responds to an otherwise harmless antigen, such as pollen, and causes the release of histamine and other vasoactive amines from basophils, eosinophils and mast cells (see Chap. 23). This response results in an acute inflammatory reaction and symptoms such as bronchospasm, wheezing, and rhinorrhea.

On first exposure to an allergen (an antigen that provokes allergic sensitization with IgE), the host responds by making antigen-specific IgE. This antigen-specific IgE then binds to the surface of basophils and mast cells. These cells have large numbers of granules containing vasoactive amines (including histamine) that are released when stimulated (see Chap. 23). Once the antigen-specific IgE is formed, the host is sensitized to that allergen.

In a type I hypersensitivity reaction, the previously sensitized person is re-exposed to the provoking allergen. The allergen binds to two adjacent IgE molecules on the surface of a basophil or mast cell, distorting the cell

membrane. This distortion initiates a series of biochemical events causing the cell granules to swell, migrate, and fuse with the cell membrane. The granular contents (vasoactive amines) are then expelled and released into the extravascular space, a process called *degranulation.*

The most important mediator is *histamine,* a short-acting vasoactive amine. Histamine causes increased capillary permeability, mucous secretion (both nasal and bronchial), smooth muscle contractions (especially of bronchioles and small blood vessels), and itching (pruritus), sometimes accompanied by redness. These symptoms last for approximately 10 minutes; the maximum reaction occurs 1 to 2 minutes after histamine release.

Clinical examples of type I reactions include systemic anaphylaxis, allergic asthma, and atopic (genetic tendency) allergies such as hay fever, allergic rhinitis, and allergies to specific allergens. Allergens can be

■ Inhaled (plant pollens, fungal spores, animal dander, house dust, grass, ragweed)
■ Ingested (foods, food additives, drugs)
■ Injected (bee venom, drugs, biological substances such as contrast dyes and adrenocorticotropic hormone)
■ Contacted (pollens, foods, environmental proteins)

Chapter 69 describes methods of allergy testing.

Anaphylaxis

Overview

Anaphylaxis, the most dramatic example of a type I hypersensitivity reaction, occurs rapidly, systemically, and affects multiple organs simultaneously within seconds to minutes after exposure to an allergen. Anaphylaxis is not common, but it can be fatal. Many substances can trigger anaphylaxis in a susceptible person (see Table 25–8).

Collaborative Management

 Assessment

Typically, a client experiencing an anaphylactic reaction first complains of feelings of uneasiness, apprehension, weakness, and impending doom. The nurse notes that the client is anxious and frightened. These feelings are followed, often quickly, by a generalized pruritus and urticaria. The nurse sees erythema and sometimes angioedema of the eyes, lips, or tongue. Frequently, discrete cutaneous wheals or urticarial eruptions appear that are intensely pruritic and sometimes merge together in a large, red blotch.

Histamine and other chemical mediators cause bronchoconstriction, mucosal edema, and excess mucus. On respiratory assessment, the nurse notes congestion, rhinorrhea, dyspnea, and increasing respiratory distress with audible wheezing.

On auscultation, the nurse detects crackles, wheezing, and diminished breath sounds. Clients may experience laryngeal edema as a "lump in the throat," hoarseness, and stridor (a crowing sound). Distress increases as the tongue and larynx become more edematous and excess mucous secretion continues. The nurse may note increas-

TABLE 25-8

Common Agents That Cause Anaphylaxis

Drugs/Foreign Proteins

- Antibiotics (penicillin, cephalosporins, tetracycline, sulfonamides, streptomycin, vancomycin, chloramphenicol, amphotericin B, others)
- Adrenocorticotropic hormone, insulin, vasopressin, protamine*
- Allergen extracts, muscle relaxants, hydrocortisone, vaccines, local anesthetics (lidocaine, procaine)*
- Whole blood, cryoprecipitate, immune serum globulin*
- Radiocontrast media*
- Opiates

Foods

- Shellfish
- Eggs
- Legumes, nuts
- Grains
- Berries
- Preservatives

Other Agents

- Pollens
- Exercise
- Heat/cold
- Other

Insects/Animals

- Hymenoptera: bees, wasps, hornets
- Fire ants
- Snake venom

* Anaphylaxis caused by these substances is probably a result of direct mast cell degranulation rather than an IgE-mediated hypersensitivity event.

ing stridor and anxiety as the airway begins to close. Respiratory failure may follow quickly as a complication of laryngeal edema, suffocation, or lower airway bronchoconstriction causing hypoxemia (insufficient oxygenation of blood) and hypercapnia (increased carbon dioxide in blood).

In performing the cardiovascular assessment, the nurse usually finds hypotension and a rapid, weak, possibly irregular pulse. These findings are due to chemical mediators causing vasodilation and increased capillary permeability with resultant leakage of intravascular fluids. The nurse notes faintness and diaphoresis, increasing anxiety, confusion, and, if the client is not treated immediately, loss of consciousness. Dysrhythmias, shock, and cardiac arrest may occur within minutes as intravascular volume is lost. Less often, the client may have abdominal cramping, diarrhea, or vomiting. Seventy percent of deaths are caused by respiratory failure or by shock and cardiac dysrhythmias.

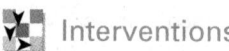 Interventions

➤ Emergency Respiratory Management

Emergency respiratory management is critical for the client having an anaphylactic reaction, because the severity of the reaction and gravity of the consequences increase with time. An airway must be established or stabilized immediately. The nurse may need to initiate cardiopulmonary resuscitation. Epinephrine (1:1000), 0.2 to 0.5 mL, should be given subcutaneously as soon as possible after a person displays symptoms of systemic anaphylaxis. This agent constricts blood vessels, increases myocardial contraction, and dilates the bronchioles. The same dose may be repeated every 15 to 20 minutes if needed. Other commonly administered drugs are listed in Chart 25-10.

Antihistamines, such as diphenhydramine (Allerdryl✦, Benadryl), 25 to 100 mg, are usually given IV, IM, or orally to treat angioedema and urticaria. This agent blocks the histamine receptor site (H_1) in vascular and bronchiolar smooth muscle. If the extent of upper airway narrowing requires it, the physician may insert a small endotracheal tube or perform an emergency tracheostomy.

If the client can breathe independently, the nurse administers oxygen, as ordered, to minimize hypoxemia. Oxygen should be started via nasal cannula at 5 to 10 L/minute or via face mask at 40% to 60% before arterial blood gas results are obtained. The nurse monitors tissue oxygen saturation using pulse oximetry. Arterial blood gas concentrations are monitored to determine oxygenation adequacy, with the goal of maintaining partial pressure of oxygen between 80 and 100 mm Hg. The nurse uses suction to remove excess mucous secretions, if indicated. The client's rate, rhythm, and depth of respirations as well as the presence of bronchospasm and abnormal breath sounds are assessed continually. The nurse or other assistive personnel elevates the client's bed to 45 degrees unless contraindicated because of hypotension.

For severe bronchospasm, the client is given aminophylline (Truphylline), 6 mg/kg IV, over 20 to 30 minutes. If the client is taking aminophylline regularly, no more than 3 mg/kg is given. Maintenance aminophylline (0.3-0.5 mg/kg/hour) is initiated. The client may be given an inhaled beta-adrenergic agonist such as metaproterenol (Alupent) or albuterol (Proventil) every 2 to 4 hours. For persistent symptoms (after 1-2 hours), corticosteroids are added to prevent the late recurrence of symptoms.

The nurse's primary role in caring for the client with anaphylaxis is to assess changes in any body system or adverse effects of drug therapy. For severe anaphylaxis, the client is admitted to a critical care unit for cardiac, pulmonary arterial, and capillary wedge pressure monitoring. The nurse carefully observes the client for fluid overload from the rapid administration of medications and IV fluids and reports changes to the physician immediately. The client may be discharged from the hospital when respiratory and cardiovascular systems have returned to baseline.

➤ Prevention

Because of the rapid onset of life-threatening symptoms and the potential for a fatal outcome, sometimes even with appropriate medical intervention, preventing anaphylaxis is paramount. The nurse teaches the client with a history of allergic reactions to avoid allergens whenever possible, to wear a medical alert bracelet, and to alert health care personnel about specific allergies. Some clients must carry an emergency anaphylaxis kit, such as a bee sting kit with injectable epinephrine, or an epinephrine injector, such as the EpiPen automatic injector (Center Laboratories). The EpiPen device is an easy-to-use, spring-

Chart 25–10

Drug Therapy for Anaphylaxis

Drug	Mechanism	Side Effects
Sympathomimetics		
• Epinephrine (Adrenalin)	• Rapidly stimulates alpha- and beta-adrenergic receptors of autonomic nervous system (alpha: vasoconstriction; beta: bronchodilation)	• Pallor, tachycardia and palpitations, nervousness, muscle twitching, sweating, anxiety, insomnia, hypertension, headache, hyperglycemia
• Isoproterenol (Isuprel)	• Stimulated beta-adrenergic receptors, relaxing bronchial muscle and dilating vessels	• Same as for epinephrine
• Ephedrine sulfate (Vatronol)	• Similar to isoproterenol, but with longer duration of action	• Same as for epinephrine
Antihistamines		
• Diphenhydramine HCl (Allerdryl❦, Benadryl)	• Competes with histamine for H_1 receptors on effector cells, thus blocking effects of histamine on bronchioles, gastrointestinal tract, and blood vessels	• Drowsiness, confusion, insomnia, headache, vertigo, photosensitivity, diplopia, nausea, vomiting, dry mouth
Corticosteroids		
• Prednisone (PO)	• Anti-inflammatory; inhibits mast cell degranulation	• Fluid and sodium retention, hypertension, cushingoid state, gastric distress, adrenal suppression, psychosis, osteoporosis, susceptibility to infection
• Hydrocortisone sodium succinate (Solu-Cortef) (IV/IM)		
• Methylprednisolone sodium succinate (Solu-Medrol) (IV/IM)		
• Beclomethasone (inhalant)		
Methlyxanthines		
• Aminophylline (Truphylline)	• Relaxes bronchial smooth muscle	• Restlessness, dizziness, palpitations, tachycardia, nausea, vomiting, epigastric distress, headache, convulsions
Vasopressors		
• Norepinephrine (Levophed)	• Raises blood pressure and cardiac output in severely decompensated states	• Headache, tachycardia, fibrillation, decreased urinary output, hypertension, metabolic acidosis
• Dopamine (Intropin)		• Arrhythmias, tachycardia, hypertension, dyspnea, nausea and vomiting, azotemia, headache
Inhaled Beta-Adrenergic Agonists		
• Metaproterenol (Alupent, Metaprel)	• Rapidly stimulates $beta_2$-receptor sites in pulmonary smooth muscle, causing bronchodilation	• Palpitations, tachycardia, dysrhythmias, hypokalemia
• Albuterol (Proventil, Ventolin)	• Same as for metaproterenol	• Same as for metaproterenol, plus painful urination, flushing of the face

loaded injector that delivers 0.3 mg of epinephrine per 2 mL dose.

The medical record of a client with a history of anaphylactic symptoms should prominently display the list of allergens to which the client is sensitive. A careful history is taken before any drug or therapeutic agent is given. Skin tests should be performed before any substance with a highly associated incidence of anaphylactic reactions, such as allergenic extract or horse serums, is administered. Physicians and nurses must be aware of common cross-reacting agents. For example, a client with a history of sensitivity to penicillin is also likely to react to cephalosporins because both have a similar biochemical structure.

If an agent must be used despite a history of allergenic reactions, precautionary measures should be taken. IV solution should be started, and intubation equipment and a tracheostomy set placed at the bedside. The substance should be given first intradermally, then subcutaneously, and then intramuscularly in increasing doses at 20- to 30-minute intervals so the initial dose by the next route does not exceed the final dose by the previous route. When carefully done, this procedure is fairly safe.

Atopic Allergy

Atopic reactions are allergic manifestations that occur in people who are genetically predisposed to respond to a variety of environmental allergens by forming immunoglobulin E (IgE). Once the person has sensitized IgE, allergic symptoms occur on re-exposure to the allergen via degranulation of mast cells. Conditions such as allergic asthma, allergic rhinitis, urticaria (hives), and eczematous dermatitis are manifested alone or in combination. Dermatitis and urticaria are described in Chapter 70 as types of skin inflammation. Asthma is discussed in Chapter 32. Allergic rhinitis is discussed in Chapter 31.

Type II: Cytotoxic Reactions
Overview

In a type II (cytotoxic) reaction, the body makes special autoantibodies directed against self cells or tissues that have some form of foreign protein attached to them. The autoantibody binds to the self cell and forms an antigen–antibody complex, or immune complex. The self cell is then destroyed by phagocytosis or complement-mediated lysis (see Chap. 23). Clinical examples of type II reactions include Coombs'-positive hemolytic anemias, thrombocytopenic purpura, hemolytic transfusion reactions (when an individual receives the wrong blood type during a transfusion), hemolytic disease of the newborn, Goodpasture's syndrome, and drug-induced hemolytic anemia.

Collaborative Management

Treatment of type II cytotoxic reactions begins with discontinuation of the offending drug or blood product. Plasmapheresis to remove autoantibodies may be beneficial. Otherwise, treatment is symptomatic. Complications such as hemolytic crisis and renal failure can be life threatening.

Type III: Immune Complex Reactions
Overview

In a type III reaction, soluble immune complexes are formed, usually with antigen excess (Fig. 25–2). These circulating immune complexes are then usually deposited in small blood vessel walls. Common sites include the kidneys, skin, joints, and other small blood vessels. The deposited immune complex activates complement, and tissue or vessel damage results.

There are many immune complex disorders (mostly connective tissue disorders) in which the type III reaction is the major mechanism of disease. For example, the clinical manifestations of rheumatoid arthritis are caused by immune complexes that lodge in joint spaces followed by destruction of tissue and, later, scarring and fibrous changes. Similarly, the clinical manifestations of systemic lupus erythematosus result from immune complex deposition in the vessels (vasculitis), the glomeruli (nephritis), the joints (arthralgia, arthritis), and other organs and tissues. In this disorder, the immune complex is composed of cellular DNA and anti-DNA antibodies. (For a detailed discussion of these and other connective tissue disorders, see Chapter 24.)

Serum sickness is a complex of symptoms that occurs after administration of a foreign serum or certain drugs, caused by collection of immune complexes deposited in blood vessel walls of the skin, joints, and kidney. The most common causes of serum sickness today are penicillin and related drugs and some animal serum antitoxins. Serum sickness used to be quite common when vaccines were made with horse or rabbit serum, but now most vaccines are made with human serum or antigen fragments. Relatively new agents that can cause serum sickness are antilymphocyte globulin and antithymocyte globulin, used to suppress the immune response in organ transplantation.

Collaborative Management

The client with serum sickness has symptoms of fever, arthralgia (achy joints), rash, lymphadenopathy (enlarged lymph nodes), malaise, and possibly polyarthritis and nephritis, usually about 7 to 12 days after administration of the causative agent. The nurse alerts the client to the possibility of serum sickness and what symptoms to look for. When administering a foreign serum to a client, the nurse is also prepared for a type I anaphylactic reaction and has emergency equipment and medications close at hand.

Serum sickness is usually self-limiting, and symptoms subside after several days. Treatment is usually symptomatic; antihistamines are given for pruritus and aspirin for arthralgias. Prednisone is given if symptoms are severe.

Type IV: Delayed Hypersensitivity Reactions
Overview

In a type IV reaction, the reactive cell is the T lymphocyte. Antibodies and complement are not involved. Sensitized T lymphocytes (from a previous exposure) respond to an antigen by producing and releasing certain lymphokines (chemical mediators) and recruit, retain, and activate macrophages to destroy the antigen. A type IV response typically occurs hours to days after exposure rather than immediately, as in a type I hypersensitivity reaction. A type IV reaction is characterized by an accu-

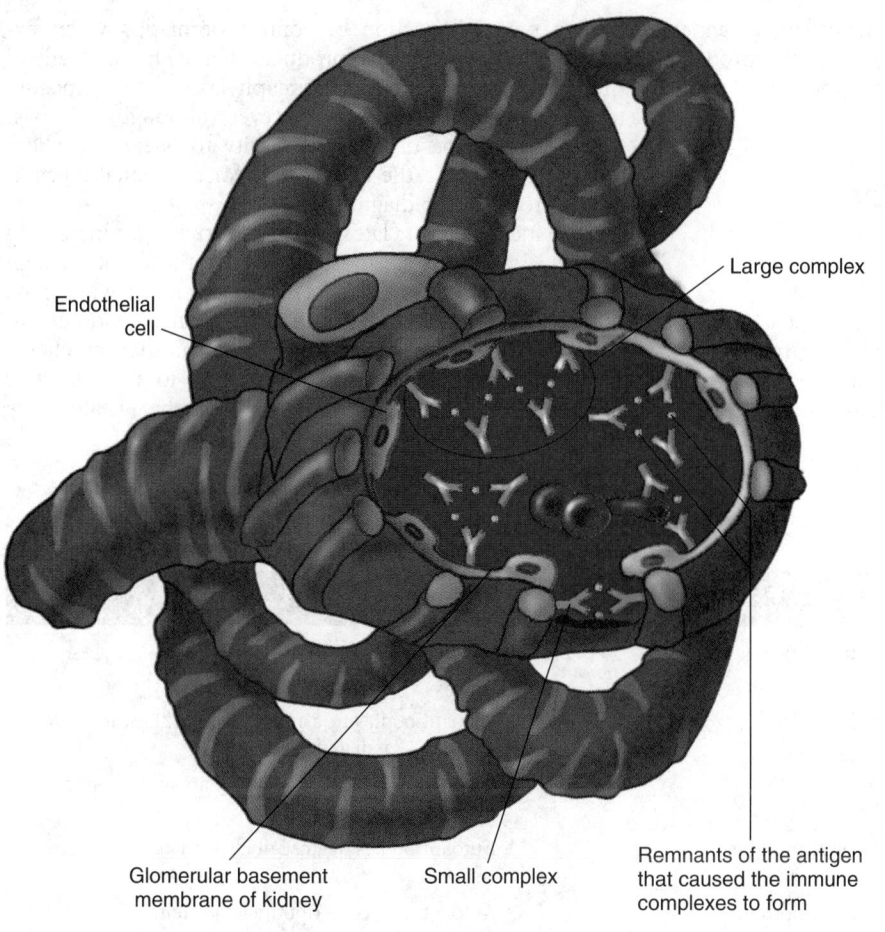

Figure 25–2. An immune complex in a type III hypersensitivity reaction.

mulation of lymphocytes and macrophages, causing edema, ischemia, and tissue destruction at the site.

An example of a type IV reaction is a positive purified protein derivative (PPD) test. In a client who had previously been exposed to tuberculosis, an intradermal injection of this agent causes sensitized T cells to accumulate at the injection site, release lymphokines, and recruit and activate macrophages. Induration and erythema at the site of the injection appear approximately 24 to 48 hours later.

Clinical examples of type IV hypersensitivity reactions include contact dermatitis, poison ivy skin rashes, local response to insect stings, allograft (tissue transplant) rejections, and granulomatous diseases in which the antigen is unknown (e.g., sarcoidosis).

Collaborative Management

Removal of the offending antigen is the major focus of management. The reaction is self-limiting in 5 to 7 days, and the client is treated symptomatically. Nursing responsibilities include monitoring the reaction site and sites distal to the reaction for circulation adequacy. Diphenhydramine is of minimal benefit for type IV reactions because histamine is not the main mediator. Corticosteroids or other anti-inflammatory agents can reduce the discomfort and resolve the reaction more quickly.

Type V: Stimulatory Reactions
Overview

This relatively new category of hypersensitivity reactions involves inappropriate stimulation of a normal cell surface receptor by an autoantibody, resulting in a continuous "turned-on" state for the cell. The classic example of a stimulatory reaction is Graves' disease, in which an autoantibody binds to the thyroid-stimulating hormone (TSH) receptor sites on the thyroid gland. This binding continually stimulates the thyroid cells to produce thyroid hormones, causing the client to have symptoms of severe hyperthyroidism (see Chap. 67), although the thyroid gland is completely normal. In a sense, the tissue responding to the autoantibody is "out of control" from the body's normal feedback system of checks and balances.

Collaborative Management

For type V reactions involving only one organ, the management focuses on removing enough of the responding (stimulated) tissue to return the function to normal. In the case of Graves' disease, thyroid tissue usually is either surgically removed or destroyed with radiation. For type V reactions in which either more than one tissue is being stimulated by the autoantibodies or the tissue is widespread, the focus of treatment is on reducing the production of autoantibodies through immunosuppression.

Mixed Hypersensitivity Reactions: Latex Hypersensitivity

It is important to remember that a client's exposure to an allergen can result in a combination of two or more types of hypersensitivity reactions. One example of such a mixed reaction is latex sensitivity. Many people experi-

ence a type IV reaction of contact dermatitis when exposed externally to latex products. Some, but not all, of these people also experience anaphylaxis when exposure to latex occurs internally. However, although the existence of one type of hypersensitivity to latex in a client appears to increase the client's risk for additional types, it is not predictive or diagnostic.

The incidence of latex hypersensitivity is increasing (Kellett, 1997). People most at risk are those with a high exposure (such as health care workers, clients with spina bifida, and people who routinely use latex condoms) to natural latex products. The nurse must question all clients regarding use of and known reactions to natural latex products. In addition, the nurse and other health care

TABLE 25–9

Autoimmune Disorders*

Disorder	Autoantigen	Comments
Systemic or Non–Organ-Specific		
Systemic lupus erythematosus	• DNA, DNA proteins	• Autoantibodies to a number of entities; immune complex–mediated damage
Rheumatoid arthritis	• IgG	• Immune complex–mediated damage in joints (arthritis, fibrosis)
Progressive systemic sclerosis	• DNA proteins	• Autoantibodies against nuclear materials; sclerosis
Mixed connective tissue disease	• DNA proteins	• Autoantibodies to ribonucleoprotein
Organ-Specific		
Autoimmune hemolytic anemia	• Erythrocytes	• Killing of antibody-coated erythrocytes
Autoimmune thrombocytopenic purpura	• Plateletes	• Killing of antibody-coated platelets or innocent bystander effect
Myasthenia gravis	• Acetylcholine receptor	• Blocking of impulse transmission by autoantibody to acetylcholine receptor on muscle
Graves' disease	• Thyroid-stimulating hormone receptor	• Stimulation by autoantibody to thyroid-stimulating hormone receptor
Rheumatic fever	• Myocardial cells	• Cross-reaction of antibody with myocardial cells
Idiopathic Addison's disease	• Adrenal cell	• Antibody- and cell-mediated adrenal cytotoxicity
Hashimoto's thyroiditis	• Thyroid cell surface	• Antibody- and cell-mediated thyroid cytotoxicity
Pernicious anemia	• Intrinsic factor/parietal cell	• Autoantibodies to intrinsic factor, intrinsic factor/B_{12} complexes, and parietal canalicula cells
Goodpasture's syndrome	• Basement membrane	• Antiglomerular basement membrane antibodies, which also cross-react with pulmonary basement membrane
Glomerulonephritis	• Glomerular basement membrane	• Autoantibodies and/or immune complex–mediated damage
Uveitis	• Uvea	• Cell-mediated and humoral damage
Vasculitis	• Unknown	• Probably primarily immune complex–mediated damage

* Other inflammatory, granulomatous, degenerative, and atrophic disorders are thought to be autoimmune because there is no more reasonable alternative explanation.

workers need to consider their own exposure and risk for hypersensitivities to natural latex products.

Autoimmunities

Overview

Autoimmunity is a process whereby a person develops and expresses immunologic reactivity, especially in the form of antibodies, against self components. For unknown reasons, certain cells or tissues of the body are recognized as non-self or no longer tolerated as self, and immune reactions occur. The responses, both antibody- and cell-mediated, are similar to normal immune responses against non-self, although inappropriate and sometimes excessive. Reasons for alterations in self-tolerance are not known, but there are multiple theories.

Autoimmunity research is ongoing, and there are few confirmed, established data. Not only is the cause of autoimmunity uncertain, but there is also a lack of consensus as to which diseases are truly autoimmune. Diseases that are generally believed to be autoimmune include systemic lupus erythematosus, polyarteritis nodosa, rheumatoid arthritis, autoimmune hemolytic anemia, rheumatic fever, and Hashimoto's thyroiditis (Table 25–9).

Connective tissue disorders, sometimes referred to as collagen disorders, are characterized by changes in connective tissue. Many of these diseases are considered autoimmune, and for most, autoantibodies have been detected. Connective tissue disorders include systemic lupus erythematosus, rheumatoid arthritis, scleroderma, and polyarteritis nodosa. Most of these tissue disorders are characterized as organ-nonspecific autoimmunities, which means that the autoantibodies and the tissue damage are not limited to a specific organ. In organ-specific autoimmunities, tissue damage occurs in a specific organ (see Chap. 24).

Collaborative Management

Treatment of autoimmunities depends on the organ or organs affected. Anti-inflammatory drugs and immunosuppressive drugs are commonly used.

Gammopathies: Multiple Myeloma

Overview

Gammopathies are relatively rare disorders involving abnormal reproduction of the lymphoid cells that produce immunoglobulins. More specifically, gammopathies are associated with increased production of an abnormal clone of immunoglobulin-secreting plasma cells derived from B lymphocytes (see Chap. 23). Several terms other than gammopathies are used to describe this group of diseases: monoclonal gammopathies, plasma cell dyscrasias, paraproteinemias, dysproteinemias, and immunoglobulinopathies.

The most common example of disease in this group is multiple myeloma. Other gammopathies are plasmacytoma, Waldenström's macroglobulinemia, heavy chain disease, and histiocytoses.

Multiple myeloma is a malignant condition in which a clone of transformed (cancer-like) plasma cells multiplies in bone marrow. The result is disruption of normal bone marrow function and eventual invasion and destruction of adjacent bone. The ability of plasma cells to make functional antibodies decreases, leaving the client immunocompromised. The cause of multiple myeloma is unknown, but genetic predisposition, oncogenic viruses, inflammatory stimuli, and chronic antigenic stimulation have all been identified as possible etiologic factors.

Essentially, an excess number of abnormal plasma cells invade the bone marrow, develop into tumors, and ultimately destroy bone. They then invade lymph nodes, liver, spleen, and kidneys. These plasma cells produce an abnormal antibody often referred to as a myeloma protein, or the Bence Jones protein, found in the blood and urine of people with multiple myeloma. Multiple myeloma occurs in middle-aged and elderly clients and in men more often than in women.

The onset of multiple myeloma is insidious, and most people remain asymptomatic until the disease is advanced. Some people are diagnosed without symptoms by Bence Jones proteinuria and an elevated total serum protein level. The major complaint is usually skeletal pain—especially in the pelvis, spine, and ribs—weakness, fatigue, and recurrent infection. Other clinical manifestations include osteoporosis (bone loss) and hypercalcemia (increased serum calcium) related to destruction of bone. If there is vertebral involvement and destruction, spinal cord compression and paraplegia may occur. Pathologic fractures are also common.

Anemia is a major problem for these clients. Anemia is due to invasion of the bone marrow by plasma cells and, therefore, a failure of normal marrow function. Thrombocytopenia (decreased serum platelets) and granulocytopenia (decreased serum granulocytes) also occur. Renal failure occurs in approximately 20% of clients as a result of increased calcium levels, severe proteinuria, and hyperuricemia (increased serum uric acid).

Collaborative Management

The diagnostic work-up shows pancytopenia (a decrease of all serum blood cells), a high total serum protein level, hyperuricemia, hypercalcemia, an elevated serum creatinine level, and Bence Jones proteinuria. Radiograph and isotope scans show the extent of bony destruction. X-ray films show bones with multiple dark lesions—a "Swiss cheese" appearance.

Treatment includes systemic chemotherapy and supportive care of complications. The chemotherapeutic agent most commonly used is melphalan (Alkeran), often with corticosteroids and cyclophosphamide (Cytoxan). Therapy with cytokines is under investigation for multiple myeloma. Supportive care is important to control symptoms and prevent complications, especially bone fractures, renal failure, and infections.

Clients need fluids (approximately 3–4 L/day) to offset the potential problems of hypercalcemia and proteinuria.

(See Chapters 16 and 27 for additional interventions in reducing the serum calcium level.)

The nurse is alert for back pain and the development of neurologic symptoms in the lower extremities. These symptoms may indicate impending spinal cord compression and should be diagnosed and treated (with surgery or radiation) as soon as possible to prevent paraplegia. The nurse teaches the client to recognize signs and symptoms of infection so infections can be diagnosed and treated early and efficiently. Blood transfusions are often required for anemia. Pain control is essential. Analgesics, orthopedic supports, local radiation, and relaxation techniques are all helpful.

CASE STUDY for the Client with AIDS

■ A 32-year-old woman is one of your home care clients with AIDS. Her medication orders include TMP 160 mg BID, SMX 800 mg BID, Ketoconazole, 200 mg QD, Didanosine, 200 mg BID.

■ Today, she complains that she is short of breath, and has sharp pains in her chest. She appears anxious. During the respiratory assessment, you find that she is dyspneic and tachypneic at rest, with a respiratory rate of 30. On auscultation, you hear crackles in her right lower lobe.

QUESTIONS:
1. When taking the client's history, what important questions should you ask?
2. What physical assessment techniques should you perform?
3. Given the respiratory findings, what should you do first?

SELECTED BIBLIOGRAPHY

Abbas, A., Lichtman, A., & Pober, J. (1997). *Cellular and molecular immunology* (3rd ed). Philadelphia: W. B. Saunders.
Anastasi, J., & Lee, V. (1994). HIV wasting: How to stop the cycle. *American Journal of Nursing, 94*(6), 18–25.
Anastasi, J., & Rivera, J. (1994). Understanding prophylactic therapy for HIV. *American Journal of Nursing, 94*(2), 36–41.
Barnes, D. (1995). HIV-1-infected long-term non-progressors: A distinct group or part of a continuum? *Journal of NIH Research, 7*(2), 19–21.
Bechtel-Boenning, C. (1996). State of the art: Antiviral treatment of HIV infection. *Nursing Clinics of North America, 31*(1), 1–13.
Bjorgen, S. (1998). Clinical snapshot: Herpes zoster. *American Journal of Nursing, 98*(2), 46–47.
*Centers for Disease Control. (1987). Public Health Service guidelines for counseling and antibody testing to prevent HIV infection and AIDS. *MMWR. Morbidity and Mortality Weekly Report, 36*(31), 509–515.
*Centers for Disease Control. (1991). Recommendations for preventing transmission of human immunodeficiency virus and hepatitis B virus to patients during exposure-prone invasive procedures. *MMWR. Morbidity and Mortality Weekly Review, 40*(RR-8), 1–9.
Centers for Disease Control and Prevention. (1997). *HIV/AIDS surveillance report*. Atlanta, GA: Author.
Coste, J., Montes, B., Reynes, J., Peeters, M., Segarra, C., Vendrell, J., Delaporte, E., & Segondy, M. (1996). Comparative evaluation of three assays for the quantitation of human immunodeficiency virus type 1 RNA in plasma. *Journal of Medical Virology, 50*(4), 293–302.

Cotran, R., Kumar, V., & Robbins, S. (1994). *Robbins' pathologic basis of disease* (5th ed). Philadelphia: W. B. Saunders.
Dowling, M. (1997). Multiple myeloma. *Professional Nurse, 12*(5), 354–357.
Emlet, C. (1997). HIV/AIDS in the elderly. *Home Care Provider, 2*(2), 69–75.
*Friedland, G., Kahl, P., Saltzman, B., Rogers, M., Feiner, C., Mayers, M., Schable, C., & Klein, R. (1990). Additional evidence for lack of transmission of HIV infection by close interpersonal (casual) contact. *AIDS, 4*, 639–644.
*Gershon, R., Vlahov, D., & Nelson, K. (1990). The risk of transmission of HIV-1 through non-percutaneous, non-sexual modes: A review. *AIDS, 4*, 645–650.
Greening, J. G. (1994). Intravenous foscarnet administration for treatment of cytomegalovirus retinitis. *Journal of Intravenous Nursing, 17*(2), 74–77.
Guyton, A., & Hall, J (1991). *Textbook of medical physiology* (9th ed.). Philadelphia: W. B. Saunders.
Hellmann, D. (1995). Vasculitis: When should you suspect it? *Emergency Medicine, 27*(2), 22–36.
*Henry, S., & Holzemer, W. (1992). Critical care management of the patient with HIV infection who has *Pneumocystis carinii* pneumonia. *Heart & Lung, 21*(3), 243–249.
Howard, B. A. (1994) Guiding allergy sufferers through the medication maze. *RN, 57*(4), 26–30.
*Imagawa, D. T., Lee, M. H., Wolinsky, S. M., Sano, K., Morales, F., Kwok, S., Shinsky, J. J., Nishanian, P. G., Giorgi, J., Fahey, J. L., Dudley, J., Visscher, B. R., & Detels, R. (1989). Human immunodeficiency virus type 1 infection in homosexual men who remain seronegative for prolonged periods. *New England Journal of Medicine, 320*(22), 1458–1489.
Kelly, A. (1994). Human immunodeficiency virus: Current trends in assessment, diagnosis, and treatment. *Journal of Intravenous Nursing, 17*(2), 83–92.
Kellett, P. (1997). Latex allergy: A review. *Journal of Emergency Nursing, 23*(1), 27–36.
Lewis, J., Doyle, K., & Sampson, D. (1995). Self-test: Caring for AIDS patients. *Nursing95, 25*(4), 76–78.
Lisanti, P. (1996). Anaphylaxis. *American Journal of Nursing, 96*(11), 51.
Lisanti, P., & Zwolski, K. (1997). Understanding the devastation of AIDS. *American Journal of Nursing, 97*(1), 26–35.
McKinnon, B. (1996). New AIDS drugs offer hope, but bring even higher costs. *Continuing Care, 15*(7), 12–14.
*McMahon, K. (1988). The integration of HIV testing and counseling into nursing practice. *Nursing Clinics of North America, 23*(4), 803–821.
Meisenhelder, J. B. (1994). Contributing factors to fear of HIV contagion in registered nurses. *Image, 26*(1), 65–69.
National Institute of Allergy and Infectious Disease. (1994, February 21). AZT reduces rate of maternal transmission of HIV. *NIAID News*. Bethesda, MD: National Institutes of Health, U.S. Public Health Service.
Nokes, K., Kendrew, J., & Longo, M. (1995). Alternative/complementary therapies used by persons with HIV disease. *Journal of the Association of Nurses in AIDS Care, 6*(4), 19–24.
Nowak, M., & McMichael, A. (1995). How HIV defeats the immune system. *Scientific American, 273*(2), 58–65.
Roitt, I. (1994). *Essential immunology* (8th ed). Boston: Blackwell Scientific Publications.
Sabo, C. E., & Carwein, V. L. (1994). Women and AIDS. *Journal of the Association of Nurses in AIDS Care, 5*(3), 15–21.
Sande, M. A., & Volberding, P. A. (1997). *The medical management of AIDS* (5th ed.). Philadelphia: W. B. Saunders.
Tierney, A. (1995). HIV/AIDS: Knowledge, attitudes and education of nurses: A review of the research. *Journal of Clinical Nursing, 4*(1), 13–21.
Ungvarski, P. (1995). Adults and HIV/AIDS: Clinical considerations for care management. *The Journal of Care Management, 1*(3), 40–55.
Ungvarski, P. (1997). Update on HIV infection. *American Journal of Nursing, 97*(1), 44–52.
Volberding, P. A. (1994). Treatment dilemmas in HIV infection. *Hospital Practice, 29*(4), 49–60.
Wang, J. F. (1997). Attitudes, concerns, and fear of acquired immune deficiency syndrome among registered nurses in the United States. *Holistic Nursing Practice, 11*(2), 36–49.

Whipple, B., & Scura, K. (1996). The overlooked epidemic: HIV in older adults. *American Journal of Nursing, 96*(2), 23–29.

Workman, M. L. (1995). Essential concepts of inflammation and immunity. *Critical Care Clinics of North America, 7*(4), 601–615.

*World Health Organization. (1991). Statistics from the World Health Organization and the Centers for Disease Control. *AIDS, 5, 1399–1403.*

SUGGESTED READINGS

Anastasi, J. K., & Lee, V. S. (1994). HIV wasting: How to stop the cycle. *American Journal of Nursing, 94*(6), 18–25.
This article describes factors underlying HIV wasting syndrome. Suggestions regarding how to conduct a nutritional assessment are presented, and interventions for nutritional support are outlined.

Sabo, C. E., & Carwein, V. L. (1994). Women and AIDS. *Journal of the Association of Nurses in AIDS Care, 5*(3), 15–21.
This article describes the issues specific to women with HIV. These include psychosocial, sociocultural factors, and female-specific clinical conditions associated with HIV infection.

Ungvarski, P. J. (1995). Adults and HIV/AIDS: Clinical considerations for care management. *The Journal of Care Management, 1*(3), 40–55.
This article describes a comprehensive model of care for persons at risk for or with HIV that includes primary, secondary, and tertiary prevention. Strategies for screening, prevention of complications, and minimization of disability are outlined.

Chapter 26

ALTERED CELL GROWTH AND CANCER DEVELOPMENT

CHAPTER HIGHLIGHTS

All people experience some form of altered cell growth. The most common forms are harmless (benign) and do not require intervention. Cancer, or malignant cell growth, is the most serious type and, without intervention, leads to death. Approximately 1.5 million people in the United States and Canada are newly diagnosed with cancer each year (American Cancer Society, 1998), making cancer a very common health problem. Some types of cancer can be prevented, and others have better cure rates if diagnosed early. The nurse is crucial in educating the public about cancer prevention and early detection methods. A strong knowledge base of the causes and consequences of cancer development can assist nurses in this role.

HISTORICAL PERSPECTIVE

Cancer is not a new disorder. There is evidence that even prehistoric humans experienced cancer. Some types of cancer are more prevalent today, especially among industrialized societies, than in centuries past. Two reasons are the increasing longevity of people in industrialized countries and increased environmental exposure to substances that stimulate cancer development.

Cancer will occur in approximately one of every three people currently living in North America (American Cancer Society, 1998), although cancer risk differs for each person. More than 10 million Americans with a history of cancer are alive today, nearly 5 million of whom can be considered cured (American Cancer Society, 1998). Terms used to describe abnormal cell growth and cancer are presented in Table 26–1.

OVERVIEW

The continuous growth of cells and tissues is expected during infancy and childhood, and many human body cells continue to "grow" by cell division (mitosis) long after development and maturation are complete. Such cells are located in tissues where constant damage or wear is likely and where continued cell growth is necessary to replace dead tissues. Cells of the skin, hair, mucous membranes, bone marrow, and linings of glandular organs (lungs, stomach, intestines, bladder, uterus) and support cells of the brain (glial cells), among others, keep the ability to divide through a person's life span. The growth of these cells is well controlled, so only the

TABLE 26–1

Terminology Commonly Associated with Abnormal Cell Growth

Term	Definition
Anaplastic	• Without shape or definition
Benign	• New cell growth not needed for normal growth or replacement that is not malignant
Carcinogenesis	• The transformation of a normal cell into a cancer cell
Doubling time	• The amount of time it takes for a tumor to double in size by mitotic cell divisions
Fibronectin	• A large, extracellular, transformation-sensitive cell-surface protein present on normal cells that allows normal cells to adhere tightly together
Gene expression	• The activation, or "turning on," of a specific gene to the extent that it synthesizes a specific protein that influences the activity of a cell or group of cells
Gene repression	• The deactivation, or "turning off," of a specific gene so that it is silent and does not synthesize a protein
Generation time	• The period of time necessary for one cell to enter and complete one round of cell division by mitosis
Initiation	• The damage of a normal cell's DNA by a carcinogen
Latency	• The period of time between when a carcinogenic agent or substance damaged the DNA of a normal cell (initiated it) and when an overt cancer is present
Malignant	• Cancerous, new growth of cells by invasion that is not needed for normal development or tissue replacement
Metastasis	• Invasive growth of cancer cells from the original tumor into distant areas
Mitosis	• Cell division by exact duplication
Morphology	• Appearance or shape
Multipotent	• An undifferentiated cell that has multiple potentials for maturation and differentiation (also called totipotent and pluripotent)
Neoplasia	• New cell growth not needed for normal body growth or replacement of dead or missing tissue
Oncogene	• Developmental gene (proto-oncogene) expressed at an inappropriate time, capable of transforming a normal cell into a cancer cell
Ploidy	• The chromosome content of a cell
Aneuploid	• Chromosome content of a cell that is greater or lesser than the normal chromosomal number for the species
Diploid (euploid)	• Normal chromosome content of a cell for the species (e.g., human cells have 46 chromosomes [23 pairs] per cell)
Primary tumor	• A tumor formed in a specific tissue as a result of a carcinogenic agent or event
Promotion	• Enhancement of cell division in a cell initiated by a carcinogen
Proto-oncogene	• A developmental gene expressed during early embryonic development
Secondary tumor	• A tumor formed as a result of breaking off from a primary tumor and spreading to distant sites (metastasis)
Transformation	• The changing of a normal cell into a cancer cell by a carcinogenic agent or event

right number of cells is always present in any tissue or organ.

Some tissues and organs stop growing by cell division after development is complete. For example, heart muscle cells no longer divide after fetal life; the number of heart muscle cells is fixed at birth. The size of the heart increases as the person grows because each of the cells gets larger, but the number of muscle cells in the heart does not. Growth that causes an organ or tissue to increase in size by enlarging individual cells is called *hypertrophy*. Growth that causes an organ or tissue to increase in size by increasing the number of cells is called *hyperplasia* (Fig. 26–1).

Any new or continued cell growth not needed for normal development or replacement of dead and damaged tissues is called *neoplasia* and is always considered abnormal even if it causes no harm. Whether the new cells are benign or malignant, neoplastic cells develop from normal cells (parent tissues or cells). Thus, cancer or any neoplastic cells were once normal cells but changed to no longer look, grow, or function normally. The strict processes controlling normal growth and function have been lost or suppressed. To understand how cancer cells grow, it is first necessary to understand the regulation and function of normal cells.

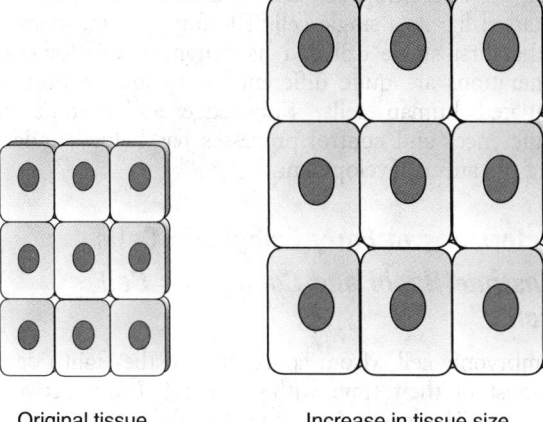 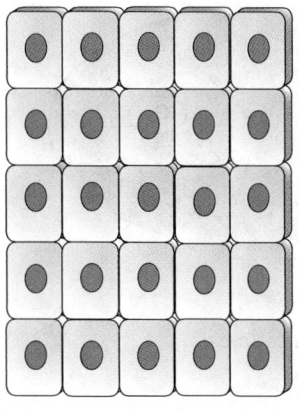

Original tissue   Increase in tissue size
by hypertrophy

Increase in tissue size
by hyperplasia

Figure 26–1. Tissue growth by hypertrophy and hyperplasia.

Biology of Normal Cells

Different types of normal cells work together to make the whole person function at an optimal level. To achieve optimal function, each individual cell must perform in a predictable manner.

Characteristics of Normal Cells

Have Limited Cell Division

Normal cells divide (undergo mitosis) for one of two reasons: (1) to develop normal tissue or (2) to replace lost or damaged normal tissue. Even when capable of mitosis, normal cells divide only when all internal body conditions and nutrition are just right to promote cell division.

Show Specific Morphology

Each normal cell type has a distinct and recognizable appearance, size, and shape, as shown in Figure 26–2.

Have a Small Nuclear–Cytoplasmic Ratio

As shown in Figure 26–2, the space that the nucleus occupies inside a normal cell is small compared with the size of the cell. The nuclear space is small in proportion to the cytoplasmic space.

Perform Specific Differentiated Functions

Every normal cell must perform at least one special function to contribute to whole body homeostasis. For example, skin cells make keratin, liver cells make bile, cardiac muscle cells contract rhythmically, nerve cells generate and conduct impulses, and red blood cells make hemoglobin to carry oxygen.

Adhere Tightly Together

Normal cells make and secrete cell-surface proteins that protrude from the cell surface, allowing cells to bind closely and tightly together. In the presence of a protein called fibronectin, normal cells composing any normal tissue are bound tightly to each other.

Are Nonmigratory

Because normal cells are tightly bound together, they do not wander from one tissue to the next (with the exception of erythrocytes and leukocytes).

Grow in an Orderly and Well-Regulated Manner

Normal cells capable of mitosis do not divide unless all internal body conditions are optimal for cell division. These conditions include the need for more cells, adequate space, and sufficient nutrients and other resources. Cell division, occurring in a well-recognized pattern, is described by the cell cycle. Figure 26–3 shows the phases of the cell cycle.

Living cells not actively reproducing are not in the cell cycle but in a reproductive resting state termed G_0. During the G_0 period, cells actively carry out specific functions but do not divide. Most normal cells spend most of their existence in the G_0 state, just like most humans spend the majority of their lives in a nonpregnant state.

Mitotic cell division makes a cell divide into two cells. These two cells are identical to each other and to the original cell that started the mitotic cell division. The

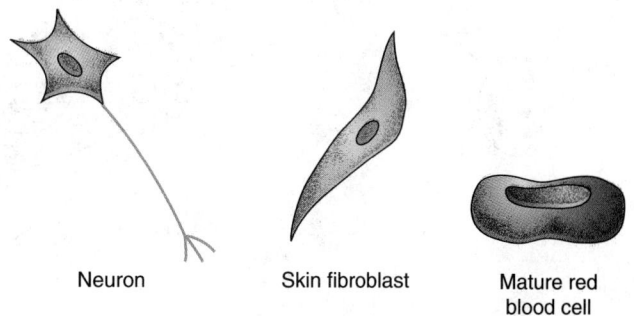

Neuron   Skin fibroblast   Mature red
blood cell

Figure 26–2. Distinctive morphology of some normal cells.

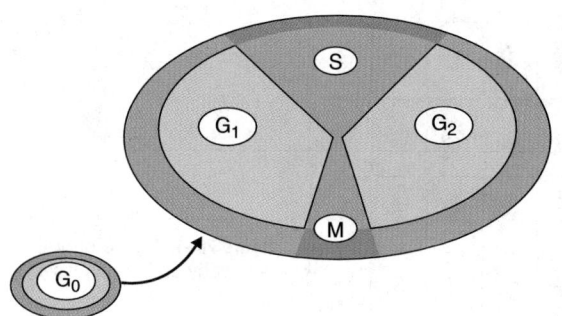

Figure 26–3. The cell cycle.

processes of entering and completing the cell cycle are rigidly controlled. Figure 26–4 shows the activities occurring during the phases of the cell cycle:

- G_1. The cell is preparing for division by taking on extra nutrients, generating more energy, and making extra membrane. The amount of cell fluid (cytoplasm) also increases.
- S. Because making one cell into two cells requires twice as much of everything, including deoxyribonucleic acid (DNA), the cell doubles its DNA content through DNA synthesis.
- G_2. The cell makes important proteins that will be used in actual cell division and in normal physiologic function after cell division is complete.
- M. The single cell splits apart into two cells (actual mitosis).

Are Contact Inhibited

Among normal cells capable of cell division, each individual cell will divide only as long as it has some surface not in direct contact with another cell. Once a normal cell is in direct contact on all surface areas with other cell membranes, it no longer undergoes mitosis. Thus, normal cell division is *contact inhibited*.

Each normal, mature cell has a specific structure and function, an interesting concept considering that all humans started life as a single cell. The function and behavior of that first single cell and its daughter cells for several generations are quite different from those of normal differentiated human cells. Knowledge about some of their differences and control processes has helped understanding of cancer development.

Characteristics of Early Embryonic Cells
Demonstrate Rapid and Continuous Cell Division

Early embryonic cells (from conception to the eighth day) spend most of their time within the cell cycle, actively reproducing. The generation time for these cells ranges from 2 to 8 hours.

Show Anaplastic Morphology

The term *anaplasia* means "without structural shape or differentiation." Early embryonic cells do not look like the mature cells they will eventually become. They all have the same anaplastic appearance, small and round (Fig. 26–5).

Have a Large Nuclear–Cytoplasmic Ratio

The nucleus of an early embryonic cell takes up most of the space inside the cell. The ratio of nuclear space to cytoplasmic space is larger than that of a normal differentiated cell.

Perform No Differentiated Functions

In the early embryonic period, cells do not have any differentiated functions. They have not yet committed to a specific maturity. Each early embryonic cell is totally flexible and can mature to become any body cell. This flexibility is called *pluripotency*, *multipotency*, or *totipotency* because each cell has an unlimited potential for maturation.

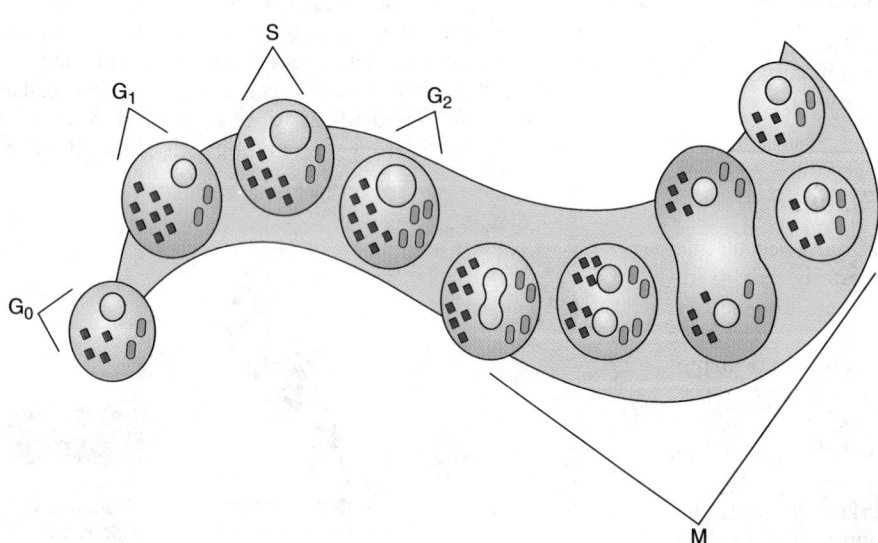

Figure 26–4. Cellular events during mitotic cell division.

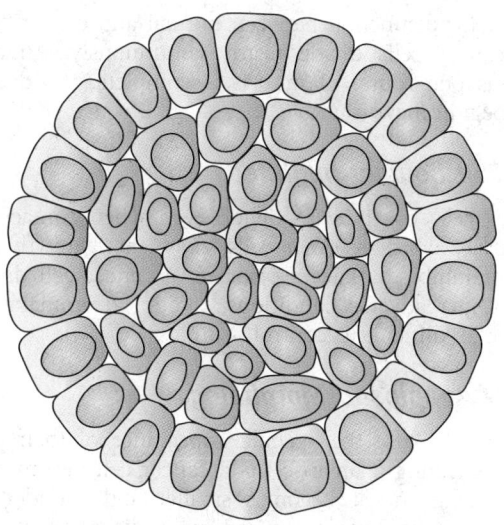

Figure 26–5. Embryonic cells at about 5 days after conception.

Adhere Loosely Together

Early embryonic cells do not make fibronectin and are not tightly bound together.

Are Able to Migrate

Because early embryonic cells are not tightly bound together, they do not remain in one place within the embryo but migrate throughout the early embryo.

Are Not Contact Inhibited

Having all sides or areas of an early embryonic cell in continuous contact with the membrane surfaces of other cells does not inhibit embryonic cell division.

Commitment

At some point in early embryonic development, cells become differentiated. In response to an unknown signal, each cell commits itself to a specific differentiated maturational outcome. The cell has not yet taken on any differentiated features or functions; rather, it positions itself within a group of cells that will eventually become only one specific organ or tissue.

Commitment involves turning off specific early embryonic genes that controlled or regulated early rapid growth, called *proto-oncogenes*. These genes have no apparent normal function at any other point in life.

After the early embryonic regulatory genes are "turned off" (repressed), other specific genes that control the expression of specific differentiated functions must be "turned on" (expressed) selectively in different cell types. For example, the gene for insulin is actively expressed only in fetal pancreatic beta cells and repressed in all other cells. This selective gene expression directs the normal growth and differentiation of specific body cells.

Biology of Abnormal Cells

Body cells do not exist in isolation but are exposed to personal and environmental changes, which can alter how the cells grow or function. When either cell growth or cell function is changed, the cells are considered abnormal. Table 26–2 compares characteristics of normal, embryonic, benign tumor, and cancer cells.

Characteristics of Benign Cells

Benign tumor cells are normal cells growing in the wrong place, at the wrong time, or at the wrong rate. Examples include moles, uterine fibroid tumors, skin tags, endometriosis, and nasal polyps.

TABLE 26–2

Characteristics of Normal and Abnormal Cells				
Characteristic	**Normal Cell**	**Embryonic Cell**	**Benign Tumor Cell**	**Malignant Cell**
Cell division	• None or slow	• Rapid, continuous	• Continuous or inappropriate	• Rapid or continuous
Appearance	• Specific morphologic features	• Anaplastic	• Specific morphologic features	• Anaplastic
Nuclear–cytoplasmic ratio	• Small	• Large	• Small	• Large
Differentiated functions	• Many	• None	• Many	• Some-none
Adherence	• Tight	• Loose	• Tight	• Loose
Migratory	• No	• Yes	• No	• Yes
Growth	• Well regulated	• Well regulated	• Expansion	• Invasion
Chromosomes	• Diploid (euploid)	• Diploid (euploid)	• Diploid (euploid)	• Aneuploid*
Mitotic index	• Low	• High	• Low	• High*

*Depends on the degree of malignant transformation.

Demonstrate Continuous or Inappropriate Cell Growth

Benign tumors are tissues unnecessary for normal function, growing too much or in the wrong place.

Show Specific Morphology

Benign tumors strongly resemble their parent tissues, retaining the specific morphologic features of parent tissue.

Have a Small Nuclear–Cytoplasmic Ratio

Just like completely normal cells, benign tumor cells have a small nucleus compared with the rest of the cell.

Perform Differentiated Functions

Not only do benign tumors look like their parent tissues, but they also perform the same differentiated functions. For example, in endometriosis, one type of benign tumor, the normal lining of the uterus (endometrium) grows in an abnormal place (such as on an ovary, on the peritoneum, or in the chest cavity). This displaced endometrium acts just like normal endometrium by increasing vascularity and tissue thickness each month under the influence of estrogen and progesterone. When these hormone levels drop and the normal endometrium sheds from the uterus, the displaced endometrium—wherever it is—also sheds.

Adhere Tightly Together

Benign tumor cells make and secrete fibronectin, and benign tumor cells bind tightly to one another. In addition, many benign tissues are "encapsulated," or surrounded with fibrous connective tissue, helping to hold the benign tissue together.

Are Nonmigratory

Benign tissues do not wander but remain tightly bound and do not invade other body tissues.

Grow in an Orderly Manner

Benign tumor cells follow normal cell growth patterns even though their growth is not needed. Growth may continue beyond an appropriate time, but the rate of growth is normal for the parent tissue. The benign tumor grows by hyperplastic expansion.

Characteristics of Malignant Cells

Cancer (malignant) cells are abnormal, serve no useful function, and are harmful to normal body tissues. The following characteristics are common in malignant tumors.

Demonstrate Rapid or Continuous Cell Division

Some cancer cells have a short generation time (2–4 hours); others have a generation time even longer than that of normal cells. Most cancer cells have a generation time similar to that of the parent tissue.

A major distinction between normal and cancer cells is that cancer cells divide nearly continuously. Almost as soon as one round of mitosis is complete, the daughter cells begin a new round.

Are Not Contact Inhibited

Cancer cells continue to divide even when contacted on all surface areas by other cells; thus, their growth is not contact inhibited. The persistence of cancer cell division, even under adverse conditions, is one factor making the disease so difficult to control.

Show Anaplastic Morphology

Cancer cells lose the specific appearance of their parent cells, becoming anaplastic. As a cancer cell becomes even more malignant, it becomes smaller and rounder. This loss of specific appearance can make diagnosis of cancer type difficult, because many types of cancer cells look alike.

Have a Large Nuclear–Cytoplasmic Ratio

The nucleus of a cancer cell is larger than that of a normal cell, and the cancer cell is small. The nucleus occupies much of the space within the cancer cell, creating a large nuclear–cytoplasmic ratio.

Lose Some or All Differentiated Functions

Along with losing the appearance of the parent cell, cancer cells lose some differentiated functions the parent tissue performed. Cancer cells serve no useful purpose.

Adhere Loosely Together

Cancer cells make little, if any, fibronectin. As a result, they adhere poorly to each other, and little pressure is needed to allow some cancer cells to break off from the primary tumor.

Are Able to Migrate

Because cancer cells do not bind tightly together and have many enzymes on their cell surfaces, they are able to slip through blood vessels and tissues and spread from the original tumor site to many other body sites. This ability to spread (metastasize) is a key characteristic of cancer cells.

Grow by Invasion

Cancer cells expand and extend into other tissues, both close by and more remote from the original tumor, by invasion or *metastasis*. Together with persistent growth, metastasis makes untreated cancer deadly.

CANCER DEVELOPMENT
Carcinogenesis/Oncogenesis

Carcinogenesis and *oncogenesis* are synonyms for cancer development. Table 26–3 summarizes key concepts about cancer development. The process of changing a cell with

TABLE 26-3

Key Concepts Related to Cancer Development

- Neoplastic cells originate from normal body cells.
- Transformation of a normal cell into a cancer cell involves mutation of the genes (DNA) of the normal cell.
- Early embryonic genes activated at an inappropriate time can cause a cell to develop into a tumor.
- Only one cell has to undergo malignant transformation for cancer to begin.
- Benign tumors grow by expansion, whereas malignant tumors grow by invasion.
- Most tumors arise from cells that are capable of cell division.
- Primary prevention of cancer involves avoiding exposure to known causes of cancer.
- Secondary prevention of cancer involves screening for early detection.
- Tobacco use is a causative or permissive factor in 30% of all malignant neoplasms.
- Tumors that metastasize from the primary site into another organ are still designated as tumors of the originating tissue.

a normal appearance and function into a cell with malignant characteristics is called *malignant transformation.* Malignant transformation occurs through the steps of *initiation, promotion, progression,* and *metastasis* (Caudell et al., 1996).

Initiation

The first step in carcinogenesis is initiation. Normal cells can become cancer cells if their proto-oncogenes are turned back on any time after early embryonic development is complete. Anything that can penetrate a cell, get into the nucleus, and damage the DNA can damage the genes, turning on genes that should remain repressed and turning off normal genes (Cooper, 1995). Substances that can change the activity of a cell's genes so the cell has malignant characteristics are called *carcinogens.* Carcinogens may be chemicals, physical agents, or viruses. Table 26–4 lists common carcinogens and the types of cancers they cause. Chapters presenting the care of clients with specific cancers discuss specific carcinogens (when known) under the heading "Etiology."

Pure carcinogens initiate mutational changes in a cell's genes and are thus called *initiators.* Initiation is an irreversible event that can lead to cancer development if it does not interfere with the cell's ability to divide.

Once a cell has been initiated, it can become a cancer cell if the cellular changes that occurred during initiation are enhanced by *promotion.* One cancer cell is not significant, however, unless it can divide. If it cannot divide, it cannot form a tumor. *If growth conditions are right, however, widespread metastatic disease can develop from just one cancer cell.*

Promotion

Once a normal cell has been initiated by a carcinogen and has cancer cell characteristics, it can become a tumor

if its growth is enhanced. The time between a cell's initiation and development of an overt tumor is called the *latency period,* which can range from months to years and depends on the type of cell initiated and the presence of promoters.

Promoters are substances that promote or enhance initiated cell growth (Weinberg, 1996). They can also shorten the latency period. Promoters may be hormones, drugs, and a wide variety of industrial chemicals.

Progression

After cancer cells have grown to the point that a detectable tumor is formed (a 1-cm tumor has at least 1 billion cells in it), other events must occur for this tumor to become a health problem. First, the tumor must establish its own blood supply. In the early stages, the center cells of the tumor receive nutrition only by diffusion from the surrounding fluids. However, after the tumor reaches 1 cm, diffusion is not efficient, and cells in the center of the tumor become hypoxic and start to die. To continue

TABLE 26-4

Known Environmental Carcinogens

Carcinogen	Associated Cancer Site or Neoplasm
Alcoholic beverages	• Liver, esophagus, mouth, pharynx, breast, colon, and rectum
Anabolic steroids	• Liver
Arsenic	• Lung, skin
Asbestos	• Lung, pleura, peritoneum, pericardium
Benzene	• Myelogenous leukemia
Chemotherapy drugs Alkylating agents Anthracycline antibiotics Antimetabolites	• Acute leukemia, lymphoma
Cyclosporine	• Non-Hodgkin's lymphoma
Diesel exhaust	• Lung
Formaldehyde	• Nasopharynx
Hair dyes	• Bladder
Ionizing radiation	• Bone marrow, thyroid, many organs
Mineral oils	• Skin
Pesticides	• Lung
Polycyclic hydrocarbons	• Lung, skin, scrotum
Polychlorinated biphenyls	• Liver, skin
Sunlight	• Skin, eyes
Tobacco	• Lung, esophagus, mouth, pharynx, larynx, pancreas, bladder, kidney, liver, stomach, colon, rectum, leukemia

to grow and survive, the tumor makes *tumor angiogenesis factor* (TAF). TAF stimulates capillaries and other blood vessels in the area to grow new branches into the tumor (Pitot, 1986). These blood vessels ensure the tumor's continued nourishment.

As tumor cells continue to divide, some of the new cells experience more change from the original initiated cancer cell. Actual colonies or subpopulations within the tumor begin to appear. These subpopulations differ from the original cancer cell. Some of the differences provide these subpopulations with advantages that allow them to live and divide no matter how the environmental conditions around them change, and are thus called "selection advantages" (Fidler & Hart, 1982). Changes that a tumor undergoes at this time allow it to become more malignant. Over time the tumor cells come to have fewer and fewer normal cell characteristics.

The original tumor formed from transformed normal cells is called the *primary* tumor. It is usually identified by the tissue from which it arose (parent tissue), such as in breast cancer or lung cancer. When primary tumors are located in vital organs, such as the brain or lungs, they can grow to such an extent that they either lethally damage the vital organ or "crowd out" healthy organ tissue and interfere with that organ's ability to perform its vital function. At other times, the primary tumor is located in soft tissue that can expand without damage as the tumor grows. One such site is the breast. The breast is not a vital organ, and even if it had a large tumor in it, the primary tumor would not cause the client's death. When the tumor spreads from the original site into vital areas, life functions can be disrupted.

Metastasis

In metastasis, cancer cells move from their original location by breaking off from the original group and establishing remote colonies. These additional tumors are called *metastatic* or *secondary tumors*. Even though the tumor is now in another organ, it is still a cancer from the original altered tissue. For example, when breast cancer spreads to the lung and the bone, it is breast cancer in the lung and bone, not lung cancer and not bone cancer. Metastasis occurs through several progressive steps, shown in Figure 26–6 (Liotta, 1992; Nicolson, 1979).

Extension into Surrounding Tissues

Tumors secrete enzymes that open up areas of surrounding tissue. Mechanical pressure, created as the tumor increases in size, forces tumor cells to invade new territory.

Penetration into Blood Vessels

The same enzymes that open up areas of surrounding tissue make large pores in the client's blood vessels, allowing tumor cells to enter blood vessels.

Release of Tumor Cells

Because tumor cells are loosely held together, clumps of cells break off the primary tumor into blood vessels for transport.

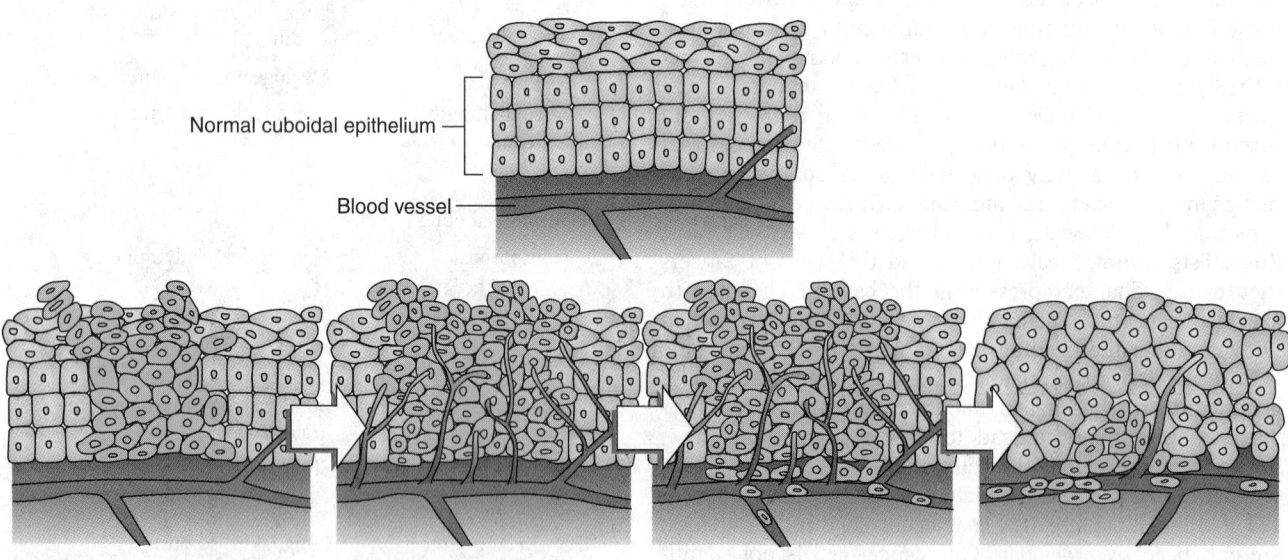

Malignant transformation
Some normal cuboidal cells have undergone malignant transformation and have divided enough times to form a tumorous area within the cuboidal epithelium.

Tumor vascularization
Cancer cells secrete tumor angiogenesis factor (TAF), stimulating the blood vessels to bud and form new channels growing into the tumor.

Blood vessel penetration
Cancer cells have broken off from the main tumor. Enzymes on the surface of the tumor cells make holes in the blood vessels, allowing cancer cells to enter blood vessels and travel around the body.

Arrest and invasion
Cancer cells clump up in blood vessel walls and invade new tissue areas. If the new tissue areas have the right conditions to support continued growth of cancer cells, new tumors (metastatic tumors) will form at this site.

Figure 26–6. The steps of metastasis.

TABLE 26–5

Common Sites of Metastasis for Different Cancer Types

Cancer Type	Sites of Metastasis
Breast cancer	• Bone* • Lung* • Liver • Brain
Lung cancer	• Brain* • Bone • Liver • Lymph nodes • Pancreas
Colorectal cancer	• Liver* • Lymph nodes • Adjacent structures
Prostate cancer	• Bone (especially spine and legs)* • Pelvic nodes
Melanoma	• Gastrointestinal tract • Lymph nodes • Lung • Brain
Primary brain cancer	• Central nervous system

*Most common site of metastasis for the specific malignant neoplasm.

Invasion of Tissue at Site of Arrest

Tumor cells circulate through the blood and enter tissues at remote sites. When conditions in the remote site are appropriate for the tumor, the cells stop circulating (arrest) and invade the surrounding tissues, creating secondary tumors. Table 26–5 lists the common sites of metastasis for specific tumor types. Three routes responsible for metastatic spread are local seeding, blood-borne metastasis, and lymphatic spread.

LOCAL SEEDING. Local seeding involves distribution of shed cancer cells in the local area of the primary tumor. In ovarian cancer, for example, cells often spill from the primary tumor into the peritoneal cavity and set up multiple seeding sites.

BLOOD-BORNE METASTASIS. Blood-borne metastasis (tumor cell release into the blood) is the most common cause of cancer spread. Combined with seeding, distribution via the bloodstream determines the area of metastases.

Many circulating tumor cells are destroyed by factors in the circulation, immune responses, or unsuitable environments in the organs in which the cells stop. Clumps of tumor cells can become trapped in capillaries. These clumps damage the capillary wall and allow tumor cells to enter the surrounding tissue.

LYMPHATIC SPREAD. Lymphatic spread is related to the number, structure, and location of lymph nodes and vessels. Primary sites rich in lymphatics are more susceptible to early metastatic spread than are areas with few lymphatics.

Cancer Classification

Terms that describe neoplasia by tissue origin and classify the tumor as benign or malignant are listed in Table 26–6. Other terms describe the tumor's biologic behavior, anatomic site, and degree of differentiation.

Approximately 100 different types of cancer arise from various tissues or organs. Figure 26–7 compares cancer

TABLE 26–6

Classification of Tumors by Tissue Type

Tissue of Origin	Benign Tumors	Malignant Tumors
Epithelial		
Glandular	Adenoma	Adenocarcinoma
Epithelial	Polyp, papilloma	Carcinoma
Connective		
Bone	Osteoma	Osteosarcoma
Fibrous	Fibroma	Fibrosarcoma
Fat	Lipoma	Liposarcoma
Smooth muscle	Leiomyoma	Leiomyosarcoma
Striated muscle	Rhabdomyoma	Rhabdomyosarcoma
Hematopoietic		
Erythrocytes		Erythroleukemia
Lymphocytes		Lymphocytic leukemia
Lymphatic tissue		Malignant lymphoma, Hodgkin's disease
Plasma cell		Multiple myeloma
Pigmented cells	Nevus	Melanoma
Neural	Neuroma	Glioblastoma

Modified from Caudell, K., Cuaron, L., & Gallucci, B. (1996). Cancer biology: Molecular and cellular aspects. In R. McCorkle, M. Grant, M. Frank-Stromborg, & S. Baird (Eds.), *Cancer nursing: A comprehensive textbook* (2nd ed., p. 154). Philadelphia: W. B. Saunders.

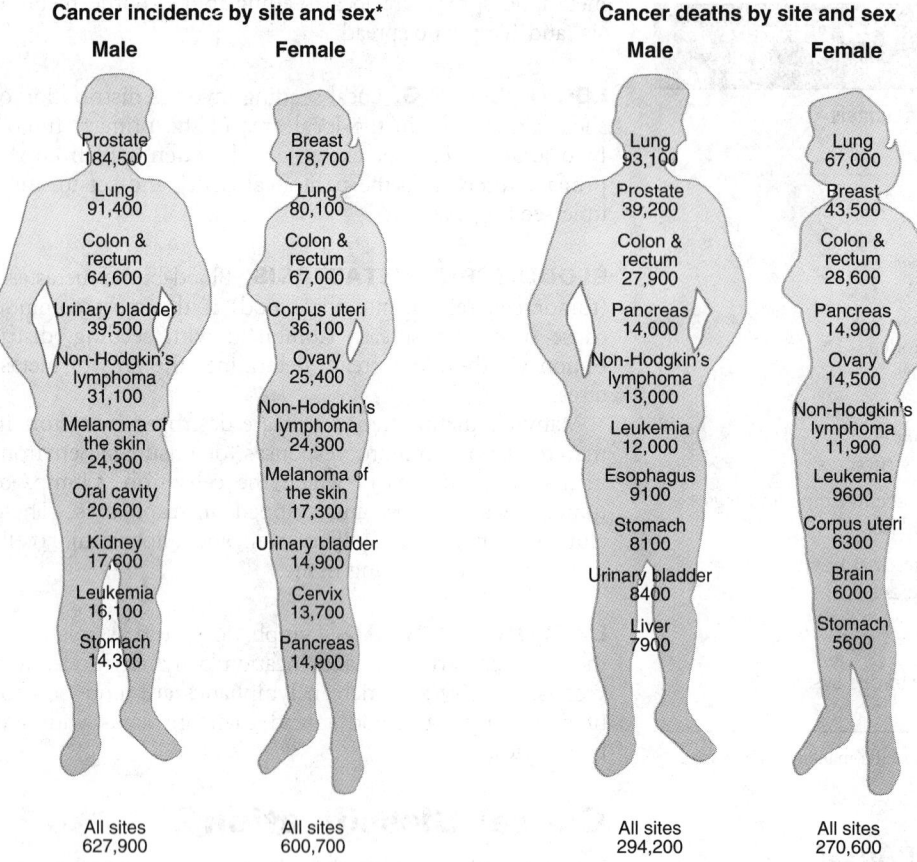

Figure 26–7. Cancer incidence and death by site and sex. (© 1998, American Cancer Society, Inc.)

distribution by site and gender. Cancers are divided into two major categories: solid and hematologic.

Solid tumors are associated with the organs from which they develop, for example, breast cancer and lung cancer. Hematologic cancers (e.g., leukemias and lymphomas) originate from blood cell–forming tissues, which communicate with all organs.

Cancer Grade and Stage

To help standardize cancer diagnosis, prognosis, and treatment, classification systems of grading and staging were developed. Grading a tumor classifies cellular aspects of the cancer. Staging of the client classifies clinical aspects of the cancer.

Grading

Some cancer cells are "more malignant" than others, varying in their aggressiveness and sensitivity to treatment. Some cancer cells barely resemble the tissue from which they arose, are aggressive, and rapidly metastasize. These cells are considered more malignant, a "high-grade tumor." On the basis of cell appearance and activity, grading compares the cancer cell with the normal parent tissue from which it arose (Caudell et al., 1996).

Different groups have established different grading systems for different kinds of cancer cells, but overall they resemble the standard system listed in Table 26–7. This system rates tumor cells; the lowest rating is given to those tumors that closely resemble normal cells and the highest to those that little resemble normal cells.

Grading the cells is the first step in confirming cancer. Grading provides one means of evaluating the client with cancer for prognosis and appropriate therapy. It also allows health care professionals to evaluate the results of management and compare local, regional, national, and international statistics.

Ploidy

Another biological feature describing cancer cells is chromosome number and appearance. Normal human cells have 46 chromosomes (23 pairs), the normal diploid number. When malignant transformation occurs, changes in the genes and chromosomes also occur. Some tumor cells gain or lose whole chromosomes and may have structural abnormalities of the remaining chromosomes. When a tumor cell has more or less than the normal diploid number, it is said to be *aneuploid*. The degree of aneuploidy generally increases with the degree of malignant transformation.

TABLE 26–7

Grading of Malignant Tumors

Grade	Cellular Characteristics
GX	• Grade cannot be determined.
GI	• Tumor cells are well differentiated and closely resemble the normal cells from which they arose. • This grade is considered a low grade of malignant change. • These tumors are malignant but are relatively slow-growing.
G2	• Tumor cells are moderately differentiated; they still retain some of the characteristics of normal cells but also have more malignant characteristics than do G1 tumor cells.
G3	• Tumor cells are poorly differentiated, but the tissue of origin can usually be established. • The cells have few normal cell characteristics.
G4	• Tumor cells are poorly differentiated and retain no normal cell characteristics. • Determination of the tissue of origin is difficult and perhaps impossible.

Staging

Staging determines the cancer's exact location and degree of metastasis present at diagnosis. Staging is important because, for most cancers, the smaller the tumor is at diagnosis and the less it has spread, the greater the chances are that treatment will result in a cure. Tumor stage also influences selection of therapy. Staging is done in three different ways:

1. Clinical Staging. This assesses the client's clinical manifestations and evaluates clinical signs for the tumor size and degree of metastasis. Clinical tests are used, and tumor cells may be obtained for biopsy, but clinical staging does not include major surgery.
2. Surgical Staging. This determines the tumor size, number, sites, and degree of metastasis by inspection at surgery.
3. Pathologic Staging. This is the most definitive type of staging. Tumor size, number, sites, and degree of metastasis are determined by pathologic examination of tissues obtained at surgery.

Some site-specific staging systems exist, such as Dukes' staging of colon and rectal cancer and Clark's levels method of staging skin cancer. The American Joint Committee on Cancer (AJCC) developed the TNM (tumor, node, metastasis) system to describe the anatomic extent of cancers. The stages guide treatment and are useful for prognosis and comparison of the end results of treatment. The TNM staging system is based on the concept that similar cancers share similar patterns of growth and extension. TNM staging systems are specific to each solid tumor site. Table 26–8 gives basic definitions for the TNM staging system. TNM staging is not useful for can-

cers that arise in the bone marrow or lymphoid tissues. Staging for these cancers is discussed in Chapter 42.

Tumor growth is discussed in terms of doubling time (the amount of time it takes for a tumor to double in size) and mitotic index (the percentage of actively dividing cells within a tumor). The smallest tumor likely to be detected by a physical examination or diagnostic test is 1 cm in diameter and contains 1 billion cells. To reach this size, a tumor will have undergone at least 30 doublings. A tumor with a mitotic index of less than 10% is a relatively slow-growing tumor; a tumor with one of 85% is fast growing. Tumors have a wide range of growth rates. Fast-growing tumors, such as lymphomas, may double in 4 weeks; an adenocarcinoma of the lung may double in 21 to 40 weeks.

Causes of Cancer Development

Carcinogenesis or oncogenesis takes years and depends on several tumor and client factors. Essentially, three interacting primary factors influence the development of cancer: environmental exposure to carcinogens, genetic predisposition, and immune function. These interactions account for variation in cancer development from one person to another, even when each person is exposed to the same hazards.

For some types of cancers, specific causes have been identified, and people at risk can avoid contact with specific agents associated with the development of that cancer type. This is called *primary prevention of cancer* and is effective in minimizing the risk for some types of cancers. For many types of cancer, however, absolute causes remain unknown. For other cancer types, even though the cause may be known, exposure cannot be avoided. These problems make primary prevention of some types of can-

TABLE 26–8

Staging of Cancer: TNM Classification

Primary Tumor (T)	
TX	• Primary tumor cannot be assessed
T0	• No evidence of primary tumor
Tis	• Carcinoma in situ
T1, T2, T3, T4	• Increasing size and/or local extent of the primary tumor
Regional Lymph Nodes (N)	
NX	• Regional lymph nodes cannot be assessed
N0	• No regional lymph node metastasis
N1, N2, N3	• Increasing involvement of regional lymph nodes
Distant Metastasis (M)	
MX	• Presence of distant metastasis cannot be assessed
M0	• No distant metastasis
M1	• Distant metastasis

Modified from American Joint Committee on Cancer. (1988). In O. H. Beahrs, D. E. Henson, R. V. Hutter, & M. H. Myers (Eds.), *Manual for staging of cancer* (3rd ed., p. 7). Philadelphia: J. B. Lippincott.

cers impossible (Mettlin & Michalek, 1996). For people with these cancers, early detection, or *secondary prevention*, can be helpful because treatment outcome is usually better with diagnosis of small tumors that have not metastasized.

Oncogene Activation

Regardless of specific cause, the mechanism of carcinogenesis appears to be the same: the activation of proto-oncogenes into oncogenes. When a normal cell is exposed to any carcinogen (initiator), the normal cell's DNA can be damaged or mutated. The mutations can cause the early embryonic genes (proto-oncogenes), which should be repressed forever, to be turned on or activated again. These genes are then oncogenes and can cause the cell to change from normal to malignant (Cooper, 1995).

About 50 different proto-oncogenes that can be activated into oncogenes have been identified so far, and scientists estimate that at least 50 more exist (Cooper, 1995; Weinberg, 1994). *These oncogenes are not abnormal genes* but are part of every cell's normal make-up and were critically important in early development. Oncogenes become a problem only if they are activated (derepressed) after development is complete, as a result of exposure to carcinogenic agents or events. Activation of some specific oncogenes causes specific cancers. Table 26–9 lists known oncogenes and the malignancies they have been

TABLE 26–9

Malignancies Associated with Altered Oncogene Activity	
Oncogene	**Malignancies**
abl	Chronic myelogenous leukemia, other leukemias
c-myc	Burkitt's lymphoma; T-cell and B-cell neoplasms; breast, stomach, and lung carcinomas
erb B	Glioblastomas, squamous cell carcinoma
erb B-2	Breast, salivary gland, ovarian carcinomas
ets	Lymphoma
hst	Breast carcinoma, squamous cell cancers
int-2	Breast carcinoma, squamous cell cancers
L-*myc*	Lung carcinomas
met	Osteosarcoma
myb	Colorectal carcinomas, leukemia
PRAD-1	Breast carcinoma, squamous cell cancers
H-*ras* K-*ras* N-*ras*	Carcinomas, sarcomas, neuroblastoma, leukemias, lymphomas
ret	Thyroid carcinomas
trk	Colorectal and thyroid carcinomas

Data from Cooper, G. (1995). *Oncogenes* (2nd ed.). Boston: Jones and Bartlett.

found to cause. Extrinsic and intrinsic factors are associated with oncogene activation.

Extrinsic Factors Influencing Cancer Development

Up to 80% of cancer in North America may be the result of environmental, or extrinsic, factors (Trichopoulos et al., 1996). Environmental carcinogens are chemical, physical, or viral agents that cause cancer. Table 26–4 lists known environmental causes of human cancer.

Chemical Carcinogenesis

Many chemicals capable of causing malignant transformation appear to have similar chemical structures. More than 20 organic and inorganic industrial chemicals, drugs, and other products used in everyday life are known to be carcinogenic, and hundreds are suspected of being so.

Some chemicals are complete carcinogens that can both initiate and promote cancer. Others are pure initiating agents, or incomplete carcinogens. Still others are only promoting agents. Some substances, such as tobacco and alcohol, appear to be only mildly carcinogenic; it takes chronic exposure to large amounts before a cancer develops. However, these two substances can act as cocarcinogens; when taken together, they enhance the carcinogenic activity of each other or other carcinogens.

Cells are not equally susceptible to chemically induced malignant transformation. Normal cells that retain the capacity for mitotic cell division are at greater risk for cancer development than are normal cells not capable of cell division. Cancers commonly arise in bone marrow, skin, lining of the gastrointestinal tract, ductal cells of the breast, and lining of the lungs. All of these cells normally undergo mitotic cell division. Cancers of nerve tissue, cardiac muscle, and skeletal muscle are rare. These cells do not normally undergo mitotic cell division.

Approximately 30% of cancers diagnosed in North America are related to tobacco use (American Cancer Society, 1998). It is the single most important source of preventable chemical carcinogenesis. Tobacco contains many different chemical compounds, including complete carcinogens and cocarcinogens. Tobacco use or ingestion can initiate and promote cancer. The risk of cancer development for a person who uses tobacco depends on his or her immune function; amount, depth, and mode of exposure; and tobacco tar content. The type of cancer that develops depends on the susceptibility of specific sites to various concentrations of tobacco and its metabolites.

Tissues associated with the greatest risk for cancer are those with direct contact with tobacco smoke. Cigarette smoking and tobacco use are also implicated in the development of cancers remote from tissues with direct contact with tobacco. Table 26–10 summarizes the association of tobacco and development of specific cancers.

Physical Carcinogenesis

Physical agents or events may cause cancer by the same mechanism as for chemical carcinogens, that is, by in-

TABLE 26–10

Malignancies Associated with Tobacco Use	
Lung	Oral cavity
Pharyngeal	Laryngeal
Esophagus	Pancreatic
Cervical	Kidney
Bladder	

Data from American Cancer Society. (1998). *Cancer Facts & Figures—1998* (Report No. 98-300M-No. 5008.98). Atlanta, GA: Author.

duction of DNA damage. Two types of physical agents suspected of causing cancer are radiation and chronic irritation (Pitot, 1986).

Radiation

Radiation is a physical agent capable of carcinogenesis. Even small doses of radiation affect cells. Some effects are temporary and reparable; others are irreversible and may be lethal to the damaged cell. The two types of radiation associated with carcinogenesis are ionizing and ultraviolet. Ionizing radiation occurs naturally in such minerals as radon, uranium, and radium. Most rocks and soil contain various concentrations of uranium and radium. Other sources of ionizing radiation include diagnostic and therapeutic x-rays and cosmic radiation. Ultraviolet (UV) radiation is the most common type of solar radiation. Other sources of UV radiation include tanning beds and germicidal lights. UV rays do not penetrate deeply, and the most common type of cancer associated with UV exposure is skin cancer.

Both ionizing and ultraviolet radiation produce gene mutations and chromosomal damage. Although radiation exposure induces cancers more frequently among cells that can divide, it can also cause cancer among nondividing cells as well.

Chronic Irritation

Chronic irritation and tissue trauma have been suspected as predisposing physical agents to cancer development, but this theory has not yet been supported directly. The incidence of skin cancer is higher in people with burn scars and other tissues that have sustained severe injury. Chronically irritated tissues may undergo frequent mitosis and, thus, are at an increased risk for spontaneous DNA mutation (Pitot, 1986).

Viral Carcinogenesis

Relatively few viruses have yet been proved to be carcinogenic to humans, although suspected to play major roles in cancer development. When viruses infect body cells, they break the DNA chain and insert their own genetic material into the human DNA chain. Breaking the DNA along with viral gene insertion mutates the normal cell's DNA and can either activate an oncogene or repress a

TABLE 26–11

Malignancies Associated with a Known Viral Origin	
Virus	**Malignancies**
Epstein-Barr virus	Burkitt's lymphoma, B-cell lymphomas, nasopharyngeal carcinoma
Hepatitis B virus	Primary liver carcinoma
Human papillomavirus	Cervical carcinoma, vulvar carcinoma, and other anogenital carcinomas
Human lymphotrophic virus type I	Adult T-cell leukemia
Human lymphotrophic virus type II	Hairy cell leukemia

Data from Cooper, G. (1995). *Oncogenes* (2nd ed.). Boston: Jones and Bartlett.

suppressor gene. Viruses capable of causing cancer are known as oncoviruses. Table 26–11 lists specific cancers of known viral origin.

Dietary Factors Related to Carcinogenesis

Epidemiologic data relate cancer development to many dietary practices or combinations of dietary practices and environmental exposures. However, the relationship of diet to carcinogenesis is poorly understood. Because dietary considerations are rarely independent of other possible carcinogenic agents, evidence of dietary contributions to cancer development is clouded. Suspected dietary factors include low crude fiber intake, high intake of red meat, and high animal fat intake. Preservatives, contaminants, preparation methods, and additives (dyes, flavorings, and sweeteners) are being assessed for possible carcinogenic effects. Chart 26–1 identifies foods considered to have high carcinogenic potential.

Chart 26–1

Health Promotion Guide: Dietary Habits to Reduce Cancer Risk

- Avoid excessive intake of animal fat.
- Avoid nitrites (prepared lunch meats, sausage, bacon).
- Minimize your intake of red meat.
- Keep your alcohol consumption to no more than one or two drinks per day.
- Eat more bran.
- Eat more cruciferous vegetables, such as broccoli, cauliflower, Brussels sprouts, and cabbage.
- Eat foods high in vitamin A (such as apricots, carrots, and leafy green and yellow vegetables) and vitamin C (such as fresh fruits and vegetables, especially citrus fruits).

Chart 26–2

Nursing Focus on the Elderly: Cancer Assessment Considerations

Cancer Type	Assessment Consideration	Cancer Type	Assessment Consideration
Colorectal cancer	• Ask the client whether bowel habits have changed over the past year (e.g., in consistency, frequency, or color). • Is there any obvious blood in the stool? • Test at least one stool specimen for occult blood during the client's hospitalization. • Encourage the client to have a baseline colonoscopy. • Encourage the client to reduce dietary intake of animal fats, red meat, and smoked meats. • Encourage the client to increase dietary intake of bran, vegetables, and fruit.	Skin cancer	• Examine skin areas for moles or warts. • Ask the client about changes in moles (e.g., color, edges, or sensation).

		Leukemia	• Observe the skin for color, petechiae, or ecchymosis.
			• Ask the client about
			    Fatigue
			    Bruising
			    Bleeding tendency
			    History of infections and illnesses
			    Night sweats
			    Unexplained fevers

Bladder cancer	• Ask the client about the presence of
	    Pain on urination
	    Blood in the urine
	    Cloudy urine
	    Increased frequency or urgency
		Lung cancer	• Observe the skin and mucous membranes for color.
			• How many words can the client say between breaths?
			• Ask the client about
			    Cough
			    Hoarseness
			    Smoking history
			    Exposure to inhalation irritants
			    Shortness of breath
			    Activity tolerance
			    Frothy or bloody sputum
			    Pain in the arms or chest
			    Difficulty swallowing

Prostate cancer	• Ask the client about
	    Hesitancy
	    Change in the size of the urine stream
	    Pain in back or legs
	    History of urinary tract infections		

Intrinsic Factors Influencing Cancer Development

Other intrinsic factors affect whether a person is likely to develop cancer, including immune function, age, and genetic predisposition.

Immune Function

The immune system protects the body from foreign invaders and non-self cells (see Chap. 23). Non-self cells include cells made in the body that are no longer normal, such as cancer cells. The part of the immune system responsible for cancer protection is cell-mediated immunity. Natural killer (NK) and helper T cells are most important to immune surveillance (Applebaum, 1992).

The instrumental role of the immune system in protecting the body from cancer is supported by cancer incidence statistics in immunosuppressed people. Children younger than 2 years and adults older than 60 years have immune systems that function at less than optimal levels, and both groups have a higher incidence of cancer compared with that of the general population. Organ transplant recipients taking immunosuppressive drugs to re-

duce the risk of organ rejection also have a higher incidence of cancer. In clients with AIDS, incidence may be as high as 70% (Pitot, 1986).

Age

Advancing age is probably the single most significant risk factor related to the development of cancer (American Cancer Society, 1991). Of all cancers, 50% occur in people older than 65 years (American Cancer Society, 1998). The higher cancer incidence in this age group may reflect

TABLE 26–12

The Seven Warning Signs of Cancer

• C   Changes in bowel or bladder habits
• A   A sore that does not heal
• U   Unusual bleeding or discharge
• T   Thickening or lump in the breast or elsewhere
• I   Indigestion or difficulty swallowing
• O   Obvious change in a wart or mole
• N   Nagging cough or hoarseness

TABLE 26–13

Malignancies Associated with Altered Suppressor Gene Activity

Suppressor Gene	Malignancies
APC	Colorectal, stomach, and pancreatic carcinomas
DCC	Colorectal carcinomas
MTS1	Melanoma; brain tumors; leukemias; sarcomas; breast, bladder, ovarian, lung, and kidney carcinomas
NF1	Neurofibroma, colon, astrocytoma
NF2	Neurofibroma, meningioma, schwannoma
p53	Breast, bladder, colorectal, esophageal, liver, lung, and ovarian carcinomas; brain tumors; sarcomas; leukemias and lymphomas
Rb	Retinoblastomas; sarcomas; breast, bladder, esophageal, and lung carcinomas
VHL	Renal cell carcinoma, pheochromo-cytoma, hemangioblastoma
WT1	Wilms' tumor

Data from Cooper, G. (1995). *Oncogenes* (2nd ed.). Boston: Jones and Bartlett.

lifelong accumulation of DNA mutations that result in cell transformation and cancer. The body may no longer be able to repair these mutations as it once did. The effectiveness of the immune system, especially cell-mediated immunity, is also reduced in the elderly, resulting in a limited ability to recognize and eliminate altered self cells. Cancer assessment considerations for the elderly are given in Chart 26–2.

Manifestations of cancer in elderly clients may be overlooked and attributed to changes that coincide with normal aging. Elders must be aware of and report symptoms, such as the seven warning signs of cancer (Table 26–12), to health care providers. Health care providers must treat these reports with respect and thoroughly investigate all manifestations suggestive of disease.

Genetic Predisposition

As previously discussed, oncogenes are primarily intrinsic factors related to carcinogenesis. Proto-oncogenes, precursors of oncogenes, are passed on from generation to generation. The development of cancer, however, depends on more than these genes. The proto-oncogene needs to be damaged or altered to allow expression of the oncogene. In some people, the location of specific proto-oncogenes is different and may allow them to be activated more easily (Cooper, 1995). In other people, the position of the oncogene may be normal, but the gene controlling the oncogene's activity, the *suppressor gene*, may be abnormal or out of place. These variations in gene location are

inheritable. Table 26–9 lists specific malignancies associated with altered oncogene activity; Table 26–13 lists specific malignancies associated with altered suppressor gene activity.

Patterns of genetic predisposition for cancer other than oncogenes have also been identified, including

- Inherited predisposition for specific cancers
- Inherited conditions associated with cancer
- Familial clustering
- Chromosomal aberrations

Table 26–14 lists different conditions associated with a genetic predisposition for cancer development.

TRANSCULTURAL CONSIDERATIONS

The incidence of cancer varies among races. American Cancer Society data, as reported by Wingo et al. (1996), show that African-Americans have a higher incidence of cancer than Caucasians do, and the death rate is higher for African-Americans. Since 1960, the overall incidence among African-Americans has increased 27%, whereas for Caucasians it has increased 12%. Cancer sites and cancer-related mortality vary along racial lines as well. Table 26–15 summarizes common cancers among Caucasian, African-American, Asian, and Hispanic populations.

When risks for cancer development are assessed, however, race and genetic predisposition cannot be considered alone. Behavior related to culture or ethnic group, geographic location, diet, and socioeconomic factors must also be assessed (Olsen & Frank-Stromborg, 1994; Palos, 1994). The American Cancer Society (1998) has reported that cancer incidence and survival are often related to socioeconomic factors, such as the availability of health care services or the belief that seeking early health care

TABLE 26–14

Conditions Associated with a Genetic Predisposition for Cancer

Condition	Specific Cancer Type
Inherited cancers*	• Retinoblastoma • Wilms' tumor
Familial clustering	• Breast cancer • Melanoma
Bloom's syndrome	• Leukemia
Familial polyposis	• Colorectal cancer
Chromosomal aberrations Down syndrome (47 chromosomes)	• Leukemia
Klinefelter's syndrome (47, XXY)	• Breast cancer
Turner's syndrome (45, XO)	• Leukemia • Gonadal carcinoma • Meningioma • Colorectal cancer

*Not all retinoblastomas or Wilms' tumors are inherited.

TABLE 26-15

Racial Differences in Cancer Development	
Race	**Common Cancer Types**
Caucasian	1. Lung
	2. Breast
	3. Colorectal
	4. Prostate
African-American	1. Lung
	2. Prostate
	3. Breast
	4. Colorectal
	5. Uterine
Asian	1. Breast
	2. Colorectal
	3. Prostate
	4. Lung
	5. Stomach
Hispanic	1. Prostate
	2. Breast
	3. Colorectal
	4. Lung

Data from American Cancer Society. (1994). *Cancer facts and figures—1994.* Atlanta, GA: Author.

has a positive effect on the outcome of cancer diagnosis (see Research Applications for Nursing).

CANCER PREVENTION
Avoidance of Known or Potential Carcinogens

A very effective means of preventing cancer development is avoidance of known or potential carcinogens. This method of prevention is appropriate when the cause of a specific cancer is known or strongly implicated and avoidance is easily accomplished. Examples of effective avoidance are using skin protection during sun exposure, avoiding tobacco, and eliminating environmental asbestos. As more causes of cancer are identified, the prevention method of avoidance will likely become even more effective.

Avoidance or Modification of Associated Factors

Absolute causes are not known for many cancers, but specific conditions or exposures appear to have an associated risk. Some examples are the increased incidence of some cancer types among people who consume alcohol; the association of a diet high in fat and low in fiber with colon cancer, breast cancer, and ovarian cancer; and the greater incidence of cervical cancer among women with many sexual partners. It is thought that avoidance or reduction of exposure to the associated condition or factor might result in decreased risks for cancer development.

Chemoprevention

A new form of cancer prevention, chemoprevention, is currently under study to determine its effectiveness. This strategy uses exogenous chemicals, such as synthetic chemicals, natural nutrients, or other substances found in plant food sources, to disrupt one or more steps important to cancer development. Such agents may be able to reverse existing damage or halt the progression of the transformation process. Chemoprevention agents have a variety of actions that disrupt at least one important step in the process of cancer development, including

- Blocking an inactive compound from becoming an active carcinogen
- Blocking the direct action of a carcinogen on DNA

▷ Research Applications for Nursing

Elderly African-American and Caucasian Women's Attitudes Toward a Cancer Diagnosis

Powe, B. (1995). Cancer fatalism among elderly Caucasians and African Americans. Oncology Nursing Forum, 22(9), 1355–1359.

The investigator of this prospective descriptive study surveyed the beliefs of elderly Caucasian and African-American women in senior citizen centers in a southern state. The majority of women were older than 70 years, and their average education was at the 8th-grade level. The survey questionnaire was developed by the investigator after an extensive literature review. Testing of the instrument revealed an alpha coefficient for reliability ranging from 0.84 to 0.87. Because the overall education level was relatively low, the questionnaire was read to the participants.

The results indicated that African-American participants had higher fatalism scores than did their Caucasian counterparts. It is suggested that people who are fatalistic about any diagnosis are less likely to seek screening or appropriate medical care and thus would reduce their chances for cure or long-term survival. The investigator suggests that educational interventions targeted to African-Americans could dispel myths and reduce fatalism, contributing to greater compliance with recommended cancer screening regimens.

Critique. Although the results showed a greater degree of fatalism among African-Americans as compared with Caucasians, educational and income levels were also predictors of fatalism. Replication of this study among people of different ethnicities but with higher educational backgrounds and socioeconomic resources could be conducted to determine whether ethnic differences in fatalistic outlook hold when other variables diminish. The survey questions were all "forced-choice" questions. Including open-ended questions may address the origin of fatalistic beliefs.

Possible Nursing Implications. Much of fatalism toward cancer is based on inaccurate information. Many people with fatalistic beliefs either have had negative experiences with cancer or are basing their opinions on out-of-date cancer statistics. Nurses must take responsibility in determining each client's beliefs regarding cancer prognosis and provide accurate, culturally sensitive information about the potential for improved cancer outcomes with different types of treatment.

TABLE 26–16

Agents Under Investigation for Chemoprevention of Cancer

Category of Prevention	Specific Agents
Prevention of carcinogen formation	Ascorbic acid (vitamin C) Tocopherol (type of vitamin E) Selenium Caffeic acid
Blocking the action of a carcinogen on DNA ("antimutagens")	Carotenoids (vitamin A derivative) Retinoids (vitamin A derivative) Ellagic acid Flavones Oltipraz Butylated hydroxyanisole
Enhancing the elimination of a carcinogen	Isothiocyanate Indole-3-carbinol
Suppression of carcinogenic action	Aspirin Retinoids Indomethacin Selenium Steroidal anti-inflammatory agents Protease inhibitors

Antipromotion activity	Carotenoids
	Retinoids
	Selenium
	Coumarin
	Piroxicam
	Indomethacin
	Calciferol (vitamin D)
	Hormone antagonists
	   Tamoxifen
	   Fenasteride

Suppression of progression	Danazol Interferon Cysteamine Vorozole

- Enhancing the rate of elimination of a carcinogen from the body
- Suppressing the activity of a carcinogen
- Suppressing the promoting activity of a carcinogen
- Suppressing the progression of a premalignant or early-stage malignancy into a more malignant state

Table 26–16 lists agents under current investigation for effectiveness in chemoprevention.

The ultimate goal of chemopreventive strategies is prevention of cancer development. Target populations for whom chemoprevention might be effective include

- Healthy people with no known specific cancer risk
- People at greater than normal risk because of increased environmental exposure or decreased immune function
- People with precancerous lesions
- People with a history of cancer

Gene Alteration as a Potential Form of Cancer Prevention

Because cancer development clearly involves gene changes, either congenital genetic abnormalities or acquired gene damage, researchers have suggested that altering damaged genes could prevent cancer development. At the present state of science, people can be screened for some gene alterations that will eventually lead to cancer. Such screening can help a genetically susceptible person either alter lifestyle factors or participate in early detection methods to identify a malignancy when cure is more likely. Although it is not yet possible to "fix" or remove an abnormal gene in humans, "gene therapy" in the future is not out of the realm of possibility.

SELECTED BIBLIOGRAPHY

*American Cancer Society. (1991). *Proceedings of the National Workshop on Cancer Control and the Older Person* (Report No. 91–3M–No. 3043). Atlanta, GA: Author.

American Cancer Society. (1998). *Cancer facts & figures—1997* (Report No. 98–300M–No. 5008.98). Atlanta, GA: Author.

Ames, B., Gold, L., & Willett. (1995). The causes and prevention of cancer. *Proceedings of the National Academy of Sciences, 92*(12), 5258–5265.

*Applebaum, J. (1992). The role of the immune system in the pathogenesis of cancer. *Seminars in Oncology Nursing, 8*(1), 51–62.

Appling, S. (1996). One in nine: Risks and prevention strategies for breast cancer. *Medical-Surgical Nursing, 5*(1), 62–64.

Baron, R., & Borgen, P. (1997). Genetic susceptibility for breast cancer: Testing and primary prevention options. *Oncology Nursing Forum, 24*(3), 461–468.

*Bishop, J. (1982). Oncogenes. *Scientific American, 246*(3), 80–92.

Bishop, J. (1995). Cancer: The rise of the genetic paradigm. *Genes and Development, 9*(11), 1309–1315.

Calzone, K. (1997). Genetic predisposition testing: Clinical implications for oncology nurses. *Oncology Nursing Forum, 24*(4), 712–718.

Caudell, K., Cuaron, L., & Gallucci, B. (1996). Cancer biology: Molecular and cellular aspects. In R. McCorkle, M. Grant, M. Frank-Stromborg, & S. Baird (Eds.), *Cancer nursing: A comprehensive textbook* (2nd ed., pp. 150–170). Philadelphia: W. B. Saunders.

Cooper, G. (1995). *Oncogenes* (2nd ed). Boston: Jones & Bartlett.

Cox, B. (1995). Cancer update 95. *Nursing 95, 25*(4), 47–49.

Daley, E. (1998). Clinical update on the role of HPV and cervical cancer. *Cancer Nursing, 21*(1), 31–35.

Dimond, E., Calzone, K., Davis, J., & Jenkins, J. (1998). Programmed instruction: The role of the nurse in cancer genetics. *Cancer Nursing, 21*(1), 57–74.

Erdos, D., & Mowad, L. (1995). Resources for helping patients to quit smoking. *Cancer Practice, 3*(4), 254–257.

Fidler, I., & Hart, I. (1982). Biologic diversity in metastatic neoplasia: Origins and implications. *Science, 217*(4564), 998.

Foltz, A., & Culhane, B. (1994). Cancer resources in the United States. *Oncology Nursing Forum, 21*(9), 1583–1593.

Frank-Stromborg, M., Heusinkveld, K., & Rohan, K. (1996). Evaluating cancer risks and preventive oncology. In R. McCorkle, M. Grant, M. Frank-Stromborg, & S. Baird (Eds.), *Cancer nursing: A comprehensive textbook* (2nd ed., pp. 213–264). Philadelphia: W. B. Saunders.

*Frank-Stromborg, M., & Olsen, S. (1993). *Cancer prevention in minority populations: Cultural implications for health care professionals.* St. Louis: C. V. Mosby.

Greco, K., & Kulawiak, L. (1994). Prostate cancer prevention: Risk reduction through life-style, diet, and chemoprevention. *Oncology Nursing Forum, 21*(9), 1504–1511.

Greenwald, P. (1996). Chemoprevention of cancer. *Scientific American, 275*(3), 96–99.

Greenwald, P., Kelloff, G., Burch-Whitman, C., & Kramer, B. (1995). Chemoprevention. *CA: A Cancer Journal for Clinicians, 45*(1), 31–49.

Grenier, L. M. (1995). Cancer information and resources for Hispanic populations. *Cancer Practice, 3*(5), 317–319.

Harrison, K., & Tempero, M. (1995). Diagnostic use of radiolabeled antibodies for cancer. *Oncology, 9*(7), 625–631.

*Liotta, L. (1992). Cancer cell invasion and metastasis. *Scientific American, 266*(2), 54–62.

McCorkle, R., Grant, M., Frank-Stromborg, M., & Baird, S. (1996). *Cancer nursing: A comprehensive textbook* (2nd ed.). Philadelphia: W. B. Saunders.

Mettlin, C., & Michalek, A. (1996). The causes of cancer. In R. McCorkle, M. Grant, M. Frank-Stromborg, & S. Baird (Eds.), *Cancer nursing: A comprehensive textbook* (2nd ed., pp. 138–149). Philadelphia: W. B. Saunders.

Misner, T., & Fuller, S. (1995). Testicular versus breast and colorectal cancer screening. *Cancer Practice, 3*(5), 310–316.

Mitelman, F. (1994). Chromosomes, genes, and cancer. *CA: A Cancer Journal for Clinicians, 44*(3), 133–135.

Morrison, C. (1996). Determining crucial correlates of breast self-examination in older women with low incomes. *Oncology Nursing Forum, 23*(1), 83–93.

*Nicolson, G. (1979). Cancer metastasis. *Scientific American, 240,* 66–79.

Olsen, S., & Frank-Stromborg, M. (1994). Cancer prevention and screening activities reported by African American nurses. *Oncology Nursing Forum, 21*(3), 487–494.

Olsen, S., & Frank-Stromborg, M. (1996). Cancer screening and early detection. In R. McCorkle, M. Grant, M. Frank-Stromborg, & S. Baird (Eds.), *Cancer nursing: A comprehensive textbook* (2nd ed., pp. 265–297). Philadelphia: W. B. Saunders.

Palos, G. (1994). Cultural heritage: Cancer screening and early detection. *Seminars in Oncology Nursing, 10*(2), 104–113.

*Pitot, H. (1986). *Fundamentals of Oncology* (2nd ed.). New York: Marcel Dekker.

Poe, M., & DeVore, L. (1996). Using the telephone for cancer information. *Cancer Practice, 4*(1), 47–49.

Powe, B. (1996). Cancer fatalism among African-Americans: A review of the literature. *Nursing Outlook, 44*(1), 18–21.

Powe, B. (1995). Cancer fatalism among elderly Caucasians and African-Americans. *Oncology Nursing Forum, 22*(9), 1355–1359.

Ruoslahti, E. (1996). How cancer spreads. *Scientific American, 275*(3), 72–77.

Soltis, M., Hubbard, S., & Kohn, E. (1996). The biology of invasion and metastasis. In R. McCorkle, M. Grant, M. Frank-Stromborg, & S. Baird (Eds.), *Cancer nursing: A comprehensive textbook* (2nd ed., pp. 190–212). Philadelphia: W. B. Saunders.

Stellman, J., & Stellman, S. (1996). Cancer and the workplace. *CA: A Cancer Journal for Clinicians, 46*(2), 70–92.

Swan, D., & Ford, B. (1997). Chemoprevention of cancer: Review of the literature. *Oncology Nursing Forum, 24*(4), 719–727.

Tomaino-Brunner, C., Freda, M., & Runowicz, C. (1996). "I hope I don't have cancer": Colposcopy and minority women. *Oncology Nursing Forum, 23*(1), 39–44.

Trichopoulos, D., Li, F., & Hunter, D. (1996). What causes cancer? *Scientific American, 275*(3), 80–87

Weinberg, R. (1996). How cancer arises. *Scientific American, 275*(3), 62–70.

Weinberg, R. (1994). Oncogenes and tumor suppressor genes. *CA: A Cancer Journal for Clinicians, 44*(3), 160–170.

Willett, W., Colditz, G., & Mueller, N. (1996). Strategies for minimizing cancer risk. *Scientific American, 275*(3), 88–95.

Wingo, P., Bolden, S., Tong, T., Parker, S., Martin, L., & Heath, C. (1996). Cancer statistics for African Americans, 1996. *CA: A Cancer Journal for Clinicans, 46*(2), 113–125.

SUGGESTED READINGS

Erdos, D., & Mowad, L. (1995). Resources for helping patients to quit smoking. *Cancer Practice, 3*(4), 254–257.

Cigarette smoking has been implicated as a cause of or major contributing factor to cancer development. This article suggests additional counseling and personal-contact interventions to be combined with alternative nicotine sources to help clients stop smoking through behavior modification.

Palos, G. (1994). Cultural heritage: Cancer screening and early detection. *Seminars in Oncology Nursing, 10*(2), 104–113.

This excellent article reviews the literature regarding culture, compliance, and cancer screening interventions. The author includes the cultures of poverty and aging as separate from the mainstream or dominant culture of the United States. A model for developing culturally appropriate cancer screening and early detection programs is also presented.

Ruoslahti, E. (1996). How cancer spreads. *Scientific American, 275*(3), 72–77.

The author makes excellent use of color diagrams and common language to describe what is known currently about metastasis. Scientific jargon is avoided when explaining the research that supports theories of cancer spread. A great article to give to clients and families.

INTERVENTIONS FOR CLIENTS WITH CANCER

Cancer, discussed in Chapter 26, is a broad term for a variety of malignant diseases originating in many different tissues and organs. The purpose of this chapter is to provide a general overview of common client problems and care issues related to the diagnosis and treatment of cancer. Specific risk factors, treatments, and side effects for each cancer type are presented in the chapters associated with the body system in which the cancer first developed. For example, melanoma is presented in Chapter 70, and breast cancer is presented in Chapter 77. Table 27–1 provides a guide to the text location of discussions of specific cancer types.

Cancer is a diagnosis that people fear and equate with death in spite of the fact that many types of cancer can be cured or controlled. A diagnosis of cancer causes psychological distress and has the potential to disrupt personal and professional relationships, finances, role identity, self-esteem, body image, and normal physiologic function. Providing care to clients and families experiencing cancer is challenging and complex. Table 27–2 lists key concepts about living with cancer.

GENERAL DISEASE-RELATED CONSEQUENCES OF CANCER
Pathophysiology

Cancer can develop in any organ or tissue, but tends to occur in some much more frequently than in others. Cancer destroys normal tissue, resulting in decreased function in that tissue or organ. Even when cancers occur in nonvital tissues or organs, they can cause death by metastasizing (spreading) into vital organs and disrupting critical physiologic processes (see Chap. 26). Left untreated, cancers produce serious health problems, such as

- Impaired immune and hematopoietic (blood-producing) function
- Altered gastrointestinal (GI) tract structure and function
- Motor and sensory deficits
- Decreased respiratory function

Not only do these impairments cause great physical and emotional distress to the client, but, without inter-

Table 27–1

Text Location of Specific Cancer Content				
Cancer Type	Chapter	Pathology/Etiology	Treatment	Nursing Care
Breast	77	1962	1963–1978	1963–1978
Lung	32	640–644	645–659	647–656
Prostate	79	2031	2032–2036	2032–2036
Colorectal	59	1410–1411	1411–1412	1412–1420
Skin	70	1743	1744–1746	1744–1746
Leukemia	42	961–963	963–978	967–978
Lymphoma	42	978–980	978–980	978–980
Ovarian	78	2013	2014–2015	2015

vention, persistent cancer invasion of normal tissues leads to death.

Impaired Immune and Hematopoietic Function

Impaired immune and hematopoietic function occurs most often in clients who have leukemia and lymphoma, but such impairment can occur with any cancer that invades the bone marrow. Tumor cells enter the bone marrow, causing decreased production of healthy white blood cells needed for normal immune function (see Chap. 23). Thus, clients who have cancer, especially leukemia, are at an increased risk for infection.

When cancer invades the bone marrow, it also decreases the number of red blood cells and platelets. These changes may be caused by the cancer itself, such as in leukemia, or by cancer treatment. In either case, the client becomes anemic and has an increased tendency to bleed.

Altered Gastrointestinal Structure and Function

Cancer can alter GI function and disturb the client's nutritional status. For example, tumors may cause obstruc-

Table 27–2

Key Points About Cancer Treatment
• With multiapproach to cancer treatment, 50% of clients with cancer can be cured. • Surgery is most effective for cancer therapy when tumors are small and well localized. • Radiation therapy is only effective on the tissues directly within the radiation path. • Side effects of radiation therapy are confined to the tissues within the radiation path. • The most common side effects of radiation therapy are skin irritation, fatigue, and altered taste sensation. • Chemotherapy is systemic therapy for cancer and affects all body tissues. • The most common side effects of chemotherapy are alopecia, nausea and vomiting, mucositis, skin changes, and bone marrow suppression. • The most life-threatening side effect of chemotherapy is bone marrow suppression.

tion or compression anywhere along the GI tract, interfering with the client's ability to ingest or digest adequate nutrients and eliminate waste products. In addition, tumors can affect a person's basal metabolic rate and increase requirements for protein, carbohydrates, and fat at the same time the person has less energy available to prepare food and eat.

Many tumors spread to the liver, causing profound damage. The liver has many important metabolic functions and helps digest and utilize proteins and fats. Altered liver function contributes to malnutrition and death among clients with cancer.

The anorexia experienced by clients with cancer often interferes with the client's ability to meet energy requirements. Cachexia (extreme body wasting and malnutrition) develops from the imbalance between food intake and energy use, and may occur in spite of what appears to be adequate nutritional intake. Changes in a client's taste can result from the cancer or the treatment and cause a decrease in appetite. A complete list of cancer-related factors that can contribute to malnutrition is presented in Table 27–3.

Nutritional support for the client with cancer, especially one undergoing cancer therapy, is complex and controversial. Often a diet high in protein and carbohydrates is ordered to assist the client to maintain his or her weight and provide nutrients needed for energy and cellular repair. However, some scientists believe that excessive intake of protein, carbohydrates, and vitamins increases the nutrition of the cancer cells and contributes to cancer progression. Clients often believe that by eating more food, especially a diet low in fat and high in fiber, grains, fruit, and vegetables, their cancer can be cured more easily. At present, no one nutritional plan meets the needs of all clients with cancer.

Motor and Sensory Deficits

Motor (movement) and sensory deficits can occur when cancers invade bone or the brain or compress nerves. In most clients with bone metastases, the primary cancer is in the prostate, breast, or lung. Bone sites most affected include the vertebrae, ribs, pelvis, and femur. The humerus, scapula, sternum, skull, and clavicle are also common metastatic sites. Bone metastases can cause fractures, spinal cord compression, and hypercalcemia,

Table 27–3

Causes of Malnutrition in Clients with Cancer

Anorexia

- Local causes
  - Pelvic or abdominal tumors
  - Hepatic metastases
  - Intestinal compression or obstruction
  - Others
- Remote causes
  - Food aversions
  - Early satiety
- Treatment-related causes
  - Postsurgical small stomach or stasis
  - Drugs, including chemotherapy
  - Radiation—local and systemic effects
- Systemic illness
  - Infection
  - Hepatitis or pancreatitis
  - Endocrinopathies
- Taste disorders
  - Drugs (e.g., metronidazole)
  - Remote effects of neoplasm and its treatment
  - Local disease and its treatment (e.g., stomatitis, naso-pharyngeal tumor, radiation, and surgery)
  - Nausea and vomiting
- Psychogenic causes
  - Depression
  - Anxiety
  - Conditioned aversions
- Intolerance of institutional food

Difficulty in Eating

- Head and neck tumors and their treatment
- Xerostomia
- Stomatitis
- Loss of teeth and dental problems
- Dysphagia and odynophagia

Maldigestion or Malabsorption

- Pancreatic insufficiency
- Bile salt deficiency
- Hypersecretory states
  - Zollinger-Ellison syndrome
  - Pancreatic cholera
  - Bowel infiltration
  - Diffuse invasion (e.g., lymphoma)
  - Local blockage
  - Fistula
- Postsurgical causes
  - Esophageal surgery (with vagotomy, gastric stasis diarrhea, and steatorrhea)
  - Gastrectomy—dumping, achlorhydria, or afferent loop syndrome
  - Small intestine resections
- Postirradiation causes
  - Enteritis (may occur as late sequela)
  - Fistula
  - Stenosis
  - Obstruction

Protein-Losing Enteropathy

Malutilization

- Cancer cachexia
- Steroids
  - Nitrogen wasting
  - Hyperglycemia
  - Calcium loss

each of which results in decreased mobility for the client.

The client may also experience sensory changes if the spinal cord is damaged by tumor compression or if nerve ganglia are compressed. When tumors metastasize to the brain, sensory, motor, and cognitive functions are severely disrupted.

The client with cancer may also experience pain. Pain does not always accompany cancer, but can be a significant problem for clients with terminal cancer. Chapter 9 provides an in-depth discussion of cancer pain causes and management.

Decreased Respiratory Function

Cancer can disrupt a client's respiratory function in several ways and often results in death. Tumors involving the airways can cause airway obstruction, for instance. If lung tissue is involved, lung capacity is decreased. Tumor growth can also press on vascular and lymphatic structures in the chest, blocking blood flow through the chest and lungs, resulting in pulmonary edema and dyspnea. Tumors also can thicken the alveolar membrane and damage pulmonary blood vessels, reducing gas exchange.

TREATMENT-RELATED CONSEQUENCES OF CANCER

The purpose of any cancer treatment is to prolong clients' survival time or improve quality of life. Although a few spontaneous regressions of malignant tumors have been reported, most clients with cancer would die within months of diagnosis without appropriate cancer therapy. Therapies for cancer include surgery, radiation, chemotherapy, hormonal manipulation, immunotherapy, and gene therapy. These therapies may be used individually or in combination to kill tumor cells. The type and amount of therapy are determined by the

- Specific type of cancer present
- Extent of the disease
- Overall health of the client

For most types of cancer, one or more regimens of therapy (protocols) have been established, based on ex-

Table 27-4

Diagnostic/Biopsy Surgeries for Cancer		
Biopsy Type	**Description**	**Problem/Limitations**
Needle	• Aspiration of cells in a fluid or in very soft tissue • Bore a "core" of solid tissue by using a long needle or making a punch, scrape, or bite.	• Sample error—may biopsy only noncancerous cells in a tissue or organ • Sample size may not be adequate for accurate testing • Procedure may spread cancer by seeding it into surrounding tissues • Procedure may damage healthy tissue
Incisional	• Wedge of suspected tissue is removed from a larger tissue mass, leaving some tumor cells remaining in the tissue.	• Sample error • Tumor seeding • Damage to healthy tissue
Excisional	• Complete removal of an entire lesion without removing any adjacent normal tissues	• Tumor seeding • Leaving micrometastasis • Damage to healthy tissue
Staging	• Multiple needle or incisional biopsies in tissues where metastasis is suspected or likely	• Tumor seeding • Sample error • Damage to healthy tissue

periments with cancer cells, animals, and other clients with cancer.

Surgery

Rationale for Cancer Treatment

Surgery for cancer involves removal of diseased tissue. If cancer is confined to the tissue removed, surgery alone can result in "cure" for that cancer. Although many cancers have spread too far at the time of diagnosis for surgery alone to be curative, surgery may still be a useful part of diagnosis, treatment, follow-up, and rehabilitation.

Mechanism of Action

Surgery is the oldest form of cancer treatment and the first method to cure cancer. Cancer surgery may be prescribed for any of the following purposes: prophylaxis, diagnosis, cure, control, palliation, determination of therapy effectiveness, and reconstruction.

Prophylaxis

Prophylactic surgery is performed when a client has either an existing "premalignant" condition or a known family history that strongly predisposes the person to the development of cancer. An attempt is made to remove the tissue or organ "at risk" and thus prevent the development of cancer. An example of prophylactic surgery for a premalignant condition is removal of a benign mole from a location where it would receive continuous irritation or exposure to sunlight.

Diagnosis (Biopsy)

Diagnostic surgery can provide histologic proof of malignancy. Usually, all or part of a suspected lesion is removed for microscopic examination and testing. Specific types of biopsies are summarized in Table 27-4.

Cure

Surgery for cure can, without additional therapy, result in a cure rate of 25% to 30%. All gross and microscopic tumor is either removed or destroyed. Types of curative surgeries are described in Table 27-5.

Control (Cytoreductive Surgery)

Cancer control, or cytoreductive surgery, is a "debulking" procedure that consists of removing part of the tumor while known gross tumor is left. This type of surgery alone cannot result in a cure, but it does decrease the number of cancer cells and increase the chances that other therapies can be successful.

Palliation

Palliative surgery aims not to cure (or even increase survival time in many instances) but to improve quality of life during the survival time. The surgeon removes tumor tissue that is causing pain, intestinal obstruction, or difficulty swallowing. What is done specifically during palliative surgery depends on the client's specific problem.

Determination of Therapy Effectiveness ("Second Look")

Second-look surgery is essentially a "rediagnosis" after treatment, performed to assess the disease status in clients who have been treated and have no symptoms of remaining or recurrent tumor. The results of this surgery serve as a basis for discontinuing or continuing specific therapy.

Reconstructive or Rehabilitative Surgery

Reconstructive-rehabilitative surgery is relatively new. People with cancer are surviving long enough to need reconstruction. This type of surgery increases function, en-

Table 27–5

Curative Surgeries for Cancer		
Surgery Type	**Description**	**Purpose/Use**
Local excision	• Removal of all identifiable tumor along with a small margin of normal tissues	• Small, localized tumors
Wide local excision (radical)	• Removal of identifiable tumor plus immediate tissue or adjacent tissue	• Small tumors with only local tissue invasion
Wide excision	• Removal of tumor, surrounding tissue, adjacent structures, and usual lymph channels draining the area	• Small to moderate-size tumors with known local invasion
Extended radical excision	• Removal of tumor, lymphatics, adjacent organs, and all tissues in the region	• Tumor infiltrate in a wide area but with no known distant metastasis

hances cosmetic appearance, or both. Examples include breast reconstruction after mastectomy, replacement of the esophagus after radiation damage, bowel reconstruction, revision of scars, release of contractures, and placement of penile implants.

Side Effects of Surgical Therapy

Unlike surgery performed for many other reasons, cancer surgery often involves the loss or loss of function of a specific body part. Sometimes whole organs are removed, such as the kidney, lung, breast, testes, arm, or tongue. Any organ loss results in reduced function. The amount of function that is lost and the degree to which the loss physically affects clients depend on the location and extent of the surgery. Some surgical procedures for cancer also may result in significant scarring or disfigurement. In addition to actual body part loss and anxiety about the chances of surviving, clients may be grieving about a loss of body image or a change in lifestyle imposed by the cancer or its treatment.

Nursing Care Needs of Clients Undergoing Surgical Therapy

Nursing care associated with surgery for cancer is not vastly different from that related to surgery for other reasons (see Chaps. 20–22). The nurse considers all the physical and psychosocial factors related to the client's ability (or that of family and significant others) to cope with the uncertainty of cancer and its treatment, along with changes in body image and role. For example, surgery involving the genitals, urinary tract, colon, and rectum may permanently damage these organs. Surgical procedures that create a urinary or fecal diversion (such as a colostomy) may disturb innervation, causing erectile impotence or ejaculatory dysfunction in men and painful intercourse (dyspareunia) in women.

Radiation

Rationale for Cancer Treatment

The purpose of all types of radiation therapy for cancer is to destroy cancer cells with minimal exposure of the normal cells to damaging actions of the radiation. The effects of radiation are seen only in those tissues in the path of the radiation beam. Some effects are apparent within days or weeks after radiation treatment; others may not be apparent for months to years after radiation therapy is completed.

Mechanism of Action

Most of the radiation used to treat malignant tumors is *ionizing* radiation. When cells are exposed to this type of radiation, atoms within the cell are "kicked out" of orbit, resulting in a tremendous release of intracellular energy. Ionizing radiation is given off naturally by some substances, such as radium and cobalt, and can also be generated by machines called linear accelerators. Naturally occurring radiation is called *gamma* radiation; radiation that is generated by machine is called *roentgen* radiation. Their effect on cells is exactly the same.

Cells damaged by radiation either die outright or become unable to divide. Cellular damage, caused by a combination of intracellular oxidation and tight binding of deoxyribonucleic acid (DNA) strands, inhibits cells' capacity to divide.

Radiation damage can occur any time a cell is exposed to radiation; it is not confined to cells actively in the cell cycle. However, cells in the cell cycle experience more damage when exposed to radiation than do nondividing cells.

Three different types of energy, or rays, are produced by gamma radiation: gamma, beta, and alpha rays (Hilderley & Dow, 1996). These rays vary in their ability to penetrate tissues and damage cells. Table 27–6 summarizes the features of these three types of gamma radiation, and Figure 27–1 shows the penetrating ability of each.

The intensity of the radiation emitted decreases with the distance from the radiation source (Fig. 27–2), the *inverse square law*. In practice, this means that the dose of radiation received at a distance of 2 inches from the radiation source is only 25% of the dose received at a distance of 1 inch from the radiation source; the dose of radiation received at 3 inches is only one-ninth the dose received at a distance of 1 inch (Hassey, 1987).

The amount of radiation aimed at or delivered to a tissue is called *exposure*, and the amount of radiation absorbed by the recipient tissue is called the *dose*. The

Table 27–6

Characteristics of Different Types of Gamma Radiation

Type of Ray	Characteristics
Gamma	• Gamma rays are very light with a low energy-transfer potential and travel at the speed of light allowing them to be concentrated and penetrate deeply into tissues. • This is the most common type of radiation used for the treatment of cancer. • This type of radiation can also cause serious, irreversible harm to tissues. • Exposure to this type of radiation must be avoided or severely limited.
Beta	• Beta rays are heavier with moderate to high speed. They have a high linear energy-transfer potential and do not penetrate tissues or other substances well. • Some beta rays are used inside the body for specific radiation therapy. • Beta rays are used in some diagnostic tests. • Beta rays pose health hazards to humans exposed to them, but exposure must be considerable for damage to occur.
Alpha	• Alpha rays are very heavy and slow. They easily transfer energy to surroundings and quickly lose their ability to penetrate tissues (0.04 mm into tissue). • Currently, alpha rays are used in laboratory tests rather than as treatment for cancer. • This type of radiation is harmful to humans only if it is ingested chronically.

dose is always somewhat less than the exposure. Three major factors determine the absorbed dose: intensity of the radiation exposure, proximity of the radiation source to the cells, and duration of exposure.

Killing Effects of Radiation

If the dose of radiation is high enough, all cells will be killed immediately, but this does not usually happen. Instead, radiation damage to the DNA is not usually apparent until the cell attempts to divide. In a population of tumor cells treated with a single exposure of radiation, all cells within the tumor absorb the radiation slightly differently; thus, their overall response to the radiation is slightly different. A few cells die immediately on exposure, and more die within the next 24 hours as they attempt to divide. Some cells become sterile as a result of this single treatment; still others repair the radiation-induced damage and continue to reproduce for many cell generations.

Because of the varying responses of all cancer cells within a given tumor, radiation for cancer therapy is administered as a series of divided doses. Small doses of radiation are delivered on a daily basis for a set period of time. Giving radiation treatment serially rather than as a single dose allows multiple opportunities to catch and destroy cancer cells that survived the initial hit of radiation while minimizing damage to normal tissues. This dose division is called *fractionation*. Standard radiotherapy is usually fractionated between 180 and 250 rad/day, multiplied by as many days as needed to achieve the total prescribed dose.

The total therapeutic dose of radiation to a tumor varies according to the size of the tumor, location of the tumor, radiation sensitivity of the tumor, and radiation sensitivity of the surrounding normal tissues. Some normal tissues are more sensitive to radiation than other normal tissues. For example, a total dose of 1200 rad might be prescribed for a primary liver tumor, but a total dose of 5000 to 6000 rad for a breast carcinoma (delivered over 25–30 separate days). If a 6000-rad dose were delivered to the liver, such extensive damage would occur to liver tissue that the client would experience liver failure and die even if the tumor were destroyed.

Two types of radiation delivery are most commonly used for cancer therapy: teletherapy and brachytherapy. The type used depends on the site of the tumor, stage of the tumor (including size and depth of the lesion), radiosensitivity of the tumor, and the client's general condition and state of health. Regardless of how administered, the optimum dose of radiation is one that cures or pro-

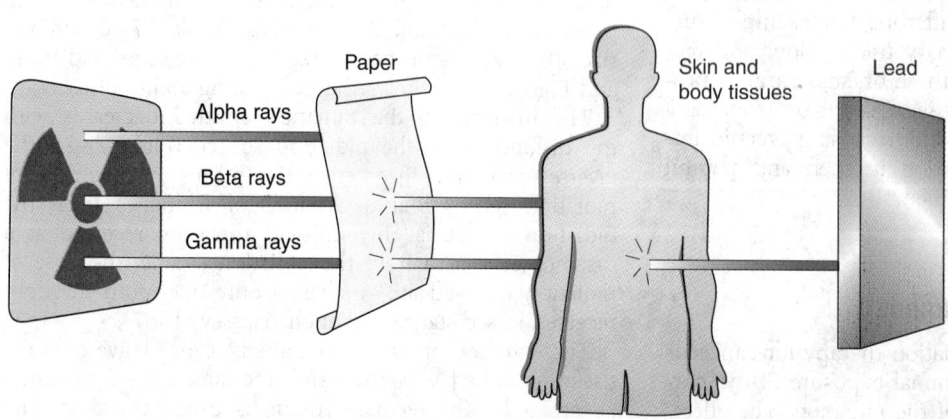

Figure 27–1. Penetrating capacity of different types of radiation.

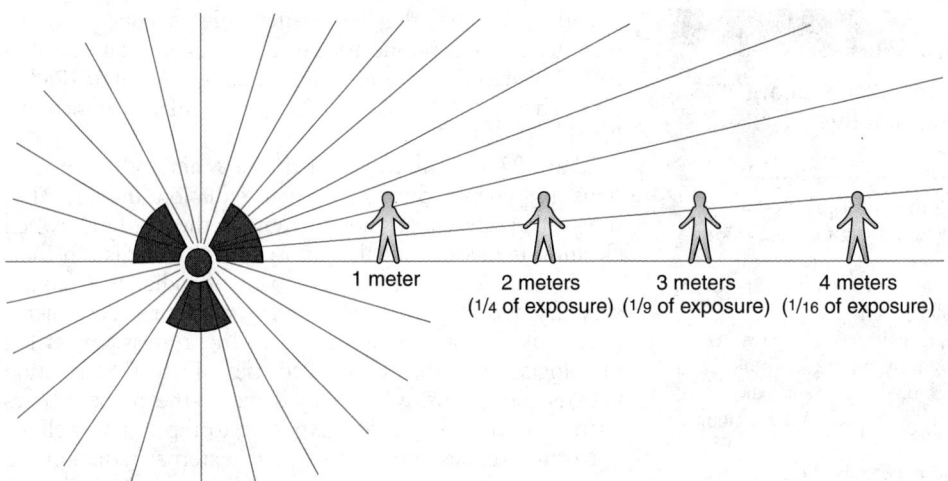

Figure 27–2. The inverse square law of radiation exposure.

1 meter

2 meters
(1/4 of exposure)

3 meters
(1/9 of exposure)

4 meters
(1/16 of exposure)

duces the desired killing effect on the cancer cells with an acceptable level of damage to normal tissues (some damage to normal tissues cannot be avoided).

Teletherapy

Teletherapy is derived from the Greek prefix "tele," meaning distant. In teletherapy, the actual radiation source is external to the client and remote from the tumor site. Because the source is external, the client never emits radiation and poses no hazard to anyone else. This type of therapy is also called *beam* radiation.

To increase the accuracy of radiation delivery to cancer cells, exact localization of the tumor is determined first. Once the pattern of radiation delivery has been established, the client must always be in exactly the same position for all treatments. The nurse makes sure that the client can get into and maintain this position with relative ease. Position-fixing devices and markings, either on the client's body or on the devices, ensure that the client assumes the proper position each day of treatment.

Brachytherapy

Brachytherapy is derived from the Greek word "brach," meaning short. In brachytherapy, the radiation source must come into direct, continuous contact with the tumor tissues for a specific period of time. The rationale is to provide a high absorbed dose of radiation in tumor tissues and a very limited absorbed low dose in surrounding normal tissues. The radiation delivered by brachytherapy has the same tissue effects as ionizing radiation delivered by external sources.

Brachytherapy involves the use of radioactive isotopes, either in solid form or within body fluids. Isotopes can be delivered to the tumor tissues in several ways. *With all types of brachytherapy, the radiation source is within the client; thus, for a period of time, the client emits radiation and can pose a hazard to others.*

UNSEALED RADIATION SOURCES. Soluble isotopes are unsealed radioactive sources administered via the oral or intravenous (IV) routes, or as an instillation into body cavities such as the peritoneal cavity and the spinal fluid space. Because the isotopes are unsealed, they are not completely confined to any one body area, although they may concentrate more in some body tissues than in others. These soluble isotopes enter body fluids, and eventually are eliminated from the body in various excreta (waste products), which are radioactive and can be harmful to other people.

An example of brachytherapy with soluble isotopes is the ingestion or injection of the radionuclide iodine 131 (an iodine base with a half-life of 8.05 days) to treat hyperthyroidism and some thyroid malignancies. The radioactive iodine concentrates in the thyroid gland, destroying the thyroid cancer cells. Most of this isotope is eliminated from the body within 48 hours. Once eliminated, neither the client nor the excreta are radioactive.

SEALED RADIATION SOURCES. The solid forms of brachytherapy involve sealed, temporary or permanent radiation sources implanted within the tumor target tissues. Most of the implants emit lower energy radiation continuously to tumor tissues. Some devices, such as seeds or needles, can be placed into the tissues and will stay in place alone. Other solid radiation sources must be held in place within the tissue or cavity by special applicators. The needles and seeds are radioactive at the time of insertion or implantation, and have already been preloaded with the radioactive isotope ("hot implantation"). Some of these devices are so small and the half-life of the isotope so short that the device is permanently left in place (most often for clients with prostate cancer). Other devices are removed and are reused in other clients.

In afterloading, the implant, without the radioactive isotope, is placed within the cavity, with special applicators that hold it in position. When placement has been ascertained and the client is in the proper environment, the implants are loaded with the radioisotope. After the prescribed dose has been delivered, the implant, radioisotopes, and position-holding applicators are removed. *With solid implants, the client emits radiation while the implant is in place, but the excreta are not radioactive* (Chart 27–1).

Chart 27–1

Nursing Care Highlight: Care of the Client with Sealed Implants of Radioactive Sources

• Assign the client to a private room with a private bath.
• Place a "Caution: Radioactive Material" sign on the door of the client's room.
• Wear a dosimeter film badge at all times while caring for clients with radioactive implants. The badge offers no protection, but measures an individual's exposure to radiation and should be used by only one individual.
• Pregnant nurses should not care for these clients; do not allow children younger than 16 or pregnant women to visit.
• Limit each visitor to one-half hour per day. Be sure visitors are at least 6 feet from the source.
• Never touch the radioactive source with bare hands. In the rare instance that it is dislodged, use a long-handled forceps to retrieve it. Deposit the radioactive source in the lead container kept in the client's room.
• Save all dressings and bed linens until after the radioactive source is removed. After the source is removed, dispose of dressings and linens in the usual manner. Other equipment can be removed from the room at any time.

Side Effects of Radiation Therapy

Because the immediate and long-term side effects for all types of radiation are limited to the tissues exposed to the radiation, side effects vary according to the site. Skin changes and hair loss (alopecia) are local but likely to be permanent, depending on total absorbed dose (Hilderley & Dow, 1996).

Depending on the dose, altered taste sensations and fatigue are two systemic side effects often noted by clients receiving external beam radiation, regardless of radiation site. Change in taste is thought to be caused by metabolites released from dead and dying cells. In particular, many clients experience an aversion to the taste of red meats. Fatigue may be related to the increased energy demands needed to repair radiation-damaged cells (Hilderley & Dow, 1996).

Radiation damage to normal tissues during cancer therapy can initiate inflammatory responses that cause tissue fibrosis and scarring. Their effects may not be apparent for many years after radiation treatment. For example, women who receive high-dose radiation therapy for uterine cancer may experience radiation-induced changes in the colon years later, resulting in constipation and obstruction.

Nursing Care of Clients Undergoing Radiation Therapy

Most clients are anxious about radiation. The nurse must be knowledgeable about its nature and be able to explain its purpose and side effects to clients and families. When clients receive concrete objective information regarding radiation therapy, they are better able to cope with the treatment and continue to participate in normal activities (see Research Applications for Nursing: Accurate Radiation Therapy Information Positively Affects Functional Level).

Chart 27–2 summarizes skin care and other precautions for clients during external radiation therapy. The nurse instructs clients not to remove the markings when cleaning the skin until the entire course of radiation therapy is completed. Skin in the path of radiation becomes very dry and may break down. The nurse instructs clients not to use lotions or ointments in these areas unless the radiologist prescribes them. Because skin in the radiation path is more sensitive to sun damage, the nurse advises clients to avoid direct skin exposure to the sun as well.

Normal tissues most sensitive to external radiation are hematopoietic (blood producing), epithelial (including

▶ Research Applications for Nursing

Accurate Radiation Therapy Information Positively Affects Functional Level

Johnson, J. (1996). Coping with radiation therapy: Optimism and the effect of preparatory interventions. Research in Nursing & Health, 19(1), 3–12.

The investigator of this prospective experimental study hypothesized that pessimistic clients undergoing radiation therapy for cancer might benefit from concrete information on self-regulation theory and that optimistic clients would benefit from instruction in self-care and coping. The interventions were audiotaped messages. The control group's tape recordings focused on radiation therapy topics not specific to the client's situation. The coping experimental group's tape recordings focused on specific strategies to deal with particular side effects of radiation therapy. The concrete objective group's tape recordings focused on exactly what would happen during radiation therapy and what types of side effects could be expected. Mood, outcome expectancies, disruption of usual activities, and clinical data were measured during and after radiation therapy.

Neither the self-care instruction nor the coping strategy intervention affected the outcome variables. The concrete objective intervention had a positive effect on function for both pessimists and optimists. The findings of this study are not consistent with similar studies conducted one and two decades ago.

Critique. The article did not indicate whether the clients were tested for their coping skills, knowledge of radiation therapy, or previous experience with cancer (their own or a close contact's) before the interventions. No pretreatment data on activity disruption were obtained. Such information could be useful in determining homogeneity of the participant groups.

Possible Nursing Implications. Although research in the area of coping indicates that some clients do not actively seek information as a coping strategy, most clients appear to benefit from honest and accurate objective information. Nurses need to provide objective concrete information regarding procedures and treatments to all clients and family members.

skin, mucous membranes, and hair follicles), and gonadal (reproductive) tissues. Some changes caused by radiation are permanent. Long-term problems experienced by clients vary with the location and dose of radiation administered. For example, radiation to the throat and upper chest can cause the client difficulty in swallowing. Head and neck radiation may damage the salivary glands and cause dry mouth. The nurse teaches clients about the types of symptoms that might be expected from the location and dose of radiation delivered.

Chemotherapy

Chemotherapy, the treatment of disease through chemical agents, has assumed a major role in managing clients with cancer. Chemotherapy as a cancer treatment is used to cure, increase mean survival time, and decrease the risk for specific life-threatening complications.

Rationale for Cancer Treatment

As described in Chapter 26, a characteristic of cancer growth is the ability of cancer cells to separate from the original tumor, spread to new areas, and establish new cancers at distant sites (metastasize). Clients with metastatic disease will die of their cancers unless treatment focuses on the metastatic cancer cells as well as the original cancer cells. Chemotherapy is useful in treating cancer because its effects are systemic and thus provide the opportunity to kill metastatic cancer cells that may have escaped local treatment. Table 27-7 indicates general responsiveness of specific cancers for chemotherapy.

Mechanism of Action

Chemotherapy can be successful in treating cancer because it has some demonstrated selectivity for cancer cells over normal cells. The killing effect of chemotherapy on cancer cells appears to be related to its ability to damage DNA and interfere with cell division. Because of this, the tumors most sensitive to chemotherapy are those that have rapid growth.

Unfortunately, chemotherapeutic agents usually are administered systemically and exert their cell-damaging (cytotoxic) effects against both healthy and cancerous cells. Normal cells most profoundly affected by systemic chemotherapy are those that undergo frequent cell division, including skin, hair, epithelial lining of the gastrointestinal (GI) tract, spermatocytes, and hematopoietic cells.

Chemotherapy includes many drugs or chemical compounds that are effective in killing cancer cells, and are classified by the specific

- Types of biologic action they exert in the cancer cell
- Period in the life of a cell during which the chemotherapeutic agent is most likely to succeed in disrupting vital cell processes

Table 27-8 lists categories and specific chemotherapeutic agents.

Antimetabolites

Antimetabolites are chemicals similar to normal metabolites (cofactors, vitamins, and nucleotides—purines and

Table 27-7

General Tumor Responsiveness to Standard Chemotherapy

Malignancies Usually Very Responsive to Chemotherapy
- Acute lymphocytic leukemia (ALL)
- Chronic lymphocytic leukemia (CLL)
- Lymphoma (Hodgkin's)
- Choriocarcinoma
- Small cell lung cancer

Malignancies Often Responsive to Chemotherapy
- Breast carcinoma
- Testicular carcinoma
- Prostatic carcinoma
- Head and neck carcinoma
- Acute myelocytic leukemia (AML)
- Chronic myelocytic leukemia (CML)

Malignancies Occasionally Responsive to Chemotherapy
- Colorectal carcinomas
- Central nervous system tumors
- Multiple myeloma
- Ovarian carcinoma
- Uterine carcinoma

Malignancies Usually Nonresponsive to Chemotherapy
- Renal cell carcinoma
- Pancreatic carcinoma
- Bladder carcinoma
- Liver carcinoma (primary)
- Non–small cell carcinomas of the lung

From Guy, J. (1991). Medical oncology—The agents. In S. Baird, R. McCorkle, & M. Grant (Eds.), *Cancer nursing: A comprehensive textbook* (pp. 266–290). Philadelphia: W. B. Saunders. Used with permission.

Table 27–8

Categories of Chemotherapeutic Agents

Generic Name	Trade Name	Usual Dose	Nadir
Antimetabolites			
Methotrexate	Mexate, Folex	3.3 mg/m^2	10–14 days
6-Mercaptopurine	Purinethol	80–100 mg/m^2	5–40 days
6-Thioguanine	Lanvis	2–3 mg/kg	1–4 weeks
5-Fluorouracil	Adrucil, Efudex, Fluoroplex	300–750 mg/m^2	9–14 days
Fludarabine	Fludara	25 mg/m^2	3–25 days
Floxuridine	FUDR	0.1–0.6 mg/kg	4–7 days
Cytarabine	Cytosar, ara-C	100–300 mg/m^2	4–7 days
Pentostatin	Nipent	4 mg/m^2	3–10 days
Gemcitabine	Gemzar	800 mg/m^2	7–12 days
Antibiotics			
Bleomycin	Blenoxane	10–20 U/m^2	7–14 days
Dactinomycin	Cosmegen	0.4–0.6 mg/m^2	14–21 days
Doxorubicin	Adriamycin, Rubex	50–80 mg/m^2	10–15 days
Daunorubicin	Cerubidine	30–60 mg/m^2	10–14 days
Idarubicin	Idamycin	12–25 mg/m^2	10–14 days
Plicamycin	Mithracin	0.025–0.030 mg/m^2	10–12 days
Mitomycin C	Mutamycin	10–20 mg/m^2	21–50 days
Mitoxantrone	Novantrone	12–14 mg/m^2	7–10 days
Alkylating Agents			
Cyclophosphamide	Cytoxan, Procytox	50–500 mg/m^2	7–14 days
Cisplatin	Platinol	25–120 mg/m^2	10–20 days
Carboplatin	Paraplatin	360 mg/m^2	21–28 days
Ifosfamide	IFEX	1.2 g/m^2	10 days
Mechlorethamine	Mustargen	0.2–0.3 mg/kg	10–14 days
Busulfan	Myleran	1–8 mg	14–21 days
Chlorambucil	Leukeran	1–4 mg/m^2	> 28 days
Melphalan	Alkeran	1–6 mg/m^2	14–21 days
Carmustine	BiCNU	200–250 mg/m^2	4–6 weeks
Lomustine	CCNU, CeeNU	130 mg/m^2	4–6 weeks
Thiotepa		0.3–0.8 mg/kg	15–30 days
Streptozocin	Zanosar	500–1500 mg/m^2	14 days
Antimitotics			
Vincristine	Oncovin, leurocristine, VCR	0.5–2.0 mg/m^2	7 days
Vinblastine	Velban, Velbe, Velsar	5–10 mg/m^2	5–11 days
Vindesine	DAVA, Eldisine	2 mg/m^2	2–7 days
Vinorelbine	Navelbine	30 mg/m^2	7–10 days
Etoposide	VP16, VePesid	50–100 mg/m^2	8–10 days
Paclitaxel	Taxol	100–250 mg/m^2	8–11 days
Teniposide	Vumon, VM-26	100–180 mg/m^2	8–10 days
Docetaxel	Taxotere	60–100 mg/m^2	8–10 days
Topoisomerase Inhibitors			
Irinotecan	Camptosar	125–150 mg/m^2	18–25 days
Topotecan	Hycamtin	1.5 mg/m^2	7–14 days
Other Agents			
Procarbazine	Matulane, Natulan	100–300 mg	14–28 days
Dacarbazine	DTIC	75–250 mg/m^2	10–14 days
Hydroxyurea	Hydrea	25 mg/kg	4–7 days
Asparaginase	Elspar	200–1000 IU/kg	4–10 days

United States Pharmacopeia (1998). Drug information for the health care professional (Vol. 1, 18th ed.). Taunton, MA: World Color Book Services.

pyrimidines) that play critical roles in essential cell processes. Most cellular reactions require metabolites to begin or continue the reaction. Antimetabolites closely resemble normal metabolites, and can be considered "counterfeit" metabolites that literally fool cancer cells into using the antimetabolites in cellular reactions. Because antimetabolites cannot function as proper metabolites, their presence impairs or prevents cell division.

Antitumor Antibiotics

Antitumor antibiotics are a class of anticancer drugs initially developed to combat bacterial infections by causing major damage on the cell's DNA and interrupting DNA or ribonucleic acid (RNA) synthesis. Exactly how the interruptions occur varies with each antibiotic.

Alkylating Agents

All alkylating agents cross-link DNA by various means. Whatever the mechanism, the double strands of DNA become more tightly bound together. This tight binding prevents proper DNA and RNA synthesis, thus resulting in inhibition of cell division.

Antimitotic Agents

Antimitotic agents are alkaloid substances made from plant sources. Their primary mechanism of action is to interfere with the proper formation of microtubules, so cells cannot complete mitosis during cell division. As a result, the cell either does not divide at all or divides only once, resulting in two daughter cells with unequal amounts of DNA that cannot continue to divide.

Miscellaneous Chemotherapeutic Agents

The actions of other chemotherapeutic agents do not fit any of the broad categories of chemotherapeutic agents and include

- Inhibition of important enzyme systems
- Competition for important substances in metabolic pathways

Combination Chemotherapy

Chemotherapy for cancer usually involves the timed administration of more than one specific anticancer drug, called *combination chemotherapy*. Using more than one drug is much more effective in killing cancer cells than using a single agent. Unfortunately, the damage caused to normal tissues also is increased with combination chemotherapy.

Table 27–9 presents one protocol (among many) of combination chemotherapy for breast cancer. The selection of drugs is based on known tumor sensitivity to the

Table 27–9

Example of One Chemotherapy Protocol for Breast Cancer		
Agent	**Dose**	**Route**
Cyclophosphamide	250–400 mg/m²	Intravenous
Methotrexate	3–5 mg/m²	Intravenous
5-Fluorouracil	500 mg/m²	Intravenous

This combination is administered every 3–4 weeks (depending on severity of immunosuppression) × six rounds.

drugs and the degree of side effects expected. For example, most chemotherapeutic drugs suppress bone marrow activity and immune function to some degree, but some agents are more profoundly immunosuppressive than others. These include busulfan, cyclophosphamide, etoposide, dactinomycin, doxorubicin, and mechlorethamine. There is also variation in the timing of drug-induced immunosuppression.

The time during which bone marrow activity and peripheral white blood cell counts are at their lowest levels after chemotherapy is the *nadir*. The nadir occurs at different times for different chemotherapeutic agents (see Table 27–8). For instance, the expected nadir after cytosine arabinoside administration is 5 to 7 days; after methotrexate, 10 to 14 days, and after mitomycin C, about 4 weeks. Combination chemotherapy is planned to avoid prescribing different drugs with nadirs at or near the same time to minimize immunosuppression.

Drug Dosage

Doses of most chemotherapeutic agents are calculated according to the type of cancer and the client's size. A few drug dosages are calculated in terms of milligrams per kilogram of body weight. More frequently, calculations are based on milligrams per square meter of total body surface area (TBSA). This parameter also takes into account the client's height and weight and is calculated as follows: the height of the client (in centimeters) divided by his or her weight (in kilograms), and the result divided by 10,000 (moving the decimal point four spaces to the left). For example, a woman who is 68 inches tall (173 cm) and weighs 143 pounds (65 kg) would have a TBSA of 11,245 cm², or 1.12 m².

Drug Schedule

Chemotherapeutic agents are administered on a regular basis, timed to maximize cancer cell kill and minimize damage to normal cells. The schedule may vary somewhat to accommodate individual client response to therapy, but usually chemotherapy is scheduled every 3 to 4 weeks for a specified number of times (on average, 6–12 times). The entire planned schedule is the *course* of chemotherapy; the individual days of administration are the *rounds*.

Drug Administration

Most chemotherapeutic drugs are administered intravenously, although other routes may be used for specific cancers (Table 27–10). Techniques and nursing care considerations for different routes are described with the specific cancer type most commonly associated with the special administration route. Chapter 17 describes various types of venous access devices, many of which are used to administer chemotherapy.

Intravenous is the most preferred route for chemotherapy because the therapeutic effects of the drugs are rapid and many of these agents are irritating or damaging to tissues. A major complication of IV administration is extravasation, or movement of the IV needle so that the

Table 27-10

Routes of Chemotherapy Administration	
Route	**Typical Cancer**
Oral	• Hodgkin's lymphoma • Leukemia (maintenance phase) • Small cell lung cancer
Intravenous	• Most solid tumors, leukemias • Lymphomas
Intra-arterial	• Hepatic tumors (primary and metastatic) • Head and neck cancers

Isolated limb perfusion	• Cancers confined to a limb
	  • Osteogenic sarcoma
	  • Ewing's sarcoma
	  • Rhabdomyosarcoma
	  • Regional melanoma

Intracavitary • Intraperitoneal • Intraventricular • Intrathecal • Intravesical	 • Ovarian cancer • Brain tumors • Brain tumors • Prophylaxis for acute lympho-cytic leukemia • Bladder tumors

drug leaks into the surrounding skin and subcutaneous tissues. The results of extravasation when the administered agents are vesicants (chemicals that cause tissue damage on direct contact) can include pain, infection, and tissue loss, sometimes necessitating surgical intervention. (See Table 27-11 for known vesicant or irritant chemotherapeutic agents.)

The most important nursing intervention for extravasation is prevention (Wood & Gullo, 1993). Most extravasations resolve without extensive treatment if less than 0.5 mL of the irritating drug has infiltrated into the tissues; if a larger amount has leaked, extensive tissue damage occurs and surgical intervention may be necessary. Immediate treatment depends on the specific agent extravasated. With some agents, cold compresses to the area are appropriate and for others, warm compresses. Antidotes may be injected into the site of extravasation. The nurse consults with the oncologist and pharmacist to determine the specific antidote needed for the agent extravasated. Chart 27-3 outlines appropriate documentation of an extravasation event.

Most chemotherapeutic agents are readily absorbed through the skin and mucous membranes. As a result, health care workers, especially nurses and pharmacists, who prepare or administer chemotherapeutic agents are at risk for absorbing these agents. Even at low doses, chronic exposure to chemotherapeutic agents can seriously affect health. Nurses and other health care professionals must use extreme caution and wear protective clothing whenever preparing, administering, or disposing of chemotherapeutic agents. The Occupational Safety and Health Administration (OSHA) and the Oncology Nursing Society have established practice guidelines and protective standards.

Side Effects of Chemotherapy

Serious side effects are associated with aggressive chemotherapy, including alopecia (hair loss), nausea and vomiting, open sores on mucous membranes (mucositis), and various skin changes. Common side effects of chemotherapy on the hematopoietic (blood-producing) system can be life threatening and are the most common reason for altering the dosage or schedule. Chemotoxic effects on the blood-forming cells of the bone marrow also produce specific side effects, including immunosuppression, anemia, and thrombocytopenia (decreased numbers of platelets).

Nursing Care of Clients Undergoing Chemotherapy

The major nursing care issue during chemotherapy is managing clients' therapy-associated distressing symptoms. For some clients, the symptoms are so disagreeable that they discontinue treatment.

Alopecia

OVERVIEW. Clients receiving chemotherapy for cancer frequently experience whole body hair loss. Some drugs, such as methotrexate, may cause only thinning of scalp hair. Others, such as doxorubicin, vincristine, and cisplatin, cause a more complete hair loss.

COLLABORATIVE MANAGEMENT. The nurse reassures clients that hair loss is temporary. Usually, hair regrowth begins about 1 month after chemotherapy is completed. The nurse cautions clients that the new hair may differ from the original hair in color, texture, and thickness.

No known treatment totally prevents alopecia. Techniques to reduce the amount of chemotherapeutic agents reaching the hair follicles during treatment have been somewhat effective in reducing it, however. These tech-

Table 27-11

Chemotherapy Tissue Vesicants and Irritants	
Vesicants	**Irritants**
Amsacrine	Bleomycin
Dactinomycin	Carmustine
Daunorubicin	Cisplatin
Doxorubicin	Dacarbazine
Epirubicin	Etoposide
Esorubicin	Fluorouracil
Idarubicin	Mitoxantrone
Mechlorethamine	Paclitaxel
Menogaril	Plicamycin
Mitomycin C	Streptozocin
Pyrazofurin	Teniposide
Vinblastine	
Vincristine	
Vindesine	
Vinorelbine	

Chart 27–3

Nursing Care Highlight: Documentation of Extravasation

- Document the date and time when extravasation was suspected or identified.
- Note the date and time when the infusion was started.
- Record the time when the infusion was stopped.
- Note the exact contents of the infusion fluid and the volume of fluid infused.
- Document the estimated amount of fluid extravasated.
- Note the needle type and size.
- Diagram the exact insertion site.
- Indicate on the diagram the location and number of venipuncture attempts.
- Record the time between the extravasation and the last full blood return.
- Identify all agents administered in the previous 24 hours through this site (list agent administered, dosage and volume, and order of administration).
- Note the client's vital signs.
- Take a photograph of the site.
- Document the administration of neutralizing or antidote agents.
- Note the application of compresses.
- Note other nursing interventions.
- Record the client's responses to nursing interventions.
- Document the physician notification (including the time).
- Document the written and oral instructions given to the client about follow-up care.
- Note any consultation request.
- Sign the documentation.

---

niques include applying ice packs and caps to the scalp or applying a scalp tourniquet during chemotherapy administration and for a few hours immediately afterward. These techniques are not endorsed by oncologists or oncology nurses because it is believed that some circulating cancer cells may escape chemotherapy, resulting in a less favorable treatment outcome.

Nurses can assist clients in selecting a type of head covering that suits their financial means and lifestyle. High-quality wigs are expensive but can look very much like the client's own hair. Many local units of the American Cancer Society offer wigs that other clients have used temporarily and have donated to be lent to other clients with cancer. Clients can disguise hair loss relatively inexpensively by the creative use of scarves and turbans, available in many fabrics, styles, and prices, or with caps.

Nausea and Vomiting

OVERVIEW. Chemotherapy-induced nausea and vomiting arises from a variety of local and central nervous system mechanisms (Fessele, 1996). Most chemotherapeutic agents are emetogenic (vomiting inducing) to some degree, depending on the dose, but agents producing the most severe nausea and vomiting include cisplatin, doxorubicin, mithramycin, nitrogen mustard, vinblastine, and

etoposide. Most of these agents induce nausea and vomiting during drug administration and for 1 to 2 days afterward. Some agents, such as cisplatin, induce delayed nausea and vomiting that can continue as long as 5 to 7 days after administration. Clients who have experienced chemotherapy-related nausea and vomiting during one round of chemotherapy may begin having the same symptoms before the next round as a result of sheer anticipation.

ELDERLY CONSIDERATIONS

It has long been thought that older clients do not tolerate chemotherapy, especially the side effects of nausea and vomiting, as well as younger clients do. At times, older clients have received lower doses of chemotherapy agents in anticipation of these side effects. More recent research indicates that older clients do not have greater nausea and vomiting than do younger clients, and should not have their chemotherapy regimens altered on this basis alone. See the accompanying Research Applications for Nursing: Older Versus Younger Clients and Chemotherapy-Induced Nausea, Vomiting, and Retching.

> ## Research Applications for Nursing

Older Versus Younger Clients and Chemotherapy-Induced Nausea, Vomiting, and Retching

Dodd, M., Onishi, K., Dibble, S., & Larson, P. (1996). Differences in nausea, vomiting, and retching between younger and older outpatients receiving cancer chemotherapy. Cancer Nursing, 19(3), 155–161.

The purpose of this descriptive, prospective study was to determine the rates of nausea, vomiting, and retching among 127 clients undergoing outpatient chemotherapy with some combination of five specific chemotherapeutic agents. Demographic, treatment, and response to treatment data were collected using the Disease and Treatment Questionnaire. Twenty-five clients were older than 65 years, and 102 were younger than 65 years. The younger clients had higher incomes and had more years of education than did older clients. The questionnaires were distributed to the clients before each cycle of chemotherapy, and were completed 24 and 48 hours after chemotherapy.

The younger clients consistently reported more difficulty with nausea, vomiting, and retching than did the older ones. Younger clients also participated in more distractive behaviors to ignore their symptoms.

Critique. There were four times as many subjects in the younger group than the older group. Cancer types experienced also differed by group. Repeating this study with more homogeneous groups of clients in terms of cancer type and number and type and dosage of chemotherapy could increase the credibility of the findings.

Possible Nursing Implications. In the belief that older clients would not be able to tolerate chemotherapy side effects, many may not be offered the same treatment options as younger clients. This limitation could have serious adverse effects on overall cancer treatment outcome.

Chart 27-4

Drug Therapy for Chemotherapy-Induced Nausea and Vomiting

Drug	Usual Dosage	Side Effects
Serotonin Antagonists		
Ondansetron (Zofran)	8 mg q8h	Constipation, diarrhea, fever, lightheadedness, drowsiness
Granisetron (Kytril)	1 mg q12h	Fever, dysrhythmias, chest pain, fainting
CNS Depressants		
Trimethobenzamide (Tigan, Benzacot, Arrestin, T-Gen)	200 mg tid or qid	Drowsiness, blurred vision, dizziness, diarrhea, headache, mental depression, tremors
Benzodiazepines		
Lorazepam (Ativan)	1–3 mg bid or tid	Amnesia, bradycardia, hypotension, muscle weakness, anemia
Phenothiazines		
Prochlorperazine (Compazine, Stemetil)	10–20 mg qid	Hypotension, CNS depression, extrapyramidal reactions, dry mouth, blurred vision
Chlorpromazine (Thorazine, Ormazine)	25–50 mg qid	Hypotension, CNS depression, extrapyramidal reactions, dry mouth, blurred vision
Antihistamines		
Diphenhydramine (Benadryl)	25–50 mg qid	Drowsiness, dry mouth, hypotension
Corticosteroids		
Dexamethasone (Decadron)	5–10 mg qd	Fluid and electrolyte imbalances, immunosuppression, GI bleeding, bruising, cushingoid symptoms

CNS = central nervous system; GI = gastrointestinal.

COLLABORATIVE MANAGEMENT. Many oral and parenteral antiemetics (agents that alleviate nausea and vomiting) are available. These agents vary in their production of side effects as well as their effectiveness in controlling chemotherapy-induced nausea and vomiting. Usually, one or more antiemetics are administered before and after chemotherapy. Drugs commonly used to control chemotherapy-induced nausea and vomiting are presented in Chart 27–4. Client response to antiemetic therapy is highly variable, and the drug combinations must be individualized for best effect.

The nurse also assists the client with chemotherapy-induced nausea and vomiting to achieve comfort through nonpharmacologic means. Progressive muscle relaxation, guided imagery, or distraction may help reduce anxiety and relieve some nausea and vomiting. The nurse also assesses the client for complications associated with excessive vomiting, such as dehydration and electrolyte imbalances.

Some facilities have created clinical pathways for clients with nausea, vomiting, and dehydration related to cancer and its treatment (see Oncology Clinical Pathway).

Mucositis

OVERVIEW. Clients undergoing chemotherapy for cancer frequently have mucositis (sores in mucous membranes) of the entire GI tract, especially in the mouth (stomatitis). Normally, the mucous membrane of the GI tract undergoes rapid cell division and replaces dead or damaged cells quickly. In chemotherapy, mucous membrane cells are killed more rapidly than they are replaced, resulting in sore formation. Mouth sores are painful and interfere with clients' desire and ability to eat. (Chart 27–5 lists nursing care highlights for clients with mucositis.)

COLLABORATIVE MANAGEMENT. Frequent mouth assessment is key in managing stomatitis and mucositis. A variety of assessment tools have been developed with varying degrees of utility. In the Research Applications for Nursing: Reliability of One Mouth Assessment Instrument for Mucositis, the efficacy of one such tool is described.

A major component in managing oral mucositis is oral hygiene. The nurse stresses the importance of good and frequent oral hygiene, including tooth cleaning and mouth rinsing. Because most clients with chemotherapy-induced mucositis also have bone marrow suppression, they must take care to avoid traumatizing the oral mucosa. The nurse instructs clients to use a soft-bristled toothbrush or disposable mouth sponges and to avoid using dental floss and water pressure gum cleaners (such as a water pick). The nurse encourages clients to rinse the mouth every hour while awake with plain water or saline. The nurse warns them against using commercial mouth-

1 - 7-3
2 - 3-11
3 - 11-7

LAST   [ ] Chemotherapy   Date _____
      [ ] Radiation   Date _____

CARE NEED	DAY 1 ADMIT DAY date ____	DAY 2 date ____	DAY 3 date ____	DAY 4 date ____
ASSESSMENTS/ TREATMENTS	Postural BP on admission & prn Weight documented I&O Baseline vital signs documented Vital signs q shift and prn Review old chart Previous admit for n/v/d date: ____ Safety/fall assessment	AM weight I&O Vital signs q shift — stable Evaluate lab results	AM weight I&O Vital signs ONLY 7-3 and 3-11 if stable	

FLUIDS/ NUTRITIONS	Start IV hydration @ admit
	1000cc D_5 ½ NS 20 KCL @ 100
	IV antiemetics
	Adjust IV fluids based on lab results within 8° of admit
	Clear liquids as tolerated
		IV fluids continue
		Start PO or PR antiemetics q 6° around-the-clock
		Cont. IV antiemetics for BREAKTHROUGH
		Clear liquids-Intake:
		  7-3 500; 3-11 400; 11-7 100
		Advance to full liquid dinner or as tolerated
			DC or HL IV by noon
			Antiemetics AC and HS PO only
			Advance to regular diet for lunch
			Fluid Intake:
			  7-3 600; 3-11 500; 11-7 100	

LAB/ DIAGNOSTICS	CBC—if not available from MD office SMA 20-SMA 7 stat	SMA-7		
ACTIVITY	Up to BR Ambulate in room 1x day/evenings	Up to BR Ambulate ½ length of hallway TID	Ambulate full length of hallway TID	
SELF-CARE	Mouth care Face/hand washing Feeding	Mouth care Self bath @ bedside Feeding	Mouth care Shower	
DISCHARGE PLANNING	Evaluate home care support Refer to Social Services if: Social Work intervention needed	Document discharge plan: Social Services or Nursing	Finalize home care needs	Discharge by 11:00 AM
TEACHING	____ Assess current knowledge of antiemetics; document on kardex	____ Medication instruction ____ Dietary consult evaluate need for diet counseling	____ Review/reinforce med instruction ____ Review/reinforce diet instruction	____ Verbalizes understanding of meds for home care and diet
	RN __ D __ E __ N Initial Signature	RN __ D __ E __ N Initial Signature	RN __ D __ E __ N Initial Signature	RN __ D __ E __ N Initial Signature

Good Samaritan Hospital
A division of Good Samaritan Community Healthcare
407-14th Ave SE, PO Box 1247, Puyallup, WA 98371-0192 (206) 848-6661

Oncology
Clinical Pathway
Nausea/Vomiting/Dehydration

Chart 27–5

Nursing Care Highlight: Mouth Care for Clients with Mucositis

- Examine the client's mouth (including the roof, under the tongue, and between the teeth and cheek) every 4 hours.
- Document the location, size, and character of fissures, blisters, sores, or drainage.
- Get an order to obtain specimens of sores or drainage for culture.
- Brush the teeth and tongue with a soft-bristled brush or sponges every 8 hours.
- Rinse the mouth with solution of ½ peroxide and ½ normal saline every 12 hours.
- Avoid use of alcohol or glycerin-based mouthwashes.
- Administer antimicrobial medications as prescribed.
- Administer topical analgesic medications as prescribed or as needed.
- Help the conscious client to "swish and spit" room-temperature tap water or normal saline as needed.
- Apply petrolatum jelly to the client's lips after each episode of mouth care and as needed.
- Assist the client in using "artificial saliva" as needed, if ordered.
- Assist the client in menu choices to avoid spicy or hard food.
- Offer complete mouth care before and after every meal.

---

washes that contain alcohol or other drying agents that may further irritate the mucosa.

Clients must keep oral hygiene equipment clean. The nurse reminds clients not to share toothbrushes with anyone. Clients can clean toothbrushes daily by running them through a home dishwasher or rinsing them with either a concentrated solution of liquid bleach or hydrogen peroxide.

Many compounds are available for pain relief from stomatitis or mucositis. Many hospitals offer their own special "swish and spit" mixtures, which usually contain a local anesthetic combined with anti-inflammatory agents. The nurse stresses that these mixtures are not to be swallowed.

Bone Marrow Suppression

OVERVIEW. Bone marrow suppression results in decreased numbers of circulating leukocytes, erythrocytes, and platelets. Decreased leukocyte numbers cause immunosuppression. Decreased erythrocytes and platelets cause hypoxia, fatigue, and increased bleeding tendency.

Immunosuppression, which places the client at extreme risk for infection, is the major dose-limiting side effect of cancer chemotherapy. Most chemotherapeutic agents suppress bone marrow function to some degree. The agents associated with severe bone marrow suppression include busulfan, cyclophosphamide, cytosine arabinoside, dactinomycin, doxorubicin, daunorubicin, etoposide, mitomycin C, nitrogen mustard, and triethylenethiophosphor-

amide. *Suppression of immune function is the most life-threatening side effect and presents the nurse with the serious challenge of providing the client with the understanding, environment, and support to withstand this potentially devastating complication.*

The clinical problems associated with immunosuppression are related primarily to a temporary reduction of circulating neutrophils and tissue macrophages, causing a decrease in the body's protective inflammatory responses to microorganism invasion. The severity and duration of the impairment are related directly to the dosage of specific chemotherapeutic agents. Although this impairment is usually temporary, with good recovery of inflammatory responses evident within weeks or months of therapy completion, the seriousness of potential infection complications makes this a major treatment concern. The infectious processes most commonly observed include those of

---

▶ Research Applications for Nursing

Reliability of One Mouth Assessment Instrument for Mucositis

Dibble, S., Shiba, G., MacPhail, L., & Dodd, M. (1996). MacDibbs mouth assessment. Cancer Practice, 4(3), 135–140.

The purpose of this descriptive, longitudinal study was to evaluate the ease of use and accuracy of the MacDibbs Mouth Assessment instrument in determining mouth changes among clients receiving radiation therapy for head and neck cancer. The MacDibbs instrument consists of a one-page check list with clients rating pain, dryness, eating, talking, swallowing, tasting, and amount of saliva; report of examination by a health care professional regarding observations and measurements of lesions and areas of color change; and results of potassium hydroxide (KOH) smears or herpes simplex virus (HSV) cultures.

Client symptom reports correlated with health care professional observations. Interrater reliability for observable signs was 100%, except for lesion size, which was thought to vary because the measuring probe was of insufficient length. Information regarding KOH smear and HSV cultures was not provided in the study. The investigators deemed the instrument to be useful in measuring radiation-induced mucositis.

Critique. Symptoms and signs total scores could be calculated separately. Although the instrument appears reliable in determining mucositis, the investigators did not offer clear-cut guidelines regarding the point at which to initiate specific treatments. Although developed for clients undergoing radiation therapy, the instrument may also have value in assessing mouth problems for clients undergoing chemotherapy. Further research is necessary to determine generalizability.

Possible Nursing Implications. The main value of this article is in pointing out the importance of having a specific mouth assessment tool to accurately document changes in oral status among clients undergoing therapy for cancer. A user-friendly assessment tool should be concise and should incorporate both client subjective symptoms and health care provider objective assessment data. The MacDibbs Mouth Assessment appears to meet these criteria.

fungal origin, yeast, some residual viral breakthrough, and a wide variety of bacteria.

Decreased numbers of circulating erythrocytes (anemia) and platelets (thrombocytopenia) result from the generalized bone marrow suppression caused by some chemotherapeutic agents. The anemia causes clients to feel fatigued, and some tissues must operate under hypoxic conditions. The cardiac and respiratory systems may be overtaxed in their effort to maintain adequate oxygenation. Thrombocytopenia increases the risk for uncontrolled bleeding. When the platelets are less than 50,000/mm³, any small trauma can lead to episodes of prolonged bleeding. When less than 20,000/mm³, clients may experience spontaneous and uncontrollable bleeding, requiring extensive transfusion therapy and other interventions to resolve.

COLLABORATIVE MANAGEMENT. Management of clients with immunosuppression aims to improve immune function and protect them from infection.

In some instances, immunosuppression can be managed medically by the administration of biological response modifiers (BRMs) to stimulate bone marrow production of immune system cells. Although not appropriate for all types of cancer, this supportive treatment can reduce clients' risk for infection during chemotherapy. However, BRMs are expensive and not consistently covered by insurance. Further discussion of this treatment is presented under Immunotherapy.

The nurse works closely with clients and other health care professionals to provide safe care to clients at risk for infection. Chart 27–6 lists specific nursing care actions to prevent infection among immunosuppressed clients. Good hand washing by all health care professionals and unlicensed assistive personnel before contact with clients is the cornerstone for prevention of infection. Health care professionals must practice asepsis (prevention of contact with microorganisms) when performing any invasive technique or procedure.

Many clients remain at home during periods of immunosuppression. The nurse teaches clients and family members precautions to take to reduce clients' chances of developing an infection (Chart 27–7).

The nurse provides a safe hospital environment for clients with thrombocytopenia, and teaches them how to avoid excessive bleeding when they are discharged before the platelet count has returned to normal. Chart 27–8 lists nursing actions to reduce clients' risk for bleeding during hospitalization. The nurse teaches clients how to prevent bleeding and what to do if bleeding should occur after discharge (Chart 27–9).

Hormonal Manipulation
Rationale for Cancer Treatment

Hormones are naturally occurring chemicals secreted by endocrine (ductless) glands and picked up by capillaries. Once in the bloodstream, hormones circulate to all body areas but exert their effects only on their specific target tissues. Some hormones make hormone-sensitive tumors

---

Chart 27–6

Nursing Care Highlight: Care of the Client with Immunosuppression

- Place the client in a private room whenever possible.
- Use good hand washing technique before touching the client or any of the client's belongings.
- Ensure that the client's room and bathroom are cleaned at least once each day.
- Do not use supplies from common areas for immunosuppressed clients. For example, keep a sleeve or box of paper cups in the client's room and do not share this box with any other client. Other articles include drinking straws, plastic knives and forks, dressing materials, gloves, and bandages.
- Limit the number of care personnel entering the client's room.
- Monitor vital signs every 4 hours; note minor temperature elevation, which may suggest early sepsis.
- Inspect the client's mouth at least every 8 hours.
- Inspect the client's skin and mucous membranes (especially the anal area) for the presence of fissures and abscesses at least every 8 hours.
- Inspect open areas, such as IV sites, every 4 hours for manifestations of infection.
- Change wound dressings daily.
- Obtain specimens of all suspicious areas for culture, and promptly notify physician.
- Assist the client in performing coughing and deep-breathing exercises.
- Encourage activity at appropriate level for the client's current health status.
- Change IV tubing daily.
- Keep frequently used equipment in the room for use by the client only (e.g., blood pressure cuff, stethoscope, thermometer).
- Limit visitors to healthy adults.
- Use strict aseptic technique for all invasive procedures.
- Monitor the white blood cell count, especially the absolute neutrophil count (ANC), daily.
- Avoid the use of indwelling urinary catheters.
- Keep fresh flowers and potted plants out of the client's room.
- Teach the client to eat a low-bacteria diet (see Chart 27–7).

---

grow more rapidly. Some tumors actually require specific hormones to divide. Therefore, altering the availability of these hormones to hormonally sensitive tumors can directly alter tumor growth rate.

Mechanism of Action
Hormones

Hormonal manipulation can help control some types of cancer for many years; however, this therapy does not lead to cure. The endocrine system usually keeps hormones within narrow ranges, and a balance is maintained. When a large amount of one hormone is administered, it

---

Chart 27-7

Education Guide: Prevention of Infection

- Avoid crowds and other large gatherings of people who might be ill.
- Do not share personal toilet articles, such as toothbrushes, toothpaste, washcloths, or deodorant sticks, with others.
- If possible, bathe daily.
- Wash the armpits, groin, genitals, and anal area at least twice a day with an antimicrobial soap.
- Clean your toothbrush daily by either running it through the dishwasher or rinsing it in liquid laundry bleach.
- Wash your hands thoroughly with an antimicrobial soap before you eat or drink, after touching a pet, after shaking hands with anyone, as soon as you come home from any outing, and after using the toilet.
- Eat a low-bacteria diet, and avoid salads, raw fruit and vegetables, undercooked meat, pepper, and paprika.
- Wash dishes between use with hot, sudsy water or use a dishwasher.
- Do not drink water that has been standing for longer than 15 minutes.
- Do not reuse cups and glasses without washing.
- Do not change pet litter boxes.
- Take your temperature at least once a day.
- Report any of the following signs or symptoms of infection to your physician immediately:
  - Temperature greater than 100°F (38°C)
  - Persistent cough (with or without sputum)
  - Pus or foul-smelling drainage from any open skin area or normal body opening
  - Presence of a boil or abscess
  - Urine that is cloudy or foul smelling or that causes burning on urination
- Take all prescribed medications as ordered.
- Do not dig in the garden or work with houseplants.

---

upsets the balance and disturbs the uptake of some other hormones. If a tumor depends on hormone A for growth and a large quantity of hormone B (structurally but not functionally related to A) is given to the client, hormone B will interfere with the tumor's uptake of hormone A or will limit the amount of hormone A produced (through competition or feedback inhibition), and tumor growth is slowed. Thus, hormonal therapy may increase survival time. Table 27-12 lists drugs commonly used in hormonal manipulation for cancer therapy.

Hormone Antagonists

Hormone antagonists, competitors for the hormones at the receptor sites, may be antibodies specific to the receptor. When hormone antagonists are administered, they bind to the specific hormone receptor of the tumor cell and prevent the needed hormone from binding to the receptor. Therefore, if a tumor requires a certain hormone to grow and the hormone can enter or activate the cell only through a receptor, hormone antagonists can slow down tumor growth.

Side Effects of Hormonal Manipulation

In women, androgens and the antiestrogen receptor drugs cause masculinizing manifestations. Chest and facial hair may develop, menstrual periods stop, and breast tissue shrinks. Women usually experience some fluid retention. For men and women receiving androgens, acne may develop, hypercalcemia is common, and liver dysfunction may occur with prolonged therapy. Women receiving estrogens or progestins have irregular but heavy menses, fluid retention, and breast tenderness. Male and female clients taking estrogen or progestins are at an increased risk for thrombus formation.

When men take estrogens, progestins, or antiandrogen receptor drugs, some feminine clinical manifestations usually develop. Facial hair thins or disappears, facial skin becomes smoother, body fat is redistributed, and gynecomastia (breast development in men) can occur. Testicular and penile atrophy occurs to some degree as well. Although sexual function may continue, achieving and maintaining an erection are much more difficult.

Chart 27-8

Nursing Care Highlight: Care of the Client with Thrombocytopenia

- Handle the client gently.
- Use a lift sheet when moving and positioning the client in bed.
- Avoid intramuscular injections and venipunctures.
- When injections or venipunctures are necessary, use the smallest-gauge needle for the task.
- Apply firm pressure to the needlestick site for 10 minutes or until site no longer oozes blood.
- Apply ice to areas of trauma.
- Test all urine and stool for the presence of occult blood.
- Observe intravenous sites every 2 hours for bleeding.
- Avoid trauma to rectal tissues:
  - Do not take temperatures rectally.
  - Do not administer enemas.
  - Administer well-lubricated suppositories and with caution.
  - Advise the client not to have anal intercourse.
- Measure the client's abdominal girth daily.
- Use an electric razor.
- Teach the client to avoid mouth trauma by
  - Using soft-bristled toothbrush or tooth sponges
  - Not flossing
  - Avoiding dental work, especially extractions
  - Avoiding hard foods
  - Making certain that dentures fit and do not rub
- Encourage the client not to blow the nose or insert objects into the nose.
- Instruct the client to avoid contact sports.
- Advise the client to wear shoes with firm soles whenever he or she is ambulating.

Education Guide: The Client at Risk for Bleeding

- Use an electric razor.
- Use a soft-bristled toothbrush, and do not floss.
- Do not have dental work done without consulting your doctor.
- Do not take aspirin or any aspirin-containing products. Read the label to be sure that the product does not contain aspirin or salicylates.
- Do not participate in contact sports or any activity likely to result in your being bumped, scratched, or scraped.
- If you are bumped, apply ice to the site for at least 1 hour.
- Notify your doctor if you
  - Experience an injury and persistent bleeding results
  - Have excessive menstrual bleeding
  - See blood in your urine or bowel movement
- Avoid anal intercourse.
- Take a stool softener to prevent straining during a bowel movement.
- Do not use enemas or rectal suppositories.
- Avoid bending over at the waist.
- Do not wear clothing or shoes that are tight or that rub.
- Avoid blowing your nose or placing objects in your nose. If you must blow your nose, do so gently without blocking either nasal passage.

Immunotherapy: Biological Response Modifiers

Biological response modifiers (BRMs) are agents or approaches that modify the client's biologic responses to tumor cells with a beneficial result (Clark & Longo, 1986). BRMs in current use or under investigation for use as cancer therapy are cytokines, small protein hormones synthesized by the various leukocytes. Cytokines synthesized by the mononuclear phagocytes (macrophages, neutrophils, eosinophils, and monocytes) are monokines; cytokines produced by lymphocytes (especially the T lymphocytes) are lymphokines. Essentially, cytokines make the immune system work better (see Chap. 23, especially Table 23–5).

Rationale for Cancer Treatment

Cytokines enhance immune system effectiveness. Immune function plays an important role in cancer prevention (see Chaps. 23 and 26). Cytokines and other BRMs are potentially therapeutic as a cancer treatment by stimulating the immune system to recognize cancer cells and take actions to eliminate or destroy them. Some BRMs may also be useful in a supporting role. Other BRMs (colony-stimulating factors) stimulate faster recovery of bone marrow function after treatment-induced suppression.

Mechanism of Action

Cytokine activity is similar to that of any other kind of peptide hormone in that one cell produces and secretes a cytokine, which then exerts its effects on other cells of the immune system. The cells responding to the cytokine may be right next to the cytokine-secreting cell or quite remote from it. The cells that change their activity in response to the cytokine are *responder* cells. For a responder cell to be able to respond to a cytokine, the membrane of the responder cell must have a specific receptor for the cytokine to bind to and initiate changes in the responder cell's activity.

Biological Response Modifiers for Cancer Therapy

Two categories of BRMs are being used as cytotoxic therapy for cancer: interleukins and interferons. These agents can stimulate some immune system cells to attack and destroy cancer cells.

INTERLEUKINS. Sixteen interleukins (ILs) have been identified (see Table 23–5), many now synthetically produced through recombinant DNA technology. Interleukins help different immune system cells recognize and destroy abnormal body cells. In particular, IL-1, -2, and -6 appear

Table 27–12

Common Agents Used for Hormonal Manipulation of Cancer	
Type of Agent	**Example**
Hormone Agonists	
Androgen	• Calusterone • Danocrine • Fluoxymesterone • Testosterone • Testolactone
Estrogen	• Conjugated estrogens • Diethylstilbestrol • Ethinyl estradiol
Progestin	• Medroxyprogesterone • Megestrol
Luteinizing-hormone releasing hormone (LHRH)	• Leuprolide • Goserelin
Hormone Antagonists	
Antiandrogens	• Flutamide • Cyproterone acetate
Antiprogestins	• Mifepristone
Antiestrogens	• Droloxifen • Idoxifene • Tamoxifen • Toremifene • Trioxifene mesylate • Zindoxifene

to "charge up" the immune system and enhance attacks on cancer cells by macrophages, natural killer (NK) cells, lymphokine-activated killer (LAK) cells, and tumor-infiltrating lymphocytes. At present, cancer treatment with interleukins is experimental, but good responses have occurred in clients with renal cell carcinoma, colorectal cancer, and melanoma.

INTERFERONS. Interferons are substances produced by cells that can protect noninfected cells from viral infection and replication. There are many types of interferons, and, although they all have similar functions, each type has unique properties and functions. The most completely characterized interferon is interferon-alpha$_{2b}$.

Although different body cells can produce interferon, leukocytes produce the most. Today, interferons are mass produced synthetically by recombinant DNA technology. Cancer-related functions of interferon include the ability to

- Slow down tumor cell division
- Stimulate the proliferation and activation of NK cells
- Help cancer cells resume a more normal appearance and revert to their previous characteristics
- Inhibit expression of oncogenes

Although interferons are approved for limited use as a cancer treatment, they have been effective to some degree in the treatment of hairy cell leukemia, renal cell carcinoma, ovarian cancer, and cutaneous T-cell lymphoma.

Biological Response Modifiers for Cancer Support

Biological response modifiers approved for use as supportive therapy during cancer treatment are the colony-stimulating factors (Table 27–13). Essentially, these factors induce more rapid recovery of the bone marrow after suppression by chemotherapy.

This effect may have two benefits. First, when bone marrow suppression is less severe or of shorter duration, clients are less at risk for life-threatening infections and anemia. Second, because the colony-stimulating factors allow more rapid bone marrow recovery, clients can re-

Table 27–13

Colony-Stimulating Factors			
Variable	Granulocyte/Macrophage Colony-Stimulating Factor (GM-CSF)	Granulocyte Colony-Stimulating Factor (G-CSF)	Erythropoietin (EPO)
Generic name	• Sargramostim	• Filgrastim	• Epoetin alfa
Brand name	• Leukine (Immunex) • Prokine (Hoechst/Roussel)	• Neupogen (Amgen)	• Epogen (Amgen) • Procrit (Ortho Biotech)
Source	• T cells (lymphokine)	• Monocytes • Fibroblasts • Endothelial epithelial cells	• Renal
Cell type affected	• All granulocytes • Neutrophils • Eosinophils • Monocytes/macrophages	• Neutrophil	• Red blood cells
Indications	• To accelerate myeloid recovery in patients with non-Hodgkin's lymphoma, ALL, and Hodgkin's disease who are undergoing autologous bone marrow transplantation	• To decrease the incidence of infection, manifested by febrile neutropenia, in patients with nonmyeloid malignancies receiving myelosuppressive anticancer drugs associated with a significant incidence of severe neutropenia with fever	• Anemia of chronic renal failure patients • Anemia in AZT-treated HIV patients
Dosage	• 250 μg/m²/day × 21 days as a 2-hour IV infusion beginning 2–4 hours after autologous bone marrow transplantation and not < 24 hours after the last dose of chemotherapy and 12 hours after the last dose of radiotherapy	• 5 μg/kg/day, SC or IV, as a single daily injection not < 24 hours after cytotoxic chemotherapy or in the 24 hours preceding chemotherapy • Give for up to 2 weeks, until the absolute neutrophil count has reached 10,000 mm³ after the expected chemotherapy-induced neutrophil nadir	• Starting dose 50–100 μg/kg TIW • IV for dialysis patients • IV or SC for nondialysis CRF patients • Individualize dose to reach the HCT target range of 30–33%

IV = intravenous; SC = subcutaneous; ALL = acute lymphocytic leukemia; AZT = zidovudine; HIV = human immunodeficiency virus; CRF = chronic renal failure; HCT = hematocrit.
Modified from Susan M. Schneider. © 1992, Susan M. Schneider, All Rights Reserved.

ceive their chemotherapy on time and may even be able to tolerate higher doses, potentially improving the curative outcome of chemotherapy. These agents must be used cautiously for malignancies in which the cancer cells may also have a BRM receptor, such as the leukemias and lymphomas.

Side Effects of Biological Response Modifier Therapy

Clients receiving interleukins at therapeutic doses experience generalized and sometimes severe inflammatory reactions. Fluid shifts and capillary leak are widespread. Tissue swelling affects the function of all major organs and can be life threatening. Clients receiving high-dose BRM therapy should be cared for in intensive care or monitoring units. These effects are limited to the period of acute drug administration and resolve spontaneously when treatment is completed.

Many of the BRMs induce general symptoms of mild inflammatory reactions during and immediately after administration, including fever, chills, rigors, and flu-like general malaise. Symptoms are worse when higher doses are given and seem to become less severe over time. Fever is treated with acetaminophen. Clients with rigors, if severe, are managed with meperidine (Demerol, pethidine).

Gene Therapy

Gene therapy as a primary or adjunct cancer treatment modality has only investigational status currently. Although response rates to date are limited, experimental successes indicate potential for gene therapy as a form of cancer treatment.

Increased Tumor Cell Susceptibility

One method of using gene therapy for cancer is to render the tumor cells more susceptible to damage or death by other treatments. Insertion of a viral enzyme gene into brain tumor cells makes the cancer cells more susceptible to being killed by antiviral agents. Other techniques involve inserting human leukocyte antigen (HLA) genes different from the client's own HLAs into the client's tumor cells. This technique makes the client's immune system cells better able to recognize the cancer cells as foreign and take steps to eliminate or destroy them. Both methods of gene therapy for cancer have shown some success in early-phase clinical trials.

Increased Immune System Cell Activity

Some immune system cells are capable of attacking and killing cancer cells (see Chap. 23). This ability is increased when more of certain cytokines, like IL-2, is present. Some gene therapy for cancer involves inserting additional genes for cytokines into the client's own immune system cells. These "charged-up" cancer-fighting immune system cells remain active in the client for up to 6 months and can participate in cancer cell–killing episodes.

Potential Uses of Gene Therapy for Cancer

Because cancer is caused by one or more changes in the genes of a normal cell, it is not unreasonable to think that gene alterations could influence a cancer cell to become normal. Areas under current research for gene therapy against cancer include

- Insertion of additional or healthy suppressor genes into cancer cells
- Insertion of chemotherapy resistance genes into normal cells so higher doses of chemotherapy can be given without affecting normal cells
- Removing damaged, mutated, or activated oncogenes
- Inserting multiple genes into cancer cells to make them more easily recognized by immune system cells and more susceptible to other treatment modalities

ONCOLOGIC EMERGENCIES

Cancer is considered a chronic disease; however, a number of acute conditions associated with cancer and its treatment can occur. These conditions, or complications, often require immediate medical intervention and are thus considered *oncologic emergencies*. Early diagnosis of such conditions is essential to avoid life-threatening situations.

Sepsis and Disseminated Intravascular Coagulation
Overview

Sepsis, or septicemia, is a condition in which microorganisms enter the bloodstream. Septic shock is a life-threatening result of sepsis and a frequent cause of death in clients with cancer. These clients are at increased risk for infection and sepsis because their white blood cell counts are often low and their immune function is usually impaired. (Chapter 39 describes the pathophysiology of sepsis and septic shock.)

Disseminated intravascular coagulation (DIC) is a condition indicating a problem with a person's blood-clotting process, triggered by many severe illnesses, including cancer. In clients with cancer, DIC is caused by sepsis (usually gram-negative infection), by release of thrombin or thromboplastin (clotting factors) from cancer cells, or by blood transfusions. DIC is most often associated with leukemia and with adenocarcinomas of the lung, pancreas, stomach, and prostate.

In clients with DIC, extensive, abnormal clot formation occurs throughout small blood vessels. The widespread clotting consumes all circulating clotting factors and platelets. This process is followed by extensive bleeding. Bleeding from many sites is the most common problem and ranges from minimal to fatal hemorrhage. Blockage of blood vessels from clots decreases blood flow to major body organs and results in pain, stroke-like signs and symptoms, dyspnea, tachycardia, oliguria (decreased urine output), and bowel necrosis (tissue death). (Chapter 39 describes the pathophysiology and collaborative management of sepsis-induced DIC.)

Collaborative Management

DIC is a life-threatening problem; the mortality rate is 70% even when appropriate therapies are instituted. Therefore, the best treatment plan for sepsis and DIC is prevention. The nurse identifies those clients at greatest risk for development of sepsis and DIC. Strict adherence to aseptic technique is practiced during invasive procedures and during manipulation of nonintact skin and mucous membranes in immunocompromised clients. The nurse teaches clients and family members the early clinical manifestations of infection and sepsis and when to seek medical assistance.

When sepsis is present and DIC is likely, treatment focuses on reducing the infection and halting the DIC process. Appropriate IV antibiotic therapy is initiated. During the early phase of DIC, anticoagulants (especially heparin) are administered to limit unnecessary clotting and prevent the rapid consumption of circulating clotting factors. When DIC has progressed to the later phase and hemorrhage is the primary problem, cryoprecipitated clotting factors are administered.

Syndrome of Inappropriate Antidiuretic Hormone
Overview

In healthy people, antidiuretic hormone (ADH) is secreted by the posterior pituitary gland only when more fluid (water) is needed in the body, such as when plasma volume is decreased (see Chap. 14). In people with certain health problems, however, ADH is secreted when not needed by the body or it is secreted inappropriately.

Cancer is the most common cause of the syndrome of inappropriate ADH (SIADH). The type of cancer most frequently associated with SIADH is carcinoma of the lung (especially small cell lung cancer), but SIADH may occur in other types of cancer as well, especially when tumors are present in the brain. Some tumors actually make and secrete ADH; others stimulate the brain to synthesize and secrete ADH. In addition, certain drugs frequently used in clients with cancer can cause the problem (most notably morphine sulfate and cyclophosphamide).

In SIADH, excessive amounts of water are reabsorbed by the kidney and put into systemic circulation. The increased water causes hyponatremia (decreased serum sodium levels) and some degree of fluid retention. Mild symptoms, including weakness, muscle cramps, loss of appetite, and fatigue, occur; serum sodium levels range from 115 to 120 mEq/L (normal range: 135–145 mEq/L). More serious signs and symptoms are related to water intoxication, including weight gain, nervous system changes (especially personality changes), confusion, and extreme muscle weakness. As the sodium level approaches 110 mEq/L, seizures, coma, and eventually death may follow unless the condition is rapidly treated.

Collaborative Management

The syndrome of inappropriate antidiuretic hormone is managed by treating the condition and the cause.

Treatment regimens for SIADH usually include fluid restriction (sometimes total fluid intake is reduced to 1 L/day), increased sodium intake, and drug therapy. A commonly used drug for this condition is demeclocycline, a form of tetracycline antibiotic, taken orally. The mechanism of action appears to be antagonistic to ADH. Because hypernatremia can develop suddenly as a result of this treatment, serum sodium levels should be monitored closely with this regimen.

The second method is to reduce or eliminate the underlying cause. The immediate institution of appropriate cancer therapy, usually either radiation or chemotherapy, can cause such tumor regression that ADH synthesis and release processes return to normal.

Spinal Cord Compression
Overview

Spinal cord compression and damage occur when a tumor directly enters the spinal cord or when the vertebral column collapses from tumor entry. Tumors may begin in the spinal cord but more commonly spread from other areas of the body, such as the lung, prostate, breast, and colon. Spinal cord compression causes back pain, usually before neurologic deficits occur. These are related to the spinal level of compression and include numbness; tingling; loss of urethral, vaginal, and rectal sensation; and muscle weakness. If paralysis occurs, it is usually permanent.

Collaborative Management

Nurses caring for clients with spinal cord compression must recognize the condition early. The nurse assesses the client for neurologic changes consistent with spinal cord compression. The nurse also teaches clients and families to recognize symptoms of early spinal cord compression and to seek medical assistance as soon as symptoms are apparent.

Treatment is largely palliative. Usually, high-dose radiation is administered to reduce the size of the tumor in the area and to relieve compression. Radiation may be given in conjunction with chemotherapy to treat the total disease. Occasionally, surgery is performed to remove the tumor from the area and rearrange the bony tissue so that less pressure is placed on the spinal cord. External back or neck braces may be prescribed to reduce the weight borne by the spinal column and reduce pressure on the spinal cord or spinal nerves.

Hypercalcemia
Overview

Hypercalcemia (increased serum calcium level), a late manifestation of extensive malignancy, occurs most often in clients with bone metastasis. Cancer in bone causes the bone to release calcium into the bloodstream. In clients with cancer in other parts of the body, especially the lung, head and neck, kidney, or lymph nodes, the tumor secretes parathyroid hormone (parathormone), causing bone to release calcium. Decreased physical mobility also contributes to or worsens hypercalcemia.

Early signs and symptoms of hypercalcemia include fatigue, loss of appetite, nausea, vomiting, constipation, and polyuria (increased urine output). More serious signs and symptoms include severe muscle weakness, diminished deep tendon reflexes, paralytic ileus, dehydration, and electrocardiographic (ECG) changes. The severity of signs and symptoms depends on how high the serum calcium level is and how quickly it developed (see also Chapter 16).

Collaborative Management

Hypercalcemia as a consequence of cancer develops very slowly for many clients, allowing the body time to adapt to this electrolyte change. As a result, the symptoms of hypercalcemia may not be evident until the serum calcium level is greatly elevated. Because adaptation does occur, treatment of hypercalcemia associated with cancer is instituted only when clinical manifestations are present.

Conservative management, such as oral hydration alone, may be enough to reduce the serum calcium to an acceptable level. When parenteral hydration is needed, normal saline is the fluid of choice.

Many drugs lower serum calcium levels, some quite dramatically (e.g., oral glucocorticoids, calcitonin, diphosphonate, gallium nitrate, mithramycin). These agents do not cure hypercalcemia but reduce the serum calcium levels temporarily. In addition, when cancer-induced hypercalcemia is life threatening or accompanied by renal impairment, dialysis can temporarily reduce serum calcium levels.

Superior Vena Cava Syndrome
Overview

Superior vena cava (SVC) syndrome occurs when the SVC is compressed or obstructed by tumor growth (Figure 27–3). SVC compression can lead to a painful and life-threatening emergency, most often in clients with lymphomas and bronchogenic carcinoma. Clients with cancer of the breast, esophagus, colon, and testes may also be affected.

The signs and symptoms associated with SVC syndrome result from blockage of blood flow in the venous system of the head, neck, and upper trunk. Early signs and symptoms generally occur in the early morning and include edema of the face, especially around the eyes (periorbital edema), and tightness of the shirt or blouse collar (Stokes' sign). As the compression worsens, the

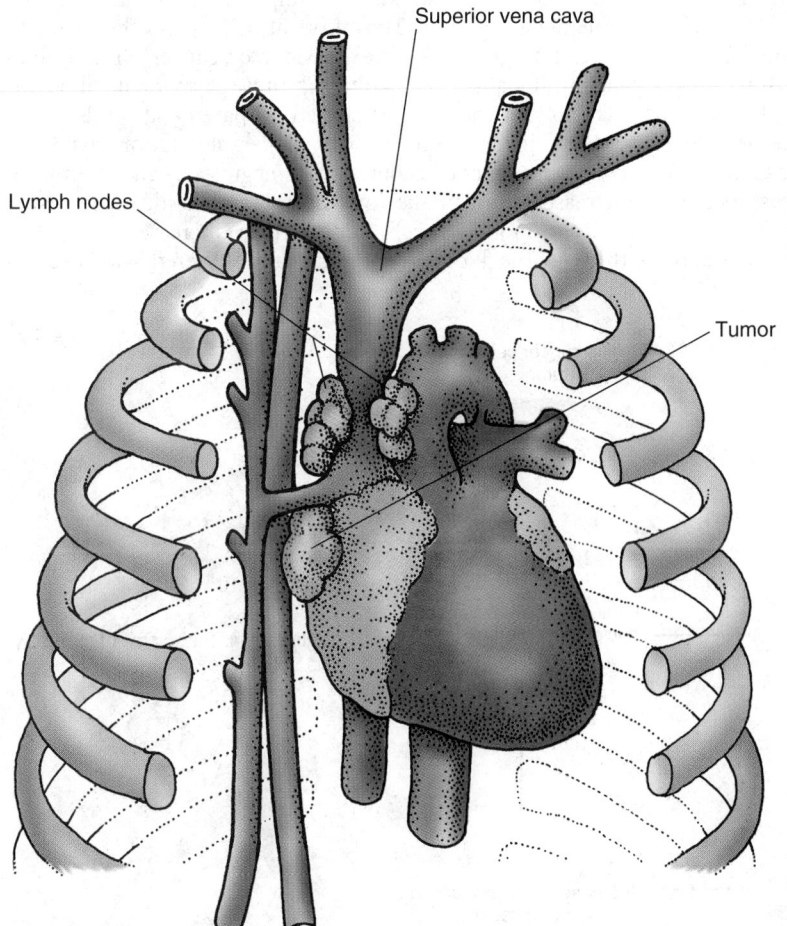

Figure 27–3. Compression of the superior vena cava in SVC syndrome.

client typically experiences edema in the arms and hands, dyspnea, erythema of the upper body, and epistaxis (nosebleeds). Late life-threatening signs and symptoms include hemorrhage, cyanosis, mental status changes from lack of blood to the brain, decreased cardiac output, and hypotension (low blood pressure). Death can result if compression is not relieved.

Collaborative Management

Superior vena cava syndrome is a late-stage manifestation; the tumor is usually widespread. High-dose radiation therapy to the mediastinal area is most frequently the treatment of choice and can provide temporary relief in about 70% of clients. Surgery is not performed for this condition because the tumor may have increased the intrathoracic pressure so high it may not be possible to close the chest after the procedure.

The best therapeutic and palliative results occur when SVC syndrome is in the early stages. The nurse assesses each client for signs and symptoms of SVC syndrome and notifies the physician.

Tumor Lysis Syndrome
Overview

In tumor lysis syndrome (TLS), large quantities of tumor cells are destroyed rapidly; their intracellular contents, including potassium and purines (DNA components), are released into the bloodstream faster than the body's homeostatic mechanisms can handle them (Figure 27–4). Unlike other oncologic emergencies, TLS is a positive sign that cancer treatment is effective. However, if TLS is severe or left untreated, it can cause severe tissue damage and death. Serum potassium levels can increase to the point of hyperkalemia, causing severe cardiac dysfunction (see Chap. 16). In addition, the large quantities of released purines are converted in the liver to uric acid and

released into systemic circulation, causing hyperuricemia. These uric acid molecules precipitate in the kidney, forming a sludge in the kidney tubules, blocking them, and leading to acute renal failure.

TLS is most commonly seen in clients receiving radiation or cancer drug therapy for cancers initially very sensitive to these therapies, including leukemia, lymphoma, small cell lung cancer, and multiple myeloma.

Collaborative Management

Prevention through hydration is the best management for TLS. Hydration alone can dilute the serum potassium level and increases the glomerular filtration rate. As a result, urine flows through the kidney at a greatly increased rate, preventing precipitation of uric acid crystals, enhancing renal excretion of potassium, and mechanically flushing out any renal tubular sludge.

For clients with tumors known to be very sensitive to cancer therapy, the nurse instructs them to drink at least 3000 mL (5000 mL is more desirable) of fluid each day on the day before, the day of, and for 3 days after the treatment. Some fluids should be alkaline to help prevent crystallization of uric acid. The nurse stresses the importance of keeping fluid intake relatively consistent throughout the 24-hour day and helps clients draw up a schedule of fluid intake.

Because some clients experience nausea and vomiting after cancer therapy and may not feel like taking oral fluids, the nurse stresses the importance of following the antiemetic regimen. The nurse also instructs the client to contact their health care provider or cancer clinic immediately if nausea and vomiting prevent adequate fluid intake so that they can be started on parenteral fluids.

For clients who become hyperkalemic or hyperuricemic, treatment becomes more aggressive. In addition to increased fluid intake (oral or parenteral), diuretics (especially osmotic types) are given to increase urine flow through the kidney. These are administered with caution

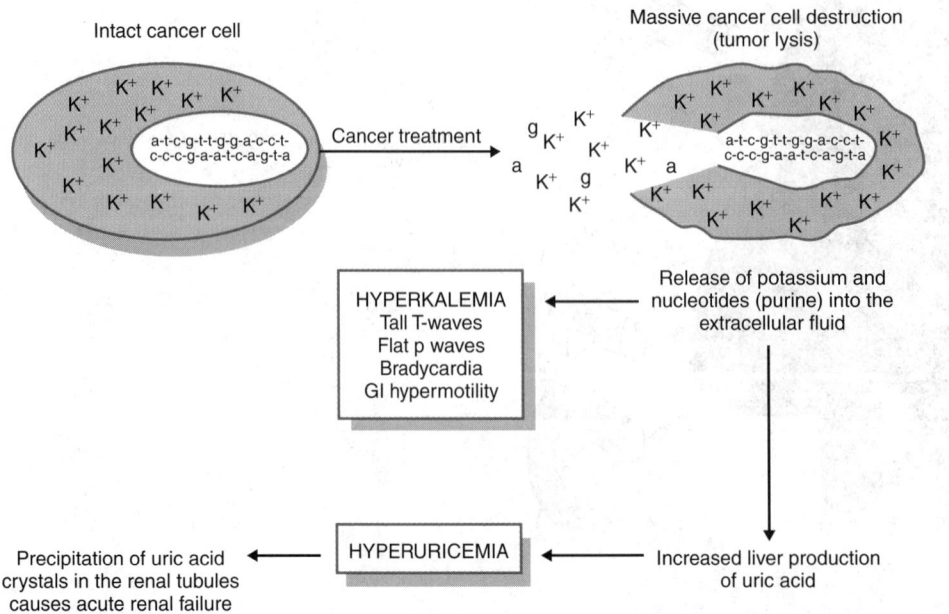

Figure 27–4. Pathology of tumor lysis syndrome.

because clients must not become dehydrated. Drugs that increase the excretion of purines, such as allopurinol (Alloprin, Zyloprim), are administered. To reduce serum potassium levels, clients may be given IV infusions containing glucose and insulin. Those clients who experience more severe and persistent hyperkalemia and hyperuricemia may require dialysis.

CANCER TREATMENT FAILURE

Although more than 50% of people diagnosed with cancer in North America this year will be cured of their disease and many others will live 2 years or longer, some clients will experience cancer treatment failure and die. The process of dying with cancer is usually long, lasting weeks or months. Clients and families require special support and assistance during this time. Chapter 12 addresses hospice care and other important physical, emotional, social, and spiritual needs of clients and families during and after the dying process.

SELECTED BIBLIOGRAPHY

*American Cancer Society. (1991). *Proceedings of the National Workshop on Cancer Control and the Older Person.* Atlanta: American Cancer Society.

American Cancer Society. (1998). Cancer facts and figures—1998 (Report No. 98-300M-No.5008.98). Atlanta: American Cancer Society.

Angel, F. E. (1995). Current controversies in chemotherapy administration. *Journal of Intravenous Nursing, 18*(1), 16–23.

Armstrong, T. S. (1994). Stomatitis. *Cancer Nursing, 17*, 403–410.

Aulas, J. (1996). Alternative cancer treatments. *Scientific American, 275*(3), 162–163.

Bender, C. (1995). Cognitive dysfunction associated with cancer and cancer treatment. *Medsurg Nursing, 4*(5), 398–400.

Bociek, R. G., & Armitage, J. (1996). Hematopoietic growth factors. *CA: A Cancer Journal for Clinicians, 46*(3), 165–184.

Boyle, D., & Engelking, C. (1995). Vesicant extravasation: Myths and realities. *Oncology Nursing Forum, 22*(1), 57–67.

Boyle, N., Bertin-Matson, K., & Bratschi, A. (1994). A patient's guide to Taxol. *Oncology Nursing Forum, 21*(9), 1569–1572.

Bryce, J. (1994). S.I.A.D.H. *Nursing 94, 24*(4), 33.

Campbell, M., & Pruitt, J. (1996). Radiation therapy: Protecting your patient's skin. *RN, 59*(1), 46–47.

Chan, B., & Ignoffo, J. (1995). Vinorelbine tartrate. *Cancer Practice, 3*(5), 320–323.

*Clark, J., & Longo, D. (1986). Biologic response modifiers. *Mediguide to Oncology, 6*, 1–10.

Clayton, K. (1997). Cancer-related hypercalcemia: How to spot it, how to manage it. *American Journal of Nursing, 97*(5), 42–49.

*Cooper, G. (1992). *Elements of human cancer.* Boston: Jones & Bartlett.

Daley, E. (1998). Clinical update on the role of HPV and cervical cancer. *Cancer Nursing, 21*(1), 31–35.

Davis, M., DeSantis, D., & Klemm, K. (1995). A flow sheet for follow-up after chemotherapy extravasation. *Oncology Nursing Forum, 22*(6), 979–983.

Dibble, S., Shiba, G., MacPhail, L., & Dodd, M. (1996). MacDibbs mouth assessment. *Cancer Practice, 4*(3), 135–140.

DiSipio, L. (1995). Relieving xerostomia from radiation therapy. *Oncology Nursing Forum, 22*(8), 1287.

*Doane, L., Fisher, L., & McDonald, T. (1990). How to give peritoneal chemotherapy. *American Journal of Nursing, 90*(4), 58–65.

Dodd, M., Onishi, K., Dibble, S., & Larson, P. (1996). Differences in nausea, vomiting, and retching between younger and older outpatients receiving cancer chemotherapy. *Cancer Nursing, 19*(3), 155–161.

Dumas, M. A. (1996). What it's like to belong to the cancer club. *American Journal of Nursing, 96*(4), 40–42.

Eckardt, J., Eckhardt, G., Villalona-Calero, M., Drengler, R., & Von

Hoff, D. (1995). New anticancer agents in clinical development. *Oncology, 9*(11), 1191–1200.

Ferrell, B., & Dow, K. H. (1996). Portraits of cancer survivorship. *Cancer Practice, 4*(2), 76–80.

Fessele, K. (1996). Managing the multiple causes of nausea and vomiting in the patient with cancer. *Oncology Nursing Forum, 23*(9), 1409–1417.

Folkman, J. (1996). Fighting cancer by attacking its blood supply. *Scientific American, 275*(3), 150–154.

*Fraser, M., & Tucker, M. (1989). Second malignancies following cancer therapy. *Seminars in Oncology Nursing, 5*(1), 43.

Gates, M., Lackey, N., & White, M. (1995). Needs of hospice and clinic patients with cancer. *Cancer Practice, 3*(4), 226–232.

Grindel, C. (1994). Fatigue and nutrition. *Medsurg Nursing, 3*(6), 475–481.

Gullo, S. (1995). Safe handling of cytotoxic agents. *Oncology Nursing Forum, 22*(3), 517–601.

Guy, J., & Ingram, B. (1996). Medical oncology—The agents. In R. McCorkle, M. Grant, M. Frank-Stromborg, & S. Baird (Eds.), *Cancer nursing: A comprehensive textbook* (2nd ed., pp. 359–394). Philadelphia: W. B. Saunders.

*Hassey, K. (1987). Principles of radiation therapy and protection. *Seminars in Oncology Nursing, 3*, 23–29.

*Hawthorne, J., Schneider, S., & Workman, M. (1992). Common electrolyte imbalances associated with malignancy. *AACN Clinical Issues in Critical Care, 3*(3), 714–723.

Hedges, C. (1994). Recognizing the patient at risk for opportunistic infections. *Medsurg Nursing, 3*(6), 445–452.

Held, J. (1995). Preventing and treating constipation. *Nursing 95, 25*(3), 28–30.

Hellman, S., & Vokes, E. (1996). Advancing current treatments for cancer. *Scientific American, 275*(3), 118–123.

Henry, D. (1996). Recombinant human erythropoietin treatment of anemic cancer patients. *Cancer Practice, 4*(4), 180–184.

Hilderley, L., & Dow, K. H. (1996). Radiation oncology. In R. McCorkle, M. Grant, M. Frank-Stromborg, & S. Baird (Eds.), *Cancer nursing: A comprehensive textbook* (2nd ed., pp. 331–358). Philadelphia: W. B. Saunders.

Hoffman, V. (1996). Tumor lysis syndrome: Implications for nursing. *Home Healthcare Nurse, 14*(8), 595–602.

Hood, L., & Abernathy, E. (1996). Biologic response modifiers. In R. McCorkle, M. Grant, M. Frank-Stromborg, & S. Baird (Eds.), *Cancer nursing: A comprehensive textbook* (2nd ed., pp. 434–457). Philadelphia: W. B. Saunders.

Houldin, A., & Wasserbauer, N. (1996). Psychosocial needs of older cancer patients. *MedSurg Nursing, 5*(4), 253–256.

Jain, R. (1994). Barriers to drug delivery in solid tumors. *Scientific American, 271*(1), 58–65.

*Jassak, P., & Sticklin, L. (1986). Interleukin-2: An overview. *Oncology Nursing Forum, 13*(6), 17–22.

Johnson, J. (1996). Coping with radiation therapy: Optimism and the effect of preparatory interventions. *Research in Nursing & Health, 19*(1), 3–12.

Johnson, M., Moroney, C., & Gay, C. (1997). Relieving nausea and vomiting in patients with cancer: A treatment algorithm. *Oncology Nursing Forum, 24*(1), 51–57.

Jones, S., & Burris, H. (1996). Topoisomerase I inhibitors: Topotecan and irinotecan. *Cancer Practice, 4*(1), 51–53.

Kaplan, R. (1994). Hypercalcemia of malignancy. *Oncology Nursing Forum, 21*(6), 1039–1046.

Karius, D., & Marriott, M. (1997). Immunologic advances in monoclonal antibody therapy: Implications for oncology nursing. *Oncology Nursing Forum, 24*(3), 483–494.

Kimmick, G., & Muss, H. (1995). Current status of endocrine therapy for metastatic breast cancer. *Oncology, 9*(9), 877–886.

Krakoff, I. (1996). Systemic treatment of cancer. *CA: A Cancer Journal for Clinicians, 46*(3), 136–141.

*Maddock, P. (1987). Brachytherapy sources and applicators. *Seminars in Oncology Nursing, 3*(1), 15.

Madeya, M. L. (1996). Oral complications from cancer therapy: Part 1. Pathophysiology and secondary complications. *Oncology Nursing Forum, 23*(7), 801–807.

Madeya, M. L. (1996). Oral complications from cancer therapy: Part 2. Nursing implications for assessment and treatment. *Oncology Nursing Forum, 23*(5), 808–821.

Martin, V., Walker, F., & Goodman, M. (1996). Delivery of cancer chemotherapy. In R. McCorkle, M. Grant, M. Frank-Stromborg, & S. Baird (Eds.), *Cancer nursing: A comprehensive textbook* (2nd ed., pp. 395–433). Philadelphia: W. B. Saunders.

Mayo, D., & Pearson, D. (1995). Chemotherapy extravasation: A consequence of fibrin sheath formation around venous access devices. *Oncology Nursing Forum, 22*(4), 675–680.

McCorkle, R., Grant, M., Frank-Stromborg, M., & Baird, S. (Eds.). (1996). *Cancer nursing: A comprehensive textbook* (2nd ed.). Philadelphia: W. B. Saunders.

McMenamin, E., McCorkle, R., Barg, F., Abrahm, J., & Jepson, C. (1995). Implementing a multidisciplinary cancer pain education program. *Cancer Practice, 3*(5), 303–309.

Miaskowski, C. (1996). Oncologic emergencies. In R. McCorkle, M. Grant, M. Frank-Stromborg, & S. Baird (Eds.), *Cancer nursing: A comprehensive textbook* (2nd ed., pp. 1183–1192). Philadelphia: W. B. Saunders.

Morse, J., & Doberneck, B. (1995). Delineating the concept of hope. *Image, 27*(4), 277–285.

Old, L. (1996). Immunotherapy for cancer. *Scientific American, 275*(3), 136–143.

Oliff, A., Gibbs, J., & McCormick, F. (1996), New molecular targets for cancer therapy. *Scientific American, 275*(3), 144–149.

Pitler, L. (1996). Hematopoietic growth factors in clinical practice. *Seminars in Oncology Nursing, 12*(2), 115–129.

Pu, A., Robertson, J., & Lawrence, T. (1995). Current status of radiation sensitization by fluoropyrimidines. *Oncology, 9*(8), 707–714.

Rhodes, V., McDaniel, R., Simms, S., & Johnson, M. (1995). Nurses' perceptions of antiemetic effectiveness. *Oncology Nursing Forum, 22*(8), 1243–1252.

Rhodes, V., Watson, P., McDaniel, R., Hanson, B., & Johnson, M. (1995). Expectation and occurrence of postchemotherapy side effects. *Cancer Practice, 3*(4), 247–253.

Richardson, A., Ream, E., & Wilson-Barnett, J. (1998). Fatigue in patients receiving chemotherapy: Patterns of change. *Cancer Nursing, 21*(1), 17–30.

Rieger, P., & Haeuber, D. (1995). A new approach to managing chemotherapy-related anemia: Nursing implications of epoetin alfa. *Oncology Nursing Forum, 22*(1), 71–81.

Rose, M., Shrader-Bogen, C., Korlath, G., Priem, J., & Larson, L. (1996). Identifying patient symptoms after radiotherapy using a nurse-managed telephone interview. *Oncology Nursing Forum, 23*(1), 99–102.

Russell, S. (1994). Septic shock: Can you recognize the clues? *Nursing 94, 24*(4), 40–48.

Schneider, S. (1994). Clinical implications for the administration of colony stimulating factors. *Journal of Orthopaedic Nursing, 13*(1), 56–62, 64.

*Strohl, R. (1992). The elderly patient receiving radiation treatment: Sequelae and nursing care. *Geriatric Nursing, 13*(3), 152–156.

Sweet, V., Servy, E., & Karow, A. (1996). Reproductive issues for men with cancer: Technology and nursing management. *Oncology Nursing Forum, 23*(1), 51–58.

Toth, B., Chambers, M., Fleming, T., Lemon, J., & Martin, J. (1995). Minimizing oral complications of cancer treatment. *Oncology, 9*(9), 851–858.

Ward, U. (1995). Biological therapy in the treatment of cancer. *British Journal of Nursing, 4*(15), 869–899.

Weintraub, F., & Neumark, D. (1996). Surgical oncology. In R. McCorkle, M. Grant, M. Frank-Stromborg, & S. Baird (Eds.), *Cancer nursing: A comprehensive textbook* (2nd ed., pp. 315–330). Philadelphia: W. B. Saunders.

Wilmoth, M., & Townsend, J. (1995). A comparison of the effects of lumpectomy versus mastectomy on sexual behaviors. *Cancer Practice, 3*(5), 279–285.

*Wood, L., & Gullo, S. (1993). IV vesicants: How to avoid extravasation. *American Journal of Nursing, 93*(4), 42–46.

Workman, M. L. (1996). Gene therapy. In R. McCorkle, M. Grant, M. Frank-Stromborg, & S. Baird (Eds.), *Cancer nursing: A comprehensive textbook* (2nd ed., pp. 458–469). Philadelphia: W. B. Saunders.

*Workman, M. L., Ellerhorst-Ryan, J., & Koertge, V. (1993). *Nursing care of the immunocompromised patient*. Philadelphia: W. B. Saunders.

Yost, L. (1995). Cancer patients and home care. *Cancer Practice, 3*(2), 83–87.

SUGGESTED READINGS

Gullo, S. (1995). Safe handling of cytotoxic agents. *Oncology Nursing Forum, 22*(3), 517–601.

> Originally published in 1988, this updated article provides gold-standard information regarding the safe handling of chemotherapeutic agents.

Madeya, M. L. (1996). Oral complications from cancer therapy: Part 1. Pathophysiology and secondary complications. *Oncology Nursing Forum, 23*(5), 801–807.

> This excellent article provides a comprehensive explanation of mucositis, stomatitis, and other oral complications of cancer therapy. The text is enhanced by color photographs of oral mucous membranes with different types of infections.

Madeya, M. L. (1996). Oral complications from cancer therapy: Part 2. Nursing implications for assessment and treatment. *Oncology Nursing Forum, 23*(5), 808–821.

> In a follow-up to the previous article, the author stresses assessment techniques and nursing interventions for mucositis, stomatitis, and other oral complications. The table on agents used to treat primary and secondary oral complications is particularly useful.

Pitler, L. (1996). Hematopoietic growth factors in clinical practice. *Seminars in Oncology Nursing, 12*(2), 115–129.

> This article provides a comprehensive, current description of how hematopoietic growth factors are being used in clinical practice. Although targeted specifically to oncology nurses, students would particularly benefit from the tables addressing monitoring and other nursing care issues.

INTERVENTIONS FOR CLIENTS WITH INFECTION

Many infections and infectious diseases are easily preventable and treatable with vaccines or appropriately used antibiotics; nevertheless, infectious diseases remain a major cause of illness and death worldwide. New, re-emerging, and drug-resistant infections are significant health threats now and into the new century. Changes in the way people live, eat, and travel have made them more vulnerable to infectious diseases. Advancing technology and invasive procedures introduce previously harmless microorganisms into the body with resulting infection. The nurse's understanding of the infectious process can help prevent or minimize the effects of infection.

INFECTIOUS PROCESS

Overview

Definitions

An infection is caused by microorganisms when they invade the body. Infections can be communicable (e.g., hepatitis and influenza) or noncommunicable (e.g., pancreatitis and cellulitis).

The process of infection requires a pathogen, or causative agent, and a susceptible host, or recipient of infection. A pathogen is any microorganism capable of producing disease in a person. People are surrounded by countless microorganisms with differing degrees of pathogenicity (ability to cause disease). *Virulence* is a term often used as a synonym for *pathogenicity*. However, virulence is related more to the frequency that a pathogen causes disease in exposed people (degree of communicability) and its ability to invade and damage a host. Virulence can also indicate the severity of the disease. Another important characteristic is invasiveness: the ability of pathogens to spread and grow in the tissues of a host after entrance.

Most microorganisms commonly live in or on the human host without causing disease. Some microbes are actually beneficial. For example, each body location harbors its own characteristic bacteria, or *normal flora*. One important function of normal flora is to compete with and prevent infection by unfamiliar microorganisms attempting to invade a body site. In some instances, microorganisms may be present in the tissues of the host and yet not cause symptomatic disease; this process is called *colonization*.

In many instances, microorganisms behave as parasites; that is, the microorganisms live at the expense of their human hosts. In this interaction with its host, the microbe gains some advantage and infection occurs. Infection is the establishment of a host-parasite interaction.

519

TABLE 28–1

Infectious Diseases that Must Be Reported to the CDC

Acquired immunodeficiency syndrome (AIDS)	*Haemophilus influenzae,* invasive disease	Psittacosis
Anthrax	Hansen's disease (leprosy)	Rabies, animal
Botulism†	Hantavirus pulmonary syndrome	Rabies, human
Brucellosis	Hemolytic-uremic syndrome, postdiarrhea†	Rocky Mountain spotted fever
Chancroid		Rubella
Chlamydia trachomatis, genital infection	Hepatitis A	Salmonellosis†
	Hepatitis B	Shigellosis†
Cholera	Hepatitis C	Streptococcal disease, invasive, group A†
Coccidioidomycosis†	Human immunodeficiency virus infection, pediatric (i.e., in persons ages <13 years)	*Streptococcus pneumoniae,* drug resistant†
Congenital rubella syndrome		Streptococcal toxic-shock syndrome†
Congenital syphilis		Syphilis
Cryptosporidiosis	Legionellosis	Tetanus
Diphtheria	Lyme disease	Toxic-shock syndrome
Encephalitis, California	Malaria	Trichinosis
Encephalitis, eastern equine	Measles	Tuberculosis
Encephalitis, St. Louis	Meningococcal disease	Typhoid fever
Encephalitis, western equine	Mumps	Yellow fever†
Escherichia coli O157:H7	Pertussis	Varicella (chicken pox)*
Gonorrhea	Plague	
	Poliomyelitis, paralytic	

* Although varicella is not a nationally notifiable disease, the Council of State and Territorial Epidemiologists recommends reporting of cases of this disease to CDC.
† Not currently published in the weekly tables.
Data from Centers for Disease Control and Prevention (1997). Summary of notifiable diseases, United States, 1996. *Morbidity and Mortality Weekly,* 45(53), iv.

Subclinical infection causes no apparent reaction in the host and thus elicits no detectable symptoms. Most often, subclinical infection can be identified only by the immune response of the host. This is demonstrated by a rise in the titer of antibody directed against the infecting agent. Clinically apparent infection in which the host-parasite interaction causes obvious injury is accompanied by one or more clinical manifestations and is known as infectious disease. Disease caused by an infectious agent may range from mild to fatal.

The Centers for Disease Control and Prevention (CDC) collects information about the occurrence and nature of infectious diseases. The CDC then makes recommendations to health care agencies for infection control and prevention. Certain diseases must be reported to health departments and the CDC (Table 28–1).

Chain of Infection

Infectious disease development depends on the chain of infection (Fig. 28–1). Transmission of infection requires the following factors:

Reservoir
Pathogen
Susceptible host
Portal of entry
Mode of transmission
Portal of exit

Preventing the spread of infection depends on breaking the chain of infection at any point. Eliminating the microorganism, providing the host with immunity, or, most often, interrupting the mode of transmission breaks the chain of infection. In health care settings, nurses and other personnel interrupt the transmission of pathogens by scrupulous hand washing, implementing barrier precautions, and using antimicrobial agents.

Reservoir

Reservoirs, or sources of infectious agents, are numerous. A reservoir is any place where the pathogen is found; it can be animate (living) or inanimate (not living). Animate reservoirs include people, animals, and insects. Inanimate reservoirs include soil, water, other environmental sources, and medical equipment, such as intravenous (IV) solutions and urine collection devices. The host's own body can be a reservoir; pathogens can colonize in skin and body substances, such as feces, sputum, saliva, and wound drainage. A person with an active infection or an asymptomatic carrier (a person who does not have a disease but harbors the infectious agent) can be a reservoir. A carrier can be incubating the pathogen before signs and symptoms develop, have a subclinical infection, be convalescing from an infection, or be a chronic carrier of the pathogen. Examples of community reservoirs are sewage or stagnant water and certain improperly cooked foods.

Pathogen

Several different classes of microorganisms produce infection (Table 28–2). Survival and continued multiplication of a pathogen are often accompanied by the production of *toxins.* Toxins are protein molecules released by bacteria to affect host cells at a distant site. *Exotoxins* are produced and released by certain bacteria into the sur-

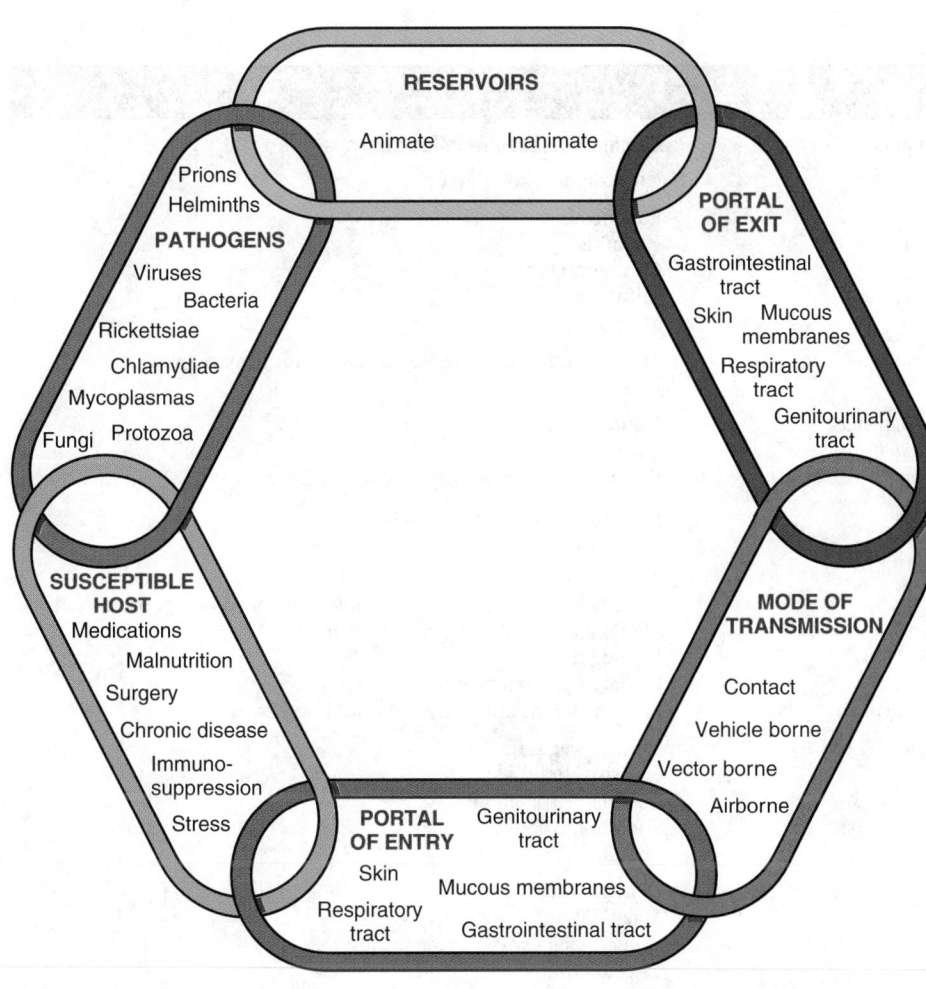

Figure 28–1. The chain of infection: the process by which pathogens are transmitted from the environment to a host, invade the host, and cause infection.

rounding environment. Botulism, tetanus, and diphtheria are attributed to exotoxins. *Endotoxins* are produced in the cell walls of certain bacteria and released only with cell lysis. Typhoid and meningococcal diseases are caused by endotoxins.

Host

Several host factors influence the development of infection (Table 28–3). The human body has an efficient system for self-protection against pathogens known as host defense (see later discussion). Breakdown of any of these defense mechanisms may increase the susceptibility of the host to infection.

Clients' immune status plays the largest role in determining their risk for infection. Congenital abnormalities as well as acquired health problems, such as acquired immunodeficiency syndrome (AIDS), can result in numerous immunologic deficiencies. Such depression of the immune system may render the host particularly susceptible to infection or cripple the host's ability to combat organisms that have gained entry.

IMMUNITY. Immunity is resistance to infection usually associated with the presence of antibodies or cells that act on specific microorganisms. *Passive immunity* is of short duration (days or months) and either natural by transpla-

cental transfer from the mother or artificial by injection of antibodies (e.g., immune globulin). *Active immunity* lasts for years and is either natural by infection or artificial by injection of the agent itself or a modified form of the agent.

ELDERLY CONSIDERATIONS

Host factors such as age may influence immunity. Because of their decreased ability to produce an adequate immune response, elderly clients are at increased risk for infection. Immunity declines in the elderly, as evidenced by decreasing T-cell and primary antibody responses (also see Chap. 23).

OTHER FACTORS. Hormonal factors play a role in the incidence and mortality rate of many infectious diseases. People with diabetes mellitus and adrenal insufficiency experience increased numbers of acute and chronic bacterial infections.

Certain environmental factors may influence clients' immune status and thus their susceptibility to or ability to fight infection. Examples include alcohol consumption, inhalation of toxic chemicals that may suppress bone marrow function, and certain vitamin deficiencies. Malnutrition, especially protein-calorie malnutrition, places clients at increased risk for infection.

TABLE 28–2

Infectious Organisms*

Organism Class	Common Examples	Common Disease Manifestations
Prions		Creutzfeldt-Jakob disease
Viruses	Poliovirus	Poliomyelitis
	Hepatitis A virus	Hepatitis
	Rhinovirus	Common cold
	Influenza A virus	Influenza
	Mumps virus	Mumps
Chlamydiae	*Chlamydia trachomatis*	Trachoma, lymphogranuloma venereum, conjunctivitis
	C. psittaci	Psittacosis (parrot fever)
Mycoplasmas	*Mycoplasma pneumoniae*	Pneumonia
	Ureaplasma urealyticum	Urethritis
	Mycoplasma hominis	Pyelonephritis, pelvic inflammatory disease
Rickettsiae	*Rickettsia rickettsii*	Rocky Mountain spotted fever
	R. prowazekii	Typhus
	Coxiella burnetii	Q fever
Bacteria	*Staphylococcus* sp.	Superficial skin infections, osteomyelitis, pneumonia, bacteremia
	Streptococcus sp.	Pharyngitis, skin infections, pneumonia
	Neisseria meningitidis	Meningitis
	Escherichia coli	Urinary tract infection
	Pseudomonas aeruginosa	Skin infection, otitis, urinary tract infection
Fungi	*Candida albicans*	Thrush, vaginitis
	Aspergillus sp.	Sinusitis, brain abscess
	Cryptococcus neoformans	Meningitis, pneumonia
	Histoplasma capsulatum	Pneumonia
	Coccidioides immitis	Pneumonia
Protozoa	*Entamoeba histolytica*	Diarrhea, colitis
	Plasmodium sp.	Malaria
	Leishmania sp.	Fever, weight loss, cutaneous lesions
	Toxoplasma gondii	Chorioretinitis, encephalitis
	Pneumocystis carinii	Pneumonia
Helminths	*Ancylostoma duodenale* (hookworm)	Anemia
	Ascaris lumbricoides (roundworm)	Intestinal obstruction
	Enterobius vermicularis (pinworm)	Anal pruritus
	Schistosoma sp. (blood flukes)	Hydronephrosis
	Taenia solium (pork tapeworm)	Epilepsy from cysticercosis

* Organisms are presented in order of increasing complexity.

Finally, certain types of medical interventions may suppress or impair the normal immune response. Corticosteroid therapy, chemotherapy for malignant neoplasms, and cytotoxic therapy specifically intended to suppress the immune response (e.g., cyclophosphamide [Cytoxan] for lupus nephritis and cyclosporine in organ transplant recipients) increase the risk of infection. Medical devices, such as percutaneous intravascular catheters, urethral catheters, and endotracheal tubes, also impair or violate normal host defense mechanisms.

Portal of Entry

Microorganisms may enter the body in a variety of ways (Table 28–4).

RESPIRATORY TRACT. A number of pathogens enter the body through the respiratory tract. Microbes in contaminated droplets are sprayed into the air when people with infected oral, nasal, or throat tissues talk, cough, or sneeze. These droplets are then inhaled by a susceptible host and either localize in the lung or are distributed via the lymphatic system or the bloodstream to other areas of the body. Microorganisms that enter the body by the respiratory tract but produce distant infection include *Mycobacterium tuberculosis,* influenza virus, and *Neisseria meningitidis* (the organism most commonly responsible for epidemic meningitis).

GASTROINTESTINAL TRACT. Some pathogens enter the body through the gastrointestinal (GI) tract. Of these, some stay in the GI tract and produce disease (e.g., enteroviruses, *Giardia,* and the organisms that cause self-limited food poisoning). Others invade the GI tract to produce local and then distant infection (e.g., *Salmonella enteritidis*). Still others produce limited GI symptoms,

TABLE 28-3

Host Factors that Influence the Development of Infection	
Host Factor	**Increased Risk of Infection**
Natural immunity	Congenital or acquired immuno-deficiencies
Normal flora	Alteration of normal flora by anti-biotic therapy
Age	Infants and elderly clients
Hormonal factors	Pregnancy, diabetes, cortico-steroid therapy, and adrenal insufficiency
Phagocytosis	Defective phagocytic function, circulatory disturbances, and neutropenia
Skin/mucous membranes/normal excretory secretions	Break in skin or mucous membrane integrity; interference with flow of urine, tears, or saliva; interference with cough reflex or ciliary action; changes in gastric secretions
Nutrition	Malnutrition or dehydration
Environmental factors	Smoking, alcohol consumption, and inhalation of toxic chemicals
Medical interventions	Invasive therapy, chemotherapy, radiation therapy, and steroid therapy; surgery

causing either a systemic infection (e.g., *Salmonella typhi*) or profound involvement of another organ (e.g., hepatitis A virus).

ELDERLY CONSIDERATIONS

Clostridium difficile can cause diarrhea, especially in the elderly, and occurs when antibiotic therapy destroys the normal flora of the bowel. When diarrhea subsides, stool cultures may still be positive for the microbe.

GENITOURINARY TRACT. A third portal of entry for microorganisms is the genitourinary tract. Urinary tract infection is one of the most common infectious diseases treated each year.

WOMEN'S HEALTH CONSIDERATIONS

Microorganisms (often normal colonic bacterial flora) colonize the perineal area, the urethral meatus, and the bladder, especially in women. The elderly woman is at an even greater risk because of decreased resistance to infection, stress incontinence, or, possibly, inability to practice proper hygiene.

SKIN/MUCOUS MEMBRANES. Some pathogens, such as *Treponema pallidum,* can enter the body through intact

skin or mucous membranes. Most enter through breaks in these normally effective surface barriers. Sometimes a medical procedure creates a break in the normal cutaneous (skin) or mucocutaneous (mucous membrane) barriers, as in catheter-acquired bacteremia (bacteria in the bloodstream) and surgical wound infections. Fragile skin of the elderly and of those on prolonged steroid therapy increases infection risk.

BLOODSTREAM. Microorganisms can gain direct access to the bloodstream. Normal skin bacteria introduced by vascular devices cause more than 31% of hospital-acquired (nosocomial) bloodstream infections (NNIS, 1996). Insects can inject organisms into the bloodstream by biting the host, causing such infections as malaria, Lyme disease, and Rocky Mountain spotted fever.

Mode of Transmission

For infection to be transmitted, a mechanism must transport the invading organism from the infected source to a susceptible host. Microorganisms are transmitted by several routes, and the same microorganism may be transmitted by more than one route. The four common routes are

Contact transmission
Airborne transmission
Vehicle transmission
Vectorborne transmission

CONTACT TRANSMISSION. Many infections are spread by contact, which may be direct or indirect. With direct contact, the source and host come into physical contact; microorganisms are transferred directly, usually through skin to skin or mucous membrane to mucous membrane. Often called person-to-person transmission, direct contact is best illustrated by the spread of sexually transmitted diseases.

Indirect contact leading to transmission of infectious agents involves transfer of microorganisms from a source to a host by passive transfer from an inanimate (not living) intermediate object (also called a fomite). Contaminated articles, especially those that may contact nonintact skin or mucous membranes, may serve as sources of infection. One example of transmission through indirect contact is transfer of hepatitis B virus from a contaminated source to a susceptible host by a contaminated needlestick.

Another method of indirect contact, *droplet spread,* involves transmission of infection through contact with infective secretions. Droplets are relatively large, usually greater than 5 μm in size. These droplets are produced when a person talks or sneezes, and they travel through the air only a short distance (usually less than 3 feet, or 1 m). Susceptible hosts may acquire infection by contact with droplets deposited on the membranes of the nose, mouth, or conjunctivae. A common example of droplet-spread infection is influenzae. Susceptible people who are closest to the infected source have the highest risk for infection with a droplet-spread organism.

TABLE 28–4

Portals of Entry of Selected Disease-Producing Organisms

Portal of Entry	Infecting Organisms	Resultant Diseases
Respiratory tract	*Neisseria meningitidis*	Meningococcal pneumonia, meningococcal meningitis, meningococcemia
	Cryptococcus neoformans	Cryptococcal meningitis, cryptococcal pneumonia
	Mycobacterium tuberculosis	Tuberculosis
	Influenza A virus	Influenza
	Streptococcus pneumoniae	Pneumococcal pneumonia
	Measles virus (rubeola)	Measles
	Legionella pneumophila	Legionnaires' disease
	Varicella-zoster virus	Chickenpox
Gastrointestinal tract	*Salmonella enteritidis*	Gastroenteritis
	Salmonella typhi	Typhoid fever
	Giardia lamblia	Diarrhea
	Clostridium botulinum	Botulism
	Poliovirus	Poliomyelitis
	Hepatitis A virus	Hepatitis A
Genitourinary tract	*Neisseria gonorrhoeae*	Gonorrhea
	Chlamydia trachomatis	Lymphogranuloma venereum, cervicitis, urethritis, endometritis
	Enterobacteriaceae (*Escherichia coli*, *Klebsiella* sp., *Serratia* sp., *Proteus* sp.)	Urinary tract infections
Intact skin or mucous membranes	Rhinovirus	Common cold
	Respiratory syncytial virus	Pneumonia, bronchiolitis, tracheobronchitis
	Schistosoma sp.	Schistosome dermatitis (swimmer's disease)
	Herpes simplex virus	Oral or genital herpes
Bloodstream	Hepatitis B virus	Hepatitis B
	Plasmodium	Malaria
	Clostridium tetani	Tetanus
	Human immunodeficiency virus	Acquired immunodeficiency syndrome

Oral-fecal transmission is another example of indirect contact for the spread of infection. Ingestion of enteric pathogens (e.g., eating food prepared by a person with hepatitis A infection who does not wash his or her hands) can cause transmission of the virus.

AIRBORNE TRANSMISSION. Airborne transmission occurs when small, airborne, infected particles leave the infected source and travel farther than 3 feet (approximately 1 m) in the air. These particles are usually contained in droplet nuclei or dust; they are most often propelled from the respiratory tract by coughing or sneezing. A susceptible person then inhales the particles directly into the respiratory tract. Tuberculosis, chickenpox, and rubeola measles are transmitted by the airborne route.

VEHICLE TRANSMISSION. Vehicle transmission occurs when infectious agents are transmitted through a common source, such as contaminated food, water, or IV fluid. Salmonellosis is an example of a frequently vehicle-transmitted disease.

VECTORBORNE TRANSMISSION. Vectorborne transmission of infection involves insects and animals that act as intermediaries between two or more hosts. For exam-

ple, ticks can transmit Rocky Mountain spotted fever and mosquitoes can spread malaria.

Portal of Exit

The portal of exit completes the chain of infection. An infecting organism exits from the once-susceptible person who has become a reservoir for infection. Exit from the host most often occurs through the portal of entry. An organism, such as *Mycobacterium tuberculosis*, enters the susceptible client's respiratory tract and exits the respiratory tract as the infected host coughs into the air. However, some organisms may exit from the infected host by several routes. For example, varicella-zoster virus can spread through direct contact with infective fluid in the chickenpox vesicles and by droplet contact.

Defense Against Infection

Several host factors influence the development of infection. Strong and intact host defenses can prevent a microbe from entering the body, or they can destroy a pathogen that has gained entry. Conversely, impaired host defenses may be unable to defend against microbial invasion, allowing entry of microorganisms that can destroy host cells and cause infection.

Host defense mechanisms may be classified as nonspecific or specific.

TABLE 28–5

Nonspecific Defenses Against Infection		
Body Tissue	**Type of Action**	**Defense Action**
Intact skin	Physical	Provides a barrier
	Chemical	Normal flora and acid pH create a hostile environment
Mucous membranes	Mechanical	Mucociliary action clears bacteria
	Chemical	Lysosomes dissolve bacterial wall
Respiratory tract	Mechanical	Mucociliary action Cough
	Chemical	Lysosome action Humidification
Gastrointestinal tract	Mechanical	Peristalsis
	Chemical	Enzymes Acid pH Normal bowel flora
Genitourinary tract	Mechanical	Flushing action of urine
	Chemical	Acid pH

Nonspecific Defenses

Nonspecific mechanisms, most often representing the first encounter an invading pathogen has with its human host, include body tissues, such as the skin and mucous membranes; phagocytosis; and inflammation (Table 28–5).

BODY TISSUES. Intact skin forms the first and most important physical barrier to the entry of microorganisms into the body. In addition to providing a mechanical barrier, the skin's slightly acidic pH (resulting from the breakdown of lipids into fatty acids), together with the normal skin flora, creates an unfriendly environment for pathogenic bacteria.

Mucous membranes, by their mucociliary action, provide some mechanical protection against pathogenic invasion. More important, however, mucous membranes are bathed in secretions that inactivate many microorganisms. Lysozymes, which are enzymes that dissolve the cell walls of some bacteria, are present in large quantities in many body secretions, particularly in nasal mucus and tears.

Other body systems provide natural barriers to infection. The respiratory tract can clear about 90% of all inhaled material by filtration in the upper airways, humidification, mucociliary transport, and expulsion by coughing. Peristaltic action mechanically empties the gastrointestinal tract of pathogenic organisms. In addition, the acid pH of the stomach, intestinal secretions, pancreatic enzymes, and bile, together with the competition from normal bowel flora, provides an environment that protects the gastrointestinal tract from invasion by harmful organisms. In the genitourinary tract, the flushing action of urine eliminates pathogenic organisms. The low pH of urine also maintains a sterile environment, although certain microorganisms, like *Escherichia coli,* can thrive in an acid medium.

PHAGOCYTOSIS. Phagocytosis occurs when a foreign substance evades the first-line mechanical barriers and enters the body. Various types of leukocytes function differently in the immune reaction, but neutrophils bear the primary responsibility for phagocytosis. This process of engulfing, ingesting, killing, and disposing of an invading organism is an essential mechanism in host defense. Phagocytic dysfunction dramatically increases a client's risk for infection and recurrent infections.

INFLAMMATION. Inflammation is another important nonspecific defense mechanism in preventing the spread of infection. Inflammation occurs when tissue becomes damaged. The damaged cells release enzymes, and polymorphonuclear leukocytes are attracted to the infected site from the bloodstream. One important enzyme, histamine, increases the permeability of the capillaries in the inflamed tissues, thus allowing fluid, proteins, and white blood cells to enter the inflamed area. Still other enzymes activate fibrinogen, which causes the leaked fluid to clot and prevents its flow away from the damaged site into unaffected tissue, essentially "walling off" the inflamed tissue. The process of phagocytosis then disposes of the invading microorganism and often the dead tissue. If the inflammation is caused by infection, the end products of inflammation form the substance commonly known as pus, which is subsequently absorbed or exits the body through a break in the skin. (See also Chapter 23 for a discussion of the inflammatory response.)

Specific Defenses

Specific defenses against infection, that is, specific responses to specific microorganisms, are provided by the antibody-mediated and cell-mediated immune systems. The antibody-mediated immune system produces antibodies directed against certain pathogens. These antibodies inactivate or destroy the invading microorganism as well as protect against future infection with that microorganism. Resistance to other microorganisms is mediated by the action of specifically sensitized T lymphocytes and is called cell-mediated immunity. The components of the immune system work both independently and together to protect against infection (see Chap. 23).

Infection Control in Health Care Agencies
Inpatient Facilities

Infection acquired in the hospital, nursing home, or other inpatient setting (not present or incubating at the time of admission) is termed *nosocomial.* Nosocomial infections can be endogenous (from the client's own flora) or exogenous (from outside the client, usually from the health care facility environment or hands of health care workers). Nosocomial infections are acquired by about 2 million inpatients annually with a cost of approximately $4.5

billion annually (NNIS, 1996). The costs associated with the additional morbidity and mortality cannot be measured. Infection control within a health care facility is designed to reduce the risk of nosocomial infection in clients or personnel and thus reduce morbidity and mortality and their associated costs. A program for infection control and prevention includes facility- and department-specific infection control policies and procedures, surveillance and analysis, client and staff education, and product evaluation and an overall emphasis on cost and quality. The program is coordinated and implemented by an infection control practitioner who is usually a nurse certified in infection control (CIC) and who also has varied experience in the clinical setting with administrative skills.

Home Care Settings

Guidelines on infection control in home care are beginning to be published. Currently, the Joint Commission on Accreditation of Healthcare Organizations (JCAHO) does not require a designated infection control practitioner or committee. Commonsense approaches to infection control in the home are used. For example, the nurse is not required to place a barrier under the nursing bag, but the bag should be placed on a clean surface. Closed sharps containers may be hand carried or hooked to the outside of the nursing bag. Home care nurses should follow CDC guidelines for protection when caring for a client with an infection (Friedman, 1997).

Methods of Infection Control

Infection or the spread of infection can be prevented or controlled in at least five ways:

> Hand washing
> Hygiene
> Sanitation
> Disinfection/sterilization
> Barriers (such as gloves)

Every health care agency employee who comes in contact with clients or client care areas is involved in some aspect of the infection control program of the agency.

Hand Washing

Hand washing is the single most effective mechanism for preventing the spread of infection. Effective hand washing takes 10 to 15 seconds and consists of wetting, soaping, lathering, applying friction under running water, rinsing, and drying adequately. Friction may be supplied by soft brushes or simply by rubbing the skin surfaces together. Friction is essential to emulsify the oils on the skin and to disperse transient bacteria and soil from the skin surface. To minimize chapped or cracked skin, nurses should rinse and dry their hands thoroughly.

A recent study found that 27% of nurses had irritant dermatitis from frequent hand washing. Lotions and other products that do not contain iodophor may help protect the skin. The most promising skin-protecting lotions apply a film to the skin for 3 or 4 hours during multiple hand washings, acting like invisible gloves. Examples of

these new products include DermaMed, HealthSafe, and Viragard (Beaumont, 1997).

Health care personnel should always wash their hands before and after direct contact with a client and immediately after contact with blood, secretions, and excretions. The use of gloves does not eliminate the need for hand washing. Some studies have shown that 20% to 34% of gloves allow bacterial penetration, and as many as 53% leak or allow bacterial penetration during use (Beaumont, 1997).

The Centers for Disease Control and Prevention (CDC) recommend the use of antiseptic solutions, such as chlorhexidine or povidone-iodine, for hand washing in the care of clients who are at high risk (e.g., immunocompromised clients). The use of these solutions is also recommended after caring for clients who are colonized or infected with multiply-resistant or other virulent organisms.

Other Infection Control Measures

Potentially harmful microorganisms are eliminated or greatly reduced through various methods. Meticulous hand washing and proper hygiene, including bathing, are important in preventing infection for both clients and health care personnel. Strict attention to health care facility sanitation and infectious waste disposal (e.g., soiled dressings) and incineration must be followed in keeping with CDC guidelines. Sterilization and disinfection procedures keep equipment and the physical environment clean. Housekeeping personnel use strong but safe cleaning disinfectants that eliminate or minimize microbes.

The nurse must try to keep infectious clients apart from those who are highly susceptible to infection. Clients who are immunocompromised or who have just had surgery will be more susceptible to infections. Keeping these clients separate helps prevent client-to-client transmission of infection.

BARRIER PRECAUTIONS. *Barriers* are items placed between the client and the health care provider. Gloves, masks, and gowns are examples. Barrier precautions, also called isolation precautions, are designed to prevent the spread of infection. These precautions have changed dramatically over the past 20 years as transmission of infections has become better understood and new infections have emerged. Additional guidelines from the CDC continue to be distributed periodically to health care facilities. The latest guidelines are reviewed by each health care facility's infection control committee and then tailored to meet the specific needs of that facility. Policies and procedures for types of barriers and precautions may vary among facilities, but the principles are the same.

UNIVERSAL PRECAUTIONS GUIDELINES. In 1987 the CDC published Universal Precautions guidelines. The guidelines address the prevention of bloodborne disease transmission. All clients' blood and certain body fluids are considered potentially infected with bloodborne disease. Feces, urine, and perspiration are not considered potential routes of bloodborne disease, unless there is visible blood. Most of the focus is on the human immunodeficiency

TABLE 28–6

Universal Precautions

These precautions are to be used with all clients to protect health care providers from bloodborne communicable diseases.

- *Gloves* should be worn for contact with blood and body fluids, nonintact skin, and mucous membranes of all clients; for handling surfaces or items soiled with blood and body fluids; and for performing venipuncture and other vascular access procedures. Gloves should be changed after each client contact.
- *Masks or protective goggles* should be worn during procedures that are likely to cause splashes of blood or body fluids.
- *Gowns or aprons* should be worn during procedures likely to result in splashes of blood or body fluids.
- *Hand washing* should be done immediately on contact with blood or other body fluids. Wash hands as soon as gloves are removed.
- *Needles and sharp instruments* should be placed in puncture-resistant containers for disposal to prevent injuries from needles or other sharp items. Needles should not be recapped, bent, or removed from the syringe.
- *Mouth-to-mouth resuscitation* should be performed with use of mouthpieces or other ventilation devices.

Data from Centers for Disease Control, (1987). Recommendations for prevention of HIV transmission in health-care settings. *Morbidity and Mortality Weekly Report, 36*(25), 3–17.

virus (HIV), which causes acquired immunodeficiency syndrome (AIDS), and hepatitis B virus (HBV). HBV is more contagious and more commonly transmitted and affects health care workers more often than HIV. Table 28–6 outlines the guidelines for Universal Precautions, and Table 28–7 notes which body fluids are the highest risk for transmission of any bloodborne disease and which are not.

The increased glove use required by universal precautions has at times promoted hand irritation problems to specific gloves and sometimes latex allergy. Hand irritation is most often due to development of sensitivity to the powder or the chemicals used in the manufacture of gloves. Switching to another brand of gloves may resolve hand irritation. The use of vinyl or other nonlatex gloves or cotton glove liners may be required. Masks not made with latex ear loops should be used for those with latex allergy. When latex allergy is suspected, medical evaluation and treatment are necessary.

BODY SUBSTANCE PRECAUTIONS. Universal Precautions were expanded by infection control experts to include other body fluids and materials rather than only those that caused bloodborne diseases. These expanded guidelines are called body substance precautions or body substance isolation (BSI). With the increased occurrence of GI microorganisms, like *Clostridium difficile,* any client's feces is considered a potential source of infection. Therefore, in addition to wearing barriers as for universal precautions, the nurse and other health care personnel should always wear gloves when coming in contact with

feces or anything contaminated with feces, like soiled linen and underpads. Gowns may also be necessary to protect the staff's uniform.

Another trend in infection control practice discourages the term *isolation,* which implies that the client is removed from everyone else. Nonprofessional health care facility employees are often afraid of isolation and fear that they will "catch" an infection from the isolated client. The terms *barrier* and *precautions* are preferred.

Whichever system for precautions is used, the nurse must be careful to prevent forced client solitude and to promote quality care. In some cases, initiating barrier precautions may be associated with untoward psychosocial effects. For the few clients who must be confined to their rooms, the constant environment of the hospital room may be difficult to tolerate. Family members may also express fear or anxiety because the client is isolated.

CDC TRANSMISSION-BASED GUIDELINES. The CDC published new isolation guidelines for hospitals in 1997 (Table 28–8) to replace the 1983 disease- and category-specific precautions. The new CDC guidelines apply available knowledge, focus on mechanisms of transmission, and combine the best aspects of previous guidelines. Included in these guidelines are standard, airborne, droplet, and contact precautions. Standard precautions, or the equivalent, should be used in the care of all clients. Airborne, droplet, and contact precautions are used in addition to standard precautions.

Standard Precautions acknowledge that all body excretions, secretions, and moist membranes and tissues, excluding perspiration, are potentially infectious. The exten-

TABLE 28–7

Transmission of Bloodborne Disease by Various Body Fluids

Body Fluids Likely to Transmit Bloodborne Disease (Universal Precautions apply)

- Blood and other body fluids containing visible blood
- Semen and vaginal/cervical secretions
- Tissues
- Cerebrospinal fluid
- Amniotic fluid
- Synovial fluid
- Pleural fluid
- Peritoneal fluid
- Pericardial fluid
- Breast milk

Body Fluids Not Likely to Transmit Bloodborne Disease (Universal Precautions do not apply unless the fluids contain visible blood)

- Feces
- Nasal secretions
- Sputum
- Vomitus
- Sweat
- Tears
- Urine
- Saliva, except in dentistry

TABLE 28-8

Transmission-Based Infection Control Precautions

Category	Precautions* In addition to Standard Precautions	Examples of Diseases in Category†

Airborne Precautions	1. Private room with monitored negative airflow (with appropriate # air exchanges & air discharge to outside or through HEPA). Keep door(s) closed
	2. Special respiratory protection:
	  • N-95† or HEPA† respirator mask for known or suspected TB
	  • Susceptible persons not to enter room of client with known or suspected measles or varicella unless immune caregivers are not available; Susceptible persons who must enter room must wear N-95 or HEPA
	3. Transport: client to leave room only for essential clinical reasons wearing surgical mask
		Diseases that are known or suspected to be:
		Measles (rubeola)
		M. tuberculosis, including multi-drug-resistant TB (MDRTB)
		Varicella (chickenpox)‡
		Zoster, disseminated (shingles)‡

Droplet Precautions	1. Private room: if not available, may cohort with client with same active infection with same microorganisms if no other infection present; maintain at least 3 feet distance from other clients if private room not available 2. Mask: required when working within 3 feet of client 3. Transport: as above	Diseases that are known or suspected to be: Diphtheria (pharyngeal) Strep. pharyngitis, pneumonia, scarlet fever (in infants or young children) Influenza Rubella Invasive disease (meningitis, pneumonia, sepsis) caused by *H influenzae* type b or *Neisseria meningitidis* Mumps Pertussis
Contact Precautions	1. Private room: if not available, may cohort with client with same active infection with same microorganisms if no other infection present 2. Wear gloves when entering room. 3. Wash hands with antimicrobial soap before leaving client's room 4. Wear gown to prevent contact with client or client contaminated items or if client has uncontrolled body fluids; remove gown before leaving room 5. Transport: client to leave room only for essential clinical reasons; during transport use needed precautions to prevent disease transmission 6. Dedicated equipment for this client only (or disinfect after use before taking from room)	Diseases that are known or suspected to be: *Clostridium difficile* Colonization or infection caused by multi-drug-resistant organisms (e.g., MRSA or VRE) Pediculosis Respiratory syncytial virus Scabies Viral hemorrhagic infections (Ebola, Lassa, or Marburg)

Modification by facilities: CDC encourages individual facilities to adapt these guidelines, still following sound epidemiologic principles (e.g., some have removed TB transmission prevention guidelines from the airborne precautions category and added the category of AFB precautions).
HEPA = high-efficiency particulate air filter; TB = tuberculosis; MRSA = methicillin-resistant *Staphylococcus aureus;* VRE = vancomycin-resistant *Enterococcus.*
* In addition to standard precautions.
† Before use: training and fit testing required for personnel.
‡ Add contact precautions for draining lesions.
(CDC, 1997)

sive protective safety measures and controls from Universal Precautions and from Body Substance Isolation are combined.

Airborne Precautions are used for clients known or suspected to have serious infections transmitted by small droplet nuclei. These nuclei can be suspended in the air for a prolonged time and are usually expelled into the air during coughing or sneezing. To prevent microbes from being spread through the ventilation system, negative airflow ventilation rooms are required. Special enclosed booths with high-efficiency particulate air (HEPA) filtration and/or ultraviolet (UV) light may be used for sputum-induction procedures. Tuberculosis, measles (rubeola), and chickenpox (varicella) are examples of airborne diseases.

Health care workers must wear HEPA respirators or

N-95 respirators to filter inspired air when entering the room of a client with known or suspected pulmonary tuberculosis. The client wears a surgical mask when leaving his or her room to filter expired air.

Droplet Precautions are used for clients known or suspected to have serious infections transmitted by large-particle droplets. These droplet-spread microbes are transmitted in the air for about 3 feet. Examples of infectious conditions requiring droplet precautions include influenza, mumps, pertussis, mycoplasma pneumonia, and meningitis caused by either *Neisseria meningitidis* or *Haemophilus influenzae* type B.

Contact Precautions are used for clients known or suspected to have serious infections transmitted by direct contact with the infected client or items in the client's environment. Clients with significant multi-drug–resistant organism infection or colonization (e.g., methicillin-resistant *Staphylococcus aureus* [MRSA] or vancomycin-resistant *Enterococcus* [VRE]), are placed on contact precautions. Some of the other infections needing contact precautions include scabies, pediculosis, respiratory syncytial virus (RSV), and *Clostridium difficile*. Information about drug-resistant infections is found in Chart 28–1.

Occupational Exposure to Sources of Infection

The Occupational Safety and Health Administration (OSHA) is a federal agency that protects all workers from injury or illness at their place of employment. Unlike the voluntary guidelines developed by the CDC, OSHA regulations are law. Employers can be disciplined or fined for noncompliance with OSHA regulations.

In 1991, Congress passed the Bloodborne Pathogens Standard prepared by OSHA (Table 28–9). Effective March 6, 1992, this legislation eliminates or minimizes occupational exposure to hepatitis B virus (HBV), human immunodeficiency virus (HIV), and other bloodborne pathogens. The standard defines whether a health care employee is at risk for occupational exposure to blood or body fluids and requires administrators to provide HBV vaccine for those employees. Engineering and work controls to reduce exposure risk are mandated. A written agency plan, annual education, and record keeping of education and vaccine are also required.

Bloodborne Pathogens

Reduction of percutaneous injuries (e.g., needlesticks) is of utmost importance to reduce transmission of bloodborne pathogens to health care personnel. OSHA mandates that sharps and needles be handled with care. Availability and consistency in the use of protective devices are vital (e.g., needleless systems). In a national survey involving 56 diversified U.S. hospitals, the rate of percutaneous injuries was 32 per 100 occupied beds for 1993 and 1994 and 22 in 1995 (Jagger & Bently, 1996). In a case-control study among health care workers occupationally exposed to HIV, CDC reported a 79% decrease in the risk for HIV seroconversion for those who took zidovudine (ZDV) after exposure, compared with exposed health care workers who did *not* take ZDV. In 1996, CDC issued provisional guidelines for postexposure prophylaxis (PEP)

Chart 28–1

Nursing Care Highlight: Drug-Resistant Infections

Prevalent Resistant Organisms:

- Aminoglycoside*-resistant *Pseudomonas*
- Methicillin-resistant *Staphylococcus aureus* (MRSA)
- Penicillin-resistant *Neisseria gonorrhoeae*
- Vancomycin-resistant *Enterococcus* (VRE)

Enabling and Contributing Factors:

- Long-term antibiotic use and misuse
- Fewer new antibiotics are being developed
- Invasive devices or procedures, especially
  - Gastric/endotracheal tubes
  - Catheters
  - Surgical drains or wounds
  - Vascular devices
- Increased exposure risk through prolonged or repeated hospital stays
- Compromised or weakened defenses
- Inadequate health care hand washing facilities or practices
- Inconsistent cleaning and decontamination of health care equipment or environment
- Food preparation or handling inconsistencies
- Delayed identification and institution of infection control precautions

CDC Control Plan Emphasizes Four Goals:

- Rapid national and international detection and response
- Applied research in disease diagnosis and prevention
- Better communication and implementation of prevention strategies
- Stronger connections among local, state, and federal public health providers to support tracking, prevention, and control programs.

Nursing Implications:

- Early identification is important. Look for
  - Signs of new or spreading infection
  - Culture and sensitivity (C&S) result that shows resistance (e.g., MRSA, VRE)
  - C&S result that matches another client's drug sensitivity pattern (possibly indicating a cluster of infections from the same source)
- Implementation of infection control measures should be done in a timely manner:
  - Consistent use of Standard or Universal Precautions.
  - Implement special additional precautions promptly (Contact Precautions).
  - Post signs and labels to notify others as per hospital policy.
  - Educate the client and family about infection control measures.
  - Notify the physician and infection control practitioner about infection.
- Appropriately administer antibiotics and teach discharged client and family about appropriate antibiotic use.

*Gentamicin, tobramycin, amikacin.
CDC = Centers for Disease Control and Prevention.

TABLE 28–9

OSHA Bloodborne Pathogens Standard

- Employers whose workers are at risk of "occupational exposure" must establish a written exposure control plan that is updated annually and available to all employees.
- Employers must implement and enforce procedures that reduce the risk of occupational exposure, including, but not limited to, Universal Precautions, hand washing, and providing supplies for avoidance of blood or other infectious materials.
- Employers must provide and launder protective garments and other equipment, such as gloves, gowns, masks, face shields, goggles, and ventilation devices. Gloves must be hypoallergenic or powderless for employees allergic to glove material.
- Employers must provide the hepatitis B vaccine to all employees at no cost to the employee within 10 days of employment. If the employee refuses the vaccine, the employer must obtain a signed statement indicating this refusal.
- Employers must provide postexposure evaluation for all employees who are exposed to blood or other infectious material.
- Employers must train employees about the hazards of blood and other infectious materials, and the bloodborne pathogens standard; this training must be done annually.

Adapted from the Occupational Safety and Health Administration, (1991)

after occupational exposure to HIV and requested that health care providers in the United States enroll all workers who receive PEP in an anonymous registry (see Research Applications for Nursing).

Tuberculosis

In addition to standards protecting workers from bloodborne diseases, OSHA is developing regulations that address protection from tuberculosis and the newer resistant strains of tuberculosis. Some states have already implemented legislation for this purpose. To prevent occupational exposure, each agency will be required to provide employee education and counseling, tuberculosis screening at the appropriate frequency, specially designed client isolation rooms, and special respirators (N-95 or HEPA) with fit testing to protect the health care worker.

Complications of Infection

Most complications of infection relate to inadequate treatment. This may range from an incorrect choice of antibiotics to poor client compliance. Some infections relapse in a subtle fashion when a client thinks he or she is slowly getting better. Noncompliance with the drug regimen (e.g., taking the medicine when the client feels like it) prevents contact of the harmful microorganism with sufficient concentrations of the antibiotic and contributes to the development of resistant organisms.

Local Complications

Serious complications of infection may result from incomplete antibiotic therapy. Local infections that could be cured without complications, such as cellulitis and pneumonia, may progress to abscess formation if appropriate drug therapy is not continued. Although adequate antibiotic therapy does not always prevent abscess, early therapy may prevent or at least limit the size of an abscess.

Systemic Complications

In addition to abscess formation, systemic complications may develop as a result of inadequate therapy. If a client's infection is not completely resolved or if it is being treated with drugs that are not effective against the offending microorganism, the pathogen may enter the bloodstream. Systemic sepsis or septicemia results. Even small local infections, if left untreated or treated inadequately, may spread locally or via the bloodstream to produce significant complications, such as leukocytosis (increased white blood cell count) or leukopenia (decreased white blood cell count) and disseminated intravascular coagulation (DIC) (see Chap. 27). After pathogens invade the bloodstream, no site is protected from invasion.

Sepsis may progress to sepsis-induced distributive shock, also known as septic shock. In septic shock, insufficient cardiac output is compounded by hypovolemia; inadequate blood supply to vital organs leads to hypoxia (lack of oxygen) and metabolic failure (see Chap. 39).

▷ Research Applications for Nursing

Hospital-wide Infections Reduced with the Implementation of a Bloodborne Pathogens Control Plan

Malone, N., & Larson, E. (1996). Factors associated with a significant reduction in hospital-wide infection rates. American Journal of Infection Control, 24(3), 180–185.

A 500-bed northwestern Arkansas hospital noted a significant reduction in total hospital nosocomial infection rates over the past 10 years from 3.6% to 2.6% in 1993. Factors that were statistically associated with this decrease were implementation of an OSHA bloodborne pathogens control plan with body substance isolation, increased glove use, and a barrier hand foam. Fewer inpatient surgeries and shorter length of stays may also have had some impact.

Critique. The authors controlled for other variables that could have had an impact on decreased infection rates. They noted that care practices, policies, and procedures in general had not changed. Client demographics and the top five causative nosocomial organisms had also not changed.

Possible Nursing Implications. Compliance with a bloodborne pathogens control plan and the new CDC transmission-based precautions should help reduce infections for both personnel and clients. Barrier hand foams are new products with potential to reduce infections and need further study.

Collaborative Management

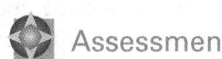 Assessment

➤ History

Careful attention to the history of a client with a possible infectious disease helps the nurse determine risk factors for infection. The age of a client, history of cigarette smoking or alcohol use, current illness or disease (such as diabetes), past and current medication use (such as steroids), familial predisposition, and poor nutritional status may place the client at increased risk for a number of infectious diseases.

The nurse also determines whether the client has been exposed to infectious agents. A history of recent exposure to someone with similar clinical symptoms (does a family member have the same symptoms?) or to contaminated food or water, as well as the time of exposure, assists in identifying a possible source for infection. Nurses may find this information helpful for determining the incubation period for the disease and thus for providing a clue to its cause.

Contact with animals, including pets, may facilitate exposure to infection. The nurse asks the client about recent contact with animals at home, at work, or in the course of leisure activities, such as hunting. The nurse also asks about recent contact with insects.

The nurse obtains a travel history from the client. Travel to areas both within and outside the client's home country may expose a susceptible client to infectious organisms not encountered in the local community.

A thorough sexual history may reveal sexual behavior associated with increased risk of sexually transmitted diseases. The nurse should obtain a history of IV drug use and a transfusion history to assess the client's risk for hepatitis B, hepatitis C, and HIV infections.

Ascertaining the type and location of symptoms may provide a key to the affected organ system. The order of onset of symptoms may also provide clues to the client's specific problem.

➤ Physical Assessment/Clinical Manifestations

Disorders caused by pathogens vary, depending on the cause and the site of infection. Common clinical manifestations are associated with specific sites of infection (Chart 28–2). Symptoms of local infection at any site include pain, swelling, heat, redness, and possibly pus. The nurse carefully inspects the skin for these symptoms.

Fever (generally a body temperature above 38° C [101° F]), chills, and malaise are primary indicators of a systemic infection. Fever may also accompany other noninfectious disorders, and infection can be present without fever. The elderly client whose normal body temperature may be 1° to 2° lower than in younger adults may manifest fever at 37° C (99° F). The nurse assesses the client for these symptoms and carefully questions the client about the history and patterns of symptoms.

Lymphadenopathy, photophobia, pharyngitis, and gastrointestinal disturbance (usually diarrhea or vomiting) are

---

Chart 28–2

Key Features of Infection of Specific Sites

Gastrointestinal Infections

Fever
Nausea and vomiting
Diarrhea
Abdominal distention

Genitourinary Infections

Dysuria
Frequency
Urgency
Hematuria
Fever
Purulent discharge
Pelvic or flank pain

Respiratory Infections

Cough
Congestion
Rhinitis
Sore throat
Sputum
Fever
Chest pain

Skin Infections

Redness
Warmth
Swelling
Drainage
Pain

Generalized Infections

Fever
Malaise
Fatigue
Muscle aches
Joint pain

---

often associated with infection. The nurse palpates the cervical and axillary lymph nodes to detect enlargement and examines the throat for redness. Other lymph nodes are also palpated for enlargement.

ELDERLY CONSIDERATIONS

In the elderly, a change in mental status may be the first, if not the only, presenting symptom. The nurse determines the client's baseline mental status for comparison. The client typically becomes increasingly confused and disoriented (Chart 28–3).

➤ Psychosocial Assessment

The client with an infectious disease often has psychosocial concerns. Typically, several diagnostic tests must be performed, and definitive identification of the microorganism responsible for the client's symptoms may be prolonged. This delay produces frustration and anxiety for

---

Chart 28-3

Nursing Focus on the Elderly: Infection

- Assess for atypical clinical manifestations of infection, such as confusion and unusual behavior. Typical manifestations, such as fever and pain, may not be present.
- Monitor renal function carefully when the client receives antibiotic therapy, especially aminoglycosides.
- Observe for and report adverse effects of antibiotic therapy because they may cause serious complications or death in an elderly client.
- Monitor for diarrhea from *Clostridium difficile* infection; obtain a specimen for culture if diarrhea occurs.
- Keep the client well hydrated because the elderly client is at high risk for dehydration.

---

the client. The nurse assesses the client's level of understanding about various diagnostic procedures and the time that may be required to obtain accurate results.

Frequently noted symptoms of infection are prolonged feelings of malaise and fatigue. The nurse assesses the client's psychological and sociologic adjustment to a decreased energy level. The nurse evaluates the client's current level of activity and the impact of these symptoms on usual family, occupational, and recreational activities.

An additional stress associated with the diagnosis of an infection is the potential spread of infection to others. The client may curtail family and social interactions for fear of spreading the illness. The nurse assesses the client's and family's levels of understanding of the infection, its mode of transmission, and mechanisms that may limit or prevent transmission. The nurse assesses the effects of the client's illness on usual interpersonal interactions.

Finally, a number of transmissible infectious diseases, especially those associated with socially unacceptable lifestyles (such as IV drug abuse), are associated with some degree of social labeling. The client may feel socially isolated and may experience guilt related to behavior that increases the risk for infection. The nurse observes carefully for signs of the client's reaction to social labels and how these feelings further affect socialization.

> *Laboratory Assessment*

The definitive diagnosis of an infectious disease requires identification of a microorganism in the tissues of an infected client. Direct examination of blood, body fluids, and tissues under a microscope in the laboratory may not yield positive identification of an organism. However, laboratory assessment usually provides helpful information about the microorganism, such as its shape, motility, and reaction to various staining agents. Even when direct microscopy does not prove diagnostic, enough information is often gathered for initiating appropriate antibiotic therapy.

Culture and Sensitivity. The most definitive procedure for identification of a microorganism is *culture,* or isolation of the pathogen by cultivation in tissue cultures or various artificial media. Specimens for culture may be

obtained from almost any body fluid or tissue. The health care provider usually decides when and where the specimen for culture is taken. The nurse often obtains the specimen when ordered.

Proper collection and handling of specimens for culture are essential for obtaining accurate results. The specimen collected by the nurse must be appropriate for the suspected infection. Material must be in sufficient quantity, freshly obtained, placed in a sterile container that adequately preserves the specimen and microorganism to be examined, and properly labeled. Chart 28-4 suggests techniques for collecting specimens for culture. The nurse always checks with the laboratory or laboratory manual for the specific procedure to be followed in a particular facility, but uses Standard Precautions for collecting and handling specimens.

After isolation of a microorganism in culture, antibiotic sensitivity testing is usually performed to determine the effects of various antibiotics on that particular microorganism. A microorganism that is killed by acceptable levels of an antibiotic is considered sensitive to that drug. An organism that is not killed by tolerable levels of an antibiotic is considered resistant to that drug. If sensitivity testing is desired, the nurse ensures that the laboratory slip is marked for a "C & S," indicating that both culture and sensitivity testing are to be performed on the specimen. Preliminary results are usually available in 24 to 48 hours, but the final results generally take 72 hours.

Serology. A less specific laboratory test for determining the presence of an infectious microorganism is a serologic test, a blood test to look for antibodies that react with a certain antigen. Serologic tests are available for virtually all classes of microorganisms. Examples of diseases for which serologic studies commonly aid diagnosis include syphilis, mononucleosis, Rocky Mountain spotted fever, Lyme disease, and cryptococcosis.

A positive serologic result does not necessarily indicate active infection but merely signifies that the client has had previous exposure to the antigen in question. Two serum specimens are typically obtained from a client: the first during the acute phase of illness, and the second 7 to 10 days later. A fourfold or greater rise in antibody titer in the second specimen indicates a recent infection.

Complete Blood Count. A complete blood count (CBC) is nearly always performed on the client with a suspected infectious disease. Five types of leukocytes (white blood cells) have been identified: neutrophils, lymphocytes, monocytes, eosinophils, and basophils. In most active infections, especially those caused by bacteria, the total leukocyte count is elevated. Various diseases are characterized by changes in the percentages of the different types of leukocytes. The differential count most often shows an increased number of immature neutrophils, or a shift to the left. A few infectious diseases, however, are associated with neutropenia (decreased neutrophils), such as malaria and infectious mononucleosis.

Erythrocyte Sedimentation Rate. The erythrocyte sedimentation rate (ESR) measures the rate at which red blood cells fall through plasma. This rate is most significantly affected by an increased number of acute phase

Chart 28–4

Nursing Care Highlight: Collection Techniques for Commonly Cultured Specimens

Specimen	Collection Method	Comments
Blood	1. Decontaminate the skin with 70% alcohol followed by 2% tincture of iodine, allowed to dry. 2. Perform venipuncture and collect 10 mL of blood (2 mL in infants). 3. Inject into sterile culture bottles—usually one vented and one unvented for anaerobic culture.	Three separate specimens are usually collected over a 24-hr period to ensure isolation of the causative organism. Avoid use of intravenous catheters because of contamination and possible false bacteremia report.
Urine Clean void	1. Clean the urethral meatus with tincture of iodine or other antiseptic solution. 2. Have the client void small amount and then collect approximately 2 mL of midstream urine specimen into a sterile container.	The specimen may be refrigerated. If not, the specimen must be delivered to the laboratory within 30 min to be useful for quantitative studies.
Indwelling catheter	1. Clean the aspiration site on catheter drainage tubing with iodine. 2. Collect a 2-mL specimen into a sterile container.	
Wound	1. Decontaminate the skin with 70% alcohol. 2. Swab an active margin of the wound with a sterile swab and place the swab into a sterile tube.	
Throat	1. Swab an inflamed area of the throat, especially areas of exudate. 2. Place the swab into sterile medium for transport.	Inform the laboratory of any suspected organism other than group A streptococcus.
Sputum	1. Collect first-morning expectorated sputum into a sterile container.	Production of an adequate specimen may be aided by saline aerosol administration or by postural drainage. Sputum specimens may also be collected via tracheal or transtracheal aspiration.
Pus (abscesses)	1. Decontaminate the skin with alcohol. 2. Coat a sterile swab rapidly with pus. 3. Insert the swab immediately into a specially prepared anaerobic transport tube.	Deliver the specimen to the laboratory immediately.
Vagina	1. Wipe the vagina clean of secretions with dry gauze. 2. Swab the exudate with a sterile swab. 3. Insert into a sterile container or into specially prepared medium.	If trichomoniasis is suspected, place the swab in a small amount of sterile saline and send to the laboratory immediately.
Rectal swab	1. Insert the swab into the rectum approximately 1 inch (2.5 cm) and rotate once. 2. Place into transport medium.	The specimen is usually sent on 3 consecutive days. The swab should show obvious soiling.
Stool	1. Collect stool in a clean waxed cardboard container.	Deliver to the laboratory immediately. The specimen is often collected on 3 consecutive days.
Intravenous catheters	1. Clean the catheter insertion site with alcohol. 2. Withdraw the catheter and cut off approximately a 5-cm tip with sterile scissors. 3. Place into a sterile container.	In general, catheter tips that are contaminated during removal will grow only a few colonies, whereas infected catheters usually show heavy growth.

reactants, which occurs with inflammation. Thus, an elevated ESR (>20 mm/hr) indicates inflammation or infection somewhere in the body. Chronic infection, most notably osteomyelitis, and chronic abscesses are commonly associated with an elevated ESR. The effectiveness of therapy is often monitored by a fall in this value.

➤ Radiographic Assessment

X-rays are often obtained to determine activity or destruction by an infectious microorganism. Radiologic studies (such as chest films, sinus films, joint films, gastrointestinal studies, and renal films) are typically obtained for diagnosis of infection in a specific body site.

A more sophisticated technique for diagnosis of an infection is computed tomography. This method is particularly helpful in assessing the presence and location of abscesses.

➤ Other Diagnostic Assessment

Another diagnostic tool for the evaluation of a client with an infectious disease is *ultrasonography*. This noninvasive procedure is particularly helpful in detecting infection that has affected the heart valves.

Scanning techniques using radioactive substances, such as gallium, can determine the presence of inflammation. Inflammatory tissue is identified by its increased uptake of the injected radioactive material.

To obtain tissue for culture, biopsy of the infected site may be necessary. Biopsy sites may include the liver, bone marrow, skin, pleura, lymph nodes, kidney, bone, or even the brain. To obtain specimens for examination, invasive procedures (such as bronchoscopy or endoscopy) or even surgery (such as open lung biopsy or laparotomy) may be necessary. These procedures are described in detail elsewhere in this text.

 Analysis

➤ Common Nursing Diagnoses and Collaborative Problems

The most common nursing diagnoses for clients with an infection or infectious disease include
1. Hyperthermia related to increased metabolic state
2. Fatigue related to increased metabolic energy production
3. Social Isolation related to effects of illness

The inclusion of other nursing diagnoses depends on the type and extent of the infection. For example, a client with pneumonia might experience ineffective airway clearance; a client with a sexually transmitted disease may have altered sexuality patterns.

➤ Additional Nursing Diagnoses and Collaborative Problems

The major collaborative problem is a client's risk for sepsis, septic shock, and disseminated intravascular coagulation (DIC).

 Planning and Implementation

➤ Hyperthermia

Planning: Expected Outcomes. The primary outcome is that the client's body temperature is expected to return to baseline.

Interventions. Fever (hyperthermia) is one way in which the body attempts to destroy pathogens. The primary concern is to provide measures to eliminate the underlying cause of hyperthermia, to destroy the causative microorganism. Interventions are implemented to reduce fever, such as antimicrobial therapy, antipyretic therapy, external cooling, and fluid administration.

Antimicrobial Therapy. The cornerstone of therapy for infectious diseases is antimicrobial drug therapy, also called antiinfective therapy. Antibiotics, antiviral agents, and antifungals are types of antimicrobials. The sulfonamides, the first antibiotic group, were used in the mid-1930s. Shortly thereafter, in the 1940s, penicillin became the primary antibiotic used systemically. Since these early days, a wide variety of antimicrobial drugs have been developed for treatment as well as prevention of infection associated with virtually every class of microorganism. Effective antibiotics are available to treat nearly all bacterial infections, but misuse of antibiotics has contributed to the development of antibiotic-resistant bacteria. A few effective antifungal agents have been developed, but these drugs generally exhibit more toxicity than do antibacterial agents. Few effective chemotherapeutic agents are currently available for treatment of infections caused by viruses.

Effective antimicrobial therapy requires delivery of the appropriate agent, sufficient dosage, proper route of administration, and sufficient duration of therapy. Fulfilling these four requirements ensures that a concentration of drug is delivered in excess of that needed to inhibit or kill the infecting microorganism. The health care provider, often in consultation with the pharmacist, decides about each requirement. The nurse needs to know the drug actions, side effects, and toxic effects and teach them to the client.

Antimicrobials act on susceptible pathogens by
■ Inhibiting cell wall synthesis (penicillins and cephalosporins)
■ Injuring the cytoplasmic membrane (antifungal agents)
■ Inhibiting biosynthesis (reproduction) (erythromycin, tetracycline, and gentamicin)
■ Inhibiting nucleic acid synthesis (actinomycin)

The nurse observes and reports side effects and toxic effects, which vary according to the specific classification of the drug. Most antibiotics can cause nausea, vomiting, and rashes along with a long list of other problems. The nurse ensures that the prescribed drug is not one to which the client is allergic. An accurate allergy history before drug therapy begins is essential.

Antipyretic Therapy. The health care provider prescribes antipyretic drugs, such as aspirin (Ancasal✦) and acetaminophen (Tylenol, AceTabs♣) to reduce hyperthermia. However, because antipyretics mask fever, monitoring the course of the client's disease may be difficult. Therefore, unless the client is extremely uncomfortable or if hyperthermia presents a significant risk (e.g., in the client with heart failure, febrile seizures, or head injury), antipyretics are not always ordered.

The nurse must be alert for waves of sweating after each dose. Sweating may be accompanied by a fall in blood pressure and subsequent return of fever. These unpleasant side effects of antipyretic therapy can often be alleviated by liberal administration of fluids and by regular scheduling of drug administration.

External Cooling. Cooling or hypothermia blankets, or ice bags and packs, are highly effective external mechanisms for reducing fever. For convenience, cooling blankets are used extensively in the hospital setting, yet there are no universal guidelines for their use.

Alternatives to cooling blankets may be used, particularly in settings other than hospitals. The nurse may sponge the client's body with tepid water or saline solution or apply cool compresses to the skin and pulse points to reduce body temperature. The nurse observes the client for shivering during any form of external cooling. Shivering indicates that the client is possibly being cooled too quickly.

Fluid Administration. In clients with fever, there is increased fluid volume loss from rapid evaporation of body fluids as well as increased perspiration. As body temperature increases, fluid volume loss increases. The nurse carefully monitors for signs of dehydration, such as increased thirst, decreased skin turgor, and dry mucous membranes, especially in the elderly. The nurse encourages increased oral fluid intake and administers IV fluids as prescribed by the health care provider (see Chapter 15 for additional information on fluid volume deficit).

➤ *Fatigue*

Planning: Expected Outcomes. The desired outcome is that the client is expected to progress from previous level of activity.

Interventions. Whether a client achieves the outcome depends on recognition and correction of factors that contribute to activity intolerance. Malaise and easy fatigability are classic clinical manifestations of an infectious process. Fever accelerates many metabolic processes, which accentuates weight loss and nitrogen wasting. The heart rate increases, and water loss may be excessive; both factors contribute to a feeling of general malaise.

Nutrition. The nurse observes the client for causative factors of malaise and easy fatigability, such as nutritional deficiencies or fluid and electrolyte imbalances. The nurse collaborates with the client and dietitian to establish a dietary program that is tolerable for the client and meets calorie and protein requirements.

Activity Management. The nurse encourages bed rest during the acute phase of the client's illness while treatment for the underlying infection is initiated. The nurse

works closely with the client to develop a progressive program for return to his or her normal level of activity. The program depends on the client's response to antibiotic therapy, as evidenced by diminished clinical manifestations of infection. Frequent rest periods are encouraged. Throughout the course of the client's illness, the nurse encourages the client to verbalize feelings of frustration and discouragement related to chronic fatigue and decreased ability to perform activities of daily living.

➤ *Social Isolation*

Planning: Expected Outcomes. The desired outcome is that the client is expected to be free of feelings of social isolation.

Interventions. Education is the major intervention for meeting this goal. The nurse develops an educational program to instruct the client and the family about the mode of transmission of infection and mechanisms that prevent its spread to others. The nurse also initiates appropriate barrier precautions.

The nurse ensures that the client and family understand the client's disease process and its cause. The nurse specifically explains the mode of transmission of the infecting microorganism, the risk for transmission to others, and mechanisms that may prevent transmission. If necessary, the nurse ensures that the client and family can state specific ways in which precautions will be instituted in the home after discharge from the hospital.

Because the client requiring precautions may feel secluded, the nurse encourages health care personnel as well as family members and friends to maintain contact with the client. The nurse reminds all personnel caring for the client that the disease—not the client—requires isolation. Family members and friends are encouraged to visit the client and to use the appropriate barrier precautions when necessary. Communication by telephone is often effective for continuing contact with loved ones. Television and radio help bring the outside world into the life of the client confined to the room.

In the nursing home setting, an outbreak of respiratory or GI infection usually requires a limit on visitors, activities, and admissions to the facility. The nurse working in a nursing home needs to be familiar with state regulations regarding handling infections in nursing homes.

 ## Continuing Care

Clients with infections may be cared for in the home, hospital, nursing home, or ambulatory care setting, depending on the type and severity of the infectious process. Infections among the elderly in nursing homes are very common (Table 28-10).

➤ *Health Teaching*

Infection Control

The nurse explains the disease and makes certain that the client understands what is causing the illness. The nurse also explains whether the pathogen causing the client's

TABLE 28-10

Factors that May Promote Infection in the Elderly Client	
Factor	**Aging-Associated Changes or Conditions**
Immune system	Decreased antibody production, lymphocytes, and fever response
Integumentary system	Thinning skin, decreased subcutaneous tissue, decreased vascularity, slower wound healing
Respiratory system	Decreased cough and gag reflexes
Gastrointestinal system	Decreased gastric acid and intestinal motility
Chronic illness	Diabetes mellitus, chronic airflow limitation, neurologic impairments
Functional/cognitive impairments	Immobility, incontinence, dementia
Invasive devices	Urinary catheters, feeding tubes, intravenous devices, tracheostomies
Institutionalization	Increased person-to-person contact and transmission

infection can be spread to family members, social contacts, or other community contacts. If the client has an infectious disease caused by a transmissible agent, the nurse describes how the pathogen causing the client's infection is transmitted.

If the client has an infectious disease that is potentially transmissible, the nurse teaches the client, family, or home caregivers the precautions for preventing transmission of infection. General household cleaning measures are often sufficient (e.g., a dishwasher for dishes, a washer and dryer for laundry). If these are not available, dishes can be sanitized with weak bleach solution (100 parts per million [ppm] available chlorine) attained by adding 30 mL (1 ounce) of bleach to 4 gallons of water. Clothing soiled with blood or other body fluids can be washed with bleach or disinfectant (e.g., Lysol). Recommended cleaning measures should be based on actual available equipment or facilities.

Drug Therapy

For the client who is discharged to the home setting to complete a course of antibiotic therapy, the nurse also explains the importance of compliance with the planned drug regimen. The nurse emphasizes the importance of both the timing of doses and the completion of the planned number of days of therapy. The nurse also teaches the client how the agents should be taken (e.g., before meals, with meals, and without other agents), and explains to the client and family the possible side effects. Side effects include those that are expected (such as gas-

tric distress after the oral administration of erythromycin) as well as more severe adverse reactions (such as rash, fever, or other systemic signs and symptoms of an acute adverse drug reaction). The nurse also teaches the client about allergic manifestations (Table 28-11) and the need for the client and family or significant other to notify the health care provider if adverse or allergic reactions occur.

In the past, many clients with severe infection were hospitalized for several weeks or more simply to receive intravenous (IV) antibiotic therapy. Since the implementation of managed care, many clients have been discharged with an IV device in place and continue to receive IV antibiotics at home or in the nursing home. Clients, a family member, or a nurse administers the drugs. When clients are discharged with an indwelling intravascular device in place, the nurse teaches them or their assisting family members how to care for it. The nurse also instructs clients to be alert for malfunction of the device as well as for signs of inflammation resulting from infection at the catheter insertion site (e.g., redness, heat, pain, swelling, and purulent discharge). Chapter 17 discusses infusion therapy in detail.

Psychosocial Support

The client with an infection is often anxious and fearful that the infection will be transmitted to family members or friends. The nurse allays these fears by teaching the client and the family ways of preventing the spread of disease. Careful attention is paid to the client's concerns. The nurse makes concrete suggestions (e.g., "Your wife can wear gloves when changing your dressing") to address specific concerns.

The client with an infectious disease associated with lifestyle behaviors, such as sexual activity or IV drug abuse, may experience guilt related to the disease. The nurse encourages the client to verbalize feelings associated with the illness and assists the client in locating support systems that may help alleviate these problems. Supportive family members, friends, or groups can help in easing the client's adjustment to illness.

TABLE 28-11

Allergic Reactions to Antibiotic Therapy
Flushing
Wheezing
Sneezing
Pruritus
Urticaria
Rashes
Maculopapular to exfoliative dermatitis
Vascular eruptions
Erythema multiforme (Stevens-Johnson syndrome)
Angioneurotic edema
Serum sickness (headache, fever, chills, hives, malaise, and conjunctivitis)
Anaphylaxis (laryngeal edema, bronchospasm, hypotension, vascular collapse, and cardiac arrest)
Death

> ### *Home Care Management*

The client with an infectious disease, such as osteomyelitis, who is discharged from the hospital to home may require continued, long-term antibiotic therapy. The nurse emphasizes the importance of a clean home environment, especially for the client who continues to be immunocompromised or who is uniquely susceptible to superinfection (i.e., reinfection or second infection of the same kind) because of antimicrobial drug therapy. Medications often need to be refrigerated. The nurse ensures that the client has access to proper storage facilities and instructs the client to check for signs of improper storage, such as discoloration of the medication.

The nurse questions the client to be sure that hand washing facilities are available in the home and provides supplies and instructions as needed.

> ### *Health Care Resources*

In unusual instances, a client who has been hospitalized for an infectious disease may not be able to return to the home setting immediately. In such circumstances, temporary placement in a long-term care facility may be advantageous. The staff nurse carefully notes the client's care requirements, medication schedules, and personal needs and preferences on the transfer documents. When possible, the staff nurse communicates directly with a nurse at the receiving facility to facilitate a smooth transition from the hospital to the intermediate care setting.

Because of the early discharge trend from hospitals, the client with severe or chronic infections may be discharged to home before completing long-term antibiotic therapy. The client may continue to receive IV antibiotic therapy at home. The ambulatory client may be asked to return to an outpatient facility every third day to have a new peripheral venous catheter placed for use as a heparin lock. Implanted ports may be used for convenience and to decrease the chance of infection at the skin site. The client's primary nurse communicates with the outpatient facility staff to effect a smooth transition from the hospital to the outpatient setting.

Home health care services are frequently used to ensure appropriate administration of antibiotics at the client's home. These home care services have proved efficient, effective, and much less expensive than hospitalization or intermediate care facilities. Occasional visits from a home care nurse may also facilitate detection of early antimicrobial failures, toxic reactions, or other side effects of therapy.

Evaluation

On the basis of the identified common nursing diagnoses, the nurse evaluates the care of the client with an infectious disease. Expected outcomes for the client with an infection include that the client

- Describes and complies with the antibiotic regimen as ordered
- Maintains baseline body temperature
- Returns to his or her usual level of activity
- Describes and implements precautions so that infection is not transmitted to others
- Exhibits no clinical manifestations of recurrence, relapse, or reinfection

SELECTED BIBLIOGRAPHY

Baker, O. G., et al. (1996). ICPs show power of prevention in efficacy efforts cost-saving projects. *Hospital Infection Control, 23*(10), 121–124.

Beaumont, E. (1997). Technology scorecard: Focus on infection control. *American Journal of Nursing, 97*(12), 51–54.

Beneson, A. S. (Ed.). (1995). *Control of Communicable Diseases Manual* (16th ed., pp. 533–545). Washington, DC: American Public Health Association.

Carter, L. W. (1994). Bacterial translocation: Nursing implications in the care of patients with neutropenia. *Oncology Nursing Forum, 21*(5), 857–867.

*Centers for Disease Control. (1987). Recommendations for prevention of HIV transmission in health care settings. *Morbidity and Mortality Weekly Report, 36*(2S), 3–17.

Centers for Disease Control and Prevention. (1994). Guidelines for preventing the transmission of *Mycobacterium tuberculosis* in health-care facilities, 1994. *Morbidity and Mortality Weekly Report, 43*, RR–13.

Centers for Disease Control and Prevention. (1996a). Update: Provisional Public Health Service recommendations for chemoprophylaxis after occupational exposure to HIV. *Morbidity and Mortality Weekly Report, 45*(22), 468–472.

Centers for Disease Control and Prevention. (1997). Summary of notifiable diseases, United States, 1996. *Morbidity and Mortality Weekly Report, 45*(53), 6.

Centers for Disease Control and Prevention and Hospital Infections Advisory Committee. (1994). Recommendations for prevention of nosocomial pneumonia. *American Journal of Infection Control, 22*(4), 267–277.

Centers for Disease Control and Prevention and HICPAC. (1994). Recommendations for preventing the spread of vancomycin resistance. *Infection Control and Hospital Epidemiology, 16*(2), 105–113.

Chiarello, L., Feinstein, S. A., Irwin, W., Murtha, R., Stanley, A. H., & Stricof, R. L. (1995). Antibiotic resistance B an emerging trend. *Practice—Infection Control & Prevention in Home Care, 2*(2), 3–4.

Cohen, F. L., & Larson, E. (1996). Emerging infectious diseases: Nursing responses. *Nursing Outlook, 44*(4), 164–168.

Emerging Infections Information Network. (1997). *Emerging/reemerging infections*. New Haven, CT: Department of Epidemiology and Public Health, Yale University.

Friedman, M. M. (1997). Joint Commission on Accreditation of Healthcare Organizations infection control requirements. *Home Healthcare Nurse, 15*(4), 236–238.

Garner, J. S., & HICPAC. (1996). *Guidelines for isolation precautions in hospitals*. Atlanta: Centers for Disease Control and Prevention.

Gould, D., & Chamberlanine, A. (1995). *Staphylococcus aureus:* A review of the literature. *Journal of Clinical Nursing, 4*(1), 5–11.

Herwaldt, L. A., Smith, S. D., & Carter, C. D. (1998). Infection control in the outpatient setting. *Infection Control and Hospital Epidemiology, 19*(1), 41–73.

Jagger, J. J., & Bently, M. (1996). Substantial nationwide drop in percutaneous injury rates detected for 1995. *Advances in Exposure Prevention, 2*(4), 1–12.

Larson, E. L. (1995). APIC guidelines for handwashing and hand antisepsis in health care settings. *American Journal of Infection Control, 23*(4), 251–269.

Malone, N., & Larson, E. (1996). Factors associated with a significant reduction in hospital wide infection rates. *American Journal of Infection Control, 24*(3), 180–185.

Mayone-Ziomek, J. M. (1997). Handwashing in critical care. *MedSurg Nursing, 6*(6), 364–369.

National Nosocomial Infections Surveillance System. (1996). *NNIS report, data summary from October 1986—April 1996, issued May 1996.* Atlanta: Hospital Infection Program, National Center for Infectious Diseases, Centers for Infectious Diseases and Prevention.

Nicolle, L. E., & Garibaldi, R. A. (1995). Infection control in long term care facilities. *Infection Control and Hospital Epidemiology, 16*(6), 348–353.

Reiss, P. J. (1996). Battling the super bug. *RN Magazine, 59*(3), 36–41.

Schumann, D. (1996). *Reducing post critical care infection. MedSurg Nursing, 5*(3), 169–176.

Sheff, B. (1998). VRE & MRSA—Putting bad bugs out of business. *Nursing 98, 28*(3), 40–44.

Shoup, A. (1995). Risk factors related to the use of latex gloves: Taking measures to minimize risk and hidden costs while maintaining quality outcomes. *QRC Advisor, 11*(9).

Smith, P. W., & Rusnak, P. G. (1997). Infection prevention and control in the long-term-care facility. *American Journal of Infection Control, 25*(6), 488–512.

Strausbaugh, L. J., Crossley, K. B., Nurse, B. A., & Thrupp, L. D. (1996). SHEA position paper: Antimicrobial resistance in long-term care facilities. *Infection Control and Hospital Epidemiology, 17*(2), 129–140.

Sutterly, L. (1995). Winning the war against antibiotic resistant infections. *Nursing Spectrum, XX,* 12–14.

Workman, M. L. (1995). Essential concepts of inflammation and immunity. *Critical Care Clinics of North America, 7*(4), 601–615.

SUGGESTED READINGS

Beneson, A. S. (Ed.). (1995). *Control of communicable diseases manual* (16th ed.). Washington, DC: American Public Health Association.

This reference book details information about specific infectious diseases. It is frequently used by infection control practitioners, epidemiologists, physicians, and nurse practitioners in all health care settings and is an excellent resource for nurses as well.

Cohen, F. L., & Larson, E. (1996). Emerging infectious diseases: Nursing responses. *Nursing Outlook, 44*(4), 164–168.

This article describes the problem of emerging and re-emerging infectious disease and the needed role of nurses in prevention of infections.

Workman, M. L. (1995). Essential concepts of inflammation and immunity. *Critical Care Clinics of North America, 7*(4), 601–615.

This article reviews the physiology of inflammation and immunity, concepts that need to be understood to provide appropriate client assessments and interventions.

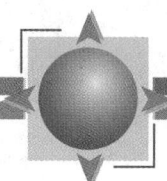

Problems of Oxygenation:

Management of Clients

with Problems of the

Respiratory Tract

ASSESSMENT OF THE RESPIRATORY SYSTEM

To assess the client with respiratory problems accurately, the nurse needs an adequate knowledge of anatomy, physiology, pathophysiology, and various diagnostic tests. Respiratory disease currently ranks as the fifth leading cause of death in the United States (Parker et al., 1997). As clients with chronic respiratory impairments live longer because of advances in diagnosis, treatment, and management, the nurse is confronted with the need for expert assessment skills to plan and implement care for increasing numbers of clients with various respiratory disorders.

ANATOMY AND PHYSIOLOGY REVIEW

The two major purposes of the respiratory system are to provide oxygen for metabolism in the tissues and to remove carbon dioxide, the waste product of metabolism. The respiratory system performs several secondary functions:

Maintaining acid-base balance
Producing speech
Facilitating the sense of smell
Maintaining body water levels
Ensuring heat balance

Upper Respiratory Tract

The upper airways consist of the nose, the sinuses, the pharynx, and the larynx (Fig. 29–1).

Nose and Sinuses

The nose, a rigid structure that is bony in the upper third and cartilaginous in the lower two thirds, contains two passages separated in the middle by the septum. The septum and interior walls of the nasal cavity are lined with mucous membranes, as is the rest of the respiratory tract. The nostrils (anterior nares), or external openings into the nasal cavities, are lined with skin and hair follicles (vibrissae). Vibrissae are the first defense mechanisms of the respiratory system, keeping foreign particles or organisms from entering the lungs. The posterior nares are openings from the nasal cavity into the nasopharynx.

Three major bony projections called *turbinates,* or conchae, arise from the lateral walls of the internal portion of the nose (Fig. 29–1). Turbinates increase the total surface area for filtering, heating, and humidifying inspired air before it passes into the nasopharynx. Inspired air entering the nose is filtered first by vibrissae in the nares. Particles not filtered out in the nares are trapped in the mucous layer of the turbinates. These particles are passed

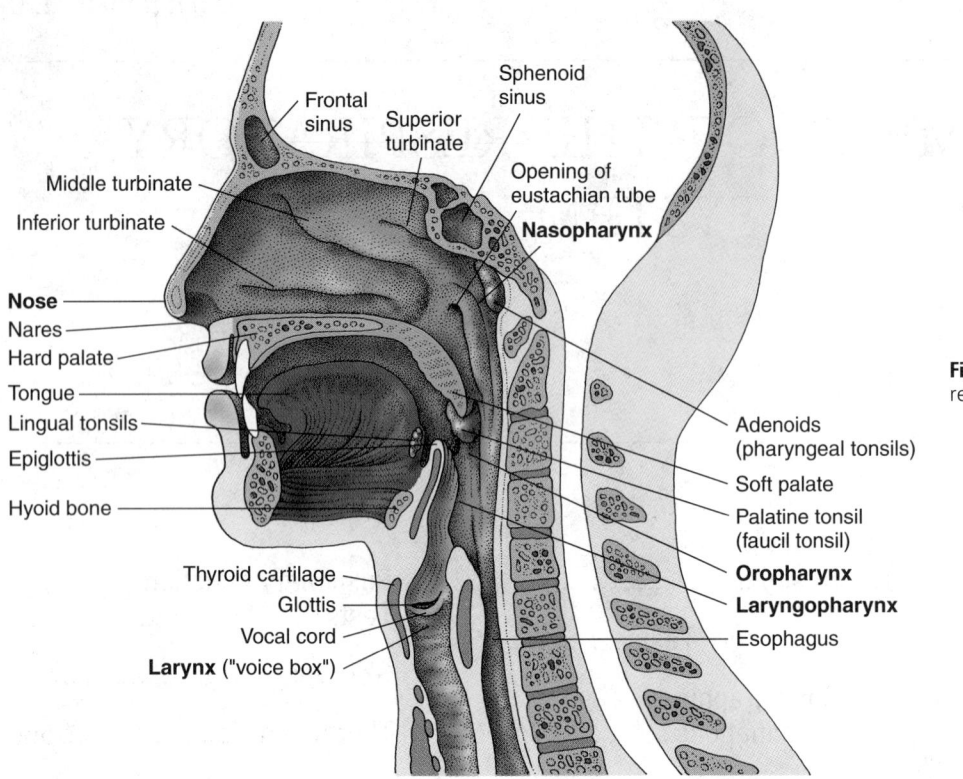

Figure 29–1. Structures of the upper respiratory tract.

posteriorly by cilia (hair-like projections) to the oropharynx, where they are swallowed or expectorated. Inspired air is humidified by contact with the mucous membrane and is warmed by exposure to heat from the vascular network. The nose is the organ of smell; olfactory receptors from cranial nerve I are located in the roof of the nose and in the superior turbinate.

The paranasal sinuses are air-filled cavities within the bones that surround the nasal passages. They are lined with ciliated epithelium. The four paranasal sinuses are shown in Figure 29–2. The sinuses provide resonance during speech.

Pharynx

The pharynx, or throat, serves as a passageway for both the respiratory and digestive tracts and is located behind the oral and nasal cavities. It is divided into the nasopharynx, the oropharynx, and the laryngopharynx (see Fig. 29–1).

Located behind the nose, the nasopharynx lies above the soft palate and contains the adenoids and the distal opening of the eustachian tube. The adenoids (pharyngeal tonsils) act as an important defense mechanism by trapping organisms entering the nose and the mouth. The eustachian tube connects the nasopharynx with the middle chamber of the ear and opens during swallowing to equalize the pressure within the middle ear.

The oropharynx is located behind the mouth below the nasopharynx. It extends from the soft palate to the base of the tongue. The palatine tonsils (also known as faucial tonsils) are located on the anterolateral borders of the

oropharynx. These tonsils also guard the body against invading organisms.

Located behind the larynx, the laryngopharynx extends from the base of the tongue to the esophagus. The laryngopharynx is the critical dividing point where solid foods and fluids are separated from air. At this point, the passageway bifurcates into the larynx and the esophagus.

Larynx

The larynx, or voice box, is located above the trachea, just below the pharynx at the root of the tongue. It is

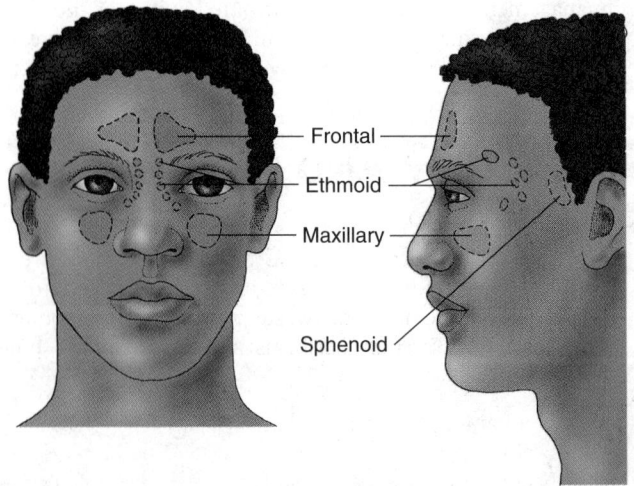

Figure 29–2. The paranasal sinuses.

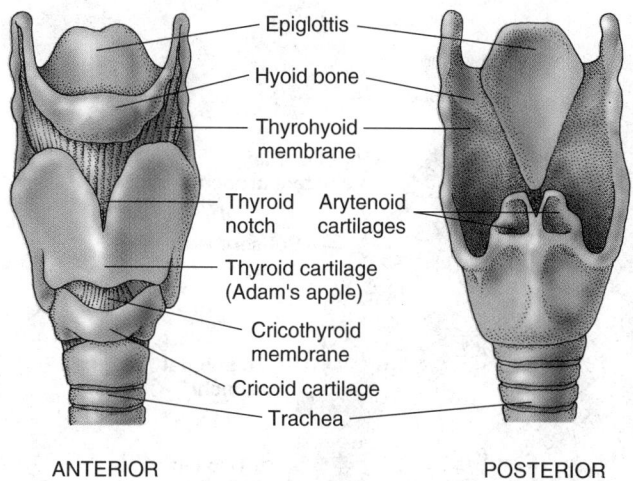

ANTERIOR   POSTERIOR

Figure 29-3. Structures of the larynx.

innervated by the recurrent laryngeal nerves. The larynx is composed of several cartilages (Fig. 29–3). The thyroid cartilage is the largest and is commonly referred to as the Adam's apple. The cricoid cartilage, which contains the vocal cords, lies below the thyroid cartilage. The cricoid cartilage is the only complete ring of cartilage in the airway. The cricothyroid membrane is below the level of the vocal cords and joins the thyroid and cricoid cartilages. This site is used in an emergency for access to the lower airways. The procedure, a cricothyroidotomy (an opening made between the thyroid and cricoid cartilage), is also called a cricothyrotomy and results in a tracheostomy. The two arytenoid cartilages, to which the posterior ends of the vocal cords are attached, are used together with the thyroid cartilage in vocal cord movement.

Inside the larynx are two pairs of vocal cords: the false and true cords. The opening between the true vocal cords is the *glottis* (Fig. 29–4). The glottis plays an important role in coughing, which is the most fundamental defense mechanism of the lungs. The *epiglottis* is a leaf-shaped, elastic structure that is attached along one edge to the top of the larynx. Its hinge-like action prevents food from entering the tracheobronchial tree (aspiration) by closing over the glottis during swallowing.

Lower Respiratory Tract

The lower airways consist of the trachea; two mainstem bronchi; lobar, segmental, and subsegmental bronchi; bronchioles; alveolar ducts; and alveoli (Fig. 29–5). The tracheobronchial tree is an inverted tree-like structure consisting of muscular, cartilaginous, and elastic tissues. This system of bifurcating tubes, which decrease in size from the trachea to the respiratory bronchioles, allows the passage of gases to and from the pulmonary parenchyma. Gas exchange takes place in the pulmonary parenchyma between the alveoli and the pulmonary capillaries.

Trachea

The trachea, commonly referred to as the windpipe, is located in front of (anterior to) the esophagus. It begins

at the lower border of the cricoid cartilage of the larynx and extends to the level of the fourth or fifth thoracic vertebra. The trachea branches into the right and left mainstem bronchi at the carina. The carina is located at the sternal angle where the manubrium joins the sternum.

The trachea is composed of 6 to 10 C-shaped cartilaginous rings. The open portion of the C is the back (posterior) portion of the trachea; it contains smooth muscle that is shared with the esophagus. Low pressure must be maintained in endotracheal and tracheostomy tube cuffs so as not to cause erosion of this posterior wall and create a tracheoesophageal fistula.

Mainstem Bronchi

The mainstem, or primary, bronchi begin at the carina. The structure of a bronchus resembles that of the trachea. The right bronchus is slightly wider, shorter, and more vertical than the left bronchus. Because of the more vertical line of the right bronchus, accidental intubation of the right bronchus is possible when an endotracheal tube is passed. Also if a foreign object is aspirated from the pharynx, it most likely enters the right bronchus.

Lobar, Segmental, and Subsegmental Bronchi

The mainstem bronchi further divide into the five secondary, or lobar, bronchi that enter each of the five lobes of the lung. Each lobar bronchus is surrounded by connective tissue, blood vessels, nerves, and lymphatics, and each branches into segmental and subsegmental divisions. The cartilage of these lobar bronchi is nearly circumferential and resists collapse. The bronchi are lined with ciliated, mucus-secreting epithelium. The cilia propel mucus up and away from the lower airway to the trachea, where it can be expectorated or swallowed.

Bronchioles

The bronchioles, branching from the secondary bronchi, subdivide into smaller and smaller tubes: the terminal and respiratory bronchioles (Fig. 29–6). These terminal and respiratory tubes are less than 1 mm in diameter. They have no cartilage and, therefore, depend entirely on the elastic recoil of the lung for patency. The terminal bronchioles contain no cilia and do not participate in gas exchange.

ANTERIOR

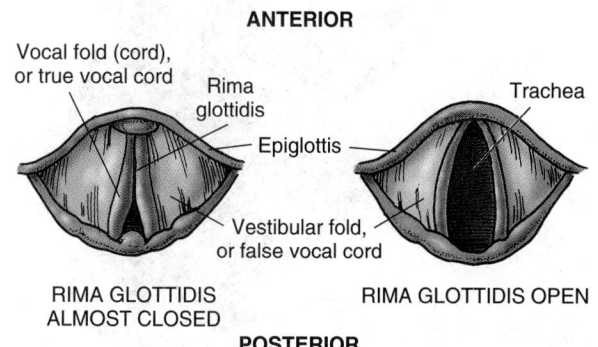

RIMA GLOTTIDIS   RIMA GLOTTIDIS OPEN
ALMOST CLOSED

POSTERIOR

Figure 29-4. Detail of the glottis (two vocal folds and the intervening space, the rima glottidis).

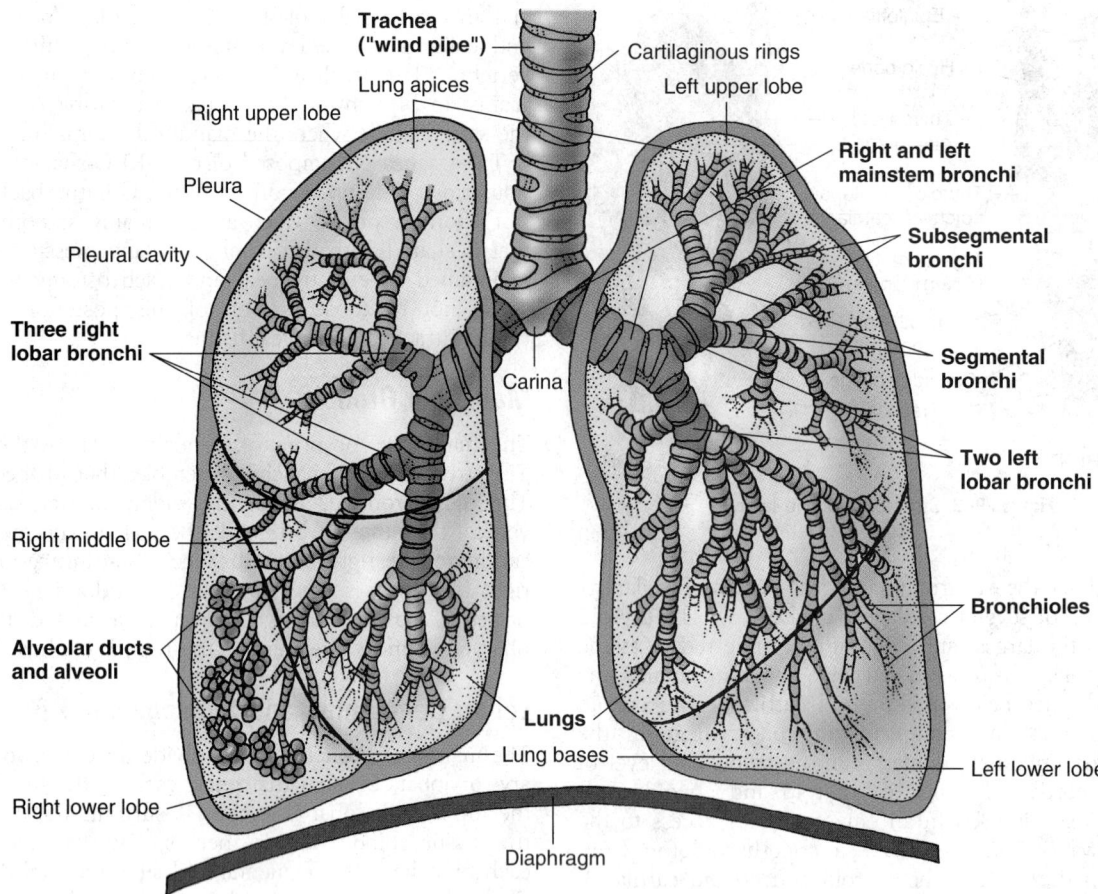

Figure 29–5. Structures of the lower respiratory tract (structural size and proportions not drawn to scale).

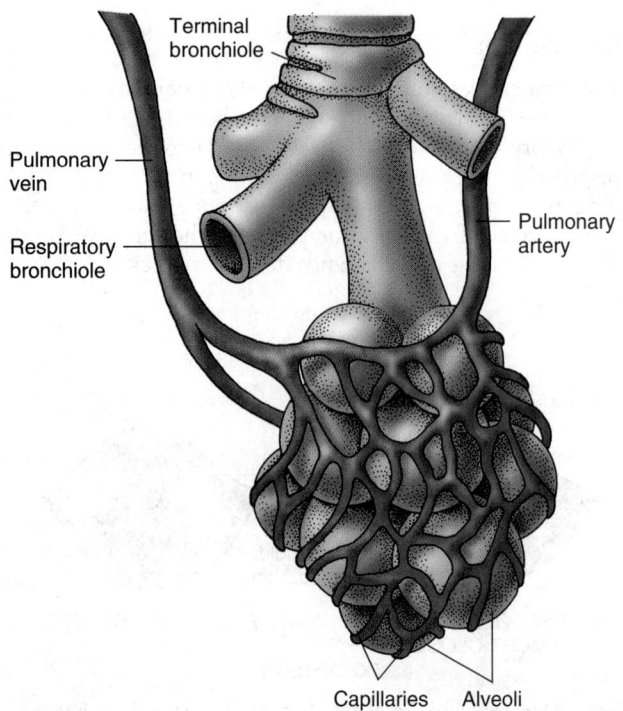

Figure 29–6. The terminal bronchioles and the acinus.

TABLE 29–1

Age Distributions and Partial Pressure of Arterial Oxygen (PaO$_2$) Values (Mean)	
Age (years)	**PaO$_2$**
40–44	95
45–49	88.6
50–54	87.1
55–59	85.1
60–64	84.8
65–69	82.3
70–74	79.1
75–79	82.9
80–84	83.4
85–90	83.2

Modified with permission from Cerveri, I., Zoia, M. C., Fanfulla, F., et al. (1995). Reference values of arterial oxygen tension in the middle-aged and elderly. *American Journal of Respiratory and Critical Care Medicine, 152,* 934–941.

Alveolar Ducts and Alveoli

Alveolar ducts, which resemble a bunch of grapes, branch from the respiratory bronchioles. Alveolar sacs arise from these ducts. The alveolar sacs contain clusters of alveoli, which are the basic units of gas exchange (see Fig. 29–6). It is estimated that the lungs contain about 300 million alveoli, surrounded by pulmonary capillaries. Because these microscopic alveoli are so numerous and share common walls, the surface area for gas exchange in the lungs is extensive. In a healthy adult, this surface area is approximately the size of a tennis court. *Acinus* is a term used to indicate all structures distal to the terminal bronchiole (e.g., respiratory bronchiole, alveolar duct, and alveolar sac).

Certain cells located in the walls of the alveoli secrete *surfactant,* a phospholipid protein that reduces the surface tension in the alveoli. Without sufficient surfactant, atelectasis (collapse of the alveoli) ultimately occurs. In atelectasis, gas exchange is reduced because the surface area is reduced.

Lungs

The lungs are sponge-like, elastic, cone-shaped organs located in the pleural cavity in the thorax. The apex of each lung extends above the clavicle; the base of each lung lies just above the diaphragm (the major muscle of inspiration). The lungs are composed of millions of alveoli and their related ducts, bronchioles, and bronchi. The right lung, which is larger than the left, is divided into three lobes: upper, middle, and lower. The left lung, which is somewhat narrower than the right lung to accommodate the heart, is divided into two lobes.

The hilum is the point at which the primary bronchus, pulmonary blood vessels, nerves, and lymphatics enter each lung. Innervation of the chest wall is via the phrenic (pleura) and intercostal (diaphragm, ribs, and muscles) nerves; innervation of the bronchi is via the vagus nerve.

Composed of two surfaces, the pleura, a continuous smooth membrane, totally encloses the lung. The parietal pleura lines the inside of the thoracic cavity, including the upper surface of the diaphragm. The visceral pleura covers the pulmonary surfaces, including the major fissures between the lobes. A thin fluid (surfactant) produced by the cells lining the pleura lubricates these two surfaces, thereby allowing them to glide smoothly and painlessly during respirations.

Blood flow through the lungs occurs via two separate systems: the pulmonary system and the bronchial system. The bronchial arteries, arising from the thoracic aorta, are part of the systemic circulation and do not participate in gas exchange. This system carries the blood necessary to meet the metabolic demands of the lungs. The pulmonary circulation is composed of a highly vascular capillary network. Oxygen-depleted blood travels from the right ventricle of the heart into the pulmonary artery, which eventually branches into arterioles that form the capillary networks. The capillaries are enmeshed around and through the alveoli, the site of gas exchange (see Fig. 29–6). Freshly oxygenated blood then travels through the venules to the pulmonary vein and on to the left atrium, where it is pumped throughout the systemic circulation.

Accessory Muscles of Respiration

Accessory muscles of respiration include the scalene muscles, which elevate the first two ribs; the sternocleidomastoid muscles, which raise the sternum; and the trapezius and pectoralis muscles, which fix the shoulders. Additionally, various back and abdominal muscles are used in disease states.

Respiratory Changes Associated with Aging

Respiratory changes that occur with aging are described in Chart 29–1. Many changes associated with elderly clients are due to a lifetime of exposure to environmental stimuli (e.g., cigarette smoke, bacteria, air pollutants, and industrial fumes and irritants) and heredity. Table 29–1 shows the results of one study demonstrating that partial pressure of arterial oxygen (PaO_2) decreases with age up to age 75 years and then increases. Partial pressure of arterial carbon dioxide ($PaCO_2$) did not increase with age.

Chart 29–1

Nursing Focus on the Elderly: Changes in the Respiratory System Related to Aging

Physiologic Change	Nursing Implications	Rationales
Chest Wall		
Anteroposterior diameter increases. Thorax becomes shorter.	Discuss the normal changes of aging.	Clients may be anxious because they must work harder to breathe.
Progressive kyphoscoliosis occurs. Chest wall compliance (elasticity) decreases.	Discuss the need for increased rest periods during exercise.	Older clients have less tolerance for exercise.
Mobility may decrease. Osteoporosis is possible.	Encourage adequate calcium intake (especially during a woman's premenopause phase).	Calcium intake helps prevent osteoporosis by building bone in younger clients.

Continued

Chart 29–1. Nursing Focus on the Elderly: Changes in the Respiratory System Related to Aging   Continued

Physiologic Change	Nursing Implications	Rationales
Alveoli		
Alveolar surface area decreases. Diffusion capacity decreases. Elastic recoil decreases. Bronchioles and alveolar ducts dilate. Ability to cough decreases. Airways close early.	Encourage vigorous pulmonary hygiene (i.e., encourage the client to turn, cough, and deep breathe), especially if the client is confined to bed or has had surgery. Encourage upright position.	There is increased potential for mechanical or infectious respiratory complications in these situations. The upright position minimizes ventilation-perfusion mismatching.
Lungs		
Residual volume increases. Vital capacity decreases. Efficiency of oxygen and carbon dioxide exchange decreases. Elasticity decreases.	Include inspection, palpation, percussion, and auscultation in lung assessments. Help client in actively maintaining health and fitness. Assess the client's respirations for abnormal breathing patterns. Encourage frequent oral hygiene.	Inspection, palpation, percussion, and auscultation are needed to detect normal age-related changes. Health and fitness helps to keep losses in respiratory functioning to a minimum. Periodic breathing patterns (e.g., Cheyne-Stokes) can occur. Oral hygiene aids in the removal of secretions.
Pharynx and Larynx		
Muscles atrophy. Vocal cords become slack. Laryngeal muscles lose elasticity and cartilage.	Have face-to-face conversations with client when possible.	Client's voices may be soft and difficult to understand.
Pulmonary Vasculature		
Increased vascular resistance to blood flow through pulmonary vascular system occurs. Pulmonary capillary blood volume decreases. Risk of hypoxia increases.	Assess the client's level of consciousness.	Clients can become confused during acute respiratory conditions.
Exercise Tolerance		
Body's response to hypoxia and hypercarbia decreases.	Assess for subtle signs and symptoms of hypoxia.	Early assessment helps to prevent complications.
Muscle Strength		
Respiratory muscle strength, especially the diaphragm and the intercostals, decreases.	Encourage pulmonary hygiene and help the client in actively maintaining health and fitness.	Regular pulmonary hygiene and overall fitness help maintain maximal functioning of the respiratory system and prevent illness.
Proneness to Infection		
Effectiveness of the cilia decreases. Immunoglobulin A decreases. Alveolar macrophages are altered.	Encourage pulmonary hygiene and help the client in actively maintaining health and fitness.	Regular pulmonary hygiene and overall fitness help maintain maximal functioning of the respiratory system and prevent illness.

Respiratory disease is a major cause of acute illness and chronic disability in elderly clients. Although respiratory function normally declines with age, there is usually little difficulty with the demands of ordinary activity. However, the sedentary elderly client often reports feeling breathless during exercise.

It is difficult to differentiate the normal changes related to aging from the pathologic changes associated with respiratory disease or exposure to pollutants. In addition, disorders of the neuromuscular and cardiovascular systems that occur with aging may cause abnormal respiration even if the lungs are normal.

HISTORY
Demographic Data

Age, sex, and race can affect the physical and diagnostic findings. Many of the diagnostic studies relevant to respiratory disorders (e.g., pulmonary function tests) use these data for determining predicted normal values.

WOMEN'S HEALTH CONSIDERATIONS

 Women have greater bronchial responsiveness (i.e., bronchial hyperreactivity) than men, especially

women smokers. Women also have larger airways than men (Paoletti et al., 1995, p. 1775–1776). Increased bronchial responsiveness is a risk factor for a more rapid decline in lung function in the elderly, particularly in former and current smokers (Villar et al., 1995).

TRANSCULTURAL CONSIDERATIONS

The largest chest volumes are found in Caucasians; the smallest volumes are found in Native Americans. The chest volumes of African-Americans are significantly larger than those of Asian-Americans but not as large as those of Caucasians (Jarvis, 1996, p. 468).

Personal and Family History
Medical and Family History

The nurse questions clients about their respiratory history (Table 29–2). The client's history as well as that of family members could be significant. The nurse obtains a family history to consider respiratory disorders with a genetic component, such as cystic fibrosis, some lung cancers, and alpha$_1$-antitrypsin deficiency (one cause of emphysema). Clients with asthma often have a family history of allergic symptoms and reactive airways. The nurse assesses for a family history of infectious disease such as tuberculosis and considers that family members may have similar environmental or occupational exposures.

Smoking History

The nurse questions the client about the use of cigarettes, cigars, pipe tobacco, and marijuana and other controlled substances, and notes whether the client has passive exposure to smoke in the home or workplace. If the client smokes, the nurse asks how long the client has smoked, how many packs a day, whether the client has quit, and how long ago the client stopped smoking. The smoking history is documented in pack-years (number of packs smoked per day multiplied by number of years). Because the client may harbor guilt or denial about this habit, the nurse assumes a nonjudgmental attitude when questioning the client.

Smoking induces anatomical changes in the large and peripheral airways, which lead to varying degrees of airway obstruction (Paoletti et al., 1995). Men who continue to smoke have a more rapid decline in their pulmonary function than do nonsmokers. After quitting for 2 years, however, the decline in function has been found to be similar to that of a nonsmoker (Burchfiel et al., 1995).

Medication Use

The nurse questions the client about medications taken for breathing problems and also about drugs taken for other conditions. Cough, for example, can be a side effect of the angiotensin-converting enzyme (ACE) inhibitors. The nurse determines which over-the-counter medications, such as cough syrups, antihistamines, decongestants, inhalants, and nasal sprays, the client is using. The nurse also assesses home remedies. The nurse asks about past medication use and why it was discontinued. For

TABLE 29–2

Important Aspects to Assess in a Respiratory System History

- Smoking history
- Childhood illnesses
  - Asthma
  - Pneumonia
  - Communicable diseases
  - Hay fever
  - Allergies
  - Eczema
  - Frequent colds
  - Croup
  - Cystic fibrosis
- Adult illnesses
  - Pneumonia
  - Sinusitis
  - Tuberculosis
  - HIV and AIDS
  - Lung disease such as emphysema and sarcoidosis
  - Diabetes
  - Hypertension
  - Heart disease
- Influenza, pneumococcal (Pneumovax) and BCG vaccinations
- Surgeries of the upper or lower respiratory system
- Injuries to the upper or lower respiratory system
- Hospitalizations
- Date of last chest x-ray, pulmonary function test, tuberculin test, or other diagnostic tests and results
- Recent weight loss
- Night sweats
- Sleep disturbances
- Lung disease and condition of family members

HIV = human immunodeficiency virus; AIDS = acquired immunodeficiency syndrome; BCG = bacille Calmette-Guérin.

example, a client may have used numerous bronchodilator metered-dose inhalers but may prefer one particular drug for relieving breathlessness.

Allergies

Data about allergies are extremely important and relevant to the respiratory history. The nurse determines whether the client has any known allergies to foods, dust, molds, pollen, bee stings, trees, grass, animal dander and saliva, or medications. The nurse asks the client to explain a specific allergic response. For example, does the client wheeze, have trouble breathing, cough, sneeze, or experience rhinitis after exposure to the allergen? Has the client ever been treated for an allergic response? If the client has received treatment, the nurse asks about the circumstances leading up to the need for treatment, the type of treatment, and the client's response to treatment.

ELDERLY CONSIDERATIONS

 Allergy is a risk factor for a more rapid decline in lung function in the elderly (Villar et al., 1995).

Travel and Area of Residence

Travel and area of residence may be relevant for a history of exposure to certain diseases. For example, histoplasmosis, a fungal disease caused by inhalation of contaminated dust, is found in the central United States, the Mississippi and Missouri river valleys, and Central America. Coccidioidomycosis, another fungal disease, is found predominantly in the western and southwestern United States, Mexico, and portions of Central America.

Diet History

An evaluation of the client's diet history may reveal allergic reactions after ingestion of certain foods or preservatives. Signs and symptoms range from rhinitis, chest tightness, weakness, shortness of breath, urticaria, and severe wheezing to loss of consciousness. The nurse notes allergies and the allergic response in a prominent location of the client's record. The nurse asks about the client's usual food intake and ascertains whether any symptoms occur with eating. Malnutrition may occur when the client has difficulty breathing during the food preparation process or during eating.

Occupational History and Socioeconomic Status

The nurse considers the home, community, and workplace for environmental factors possibly causing or contributing to the client's lung disease. Occupational pulmonary diseases include pneumoconiosis (resulting from the inhalation of dust such as coal dust, stone dust, and silicone dust), toxic lung injury, and hypersensitivity disease (as from latex). The occupational history includes exact dates of employment and a brief job description. Exposure to industrial dusts (both organic and inorganic) or noxious chemicals found in smoke and fumes may cause respiratory disease. Some of the most susceptible clients include coal miners, stonemasons, cotton handlers, welders, potters, plastic and rubber manufacturers, printers, farm workers, and steel foundry workers.

The nurse obtains information about the client's home and living conditions, such as the type of heat used (e.g., gas heater, wood-burning stove, fireplace, and kerosene heater) and exposure to environmental irritants (e.g., noxious fumes, chemicals, animals, birds, and air pollutants). The nurse also asks about the client's hobbies and leisure activities. Pastimes such as painting, working with ceramics, model airplane building, furniture refinishing, or woodworking may have exposed the client to harmful chemical irritants.

Current Health Problem

Whether the pulmonary problem is acute or chronic, the client's chief complaint is likely to include cough, sputum production, chest pain, and shortness of breath at rest or on exertion. During the interview, the nurse explores the history of the present illness, preferably in a chronological order. This analysis includes the following:

Onset
Duration
Location
Frequency
Progressing and radiating patterns
Quality and number of symptoms
Aggravating and relieving factors
Associated signs and symptoms
Treatments

Cough

Cough is the cardinal sign of respiratory disease. The nurse asks the client how long the cough has persisted (e.g., 1 week, 3 months). The nurse also asks whether it occurs at a specific time of day (e.g., on awakening in the morning, as is common in smokers) or in relation to any physical activity. The nurse determines whether the cough is productive or nonproductive, congested, dry, tickling, or hacking.

Sputum Production

An important symptom associated with coughing is sputum production. The nurse notes the duration, color, consistency, odor, and amount of sputum. Sputum may be clear, white, tan, gray, or, if infection is present, yellow or green.

The nurse describes sputum consistency as thin, thick, watery, or frothy. Smokers with chronic bronchitis have mucoid sputum because of chronic stimulation and hypertrophy of the bronchial glands (George et al., 1995). Voluminous, pink, frothy sputum is characteristic of pulmonary edema. Pneumococcal pneumonia is often associated with rust-colored sputum, and foul-smelling sputum is often found in anaerobic infections such as lung abscess. Blood in the sputum (hemoptysis) is most commonly noted in clients with chronic bronchitis or bronchogenic carcinoma. Clients with tuberculosis, pulmonary infarction, bronchial adenoma, or lung abscess may expectorate grossly bloody sputum.

Sputum can be quantified by describing its production in terms of measurements such as teaspoon, tablespoon, and cups or fractions of cups. Normally, the tracheobronchial tree can produce up to 3 ounces (90 mL) of sputum per day. The nurse determines whether sputum production is increasing, possibly from external stimuli (such as an irritant in the work setting) or from an internal cause (such as chronic bronchitis or a pulmonary abscess).

Chest Pain

A detailed description of chest pain helps the nurse differentiate pleural, musculoskeletal, cardiac, and gastrointestinal pain. Because perception of pain is purely subjective, the nurse analyzes pain in relation to the characteristics described in the history of the present illness. Coughing, deep breathing, or swallowing usually makes chest wall pain worse. (Chapter 9 discusses pain in detail.)

TABLE 29–3

Correlation of Dyspnea Classification with Performance of Activities of Daily Living (ADLs)

Classification	Activities of Daily Living Key
Class I: No significant restrictions in normal activity. Employable. Dyspnea occurs only on more than normal or strenuous exertion.	• *4:* No breathlessness, normal.
Class II: Independent in essential ADLs but restricted in some other activities. Dyspneic on climbing stairs or on walking on an incline but not on level walking. Employable for only sedentary job or under special circumstances.	• *3:* Satisfactory, mild breathlessness. Complete performance is possible without pause or assistance, but not entirely normal.
Class III: Dyspnea commonly occurs during usual activities, such as showering or dressing, but the client can manage without assistance from others. Not dyspneic at rest; can walk for more than a city block at own pace but cannot keep up with others of own age. May stop to catch breath partway up a flight of stairs. Is probably not employable in any occupation.	• *2:* Fair, moderate breathlessness. Must stop during activity. Complete performance is possible without assistance, but performance may be too debilitating or time consuming.
Class IV: Dyspnea produces dependence on help in some essential ADLs such as dressing and bathing. Not usually dyspneic at rest. Dyspneic on minimal exertion; must pause on climbing one flight, walking more than 100 yards, or dressing. Often restricted to home if lives alone. Has minimal or no activities out of home.	• *1:* Poor, marked breathlessness. Incomplete performance; assistance is necessary.
Class V: Entirely restricted to home and often limited to bed or chair. Dyspneic at rest. Dependent on help for most needs.	• *0:* Performance not indicated or recommended; too difficult.

Dyspnea

The perception of difficulty in breathing (breathlessness) is subjective and varies among clients, and a client's perception may not be consistent with the severity of the presenting problem. For that reason, the nurse determines the type of onset (slow or abrupt), the duration (number of hours, time of day), relieving factors (changes of position, medication use, activity cessation), and evidence of audible sounds (wheezing, crackles, stridor).

The nurse tries to quantify dyspnea by determining whether this symptom interferes with activities of daily living (ADLs) and, if so, how severely. For example, is the client breathless while dressing, showering, shaving, or eating? Does dyspnea on exertion occur after the client walks one block or climbs one flight of stairs? Table 29–3 correlates dyspnea classifications with ADL performance. The nurse also may use a dyspnea assessment scale to assess dyspnea (see Chap. 32).

The nurse inquires about paroxysmal nocturnal dyspnea (PND) and orthopnea, which are commonly associated with chronic pulmonary disease and left ventricular failure. In PND, the client has a sudden onset of difficulty breathing that is severe enough to awaken the client from sleep. The term *orthopnea* is used when the client needs to be in an upright position to have easier breathing.

PHYSICAL ASSESSMENT
Nose and Sinuses

The nurse inspects the client's external nose for deformities or tumors and the nostrils for symmetry of size and shape. Nasal flaring may indicate increased respiratory effort. To observe the interior nose, the nurse asks the client to tilt the head back for a penlight examination. The nurse may use a nasal speculum and nasopharyngeal mirror for a more thorough examination of the nasal cavity.

The nurse inspects for color, swelling, drainage, and bleeding. The mucous membrane of the nose normally appears redder than the oral mucosa, but it may appear pale, engorged, and bluish gray in clients with allergic rhinitis. The nurse checks the nasal septum for evidence of bleeding, perforation, or deviation. Some degree of septal deviation is common in most adults and appears as an S shape, inclining toward one side or the other. A perforated septum is noted if the light shines through the perforation into the opposite nostril; it is often found in cocaine users. Nasal polyps, a frequent cause of obstruction, appear as pale, shiny, gelatinous structures attached to the turbinates (see also Chap. 31).

The nurse occludes one nare at a time to check whether air moves through the nonoccluded nare easily. The nurse also palpates the nose and the paranasal sinuses to detect tenderness or swelling. Only the frontal and maxillary sinuses are readily accessible to clinical examination because the ethmoid and sphenoid sinuses lie deep within the skull (see Fig. 29–2). Using the thumbs, the nurse checks for sinus tenderness by pressing upward on the frontal and maxillary areas; both sides are assessed simultaneously. Tenderness in these areas suggests inflammation or acute sinusitis. Slight tapping with the plexor over the sinuses also will elicit tenderness if inflamed.

The nurse may use transillumination of the sinuses to detect sinusitis. A darkened room and a penlight are needed for this procedure. Normally, the nurse sees a faint glow of light through the bone outlining the sinus. Transillumination is absent or decreased in sinusitis. Computed tomographic (CT) scans and x-rays of the sinuses are more definitive tools for detecting inflammation or sinusitis.

Pharynx, Trachea, and Larynx

Examination of the pharynx begins with inspection of the external structures of the mouth. Chapter 55 describes a complete physical assessment of the oral cavity, and Chapter 56 discusses disorders of the oral cavity.

Using a tongue depressor, the nurse presses down one side of the tongue at a time (to avoid stimulating the client's gag reflex) to examine the structures of the posterior pharynx. As the client says "ah," the nurse notes the rise and fall of the soft palate and uvula and observes for color and symmetry, evidence of mucopurulent discharge (postnasal drainage), edema or ulceration, and tonsillar enlargement or inflammation.

The nurse inspects the neck for symmetry, alignment, masses, swelling, bruises, and the use of accessory neck muscles in breathing. The nurse palpates lymph nodes for size, shape, mobility, consistency, and tenderness. Tender nodes are usually movable and suggest inflammation. Malignant nodes are often hard and fixed to the surrounding tissue.

The nurse gently palpates the trachea for deviation, mobility, tenderness, and masses. Firm palpation may elicit coughing or gagging. The space on either side of the

trachea should be equal. Many pulmonary disorders cause the trachea to deviate from the midline. Tension pneumothorax, large pleural effusion, mediastinal mass, and neck tumor push the trachea away from the affected area, whereas pneumonectomy, fibrosis, and atelectasis cause a pull toward the affected area. Decreased tracheal mobility may occur with carcinoma or fibrosis of the mediastinum.

The larynx is usually examined by a specialist with a laryngoscope. The nurse may observe an abnormal voice, especially hoarseness, when there are abnormalities of the larynx.

Lungs and Thorax

Before examining the thorax, the nurse becomes familiar with anatomic landmarks. Identifying the location of physical assessment findings depends on accurate numbering of the ribs, intercostal spaces, and vertebrae and on accurate use of imaginary lines drawn on the chest (Fig. 29–7).

Inspection

Inspection of the chest begins with assessment of the anterior and posterior thorax, with the client in a sitting position, if possible. The client should be undressed to the waist and draped for privacy and warmth. The chest is observed by comparing one side with the other. The nurse works from the top (apex) and moves downward toward the base. The nurse inspects for discoloration, scars, lesions, masses, and spinal deformities such as kyphosis, scoliosis, and lordosis.

The nurse notes the rate, rhythm, and depth of inspirations as well as symmetry of chest movement. An im-

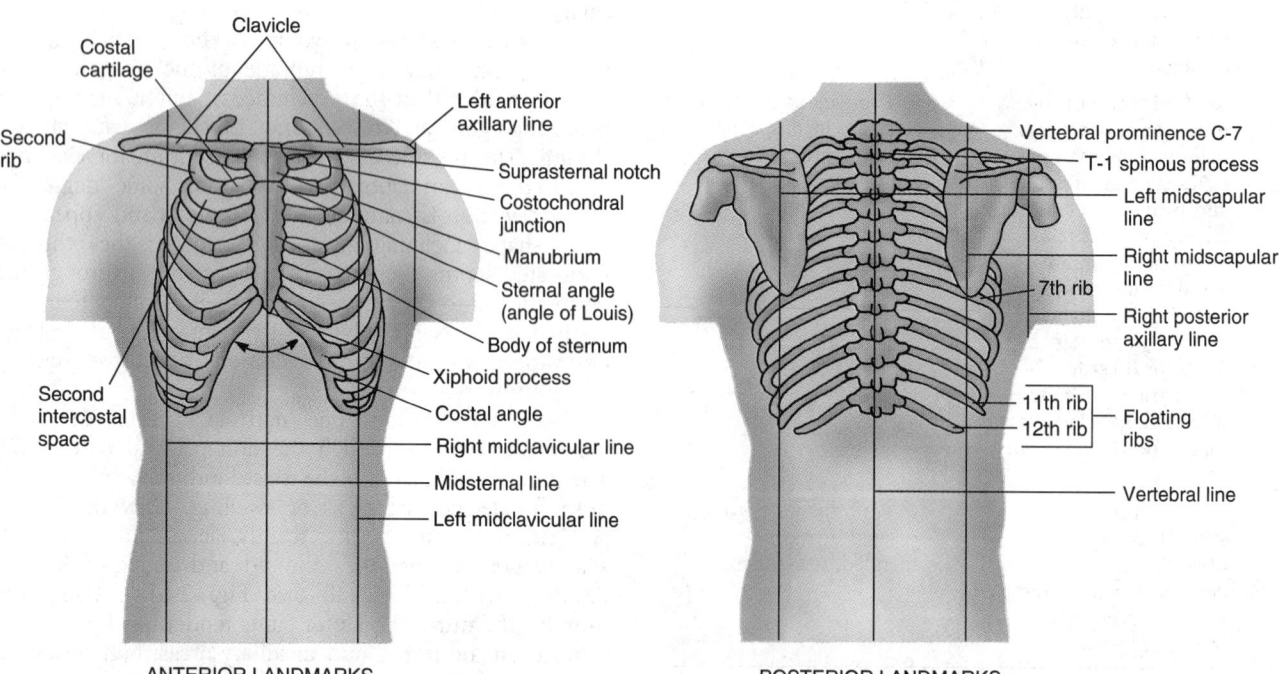

ANTERIOR LANDMARKS   POSTERIOR LANDMARKS

Figure 29–7. Anterior and posterior thoracic landmarks.

paired movement or unequal expansion may indicate underlying disease of the lung or the pleura. The nurse observes the type of breathing, such as pursed-lip or diaphragmatic breathing, and the use of accessory muscles. In observing respiration, the nurse notes the duration of the inspiratory (I) and expiratory (E) phases. The ratio of these phases (the I/E ratio) is normally 1:2. A prolonged expiratory phase indicates obstruction of air outflow and is frequently seen in clients with chronic airflow limitation (CAL).

The nurse notes the client's chest configuration and compares the anteroposterior (AP) diameter with the lateral diameter. This ratio normally ranges from 1:2 to about 5:7, depending on the client's body build. The ratio approximates 1:1 in the client with emphysema, thus giving the client the typical barrel chest appearance (see Fig. 32–5).

Normally, the ribs slope downward. However, clients with air trapping in the lungs caused by chronic asthma or emphysema have little or no slope to the ribs (i.e., the ribs are more horizontal).

The nurse also checks for abnormal retractions of the intercostal spaces during inspiration, which indicate airflow obstruction. These retractions may be due to fibrosis of the underlying lung, severe acute asthma, emphysema, or tracheal or laryngeal obstruction.

Palpation

After inspection, the nurse palpates the chest. Palpation enables the nurse to assess symmetry of respiratory movement and observable abnormalities, to identify areas of tenderness, and to elicit vocal or tactile fremitus (vibration).

In palpation, the nurse assesses thoracic expansion by placing the thumbs posteriorly on the spine at the level of the ninth ribs; the fingers are extended laterally around the rib cage. As the client inhales, both sides of the chest should move upward and outward together in one symmetric movement; the nurse's thumbs thus move apart. On exhalation, the thumbs should come back together as they return to the midline. Splinting or decreased movement on one side (unilateral or unequal expansion) may be due to pleuritic pain, trauma, or pneumothorax (air in the pleural cavity). Respiratory lag or impairment of thoracic movement may also indicate the presence of a pulmonary mass, pleural fibrosis, atelectasis, pneumonia, or a lung abscess.

The nurse palpates the thorax for any abnormalities found on inspection (e.g., masses, lesions, bruises, and swelling). The nurse also palpates for tenderness, particularly if the client has reported pain. *Crepitus,* or subcutaneous emphysema, is a crackling sensation felt beneath the fingertips and should be noted, especially around a wound site or if a pneumothorax is suspected. Crepitus indicates that air is trapped within the tissues.

Vocal fremitus is a vibration of the chest wall produced when the client speaks; when palpated, it is termed *tactile fremitus.* To elicit tactile fremitus, the nurse places the palm or the base of the fingers against the client's chest wall and instructs the client to say the number 99. The nurse compares vibrations (with the same hand) from one side of the chest with those from the other side, moving from the apices to the bases. Palpable vibrations are transmitted from the tracheobronchial tree, along the solid surface of chest wall, to the nurse's hand.

The nurse notes symmetry of the vibrations and areas of enhanced, diminished, or absent fremitus. Fremitus is decreased if the transmission of sound waves from the larynx to the chest wall is slowed. This situation can occur when the pleural space is filled with air (pneumothorax), fluid (pleural effusion), or solid tissue (pleural thickening). Fremitus is increased over large bronchi because of their proximity to the chest wall. Disease processes such as pneumonia and abscesses decrease the distance vibrations must travel to reach the chest wall, also resulting in increased tactile fremitus.

Percussion

The nurse uses percussion to assess for pulmonary resonance, the boundaries of organs, and diaphragmatic excursion. Percussion involves tapping the chest wall, which sets the underlying tissues into motion and produces audible sounds. The nurse places the distal joint of the middle finger of the less dominant hand firmly on the surface over the intercostal space to be percussed. No other part of the nurse's hand touches the client's chest wall because it absorbs the vibrations. The nurse uses the middle finger of the dominant hand to deliver quick, sharp strikes to the distal joint of the positioned finger (Fig. 29–8). The nurse maintains a loose, relaxed wrist while delivering the taps with the tip of the finger, not the finger pad. The nurse repeats this technique two or three times and listens to the intensity, pitch, quality, and duration of the sound produced. Long fingernails may limit the ability to percuss.

Percussion produces five distinguishable notes as described in Table 29–4. These sounds assist the nurse in determining the density of the underlying structures (i.e., whether the lung tissue contains air or fluid or is solid). Percussion of the thorax is performed over the rib intercostal spaces because percussing the sternum, ribs, or scapulae yields sound indicating solid bone. Percussion penetrates only 2 to 3 inches (5–7 cm), so deeper lesions are not detected with this technique.

The percussion technique begins with the client sitting in an upright position. The nurse assesses the posterior thorax first and proceeds systematically, beginning at the apex and working toward the base. The apex of the lung extends about ¾ to 1½ inches (2–4 cm) above the clavicle anteriorly. Posteriorly, there is approximately a 2-inch (5 cm) width of lung tissue at the apex.

The nurse assesses diaphragmatic excursion by instructing the client to "take a deep breath and hold it" while percussing downward until dullness is noted at the lower border of the lung. Normal resonance of the lung stops at the diaphragm, where the sound becomes dull, and this site is marked. The nurse repeats the process after instructing the client to "let out all your breath and hold." The difference between the two markings or sounds is the diaphragmatic excursion, which may range from 1 to 2 inches (3–5 cm). The diaphragm is normally higher on the right because of the location of the liver. Diaphrag-

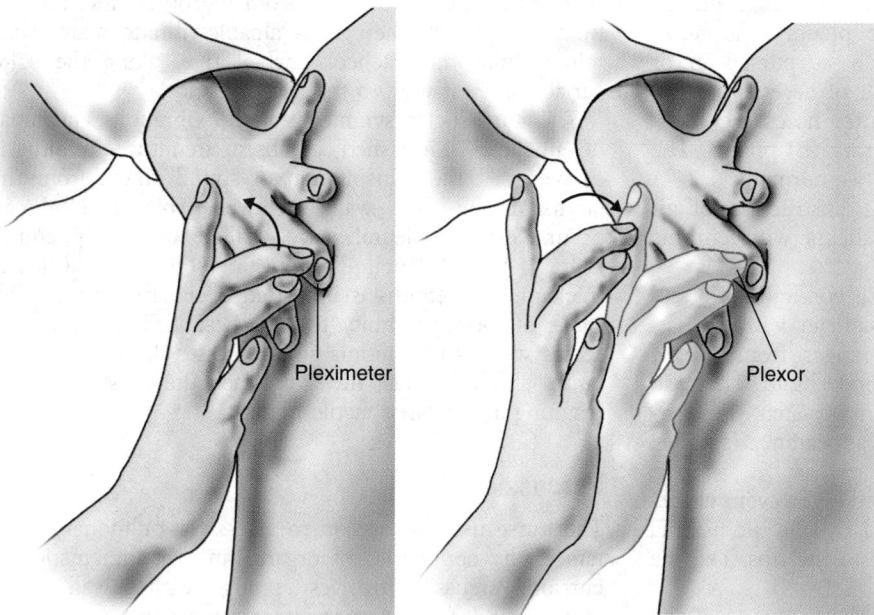

Pleximeter

Plexor

Figure 29–8. Percussion technique.

matic excursion may be decreased or absent in clients with pleurisy, diaphragm paralysis, or emphysema.

The nurse continues assessment of the thorax with percussion of the anterior and lateral chest. The percussion note changes from resonance of the normal lung to dullness at the borders of the heart and the liver. If a dull percussion note is found over lung tissue, the nurse expects that fluid or solid material is replacing the normal air-containing lung (as occurs in pneumonia, pleural effusion, fibrosis, atelectasis, and tumor).

Auscultation

Auscultation includes listening for normal breath sounds, adventitious sounds, and voice sounds. Auscultation provides information about the flow of air through the tracheobronchial tree and helps the listener identify fluid, mucus, or obstruction in the respiratory system. The diaphragm of the stethoscope is designed to detect high-pitched sounds.

The auscultation procedure begins with the client sit-

TABLE 29–4

Characteristic Features of the Five Percussion Notes

Note	Pitch	Intensity	Quality	Duration	Findings
Resonance	• Low	• Moderate to loud	• Hollow	• Long	• Resonance is characteristic of normal lung tissue.
Hyperresonance	• Higher than resonance	• Very loud	• Booming	• Longer than resonance	• Hyperresonance indicates the presence of trapped air, so it is commonly heard over an emphysematous or asthmatic lung and occasionally over a pneumothorax.
Flatness	• High	• Soft	• Extreme dullness	• Short	• An example location is the sternum. Flatness percussed over the lung fields may indicate a massive pleural effusion.
Dullness	• Medium	• Medium	• Thud-like	• Medium	• An example location is over the liver and the kidneys. Dullness can be percussed over atelectatic lung or consolidated lung.
Tympany	• High	• Loud	• Musical, drum-like	• Short	• Examples are the cheek filled with air and the abdomen distended with air. Over the lung, a tympanic note usually indicates a large pneumothorax.

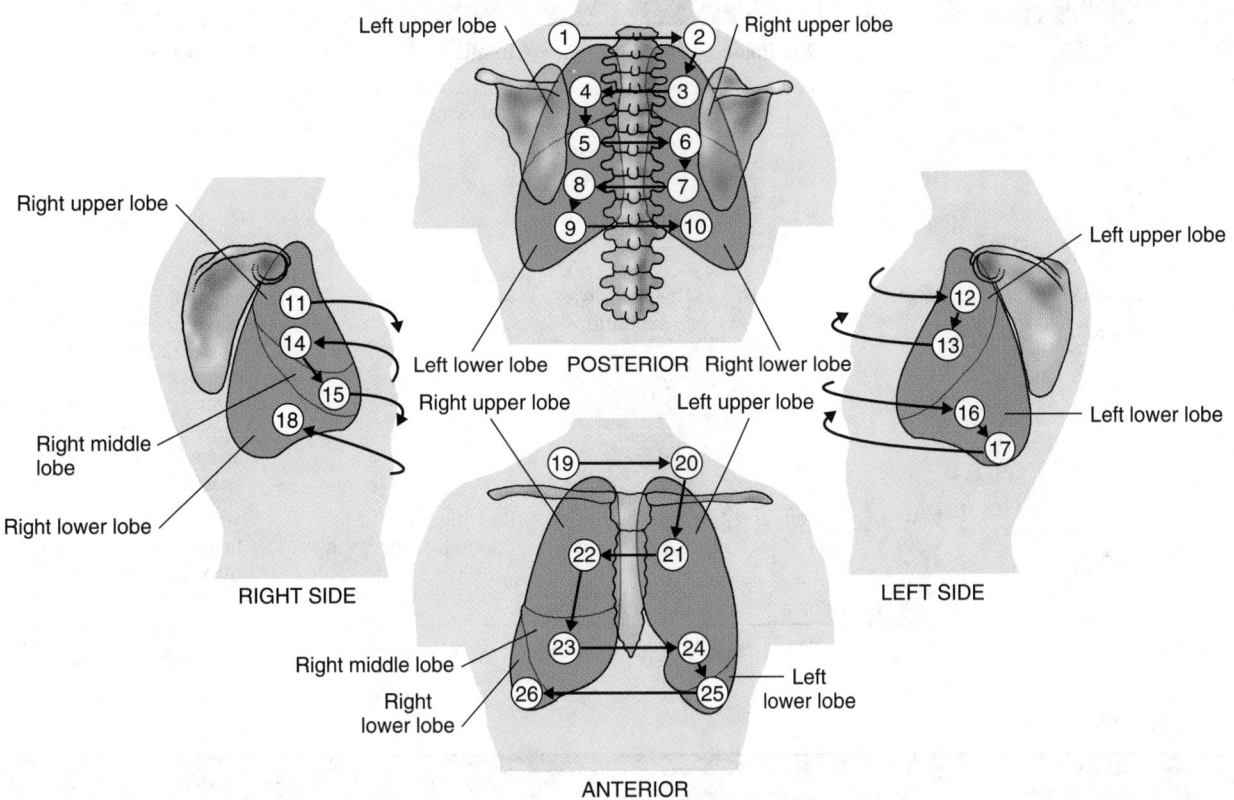

Figure 29–9. Sequence for percussion and auscultation.

ting in an upright position. With the stethoscope pressed firmly against the chest wall (clothing can distort or muffle sounds), the nurse instructs the client to breathe slowly and deeply through an open mouth. Breathing through the nose would set up turbulent sounds that are transmitted to the lungs. The nurse uses a systematic approach beginning at the apices and moving down through the intercostal spaces to the bases (Fig. 29–9). The nurse avoids listening over bony structures while auscultating the thorax posteriorly, laterally, and anteriorly. The nurse listens to a full respiratory cycle, noting the quality and intensity of the breath sounds. The nurse observes the client for signs of lightheadedness or dizziness caused by hyperventilation during auscultation and allows the client to breathe normally for a few minutes if these symptoms occur.

Normal Breath Sounds

Normal breath sounds are produced as air vibrates while passing through the respiratory passages from the larynx to the alveoli. Breath sounds are identified by their location, intensity, pitch, and duration within the respiratory cycle (e.g., early or late inspiration and expiration). Normal breath sounds are known as bronchial (or tubular), bronchovesicular, and vesicular (Table 29–5). The nurse describes these sounds as normal, increased, decreased (diminished), or absent.

When bronchial breath sounds are heard peripherally, they are abnormal. This increased sound occurs when there is transmission of centrally generated bronchial sounds to an area of increased density such as in clients with atelectasis, tumor, or pneumonia. Bronchovesicular breath sounds, when audible in an abnormal location, may indicate normal aging or an abnormality such as pulmonary consolidation and chronic airway disease.

Adventitious Breath Sounds

Adventitious sounds are additional breath sounds superimposed on normal sounds and indicate pathologic changes in the tracheobronchial tree. Table 29–6 classifies and describes the adventitious sounds: crackle, wheeze, rhonchus, and pleural friction rub (American College of Chest Physicians and the American Thoracic Society Joint Committee on Pulmonary Nomenclature, 1975; Mikami et al., 1987). Various subclassifications of these categories exist. Adventitious sounds vary in pitch, intensity, duration, and the phase of the respiratory cycle in which they occur. The terms for adventitious sounds vary among respiratory care practitioners. The nurse is encouraged to document exactly what is heard on auscultation instead of relying on numerous labels.

Voice Sounds

If the nurse discovers abnormalities during the physical assessment of the lungs and thorax, the client is assessed for vocal resonance. Auscultation of voice sounds through the normally air-filled lung produces a muffled, unclear sound because sound vibrations travel poorly through air. Vocal resonance is increased when the sound must travel

TABLE 29–5

Characteristics of Normal Breath Sounds

	Pitch	Amplitude	Duration	Quality	Normal Location
Bronchial (Tubular, tracheal)	High	Loud	Inspiration < expiration	Harsh, hollow, tubular, blowing	Trachea and larynx
Bronchovesicular	Moderate	Moderate	Inspiration = expiration	Mixed	Over major bronchi where fewer alveoli are located: posterior, between scapulae especially on right; anterior, around upper sternum in first and second intercostal spaces
Vesicular	Low	Soft	Inspiration > expiration	Rustling, like the sound of the wind in the trees	Over peripheral lung fields where air flows through smaller bronchioles and alveoli

From Jarvis, C. (1996). *Physical examination and health assessment* (2nd ed.). Philadelphia: W. B. Saunders, p. 479. Used with permission.

TABLE 29–6

Characteristic Features of Adventitious Breath Sounds

Adventitious Sound	Occurrence in the Respiratory Cycle	Character	Association
Discontinuous			
Fine crackles Fine rales High-pitched rales	• Either early or late inspiration	• Popping, discontinuous sounds caused by air moving into previously deflated airways; sounds like hair being rolled between fingers near the ear • "Velcro" sounds late in inspiration usually associated with restrictive disorders	Asbestosis Atelectasis Interstitial fibrosis Bronchitis Pneumonia Chronic pulmonary diseases
Coarse crackles Low-pitched crackles	• More common on expiration, but may be present early in inspiration	• Lower pitched, coarse, discontinuous rattling sounds caused by fluid or secretions in large airways; likely to change with coughing or suctioning	Bronchitis Pneumonia Tumors Pulmonary edema
Continuous			
Wheeze	• Audible during either inspiration or expiration, or both	• Squeaky, musical, continuous sounds associated with air rushing through narrowed airways; may be heard without a stethoscope • Arise from the small airways • Usually do not clear with coughing	Inflammation Bronchospasm Edema Secretions Pulmonary vessel engorgement (as in cardiac "asthma")
Rhonchus (rhonchi)	• Audible during both inspiration and expiration, but commonly more prominent on expiration	• Lower-pitched, coarse, continuous snoring sounds • Arise from the large airways	Thick tenacious secretions Sputum production Obstruction by foreign body Tumors
Pleural Friction Rub	• Heard during both inspiration and expiration, generally at the end of inspiration and the beginning of expiration	• Loud, rough, grating, scratching sounds caused by the inflamed surfaces of the pleura rubbing together; often associated with pain on deep inspirations • Heard in lateral lung fields	Pleurisy Tuberculosis Pulmonary infarction Pneumonia Lung cancer

through a solid or liquid medium, as it does in clients with a consolidated area of the lung, pneumonia, atelectasis, pleural effusion, tumor, or abscess.

BRONCHOPHONY. This is the abnormally loud and clear transmission of voice sounds through an area of increased density. For assessment of bronchophony, the client repeats the number 99 while the nurse systematically auscultates the thorax.

WHISPERED PECTORILOQUY. This is much more sensitive than bronchophony and is perceived by having the client whisper the number sequence *one, two, three.* Normally, whispered words sound faint and indistinct; if they are heard loudly and distinctly, the nurse suspects consolidation of lung tissue.

EGOPHONY. This is another form of abnormal vocal resonance and has a high-pitched, bleating, nasal quality. The nurse instructs the client to repeat the letter *E* and auscultates the thorax. Egophony exists when this letter is heard as a flat, nasal sound of *A* through the stethoscope. This abnormal sound indicates an area of consolidation, pleural effusion, or abscess.

PSYCHOSOCIAL ASSESSMENT

The nurse assesses aspects of the client's lifestyle that may significantly affect respiratory function. Some respiratory conditions may be exacerbated by stress. The nurse questions the client about present life stresses and usual coping mechanisms.

Chronic respiratory illnesses may cause changes in family roles and relationships, social isolation, financial problems, and unemployment or disability. By discussing coping mechanisms, the nurse assesses the client's reaction to these psychosocial stressors and discovers strengths as well as ineffective behaviors. For example, the client may react to stress with dependence on family members, withdrawal, or noncompliance with interventions. After completing the psychosocial assessment, the nurse assists the client in determining the support systems available to help cope with respiratory impairment.

DIAGNOSTIC ASSESSMENT
Laboratory Tests
Blood Tests

Several laboratory tests (Chart 29–2) are relevant to the care of clients with respiratory disorders. A red blood cell count (also see Chap. 41) provides data regarding the transport of oxygen from the lungs. A hemoglobin deficiency directly affects tissue oxygenation because hemoglobin transports oxygen to the cells and could cause hypoxemia.

Arterial blood gas (ABG) analysis assesses oxygenation (arterial oxygen pressure [PaO_2]), alveolar ventilation (arterial carbon dioxide pressure [$PaCO_2$]), and acid-base balance. Blood gas studies (also see Chap. 18) provide valuable information for monitoring treatment results, adjusting oxygen therapy, and evaluating the client's responses to treatment and therapy as during weaning from mechanical ventilation.

Sputum Tests

Sputum specimens obtained by expectoration or tracheal suctioning assist in the identification of pathogenic organisms or abnormal cells such as in a malignancy or a hypersensitivity state. Sputum culture and sensitivity analyses identify bacterial infection with either gram-negative or gram-positive organisms and determine the vulnerability to specific antibiotics. Cytologic examination is performed on sputum to help diagnose and specify malignant lesions by identifying cancer cells. Benign conditions, such as a hypersensitivity state, may also be identified by cytologic testing. Eosinophils and Curschmann's spirals (a mucous form) are often found by cytologic study in clients with allergic asthma.

Radiographic Examinations
Standard Radiography

Chest x-rays are taken for clients with respiratory tract disorders to evaluate the present status of the chest and to provide a baseline for comparison with future changes. Standard chest x-rays are taken from posteroanterior (PA; back to front) and left lateral (LL) projections. Portable chest x-rays (taken anteroposterior, or AP, front to back) cost more, and the films produced are of lower quality and are more difficult for the radiologist to interpret.

Chest x-rays can be used to assess pathologic changes in the lung such as those occurring in clients with pneumonia, atelectasis, pneumothorax, and tumor. The presence of pleural fluid and the position and placement of an endotracheal tube or other invasive catheters also can be detected by chest radiography. However, these films have limitations; they may appear normal even in a severe form of certain diseases, such as chronic bronchitis, asthma, and emphysema.

Sinus and facial x-rays are taken to assess the fluid levels in the sinus cavities to assist in the diagnosis of acute or chronic sinusitis.

Digital Chest Radiography

By using a computer, bone images can be eliminated from the chest x-ray, thereby creating better views of nonbone images. The test is useful in detecting lung lesions.

Tomography

Tomography is valuable in the assessment of the client with a respiratory disorder because pulmonary densities, tumors, and lesions can be seen. Positron emission tomography (PET) is useful for studying ventilation-perfusion relationships in the lung. Computed tomography (CT) provides consecutive 10-mm cross-sectional views of the thorax and produces a three-dimensional assessment of the lungs and the thorax.

Chart 29–2

Laboratory Profile: Respiratory Assessment

Test	Normal Range for Adults	Significance of Abnormal Findings
Blood Studies		
Complete blood count		
Red blood cells	Females: 18–44 years: 3.8–5.1 million/mm³ 45–64 years: 3.8–5.3 million/mm³ 65–74 years: 3.8–5.2 million/mm³ Males: 18–44 years: 4.3–5.7 million/mm³ 45–64 years: 4.2–5.6 million/mm³ 65–74 years: 3.8–5.8 million/mm³	*Elevated levels* (polycythemia) may be due to the excessive production of erythropoietin, which occurs in response to a hypoxic stimulus, as in CAL and from living at high altitude. *Decreased levels* indicate possible anemia, hemorrhage, or hemolysis.
Hemoglobin, total	Females: 18–44 years: 11.7–15.5 g/dL, or 117–155 g/L 45–64 years: 11.7–16 g/dL, or 117–160 g/L 65–74 years: 11.7–16.1 g/dL, or 117–161 g/L Males: 18–44 years: 13.2–17.3 g/dL, or 132–173 g/L 45–64 years: 13.1–17.2 g/dL, or 131–172 g/L	Same as for red blood cells
Hematocrit	Females: 18–44 years: 35%–45% 45–74 years: 35%–47% Males: 18–44 years: 39%–49% 45–64 years: 39%–50% 65–74 years: 37%–51%	Same as for red blood cells
White blood cell count (leukocyte count, WBC count)	Total: 4.5–11.0 × 10³ cells/μL, or 7.4 IRU African-Americans: 3.6–10.2 × 10³ cells/μL	*Elevations* indicate possible acute infections or inflammations, pneumonia, meningitis, tonsillitis, or emphysema. *Decreased levels* may indicate an overwhelming infection, an autoimmune disorder, or immunosuppressant therapy.
Differential white blood cell (leukocyte) count		
Neutrophils	1.8–7.7 × 10³ cells/μL; 18%–77% of total African-Americans: slightly lower	*Elevations* indicate possible acute bacterial infection (pneumonia), CAL, or inflammatory conditions (smoking). *Decreased levels* indicate possible viral disease (influenza).
Eosinophils	0–0.7 × 10³ cells/μL; 0%–7% of total	*Elevations* indicate possible CAL, asthma, or allergies. *Decreased levels* in pyogenic infections
Basophils	0–0.15 × 10³ cells/μL; 0%–1.5% of total	*Elevations* indicate possible inflammation; seen in chronic sinusitis, hypersensitivity reactions. *Decreased levels* may be seen in an acute infection.

Continued

Fat, cystic, and solid tissue can be distinguished with CT. By adding an intravenously (IV) injected contrast agent, vessels and other soft tissue structures can be identified. CT is especially valuable in studying the mediastinum, the hilar region, and the pleural space. The newer high-resolution CT (HRCT) uses 1.5-mm to 2-mm "slices" to assist in the assessment of bronchial abnormalities, interstitial disease, and emphysema. Nursing interventions for clients undergoing CT include education about the procedure and determination of the client's sensitivity to the contrast medium.

Ventilation and Perfusion Scanning

A ventilation and perfusion scan (also known as a V̇/Q̇ scan) identifies the areas of the lung being ventilated and the distribution of pulmonary blood. It is used primarily to confirm or rule out a diagnosis of pulmonary embolism.

Chart 29–2. Laboratory Profile: Respiratory Assessment   Continued

Test	Normal Range for Adults	Significance of Abnormal Findings
Lymphocytes	$1.5–4.0 \times 10^3$ cells/μL; 15%–40% of total	*Elevations* indicate possible viral infection, pertussis, and infectious mononucleosis. *Decreased levels* may be seen during corticosteroid
Monocytes	$0–0.8 \times 10^3$ cells/μL; 0%–8% of total	*Elevations:* see Lymphocytes; also may indicate active tuberculosis. *Decreased levels:* see Lymphocytes.
Arterial blood gases		
PaO_2	83–100 mmHg Elderly: values may be lower	*Elevations* indicate possible excessive oxygen administration. *Decreased levels* indicate possible CAL, chronic bronchitis, cancer of the bronchi and lungs, cystic fibrosis, respiratory distress syndrome, anemias, atelectasis, or any other cause of hypoxia.
$PaCO_2$	Females: 32–45 mmHg Males: 35–48 mmHg	*Elevations* indicate possible CAL, pneumonia, anesthesia effects, or use of opioids (respiratory acidosis). *Decreased levels* indicate hyperventiation/respiratory alkalosis.
pH	Up to 60 years: 7.35–7.45 60–90 years: 7.31–7.42 >90 years: 7.26–7.43	*Elevations* indicate metabolic or respiratory alkalosis. *Decreased levels* indicate metabolic or respiratory acidosis.
HCO_3^-	22–26 mEq/L	*Elevations* indicate possible respiratory acidosis as compensation for a primary metabolic alkalosis. *Decreased levels* indicate possible respiratory alkalosis as compensation for a primary metabolic acidosis.
SaO_2	94%–98% Elderly: values may be slightly lower	*Decreased levels* indicate possible impaired ability of hemoglobin to release oxygen to tissues.
Sputum studies		
Gram's stain	Negative	Presence of gram-positive or gram-negative bacteria indicates the type of microorganism that is causing the respiratory infection.
Culture and sensitivity	Negative	Presence of microorganisms indicates possible respiratory infections (e.g., pneumonia or bronchitis).
Acid-fast stain	No acid-fast bacilli	Presence of bacilli indicates possible tuberculosis.
Cytologic tests	Negative	Presence of abnormal cells indicates possible malignancy.

CAL = Chronic airflow limitation (formerly referred to as chronic obstructive pulmonary disease [COPD]); IRU = international recommended unit; PaO_2 = partial pressure of arterial oxygen; $PaCO_2$ = partial pressure of arterial carbon dioxide; HCO_3^- = bicarbonate ion; SaO_2 = arterial oxygen saturation.

To perform the study, the physician first injects a radionuclide with the client in a supine position and then takes six perfusion views: anterior, posterior, right and left lateral, and two obliques. If the perfusion scan is normal, there is no reason to continue with the ventilation scan. Otherwise, the client inhales a radioactive gas or a radioaerosol and the lung is scanned continuously as the substance is making its way into the lungs (the wash-in phase), once the substance has reached equilibrium within the lungs, and then during the time the substance is leaving the lungs (the wash-out phase).

The nurse teaches the client about the procedure and explains that the radioactive substance will clear from the body in approximately 8 hours.

Bronchography

Bronchography is now considered an archaic technique for evaluation of the bronchial tree (Bordow & Moser, 1996, p. 7).

Other Noninvasive Diagnostic Tests

Pulse Oximetry

Pulse oximetry identifies hemoglobin saturation. Usually, hemoglobin is almost 100% saturated with oxygen. The pulse oximeter uses a wave of infrared light and a sensor placed on the client's finger, toe, nose, earlobe, or forehead. Ideal normal pulse oximetry values are 95% to 100%; in elderly clients, values may be a little lower. So as not to be confused with the PaO_2 values from arterial blood gases, the pulse oximetry reading is recorded as the SaO_2, or SpO_2.

A pulse oximetry reading can alert the nurse to desaturation before clinical signs occur (e.g., dusky skin, pale mucosa, and nail beds). The nurse, however, considers client movement, hypothermia, decreased peripheral blood flow, ambient light (sunlight, infrared lamps), decreased hemoglobin, and edema as possible causes for low readings. Positioning or covering of the sensor could yield better accuracy if ambient light was present.

The nurse may consider results lower than 91% (and certainly below 86%) an emergency, necessitating immediate treatment. If the SaO_2 is below 85%, the body's tissues have a difficult time becoming oxygenated. An SaO_2 of less than 70% is certainly life threatening in the typical person, but values below 80% may be life threatening in others. Pulse oximetry readings are the least accurate at the lower values.

Pulmonary Function Tests

Pulmonary function tests (PFTs) evaluate lung function and dysfunction and include studies such as lung volumes and capacities, flow rates, diffusion capacity, gas exchange, airway resistance, and distribution of ventilation. The physician interprets the results by comparing the client's data with normal findings predicted according to age, sex, race, height, and weight. Smoking has a definite effect on PFTs, but studies have shown that smoking cessation is beneficial to the lungs (see Research Applications for Nursing).

PFTs are useful in screening clients for pulmonary disease even before the onset of signs or symptoms. Serial testing gives objective data that may be used as a guide to treatment (e.g., changes in pulmonary function can support a decision to continue, change, or discontinue a specific therapy). Preoperative evaluation with pulmonary function tests may identify the client at risk for postoperative pulmonary complications. One of the most common reasons for performing such tests is to determine the cause of breathlessness. When performed while the client exercises, PFTs help to determine whether dyspnea is caused by a pulmonary or a cardiac dysfunction or by muscle deconditioning. These tests are also useful for determining the effect of the client's occupation on pulmonary function and evaluating any related disability for legal purposes.

CLIENT PREPARATION. The nurse prepares the client for PFTs by explaining the purpose and value of the tests for planning the client's care. The client is advised not to smoke for 6 to 8 hours before testing. According to institutional policy and procedure, the nurse withholds bronchodilator medication for 4 to 6 hours before the test. Frequently, the client with respiratory impairment fears further breathlessness and is usually anxious before these so-called "breathing" tests. The nurse helps to alleviate apprehension by describing what the client will experience during and after the testing.

PROCEDURE. PFTs can be performed at the client's bedside or in the respiratory laboratory. The client is asked to breathe through the mouth only. A nose clip may be used to prevent air from escaping. The client performs different breathing maneuvers while measurements (Fig. 29–10) are obtained. Table 29–7 describes the most frequently used PFTs and their purpose.

FOLLOW-UP CARE. Because numerous breathing maneuvers are performed during pulmonary function tests, the nurse observes the client for increased dyspnea or bronchospasm after such studies. The nurse notes whether bronchodilator medication was administered during testing and alters the client's medication schedule as indicated.

Exercise Testing

Exercise, or activity in general, increases metabolism and gas transport as energy is generated. Five reasons for exercise testing are listed in Table 29–8. The tests are performed on a treadmill or bicycle or by a self-paced 12-minute walking test. The normal client's exercise is limited by hemodynamic factors, whereas the pulmonary client's limitation is ventilatory capacity or pulmonary

---

▶ Research Applications for Nursing

Cessation of Smoking Has an Effect on Pulmonary Function

Burchfiel, C. M., Marcus, E. B., Curb, J. D., et al. (1995). Effects of smoking and smoking cessation on longitudinal decline in pulmonary function. American Journal of Respiratory and Critical Care Medicine (151), 1778–1785.

In this study the effects of smoking and smoking cessation on the rate of FEV_1 decline over 6 years were examined in 4451 men between the ages of 45 and 68 years.

The researchers found that the men who continued to smoke had steeper rates of decline than those who had never smoked. The duration of their smoking habit was significantly associated with the rate of decline, but pack-years was of only borderline significance.

In the first 2 years for men who had quit smoking, the rate of decline was the same as those who continued to smoke, but after those 2 years, the rate of decline was similar to those who had never smoked. Even the men who were smokers and had impaired pulmonary function showed a slower rate of decline after smoking cessation.

Critique. Only men from a limited geographic area were studied, which could limit the generalization of these results to the broader population.

Possible Nursing Implications. With knowledge from this and other research studies, the nurse can become more involved with public education regarding smoking and smoking cessation at the community and national levels. The nurse can lobby for more research funds to be devoted to duplicating studies such as this one in women.

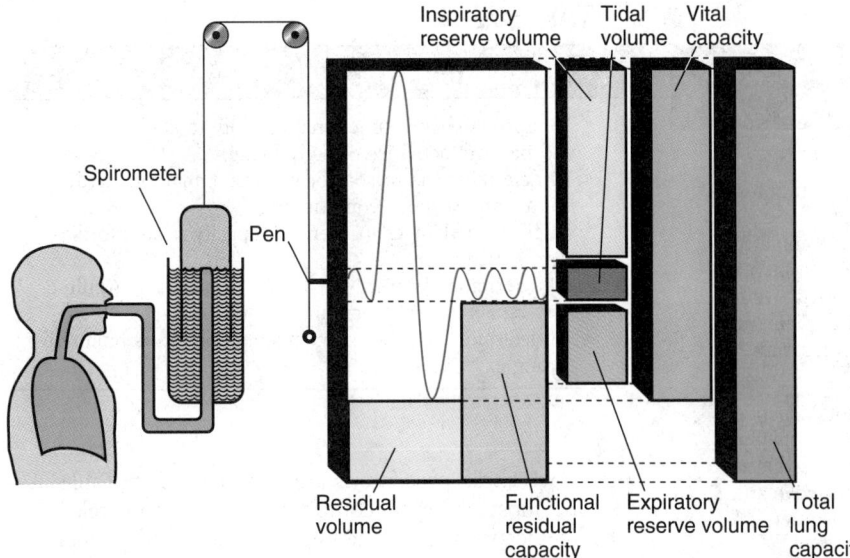

Inspiratory reserve volume
Tidal volume
Vital capacity
Spirometer
Pen
Residual volume
Functional residual capacity
Expiratory reserve volume
Total lung capacity

Figure 29-10. Common measurements in pulmonary function testing. Adapted from Luce, J. M., Pierson, D. J., & Tyler, M. L. (1993). *Intensive respiratory care* (2nd ed.). Philadelphia: W. B. Saunders).

gas exchange compromise, or both. The nurse explains exercise testing to the client and assures the client of close monitoring by trained professionals throughout the testing.

Skin Tests

Skin tests are used in combination with other diagnostic data to identify various infectious diseases (such as tuberculosis), viral diseases (such as mononucleosis and mumps), and fungal diseases (such as coccidioidomycosis and histoplasmosis). The presence of allergic hypersensitivity and the status of the immune system can be demonstrated through skin testing. Exposure to the allergen or organism used in testing produces a specific reaction (delayed hypersensitivity reaction) of the client's immune system. (For further discussion, see Chapters 23 and 25.)

CLIENT PREPARATION. To ensure cooperation and to alleviate anxiety, the nurse explains the purpose of skin testing and the procedure to the client. The client is questioned about a history of hypersensitivity to any of the local antigens used or a previous reaction to skin tests. The nurse also informs the client what is expected after testing is completed; for example, to prevent infection or abscess formation, the client is warned not to scratch the testing site. The client is also instructed to refrain from washing test or injection sites that have been circled with a marking pen for identification.

PROCEDURE. The actual procedure depends on the specific purpose of the test and the institution's policy. An intradermal injection technique causes a wheal to form after injection of the antigen. It is vital that the nurse perform the procedure correctly because incorrect antigen administration is responsible for erroneous results. The nurse ensures that the chosen test site is free from excessive body hair, dermatitis, and blemishes. A severe anaphylactic response can occur in clients who are hypersensitive to the test antigens. The nurse must recognize

and be prepared to treat reactions as described in Chapter 25.

FOLLOW-UP CARE. The reaction at injection sites is interpreted 24 to 72 hours after administration of the test antigen. If the testing is done as an outpatient procedure, the nurse instructs the client when to return to have the results read. The nurse documents the amount of induration (hard swelling) in millimeters and the presence of erythema and vesiculation (formation of small blister-like elevations).

Magnetic Resonance Imaging

Magnetic resonance imaging (MRI) assists in the diagnosis of respiratory system disorders by providing information about the type and condition of the tissues being imaged along any plane inside the body: vertically, horizontally, and diagonally. This costly procedure requires little client preparation other than the removal of all metal objects. Because of the powerful magnets used in MRI, clients with pacemakers, aneurysm clips, inner-ear implants, cardiac valves, or metallic foreign objects in the body are not candidates for MRI. The nurse informs the client of possible claustrophobia and discomfort from lying inside the magnet's small cylinder on a hard, cool table. The nurse instructs the client in the use of relaxation techniques and imagery to help decrease these sensations. In some cases, however, sedation may be necessary. In addition, the nurse informs the client that the noises heard during the examination are the natural, rhythmic sounds of radiofrequency pulses, which may range from barely audible to noticeable.

Other Invasive Diagnostic Tests
Endoscopic Examinations

Endoscopic diagnostic studies to assess respiratory disorders include bronchoscopy, laryngoscopy, and mediasti-

TABLE 29–7

Characteristics and Purposes of Pulmonary Function Tests	
Test	**Purpose**
FVC (forced vital capacity) records the maximal amount of air that can be exhaled as quickly as possible after maximal inspiration.	• FVC gives an indication of respiratory muscle strength and ventilatory reserve. FVC is often reduced in obstructive disease because of air trapping and in restrictive disease.
FEV_1 (forced expiratory volume in 1 sec) records the maximal amount of air that can be exhaled in the first second of expiration.	• FEV_1 is effort dependent and declines normally with age. It is reduced in certain obstructive and restrictive disorders.
FEV_1/FVC is the ratio of expiratory volume in 1 sec to FVC.	• This ratio provides a much more sensitive indication of obstruction to airflow. This ratio is the hallmark of obstructive pulmonary disease. It is normal or increased in restrictive disease.
$FEF_{25\%-75\%}$ records the forced expiratory flow over the 25%–75% volume (middle half) of the FVC.	• This measure provides a more sensitive index of obstruction in the smaller airways.
FRC (functional residual capacity) is the amount of air remaining in the lungs after normal expiration. FRC requires use of the helium dilution technique.	• Increased FRC indicates hyperinflation of air trapping, which may result from obstructive pulmonary disease. FRC is normal or decreased in restrictive pulmonary diseases.
TLC (total lung capacity) is the amount of air in the lungs at the end of maximal inhalation.	• Increased TLC indicates air trapping associated with obstructive pulmonary disease. Decreased TLC indicates restrictive disease.
RV (residual volume) is the amount of air remaining in the lungs at the end of a full, forced exhalation.	• RV is increased in obstructive pulmonary disease such as emphysema.
DLCO (diffusion capacity of carbon monoxide) reflects the surface area of the alveolocapillary membrane. The client inhales a small amount of CO, holds for 10 sec, then exhales. The amount inhaled is compared with the amount exhaled.	• DLCO is reduced whenever the alveolocapillary membrane is diminished, as occurs in emphysema, pulmonary hypertension, and pulmonary fibrosis. It is increased with exercise and in conditions such as polycythemia and congestive heart disease.

TABLE 29–8

Five Indications for Exercise Testing
• To assess a client's functional capacity (ability to work and perform activities of daily living)
• To determine the reason for exercise limitation: cardiac, pulmonary, or poor conditioning
• To evaluate changes in exercise capacity related to disease or treatment
• To determine the basis for the development of a pulmonary rehabilitation program
• To determine whether supplemental oxygen is required during exercise

noscopy. These procedures are summarized in Table 29–9. The most common complications are those related to the medications and bleeding. Cardiac dysrhythmias are rare in the absence of hypoxemia.

Thoracentesis

Thoracentesis is the aspiration of pleural fluid or air from the pleural space. This procedure is used for diagnosis or treatment. Microscopic examination of the pleural fluid helps make a diagnosis. Pleural fluid may be drained to relieve pulmonary compression and the resultant respiratory distress caused by cancer, empyema, pleurisy, or tuberculosis. To assist in further assessment of the parietal pleura, thoracentesis is often followed by pleural biopsy. Thoracentesis also allows the instillation of medications into the pleural space, which may be necessary to prevent further fluid formation in certain cases of pleural effusion caused by lung cancer.

CLIENT PREPARATION. Adequate client preparation is essential before thoracentesis to ensure the client's cooperation during the procedure and to prevent complications. The nurse tells the client to expect a stinging sensation from the local anesthetic agent and a feeling of pressure when the needle is inserted. The nurse reinforces the importance of the client's not moving (avoiding coughing, deep breathing, or sudden movement) during the procedure to avoid puncture of the visceral pleura or lung.

Figure 29–11 illustrates appropriate positions for thoracentesis. These positions widen the intercostal spaces and permit the physician to have easy access to where the pleural fluid gravitates. The nurse properly positions and physically supports the client. Pillows are used to make the client comfortable and to provide physical support.

Before the procedure, the nurse checks the client's history for hypersensitivity to local anesthetic agents and checks to make sure the client has signed an informed consent. The entire chest or back is exposed, and the aspiration site is shaved if necessary. The actual site depends on the volume and location of the effusion, which are determined by radiography and physical examination procedures such as percussion.

PROCEDURE. Thoracentesis is usually done at the bedside, although ultrasonography or computed tomography

TABLE 29–9

Care of the Client Undergoing Endoscopic Tests for Respiratory Disorders

Procedure	Purpose and Description	Nursing Interventions	Rationale
Bronchoscopy	• To assess airway anatomy for tumors, obstruction, and atelectasis • To assist in the diagnosis of infection or cancer by biopsy of lesions; biopsy techniques include the brush biopsy and needle aspiration • To remove thick secretions, mucus plugs, or foreign bodies • A flexible fiberoptic bronchoscope is inserted through the mouth, nose, endotracheal tube, or tracheostomy tube. The procedure may be done in the operating room or the radiology department. Oxygen administration and blood pressure monitoring are standard procedures.	• Allow the client nothing by mouth for several hours before the test. • Assess for allergies to iodine, local anesthetics, or pretest medications. • Place pulse oximeter • Administer pretest medications (atropine, diazepam) as ordered. • Prepare the client for topical anesthetic administration into the oropharynx. • Remove the client's dentures if present. • After the procedure, monitor the client's vital signs for 15 min until stable and monitor for hemoptysis. • After the procedure, allow the client nothing by mouth until the gag reflex returns. • Discourage smoking, talking, and coughing for several hours.	• The client may aspirate gastric contents if vomiting occurs. • A knowledge of allergies helps prevent allergic reactions. • For continuous monitoring throughout the procedure. • Pretest medications help decrease secretions and reduce anxiety. • Explanations about the effects of the anesthetic agent (numbness and gagging) help to decrease anxiety. • Injury may occur if dentures are left in place. • Assessment helps the nurse detect respiratory distress and signs of complications related to the procedure. • Allowing the client nothing by mouth reduces the possibility of aspiration. • Throat irritation is decreased by avoiding these activities.
Laryngoscopy	• *Direct:* To detect or remove lesions or foreign bodies in the larynx or to diagnose cancer by removing tissue for biopsy or samples for culture. A fiberoptic laryngoscope is used. • *Indirect:* To assess the function of the vocal cords or to obtain tissue for biopsy. Observations are made during rest and phonation by using a laryngeal mirror, head mirror, and light source.	• Allow the client nothing by mouth for several hours before the test. • Assess the client for allergies to iodine, contrast media, or local anesthetics. • Administer pretest medications (atropine, diazepam) as ordered. • Assess the client for fears concerning the procedure. Assure the client that he or she will be monitored for any respiratory problems. • For indirect laryngoscopy, assist the client to sit in an upright position and encourage normal breathing. • After the procedure, allow the client nothing by mouth until the gag reflex returns. • Encourage coughing and fluid intake. • Assess vital signs frequently for 24 hr. Assess the client for bleeding. • After the procedure, administer lozenges or gargles as ordered.	• Aspiration is possible if vomiting occurs. • A knowledge of allergies helps prevent allergic reactions. • Pretest medications help decrease secretions and reduce anxiety. • Reassurance helps decrease fears about not being able to breathe during the procedure. • An upright sitting position facilitates the passage of the laryngeal mirror into the mouth. • The client may aspirate gastric contents if vomiting occurs. • Hydration and coughing promote the expectoration of secretions. • Frequent monitoring of vital signs enables the nurse to detect changes such as dyspnea. • Lozenges and gargles help to relieve sore throat.

Table continued on following page

TABLE 29–9

Care of the Client Undergoing Endoscopic Tests for Respiratory Disorders *Continued*

Procedure	Purpose and Description	Nursing Interventions	Rationale
Mediastinoscopy	• To inspect and remove samples for biopsy of lymph nodes that drain the lung • To detect metastasis of lung cancer • To obtain tissue for biopsy for diagnosis of tuberculosis or sarcoidosis • The procedure is done in the operating room with the client given local or general anesthesia; a suprasternal incision is used.	• Explain preoperative measures and the procedure to the client. • Postoperatively, assess the client for bleeding, pneumothorax, and vocal cord paralysis. • Assess the client for pain, and administer analgesics as ordered.	• Explanations about the anticipated procedure help to decrease anxiety. • Ongoing assessment for complications helps to ensure prompt treatment. • Medication decreases discomfort associated with the procedure.

may be used to guide it. After draping the client and cleaning the skin with a germicidal solution, the physician uses aseptic technique and injects a local anesthetic agent into the selected intercostal space. The nurse keeps the client informed of the procedure while observing for shock, pain, nausea, pallor, diaphoresis, cyanosis, tachypnea, and dyspnea. The physician advances the short 18- to 25-gauge thoracentesis needle with a syringe attached into the pleural space. Gentle suction is applied as the fluid in the pleural space is slowly aspirated. A vacuum collection bottle is sometimes necessary to remove larger volumes of fluid. To prevent reexpansion pulmonary

edema, no more than 1000 mL of fluid is removed at one time (Bordow & Moser, 1996, p. 57). If a pleural biopsy is to be performed, a second, larger needle with a cutting edge and collection chamber is used (Luce et al., 1993, p. 95). After the physician withdraws the needle, pressure is applied to the puncture site, followed by the application of a small sterile dressing.

FOLLOW-UP CARE. After thoracentesis, the physician orders a chest x-ray to rule out possible pneumothorax and subsequent mediastinal shift. The nurse monitors the client's vital signs and auscultates breath sounds while

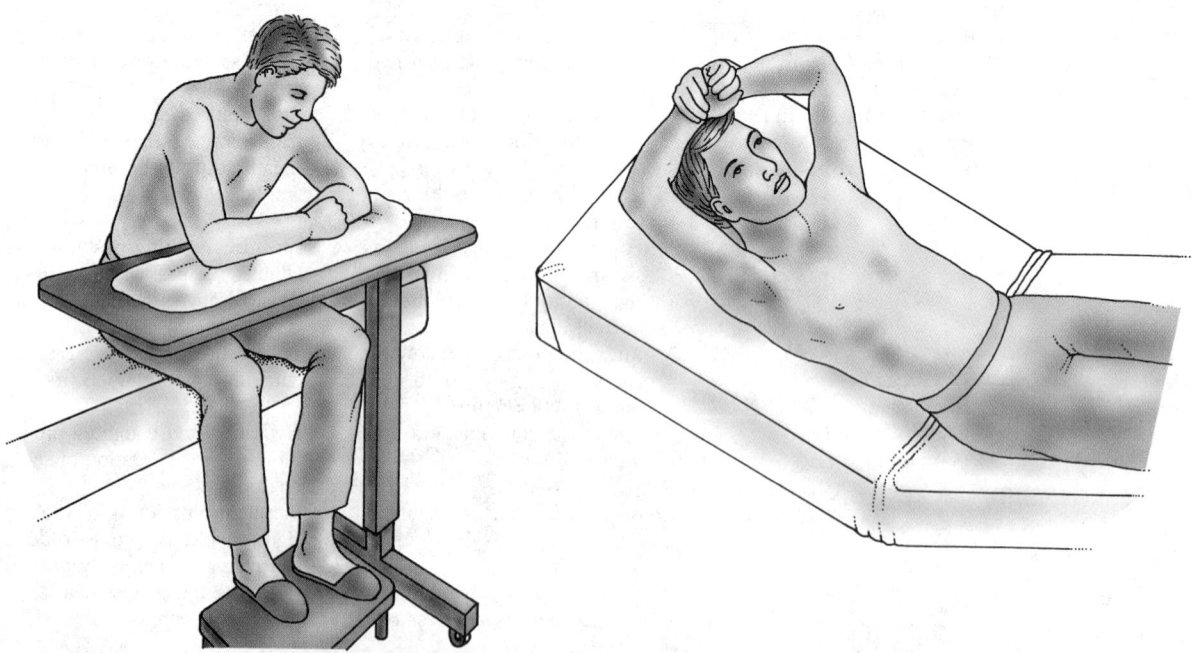

Sitting on the edge of a bed with the feet supported. The arms and shoulders are elevated, and the head is resting on the overbed table, which is padded with pillows or bath blankets.

Sitting in bed in semi-Fowler's position with the arm on the side on which the procedure will be performed raised above the head. The other arm may be used to hold the one arm as still as possible.

Figure 29–11. Positions for thoracentesis.

noting absent or diminished sounds on the affected side. The nurse observes the puncture site and dressing for leakage or bleeding. The nurse also assesses for other complications after thoracentesis, such as reaccumulation of fluid in the pleural space, subcutaneous emphysema, pyrogenic infection, and tension pneumothorax. The client is encouraged to breathe deeply to promote reexpansion of the lung. The nurse documents the procedure in the client's chart and notes the client's tolerance, the volume and character of the fluid removed, any specimens sent to the laboratory, the location of the puncture site, and respiratory assessment findings before, during, and after the procedure.

Lung Biopsy

Lung biopsy is performed to obtain tissue for histologic analysis, culture, or cytologic examination. The physician uses tissue samples to make a definite diagnosis regarding the type of malignancy, infection, inflammation, or other type of lung disease. Biopsy procedures include transbronchial biopsy (TBB) and transbronchial needle aspiration (TBNA), both performed in conjunction with bronchoscopy; transthoracic needle aspiration (percutaneous approach for areas not accessible by bronchoscopy); and open lung biopsy (in the operating room).

CLIENT PREPARATION. The nurse prepares the client by explaining what the client can expect before and after the biopsy. The client may have predetermined ideas about the outcome. The terms *biopsy* and *cancer* may be closely associated in the client's mind, so the nurse explores the client's feelings and fears before and after the procedure. To reduce discomfort and anxiety, the physician may prescribe an analgesic or sedative before the procedure. The nurse informs the client undergoing percutaneous biopsy that discomfort is minimized by the administration of a local anesthetic agent, but that the client may experience a sensation of pressure during insertion of the needle and aspiration of the tissue. For an open lung biopsy, the usual preoperative preparations apply.

PROCEDURE. Percutaneous lung biopsy may be performed in the client's room or in the radiology department after an informed consent has been obtained. Fluoroscopy, CT, or ultrasonography is frequently used to better visualize the area undergoing biopsy and to guide the procedure. Positioning of the client is similar to that for thoracentesis. The physician cleans the skin with an antibacterial agent and then administers a local anesthetic agent. Under sterile conditions, the physician inserts a spinal-type 18- to 22-gauge needle through the skin into the desired area (e.g., tissue, nodule, or lymph node) and obtains the tissue needed for microscopic examination. The nurse then applies a dressing.

Open lung biopsy is performed in the operating room. The client undergoes thoracotomy where lung tissue is exposed. At least two tissue specimens are taken (usually from an upper lobe and a lower lobe site). The surgeon places a chest tube to remove air and fluid so the lung can reinflate and then closes the chest.

FOLLOW-UP CARE. The nurse monitors the client's vital signs and breath sounds every 4 hours for 24 hours and assesses for signs of respiratory distress (e.g., dyspnea, pallor, diaphoresis, and tachypnea). Pneumothorax is the major complication after needle biopsy and open lung biopsy, so it is important for the nurse to report untoward signs and symptoms promptly. The nurse also monitors for hemoptysis, which may be scant and transient, or, in rare cases, for frank bleeding from vascular or lung trauma during the procedure.

SELECTED BIBLIOGRAPHY

*American College of Chest Physicians and the American Thoracic Society Joint Committee on Pulmonary Nomenclature. (1975). Pulmonary terms and symbols. *Chest, 67,* 583–593.

*Avalos-Bock, S. (1994). Getting a rise out of tuberculosis with the P.P.D. skin test. *Nursing, 24*(8), 51–53.

Bates, B. (1995). *A guide to physical examination and history taking* (6th ed.). Philadelphia: J. B. Lippincott.

Bordow, R. A., & Moser, K. M. (1996). *Manual of clinical problems in pulmonary medicine* (4th ed.). Boston: Little, Brown.

Burchfiel, C. M., Marcus, E. B., Curb, J. D., et al. (1995). Effects of smoking and smoking cessation on longitudinal decline in pulmonary function. *American Journal of Respiratory and Critical Care Medicine, 151,* 1778–1785.

*Carrieri-Kohlman, V., Douglas, M., Gormley, J., & Stulborg, M. (1993). Desensitization and guided mastery: Treatment approaches for the management of dyspnea. *Heart & Lung, 22*(3), 226–234.

Carroll, P. (1997). Pulose oximetry at your fingertips. *RN, 60*(2), 22–27.

Cerveri, I., Zoia, M. C., Fanfulla, F., et al. (1995). Reference values of arterial oxygen tension in the middle-aged and elderly. *American Journal of Respiratory and Critical Care Medicine, 152,* 934–941.

*Clemente, C. D. (Ed.). (1985). *Gray's anatomy of the human body* (30th ed.). Philadelphia: Lea & Febiger.

*Davis, D., & Scarpa, N. (1991). Transbronchial needle aspiration. *Gastroenterology Nursing, 14*(2), 80–84.

George, R. B., Light, R. W., Matthay, M. A., & Matthay, R. A. (1995). *Chest medicine: Essentials of pulmonary and critical care medicine* (3rd ed.). Baltimore: Williams & Wilkins.

*Gift, A. G. (1990). Dyspnea. *Nursing Clinics of North America, 25*(4), 955–965.

Guyton, A. C. (1996). *Textbook of medical physiology* (9th ed.). Philadelphia: W. B. Saunders.

Jarvis, C. (1996). *Physical examination and health assessment* (2nd ed.). Philadelphia: W. B. Saunders.

*Kernicki, J. G. (1993). Differentiating chest pain: Advanced assessment techniques. *Dimensions of Critical Care Nursing, 12*(2), 66–76.

*Kersten, L. D. (1989). *Comprehensive respiratory nursing: A decision making approach.* Philadelphia: W. B. Saunders.

Kirton, C. A. (1996). Assessing breath sounds. *Nursing, 26*(6), 50–51.

*Kuhn, J. K., & McGovern, M. (1992). Respiratory assessment of the elderly. *Journal of Gerontological Nursing, 18*(5), 40–43.

*Lehrer, S. (1993). *Understanding lung sounds* (2nd ed.). Philadelphia: W. B. Saunders.

Levitzky, M. G. (1995). *Pulmonary physiology* (4th ed.). New York: McGraw-Hill.

*Luce, J. M., Pierson, D. J., & Tyler, M. L. (1993). *Intensive respiratory care* (2nd ed.). Philadelphia: W. B. Saunders.

Matteson, M. A., McConnell, E. S., & Linton, A. D. (1997). *Gerontological nursing: Concepts and practice* (2nd ed.). Philadelphia: W. B. Saunders.

*Mikami, R., Murao, M., Cugell, D. W., et al. (1987). International Symposium on Lung Sounds: Synopsis of proceedings. *Chest, 92,* 342–345.

*Nield, M., & Kim, M. J. (1991). The reliability of magnitude estimation for dyspnea measurement. *Nursing Research, 40*(1), 17–19.

Paoletti, P., Carrozzi, L., Viegi, G., et al. (1995). Distribution of bronchial responsiveness in a general population: Effect of sex, age, smoking, and level of pulmonary function. *American Journal of Respiratory and Critical Care Medicine, 151,* 1770–1777.

Parker, S. L., Tong, T., Bolden, S., & Wingo, P. A. (1997). Cancer statistics, 1997. *CA-A Cancer Journal for Clinicians, 47*(1), 5–27.

*Report of the American College of Chest Physicians and the American Thoracic Society Ad Hoc Subcommittee on Pulmonary Nomenclature. (1977). *ATS News, 3,* 5–6.

Springhouse Corp. (1995). A quick look at common respiratory patterns. *Nursing, 25*(1), 32L.

Tietz, N. W. (1995). *Clinical guide to laboratory tests* (3rd ed.). Philadelphia: W. B. Saunders.

Villar, M. T. A., Dow, L., Coggon, D., et al. (1995). The influence of increased bronchial responsiveness, atopy, and serum IgE on decline in FEV1. *American Journal of Respiratory and Critical Care Medicine, 151,* 656–662.

*Wilkins, R., Hodghin, J., & Lopez, B. (1988). *Lung sounds: A practical approach.* St. Louis: C. V. Mosby.

*Williams, T. F. (Ed.). (1984). *Rehabilitation in the aging.* New York: Raven.

SUGGESTED READINGS

Avalos-Bock, S. (1994). Getting a rise out of tuberculosis with the P.P.D. skin test. *Nursing, 24*(8), 51–53.
    The article includes clear photographs showing the steps to take in placing a P.P.D. Interpretation of results, even for high-risk groups, is included. Proper documentation of the test and results is addressed.

Carroll, P. (1997). Pulse oximetry at your fingertips. *RN, 60*(2), 22–27.
    This clear and concise article covers a number of items related to determining a client's state of oxygenation, including dissolved oxygen versus bound oxygen, the importance of knowing the client's hemoglobin to interpret the pulse oximetry reading accurately, and an explanation of technical factors such as motion and ambient light that can affect readings. The formula for calculating a client's overall oxygen-carrying capacity is included, as is an explanation of the graphic relationship between the PaO_2 and the oxygen saturation.

Springhouse Corp. (1995). A quick look at common respiratory patterns. *Nursing, 25*(1), 32L.
    This one-page chart identifies the characteristics of eight different respiration patterns, including Cheyne-Stokes respirations, cluster breathing, and apneustic breathing. A drawing accompanies each pattern.

Chapter 30

INTERVENTIONS FOR CLIENTS WITH OXYGEN OR TRACHEOSTOMY

CHAPTER HIGHLIGHTS

Oxygen Therapy

Overview

Oxygen (O_2) is a potent drug prescribed by the physician for relief of symptoms of hypoxemia (low levels of oxygen in the blood) and its resultant hypoxia (decreased tissue oxygenation). The usual oxygen content of atmospheric air is approximately 21%; supplemental oxygen is prescribed when oxygen needs of the body cannot be met on "room air" alone. Oxygen is used for both episodic (acute) and subacute or chronic respiratory conditions associated with decreased partial pressure of arterial oxygen (PaO_2) levels. Oxygen therapy is indicated in conditions outside the respiratory system such as increased oxygen demand, decreased oxygen-carrying capability of the blood, and decreased cardiac output. Conditions that increase oxygen demand include sepsis, fever, and the increased workload of dyspnea. Insufficient amounts of hemoglobin or altered hemoglobin quality result in the inability of the hemoglobin to carry enough oxygen to the tissues.

The goal of oxygen therapy is to use the lowest fraction of inspired oxygen (FIO_2) to produce the most acceptable oxygenation without causing the development of harmful side effects. Although oxygen improves the PaO_2 level, it does not cure the condition or stop the disease process.

The average client requires an oxygen flow of 2–4 L/minute via nasal cannula or up to 40% via Venturi mask. The client who is hypoxemic and also has chronic hypercarbia requires lower levels of oxygen delivery, usually 1–2 L/minute via nasal cannula. A low arterial oxygen level is this client's primary drive for breathing.

Collaborative Management

 Assessment

Arterial blood gas (ABG) analysis is the best tool for determining the need for oxygen therapy and for evaluating its effects. Oxygen need can also be determined by noninvasive monitoring, such as pulse oximetry.

 Interventions

The nurse administers oxygen as per physician order or approved protocol. Before initiating oxygen therapy and while caring for a client receiving oxygen therapy, the nurse is knowledgeable about associated hazards and complications. For a particular client, the nurse also knows the rationale and the expected outcome related to oxygen therapy.

➤ *Hazards and Complications of Oxygen
Therapy*

Oxygen therapy is associated with several hazards and complications. Understanding these hazards and complications, the nurse can detect early signs and symptoms.

Combustion. Oxygen itself does not burn, but it supports combustion. Therefore, a fire burns more readily in the presence of oxygen. The nurse takes special precautions, including posting a sign on the door of the client's room. During the administration of oxygen, smoking is prohibited in the client's room, including at home. All electrical equipment must be grounded (i.e., with three prongs having a green or red dot on the plate). Frayed cords must be repaired because they can cause a spark that can ignite a flame. Any type of flammable solution containing alcohol or oil is prohibited from the room when oxygen is in use.

Oxygen-Induced Hypoventilation. The nurse assesses for oxygen-induced hypoventilation in the client whose principal respiratory drive is hypoxia (hypoxic drive), as in the client with chronic lung disease who also has hypercarbia. Arterial carbon dioxide level ($PaCO_2$) for these clients gradually rises over time. The central chemoreceptors in the brain (medulla) are normally sensitive to high $PaCO_2$ levels, which stimulate breathing and cause an increased respiratory rate. When the $PaCO_2$ increases above 60–65 mmHg, however, this normal mechanism shuts off. At that point, peripheral chemoreceptors found in the carotid and aortic arch bodies become the major stimulus for breathing. These peripheral receptors are sensitive to low PaO_2 levels. When PaO_2 drops below 55–60 mmHg, these receptors signal the brain to increase the respiratory rate or depth, which results in a hypoxic drive to breathe (Fig. 30–1).

The hypoxic drive occurs only in the presence of severely elevated $PaCO_2$ levels (i.e., in the client who has hypoxemia *and* hypercarbia). When the client with PaO_2 levels less than 55–60 mmHg (and $PaCO_2$ levels greater than 60–65 mmHg) receives oxygen therapy, the PaO_2 level increases. The hypoxic drive, however, the only stimulation for breathing, is eliminated. As a result, the client experiences respiratory depression that could lead to apnea or respiratory arrest. (The client being ventilated mechanically will not be at risk for this complication.)

The physician prescribes oxygen therapy at the lowest liter flow (usually 1–2 or 3 L/minute) necessary to treat the hypoxemia without raising the $PaCO_2$. A system that delivers precise oxygen concentrations in low amounts, such as a nasal cannula or Venturi mask, is preferred for this client.

The nurse closely monitors the respiratory rate and depth while the client is receiving oxygen. This monitoring is especially important when it is the first time the client has received oxygen or when the $PaCO_2$ levels are not known. Signs and symptoms of hypoventilation are seen during the first 30 minutes of oxygen administration; the client's color improves (from ashen or gray to pink) related to an increase in the PaO_2 level before the apnea or respiratory arrest occurs from the loss of the hypoxic drive. The nurse, therefore, questions oxygen orders for clients at risk for oxygen-induced hypoventilation, apnea, and respiratory arrest.

Oxygen Toxicity. Oxygen toxicity is related to the concentration of oxygen delivered, duration of oxygen therapy, and degree of lung disease present before oxygen therapy is started. In general, an oxygen concentration greater than 50% administered continuously for more than 24–48 hours may damage the lungs.

The pathophysiologic mechanism and clinical manifestations of lung injury associated with oxygen toxicity are the same as those for adult respiratory distress syndrome (ARDS) (see Chap. 34). The nurse observes for initial symptoms, which include nonproductive cough, substernal chest pain, gastrointestinal (GI) upset, and dyspnea. As exposure to high concentrations of oxygen continues, the symptoms become more severe and are accompanied by decreased vital capacity, decreased compliance (which results in more dyspnea), crackles, and hypoxemia. Prolonged exposure to high concentrations of oxygen causes structural damage to the lungs. Atelectasis, pulmonary edema, pulmonary hemorrhages, and hyaline membrane formation result. Mortality depends on the ability of the health care team to correct the underlying disease process and to decrease the oxygen amount delivered.

The toxic effects of oxygen are difficult to treat; hence, the physician orders the lowest concentration of oxygen required by the client to prevent oxygen toxicity. The nurse closely monitors arterial blood gases during oxygen administration and notifies the physician of PaO_2 levels greater than 100 mmHg. The nurse also monitors the prescribed oxygen concentration and length of time of administration to identify the client at higher risk. High concentrations of oxygen are avoided unless absolutely necessary. The addition of continuous positive airway pressure (CPAP) with an oxygen mask, bilevel positive airway pressure (Bi-Pap) or positive end-expiratory pres-

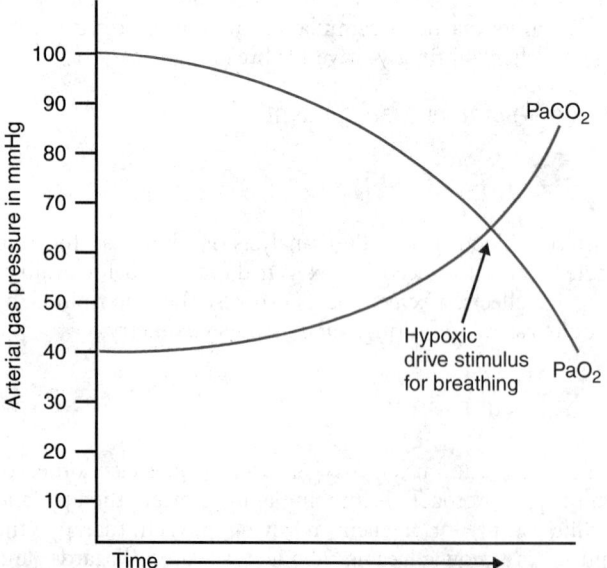

Figure 30–1. Arterial gas changes in chronic lung disease, showing the point at which the hypoxic drive becomes the stimulus for breathing.

sure (PEEP) on the mechanical ventilator (see Chap. 34) may reduce the amount of oxygen needed. As soon as the client's clinical condition allows, the physician decreases the prescribed amount of oxygen.

Absorption Atelectasis. Nitrogen normally plays a large role in the maintenance of patent airways and alveoli. Making up 79% of room air, it prevents alveolar collapse. When high concentrations of oxygen are delivered, nitrogen is washed out, oxygen diffuses from the alveoli into the pulmonary circulation, and the alveoli collapse. Collapsed alveoli cause atelectasis, called absorption atelectasis, which the nurse detects by auscultation. The nurse monitors the client closely for crackles and decreased breath sounds every 1–2 hours when the client is initially placed on oxygen therapy and frequently thereafter.

Drying of the Mucous Membranes. When an oxygen flow rate higher than 2 L/minute is needed, the nurse adds humidification upon order (Fig. 30–2). The nurse ensures that a constant mist of humidification escapes from the vents of the delivery system during inspiration and expiration. A sufficient amount of sterile water must be in the humidification container, and an adequate flow rate must be maintained so that proper humidification is delivered to the client. Condensation often forms in the tubing and is removed as needed by disconnecting the tubing and emptying the water into an appropriate receptacle. Some manufacturers place a water trap that hangs from the tubing so the nurse can drain the condensation without disconnecting. For prevention of bacterial contamination, the nurse never drains the fluid back into the humidification container. The nurse checks the water level and changes the humidifier as needed.

Oxygen can also be humidified via a nebulizer in mist form (aerosol). A heated nebulizer raises the humidity even more and is used when oxygen is administered via an artificial airway. Usually the upper airway passages have sufficient warming ability, but these passages are bypassed when an artificial airway is in use.

Infection. As mentioned, the humidification system may be a source of bacteria. *Pseudomonas aeruginosa* is frequently the organism involved. Oxygen delivery equipment such as cannulas and masks can also harbor organisms. The nurse changes equipment as per policy or protocol, which can range from 24 hours for humidification systems to every 7 days or whenever necessary for cannulas and masks.

Oxygen Delivery Systems. Oxygen can be delivered by numerous systems. Regardless of the type of delivery system used, the nurse needs to understand its indications, advantages, and disadvantages. Knowing the rationale for the oxygen delivery system used for a particular client, the nurse uses the equipment properly and ensures appropriate equipment maintenance. The type of delivery system depends on the following:

- Oxygen concentration required by the client
- Oxygen concentration achieved by a delivery system
- Importance of accuracy and control of the oxygen concentration
- Client comfort
- Expense to the client
- Importance of humidity
- Client mobility

Oxygen delivery systems are classified according to the rate at which oxygen is delivered. There are two systems: low-flow systems and high-flow systems. Low-flow systems do not provide enough oxygen to meet the total inspiratory effort of the client. Part of the tidal volume is supplied by the client's inspiring room air. The total concentration of oxygen received depends on respiratory rate and tidal volume. In contrast, high-flow systems provide a flow rate that is adequate to meet the entire inspiratory effort and tidal volume of the client regardless of the respiratory pattern. High-flow systems are used for critically ill clients and when it is particularly important to know the precise concentration of oxygen being delivered.

If the client requires a mask but is able to eat, the nurse requests an order for a nasal cannula at an appropriate liter flow for mealtimes only. The nurse replaces the mask after the meal is completed. To increase the client's mobility, up to 50 feet of connecting tubing can be used with proper connecting pieces. Other nursing interventions are listed in Chart 30–1.

Low-Flow Oxygen Delivery Systems

Low-flow delivery systems include the nasal cannula, simple face mask, partial rebreather mask, and non-rebreather mask (Table 30–1). These systems are inexpensive, easy to use, and fairly comfortable for the client. A major disadvantage is that the actual amount of oxygen obtained per liter is variable and depends on the client's breathing pattern. The oxygen delivered by the system is diluted with room air (21%), which lowers the amount of oxygen the client actually receives.

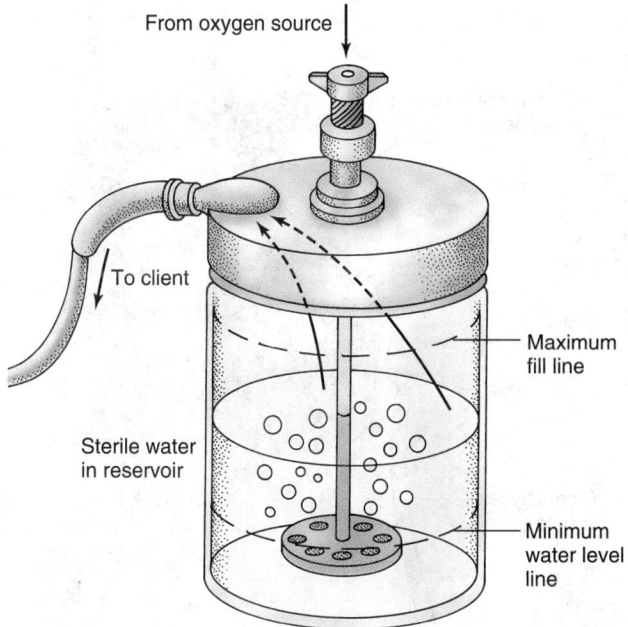

From oxygen source

To client

Maximum fill line

Sterile water in reservoir

Minimum water level line

Figure 30–2. A bubble humidifier bottle used with oxygen therapy.

Chart 30–1

Nursing Care Highlight: The Client Receiving Oxygen Therapy

- Check the physician's order with the type of delivery system and liter flow or percentage of oxygen actually in use.
- Obtain an order for humidification if oxygen is being delivered at 2 L/minute or more.
- Be sure the oxygen and humidification equipment is functioning properly.
- Check the skin around the client's ears, back of the neck, and face every 4 to 8 hours for pressure points and signs of irritation.
- Provide mouth care every 8 hours and as needed; assess nasal and oral mucous membranes for cracks or other signs of dryness.
- Pad the elastic band and change its position frequently to prevent skin breakdown.
- Cleanse cannula or mask by rinsing with clear warm water every 4 to 8 hours or as needed.
- Cleanse skin under tubing, straps, and mask every 4 to 8 hours or as needed.
- Lubricate the client's nostrils, face, and lips with water-soluble jelly to relieve the drying effects of oxygen.
- Position the tubing so it does not pull on the client's face, nose, or artificial airway.
- Ensure that there is no smoking and that no candles or matches are lit in the immediate area.
- Assess and document the client's response to oxygen therapy.
- Provide the client with ongoing teaching and reassurance to enhance the client's compliance with oxygen therapy.

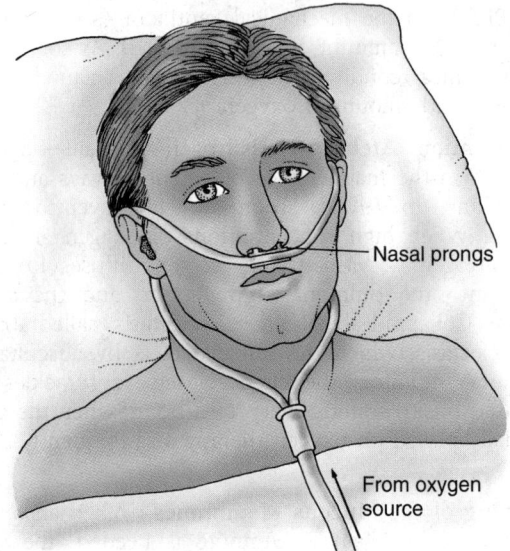

Figure 30–3. A nasal cannula (prongs).

Nasal Cannula. The nasal cannula, or nasal prongs (Fig. 30–3), is used at flow rates of 1–6 L/minute. Approximate oxygen concentrations of 24% (at 1 L/minute) to 44% (at 6 L/minute) can be achieved. Flow rates greater than 6 L/minute do not significantly increase oxygenation because the anatomic reserve or dead space (oral and nasal cavities) is full. In addition, high flow rates increase mucosal irritation. With the use of a nasal cannula, an effective oxygen concentration can be delivered to both nose breathers and mouth breathers.

The nasal cannula is frequently used for the client with chronic lung disease and for long-term maintenance of clients with other illnesses. The client who retains carbon dioxide rarely receives oxygen at a rate higher than 2–3 L/minute because of the concern of apnea or respiratory arrest. The nurse places the nasal prongs in the nostrils, with the openings facing the client.

Simple Face Mask. A simple face mask is used to deliver oxygen concentrations of 40% to 60% for short-term oxygen therapy or in an emergency (Fig. 30–4). A minimal flow rate of 5 L/minute is needed to prevent the rebreathing of exhaled air. The nurse gives special attention to skin care and to the proper fitting of the mask so that inspired oxygen concentration is maintained.

Partial Rebreather Mask. A partial rebreather mask provides oxygen concentrations of 60% to 75%, with flow rates of 6–11 L/minute. It consists of a mask with a reservoir bag but no flaps (Fig. 30–5). The client first rebreathes one third of the exhaled tidal volume, which is high in oxygen, thus providing a high FIO_2. The nurse ensures that the bag remains slightly inflated at the end of inspiration; otherwise, the client will not be getting the desired oxygen prescription. If needed, the nurse calls the respiratory therapist for assistance.

Non-Rebreather Mask. A non-rebreather mask provides the highest concentration of the low-flow systems and can deliver an FIO_2 greater than 90%, depending on the client's ventilatory pattern. The non-rebreather mask

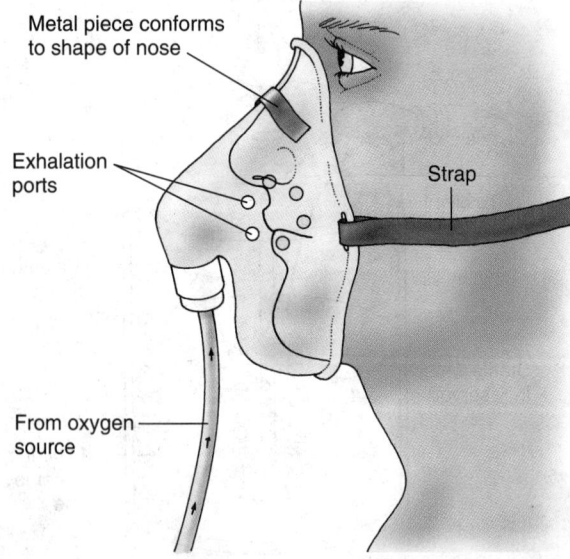

Figure 30–4. A simple face mask used to deliver oxygen.

TABLE 30–1

Comparison of Low-Flow Oxygen Delivery Systems

System	FIO$_2$ Delivered	Nursing Interventions	Rationale
Nasal cannula	24%–40% FIO$_2$ at 1–6 L/min ≈24% at 1 L/min ≈28% at 2 L/min ≈32% at 3 L/min ≈36% at 4 L/min ≈40% at 5 L/min ≈44% at 6 L/min	• Ensure that prongs are in the nares properly. • Provide water-soluble jelly to nares PRN. • Assess the patency of the nostrils. • Assess the client for changes in respiratory rate or depth.	• A poorly fitting nasal cannula leads to hypoxemia and skin breakdown. • This substance prevents mucosal irritation related to the drying effect of oxygen; promotes comfort. • Congestion or a deviated septum prevents effective delivery of oxygen through the nares. • The respiratory pattern affects the amount of oxygen delivered. A different delivery system may be needed.
Simple face mask	40%–60% FIO$_2$ at 5–8 L/min; flow rate must be set at least 5 L/min to flush mask of carbon dioxide ≈40% at 5 L/min ≈45%–50% at 6 L/min ≈55%–60% at 8 L/min	• Be sure mask fits securely over nose and mouth. • Assess skin and provide skin care to the area covered by the mask. • Monitor the client closely for risk of aspiration. • Provide emotional support to the client who feels claustrophobic. • Suggest to physician to switch the client from a mask to the nasal cannula during eating.	• A poorly fitting mask reduces the FIO$_2$ delivered. • Pressure and moisture under the mask may cause skin breakdown. • The mask limits the client's ability to clear the mouth, especially if vomiting occurs. • Emotional support decreases anxiety, which contributes to a claustrophobic feeling. • Use of the cannula prevents hypoxemia during eating.
Partial rebreather mask	60%–75% at 6–11 L/min, a liter flow rate high enough to maintain reservoir bag two thirds full during inspiration and expiration	• Make sure that the reservoir does not twist or kink, which results in a deflated bag. • Adjust the flow rate to keep the reservoir bag inflated.	• Deflation results in decreased oxygen delivered and rebreathing of exhaled air. • The flow rate is adjusted to meet the pattern of the client.
Non-rebreather mask	80%–95% FIO$_2$ at liter flow to maintain reservoir bag two thirds full	• Interventions as for partial rebreather mask; this client requires close monitoring. • Make sure that valves and rubber flaps are patent, functional, and not stuck. Remove mucus or saliva. • Closely assess the client on increased FIO$_2$ via non-rebreather mask. Intubation is the only way to provide more precise FIO$_2$.	• Rationales as for partial rebreather mask. • Monitoring ensures proper functioning and prevents harm. • Valves should open during expiration and close during inhalation to prevent dramatic decrease in FIO$_2$. Suffocation can occur if the reservoir bag kinks or if the oxygen source disconnects. • The client may require intubation.

is most frequently used for a client with deteriorating respiratory status who might soon require intubation.

The non-rebreather mask has a one-way valve between the mask and the reservoir and two flaps over the exhalation ports (Fig. 30–6). The valve allows the client to draw all needed oxygen from the reservoir bag, and the flaps prevent room air from entering through the exhalation ports. During exhalation, air leaves through these

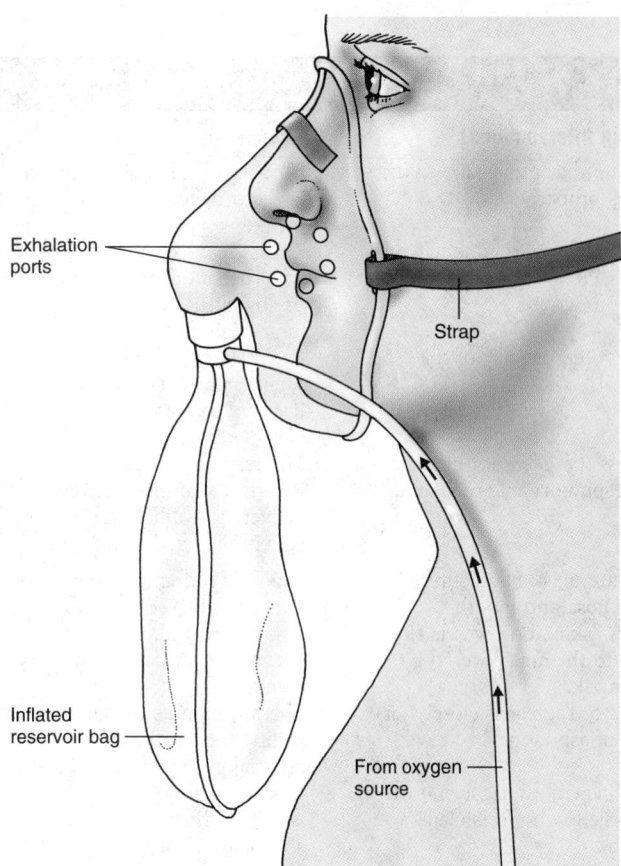

Figure 30–5. A partial rebreather mask.

exhalation ports while the one-way valve prevents exhaled air from re-entering the reservoir bag. It is crucial for the nurse to ensure that the valve and flaps are intact and functional during each breath. Some manufacturers include only one flap on the mask, or one of the exhalation flaps may be removed for safety purposes. If the oxygen source should fail or be depleted when both flaps are in place, the client would not be able to breathe in room air. The nurse assesses for this safety feature.

High-Flow Oxygen Delivery Systems

High-flow systems (Table 30–2) include the Venturi mask, aerosol mask, face tent, tracheostomy collar, and T-piece. These devices deliver a consistent and accurate oxygen concentration that meets the client's inspiratory effort when properly fitted. A high-flow system provides oxygen concentrations of 24% to 100% at 8–15 L/minute.

Venturi Mask. The Venturi mask (commonly called Venti mask) delivers the most accurate oxygen concentration. Its operation is based on a mechanism that pulls in a specific proportional amount of room air for each liter flow of oxygen. An adaptor is located between the bottom of the mask and the oxygen source (Fig. 30–7). Adaptors with holes of different sizes allow only specific amounts of air to mix with the oxygen. Precise delivery of oxygen results. Each adaptor also specifies the flow rate with which it is to be used; for example, to deliver 24% of oxygen, the flow rate must be 4 L/minute. Another type

of Venturi mask has one adaptor with a dial the nurse uses to select the amount of oxygen desired. Humidification is not necessary with the Venturi mask. The Venturi system is the best one for the client with chronic lung disease because it delivers a precise oxygen concentration.

Other High-Flow Systems. The face tent, aerosol mask, tracheostomy collar, and T-piece are often used to administer high humidity. A dial on the humidification source regulates the oxygen concentration being delivered. A face tent fits over the client's chin, with the top extending halfway across the face. The oxygen concentration varies, but the face tent is useful instead of a tight-fitting mask for the client who has facial trauma and burns. An aerosol mask is used for the client who requires high humidity after extubation or upper airway surgery or for the client who has thick secretions. The tracheostomy collar can be used to deliver high humidity and the desired oxygen to the client with a tracheostomy. A special adaptor, called the T-*piece,* can be used to deliver any desired FIO_2 to the client with a tracheostomy, laryngectomy, or endotracheal tube (Fig. 30–8). The flow rate is regulated so that the aerosol does not disappear on the exhalation side of the T-piece.

Transtracheal Oxygen Therapy

Transtracheal oxygen (TTO) is a long-term method of delivering oxygen directly into the lungs. The physician

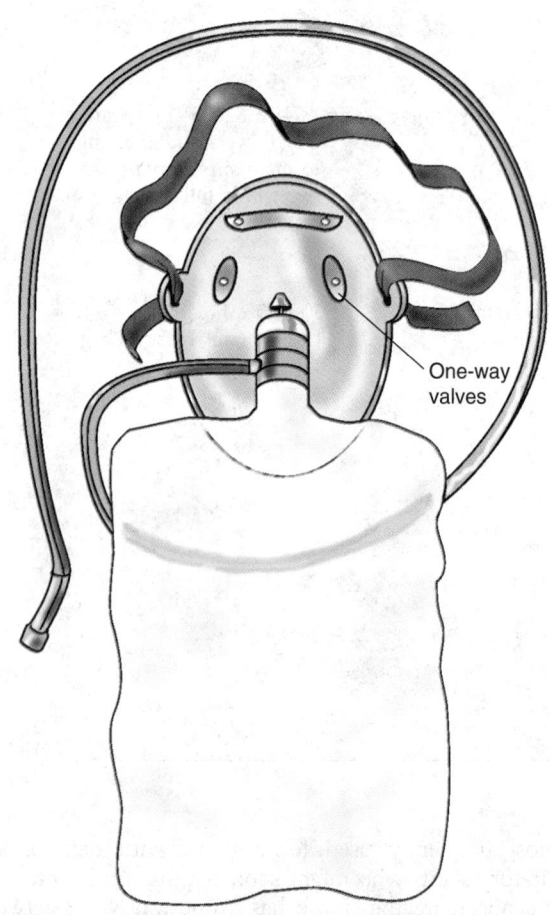

Figure 30–6. A non-rebreather mask.

TABLE 30–2

Comparison of High-Flow Oxygen Delivery Systems

System	FIO₂ Delivered	Nursing Interventions	Rationale
Venturi mask (Venti mask)	24%–55% FIO_2 with flow rates as recommended by the manufacturer, usually 4–10 L/min; provides high humidity	• Perform constant surveillance to ensure accurate flow rate for specific FIO_2. • Keep the orifice for the Venturi adaptor open and uncovered. • Provide a mask that fits snugly and tubing that is free of kinks. • Assess the client for dry mucous membranes. • Change to a nasal cannula during mealtimes.	• An accurate flow rate ensures FIO_2 delivery. • If the Venturi orifice is covered, the adaptor does not function and oxygen delivery varies. • FIO_2 is altered if kinking occurs or if the mask fits poorly. • Comfort measures may be indicated • Oxygen is a drug that needs to be given continuously.
Aerosol mask, face tent, tracheostomy collar	24%–100% FIO_2 with flow rates of at least 10 L/min; provides high humidity	• Assess that aerosol mist escapes from the vents of the delivery system during inspiration and expiration. • Empty condensation from the tubing. • Change the aerosol water container as needed.	• Humidification should be delivered to the client. • Emptying prevents the client from being lavaged with water and promotes an adequate flow rate. • Adequate humidification is ensured only when there is sufficient water in the canister.
T-piece	24%–100% FIO_2 with flow rates of at least 10 L/min; provides high humidity	• Empty condensation from the tubing. • Keep the exhalation port open and uncovered. • Position the T-piece so that it does not pull on the tracheostomy or endotracheal tube. • Make sure the humidifier creates enough mist. A mist should be seen during inspiration and expiration.	• Condensation interferes with flow rate and may drain into the tracheostomy if not emptied. • If the port is occluded, the client can suffocate. • The weight of the T-piece pulls on the tracheostomy and causes pain or erosion of skin at the insertion site. • An adequate flow rate is needed to meet the inspiration effort of the client. If not, FIO_2 is decreased.

passes a small, flexible catheter into the trachea via a small incision (Fig. 30–9A) with use of local anesthesia. TTO allows better compliance and avoids the irritation that nasal prongs cause. Clients also report it to be more cosmetically acceptable. A TTO team provides formal client education, including the purpose of TTO and care of the catheter. The physician prescribes a TTO flow rate for rest and for activity and a flow rate for the nasal cannula. The average client will have a 55% reduction of required oxygen flow at rest and a 30% decrease with activity.

SCOOP is one brand of catheter made by Transtracheal Systems. All SCOOP oxygen catheters (Fig. 30–9B) are made of kink-resistant thermoplastic polyurethane. Two opposing barium stripes provide x-ray visibility on the otherwise clear catheter. The outside diameter is 9 French (Fr). Overall length is 20 cm with a standard internal length of 11 cm. Nonstandard catheter lengths are also

available. The physician determines proper length after viewing the postprocedure x-ray with an 11-cm Pre-SCOOP stent in place. Oxygen is attached to the catheter using a SCOOP oxygen hose with a Luer taper connection. Catheters are sterilely packaged individually or in pairs and contain a cleaning rod(s), lubricating jelly, physician and client instructions, and a registration card.

 Continuing Care

➤ *Criteria for Home Oxygen Therapy*

The client must be clinically stable and optimally treated before the need for home oxygen is considered. For Medicare to cover the cost of continuous oxygen therapy, the client must have severe hypoxemia. For reimbursement purposes, severe hypoxemia is generally defined as a PaO_2

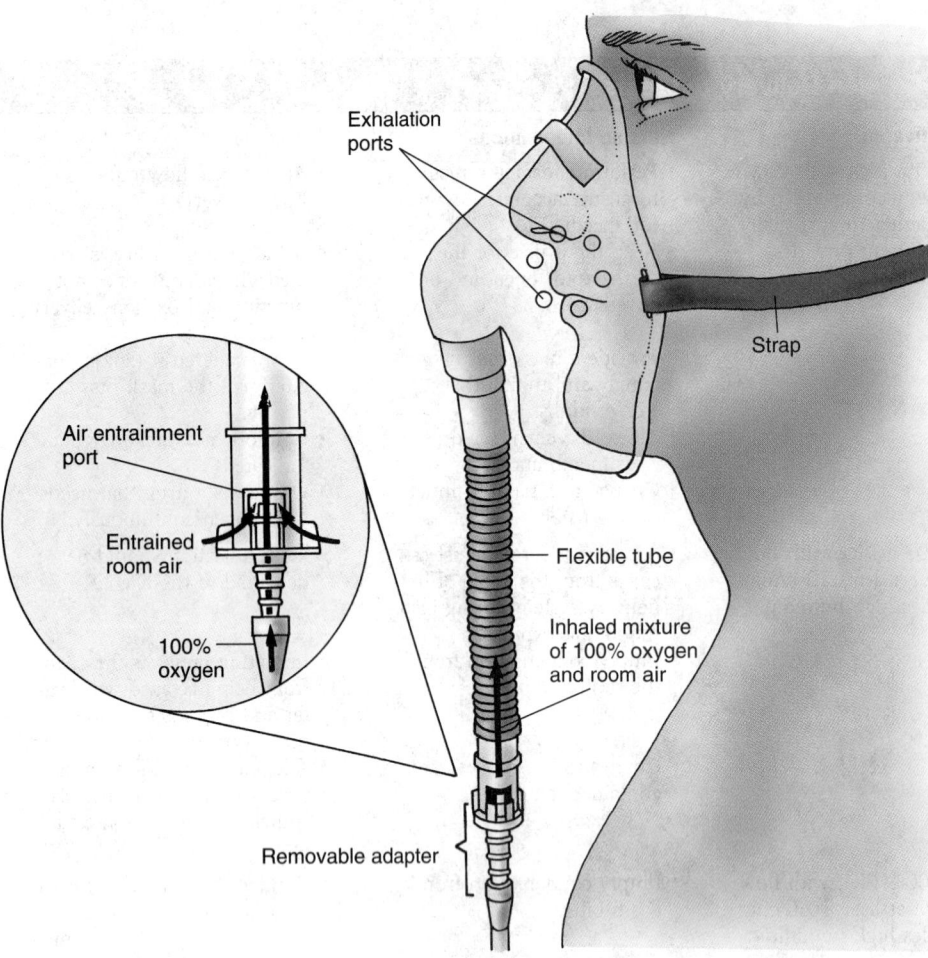

Exhalation ports

Strap

Air entrainment port

Entrained room air

100% oxygen

Flexible tube

Inhaled mixture of 100% oxygen and room air

Removable adapter

Figure 30–7. A Venturi mask for precise oxygen delivery.

level of less than 55 mmHg or an arterial oxygen saturation of less than 85% on room air and at rest. A variation of this criterion is a PaO_2 value of 56–59 mmHg or an arterial oxygen saturation value of 86% to 89% with a secondary diagnosis of symptomatic congestive heart failure, cor pulmonale as seen on an electrocardiogram, or erythrocytosis with a hematocrit of 56%. Specific criteria

Flexible tubing from oxygen source

T-piece adapter

Reservoir tube

15-mm adapter

Endotracheal tube

Figure 30–8. A T-piece apparatus for attachment to an endotracheal or tracheostomy tube.

are also established for coverage of nocturnal oxygen and portable oxygen therapy. Medicare guidelines are continually changing; therefore, it is important for the nurse to be aware of these criteria and the documentation required to meet the standards.

➤ Teaching About Home Oxygen Therapy

After the need for home oxygen therapy is verified, the nurse begins a teaching plan about oxygen therapy. The client, with the nurse's assistance, selects a durable medical equipment (DME) company to deliver oxygen equipment and a community health nursing agency for follow-up care in the home. The physician re-evaluates the client's need for oxygen therapy approximately 6 months after discharge from the health care facility and yearly thereafter.

While providing discharge planning and teaching, the nurse is sensitive to the client's psychological adjustment to oxygen therapy. The nurse encourages the client to share feelings and concerns. The client may be concerned about social acceptance and misconceptions of friends. The nurse helps the client realize that compliance with oxygen therapy is important so that normal activities of daily living (ADLs) and events that bring enjoyment can be continued.

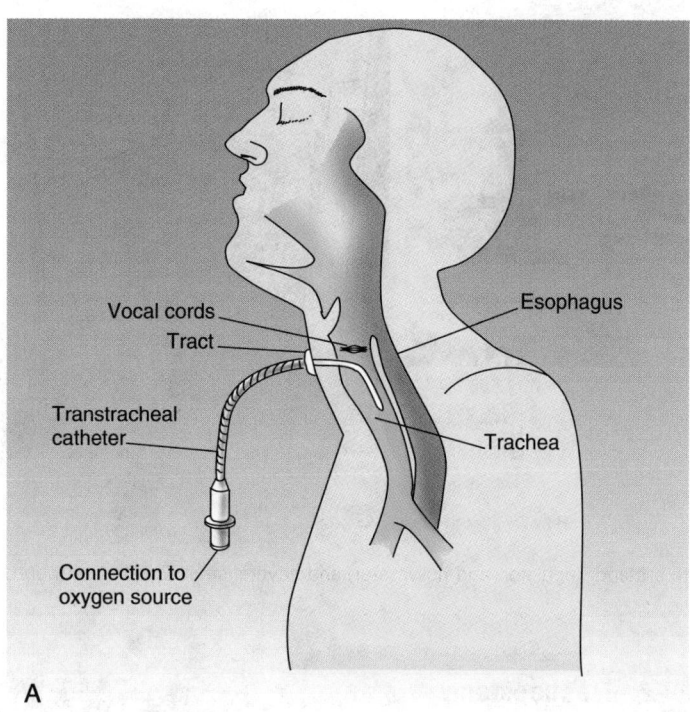

A

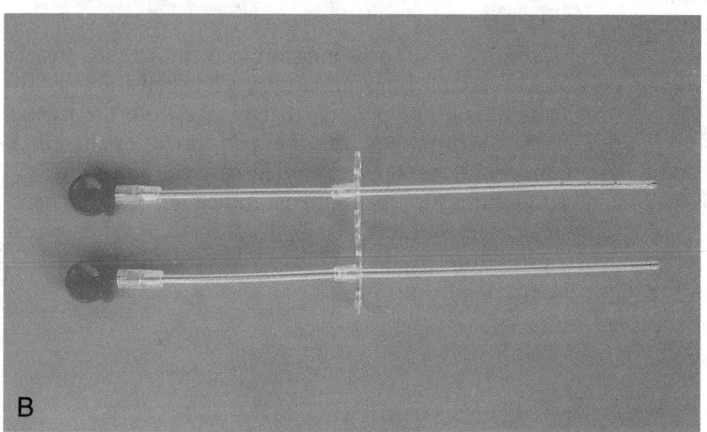

B

Figure 30–9. *A,* Example of transtracheal oxygen delivery. *B,* SCOOP-2 (*top*) and SCOOP-1 (*bottom*) transtracheal oxygen catheters. (*B,* Courtesy of Transtracheal Systems, Inc., Englewood, Co.)

➤ Equipment for Home Oxygen Therapy

The nurse or respiratory therapist teaches the client about the equipment needed for home oxygen therapy:

- Oxygen source
- Oxygen delivery device
- Humidification source
- Safety aspects of using and maintaining the equipment

Home oxygen is provided in one of three ways:

- Compressed gas in a tank or a cylinder
- Liquid oxygen in a reservoir
- An oxygen concentrator

Compressed gas in an oxygen tank (green) is the most common oxygen source. The large H cylinder is used as a stationary source; the small E tank is available for transporting the client (Fig. 30–10). As a safety precaution, the tanks must always be in a stand or rack. A tank that is accidentally knocked over could explode. Even smaller (and lighter) D or C cylinders are available for the client to carry. An oxygen tank is economical, and pure oxygen can be delivered at a wide range of flow rates.

The second type of home oxygen, liquid oxygen, is oxygen gas that has been liquefied by cooling to −300° F (−147° C); thus, a concentrated amount of oxygen is available in a lightweight and easy-to-carry container similar to a Thermos bottle (Fig. 30–11). This type of oxygen lasts longer than oxygen in a conventional tank of the same size; however, it is expensive, and the oxygen evaporates if it is not used continuously.

The last type of home oxygen source is the oxygen concentrator, which is a machine that removes nitrogen, water vapor, and hydrocarbons from room air. It is sometimes referred to as an oxygen extractor. Oxygen is concentrated from room air and is delivered at more than 90%. The concentrator is the least expensive of the systems but is not portable and is often noisy.

Humidification is rarely needed for any of these oxygen systems. Nevertheless, humidification may help when the physician prescribes a flow rate higher than 2 L/minute.

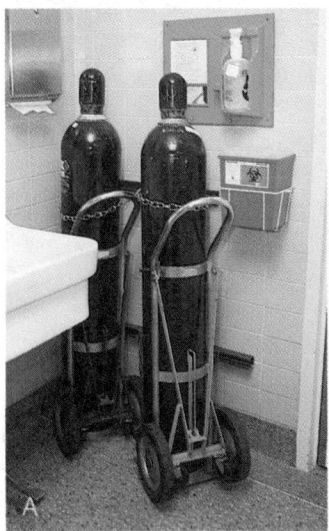
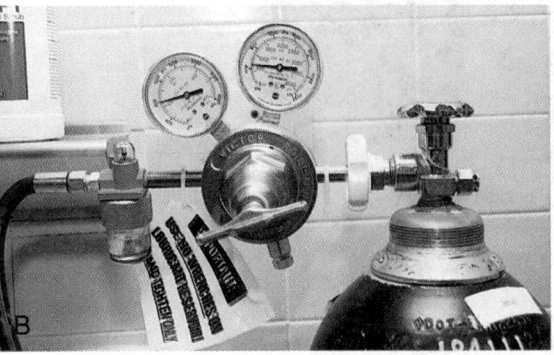
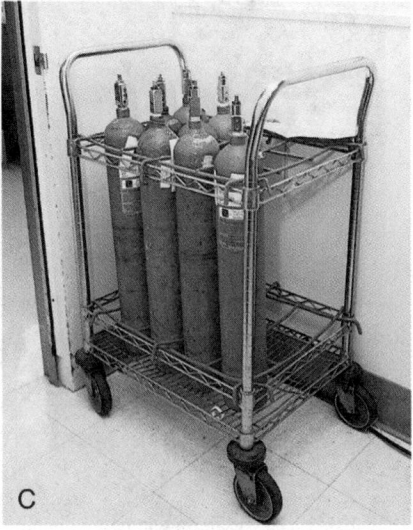

Figure 30–10. Comparison of a large H oxygen cylinder (*left*), with a stand, regulator, and flowmeter, and several small E cylinders (*right*).

In any of the three home oxygen systems, an oxygen-conserving reservoir-type nasal cannula can be used to reduce oxygen flow requirements by approximately 50%. Two types currently available are the mustache type and the pendant type. Attached to the tubing is a reservoir where exhaled oxygen is stored and then redelivered back to the client on the next inhalation. The reservoir sits on top of the upper lip (mustache type) or hangs around the neck (pendant type).

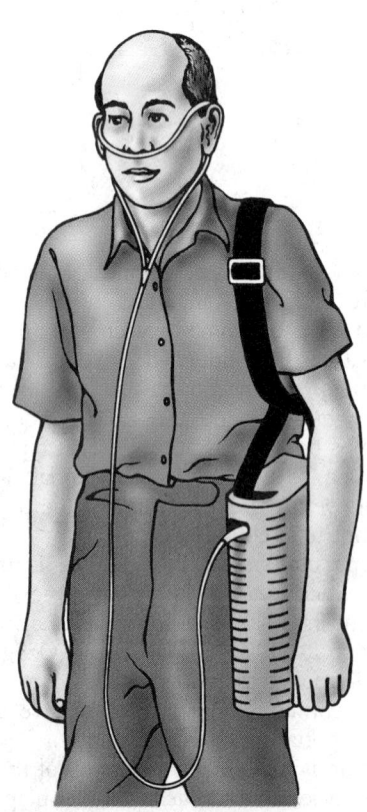

Figure 30–11. Liquid oxygen.

Tracheostomy

Overview

Tracheotomy is a surgical incision into the trachea for the purpose of establishing an airway. Tracheostomy is the (tracheal) stoma, or opening, that results from the tracheotomy. A tracheostomy can be performed as an emergency procedure or as a scheduled surgical procedure and can be temporary or permanent. Indications for tracheostomy are listed in Table 30–3. Tracheostomy as an emergency procedure for upper airway obstruction is covered in Chapter 31.

Collaborative Management

 Assessment

Assessment of the natural airway is covered in Chapter 31, as is assessment for upper airway obstruction. Assessment of a client with a tracheostomy is related to interventions that comprise nursing care for that client.

TABLE 30–3

Indications for Tracheostomy
• Acute airway obstruction when oral or nasal intubation is not feasible
• Airway protection (e.g., after head and neck cancer surgery)
• Prolonged intubation or need for mechanical ventilation
• Decreased airway dead space in combination with other indicators
• Control of pulmonary secretions refractory to conventional methods
• Airway reconstruction after laryngeal trauma or laryngeal cancer surgery
• Obstructive sleep apnea refractory to conventional therapy

Interventions

Once the determination of need for tracheostomy has been established, the nurse prepares the client for surgery.

Preoperative Care. The preoperative care for the client undergoing a tracheostomy is similar to that for a client scheduled for a laryngectomy (see Chap. 31). The nurse focuses on the client's knowledge deficits through teaching and discusses tracheostomy care, communication, and speech.

Operative Procedures. Initially, the anesthesiologist or nurse anesthetist extends the neck and places an endotracheal (ET) tube to maintain the airway. The surgeon then makes an incision through the anterior skin of the neck, dissects the subcutaneous tissue for exposure, separates the thyroid, and identifies the thyroid artery and tracheal rings. Another incision is made through the second and third or third and fourth tracheal rings to enter the trachea (Fig. 30–12). The types of incisions and specific techniques vary, depending on the surgeon's preference and the reason for the surgery.

After the surgeon enters the trachea, the ET tube is carefully removed while the tracheostomy tube is inserted. The surgeon secures the tracheostomy tube in place with sutures and tracheostomy ties and orders a chest x-ray to ensure proper placement of the tube. In clients who cannot be intubated, tracheostomy can be done with the client awake under local anesthesia.

Postoperative Care. Immediate postoperative nursing care focuses on ensuring a patent airway, confirming the presence of bilateral breath sounds, recovering the client from anesthesia, and assessing for complications from the procedure.

Complications. Six major complications may arise in the postoperative period: tube obstruction with secretions, tube dislodgment or accidental decannulation, pneumo-

thorax, subcutaneous emphysema, bleeding, and infection. Table 30–4 summarizes signs and symptoms, management, and prevention of other serious complications of tracheostomy.

Tube Obstruction. By helping the client with coughing and deep breathing, providing inner cannula care, humidifying the oxygen source, and suctioning, the nurse prevents secretions from obstructing the tube. If tube obstruction occurs as a result of cuff prolapse over the end of the tracheostomy tube, the physician repositions or replaces the tube. Specific signs and symptoms of obstruction include difficulty in breathing; noisy respirations from the tracheostomy; difficulty in inserting a suction catheter; thick, dry secretions; and unexplained peak pressures if a mechanical ventilator is in use.

Tube Dislodgment or Accidental Decannulation. The nurse prevents tube dislodgment and decannulation by securing the tube in place, thus minimizing manipulation and traction on the tube from oxygen or ventilator tubing or accidental pulling by the client. Tube dislodgment in the first 72 hours after surgery is a medical emergency because the tracheostomy tract has not matured and tissue planes are not well defined. Attempts at replacement of a fresh tracheostomy in this time frame can lead to cannulation of subcutaneous tissue planes instead of the trachea itself. In this situation, the nurse attempts to ventilate the client using a manual resuscitation bag while another nurse calls the resuscitation team for help.

The nurse ensures that a tracheostomy tube of the same type (including an obturator) and size (or one size smaller) is at the client's bedside at all times, along with a tracheostomy insertion tray. If decannulation occurs after 72 hours, the nurse extends the client's neck and opens the tissues of the stoma to secure the airway. With the obturator inserted into the tracheostomy tube, the nurse quickly and gently replaces the tube and removes the obturator. The nurse checks for airflow through the tube and for bilateral breath sounds. If unable to secure the airway, the nurse notifies a more experienced nurse or physician for assistance. The nurse attempts to ventilate via a bag-valve mask. If the client is in distress and further attempts to secure the airway fail, the nurse calls the resuscitation team, including an anesthesiologist, for assistance.

Pneumothorax. Pneumothorax (air in the chest cavity) can develop during the tracheostomy procedure if the thoracic cavity is accidentally entered. When pneumothorax occurs, it does so medially and superiorly at the apex of the lung. Chest x-ray after placement is used to assess for pneumothorax.

Subcutaneous Emphysema. When there is an opening (rent) in the trachea, air escapes into fresh tissue planes of the neck, causing subcutaneous emphysema. Air can also progress throughout the chest and axilla into the face. The nurse inspects and palpates for air under the skin of a client with a new tracheostomy.

Bleeding. A small amount of bleeding from the tracheostomy incision can be expected for the first few days,

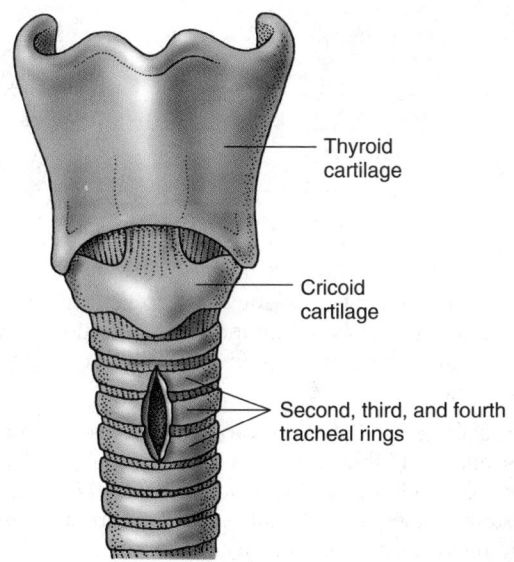

Figure 30–12. A vertical tracheal incision for a tracheostomy.

Thyroid cartilage

Cricoid cartilage

Second, third, and fourth tracheal rings

TABLE 30-4

Complications of Tracheostomy

Complications and Description	Signs and Symptoms	Management	Prevention
Tracheomalacia: constant pressure exerted by the cuff causes tracheal dilation and erosion of cartilage.	• An increased amount of air is required in the cuff to maintain the seal. • A larger tracheostomy tube is required to prevent an air leak at the stoma. • Food particles are seen in tracheal secretions. • The client does not receive tidal volume on the ventilator.	• No special management is needed unless bleeding occurs.	• Use an uncuffed tube as soon as possible. • Monitor cuff pressure and air volumes closely and detect changes.
Tracheal stenosis: narrowed tracheal lumen is due to scar formation from irritation of tracheal mucosa by the cuff.	• Stenosis usually seen after the cuff is deflated or the tracheostomy tube is removed. • The client has increased coughing; inability to expectorate secretions; or difficulty in breathing or talking.	• Tracheal dilation or surgical intervention is used.	• Prevent pulling of and traction on the tracheostomy tube. • Properly secure the tube in the midline position. • Maintain proper cuff pressure. • Minimize oronasal intubation time.
Tracheoesophageal fistula (TEF): excessive cuff pressure causes erosion of the posterior wall of the trachea. A hole is created between the trachea and the anterior esophagus. The client at highest risk also has a nasogastric tube present.	• Similar to tracheomalacia: • Food particles are seen in tracheal secretions. • Increased air in cuff is needed to achieve a seal. • The client has increased coughing and choking while eating. • The client does not receive the set tidal volume on the ventilator.	• Manually administer oxygen by mask to prevent hypoxemia. • A small soft feeding tube is used instead of a nasogastric tube for tube feedings. A gastrostomy or jejunostomy may be performed. • Monitor the client with a nasogastric tube closely; assess for TEF and aspiration.	• Maintain cuff pressure • Monitor the amount of air needed for inflation and detect changes. • Progress to deflated cuff or cuffless tube as soon as possible.
Trachea-innominate artery fistula: a malpositioned tube causes its distal tip to push against the lateral wall of the tracheostomy. Continued pressure causes necrosis and erosion of the innominate artery. **This is a medical emergency.**	• The tracheostomy tube pulsates in synchrony with the heart beat. • There is exsanguination from the stoma. • This is a life-threatening complication.	• Remove the tracheostomy tube immediately. • Apply direct pressure to the innominate artery at the stoma site. • Prepare the client for immediate repair surgery.	• Correct the tube size, length, and midline position. • Prevent pulling or tugging on the tracheostomy tube. • Immediately notify the physician of pulsating tube.

but constant oozing warrants surgical intervention, cauterization, or ligation of vessels. With physician order, the nurse wraps petroleum (Vaseline)-covered gauze around the tube and packs it gently into the wound to apply pressure to the bleeding sites.

Infection. While in the hospital, the nurse uses sterile technique to prevent infection during suctioning and tracheostomy care and assesses the stoma site for purulent drainage, redness, pain, swelling, or cellulitis. Tracheostomy dressings may be used to keep the stoma clean and dry; moist dressings provide an excellent medium for bacterial growth. Prevention and early detection of a local infection are, therefore, important. Diligent wound care prevents most local infections.

Tracheostomy Tubes. A variety of tracheostomy tubes are available (Table 30-5 and Fig. 30-13). The one chosen depends on the specific needs of the client. Tracheostomy tubes are available in numerous sizes and are made of various types of materials, such as plastic or metal. The tubes may be disposable or reusable. A tra-

TABLE 30–5

Types of Tracheostomy Tubes

Type	Description	Type	Description
Double-lumen tube	• The double-lumen tube has three major parts: • Outer cannula—fits into the stoma and keeps the airway open. The face plate indicates the size and type of tube and has small holes on both sides for securing the tube with tracheostomy ties. • Inner cannula—fits snugly into the outer cannula and locks into place. Provides the universal adaptor for use with the ventilator and other respiratory therapy equipment. Some may be removed, cleaned, and reused; others are disposable. • Obturator—is a stylet with a blunt end used to facilitate direction of the tube when inserting or changing a tracheostomy tube. It is removed immediately after tube placement and is always kept with the client and at the bedside in case of accidental decannulation.	Fenestrated tube	• The fenestrated tube has a precut opening (fenestration) in the upper posterior wall of the outer cannula. It is used to wean the client from a tracheostomy by ensuring that the client can tolerate breathing through his or her natural airway before the entire tube is removed. This tube allows the client to speak.
		Cuffed fenestrated tube	• The cuffed fenestrated tube facilitates mechanical ventilation and speech. It is often used for clients with spinal cord paralysis or neuromuscular disease who do not require ventilation all the time. When not on the ventilator, the client can have the cuff deflated and the tube capped for speech. A cuffed fenestrated tube is never used in weaning from a tracheostomy because the cuff, even fully deflated, may partially obstruct the airway.
Single-lumen tube	• The single-lumen tube is a long tube used for clients with long or extra thick necks. Often called a "bull neck trach" because of the long distance from the skin to the trachea or the longer length of the trachea in large people. More intensive nursing care is required with this tube because there is no inner cannula to ensure a patent lumen.	Metal tracheostomy tube	• The metal tracheostomy tube is used for permanent tracheostomy. It is a cuffless double-lumen tube and can be cleaned and reused indefinitely. A special adaptor attaches a manual resuscitation bag. Popular types are the Jackson and Holinger tubes.
Cuffed tube	• A cuff, when inflated, seals the airway. Used with mechanical ventilation, in preventing aspiration of oral or gastric secretions, or for tube feeding. A pilot balloon attached to the outside of the tube indicates the presence or absence of air in the cuff.	Talking tracheostomy tube	• The talking tracheostomy tube provides a means of communication for the client who is using a ventilator on a long-term basis. An extra air channel allows air to flow up through the vocal cords so that the client can speak with the cuff inflated. The air can cause drying of the vocal cords from constant dry airflow. Examples are the Pitt Trach Speaking Tube (National Catheter Corporation) and Communitrach (Implant Technologies, Inc.).
Cuffless tube	• The cuffless tube is a plastic, silicone-like (Silastic), or metal tube, usually double lumen. Used for long-term airway management in those clients who require a tracheostomy, who can protect themselves from aspiration, and who do not require mechanical ventilation. Many people can speak with this tube in place.		

cheostomy tube may or may not have a cuff. It also may have an inner cannula that can be either disposable or reusable. For clients receiving mechanical ventilation, a cuffed tube is used in acute care settings. A noncuffed tube is used for airway maintenance when mechanical ventilation is not required or when the client is being discharged.

For tubes with an inner cannula, the nurse inspects, suctions, and cleans the inner cannula. During the immediate postoperative period, the nurse may provide cannula care frequently as needed, perhaps every 30–60 minutes. Thereafter, care is usually determined by the client's needs and agency policy. In planning for self-care, the nurse teaches the client to remove the inner cannula and

Slots for
attachment   Face   Outer   Disposable
of tube ties   plate   cannula   inner cannula

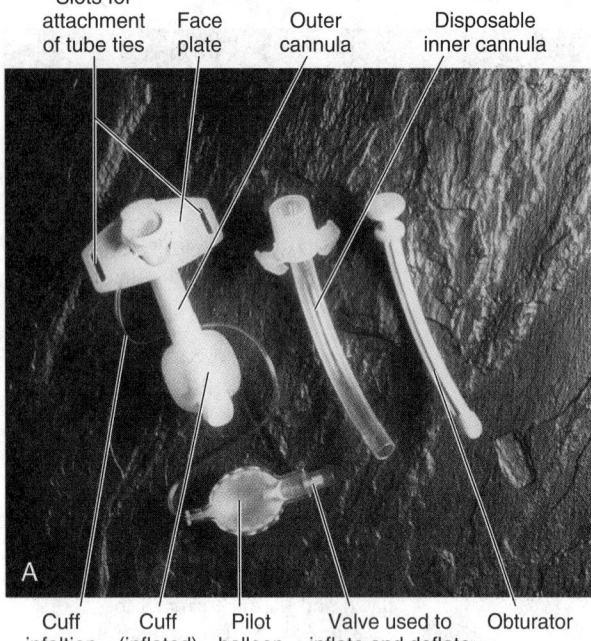

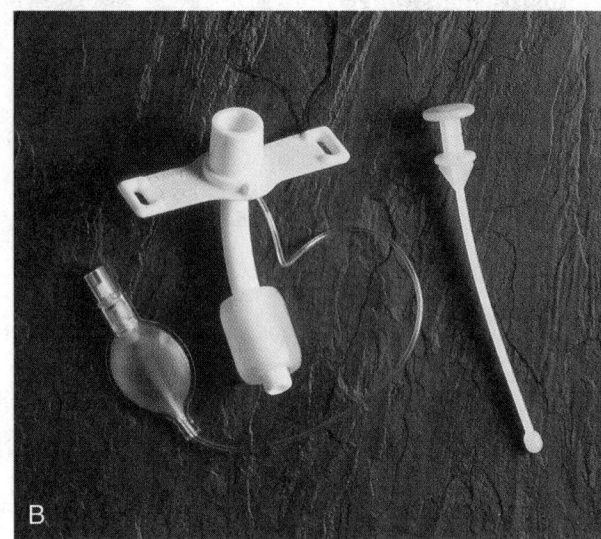

Cuff   Cuff   Pilot   Valve used to   Obturator
infaltion   (inflated)   balloon   inflate and deflate
tube   cuff and measure
                                          cuff pressure

Fenestration

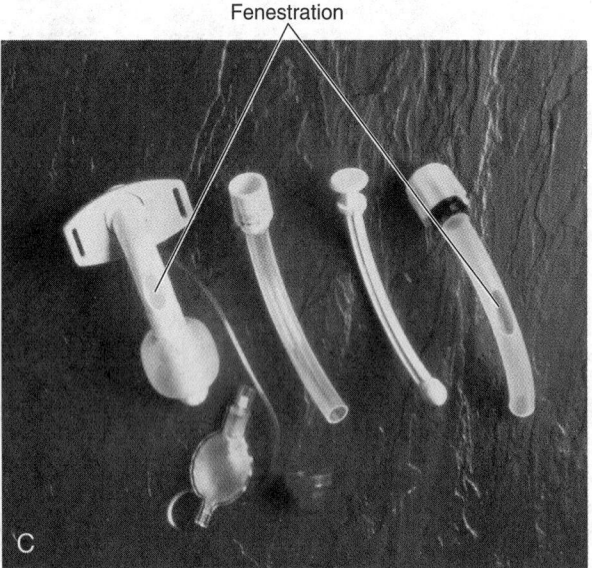

Figure 30–13. Tracheostomy tubes. *A*, Dual-lumen cuffed tracheostomy tube with disposable inner cannula. *B*, Single-lumen cannula cuffed tracheostomy tube. *C*, Dual-lumen cuffed fenestrated tracheostomy tube. (Courtesy of Mallinckrodt, Inc., Shiley Tracheostomy Products, St. Louis, MO.)

check for cleanliness. As teaching progresses, the nurse also instructs the client about suctioning and tracheostomy cleaning.

Because movement of breathing and swallowing moves the tube, a cuffed tube may not always be entirely protective against aspiration. Additionally, the pilot balloon does not reflect whether the correct amount of air is present in the cuff.

A fenestrated tube can function in many different ways. When the inner cannula is in place, the fenestration is covered over (closed), and the tube functions as a double-lumen tube. With the inner cannula removed and the plug or red decannulation stopper locked in place, air can then pass through the fenestration as well as around

the tube and up through the natural airway. The client can cough and speak, becoming reaccustomed to breathing through the upper air passages. If the client has trouble with any of these maneuvers, the nurse and physician evaluate the client for proper tube placement, patency, size, and fenestration. The nurse does not cap the tube until the problem is identified and corrected. A fenestrated tube may or may not have a cuff.

With a cuffed fenestrated tube, some air flows through the natural airway when the client is not depending on mechanical ventilation. The nurse always deflates the cuff before capping the tube with the decannulation cannula; otherwise, the client has no airway (Fig. 30–14).

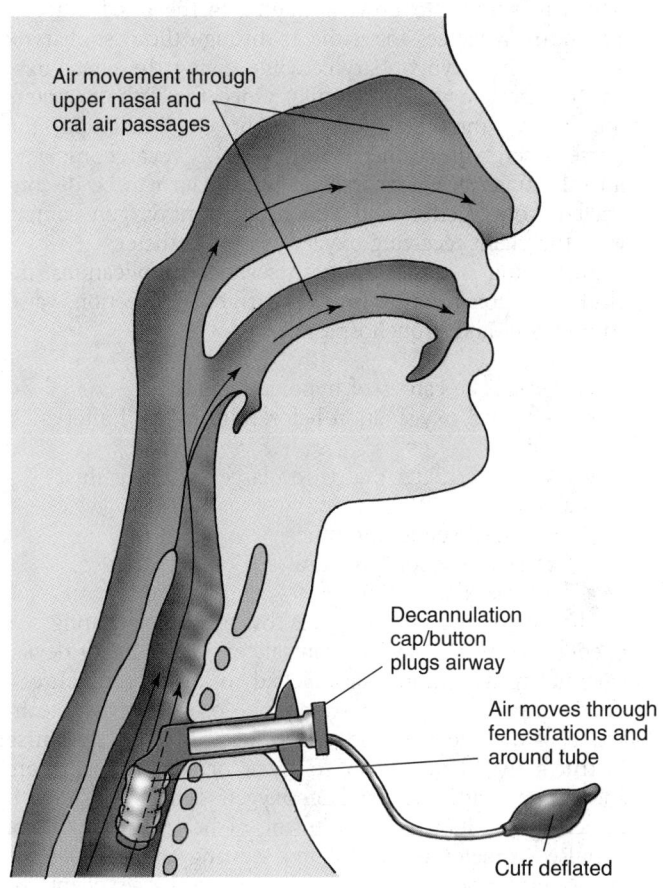

Air movement through upper nasal and oral air passages

Decannulation cap/button plugs airway

Air moves through fenestrations and around tube

Cuff deflated

Figure 30-14. Breathing through a fenestrated tracheostomy tube with a cap in place and the cuff deflated.

Prevention of Tissue Damage. Tissue damage can occur at the point where the inflated cuff presses against the tracheal mucosa. Mucosal ischemia occurs when the pressure of the cuff exerted on the mucosa exceeds the capillary perfusion pressure. Arterial capillary perfusion pressure is 30 mmHg; venous capillary perfusion pressure is 18 mmHg; and lymphatic perfusion pressure is 5 mmHg. To reduce the incidence of tracheal damage, the nurse ensures a cuff pressure between 14 and 20 mmHg.

Most cuffs are designed to use a high volume of air while maintaining a low pressure on the tracheal mucosa. The nurse inflates the cuff to provide an adequate seal between the trachea and the cuff while creating the least amount of pressure. There are two methods of cuff inflation: the minimal leak technique (for cuffs without pressure relief valves) and the occlusive technique (for cuffs with pressure relief valves).

The nurse checks cuff pressures each shift, especially with the minimal leak technique, and maintains it at 14–20 mmHg. In rare situations, cuff pressure is increased to maintain ventilator volumes when peak pressures are greater than 50 mmHg and positive end-expiratory pressure (PEEP) is greater than 10 mmHg. Manufacturers provide guidelines for the approximate recommended volumes allowed for each tracheostomy cuff size. Most cuffs are sufficiently inflated with less than 10 mL of air.

Although a high cuff pressure causes tracheal damage, other factors contribute to the severity of damage. The client's condition determines, to a degree, susceptibility to tissue damage. The client who is malnourished, hypoten-

sive, dehydrated, hypoxic, elderly, or receiving corticosteroids is unable to promote adequate tissue healing and is vulnerable to further tissue damage. Duration of intubation, extent and technique of suctioning, and stabilization of the tube against friction and movement are important factors that determine the extent of tracheal mucosa damage. The nurse minimizes local airway damage through the maintenance of proper cuff pressures, stabilization of the tube, judicious suctioning, and prevention and treatment of malnutrition, hemodynamic instability, or hypoxia.

Humidification and Warming of Air. The tracheostomy tube bypasses the upper air passages of the nose and mouth, which normally humidify, warm, and filter the air before it reaches the lower part of the respiratory tract. If humidification and warming are not adequate, tracheal damage can result from extremes in humidity and air temperature. In addition, thick, dried secretions can occlude the proximal and distal airway.

To prevent these complications, the nurse provides a humidification source, as ordered. The nurse then assesses, on an ongoing basis, for a fine mist emerging from the tracheostomy collar or T-piece during inspiration and expiration. To increase the amount of humidification delivered, the respiratory therapist attaches a warming device to the humidification source. At the same time, a temperature probe is placed in the tubing circuit. Temperature is constantly monitored and is generally maintained between 37° and 38° C (98.6° F–100.4° F), but no greater than 40° C (104° F). The nurse monitors the client's temperature by feeling the tubing during client care and by checking the temperature probe. In addition, the nurse ensures adequate hydration, which also helps to liquefy secretions.

Suctioning. Suctioning (Chart 30–2) maintains a patent airway and promotes gas exchange by removing secretions from the client who cannot adequately cough. The nurse assesses the client's need for suction, indicated by audible or noisy secretions, crackles or rhonchi on auscultation, restlessness, increased pulse or respiratory rates, presence of mucus in the artificial airway, client requests for suctioning, or an increase in the peak airway pressure on the ventilator.

Suctioning is most often through an artificial airway but can be accomplished either through the nose or mouth. Suctioning of both routes is considered routine for the client with retained secretions.

The technique of suctioning through the nose is associated with similar complications as suctioning through an artificial airway. Entry through the nasal vault into the nasopharynx can be painful. Slow, careful placement of the catheter, with a good understanding of the nasopharyngeal anatomy, can make the procedure less traumatic. The nurse may place a nasopharyngeal airway through

which to suction to prevent trauma to the nasal mucosa. The nurse advances the catheter through the nasopharynx and into the laryngopharynx while giving the client oxygen by mask or nasal cannula. Once the catheter enters the larynx, the client may cough. On inhalation, the nurse inserts the catheter through the vocal cords and into the trachea. Occasionally, the catheter can be disconnected from suction and attached to an oxygen source, with the client receiving oxygen via the catheter.

Suctioning is associated with several complications, including hypoxia, tissue (mucosal) trauma, infection, vagal stimulation, and bronchospasm.

Hypoxia. The causes of hypoxia include
- Ineffective oxygenation before, during, and after suctioning
- Use of a catheter that is too large for the artificial airway
- Prolonged suctioning time
- Excessive suction pressure
- Too-frequent suctioning

The nurse prevents hypoxia by hyperoxygenating the client with 100% oxygen from an oxygen-delivery device (manual resuscitation bag attached to an oxygen source). Suctioning can be done by a one- or two-person technique. If the client is able to take deep breaths, the nurse instructs the client to do so three or four times before suctioning, with the existing oxygen delivery system. If possible, simultaneous monitoring of heart rate or use of a pulse oximeter is helpful in assessing tolerance of the suctioning procedure. The nurse assesses the client for signs and symptoms of hypoxia (e.g., increased heart rate and blood pressure, oxygen desaturation, cyanosis, restlessness, anxiety, and cardiac dysrhythmias). Oxygen desaturation below 90% as determined by pulse oximetry indicates hypoxemia. If hypoxia occurs, the nurse terminates the suctioning procedure. Using the 100% oxygen-delivery system, the nurse reoxygenates the client until baseline parameters are achieved.

The nurse prevents hypoxia by using a catheter of the correct size. The size should not exceed half of the size of the tracheal lumen. In adults, the standard catheter size is 12 or 14 Fr. Adequate catheter size facilitates efficient removal of secretions without causing hypoxemia.

Tissue Trauma. The mucosa of the respiratory tract is extremely fragile, and frequent suctioning, prolonged suctioning time, excessive suction pressure, and nonrotation of the catheter cause damage. The nurse prevents tissue trauma by suctioning only when indicated. The nurse lubricates the catheter with sterile water or saline before insertion and suctions only during the withdrawal of the catheter. Use of a twirling motion during withdrawal prevents excessive grabbing of the mucosa.

In addition, the nurse applies suction intermittently for only 10–15 seconds. The nurse can estimate this time frame by holding his or her own breath and counting to 10 or 15 during suctioning. At the end of the 15 seconds, the suctioning procedure is finished. Fifteen seconds does not seem long to a healthy person, but most clients requiring suctioning have respiratory compromise and cannot tolerate more than 15 seconds of suctioning.

Chart 30–2

Nursing Care Highlight: Suctioning the Artificial Airway

1. Assess the need for suctioning (routine unnecessary suctioning causes mucosal damage, bleeding, and bronchospasm).
2. Wash hands. Don protective eyewear. Maintain Standard Precautions or body substance precautions.
3. Explain to the client that sensations such as shortness of breath and coughing are to be expected but that any discomfort will be very short in duration.
4. Check the suction source. Occlude the suction source, and adjust the pressure dial to between 80 and 120 mmHg to prevent hypoxemia and trauma to the mucosa.
5. Set up a sterile field.
6. Preoxygenate the client with 100% oxygen for 30 seconds to 3 minutes (at least three hyperinflations) to prevent hypoxemia. Keep hyperinflations synchronized with inhalation.
7. Quickly insert the suction catheter until resistance is met. Do not apply suction during insertion.
8. Withdraw the catheter 0.4 to 0.8 inch (1–2 cm), and begin to apply suction. Use intermittent suction and a twirling motion of the catheter during withdrawal. Never suction longer than 10 to 15 seconds.
9. Hyperoxygenate for 1 to 5 minutes or until the client's baseline heart rate and oxygen saturation are within normal limits.
10. Repeat as needed for up to three total suction passes.
11. Suction mouth as needed, and provide mouth care.
12. Describe secretions, and document client's responses.

Infection. Each catheter pass introduces bacteria into the trachea. In the hospital, the nurse uses sterile technique for suctioning and for all suctioning equipment, including suction catheters, gloves, and saline or water. After suctioning the artificial airway, the nurse then suctions the client's mouth. Oral suction equipment is never used for suctioning an artificial airway because the mouth is contaminated with bacteria, which are necessary for digestion, but could be introduced into the lungs. Home suctioning procedures emphasize clean technique because the number of virulent organisms in the home environment is lower than in the hospital.

Vagal Stimulation and Bronchospasm. Vagal stimulation results in severe bradycardia, hypotension, heart block, ventricular tachycardia, or asystole. If vagal stimulation occurs, the nurse stops suctioning immediately and oxygenates the client manually with 100% oxygen. Bronchospasm sometimes occurs when the catheter passes into the airway. The client may require a bronchodilator to relieve the bronchospasm and respiratory distress.

Tracheostomy Care. Tracheostomy care (Chart 30–3) keeps the tracheostomy tube free of obstructing secretions, maintains a patent airway, and provides wound care. This procedure is performed whether or not the client is able to clear secretions. The nurse performs tracheostomy care according to agency policy, usually every shift and as needed.

Before proceeding with tracheostomy care, the nurse assesses the client as shown in Chart 30–4. The extent of both suctioning and tracheostomy care depends entirely

---

Chart 30–4

Focused Assessment of the Client with a Tracheostomy

- Note the quality, pattern, and rate of breathing:
  - Within client's baseline?
    Tachypnea can indicate hypoxia.
    Dyspnea can indicate secretions in airway.
- Assess for any cyanosis, especially around the lips, which could indicate hypoxia.
- Check the client's pulse oximetry reading.
- If oxygen is ordered, is the client receiving the correct amount, with the correct equipment and humidification?
- Assess the tracheostomy site:
  - Note the color, consistency, and amount of secretions in the tube or externally.
  - If the tracheostomy is sutured in place, is there any redness, swelling, or drainage from suture sites?
  - If the tracheostomy is secured with ties, what is the condition of the ties? Are they moist with secretions or perspiration? Are the secretions dried on the ties? Is the tie secure?
  - Assess the condition of the skin around the tracheostomy and neck. Be sure to check underneath the neck for secretions that may have drained to the back. Check for any breakdown related to pressure from the ties or from excess secretions.
  - Assess behind the face plate for the size of the space between the outer cannula and the client's tissue. Are any secretions collected in this area?
- If the tube is cuffed, check cuff pressure.
- Auscultate the lungs.
- Is a second (emergency) tracheostomy tube and obturator available?

Chart 30–3

Nursing Care Highlight: Tracheostomy Care

1. Assemble the necessary equipment.
2. Wash your hands. Maintain Standard Precautions or body substance precautions.
3. Suction the tracheostomy tube if necessary.
4. Remove old dressings and excess secretions.
5. Set up a sterile field.
6. Remove and clean the inner cannula. Use half-strength hydrogen peroxide to clean the cannula, and sterile saline to rinse it. If the inner cannula is disposable, remove the cannula and replace it with a new one.
7. Clean the stoma site and then the tracheostomy plate with half-strength hydrogen peroxide followed by sterile saline. Ensure that none of the solutions enters the tracheostomy.
8. Change tracheostomy ties if they are soiled. Secure new ties in place before removing soiled ones to prevent accidental decannulation. If a knot is needed, tie a square knot that is visible on the side of the neck. One or two fingers should be able to be placed between the tie tape and the neck.
9. Document the type and amount of secretions and the general condition of the stoma and surrounding skin. Document the client's response to the procedure and any teaching or learning that occurred.

---

on the needs of the client. The need for suctioning and tracheostomy care is determined by the amount and consistency of secretions, medical diagnosis (specifically pulmonary diseases), ability of the client to cough and deep breathe, need for mechanical ventilation, and wound care required. The nurse inspects the inner lumen of a single-lumen tube with a flashlight or penlight to assess for the presence of secretions.

The nurse changes tracheostomy ties once a day to keep them clean and to avoid having them act as a medium for infection. A properly secured tie allows space for only one or two fingers to be placed between the tie and the neck. Tube movement causes irritation and coughing, which, in turn, may cause decannulation. Keeping the tube secure while changing the ties to prevent accidental decannulation is imperative. One way to accomplish this safely is to keep the old ties on the tube while changing ties, but a secure hand on the tube is the most reliable method of tube stabilization. The nurse includes the client in this process as a step toward self-care. Figure 30–15 demonstrates a correct technique for applying a tracheostomy dressing.

Bronchial and Oral Hygiene. Bronchial hygiene promotes a patent airway, prevents pulmonary infections,

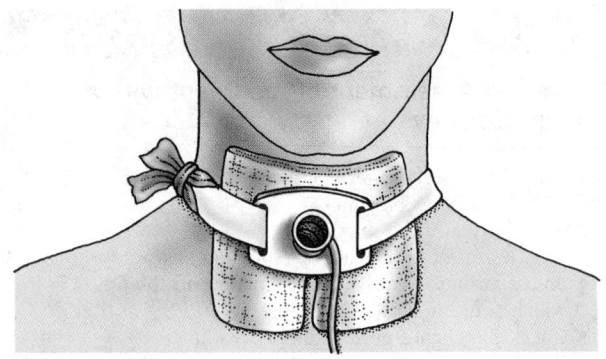

Figure 30–15. Placement of precut gauze and tie around a tracheostomy tube.

and stimulates the pulmonary system. The nurse turns and repositions the client every 1–2 hours, supports out-of-bed activities, and encourages ambulation. These interventions promote lung expansion and gas exchange and facilitate the mobilization of secretions. Coughing and deep breathing, combined with the chest physical therapy techniques of percussion, vibration, and postural drainage, are powerful measures in promoting pulmonary care (see Chap. 32).

Frequent oral hygiene is important not only to ensure a patent airway but also to prevent bacterial overgrowth and dental caries and to promote client comfort. The nurse maintains standard or body substance precautions during the procedure. Cleansing the mouth with glycerin swabs and mouthwash, which contains significant amounts of alcohol, are contraindicated because these interventions dry the oral mucosa, change its pH, and promote bacterial growth. The nurse instead uses a toothette or soft-bristle brush moistened in water for mouth care. Hydrogen peroxide solutions can help to remove crusted materials but may break down granulating tissue and are used only with a physician's order.

During oral care, the nurse examines the mouth for any alterations in mucosal integrity, dental abnormalities, and alterations in tissue integrity. Ulcers (aphthous or herpes simplex), bacterial or fungal (*Candida*) growth, or other infections are treated medically. Application of lip balms or water-soluble jelly can prevent cracked lips and further skin breakdown and can help keep the client comfortable. Providing mouth care is a simple but very effective method of promoting oral health, comfort, and aesthetic appearance. Offering an opportunity for the client or family member to perform mouth care encourages participation in care and increases the client's self-esteem.

Nutrition. Swallowing can be a major problem for the client with a tracheostomy tube in place. In a normal swallow, the larynx elevates and moves forward to protect itself from the passing stream of food and saliva. Laryngeal elevation also assists in the opening of the cricopharyngeal muscle, the upper esophageal sphincter. The tracheostomy tube sometimes tethers the larynx in place, rendering it unable to execute this motion efficiently. The result is difficulty in swallowing. Likewise, when the tracheostomy tube cuff is inflated, it can balloon posteriorly and interfere with the passage of food through the esophagus. The common wall of the posterior trachea (trachealis muscle) and the anterior esophagus is very thin, allowing this pushing phenomenon.

Provided that the tracheostomy tube is not capped, the nurse usually inflates the cuff during feeding to prevent aspiration. The nurse then instructs the client to keep the head of the bed elevated for at least 30 minutes after feeding and keeps the cuff inflated for the same period. Clients who are cognitively intact, however, may adapt to eating normal food when the tracheostomy tube is small and the cuff is not inflated.

Speech and Communication. The client will be able to speak when there is a cuffless tube, when a fenestrated tracheostomy tube is in place, and when the fenestrated tube is capped or covered. Until one of the methods for natural vocalization is feasible, the nurse establishes and teaches alternative communication methods that are easy for the client to use. A writing tablet, "magic slate," communication board with pictures and letters, hand signals, or a computer, as well as a call light within reach, is essential to promote communication and decrease the client's frustration from not being able to speak or be understood. The nurse moves the client closer to the nurses' station and marks the central call light system with indicators to communicate that the client cannot speak. Questions phrased for "yes" or "no" answers help the client respond efficiently.

The inability to talk is a major stressor for the client. Every effort to facilitate communication and speech is important. When the client can tolerate cuff deflation, the client places a finger over the tracheostomy tube on exhalation. This forces air up through the larynx, vocal cords, and mouth and allows for articulation. During the process of decannulation, when the fenestrated tube is "capped," the client experiences a very positive but secondary benefit of speech without the need to cover the tube.

Emotional Care. Addressing psychologic concerns is an important aspect of nursing care of clients recovering from a tracheostomy. While providing physical care to the client, the nurse keeps in mind the emotional impact of an artificial airway. Acknowledging the client's frustration in communication and allowing sufficient time for communication are critically important. When speaking to the client, the nurse uses a normal tone of voice. The tracheostomy tube has not altered the client's ability to hear or understand.

Body Image. The client experiences a change in body image because of deformity, the presence of a stoma or artificial airway, speech changes, a change in the method of eating, and possibly difficulty with speech. The nurse helps the client to set realistic goals, starting with involvement in self-care.

The nurse and family must make all attempts to ease the client into a more normal social environment. The nurse provides encouragement and positive reinforcement while demonstrating acceptance and caring behaviors. The family may benefit from counseling sessions that the nurse initiates in the hospital.

After surgery, the client may feel reserved and socially isolated. To cover the tracheostomy tube the client can wear loose-fitting shirts or scarves. (See Chapter 10 for a detailed discussion of body image, including additional nursing interventions.)

Weaning. Weaning the client from a tracheostomy tube entails a gradual decrease in the tube size and ultimate removal of the tube. The nurse carefully monitors this process, especially after each change. The physician or a specially trained nurse performs the steps in the process.

First, the cuff is deflated as soon as the client can manage secretions and does not require mechanical ventilation. This change allows the client to breathe through the tube and also through the upper airway. Next, the tube is changed to an uncuffed tube; then the size of the tube is gradually decreased. When a small fenestrated tube is placed (No. 4 or No. 6, depending on the size of the airway), the tube is capped so that all air passes through the upper airway and the fenestra, with none passing through the tube. The tube is removed after the client tolerates more than 24 hours of capping. The nurse places a dry dressing over the stoma, which then gradually heals on its own. A small scar remains.

Another device used for the transition from tracheostomy to natural breathing is a tracheostomy button. The button maintains patency of the stoma and facilitates spontaneous breathing. The Kistner tracheostomy tube and Olympic tracheostomy button are examples of this type of device. To function, they must fit properly. A disadvantage of these buttons is the possibility of decannulation: the tube dislodges from the trachea but remains in the anterior subcutaneous tissues of the neck.

 Continuing Care

By the time of discharge from the hospital, the client should be able to provide self-care, which may include tracheostomy care, nutritional care, suctioning, and methods of communication. Although education begins during preoperative teaching sessions, most self-care is taught in the hospital. The nurse teaches the client and family how to care for the tracheostomy tube. The nurse reviews airway care, including cleaning and inspecting for signs of infection. The nurse teaches clean suction technique and reviews the client's plan of care.

The nurse instructs the client to use a shower shield over the tracheostomy tube when bathing to prevent water from entering the airway. To shield the airway during the day, the client may wear a protective cover. Covering the permanent opening has several benefits: filtering the air entering the stoma, keeping humidity in the airway, and enhancing aesthetic appearance. To protect the airway and increase humidity, the nurse instructs the client to cover the airway with cotton or foam. Attractive coverings are available in the form of cotton scarves, crocheted bibs, and jewelry. Using colored seam binding for tracheostomy ties after the stoma has matured may enhance the client's overall body image. The client's shirt or dress color can be matched or coordinated with seam bindings of various colors. The nurse also teaches the client to increase humidity in the home.

The nurse may teach the client to instill normal saline into the artificial airway 10–15 times a day as ordered. The client continues the selected method of alternative communication that began in the hospital and wears a medical alert (Medic-Alert) bracelet.

The client should feel safe and secure with the extended plan of care. The multidisciplinary care team assesses the client's specific discharge needs and makes appropriate referrals to home care agencies and durable medical equipment companies (for suction equipment and tracheostomy supplies). Clinic or physician follow-up visits occur early after discharge, but the home care nurse also becomes a very important resource for the client and family. The home care nurse initiates, with physician order, and coordinates the services of professionals such as nutritionists, nurses, speech pathologists, and social workers. The home care or hospital nurse informs the client and family of community organizations that can offer support and friendships. When the client has problems paying for health care services, equipment supply, and prescriptions, the visiting nurse agency may be helpful in directing the client to available resources.

SELECTED BIBLIOGRAPHY

*Albarren, J. W. (1991). A review of communication with intubated patients and those with tracheostomies within an intensive care environment. *Intensive Care Nursing, 7*(3), 179–186.

*American Association of Respiratory Care. (1991). Clinical practice guideline: Oxygen therapy in the acute care hospital. *Respiratory Care, 36*(12), 1410–1413.

*Ball, R. A. (1994). Review. Liquid oxygen: A new look for an old companion. *JEMS: Journal of Emergency Medical Services, 19*(3), 85–86.

*Bolgiano, C. S., Bunting, K., & Shoenberger, M. M. (1990). Administering oxygen therapy: What you need to know. *Nursing90, 20*(6), 47–51.

Celia, L. M. (1995). Consultation stat. Supplying oxygen when a trach tube is dislodged. *RN, 58*(4), 61.

Crimlisk, J. T., Horn, M. H., Wilson, D. J., et al. (1996). Artificial airways: A survey of cuff management practices. *Heart and Lung: Journal of Acute and Critical Care, 25*(3), 225–235.

Eisenhauer, B. (1996). Action stat. Dislodged tracheostomy tube. *Nursing96, 26*(6), 25.

Hatfield, B. O. (1997). Cost effective trache teaching. *RN, 60*(3), 48–49.

*Kersten, L. D. (1989). *Comprehensive respiratory nursing: A decision making approach.* Philadelphia: W. B. Saunders.

Ladyshewsky, A., & Gousseau, A. (1996). Successful tracheal weaning. *Canadian Nurse, 92*(2), 35–38.

*Mapp, C. (1988). Trach care: Are you aware of all the dangers? *Nursing88, 18*(7), 34–43.

Mathews, P. J. (1995). Safely delivering a breath of fresh air. *Nursing95, 25*(5), 66–69.

McConnell, E. A. (1997). Administering oxygen by mask. *Nursing97, 21*(9), 26.

*Montanari, J., & Spearing, C. (1986). The fine art of measuring tracheal cuff pressure. *Nursing86, 16*(7), 46–49.

*Openbrier, D. R., Fuoss, C., & Mall, C. (1988). What patients on home oxygen therapy want to know. *American Journal of Nursing, 88*(2), 198–202.

*Openbrier, D. R., Hoffman, L., & Wesmiller, S. (1988). Home oxygen therapy. *American Journal of Nursing, 88*(2), 192–197.

Pfister, S. M. (1995). Home oxygen therapy: Indications, administration, recertification, and patient education. *Nurse Practitioner: American Journal of Primary Health Care, 20*(7), 44, 47–52, 54–56.

Provine, B. (1996). Consultation corner. Education about tracheostomy care. *Perspectives in Respiratory Nursing, 7*(2), 6.

*Schuring, L. T., Pollock, K., Cyr, M., et al. (1994). Otorhinolaryngology–head and neck nursing practice guidelines: Tracheostomy. *Otorhinolaryngology–Head and Neck Nursing, 12*(4), 26–29.

Somerson, S. J., Husted, C. W., Somerson, S. W., et al. (1996). Mastering emergency airway management. *American Journal of Nursing, 96*(5), 24–31.

*Tayal, V. S. (1994). Tracheostomies. *Emergency Medicine Clinics of North America, 12*(3), 707–727.

*Weiletz, P. B., & Dettenmeier, P. A. (1994). Test your knowledge of tracheostomy tubes. *American Journal of Nursing, 94*(2), 46–50.

SUGGESTED READINGS

Eisenhauer, B. (1996). Action stat. Dislodged tracheostomy tube. *Nursing96, 26*(6), 25.

This brief article reviews emergency measures for the nurse to take when a client's new tracheostomy tube visually appears to be in place but is actually dislodged. Assessment and rationale for interventions are included.

Mathews, P. J. (1995). Safely delivering a breath of fresh air. *Nursing95, 25*(5), 66–69.

This photoguide addresses specific steps to follow when using a portable "E" cylinder for transport. Included are safety measures, determining the amount of oxygen in the tank, using the wrench key, and bleeding the tank. Also included is a calculation the nurse can use to determine how many minutes the oxygen in the tank will last.

Chapter 31

INTERVENTIONS FOR CLIENTS WITH NONINFECTIOUS PROBLEMS OF THE UPPER RESPIRATORY TRACT

The upper respiratory tract includes the structures of the nose, sinuses, oropharynx, larynx, and trachea. Many common acute and chronic disorders affect the upper airways. The nurse encounters clients with diseases of the upper respiratory system across the health care continuum, in homes, clinics, primary care practitioners' offices, emergency departments, and hospitals and nursing homes. The major nursing priority for clients with disorders of the upper respiratory tract is to maintain a patent and functioning airway.

NONINFECTIOUS DISORDERS OF THE NOSE AND SINUSES
Fracture of the Nose

Overview

Nasal fractures commonly occur from injuries received during falls, participation in sports, or trauma related to violence or motor vehicle accidents. Usually, if the bone or cartilage is not displaced, no serious complications result from the fracture, and treatment may not be necessary. Displacement, however, can cause airway obstruc-

tion or cosmetic deformity and is a potential source of infection.

Collaborative Management

 Assessment

The nurse notes and documents nasal deviation, misaligned nasal bridge, change in nasal breathing, crepitus on palpation, midface ecchymosis, and pain. Blood or clear (cerebrospinal) fluid rarely drains from one or both nares, but such drainage could indicate a skull fracture. Radiographic examination is not always useful in nasal fractures, but is very important in evaluating the client for other concurrent facial fractures.

 Interventions

The physician performs a simple closed reduction of the fracture using local or general anesthesia within the first 24 hours after injury. After 24 hours, the fracture is more difficult to reduce because of edema and scar formation.

585

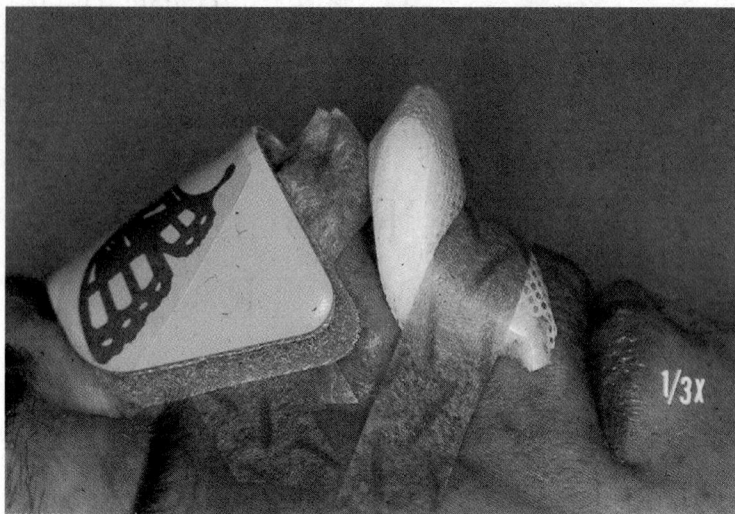

Figure 31–1. Immediate postoperative appearance of a client who has undergone rhinoplasty. Note the splint and gauze drip pad. From Tardy, M. E. (1997). *Rhinoplasty: The art and the science* (p. 207). Philadelphia: W. B. Saunders. Used with permission.

Simple closed fractures need not be surgically treated; treatment focuses on pain relief and local cold compresses to decrease swelling.

➤ *Rhinoplasty*

For severe fractures or those that do not heal properly, a reduction and rhinoplasty may be required. Rhinoplasty is a surgical reconstruction of the nose for cosmetic purposes and for functional improvement of airflow. The client returns from surgery with packing in both nostrils to prevent bleeding and to provide a *stent* (object that provides support and structure) for the reconstructed nose. The ½-inch gauze packing is typically treated with an antibiotic ointment, such as bacitracin (Bacitrin) to reduce the risk of infection. The client typically has a "mustache" dressing, or drip pad, usually a folded 2 × 2-inch gauze pad, placed under the nose. A splint or cast may cover the nose for additional alignment and protection (Fig. 31–1). The nurse or client changes the drip pad as necessary.

Postoperatively, the nurse observes the client for edema and bleeding and takes vital signs every 4 hours until discharge. The nurse assesses how often the client swallows. Repeated swallowing may indicate posterior nasal bleeding. The nurse examines the pharynx with a penlight for bleeding and, if bleeding is present, notifies the physician. The client with uncomplicated rhinoplasty with or without related surgical procedures (brow-lifts, blepharoplasties, face-lifts) is usually sent home the day of surgery. The client and family or significant other are instructed in routine care.

The nurse or family member places the client in a semi-Fowler's position and instructs the client to move slowly and to rest as much as possible. Cool compresses are applied to the nose, eyes, or face to reduce swelling and prevent excessive discoloration. Once the effects of anesthesia are eliminated and the physician has so ordered, the client may eat soft foods. An oral fluid intake of at least 2500 mL/day is encouraged. To prevent bleeding, the nurse also instructs the client to limit the Valsalva maneuver, such as forceful coughing or straining at stool, for the first few days after removal of the nasal packing. Laxatives or stool softeners may be appropriate to facilitate defecation. The client is instructed to avoid aspirin and nonsteroidal antiinflammatory drugs during this time to prevent the possibility of bleeding. The physician may order prophylactic antibiotics to prevent postoperative infection and pain medication to relieve discomfort. The nurse explains to the client that edema and discoloration usually last for several weeks and that the final surgical result will be evident in 6–12 months.

➤ *Nasoseptoplasty*

Nasoseptoplasty, or submucous resection (SMR), may be necessary to straighten a deviated septum when chronic symptoms (e.g., a "stuffy" nose) or discomfort occurs. A slight deviation of the nasal septum is present in most adults and causes no symptoms. Major deviations may obstruct the nasal passages or interfere with airflow and sinus drainage. The surgeon removes the deviated section of the cartilage and bone. The amount resected depends on the type and degree of deformity.

Nursing care is similar to that for the client with a rhinoplasty. Nasoseptoplasty is often an outpatient procedure; the nurse reviews written instructions with the client on discharge.

Epistaxis

Overview

Because of the rich capillary network within the nose, epistaxis (nosebleed) is a common problem. Nosebleeds may occur as a result of trauma, hypertension, blood dyscrasia (e.g., leukemias), inflammation, tumor, decreased humidity, excessive nose blowing, and nose picking. Men are usually affected more than women, and the elderly tend to bleed most often from the posterior portion of the nose.

Chart 31–1

Nursing Care Highlight: Emergency Care of a Nosebleed

1. Position the client in an upright position, leaning forward, to prevent blood from entering the stomach and possible aspiration.
2. Reassure the client and attempt to keep him or her quiet to reduce anxiety and blood pressure.
3. Apply direct lateral pressure to the nose for 5 minutes, and apply ice or cool compresses to the nose and face if possible.
4. Maintain standard or body substance precautions.
5. If nasal packing is necessary, loosely pack both nares with gauze or nasal tampons.
6. To prevent rebleeding from dislodging clots, instruct the client not to blow the nose for several hours after the bleeding stops.
7. Seek medical assistance if these measures are ineffective or if the bleeding occurs frequently.

Collaborative Management

 ### Assessment

The client may be holding a tissue or gauze pad up to the nares while explaining to the nurse what happened. Often the client will report that the bleeding started after sneezing or blowing the nose. The nurse notes the amount and color of the blood and takes vital signs. The nurse also assesses and documents the number, duration, and causes of previous bleeding episodes.

 ### Interventions

Chart 31–1 summarizes first aid for the client with a nosebleed. If the nosebleed does not respond to these interventions, medical attention is needed. The physician cauterizes the affected capillaries with silver nitrate or electrocautery, followed by anterior packing. Anterior packing is very effective in controlling bleeding from the anterior nasal cavity.

When bleeding originates in the posterior nasal region, the physician uses a posterior pack to stop the bleeding. A string is attached to a large gauze pack and then threaded through the nose and out the mouth. The physician positions the pack in the posterior nasal cavity above the pharynx, and then tapes the string to the client's cheek to prevent movement of the pack. This procedure is uncomfortable and may cause airway obstruction if the pack slips.

The nurse observes the client for respiratory distress and for tolerance of the packing. The physician may prescribe humidification and oxygen as well as bed rest and antibiotics. To maintain gag and cough reflexes and optimal level of consciousness, the client should not receive any sedatives and only limited pain medication. The nurse provides oral care and ensures adequate hydration, which is important because of mouth breathing. The nurse uses pulse oximetry or a cardiac monitor to observe for hypoxemia and hypercapnia. After 2–5 days, the physician removes the packing. Petroleum jelly can be applied to the nares for lubrication and comfort. Nasal saline solution and humidification may be helpful to add moisture and prevent crusting and rebleeding. At discharge the client should continue gentle saline irrigations and lubrication to the nasal cavity to prevent further crusting and subsequent rebleeding.

Nasal Polyps

Overview

Nasal polyps are benign, grape-like clusters of mucous membrane and loose connective tissue. Polyps typically occur bilaterally and are often caused by irritation to the nasal mucosa or sinuses, allergies, or infection (chronic sinusitis). If polyps become too large, airway obstruction may result.

Collaborative Management

Benign nasal polyps are treated medically with nasally inhaled steroids in conjunction with removal of the polyps. Surgical removal (polypectomy) can be accomplished with either local or general anesthesia. The nurse observes the client for postoperative bleeding. The nostrils are usually packed with gauze for 24 hours postoperatively. Nasal polyps tend to recur if not completely resected.

Inverting papilloma is a rare, histologically benign condition consisting of a space-occupying lesion that erodes nasal and maxillary skeletal structures. Often initially diagnosed as benign polyps, inverting papillomas grow by pressure into other adjacent structures. Extensive sinus and nasal surgery is necessary for complete removal. If these papillomas are completely resected, they do not recur.

Juvenile angiofibromas are similar in growth pattern but histologically different from other polyps. These tumors usually occur in adolescent males and may undergo resolution when the client reaches adulthood. These may be resected by traditional nasal surgery; more invasive tumors may require skull base resections.

Cancer of the Nose and Sinuses

Overview

Tumors of the nasal cavities and sinuses are relatively uncommon and may be benign or malignant. Malignant lesions of these areas can occur at all ages, but the peak incidence is 40 to 45 years in males and 60 to 65 years in females. There is a higher incidence of nasopharyngeal cancer in Asian-Americans.

Collaborative Management

 Assessment

The onset of sinus malignancies is insidious, and symptoms resemble sinusitis. Therefore, clients may have relatively advanced disease at diagnosis. Persistent nasal obstruction, drainage, bloody discharge, and pain that does not improve after treatment of sinusitis suggest nasal or sinus malignancy. Cervical lymph node enlargement usually occurs on the side with greater tumor mass.

 Interventions

Radiation therapy is the primary treatment for nasopharyngeal cancers. Surgical resection may be indicated in radiation therapy failures. Chemotherapy has not proved to be effective. The specific surgical procedure depends on the amount of tumor, its anatomic location, and degree of tissue invasion. The primary deficit is change in body image, speech, and alteration in nutrition, especially when the maxilla and floor of the nose are involved in the resection.

The nurse provides general postoperative care (see Chap. 22), including maintenance of a patent airway, wound care, strict attention to nutrition, and tracheostomy care (if necessary). (Tracheostomy care is covered in Chapter 30.) The nurse provides meticulous mouth and maxillary cavity care with saline irrigations for the client, using a water pick (e.g., Water Pik) or a syringe. The nurse also assesses for alterations in comfort and for infection. Optimal nutrition is essential during the perioperative period for adequate healing.

Facial Trauma

Overview

Facial trauma is defined by the specific bones (i.e., mandibular, maxillary, zygomatic, orbital, or nasal fractures) and the side of the face involved. Mandibular (lower jaw) fractures can occur at any location of the mandible and make up the majority of facial fractures. Le Fort I is a nasoethmoid complex fracture. Le Fort II is a transverse maxillary and nasoethmoid complex fracture. Le Fort III is a combination of I and II plus an orbital zygoma fracture, often called "craniofacial disjunction" because it leaves the midface with no connection to the skull. Because the face is very vascular, there is often much bleeding with facial trauma.

Collaborative Management

 Assessment

The priority in the management of facial trauma is assessment for a patent airway. Signs and symptoms of an upper airway obstruction include stridor, shortness of breath, dyspnea, anxiety, restlessness, hypoxia, hypercar-

bia, decreased oxygen saturation, cyanosis, and loss of consciousness. After establishing the airway, the nurse assesses the amount and site of soft-tissue trauma, bleeding, and palpable fractures. Additional findings on assessment include edema of soft tissue, asymmetry, pain, or leakage of cerebrospinal fluid through the ears or nose, or both, indicating temporal bone or basilar skull fracture. Because orbital and maxillary fractures can entrap the eye, the nurse assesses vision and extraocular movement (EOM) and also observes for neurologic changes (see Chap. 43). Because spinal cord trauma and skull fractures often occur in conjunction with facial trauma, cranial computed tomography, facial series, and cervical spine films are then obtained.

 Interventions

The nurse's priority is to establish and maintain a patent airway. The nurse must anticipate the need for emergent intubation, tracheotomy, or cricothyroidotomy. When the client arrives at a trauma center, care focuses on controlling hemorrhage, establishing an airway, and assessing for the extent of injury. If signs and symptoms of shock are present (see Chap. 39), fluid resuscitation and identification of bleeding sites must be initiated immediately.

In head and neck trauma, the nurse must be astute in trauma and critical care nursing. Time is paramount in stabilizing the client. Early treatment and response of the appropriate services, including the trauma team, maxillofacial surgeon, general surgeon, otolaryngologist, plastic surgeon, and dentist, optimize the client's posttrauma recovery. (Consult a specialized trauma book for more information about trauma care.)

Stabilization of the fractured segment of a mandibular fracture allows the teeth to heal in proper alignment or occlusion. The client remains in fixed centric occlusion for 6–10 weeks. Antibiotic therapy may be prescribed because of oral wound contamination. Delay in treatment, infection of the adjacent tooth, and poor oral care may result in infection in the mandibular segment. The client may then require surgical debridement, intravenous (IV) antibiotic therapy, and an extended period in fixation.

Facial fractures are now most often repaired with microplating surgical systems. These shaping plates fix the bone fragments in place until osteoneogenesis occurs. Large areas of skull can be replaced with BoneSource. The osteoblasts and osteoclasts grow into the BoneSource and rematrix into a stabilized bone support. In the United States, the plates remain in place permanently; in Europe the plates are removed after healing has occurred.

Intermaxillary fixation (IMF) is a common method of securing a mandibular fracture. The physician can repair nondisplaced aligned fractures in a clinic or office using local dental anesthesia. General anesthesia is used for repair of displaced or complex fractures or fractures that occur with other facial bone fractures.

If the mandibular fracture is repaired with titanium plates, the nurse teaches the client oral care, soft-diet restrictions, and follow-up care with a dentist. The plates are permanent and do not interfere with magnetic resonance imaging (MRI) studies.

Postoperatively, the nurse teaches oral care with an irrigating device, such as a Water Pik. If the client is in inner maxillary fixation, the nurse teaches self-care with wires in place, including a dental liquid diet. The nurse also explains the proper method of cutting the wires if emesis occurs. The client keeps wire cutters nearby at all times in preparation for this emergency. The nurse instructs the client to return to the physician for rewiring as soon as possible to reinstitute fixation.

Nutrition is important for any client with fractures. Because of oral fixation, pain, and surgery, clients may not attend to their nutritional needs. Dietary consultations are important for teaching and support.

NONINFECTIOUS DISORDERS OF THE ORAL PHARYNX AND TONSILS
Obstructive Sleep Apnea
Overview

Sleep apnea is breathing disruption during sleep lasting at least 10 seconds and occurring a minimum of five times in an hour. Although sleep apnea can have a neurologic or central origin, the most common form of adult sleep apnea occurs as a result of upper airway obstruction. Factors that contribute to sleep apnea include obesity, a large uvula, short neck, smoking, enlarged tonsils or adenoids, and oropharyngeal edema. Men are more commonly affected than women, and the incidence increases with age.

During sleep, with relaxation of skeletal muscles and displacement of the tongue and neck structures, the upper airway is obstructed even though chest wall movement is unimpaired. The apnea increases the arterial carbon dioxide level and decreases the pH. These blood gas changes stimulate neural activity. The sleeper is aroused spontaneously after 10 or more seconds of apnea and corrects the obstruction, resulting in a resumption of respiration. Upon resumption of sleep, the cycle begins again, sometimes as often as every 5 minutes.

This cyclic pattern of disrupted sleep prevents the person from reaching the prolonged state of deep sleep necessary for maximum rest. As a result, the person may have excessive daytime sleepiness, an inability to concentrate, and irritability. Some people experience *narcolepsy*, an uncontrollable and dangerous state of unintentional daytime sleep, while performing daytime activities.

Collaborative Management

 Assessment

Clients who have excessive daytime sleepiness or complaints of "waking up tired," particularly if they are known to snore heavily, may have sleep apnea. Sleep apnea can be diagnosed in some clients through the observation of family members while the client sleeps in a supine position. A complete health assessment should be

performed on any client for whom excessive daytime sleepiness is a problem.

 Interventions

For mild sleep apnea, a change in sleeping position or weight loss may be all that is required to reduce or correct the problem. Simple position-fixing devices that prevent subluxation of the tongue and neck structures also may be effective in preventing obstruction. For more severe sleep apnea, nonsurgical or surgical methods to prevent obstruction may be necessary.

A common nonsurgical method to prevent airway collapse is the use of continuous positive airway pressure (CPAP) ventilation through a face mask during sleep. A small electric compressor delivers positive pressure at an individually determined setting. Proper fit of the mask over the nose and mouth is key to successful treatment. Although intrusive, this method is well accepted by clients after an initial adjustment period.

Surgical intervention for sleep apnea may involve a simple adenoidectomy or uvulectomy, or it may require remodeling of the entire posterior oropharynx (uvulopalatopharyngoplasty). Both conventional and laser surgeries are applied for this purpose.

Oropharyngeal Cancer

Clients with cancer of the mouth, tongue, tonsils, and pharynx present special nursing needs related to airway maintenance, communication, nutrition, and self-image. (Chapter 56 provides an in-depth discussion of the collaborative management of clients with oropharyngeal cancer.)

NONINFECTIOUS DISORDERS OF THE LARYNX
Vocal Cord Paralysis
Overview

Vocal fold (cord) paralysis may result from injury, trauma, or disease affecting the larynx, the laryngeal nerves, or the vagus nerve. Prolonged intubation with an endotracheal (ET) tube may cause temporary or, rarely, permanent paralysis. Laryngeal paralysis may occur in clients with central neurologic disorders. Damage to the vagus nerve (by chest injury) or brain stem may lead to nerve dysfunction. The superior and recurrent laryngeal nerves may be damaged in disorders or trauma involving the chest, esophagus, or thyroid. Paralysis of both vocal cords may result from direct traumatic injury or bilateral cerebrovascular accident (CVA), especially involving the brain stem or after total thyroidectomy.

Collaborative Management

 Assessment

Vocal fold paralysis may be unilateral or bilateral. When only one vocal cord is involved, as is commonly the case,

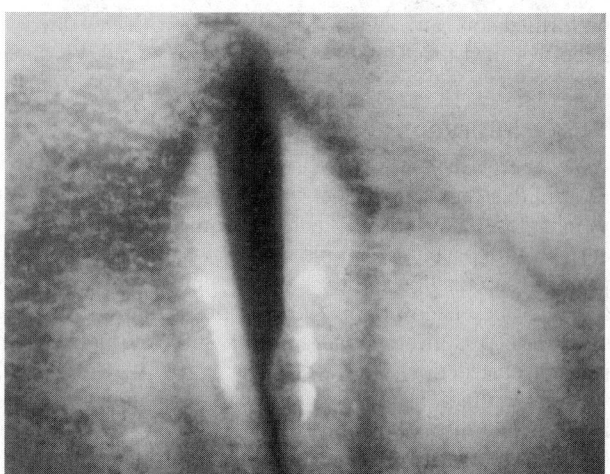

Figure 31–2. Unilateral left vocal cord nodule caused by contact and voice abuse, often seen after viral illnesses. Differential diagnosis includes cancer and trauma. The origin of the nodule may be scar tissue, bacteria, or viruses.

the airway usually remains patent, but voice use may be affected. Symptoms of abducted bilateral vocal cord paralysis include hoarseness; a breathy, weak voice; and aspiration of food. Bilateral adducted vocal cord paralysis presents with airway obstruction and dyspnea and is a medical emergency if the symptoms are severe and the client is unable to compensate. Stridor is the major presenting symptom. The client with vocal cord dysfunction is at risk for aspiration because of the inability to protect the airway by normal vocal cord closure.

Interventions

The nurse assesses for airway compromise and symptoms of upper airway obstruction. Securing a patent airway is the primary intervention. The nurse positions the client in a high Fowler's position to aid in breathing and proper alignment of airway structures. Dyspnea with stridor indicates an inadequate airway, and the nurse immediately notifies the physician. Emergent endotracheal intubation, cricothyroidotomy, or tracheostomy may be necessary.

Many surgical procedures have been used to improve the voice. In one procedure for abducted vocal cord paresis, polytef (Teflon) is injected into the affected cord so that it will enlarge toward the unaffected cord, improving approximation.

Additional nursing interventions include teaching clients to hold their breath during swallowing. This intervention allows the larynx to elevate, close, and divert the food stream posteriorly into the esophagus during swallowing. The nurse evaluates clients for aspiration of liquids and saliva related to vocal cord dysfunction. Signs and symptoms include immediate coughing on swallowing of liquids, a "wet"-sounding voice, and fever. Chest x-rays and laryngeal and chest auscultation are also useful

to diagnose the signs and symptoms of aspiration pneumonia.

Nodules and Polyps of the Vocal Cords

Overview

Nodules often appear at the point where the vocal cords touch during voicing. Nodules are hypertrophied fibrous tissue (Fig. 31–2) resulting from overuse of the voice or after an infectious process. The populations most affected are teachers, coaches, sports fans, singers, and people who use their voices in noisy environments.

Vocal cord polyps (Fig. 31–3) are chronic edematous masses. Polyps occur most commonly in adults who smoke, have many allergies, or live in dry climates. Vocal cysts also may occur.

Collaborative Management

Both nodules and polyps are painless, but they produce hoarseness because of the loss of coordinated approximation of the vocal cords and vocal wave (Fig. 31–4).

Nursing management of the client with vocal cord nodules or polyps is aimed at client and family education. The nurse teaches the client about the hazards of tobacco use, smoking cessation programs, and the importance of voice rest. Conservative treatment includes not whispering and avoiding heavy lifting. Stool softeners are used to avoid excessive Valsalva maneuvers to close the glottis.

Humidification and specialized speech therapy help to reduce the intensity of speech. Speech therapy is a primary treatment for behavioral voice changes. A conservative approach using speech therapy may make surgery unnecessary.

If hoarseness or the presenting voice disturbance is not relieved by voice rest or speech therapy, the physician may excise the nodules or polyps under direct laryngos-

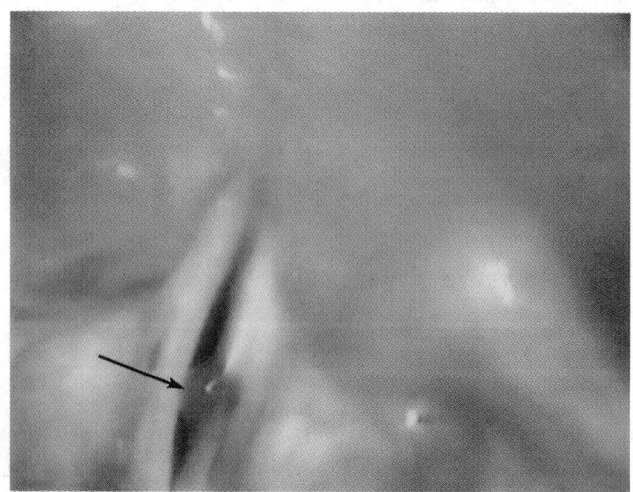

Figure 31–3. A hemorrhagic vocal cord polyp.

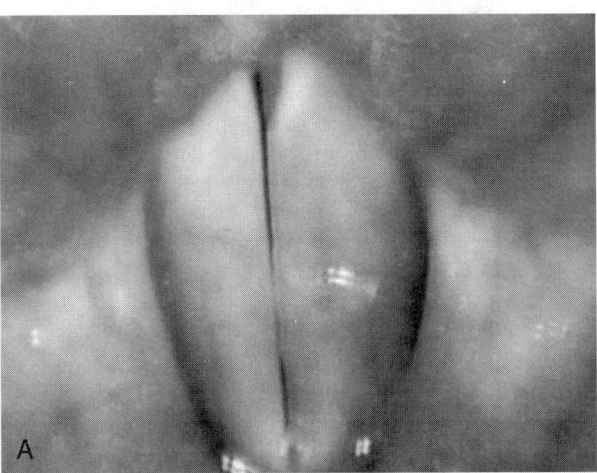
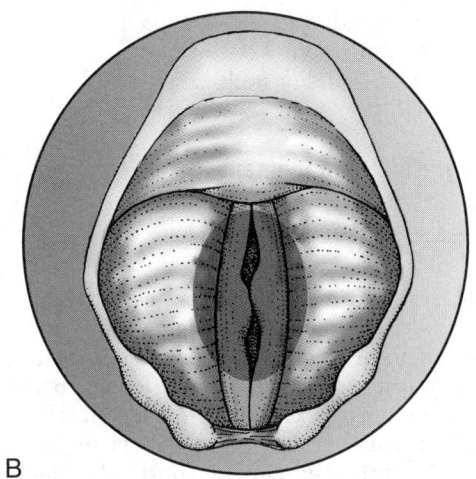

Figure 31–4. *A,* Close-up view of normal vocal folds in phonation. Saying the letter *E* in a high pitch allows the examiner to evaluate the total movement of the cords in all pitch ranges and evaluate membrane contact. *B,* Vocal cord nodules and polyps prevent approximation of the vocal cords. Hoarseness results.

copy. Laser and surgical resection are used to excise or strip the mucous membrane of the affected cord. If both cords are involved, one cord is usually allowed to heal before surgery is performed on the other cord.

After surgery, the client must maintain complete voice rest for about 14 days to promote healing. Alternative methods of communication, such as a slate board, pen and paper, "magic slate," or alphabet board are used. The nurse places a sign on the client's door, over the bed, and on the intercom system to help implement this important nursing intervention. Education is imperative before the operation and before the client returns home because these procedures are often performed in an outpatient setting.

Laryngeal Trauma

Overview

Laryngeal trauma is a result of crushing or direct blow injury, fracture, or intrinsic injury such as that induced by prolonged endotracheal intubation.

Collaborative Management

Symptoms of laryngeal trauma include dyspnea, aphonia, hoarseness, and subcutaneous emphysema. Bleeding from the airway (hemoptysis) may occur, depending on the location of the trauma. The physician performs a direct visual examination by laryngoscopy or fiberoptic laryngoscopy, of the larynx to determine the exact nature of the injury.

Management of clients with laryngeal injuries consists of assessing and frequent monitoring of vital signs (every 15–30 minutes), including respiratory status and pulse oximetry. The nursing priority is to maintain a patent airway. The nurse places oxygen and humidification as ordered to maintain adequate oxygen saturation. If the client has respiratory difficulty, as evidenced by signs

such as increasing tachypnea, anxiety, sternal retraction, shortness of breath, dyspnea, restlessness, decreased oxygen saturation, decreased level of consciousness, nasal flaring, and stridor, the nurse stays with the client and instructs other trauma team members to prepare for emergency cricothyroidotomy (cricothyrotomy) or tracheostomy.

For lacerations of the mucous membranes, cartilage exposure, and paralysis of the cords, surgical intervention is necessary. Laryngeal repair is performed as soon as possible to prevent laryngeal stenosis and to cover any exposed cartilage. An artificial airway may be indicated. Maintenance of a patent airway is the utmost priority.

OTHER UPPER AIRWAY DISORDERS
Upper Airway Obstruction

Overview

Upper airway obstruction is a life-threatening emergency defined as any significant interruption in airflow through the nose, mouth, pharynx, or larynx. Early recognition is essential to prevent further complications, including respiratory arrest. Some potential causes of upper airway obstruction are

- Tongue edema (surgery, trauma)
- Occlusion by the tongue (e.g., with loss of protective reflexes, loss of pharyngeal muscle tone, unconsciousness, and coma)
- Laryngeal edema
- Peritonsillar and pharyngeal abscess
- Head and neck carcinoma
- Thick secretions in the airway
- Cerebral disorders (i.e., cerebrovascular accident [CVA])
- Smoke inhalation edema

- Facial, tracheal, and/or laryngeal trauma
- Foreign body aspiration
- Burns of the head and/or neck area
- Anaphylaxis

Collaborative Management

 Assessment

Prompt nursing and medical care are essential to prevent a partial airway obstruction from progressing to a complete obstruction. A client with a partial obstruction (e.g., caused by limited edema or a small foreign body) may have few symptoms. Unexplained or persistent recurrent symptoms warrant evaluation even though the symptoms are vague. To rule out any potentially life-threatening condition, such as a tumor, foreign body, or infection, the physician orders diagnostic procedures, such as chest x-ray, lateral neck films, direct laryngoscopic examination, and computed tomography. Upper airway obstruction can be a frightening experience for the client and family.

The nurse observes for signs of hypoxia and hypercapnia, restlessness, increasing anxiety, sternal retractions, "seesawing" chest, abdominal movements, or a feeling of impending doom related to actual air hunger. The nurse performs pulse oximetry for the ongoing monitoring of oxygen saturation and assesses for stridor, cyanosis, and changes in level of consciousness.

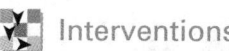 Interventions

The nurse assesses for the cause of the obstruction. When obstruction is due to the tongue falling back or to the accumulation of secretions, the nurse places the client's head and neck in a slightly extended position, inserts an oral airway, and may use suction to remove obstructing secretions. If the airway obstruction results from a foreign body, the nurse performs abdominal thrusts (Fig. 31–5).

Upper airway obstruction may necessitate emergency procedures, such as a cricothyroidotomy, endotracheal intubation, or tracheostomy. These procedures are often preceded or followed by direct laryngoscopy to evaluate the cause of obstruction. The physician uses direct laryngoscopy in a controlled situation as the treatment of choice for removal of foreign bodies.

➤ *Cricothyroidotomy*

Cricothyroidotomy is a life-saving emergency procedure and is usually performed outside the hospital by emergency medical personnel or in the emergency department by a physician. A cricothyroidotomy is a stab wound at the cricothyroid membrane between the thyroid cartilage and the cricoid cartilage ring (see Fig. 29–3). Any hollow tube—but preferably a tracheostomy tube—can be placed through this opening to keep the new airway open until a formal tracheotomy can be performed. This proce-

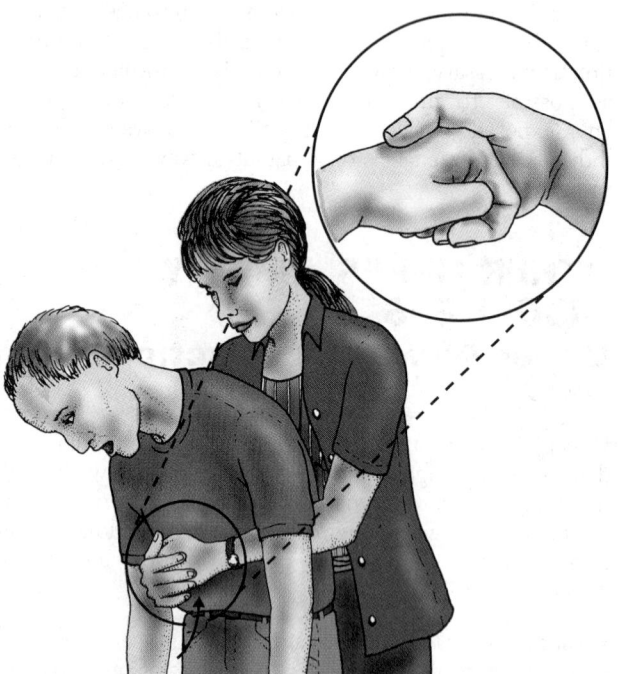

With the **conscious victim standing or sitting,** place your fist between the victim's lower rib cage and navel. Wrap the palm of your other hand around your fist. A quick inward, upward thrust expels the air remaining in the victim's lungs and with it the foreign body. If the first thrust is unsuccessful, repeat several thrusts in rapid succession until the foreign body is expelled or until the victim loses consciousness.

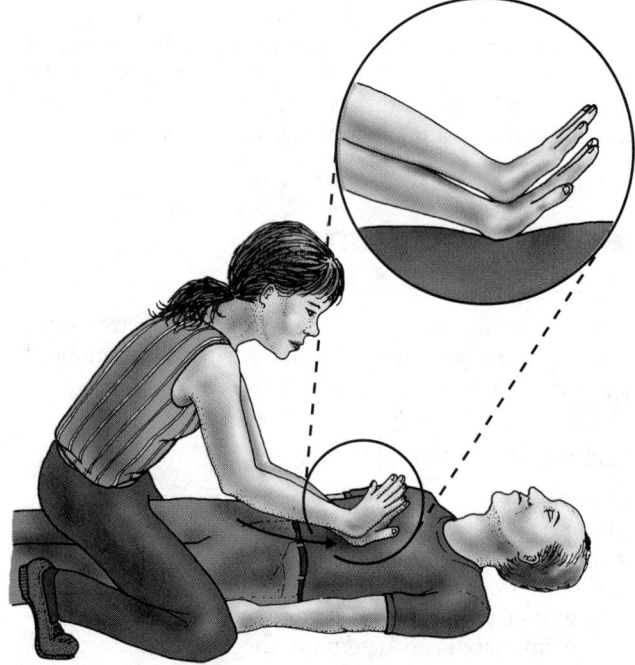

With the **unconscious victim lying supine,** straddle the victim's thighs. Place your hands one over the other as shown, with the heel of the bottom hand just above the victim's navel. Quickly thrust inward and upward, toward the victim's head.

Figure 31–5. The abdominal thrust maneuver (formerly referred to as the Heimlich maneuver) for relief of upper airway obstruction caused by a foreign body.

dure is warranted when it is the only way to secure an airway for the client. Alternatively, the physician can make an incision by inserting a 14-gauge needle immediately into the cricoid space to allow air into and out of the lungs, thus bypassing the obstruction.

➤ Endotracheal Intubation

To accomplish endotracheal intubation, a tube is inserted into the trachea via the nose (nasotracheal) or mouth (orotracheal) by a physician, a nurse anesthetist, or another specially trained nurse.

➤ Tracheostomy

Tracheostomy is usually an elective procedure that takes about 5–10 minutes to perform. The procedure takes place in the operating room (preferably) with the client under local or general anesthesia, or it can be done at the bedside. Infrequently, an awake tracheostomy with local anesthesia is done if the concern is losing the airway during induction of anesthesia. An emergency tracheostomy is reserved for the client who cannot be immediately intubated with an oral or nasal endotracheal tube. The airway can be established in less than 2 minutes in an emergency situation. (Care of the client with a tracheostomy is discussed in detail in Chapter 30.)

The client receiving mechanical ventilation as part of the treatment for upper airway obstruction or respiratory failure may require elective tracheostomy after 7 or more days of continuous oral or nasal intubation. The procedure is then performed to prevent laryngeal injury by the endotracheal tube (ET).

Neck Trauma

Overview

Injuries to the neck are most often caused by a knife, gunshot, or traumatic accident. Clients with neck trauma may have multiple injuries, including cardiovascular, respiratory, gastrointestinal, and neurologic damage. The final outcome of this type of injury depends on the initial assessment and management. (Consult a critical care or emergency textbook as well as Chapter 47 for more in-depth information. Advanced cardiac life support courses are also valuable.)

Collaborative Management

 Assessment

The priority in the management of neck trauma is assessment for a patent airway. The nurse then assesses the cardiovascular system for signs of internal or external bleeding or impending shock.

The nurse performs a baseline neurologic assessment for mental status, sensory level, and motor function. Injury to the carotid artery may result in death, stroke, or paralysis related to interruption of blood to the brain. The physician may order a carotid angiogram (see Chap. 35) to rule out vascular injuries.

Injuries involving the esophagus also may occur with neck trauma. The nurse assesses for chest pain and tenderness, oral bleeding, and crepitus. The physician may order a barium or meglumine diatrizoate (Gastrografin) swallow to rule out esophageal perforation injury.

 Interventions

Cervical spine injuries often occur at the same time as a neck injury (see Chap. 45). The nurse and emergency personnel must take great care not to exacerbate these injuries by causing neck movement while establishing the airway. The nurse prepares to assist in emergency intubation, cricothyrotomy, or tracheostomy to establish a patent airway. (Interventions for clients in shock are detailed in Chapter 39.)

Head and Neck Cancer
Overview

Head and neck cancer interferes with breathing, eating, facial appearance, self-image, speech, and communication. This form of cancer can be a devastating disease even if it is successfully treated. The nurse is challenged in caring for the client with these complex problems. The client can receive appropriate care only through accurate identification of the location and size of the original tumor. An interdisciplinary health care team approach is essential to address the entire spectrum of needs for these clients.

Head and neck cancer can be a curable disease when treated early. The prognosis for those who have more advanced disease at diagnosis depends on the extent and location of the tumor. Untreated cancer of the head and neck is a fatal disease, and the untreated client will usually die within 2 years of diagnosis.

Pathophysiology

Most head and neck cancers (80%) are squamous cell (mucosal epithelial) carcinomas (Fig. 31–6), usually requiring several years to develop. Many head and neck tumors present as malignant ulcerations with underlying infiltration.

Initially, the mucosa is subjected to an irritating substance and transforms itself into a tougher mucosa (squamous metaplasia) by increasing the mucosal thickness (acanthosis or hyperplasia) or by developing a keratin layer (keratosis). At the same time, cellular gene changes lead to the proliferation of atypical or dysplastic epithelial cells that eventually become malignant. These atypical lesions may then take the form of white, patchy lesions or red, velvety patches. Head and neck carcinoma is often diagnosed on the basis of white, patchy mucosal lesions called *leukoplakia*, or red patches called *erythroplasia*.

Growth and spread of the carcinoma depend on the site of the primary tumor. Spread is predominantly to adjacent anatomic areas like mucosa, muscle, and bone. Systemic dissemination through the circulatory and lymphatic systems may also occur. When metastasis occurs, it is most commonly to the lungs or liver.

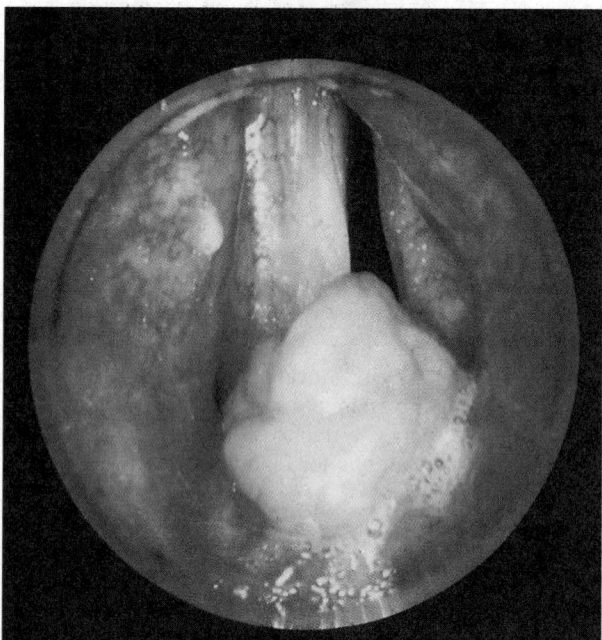

Figure 31–6. Laryngeal cancer is frequently caused by the combination of alcohol and tobacco. This laryngoscopic photograph shows a large granular cell tumor of the true vocal cord. From Wenig, B. M. (1993). *Atlas of head and neck pathology.* Philadelphia: W. B. Saunders. Used with permission.

The histologic description of squamous cell cancers includes carcinoma in situ, well-differentiated carcinoma, moderately differentiated carcinoma, or poorly differentiated carcinoma. Most head and neck cancers are of squamous origin, but they also can be of salivary gland or thyroid (papillary or follicular) origin. They can also be epidermoid, adenoid cystic, malignant melanoma, or adenocarcinoma. These tumors are treated by various methods directed by the type of tumor and its known response to therapies.

Etiology

Numerous risk factors have been identified as contributing to the development of head and neck cancer. The two most important risk factors are tobacco and alcohol use and especially the combination of the two. Other risk factors include chewing tobacco, pipe smoking, marijuana, voice abuse, chronic laryngitis, exposure to industrial chemicals or hardwood dust, and complete neglect of oral hygiene.

Incidence/Prevalence

The frequency of occurrence of head and neck carcinoma is increasing. The American Cancer Society (ACS) estimates 42,100 newly diagnosed cases of oral and laryngeal cancers per year, accounting for more than 4% of all carcinomas and more than 11,000 deaths per year (American Cancer Society, 1998). About three times more males are affected than females, and most head and neck cancers occur in people older than 60 years.

TRANSCULTURAL CONSIDERATIONS

 The rate of death for men of all races from cancer of the larynx has not changed over three decades, but there has been a 110% increase in the non-Caucasian population, up from 2.3 to 4.9 cases. Death rates for women with oral or laryngeal cancers have increased for all races over the past three decades.

Collaborative Management

Assessment

➤ History

The client with head and neck cancer may have difficulty speaking because of hoarseness, shortness of breath, tumor bulk, and pain. The nurse is sensitive to these difficulties during the interview.

The nurse questions the client about tobacco and alcohol use, history of recurrent acute or chronic laryngitis or pharyngitis, oral sores, and lumps in the neck. The client's smoking history is calculated in *pack-years* (the number of packs smoked per day times the number of years the client has smoked). The nurse asks about alcohol intake (how many drinks per day and for how many years). Questions of this nature may be uncomfortable for both the client and the nurse but are an important part of the history. The nurse also asks whether the client has been exposed to any environmental or occupational pollutants.

The nurse assesses problems related to risk factors. For example, nutrition may be poor because of alcohol intake and impairment of liver function. The nurse assesses dietary habits and any reported weight loss. The nurse notes a history of chronic lung disease, which has an impact on the client's breathing pattern and is an important operative risk factor.

➤ Physical Assessment/Clinical Manifestations

Table 31–1 summarizes the warning signs of head and neck cancer. With laryngeal cancer, hoarseness may occur because of tumor bulk and a lack of ability to approximate vocal cords in a normal fashion during phonation (see Fig. 31–7 for common sites of laryngeal cancer). Lesions of the true vocal cords are the earliest form of laryngeal cancer. A careful evaluation is important for anyone who has a history of hoarseness, sores in the mouth, or a lump in the neck for a period of 3–4 weeks or longer.

The techniques of inspection and palpation of the head and neck are an important part of the physical examination. A nurse who is specially trained may perform a laryngeal examination, which includes the use of the laryngeal mirror or fiberoptic laryngoscope. Lesions may be visible on direct inspection, and the nurse palpates the neck for tumor nodal involvement. A cranial nerve assessment (see Chap. 43) is also valuable because some tumors have an affinity for dissemination along these nerves as well as direct tumor invasion.

TABLE 31-1

Warning Signs of Head and Neck Cancer

- Pain
- A lump in the mouth, throat, or neck
- Difficulty in swallowing
- Color changes in the mouth or tongue to red, white, gray, dark brown, or black
- An oral lesion or sore that does not heal in 2 weeks
- Persistent or unexplained oral bleeding
- Numbness of the mouth, lips, or face
- Change in the fit of dentures
- Burning sensation when drinking citrus juices or hot liquids
- Persistent, unilateral ear pain
- Hoarseness or change in voice quality
- Persient or recurrent sore throat
- Shortness of breath
- Anorexia and weight loss

➤ *Psychosocial Assessment*

The typical client with head and neck carcinoma has a long-standing history of cigarette or alcohol use, or both. The client or family may experience denial, guilt, blame, or shame once the diagnosis is suspected. The nurse assesses the availability and adequacy of support systems and coping mechanisms. Because the client frequently requires extensive assistance at home after treatment, assessment and documentation of social and family support are essential. The nurse consults the social worker for assistance as needed. Because of the importance of preoperative and postoperative teaching, the nurse also evaluates cognitive functioning (see Chap. 43), level of education, and literacy of the client and family.

The nurse notes any family history of cancer as well as the client's age, gender, occupation, interests, and ability to perform the activities of daily living. The nurse investigates whether the client's occupation requires continual oral communication, whether the client will need retraining in other vocational areas, or whether the client will be able to resume the same job after treatment.

➤ *Laboratory Assessment*

Routine diagnostic laboratory tests include a complete blood count, bleeding times, urinalysis, and SMA-20. The nurse is alert to decreased hemoglobin or hematocrit values and an increased alkaline phosphatase level. Decreased protein and albumin levels indicate a loss of protein stores and define nutritional risks often seen in the alcoholic client. Renal and liver function tests are performed to rule out metastatic disease and to evaluate the client's ability to metabolize medications and chemotherapeutic agents.

➤ *Radiographic Assessment*

Many types of radiographic studies, including x-rays of the skull, sinuses, neck, and chest, are useful in diagnosing metastases, second primary tumors, and the extent of

tumor invasion. Computed tomography (CT) of the head and neck, with or without contrast media, helps evaluate the tumor's exact location.

➤ *Other Diagnostic Assessment*

Magnetic resonance imaging (MRI) can differentiate normal from diseased tissue. MRI is more sensitive than CT in defining the extent of soft-tissue invasion.

The brain, bone, and liver may also be evaluated with nuclear imaging, bone scans, SPECT (single photon emission computed tomography) and PET (positron emission tomography) scans. These tests help locate additional tumor sites.

Other diagnostic tests include direct and indirect laryngoscopy, tumor mapping, and biopsy. Panendoscopy is performed with general anesthesia to define the extent of the tumor. This procedure includes laryngoscopy, nasopharyngoscopy, esophagoscopy, and bronchoscopy. Anatomic tumor mapping uses biopsy to outline and identify tumor location. At the time of the panendoscopy, the biopsy confirms the diagnosis and determines the tumor type, histologic presentation, and defined location. Tumor staging by the TNM classification (see Chap. 26 and Table 26–8) is done at this time.

▼ Analysis

➤ *Common Nursing Diagnoses and Collaborative Problems*

The primary collaborative problem is High Risk for Ineffective Breathing Pattern related to impaired airway from

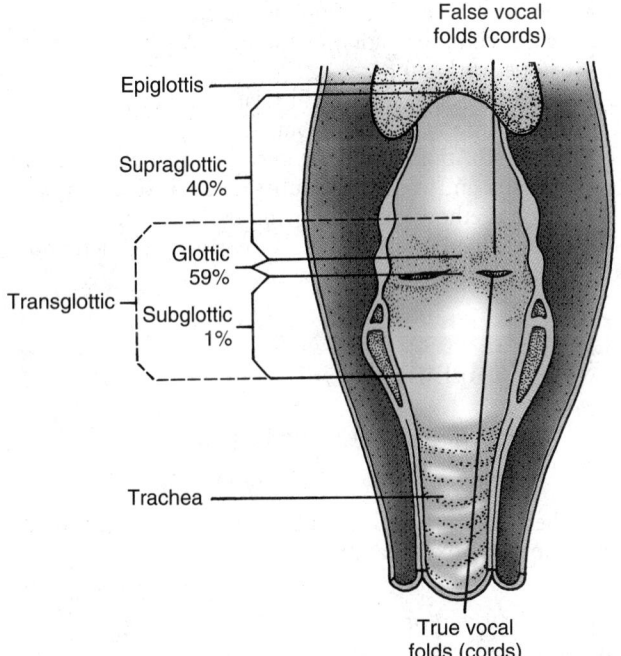

Figure 31–7. Sites and incidence of primary laryngeal tumors.

the disease process (i.e., tumor invasion or obstruction, edema, and chronic lung disease).

The priority nursing diagnoses for clients with head and neck carcinomas are

1. Risk for Aspiration related to edema, anatomic changes, or alteration of protective oropharyngeal reflexes
2. Anxiety related to fear of the unknown
3. Body Image Disturbance related to tumor and treatment modalities

➤ Additional Nursing Diagnoses and Collaborative Problems

In addition to the common nursing diagnoses and collaborative problems, the client may present with one or more of the following:

- Pain related to tumor invasion of tissues and nerves and surgical intervention
- Altered Nutrition: Less than Body Requirements related to dysphagia, anxiety, tumor process, surgical resection, or chronic alcohol intake
- Impaired Verbal Communication related to tumor invasion, associated aphonia, hoarseness, pain, and/or surgical resection
- Altered Cerebral Tissue Perfusion related to wound breakdown, recurrent tumor, and resultant interruption of arterial blood flow from carotid rupture
- Impaired Tissue Integrity related to altered circulation, nutritional deficit, tumor invasion, radiation, chemical factors (body secretions or substances), or surgical wound
- Impaired Skin Integrity related to altered circulation, nutritional deficit, tumor invasion, radiation, chemical factors (body secretions or substances), or surgical wound
- Ineffective Individual Coping related to altered body image, communication method, and/or ineffective social network support
- Impaired Social Interaction related to body image disturbance and lifestyle practices
- Impaired Adjustment related to self-care of the tracheostomy and nasogastric tubes, alternative communication methods, and body image disturbance
- Knowledge Deficit related to treatment regimen and unfamiliarity with information resources

 Planning and Implementation

➤ Ineffective Breathing Pattern

Planning: Expected Outcomes

The client is expected to attain or maintain adequate ventilation and oxygenation.

Interventions

The goal of treatment is removal or eradication of the cancer with preservation of as much normal function as possible. The physician presents available treatment op-

tions to the client. Modalities may be used alone or in combination. When planning treatment options, the physician considers general physical condition, nutritional status, age, effects of the tumor on body function, and, most importantly, the client's personal choice. Before recommending extensive surgery, the physician considers the client's ability to manage his or her own care postoperatively.

The treatment of laryngeal cancer may range from radiation therapy, for a small specific area or tumor, to total laryngopharyngectomy, with bilateral neck dissections followed by radiation therapy. The specific treatment depends on the extent and location of the lesion. Voice conservation procedures are elected only if they can be accomplished without risking incomplete removal of the tumor. The nurse focuses on the client's total needs, including preoperative preparation, competent in-hospital care, discharge planning and teaching, and extensive outpatient rehabilitation.

Nonsurgical Management. The nurse monitors the client's respiratory system by assessing respiratory rate, breath sounds, pulse oximetry, arterial blood gas values, and results of pulmonary function tests. Signs of respiratory distress may indicate narrowing of the airway related to tumor growth, edema, or both. The nurse positions the client for optimal air exchange. The nurse educates the client and family about the use of Fowler's and semi-Fowler's positions. The client may breathe more comfortably by sitting upright in a reclining chair. Chapters 9 and 12 and texts on hospice care can provide additional information on palliation and pain control for the client who elects no therapy and for the client whose therapy has not been effective.

Radiation Therapy. Radiation treatment of small cancers in specific locations offers a cure rate of 80% and greater. Treatment of larger cancers offers a lower cure rate when radiation is used as a single-modality therapy. Standard therapy uses 5000–7500 rad usually over 6 weeks in daily or twice-daily doses. The physician may recommend radiation alone or in combination with surgery. Because radiation therapy causes alterations in tissue healing, it might not be recommended preoperatively. Radiation therapy is commonly an outpatient procedure (see Chap. 27). During and for a few weeks after radiation therapy, the client will have uncomfortable side effects.

Hoarseness becomes worse. The nurse reassures the client and family that vocalization will improve to at least pretreatment levels within 4–6 weeks after completion of radiation therapy. The client is encouraged to use voice rest and alternative means of communication until the effects of radiation have subsided.

Most clients have a sore throat and difficulty swallowing during radiation therapy. Gargling with saline or sucking ice may decrease discomfort. Pain medication is ordered as needed.

The skin at the site of radiation becomes red and tender, and it may peel during therapy. The client must avoid exposing this area to sun, heat, cold, and abrasive treatments such as shaving. The nurse instructs the client to wear protective clothing made of soft cotton and to wash this area gently with a mild soap, such as Dove. The client should use only lotions or powders prescribed by the radiologist until the area has healed.

If the salivary glands are in the path of radiation, the client will have a dry mouth. This side effect is long term and may be permanent. Heavy fluid intake, particularly of water, and a humidified atmosphere can help relieve the discomfort. Some clients benefit from the use of artificial saliva.

Chemotherapy. Chemotherapy is not usually used alone for cancers of the head and neck. At times, it is an adjuvant to surgery or radiation. The most commonly used chemotherapeutic agents for cancer of the neck include methotrexate (Mexate), vincristine (Oncovin), bleomycin (Blenoxane), and cisplatin (Platinol). Methotrexate may be used for patients who cannot undergo rigorous surgery, radiation, or chemotherapy. Often terminal patients receive methotrexate for control (not cure) of the disease, and for assistance in pain control. (Chapter 27 includes general care needs of clients receiving chemotherapy.)

Surgical Management. Tumor size and location (TNM classification) defines the extent of surgical intervention for cancer of the head and neck. The method of reconstruction is also determined by the tumor size and amount of tissue to be resected and reconstructed. Surgical procedures for head and neck cancers include laryngectomy (total and partial), tracheostomy, and oropharyngeal cancer resections.

Laryngectomy and Related Surgical Procedures. The major types of resections for laryngeal cancer include cordal stripping, *cordectomy* (excision of a vocal cord), partial laryngectomy, and total laryngectomy. If neck lymph nodes are involved or if the tumor carries with it a known high rate of nodal spread, the surgeon performs a nodal neck dissection in conjunction with removal of the primary tumor. A pathologist evaluates the resected lymph nodes for tumor invasion.

Preoperative Care. As the client advocate, the nurse teaches the client and family about the tumor. The physician explains the surgical procedure and obtains the client's informed consent. The nurse discusses and interprets the implications of such consent.

The nurse explains about self-care of the airway, compensatory methods of communication, suctioning, pain control methods, the critical care environment (including ventilators and critical care routines), nutritional support, feeding tubes, and goals for discharge. The client must learn new methods of speech postoperatively. The nurse prepares the client for this change through preoperative teaching and establishes with the client an alternative form of communication (e.g., pen and pencil, "magic slate," picture or alphabet board) before surgery.

The explanations of routines and outcomes of care are very important because these discussions are used to plan the hospitalization and rehabilitation. Multidisciplinary teams of speech pathologists, social workers, dietitians, and occupational and physical therapists, along with the nurses and physicians, are vitally important in the preoperative evaluation and preparation of clients with cancer. (Chapter 20 describes general preoperative assessment and education in detail.)

Operative Procedures. Hemilaryngectomy (vertical or horizontal) and supraglottic laryngectomy are types of partial voice conservation laryngectomies. Table 31–2 presents more specific information on the various surgical procedures.

To protect the airway, a temporary or permanent tracheostomy is usually performed with a partial laryngectomy. With a total laryngectomy, the upper airway is separated from the pharynx and esophagus, and the trachea is brought out through the skin in the neck and sutured in place, creating a stoma. This airway opening is *always* permanent and is referred to as a laryngectomy stoma.

Neck dissection includes removal of tumor-involved lymph nodes, the sternocleidomastoid muscle, the jugular vein, the 11th cranial nerve, and surrounding involved soft tissue. Because the 11th cranial nerve—the spinal accessory nerve—is resected during the nodal dissection, shoulder drop will be present postoperatively. Physical therapy exercises are imperative and help the client ease

TABLE 31–2

Surgical Procedures for Laryngeal Cancer and Their Effect on Voice Quality

Procedure	Description	Resulting Voice Quality
Laser surgery	• Tumor reduced or destroyed by laser beam through laryngoscope	• Normal/ hoarse
Transoral cordectomy	• Tumor (early lesion) resected through laryngoscope	• Normal (high cure rate)/ hoarse
Laryngofissure	• No cord removed (early lesion)	• Normal (high cure rate)
Supraglottic partial laryngectomy	• Hyoid bone, false cords, and epiglottis removed • Neck dissection on affected side performed if nodes involved	• Normal/ hoarse
Hemilaryngectomy or vertical laryngectomy	• One true cord, one false cord, and one half of thyroid cartilage removed	• Hoarse voice
Total laryngectomy	• Entire larynx, hyoid bone, strap muscles, one or two tracheal rings removed • Nodal neck dissection if nodes involved	• No natural voice

the shoulder drop by increasing the use of other muscle groups.

Postoperative Care. Head and neck surgical procedures often last 8 hours or longer. Because of the duration of anesthesia and the amount of resection and reconstruction, the client may spend the immediate postoperative period in the surgical intensive care unit. The nurse monitors the client's airway patency, vital signs, hemodynamic status, and comfort level. The nurse is also alert to the possibility of postoperative hemorrhage and other general complications of anesthesia and surgery (see Chap. 22). Vital signs are monitored every hour for the first 24 hours and then every 2 hours until the client is stable. After the client is transferred from the critical care unit, vital signs can be monitored every 4 hours or according to agency policy. The client is generally out of bed by the second postoperative day.

Complications after a head and neck cancer resection include airway obstruction, hemorrhage, wound breakdown, and tumor recurrence. The priorities in postoperative head and neck cancer care include airway maintenance and ventilation; wound, flap, and reconstructive tissue care (see Client Care Plan); pain management; nutrition; and psychological adjustment, including speech therapy.

Airway Maintenance and Ventilation. In the immediate postoperative period, clients may need ventilatory assistance because of a long-term smoking history, chronic lung disease, or long duration of anesthesia. Although many clients also have chronic lung disease, weaning usually is not difficult because the thoracic and abdominal cavities are not entered during the surgical procedure and because the cough mechanism is intact. When weaned from the ventilator, clients typically use a tracheostomy collar (over the artificial airway or open stoma) with oxygen and humidification to help mobilize mucous secretions. Secretions may remain blood tinged for 1–2 days. The nurse maintains body substance precautions and reports any increase in bleeding to the physician. Humidification helps to remove crusts and prevent obstruction of the tube with secretions. Sterile saline instillation of 5–10 mL every 2 hours or as needed may also be ordered.

Clients who have had a total laryngectomy and need an appliance to prevent scar tissue contracture at the skin tracheal border use a laryngectomy tube. This tube is similar to a conventional tracheostomy tube but is shorter and fatter with a larger lumen and a more acute angle (Fig. 31–8). Laryngectomy tube care is similar to tracheostomy tube care (see Chap. 30), except that clients can change the laryngectomy tube on a daily or an as-needed basis. A laryngectomy button is similar to a laryngectomy tube but is made of a silicone-like substance (Silastic), has a single lumen, and is very short. A button is very comfortable for laryngectomy patients, is easily removed for cleaning, and is available in various sizes and lengths for a custom fit. The nurse provides a "magic slate" or paper and pencil for communication because clients have no immediate oral communication capabilities other than mouthing words.

Coughing, deep breathing, and saline instillation are often totally effective in clearing secretions. The lack of

surgical interruption in the thoracic cavity or abdomen improves the ability to cough. The nurse instructs clients in the proper techniques for coughing and deep breathing (see Chap. 20) to clear secretions.

Oral secretions can be suctioned with a Yankauer or tonsillar suction. The nurse teaches clients to suction away from the side of an oral cavity cancer resection to preserve continuity of the wounds immediately after surgery. The nurse teaches clients self-care by providing this catheter for suctioning oral airway secretions. Using a table mirror for visibility, clients can participate in their own care. The nurse provides a clean environment for the catheter.

Stoma care after total laryngectomy is a combination of wound care and airway care. Careful inspection of the stoma with a flashlight is routine. The nurse cleans the suture line with half-strength hydrogen peroxide to prevent secretions from forming crusts and obstructing the airway. Suture line care is performed every 1–2 hours initially, advancing to every 4 hours by the fifth postoperative day. The mucosa of the stoma and trachea should be bright and shiny without crusts, similar to the appearance of the buccal mucosa.

Wound, Flap, and Reconstructive Tissue Care. Commonly used reconstructive flaps are pectoralis major myocutaneous flaps, island flaps, rotation flaps, trapezius flaps, split-thickness skin grafts (STSGs), and free flaps with microvascular anastomosis (scapula, fibula, or radial forearm free flaps). These flaps may be used for reconstruction

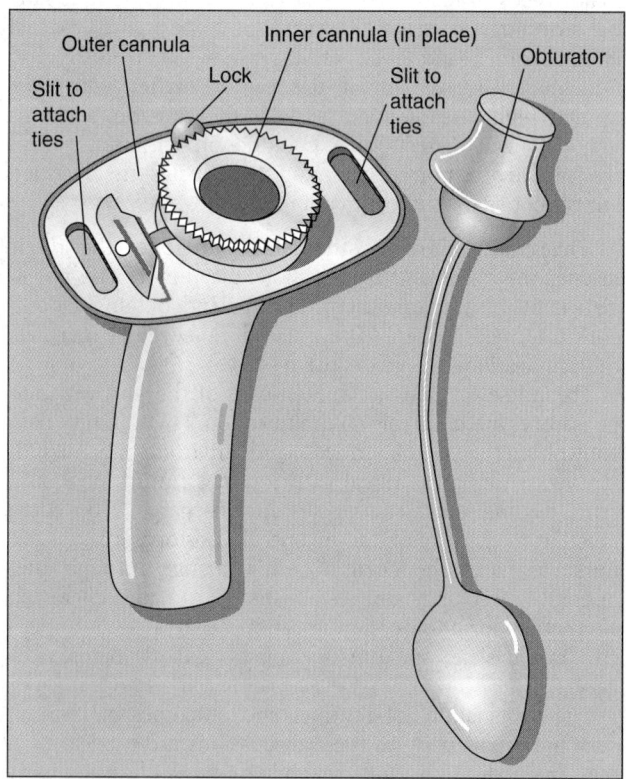

Figure 31–8. A laryngectomy tube. Note that the outer cannula is shorter and has a diameter wider than that of a tracheostomy tube.

Client Care Plan

The Client Who Has Had Head and Neck Surgery

Nursing Diagnosis No. 1: Ineffective Airway Clearance related to impaired airway from disease process (i.e., tumor invasion/obstruction, edema, chronic lung disease) and surgical intervention

Expected Outcomes	Nursing Interventions	Rationale
The client is expected to attain and/or maintain a patent airway. Lung sounds are expected to be maintained at the client's baseline or improved. Breathing efforts are expected to be without distress.	■ Monitor airway patency. ■ Assess for signs and symptoms of respiratory distress. ■ Place client in semi-Fowler's or Fowler's position as soon as possible postoperatively. ■ Suction client via the artificial airway frequently postoperatively (q30–60 minutes and advance to q2h and as needed). ■ Suction oral cavity as ordered using a Yankauer tonsillar tip catheter. ■ Inspect and clean laryngectomy stoma q2h and as needed. Use cotton-tipped applicators with peroxide and saline. ■ Perform laryngectomy tube care q4h, and advance to q shift, as needed, if ordered. ■ Have the client cough and deep breathe; if ordered, instill saline as needed. ■ Place an appropriate-sized laryngectomy set at bedside. ■ Document assessment findings and the client's response to interventions.	■ Ongoing assessment promotes early detection and treatment of complications. ■ Positioning makes breathing easier and facilitates oxygenation, secretion removal, and airway patency. ■ Suctioning and tube (if present) care promote removal of secretions that could obstruct airway. ■ A laryngectomy tube prevents scar tissue contracture and maintains airway. ■ Peroxide removes crusts and secretions. ■ Suction and cleaning procedures help to prevent obstruction and infection and promote healing. ■ Pulmonary hygiene exercises prevent pooling of secretions and promote oxygenation and ventilation. ■ Having duplicate equipment readily available enables prompt response in the event of distress or if urgent replacement of the tube is required (i.e., if the tube accidentally comes out). ■ Documentation provides an ongoing, permanent record of the client's progress and care requirements.

Nursing Diagnosis No. 2: Impaired Tissue Integrity and Impaired Skin Integrity related to the surgical wound

Expected Outcomes	Nursing Interventions	Rationale
The client's surgical wound area is expected to remain intact and heal without complications.	■ Assess wound integrity, capillary refill, and color q1–2 h for 48 hr. ■ Strip surgical drains q1–2h to ensure correct functioning. ■ Record each drain amount separately at least q shift.	■ Ongoing assessment promotes early detection and treatment of complications. ■ An accumulation of drainage beneath the skin or reconstructive flaps impairs tissue nutrition, resulting in vascular insufficiency and tissue breakdown.

(Continued)

Client Care Plan

Expected Outcomes	Nursing Interventions	Rationale
	■ Avoid constricting dressings, ties, or oxygen tubing around the suture lines or reconstructive flaps.	■ Pressure on altered or operated skin and tissue causes alteration in circulation.
	■ Keep wound clean and dry; perform routine care as ordered.	■ Appropriate wound care promotes healing and prevents complications.
	■ Ensure adequate nutrition by the enteral or parenteral feeding method.	■ Nutrition is imperative for tissue nutrition and healing.
	■ Document assessment findings and the client's response to interventions.	■ Documentation provides an ongoing, permanent record of care.

Nursing Diagnosis No. 3: Risk for Impaired Tissue Integrity and Impaired Skin Integrity related to tumor resection, wound breakdown, altered circulation, nutritional deficit, and chemical factors (body secretions or substances)

Expected Outcomes	Nursing Interventions	Rationale
The client's wound is expected to remain intact without complications of infection, bleeding, dehiscence, or fistula.	■ Monitor for signs of infection (e.g., redness, pus, suture line separation, increasing white blood cell count, fever, malaise).	■ Ongoing assessment promotes early detection and treatment of complications.
	■ Assess for saliva or refluxed enteral feeding in wound secretions.	■ Feedings or saliva in the wound represents a pharyngocutaneous fistula and wound infection.
	■ Provide wound care, as ordered, q2–4h	■ Aggressive nursing care keeps the wounds clean and free of cellular debris and promotes granulation tissue formation and healing.
	■ Maintain adequate nutrition via enteral or parenteral route, as ordered.	■ Adequate nutrition helps to prevent wound breakdown and promotes healing.

Nursing Diagnosis No. 4: Risk for Altered (Cerebral) Tissue Perfusion related to wound breakdown, recurrent tumor, and resultant interruption of arterial blood flow from carotid rupture

Expected Outcomes	Nursing Interventions	Rationale
The client's carotid artery is expected to remain intact without bleeding complications. If bleeding occurs, the client is expected to suffer minimal or no residual complications (i.e., stroke, cerebral insufficiency, cardiac damage).	■ Maintain carotid precautions if the carotid artery is exposed: 　■ Keep the carotid artery and dressing wet with *sterile* saline at all times, as ordered by the physician. 　■ Change dressings q2h to maintain a wet-to-wet dressing.	■ Keeping the carotid dressing clean and moist prevents drying and infection, which could cause bleeding, and promotes granulation of tissue over the carotid artery.

(Continued)

Client Care Plan

Expected Outcomes	Nursing Interventions	Rationale
	■ Move client to room closest to the nursing station or to the intensive care unit. ■ Place two large-gauge IV catheters, as ordered. ■ Keep dressing supplies, sterile saline, gloves, and IV solution (lactated Ringer's) at the bedside. ■ Be sure client has had a type and cross-match for blood ordered. ■ Alert operating room of any client receiving carotid precautions. ■ Monitor for and report any bleeding to the physician.	■ Being prepared for a carotid bleed may result in a more positive outcome. ■ Ongoing assessment promotes early detection and treatment of complications. ■ A small amount of bright red bleeding that stops spontaneously may herald a true carotid bleed.
	■ Discuss with client and family the potential for carotid rupture along with prevention, precautions, preparations, and goals of care.	■ Client and family education helps promote understanding, acceptance, and participation in the plan of care.

	■ If carotid bleeding occurs:
	  ■ Apply immediate direct pressure to the artery and **do not remove pressure.**
	  ■ Call for assistance!
	  ■ Direct another nurse to call the physician **immediately.**
	  ■ Secure the client's airway.
	  ■ Institute intravenous hydration as per standing order.
	  ■ If possible, talk to the client during emergency care.
	  ■ Transport to the operating room and **do not remove pressure** during transport.
		■ Direct pressure applied to the arterial bleeding site prevents rapid blood loss.
		
		■ Assistance will be needed for this emergency situation.
		
		■ A patent airway will help to ensure oxygenation.
		
		■ Talking to the client provides reassurance.

after any type of head and neck resection. After neck dissection, the surgeon places an STSG over the exposed carotid artery before covering it with skin flaps or reconstructive flaps.

The first 24 hours are critical. The nurse evaluates all flaps every hour for the first 72 hours, monitoring capillary refill, color, and Doppler activity of the major feeding vessel. Any changes are reported to the surgeon immediately because surgical intervention may be indicated. The nurse positions the client to protect the vascular supply of the reconstructed flaps.

Hemorrhage. Hemorrhage is a possible postoperative complication for all clients undergoing surgery, but it is uncommon in clients with laryngectomy. The physician often places a closed surgical drain (see Chap. 22) in the neck area to collect blood and drainage for approximately 72 hours postoperatively. The drain also helps to maintain the position of the reconstructed skin flaps. Any drain obstruction or equipment malfunction may cause a build-up of blood or serum under the flaps. This accumulation jeopardizes the blood supply of the flaps by interfering with both arterial supply and venous drainage.

Malfunction of the drains may necessitate a surgical procedure to remove accumulated clots.

Wound Breakdown. Wound breakdown is a frequent complication because of poor nutrition, wound contamination from the oral cavity, and previous radiation therapy. A history of alcohol use further complicates the nutritional status.

The nurse treats such wound breakdown with packing and local care as ordered to keep the wound clean and stimulate the growth of healthy granulation tissue. Wounds may be extensive, and the carotid artery may be exposed under the dehisced wounds. At the initial surgical resection, STSGs are placed over the carotid for protection in the event of such a wound dehiscence. As the wound heals, granulation tissue covers the artery and prevents rupture. If granulation is slow and the carotid artery is at risk, another surgical flap may be raised to cover the carotid artery and close the wound.

If the carotid artery ruptures because of drying or infection, the nurse places *immediate constant pressure* over the site and secures the airway. The client, still with direct manual pressure on the carotid artery, is *immediately* transported to the operating room for carotid resection. Carotid artery rupture has a high risk of stroke and death. Immediate nursing response can save the client's life.

Pain Management. After cancer surgery, the client's pain should be controlled, and the client should still be able to participate in care. Morphine (Statex✦) often is given by intravenous (IV) bolus and continuously for the first days after surgery. As the client progresses, acetaminophen with codeine and then acetaminophen alone can be given, all by feeding tube. Oral medications for pain and discomfort are started only after the client can tolerate oral nutrition. After discharge, the client still requires pain medication, especially if he or she is receiving radiation therapy. An adjunct to the pain regimen may be liquid nonsteroidal antiinflammatory drugs (NSAIDs); these drugs provide excellent pain relief and can be used in conjunction with opioid analgesics (see also Chap. 9). Amitriptyline (Elavil) or similar medications may also be used as an adjunct to pain medication administration for the lancinating pain of nerve root involvement.

Nutrition. A nasogastric, gastrostomy, or jejunostomy tube is placed intraoperatively for nutritional support while the aerodigestive tract heals. Initially, however, the client receives IV fluids (see Chap. 17) or parenteral nutrition (see Chap. 64) until the gastrointestinal tract has recovered from the effects of anesthesia. After that, nutrients may be administered via the feeding tube. The nutritional support team or dietitian assesses the client preoperatively and is available for consultations after surgery. A standard postoperative therapeutic goal is 35–40 kcal/kg of body weight. Protein and insensible water loss must also be very carefully calculated.

The nasogastric tube (the most commonly used tube type) usually remains in place for about 10 days after surgery. Before removing the tube, the nurse assesses the client's ability to swallow if the client is to receive nutrition by mouth. A client cannot aspirate after an uncomplicated total laryngectomy because the airway and esophagus are separated completely. The nurse reassures the client that aspiration will not occur and stays with the client during the first few swallowing attempts. The nurse anticipates that swallowing may be uncomfortable at first and may administer analgesics as ordered.

Speech Rehabilitation. Because the client's voice and speech can be expected to be altered after surgery, the speech pathologist and nurse discuss the principles of speech therapy with the client and family early in the course of the treatment plan. The differences will depend on the type of surgical resection (see Table 31–2). Speech production varies with client practice, amount of resection, and radiation effects, but the client's speech can be very understandable.

The speech rehabilitation plan for the client undergoing total laryngectomy consists initially of writing, then using an artificial larynx, and then learning esophageal speech. The client needs support and encouragement from the speech pathologist, hospital team, and family while relearning to speak. This process can be time consuming and necessitates concentration each time the client speaks. Having a laryngectomee from one of the local self-help organizations visit the client and family is often beneficial. The International Association of Laryngectomees is very active and supportive, as is the American Cancer Society Visitor Program.

Esophageal Speech. Most total laryngectomees attempt esophageal speech. Clients produce esophageal speech by "burping" the air swallowed or injected through the pharyngoesophageal (P-E) segment and articulate words in the mouth. The voice produced is a monotone; it cannot be raised or lowered and carries no pitch. Clients must have adequate hearing, or esophageal speech will be difficult because they use the mouth to shape the words as they hear them. Hearing-impaired clients may require hearing aids. In the English language, the vocal cords are necessary for 15 consonants; the remaining 10 consonants can be formed by shaping the mouth.

Initially, gastrointestinal bloating occurs as a result of swallowing air for esophageal speech. Antacids may help to diminish bloating sensations. Esophageal speech also helps to strengthen the respiratory and abdominal musculature, which aids the client in expectorating secretions and in breathing.

Mechanical Devices. Clients who cannot attain esophageal speech can use mechanical devices called electrolarynges. Most are battery-powered devices placed against the side of the neck or cheek. The air inside the mouth and pharynx is vibrated, and the client articulates as usual. Another external device (Cooper Rand), also battery powered, consists of a plastic tube, placed within the client's mouth, that vibrates on articulation.

Tracheoesophageal Fistula. A tracheoesophageal fistula (TEF) may be used if esophageal speech is insufficient for communication and if the client meets strict criteria. A surgical fistula is created between the trachea and the esophagus either at the time of the laryngectomy or in the postoperative period (Fig. 31–9). The surgeon places a

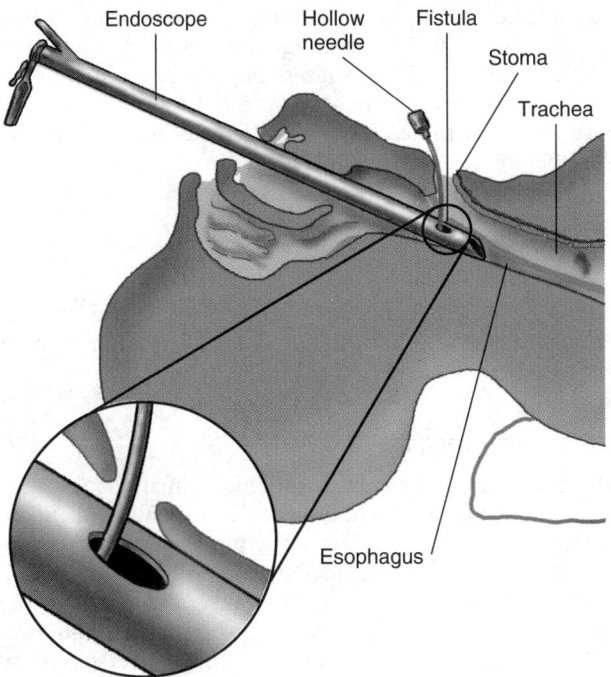

Figure 31–9. One method of creating a tracheoesophageal fistula.

catheter into the laryngectomy stoma and surgically creates a fistula into the esophagus. Usually, the catheter is then sutured to the neck to prevent accidental dislodgment. After the fistula heals, a silicone prosthesis, such as the Blom-Singer prosthesis (Fig. 31–10), is inserted in place of the catheter. The client covers the stoma and the opening of the prosthesis with a finger or opens and closes the opening with a special valve to divert air from the lungs, through the trachea, into the esophagus, and out of the mouth. Lip and tongue movement, not the prosthesis itself, produces speech.

Surgical Procedures for Other Head and Neck Cancers. The major types of resections, defined by the tumor location of the oropharyngeal cancer, are called composite resections. Composite resections are a combination of surgical procedures that include partial or total glossectomies, partial mandibulectomies, and, if required, nodal neck dissections. Tracheostomy may be planned to provide an adequate airway. (More information on oral cancer is found in Chapter 56.)

Tracheostomy. A tracheostomy can be performed as an emergency procedure or as a scheduled surgical procedure. A tracheotomy is a surgical incision into the trachea for the purpose of establishing an airway. Tracheostomy is the (tracheal) stoma, or opening, that results from the tracheotomy. The tracheostomy can be temporary or permanent. (Chapter 30 presents in detail the nursing care requirements of a client with a tracheostomy.)

➤ High Risk for Aspiration

Planning: Expected Outcomes

The client is expected not to aspirate food, gastrointestinal contents, or oral secretions into the lungs.

Interventions

Depending on tumor size and location or type of tumor resection, the client may aspirate during eating. This inci-

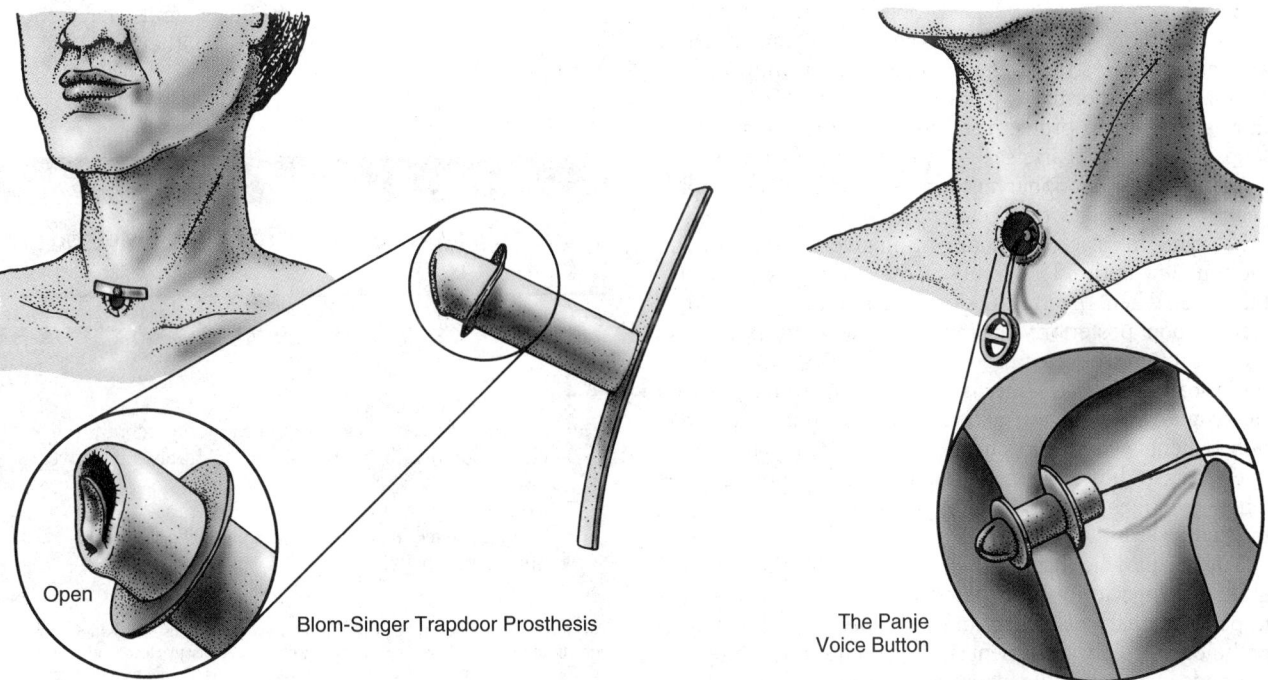

Figure 31–10. Examples of tracheoesophageal prostheses.

dent can result in life-threatening pneumonia, weight loss, further hospitalization, and increased costs.

Because of anatomic or surgical changes in the upper respiratory tract and altered swallowing mechanisms, the client with head and neck cancer is at risk for aspiration. The presence of a nasogastric (NG) feeding tube may further increase the potential for aspiration because of the incompetent lower esophageal sphincter (LES). The one exception is the client who has had a total laryngectomy; because the airway is separated from the esophagus, making aspiration impossible, such a person is not at risk.

A dynamic swallow study evaluates a client's ability to protect the airway from aspiration and helps to determine the appropriate method of swallow rehabilitation. Bedside clinical assessment of swallowing is important but carries with it a high rate of inaccuracy. In many cases, the physician must institute enteral feedings either because of the client's inability to swallow or because of continued aspiration potential.

When an NG tube is in place, the nurse helps to prevent aspiration through routine reflux precautions, including elevating the head of the bed and strictly adhering to tube feeding regimens, including no bolus feedings at night. The nurse checks residual feeding amounts before each bolus feeding (or every 4–6 hours with continuous feeding) and evaluates the client's tolerance of the tube feeding. If the residual volume is too high (<100 mL), the nurse withholds the feeding and notifies the physician. The nurse adds food coloring to the tube feeding and observes tracheal secretions. If aspiration occurs, secretions may be the color of the food coloring. Methylene blue is not used today as an additive to tube feedings because it is systemically excreted through the lungs and can appear in pulmonary secretions. (See Chapter 64 for other interventions related to NG tubes and tube feedings.)

Swallowing can be a major problem for the client with a tracheostomy tube in place, but if the cranial nerves and anatomical structures are intact, swallowing can be normal. In a normal swallow, the larynx elevates and moves forward to protect itself from the passing stream of food and saliva. Laryngeal elevation also assists in the opening of the cricopharyngeal muscle, the upper esophageal sphincter. The tracheostomy tube sometimes tethers the larynx in place, rendering it unable to execute this motion efficiently. The result is difficulty in swallowing. Likewise, when the tracheostomy tube cuff is inflated, it can balloon posteriorly and interfere with the passage of food through the esophagus. The common wall of the posterior trachea (trachealis muscle) and the anterior esophagus is very thin, allowing this pushing phenomenon. Clients with head and neck cancer who are cognitively intact, however, may adapt to eating normal food when the tracheostomy tube is small and the cuff is not inflated.

The client who has had a subtotal, vertical, or supraglottic laryngectomy, *must* be observed for aspiration. It is imperative that the nurse and the speech and language pathologist teach the client the procedure for alternate methods of swallowing without aspirating. Especially effective after partial laryngectomy or base-of-tongue resec-

tion is the "supraglottic method" of swallowing (Chart 31–2). To reinforce teaching and learning, the nurse places a chart in the client's room detailing the steps. A dynamic swallow study is performed to evaluate the client's ability to protect the airway and to guide rehabilitation therapy for swallowing.

> ➤ Anxiety

Planning: Expected Outcomes

The client is expected to verbalize decreased anxiety through increased knowledge and understanding about the specific, individualized treatment plan.

Interventions

The client may benefit from multidisciplinary conferences with the physician, clinical nurse specialist, dietitian, speech and language pathologist, physical therapist, psychologist, social worker, discharge planning nurse, as well as the general nursing staff. The nurse explores with the client the reason for anxiety (e.g., fear of the unknown, lack of preoperative teaching, fear of pain, fear of airway compromise, fear of hospitalization, and loss of control). Many times the client and family can benefit from further information. Before the client is scheduled for surgery and while the client is still at home, home care nurses or community-sponsored associations, such as the American Cancer Society, may be able to alleviate the fears of the client and family about the disease process and surgical interventions.

The nurse administers antianxiety agents, such as diazepam (Valium), with caution because of the possibility of hypercarbia and hypoxia in an already compromised client. The location of the tumor and any other concurrent lung disease may be causing some degree of airway obstruction. For anxiety in this client, the physician prescribes drug therapy judiciously and may choose lorazepam (Ativan, Novo-Lorazem✢) rather than a solely sedating agent.

Chart 31–2

Education Guide: The Supraglottic Method of Swallowing

1. Position yourself in an upright, preferably out-of-bed, position.
2. Clear your throat.
3. Take a deep breath.
4. Place ½ to 1 teaspoon of food into your mouth.
5. Hold your breath or "bear down" (Valsalva maneuver).
6. Swallow twice.
7. Release your breath, and clear your throat.
8. Swallow twice again.
9. Breathe normally.

This method exaggerates the normal protective mechanisms of cessation of respiration during the swallow. The double swallow attempts to clear food that may be pooling in the pharynx, vallecula, and piriform sinuses. This method is used only after a dynamic radiographic swallow study has demonstrated that it is appropriate and safe for the client.

➤ *Body Image Disturbance*

Planning: Expected Outcomes

The client is expected to state understanding and, in time, acceptance of body image changes and returns to the previous lifestyle within the limits of the disease.

Interventions

The client with head and neck cancer experiences a permanent change in body image because of deformity, the presence of a stoma or artificial airway, speech changes, and a change in the method of eating. The client may be aphonic (unable to speak) or may have permanent hoarseness or speech deficits. The nurse helps the client to set realistic goals, starting with involvement in self-care. The nurse teaches alternative communication methods so that the client can functionally communicate in the hospital and after discharge.

The nurse and family must make all attempts to ease the client into a more normal social environment. The nurse provides encouragement and positive reinforcement while demonstrating acceptance and caring behaviors. The family may benefit from counseling sessions that the nurse initiates in the hospital.

After surgery, the client may feel reserved and socially isolated because of the change in voice and facial appearance. To cover the laryngectomy stoma, the tracheostomy tube, and postoperative changes related to surgery, the client can wear loose-fitting, high-collar shirts or sweaters (e.g., turtleneck), scarves, and jewelry. Cosmetics may aid in covering any disfigurement. Most surgeons try to place the surgical incisions in the client's natural skin fold lines if doing so does not pose a risk for cancer recurrence. (See Chapter 10 for a detailed discussion of body image, including additional nursing interventions.)

➤ Continuing Care

If no complications occur, the client is usually ready to be discharged home or to an extended care facility within 2 weeks. At the time of discharge, the client should be able to provide self-care, which may include tracheostomy or stoma care, nutrition, wound care, and methods of communication.

The client and family may feel more secure about discharge if they receive a referral to a community health agency familiar with the care of the client recovering from head and neck cancer. The multidisciplinary team assesses the client's specific discharge needs and makes the appropriate referrals to home care agencies, including such professionals as nutritionists, nurses, physical therapists, speech pathologists, and social workers. The nurse coordinates the scheduling for chemotherapy or radiation therapy with the client and family.

➤ *Health Teaching*

Although education begins during preoperative teaching sessions, most self-care is taught in the hospital. The nurse teaches the client and family how to care for the stoma or tracheostomy or laryngectomy tube, depending

Chart 31–3

Education Guide: Home Laryngectomy Care

- Avoid swimming, and use care when showering or shaving.
- Lean slightly forward and cover the stoma when coughing or sneezing.
- Wear a stoma guard or loose clothing to cover the stoma.
- Clean the stoma with mild soap and water. Lubricate the stoma with non-oil-based ointment as needed.
- Increase humidity by using saline in the stoma as instructed, a bedside humidifier, pans of water, and houseplants.
- Obtain and wear a Medic-Alert bracelet and emergency care for life-threatening situations.

on the type of surgery performed. The nurse reviews incision and airway care, including cleaning and inspecting for signs of infection. The nurse teaches clean suction technique and reviews the client's plan of care.

Chart 31–3 summarizes the highlights of self-care for the client discharged after laryngeal cancer surgery. Many of the highlights are also applicable to someone discharged after any resection for head and neck cancer.

Stoma Care. To prevent water from entering the airway, the nurse instructs the client to use a shower shield over the tracheostomy tube or laryngectomy stoma when bathing. To shield the airway during the day, the client may wear a protective cover or stoma guard.

For the client with a permanent stoma after laryngectomy or for the client with a permanent tracheostomy, covering the permanent opening has a double benefit: filtering the air entering the stoma while keeping humidity in the airway and enhancing aesthetic appearance. To protect the airway and increase humidity, the nurse instructs the client to cover the airway with cotton or foam. Attractive coverings are available in the form of cotton scarves, crocheted bibs, and jewelry. Using colored seam binding for tracheostomy ties after the stoma has matured may enhance the client's overall body image. The client's shirt or dress color can be matched or coordinated with seam bindings of various colors. The nurse also teaches the client how to increase humidity in the home. The nurse may teach the client to instill normal saline into the artificial airway 10–15 times a day as ordered.

Communication. The client continues the selected method of alternative communication that began in the hospital. The client wears a medical alert (Medic-Alert) bracelet and carries a special identification card (Fig. 31–11). For the client who had a laryngectomy, this card is available from the local chapter of the International Association of Laryngectomees. The card instructs the reader in providing an emergency airway or resuscitating the client who has a stoma.

Smoking Cessation. A difficult but important issue for the client after head and neck cancer surgery is smok-

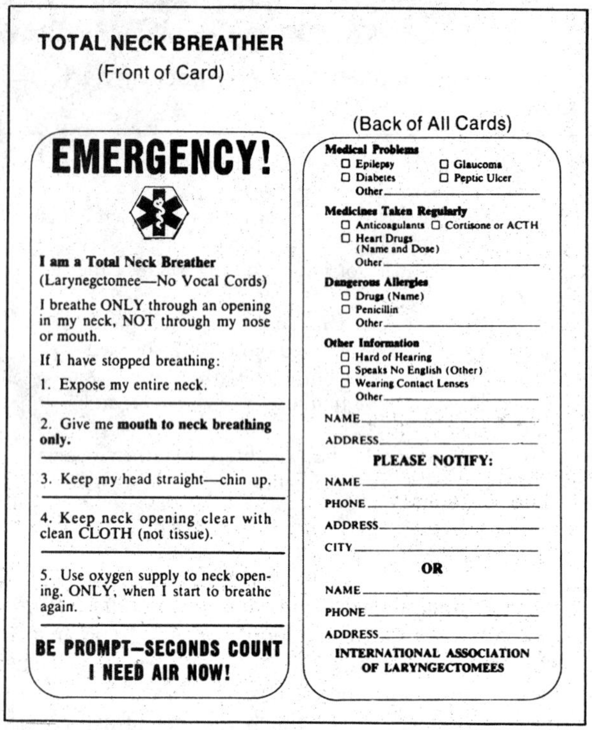

Figure 31-11. Emergency wallet card for identification of laryngectomy.

ing cessation. Smoking plays a major role in the development of head and neck cancer. The nurse stresses to the client that smoking cessation can reduce the risk for developing additional malignancies and increase the rate of healing from surgery. Chemical and psychological assistance is available for smoking cessation.

► Psychosocial Preparation

The many physical changes resulting from a laryngectomy influence clients' physical, social, and emotional functioning. Many clients perceive changes in their quality of life (the Research Application for Nursing examines the effectiveness of a quality of life assessment tool among people undergoing head and neck surgery for cancer). The nurse begins to prepare the client and family for these changes, but another client who has adjusted to these changes is usually more effective in helping clients adjust.

Clients who are discharged with a permanent stoma, tracheostomy tube, nasogastric tube, and wounds experience an alteration in body image. The nurse stresses the importance of returning to a normal lifestyle as much as possible. About half of these clients return to full-time employment. The remainder work part time or apply for disability income. Most clients can resume many of their usual activities within 4-6 weeks after surgery or longer after a combination of radiation therapy and surgery. Clients may be frustrated at times while trying to adjust to changes in smell, taste, and communication during this time.

The client with a total laryngectomy cannot produce sounds during laughing and crying, and mucous secre-

tions may appear unexpectedly when these emotions or coughing or sneezing occurs. The mucus can be embarrassing, and the client needs to be prepared to cover the stoma with a handkerchief or gauze. The client who has undergone composite resections will have difficulty with speech and swallowing. This client may have tracheostomy and feeding tubes to deal with in public places.

► Home Care Management

Extensive home care preparation is required for the client with a laryngectomy for cancer. The convalescent period is long, and airway management is complicated. The client or family must be able to take an active role in client care.

General cleanliness of the home is assessed. If the client has severe or long-standing respiratory problems, adjustments in the home to allow for one-floor living may be necessary. Increased humidification is needed. A hu-

► Research Applications for Nursing

A New Functional Status/Quality of Life Scale

Baker, C. A. (1995). Functional status scale for measuring quality of life outcomes in head and neck cancer patients. Cancer Nursing, 18(6), 458–466.

The purpose of this study was to determine the validity and reliability of a newly developed functional status scale measuring quality of life among clients with head and neck cancer. The scale was initially developed with the input of 115 clients with head and neck cancer and reflects the concerns and terminology used by this population. Forced choices included 10 physical activities and 5 subjective symptom areas (such as pain, fatigue, appearance). An open-ended question concluded the questionnaire. The scale was tested with 172 clients with head and neck cancer and 30 clients with other types of cancer.

Psychometric testing indicates excellent discriminate validity and moderate to strong convergent validity with other measures of performance. Reliability was established at 0.88 (Cronbach's α). The scale was sensitive to the population for which it was developed.

Critique. The study was well designed and involved a sufficient number of participants. Incorporation of an open-ended question increased the sensitivity and specificity of the instrument. Longitudinal studies with this scale are needed to determine its usefulness in identifying within-participant changes in functional status over time.

Implications for Nursing. Clients with different types of cancer have different residual problems and concerns. Many functional status/quality of life measures, although designed and tested with one client population, are regarded generally as appropriate for clients with any cancer type. Client concerns, however, have probably been misunderstood and not addressed because instruments and scales have not been sufficiently sensitive to the target population. To identify and meet the needs of clients with special problems, nurses must use instruments appropriate to the population in need.

Chart 31–4

Focused Assessment for Home Care Clients After Laryngectomy

- Assess respiratory status.
  - Observe rate and depth of respiration.
  - Auscultate lungs.
  - Check patency of airway.
  - Examine the tracheostomy exudate for amount, color, and character.
  - Examine nail beds and mucous membranes for evidence of cyanosis.
  - Take a pulse oximetry reading.
- Assess condition of wound.
  - Remove dressings (noting condition of dressings).
  - Cleanse the wound.
  - Compare with previous notations of wound condition:
    Presence, amount, and nature of exudate
    Presence/absence of cellulitis
    Presence/absence of odor
- Assess client's psychosocial functioning.
  - Ask the client about passing the time, visitors, and trips outside the house.
  - Observe whether the client communicates responses directly or whether a family member speaks for the client.
  - Observe client and family member interactions.
  - Determine what method of communication the client has selected and observe the client's skill with it.
  - Is the client wearing pajamas or the client dressed?
- Take the client's temperature.
- Assess client's understanding of illness and compliance with treatment.
  - Signs and symptoms to report to health care provider
  - Medication plan (correct timing and dose)
  - Ambulation or positioning schedule
  - Dressing changes/skin care
  - Diet modifications (24-hr diet recall)
  - Skill in tracheostomy or dressing care
- Assess client's nutritional status.
  - Change in muscle mass
  - Lackluster nails/sparse hair
  - Recent weight loss >10% of usual weight
  - Impaired oral intake
  - Difficulty swallowing
  - Generalized edema

---

midifier add-on to a forced-air furnace can be obtained. If the cost is not manageable or if the home is heated by radiators, a room humidifier or vaporizer may be appropriate.

A home care nurse is involved with the client's care after discharge and becomes a very important resource for the client and family. The home care nurse assesses the client and home situation for problems in self-care, complications, adjustment, and adherence to medical regimen. Chart 31–4 lists assessment areas for the client in the home after laryngectomy. The nurse reinforces health care teaching, self-care teaching, and smoking cessation regimens.

► *Health Care Resources*

The home care or hospital nurse informs the client and family of community organizations, such as the American Cancer Society, and local laryngectomee clubs, which can offer support, accurate information, and friendships. When the client has problems paying for health care services, equipment supply and prescriptions, a visiting nurse agency may be helpful in directing the client to available resources.

In many areas, the local unit of American Cancer Society or the Canadian Cancer Society can help provide dressing materials and nutritional supplements to the client in need. This organization may also provide transportation to and from follow-up visits or radiation therapy.

 Evaluation

On the basis of the identified nursing diagnoses, the nurse evaluates the entire plan of care for the client with head and neck cancer. The expected outcomes are that the client

- Maintains a patent airway
- Attains or maintains clear lung sounds in all lung fields
- Demonstrates an understanding of head and neck cancer and its treatment
- Performs self-care of the artificial airway and wound
- Performs the activities of daily living (ADLs) independently or with minimal assistance
- States that levels of anxiety are reduced
- Resumes as normal a lifestyle as possible through rehabilitation
- States understanding of and adapts to body image changes
- Attains or maintains adequate nutrition
- Does not aspirate gastric contents or food
- Complies with smoking and alcohol cessation

 CASE STUDY for the Client with Vocal Cord Paralysis

■ You are making a home visit to a 64-year-old man with terminal lung cancer who is receiving hospice services at home. When you arrive, the client's wife tells you that she thinks he has a cold because his voice is hoarse and he has been coughing ever since breakfast 20 minutes ago. On initial assessment, you find the client to be able to talk, but his voice is raspy and does not get louder with increased effort. He is somewhat anxious and says he is coughing because "some crumbs went down the wrong way." The color of his lips and nail beds is good. His respiratory rate and depth are within the range found at the last visit 2 days ago.

QUESTIONS:

1. What assessment information do you need to document?
2. What additional assessment data do you need to document?
3. What priority nursing actions do you need to implement?
4. What expected outcomes would be specific to this situation?

SELECTED BIBLIOGRAPHY

*American Cancer Society. (1990). Cancer of the larynx. *Ca: A Cancer Journal for Clinicians, 40*(3), 133–183.

American Cancer Society. (1998). *Cancer facts and figures, 1998.* Atlanta: American Cancer Society. (98–300M, No. 5008.98)

*Baker, C. A. (1992). Factors associated with rehabilitation in head and neck cancer. *Cancer Nursing, 15*(6), 395–400.

Baker, C. A. (1995). Functional status scale for measuring quality of life outcomes in head and neck cancer patients. *Cancer Nursing, 18*(6), 458–466.

*Bartkiw, T. P., & Pynn, B. R. (1993). Close-up on mandible fracture. *Nursing 93, 23*(12), 45.

Boucher, M. (1996). When laryngectomy complicates care. *RN, 59*(8), 40–45.

Clark, L. (1995). A critical event in tracheostomy care. *British Journal of Nursing, 4*(12), 676, 678–681.

Dropkin, M. L. (1997). Coping with disfigurement/dysfunction and length of hospital stay after head and neck cancer surgery. *ORL Head and Neck Nursing, 15*(1), 22–26.

Fetzer, S. (1998). Laryngeal mask airway: Indications and management for critical-care. *Critical Care Nurse, 18*(1), 83–87.

Friedman, C. D., & Costantino, P. (1994). General concepts in craniofacial skeletal augmentation and replacement. *Otolaryngologic Clinics of North America, 27*(5), 847–857.

Garp, M. (1998). Pulse oximetry. *Critical Care Nurse, 18*(1), 94–99.

*Grant, M., Rhiner, M., & Padilla, G. (1989). Nutritional management in the head and neck cancer patient. *Seminars in Oncology Nursing, 5*(3), 195–204.

Hecht, J., Emmons, K., Brown, R., Everett, K., Farrell, N., Hitchcock, P., & Sales, S. (1994). Smoking interventions for patients with cancer: Guidelines for nursing practice. *Oncology Nursing Forum, 21*(10), 1657–1666.

Hooper, M. (1996). Nursing care of the patient with a tracheostomy. *Nursing Standard, 10*(34), 40–43.

Madeya, M. (1996a). Oral complications from cancer therapy: Part 1. Pathophysiology and secondary complications. *Oncology Nursing Forum, 23*(5), 801–807.

Madeya, M. (1996b). Oral complications from cancer therapy: Part 2. Nursing implications for assessment and treatment. *Oncology Nursing Forum, 23*(5), 808–819.

Perera, F. P. (1996). Uncovering new clues to cancer risk. *Scientific American, 275*(3), 54–62.

Phillips, S. (1997), Obstructive sleep apnea: Diagnosis and management. *Nursing Standard, 11*(17), 43–46.

Reese, J. (1996). Head and neck cancers. In R. McCorkle, M. Grant, M. Frank-Stromborg, & S. Baird (Eds.). *Cancer nursing: A comprehensive textbook* (2nd ed., pp. 773–795). Philadelphia: W. B. Saunders.

Shellenbarger, T., & Narielwala, S. (1996). Caring for the patient with laryngeal cancer at home. *Home Healthcare Nurse, 14*(2), 80–90.

*Weber, M., & Reimer, M. (1993). Laryngectomy: Grieving disfigurement and dysfunction. *The Canadian Nurse, 89*(3), 31–34.

*Weimert, T. A. (1992). Common ENT emergencies: The acute nose and throat, part 2. *Emergency Medicine, 24*(6), 26–28, 31–32, 34–36.

SUGGESTED READINGS

Hecht, J., Emmons, K., Brown, R., Everett, K., Farrell, N., Hitchcock, P., & Sales, S. (1994). Smoking interventions for patients with cancer: Guidelines for nursing practice. *Oncology Nursing Forum, 21*(10), 1657–1666.

This excellent article describes the physiologic benefits of smoking cessation on different body systems. The information is research based and includes a discussion of the health impact of continued smoking during cancer treatment. Nursing interventions include pharmacologic and nonpharmacologic strategies for assisting the client with smoking cessation.

Madeya, M. (1996). Oral complications from cancer therapy: Part 2. Nursing implications for assessment and treatment. *Oncology Nursing Forum, 23*(5), 808–819.

The author describes the most common oral complications from cancer therapy and presents them as nursing diagnoses. Clear and detailed interventions are listed in outline form for each diagnosis. Questions for self-assessment or continuing education credit follow the article.

Shellenbarger, T., & Narielwala, S. (1996). Caring for the patient with laryngeal cancer at home. *Home Healthcare Nurse, 14*(2), 80–90.

Clients with laryngeal cancer have many needs and complicated care regimens. This article presents organized assessment tips and intervention strategies for assisting these clients and families in the home.

Chapter 32

INTERVENTIONS FOR CLIENTS WITH NONINFECTIOUS PROBLEMS OF THE LOWER RESPIRATORY TRACT

Lower airway disorders account for much morbidity and mortality. Some disorders may be aggravated by environmental irritants; others have a familial tendency. The major nursing diagnoses include impaired gas exchange, ineffective breathing pattern, and ineffective airway clearance. For the elderly client with a respiratory disorder, some general nursing considerations are listed in Chart 32-1.

CHRONIC AIRFLOW LIMITATION

Overview

Chronic airflow limitation is the term for a group of chronic lung diseases, including pulmonary emphysema, chronic bronchitis, and bronchial asthma. Emphysema and chronic bronchitis are characterized by bronchoconstriction and dyspnea; these conditions have little reversibility. Unlike emphysema and chronic bronchitis, asthma is primarily an inflammatory process characterized by *re-*versible airflow obstruction and wheezing. The terms chronic obstructive pulmonary disease (COPD) and chronic airflow limitation (CAL) are often used interchangeably.

More than 1 million people between the ages of 40 and 65 are sufficiently disabled from COPD to receive regular disability income from Social Security (Bordow & Moser, 1996). Better prevention and rehabilitation will help maintain optimal functioning and improve overall health.

The onset of respiratory failure is a major event in the life of a client with CAL. More than half of the clients diagnosed with CAL will die within 10 years of diagnosis. Health care professionals have an obligation to assist clients in formulating directives before respiratory decompensation. Advanced directives provide clients with the opportunity to specify their health care wishes.

Pathophysiology

Most clients with respiratory problems present with two or more diseases (e.g., emphysema and chronic bronchitis) simultaneously, but each condition has its own pathophysiologic process (Fig. 32–1).

Pulmonary Emphysema

Pulmonary emphysema is characterized by the destruction of alveoli, loss of elastic recoil, and narrowing of small airways (bronchioles), resulting in increased resting lung volumes, increased airflow resistance, alveolar hyperinflation, and diaphragm flattening. These changes are reflected in the client by increased respiratory rate and dyspnea.

Specific Pathologic Changes

Four pathologic changes occur in the client (see Fig. 32–1):

- Loss of lung elasticity. Proteases (lung enzymes) alter or destroy the alveoli and the small airways by breaking down elastin. As a result, the alveolar sacs lose their elasticity, and the small airways collapse or narrow. Some alveoli are destroyed, whereas others remain enlarged.
- Hyperinflation of the lung. The enlarged alveoli prevent the lung from returning to its normal resting state during expiration.
- Formation of bullae. The alveolar walls deteriorate and connect to form bullae (air-filled spaces) that can be seen on x-ray examination.
- Small airway collapse and air trapping. As the client forcibly attempts to exhale air trapped in the enlarged alveoli, positive intrathoracic pressures collapse the small airways.

EFFECTS OF PATHOLOGIC CHANGES ON BREATHING. Emphysema, like other CAL diseases, increases the work of breathing. In moderate to severe emphysema, the work of breathing is increased because the hyperinflated lung causes the diaphragm to flatten (Fig.

32–2). The flattened diaphragm requires the use of accessory respiratory muscles, such as neck and abdominal muscles, during expiration when the diaphragm must rise against gravity. A healthy person uses about 65% diaphragm and 35% accessory muscles to breathe; the client with emphysema uses about 30% diaphragm and 70% accessory muscles to breathe. The client needs more oxygen for more muscle use and so may experience an "air hunger" sensation. The client usually starts inspiration before expiration is completed, resulting in dyspnea with an inefficient and uncoordinated pattern of breathing.

EFFECTS OF PATHOLOGIC CHANGES ON GAS EXCHANGE. The increased work of breathing may affect gas exchange, although arterial blood gas (ABG) values are not usually affected until the client has advanced disease. Then carbon dioxide is often produced faster than the body can eliminate it, which causes carbon dioxide retention and chronic respiratory acidosis (see Chap. 19). The client with late-stage emphysema has a low arterial blood oxygen concentration (PaO_2) as well because it is difficult for oxygen to move from diseased lung tissue into the bloodstream.

CLASSIFICATION OF EMPHYSEMA. Emphysema is classified according to the pattern of destruction and dilation of the gas-exchanging units (acini) of the lung. Emphysema can be divided into panlobular, centrilobular, and paraseptal types (see Fig. 32–1). Each type can occur alone or in combination in the same lung.

Panlobular (panacinar) emphysema (PLE) involves destruction of the entire alveolus uniformly. Panacinar emphysema is a diffuse disease that is usually more severe in the lower lung area. This type of emphysema is seen with homozygous alpha$_1$-antitrypsin (ATT) deficiency.

In centrilobular (centriacinar) emphysema (CLE), openings develop in the respiratory bronchioles and allow spaces to develop as tissue walls disintegrate. Although this is a diffuse disease, the upper lung sections are most severely affected. This type of emphysema is often seen in long-standing cigarette smokers.

In paraseptal, distal acinar emphysema, the disease is confined to the distal portion of the acinus; only alveolar ducts and alveoli are involved. This disease type tends to be localized and is associated with the formation of bullae. Spontaneous pneumothorax, with the formation of blebs, can result in the diseased lung area. Spontaneous pneumothorax is a collapse of a portion of the lung because of an opening from the lung side into the pleural space. A bleb is a collection of air within the pleura that is generally less than 1–2 cm.

Alpha$_1$-antitrypsin deficiency is a genetic abnormality that leads to emphysema. Less than 1% of clients with emphysema have this type. The physician or Nurse Practitioner suspects ATT in the client who presents with an onset of dyspnea, cough, wheeze, and increased mucus production at an early age (younger than 50 years). ATT, a serum protein produced by the liver, is found in the lungs. Its primary function is to inhibit neutrophil elastase. Diagnosis is made by analysis of the serum ATT levels and Pi typing (serum protease inhibitor phenotyping).

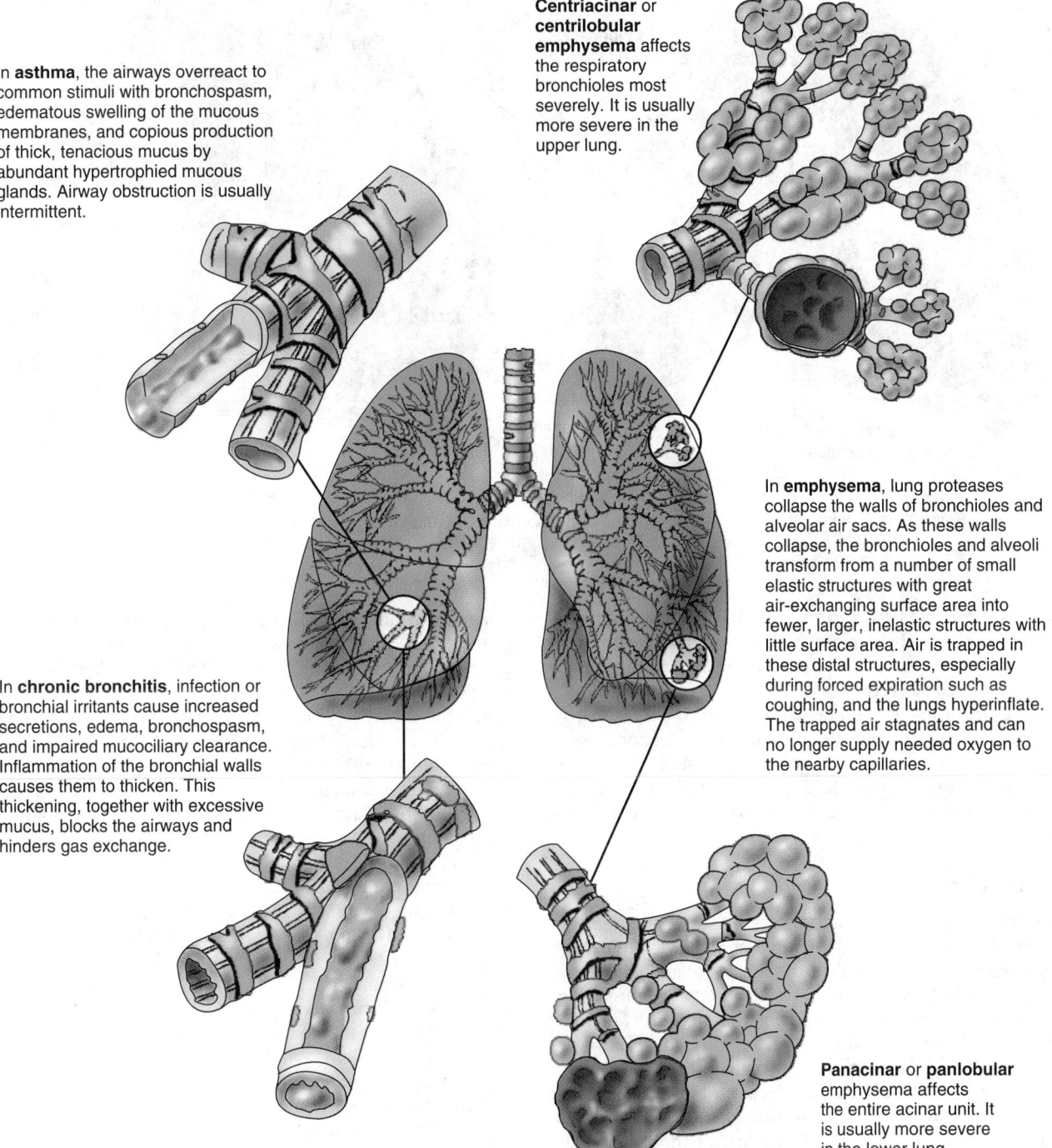

In **asthma**, the airways overreact to common stimuli with bronchospasm, edematous swelling of the mucous membranes, and copious production of thick, tenacious mucus by abundant hypertrophied mucous glands. Airway obstruction is usually intermittent.

Centriacinar or **centrilobular emphysema** affects the respiratory bronchioles most severely. It is usually more severe in the upper lung.

In **emphysema**, lung proteases collapse the walls of bronchioles and alveolar air sacs. As these walls collapse, the bronchioles and alveoli transform from a number of small elastic structures with great air-exchanging surface area into fewer, larger, inelastic structures with little surface area. Air is trapped in these distal structures, especially during forced expiration such as coughing, and the lungs hyperinflate. The trapped air stagnates and can no longer supply needed oxygen to the nearby capillaries.

In **chronic bronchitis**, infection or bronchial irritants cause increased secretions, edema, bronchospasm, and impaired mucociliary clearance. Inflammation of the bronchial walls causes them to thicken. This thickening, together with excessive mucus, blocks the airways and hinders gas exchange.

Panacinar or **panlobular** emphysema affects the entire acinar unit. It is usually more severe in the lower lung.

Figure 32–1. The pathophysiology of chronic airflow limitation (CAL).

Acute and Chronic Bronchitis

Bronchitis results from exposure to infectious or noninfectious irritants, especially tobacco smoke. The irritant produces an inflammatory response, which causes vasodilation, congestion, mucosal edema, and bronchospasm. Unlike emphysema, bronchitis affects the small and large airways rather than the alveoli. Airflow may or may not be limited.

Acute bronchitis can occur as a single episode or can represent an acute exacerbation of chronic bronchitis. An upper respiratory infection, usually viral, often precedes the acute bronchitis episode.

Chronic bronchitis is chronic inflammation of the airways. Chronic inflammation results in mucous gland hypertrophy and hyperplasia, which produce increased viscid mucus. The bronchial walls thicken (often to twice the normal thickness) and impair airflow. This thickening, together with production of excessive mucus, blocks some of the smaller airways and narrows larger ones. Small airways (bronchioles) are often affected before the large

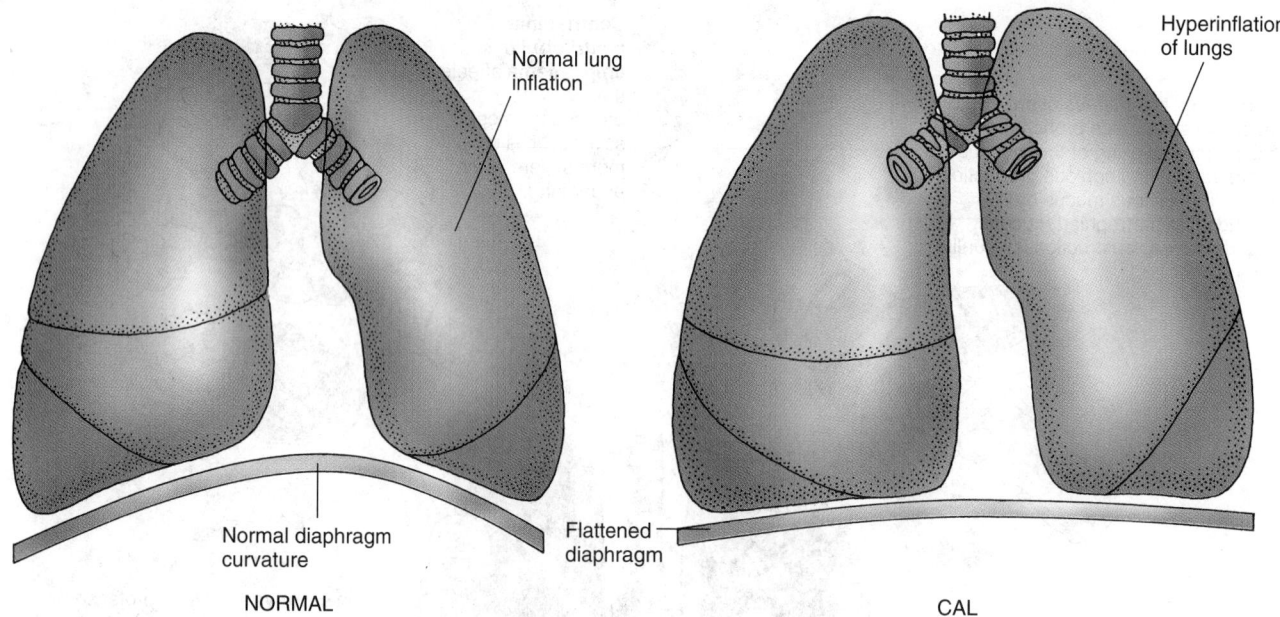

Figure 32–2. Diaphragm shape and lung inflation in the normal client and in the client with chronic airflow limitation (CAL).

airways (bronchi) become involved. The physician diagnoses chronic bronchitis when a client has had a cough or sputum production on most days for at least 3 months of a year for 2 consecutive years.

Chronic bronchitis hinders airflow and gas exchange because of mucous plugs and secondary infections. As a result, the arterial blood oxygen concentration (PaO_2) decreases, causing hypoxemia, and the arterial blood carbon dioxide concentration ($PaCO_2$) increases, causing respiratory acidosis.

Bronchial Asthma

Bronchial asthma is characterized by reversible airflow obstruction, airway inflammation, and airway hyperresponsiveness. It is primarily a disease of inflammation that precipitates bronchospasm and can be fatal. Asthma, like bronchitis, affects the airways, not the alveoli. Therefore, asthma does not typically lead to emphysema; however, asthma may coexist with emphysema and bronchitis.

Asthma can present in any decade of life, but in approximately half of those with asthma, the disease developed before age 10 years. At least half of those in whom asthma develops in childhood will have remission as adults. Asthma is more common in urban than in rural settings and appears to be higher in minority populations (Bordow & Moser, 1996).

Bronchial hyperresponsiveness is a cardinal feature of asthma. Once the client is exposed to the stimulus, chemical mediators are immediately released. Within minutes of being exposed, the client experiences dyspnea, wheezing, cough, and mucus production.

Asthma is the result of acute- and late-phase reactions. The acute-phase reaction is the result of an immediate hypersensitivity to the allergen, which stimulates the mast cell to release histamine and other cell mediators. This reaction results in smooth muscle contraction, vascular leakage, flushing (vasodilation), hypotension, mucus secretion, and pruritus. Levels of allergen exposure influence the prevalence of airway hyperresponsiveness. The late-phase response occurs within 2–8 hours after the early-phase reaction. Onset of the late phase is associated with inflammation. Eosinophils, neutrophils, and basophils infiltrate the tissues and result in inflammation. Long-term inflammation is associated with fiber deposition. The obstruction is less responsive to bronchodilator therapy, and airway reactivity increases.

Initial approaches to the client diagnosed with asthma include monitoring of peak expiratory flow rates to determine a pattern of obstruction. The client attempts to control the environmental exposure to allergens and irritants and is established on a pharmacologic plan to control the symptoms.

Because inflammation plays the key role in asthma, antiinflammatory therapy is the cornerstone for the control of asthma. Beta agonists and other bronchodilator medications help control symptoms but have no effect on the underlying disease and do not alter inflammation or bronchial hyperreactivity.

TYPES OF ASTHMA. Asthma can be divided into extrinsic and intrinsic types. Extrinsic asthma (immunoglobulin E [IgE]–mediated), the allergic form of bronchial asthma, is seen more in children than in adults. By contrast, intrinsic asthma is the nonallergic form of the disease. Many factors, often a viral upper respiratory infection, can cause an attack. Some researchers believe intrinsic asthma develops from a hypersensitivity to the viruses causing the infection.

Nocturnal asthma is associated with circadian rhythms. The client often awakens with the worst symptoms between 3 and 5 AM. It is believed that half of all asthma deaths are due to this form of the disease.

PATTERNS OF DISEASE. In adults, asthma attacks are usually separated by symptom-free intervals but may also occur on a continuous basis. The airways of the person with asthma are overreactive and ready to respond to various stimuli. In those people with intrinsic asthma, changes in the environment may precipitate a wheezing episode. Common agents or stimuli include exercise, fog, smog, smoke (both first- and second-hand smoke), odors, aerosols, and upper respiratory tract infections. Pollen, mold spores, animal dander, and arthropods such as house dust mites and cockroaches usually produce bronchoconstriction only in the client with extrinsic (allergic) asthma. Certain foods or medications may be involved in the allergic form of asthma as well (Chart 32–2). Emotional excitement, anxiety, hormonal changes, and fatigue are not causes of asthma but may aggravate, initiate, or accompany an episode of wheezing or dyspnea.

PATHOLOGY OF BRONCHOCONSTRICTION. Inhaled agents stimulate the contraction of airway smooth muscle by different mechanisms. Some agents cause bronchoconstriction by directly stimulating the smooth muscle, and some cause smooth muscle contraction indirectly by affecting neural pathways. Three neural pathways have been studied in environmentally produced bronchoconstriction: muscarinic, alpha-adrenergic, and neuropeptide.

Chart 32–2

Education Guide: Asthma

- Avoid potential environmental asthma triggers, such as smoke, fireplaces, dust, mold, and weather changes (especially warm to cold, or sudden barometric changes).
- Avoid medications that could trigger asthma, for example, aspirin, nonsteroidal anti-inflammatory drugs (NSAIDs), and beta-blockers.
- Avoid food that has been prepared with monosodium glutamate (MSG) or metabisulfite.
- If you experience symptoms of exercise-induced asthma, use your bronchodilator inhaler 30 minutes before exercise to prevent or reduce bronchospasm.
- Be sure you know the proper technique and correct sequence when you use metered-dose inhalers.
- Be sure to get adequate rest and sleep.
- Reduce stress and anxiety; learn relaxation techniques; adopt coping mechanisms that have worked for you in the past.
- Wash all bedding with hot water to destroy the dust mite.
- Monitor your peak expiratory flow rates as you were instructed.
- Seek immediate emergency care if you experience any of the following:
  - Gray or blue fingertips or lips
  - Difficulty breathing, walking, or talking
  - Retractions of the neck, chest, or ribs
  - Nasal flaring
  - Failure of medications to control worsening symptoms
  - Peak expiratory flow rates declining steadily after treatment, or a flow rate 50% below your usual flow rate

---

The non-neural mechanisms of bronchoconstriction involve humoral cells: macrophages, eosinophils, and mast cells. Macrophages are present throughout the tracheobronchial tree. Eosinophils are the principal inflammatory cell in the pathophysiologic process of asthma. The extent of eosinophils in the sputum, peripheral circulation, and airway tissues correlates with severity of the disease. Mast cells in the lung release histamine and slow-reacting substance of anaphylaxis during allergic reactions, especially those caused by pollen.

Complications of Chronic Airflow Limitation

HYPOXEMIA. The client experiences subtle changes as hypoxemia ensues. Initially, the client may experience mood changes, be unable to concentrate, and be forgetful. Restlessness is common. Tachycardia and cyanosis are later signs of hypoxemia.

RESPIRATORY ACIDOSIS. Rising carbon dioxide levels in the arterial blood ($PaCO_2$) result in respiratory acidosis. Common signs of carbon dioxide retention (hypercapnia) include increased drowsiness and lethargy, headache, fatigue, dizziness, and tachypnea with hyperventilation.

RESPIRATORY INFECTIONS. The client with chronic airflow limitation (CAL) is susceptible to respiratory infections. The organisms frequently associated with bacteria infections include *Streptococcus pneumoniae, Haemophilus influenzae,* and *Moraxella catarrhalis.* Acute respiratory infections cause increased production of mucus, increased irritability of bronchial smooth muscle, and edema of the involved mucosa. Airflow is limited; the work of breathing increases; and dyspnea results. A bacterial cause cannot be identified in most acute respiratory illnesses. However, severely compromised and debilitated clients with CAL are treated with antibiotics even when an organism has not been isolated (called empirical therapy). Some physicians prescribe antibiotics on an as-needed basis; the client self-administers the antibiotic according to changes in sputum appearance, which may indicate infection.

CARDIAC FAILURE. Cardiac failure, especially cor pulmonale (right-sided ventricular heart failure caused by pulmonary disease), must be considered in a client with worsening dyspnea. This complication is most frequently associated with chronic bronchitis, but the client with advanced emphysema is also likely to develop this problem. Detection of cor pulmonale (also called pulmonary heart disease) is difficult because its clinical signs are generally masked by those of the underlying lung disease. Signs and symptoms are listed in Chart 32–3.

Chronic airflow limitation (CAL) places a heavy workload on the right side of the heart, which is responsible for pumping blood into the lungs. As the disease progresses, the amount of oxygen in the blood decreases, causing major blood vessels in the lung to constrict. To pump blood through these narrowed vessels, the right side of the heart must generate high pressures. In re-

---

Chart 32–3

Key Features of Pulmonary Heart Disease (Cor Pulmonale)

- Hypoxia and hypoxemia
- Increasing dyspnea
- Fatigue
- Weakness
- Enlarged and tender liver
- Warm cyanotic extremities with bounding pulses
- Cyanotic lips
- Distended neck veins
- Right ventricular enlargement (hypertrophy)
- Lower sternal or epigastric pulsations
- Gastrointestinal disturbances, such as nausea or anorexia
- Dependent edema
- Metabolic and respiratory acidosis
- Pulmonary hypertension

---

sponse to this heavy workload, the right chambers of the heart enlarge and thicken, causing right-sided heart failure, or cor pulmonale. Heart failure is frequently a cause of death in clients with CAL. (Treatment for right-sided heart failure is discussed in Chapter 37.)

CARDIAC DYSRHYTHMIAS. Clients with CAL frequently experience cardiac dysrhythmias. These dysrhythmias may be a result of hypoxemia (from decreased oxygen to the heart muscle), other cardiac disease, the effect of drugs, or respiratory acidosis. Treatment for dysrhythmias is described in Chapter 36.

STATUS ASTHMATICUS. Status asthmaticus is a major complication associated with bronchial asthma. It is a severe, potentially life-threatening acute episode of airway obstruction that tends to intensify once it begins and often does not respond to common therapy. The client arrives in the emergency department of the hospital with extremely labored breathing and wheezing. Use of accessory muscles for breathing and distention of neck veins are commonly noted. If the condition is not reversed, the client can experience cor pulmonale, pneumothorax, and eventual cardiac or respiratory arrest. The physician immediately orders intravenous (IV) fluids, potent bronchodilators, steroids (to decrease inflammation), epinephrine, and oxygen in an attempt to reverse the acute condition. The nurse also prepares for emergency intubation. When wheezing diminishes, management is similar to that for any client with CAL.

Etiology

Cigarette Smoking

Smoking is the most important risk factor for CAL. The client with an 8 pack-year history usually has obstructive lung changes but no signs and symptoms of disease. The client with a 20 pack-year history or longer typically has

CAL. Pulmonary function studies reveal a forced expiratory volume in 1 second/forced vital capacity ratio (FEV_1/FVC) lower than 70% of predicted.

TRANSCULTURAL CONSIDERATIONS

The prevalence of smoking remains higher among African-Americans, blue-collar workers, and less educated people than in the overall population of the United States. Approximations of smoking prevalence range from 37% among the least educated people to 14% among the most educated. Smoking prevalence is highest among Northern Plains Native Americans (42%–70%) and Alaskan Natives (56%). The overall prevalence of smoking for both men and women has decreased over the past two decades, but the decrease for women has been proportionately less than for men. The prevalence of smoking is approximately 28% for men and 23% to 25% for women (National Center for Health Statistics, 1996).

The harmful effects of tobacco result in part because inhaled smoke stimulates excess release of the enzyme elastase protease from cells normally found in the lung. The elastase protease breaks down elastin, the major component in alveoli. By impairing the action of cilia, smoking also inhibits the cilia from clearing the tracheobronchial tree of mucus, cellular debris, and fluid.

In addition to the increased risk of CAL from active smoking, much attention has been given to passive smoking, or second-hand smoke. Although a person may not smoke, exposure to smoke, particularly in a small or confined space, may contribute to the development of upper and lower respiratory tract problems, including CAL. As a result of this finding, cigarette smoking is often considered an environmental hazard.

Family History

Emphysema and chronic bronchitis occur in families more often than would be expected by chance. This finding may be related to family smoking habits. However, in some people, a genetic defect results in decreased levels of the substance alpha$_1$-antitrypsin (ATT), which normally works to inhibit or prevent proteases from breaking down the elastic tissue (alveoli) of the lungs. When the amount of ATT is decreased, more damage can be done by the proteases.

Asthma and cystic fibrosis also have a strong familial association. Asthma, especially extrinsic asthma, tends to occur in families. Intrinsic asthma may occur in clients with a family or personal history of allergies. Cystic fibrosis, an inherited autosomal recessive disease, is often discussed in relation to CAL.

Although cystic fibrosis involves many organs besides the lungs (sweat glands and the pancreas), it is the main cause of chronic lung disease in children. Disease in these clients is now being diagnosed earlier, and they are living into their 30s and even 40s. Cystic fibrosis is no longer just a disease affecting children. Treatment is aimed at clearing secretions, preventing airway obstruction, and preventing and treating infection. (More information on cystic fibrosis can be found in current pediatric textbooks.)

ELDERLY CONSIDERATIONS

 Asthma in the aged is believed to be associated with a beta-adrenergic receptor dysfunction. This hypothesis may explain the decreased response to beta-adrenergic medications in treating bronchospasm. Older asthmatics who were former smokers are found to have higher IgE levels than their nonsmoking peers.

Air Pollution

The effect of air pollution appears now to be additive to tobacco exposure. Air pollution alone plays only a relatively small role in the client with emphysema and chronic bronchitis. For the client with asthma, however, increased air pollution can cause an asthma attack.

Incidence/Prevalence

The prevalence of chronic bronchitis and emphysema has been estimated at about 13.5 million and 2 million, respectively, in the United States. Another 12 million suffer from asthma, and 10 million have acute bronchitis (Benson & Marano, 1994). Since 1979, the number of people, especially elderly women, who suffer from these conditions has rapidly increased. In 1995 alone, 102,899 deaths were caused by COPD/CAL and its associated conditions. COPD/CAL is ranked as the fourth leading cause of death for females of all ages and the fifth for males (Parker et al., 1997). More than 30,000 children and young adults are affected by cystic fibrosis.

WOMEN'S HEALTH CONSIDERATIONS

In 1993, for women between the ages of 35 and 54, COPD/CAL was the ninth leading cause of death. It was the third leading cause of death in women between the ages of 55 and 74 and the fifth leading cause after age 74 (Parker et al., 1997).

Chronic airflow limitation (CAL) is responsible for a greater restriction of activity than is any other major disease category. For example, nearly 20% of people with asthma have some limitation in their daily activities. Although CAL is seen more in men, the incidence among women is increasing. The highest incidence of bronchitis is seen after age 40, and for emphysema, after age 50. Asthma is seen in the young adult as well.

Collaborative Management

◆ Assessment

➤ *History*

Risk Factors. The nurse considers age, sex, occupational history and ethnic-cultural background when taking a history from a client who has, or is suspected of having, chronic airflow limitation (CAL). Each of these factors can place the client at risk for CAL. For example, CAL is seen more often in the elderly male client. The nurse also reviews family history because certain types of CAL dis-

eases, especially extrinsic asthma and panlobular emphysema, occur in families.

The nurse obtains a thorough smoking history, if appropriate. Tobacco abuse tends to be the greatest risk factor, but the effects of cigarette smoking vary from person to person. The nurse takes a careful smoking history, which includes
- Length of time the client has smoked
- Number of packs or amount of tobacco smoked daily
- Type of cigarette or other tobacco smoked (for tar and nicotine content)
- Family history of lung disease

The nurse then quantifies this information into pack-years (for cigarette smokers) as follows:

Years of smoking × packs smoked per day = pack-years

Nature of Disease Presentation. The nurse asks the client to discuss the chief complaint and pays particular attention to the client's ability to answer questions. Can the client give clear answers and state them in complete sentences? Or is breathlessness so severe that the client gives one- or two-word answers to the questions?

Cough, dyspnea, and wheezing are the three classic signs and symptoms of CAL, although they occur in various combinations and intensity. The nurse questions the client about each of these symptoms. Early signs and symptoms of CAL include mild shortness of breath, especially on exertion (also known as dyspnea on exertion, or DOE), and a slight cough in the morning. A long-term cough is associated most often with chronic bronchitis. The nurse determines the coughing pattern by asking the client
- When, if ever, are you troubled by coughing?
- How does the cough sound? Is it dry? Hacking? Loose?
- Is the cough worse in the morning or at night?
- Is the cough worse after you smoke or are exposed to irritants?

The client's cough may be productive or nonproductive of sputum. If the cough is productive, the nurse asks whether sputum is clear or colored and how much is expectorated each day. The sputum should be clear. The nurse also asks the client to recall the time of day when most sputum is expectorated. Smokers typically have a productive cough when they get up in the morning; nonsmokers generally do not. The nurse asks whether sputum production has increased or changed.

Shortness of breath and coughing may be much worse when the client with CAL experiences an acute respiratory tract infection. The sputum usually turns from clear to yellow or green as a result of the infection, and wheezing is likely to occur. Wheezing is more commonly associated with asthma.

The nurse determines how long any of the signs and symptoms have been present, whether they are intermittent or continuous, and whether they have become progressively worse over time. The nurse realizes the client usually has an accurate perception of the severity of the symptoms; the client with asthma describes signs and symptoms as intermittent; the client with chronic bronchitis and emphysema describes signs and symptoms as continuous and worsening.

In addition to determining the onset, duration, and severity of the classic symptoms of CAL, the nurse always asks the client about the relationship between activity tolerance and dyspnea. The client is asked to compare activity level and shortness of breath with those of a month ago and a year ago. Likewise, the nurse asks about any difficulty with eating and sleeping. Many clients sleep in a semisitting position because breathlessness prevents them from lying down (thereby causing orthopnea).

The nurse or assistive personnel weighs the client on admission and compares this weight with previous weights in collaboration with the nutritionist. The client with CAL has increased metabolic requirements associated with the increased work of breathing. The increased metabolic requirements plus bothersome dyspnea and mucus production often result in poor food intake and inadequate nutrition. The nurse and nutritionist ask the client to recall a typical day's meals and fluid intake. The nurse determines whether the client uses any breathing exercises (such as pursed-lip breathing) during dyspneic episodes to help make eating easier and asks for a demonstration. The nurse, physical therapist, and occupational therapist obtain additional information about the client's usual daily activities and any difficulty with sleeping, bathing, dressing, or sexual activities.

► Physical Assessment/Clinical Manifestations

Regardless of the client's specific chronic airflow limitation (CAL) disease, the nurse observes the client's general appearance. Is the client calm or extremely anxious? The chest is inspected to determine the breathing rate and pattern. The client with respiratory muscle fatigue typically breathes with rapid, shallow respirations and may have paradoxical respirations or use accessory muscles in the abdomen or neck. The respiratory rate could be as high as 40–50 breaths per minute. Three breathing patterns commonly seen in the client with respiratory muscle fatigue are abdominal paradox, respiratory alternans, and asynchronous breathing (Table 32–1).

The nurse systematically palpates the client's anterior chest, feeling for areas of tenderness and abnormal retractions and for symmetric chest expansion. In the client with emphysema, the nurse expects to find limited excur-

sion (movement) of the diaphragm because it is typically flattened and below its usual resting state. In palpating the posterior chest for tactile fremitus (vibrations felt while the client speaks), the nurse notes decreased fremitus when the client says "99" because vibrations are not transmitted through obstructed airways.

The nurse percusses the chest, anteriorly and posteriorly, for hyperresonance in the client with emphysema related to trapped air in the alveoli. On percussion of the anterior chest, hyperresonance is often easily identified over the area of usual cardiac dullness.

The nurse then auscultates the chest to determine the depth of inspiration and to listen for adventitious breath sounds. Crackles are associated with emphysema and chronic bronchitis; wheezes are most commonly heard in a client with asthma. The nurse notes the pitch and location of the sound as well as the point in the respiratory cycle at which the sound is heard. A silent chest may indicate airflow obstruction or pneumothorax.

In addition to assessing breathing patterns and breath sounds, the nurse assesses for signs and symptoms of CAL complications. The nurse can detect early signs of hypoxemia by assessing the client's level of consciousness every 8 hours. With a concurrent respiratory infection, the client may have fever and sputum changes. Because cardiac complications are likely, the nurse determines heart rate and rhythm. The nurse assesses for swelling of the feet and ankles (dependent edema) or other signs and symptoms of right-sided heart failure (see Chart 32–3 and Chap. 37). The nurse also assesses for signs and symptoms of specific CAL diseases.

Emphysema. The most common clinical manifestation experienced by the client with emphysema is dyspnea. As the disease progresses, dyspnea worsens. Although the focus of discussions among health care professionals about dyspnea is varied, most agree there is both a subjective and an objective component to dyspnea.

The nurse assesses the degree of dyspnea by questioning the client, but this may aggravate the problem. Another approach the nurse can use is an assessment tool called a Visual Analog Dyspnea Scale (VADS). The VADS is a straight line with verbal anchors at the beginning and end of a 100-mm line. The nurse asks the client to place a mark on the line to indicate breathing difficulty. The Modified Borg Scale, a 10-point scale that rates breathlessness from nothing at all to maximal, is also used to rate perceived breathlessness. Figure 32–3 illustrates an assessment guide that combines subjective and objective assessments. The nurse uses these scales to assess dyspnea, determine the effectiveness of bronchodilator and other therapy, and pace the client's activities.

In advanced disease, the client becomes orthopneic; that is, the client must be in a sitting position, often leaning forward with arms over several pillows or an overbed table (Fig. 32–4) to breathe easier. The nurse observes for orthopnea.

The nurse also assesses for cough, which may produce only minimal sputum, and examines the client's chest, which usually has an altered shape known as a barrel chest (Fig. 32–5). In a client with a barrel chest, the ratio between the anteroposterior (AP) diameter of the chest

TABLE 32–1

Three Breathing Patterns Commonly Seen in Clients with Respiratory Muscle Fatigue

- Abdominal paradox: the diaphragm is nonfunctional; inspiration is accomplished by the intercostal and abdominal accessory muscles
- Respiratory alternans: diaphragmatic breathing alternates with abdominal paradox; may serve to rest the diaphragm
- Asynchronous breathing: the chest wall motion is unorganized; reflects the uncoordinated activity of fatigued muscles

Dyspnea Assessment Guide

Direct Measure of Dyspnea

Indicate the amount of shortness of breath you are having at this time by marking the line.

shortness of breath as bad as can be

no shortness of breath

Subjective Symptoms

On a scale of 0–4 with 0 indicating no distress and 4 indicating much distress, how much are you presently distressed by: *(circle answer)*.

poor appetite	0	1	2	3	4
worn out or weak	0	1	2	3	4
suffocation	0	1	2	3	4
tightness	0	1	2	3	4
congestion	0	1	2	3	4
a feeling of panic or anxiety	0	1	2	3	4

Objective Sign

Rise of the clavicle during inspiration:
    ABSENT = not detected
    MILD = seen but not pronounced
    SEVERE = pronounced

Figure 32–3. A dyspnea assessment tool. (Redrawn from Gift, A. G. [1989]. A dyspnea assessment guide. *Critical Care Nurse, 9*[8], 79.)

and its lateral (transverse) diameter is 2:2 rather than the normal ratio of 1:2. This change in shape results from hyperinflation of alveoli and flattening of the diaphragm, which are typical of emphysema.

Because arterial oxygen levels do not change remarkably until the terminal stage, the client with emphysema is not usually cyanotic until then. Instead, the nurse observes a pinkish skin color (most easily observed if the client has light-colored skin). The client also appears cachectic, is typically malnourished, and complains of a chronic cough and worsening dyspnea. Hypercarbia (increased $PaCO_2$ levels) usually becomes a concern in advanced disease.

Inadequate nutrition in clients with CAL, particularly elderly clients with emphysema, has been documented since the early 1960s. Malnutrition in the elderly client with CAL is a vicious cycle. The dyspnea, fatigue, abdominal bloating, and sputum production prevent the client from wanting to prepare or eat a meal. However, in malnutrition, lung tissue and respiratory muscle further deteriorate, which makes breathing even more difficult.

In addition to promoting structural changes, malnutrition impairs the immune system. The client is then more likely to experience a respiratory infection, which can be life threatening in the presence of CAL. This problem is particularly critical for the elderly client, who typically has a compromised immune system as a normal change associated with aging.

Chronic Bronchitis. The bronchitic client typically has a cyanotic, or blue-tinged, dusky appearance and complains of excessive sputum production. The nurse observes the client for cyanosis, delayed capillary refill, and clubbing of the fingers (Fig. 32–6), which indicate chronically decreased arterial oxygen levels. Clubbing is most often associated with a compensatory polycythemia. There is less hypercarbia than would be expected for the degree of hypoxemia present.

Bronchial Asthma. During an asthma attack, the nurse assesses the client for dyspnea, audible wheezing, and coughing. Breath sounds reveal inspiratory and expiratory wheezes. The cough is usually productive if the client also has an upper respiratory tract infection. The client complains of chest tightness and a feeling of suffocation. Between attacks, the client's signs and symptoms usually disappear.

➤ *Psychosocial Assessment*

Like any chronic disease, chronic airflow limitation (CAL) affects all aspects of a person's life: social, economic, and psychological.

Social Effects. CAL can affect socialization in two ways:
1. Friends may avoid the client because of annoying coughs, excessive sputum, or dyspnea.
2. The client may choose to be isolated because dyspnea interferes with the ability to socialize with friends.

The nurse questions the client about interests and hobbies but cautions the client to avoid exposure to irritants, such as aerosols, smoke, the harsh chemicals used to build or refinish furniture, and occupational exposures.

The client is questioned about home conditions. The nurse determines whether the client lives near a constant source of air pollution, such as a chemical factory or a freeway. Crowded living conditions promote the transmission of communicable respiratory diseases. Exposure to such animals as cats, dogs, and hamsters may cause allergic responses or asthma attacks.

Economic Effects. The client's economic status may be affected by the disease if both income and health insurance coverage are concerns. If the client is the head of the household, severe CAL may require a role reversal with the spouse or mate. This change may have a negative impact on the client's self-image. When the client is employed, the nurse asks about on-the-job exposure to cigarette smoke or to other substances that may irritate the respiratory system. Pulmonary medications, especially the metered-dose inhalers, are expensive, and many clients on limited incomes may use these medications only during exacerbations of the disease and not on a scheduled basis.

Psychological Effects. The nurse assesses the psychological impact of CAL and the client's ability to cope with chronic disease. Anxiety and fear related to episodes of

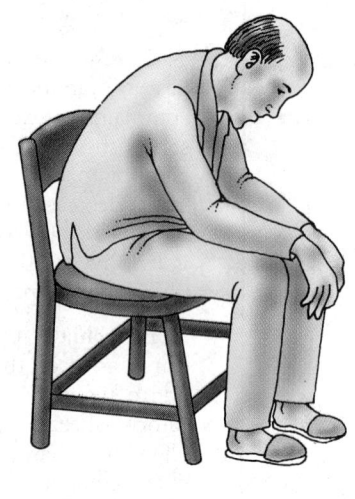

Figure 32–4. Orthopnea positions that clients with chronic airflow limitation (CAL) can assume to ease the work of breathing.

Sitting on the edge of a bed with the arms folded and placed on two or three pillows positioned over a nightstand.

Sitting in a chair with the feet spread a shoulder-width apart and leaning forward with the elbows on the knees. Arms and hands are relaxed.

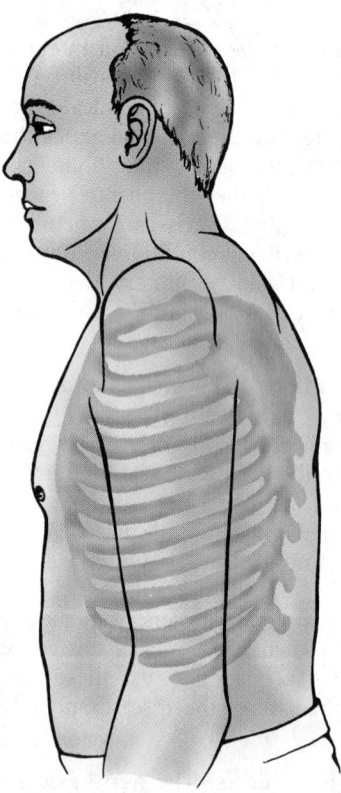

Figure 32–5. Typical barrel chest in a client with chronic airflow limitation (CAL).

dyspnea and feelings of breathlessness directly influence the client's ability to participate in a full life. Work, family, social, and sexual roles can be affected. The nurse asks whether the client is aware of support groups sponsored by the American Lung Association (ALA). Various hospitals and physicians' offices also offer group support. Those clients with access to the Internet will find many consumer-oriented educational programs.

➤ *Laboratory Assessment*

Arterial blood gas (ABG) values identify abnormalities of oxygenation, ventilation, and acid-base status. To assess

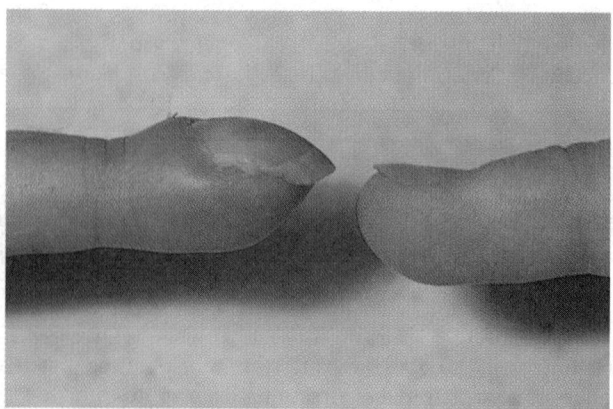

Figure 32–6. Late digital clubbing (on left) compared to a normal digit (on right). (From Swartz, M. H. [1998]. *Textbook of physical diagnosis: History and examination.* Philadelphia: W. B. Saunders Co.)

changes in the client's status over time, the nurse and respiratory therapist compare serial, or repeated, ABG values. Once baseline ABGs are obtained, pulse oximetry can gauge the client's response to treatment. In general, as CAL progresses, the amount of oxygen in the blood decreases (causing hypoxemia) and the amount of carbon dioxide in the blood increases (causing hypercarbia). Chronic respiratory acidosis (increased $PaCO_2$) then results; metabolic alkalosis (increased arterial bicarbonate) occurs as compensation. Not all clients with CAL are carbon dioxide retainers, even when hypoxemia is present. Carbon dioxide is more easily diffused across the alveolar membrane than oxygen. Hypercarbia is mostly a problem in advanced emphysema (because the alveoli are affected) and during exacerbations of emphysema rather than bronchitis (where airways are affected).

Sputum samples are collected for culture from clients who exhibit signs of an acute respiratory tract infection while hospitalized. When in the ambulatory care setting, sputum cultures are rarely obtained; the client is treated on the basis of signs and symptoms and the usual cause of bacterial organisms. A bacterial cause cannot be identified in most acute respiratory illnesses. A white blood cell count may help identify leukocytosis present in a bacterial infection.

Other blood tests that may be indicated in clients with CAL include hemoglobin and hematocrit to determine polycythemia (a compensatory increase in red blood cells in the chronically hypoxic client). The eosinophil count on the white blood cell differential is often increased in the client with extrinsic (allergic) asthma.

Initial screens for hypophosphatemia, hyperkalemia, hypocalcemia, and hypomagnesemia are important because they are associated with diminished diaphragmatic function. In clients suspected of alpha$_1$-antitrypsin (ATT) deficiency, a serum AAT and Pi typing should be performed.

▶ Radiographic Assessment

The physician orders PA and lateral chest x-rays to rule out other chest diseases and to determine the progress of clients with respiratory tract infections and chronic disease. In clients with advanced emphysema, chest x-rays usually show marked hyperinflation and flattened diaphragms. Chest x-rays, however, may not be helpful in the diagnosis of early or moderate disease.

▶ Other Diagnostic Assessment

Chronic airflow limitation is classified from mild to severe on the basis of results of pulmonary function tests (PFTs). Airflow rates and lung volume measurements help distinguish airway disease from restrictive patterns typical of interstitial lung disease. The three major components of PFTs are measurements that determine lung volumes, flow volume curves, and diffusion capacity. Each test is performed before and after the client inhales a bronchodilator agent. In the client with asthma, an improvement in abnormal results is usually observed after inhalation of a bronchodilator. If no reversibility is seen after bronchodilator treatment, however, the diagnosis of asthma cannot be excluded.

Lung volume measurements most relevant to CAL are vital capacity (VC), residual volume (RV), and total lung capacity (TLC). Although most of the measured lung volumes or capacities change to some degree with chronic lung disease, RV usually increases markedly. This increase reflects the trapped, stagnant air remaining in the lungs.

Flow volume curves measure the client's ability to move air into and out of the lung. The rate of airflow out of the lungs during a rapid, forceful, and complete expiration from TLC to RV (forced expiratory volume, or FEV) indirectly measures the flow-resistive properties of the lung. A diagnosis of chronic lung disease is based primarily on the FEV$_1$ (the FEV in the first second of expiration). FEV$_1$ can also be expressed as a percentage of the forced vital capacity (FVC). As the disease progresses, the ratio of FEV$_1$ to FVC becomes smaller.

The third part of pulmonary function testing is diffusion, formerly called the "diffusing" capacity of the lung. This test measures how well a test gas (carbon monoxide) diffuses across the alveolar-capillary membrane and combines with the hemoglobin of red blood cells. In emphysema, the decrease in diffusion ability results from the destruction of alveolar walls, leading to a significant decrease in surface area for diffusion of gas into the blood. In asthma and bronchitis, even though lung volumes are increased, the diffusion capacity is usually normal.

Pulmonary function tests are further discussed in Chapter 29 and outlined in Table 29–7. Typical pulmonary function findings in CAL are given in Table 32–2.

Clients with CAL may have a decreased oxygen saturation, often as low as 91%. Pulse oximetry results lower than 90% (and certainly below 86%) may be considered an emergency necessitating immediate treatment. Chapter 29 contains more information on pulse oximetry.

Peak expiratory flow meters are monitors used by the client, nurse, and respiratory therapist to determine the effectiveness of the prescribed treatment to alleviate obstruction. Peak flow rates will increase as the client's obstruction resolves. The client is often taught to continue to self-monitor the peak expiratory flow rates at home and adjust medications accordingly.

 Analysis

▶ Common Nursing Diagnoses and Collaborative Problems

The most common nursing diagnoses for clients with chronic airflow limitation (CAL) are
1. Impaired Gas Exchange related to alveolar membrane changes, diminished airway size, airflow limitation, respiratory muscle fatigue, excess mucus production
2. Ineffective Breathing Pattern related to airflow obstruction (narrowed airways), diaphragm flattening, fatigue, and decreased energy
3. Ineffective Airway Clearance related to excessive secretions, fatigue, and decreased energy, ineffective cough
4. Altered Nutrition: Less than Body Requirements related to dyspnea, excessive secretions, anorexia, and fatigue

TABLE 32–2

Pulmonary Function Findings in Chronic Airflow Limitation

Test	Findings
Residual volume (RV): the volume of gas remaining in the lungs after a maximal expiration	• Loss of elastic recoil causes RV to be increased in emphysema and chronic bronchitis because of the narrowing and obstruction of airways.
Total lung capacity (TLC): the total amount of gas in the lungs at the end of a maximal inspiration	• TLC is increased in emphysematous clients because of loss of elastic recoil. TLC is normal in clients with chronic bronchitis.
Vital capacity (VC): the maximal amount of gas that can be expired after a maximal inspiration	• VC may be normal or decreased in the client with CAL.
Forced vital capacity (FVC): VC that is produced from a maximal forced expiratory effort.	• FVC is often increased in CAL clients secondary to air trapping.
Forced expiratory volume (FEV$_1$, FEV$_2$): volume of air that is exhaled during a specified time (in seconds) while measuring FVC	• FEV mainly reflects resistance in large airways and is usually reduced in the client with CAL.
Functional residual capacity (FRC): the amount of gas remaining in the lungs at the end of a tidal expiration	• FRC is increased in clients with chronic bronchitis if obstruction is severe.
Diffusion: measure of carbon monoxide uptake across the alveolar-capillary membrane	• The diffusion value is decreased in severe emphysema. Chronic bronchitis has little effect on diffusion.

5. Anxiety related to loss of control during dyspneic episodes or asthma attacks, dyspnea, change in health status, and situational crisis
6. Activity Intolerance related to fatigue, dyspnea, and an imbalance between oxygen supply and demand

A common collaborative problem for clients with COPD/CAL is potential for pneumonia or other respiratory infections.

> ➤ *Additional Nursing Diagnoses and Collaborative Problems*

In addition to the common diagnoses, the client with CAL may also have other associated problems, which may include

- Fatigue related to change in metabolic energy, hypoxemia
- Knowledge Deficit (disease process, prescribed treatments, activity limitations) related to unfamiliarity with information resources
- Altered Sexuality Patterns related to extreme fatigue
- Inability to Sustain Spontaneous Ventilation related to respiratory muscle fatigue
- Ineffective Management of Therapeutic Regimen related to knowledge deficits, decreased support systems, or economics.
- Sleep Pattern Disturbance related to dyspnea, unfamiliar environment (hospitalization)
- Altered Thought Processes related to hypoxemia, sleep deprivation
- Powerlessness related to difficulty in performing self-care, illness-related regimen
- Ineffective Individual Coping related to effects of chronic illness, loss of control over body function, major changes in lifestyle, situational crisis, knowledge deficit regarding therapeutic regimen/disease process/prognosis

- Altered Role Performance related to change in health status, role loss

Other collaborative problems for clients with COPD/CAL include potential for status asthmaticus, potential for acute exacerbation of disease, potential for respiratory failure, and potential for right heart failure.

 Planning and Implementation

> ➤ *Impaired Gas Exchange*

The client should attain and maintain PaO$_2$ (or oxygen saturation) and PaCO$_2$ levels within normal ranges or within the client's chronic baseline values. The *minimum* goal for most clients is a PaO$_2$ of 55–60 mmHg and an oxygen saturation between 91% and 95%, but this goal varies according to the client's age and disease process.

Also expected is that the client will

- Demonstrate a decrease in tachypnea, dyspnea, and confusion (from the hypoxemia)
- State that fatigue is reduced
- Demonstrate techniques and methods that support improved oxygenation without carbon dioxide retention

Some facilities have created clinical pathways to guide the planning of care for the client with asthma or for the client with an exacerbation of COPD/CAL.

 Interventions

The nurse assesses the client at frequent intervals (every 2 hours), especially during the acute phase of the illness. The nurse provides the prescribed oxygen, assesses the client's response to treatment, and intervenes to prevent complications. Additional interventions can be found in the Client Care Plan regarding CAL.

Client Care Plan

The Client with Chronic Airflow Limitation

Nursing Diagnosis No. 1: Impaired Gas Exchange related to alveolar membrane changes, airflow limitation, respiratory muscle fatigue, excess production of mucus, and intrapulmonary shunting

Expected Outcomes	Nursing Interventions	Rationale
The client demonstrates correct use of techniques and methods that support improved oxygenation.	■ Assess oxygenation of the client, including a. Level of consciousness b. Pulse oximetry c. Breathing pattern, rate, and depth; chest expansion; dyspnea, nasal flaring; pursed-lip breathing; prolonged expiratory phase; and use of accessory muscles d. Peak expiratory flow rate ■ Instruct client and monitor proper placement of oxygen devices (e.g., nasal cannula). ■ Teach energy conservation techniques: a. Encourage sitting for most activities, such as peeling potatoes or talking on the telephone. b. Teach the client never to hold his or her breath while performing activities. c. Be aware that activities involving the arms may increase dyspnea. d. Plan rest between periods of activity. ■ Instruct the client in the following: a. Pursed-lip breathing b. Diaphragmatic breathing c. Relaxation therapy d. Controlled cough techniques ■ Formulate a plan with the client and family for pacing activities of daily living.	■ Information will provide answers to questions of hypoxemia. ■ Clients with hypoxemia will desaturate rapidly within minutes once oxygen is removed. ■ Increased activity and work of breathing will increase oxygen consumption. These techniques assist the client in oxygen conservation. ■ These techniques assist the client with better ventilation. ■ Planned activities are better controlled and provide better data for evaluation.
The client demonstrates correct technique to normalize $PaCO_2$.	■ Assess the quality and quantity of sputum: color, consistency, amount, and odor. ■ Maximize the effect of medical interventions by proper sequence of respiratory treatments and by judicious use of bronchodilators and steroids.	■ Increased mucus and inflammation can cause airflow limitation. ■ These interventions result in decreased airflow limitation.

(Continued)

Client Care Plan

Expected Outcomes	Nursing Interventions	Rationale
	■ Instruct and monitor client's technique with metered-dose inhalers. ■ Teach potential hazard of excessive inspired oxygen to clients and family. ■ Teach signs and symptoms of hypercapnia: 　a. Headache 　b. Drowsiness and fatigue	■ Correct technique, sequence, and use are key to effective treatment. ■ Clients with chronic hypercapnia have blunted CO_2 drives to breathe. ■ Acute hypercapnia can result in respiratory failure.

Nursing Diagnosis No. 2: Ineffective Breathing Pattern related to airflow obstruction (narrowed airways), fatigue, and decreased energy from respiratory muscle fatigue

Expected Outcomes	Nursing Interventions	Rationale
The client will demonstrate a breathing pattern that decreases the work of breathing.	■ Assess respiratory rate, depth, and rhythm at least every shift. ■ Assist the client in maintaining proper positioning during dyspneic episodes: 　a. Sitting up and leaning on overbed table 　b. Sitting up and resting with elbows on knees 　c. Standing and leaning against the wall ■ Teach pursed-lip and diaphragmatic breathing techniques. ■ Teach energy conservation techniques. ■ Initiate respiratory muscle training, if appropriate. ■ Identify in writing various factors that elicit an anxious response. ■ Help the client to formulate a plan for coping with dyspneic and wheezing episodes. ■ Allow the client to verbalize feelings. ■ Teach the client various interventions for anxiety: 　a. Relaxation techniques 　b. Biofeedback ■ Refer the client for professional counseling if necessary.	■ Assessment provides the nurse with baseline information. ■ These positions can decrease the work of breathing. ■ These breathing techniques facilitate increased expiratory flow. ■ Respiratory muscles fatigue easily in CAL clients. ■ Inspiratory muscle training can assist in strengthening the diaphragm. ■ This process gives the client control of his or her situation. ■ A plan prepares the client for episodes of anxiety. ■ Verbalization tends to prevent or decrease anxiety. ■ Interventions decrease stress. ■ Counseling assists the client with self-analysis and coping techniques.

Client Care Plan

Nursing Diagnosis No. 3: Ineffective Airway Clearance related to excessive secretions, fatigue and decreased energy, and ineffective cough

Expected Outcomes	Nursing Interventions	Rationale

The client will demonstrate effective airway clearance techniques and will attain optimal lung sounds.	■ Assess sputum for color, amount, consistency, and odor.
	■ Assess the client's ability to expectorate sputum with ease.
	
	■ Assess breath sounds at least every 8 hours.
	■ Monitor and encourage adequate fluid intake daily.
	
	■ Position the client to prevent aspiration.
	■ Teach a method of controlled cough.
	
	■ Suction as necessary to remove secretions.
	■ Teach postural drainage and chest physiotherapy techniques, if ordered:
	  a. Assess level of consciousness.
	  b. Observe for hypoxemia.
	  c. Assess breath sounds for wheezes caused by bronchospasm.
		■ Secretions can obstruct airways.
		■ Observe the client's cough efforts to determine best technique.
		■ Assessment provides vital information of respiratory status.
		■ Dehydration impairs ciliary action; hydration helps to liquify secretions.
		■ Aspiration is the leading cause of pneumonia in the elderly.
		■ This technique will produce the best results with the least effort.
		■ Suctioning is based on breath sound assessment.
		■ Chest physiotherapy can cause hypoxemia and bronchospasm.

If the client's condition continues to deteriorate despite treatment, more aggressive therapy is required. Intubation and mechanical ventilation may be necessary for clients in respiratory failure, including those who are unable to sustain spontaneous ventilation. Chapter 34 discusses mechanical ventilation in detail.

Maintaining Airway Patency. The nurse's first intervention to improve gas exchange is to maintain a patent airway. The nurse maintains the client's head, neck, and chest in alignment, assists the client in liquefying secretions, and clears the airway of secretions. (More information on airway obstruction can be found in Chapter 31.)

Oxygen Therapy. Oxygen (O_2) is a potent drug prescribed by the physician for relief of symptoms of hypoxemia (low levels of oxygen in the blood) and its resultant hypoxia (decreased tissue oxygenation). Arterial blood gas (ABG) analysis is the best tool for determining the need for oxygen therapy and for evaluating its effects. Oxygen need can also be determined by noninvasive monitoring, such as pulse oximetry.

The average client requires an oxygen flow of 2–4 L/minute via nasal cannula or up to 40% via Venturi mask.

The client who is hypoxemic and also has chronic hypercarbia requires lower levels of oxygen delivery, usually 1–2 L/minute via nasal cannula. A low arterial oxygen level is this client's primary drive for breathing. More information on oxygen therapy can be found in Chapter 30.

Drug Therapy. The physician or Nurse Practitioner uses six main classes of drugs in managing a client with COPD/CAL:
■ Bronchodilators
■ Anticholinergics
■ Corticosteroids
■ Cromolyn sodium/nedocromil
■ Mucolytics
■ Leukotriene modifiers
Chart 32–4 summarizes these drugs.

Stepped therapies have been recommended for clients with asthma and chronic bronchitis or emphysema (Tables 32–3 and 32–4). The key elements of stepped therapy include pharmacologic therapy, monitoring (i.e., peak expiratory flow rates in the client with asthma), and control of environmental irritants and allergens. The expected outcomes of stepped therapy are for the client to have more awareness of the disease and to increase participa-

Chart 32–4

Drug Therapy for Chronic Airflow Limitation (CAL)

Drug	Usual Dosage	Nursing Interventions	Rationale
Bronchodilators			
Sympathomimetics (adrenergics, beta stimulants)			
Metaproterenol (Metaprel, Alupent)	• MDI: 2–4 puffs q4–6hr • PO: 20 mg tid • Aerosol: 0.2–0.3 mL q4–6hr	• Instruct the client to use the bronchodilator inhaler before the steroid inhaler (if ordered). • Teach the client the correct method of using the inhaler and observe the client's technique.	• Use of the beta-2 agent inhaler first opens the airways and facilitates deeper penetration of the steroid. • Correct technique ensures proper inhalation. Sequencing the steps in using an inhaler can be tricky for children and the elderly. Two critical variables are the speed of inhalation and the duration of breath holding.
Albuterol (salbutamol, Proventil, Ventolin)	• MDI: 2–4 puffs q4–6hr • PO: 2–4 mg q6–8hr • Aerosol: 0.5 mL q4–6hr	• Observe the client for fine finger tremors.	• The nurse observes the client to detect side effects of this selective beta-2 agent.
Pirbuterol (Maxair)	• MDI: 1–2 puffs q4–6hr	• Observe the client for tremors, nervousness, insomnia, headache, nausea, tachycardia, and palpitations.	• The nurse observes the client to detect side effects. The drug stimulates beta-adrenergic receptors in the heart and lungs.
Salmeterol xinafoate (Serevent)	• MDI: 2 puffs q12hr	• Do not use to relieve acute symptoms. • Give 30 min before exercise or HS	• The drug is a long-acting bronchodilator. • Serevent is used to prevent exercise-induced or nocturnal symptoms.
Isoetharine (Bronkosol)	• MDI: 2–4 puffs q3–6hr • Nebulizer: 0.5 mL diluted 1:3 with saline	• Observe the client for tachycardia, palpitations, headache, and blood pressure alterations.	• Same as for pirbuterol.
Epinephrine (Adrenalin, Primatene Mist, Bronkaid Mistometer✦, Dysne-Inhal✦)	• MDI: 2–3 puffs q2–4hr • SC or IM: 0.2–0.5 mL of 1:1000 solution; may repeat in 10–15 min • IV: 0.1–0.25 mL of 1:1000 solution	• Observe the client for anxiety, tremors, and palpitations. • Assess the client for a history of hyperthyroidism and ischemic heart disease.	• The nurse observes the client to detect side effects. The drug is fast acting, with an onset of about 20 min. • The nurse observes the client to detect possible contraindications.
Isoproterenol (Isuprel, Medihaler-Iso)	• MDI: 1–2 puffs 4–6 times/day	• Monitor the client for palpitations.	• The nurse monitors the client to detect severe cardiac dysrhythmias, especially with IV administration.
Terbutaline (Brethine, Brethaire, Bricanyl)	• MDI: 2–4 puffs q4–8hr • PO: 5 mg q8hr • SC: 0.25 mg, not to exceed 0.5 mg q4hr	• Monitor the client for palpitations and tachycardia.	• The nurse monitors the client to detect these infrequent side effects. The drug has a more selective beta-2 action, slower onset, and longer duration than do other sympathomimetics.
Methylxanthines			
Aminophylline (contains 80% theophylline; Corophyllin✦)	• IV loading dose: 5–7 mg/kg over 20–40 min • IV maintenance dose: 0.5–1.2 mg/kg/hr	• Monitor drug levels.	• Monitoring blood levels detects possible toxicity. The drug has a narrow therapeutic range of 10–20 μg/mL. (Some clients do well at levels of 5–12 μg/mL.)

Chart 32–4. Drug Therapy for Chronic Airflow Limitation (CAL) Continued

Drug	Usual Dosage	Nursing Interventions	Rationale
		• Observe the client for nausea and vomiting, diarrhea, tachycardia, palpitations, dizziness, and restlessness. • Space doses equally throughout a 24-hr period. • Give in saline or 5% dextrose/water by infusion pump. • Avoid caffeine intake.	• The nurse observes the client to detect side effects and potential toxic effects, most of which are dose related. • Spacing of doses ensures even coverage throughout the day. • Infusion is constant, steady, and controlled. • Avoidance of caffeine reduces other sources of sympathetic stimulation.
Theophylline (Slo-Phyllin, Theo-Dur, Theobid, Uniphyl, Uni-Dur, Slo-bid Gyrocaps, Acet-Am♣)	• PO: initially: 10–12 mg/kg/day, increased by 25% at 3-day intervals until a maximal oral dose of 13 mg/kg/day in 2–4 divided doses (usually 400–800 mg/day) is reached; Uni-Dur is once a day.	• Same as for aminophylline. • Administer with food, such as milk and crackers. • Instruct client to take medication even when feeling good. • Know whether the medication is the immediate-release form or the timed-release form.	• Taking the drug with food prevents gastrointestinal irritation. • A therapeutic blood level is maintained. • Sustained-release preparations give better coverage than regular preparations, which makes them ideal for clients who awaken at night with shortness of breath.
Anticholinergics (give 5 min after the sympathomimetic)			
Ipratropium bromide (Atrovent)	• MDI: 2–3 puffs qid, up to 6–8 puffs 3–4 times per day in acute exacerbation	• Instruct the client to close eyes while activating inhaler if not using spacer. • Monitor the client for cough, dry mouth, headache, nausea, blurred vision, nervousness, palpitations.	• Medication in the eyes will cause temporary blurring of vision. • The nurse monitors the client to detect side effects.
Atropine	• Aerosol: 0.2% (1 mg) 0.5% (2.5 mg) 5–10 mg q6–8hr (long-term maintenance) 2.5–5 mg q4–6hr (acute severe asthma)	• Monitor for troublesome anticholinergic side effects (i.e., drying of mucous secretions, decreased mucociliary transport tachycardia, glaucoma, prostatism, and urinary retention).	• The nurse monitors the client to detect side effects.
Corticosteroids (give 5 minutes after the anticholinergic)			
Prednisone (Deltasone, Apo-Prednisone♣, Winpred♣) Methyl-prednisolone (Solu-Medrol, Medrol♣)	• PO, IV: dosage varies	• Instruct the client about the side effects of long-term steroid use, such as hyperglycemia, osteoporosis, increased fat production and weight gain, immunologic impairment, reduced inflammatory response, increased gastric acidity • Monitor serum potassium levels for hypokalemia. • Instruct the client to take medication with food. • Instruct the client never to discontinue steroid use suddenly.	• The nurse warns the client of possible side effects, many of which are irreversible but must be treated. • Systemic steroids cause potassium loss with sodium and water retention. • Food minimizes gastric irritation. • Sudden discontinuation of steroids precipitates adrenal crisis and shock.
Beclomethasone (Vanceril, Beclovent, Rotacaps♣)	• MDI: 2–4 puffs tid–qid	• Observe the client's mouth daily for the bright, fire red or cherry color of oral candidiasis.	• Oral candidiasis is a complication of inhaled steroids.

Continued

Chart 32-4. Drug Therapy for Chronic Airflow Limitation (CAL)   Continued

Drug	Usual Dosage	Nursing Interventions	Rationale
		• Instruct the client in the proper sequencing of sympathomimetic and steroid inhalers, if appropriate, and observe the client's technique.	• Proper sequencing and technique promote optimal distribution of the steroid.
		• Instruct the client to drink 8 ounces of water after inhaling steroids or gargle and rinse mouth after use.	• Drinking water washes away excess medication from the back of the throat and thus minimizes the growth of *Candida*.
		• Provide reservoir spacer.	• A spacer decreases oropharyngeal deposition of the drug.
Triamcinolone (Azma-cort)	• MDI: 2–6 puffs tid–qid • Maximum: 16 puffs/day	• Same as for beclomethasone.	
Flunisolide (AeroBid)	• MDI: 2–4 puffs bid	• Same as for beclomethasone.	
Fluticasone (Flovent)	• MDI: 2–4 puffs bid	• Same as for beclomethasone.	
Cromolyn and nedocromil			
Nedocromil (Tilade)	• MDI: 2 puffs q6–12hr	• Monitor for headache, unpleasant taste in the mouth, runny nose, and nausea. • Instruct client to stop medication and call physician if bronchospasm or continued coughing occurs. • Instruct the client that the drug must be used even when symptom free.	• The nurse observes the client for side effects. • The client may be sensitive to propellants in the MDI. • The medication is not effective during acute episodes.
Cromolyn Sodium (Intal, Gastrocrom, Rynacrom✦) (Intal, Rynacrom✦)	• MDI: 1 or 2 puffs qid • Aerosol • PO: 200 mg qid before meals and HS	• Observe the client for maculopapular rash and urticaria. • Instruct the client that cromolyn is a prophylactic drug. • Inform the client that an optimal response may not occur before 2 months of daily use.	• The nurse observes the client to detect rare side effects. • Encourage the client to seek other treatment during an acute attack. • Continued use is promoted until the drug takes effect.
Mucolytics			
Acetylcysteine (Mucomyst, Airbron✦)	• Aerosol (nebulizer): 3–5 mL (20%) 3–4 times daily 6–10 mL (10%) 3–4 times daily	• Observe the client for nausea and bronchospasm.	• The nurse observes the client to detect common side effects.
Dornase alfa (Pulmozyme)	• Aerosol (nebulizer): 2.5 mg once daily	• Observe the client for pharyngitis, voice alterations, laryngitis, conjunctivitis, rash, urticaria.	• The nurse observes the client to detect common side effects.
Iodinated glycerol (Organidin)	• PO: 60 mg qid	• Instruct the client to have T_3 and T_4 tests done before starting therapy and then at the 3-month follow-up examination.	• The iodine content can cause hypothyroidism.
Leukotriene Modifiers			
Zafirlukast (Accolate)	• PO: 20 mg bid 1 hr before or 2 hr after meals	• Do not use to relieve acute symptoms	• Accolate will not reverse acute bronchospasm.
Zileuton (Zyflo)	• PO: 600 mg qid	• Monitor liver enzymes.	• A serious side effect is the elevation of liver enzymes.

MDI = metered-dose inhaler; T_3 = triiodothyronine; T_4 = thyroxine.

TABLE 32-3

Pharmacologic Stepped Approach to Treating Asthma Symptoms	
Asthma Symptoms	**Treatment**
Step 1: mild intermittent	• Beta-2 agonist (short acting), 1–2 puffs prn rescue treatment < 3×/wk
Step 2: mild persistent	• Add inhaled, cromolyn sodium or nedocromil, or leukotriene antagonist • May add long-acting beta-2 agonist (client >12 years) • Client adjusts doses according to peak expiratory flow rates
Step 3: moderate persistent	• Daily inhaled corticosteroid • May add nedocromil or theophyllin
Step 4: severe persistent	• Add corticosteroids PO or IV PO dose: 40–60 mg/day for up to 2 weeks. • Wean to low dose or inhaled corticosteroid

tion symptom management. When adequate symptom control has been achieved for a few months, "stepping down" may be attempted.

Bronchodilators. The preferred technique for administration of bronchodilators is via the metered-dose inhaler (MDI) because it delivers the drug directly to the lung. Side effects are reduced because only a limited amount of the drug gets into the general circulation. The bronchodilators are divided into sympathomimetics and methylxanthines.

Sympathomimetics. The sympathomimetic drugs, or adrenergic bronchodilators, are drugs that mimic, or act like, the sympathetic nervous system. These drugs cause bronchodilation through activation of the enzyme adenylate cyclase, which converts adenosine triphosphate (ATP) to adenosine 3′,5′-cyclic monophosphate (cAMP), the body's own natural bronchodilator.

In choosing a specific drug, the physician considers the beta-adrenergic activity of each drug. Beta$_1$-receptors are located in the heart, whereas beta$_2$-receptors are located in the lung. The more selective beta$_2$-adrenergic drugs (e.g., metaproterenol [Alupent], albuterol [Proventil, Ven-

tolin], and terbutaline [Brethine]) generally do not stimulate the heart directly, have a faster onset of action, and are longer in duration. The long-acting form is preferred for the client with symptoms of nocturnal asthma or requiring step 2 therapy for asthma. Many of the sympathomimetics can be administered in an inhaled form (Chart 32-5).

The rapidly metabolized, short-acting sympathomimetic drugs are first line for acute exacerbations of asthma and for prevention of exercise-induced bronchospasm. Their effect, however, is often minimized in the elderly. The nurse teaches the client with asthma to use the beta$_2$-adrenergic inhaler (rather than the anticholinergic) at the onset of symptoms because of the more rapid onset of action.

Methylxanthines. Methylxanthines act to increase the levels of cAMP. Other actions include the antagonism of adenosine and prostaglandins, both natural bronchoconstrictors.

Aminophylline. In an acute flare-up of asthma or severe bronchospasm caused by any type of CAL, the physician may prescribe a loading dose of intravenous (IV) amino-

TABLE 32-4

Pharmacologic Stepped Approach to Treating Chronic Bronchitis and Emphysema	
Step 1: mild symptoms	• Beta-2 agonist, 1–2 puffs q2–6 hr, prn (not to exceed 8–12 puffs in 24 hr)
Step 2: mild to moderate symptoms daily	• Ipratropium bromide 2–6 puffs q6–8 hr • Beta-2 agonist, 1–4 puffs for rescue treatment or as regular supplement
Step 3: unsatisfactory response to step 2	• Add theophylline 200–400 mg, bid or 400–800 mg HS (nocturnal bronchospasms) or albuterol SR 4–8 mg bid or HS only
Step 4: unsatisfactory response to step 3	• Add prednisone 40 mg/day for 10–14 days *Wean when improvement noted to low daily or QOD dose *Place on steroid metered-dose inhaler if has bronchial hyperreactivity *Stop steroids if no improvement noted
Step 5: severe exacerbation	• Beta-2 agonist with spacer, 6–8 puffs q½–2hr • Ipratropium bromide with spacer, 6–8 puffs q3–4hr • Theophylline IV • Methylprednisolone 50–100 mg IV STAT, then q6–8hr. Wean as soon as possible. • Antibiotics if indicated • Mucokinetic agents if sputum tenacious

Chart 32-5

Education Guide: How to Use an Inhaler Correctly*

Without a Spacer (Preferred Technique)

1. Before each use, remove the cap and shake the inhaler according to the instructions in the package insert.
2. Tilt your head back slightly and breathe out fully.
3. Open your mouth and place the mouthpiece 1 to 2 inches away.
4. As you begin to breathe in deeply through your mouth, press down firmly on the canister of the inhaler to release one dose of medication.
5. Continue to breathe in slowly and deeply (usually over 3 to 5 seconds).
6. Hold your breath for at least 10 seconds to allow the medication to reach deep into the lungs, then breathe out slowly.
7. Wait at least 1 minute between puffs.
8. Replace the cap on the inhaler.
9. At least once a day, remove the canister and clean the plastic case and cap of the inhaler by thoroughly rinsing in warm, running tap water.

Without a Spacer (Alternative Method)

1. Follow steps 1 and 2 above.
2. Place the mouthpiece into your mouth, over your tongue, and seal your lips tightly around it.
3. Follow steps 4 to 9 above.

With a Spacer

1. Before each use, remove the caps from the inhaler and the spacer.
2. Insert the mouthpiece of the inhaler into the non-mouthpiece end of the spacer.
3. Shake the whole unit vigorously 3 or 4 times.
4. Place the mouthpiece into your mouth, over your tongue, and seal your lips tightly around it.
5. Press down firmly on the canister of the inhaler to release one dose of medication into the spacer.
6. Breathe in slowly and deeply. If the spacer makes a whistling sound, you are breathing in too rapidly.
7. Remove the mouthpiece from your mouth and, keeping your lips closed, hold your breath for at least 10 seconds, then breathe out slowly.
8. Wait at least 1 minute between puffs.
9. Replace the caps on the inhaler and the spacer.
10. At least once a day, clean the plastic case and cap of the inhaler by thoroughly rinsing in warm, running tap water; at least once a week, clean the spacer in the same manner.

*Avoid spraying in the direction of the eyes.

phylline. Maintenance doses may need to be higher for heavy smokers.

Theophylline. Theophylline is useful in managing severe bronchospasms and in treating nocturnal symptoms. It is usually given orally in immediate- or sustained-release preparations. The drug is well absorbed orally, with peak serum concentrations occurring in 1–2 hours. Achieving a therapeutic level can be challenging because various conditions influence the serum concentration (Table 32–5). The physician or Nurse Practitioner makes adjustments in dosage based on the client's clinical response to therapy.

Over-the-Counter (OTC) Bronchodilators. The Food and Drug Administration (FDA) believes people should have ready access to certain bronchodilator drug products. A potential for abuse exists, particularly when these preparations are taken with prescription drugs. The nurse teaches clients that OTC preparations contain active ingredients, usually epinephrine, ephedrine, and theophylline, and are to be respected. The nurse asks whether the client routinely uses OTC preparations and cautions the client about potential abuse.

Anticholinergics. Most of the autonomic nerves in the airways are branches of the vagus nerve. They are predominantly located in the large and medium-sized airways. Release of acetylcholine at these sites results in smooth muscle contraction. An anticholinergic agent, then, acts as a bronchodilator. It is most useful in the elderly and those clients with chronic bronchitis and emphysema, whereas beta-2 agonists are more useful in the treatment of asthma.

Corticosteroids. Steroid preparations reduce inflammation in the throat and lungs but also act to stimulate cAMP production and cause bronchodilation. They are known to decrease the production of cysteinyl leukotrienes, which are involved in the early- and late-phase asthmatic response, thus reducing the levels of preinflam-

TABLE 32-5

Factors that Influence Theophylline Clearance	
Factors that Decrease Clearance (Resulting in Increased Drug Levels)	**Factors that Increase Clearance (Resulting in Decreased Drug Levels)**
Diseases	
• Renal failure	• Hyperthyroidism
• Cirrhosis or other liver abnormalities	
• Congestive heart failure	
• Alcoholism	
• Upper respiratory tract infections	
• Hypothyroidism	
Drugs	
• Caffeine	• Isoproterenol (Isuprel)
• Allopurinol (Zyloprim)	• Rifampin (Rifadin, Rofact♣)
• Erythromycin (E-Mycin, Apo-Erythro♣)	• Phenobarbital (Luminal♣)
• Cimetidine (Tagamet)	• Phenytoin (Dilantin)
• Oral contraceptives	
• Ciprofloxacin (Cipro)	
• Calcium channel blockers	
Other factors	
• Older age, elderly	• Cigarette smoking

matory cytokines. When long-term oral use is necessary, alternate-day therapy minimizes adrenal suppression and other side effects. See Chapter 66 for more information on steroids and steroid side effects.

An advantage of the aerosol route of administration is equivalent or greater bronchodilation and protection with fewer systemic side effects. However, at doses greater than 1000 μg of inhaled steroid, systemic symptoms have been seen, including bone loss, thinning skin, and purpura.

If the physician has prescribed both an inhaled bronchodilator and an inhaled steroid for administration at the same time, the nurse instructs the client to use the bronchodilator first. With dilation of the large airways, a greater portion of the steroid preparation reaches the peripheral airways.

The client with asthma who is using stepped therapy will monitor peak expiratory flow rates in the early morning and in the evening. If the difference in the expiratory flow rates exceeds 20%, the client adjusts the treatment dosage of oral or inhaled corticosteroid to that recommended by the health care provider.

Cromolyn Sodium and Nedocromil. Cromolyn sodium (Intal) or nedocromil (Tilade) can be used prophylactically in clients with asthma whose symptoms are not controlled adequately by bronchodilators or as a first-line treatment before bronchodilators are given. It is not useful during acute attacks. The desired effects of cromolyn are to reduce the severity and frequency of asthma attacks and to reduce the need for bronchodilators and steroids. Cromolyn probably acts by strengthening the mast cell membrane to prevent release of histamine and thereby decreases bronchospasm in the allergic asthmatic. Nedocromil sodium works much like cromolyn but may have additional anti-inflammatory effects. It is thought to be more useful in the elderly and reduces the airway response in the nonallergic asthmatic. Cromolyn is administered via metered-dose inhaler (MDI) or as solution in a nebulizer, usually four times a day.

Cromolyn, nedocromil, and beta-2 agonists are the preferred treatment for exercise-induced bronchospasm. Although corticosteroids can reduce or prevent exercised induced bronchospasm, they may take several weeks to become effective.

Mucolytics. The physician orders mucolytic agents for clients with thick, tenacious (sticky) mucous secretions. Nebulizer treatments with normal saline or with a mucolytic agent like acetylcysteine (Mucomyst) and normal saline help to thin secretions and facilitate expectoration.

Leukotriene Modifiers. This new therapy is indicated as adjunct therapy for the prophylaxis and chronic treatment of early- and late-phase asthmatic response. These drugs either block the leukotrienes released in response to the allergen (zafirlukast), or inhibit leukotriene formation (zileuton). They are not bronchodilators and should not be used to treat acute asthma episodes.

Lung Volume Reduction. Lung volume reduction (LVR) is used in the treatment of end-stage emphysema. LVR was first introduced in 1957 and again reintroduced in 1990. Currently, it is considered most appropriate for those clients with pure emphysema.

Criteria used for selection of patients include evidence of bullous or nonbullous emphysema, disabling dyspnea, postbronchodilator FEV_1 less than 35% predicted, residual volumes greater than 200% predicted, total lung capacity greater than 120% predicted, and an ability to perform in a preoperative pulmonary rehabilitation program (Naunheim & Ferguson, 1996). The purpose of LVR is to resect the dysfunctional areas of the lung, thus reducing the amount of trapped air. The results are reduced dyspnea and improved functional status, spirometric indexes, and oxygen saturation. Additional interventions introduced in 1989 include single lung transplantation. Although this option is available, its actual use is limited.

➤ Ineffective Breathing Pattern

Planning: Expected Outcomes. The client should achieve an effective breathing pattern that decreases the work of breathing. Specific outcomes may be for the client to have
- A respiratory rate, depth, and timing within normal limits
- A respiratory rhythm within normal limits for the client's age
- Synchronous thoracoabdominal movement
- Use of accessory muscles appropriate to activity level
- Increased activity tolerance

Interventions. Before any interventions can be implemented, the nurse, physician, physical therapist, and respiratory therapist assess the client to determine the breathing pattern, especially the rate, rhythm, depth, and use of accessory muscles. The client with chronic airflow limitation (CAL) relies more on accessory muscles than on the diaphragm for ventilation. However, these muscles are less efficient than the diaphragm; consequently, the client experiences increased work of breathing. The nurse determines whether there are any contributing factors to the increased work of breathing, such as respiratory tract infection. Interventions are aimed at improving the client's breathing efforts and decreasing the work of breathing (see Client Care Plan addressing CAL).

Breathing Techniques. Diaphragmatic or abdominal and pursed-lip breathing maneuvers may be beneficial interventions for managing dyspneic episodes. The client uses these techniques, shown in Chart 32–6, during all activities. The amount of stagnant air in the lung is minimized, and the client gains confidence and control in managing dyspnea.

Diaphragmatic or Abdominal Breathing. In diaphragmatic breathing, the client attempts consciously to increase diaphragmatic movement. Lying on the back allows the abdomen to relax.

Pursed-Lip Breathing. The technique of pursed-lip breathing uses the mild resistance of partially opposed lips to prolong exhalation and to increase airway pressure, thereby delaying dynamic compression of airways and minimizing the effects of air trapping. Many clients with CAL learn this technique on their own. Pursed-lip breathing can be used during diaphragmatic or abdominal

Chart 32–6

Education Guide: Breathing Exercises

Diaphragmatic or Abdominal Breathing

- Lie on your back with your knees bent.
- Place your hands or a book on your abdomen to create resistance.
- Begin breathing from your abdomen while keeping your chest still. You can tell if you are breathing correctly if your hands or the book rises and falls accordingly.

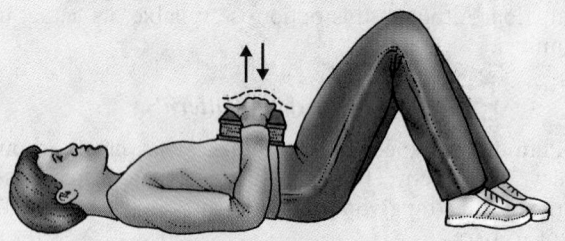

Pursed-Lip Breathing

- Close your mouth and breathe in through your nose.
- Purse your lips as you would to whistle. Breathe out slowly through your mouth, without puffing your cheeks. Spend at least twice the amount of time it took you to breathe in. Use your abdominal muscles to squeeze out every bit of air you can.
- Remember to use pursed-lip breathing during any physical activity. Always inhale before beginning the activity and exhale while performing the activity. Never hold your breath.

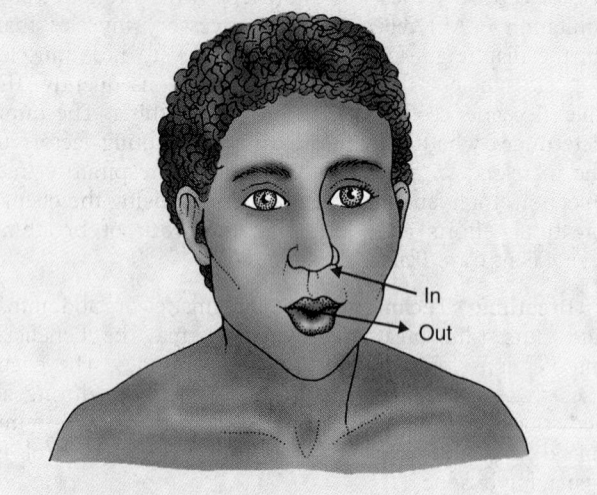

breathing. The nurse teaches both of these breathing techniques when the client is free from dyspnea.

Positioning. The nurse assists the client to an upright position, with the head of the bed elevated to promote easier breathing patterns. The client uses various positions to assist in alleviating dyspnea (see Fig. 32–4). In one position, the client sits on the edge of the bed with the arms resting on two or three pillows on an overbed table. If extra pillows are not available, the client may lean on a

table or rest on the elbows. These positions promote increased chest expansion, relax the chest muscles, and place the diaphragm in the proper position to contract while conserving energy by supporting the client's arms and upper body. The client may also find this position particularly helpful during an acute attack when tired but too short of breath to lie back.

The client uses the standing position (Fig. 32–7) when there is no place to sit. Clients with CAL use a greater proportion of their accessory muscles for breathing. Supporting the thorax, therefore, allows these muscles to work better.

Exercise Conditioning. Clients suffering from exercise-induced shortness of breath respond to dyspnea by limiting their activity, even basic activities of daily living (ADLs). Over time, the muscles of respiration and the general large muscle groups weaken, becoming less efficient in their use of oxygen. The result is increased dyspnea with lower activity levels. (Table 29–3 summarizes the relationship between dyspnea and the performance of daily activities.)

Exercise conditioning is part of a complete pulmonary rehabilitation program. Conditioning of the large muscle groups (indirect) or retraining of the respiratory muscles (direct) can be done. The indirect approach is accomplished through any general exercise program.

Two direct techniques currently used are isocapneic hyperventilation and resistive breathing. Isocapneic hyperventilation is designed to increase endurance. The client hyperventilates into a machine that controls the concen-

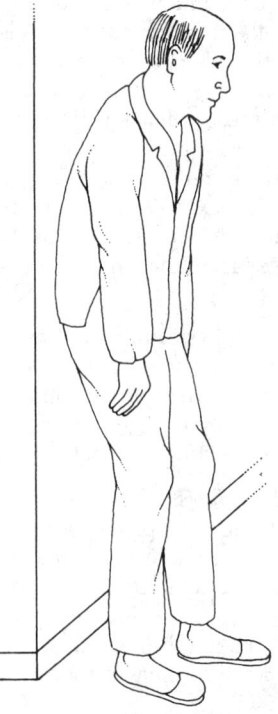

Figure 32–7. The standing position that is used to help clients with chronic airflow limitation (CAL) to breathe. The client stands with the back and hips against a wall and with the feet about 30 cm (12 inches) from the wall. The shoulders are relaxed and bent slightly forward.

trations of oxygen and carbon dioxide. In resistive breathing, the client breathes against a set resistance. Resistive breathing theoretically trains respiratory muscles for both strength and endurance. Retraining of the respiratory muscles is currently done predominantly in research settings.

Energy Conservation. Energy conservation is the planning and placing of activities for maximal tolerance and minimal discomfort. Once the FEV_1 falls below 50% predicted, the client's ability to perform ADLs is disturbed. The nurse or therapist (physical or occupational) begins by asking the client to describe a typical daily schedule. Then each activity is divided into its smaller parts to determine whether that task can be performed in a different way or at a different time of the day. The nurse assists the client in planning and pacing activities for the day. Rest periods are paced between activities. It is helpful for the nurse and the client to develop a chart outlining the day's activities and planned rest periods. Once a day, the nurse and client review the previous day's plan and make adjustments as indicated to promote energy conservation and yet provide activity.

The nurse reminds the client to avoid working with the arms raised. Activities involving the arms decrease exercise tolerance because the accessory muscles of respiration are then used to stabilize the shoulders. Many activities involving the arms can be done sitting at a table leaning on the elbows.

The nurse reminds the client to adjust work heights. Improper working height causes back strain and fatigue. The best work height for a table top is 5 cm (2 inches) below the bent elbow. Rapid, jerky arm motions cause shortness of breath and fatigue and put an extra strain on the heart. Clients should be reminded to keep arm motions smooth and flowing. Long-handled dustpans, sponges, and feather dusters minimize bending and reaching.

The nurse gives suggestions to the client about the organization of work spaces so that items used most often are within easy reach. Measures like dividing laundry or groceries into small parcels that can be handled easily, using disposable plates to save washing time, and letting dishes dry in the rack also conserve energy. The nurse suggests that clients straighten bed covers before getting out of bed for easier bed making. Talking requires energy and use of the lungs; therefore, the nurse instructs the client not to talk when engaged in other activities that require energy, such as walking. In addition, the nurse instructs the client that the key to any activity is to remember to avoid holding the breath and always to exhale while performing any activity.

Ineffective Airway Clearance

Planning: Expected Outcomes. The client should attain optimal lung sounds. Additional outcomes include that the client will
- Maintain a patent airway
- Demonstrate an effective cough
- Remain free from aspiration
- Implement the stepped therapy approach to control of symptoms

Interventions. The client with chronic bronchitis and advanced emphysema often has difficulty with removal of secretions, which results in compromised breathing and inadequate oxygenation. In addition to impairing breathing, excessive mucus predisposes the client to respiratory infections. The nurse auscultates breath sounds routinely as part of physical assessment but also before and after interventions as part of the evaluation for ineffective airway clearance. Careful use of drugs combined with controlled coughing, hydration, and postural drainage may help in airway clearance. If these measures fail, a tracheostomy may be required on a temporary or permanent basis.

Controlled Coughing. Because clients with chronic airflow limitation (CAL) produce more mucus than healthy people, they may benefit from specific coughing at certain times of the day. The nurse teaches the client to cough on arising early in the morning to eliminate mucus that collected during the night. Coughing to expectorate mucus before mealtimes may facilitate a more pleasant meal, and coughing before bedtime may ensure clear lungs for an uninterrupted night's sleep.

To cough effectively, the client sits in a chair or on the side of a bed with feet placed firmly on the floor. The nurse instructs the client to turn the shoulders inward and to bend the head slightly downward, hugging a pillow against the stomach. The pillow helps decrease chest discomfort.

The nurse then instructs the client to take a few diaphragmatic breaths (see Charts 20–5 and 32–6). After the third to fifth deep breath (in through the nose, out through pursed lips), the nurse instructs the client to bend forward slowly while producing two or three strong coughs from the same breath. The first cough moves the secretions; the second and third coughs facilitate expectoration. The nurse notes the color, consistency, odor, and amount of secretions. On return to a sitting position, the client takes a comfortable deep breath. The entire coughing procedure is repeated at least twice. After coughing exercises, the nurse allows the client to rest and then assists in providing mouth care.

Chest Physiotherapy and Postural Drainage. Chest physiotherapy (PT) with postural drainage (Fig. 32–8) is a technique that assists in mobilizing secretions from peripheral to central airways, in re-expanding lung tissue, and in promoting efficient use of the respiratory muscles. Chest PT combines chest percussion with vibration to loosen secretions. Postural drainage uses specific positions and gravity to assist in removing bronchial secretions. Postural drainage with chest PT may be helpful for select CAL clients with excessive secretions and airway clearance problems but should not be used routinely on all CAL clients.

Suctioning. Suctioning is based on the auscultation of adventitious breath sounds and is not performed on a routine schedule. For the client with a weak cough, weak pulmonary musculature, and inability to expectorate effectively, the nurse or respiratory therapist performs nasotracheal suctioning. The nurse assesses the client for dyspnea and tachycardia or other dysrhythmias during the

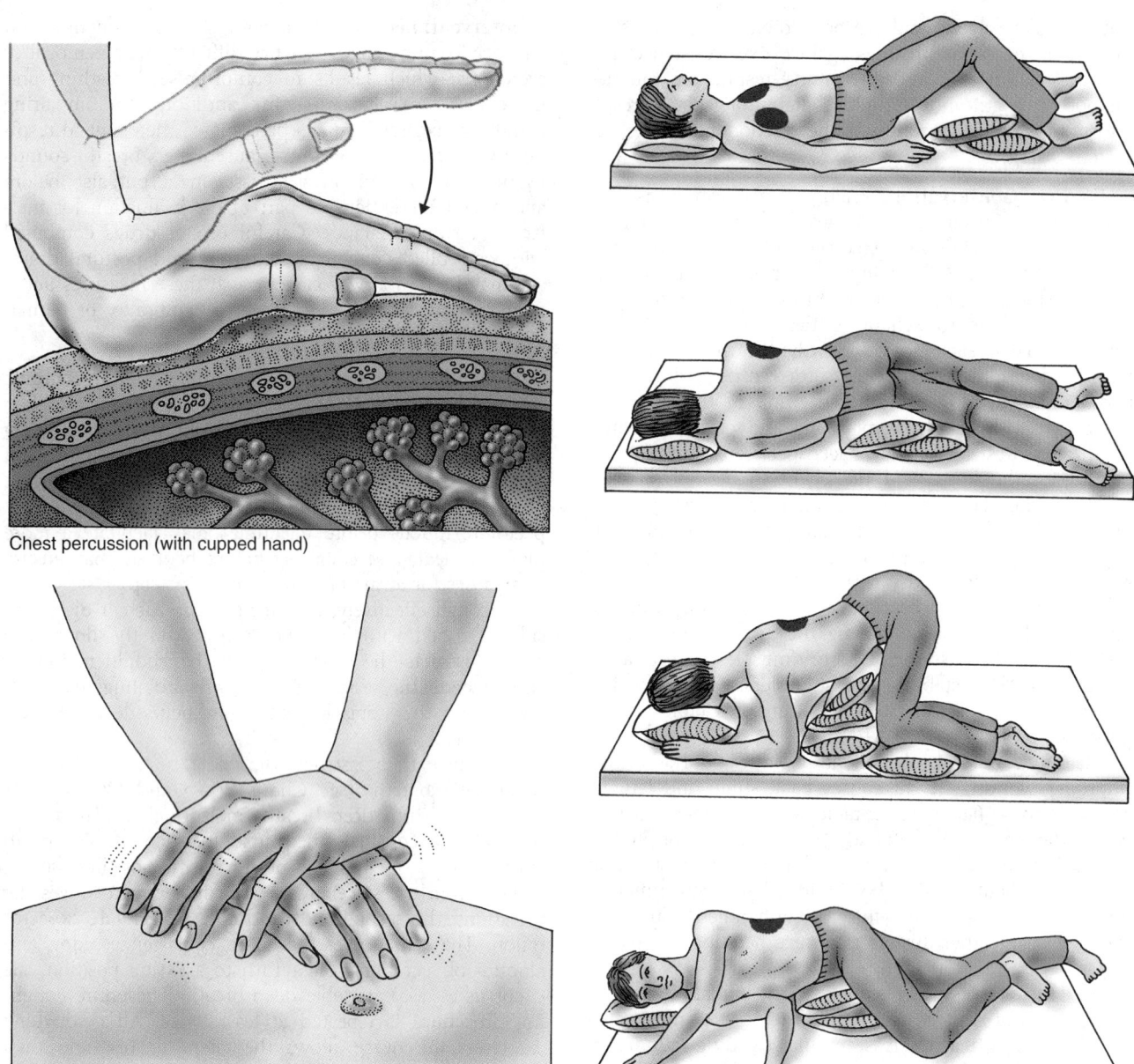

Chest percussion (with cupped hand)

Chest vibration

Figure 32–8. Chest physiotherapy (chest PT) and postural drainage. *Left,* Percussion and vibration techniques. The nurse may use one or two hands with vibration, which is performed when the client exhales or coughs. *Right,* Positions for postural drainage of respiratory secretions.

suctioning procedure and for improved breath sounds afterward. (Chapter 30 discusses suctioning in detail.)

Positioning. When the client can tolerate sitting in a chair, the nurse assists the client out of bed for 1-hour periods two to three times a day. This intervention helps mobilize secretions and also places the diaphragm in a position to provide more effective ventilation of the lungs.

Hydration. Unless hydration is medically contraindicated, the nurse teaches clients with CAL to drink 2–3 L/day to maintain adequate hydration, which helps liquefy secretions. Humidifiers may be useful for clients living in a dry climate or who complain of dry heat during the winter. The nurse instructs the client to clean the humidifier daily to prevent the growth of mold spores.

➤ *Altered Nutrition: Less than Body Requirements*

Planning: Expected Outcomes. The client should achieve and then maintain a body weight within 10% of ideal.

Interventions. Clients with acute or chronic lung disease often complain of food intolerance, nausea, early satiety, loss of appetite, and meal-related dyspnea. In addition, the increased work of breathing raises calorie and protein requirements. These situations lead to protein-calorie malnutrition for many clients with chronic airflow limitation (CAL). Malnourished clients lose total body mass, respiratory muscle mass, respiratory muscle strength, lung elasticity, and alveolocapillary surface area, which contributes to an ineffective breathing pattern.

The nurse identifies clients at risk or those experiencing this complication and initiates dietary consultation. The nurse and nutritionist monitor the client's weight and other indicators of nutrition, such as skin condition and serum pre-albumin levels.

Dyspnea Management. Shortness of breath is the most common complaint related to eating. The nurse teaches the client that shortness of breath during mealtimes can be minimized by resting before meals. The biggest meal of the day is planned for the time when the client is most hungry. Four to six small meals a day may be preferred. The nurse suggests the use of pursed-lip and abdominal breathing to alleviate dyspnea. A bronchodilator used 30 minutes before the meal may be helpful if the meal-related dyspnea is due to bronchospasm or secretions.

Food Selection. Abdominal bloating and a feeling of fullness often prevent the client from eating a complete meal. In the acute care setting, the client may need assistance in choosing menus; the nurse reminds the client to choose foods that are easy to chew and not gas forming. Dry foods stimulate coughing, and foods like milk and chocolate may increase the thickness of saliva and secretions. The nurse advises avoidance of these foods in the symptomatic client. The nurse also teaches the client to avoid caffeinated beverages; they promote diuresis and contribute to dehydration and increased nervousness.

The nurse and nutritionist explore the types of high-calorie foods that the client likes. Dietary supplements such as Pulmocare are specifically designed to provide nutritional supplementation with reduced CO_2 production. If the client has early satiety, the nurse recommends that the client avoid drinking fluids before and during the meal.

Assistance with Feeding. The nurse assists in feeding of the client who tires easily. Most clients do not have the energy to feed themselves when they are working hard to breathe. Many times, clients do not have the urge to eat. The nurse tries various interventions to deal with the anorexia. Sucking on hard candy or chewing gum before meals to begin salivation and stimulate taste buds may help. The nurse also offers to assist the client with oral hygiene before meals.

➤ *Anxiety*

Planning: Expected Outcomes. The client should demonstrate decreased anxiety, be able to identify factors that contribute to anxious behaviors, and identify activities that tend to decrease anxious behaviors.

Interventions. Anxiety plays a major role in clients with CAL. Emotional upset can trigger or aggravate wheezing episodes in clients with asthma. The resultant dyspnea increases anxiety even more. Clients with emphysema and chronic bronchitis typically experience increased anxiety during acute dyspneic episodes, especially if they feel they are choking on excess secretions. Anxiety has been shown to cause dyspnea, which then affects

clients' functional status (see Research Applications for Nursing).

Psychological Interventions. If a client's symptoms are worsened because of anxiety, it is important that the client understand this effect and have a clear plan prepared in advance for dealing with anxiety. The nurse and the client together develop a written plan that states exactly what the client should do if symptoms flare. Having a plan gives the client confidence and control in knowing exactly what to do, which often helps reduce anxiety.

For example, the nurse helps clients to think of themselves not as asthmatics but as people who have asthma. The client is encouraged to discuss feelings and concerns with the nursing staff and other members of the health care team. The nurse explores other alternative psychological approaches to help the client control dyspneic episodes and panic attacks. Examples include relaxation techniques (see Chap. 8), hypnosis therapy, and biofeedback. Biofeedback helps the client determine the impact of various stimuli on symptoms. The client ultimately learns to relax and control these stimuli to avoid the aggravating symptoms.

The client uses pursed-lip and diaphragmatic breathing techniques in conjunction with relaxation therapy. The nurse instructs the client in the various techniques and assesses the client's understanding and performance of the

➤ Research Applications for Nursing

Psychologic Factors Influence Functional Status in COPD

Weaver, T. E., Richmond, T. S., & Narsavage, G. L. (1997). An explanatory model of functional status in chronic obstructive pulmonary disease. Nursing Research, 46(1), 26–32.

This study examined which variables influenced the functional status of 104 clients with chronic obstructive pulmonary disease (COPD). All clients were diagnosed with emphysema, bronchitis, or COPD; 82% were male; 70% were married; the mean age was 65.6 years; and the mean duration of illness was 11.6 years. Functional status was measured using the Pulmonary Functional Status Scale (PFSS), which defines functional status in terms of physical, mental, and social functioning in everyday life. Exercise capacity, dyspnea, and depressed mood were found to influence functional status directly. Dyspnea, depression, and pulmonary function indirectly influenced functional status through exercise capacity. Self-esteem and anxiety indirectly influenced functional status through depressed mood.

Critique. This well-designed study has few limitations. The majority of the subjects were males, and no data were included to address whether any differences exist between men and women. The PFSS tool includes the "everyday tasks" of grocery shopping, household tasks, and meal preparation and would be more common to women than men.

Possible Nursing Implications. To improve functional status of clients with COPD, the nurse should focus on interventions that will improve exercise capacity, reduce dyspnea and anxiety, and elevate the client's depressed mood.

techniques. The client practices the techniques daily and uses the techniques during panic attacks or episodes of dyspnea.

Family, friends, and support groups can be quite helpful. Professional counseling, if recommended, should be viewed as a positive suggestion; in no way should the client view this need as a failure to cope. The nurse helps the client understand that talking with a professional counselor can assist in identifying potential techniques that can help in maintaining control over the dyspnea and feelings of panic.

Drug Therapy. Some clients may benefit from drugs that reduce anxiety. These drugs are particularly helpful for some clients with asthma during an attack.

➤ *Activity Intolerance*

Planning: Expected Outcomes. The client should
- Perform activities of daily living (ADLs) without assistance or with limited assistance
- Adjust the daily schedule, making minimal changes in usual routine or lifestyle
- Perform activities, including walking for short distances, without experiencing dyspnea or tachycardia
- Participate in family or social activities as desired

Interventions. The client with emphysema and chronic bronchitis typically experiences chronic fatigue. While in the acute phases of the illness, the client may require extensive assistance with ADLs, like bathing and grooming. As the client's acute episode resolves, the nurse encourages the client to pace activities and provide as much self-care as possible. The nurse instructs the client not to rush through morning activities because rushing is likely to increase dyspnea, fatigue, and also, potentially, hypoxemia in the client requiring oxygen. As the client gradually increases activity, the nurse continually assesses the physiologic response by noting skin color changes, pulse rate and regularity, and blood pressure and work of breathing. If the physician has ordered supplemental oxygen, it should be used continually, particularly during periods of increased energy use such as bathing or walking for short periods. (Other interventions, such as energy conservation, are discussed under Ineffective Breathing Pattern.)

➤ *Potential for Pneumonia or Other Respiratory Infection*

Planning: Expected Outcomes. The client should not experience secondary respiratory infection and should recognize early signs and symptoms of infection. The client should then seek prompt treatment.

Interventions. Pneumonia is one of the most common complications of COPD/CAL. Clients who have excessive secretions or have artificial airways are at increased risk for respiratory infections. The risk is greatly increased in the elderly. The nurse teaches clients to avoid large crowds of people, such as in a shopping center. The nurse also teaches clients the importance of receiving an annual influenza vaccine ("flu shots") and a pneumococcal vaccination (as frequently as recommended by the physi-

cian or Nurse Practitioner) to prevent these potentially deadly diseases. The highest mortality from these diseases is in elderly clients with CAL. (See Chapter 33 for more information on pneumonia and influenza.)

 ## Continuing Care

➤ *Health Teaching*

Clients with a chronic, disabling disease like CAL need to know as much about the disease as possible so they can better manage it and themselves. Specifically, clients and family members or significant others should be able to discuss medications, signs and symptoms of infection, avoidance of respiratory irritants, diet therapy regimen, and activity progression. They need to identify and avoid stressors that can exacerbate the disease. The nurse stresses the importance of communication between clients and their family. Spouses or family members frequently avoid any communication they believe will upset the client. Family therapy may be needed to facilitate communication techniques.

The nurse instructs clients in techniques of breathing, including pursed-lip breathing, diaphragmatic breathing, positioning, relaxation therapy, energy conservation, and coughing and deep breathing. Figure 32–9 is a sample CAL client education checklist used for discharge teaching. Education related to specific interventions has been discussed under the various nursing diagnoses. Two factors may interfere with teaching hospitalized clients: the shortened length of stay coupled with a multitude of topics to discuss and clients' level of tolerance and dyspnea. It may be unrealistic to cover all of the topics in the education checklist during a single hospitalization. The primary nurse or case manager will coordinate teaching with the home health or clinic staff.

Hypoxemic clients can benefit from long-term use of oxygen at home. As with other therapies, the physician's decision to prescribe home oxygen is made with calculated analysis. The physician may prescribe oxygen only during periods of exercise or sleep if hypoxemia occurs only during these times. Continuous, long-term administration of oxygen can reverse tissue hypoxia and decrease pulmonary vascular resistance; it can also improve cognitive ability and well-being. (More information on oxygen therapy is found in Chapter 30.)

➤ *Home Care Management*

Most clients are treated in the ambulatory care setting and cared for at home. The client with chronic airflow limitation (CAL) in whom pneumonia or a severe exacerbation of the disease develops is usually treated and discharged from the hospital to a previous home setting. For clients with advanced disease, however, 24-hour care may be needed for ADLs and for monitoring clients for acute episodes or progression of the illness. Clients may not be able to enjoy work or recreational activities because of spending all available energy on the work of breathing. If arrangements for home care are not possible, clients may need to be transferred to a long-term care setting.

Most clients can benefit from a structured pulmonary

Checklist for CAL Client Education

	Date	Signature

The Client Has Received the Following Education:

A. Basic anatomy and physiology of the respiratory system
    1. Structures composing the respiratory system
    2. Functions of the respiratory passageways
B. Pathophysiology related to condition
    1. Name of lung disease
    2. Generalized physiologic effects
    3. Generalized psychosocial effects
C. Medications
    1. Medication safety
    2. Name of each medication
    3. Action of each medication
    4. Dosage
    5. How to take each medication
    6. How to use a metered dose inhaler with or without a "spacer"
    7. Recognition of side effects
    8. Importance of carrying a medication list and a medical alert
      (Medic Alert) bracelet or card
D. Respiratory therapy interventions and bronchial hygiene
    1. Proper care and cleaning of home equipment, i.e., oxygen, cannulas, nebulizers
    2. Sequence of treatments
    3. Adequate hydration
    4. Postural drainage and chest physiotherapy (optional and only with excessive secretions)
    5. Prevention of respiratory tract infection:
       a. Avoid exposure to crowds and people with respiratory tract infections
       b. Signs and symptoms of respiratory tract infection
       c. Use of prescribed antibiotics with as needed (prn) schedule
       d. Influenza immunization; pneumococcal immunization
       e. Use of measures to promote oronasal hygiene
E. Management of dyspnea
    1. Controlled cough maneuver
    2. Pursed-lip breathing
    3. Diaphragmatic breathing
    4. Positioning techniques
    5. Stress management and relaxation techniques
F. Adaptation of a daily routine
    1. Daily schedule of graded exercises
    2. Walking exercise on level ground
    3. Stair climbing
    4. Activities of daily living: adjust activities according to individual fatigue patterns
G. Nutrition
    1. Type of diet prescribed
    2. Balanced diet: meat, dairy, grain, fruit and vegetables: 2:2:4:4 ratio
    3. Low salt intake
H. Control of environment
    1. Environmental problems related to pulmonary disease
    2. Ways to make the environment conducive to living with pulmonary disease
       a. Avoid irritants and use air purification system
       b. Use mask when exposed to dusts and cold air
       c. Stay indoors with air conditioning operating when air quality is poor
       d. Check air quality telephone recording
I. Smoking
    1. Rationale for smoking cessation
    2. Suggest ways to stop smoking
J. Body image and human sexuality
    1. Alterations in self-esteem and body image related to pulmonary disease
    2. Communication in human relationships.
    3. Alterations in sexual relationships related to pulmonary disease
K. Available community resources
    1. Discharge planning; referral to home care professionals
    2. Available community services: Meals on Wheels; American Lung Association;
      American Heart Association; American Cancer Society

Figure 32–9. A checklist for education of the client with chronic airflow limitation (CAL).

TABLE 32-6

Areas of Focus in a Pulmonary Rehabilitation Program
• Education
• Exercise conditioning
• Energy conservation
• Breathing retraining
• Bronchial hygiene
• Dietary counseling
• Vocational training
• Psychological counseling

rehabilitation program (Table 32–6). Pulmonary rehabilitation programs vary, but the overall goal of these multidisciplinary programs is to increase a person's ability to compensate for and live with CAL. In collaboration with the physician, the nurse refers clients with CAL to a pulmonary rehabilitation program before illness becomes severe. Clients with the least severe functional abnormality benefit the most.

The nurse works with the hospital discharge-planning nurse or case manager to obtain the necessary equipment for care at home. Often the case manager coordinates the necessary resources to facilitate a smooth transition back to the community and ensures appropriate follow-up in the community. Client needs may include oxygen therapy, a hospital-type bed, a nebulizer, a tub transfer bench, and arrangements for a home health nurse to continue monitoring the health status, review medication compliance, and evaluate home care needs.

The client with CAL faces a lifelong disease with remissions and exacerbations. The nurse explains to both the client and the family that the client may experience periods of anxiety, depression, and ineffective coping. The client who was a smoker also may have self-directed anger, particularly if the client recognizes that smoking contributed to the disease.

Financial concerns often increase the client's and family's anxiety and interfere with disease management. The client's condition may worsen to the point that the client cannot work. Disability benefits through Social Security or private disability insurance plans can help ease the financial burden. Medicare or other health insurers may assist with payment for home oxygen therapy and nebulizer treatments. The nurse collaborates closely with the social worker or discharge-planning nurse to help the client make the necessary arrangements.

➤ *Health Care Resources*

The nurse provides appropriate referrals as necessary. Home care visits may be warranted, particularly if the client must use home oxygen therapy for the first time. Referral to assistance programs, such as Meals on Wheels, can be extremely helpful. The nurse provides the client with a list of various support groups and Better Breathing groups sponsored by the American Lung Association. If the client is having difficulty with smoking cessation and

indicates the need for assistance, the nurse makes the appropriate referrals.

 Evaluation

The nurse evaluates the care of the client with CAL on the basis of the identified nursing diagnoses. The expected outcomes are that the client

■ Attains and maintains ventilation parameters (PaO_2, $PaCO_2$) within the normal range for the client
■ Adheres to the prescribed pharmacologic therapy
■ Demonstrates lung sounds optimal for the client
■ Demonstrates breathing techniques of pursed-lip breathing and abdominal or diaphragmatic breathing
■ Demonstrates positioning techniques to use during dyspneic episodes
■ Identifies various methods of conserving energy
■ Maintains a patent airway by removing excessive secretions
■ Demonstrates controlled coughing
■ Increases or maintains fluid intake
■ Attains and maintains body weight within 10% of ideal
■ States methods of reducing anxiety
■ Identifies personal strengths rather than focusing on limitations
■ Performs self-care independently or with minimal assistance for as long as possible
■ States the need to avoid irritants and sources of infection
■ Participates in social and family activities as desired
■ Maintains employment or same level of activity
■ Decreases exacerbations of symptoms
■ Decreases use of emergency room treatment
■ Decreases hospitalizations

SARCOIDOSIS

Overview

Sarcoidosis is a multisystem granulomatous disorder of unknown cause that can affect virtually any organ. It is one of a group of diseases within a broader classification of pulmonary diseases called interstitial lung disease. Interstitial lung disease is used interchangeably with the term *fibrotic lung disease*. The hallmark of sarcoidosis is noncaseating granuloma. The granulomas of sarcoidosis can occur in almost any organ or tissue of the body but most frequently affected are the lung, liver, spleen, lymph nodes, eyes, small bones of the hands and feet, and skin.

The disease often presents in young adults. It peaks between age 20 and 30 years and again between 45 and 65 years. Physical findings include bilateral hilar adenopathy, pulmonary infiltrates, skin lesions, and eye lesions. The first presentation may be an abnormal chest radiograph in an asymptomatic client. The most common symptoms include nonproductive cough, dyspnea, and chest discomfort. Fortunately, in most clients, the illness resolves spontaneously. Others may experience pulmonary fibrosis and severe systemic disease.

The organ most frequently involved is the lung. More than 90% of the clients affected will have lung or intrathoracic lymph node involvement. Pulmonary sarcoidosis is a chronic disorder of the alveolar structure that develops over time in a step-by-step manner. Growths called granulomas characterize the disease. Granulomas are composed of lymphocytes, macrophages, epithelioid cells, and giant cells.

It is currently believed that the development of pulmonary sarcoidosis involves the activation of T lymphocytes; the stimulus for this activation is unknown. However, normal resident immune cells (the T lymphocytes) recruit additional immune cells, probably by releasing chemotactic factor. Monocytes are then attracted to the T lymphocytes. Monocytes are precursors of macrophages, epithelioid cells, and the multinucleated giant cells that compose the granuloma. *Alveolitis* is the term that describes this process of accumulation of inflammatory immune cells in the alveoli.

It is believed that the T lymphocytes are primarily responsible for granuloma formation and that the activated macrophages are primarily responsible for interstitial fibrosis because of their ability to recruit and increase the number of fibroblasts. The fibrosis results in a loss of lung compliance (elasticity) and a loss of functional ability to exchange gases. Cor pulmonale (right-sided cardiac failure) is often present because the heart can no longer pump against the noncompliant, fibrotic lung.

Collaborative Management

 Assessment

A diagnosis of sarcoidosis is suspected in clients who present with symptoms of cough and dyspnea and have incidental abnormal chest radiograph findings but are otherwise asymptomatic. Sarcoidosis is considered a disease of exclusion. The most important diseases to exclude are infections and neoplasms.

Sarcoidosis is staged on the basis of radiograph criteria:
- Stage 0: normal chest x-ray
- Stage 1: bilateral hilar adenopathy
- Stage 2: bilateral hilar adenopathy with diffuse parenchymal infiltrates
- Stage 3: diffuse infiltrates with adenopathy
- Stage 4: lung fibrosis

Stage 2 radiograph findings are considered a reliable sign of sarcoidosis. A client who presents with a stage 0 or 1 radiograph may have a high-resolution computed tomographic (CT) scan to detect any parenchymal involvement. For all those diagnosed with sarcoidosis, two thirds will have resolution of the disease.

Pulmonary function studies often show a restrictive pattern of decreased lung volumes and impaired diffusing capacity. Irreversible lung changes develop in 10% to 15% of clients. In those in whom severe restrictive disease develops, pulmonary hypertension may develop in response to the severe disease.

Fiberoptic bronchoscopy (see Chap. 29) allows researchers to sample the epithelial fluid of the lower respiratory tract to investigate the alveolitis of clients with active disease. This test confirms that pulmonary sarcoidosis is a disease associated with an intense cellular immune response in the alveolar structure.

TRANSCULTURAL CONSIDERATIONS

 In the United States, sarcoidosis affects African-Americans 10 times more frequently than Caucasians. The overall prevalence is similar in women and men, but it is twice as common in women of childbearing age as in women of other ages. A distinctive feature of sarcoidosis is its age distribution: most cases develop in people between 20 and 40 years of age. Other countries with high prevalence include Scandinavian countries, England, and Japan.

Interventions

The goal of therapy is to lessen symptoms and prevent fibrosis. Indications for treatment vary. If the client is asymptomatic and has no abnormal pulmonary function, no treatment is given. Indications for treatment include clinical symptoms; decrease in total lung capacity, diffusing capacity, or forced vital capacity; extrapulmonary involvement; and hypercalcemia.

Corticosteroids are the cornerstone of therapy. Protocols may vary from 40–60 mg/day with tapering doses over 6–8 weeks to a maintenance dose of 10–15 mg for 6 months. Further therapy will occur over 12 months. Follow-up and monitoring includes review of symptoms, pulmonary function studies, chest x-rays, complete blood count, serum creatinine, serum calcium, and urinalysis. The nurse and pharmacist teach the client and family about side effects of steroid therapy and other aspects of the client's physical care as indicated and appropriate.

IDIOPATHIC PULMONARY FIBROSIS

Overview

Idiopathic pulmonary fibrosis is the second major form of the interstitial pulmonary disease. Unlike sarcoidosis, it is a highly lethal interstitial lung disease. Most clients have progressive disease with few remission periods. Remission in this disease is rare. Outcomes are fairly predictive at the end of 1 year.

Pulmonary fibrosis has been described as a model of excessive wound healing. Once lung injury occurs, an inflammatory process ensues. The initial response is predominantly neutrophilic followed by a predominance of lymphocytes and macrophages. There is an exudation of serum proteins into the alveolar space, resulting in collapse of alveolar units and healing by fibrosis. Normal lung tissue can be found interspersed between areas of fibrosis.

Although the cause of pulmonary fibrosis is unknown, factors such as cigarette smoking and exposure to metal dust, organic dust, and wood fires has been shown to be predictors of the disease.

TRANSCULTURAL CONSIDERATIONS

 Between 1979 and 1991, there was an increase in mortality rates for both men and women with pulmonary fibrosis. Mortality rates were lowest in the Midwest and Northeast and highest in the West and Southeast. Rates were also higher for the older aged. The age-adjusted rate for the period 1979 through 1991 was 33.0 per 1,000,000.

Collaborative Management

Assessment

The onset of symptoms can be insidious, with initial symptoms of dyspnea. Pulmonary function studies reveal decreased forced vital capacities. As the fibrosis progresses, the client becomes more dyspneic, and hypoxemia becomes severe. These clients will eventually require high levels of oxygen and often remain hypoxemic on these high oxygen levels.

The nurse obtains a complete history and performs a complete respiratory assessment. Dyspnea is measured, and hypoxemia is assessed. Particular attention is paid to any recent exposure to an occupational or environmental agent. (More details as to occupational causes of fibrosis are described under Occupational Pulmonary Disease.)

Interventions

The physician usually prescribes corticosteroids for treatment. Most clients are also treated with a cytotoxic drug such as cyclophosphamide (Cytoxan, Neosar, Procytox✦), azathioprine, chlorambucil (Leukeran), or methotrexate (Folex), which by themselves can cause lung injury. Of the clients who respond to therapy, initiation of therapy early in the disease process is critical. Current therapy and research are aimed at agents that inhibit cytokines, growth factors, and oxidant injury in the lung. Gene therapy is also being explored. Single-lung transplantation is considered an option. However, the selection criteria, cost, and availability of organs make this option unlikely for most candidates.

The client and family will require support and assistance with community resources once the diagnosis is made. The goal of therapy is to minimize the fibrotic process and control symptoms. The nurse and health care team begins by assisting the client and family in understanding the disease process and yet maintaining hope for control of the fibrosis. It is important to prevent further lung insult from respiratory infections. The client and family are educated regarding the signs and symptoms of infection and encouraged to avoid respiratory irritants, crowds, and those with known infections.

Home oxygen is often required once the diagnosis is made because by the time the client becomes symptomatic significant fibrosis has already occurred. The nurse and respiratory therapist begin education regarding oxygen use and stress the importance of using the oxygen as a continuous therapy. The occupational therapist is most helpful in assessing ADL limitations and recommending adaptive equipment to assist in energy conservation, which will minimize oxygen consumption and decrease work of breathing. As with other restrictive lung diseases, these clients have rapid respirations associated with decreased lung compliance. The nurse supports the client's need to be as independent as possible and yet encourages the client to pace activities and accept assistance as needed.

The social worker meets with the family to answer questions regarding community resources and provide assistance with applications regarding disability, if applicable. The disease can be economically devastating to a family because the client is often unable to continue work. Home health nurses may be arranged to assist in continued monitoring of the client's health status and oxygen needs.

In the later stages of the disease, the focus is to minimize the sensation of shortness of breath, which is often accomplished with the use of morphine, either oral or intravenous. The home health nurse can assist the physician in regulating the medication to control the symptoms.

The physician and Nurse Practitioner keep the client informed of the disease process and assist the client with identification of advanced health care wishes. The client and family are provided information regarding hospice, which provides support and coordination of resources to meet the needs of the client and family when the prognosis is less than 6 months.

OCCUPATIONAL PULMONARY DISEASE

Overview

Exposure to occupational or environmental fumes, dust, vapors, gases, bacterial or fungal antigens, and allergens can result in a variety of respiratory disorders. Depending on the degree, frequency, and intensity of exposure, the smoking history, and underlying pulmonary disease, clients may experience acute reversible effects or chronic pulmonary disease.

With a greater focus on ambulatory care, nurses and other health care providers are refocusing and retooling their education to care of the client outside the hospital setting. Many occupational diseases have an onset of symptoms long after their initial exposure to the offending agent. Through skilled history taking, the nurse investigates the many nuances of respiratory symptoms associated with the work environment over a lifetime.

OCCUPATIONAL ASTHMA. Occupational asthma (OA) is the most common form of occupational lung disease in the United States. OA differs from other forms of asthma in that it is associated with variable airway narrowing related to an exposure in the working environment and not to stimuli outside the workplace. These clients usually have no childhood or family history of the disease. In some cases, symptoms may develop after several years of exposure. OA may be difficult to recognize because the client may continue to experience respiratory distress when away from the work setting.

With the rapid development of the chemical industry, large numbers of inorganic and organic substances have been found to cause asthma by direct bronchial irritation. Aside from chemical irritants, enzymes used in food processing, detergent, and pharmaceutical industries may be asthma-inducing agents. Plant- and animal-derived materials also may be sources of irritation.

Occupational asthma is divided into two types, which are differentiated by onset of symptoms. The most common type is OA with a latency period. The disease develops after a period of exposure, which can vary from a few weeks to several years. Included are all instances induced by immunoglobulin E (IgE)–dependent agents. These agents are classified as high molecular weight and low molecular weight.

The IgE-dependent agents with high molecular weights include cereals, animal-derived allergens, enzymes such as those in detergents, gums used in carpets, latex found in gloves, seafoods, and pharmaceuticals. The low-molecular-weight agents act as haptens and induce specific IgE antibodies by combining with a body protein. The most commonly occurring low-molecular-weight agent is toluene diisocyanate, which is used in the manufacture of polyurethane foam and coatings. Other agents that cause OA include wood dust, anhydrides used in plastic and epoxy resins, amines found in shellacs, flux, chloramine-T found in janitors' cleaners, dyes used in textiles, persulfate used by hairdressers, formaldehyde and glutaraldehyde used by hospital staff, acrylate found in adhesives, metal, and drugs.

Clients diagnosed with latency OA related to a specific allergen will have a permanent impairment or disability, which is observed when performing pulmonary function testing using a bronchial provocation test to stimulate hyperresponsiveness. These clients will demonstrate airflow limitation.

The second type of OA does not have a latency period. In the past it was referred to as reactive airways dysfunction syndrome (RADS), but it is more frequently referred to as *irritant-induced asthma*. This terminology recognizes that similar effects and outcomes also occur in clients with multiple exposures but with lower levels of concentration of the offending agent. The client who experiences this type of OA may have been near a chemical spill. Onset of symptoms occurs within 24 hours. The most commonly occurring precipitating agents include chlorine, ammonia, and phosgene. Exposure to massive concentrations of the chemical can result in pulmonary edema, adult respiratory distress syndrome (ARDS), and death.

Pathologic changes associated with irritant-induced asthma include desquamation of the epithelial layer, thickening of the basement membrane, and inflammation of cells of the bronchial mucosa. T lymphocytes and activated eosinophils can be found in the bronchial mucosa.

Symptoms often persist for 3 months but can occur for years or even permanently after the exposure. These symptoms frequently include cough, wheeze, and dyspnea. Some clients report a burning sensation in the throat and nose and chest discomfort.

PNEUMOCONIOSIS. Pneumoconiosis is the lodging of any inhaled dust in the lungs. Two types of pneumoconiosis are silicosis and coal miners' pneumoconiosis.

Silicosis, a chronic fibrosing disease of the lungs, is produced by excessive inhalation of free crystalline silica dust. Mining and quarrying are associated with a high incidence of silicosis. Hazardous exposure to silica dust also occurs in foundry work, tunneling, sandblasting, pottery making, stone masonry, and manufacture of glass, tile, and bricks. The finely ground silica used in soaps, polishes, and filters is especially dangerous.

Chronic silicosis results from exposure to low concentrations of silica dust for 20 years or more. The formation of selective nodules in the pulmonary parenchyma is characteristic. This process may be accompanied by progressive massive fibrosis.

Uncomplicated, or simple, silicosis is often entirely asymptomatic and causes only mild ventilating restriction and evidence of fibrosis on an x-ray. Clients with chronic complicated disease experience significant dyspnea on exertion, marked reduction in lung volume, and massive fibrosis of the upper lobes. Malaise, anorexia, and weight loss may be present with an outcome of respiratory failure.

Coal Miners' Pneumoconiosis. Chronic pneumoconiosis of coal miners also results in massive pulmonary fibrosis as a result of deposition of coal dust in the lung. There is an additive effect of cigarette smoking to inhalation of coal dust. Symptoms are related to the amount and frequency of exposure. Initial symptoms are similar to bronchitis with eventual development of centrilobular emphysema.

DIFFUSE INTERSTITIAL FIBROSIS. *Asbestosis* refers to diffuse interstitial fibrosis caused by exposure to asbestos. There is generally a considerable latency period between the initial exposure and the onset of clinical manifestations of fibrosis, often 10–20 years. People who are at risk for asbestosis are asbestos miners and millers and those employed in the building trades and shipyards, carpenters and electricians, loggers, insulation workers, pipe fitters, steamfitters, sheet metal workers, and welders.

Asbestos causes a diffuse pleural thickening with diaphragmatic calcification. Presence of calcified pleural plaques on a chest radiograph is the most common manifestation of asbestos exposure. Pulmonary function abnormalities usually indicate a restrictive ventilatory defect. Removal of the worker from exposure does not necessarily prevent the effects of the disease. The chances of arresting the disease are best in its early stages. Clients with this disease frequently have respiratory infections.

Malignant asbestosis includes bronchial cancers and malignant mesotheliomas of the pleura and peritoneum.

Talcosis is a pulmonary fibrosis that occurs after years of exposure to high concentrations of talc dust. Significant exposures can occur during the manufacture of paints, ceramics, asphalt, roofing materials, cosmetics, and rubber goods. The clinical picture of the client closely resembles that of asbestosis.

Berylliosis is a chronic granulomatous disorder of the lungs caused by inhalation of beryllium. The typical exposure history includes involvement in an operation in which metals are heated to fumes (e.g., welding, burning, or casting) or are machined to dust. Clients with beryl-liosis exposure may be screened with a peripheral blood lymphocyte proliferation test. Results will be elevated in those with chronic beryllium disease or with exposure to beryllium, who are more likely to progress to advanced irreversible disease than are those with sarcoidosis of unknown cause.

EXTRINSIC ALLERGIC ALVEOLITIS. A granulomatous inflammatory reaction, extrinsic allergic alveolitis is a hypersensitivity pneumonitis caused by an immunologic response to inhaled organic dust or chemicals containing bacteria or fungal antigens. Three of the most common forms of this disease include farmer's lung, bird fancier's lung, and machine operator's lung.

Farmer's lung is caused by the inhalation of fungal antigens found in molding hay and straw. The client will complain of a dry cough and experience minimal wheezing, if any.

Bird fancier's lung results from inhalation of antigens found in bird excreta. The nurse suspects this condition if the client presents with flu-like symptoms after exposure to the antigen and recovers within 48 hours after removal from the source. The chest radiograph may show a ground-glass pattern. Pulmonary function studies reveal reduced lung volumes and impaired gas transfer.

Machine operator's lung is caused by exposure to metal working fluid. The fluid, which is recirculated at a high pressure, creates an aerosol, which may contain a bacterial antigen. Once inhaled, a hypersensitivity pneumonitis ensues. The client may report dyspnea, cough, fatigue, fever, or weight loss. Chest radiograph may show interstitial infiltrates.

Collaborative Management

 Assessment

An occupational cause should be investigated for all clients with new-onset asthma. The health care team screens the client for all known causes of occupational asthma. Because there may or may not be a latency period between exposure and onset of symptoms, the nurse obtains a thorough history of occupational exposure, onset of symptoms associated with the work environment, symptoms while away from work, dose exposure, frequency of exposure, history of smoking, history of lung disease, and use of a protective device. The client with occupational asthma with a latency period should be removed from the site of exposure, transferred to a job without exposure, and treated with medications for asthma.

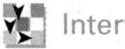 Interventions

Prevention is extremely important for avoiding pulmonary disability caused by occupationally related disease. The nurse or other public health advocate stresses the importance of using special respirators and ensuring adequate ventilation when working in potentially harmful environ-

ments. When assessing the client with respiratory distress, the nurse ascertains whether symptoms are acute or chronic. If the client is having an allergic reaction, the nurse stresses avoidance of the allergen. Nursing care is similar to care of the client with asthma not caused by the workplace environment. The nurse refers the client to a social worker, who provides information regarding compensation and pension.

Nursing interventions for clients experiencing occupational pulmonary restrictive disease are related to the effects of decreased chest wall compliance, vital capacity, and total lung volume. These deficits are related to the fibrotic process, which restricts lung expansion. Most nursing diagnoses appropriate for clients with chronic airflow limitation (CAL) apply to these clients. Hypoxemic clients require supplemental oxygen. In addition, respiratory therapies to promote sputum clearance are essential.

LUNG CANCER

Overview

Lung cancer is the leading cause of cancer-related deaths worldwide. Lung cancer accounts for 25% of all cancer deaths. The overall 5-year survival rate for all clients with lung cancer is 12.5%. Metastatic disease is often present, and only 14% of clients have localized disease at the time of diagnosis (Parker et al., 1997). The prognosis for lung cancer remains poor. Cancer of the lung is essentially incurable unless surgical resection can be accomplished. Treatment of lung cancer is often aimed toward relieving symptoms (palliation) rather than cure because of the presence of metastasis. It has been estimated that 85% of lung cancers might be prevented through the elimination of cigarette smoking. (Chapter 26 further discusses causes of cancer development.) Therefore, the nurse plays a major role in public education to prevent the initiation of smoking. The nurse also uses interventions that improve the quality of life for clients with lung cancer.

Pathophysiology

More than 90% of all primary lung cancers arise from the bronchial epithelium. These cancers are collectively called bronchogenic carcinomas. Lung cancers are classified according to their histologic cell type as

■ Small cell or oat cell
■ Epidermoid or squamous cell
■ Adenocarcinoma
■ Large cell

The last three types are often referred to as non–small cell lung cancers (NSCLC). All of the bronchogenic carcinomas can be further divided into more specific subtypes, such as a variant of adenocarcinoma known as bronchioloalveolar carcinoma (Travis et al., 1996). Approximately 60% of clients with NSCLC will have metastasis at the time of diagnosis, which eliminates surgery as a curative treatment modality (Carney, 1996). Major tumor cell types are summarized in Table 32–7.

TABLE 32–7

Differential Features of the Major Types of Lung Cancer

Type	Approximate Incidence	Characteristics	Treatment
Small cell (oat cell)	• 20%	• Centrally located tumors (80%), rapidly growing, most malignant type • High rate of metastasis via the lymph and circulatory systems with early extrathoracic involvement • Associated with paraneoplastic syndromes • Prognosis poor; survival usually not more than 2 yr with treatment	• Combination chemotherapy is the initial treatment of choice • Surgical resectability poor • Palliative endobronchial laser therapy to relieve obstruction • Radiation not recommended for metastatic disease
Non-small cell Epidermoid (squamous cell)	• 30%	• Frequently originates in a central or hilar location and at the bifurcation points of segmental bronchi • In a peripheral location, cavities may form in lung tissue • Strong association with cigarette smoking • Slower growing, less invasive; metastasis often limited to the thorax, including regional nodes, pleura, and chest wall • Commonly associated with obstructive symptoms and pneumonias; client presents with chest pain, cough, dyspnea, and hemoptysis	• Surgical resectability good if stage I or stage II • Chemotherapy and radiation therapy may be used to palliate symptoms
Adenocarcinoma	• 30%–35%	• Tumors are located peripherally • Slow growing • Hematogenous spread occurs frequently and usually early in the course of the disease • High frequency of metastasis to brain; other sites include adrenals, liver, bone, and kidneys • Predominant type in nonsmokers; most frequent type of lung cancer found in women • Often arises in previously scarred or fibrotic lungs	• Surgical resectability good if stage I or stage II • Moderately good response to chemotherapy • Radiation therapy used to palliate pulmonary and metastatic disease
Large cell	• 11%	• Peripheral, subpleural lesions with necrotic surfaces or cavities • Often form larger tumor masses than adenocarcinoma • Slow growing • Metastasis is similar to that for adenocarcinoma with addition of gastrointestinal tract • Prognosis poor	• Surgical resectability good if stage I or stage II • Chemotherapy has limited benefit • Palliative radiation therapy

Metastasis

Lung cancers metastasize (spread) by direct extension, lymphatic invasion, and blood-borne avenues. Bronchial tumors can spread by direct invasion and grow to occlude the bronchus partially or completely. Invasion of the bronchial wall and encircling or obstruction of the airway can also occur. Pulmonary spread can compress lung structures other than the airway, including the alveoli, nerves, blood vessels, and lymph vessels.

The patterns of metastasis depend on the type of tumor cell and the anatomic location of the tumor. Lymphatic spread is usually associated with embolization and invasion by tumor. The mediastinal, paratracheal, and central hilar lymph nodes are most commonly involved. Lower lobe tumors tend to metastasize diffusely more often by lymph channels than do tumors located in other portions of the lung.

Hematogenous (blood-borne) metastasis of lung cancer is due to invasion of the pulmonary venous system. Tumor emboli spread to other, distant areas of the body. Distant sites of metastasis include the bone (lower thoracic and upper lumbar vertebrae and long bones; 19%–33%), adrenal glands (18%–38%), abdominal lymph

TABLE 32–8

Endocrine Paraneoplastic Syndromes Associated with Lung Cancer	
Ectopic Hormone	**Manifestation**
Adrenocorticotropic hormone (ACTH)	• Cushing's syndrome
Antidiuretic hormone	• Syndrome of inappropriate antidiuretic hormone (SIADH)
Follicle-stimulating hormone (FSH)	• Gynecomastia
Parathyroid hormone	• Hypercalcemia
Ectopic insulin	• Hypoglycemia

TABLE 32–9

Nonendocrine Paraneoplastic Syndromes Associated with Lung Cancer	
Tissue/System	**Manifestation**
Connective tissue	• Arthralgia • Digital clubbing
Hematologic system	• Anemia • Leukocytosis • Thrombocytopenia purpura • Polycythemia • Thrombocytosis
Neuromuscular system	• Peripheral neuropathy • Carcinomatous myopathy • Cortical cerebellar degeneration • Seizure • Polymyositis • Myasthenia-like syndrome
Integumentary system	• Dermatomyositis • Scleroderma • Acanthosis nigricans
Vascular system	• Thrombophlebitis • Nonbacterial endocarditis
Renal system	• Arterial thrombosis • Nephrotic syndrome • Proteinuria

nodes (29%), brain (15%–43%), kidney (16%–23%), and liver (33%–40%).

Additional pathophysiologic manifestations, known as paraneoplastic syndromes, complicate certain lung cancers. The paraneoplastic syndromes are caused by various hormones, antigens, or enzymes. Small cell carcinomas are most commonly associated with paraneoplastic syndromes. Tables 32–8 and 32–9 list the endocrine and nonendocrine paraneoplastic syndromes, respectively, that may be associated with lung cancer.

Staging

The staging of lung cancer is based on the TNM system (T, primary tumor; N, regional lymph nodes; M, distant metastasis). The TNM staging system determines the anatomic extent of the disease and predicts prognosis. The TMN system is further described in Chapter 26.

Staging groups are used clinically because of the significant relationship between the extent of the disease and survival rates. Table 32–10 describes stage grouping for lung cancers. Figure 32–10 shows the various anatomic stages of lung cancer (Mountain et al., 1991).

Etiology

Exposure

Lung cancers have been associated with repeated exposure to substances that cause chronic tissue irritation or inflammation. Cigarette smoking is the major risk factor and is responsible for 85% of all lung cancer deaths (Shottenfeld, 1996).

TABLE 32–10

TMN Stage Grouping for Lung Cancer			
Occult carcinoma	TX	N0	M0
Stage 0	Tis	Carcinoma in situ	
Stage I	T1	N0	M0
	T2	N0	M0
Stage II	T1	N1	M0
	T2	N1	M0
Stage IIIa	T3	N0	M0
	T3	N1	M0
	T1–3	N2	M0
Stage IIIb	Any T	N3	M0
	T4	Any N	M0
Stage IV	Any T	Any N	M1

From Mountain, C. F., Greenberg, M. D., & Fraire, A. E. (1991). Tumor stages in non-small cell carcinoma of the lung. *Chest, 99*(5), 1258.

STAGE I
(No lymph node involvement)

STAGE II
(Intrapulmonary and/or hilar nodes involved)

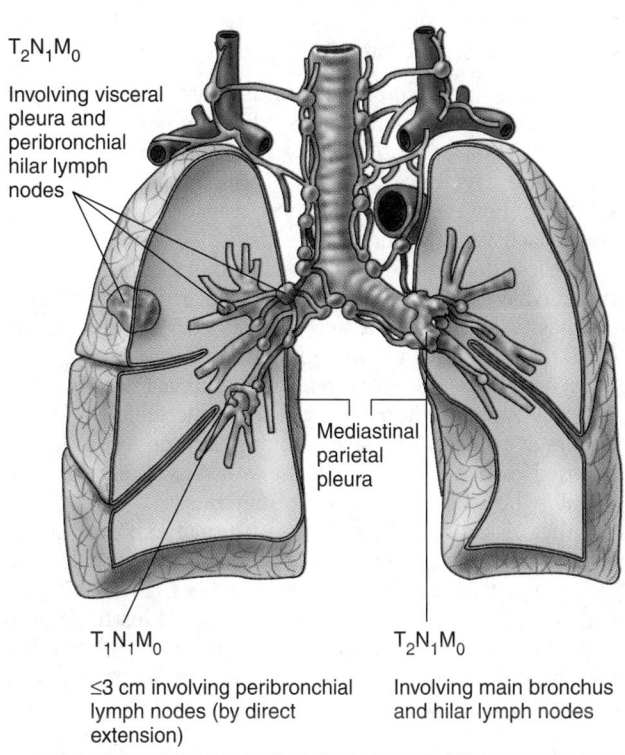

$T_2N_1M_0$

Involving visceral
pleura and
peribronchial
hilar lymph
nodes

Mediastinal
parietal
pleura

$T_2N_0M_0$

Involving
visceral
pleura

$T_2N_0M_0$

Involving mainstem
bronchus >2 cm
distal to carina

$T_1N_0M_0$

Peripheral "coin"
lesion

$T_1N_1M_0$

≤3 cm involving peribronchial
lymph nodes (by direct
extension)

$T_2N_1M_0$

Involving main bronchus
and hilar lymph nodes

Mediastinal
parietal
pleura

STAGE III-a

STAGE III-b

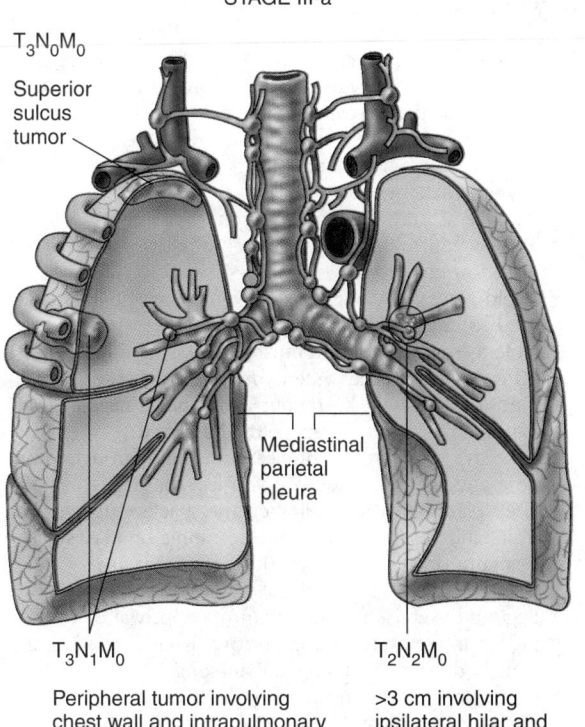

$T_3N_0M_0$

Superior
sulcus
tumor

Mediastinal
parietal
pleura

$T_3N_1M_0$

Peripheral tumor involving
chest wall and intrapulmonary
lymph nodes

$T_2N_2M_0$

>3 cm involving
ipsilateral hilar and
mediastinal lymph nodes

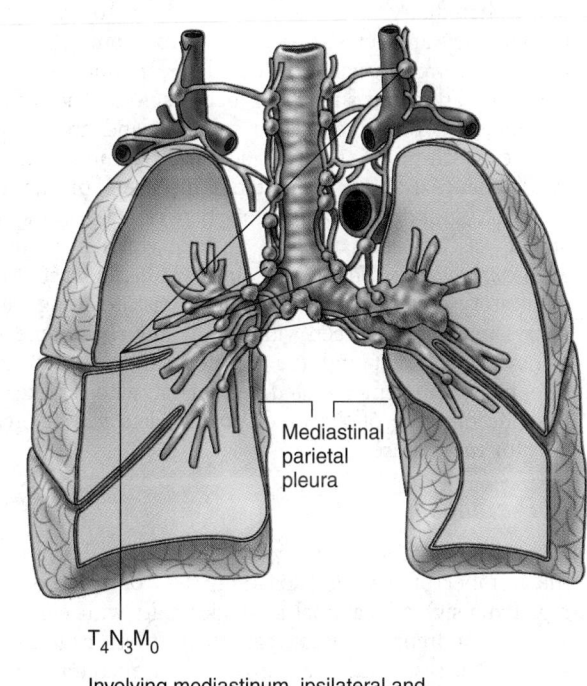

Mediastinal
parietal
pleura

$T_4N_3M_0$

Involving mediastinum, ipsilateral and
contralateral mediastinal lymph nodes, contralateral
hilar nodes, supraclavicular lymph nodes

Figure 32–10. Anatomic staging of lung cancer. (Redrawn from Mountain, C. F., Greenberg, M. D., & Fraire, A. E. [1991]. Tumor stages in non-small cell carcinoma of the lung. *Chest, 99*[5], 1258.)

Increased risk for lung cancer is directly related to

- Total exposure to cigarette smoke as determined by the number of years of smoking
- Number of cigarettes smoked per day
- Depth of inhalation
- Tar and nicotine content of cigarettes

Pipe and cigar smoking also increase risk. The incidence of lung cancer decreases when smoking stops and, after 15 years of smoking cessation, approaches that of those who have never smoked. Approximately 48,000 ex-smokers, however, develop lung cancer in the United States each year (Minna, 1996).

Studies demonstrate that nonsmoking spouses of a smoker have a higher risk for lung cancer from inhalation of "passive" smoke. Passive smoke, also referred to as sidestream smoke and environmental tobacco smoke, contains many of the carcinogens found in actively inhaled, or "mainstream," tobacco smoke (Schottenfeld, 1996). Others at risk from passive smoking include those heavily exposed to passive smoke in the workplace, among them people who work in bars and restaurants.

Other risk factors include occupational exposure to asbestos, beryllium, chromium, coal distillates, cobalt, iron oxide, mustard gas, petroleum distillates, radiation, tar, nickel, and uranium. Atmospheric and industrial pollution that contains benzopyrenes and hydrocarbons has also been associated with an increased incidence of lung cancer.

Other Etiologic Factors

Some hereditary conditions predispose to cancer, although they are not strongly linked to bronchogenic carcinoma. However, evidence for adenocarcinoma and alveolar cell carcinoma suggests genetic factors. These factors do not seem to be related to smoking and are found in families with other tumors, acquired immunodeficiency syndrome (AIDS), or inheritable disorders of the lung. Research supports a correlation between a specific gene and a predisposition to lung cancer, which may thus be an inherited trait (Shell et al., 1996). Clients with chronic respiratory diseases are also at higher risk for lung cancer. A possible link between vitamin A and β-carotene deficiency in the diet and the development of lung cancer also has been demonstrated. A person who smokes and has one or more of the predisposing factors is at greatest risk for the disease.

Prevention

Primary prevention for lung cancer is directed at reducing the number of new and existing cases of tobacco smoking. Extensive educational strategies start with elementary school children to discourage them from beginning to smoke. Nurses are actively involved in encouraging nonsmokers not to begin to smoke, in promoting smoking cessation programs, and in establishing a smoke-free environment. For example, nurses from the Canadian Cancer Society's Industrial Education Program visit places of employment to educate workers about the dangers of smoking. This avenue of education has also been successfully used in the United States. Smoking cessation programs

for assisting those who smoke are available in most geographic areas. Chart 32–7 reviews interventions to help a person stop smoking. The nurse encourages nonsmokers to avoid passive or sidestream smoking by avoiding environmental exposure. Smoke-free environments or areas have been established in most public places.

The nurse also educates workers about safety precautions, such as wearing specialized masks and protective clothing to reduce occupational hazards. The nurse encourages people who are at high risk through smoking history, occupational hazards, or possible genetic background to seek frequent health examinations.

Incidence/Prevalence

Lung cancer is a major health problem throughout the world. Estimates for 1997 were approximately 178,100 new cases of lung cancer and 160,400 deaths from this

---

Chart 32–7

Health Promotion Guide: Suggestions to Help You Stop Smoking

- Make a list of the reasons that you want to stop smoking (e.g., your health and the health of those around you, saving money, social reasons).
- Set a date to stop smoking and keep it. Decide whether you are going to begin to cut down on the amount you smoke or are going to stop "cold turkey." Whatever way you decide to do it, keep this important date!
- Ask for help from those around you. Find someone who wants to quit smoking and "buddy up" for support. Look for assistance in your community, such as formal smoking cessation programs, counselors, and certified acupuncture specialists or hypnotists.
- Consult your physician about nicotine replacement therapy (i.e., patches or gum).
- Remove ashtrays and lighters from view.
- Talk to yourself! Remind yourself of all the reasons you want to quit.
- Avoid places that might tempt you to smoke. If you are used to having a cigarette after meals, get up from the table as soon as you are finished eating. Think of new things to do at times when you used to smoke.
- Find activities that keep your hands busy: needlework, painting, gardening, even holding a pencil.
- Take five deep breaths of clean, fresh air through your nose and out your mouth if you feel the urge to smoke.
- Keep plenty of healthy, low-calorie snacks, such as fruits and vegetables, on hand to nibble on. Try sugarless gum or mints as a substitute for tobacco.
- Drink at least eight glasses of water a day.
- Begin an exercise program with the approval of your physician. Be aware of the positive, healthy changes in your body since you stopped smoking.
- Plan a special way to reward yourself with the money that you save from not smoking.
- List the many reasons why you are glad that you quit. Keep that list handy as a reminder of the positive things you are doing for yourself.
- Think of each day without tobacco as a major accomplishment. It is!

disease in the United States. Lung cancer represents 13% of new cancers in both men and women. Deaths from lung cancer account for 32% of cancer deaths in men and 25% of cancer deaths in women (Parker et al., 1997). In 1986, deaths from lung cancer in women began to exceed deaths from all other cancers, including breast cancer. Researchers attribute this change to a causal relationship with cigarette smoking.

TRANSCULTURAL CONSIDERATIONS

 Lung cancer occurs more frequently and with higher mortality in non-Caucasians. Lung cancer is the most common newly diagnosed cancer in African-Americans (Parker et al., 1997). The impact of industrial factors on the geographic variation in lung cancer rates is pronounced. Mortality rates are higher in countries with significant paper and petroleum industries.

Collaborative Management

Assessment

➤ History

Risk Factors. The nurse extensively questions the client about risk factors, including smoking and occupational hazards in the workplace, and warning signals (Table 32–11). A detailed history of the duration, frequency, and intensity of exposure is elicited. Cigarette smoking history is described in terms of *pack-years*. For example, a person who has smoked two packs per day for 22 years has a 44 pack-year smoking history.

Hoarseness and Cough. When obtaining the history, the nurse notes vague but persistent subjective complaints. Hoarseness, caused by laryngeal nerve invasion, is an early sign of lung cancer. In addition, the nurse asks whether changes in position affect hoarseness, because a recumbent position often exacerbates this sign. The nurse questions the client about any persistent cough or change

TABLE 32–11

Warning Signals Associated with Lung Cancer

- Hoarseness
- Change in respiratory pattern
- Persistent cough or change in cough
- Blood-streaked sputum
- Rust-colored or purulent sputum
- Frank hemoptysis
- Chest pain or chest tightness
- Shoulder, arm, or chest wall pain
- Recurring episodes of pleural effusion, pneumonia, or bronchitis
- Dyspnea
- Fever associated with one or two other signs
- Wheezing
- Weight loss
- Clubbing

in cough and whether the cough is productive of sputum. The nurse also notes a history of any change in respiratory pattern, shortness of breath, or hemoptysis.

Pain. The nurse assesses for chest pain or discomfort, which can occur at any stage of tumor development. Chest pain may be localized or unilateral and can range from mild to severe. The nurse assesses for any vague sensation of fullness, tightness, or pressure in the chest, which may suggest obstruction. A piercing chest pain or pleuritic pain may accompany inspiration. Subscapular pain radiating to the arm commonly results from tumor invasion in advanced disease.

➤ Physical Assessment/Clinical Manifestations

Clinical manifestations associated with lung cancer are often nonspecific and noted late in the disease process. Clinical signs and symptoms depend on the type of primary tumor. Persistent chills, fever, and cough may be related to persistent pneumonitis, indicating obstruction of the bronchi.

Sputum. The nurse assesses sputum quantity and quality. Blood-tinged sputum may be associated with bleeding from a malignant tumor. Hemoptysis is a later finding in the course of the disease. If infection or necrosis is present, sputum may be purulent and copious. The nurse also elicits any history of fever indicative of infection.

Breathing Patterns. The nurse assesses breathing patterns, which may be labored or painful. An obstructive breathing pattern may be evident; expiration is prolonged and labored and alternates with periods of shallow breathing. Rapid, shallow breathing suggests pleuritic chest pain and an elevated diaphragm. Inspiratory efforts may be diminished in advanced disease. The nurse assesses for abnormal retractions, the use of accessory muscles, flared nares (which could be signs of hypoxemia), and stridor (which can indicate obstruction by tumor). The nurse also observes for asymmetry of diaphragmatic movement on inspiration. Bronchial obstruction or pressure in the carina, mediastinum, or trachea may produce dyspnea or wheezing. The nurse assesses the client's level of dyspnea at rest and with activity. The nurse also notes the compensatory mechanisms the client uses to overcome this difficulty. Pursed-lip breathing and orthopnea are common compensatory mechanisms.

Fremitus. On palpation of the chest wall, the nurse may find areas of tenderness or masses. Changes in tactile fremitus (vibrations felt on the chest wall) indicate areas of consolidation (the process whereby air spaces in the lung are replaced with solid material, such as tumor or fluid). Fremitus is decreased or absent when the bronchus is obstructed or the pleural space is occupied by a tumor. Palpation of the trachea may reveal deviation from midline, or "shifting," related to a thoracic mass.

Masses. By percussion of the chest wall, the nurse examines for areas of dullness or obvious masses. With diaphragmatic excursion, resonance usually occurs around the 10th rib.

Breath Sounds. The nurse auscultates the chest to determine changes in breath sounds directly related to the presence of a tumor. Wheezes indicate partial obstruction of airflow in passages narrowed by tumors. Decreased or absent breath sounds are an ominous sign. Absent breath sounds indicate impairment of air passages from obstruction by a tumor or replacement of lung tissue with a solid tumor or fluid. Auscultation of vocal fremitus (i.e., bronchophony, pectoriloquy, and egophony [see Chap. 29]) reveals changes in the sound normally heard. Increased loudness or sound intensity indicates consolidation or compression of the pleural tissue by tumor. Auscultation of a pleural friction rub suggests an inflammatory response to an invading tumor.

Cardiac Status. The nurse notes distant heart sounds, which may indicate cardiac tamponade related to an extended tumor. Dysrhythmias may be present as a result of hypoxemia. The nurse may also observe cyanosis of the lips and fingertips or clubbing (see Fig. 32–6).

Late Signs and Symptoms. Late manifestations of lung cancer may include nonspecific systemic symptoms, such as fatigue, recent weight loss, anorexia, dysphagia, and nausea and vomiting. Superior vena cava syndrome may result from intrathoracic spread of the malignant tumor; this syndrome constitutes an emergency (see Chap. 27). Lethargy and somnolence may develop; therefore, the nurse performs a baseline neurologic assessment. Bowel and bladder tone and function may be affected by tumor spread to the spine and spinal cord.

➤ Psychosocial Assessment

To complete the psychosocial assessment of the client with lung cancer, the nurse evaluates various parameters, including

- Age
- Occupation
- Previous experience with illness
- Marital status
- Dependents
- Support systems
- Usual coping mechanisms

Symptoms associated with lung cancer, especially dyspnea, often add to the client's fear and anxiety. Clients with a history of cigarette smoking may experience guilt and shame. The nurse conveys acceptance of the client and interacts in a nonjudgmental way.

Societal awareness of the poor prognosis of lung cancer poses many challenges for the client and family. Few clients with the diagnosis of lung cancer are candidates for curative therapy. Most are given palliative treatment limited to relief of symptoms. Overall survival time is only moderately lengthened. Fear of abandonment and separation is common in clients with lung cancer.

The client and family will undergo a rapid course in which the nurse

- Supports the client and family through the diagnosis and treatment phases
- Assesses the client's emotional response to the diagnosis of lung cancer
- Listens carefully to the client's and family's concerns

Family members play an important role in the physical and psychosocial care of the client. Family members and significant others can help alleviate the client's anxiety, anticipate needs, and act as liaisons between the staff and the client. The nurse recognizes that the family and significant others also have unmet psychosocial needs and assists them in expressing their needs and concerns.

The nurse identifies resources to assist the client and family in the treatment phase, through the progression of illness, and during anticipatory and actual bereavement. The nurse assesses the grief response as the client and family react to their situation and adjusts care accordingly. A holistic approach includes spiritual counseling and crisis intervention, which are incorporated into the multidisciplinary treatment plan as needed (Georgesen & Dungan, 1996). (Chapter 12 covers grief and loss in detail.)

➤ Laboratory Assessment

A definitive diagnosis of lung cancer is made by isolation of malignant cells. Cytologic examination of early morning sputum specimens may identify tumor cells. However, even with a lung tumor, malignant cells may not be obtained in sputum. With pleural effusion, fluid can be obtained for cytologic examination by thoracentesis.

➤ Radiographic Assessment

Pulmonary lesions are frequently seen on chest x-ray, but tomograms and computed tomography (CT) are used to identify the lesions clearly. CT scan identifies and localizes the extent of masses in the chest, including mediastinal and lymph node involvement.

➤ Other Diagnostic Assessment

Fiberoptic bronchoscopy is extremely important in the diagnosis of lung cancer. It provides direct visibility of the tracheobronchial tree. Specimens and bronchial brushings can thus be obtained, especially when lesions are located endobronchially or are close to an airway. Transthoracic and transbronchial needle biopsy also may be used in an attempt to obtain malignant cells.

A thoroscopy may be performed for diagnostic and therapeutic indications through a video-assisted thoroscope entering the chest cavity via small incisions through the chest wall. This procedure allows direct visibility of the pulmonary tissue and leads to a definitive diagnosis (Davidson & Colt, 1997).

To identify metastasis in mediastinal lymph nodes, the physician may perform mediastinoscopy by inserting a scope through a small anterior chest incision at the suprasternal notch. Mediastinoscopy is an important staging tool for determining the extent of the lung cancer and formulating a treatment plan. If scalene (near the first rib) or supraclavicular lymph nodes are palpable, biopsy of these nodes also may be performed.

To determine a definitive diagnosis and assess overall pulmonary status, other diagnostic studies may be needed, including percutaneous needle biopsy, direct surgical biopsy, and thoracentesis with pleural biopsy. A magnetic resonance imaging (MRI) study may be ordered to identify possible invasion or compression of vascular structures by tumor. Radionuclide scans of the liver, spleen, brain, and bone may be used to assess metastasis of lung cancer. Pulmonary function studies and arterial blood gas analysis may be included to determine the client's overall respiratory status.

 Analysis

➤ *Common Nursing Diagnoses*

Three nursing diagnoses are common in clients with lung cancer:

1. Impaired Gas Exchange related to decreased lung capacity secondary to tissue destruction
2. Ineffective Airway Clearance related to tumor obstruction and increased tracheobronchial secretions
3. Pain related to tumor pressure on surrounding tissues and erosion of tissues

➤ *Additional Nursing Diagnoses and Collaborative Problems*

In addition to the common diagnoses, the client may present with one or more of the following diagnoses:

- Ineffective Breathing Pattern related to decreased energy, fatigue, pain, tracheobronchial obstruction, anxiety
- Activity Intolerance related to imbalance between oxygen supply and demand, dyspnea, fatigue, generalized weakness, weight loss, malnourishment, pain, depression
- Fluid Volume Excess related to compromised antidiuretic hormone regulating mechanism
- Risk for Injury related to metabolic imbalances (e.g., hypercalcemia)
- Fatigue related to increased metabolic energy production, overwhelming emotional demands, states of discomfort, altered body chemistry (e.g., chemotherapy)
- Risk for Trauma related to weakness
- Altered Nutrition, Less than Body Requirements related to the active disease process (increased metabolism), anorexia, nausea, vomiting
- Decreased Cardiac Output related to electrical malfunction secondary to hypoxic dysrhythmias
- Impaired Physical Mobility related to decreased strength and endurance, fatigue, intolerance to activity, dyspnea
- Anticipatory Grieving related to actual or potential loss of health status
- Anxiety related to change in health status, situational crisis, threat of death, loss of control
- Fear related to pain, threat of death, effects of loss of body part or function
- Altered Role Performance related to change in health status, role loss
- Ineffective Family Coping related to effects of major life events, effects of impending death of family member, temporary family disorganization and role changes, effects of acute or chronic illness

- Ineffective Individual Coping related to effects of acute or chronic illness, loss of control over body part or function, major changes in lifestyle, situational crisis, knowledge deficit regarding therapeutic regimen/disease process/prognosis
- Potential for Superior Vena Cava Syndrome

➤ *Impaired Gas Exchange*

Planning and Implementation. The major goal is that the client will be adequately oxygenated, as evidenced by decreased symptoms of hypoxia (such as dyspnea) and decreased signs of hypoxemia (i.e., acceptable blood gas or pulse oximetry results).

Interventions. The nurse evaluates the hypoxemic client's respiratory status as often as indicated, perhaps every 2–4 hours. Color of the skin, lips, ear lobes, and nail beds is noted. The nurse also assesses for signs of respiratory distress, such as dyspnea and use of accessory muscles for breathing. The client in obvious distress is further evaluated by pulse oximetry and arterial blood gas studies.

Nonsurgical Management

Oxygen Therapy. If the client is hypoxemic, the nurse provides supplemental oxygen via mask or nasal cannula as ordered. Even if the client is not overtly hypoxemic, the physician may order oxygen as needed to relieve dyspnea (difficulty breathing) and anxiety in the lung cancer client. (See Chapter 30 for nursing care associated with oxygen therapy.)

Drug Therapy. If the client is experiencing bronchospasm, the physician may prescribe bronchodilators (as for clients with asthma) and corticosteroids to decrease bronchospasm, inflammation, and edema.

Chemotherapy. Chemotherapy is frequently the treatment of choice for lung cancers, especially small cell lung cancer, and as adjuvant therapy in combinations with surgery or in the presence of metastasis for non–small cell lung cancer. Chemotherapy may also be used in conjunction with surgical treatment modalities. Chemotherapeutic agents commonly administered for the treatment of lung cancer include combinations such as

- Cyclosphosphamide, doxorubicin, and vincristine or etoposide
- Etoposide and cisplatin or carboplatin
- Ifosfamide, carboplatin, and etoposide
- Mitomycin, vinblastine, and cisplatin

Recent combination drug regimens using paclitaxel (Taxol) or vinorelbine (Navelbine) with some of these agents are yielding promising results in the treatment of lung cancer (Le Chevalier, 1996). New drug regimens containing taxines, gemcitabine, and topoisomerase 1 inhibitors are on the front line of lung cancer research (McVie, 1996).

The nurse understands the mode of action for each chemotherapeutic agent and takes measures to control common side effects (Table 32–12). The nurse supports the client and family throughout the course of chemotherapy. The nurse educates the client and family about this

TABLE 32–12

Side Effects of Chemotherapeutic Agents Used in the Treatment of Lung Cancer

Drug	Side Effects				Specific Toxic Effects
	Alopecia	Nausea and Vomiting	Bone Marrow Suppression	Diarrhea	
Cisplatin (Platinol)	+	++++	+++	−	• Constipation • Nephrotoxic effects • Ototoxic effects • Hypophosphatemia
Cyclophosphamide (Cytoxan, Procytox✦)	++	++	++	+	• Hemorrhagic cystitis • Syndrome of inappropriate antidiuretic hormone (SIADH) • Hyperpigmentation
Doxorubicin (Adriamycin)	+++	++	+++	+	• Tissue vesicant • Cardiotoxic effects • Mucositis • Hyperpigmentation
Etoposide (VP-16, Vepesid)	+++	+++	++++	−	• Constipation • Postural hypotension
Methotrexate (MTX)	+	++	+++	+	• Mucositis
Mitomycin-C (Mutamycin)	+++	++	+++	+	• Tissue vesicant • Pulmonary injury
Procarbazine (Matulane)	+	+++	+++	+++	• Postural hypotension • Myalgia • Arthralgia
Vinblastine (VLB, Velban)	+	+++	+	−	• Tissue vesicant • Pain at tumor site • Jaw pain • Neurotoxic effects • Loss of deep tendon reflexes

treatment modality and explains how to prevent and manage potential side effects. (See Chapter 27 for further discussion of chemotherapeutic agents and associated nursing care.)

Immunotherapy. Many clients with lung cancer are immunocompromised (unable to defend adequately against potentially harmful substances). Treatment is directed at enhancing an effective immune response, which favorably affects the course of the disease. Immunotherapeutic agents (cytokines) that are "growth factors" are most commonly administered. Cytokines decrease the time that the client is neutropenic (has a low white-blood-cell count) and allow continuation of chemotherapy (also see Chaps. 23 and 27).

Radiation Therapy. Radiation therapy can be an effective primary treatment for localized, unresectable, intrathoracic lung tumors. Radiation therapy also can be helpful for palliation of hemoptysis, obstruction of the bronchi and great veins (superior vena cava syndrome), dysphagia related to esophageal compression, and pain resulting from bone metastasis. Preoperative irradiation

may be attempted to shrink a tumor and promote resectability. After surgical resection of primary tumors, radiation has successfully reduced residual pleural or mediastinal disease. Because of the high frequency of brain metastasis with small cell carcinoma and adenocarcinoma, prophylactic brain radiation may be recommended for clients with these types of lung cancer.

Laser Therapy. Neodymium-yttrium aluminum garnet (YAG) lasers and (rarely) carbon dioxide lasers have been used for palliation of endobronchial obstruction in clients with benign or malignant tumors that are accessible by bronchoscopy. The surgeon debulks the obstructive portion of the tumor, and the airway is reopened. Laser therapy does not produce systemic or toxic effects and is well tolerated by most clients.

Thoracentesis and Pleurodesis. Malignant pleural effusions can be a common problem for clients with lung cancer. Effusions can be caused by involvement of the visceral or parietal pleura by tumor and also by mediastinal lymphatic obstruction or obstructive pneumonitis. The goal of treatment is to remove pleural fluid and prevent its accumulation (Fox, 1994). Thoracentesis (see Chap. 29) removes fluid from the intrapleural space and relieves immediate signs and symptoms of hypoxia.

Fluid can rapidly reaccumulate in the pleural space, and the client may again experience respiratory compromise within a few days. Repeated thoracentesis can create pain and anxiety and can place the client at risk for further complications. As an alternative to repeated thoracentesis, the physician inserts a chest tube to drain the fluid and instills a sclerosing agent, an irritant that causes inflammation and results in fibrosis of tissue. Doxycycline, thiotepa, bleomycin, minocycline, nitrogen mustard, and 5-fluorouracil as well as talc have been used for this treatment. Clinical studies have demonstrated talc to be the most effective and cost-effective sclerosing agent (Sahn, 1996). The aim of thoracentesis and intrapleural administration of one of these agents is to create a *pleurodesis,* which causes adherence of the pleura to the chest wall. Thus, the potential space is eliminated, and reaccumulation of effusion is prevented.

Before pleurodesis, the nurse medicates the client with an analgesic or sedative, as ordered. The physician anesthetizes the pleural surfaces by injecting 1% lidocaine through the chest tube. The physician instills the sclerosing agent; then the nurse or physician clamps the chest tube to prevent drainage of the agent. The physician may order that the client be rotated through various positions at 15- to 30-minute intervals. However, limited research has demonstrated that dispersion of the sclerosing agent is not enhanced by rotation of the client's position (Scott et al., 1993). Chart 32–8 reviews nursing care of the client undergoing pleurodesis.

Surgical Management

Surgery is the treatment of choice for stage I and stage II non–small cell lung cancer (see Fig. 32–10). Total resection of a non–small cell primary bronchogenic tumor is undertaken in hope of achieving a cure. If complete resectability is not possible, the surgeon removes the bulk of the tumor and decreases the possibility of metastatic extension. The choice of surgical procedure depends on the findings of the staging process and the client's overall health and functional status.

Thoracotomy. A thoracotomy is an opening into the thoracic cavity to locate tumors, perform a biopsy, or identify sites of bleeding or injury. Thoracotomy is most often performed to remove all or a portion of the lung.

Preoperative Care. The goals of preoperative care are to relieve anxiety and promote the client's participation (see Chap. 20 for routine preoperative care). The nurse uses interventions to relieve the client's anxiety related to the diagnosis of lung cancer, postoperative management, and loss of a portion or all of a lung. The nurse encourages the client to express fears and concerns, reinforces the physician's explanation of the surgical procedure, and provides education related to the postoperative course. The nurse teaches the client the anticipated location of the surgical incision, if known; shoulder exercises; and about the chest tube and drainage system (except after pneumonectomy).

Chart 32–8

Nursing Care Highlight: The Client Undergoing Pleurodesis

- Reinforce explanation of the pleurodesis and inform the client that medication will be provided to promote comfort before the procedure. (The physician may administer IV analgesia/sedation immediately before the procedure.)
- Ensure that the chest tube is clamped after instillation of the sclerosing agent.
- Monitor vital signs and respiratory status at the completion of the procedure and then at least every 30 min until the effects of the IV medication have dissipated.
- Thereafter, monitor vital signs every 4 hr for 24 hr. (The client may experience a low-grade fever. Pleurodesis creates pleuritis between the visceral and parietal layers, thus preventing reaccumulation of fluid.)
- If a rotation schedule is ordered, assist the client to the correct position for appropriate time frames and provide reassurance.
- Unclamp the chest tube after completion of the rotation schedule or at the specified time ordered by the physician.
- Assess chest tube drainage and document the amount and character of the drainage.
- Perform a complete respiratory assessment every 8 hr and observe for signs and symptoms of distress, including those of pneumothorax.
- Analgesics may be administered as needed to promote the client's comfort.
- When drainage has decreased (<150 mL in 12–24 hr), the physician may remove the chest tube. Maintain an occlusive dressing at the insertion site for a minimum of 48 hr.

Operative Procedures. Three types of incisions can be made:

- Posterolateral thoracotomy
- Anterolateral thoracotomy
- Median sternotomy

A posterolateral thoracotomy incision begins in the submammary fold of the anterior chest, is drawn down below the scapular tip and along the course of the ribs, and then curves posteriorly and upward as far as the spine of the scapula. An anterolateral thoracotomy involves an incision below the breast and above the costal margins. This incision extends from the anterior axillary line and then turns downward to avoid the axillary apex. A median sternotomy is a straight incision from the suprasternal notch to the area below the xyphoid process. The sternum must be transected with an electric or air-driven saw.

Postoperative Care. General care of the client after thoracotomy is reviewed in the Client Care Plan concerning lung cancer. Postoperative management of clients who have undergone thoracotomy requires closed-chest drainage to drain air and blood that may accumulate in the pleural space. A chest tube, a drain placed in the pleural

Text continued on page 654

The Client Who Has Had a Thoracotomy for Lung Cancer

Nursing Diagnosis No. 1: Impaired Gas Exchange related to ventilation-perfusion imbalance secondary to removal of all or part of a lung and ineffective airway clearance

Expected Outcomes	Nursing Interventions	Rationale
The client will have adequate lung expansion and mobilization of secretions.	▪ Perform complete respiratory assessment every 2 hr. Assess breath sounds; rate, depth, and pattern of respirations; signs and symptoms of hypoxia, including restlessness and irritability; and position of mediastinum.	▪ Ongoing astute assessments alert the nurse to subtle and early signs and symptoms of changes in respiratory status.
The client's blood gases and pulse oximetry will be within normal range.	▪ Monitor vital signs, pulse oximetry, and arterial blood gases as ordered. Report abnormalities to the physician.	▪ Prompt reporting of abnormalities enable the physician to institute early treatment and prevent further complications.
	▪ Administer oxygen therapy as ordered.	▪ Supplemental oxygen will help correct hypoxemia.
	▪ Maintain patency and integrity of the chest tube and drainage system, if present.	▪ A properly functioning chest drainage system promotes adequate drainage of blood and air that may accumulate in the pleural space, allowing re-expansion of the lung.
	▪ Assess for and report signs and symptoms of air leak from the chest tube or hemorrhage.	▪ Prompt reporting of abnormalities helps prevent further complications.
	▪ Perform pain assessment and administer analgesics as ordered. (Observe for signs and symptoms of respiratory depression related to opioids.)	▪ Effective pain management promotes the client's participation in deep breathing and mobility, thus fostering optimal respiratory effort.
	▪ Reposition the client every 2 hr. Check order for positioning carefully and seek clarification if necessary. (Do not place the client on the operative side after pneumonectomy.)	▪ Repositioning promotes lung expansion.
	▪ Encourage the client to perform deep-breathing exercises every 2 hr and to use incentive spirometry devices as soon as he or she is physically able.	▪ Breathing exercises promote lung expansion and help prevent atelectasis and pneumonia.
	▪ Coach in effective coughing technique if secretions are present. Assist to high-Fowler's position with knees bent and feet flat on bed. Instruct the client to obtain maximal inspiration and to hold the breath for 2 sec; follow by having the client cough twice with the mouth open, pause, and then inhale through the nose and rest.	▪ Effective coughing improves airway clearance and prevents stasis of secretions.

Client Care Plan

Expected Outcomes	Nursing Interventions	Rationale
	■ Assist the client to remove and properly dispose of secretions.	■ Proper disposal of secretions is required for infection control purposes.
	■ Assist the client to sit in a chair, when ordered, and monitor tolerance.	■ Lung expansion is enhanced when the client is able to be out of bed.

Nursing Diagnosis No. 2: Pain related to tissue trauma as a result of surgery, inflammation of incised muscles, and presence of chest tubes

Expected Outcomes	Nursing Interventions	Rationale
The client will be as pain-free and alert as possible.	■ Perform a complete pain assessment using designed pain level scale (i.e., 0 = no pain, 5 = severe pain).	■ Obtain the baseline pain assessment rating and use it for comparison with the routine pain assessment score to determine the effectiveness of pain management interventions.
	■ Assist with incisional splinting during deep-breathing exercises, with turning, and in anticipation of cough stimulation.	■ Splinting promotes the client's comfort and participation in measures that promote respiratory function.
	■ Secure the chest tube to prevent excessive discomfort resulting from movement of the tube.	■ Nonpharmacologic nursing interventions are instrumental in helping the client to achieve optimal comfort.
	■ Promote optimal comfort through proper positioning, hygiene, gentle massage, and relaxation techniques.	
	■ Administer analgesics as ordered. Plan activities to coincide with peak of analgesic effectiveness. Observe for signs and symptoms of respiratory depression associated with opioids.	■ The client's participation in respiratory excursion activities will be increased with effective pain management.
	■ Use diversional activities as appropriate.	
	■ Document the client's response to the pain control regimen and seek adjustment as needed.	■ Ongoing assessment and evaluation of the effectiveness of the pain control regimen are essential to the client's optimal comfort.

(Continued)

Client Care Plan

Nursing Diagnosis No. 3: Activity Intolerance related to restricted arm and shoulder movement

Expected Outcomes	Nursing Interventions	Rationale
The client will maintain normal arm and shoulder movement and function as evidenced by the ability to perform range-of-motion exercises on the operative side.	■ Educate the client about the possible complication and prevention of "frozen shoulder syndrome." ■ Monitor and report restricted arm and shoulder movement postoperatively. ■ Perform passive range-of-motion exercises to the affected arm and shoulder 2 times every 4 hr during the first 24 hr postoperatively and then 10 times every 2 hr. ■ Instruct the client in active range-of-motion exercises beginning the second day after surgery. ■ Encourage the client to use the affected arm for activities of daily living and place frequently used items on the same side of the bed as the operative side to facilitate reaching and gentle stretching. ■ Administer analgesic as needed to promote active participation in exercises. ■ Offer encouragement and support for the client's progress.	■ The client is more likely to actively participate in preventive measures when he or she is knowledgeable about this potential postoperative complication. ■ Ongoing assessments help detect early signs of complications. ■ Exercising maintains strength, facilitates mobility, and prevents fixation. ■ Active participation by the client promotes well-being, autonomy, and independence. ■ Effective levels of analgesia allow the client to perform prescribed exercises and prevent complications. ■ Positive reinforcement enables the client to continue the rehabilitation process.

Nursing Diagnosis No. 4: Body Image Disturbance related to actual change in body structure and function

Expected Outcomes	Nursing Interventions	Rationale
The client will verbalize feelings about loss of all or part of a lung and identify ways in which to compensate for altered lung capacity.	■ Establish a therapeutic nurse-client relationship by building trust and confidence. ■ Encourage expression of feelings and concerns related to lung cancer diagnosis, grief about loss of lung, and effects on lifestyle. ■ Support a realistic hope of regaining aspects of usual activities.	■ Sincere behaviors that display concern and caring enable the client to feel comfortable and at ease with the nurse. ■ Ventilation of feelings and concerns can serve as an effective coping strategy and assist the client to express needs. ■ Hope is a universal coping mechanism and can enable the client to attain activity potential within the present physical limitations.

Client Care Plan

Expected Outcomes	Nursing Interventions	Rationale
	■ Assist the client to identify activities that can be performed with present lung capacity.	■ Identification of activities that can be performed by the client encourages independence and increased self-esteem.
	■ Identify measures to promote increased endurance and participation in activities (i.e., carefully schedule activities, ensure rest periods and proper nutrition).	■ Energy conservation and health promotion activities assist the client to achieve optimal physical activity.
	■ Provide support for accomplishments and encourage the concept of slow progression without compromising respiratory status.	■ Positive reinforcement of achievements enhances body image and self-esteem.

Nursing Diagnosis No. 5: Knowledge Deficit related to care after hospitalization

Expected Outcomes	Nursing Interventions	Rationale
The client will verbalize follow-up care and signs and symptoms to report to the primary care provider.	■ Review the discharge instructions with the client, including follow-up visit, medications, permitted activities, and arm and shoulder exercises.	■ Ensuring that the client understands required information before discharge promotes the client's participation in the treatment plan and minimizes anxiety after discharge.
	■ Instruct the client to report signs and symptoms of fever, cough and sputum production, increased discomfort, or dyspnea to the primary care provider (physician or nurse).	■ Early detection and treatment of possible respiratory infection or other respiratory complications can reduce the extent of the complication.
	■ Encourage the client to pace tolerable activities and rest periods.	■ When the client understands how to balance and limit activities, complications can be prevented.
	■ Reinforce that heavy lifting is to be avoided for 6 months and to stop any activity that provokes excessive dyspnea or discomfort.	
	■ Review and educate the client about additional proposed treatment as indicated (chemotherapy, radiation therapy).	■ Education related to further treatment modalities fosters the client's understanding of and compliance with the treatment plan and can reduce anxiety and possible misconceptions.
	■ Refer the client to appropriate community resources, if indicated (e.g., home health agency, American Cancer Society, American Lung Association).	■ Community resources are an additional avenue for information and support.

space to restore intrapleural pressure, allows re-expansion of the lung. The chest tube also prevents air and fluid from returning to the chest. The drainage system consists of

- One or more chest tubes or drains
- A collection container placed below the chest level
- A water seal to keep air from entering the chest

The tip of the tube used to drain air is usually placed anteriorly near the lung apex. The tube that drains liquid is placed laterally near the base of the lung. After lung resection, two tubes, anterior and posterior, are used. The puncture wounds are covered with airtight dressings.

The chest tube is connected to approximately 6 feet of tubing that leads to a collection device placed several feet below the chest. The tubing allows the client to turn and move easily. Positioning the collection device below the chest allows gravity to drain the pleural space. When two chest tubes are inserted, they are usually joined by a Y-connector near the client's body; the 6 feet of tubing are attached to the Y-connector.

The chest drainage system has a separate water seal mechanism that acts as a one-way valve. In setting up current chest drainage systems, the nurse adds a specified amount of sterile saline to the water seal chamber. (In older systems, the end of the tubing was placed beneath the surface of a sterile saline solution to create the water seal.) The water seal closes the open end of the system (or the end of the tubing) from the atmosphere. When the positive pressure in the lungs during exhalation pushes air out of the pleural space through the tubing, the air bubbles into the saline and cannot re-enter the chest.

Earlier chest drainage consisted of one-, two-, and three-bottle systems. Technology has greatly improved these bulky glass bottle systems through the availability of one-piece disposable chest drainage devices. The Pleur-Evac system, one of the most widely distributed, uses a one-piece disposable, molded plastic unit with three chambers. This system duplicates the older three-bottle system. From right to left, the system contains chambers for drainage, a water seal, and suction control (Fig. 32–11). The plastic devices reduce the risk of breakage or contamination of the drainage system and allow the client increased mobility. All systems are vented so that incoming pleural air cannot build up, thereby preventing further air entry into the chest. Suction may be added, as ordered.

In one system, a knob on the collection device can be set to the ordered amount of suction. The wall suction source dial is then turned until a small orange floater valve appears in a certain window (Fig. 32–12). When the orange valve is in the window, the right amount of suction has been applied. With this system, the nurse notes the absence of bubbling in the chamber, which is normal for this so-called dry suction system.

The nurse routinely checks to ensure the sterility and patency of the system. The nurse tapes the tubing junctions to prevent accidental disconnections and maintains an occlusive dressing at the chest tube insertion site. To cover the insertion site immediately if the chest tube becomes accidentally dislodged, sterile gauze is kept at the bedside. The nurse keeps heavily padded clamps at the bedside for use if the drainage system is inadvertently interrupted or to facilitate changing of the drainage system when necessary. The nurse carefully positions the drainage tubing to prevent kinks and large loops of tubing, which can impede drainage and lung re-expansion. Vigorous stripping of the chest tube should be avoided. Gentle milking of the tube, however, may prevent obstruction by moving any blood clots.

The nurse assesses the client's respiratory status and notes the amount and type of drainage. Immediately after surgery, the nurse records hourly the amount of drainage. Drainage of more than 100 mL/hr is considered excessive, and the physician is notified. After the first 24 hours, the nurse usually assesses drainage and the drainage system minimally every 8 hours.

The nurse checks the water seal chamber for unexpected bubbling created by an air leak in the system. Bubbling is anticipated during forceful expiration or coughing because air in the chest is being expelled. Continuous bubbling indicates an air leak and requires an effort to identify its source. On the physician's order, the nurse gently applies a padded clamp on the drainage tubing close to the occlusive dressing. If the bubbling stops, the air leak may be at the chest tube insertion site or within the chest. Further assessment of the insertion site and chest tube position is necessary, and the nurse consults the physician for identified problems. Air bubbling that does not cease when the nurse applies a padded clamp indicates that the air leak is between the clamp and the drainage system. For ensuring patency and sterility of the system, this tubing and drainage device should be replaced, as ordered.

The nurse also checks for rising and falling of fluid in the water seal as the client breathes in and out. These fluctuations act like a manometer by representing the pressure changes in the pleural space, and they reliably indicate overall respiratory effort. Fluctuations of 5–10 cm (2–4 inches) during normal breathing are common. The absence of fluctuations could mean the tubing is obstructed by a kink, the client is lying on the tubing, or dependent fluid has filled a loop of tubing. Expanded lung tissue can also block the chest tube eyelets during expiration, or no more air may be leaking into the pleural space.

Suction can be added to current collection systems on physician's order. Suction enhances the pressure difference between the pleural space and the drainage system, causing the pressure to drop inside the system by 15–20 cm. In some systems, the ordered amount of suction, often a negative 20 cm, is determined by the height of the saline in the water seal chamber. When suction is added, air is pulled down into the water seal chamber. When the depth of the saline solution is 20 cm, 20 cm of water creates the negative pressure required to pull air to the bottom of the chamber, where it bubbles out into the solution. While suction is applied, the nurse notes gentle bubbling in the chamber. The depth of the saline determines the maximal suction level for the system. Increasing the suction source causes more bubbling, but it cannot increase the effective suction because the outside air offsets any further air removal. When vigorous bubbling is noted, an air leak may be present. Bubbling also en-

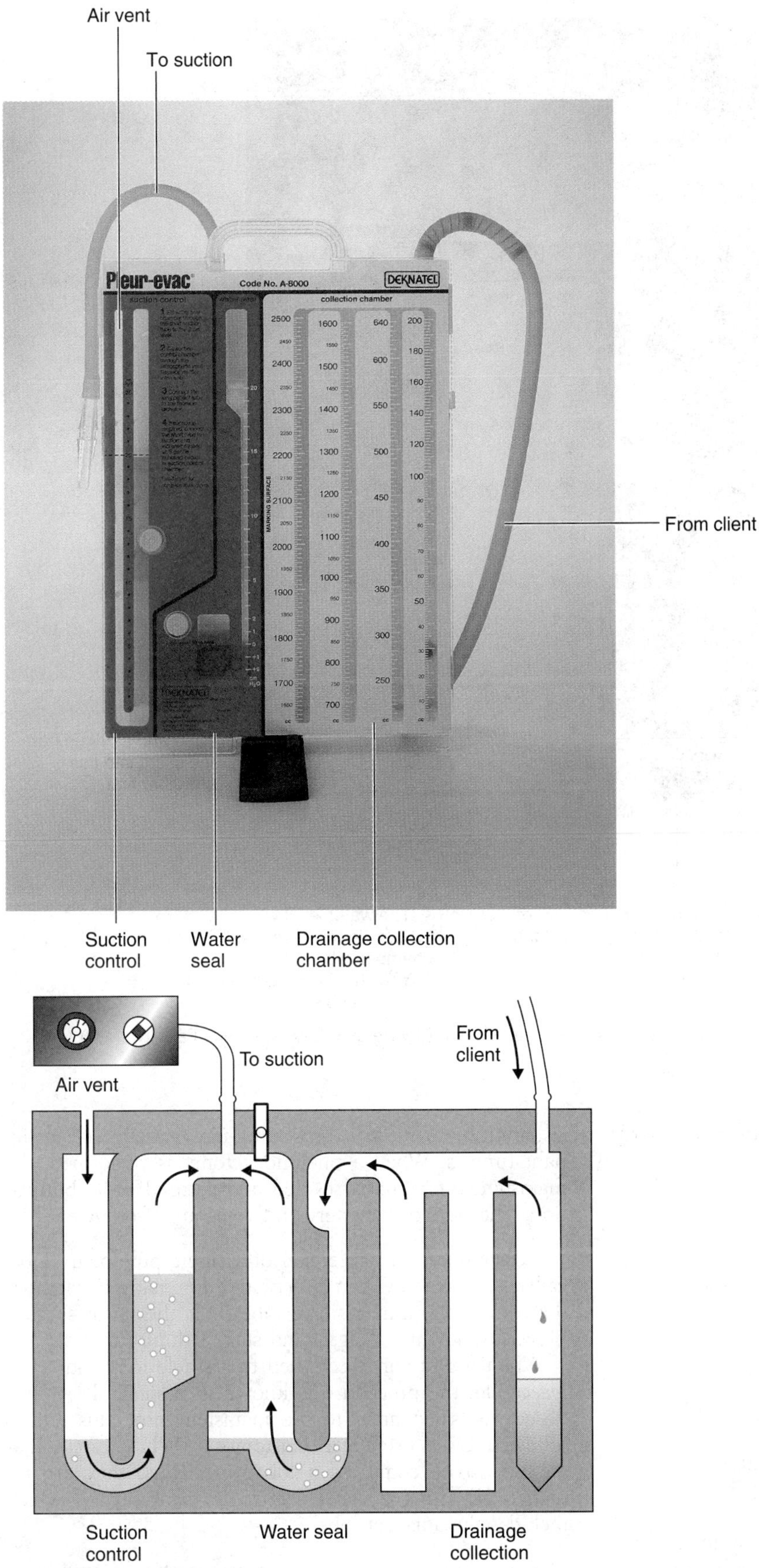

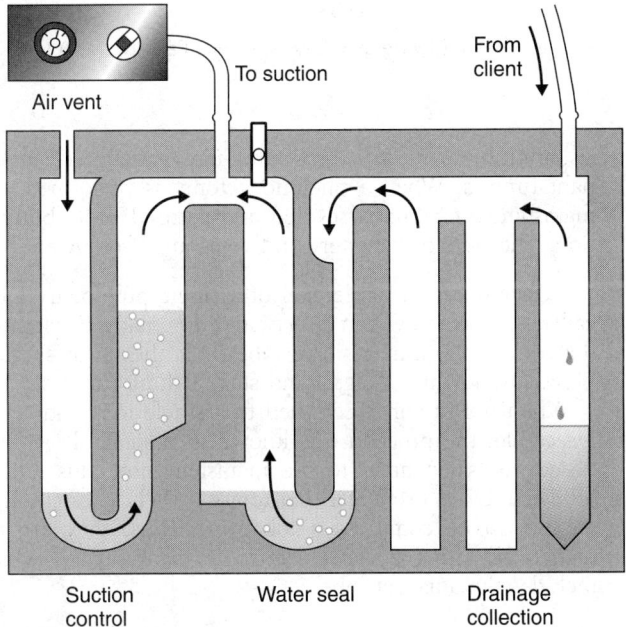

Air vent
To suction
Pleur-evac
Code No. A-8000
DEKNATEL
collection chamber
From client
Suction control
Water seal
Drainage collection chamber
To suction
Air vent
From client
Suction control
Water seal
Drainage collection

Figure 32–11. *Top,* The Pleur-Evac drainage system, a commercial three-bottle chest drainage device. *Bottom,* Schematic of the drainage device.

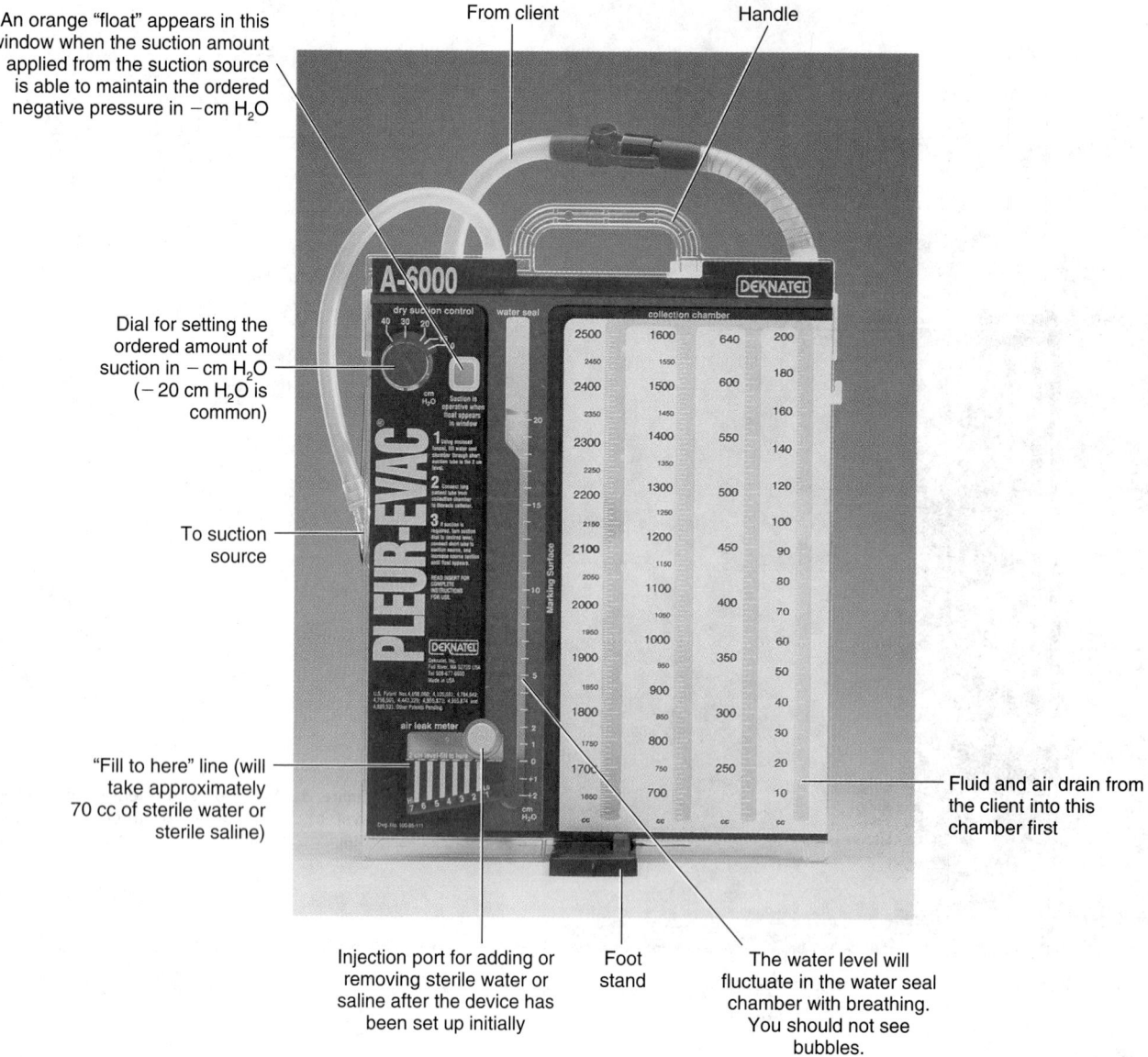

An orange "float" appears in this window when the suction amount applied from the suction source is able to maintain the ordered negative pressure in −cm H₂O

From client

Handle

Dial for setting the ordered amount of suction in −cm H₂O (−20 cm H₂O is common)

To suction source

"Fill to here" line (will take approximately 70 cc of sterile water or sterile saline)

Injection port for adding or removing sterile water or saline after the device has been set up initially

Foot stand

The water level will fluctuate in the water seal chamber with breathing. You should not see bubbles.

Fluid and air drain from the client into this chamber first

Figure 32–12. The A-6000 dry suction control Pleur-Evac chest drainage system. (Courtesy of Deknatel, Inc., Fall River, MA.)

hances evaporation, so that the nurse adds more sterile saline in the chamber as needed.

Other Procedures

Preoperative Care. The preoperative care for the client undergoing these surgical procedures is the same as for the client having a thoracotomy.

Operative Procedures

Pneumonectomy. Pneumonectomy, removal of an entire lung, is required for
- Large, centrally located bronchogenic tumors
- Involvement of a mainstem bronchus
- Invasion of the main pulmonary artery

Less frequent indications for pneumonectomy include extensive unilateral tuberculosis (TB), extensive bronchiecta-

sis, multiple lung abscesses, and rare varieties of malignant tumors. When a pneumonectomy is performed, the mainstem bronchus is severed and sutured at its bifurcation. The pulmonary artery and veins are also ligated.

Lobectomy. The resection of a single pulmonary lobe, called a lobectomy, can be curative for many carcinomas that develop within a single lobe. It is the usual surgical procedure for most stage I and stage II lung cancers.

When the tumor is confined to a single lobe and easily resectable, the procedure is known as a *simple lobectomy*. Resection is extended to the mainstem bronchus and is followed by a bronchial anastomosis. When carcinomas are within or compress a lobar bronchus, they are removed by using a *sleeve lobectomy (bilobectomy)*, which includes the adjacent lobe.

Resection. A limited pulmonary resection is any surgical resection of the lung that does not involve a complete lobectomy. A *limited resection* is considered only when the lung tumor is in stage I, the tumor size is 3 cm or less, and the client's pulmonary status is compromised. A lung resection may be used if the client cannot tolerate a lobectomy or pneumonectomy.

A *segmental resection (segmentectomy)* is a pulmonary resection that includes the bronchus, pulmonary artery and vein, and lung parenchyma of the involved lung segment or segments, which are divisions of lobes. A *wedge resection* is removal of the peripheral portion of small localized areas of disease.

Postoperative Care. After pneumonectomy, the pleural cavity on the affected side is an empty space. The physician sometimes inserts a clamped chest tube for only a day because serous fluid may then accumulate in the empty space and create adhesions, which reduce mediastinal shift toward the affected side. Closed-chest drainage is not usually used.

Possible complications of a pneumonectomy can include empyema and the development of a bronchopleural fistula. The nurse is careful not to turn the client onto the operative side immediately after a pneumonectomy. Positioning on the operative side can place increased stress on the bronchial stump incision and risk disruption of the suture line.

After lobectomy, the remaining lung tissue expands to fill in the portion of lung space previously occupied by the removed lung tissue. A chest tube is usually inserted for postoperative closed drainage. Nursing care after lobectomy or lung resection is the same as for the client undergoing thoracotomy (see the Client Care Plan concerning lung cancer). The nurse continues to assess respiratory status and observes for general postoperative complications (see Chap. 22).

> ### ➤ *Ineffective Airway Clearance*

Planning: Expected Outcomes. The client should
▪ Breathe without dyspnea or discomfort
▪ Maintain a patent airway

Interventions. The client who produces copious secretions may benefit from the use of a humidifier and a vaporizer, which provide moisture to loosen the secretions. The nurse suctions the client, as indicated and as ordered, to clear secretions from the airway. If the client also has an underlying chronic lung disease, beta agonists and inhaled steroids may relieve symptoms. In moderately advanced disease, postural drainage and chest physiotherapy may help.

The client with lung cancer fatigues easily and is often most comfortable resting in a semi-Fowler's position. Dyspnea can be reduced with supplemental oxygen, use of a morphine drip, and positioning for comfort and to facilitate drainage of secretions. The severely dyspneic client may be most comfortable sitting in a lounge or a reclining chair. The nurse monitors the amount of blood loss in the client with hemoptysis. Because blood is an excellent medium for bacterial growth, the nurse is alert for signs and symptoms of infection. The nurse and phy-

sician work closely together to provide a regimen effective in relieving pain, discomfort, and dyspnea.

> ### ➤ *Pain*

Planning: Expected Outcomes. The client should experience relief or reduction of pain and discomfort.

Interventions. The client with lung cancer may experience chest pain and possibly subscapular pain radiating to the arm. With bone metastasis, the client may also experience bone pain. The nurse performs a complete pain assessment with attention to
▪ Onset, intensity, quality, duration, and client's description of the pain
▪ Discomfort
▪ Accompanying symptoms
▪ Factors that alleviate the pain
▪ Factors that increase the intensity of the pain
The nurse needs to identify ways in which to correlate the nursing assessment of pain with the client's self-reporting. Accurate interpretation of the client's perception of the pain experience leads to improved pain management, minimized suffering, and optimal functioning of the client with lung cancer (Wilkie et al., 1995). The nurse intervenes with nonpharmacologic measures, such as positioning, hot or cold compresses, distractions, and guided imagery. The nurse administers prescribed analgesic medications, as ordered, to foster pain relief. Oral, parenteral, transdermal opioid analgesics or an intravenous opioid infusion may be used for more severe pain in clients with advanced disease. The nurse observes the clients' respiratory status for changes when administering potentially respiration-depressing medications. Clients experiencing pain usually have advanced disease and a limited prognosis. Ongoing assessment and evaluation of the effectiveness of the pain control regimen is a primary nursing responsibility (Kodiath & Kodiath, 1995). The nurse's goal is to assist the client to be as pain free and as comfortable as possible.

Continuing Care

> ### ➤ *Health Teaching*

Symptom Management

The nurse reviews any limitations of physical activity with the client and family and prescribes an acceptable activity level. Nurses provide instruction on dealing with dyspnea and explain positions that facilitate easier breathing, such as leaning forward and sitting in a chair. The nurse emphasizes the need to prevent exposure to others with infections and outlines signs and symptoms that should be reported to health care professionals. The nurse instructs the family to call the physician when the prescribed pain medications or respiratory therapy is not providing comfort and when the client is not receiving adequate relief from dyspnea. The nurse also provides specific information about medications as well as safety precautions for the use of oxygen.

Psychosocial Preparation

Psychosocial interventions differ, depending on the prognosis. The client with resectable carcinoma of the lung can be encouraged to have an optimistic outlook and gradually to resume normal activities. The nurse continues to help the client and family with their fear of death and their anxiety related to the cancer diagnosis as well as the client's uncertain future health.

The client whose prognosis is poor is one who, with the family, is facing death. The nurse facilitates the expression of fears and concerns, encourages the client and family to maintain open lines of communication, and stresses the quality of life defined by the client. The nurse's continued support and understanding can help the client and family through this difficult time. The nurse, case manager, or social worker makes referrals to community hospice and home care agencies as indicated. (Chapter 12 presents nursing interventions for people experiencing loss and grief.)

Home Care Management

Clients and their families usually have significant needs upon the client's discharge from the acute care setting. The nurse works with the client and family before discharge to identify their expected needs. Appropriate referrals are made to community agencies, including home health nursing or hospice programs as indicated. The nurse coordinates arrangements for oxygen and other respiratory therapy to be available if needed by the client at home.

Health Care Resources

For the client in the terminal phase of lung cancer, a referral to a hospice program can be beneficial. The discharge-planning nurse, case manager, or social worker can assist in making these arrangements. Hospice programs provide support to the terminally ill client and the family by meeting physical and psychosocial needs, adjusting the palliative care regimen as needed, making home visits, and providing volunteers for errands and respite care. The American Cancer Society may also be able to provide assistance through support groups for clients and families or through the use of equipment, such as a hospital bed.

 Evaluation

In evaluating the care of the client with lung cancer, the nurse expects that the client will
- Maintain a patent airway
- State that pain or discomfort is reduced or alleviated
- Breathe without severe dyspnea
- Maintain acceptable arterial blood gas levels
- Resolve the reality of the diagnosis and prognosis
- State an understanding of the treatment plan
- Experience no major complications from radiation therapy, chemotherapy, or surgery

---

 CASE STUDY for the Client with Lung Cancer

▪ G.F. is a 62-year-old married man with three independent children. He was initially seen by his family physician and treated for an upper respiratory tract infection. His symptoms did not resolve, and further diagnostic tests were initiated. G.F. presents now with a 6-week history of right shoulder pain and dyspnea on exertion, cough productive of yellow sputum, a 7-pound weight loss over the last 4 weeks, and intermittent diaphoresis.

MEDICAL HISTORY

No chronic illness
Pneumonia: 1992
Bronchitis: "every year or so"
No current medications
Alcohol: social
Tobacco: quit smoking 4 years ago, prior 40-pack-year history

FAMILY HISTORY

Father: deceased, age 68, emphysema
Mother: deceased, age 72, myocardial infarction
Brother: alive, age 64, hypertension
Sisters: alive, ages 59, 66; no chronic illness

PHYSICAL EXAMINATION

▪ Well-developed, alert, and oriented male in no acute distress. Vital signs: afebrile; pulse, 124; respirations, 24; blood pressure, 138/72. Neck exam revealed three right-sided supraclavicular lymph nodes measuring approximately 1–2 cm in diameter. Auscultation of the chest: lungs clear on the left and rhonchi on the right. The abdomen was soft, nondistended with positive bowel sounds in all quadrants, and no hepatosplenomegaly. The extremities were without clubbing, cyanosis, or edema. Right shoulder and axilla tenderness was noted.

DIAGNOSTIC STUDIES

▪ Chest computed tomography (CT) revealed a 3-cm mass in the apex of the right lung with invasion into the right axilla. Additionally, tracheobronchial and mediastinal lymph node enlargement was noted. Bone scan: normal. CT of head: mild atrophy without lesions. CT-guided fine needle biopsy: Tissue samples revealed adenocarcinoma of the lung, classified as non–small cell lung carcinoma. Staging bronchoscopy and mediastinoscopy: Bronchoscopy demonstrated no evidence of endobronchial lesions, and mediastinoscopy showed additional mediastinal lymph node involvement measuring greater than 1.5 cm. Histologic staging: stage IIIb T2, N3, M0.

QUESTIONS:

1. On the basis of G.F.'s staging, what treatment is most likely to be recommended?
2. In preparing G.F. for treatment, what areas does the nurse need to include in the teaching plan?
3. To what resources can the nurse direct G.F.?

CASE STUDY for the Client with Chronic Airflow Limitation

■ A 55-year-old man arrives at your primary care clinic with complaints of persistent cough, shortness of breath, and occasional wheezing. His symptoms have become progressively worse over the past 2 weeks. The client's medical history includes hypertension. Social history includes tobacco abuse for 15 years, and the client currently smokes one pack of cigarettes per day.

Current medications include daily vitamins and atenolol, 50 mg per day. Vital signs are blood pressure, 130/78; pulse, 96; and respirations, 26. The client denies any sputum production, fever, and chills.

QUESTIONS:

1. While obtaining a history from your client, what important questions do you want to ask?
2. What initial physical assessments do you want to perform?
3. What are some possible diagnoses related to the symptoms?
4. What interventions may be ordered or implemented to minimize or treat the client's symptoms?
5. What are some key educational interventions related to health promotion or disease prevention that you will consider and or implement?

SELECTED BIBLIOGRAPHY

Aboussouan, L. S. (1996). Acute exacerbations of chronic bronchitis. *Postgraduate Medicine, 99*(4), 89–102.

Alberts, W. M., & Brooks, S. M. (1995). Occupational asthma. *Postgraduate Medicine, 97*(6), 93–104.

*American Thoracic Society. (1991). Standards of nursing care for adult patients with pulmonary dysfunction. *American Review of Respiratory Disease, 144*(1), 231–236.

American Thoracic Society. (1995). Standards for the diagnosis and care of patients with chronic obstructive pulmonary disease. *American Journal of Respiratory and Critical Care Medicine, 152*(5), S78–S121.

Baldini, E. H. (1997). Palliative radiation therapy for non–small cell lung cancer. *Hematology/Oncology Clinics of North America, 11*(20), 303–319.

Ball, P. (1995). Epidemiology and treatment of chronic bronchitis and its exacerbations. *Chest, 108*(2), 43S–52S.

Benson, V., & Marano, M. A. (1994). *Current estimates from the National Health Interview Survey* (DHHS Pub. No. [PHS] 94–1517). Hyattsville, MD: National Center for Health Statistics.

Berg, D. T. (1997). New chemotherapy treatment options and implications for nursing care. *Oncology Nursing Forum Suppl, 24*(1), 5–12.

Blackmon, G. M., & Raghu, G. (1995). Pulmonary sarcoidosis: A mimic of respiratory infection. *Seminars of Respiratory Infections, 10*(3), 176–186.

Bone, R. C. (1996). Goals of asthma management. A step care approach. *Chest, 109*(4), 1056–1065.

Bordow, R. A., Moser, K. M. (1996). Manual of clinical problems in pulmonary medicine (4th ed.). Philadelphia, PA: Lippincott-Raven.

Bunn, P. A. (1996a). Combination paclitaxel and platinum in the treatment of lung cancer: U.S. experience. *Seminars in Oncology Suppl, 23*(6), 9–16.

Bunn, P. A. (1996b). Current therapy for small cell lung cancer. *Seminars in Oncology Suppl, 23*(6), 1–5.

Busse, W. W. (1996). Long and short acting beta₂-adrenergic agonists. *Archives of Internal Medicine, 156*, 1514–1520.

*Busse, W. W., Lemanske, R. F., & Dick, E. C. (1992). The relationship of viral respiratory infections and asthma. *Chest, 101*(6), 385s–388s.

Carney, D. N. (1996). Non–small cell lung cancer: Slow but definite progress. *Seminars in Oncology, 23*(6), 5–6.

*Carrieri-Kohlman, V., Douglas, M. K., Gormley, J. M., & Stulbarg, M. S. (1993). Desensitization and guided mastery: Treatment approaches for the management of dyspnea. *Heart and Lung, 22*(3), 226–234.

Carroll, P. (1995). Chest tubes made easier. *RN, 58*(12), 46–55.

Celli, B. R. (1995). Pulmonary rehabilitation in patients with COPD. *American Journal of Respiratory and Critical Care Medicine, 152*, 861–864.

Celli, B. R. (1996). Current thoughts regarding treatment of chronic obstructive pulmonary disease. *Medical Clinics of North America, 80*(3), 589–609.

Chan-Yeung, M. (1995). Assessment of asthma in the workplace. *Chest, 108*(4), 1084–1117.

Chang, J. T., Moran, M. B., Cugell, D. W., & Webster, J. R. (1995). COPD in the elderly. *Chest, 108*(3), 736–740.

Chapman, K. R. (1996). Therapeutic approaches to chronic obstructive pulmonary disease: An emerging consensus. *American Journal of Medicine, 100*(Suppl. 1A), 1A-5S–1A-10S.

Chestnutt, A. N. (1995). Enigmas in sarcoidosis. *Western Journal of Medicine, 162*(6), 519–526.

Chiocca, E., & Russo, L. (1997). Action stat: Acute asthma attack. *Nursing97, 26*(7), 43.

Cockcroft, D. W., & Dosman, J. A. (1996). Obstructive lung diseases, part II. *The Medical Clinics of North America.*

Cockcroft, D. W., & Kalra, S. (1996). Outpatient asthma management. *Medical Clinics of North America, 80*(4), 701–718.

Couser, J. I., Guthmann, B. A., Hamadeh, M. A., & Kane, C. S. (1995). Pulmonary rehabilitation improves exercise capacity in older elderly patients with COPD. *Chest, 107*(3), 730–734.

Davidson, J. E,. & Colt, H. G. (1997). Thoracoscopy: Nursing implications for optimal patient outcomes. *Dimensions of Critical Care Nursing, 16*(1), 20–28.

*DeLetter, M. C. (1991). Nutritional implications for chronic airflow limitation patients. *Journal of Gerontological Nursing, 17*(5), 21–26.

DeRemee, R. (1995). Concise review for primary-care physicians. *Mayo Clinic Procedures, 70*, 177–181.

Dosman, J. A., & Cockcroft, D. W. (1996). Obstructive lung diseases, part I. *The Medical Clinics of North America.*

Dow, J. S., & Mest, C. G. (1997). Psychosocial interventions for patients with chronic obstructive pulmonary disease. *Home Healthcare Nurse, 15*(6), 414–420.

Emmons, K. M., & Kawachi, I. Tobacco control: A brief relief of its history and prospects for the future. *Hematology/Oncology Clinics of North America, 11*(2), 177–195.

*Faryniarz, K., & Mahler, D. (1990). Writing an exercise prescription for patients with COPD. *Journal of Respiratory Diseases, 11*(7), 638–648.

Fieler, V. K., Wlasowicz, G. S., Mitchell, M. L., Jones, L. S., & Johnson, J. E. (1996). Information preferences of patients undergoing radiation therapy. *Oncology Nursing Forum, 23*(10), 1603–1608.

Fiocco, M., & Krasna, M. J. (1997). The management of pleural and pericardial effusions. *Hematology/Oncology Clinics of North America, 11*(20), 253–265.

Fishman, A. P. (1994). Pulmonary rehabilitation research. *American Journal of Respiratory and Critical Care Medicine, 149*, 825–833.

Fox, J. M. (1994). Malignant pleural effusion. *MEDSURG Nursing, 3*(5), 353–360.

*Frank-Stromborg, M., & Rohan, K. (1992). Nursing's involvement in primary and secondary prevention of cancer: Nationally and internationally. *Cancer Nursing, 15*(2), 79–108.

Garshick, E., Schenker, M., & Dosman, J. (1996). Occupationally induced airways obstruction. *Medical Clinics of North America, 80*(4), 851–878.

Gazarian, P. K. (1997). Teaching your patient to use a metered-dose inhaler: The direct route for asthma therapy. *Nursing97, 27*(10), 52–54.

Georgesen, J., & Dungan, J. M. (1996). Managing spiritual distress in patients with advanced cancer pain. *Cancer Nursing, 19*(5), 376–383.

Gianaris, P. G., & Golish, J. A. (1994). Changing strategies in the management of asthma. *Postgraduate Medicine, 95*(5), 105–110.

Gibbons, M. (1996). Rx for asthma: Are providers following the NHLBI strategy? *ADVANCE for Nurse Practitioners, 4*(7), 45–47.

*Gift, A. G., & Cahill, C. (1990). Psychophysiologic aspects of dyspnea in chronic obstructive pulmonary disease: A pilot study. *Heart and Lung, 19*(3), 252–257.

*Gift, A. G., Moore, T., & Soeken, K. (1992). Relaxation to reduce dyspnea and anxiety in COPD patients. *Nursing Research, 41*(4), 242–246.

Glover, J., & Miaskowski, C. (1994). Small cell lung cancer: Pathophysiologic mechanisms and nursing implications. *Oncology Nursing Forum, 21*(1), 87–97.

Goldstein, R. H., & Fine, A. (1995). Potential therapeutic initiatives for fibrogenic lung disease. *Chest, 108*(3), 848–855.

Gray-Donald, K., Gibbons, L., Shapiro, S. H., Macklem, P. T., & Martin, J. G. (1996). Nutritional status and mortality in chronic obstructive pulmonary disease. *American Journal of Respiratory and Critical Care Medicine, 153,* 961–966.

Hanson, M. J. S. (1997). The theory of planned behavior applied to cigarette smoking in African-American, Puerto Rican, and non-Hispanic white teenage females. *Nursing Research, 46*(3), 155–162.

*Houston, S. J., & Kendall, J. A. (1992). Psychosocial implications of lung cancer. *Nursing Clinics of North America, 27*(3), 681–690.

Hunninghake, G. W., & Kalica, A. R. (1995). Approaches to the treatment of pulmonary fibrosis. *American Journal of Respiratory and Critical Care Medicine, 151,* 915–918.

Imbruce, R. P., & Selevan, J. (1997). Pharmacoeconomics and the quality of life in the diagnosis and management of asthma: What is your FEEVY? *The Journal of Care Management, 3*(Suppl., 3), 1–10.

Kanner, R. E. (1996). Early intervention in chronic obstructive pulmonary disease. *Medical Clinics of North America, 80*(3), 523–544.

*Kersten, L. D. (1989). *Comprehensive respiratory nursing: A decision making approach.* Philadelphia: W. B. Saunders.

Knoell, D. L., & Wewers, M. D. (1995). Clinical implications of gene therapy for alpha$_1$-antitrypsin deficiency. *Chest, 107*(2), 535–545.

Kodiath, M. F., & Kodiath, A. (1995). A comparative study of patients who experience chronic malignant pain in India and the United States. *Cancer Nursing, 18*(3), 189–196.

*Kronenberg, R. S., & Griffith, D. E. (1993). Chronic bronchitis: Key points in evaluation. *Postgraduate Medicine, 94*(8), 93–100.

Langhorne, M. (1996). Chemotherapy. In S. E. Otto (Ed.), *Oncology nursing* (pp. 530–572). St. Louis, MO: C. V. Mosby.

Lareau, S. C. (1996). Functional status instruments: Outcome measure in the evaluation of patients with chronic obstructive pulmonary disease. *Heart and Lung, 25*(3), 212–224.

Lazarus, S. C., & Lofholm, P. W. (1996). *Asthma management: Optimizing the healthcare team.* Laguana, CA: The Institute of Medical Studies.

Le Chevalier, T. (1996). New directions in anticancer chemotherapy. *Seminars in Oncology, 23*(6), 1–2.

Lee, J. D., & Ginsberg, R. J. (1997). The multimodality treatment of stage III a/b non–small cell lung cancer. *Hematology/Oncology Clinics of North America, 11*(20), 279–299.

Lemiere, C., Malo, J., & Gautrin, D. (1996). Nonsensitizing causes of occupational asthma. *Medical Clinics of North America, 80*(4), 749–774.

*Lordi, G. M., & Reichman, L. B. (1993). Pulmonary complications of asbestos exposure. *American Family Physician, 48*(8), 1471–1477.

*Make, B. (1991). COPD: Management and rehabilitation. *American Family Physician, 43*(4), 1315–1324.

Manning, D., Etzel, R., & Parrish, G. (1996). Pulmonary fibrosis deaths in the United States, 1979–1991. *American Journal of Respiratory and Critical Care Medicine, 153,* 1548–1552.

Mathews, P. J. (1997). Using a peak flowmeter. *Nursing97, 27*(6), 57–59.

*McDowell, K. (1993). Drugs for acute bronchitis: An up-to-date guide. *Nursing93, 23*(5), 32I–32L.

McGregor, R. J., & Schakenbach, L. H. (1996). Lung volume reduction surgery: A new breath of life for emphysema patients. *MEDSURG Nursing, 5*(4), 245–252.

McMillian, S. C. (1996). Pain and pain relief experienced by hospice patients with cancer. *Cancer Nursing, 19*(4), 298–307.

McVie, J. G. (1996). Non–small cell lung cancer: Meta-analysis of efficacy of chemotherapy. *Seminars in Oncology, 23*(3), 12–14.

Middleton, A. D. (1997). Managing asthma: It takes team work. *American Journal of Nursing, 97*(1), 39–43.

Minna, J. A. (1996). Molecular biology overview. In H. I. Pass, J. B. Mitchell, D. H. Johnson, & A. T. Turrisi (Eds.), *Lung cancer* (pp. 143–148). Philadelphia, PA: Lippincott-Raven.

Miracle, V., & Miller, D. (1997). Lung volume reduction surgery: Making room for easier breathing. *Nursing97, 27*(6), 65–68.

*Mountain, C. F., Greenberg, S. D., & Fraire, A. E. (1991). Tumor stage in non–small cell carcinoma of the lung. *Chest, 99*(5), 1258–1259.

Nagai, S., & Izumi, T. (1995). Pulmonary sarcoidosis: Population differences and pathophysiology. *Southern Medical Journal, 88*(10), 1001–1010.

*National Center for Health Statistics. (1993). *Health United States, 1992 and healthy people 2000 review* (DHHS Pub. No. [PHS] 93–1232). Hyattsville, MD: Public Health Service.

National Center for Health Statistics. (1996). *Health, United States, 1995* (DHHS Pub. No. [PHS] 96–1232). Hyattsville, MD: Public Health Service.

*National Institute of Health. (1997). *Guidelines for the diagnosis and management of asthma. Expert panel report* 2(97–4051). Bethesda, MD: U.S. Department of Health and Human Services.

Naunheim, K. S., & Ferguson, M. K. (1996). The current status of lung volume reduction operations for emphysema. *Annals of Thoracic Surgery, 62,* 601–612.

Nally, A. T. (1996). Critical care of the patient with lung cancer. *AACN Clinical Issues, 7*(1), 79–94.

*Nelson, D. M. (1992). Interventions related to respiratory care. *The Nursing Clinics of North America, 27*(2), 301–323.

Nelson, H. S. (1995). Beta adrenergic bronchodilators. *New England Journal of Medicine, 333*(8), 499–506.

*O'Donnell, D. E., Webb, K. A., & McGuire, M. A. (1993). COPD: Benefits of exercise training. *Geriatrics, 48*(1), 59–69.

Parker, S. L., Tong, T., Bolden, S., & Wingo, P. A. (1997). Cancer statistics, 1997. *CA: A Cancer Journal for Clinicians, 47*(1), 5–27.

*Petty, T. (1990). *Treatment of asthma in the 1990's.* Princeton, NJ: Excerpta Medica.

*Piirila, P. (1992). Changes in crackle characteristics during the clinical course of pneumonia. *Chest, 102*(1), 176–183.

*Reed, P. G. (1991). Preferences for spiritually related nursing interventions among terminally ill and nonterminally ill hospitalized adults and well adults. *Applied Nursing Research, 4*(3), 122–128.

Reid, D. W., & Samrai, B. (1995). Respiratory muscle training for patients with chronic obstructive pulmonary disease. *Physical Therapy, 75*(11), 996–1005.

*Reinke, L. F., & Hoffman, L. A. (1992). Breathing space: How to teach asthma co-management. *American Journal of Nursing, 92*(10), 40–51.

Rogers, R. M., Sciurba, F. C., & Keenan, R. J. (1996). Lung reduction surgery in chronic obstructive lung disease. *Medical Clinics of North America, 80*(3), 623–644.

Sahn, S. (1996). Chemical pleurodesis for malignant effusions: What is the best agent? *Pulmonary Perspectives, 13*(1), 1–3.

Sarna, L., & Ganley, J. (1995). A survey of lung cancer patient-education. *Oncology Nursing Forum, 22*(10), 1545–1550.

Schottenfeld, D. (1996). Epidemiology of lung cancer. In H. I. Pass, J. B. Mitchell, D. H. Johnson, & A. T. Turrisi (Eds.), *Lung cancer* (pp. 305–321). Philadelphia, PA: Lippincott-Raven.

*Scott, R., Dryzer, M. D., Strange, C., & Sahn, S. A. (1993). A comparison of rotation and non-rotation in tetracycline pleurodesis. *Chest, 104*(6), 1763–1766.

Shell, J. A., Bulson, K. R., & Vanderlugt, L. F. (1996). Lung cancers. In S. E. Otto (Ed.), *Oncology nursing* (pp. 312–346). St. Louis, MO: C. V. Mosby.

Sherman, C. B. (1995). Late-onset asthma: Making the diagnosis, choosing drug therapy. *Geriatrics, 50*(12), 24–33.

Silverman, E. K., & Speizer, F. E. (1996). Risk factors for the development of chronic obstructive pulmonary disease. *Medical Clinics of North America, 80*(3), 501–522.

Snider, G. L. (1996). Reduction pneumoplasty for giant bullous emphysema. *Chest, 109*(2), 540–548.

Taylor, D. R., Sears, M. R., & Crockcroft, D. W. (1996). The beta-agonist controversy. *Medical Clinics of North America, 80*(4), 719–748.

Travis, W. D., Linder, J., & Mackay, B. (1996). Classification, histology, cytology, and electron microscopy. In H. I. Pass, J. B. Mitchell, D. H.

Johnson, & A. T. Turrisi (Eds.), *Lung cancer* (pp. 359–395). Philadelphia, PA: Lippincott-Raven.

*Vork, K. L., & Olson, D. K.(1990). Asbestos review and update. *American Association of Occupational Health Nurses, 38*(4), 160–164.

Walker-Coleman, S. (1996). Oncologic pharmacology: Selected topics for critic care. *AACN Clinical Issues, 7*(1), 46–64.

*Weaver, T. E., & Narsavage, G. L. (1992). Physiological and psychological variables related to functional status in chronic obstructive pulmonary disease. *Nursing Research, 41*(5), 286–291.

Weaver, T. E., Richmond, T. S., & Narsavage, G. L. (1997). An explanatory model of functional status in chronic obstructive pulmonary disease. *Nursing Research, 46*(1), 26–31.

*Webster, J. R., & Kadah, H. (1991). Unique aspects of respiratory disease in the aged. *Geriatrics, 46*(7), 31–43.

Weinberger, M., & Hendeles, L. (1996). Theophylline in asthma. *New England Journal of Medicine, 334*(21), 1380–1388.

Weinmann, G. G., & Hyatt, R. (1996). Evaluation and research in lung volume reduction surgery. *American Journal of Respiratory and Critical Care Medicine, 154,* 1913–1918.

Wilkie, D. J., Williams, A. R., Grevstad, P., & Mekwa, J. (1995). Coaching persons with lung cancer to report sensory pain. *Cancer Nursing, 18*(1), 7–15.

Wilson, R. (1995). Outcome predictors in bronchitis. *Chest, 108*(2), 53S–57S.

Witta, K. (1997). COPD in the elderly. *ADVANCE for Nurse Practitioners, 5*(7), 18–20, 22–23, 27, 72.

Wright, L., & Martin, R. (1995). Nocturnal asthma and exercise-induced bronchospasm. *Postgraduate Medicine, 97*(6), 83–90.

*Yeaw, E. M. J. (1992). Good lung down? *American Journal of Nursing, 92*(3), 27–32.

SUGGESTED READINGS

Dow, J. S., & Mest, C. G. (1997). Psychosocial interventions for patients with chronic obstructive pulmonary disease. *Home Healthcare Nurse, 15*(6), 414–420.

This article focuses on the emotional impact of chronic obstructive pulmonary disease (COPD). Levin's theoretical framework for promoting wholeness is applied to the client with COPD. Personal and social integrity is discussed, as are client and family assessments. The article concludes with a discussion of specific nursing interventions and various obstacles to coping.

Mathews, P. J. (1997). Using a peak flowmeter. *Nursing97, 27*(6), 57–59.

This brief article includes information on the different types of flowmeters and has step-by-step directions on how to use a flowmeter. Baseline parameters as well as the green, yellow, and red zones are defined. Photographs enhance the article.

Middleton, A. D. (1997). Managing asthma: It takes team work. *American Journal of Nursing, 97*(1), 39–43.

The article begins with a review of the pathologic process involved in the early- and late-phase responses to an allergen or irritant in asthma. Exacerbations of the disease; peak-flow monitoring and management; and bronchodilator and antiinflammatory medications are discussed. A chart outlining the stepwise approach to asthma management from the National Heart, Lung, and Blood Institute is included.

Chapter 33

INTERVENTIONS FOR CLIENTS WITH INFECTIONS OF THE RESPIRATORY SYSTEM

DISORDERS OF THE NOSE AND SINUSES

Rhinitis

Overview

Rhinitis is an inflammation of the nasal mucosa and is the most common disorder to affect the nose and sinuses of adults. The cause of rhinitis often involves an interplay of viruses, bacteria, and allergens.

Acute rhinitis may be caused by allergens, bacteria, or viruses. Allergic rhinitis, frequently called "hay fever" or "allergies," is commonly initiated by sensitivity reactions to allergens, especially plant pollens or molds. Acute episodes tend to be seasonal; that is, they disappear after a few weeks and recur at the same time the following year. Chronic rhinitis, or perennial rhinitis, presents intermittently or continuously when a person is exposed to certain allergens, such as dust, animal dander, wool, and foods (e.g., seafood). Rhinitis also can occur after excessive use of nose drops or sprays (rhinitis medicamentosa) as a rebound effect causing nasal congestion or after nasal inhalation of cocaine.

Acute viral rhinitis (coryza, or the common cold) is caused by any one of at least 200 viruses. It usually spreads from one person to another via droplet nuclei from sneezing or coughing and is most contagious in the first 2–3 days after symptoms appear. The condition is self-limiting unless a complication such as otitis media, sinusitis, bronchitis, or pneumonia occurs. Complications are most likely seen in young, elderly, or immunosuppressed people, especially if they live or work in crowded conditions or in group settings such as a long-term care facility.

Collaborative Management

 Assessment

In both acute and chronic allergic rhinitis, the offending substance causes a release of vasoactive mediators (e.g., histamine, serotonin, bradykinin, and prostaglandin), which induce vasodilation and increased capillary permeability. Edema and swelling of the nasal mucosa result, and the client complains of headache, nasal irritation, sneezing, nasal congestion, rhinorrhea (watery drainage from the nose), and itchy, watery eyes. (Chapter 23 further describes the physiologic mechanisms that occur in allergic reactions of the hypersensitivity type.)

In addition to the clinical manifestations observed in clients with allergic rhinitis, clients with viral infections often present with fatigue; a sore, dry throat; and, at times, a low-grade fever with chills.

 Interventions

Management of the client with any type of rhinitis includes symptomatic relief and client education. The physician prescribes appropriate drug therapy, and the nurse instructs the client as indicated. Drugs, including antihistamines and decongestants, are commonly given but must be used with caution in the elderly because of side effects such as vertigo, hypertension, urinary retention, and insomnia. These medications work by causing vasoconstriction and, subsequently, by decreasing edema. Antipyretics are administered if fever is present in the client with viral rhinitis. Antibiotics are not usually prescribed because these agents do not kill the offending virus. Decreasing or discontinuing the offending drug is the treatment for rhinitis medicamentosa.

The nurse instructs the client about the importance of rest (8–10 hours a day), and fluid intake of at least 2000 mL/day (about eight glasses) unless otherwise contraindicated (e.g., as with congestive heart failure, chronic renal failure). Humidification of air helps to relieve congestion; the nurse suggests inhaling steam from a pan of boiled water after removing it from the heat. Hot shower water produces the same effect. The nurse also instructs the client to avoid people who are susceptible to infection for 2–3 days after symptoms begin. Thorough hand washing is another important precaution, especially after the client cleans the nose or sneezes. An uncomplicated cold typically subsides within 7 days.

The client with recurrent allergic rhinitis can undergo allergy testing to determine the cause, and desensitization may help to prevent future episodes. The client may be able to avoid the offending substance. (Chapter 23 further discusses allergies.)

Sinusitis

Overview

Sinusitis is an inflammation of the mucous membranes of one or more of the sinuses. Acute sinusitis results in the obstruction of the flow of secretions from the sinuses, which may subsequently become infected. The disorder frequently accompanies or follows acute or chronic allergic rhinitis. It can also occur in conjunction with other influencing factors, including a deviated nasal septum, polyps, tumors, chronically inhaled air pollutants or cocaine, facial trauma, nasotracheal intubation, dental infection, or cystic fibrosis. In chronic sinusitis, the mucous membrane becomes permanently thickened from prolonged or repeated inflammation or infection.

The causative organism in sinus infection is usually *Streptococcus pneumoniae, Haemophilus influenzae, Diplococ-*

cus, or *Bacteroides.* Anaerobic infections also can cause sinusitis. Sinusitis most often develops in the maxillary and frontal sinuses. Complications include cellulitis, abscess, and meningitis.

Diagnosis is made on the basis of the client's history, signs and symptoms. Endoscopic examination and computed tomography (CT) of the client's sinuses may be performed.

Collaborative Management

 Assessment

The clinical manifestations of sinusitis include nasal swelling and congestion, headache, facial pressure, pain (usually aggravated by movement of the head to a dependent position), tenderness on percussion over involved area, low-grade fever, cough, and purulent or bloody nasal drainage.

 Interventions

➤ Nonsurgical Management

The treatment for sinusitis includes the use of broad-spectrum antibiotics (e.g., amoxicillin), analgesics for pain and fever (e.g., acetaminophen [Tylenol, Atasol✦]), decongestants (e.g., phenylephrine [Neo-Synephrine], astemizole [Hismanal]), steam humidification, hot, wet packs over the sinus area, and nasal saline irrigations. The nurse instructs the client to increase free water intake to more than ten glasses of water or juice per day unless medically contraindicated. When this treatment plan is not successful, the physician orders additional evaluation with sinus films and CT. Surgical intervention may be necessary.

➤ Surgical Management

Antral Irrigation. Antral irrigation, also known as maxillary antral puncture and lavage, is an outpatient surgical procedure. After local anesthesia, a large-gauge needle is inserted under the inferior turbinate of the nose and into the maxillary sinus on the affected side. Fluid or purulent material from the sinus is withdrawn. The sinus is then irrigated with saline solution, an antibiotic solution, or both.

Other Surgical Procedures. If antral irrigation is not successful, other surgical procedures may be used to open the sinus cavities in clients with chronic sinusitis. In the Caldwell-Luc procedure, the surgeon makes an incision in the anterior wall of the maxillary sinus under the upper lip. The infected mucosa in the maxillary sinus is removed. With the nasal antral window procedure, the surgeon creates an opening in the anterior portion of the inferior turbinate to allow for unobstructed drainage through the nares. With either procedure, the client may have difficulty eating for a few days postoperatively because of pain and swelling. Chart 33–1 covers nursing care for clients undergoing these procedures.

When the ethmoid sinuses need to be opened, the surgeon uses an external approach for better visibility and

---

Chart 33–1

Nursing Care Highlight: Postoperative Care for Clients with Sinus Surgery

- Position the client in the semi-Fowler's position to promote drainage and prevent swelling.
- Perform gentle oral hygiene to promote healing and prevent injury to the surgical incision.
- Use ice compresses as ordered for 24 hours.
- Change the "mustache" dressing under the nose as needed, and record the type and amount of drainage.
- Instruct the client to eat soft foods and increase fluid intake.
- Instruct the client to limit the Valsalva maneuver (no coughing, blowing the nose, or straining at stool) for at least 2 weeks postoperatively to prevent bleeding and tissue damage.

---

preservation of structures. The surgical incision is made along the side of the nose from the middle of the eyebrow (Weber-Ferguson incision).

Endoscopic Sinus Surgery. Endoscopic sinus surgery has become a revolutionary method of diagnosing and treating sinus disorders. Direct inspection of the sinuses through a sinus endoscope is an improved surgical procedure for refractory sinus disorders. Completed with the client under general anesthesia in an outpatient surgical center, the procedure takes only minutes. The client goes home the same day and can return to work in 4–5 days. Nasal mucosa may take up to 4–6 weeks to heal. The nurse instructs the client in frequent use of saline nasal sprays to prevent intranasal and sinus crusting and promote healing.

DISORDERS OF THE ORAL PHARYNX AND TONSILS

Pharyngitis

Overview

Pharyngitis is an inflammation of the mucous membranes of the pharynx. It may precede acute rhinitis or sinusitis, or these conditions may occur simultaneously with pharyngitis.

Acute pharyngitis has multiple causes (Table 33–1). The most common bacterial organism causing pharyngitis is group A beta-hemolytic *Streptococcus*, but most adult cases are caused by a virus. The incidence of streptococcal infection rises between late fall and spring, especially in the colder climates.

Collaborative Management

 Assessment

Pharyngitis is characterized by soreness and dryness in the throat, pain, pain on swallowing (odynophagia), difficulty in swallowing (dysphagia), and fever. Viral and bac-

terial pharyngitis is often difficult to differentiate on physical assessment. When inspecting the mucous membranes of a throat infected with either virus or bacteria, the nurse may note a mild to severe hyperemia (redness) with or without enlarged erythematous tonsils and with or without exudate. The nurse asks about nasal discharge, which can vary from thin and watery to thick and purulent. Cervical lymphadenopathy may be present in either viral or bacterial pharyngitis. With a parapharyngeal (or tonsillar) abscess, the client may have a characteristic "hot potato" voice, a thickened voice of poor quality.

Clinical studies indicate that streptococcal or other bacterial infections are more often associated with enlarged erythematous tonsils with exudate, purulent nasal discharge, and cervical lymphadenopathy. Chart 33–2 outlines the clinical manifestations of viral versus bacterial pharyngitis. Viral pharyngitis is communicable for 2–3 days; symptoms usually subside within 3–10 days after onset. The disease is usually self-limiting.

Bacterial pharyngitis, such as group A streptococcal infection, however, can lead to dangerous medical complications (Table 33–2). The two most serious complications, acute glomerulonephritis (Chap. 74) and rheumatic fever carditis (Chap. 37), occur in 1% to 3% of cases. Acute glomerulonephritis generally occurs 7–10 days after the acute infection, and rheumatic fever may develop 3–5 weeks after an acute streptococcal infection.

Throat cultures are important to diagnosing viral from

TABLE 33–1

Causes of Pharyngitis

Bacterial Causes

- *Streptococcus*
- *Staphylococcus*
- *Haemophilus influenzae*
- Pneumococcus
- *Corynebacterium diphtheriae*
- *Neisseria gonorrhoeae*

Viral Causes

- Adenovirus
- Rhinovirus
- Epstein-Barr virus
- Cytomegalovirus (CMV)
- Influenza virus
- Parainfluenza virus
- Herpesvirus
- Coxsackievirus A
- Echovirus

Other Causes

- *Chlamydia*
- *Mycoplasma pneumoniae*
- *Candida*
- Physical and chemical causes
  - Alcohol
  - Tobacco
  - Heat
  - Irritants
  - Dehydration
  - Trauma

Chart 33–2

Key Features of Acute Viral and Bacterial Pharyngitis

Feature	Viral Pharyngitis	Bacterial Pharyngitis
Temperature	• Low-grade or no fever	• High temperature (above 101° F [38° C], and usually 102°–104° F [38.5°–40° C])
Ear manifestations	• Retracted and/or dull tympanic membrane	• Retracted and/or dull tympanic membrane
Throat manifestations	• Scant or no tonsillar exudate • Slight erythema of pharynx and tonsils	• Severe hyperemia of pharyngeal mucosa, tonsils, and uvula • Erythema of tonsils with yellow exudate
Neck manifestations	• Possible lymphadenopathy	• Anterior cervical lymphadenopathy and tenderness
Skin manifestations	• No rash	• Possible scarlatiniform rash • Possible petechiae on chest and/or abdomen
Dysphagia, odynophagia	• Present	• Present
Other symptoms	• No cough • Rhinitis • Mild hoarseness • Headache	• No cough • Voice characterized by pain on voicing and slurred speech • Arthralgia • Myalgia
Laboratory data	• Complete blood count usually normal • White blood cell count usually lower than 10,000/mm^3 • Negative throat culture results	• Complete blood count abnormal • White blood cell count usually higher than 12,000/mm^3 • Throat culture results positive for beta-hemolytic streptococcus
Onset	• Gradual	• Abrupt

group A beta-hemolytic streptococcal infection, but results are not entirely accurate; both false-negative and false-positive results occur. To obtain a specimen, the nurse or physician rubs a cotton swab over each tonsillar area and over the posterior pharynx. The cotton swab is then

TABLE 33–2

Complications of Group A Streptococcal Infection

- Rheumatic fever
- Acute glomerulonephritis
- Peritonsillar abscess
- Retropharyngeal abscess
- Otitis media
- Sinusitis
- Mastoiditis
- Bronchitis
- Pneumonia
- Scarlet fever

streaked on a blood agar plate, which is incubated for 24 hours. An easier and faster method for determining the type of infection is a test using latex agglutination for group A streptococcal antigen; results are ready in 10 minutes, allowing rapid initiation of treatment. The incidence of sequelae of streptococcal infection should decrease with faster testing and treatment.

A complete blood count is performed when the client's condition is severe or not improving. The client may exhibit extremely high temperatures, lethargy, or signs and symptoms of complications. A complete blood count may indicate other causes of pharyngitis.

When taking a history, the nurse inquires about the client's recent contacts (within the last 10 days) with people who have been ill. Of particular importance is whether the client has been ill with symptoms of a cold or upper respiratory tract infection recently or in the past. Documenting previous streptococcal infections is essential. The nurse also notes a history of rheumatic fever, valvular heart disease, streptococcal infections, or penicillin allergy. Because diphtheria (*Corynebacterium diphtheriae*) can cause pharyngitis, the nurse questions and documents whether the client has had a diphtheria immunization.

Interventions

Most sore throats in adults are viral and do not warrant the use of antibiotics. The treatment plan includes rest, increased fluid intake, humidification of the air, analgesics for pain, warm saline throat gargles, and throat lozenges containing mild anesthetics.

The management of bacterial pharyngitis involves the use of antibiotics and the same supportive care provided for viral pharyngitis. For streptococcal infection, the physician typically prescribes an oral penicillin preparation. If the client is allergic to penicillin, erythromycin is the alternative. The nurse counsels the client on the importance of completing the entire antibiotic prescription, even if symptoms subside. If the client cannot tolerate the medication, the nurse notifies the physician so that a change in the antibiotic regimen can be made. If compliance is a concern or the client cannot swallow pills, long-acting benzathine penicillin, 1.2 million units, can be administered intramuscularly in a single dose to eradicate the organism. The client should be re-evaluated if there is no improvement in 3 days or if the symptoms are still present after completion of the antibiotic course.

The nurse instructs the client in the proper procedure for taking an oral temperature reading. This reading should be taken in the morning and in the evening until convalescence is complete. The client is not contagious after 24 hours of treatment. Family members or significant others who experience a sore throat should be evaluated, and a throat culture may be indicated.

Tonsillitis

Overview

Tonsillitis is an inflammation and infection of the tonsils and the lymphatic tissue located on each lateral side of the oropharynx (where the palatine, or faucial, tonsils are located). The tonsils consist of lymphatic tissue shaped like a small almond. Each tonsil is covered by a mucous membrane. These lymphatic tissues filter microorganisms, thus functioning as a protective mechanism for the respiratory and gastrointestinal tracts.

Tonsillitis is a contagious airborne infection. Acute or chronic tonsillitis can occur in any age group, but 5- to 10-year-old children are affected most often. The infection is usually more severe when it occurs in adolescents or adults.

The acute form usually lasts 7–10 days and is most often caused by a bacterial organism. The most common organism is *Streptococcus*. Other bacterial pathogens include *Staphylococcus aureus*, *H. influenzae,* and *Pneumococcus.* Viruses may also cause tonsillitis. Chronic tonsillitis usually results from either an acute infection that did not resolve or from recurrent infections.

Collaborative Management

◆ Assessment

Chart 33–3 summarizes the signs and symptoms of acute tonsillitis. Diagnostic studies are performed to rule out

---

Chart 33–3

Key Features of Acute Tonsillitis

- Sudden onset of a mild to severe sore throat
- Fever
- Muscle aches
- Chills
- Dysphagia, odynophagia (painful swallowing of food)
- Pain in the ears
- Headache
- Anorexia
- Malaise
- "Hot potato" voice (thickened voice of poor quality)
- Tonsils visually swollen and red with pus
- Tonsils may be covered with a white or yellow exudate
- Purulent drainage may be expressed upon pressing a tonsil
- Uvula visually edematous or inflamed
- Cervical lymph nodes usually tender and enlarged

---

other causes of the sore throat and fever (such as acute pharyngitis). A complete blood count, throat culture and sensitivity (C & S) studies, monospot test, and chest x-ray (if respiratory symptoms are present) may be ordered for a client with suspected tonsillitis. In bacterial infections, the white blood cell count is elevated. Throat culture and sensitivity studies identify the causative bacterial organism and direct the choice of regimen.

 Interventions

The physician orders systemic antibiotics (usually penicillin or erythromycin) for 7–10 days. Warm saline throat gargles, analgesics, antipyretics, and lozenges with topical anesthetic ingredients may provide symptomatic relief.

Indications for surgical intervention include
- Recurrent acute infections or chronic infections that have not responded to antibiotic therapy
- Peritonsillar abscess
- Infected hypertrophy of the tonsils or adenoids that obstructs the airway

The indication for surgery becomes stronger with evidence of repeated group A beta-hemolytic streptococcal infections. Surgery is generally not indicated if the client is experiencing an acute tonsillar infection (except with an acute peritonsillar abscess) or has a blood dyscrasia such as aplastic anemia, hemophilia, or leukemia.

The most common surgical procedure to remove the tonsils is dissection and snare. The adenoids are removed with an adenoid curette or adenotome. A tonsillectomy and adenoidectomy (T&A) is usually performed with the client under general anesthesia but is performed infrequently in adults. Postoperatively, the nurse focuses care on the following nursing diagnoses:
- Risk for Injury related to ineffective airway clearance
- Pain related to surgery and edema
- Fluid Volume Deficit related to bleeding

Peritonsillar Abscess

Overview

Peritonsillar abscess (PTA), or *quinsy*, is a complication of acute tonsillitis. The acute infection spreads from the tonsil to the surrounding peritonsillar tissue, which forms an abscess. It is one of the most common abscesses of the head and neck area. The common cause of PTA is group A beta-hemolytic streptococcus. Anaerobic organisms also may be the cause.

Collaborative Management

 Assessment

At physical examination, signs of infection are pronounced. Pus forms behind the tonsil and causes a marked asymmetric swelling and deviation of the uvula. Because of the swelling, the client may experience drooling, severe throat pain that may radiate to the ear, a voice change, and difficulty swallowing. The client may also exhibit a tonic contraction of the muscles of mastication (trismus) and complain of difficulty breathing.

 Interventions

The nurse instructs the client about comfort measures such as warm saline gargles or irrigations, an ice collar, analgesics, and the importance of completing the antibiotic regimen. The client should improve in 24–48 hours. Outpatient management using percutaneous needle aspiration and antibiotic therapy may be indicated. Hospitalization is required when the client's airway is in jeopardy or when the infection is refractory to conventional antibiotic therapy. Incision and drainage (I&D) of the abscess, plus additional antibiotic therapy, may be indicated. A tonsillectomy may be performed to prevent recurrence.

DISORDERS OF THE LARYNX AND LUNGS

Laryngitis

Overview

Laryngitis is an inflammation of the mucous membranes lining the larynx and may or may not include edema of the vocal cords. It is commonly associated with upper respiratory tract infections, and can be an entity itself or a symptom of a related disease process. Etiologic factors include exposure to irritating inhalants and pollutants, including chemical agents, tobacco, alcohol, and smoke; overuse of the voice; inhalation of volatile gases such as glue, paint thinner, and butane; or intubation.

Collaborative Management

 Assessment

The nurse assesses the client for acute hoarseness, dry cough, and dysphagia. Complete but temporary voice loss (*aphonia*) also may occur. The physician performs a laryngeal examination to assist in the diagnosis. A laryngeal mirror is used to examine the larynx and to differentiate inflammation, polyps, edema, or tumor. The physician may further order radiography and CT and fiberoptic laryngoscopic examination. Most clients are referred to an ear, nose, and throat (ENT) specialist for any suspected disorder other than acute laryngitis.

 Interventions

Nursing management is aimed toward relief of presenting symptoms and the introduction of further preventive measures. Treatment consists of voice rest, steam inhalations, increased fluid intake, and topical throat lozenges. The physician may order antibiotic therapy and bronchodilators when sinusitis, bronchitis, or a bacterial upper respiratory tract infection is also present. The nurse informs the client and family about immediate acute care therapies, infection prevention, and avoidance of alcohol, tobacco, and pollutants.

Preventive therapy is aimed toward increasing the client's and family's awareness of the hazards of tobacco and alcohol use. The nurse also emphasizes the activities that place an added strain on the larynx, such as singing, cheering, public speaking, heavy lifting, and whispering. Speech therapy is often the treatment of choice for vocal cord injuries and should be implemented for any voice disorder. For recurrent bouts of laryngitis, further medical and speech therapy evaluation are necessary.

Influenza

Influenza, or "flu," is an acute viral respiratory infection that can occur in adults of all ages. Because influenza is highly contagious, epidemics are common and can lead to complications like pneumonia or death, especially in elderly and immunocompromised clients. Hospitalization may be required. Influenza may be caused by one of several viruses, usually referred to as A, B, and C. The client with this disorder typically complains of severe headache, muscle aches, fever, chills, fatigue, weakness, and anorexia. Clinical manifestations associated with the respiratory system, such as a sore throat, cough, and rhinorrhea (watery discharge from the nose), generally follow the initial symptoms for a week or more. Most clients continue to complain of general malaise for 1–2 weeks after the acute episode has resolved.

Treatment of influenza is symptomatic because antibiotics are ineffective against viral infections. The nurse recommends that the client remain in bed for several days and drink copious amounts of fluids unless contraindicated by some other physical condition, such as chronic renal failure or congestive heart failure. Saline gargles may ease sore throat pain; when ordered, antihistamines may reduce the rhinorrhea. Other palliative measures are the same as those for acute rhinitis.

During the past two decades, vaccinations for the prevention of influenza have been developed and widely administered. With advanced refinement of the vaccine, allergic reaction is rare. The vaccine is altered every year on the basis of specific viral strains that are likely to pose a problem during the influenza season, that is, late fall and winter. It is highly recommended that persons older than 65 years, those with chronic illness or immune compromise, those living in institutions, and health care personnel in direct care of clients receive the vaccine each year, typically during October or November.

Pneumonia

Overview

Pneumonia is an inflammatory process that results in edema of interstitial lung tissue and extravasation of fluid into alveoli, causing hypoxemia. It can be caused by infectious or noninfectious irritating agents, such as inhaled fumes or aspirated food or fluids. Pneumonias are classified as community acquired (which includes the community proper and extended care facilities) or nosocomial (hospital acquired). In the past, antibiotics have reduced the mortality of pneumonia, but the recent emergence of new pathogens and resistant organisms has the health care community concerned.

Pathophysiology

The inflammation in pneumonia occurs in the interstitial spaces, the alveoli, and often the bronchioles. The pneumonic process begins in infectious pneumonia when pathogens successfully penetrate the airway mucus and multiply in the alveolar spaces. To do this, they must survive the lung's many defenses against microbial invasion. As the pathogenic organisms multiply, edematous fluid forms, and other evidence of inflammation becomes apparent. White blood cells migrate into the alveoli and cause thickening of the alveolar wall. Red blood cells and fibrin extravasate into the alveoli. Fluid fills the alveoli, which protects the organisms from phagocytosis and facilitates the movement of organisms to other alveoli. In this way, the infection spreads. If the invading organisms obtain access to the bloodstream, septicemia results; if the infection extends into the pleural cavity, an empyema results. (Chapter 23 discusses inflammation in detail and Chapter 28 has more on the infectious process.)

The fibrin and edema of inflammation stiffen the lung, thus causing decreased lung compliance and a decline in the vital capacity (VC) of the lung. Decreased production of surfactant further reduces compliance and leads to atelectasis. Some of the venous blood coming into the lungs passes through the underventilated area. This unoxygenated blood then travels to the left side of the heart. As a result, arterial oxygen tension falls, causing hypoxemia (insufficient oxygen in the blood).

Systemically, fever results from the infection. The client may develop shaking chills in an attempt to increase heat production and raise the metabolic rate. Hypoxemia and an increase in metabolic demand cause secondary tachypnea with tachycardia. Blood pressure may fall as a result of peripheral vasodilation and decreased circulating blood volume secondary to dehydration. Cardiac function may be compromised by hypoxemia and enhanced metabolism. Congestive heart failure or shock may result, and cardiac irritability may be enhanced because of inadequate tissue oxygenation, thus causing dysrhythmias.

Pneumonia may occur as lobar pneumonia with consolidation (solidification, lack of air spaces) in a segment or an entire lobe of the lung, or as bronchopneumonia, with diffuse patches around the bronchi. The extent of pulmonary involvement after the microbial invasion depends on the defenses of the host. In an immunocompromised host, bacteria can multiply. Tissue necrosis results when multiplying anaerobic organisms form an abscess that perforates the bronchial wall.

Etiology

In general, individuals develop pneumonia when their defense mechanisms are unable to combat the virulence of the invading organisms. Organisms from the environment, invasive devices, equipment and supplies, staff, or other people can invade the body. Risk factors are listed in Table 33–3. Bacteria, viruses, mycoplasmas, fungi, rickettsiae, protozoa, and helminths (worms) can all cause pneumonia; the most common organisms are listed in Table 33–4. Noninfectious causes of pneumonia include inhalation of toxic gases, chemicals, smoke, and aspiration of water, food, fluid, and vomitus.

Prevention is aimed at immunizing against the causative agent when possible and reducing the other risks of infection or exposure.

There are different serotypes of the pneumoniae organism, the most common being 6B, 23F, 14, 9V, 19A and 19F. All of these serotypes are included in the 23-valent pneumococcal vaccine that has been available since 1983. Client education is an important factor in the prevention of pneumonia (Chart 33–4), as is making the vaccines readily available to those most at risk.

TABLE 33–3

Risk Factors Associated with Pneumonia
Community-Acquired Pneumonias
Elderly
No history of pneumococcal vaccination
No history of having received the influenza vaccine in the previous year
Chronic or other co-existing condition
Recent history of, or exposure to, viral or influenza infections
History of tobacco or alcohol use
Nosocomial Pneumonias
Elderly
Chronic lung disease
Gram-negative colonization of the oropharynx and stomach
Altered level of consciousness
Aspiration
Endotracheal, tracheostomy, or nasogastric tube
Poor nutritional status
Immunocompromised status (from disease, medications)
Medications that increase gastric pH (H$_2$ blockers, antacids) or alkaline tube feedings
Mechanical ventilation

TABLE 33-4

Common Organisms Causing Pneumonia*

Community-Acquired Pneumonias

- *Streptococcus pneumoniae* (Gram positive)
- *Staphylococcus aureus* (Gram positive)
- *Haemophilus influenzae* (Gram negative)
- *Legionella pneumophila* (Gram negative)
- *Mycoplasma pneumoniae* (smallest free-living organism)
- *Chlamydia pneumoniae* (parasite)

Nosocomial Pneumonias

- *Staphylococcus aureus* (Gram positive)
- *Pseudomonas aeruginosa* (Gram negative)
- *Enterobacter* (Gram negative)
- *Klebsiella* (Gram negative)
- *Haemophilus influenzae* (Gram negative)
- *Acinetobacter* (Gram negative)
- *Candida albicans* (fungus)

*Because of various factors influencing the incidence of the pathogenic causes of pneumonia, these organisms are listed loosely in order of incidence.

The nurse follows strict hand washing and aseptic techniques to avoid the spread of organisms. Respiratory therapy equipment is well maintained and is decontaminated or changed as recommended. Sterile water rather than tap water is used in gastrointestinal tubes, and aspiration precautions are initiated as indicated. Specific interventions to prevent aspiration are discussed in Chapters 31 and 47.

Chart 33-4

Health Promotion Guide: Preventing Pneumonia

- Know whether you are at risk for pneumonia.
- Have the annual influenza vaccine after discussing appropriate timing of the vaccination with your primary health care provider.
- Discuss the usually once-in-a-lifetime pneumococcal vaccine with your primary health care provider and have the vaccination as recommended.
- Avoid crowded public areas during flu and holiday seasons.
- Cough, turn, move about, and perform deep-breathing exercises as directed by your nurse or other health care professional.
- If you are using respiratory equipment at home, clean the equipment as you have been taught.
- Avoid indoor pollutants, such as dust, secondhand (passive) smoke, and aerosols.
- If you don't smoke, don't start.
- If you smoke, seek professional help on how to stop, or at least decrease, your habit.
- Be sure to get enough rest and sleep on a daily basis.
- Eat a healthy, balanced diet and take in a sufficient amount of nonalcoholic fluids each day.

TRANSCULTURAL CONSIDERATIONS

A national health objective for the year 2000 is to vaccinate 60% of those at risk for pneumococcal disease and influenza; yet in 1995, only 35% of those older than 64 reported ever having received the pneumococcal vaccine, whereas 58% reported having received the influenza vaccine in the previous year. These percentages represent substantial increases since 1993. Of those older than 64, the highest levels of vaccination were found in women and Caucasians (Centers for Disease Control and Prevention [CDC], 1997a).

Incidence/Prevalence

There are 2–4 million cases of pneumonia per year in the United States; highest incidence occurs in those younger than 5 years, the elderly, nursing home residents, hospitalized clients, and those being mechanically ventilated (Craven & Steger, 1995; Mandell, 1995). During late fall and winter, a higher incidence of community-acquired pneumonia is likely because this illness frequently follows viral or influenza infection. Hospital-acquired pneumonia is the second most common nosocomial infection (Craven & Steger, 1995; Calianno, 1996).

Pneumonia and influenza as a combined cause of death rank sixth in the United States, and the combination is the number one cause of death from infection (King & Pippin, 1997). Nosocomial pneumonia has a 20% to 50% mortality; the highest incidence is in those with *Pseudomonas aeruginosa*, *Acinetobacter*, other "high-risk" organisms, or secondary bacteremia. Mortality also is higher in individuals who experience complications (Table 33–5). Over the past few years, interventions for pneumonia have become more aggressive in order to try to reduce the high incidence of death from this disorder.

ELDERLY CONSIDERATIONS

Pneumonia and influenza constitute the third leading cause of death for clients older than 85 years. For clients older than 64 years, the death rate between 1979 and 1992 increased 44%, from 145.6 deaths per 100,000 population to 209.1 (CDC, 1995c).

TABLE 33-5

Common Complications of Pneumonia

Hypoxemia	• Arterial oxygen <55 mmHg
Ventilatory failure	• Lungs unable to move gas in and out of lungs mechanically, resulting in hypoxemia and hypercapnia
Atelectasis	• Collapse of the affected alveoli and associated lobes of the lungs
Pleural effusion	• Collection of fluid in the pleural space (usually sterile fluid that resolves)
Pleurisy	• Pain caused by friction between layers of pleura

Collaborative Management

 Assessment

➤ History

In preparing to take the history from the client who may have pneumonia, the nurse considers risk factors consistent with infection (see Table 33–3). The nurse collects essential data from the client or a family member if the client is too dyspneic. The nurse documents data on the following:

- Age
- Living, work, or school environment
- Diet, exercise, and sleep routines
- Swallowing problems
- Nasogastrointestinal tube
- Tobacco and alcohol use
- Past and current use of medications
- History of drug addiction or intravenous (IV) drug use

The nurse lists the client's past illnesses, particularly those with a respiratory origin, and determines whether the client has been exposed to influenza or pneumonia or has experienced a recent viral episode. In addition, the nurse notes a history of any rashes, insect bites, or exposure to animals.

If the client has chronic respiratory problems, the nurse asks whether respiratory equipment is used in the home. It is essential to determine whether the client's cleaning regimen is adequate to prevent infection. The nurse also notes prior inoculations with influenza or pneumococcal vaccine.

➤ Physical Assessment/Clinical Manifestations

The nurse first observes the general appearance of the client, who may present with flushed cheeks, bright eyes, and an anxious expression. The client may have chest or pleuritic pain or discomfort, myalgia, headache, chills, fever, cough, tachycardia, dyspnea, tachypnea, and sputum production. Severe chest muscle weakness also may be present from sustained coughing.

The nurse observes the client's breathing pattern, position, and use of accessory muscles. The acutely compromised client is uncomfortable in a lying position and sits upright, balancing with the hands. The nurse assesses the client's cough and the amount, color, consistency, and odor of sputum produced for diagnostic clues about the offending pathogen.

Upon auscultation, the nurse hears crackles when there is fluid in interstitial and alveolar areas. Wheezing may be heard as a result of inflammation and exudate in the airways. Bronchial breath sounds are heard over areas of density or consolidation. Tactile fremitus is increased over areas of pneumonia, and percussion is dulled in these areas. Chest expansion may be diminished or unequal on inspiration. (Chapter 29 discusses respiratory assessment in more detail.)

In evaluating vital signs, the nurse compares the results with baseline values. The client who has pneumonia is likely to be hypotensive with orthostatic changes. A rapid, weak pulse may indicate hypoxemia, dehydration, or impending shock.

The nurse also inspects the skin for a rash, which may occur with *Mycoplasma* infection, cytomegalovirus infection (CMV), or Rocky Mountain spotted fever. The pathophysiology of selected clinical manifestations of pneumonia is summarized in Table 33–6.

ELDERLY CONSIDERATIONS

The nurse is aware of risk and predisposing factors (see Table 33–3). The elderly often have weakness, fatigue, lethargy, confusion, and poor appetite. Fever and cough may be absent, but hypoxemia is usually present.

➤ Psychosocial Assessment

The client with pneumonia experiences pain, fatigue, and dyspnea, which promote anxiety. The nurse assesses anxiety by looking at the client's facial expression and general tenseness of facial and shoulder muscles. The nurse listens to the client carefully and uses a calm, slow approach to assessment. Because of airway obstruction and muscle fatigue, the client with dyspnea speaks in broken sentences. The nurse gauges the length of the interview on the degree of dyspnea or breathing discomfort the client experiences.

TABLE 33–6

Pathophysiology of Selected Clinical Manifestations of Pneumonia	
Clinical Manifestation	**Pathophysiology**
Increased respiratory rate/dyspnea	• Stimulation of chemoreceptors • Increased work of breathing as a result of decreased lung compliance • Stimulation of J receptors • Anxiety • Pain
Hypoxemia	• Alveolar consolidation • Capillary shunting
Cough	• Fluid accumulation in the subepithelial mechanoreceptors in the trachea, bronchi, and bronchioles
Purulent, blood-tinged, or rust-colored sputum	• A result of the inflammatory process in which fluid from the pulmonary capillaries and red blood cells moves into the alveoli
Fever	• Phagocytes release endogenous pyrogens that cause the hypothalamus to increase body temperature
Pleuritic chest discomfort	• Inflammation of the parietal pleura causes pain on inspiration

➤ *Laboratory Assessment*

Sputum is obtained from the client and examined by Gram's stain, culture, and sensitivity testing. A sputum sample is easily obtained from the client who can cough into a specimen container. Extremely ill clients may require nasotracheal suctioning by the nurse or suctioning via a tracheostomy or endotracheal tube. In these situations, the nurse obtains a sputum specimen via sputum trap (Fig. 33–1) while suctioning. The responsible organism, however, may not be identified in as many as 50% of the cases. Sensitivity testing determines how resistant or sensitive the organism is to various anti-infective agents.

A complete blood count (CBC) is obtained to identify leukocytosis, which is a common finding, except in the elderly. Blood cultures may be performed to determine whether the organism has invaded the bloodstream. Assessment for human immunodeficiency virus (HIV) may be performed. Urine may be examined for hematuria, pyuria, and the presence of protein, which may occur in the septic client with pneumonia.

Arterial blood gases (ABGs) determine baseline arterial oxygen and carbon dioxide levels and help identify a need for supplemental oxygen. Serum electrolyte, blood urea nitrogen (BUN), and creatinine levels also are assessed. An increased BUN value may occur as a result of increased catabolism and a diminished glomerular filtration rate. Electrolyte changes occur with dehydration, a result of fever and malaise.

➤ *Radiographic Assessment*

In general, pneumonia appears on chest x-ray as an area of increased density. It may involve a lung segment, a lobe, one lung, or both lungs. In the elderly, the chest x-ray is essential for early diagnosis of pneumonia because their symptoms are often vague.

➤ *Other Diagnostic Assessment*

The nurse obtains oxygen saturation values by using pulse oximetry. This noninvasive test (see Chap. 29) helps detect hypoxemia. The physician may order invasive tests such as transtracheal aspiration, bronchoscopy, or direct needle aspiration of the lung to obtain lower airway specimens in selected clients; thoracentesis is most often used in those clients with pleural effusion.

 Analysis

➤ *Common Nursing Diagnoses and Collaborative Problems*

Two of the nursing diagnoses commonly identified for the client with pneumonia include
1. Impaired Gas Exchange related to effects of alveolo-capillary membrane changes
2. Ineffective Airway Clearance related to effects of infection, excessive tracheobronchial secretions, fatigue and decreased energy, chest discomfort, and muscle weakness

A common collaborative problem for the client with pneumonia is potential for sepsis related to an infectious organism.

➤ *Additional Nursing Diagnoses and Collaborative Problems*

In addition to the common diagnoses, the client may present with associated problems, which could include those listed for the client with chronic airflow limitation (see Chap. 32). Other nursing diagnoses include
- Pain related to effects of inflammation of parietal pleura, coughing
- Hyperthermia related to an increased metabolic rate, dehydration
- Fluid Volume Deficit related to fever, infection, increased metabolic rate
- Ineffective Breathing Pattern related to fatigue, decreased energy, pain, the inflammatory process, and anxiety
- Sleep Pattern Disturbance related to pain, dyspnea, unfamiliar environment (hospitalization)

An additional collaborative problem is potential for pleural effusion related to spread of the infection.

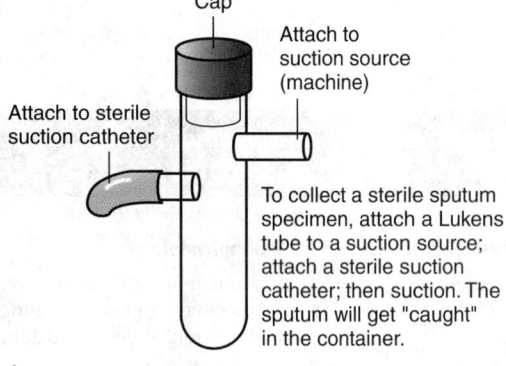

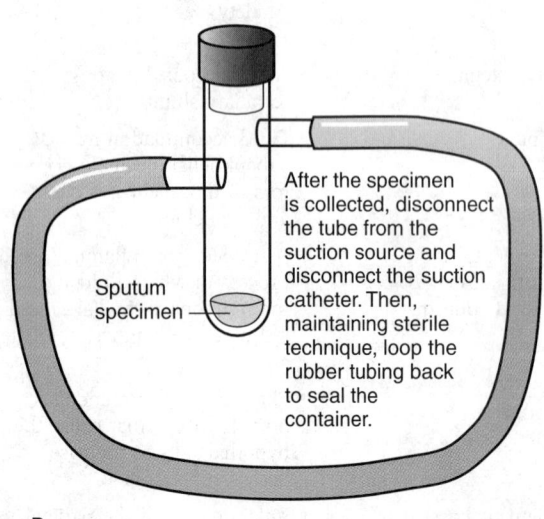

Figure 33–1. Method of collecting a sterile sputum specimen using a Lukens tube.

➤ Impaired Gas Exchange

Planning: Expected Outcomes. For the client with impaired gas exchange, the major expected outcome is to attain or maintain partial pressure of arterial oxygen and carbon dioxide (PaO_2 and $PaCO_2$, respectively) and oxygen saturation values within baseline ranges. Other expected outcomes are similar to those for the client with chronic airflow limitation (CAL).

Interventions. For the client with pneumonia, interventions to treat and manage impaired gas exchange are similar to those for the client with CAL (see Chap. 32). In pneumonia, the gas exchange affected most is oxygen; therefore, hypoxemia is the primary problem. Carbon dioxide retention is not as common in pneumonia as it is, for example, in chronic emphysema.

Incentive spirometry, also referred to as sustained maximal inspiration, is a type of bronchial hygiene used in pneumonia. The objective is to improve inspiratory muscle performance and to prevent or reverse atelectasis. The nurse obtains an incentive spirometer and instructs the client to exhale fully, then place the mouthpiece in the mouth, and take a long, slow, deep breath for 3–5 seconds. The nurse evaluates the client's technique and records the volume of air inspired. The client performs 5–10 breaths per session every hour while awake. Chapter 20 has more information on incentive spirometry.

➤ Ineffective Airway Clearance

Planning: Expected Outcomes. For the client with ineffective airway clearance, the major expected outcome is that the client will have optimal breath sounds. The goal may be to have clear lungs in all lobes upon auscultation or to have, minimally, improved breath sounds. Other goals are similar to those for the client with chronic airflow limitation (CAL).

Interventions. For the client with pneumonia, interventions for the treatment and management of ineffective airway clearance are similar to those for the client with CAL. Because of fatigue, muscle weakness, chest discomfort, and excessive secretions, the client with pneumonia often has difficulty clearing secretions. The nurse helps the client to cough and deep breathe at least every 2 hours. The alert client may use an incentive spirometer to facilitate deep breathing and stimulate coughing. Chest physiotherapy (CPT or chest PT), which was once thought to be useful for clearing secretions in the client with pneumonia, is no longer recommended in uncomplicated pneumonia. Whereas dehydration should be avoided, there is no evidence that hydration helps to clear secretions. Adequate hydration may help in thinning secretions and making them easier to remove. To ensure adequate hydration when fever and tachypnea are present, the nurse monitors intake and output.

The physician prescribes bronchodilators, especially beta-2 agonists (see Chart 32–4), when bronchospasm is part of the disease process. They are usually administered initially by aerosol nebulizer and then by metered-dose inhaler (see Chart 32–5). The use of mucolytic agents and expectorants has been found to be of marginal value

in the treatment of pneumonia. Inhaled steroid preparations are generally not used with acute pneumonia except when the client also has bronchial asthma or respiratory failure.

➤ Potential for Sepsis

Planning: Expected Outcomes. For the client with sepsis, the major expected outcome is to be free of the invading organism and to return to a prepneumonia health status.

Interventions. The key to effective treatment of pneumonia is identification and eradication of the organism causing the infection. Anti-infectives are given for all types of pneumonias except those caused by viruses. The physician prescribes anti-infective therapy depending on the organism suspected or identified, whether the pneumonia is community acquired or hospital acquired, and whether the client has other contributing factors (Table 33–7). Treatment is often initiated empirically (based on prior experience) and may be continued empirically if the specific organism is not identified.

Aerosolized pentamidine may be used in the treatment and prevention of *Pneumocystis carinii* pneumonia (PCP). Pentamidine has antiprotozoal activity and is administered via a specialized nebulizer (Respirgard II), which nebulizes the medication into particles small enough to be delivered to the alveoli. When penicillin-resistant strains of *S. pneumoniae* have been identified, treatment consists of high-dose penicillin, a third-generation cephalosporin, meropenem (Merrem) or vancomycin (Vancocin) (King & Pippin, 1997).

The client may be able to be switched from intravenous to oral therapy in 2 or 3 days depending on the response (e.g., stable clinical condition, afebrile). The course of anti-infective therapy varies with the pharmacodynamics of the drug and the organism(s) involved but generally ranges from a low of 5 days for a client with uncomplicated community-acquired pneumonia to up to 21 days for the immunocompromised client.

 Continuing Care

The client needs to continue the anti-infective medications as prescribed by the physician or primary care provider. The nurse reinforces, clarifies, and provides additional information to the client and family as indicated. In addition, the nurse assists the client in overcoming any barriers to completing the medication prescription. The nurse also recognizes the importance of preventing further episodes of pneumonia and initiates applicable interventions.

➤ Health Teaching

The most important aspect of education for the client and family is the avoidance of upper respiratory tract infections and viruses. The client must avoid crowds, especially in the fall and winter when viruses are prevalent; persons who have a cold or flu; and exposure to irritants such as smoke. The influenza vaccine is recommended

TABLE 33–7

Drug Therapy for Pneumonia	
Community-Acquired Pneumonias*	**Nosocomial Pneumonias ‖**
Without comorbidity and client age <61 years	**Gram-negative infections**
Macrolide† or tetracylcine (doxycycline [Vibramycin])	Ceftazidime
With comorbidity and/or client age >59 years	Cefoperazone
Second- or third-generation cephalosporin or trimethoprim-sulfamethoxazole (Bactrim, Septra) or beta-lactam/beta-lactamase inhibitor§ with the possible addition of erythromycin (or other macrolide) or doxycycline	Aztreonam
	Amoxicillin/clavulanic acid
	Ciprofloxacin
	For *Pseudomonas* coverage:
	Ticarcillin
	Azlocillin
Less severe, requiring hospitalization or for those who are moderately ill	Ceftazidime
	Cefoperazone
Second- or third-generation cephalosporin or beta-lactam/beta-lactamase inhibitor with the possible addition of erythromycin (or other macrolide) or doxycycline	**Gram-positive infections**
	Ticarcillin/clavulanate
	Vancomycin
Severe, requiring hospitalization	Imipenem-cilastatin
Third-generation cephalosporin with anti-*Pseudomonas* activity or other antipseudomonal agents such as imipenem/cilastatin (Primaxin) or ciprofloxacin (Cipro), with the possible addition of an aminoglycoside and erythromycin (or other macrolide)	

*Modified from Niederman, 1993, and King, 1997.
†Macrolides include erythromycin, azithromycin (Zithromax), clarithromycin (Biaxin), dirithromycin (Dynabac).
‖ Modified from Bergone-Be're'zen, 1995.
§Such as amoxicillin-clavulanate (Augmentin).

annually, and the pneumococcal vaccine currently once in a lifetime (may be more often in some high-risk cases). A balanced diet and adequate fluid intake are essential. The nurse reviews all medication with the client and family and emphasizes completing anti-infective therapy. The nurse instructs the client to notify the physician if chills, fever, persistent cough, dyspnea, wheezing, hemoptysis, increased sputum production, chest discomfort, or increasing fatigue reoccurs or if symptoms fail to resolve. The client is instructed to get plenty of rest and gradually to increase exercise.

► Home Care Management

No special structural changes are needed in the home. If the home consists of more than one story, the client may prefer to stay on the first floor for a few weeks because stair climbing may increase fatigue and dyspnea. Bath and hygiene needs may be met by using a bedside commode if a bathroom is not located on the first level. Home care needs will depend on the client's level of fatigue, dyspnea, and family and social support.

The prolonged convalescent phase of the disease process, particularly in the elderly client, can be frustrating and perhaps depressing. Fatigue, weakness, and a residual cough can last for weeks. Some clients fear that they will never return to a "normal" level of functioning. It is important that the nurse prepare the client for the course of the disease and offer reassurance so that complete recovery will occur. Initially after discharge, the client may benefit from a home health nursing assessment as outlined in Chart 33–5.

► Health Care Resources

Clients who smoke are taught that smoking is a risk factor for pneumonia. The nurse provides information on smoking cessation classes through the American Lung Association (ALA) and American Cancer Society. The physician or nurse practitioner may prescribe nicotine patches. The physician and nurse warn the client of the danger of myocardial infarction if smoking is continued while using the patches. The client should be enrolled in a smoking cessation program to assist in the nicotine withdrawal process in conjunction with using nicotine patches. The nurse also can give the client information booklets on pneumonia provided by the ALA. A client who has not already been vaccinated against influenza or pneumococcal pneumonia should be encouraged to take this preventive measure when the pneumonia has resolved.

 Evaluation

On the basis of the identified nursing diagnoses and collaborative problems, the nurse evaluates the care of the client with pneumonia. The expected outcomes are that the client

---

Chart 33-5

Nursing Care Highlight: Focused Assessment for the Client Recovering from Pneumonia

Ascertain whether the client has had any of the following:

- Chills
- Fever
- Persistent cough
- Dyspnea
- Wheezing
- Hemoptysis
- Increased sputum production
- Chest discomfort
- Increasing fatigue
- Any other symptoms that have failed to resolve

Assess the client for the following:

- Fever
- Diaphoresis
- Cyanosis, especially around the mouth or conjunctiva
- Dyspnea, tachypnea, or tachycardia
- Adventitious or abnormal breath sounds
- Weakness

■ Attains and/or maintains a PaO_2, $PaCO_2$, and oxygen saturation values within baseline ranges
■ Has optimal breath sounds, either clear lungs in all lobes on auscultation, or, minimally, improved breath sounds
■ Is free of the invading organism
■ Returns to his or her prepneumonia health status

Pulmonary Tuberculosis

Overview

In 1900, tuberculosis (TB) was the leading cause of death in the United States and Europe. After significant reduction in its incidence, TB has been on the rise, especially in clients with HIV and acquired immunodeficiency syndrome (AIDS), but it may be stabilizing currently. Continuous assessment and intervention to prevent and treat the disease must continue. Increasing poverty, numbers of homeless people and people with AIDS, and resistant strains of the TB organism (multi-drug-resistant TB [MDR-TB]) present new challenges to the control and eradication of TB.

Pathophysiology

Tuberculosis is a highly communicable disease caused by *Mycobacterium tuberculosis*. The tubercle bacillus is transmitted via aerosolization (i.e., an airborne route). When an infected person coughs, laughs, sneezes, or sings, droplet nuclei are produced, become airborne, and may be inhaled by others. When the tubercle bacillus reaches a susceptible site (bronchi or alveoli), it multiplies freely. An exudative response occurs, causing a nonspecific pneumonitis. With the development of acquired immunity, further multiplication of bacilli is controlled in most

initial lesions. The lesions typically resolve and leave little or no residual. However, a small percentage of individuals who are initially infected will acquire the disease (5% to 15%). The greatest risk of acquiring the disease for the non-HIV-infected person is in the first 2 years after infection.

Cell-mediated, or type IV, immunity develops 2-10 weeks after infection and is manifested by a significant reaction to a tuberculin test. A primary infection may be microscopic in size and may never appear on an x-ray. The process of infection occurs as follows:

■ The granulomatous inflammation created by the tubercle bacillus in the lung becomes surrounded by collagen, fibroblasts, and lymphocytes.
■ Caseation necrosis (necrotic tissue being turned into a granular mass) occurs in the center of the lesion. If this area becomes evident on x-ray, it is called Ghon tubercle, or the primary lesion.

Areas of caseation then undergo resorption, hyaline degeneration, and fibrosis. These necrotic areas may calcify (calcification) or may liquefy (liquefaction). If liquefaction occurs, the liquid material then empties into a bronchus, and the evacuated area becomes a cavity (cavitation). Bacilli continue to proliferate in the necrotic cavity wall and spread via the tracheobronchial lymph nodes into new areas of the lung.

A lesion also may progress by direct extension if bacilli multiply rapidly with marked exudative response to the inflammation. These lesions may extend through the pleura, which results in tuberculous pleural effusion with a small number of organisms. Pericardial effusions also may occur.

Miliary, or hematogenous, TB occurs when a large number of organisms enter the bloodstream and the disease becomes disseminated. Many tiny, discrete nodules scattered throughout the lung are typically seen on chest x-ray. The brain, meninges, liver, and kidney (see Chap. 74), or bone marrow are commonly involved as a result of dissemination.

Initial infection is seen more often in the middle or lower lobes of the lung. The regional lymph nodes, particularly the hilar and paratracheal nodes, are commonly involved. There is usually an asymptomatic interval after the primary infection that lasts for years, or less commonly, decades, before clinical symptoms develop. Although infected, an individual is not infectious to others until symptoms of disease occur.

Secondary TB occurs in a previously infected individual and most often represents reactivation (sometimes inaccurately termed reinfection) of the primary disease. Presumably, reactivation occurs whenever defenses are lowered, which may be part of the reason the elderly are susceptible to the development of TB. The upper lobes are the most common site of reactivation and are referred to as Simon's foci. The TB classification adopted and revised by the ALA is shown in Table 33-8.

Etiology

The organism *Mycobacterium tuberculosis* is a nonmotile, slow-growing, nonsporulating, acid-fast rod that secretes

TABLE 33–8

American Lung Association Classification of Tuberculosis (TB)
0 No TB exposure, not infected
1 TB exposure, no evidence of infection
2 TB infection, no disease
3 TB: clinically active (clients with completed diagnostic evidence of TB: both a significant reaction to tuberculin skin test and clinical or x-ray evidence of TB)
4 TB: not clinically active (clients with history of TB or with abnormal chest x-ray but no significant tuberculin skin test reaction or clinical evidence)
5 TB: suspect (diagnosis pending) (used during diagnostic testing of suspect clients, for no longer than a 3-month period)

niacin. The tubercle bacillus is transmitted via aerosolization.

People who are most commonly infected are those having repeated close contact with an infectious person who has not yet been diagnosed with TB. After the infectious person has received proper medication for 2–3 weeks, and clinical signs of improvement are seen (including reduction of acid-fast bacilli [AFB] in the sputum), the risk of transmission is greatly reduced.

Incidence/Prevalence

Figures for 1981 reveal that TB only accounted for 0.8% of deaths in the United States and that the incidence of TB was declining steadily. From 1985 on, however, the number of new TB cases have increased to more than 20,000 annually, largely thought to be related to the onset of the new disease of the time, HIV infection. Ten million persons are estimated to be infected with TB in the United States. The World Health Organization estimates that there are 10 million new cases each year with 2–3 million deaths per year worldwide. The highest at-risk populations currently include

- Those in constant, frequent contact with an untreated individual
- Those with immune dysfunction or HIV
- Those living in crowded areas such as long-term care facilities, prisons, mental health facilities
- The elderly, the homeless, and minorities
- Those who abuse intravenous drugs or alcohol
- Those from a lower socioeconomic group

TRANSCULTURAL CONSIDERATIONS

Groups known to have higher incidence of TB include African-Americans, Asians and Pacific Islanders, Native Americans and Alaskan Natives, Hispanics, and foreign-born persons from Asia, Africa, the Caribbean, and Latin America.

Collaborative Management

 Assessment

Early detection of TB depends on subjective findings rather than presentation of symptoms. TB has an insidious onset, and many clients are not aware of symptoms until the disease is well advanced. A diagnosis of TB should be considered for any client with a persistent cough or other symptoms compatible with TB such as weight loss, anorexia, night sweats, hemoptysis, shortness of breath, fever, or chills.

► History

A thorough history includes assessment of past exposure to TB. The nurse inquires about the client's country of origin and travel to foreign countries in which there is a high incidence of TB. It is important to note whether the client has had previous tests for TB and what the results were. In addition, the nurse asks whether the client has had bacille Calmette-Guérin (BCG) vaccine, a vaccine containing attenuated tubercle bacilli that is given routinely in many foreign countries to produce increased resistance to TB. Anyone who has received BCG will have a positive skin test and should be evaluated for TB with a chest x-ray. The BCG vaccine has minimal effectiveness and is not recommended by the CDC.

► Physical Assessment/Clinical Manifestations

The client with TB typically has progressive fatigue, lethargy, nausea, anorexia, weight loss, irregular menses, and a low-grade fever, which may have been present for weeks or months. Fever also may be accompanied by night sweats. The client finally notices a cough and the production of mucoid and mucopurulent sputum, which is occasionally streaked with blood. Chest tightness and a dull, aching chest pain may accompany the cough. Physical examination of the chest does not provide conclusive evidence of TB. The nurse may hear dullness with percussion over involved parenchymal areas, bronchial breath sounds, crackles, and increased transmission of spoken or whispered sounds. Partial obstruction of a bronchus because of endobronchial disease or compression by lymph nodes may produce localized wheezing.

► Diagnostic Assessment

Sputum culture of *M. tuberculosis* confirms the diagnosis. Three samples are usually obtained for an acid-fast smear. After medications are started, sputum samples are obtained again to determine the effectiveness of therapy. Most clients have negative cultures after 3 months, perhaps even earlier.

In the future, we can expect to see polymerase chain reaction (PCR) assays performed for rapid identification of mycobacteria. This process allows amplification of mycobacterial deoxyribonuclease acid and identification of the mycobacteria within hours instead of days to weeks. This test will allow for earlier diagnosis and treatment of the client with TB.

The tuberculin test (Mantoux's test) result is the most

reliable determinant of infection with TB. A small amount (0.1 mL) of intermediate-strength purified protein derivative (PPD) containing 5 tuberculin units is given intradermally in the forearm. An area of induration (not redness) measuring 10 mm or more in diameter 48–72 hours after injection indicates the person has been exposed to and infected with TB. A positive reaction does not mean that active disease is present but indicates exposure to TB or the presence of inactive (dormant) disease. For persons with HIV infection, a reaction of 5 mm or greater is considered positive. A negative skin test does not rule out TB disease or infection. People with HIV infection are more likely to have false-negative results as a result of an impaired immune system.

Once a person's skin test is positive, chest x-ray is essential to rule out clinically active TB or to detect old, healed lesions. Caseation and inflammation may be seen on the x-ray if the disease is active.

Routine, repeat skin tests and chest x-rays are no longer recommended in these clients. They should be instructed to seek medical attention if they experience symptoms suggestive of TB. The radiographic presentation in HIV-infected clients, however, may be unusual. Such clients may have infiltrates in any lung zone, often associated with hilar adenopathy, or may have a normal chest x-ray.

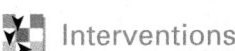 Interventions

Combination drug therapy is the most effective method of treating the disease and preventing transmission. Active TB is treated with a combination of drugs to which the organism is susceptible. Therapy is continued until the disease is under control. The use of multiple-drug regimens destroys organisms as quickly as possible and minimizes the emergence of drug-resistant organisms. Current therapy (Chart 33–6) uses isoniazid (INH) and rifampin throughout the therapy; pyrazinamide is added for the first 2 months. This protocol permits shortening of the therapy from 6–12 months to 6 months for most clients. Ethambutol and streptomycin are frequently added as the fourth drug to the treatment regimen. An early report using aerosolized interferon-gamma shows promise as additional treatment for multi–drug-resistant TB (see Research Applications for Nursing).

The nurse's major role is teaching clients about drug therapy. The nurse recognizes that the anxious client may not absorb information well. The nurse repeats the information and obtains the assistance of family members if they are available. In instructing, the nurse uses teaching aids such as those available through the ALA. The client should be able to describe the treatment regimen and major side effects for which to call the health care agency and physician.

Tuberculosis is frequently treated outside the acute care setting, so the client convalesces in the home setting. In this setting, airborne precautions are not necessary because family members have already been exposed; all members of the household need to undergo TB testing, however. The nurse instructs the client to cover the mouth and nose when coughing or sneezing, to confine used tissues to plastic bags, and to wear a mask when in contact with crowds until medication is effective in suppressing the infection.

The nurse informs the client that examinations of sputum are needed every 2–4 weeks once drug therapy is initiated. When results of three sputum cultures are negative, the client is considered to be no longer infectious and can usually return to former employment. The nurse reminds the client to avoid excessive exposure to silicone or dust because these substances can cause further lung damage.

The nurse places a hospitalized client with active TB in Airborne Precautions (see Chap. 28) in a well-ventilated room that exhausts to the outside. The room should have at least six exchanges of fresh air per minute and should be ventilated to the outside if possible. The nurse wears a N95 or HEPA respirator (Fig. 33–2) when caring for the client. Standard Precautions are implemented when there is risk of hand and clothing contamination, by using appropriate barrier protection (i.e., gowns and gloves). The nurse performs thorough hand washing before and after caring for the client. Precautions are discontinued when the client is no longer considered infectious.

Clients may prevent nausea related to the medications by taking the daily dose at bedtime. Antinausea drugs may also prevent this symptom. The nurse instructs the client about the need for adequate nutrition and a well-balanced diet to promote healing. The nurse recommends an increased intake of foods that are rich in iron, protein, and vitamin C. The nurse consults the nutritionist for specialized needs. The nurse should know the client's ideal body weight so that progress toward the goal can be evaluated. (See Chapter 64 for further discussion of nutrition.)

The client with TB notices changes in physical stamina, which may be frightening. The client also faces concerns about the prognosis of the disease. The nurse is realistic in offering a positive outlook for the client who complies with the medication regimen and suggests that fatigue will diminish as the treatment progresses. With current resistant strains of TB, however, the nurse must emphasize that noncompliance with medication could lead to an infection that is difficult to treat or has total drug resistance. The nurse listens carefully to the client's concerns throughout the treatment and responds in a supportive manner. The client's return to work and usual daily routines is likely to reduce anxiety.

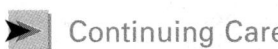 Continuing Care

➤ Health Teaching

The nurse instructs the client to follow the drug regimen exactly as prescribed and always to have a supply of medication on hand. The nurse stresses side effects and ways of minimizing them to ensure compliance. The nurse reminds the client with TB that the disease is usually no longer communicable after medication has been taken for 2–3 consecutive weeks and clinical improvement is seen. However, the client must continue with the prescribed medication for 6 months or longer as ordered.

Chart 33–6

Drug Therapy for Tuberculosis

Drug	Usual Dosage	Nursing Interventions	Drug Action/Rationale for Use
Isoniazid (INH)	• 5 mg/kg PO, IM (max 300 mg) daily; 15 mg/kg (max 900 mg) biweekly	• Observe for drug interactions. It may inhibit drug metabolism of phenytoin, carbamazepine, primidone, and warfarin. • Instruct the client to take on empty stomach and avoid antacids. • Monitor for signs of hepatitis and neurotoxicity effects.	• Isoniazid inhibits synthesis of mycolic acids and acts to kill actively growing organisms in the extracellular environment and inhibits growth of dormant organisms in the macrophages and caseating granulomas.
Rifampin (RIF)	• 10 mg/kg PO (max 600 mg) daily or biweekly	• Instruct the client that secretions, including urine, will be orange in color and will permanently discolor soft contact lenses. • Observe for drug interactions. It may enhance elimination of theophylline, steroids, opioids, oral hypoglycemics, warfarin, and occasionally vitamin D. • Observe for hepatotoxic effects. • RIF decreases effectiveness of oral contraceptives.	• Rifampin has the unique ability to kill slower growing organisms that reside in the caseating granuloma and macrophage.
Pyrazinamide (PZA)	• 15–30 mg/kg PO (max 2000 mg) daily; 50 mg/kg biweekly	• Observe for hepatotoxic effects.	• Pyrazinamide is the most active drug at killing mycobacteria present in macrophages. The acidic environment in the macrophage inhibits most agents.
Ethambutol (EMB)	• 15 mg/kg daily PO; 50 mg/kg biweekly	• Obtain baseline visual acuity and color discrimination, especially to the color green. Repeat testing q1–2 months.	• Ethambutol inhibits bacterial RNA synthesis. It is slow acting and must be used in combination with other bactericidal agents.
Streptomycin (SM)	• 1000 mg IM, or IV over 1 hr, daily for 2 months followed by biweekly injections until treatment is completed	• Obtain baseline audiometric test q1–2 months. It can impair the 8th cranial nerve. Elderly clients are especially susceptible.	• Streptomycin is an aminoglycoside antibiotic that is active against extracellular organisms only.
Amikacin	• 15 mg/kg daily IM, IV (usual dose 1 g)	• Ensure adequate hydration, monitor renal function, and hearing. Amikacin can lead to renal toxicity and ototoxicity.	• Amikacin is an aminoglycoside antibiotic that can be used if streptomycin is not available.

Current treatment recommendations:

INH + RIF + PZA + EMB or SM (induction phase)—2 months. Daily dosing. Ethambutol or streptomycin is included in the initial phase until drug susceptibility is determined.

INH + RIF (continuation phase)—4 months. Daily or 2–3 times/week dosing.

Continue treatment for at least 6 months, and 3 months beyond the time when the result of sputum culture converts to negative.

Clients with a drug resistance, co-existing HIV infection, or inability to take certain antituberculosis drugs require longer duration therapy (i.e., 9 total months, and at least 6 months after culture conversion).

Current treatment information and data from the official ATS statement. A joint statement of the ATS, American Academy of Pediatrics, the Centers for Disease Control, and the Infectious Disease Society of America. (1992). Control of tuberculosis in the United States. *American Review of Respiratory Disease, 146*(6), 1623–1633; U. S. Department of Health and Human Services, Recommendations of the Advisory Council for the Elimination of Tuberculosis. (1993). Initial therapy for tuberculosis in the era of multidrug resistance. *Morbidity and Mortality Weekly Report, 42*(RR-7), 1–8.

▷ Research Applications for Nursing

Aerosolized Interferon May Be of Benefit in Treating Multi–Drug-Resistant Tuberculosis

Condos, R., Rom, W. N., & Schluger, N. W. (1997). Treatment of multi–drug-resistant pulmonary tuberculosis with interferon-gamma via aerosol. Lancet, 349, 1513–1515.

Because interferon-gamma is a cytokine that can activate alveolar macrophages, cells important to immunity against *M. tuberculosis,* these researchers wanted to study its efficacy on severe, advanced multi–drug-resistant TB (MDR-TB). They selected five persons who had been receiving conventional directly observed TB drug therapy between 5 and 24 months and whose sputum smears and cultures were still positive. Each participant received 500 μg of recombinant human interferon-gamma three times a week for 4 weeks. Each person continued on their conventional therapy during the 4-week study period.

At the end of the study period, four of the five participants had become sputum-smear negative. The fifth had a significant reduction in the grade of the sputum smear and became negative 1 month later. Poststudy computed tomography results showed improvement compared with prestudy results. Body weight stabilized or increased in all participants during the study phase. All participants except one became sputum-smear positive after therapy with interferon was stopped.

Critique. Only five persons were studied, which limits the applicability of this treatment modality. One participant had diabetes and was HIV positive, which makes the group of five less homogeneous.

Possible Nursing Implications. The nurse who is aware of the latest research is able to contribute to the collaborative process in determining therapy for clients. The nurse communicates that muscle aches and cough were the minor adverse effects observed in this study. The nurse explains new therapies to clients and their families.

Directly observed therapy (DOT), where the nurse watches the client swallow the medications, may be indicated in some situations. This practice contributes to more treatment successes, less relapses, and less drug resistance.

The client who has experienced weight loss and severe lethargy should gradually resume usual activities. The client must maintain proper nutrition to prevent recurrence of infection.

To help the client encountering others with concerns about the contagious aspect of the infection, the nurse provides the client with information about TB. A key to preventing the transmission of TB is the identification of those in close contact with the infected person so that they can be tested and treated as necessary. Public health professionals have an important role in this aspect of care. When contacts have been identified, these people are assessed with a tuberculin test and possibly a chest x-ray to determine infection with TB. Multidrug therapy

may be indicated. In addition, certain high-risk contacts receive prophylactic therapy, usually with isoniazid (INH).

▷ Home Care Management

Most clients with TB are managed outside the hospital. However, clients may be diagnosed with TB while in the hospital if pneumonia is suspected or other possible complications exist. Discharge may be delayed if the living situation is considered high risk or if the client is likely to be noncompliant. The nurse may consult with the social service worker in the hospital or the community health nursing agency to ensure the client's discharge to the appropriate environment with continued supervision. The home health nurse follows potentially infected people in the home environment because treating and then returning the client to the same environment only to become reinfected would be futile.

▷ Health Care Resources

The nurse instructs the client to receive follow-up care by a physician for at least 1 year during active treatment. In addition, the ALA, an organization that uses volunteers, can provide free information to the client about the disease and its treatment. Alcoholics Anonymous and other health care resources for clients with alcoholism are available as well, if needed. The nurse assists the client who uses drugs to locate an appropriate drug treatment program.

Lung Abscess

Overview

A lung abscess is a localized area of lung destruction caused by liquefaction necrosis, which is usually related

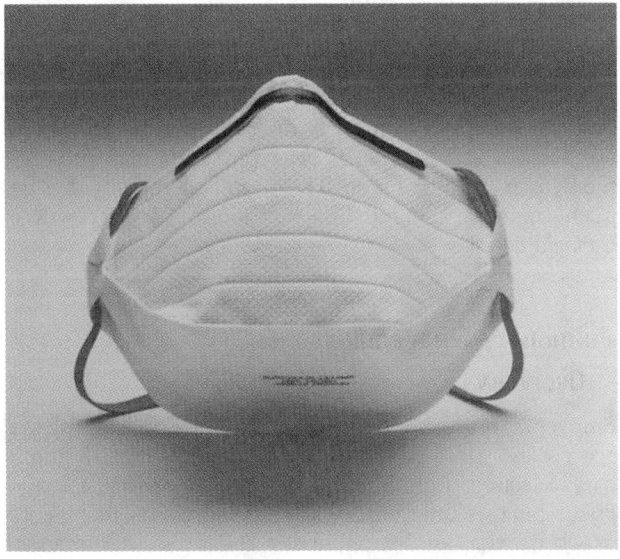

Figure 33–2. A HEPA respirator used in the care of clients with active or "rule-out" tuberculosis. (Courtesy of Uvex Safety, Smithfield, RI.)

to pyogenic bacteria. Clients who have this problem often have a history of pneumonia, possibly complicated by aspiration of oropharyngeal contents or proximal obstruction as a result of tumor or foreign body. Other causes of aspiration leading to abscess include alcoholism that causes loss of consciousness, seizure disorders or other neurologic deficits, and swallowing disorders. An obstruction of a bronchus may cause a necrotizing process in the distal lung that eventually becomes an abscess. Multiple abscesses and cavities commonly form in clients with TB or fungal infections of the lung. Immunosuppressed clients, such as those receiving chemotherapy, or those with a disease like leukemia or AIDS, are particularly susceptible to fungal infections. Most common organisms are anaerobic bacteria, *Staphylococcus* or other gram-positive organism, or gram-negative or opportunistic infections such as fungi.

Collaborative Management

 Assessment

The nurse notes a client's recent history of influenza, pneumonia, febrile illness, cough, and foul-smelling sputum production. In addition, the nurse inquires about the sputum color and odor, and about any pleuritic chest pain (a stabbing pain, especially when taking a deep breath). The client is often febrile, pale, fatigued, and cachectic. The nurse may note decreased breath sounds on auscultation and dullness on percussion in the involved area. Bronchial breath sounds and crackles are frequently heard over the site of the lesion. The physician orders a chest x-ray and sputum samples to assist in the diagnosis.

 Interventions

Nursing diagnoses and interventions identified for the client with pneumonia also apply to the client with a lung abscess. Medical treatment is directed toward drainage of the abscess and antibiotics. The physician may prescribe more than one antibiotic. The nurse, then, provides frequent mouth care and observes for oral overgrowth of *Candida albicans*.

Pulmonary Empyema

Overview

Empyema refers to a collection of pus in the pleural space. The most common cause of empyema is pulmonary infection, lung abscess, or infected pleural effusion. Pneumonia or lung abscess can spread across the pleura, or obstruction of lymph nodes can cause a retrograde flood of infected lymph into the pleural space. In addition, an intrahepatic or subphrenic abscess can spread through the diaphragm's lymphatic system. Thoracic sur-

gery and chest trauma are common predisposing conditions in which bacteria are introduced directly into the pleural space. Blood from trauma may accumulate in the pleural space. Incomplete evacuation of this blood presents a culture medium for bacterial growth.

Collaborative Management

 Assessment

Important history findings include recent febrile illness (including pneumonia), chest pain, dyspnea, cough, and trauma. The nurse notes the characteristics of the sputum. On physical assessment, the nurse may observe diminished chest wall motion. If a pleural effusion is present, the nurse notes decreased or absent fremitus on palpation, a flat percussion note on percussion, and decreased breath sounds on auscultation. With compression of lung tissue adjacent to the effusion, the nurse auscultates bronchial breath sounds, egophony, and whispered pectoriloquy.

Some clients have fever, chills, night sweats, and weight loss. If there is cardiorespiratory compromise, the client may be hypotensive because of a mediastinal deviation; the nurse may note a displacement of the PMI (point of maximal impulse) on auscultation of the heart.

The physician orders a chest x-ray and obtains a sample of the pleural fluid via thoracentesis (see Chap. 29) for help in making the diagnosis. Empyema fluid is thick, opaque, exudative, and intensely foul smelling. The pleural fluid is sent to the laboratory and is analyzed for color, red blood cell count, white blood cell count and differential, glucose and protein levels, lactate dehydrogenase (LDH), and pH. Gram and acid-fast stains of the smears and cytology studies also are done. A protein concentration higher than 3 g/100 mL of pleural fluid indicates an exudative process.

 Interventions

Therapy for empyema is based on emptying the empyema cavity, reexpanding the lung, and controlling the infection. The physician usually treats the client with antibiotics appropriate for the isolated pathogen. In addition, closed-chest drainage (see Chap. 32) is used to promote lung expansion. The physician places one or more chest tubes in the inferior parts of the empyema sac. Underwater seal drainage is used without suction initially, but negative pressure may be added if the lung fails to expand. The physician removes the tube when the lung is fully expanded; and the infectious process is under control. Open thoracotomy and decortication (removal) of a portion of the pleura may be needed for thick pus or marked pleural thickening. Nursing considerations are the same as those for clients with a pleural effusion, pneumothorax, or infection.

CASE STUDY for the Client with Tuberculosis

■ Ms. Chapel is a 25-year-old inner-city woman with AIDS. She is hospitalized now for active TB. She has four young children at home who are currently being cared for by her mother, a 42-year-old unemployed woman with diabetes.

QUESTIONS:

1. In what kind of isolation must Ms. Chapel be placed and why?
2. Sputum cultures for acid-fast bacilli (AFB) are ordered. When is the best time to collect sputum? Can you still send sputum to the laboratory that contains saliva?
3. Before Ms. Chapel is discharged to home, what interventions need to be done at home in preparation for her return?

SELECTED BIBLIOGRAPHY

Afessa, B., Greaves, W. L., & Frederick, W. R. (1995). Pneumococcal bacteremia in adults: A 14-year experience in an inner-city university hospital. *Clinical Infectious Diseases, 21,* 345–351.

American College of Chest Physicians. (1995). Institutional control measures for tuberculosis in an era of multiple drug resistance (consumers statement). *Chest, 108,* 1690–1710.

*American Thoracic Society. (1990). Diagnostic standards and classification of tuberculosis. *American Review of Respiratory Disease, 142(3),* 725–735.

*American Thoracic Society. (1992). Control of tuberculosis in the United States (the official ATS statement). *American Review of Respiratory Disease, 146(6),* 1623–1633.

*Badhwar, A. K., & Druce, H. M. (1992). Allergic rhinitis. *Medical Clinics of North America, 76(4),* 789–804.

*Benson, V., & Marano, M. A. (1994). *Current estimates from the National Health Interview Survey* (DHHS Pub. No. [PHS] 94-1517). Hyattsville, MD: National Center for Health Statistics.

Bergone-Be're'zen, E. (1995). Treatment and prevention of nosocomial pneumonia. *Chest, 108(2),* 26S–34S.

Blumberg, H. M., Watkins, D. L., & Berschling, J. D. (1995). Preventing the nosocomial transmission of tuberculosis. *Annals of Internal Medicine, 122(9),* 658–663.

*Boutotte, J. (1993). TB the second time around. *Nursing93, 23(5),* 42–50.

*Brown, R. (1993). Community-acquired pneumonia: Diagnosis and therapy of older adults. *Geriatrics, 48(2),* 43–50.

Calianno, C. (1996). Nosocomial pneumonia. *Nursing96, 26(5),* 34–40.

*Campbell, G. D. (1994). Overview of community-acquired pneumonia: Prognosis and clinical features. *Medical Clinics of North America, 78,* 1035–1048.

*Cantwell, M. F., Snider, D. E., Cauthen, G. M., et al. (1994). Epidemiology of tuberculosis in the United States, 1985 through 1992. *Journal of the American Medical Association, 272(7),* 535–539.

*Caruthers, D. (1990). Infectious pneumonia in the elderly. *American Journal of Nursing, 90(2),* 56–60.

*Centers for Disease Control. (1993a). Estimates of future global tuberculosis morbidity and mortality. *Morbidity and Mortality Weekly Report, 42(NO–49),* 961–965.

*Centers for Disease Control. (1993b). Recommendations of the Advisory Council for the elimination of tuberculosis: Initial therapy for tuberculosis in the era of multidrug resistance. *Morbidity and Mortality Weekly Report, 42(RR–7),* 1–8.

*Centers for Disease Control. (1994). Guidelines for preventing the transmission of tuberculosis in health care settings. *Morbidity and Mortality Weekly Report, 43(RR–13),* 1–32.

Centers for Disease Control. (1995a). Increasing pneumonoccal vaccination rates—United States, 1993. *Morbidity and Mortality Weekly Report, 44(40),* 741–744.

Centers for Disease Control. (1995b). Influenza and pneumonoccal vaccination coverage levels among adults aged > 64 years—United States, 1973–1993. *Morbidity and Mortality Weekly Report, 44(27),* 506–507, 513–515.

Centers for Disease Control. (1995c). Pneumonia and influenza death rates—United States, 1979–1994. *Morbidity and Mortality Weekly Report, 44(28),* 535–537.

Centers for Disease Control and Prevention. (1996). Tuberculosis morbidity—United States, 1995. *Morbidity and Mortality Weekly Report, 45(NO–18),* 365–370.

Centers for Disease Control and Prevention. (1997a). Pneumonoccal and influenza vaccination among adults aged ≥ 65 years—United States, 1995. *Morbidity and Mortality Weekly Report, 46(39),* 913–919.

Centers for Disease Control and Prevention. (1997b). Recommendations of the Advisory Committee on immunization practices: Prevention of influenza. *Morbidity and Mortality Weekly Report, 46(RR–9),* 1–24.

Centers for Disease Control and Prevention. (1997c). Recommendations of the Advisory Committee on immunization practices: Prevention of pneumococcal disease. *Morbidity and Mortality Weekly Report, 46(RR–8),* 1–24.

Centers for Disease Control and Prevention. (1997d). Tuberculosis morbidity—United States, 1996. *Morbidity and Mortality Weekly Report, 46(30),* 695–700.

Cohen, M. L., Doeman, N. J., Kauffman, C. A., et al. (1995). Antimicrobial resistance: Are the pathogens winning? *Patient Care, 29(9),* 56–60, 63–64, 67–69.

Condos, R., Rom, W. N., & Schluger, N. W. (1997). Treatment of multidrug-resistant pulmonary tuberculosis with interferon-gamma via aerosol. *Lancet, 349,* 1513–1515.

Craven, D. E., & Steger, K. A. (1995). Epidemiology of nosocomial pneumonia: New perspectives on an old disease. *Chest, 108(2),* 1S–16S.

Crespo, J. (1995). Cost considerations of implementing OSHA tuberculosis regulations. *MEDSURG Nursing, 4(5),* 353–357.

Douville, L. (1995). Pharmacologic highlights: Management of acute sinusitis. *Journal of the American Academy of Nurse Practitioners, 7(8),* 407–411.

*Elpern, E. H., & Girzadas, A. M. (1993). Tuberculosis update: New challenges of an old disease. *MEDSURG Nursing, 2(3),* 176–183.

*Esler, R., Bentz, P., Sorensen, M., & Van Orsow, T. (1994). Patient-centered pneumonia care: A case management success story. *American Journal of Nursing, 94(11),* 34–38.

*Fedson, D. (1992). Clinical practice and public policy for influenza and pneumococcal vaccination of the elderly. *Clinics in Geriatric Medicine, 8(1),* 183–199.

Felmingham, D. (1995). Antibiotic resistance: Do we need new therapeutic approaches? *Chest, 108(2),* 70S–78S.

Finklestein, L., & Petrec, C. A. (1996). Sputum testing for TB: Getting good specimens. *American Journal of Nursing, 96(2),* 14.

*Gantz, N. M., & Sogg, A. J. (1992). An update on sinusitis. *Patient Care, 26(8),* 141–143, 147–148, 157–163.

Grimes, D. E., & Grimes, R. M. (1995). Tuberculosis: What nurses need to know to help control the epidemic. *Nursing Outlook, 43(4),* 164–173.

Hahn, M. S. (1995). Tuberculosis today. *ADVANCE for Nurse Practitioners, 3(10),* 19–23.

Haney, P. E., Raymond, B. A., Hernandez, J. M., et al. (1996). Tuberculosis makes a comeback. *AORN Journal, 63(4),* 705, 707, 709.

Hect, A. (1995). Diagnosis and treatment of pneumonia in the nursing home. *Nurse Practitioner, 20(5),* 24, 27–28, 35–39.

Hopkins, M. L., & Schoener, L. (1996). Tuberculosis and the elderly living in long-term care facilities. *Geriatric Nursing, 17(1),* 27–32.

*Howard, B. A. (1994). Guiding allergy sufferers through the medication maze. *RN, 57(4),* 26–30.

Howse, E. (1996). Pharmacy practice. *Mycobacterium tuberculosis:* Implications for home health care. *Home Health Care Management & Practice, 8(3),* 69–74.

*Jacobs, R. F. (1994). Multiple-drug-resistant tuberculosis. *Clinical Infectious Diseases, 19(1),* 1–8.

*Janzen, V. D. (1987). Rhinological disorders in the elderly. *Journal of Otolaryngology, 15,* 228–230.

*Josephson, J. S., & Rosenberg, S. I. (1994). Sinusitis. *Clinical Symposia, 46*(2), 2–32.

Jovell, R. J., & Salfinger, M. (1996). Molecular fingerprinting of mycobacterium tuberculosis: A new diagnostic tool enhances TB control programs. *RT: Journal for Respiratory Care Practitioners, 9*(3), 66, 68, 70.

King, D. E., & Pippin, H. J. (1997). Community-acquired pneumonia in adults: Initial antibiotic therapy. *American Family Physician, 56*(2), 544–550.

Krouse, H. J., Parker, C. M., Purcell, R., et al. (1997). Powered functional endoscopic sinus surgery. *AORN Journal, 66*(3), 405, 408, 410–411, 413–414.

Lancaster, E., & Grimes, D. E. (1996). Tuberculosis: What nurses need to know to help control the epidemic (letter). *Nursing Outlook, 44*(2), 103–104.

Leibowitz, R. E. (1995). Critical care and tuberculosis. *Critical Care Nursing Clinics of North America, 7*(4), 661–666.

Leiner, S., & Mays, M. (1996). Diagnosing latent and active pulmonary tuberculosis: A review for clinicians. *Nurse Practitioner, 21*(2), 86, 88, 91–92.

Mandell, L. A. (1995). Community-acquired pneumonia. *Chest, 108*(2), 35S–42S.

Mayer, S. (1995). A sensitive issue . . . Detecting rhinitis. *Nursing Times, 91*(5), 23.

McAnulty, J. M., Fleming, D. W., et al. (1995). Missed opportunities for tuberculosis prevention. *Archives of Internal Medicine, 155*(7), 713–716.

*McCall, M. (1993). It killed George, or managing the peritonsillar abscess patient effectively. *ORL Head and Neck Nursing, 11*(1), 10–12.

*McCue, J. D. (1993). Pneumonia in the elderly. *Postgraduate Medicine, 94*(95), 39–40, 43–48, 51.

Mead, M. (1996). A guide to acute and chronic sinusitis. *Practice Nurse, 11*(10), 732–733.

Menzies, D., Fanning, A., & Yuan, G. (1995). Tuberculosis among health care workers. *New England Journal of Medicine, 332*(2), 92–98.

*Messner, R. L., & Zink, K. (1992). Nosocomial pneumonia: Combating a hospital menace. *RN, 55*(6), 48–53.

*Moran, G. J. (1994). Recognizing and minimizing the risks: Part 1. Multidrug-resistant TB. *Emergency Medicine, 26*(14), 36–42.

*Nadell, E. A. (1993). Environmental control of tuberculosis. *Medical Clinics of North America, 77*(6), 1315–1333.

*National Center for Health Statistics. (1993). *Health United States, 1992 and healthy people 2000 review* (DHHS Pub. No. [PHS] 93–1232). Hyattsville, MD: Public Health Service.

*Niederman, M. S., Bass, J. B., Campbell, G. D., et al. (1993). Guidelines for the initial mamagement of adults with community-acquired pneumonia: Diagnosis, assessment of severity, and initial antimicrobial therapy. Official American Thoracic Society statement. *American Review of Respiratory Disease, 148*, 1418–1426.

*Niederman, M. S., Sarosi, G. A., & Glassroth, J. (1994). *Respiratory infections: A scientific basis for management.* Philadelphia: W. B. Saunders Co.

*Norman, P. S. (1991). Allergic rhinitis: Combined therapy improves control. *Consultant, 31*(8), 25–29.

*Pattern, B. C., & Holt, J. (1992). When your patient is allergic. *American Journal of Nursing, 92*(9), 58–61.

Petroff, P. F. (1997). Computer assisted endoscopic sinus surgery. *AORN Journal, 66*(3), 416, 418–420, 422–425.

*Piirila, P. (1992). Changes in crackle characteristics during the clinical course of pneumonia. *Chest, 102*(1), 176–183.

*Rubin, F. L. (1993). Viral pneumonias: The increasing importance of a high index of suspicion. *Postgraduate Medicine, 93*(7), 57–60, 63–64.

*Sanford, J. P. (1994). Combating drug-resistant pneumonococcal infections. *Hospital Practice, 29*(10), 31–37.

*Schwartz, R. (1994). The diagnosis and management of sinusitis. *Nurse Practitioner, 19*(12), 58–63.

Shehata, M. A. (1996). Atrophic rhinitis. *Medical Journal of Otolaryngology, 17*(2), 81–86.

Shulkin, D. J., & Brennan, P. J. (1995). The cost of caring for patients with tuberculosis: Planning for a disease on the rise. *American Journal of Infection Control, 23*(1), 1–4.

*Slavin, R. G. (1991). Management of sinusitis. *Journal of the American Geriatrics Society, 39*(2), 212–217.

Stamp, D., & Arnold, M. S. (1995). Tuberculosis in home care: Complying with OSHA. *Caring, 14*(2), 16–18, 20–22.

*Stead, W. W., Senner, J. W., Reddick, W. T., et al. (1990). Racial differences in susceptibility to infection by *Mycobacterium tuberculosis.* *New England Journal of Medicine, 322*(7), 422–427.

*Strolley, J. M., & Buckwalter, K. C. (1991). Iatrogenesis in the elderly. Nosocomial infections. *Journal of Gerontological Nursing, 17*(9), 30–34.

Telzak, E., & Sepkowitz, K. (1995). Multidrug-resistant tuberculosis in patients without HIV infection. *New England Journal of Medicine, 333*(14), 907–911.

*Walsh, K. (1994). Guidelines for the prevention and control of tuberculosis in the elderly. *Nurse Practitioner, 19*(11), 79–84.

Wiseman, K. C. (1995). Tuberculosis: An old disease with a new face. *American Nephrology Nurses' Association Journal, 22*(6), 541–556.

*Wisinger, D. (1993). Bacterial pneumonia: *S. pneumoniae* and *H. influenzae* are the villains. *Postgraduate Medicine, 93*(7), 43–46, 49–50, 52.

Wolf, L. (1995). A tuberculosis control plan for ambulatory care centers. *Nurse Practitioner, 20*(6), 34, 36, 39–40.

Wurtz, R., Lee, C., Lama, J., et al. (1996). A new class of close contacts: Home health care workers and occupational exposure to tuberculosis. *Home Health Care Management & Practice, 8*(2), 28–31.

*Yoshikawa, T. T. (1992). Tuberculosis in aging adults. *Journal of the American Geriatrics Society, 40*(2), 178–187.

SUGGESTED READINGS

Calianno, C. (1996). Nosocomial pneumonia. *Nursing96, 26*(5), 34–40.
The article begins with data regarding the incidence, severity, and increased length of hospital stay related to nosocomial pneumonia. The CDC criteria for definition of nosocomial pneumonia are listed. Specifics related to the elderly are emphasized. The authors then review the organisms associated with aspiration and inhalation, followed by preventive measures for bacterial, viral, and fungal causes of nosocomial pneumonia.

Hopkins, M. L., & Schoener, L. (1996). Tuberculosis and the elderly living in long-term care facilities. *Geriatric Nursing, 17*(1), 27–32.
This article begins with reporting the incidence of tuberculosis in the elderly and discusses reasons why the elderly are at risk for TB. The article then focuses on TB identification, diagnosis, and intervention for those in long-term care settings. Screening protocols, prevention, and disease control are covered. Differences in skin testing for the elderly are explained.

Petroff, P. F. (1997). Computer assisted endoscopic sinus surgery. *AORN Journal, 66*(3), 416, 418–420, 422–425.
This article explains how applying advanced computer imaging modalities has increased the accuracy of endoscopic surgery on the sinuses and has decreased complications. As an ambulatory surgery procedure, the author proceeds to outline, step by step, the sequence of events from 1 day preoperatively to postoperative recovery and discharge. Of particular interest is the coordination of care aspects from all team members in all involved departments.

Chapter 34

INTERVENTIONS FOR CRITICALLY ILL CLIENTS WITH RESPIRATORY PROBLEMS

Acute or chronic respiratory problems can progress rapidly and become life-threatening emergencies. Even with prompt treatment, such problems often lead to death. Although the elderly experience critical respiratory problems or complications more frequently, any person can sustain an acute injury or disorder resulting in severe respiratory impairment. The client who has difficulty breathing is anxious and fearful. The nurse must be prepared to manage the client's physical and emotional needs during respiratory emergencies.

Pulmonary Embolism

Overview

A pulmonary embolism is a collection of particulate matter (solids, liquids, or gaseous substances) that enters systemic venous circulation and lodges in the pulmonary vasculature. Large emboli obstruct pulmonary circulation, leading to decreased systemic oxygenation, pulmonary tissue hypoxia, and potential death. Any substance can cause an embolism, but a blood clot is the most common.

Pathophysiology

Pulmonary embolism (PE) is the most common acute pulmonary disease (90%) among hospitalized clients. In most people with a PE, a blood clot from a deep venous thrombosis (DVT) breaks loose from one of the veins in the lower extremities or the pelvis. The thrombus detaches, travels through the vena cava and right side of the heart, and then lodges in a smaller blood vessel off the pulmonary artery. Platelets accumulate behind the embolus, triggering the release of serotonin and thromboxane A_2, which causes vasoconstriction. Widespread pulmonary vasoconstriction and pulmonary hypertension impair ventilation and perfusion. Deoxygenated blood shunts into the arterial circulation to produce hypoxemia. Approximately 12% of clients with PE do *not,* however, have hypoxemia.

Etiology

Major risk factors for DVT leading to pulmonary embolism include

- Prolonged immobilization
- Surgery
- Obesity
- Advancing age
- Hypercoagulability
- History of thromboembolism

In addition, smoking, pregnancy, estrogen therapy, congestive heart failure, stroke, malignant neoplasms (particularly of the lung or prostate), Trousseau's syndrome, and major trauma increase the risk for DVT and pulmonary embolism.

Fat, oil, air, tumor cells, amniotic fluid, foreign objects (like broken intravenous [IV] catheters), injected particles, and infected fibrin clots or pus can gain access to the venous system and cause pulmonary embolism. Fat emboli from fracture of a long bone and oil emboli from lymphangiography do not impede blood flow; rather, they result in vascular injury and adult respiratory distress syndrome (ARDS). Amniotic fluid embolus is associated with a mortality rate of 80% to 90%; it occurs in 1 per 20,000 to 30,000 deliveries and can be a complication of abortion or amniocentesis. Septic emboli commonly arise from a pelvic abscess, an infected IV catheter, and nonsterile injections of illegal drugs. The problem with septic emboli lies in the toxic effects of the infection more than in the vascular occlusion.

Incidence/Prevalence

Pulmonary embolism affects at least 500,000 people a year in the United States, approximately 10% of whom die. Many die within 1 hour of onset of symptoms or before the diagnosis has even been suspected.

Collaborative Management

 Assessment

➤ History

The nurse questions any client with sudden onset of respiratory difficulty about the risk factors for pulmonary embolism, especially a history of deep venous thrombosis, recent surgery, or prolonged immobilization.

➤ Physical Assessment/Clinical Manifestations

Respiratory Manifestations. Chart 34–1 outlines the key features of PE. The nurse assesses the client for dyspnea accompanied by tachypnea, tachycardia, and pleuritic chest pain (sharp, stabbing-type pain on inspiration). These symptoms are found in 80% of clients diagnosed with PE. Other symptoms vary considerably depending on the severity and the type of embolism. Breath sounds may be normal, but crackles occur in 50% of clients with PE. The nurse typically notes a dry cough. Hemoptysis may result from pulmonary infarction.

Cardiovascular Manifestations. The nurse assesses for distended neck veins, syncope, cyanosis, and hypotension. Hypotension associated with massive emboli indicates acute pulmonary hypertension. Auscultation of heart

---

Chart 34–1

Key Features of Pulmonary Embolism

Symptoms
- Dyspnea, sudden onset
- Pleuritic chest pain
- Apprehension
- Feeling of impending doom
- Cough
- Hemoptysis

Signs
- Tachypnea
- Crackles
- Pleural friction rub
- Tachycardia
- S_3 or S_4 heart sound
- Diaphoresis
- Fever, low grade
- Petechiae over chest and axillae

---

sounds may reveal an S_3 or S_4 sound with an altered pulmonic component of S_2.

Electrocardiogram findings are abnormal, nonspecific, and transient. T-wave changes and ST-segment abnormalities develop in 50% of clients, but left- and right-axis deviations occur with equal frequency.

Miscellaneous Manifestations. A low-grade fever may be present. Petechiae may be present on the skin over the chest and in the axillae. Some clients have more vague symptoms resembling the flu, such as nausea, vomiting, and general malaise.

➤ Laboratory Assessment

The hyperventilation from hypoxia and pain initially leads to respiratory alkalosis, which the nurse confirms with low partial pressure of arterial carbon dioxide ($PaCO_2$) values on arterial blood gas (ABG) analysis. The alveolar-arterial (A-a) gradient is increased. As blood continues to be shunted without picking up oxygen from the lungs, the $PaCO_2$ level starts to rise, leading to respiratory acidosis. Later, metabolic acidosis results from tissue hypoxia.

Arterial blood gas studies and pulse oximetry may reveal hypoxemia, but these results alone are not sufficient for the diagnosis of PE. A client with a small embolus may not be hypoxemic, and PE is not the only cause of hypoxemia.

➤ Radiographic Assessment

Radiographic assessment alone is never diagnostic of a pulmonary embolism. Chest x-ray may show some pulmonary infiltration around the embolism site; however, the chest x-ray most frequently is normal.

➤ Other Diagnostic Assessment

One of the most important studies to determine PE is the ventilation-perfusion ($\dot{V}/\dot{Q}$) lung scan. A negative perfusion scan rules out PE. If the $\dot{V}/\dot{Q}$ scan is inconclusive, pulmonary angiography, the most definitive and specific test for PE, may be done.

In a few clients, the physician performs thoracentesis (see Chap. 29) or transesophageal echocardiography (TEE; see Chap. 35) for help in detecting PE. The physician often orders Doppler ultrasound studies or impedance plethysmography (IPG) to document the presence of DVT and to support a diagnosis of PE.

➤ Psychosocial Assessment

Because the onset of symptoms is usually abrupt, the client with PE generally is extremely anxious and fearful. Hypoxemia may cause the client to have a sense of impending doom and increased restlessness. The emergent nature of the disorder and the subsequent admission to an intensive care unit (ICU) may increase the client's anxiety and fear of death.

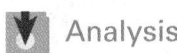 Analysis

➤ Prevention

Although pulmonary embolism (PE) can occur in apparently healthy people and may have no warning, it occurs more frequently in some situations. Thus, prevention of conditions contributing to PE is a major nursing concern. Preventive actions for PE are those that also prevent venous stasis and DVT. These actions are listed in Chart 34–2.

The physician may order small doses of prophylactic heparin administered subcutaneously every 8 hours. Heparin prevents hypercoagulation in clients immobilized for a prolonged period after surgery or restricted to bed rest. Adequate fluid intake and avoidance of oral contraceptives are also preventive. (Further information on the prevention of DVT is found in Chapter 20.)

When a client complains of the acute onset of dyspnea with associated pleuritic chest pain, the nurse notifies the physician immediately. The nurse attempts to reassure the client and assists the client to a position of comfort with the head of the bed elevated. The nurse prepares for oxygen administration and blood gas analysis while con-

---

Chart 34–2

Nursing Care Highlight: Prevention of Pulmonary Embolism

- Initiating passive and active range-of-motion exercises for the extremities of immobilized and postoperative clients
- Ambulating postoperative clients soon after surgery
- Using antiembolism and pneumatic compression stockings and devices postoperatively
- Avoiding the use of tight garters, girdles, and constricting clothing
- Preventing pressure under the popliteal space (such as with a pillow)

---

tinuing to monitor and assess the client for additional signs and symptoms.

➤ Common Nursing Diagnoses and Collaborative Problems

The primary collaborative problem for the client with pulmonary embolism is Hypoxemia related to imbalanced ventilation-perfusion.

The priority nursing diagnoses to consider when caring for a client with pulmonary embolism are
1. Decreased Cardiac Output related to acute pulmonary hypertension
2. Anxiety related to hypoxemia and life-threatening illness
3. Risk for Injury (bleeding) related to anticoagulation–thrombolytic therapy

➤ Additional Nursing Diagnoses and Collaborative Problems

In addition to the common nursing diagnoses and collaborative problems, one or more of the following may apply:

- Activity Intolerance related to hypoxemia
- Ineffective Gas Exchange related to disrupted pulmonary perfusion
- Fatigue related to ineffective gas exchange
- Altered Oral Mucous Membrane related to oxygen therapy
- Acute Confusion related to hypoxemia
- Sleep Pattern Disturbance related to ICU environment

 Planning and Implementation

Hypoxemia

Planning: Expected Outcomes. As a result of interventions, the client is expected to have adequate oxygenation in all major organs.

Interventions. Nonsurgical approaches to management of PE are most common. In some cases, surgical approaches may be needed in addition to drug therapy.

Nonsurgical Management. Management of pulmonary embolism aims to increase alveolar gas exchange, improve pulmonary perfusion, eliminate the embolism, and prevent complications. Interventions include oxygen therapy, monitoring, and anticoagulation–antithrombolytic therapy.

Oxygen Therapy. Oxygen therapy is important for the client with PE (see Chap. 30). The severely hypoxemic client may require mechanical ventilation and close monitoring with ABGs. In less severe cases, oxygen may be administered by nasal cannula or mask. Pulse oximetry is useful in monitoring arterial oxygen saturation, which reflects the degree of hypoxemia.

Monitoring. The nurse assesses the client continually for any changes in status. The nurse assesses vital signs, lung sounds, and cardiac and respiratory status at least every 1 to 2 hours, noting increasing dyspnea, dysrhyth-

---

Chart 34–3

Drug Therapy for Pulmonary Embolism

Drug	Usual Dosage	Nursing Interventions	Rationale
Heparin sodium (Hepalean♥)	• 5000–10,000 units IVP initially; then dose adjustment is based on PTT, 1300 units/hr on continuous drip or, less preferably, intermittent infusion	• Monitor PTT. • Know expected therapeutic PTT range for each client. • Report PTT results. • Monitor client for bleeding or bruising. • Rebolus every time infusion is increased. • Do not use with salicylates. • Monitor platelets daily for thrombocytopenia. • Have the antidote, protamine sulfate, available. • Avoid puncture sites and apply pressure to venipuncture and IM injection sites. • Avoid use of firm toothbrushes, straight razors, and rectal thermometers.	• Ongoing assessment helps detect side effects and prevent complications. • Reporting enables the physician to begin early treatment of a prolonged PTT. • An increased anticoagulation effect can occur with salicylates. • White clot syndrome, a type of arterial thrombosis, can occur. • Being prepared for an emergency helps prevent further complications. • Pressure at puncture sites helps promote clotting. • Safety measures help prevent bleeding.
Warfarin sodium (Coumadin, Warfilone sodium♥)	• 10–15 mg PO for 3 days initially; then dose adjustment is based on INR, usually 5–10 mg PO daily	• Monitor INR. • Know expected therapeutic INR range for each client. • Report INR results. • Monitor the client for bleeding or bruising. • Monitor for fever and skin rash. • Consult the pharmacist about potential drug interactions. • Have the antidote, vitamin K, available. • Apply pressure to venipuncture and IM injection sites. • Avoid use of firm toothbrushes, straight razors, and rectal thermometers. • Teach the client which foods are high in vitamin K.	• Ongoing assessment helps detect side effects and prevent complications. • Reporting enables the physician to begin early treatment of a prolonged INR. • Adverse drug reaction can occur. • There are many drug interactions with warfarin. • Being prepared for an emergency helps prevent further complications. • Pressure at puncture sites helps promote clotting. • Safety measures help prevent bleeding. • Food sources of vitamin K will alter INR.

Continued

---

mias, distended neck veins, and pedal or sacral edema. The nurse also notes the presence of crackles and adventitious sounds on auscultation of the lungs along with cyanosis of the lips, conjunctiva, oral mucous membranes, and nail beds.

Anticoagulation–Thrombolytic Therapy. The physician usually orders anticoagulation to keep the embolus from enlarging and prevent the formation of new clots. Active bleeding, stroke, and recent trauma are some contraindications to the use of anticoagulants. Before proceeding,

the physician evaluates each client for risks and determines the risk versus the benefit of therapy.

Heparin is commonly used unless the PE is massive or is accompanied by hemodynamic instability. A thrombolytic enzyme agent may then be used to break up the existing clot. The physician and nurse review the client's partial thromboplastin time (aPTT; also called PTT) before therapy is initiated, every 4 hours when therapy is initiated, and then usually daily thereafter. Therapeutic PTT values usually range between 1½ and 2½ times the control value.

CHART 34–3. Drug Therapy for Pulmonary Embolism   Continued

Drug	Usual Dosage	Nursing Interventions	Rationale
Alteplase (tissue plasminogen activator, recombinant; tPA; Activase)	• 100 mg IV infusion over 2 hr	• Assess for internal and external bleeding. • Reconstitute with sterile water without preservative immediately before use. • Administer with caution to clients who had been receiving aspirin, dipyridamole, heparin, or other anticoagulants.	• Bleeding is the most common adverse effect. • Recommended preparation ensures drug stability. • Other drugs with anticoagulation effects increase the risk of bleeding.
Streptokinase	• 250,000–1,500,000 IU by IV infusion over 30 min as loading dose, then 100,000 IU/hr over 24–72 hr via continuous IV infusion pump	• Draw blood samples for PTT and INR before starting infusion. • Reconstitute and further dilute with sterile normal saline; roll to mix—do not shake. • Monitor the client for internal and external bleeding. • Avoid IM injections, venipunctures, other invasive procedures, or excessive handling of the client during therapy.	• The rate of infusion depends on blood studies. • Recommended preparation ensures drug stability. • Bleeding is a common adverse effect. • Safety measures help prevent bleeding. • Bruising is common.
Urokinase	• 4400–6000 IU/kg by IV infusion as a priming dose, then 4400 IU/kg/hr for 12–24 hr via continuous IV infusion pump	• Reconstitute with sterile water, then further dilute; total volume should not exceed 200 mL. • Monitor the client for internal and external bleeding. • Avoid IM injections, venipunctures, other invasive procedures, or excessive handling of the client during therapy.	• Recommended preparation ensures drug stability. • Bleeding is a common adverse effect. • Safety measures help prevent bleeding. • Bruising is common.

IVP = intravenous push, or bolus; PTT = partial thromboplastin time; IU = international units; INR = international normalized ratio; IV = intravenous; IM = intramuscular; PO = orally.

Heparin therapy usually continues for 5 to 10 days. The physician starts most clients on oral anticoagulants, such as warfarin (Coumadin, Warfilone✦), on the third day of heparin use. Therapy with both heparin and warfarin continues until the client has an international normalized ratio (INR) of 2.0 to 3.0. Heparin is then discontinued. The nurse and physician monitor the client's INR daily. The physician usually continues warfarin for 3 to 6 weeks, but particular clients at high risk may take warfarin indefinitely. Charts 34–3 and 34–4 present the drugs used and laboratory tests monitored. (Anticoagulants and associated nursing care are also discussed in Chapter 38.)

Surgical Management. Two surgical procedures for the management of pulmonary embolism are embolectomy and inferior vena caval interruption.

Embolectomy. When thrombolytic enzyme therapy is contraindicated in a client with massive or multiple large pulmonary emboli with shock, surgical embolectomy may be necessary. Embolectomy removes the embolus or emboli from the pulmonary arteries.

Inferior Vena Caval Interruption. The physician considers placing a vena caval filter as a lifesaving measure and to prevent further emboli formation for some clients. Candidates for this procedure include clients with an absolute contraindication to anticoagulation, recurrent or major bleeding while receiving anticoagulants, septic PE, and those undergoing pulmonary embolectomy. The physician orders a pulmonary angiogram before placing the filter. (Placement of a vena caval filter is detailed in Chapter 38.)

Decreased Cardiac Output

Planning: Expected Outcomes. As a result of intervention, the client is expected to have adequate circulation.

Interventions. In addition to the interventions used for hypoxemia induced by pulmonary embolism, IV fluid therapy and drug therapy aim to increase cardiac output.

Intravenous Fluid Therapy. Intravenous access is initiated and maintained for fluid and drug therapy. Fluid therapy involves administration of crystalloid solutions to restore plasma volume and prevent shock (see Chap. 39). Clients with pulmonary embolism receiving IV fluids should undergo continuous cardiac monitoring and monitoring of pulmonary wedge pressures because the increased fluids can worsen pulmonary hypertension and contribute to right-sided heart failure.

Drug Therapy. When IV therapy alone is not effective in improving cardiac output, drug therapy with agents that increase myocardial contractility (positive inotropic

---

Chart 34–4

Laboratory Profile: Blood Tests Used to Monitor Anticoagulation Therapy

Test	Normal Range for Adults	Significance of Abnormal Findings
Partial thromboplastin time (PTT, aPTT [APTT])	• Normal values for each local laboratory may vary. • When activator reagents are used by the laboratory, the normal clotting time is shortened. • Common normal ranges are 20–30 sec in some laboratories, or 30–40 sec in others. • Therapeutic range for PE is 1.5–2.5 times the normal value (e.g., if normal is 20–30 sec, then therapeutic range is 40–75 sec).	*Subtherapeutic times* may signify that the client is not receiving enough heparin to prevent extension of the blood clot. An increase in the dosage or rate of infusion is usually indicated. *Therapeutic times* mean that the clotting time is increased from normal, but this increase is indicated in the case of PE. *Prolonged times* in clients with PE (i.e., >75 sec) indicate that the client is at risk of serious spontaneous bleeding. Heparin is usually held or decreased until the PTT drops back into the therapeutic range.
Prothrombin time (protime, PT)	• 11–12.5 sec • Therapeutic range for anticoagulant therapy in PE is 1.5–2 times the normal or control value in seconds. • Control values can vary day to day because reagents used may vary. • If INR values are reported with the PT, therapeutic range for PE is 2.5–3.0, or 3.0–4.5 for recurrent PE.	*Subtherapeutic values* may signify that the client is not receiving enough warfarin. An increase in the dosage is usually indicated. *Therapeutic values* mean that the protime is increased from normal, but this increase is indicated in the case of PE. *Prolonged values* in the treatment of PE indicate that the client is at risk for bleeding. The warfarin dose is usually decreased or held, the client is instructed to eat foods high in vitamin K, or an injection of vitamin K may be given.

PE = pulmonary embolism; INR = international normalized ratio; aPTT or APTT = activated partial thromboplastin time.

---

agents) may be prescribed. Such agents include amrinone (Inocor) and dobutamine (Dobutrex). The nurse assesses the client's cardiac status hourly during therapy with inotropic agents.

Anxiety

Planning: Expected Outcomes. The client is expected to express a reduction in level of anxiety.

Interventions. The client with PE is anxious and fearful for a variety of physiologic and psychological reasons. Interventions for reducing anxiety in clients with PE include oxygen therapy (see interventions for hypoxemia), communication, and drug therapy.

Communication. The nurse acknowledges the anxiety and the client's perception of a life-threatening situation. Speaking calmly and clearly, the nurse assures the client that appropriate measures are being taken. When administering a drug, changing the client's position, taking vital signs, or obtaining assessment data, the nurse explains the rationale to the client and shares information appropriately.

Drug Therapy. If the client's anxiety increases or prevents adequate rest, an antianxiety drug may be prescribed. Unless the client is intubated and mechanically ventilated, agents that have a sedating effect are avoided.

Risk for Injury (Bleeding)

Planning: Expected Outcomes. The client is expected to remain free from bleeding.

Interventions. As a result of anticoagulation or thrombolytic therapy, the client's ability to initiate and continue the blood-clotting cascade when injured is seriously impaired and the client is at great risk for bleeding. The nurse's major objectives are to protect the client from situations that could lead to bleeding and to monitor closely the amount of bleeding that is occurring.

The nurse assesses the client frequently for evidence of bleeding in the form of oozing, confluent ecchymoses, petechiae, or purpura. All stools, urine, nasogastric drainage, and vomitus are examined visually for the appearance of blood and are tested for occult blood. The nurse measures any blood loss as accurately as possible. The nurse measures the client's abdominal girth every 8 hours. Increases in abdominal girth can indicate internal hemorrhage. Bleeding precautions are instituted (Chart 34–5).

The nurse monitors laboratory values daily. The complete blood count (CBC) results are reviewed daily to determine the client's risk for bleeding as well as to determine whether actual blood loss has occurred. If the client sustains a severe blood loss, packed red blood cells may be ordered (see transfusion therapy in Chapter 42).

Chart 34–5

Nursing Care Highlight: Bleeding Precautions

- Handle the client gently.
- Use a lift sheet when moving or positioning the client in bed.
- Avoid intramuscular injections and venipunctures.
- When injections are necessary, use the smallest gauge needle appropriate for the task.
- Apply firm pressure to the needlestick site for 10 minutes or until the site no longer oozes blood.
- Apply ice to areas of trauma.
- Test all urine and stool for the presence of occult blood.
- Check intravenous sites every 2 hours for bleeding.
- Avoid trauma to rectal tissue:
  - Do not take temperatures rectally.
  - Do not give enemas.
  - Administer well-lubricated suppositories with caution.
- Measure abdominal girth daily.
- If the client is to be shaved, use an electric razor.
- Use a soft-bristled toothbrush or tooth sponge for oral care.
- Inspect the mouth and gums for bleeding every 4 hours.
- Pad the side rails of the bed.
- Encourage the client not to blow the nose or insert objects into the nose.
- If the client is to ambulate, ensure that the footwear has a firm sole.

may require some or much assistance with activities of daily living.

➤ Health Care Resources

For clients continuing with anticoagulation therapy, a home care nurse usually visits at least once per week to draw blood and perform an assessment (see Chart 34–7 for a focused assessment guide). Clients with severe dyspnea may require intermittent or continual home oxygen therapy. Respiratory therapy treatments can be performed in the home. The nurse or case manager coordinates arrangements for oxygen and other respiratory therapy to be available if needed by clients at home.

 Evaluation

On the basis of the identified nursing diagnoses and collaborative problems, the nurse evaluates the entire plan of

 Continuing Care

The client with a PE usually is discharged after the embolism has been resolved but may continue anticoagulation therapy.

➤ Health Teaching

The client with PE may continue anticoagulation therapy for weeks, months, or years after discharge, depending on the contributing factors. The nurse teaches the client and family about bleeding precautions, activities to reduce the risk for deep venous thrombosis and recurrence of PE, signs and symptoms of complications, and the importance of follow-up care (Chart 34–6).

➤ Home Care Management

Some clients will be discharged home with minimal risk for recurrence and no permanent physiologic changes. Other clients may have extensive lung damage and require lifestyle modifications.

Clients with extensive lung damage may have activity intolerance and become fatigued easily. The living arrangements may need to be modified so that clients can spend all or most of the time on one floor and avoid stair climbing. Depending on the degree of impairment, clients

Chart 34–6

Education Guide: The Client After Pulmonary Embolism

- Use an electric razor.
- Use a soft-bristled toothbrush and do not floss.
- Do not have dental work done without consulting your health care provider.
- Do not take aspirin or aspirin-containing products. Read the labels of all over-the-counter medications to be sure that the product does not contain aspirin or salicylates.
- Do not participate in contact sports or in any activity in which you might be bumped, scraped, or scratched.
- Apply ice immediately to any site of injury.
- Avoid anal intercourse.
- Take a stool softener to prevent straining during a bowel movement.
- Do not use enemas or rectal suppositories.
- Do not wear clothing that is tight or rubs.
- Avoid bending over at the waist.
- Avoid positions in which your knees are bent for any length of time.
- Wear elastic stockings as prescribed.
- Avoid prolonged sitting or standing.
- Avoid blowing your nose or placing objects in your nose. If you must blow your nose, do so gently without blocking either nasal passage.
- Take the prescribed dosage of medication at the precise time it was ordered to be given.
- Do not stop taking the medication abruptly or without a physician's order.
- Notify your doctor if you
  - Have an injury and persistent bleeding results.
  - Have excessive menstrual bleeding.
  - See blood in your urine or bowel movement.
  - Notice large bruises or areas of small red or purple marks over the skin.

care for the client with PE. The expected outcomes are that the client

- Attains and maintains adequate gas exchange and oxygenation
- Does not experience hypovolemia and shock
- Remains free from bleeding episodes
- States that levels of anxiety are reduced

Chart 34–7

Focused Assessment for Home Care Clients After Pulmonary Embolism

- Assess respiratory status.
  - Observe rate and depth of respiration.
  - Auscultate lungs.
  - Examine nail beds and mucous membranes for evidence of cyanosis.
  - Take a pulse oximetry reading.
  - Ask the client if chest pain or shortness of breath is experienced in any position.
  - Ask the client about the presence of sputum and its color and character.
- Assess cardiovascular status.
  - Take vital signs; including apical pulse, pulse pressure; assess presence or absence of orthostatic hypotension and quality and rhythm of peripheral pulses.
  - Take blood pressure in both arms.
  - Note presence or absence of peripheral edema.
  - Examine hand vein filling in the dependent position.
  - Examine neck vein filling in the recumbent and sitting positions.
- Assess lower extremities for deep venous thrombosis.
  - Examine lower legs and compare with each other for
    General edema
    Calf swelling
    Surface temperature
    Presence of red streaks or cord-like palpable structure
  - Measure calf circumference.
  - Ask the client to dorsiflex and plantarflex each foot. Note the ease with which the client can do this and ask whether pain is experienced in either position.
  - Gently squeeze the calf of each leg laterally and from front to back. Ask the client whether pain or tenderness is experienced with either maneuver.
- Assess for evidence of bleeding.
  - Examine the mouth and gums for oozing or frank bleeding.
  - Examine all skin areas for bruising or petechiae.
  - If the client voids during the visit, test the urine for occult blood.
- Assess cognition and mental status.
  - Level of consciousness
  - Orientation to time, place, and person
  - Can the client accurately read a seven-word sentence containing no words greater than three syllables?
- Assess client's understanding of illness and compliance with treatment.
  - Signs and symptoms to report to health care provider
  - Medication plan (correct timing and dose)
  - Bleeding precautions
  - Prevention of deep venous thrombosis

Acute Respiratory Failure

Overview

Pathophysiology

Acute respiratory failure is categorized according to abnormal blood gases. The critical values are partial pressure of arterial oxygen (PaO_2) less than 60 mmHg, arterial oxygen saturation, (SaO_2) less than 90%, or $PaCO_2$ greater than 50 mmHg with accompanying acidemia (pH < 7.30). Acute respiratory failure is further classified as ventilatory failure, oxygenation failure, or combination of both ventilatory and oxygenation failure. Whatever the underlying disorder, the client in acute respiratory failure is always hypoxemic.

Ventilatory Failure

Ventilatory failure is the type of ventilation-perfusion ($\dot{V}/\dot{Q}$) mismatching in which perfusion is normal but ventilation is inadequate. Ventilatory failure occurs when the thoracic pressure cannot be changed sufficiently to permit appropriate air movement in and out of the lungs. As a result, insufficient oxygen reaches the alveoli and carbon dioxide is retained. Both problems lead to hypoxemia.

Ventilatory failure is usually the result of one or more of the following three mechanisms: a mechanical abnormality of the lungs or chest wall, a defect in the respiratory control center in the brain, or an impairment in the function of the respiratory muscles. Ventilatory failure is usually defined by a $PaCO_2$ level above 45 mmHg in clients who have otherwise healthy lungs.

Oxygenation Failure

In oxygenation failure, thoracic pressure changes are normal, and the lungs can move air sufficiently but cannot oxygenate the pulmonary blood properly. Oxygenation failure can result from the type of $\dot{V}/\dot{Q}$ mismatch in which ventilation is normal but perfusion is decreased.

Combined Ventilatory and Oxygenation Failure

Combined ventilatory and oxygenation failure involves insufficient respiratory movements (hypoventilation). Gas exchange at the alveolar-capillary membrane is inadequate, so that too little oxygen reaches the blood and carbon dioxide is retained. The condition may or may not include poor pulmonary circulation. When pulmonary circulation is not adequate, $\dot{V}/\dot{Q}$ mismatching occurs and both ventilation and perfusion are inadequate. This type of respiratory failure results in a more profound hypoxemia than either ventilatory failure or oxygenation failure alone.

Etiology

Ventilatory Failure

Numerous diseases and conditions can result in ventilatory failure. Causes of ventilatory failure are categorized

TABLE 34-1

Common Causes of Ventilatory Failure	
Category	**Disorder**

Extrapulmonary	• Neuromuscular disorders
	  • Multiple sclerosis
	  • Myasthenia gravis
	  • Guillain-Barré syndrome
	  • Poliomyelitis
	• Spinal cord injuries affecting nerves to intercostal muscles
	• Central nervous system dysfunction
	  • Cerebrovascular accident (CVA)
	  • Cerebral edema
	  • Increased intracranial pressure
	  • Meningitis
	• Chemical depression
	  • Opioid analgesics
	  • Sedatives
	  • Anesthetic agents
	• Kyphoscoliosis
	• Massive obesity
	• Sleep apnea
	• External obstruction/constriction

Intrapulmonary	• Airway disease
	  • Chronic obstructive pulmonary disease
	  • Asthma
	• Ventilation-perfusion ($\dot{V}/\dot{Q}$) mismatching
	  • Pulmonary embolism
	  • Pneumothorax
	  • Adult respiratory distress syndrome (ARDS)
	• Amyloidosis
	• Pulmonary edema
	• Interstitial fibrosis

as either *extrapulmonary* (involving nonpulmonary tissues but affecting respiratory function) or *intrapulmonary* (disorders of the respiratory tract). Table 34–1 lists common extrapulmonary and intrapulmonary causes of ventilatory failure.

Oxygenation Failure

Many diseases and disorders of the lung can cause oxygenation failure. Mechanisms include impaired diffusion of oxygen at the alveolar level, right-to-left shunting of blood in the pulmonary vessels, ventilation-perfusion mismatching, breathing air with a low partial pressure of oxygen (a rare problem), and abnormal hemoglobin that fails to absorb the oxygen. In one type of ventilation-perfusion ($\dot{V}/\dot{Q}$) mismatching, areas of the lungs are still being perfused, but gas exchange is not able to occur, which leads to hypoxemia. An extreme example of $\dot{V}/\dot{Q}$ mismatching is a right-to-left shunt. A normal shunt is less than 5% of cardiac output. With right-to-left shunt, increased amounts of venous blood are not oxygenated, and 100% oxygen does not correct the deficiency. A clas-

sic cause of such a $\dot{V}/\dot{Q}$ mismatch is ARDS. Table 34–2 lists specific causes of oxygenation failure.

Combined Ventilatory and Oxygenation Failure

A combination of ventilatory failure and oxygenation failure occurs in clients who have abnormal lungs, as in all forms of chronic airflow limitation (CAL; i.e., chronic bronchitis, emphysema, and asthma). The bronchioles and alveoli are diseased (causing oxygenation failure), and the work of breathing increases until the respiratory muscles are unable to continue (causing ventilatory failure). Acute respiratory failure results. This process can also occur in clients who have cardiac failure as well as respiratory failure. This is a very dangerous situation because the cardiac system cannot compensate for the decreased oxygen by increasing the cardiac output.

Collaborative Management

 Assessment

The nurse assesses for dyspnea, the hallmark of respiratory failure. With use of a dyspnea assessment guide (Fig. 34–1), if one is available, the nurse objectively evaluates the dyspnea. Depending on the process, nature, and course of the underlying condition, the client may or may not be aware of dyspnea. In addition, the client needs to be alert enough to perceive the sensation of difficult breathing.

Dyspnea tends to be more intense when it develops rapidly. Slowly progressive respiratory failure may first manifest as dyspnea on exertion (DOE) or when lying down. The client notes orthopnea, finding it is easier to breathe in an upright position. In the client with CAL, a minor increase in dyspnea from the baseline condition may represent severe gas exchange abnormalities.

The nurse assesses for a change in the client's respiratory rate or pattern, a change in lung sounds, and the signs and symptoms of hypoxemia and hypercapnia (see Chap. 33). Pulse oximetry may indicate decreased oxygen

TABLE 34-2

Common Causes of Oxygenation Failure

• Low atmospheric oxygen concentration
  • High altitudes
  • Smoke inhalation
  • Carbon monoxide poisoning
• Pneumonia
• Abnormal hemoglobin
• Pulmonary embolism
• Pulmonary edema
• Interstitial pneumonitis-fibrosis
• Adult respiratory distress syndrome (ARDS)
• Mechanical obstruction
• Congestive heart failure
• Hypovolemic shock
• Hypoventilation

Dyspnea Assessment Guide

Indicate the amount of shortness of breath you are having at this time by marking the line.

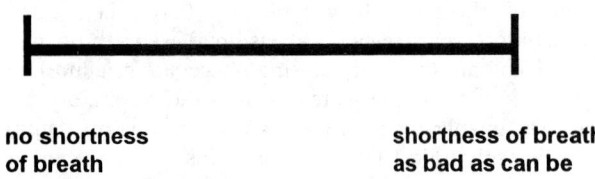

| no shortness of breath | shortness of breath as bad as can be |

Figure 34–1. A dyspnea assessment tool. Modified from Gift, A. (1989). A dyspnea assessment guide. *Critical Care Nurse,* 9(8), 79. Used with permission.

saturation, but an arterial blood gas (ABG) analysis is needed for adequate assessment of oxygenation status. The health care provider reviews the ABG studies to identify the degree of hypercapnia and hypoxemia.

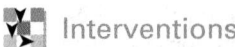 Interventions

The physician orders oxygen therapy for the client with acute respiratory failure to keep the PaO_2 level above 60 mmHg while treating the underlying cause of the respiratory failure. (Oxygen therapy is discussed in detail in Chapter 30.) If supplemental oxygen cannot maintain acceptable PaO_2 levels, the physician may order mechanical ventilation.

The nurse or assistive nursing personnel helps the client find a position of comfort that allows easier breathing. To decrease the anxiety commonly associated with dyspnea, the nurse assists the client with interventions such as relaxation, guided imagery, and diversion. Energy-conserving measures, such as minimal self-care and no unnecessary procedures, are instituted. The physician may order pulmonary medications administered systemically or by metered-dose inhaler (MDI) to open the bronchioles and promote gas exchange. The nurse instructs the client about the use of the inhaler and about the medications. Deep breathing and other breathing exercises are encouraged. (See Chapter 33 for further discussion of interventions for dyspnea and hypoxemia.)

Adult Respiratory Distress Syndrome

Overview

Adult respiratory distress syndrome (ARDS) is a form of acute respiratory failure characterized by

- Refractory hypoxemia
- Decreased pulmonary compliance
- Dyspnea
- Noncardiogenic bilateral pulmonary edema
- Dense pulmonary infiltrates (ground-glass appearance)

Adult respiratory distress syndrome usually occurs after an acute catastrophic event in people with no previous pulmonary disease. The mortality rate is 50% to 60%. Terminology for ARDS includes the current term *noncardiogenic pulmonary edema* and the former term *shock lung.*

Pathophysiology

Despite diverse causes leading to injury of the lung in ARDS, no common pathway has been found in its development, although the principal clinical manifestations are similar. In some forms of ARDS, the pathophysiologic mechanism is understood; in many others, it is not. The major site of injury in the lung is the alveolar-capillary membrane, which is normally permeable to only small molecules. The alveolar-capillary membrane can be injured intrinsically (causing sepsis, pulmonary embolism, or shock) or extrinsically (causing aspiration or inhalation injury). The interstitium of the lung normally remains relatively dry, but in clients with ARDS, increased extravascular lung fluid contains a high concentration of proteins.

Other significant changes occur in the alveoli and respiratory bronchioles. The type II pneumocyte is responsible for producing surfactant, a substance that maintains the elasticity of lung tissue and prevents alveolar collapse on expiration. Surfactant activity is reduced in ARDS either because of destruction of the type II pneumocyte or inactivation or dilution of surfactant. Consequently, the alveoli become unstable and tend to collapse unless they are filled with fluid from the interstitial space. These alveoli can no longer participate in gas exchange. As a result, interstitial edema forms around terminal airways, which are compressed and obliterated. Lung volume is further reduced, and there is even less compliance (elasticity). As the leak expands, fluid, protein, and blood cells collect in the interstitium and alveoli. Lymph channels are compressed and ineffective. Poorly ventilated alveoli receive blood. Thus, the shunt fraction increases, and hypoxemia and ventilation-perfusion ($\dot{V}/\dot{Q}$) mismatching result.

Etiology

Adult respiratory distress syndrome is associated with a number of causative factors (Table 34–3). Some causes involve direct injury to lung tissue; others do not directly involve the respiratory system. Serious nervous system injury, such as trauma, cerebrovascular accidents, tumors, and sudden increases in cerebrospinal fluid pressure, may cause massive sympathetic discharge. Systemic vasoconstriction results with redistribution of large volumes of blood into the pulmonary circuit. The marked elevation of hydrostatic pressure, then, probably causes lung injury. Processes that produce cerebral hypoxia, such as shock and ascent to high altitudes, may operate by a similar mechanism.

Some factors produce ARDS by direct injury to the lung. For example, aspiration of gastric contents leads to mechanical obstruction or produces an acid burn to the airway when the pH of the gastric contents is less than 2.5. In such a direct injury, rapid necrosis of the alveolar type I pneumocyte occurs. The injured capillary endothe-

TABLE 34-3

Common Causes of Adult Respiratory Distress Syndrome (ARDS)

- Shock
- Trauma
- Serious nervous system injury
- Pancreatitis
- Fat and amniotic fluid emboli
- Pulmonary infections
- Sepsis
- Inhalation of toxic gases (smoke, oxygen)
- Pulmonary aspiration
- Drug ingestion (e.g., heroin, opioids, aspirin)
- Hemolytic disorders
- Multiple blood transfusions
- Cardiopulmonary bypass
- Near-drowning (especially in fresh water)

lium allows protein and cellular elements to escape from the intravascular space. Radiation, near-drowning, and inhalation of toxic gases similarly injure the alveolar and capillary endothelium. In addition, trauma, sepsis, drowning, and burns cause the release of thromboplastins, which form fibrin clots in the peripheral blood. The clots, together with platelets and leukocytes, are filtered out in the lung. In many cases of ARDS, especially after trauma, production of plasminogen activation inhibitors by the liver is enhanced. Fibrinolysis is prevented, and microemboli remain in the lung. Disseminated intravascular coagulation (DIC) plays a role in some clients.

Incidence/Prevalence

Because of varying definitions, the incidence of ARDS is unknown, although a 1993 estimate suggested that more than 100,000 cases of ARDS occur yearly in the United States. Its high rank on the list of common diseases may be a result of the improved treatment of other catastrophic illnesses.

A major goal in the prevention of ARDS is early recognition of clients at high risk for the syndrome. Because clients with aspiration of gastric contents are at great risk, the nurse closely assesses and monitors elderly clients receiving tube feeding and clients with neurologic deficits and altered swallowing and gag reflexes. The nurse and assistive personnel meticulously follow all infection control guidelines, including hand washing, invasive catheter and wound care, and body substance precautions. In addition, the nurse carefully observes clients who are being treated for any of the diseases or disorders associated with ARDS.

Collaborative Management

 Assessment

The nurse assesses the client's respirations and notes whether increased work of breathing is evident, as indicated by hyperpnea, grunting respiration, cyanosis, pallor,

and retraction intercostally (between the ribs) or suprasternally (above the ribs). The nurse notes the presence of diaphoresis and any change in mental status. No abnormal lung sounds are present on auscultation because the edema of ARDS occurs first in the interstitial spaces and not in the airways. To assess for hypotension, tachycardia, and dysrhythmias, the nurse monitors vital signs frequently.

The primary laboratory study for establishing the diagnosis of ARDS is a lowered PaO_2 value, determined by arterial blood gas (ABG) measurements. The client with ARDS is poorly responsive to high concentrations of oxygen (*refractory hypoxemia*). Because a widening alveolar oxygen gradient (increased fraction of inspired oxygen [FIO_2] does not yield corresponding increased PaO_2 levels) develops with increased shunting of blood, the client has a progressive need for higher concentrations of oxygen. A large difference between the predicted and actual alveolar oxygen tension indicates shunting. The physician orders sputum cultures to isolate any organisms causing an infection that must be treated. Because decreased mortality depends on aggressive therapy, sputum may be obtained through bronchoscopy with protective brushings and by transtracheal aspiration.

The chest x-ray shows the diagnostic diffuse haziness or "whited-out" (ground-glass) appearance of the lung. An electrocardiogram rules out cardiac abnormalities and usually reveals no specific changes. The placement of a Swan-Ganz hemodynamic monitoring catheter is a diagnostic tool: in the client with ARDS, the pulmonary capillary wedge pressure (PCWP) is usually low to normal. This pressure differs from the client with cardiogenic pulmonary edema in whom the PCWP is higher than 15 mmHg.

 Interventions

Clients with adult respiratory distress syndrome (ARDS) usually require endotracheal intubation and mechanical ventilation with positive end-expiratory pressure (PEEP) or continuous positive airway pressure (CPAP). Sedation and paralysis may be necessary for adequate ventilation and for reducing oxygen requirements. Because one of the side effects of PEEP is tension pneumothorax, the nurse assesses lung sounds frequently and maintains a patent airway with suctioning. Positioning may be important in promoting gas exchange. (See the Research Applications for Nursing for a discussion of the prone position.)

➤ Drug and Fluid Therapy

Corticosteroids are seldom used in the treatment of ARDS, although they may impair neutrophil mobilization and stabilize the capillary membrane. Their efficacy, however, has not been determined. Antibiotics are used to treat infections with organisms identified by culture.

Many interventions are under investigation, but none have been shown to be effective in decreasing mortality. Some of these interventions include mediators (vitamins C and E, interleukin, prostacycline, aspirin), nitric oxide, surfactant replacement, and prone positioning.

▷ Research Applications for Nursing

Prone Position Improves Oxygenation in Clients with ARDS

Vollman, K. M., & Bander, J. (1996). Improved oxygenation in patients with acute respiratory distress syndrome. Intensive Care Medicine, 22(10), 1105–1111.

In clients with adult respiratory distress syndrome (ARDS) on mechanical ventilation, high tidal volumes, increased levels of inspired oxygen (O_2), and positive end-expiratory pressure (PEEP) are instituted to decrease shunt and improve oxygenation. More studies are indicating that the prone position improves oxygen and allows fraction of inspired oxygen (FIO_2) and pressures to be decreased. Contraindications to prone positioning include skin trauma from the turning maneuver and accidental disconnection or removal of tubes and catheters.

In this study, the primary author, a nurse, evaluated a device she developed to facilitate proning. Fifteen clients with ARDS were studied in this prospective controlled trial conducted in two medical intensive care units (ICUs). Oxygenation was better with clients in the prone position than in the supine position. Overall, there was a decrease in the alveolar-arterial (A–a) gradient of 21 mmHg when clients were prone. Responders were classified as those showing at least a 7-mmHg improvement in partial pressure of arterial oxygen (PaO_2). There were significant differences between responders and nonresponders (but not in positions) between PaO_2, partial pressure of arterial carbon dioxide ($PaCO_2$), baseline data, pulmonary artery pressures, peak inspiratory pressures on the ventilator, ICU length of stay, and time on mechanical support. No client suffered adverse hemodynamic effects, airway dislodgment, or loss of intravascular catheters during position changes. An important aspect of the turning frame is that the abdomen is not restricted.

Critique. The study sample was small and limited to a medical ICU population. The turning maneuvers were randomly assigned, and clients were used as their own controls. This study represents an important beginning to evaluate the effects of proning as well as the use of a positioning device to facilitate the maneuver.

Possible Nursing Implications. Oxygenation was found to increase in the prone position. Prone-positioned clients with ARDS may be treated with lower levels of O_2 and PEEP to maintain adequate gas exchange. Nurses have been reluctant to place clients in the prone position because of the difficulty entailed. Physicians are reluctant to request proning because of the complications that can arise, including unplanned extubation. If turning is achieved relatively easily, nurses and physicians may perform the maneuver more frequently. Use of the turning device may facilitate this nursing action and improve client outcome.

The optimal type of fluid therapy for the client with ARDS remains unknown. A colloidal solution may be effective for intravascular volume expansion. However, the value of colloid therapy is unknown. Fluid volume should be titrated to maintain adequate cardiac output and tissue perfusion. Judicious diuresis may help decrease extravascular lung fluid, but care should be taken to prevent overall dehydration and hypotension.

▷ Nutrition Therapy

Clients with ARDS are at risk for malnutrition, which further compromises the respiratory system. An altered immune response as well as an altered ventilatory response to hypoxemia may occur with undernourished clients. Diaphragmatic functioning is also altered. Therefore, enteral nutrition in the form of tube feeding or parenteral nutrition in the form of hyperalimentation is instituted as soon as possible.

▷ Case Management

Case management of the client with ARDS focuses on the phases of ARDS rather than day-to-day care. The course of ARDS and its management are divided into four phases.

- Phase 1: includes early changes with the client exhibiting dyspnea and tachypnea. Early interventions focus on supporting the client and providing oxygen.
- Phase 2: patchy infiltrates from increasing pulmonary edema. Interventions include mechanical ventilation and prevention of complications.
- Phase 3: occurs over days 2 to 10, and the client exhibits progressive refractory hypoxemia. Interventions focus on maintaining adequate oxygen transport, preventing complications, and supporting the failing lung until it has had time to heal.
- Phase 4: pulmonary fibrosis–pneumonia with progression; occurs after 10 days. This phase is irreversible and is frequently referred to as "late" or "chronic" ARDS. Interventions focus on preventing sepsis, pneumonia, and multiple organ failure (multiple organ dysfunction syndrome [MODS]) as well as weaning the client from the ventilator. Clients in this phase may be ventilator dependent for weeks to months. Clients may be cared for in specialized units or facilities that focus on rehabilitation and long-term weaning. Some clients may not be weanable and go home ventilator dependent (see Clinical Pathway).

Client Requiring Intubation and Ventilation
Overview

Through the use of mechanical ventilation, clients who have severe derangements of gas exchange may be supported until the underlying process has resolved or has been adequately treated. Thus, mechanical ventilation is nearly always a temporary life-support technique. The need for ventilatory support may, however, be lifelong, especially for those with chronic, progressive neuromuscular diseases that preclude effective spontaneous ventilation.

Mechanical ventilation is most commonly used for clients with hypoxemia and progressive alveolar hypoventilation with respiratory acidosis. The hypoxemia is usually due to intrapulmonary shunting of blood when external devices cannot provide sufficiently high FIO_2. Mechanical ventilation is also indicated

- For clients who need respiratory support after surgery
- For clients who are barely maintaining adequate gas

exchange at the cost of expending energy with high work of breathing
■ For clients who require general anesthesia or heavy sedation to allow diagnostic or therapeutic interventions

Collaborative Management

 Assessment

The nurse assesses the client about to undergo intubation in the same way as for other clients with respiratory problems. Once mechanical ventilation has been initiated, the nurse assesses the respiratory system on an ongoing basis. The nurse monitors and assesses for complications related to the artificial airway or ventilator as well as for those related to mechanical ventilation.

Interventions

➤ Endotracheal Intubation

Clients who need mechanical ventilation require an artificial airway. The most common type of artificial airway for establishing and maintaining the airway on a short-term basis is the endotracheal (ET) tube. If the client requires an artificial airway for longer than a specified period, usually longer than 10 to 14 days, the physician considers a tracheostomy (see Chap. 30) to avoid mucosal and vocal cord damage.

The goals of intubation include maintaining a patent airway, reducing the work of breathing, providing a means to remove secretions, and providing ventilation and oxygen. Major indications for intubation are listed in Table 34–4.

Endotracheal Tube. An ET tube is a long polyvinyl chloride tube that is passed through the mouth or nose and into the trachea (Fig. 34–2). When properly positioned, the tip of the ET tube rests approximately 2 to 3 cm (0.8 to 1.2 inches) above the carina (where the trachea divides into the right and left mainstem bronchi).

TABLE 34–4

Major Indications for Intubation
• Airway protection when the client loses reflexes because of anesthesia, medications, disease, or decreased level of consciousness • To provide positive pressure or high oxygen concentration • Bypass airway obstruction • Facilitating pulmonary hygiene • Suctioning of secretions when the client cannot handle secretions (as in diseases of chronic airflow limitation)

Oral intubation is the easiest and quickest method of establishing of an airway; therefore, it is also performed as an emergency procedure. The nasal route is reserved for elective intubation, for some facial or oral traumas and surgeries, and when oral intubation is not possible. This route is contraindicated if the client has a blood dyscrasia. An experienced, specially trained professional, such as an anesthesiologist, nurse anesthetist, or pulmonologist (MD), performs the intubation.

An ET tube has several parts (see Fig. 34–2). The shaft of the tube contains a radiopaque vertical line for the length of the tube, which permits demonstration of correct placement by chest x-ray. Short horizontal lines (depth markings) are used to designate correct placement of the tube at the nares or mouth (at the incisor tooth) and to identify how far the tube has been inserted.

The cuff at the distal end of the tube, with proper inflation, produces a seal between the trachea and the cuff. The seal prevents aspiration and ensures delivery of a set tidal volume when mechanical ventilation is used. When the cuff is inflated to an adequate sealing volume, no air can pass through the cuff to the vocal cords, nose, or mouth; therefore, the client is not able to talk when the cuff is inflated. The cuff should be inflated to a

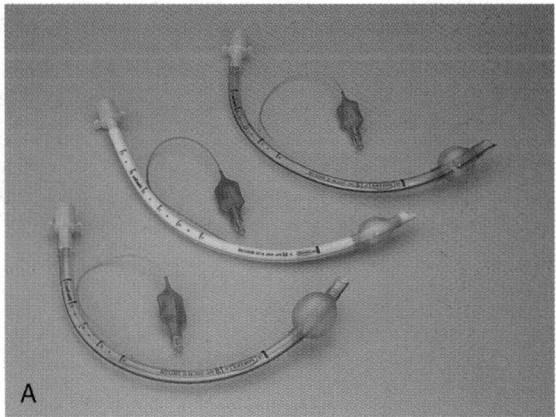

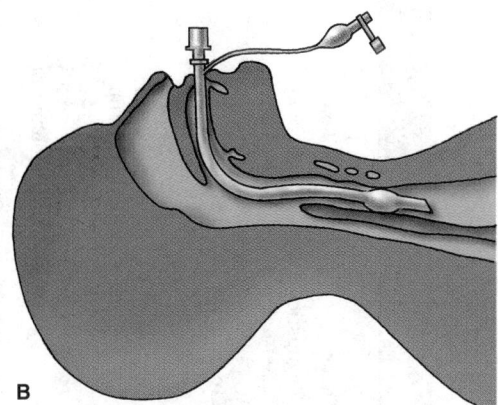

Figure 34–2. *A,* Endotracheal tubes. (Courtesy of Sims Porter, Inc.) *B,* Correct placement of an oral endotracheal tube.

Clinical Pathway for Ventilator Dependent Clients with Tracheostomy or Endotracheal Tube

Focus	Phase I Acute Ventilatory Support	Phase II Ventilatory Support	Phase III Weaning	Phase IV Resolution
Diagnostic Tests, Labs & Procedures	Arterial blood gas (ABG) CXR SMA-7 Sputum culture & sens after 72 hrs ETT Blood cultures as needed Phosphorus 4 times daily if on TF or TPN for 1st week Pre-albumin prn Pulse oximetry Complete blood count (CBC) SAM-12 ECG	Pulmonary mechanics ECG prn CBC CXR SMA-7 SMA-12 weekly ABG prn Pulse oximetry 24-hr urine nitrogen prn (if no renal failure) Pre-albumin prn	Pulmonary mechanics ECG prn CBC CXR SMA-7 SMA-12 weekly ABG prn Pulse oximetry 24-hr urine urea nitrogen prn (if no renal failure) Pre-albumin prn	Pulmonary mechanics Pulse oximetry prn
Consults	Pulmonologist consultation if intubated after 72 hours or if re-intubation is required Assess need for swallow/speech consultation Nutritional support dietitian Respiratory care clinician Social worker: Supportive counseling/crisis intervention	Physical medicine and rehabilitation Physical therapy Occupational therapy Swallow/speech consultation Social worker: Supportive counseling/crisis intervention Social worker assesses client's and family's resource needs.	Physical medicine and rehabilitation Social worker: Supportive counseling Social worker to evaluate client for placement options	
Treatments	SVO$_2$ prn Mechanical ventilation Respiratory treatments Secretion management Tracheostomy after ETT in place × 7 days GI protection (histamine blockers/carafate) Sedation prn IV medications Diuretics prn Packed cells prn Vasopressors Antibiotics prn Vasoactive infusions Paralytics prn Daily weight I & O hourly Special bed prn Suction prn Foley Swallow/dysphagia assessment	Respiratory treatments Packed cells prn Secretion management Antibiotic prn Sedation prn Diuretics prn Tracheostomy care Daily weight Suction prn I & O Foley Evaluate need for permanent IV access	Respiratory treatments Packed cells prn Secretion management Antibiotic prn Diuretics prn Tracheostomy care Daily weight Suction prn I & O D/C Foley prn If prolonged TFs, evaluate need for PEG Evaluate continued need for IV access	Tracheostomy collar Decannulator Extubator Continue vent & slow wean Daily weight I & O every 8 hours Suction prn

Diet	Nutritional assessment TPN/TF TF preferred	If on TPN, transition to TF Reassess nutritional status every 10 days	Transition to PO diet if no dysphagia Reassess nutritional status every 10 days	Continue PO diet or TF
Activity	Bedrest Passive range of motion every 4 hours Increase activity as tolerated	Up on side of bed with assistance Foot support Up in chair if tolerated Active range of motion	Up in chair 3× daily Increase ambulation	Up in chair 3× daily for increased time Increased ambulation Increased client involvement in self-care activities
Treatment	Establish a communication mode with the client. Orient client to environment. Orient family to environment, procedures, client's current condition and prognosis, care needs, and hospital policy.	Keep client and family updated about the client's condition, new and continuing procedures, treatment plans, and changes in care needs.	Teach the client and family about weaning procedures and expected responses.	Keep the client and family informed re progress, changes in treatment plan, expected responses, new equipment or personnel.
Discharge Planning	Family members and social worker: Assessment of resources and a discharge plan appropriate and individualized to the expected outcomes for the ventilator-dependent client.	Inform social worker of client's progress. Social worker to assess client's and family's resource needs; explore rehabilitation and long-term insurance coverage.	Keep social worker updated about client progress. Social worker to evaluate client for placement options. Social worker to initiate referrals.	Social worker to finalize client's transportation and disposition. Social worker to finalize arrangements for needed equipment, home health services, and follow-up care.

CBC = complete blood count, CXR = chest x-ray, ECG = electrocardiogram, ETT = endotracheal tube, I & O = intake and output, O = oral, TF = tube feeding, TPN = total parenteral nutrition, PEG = percutaneous endoscopic gastronomy, prn = as needed.

pressure of 20 to 25 cm H_2O using minimal-leak or no-leak techniques.

The pilot balloon with a one-way valve permits air to be inserted into the cuff and yet prevents air from escaping. This balloon is used as a general guideline for determining the absence or presence of air in the cuff; it will not tell how much or how little air is present.

The universal adaptor, which is 15 mm in diameter, enables attachment to ventilator tubing or other types of oxygen delivery systems. The tubing size is indicated on the adaptor or the shaft of the tube. Adult tube sizes range from 5 to 10 mm. Sizes used are 8.0 to 9.0 for large adults, 7.0 to 8.0 for medium-size adults, and 6.0 to 7.0 for small adults.

Preparing for Intubation. The nurse and assistive nursing personnel know the proper procedure for summoning intubation personnel to the bedside in an emergency situation. The nurse explains the procedure to the client as clearly as possible under the circumstances. Basic life-support measures, such as the establishment of a patent airway and the administration of 100% oxygen via a resuscitation (Ambu) bag with a face mask, are crucial to the client's survival until help arrives. The coordination for resuscitation with a bag and mask device can be cumbersome; therefore, practice is necessary.

In an emergency, the nurse or assistive personnel brings the code (or "crash") cart, respiratory equipment box, and suction equipment (which is often already on the code cart) to the bedside. The nurse maintains a patent airway through positioning and the insertion of an oral airway until the client is intubated. During intubation, the nurse continuously monitors for changes in the client's vital signs, signs of hypoxia or hypoxemia, dysrhythmias, and aspiration. The nurse also ensures that each intubation attempt lasts no longer than 30 seconds, preferably less than 15 seconds. After 30 seconds, oxygen via mask and manual resuscitation bag is provided to prevent hypoxia and potential cardiac arrest. The nurse suctions as necessary.

Verifying Tube Placement. Immediately after an ET tube is inserted, its placement must be verified. The most accurate way of verifying placement is by checking end-tidal CO_2 concentration, if available. The nurse assesses for bilateral equal breath sounds, bilateral equal chest excursion, and air emerging from the ET tube. If breath sounds and chest wall movement are absent on the left side, the tube may be in the right mainstem bronchus. The person intubating the client should be able to reposition the tube without repeating the entire intubation procedure.

The nurse auscultates over the stomach to rule out esophageal intubation. If the tube is in the stomach, the nurse hears louder breath sounds over the stomach than over the chest and notes abdominal distention. The nurse continuously monitors chest wall movement and breath sounds until tube placement is verified by chest x-ray.

Stabilizing the Tube. The nurse, respiratory therapist, or anesthesia personnel stabilize the ET tube at the mouth or nose. The tube is marked at the level at which it touches the incisor tooth or naris. Two persons working

together use a head halter technique to secure the tube. Chart 34–8 outlines the steps in the procedure.

An oral airway may also need to be inserted to keep the client from biting an oral tube. Ongoing nursing care requires an oral tube to be moved to the opposite side of the mouth daily. This common maneuver is thought to help prevent pressure and necrosis of the lip and mouth area, prevent nerve damage, and facilitate a thorough inspection and cleaning of the mouth. One person stabilizes the tube at the correct position and prevents head movement while a second person applies the tape. After the procedure is completed, the nurse verifies the presence of bilateral and equal breath sounds and the level of the tube.

Nursing Care. The nurse assesses tube placement, cuff pressure, breath sounds, and chest wall movement regularly. The nurse prevents pulling or tugging on the tube by the client to prevent dislodgment or "slipping" of the tube and checks the pilot balloon to ensure the cuff is inflated. Suctioning, coughing, and speaking attempts by the client place extra stress on the tube and also can cause dislodgment. Head flexion moves the tube away from the carina; head extension moves the tube closer to the carina. Rotation of the head also causes the tube to move. Mouth secretions and tongue movement can loosen the tape and allow malposition of the tube. When other measures fail, the nurse applies soft wrist restraints, as ordered, for the client who is voluntarily or involuntarily pulling on the tube. This intervention is a last resort to prevent accidental extubation. Adequate sedation (chemical restraint) may be necessary to decrease agitation or extubation. The nurse obtains permission for restraints from the client or family after explaining the rationale. More information on management of the artificial airway is found in Chapter 30.

Complications of an ET or nasotracheal tube can occur at each stage of the process: during placement, while in place, during extubation, or after extubation (either early or late). Trauma and complications can occur to the face; eye; nasal and paranasal areas; oral, pharyngeal, bronchial, tracheal, and pulmonary areas; esophageal and gastric areas; and cardiovascular, musculoskeletal, and neurologic systems.

➤ *Mechanical Ventilation*

Mechanical ventilation to support and maintain a client's respiratory function is widely used on medical-surgical units, in nursing homes, and in the home setting as well as in critical care units. The nurse plays a pivotal role in the coordination of care and the prevention of complications. Chart 34–9 reviews nursing care of the client during mechanical ventilation.

The goals of mechanical ventilation are to improve oxygenation and ventilation and decrease the amount of oxygen and work needed to accomplish an effective breathing pattern. Mechanical ventilation is used to support the client until lung function is adequate or until the acute episode has passed. A ventilator does not cure diseased lungs; it provides ventilation until the lungs are able to resume the process of breathing. Therefore, the nurse must remember why the client is using the ventilator so

Chart 34–8

Nursing Care Highlight: Taping an Oral and Nasal Endotracheal Tube

Little evidence is available to provide clinical direction on the best method to secure endotracheal (ET) and nasotracheal tubes. However, adhesive tape is the easiest, cheapest, and most frequently used.

Adhesive tape may be irritating to the skin, and frequent tape changes may disrupt the skin integrity. An additional reported complication is nosocomial cutaneous mucormycosis occurring around the surgical tape securing the ET tube. Protecting the skin, especially on the face, is a high priority for patients and nurses. This must be balanced against making sure the ET tube is not dislodged. A simple yet effective method of securing the oral and nasotracheal tube is demonstrated here.

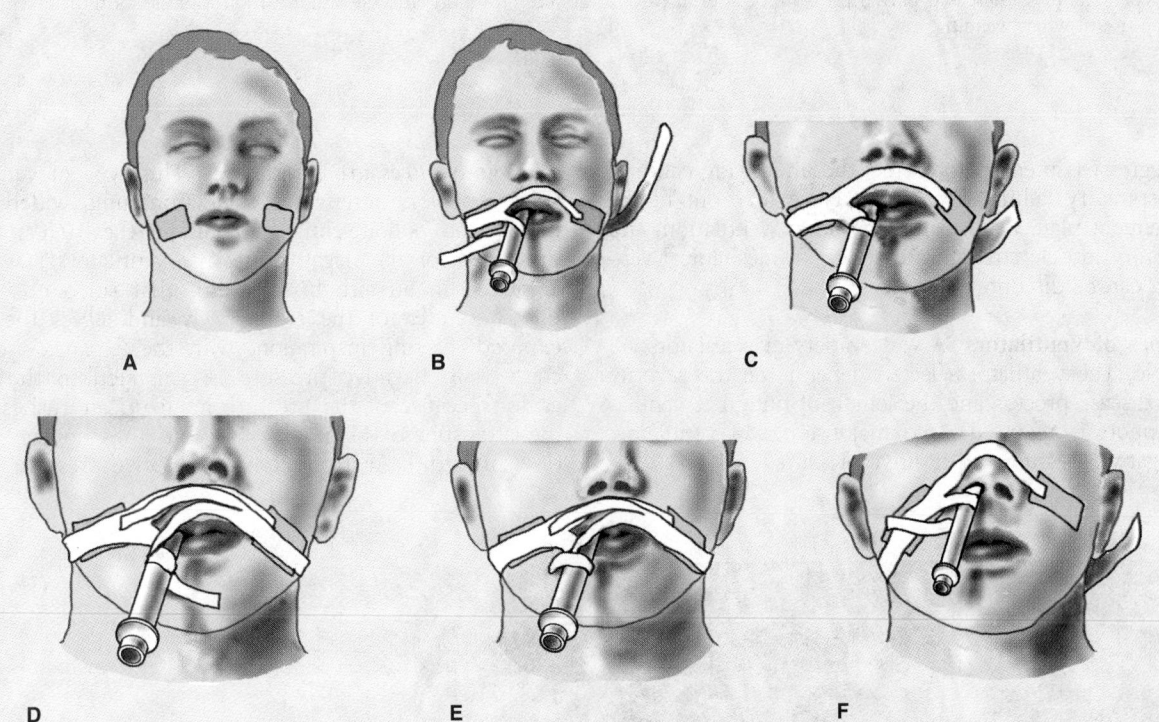

1. Prepare the skin by shaving the cheeks and upper lip, if possible.
2. Protect the skin by applying tincture of benzoin to the skin and ET tube and allow to dry (Mastisol may also be used, but Detachol **must** be used before removing the tape); then apply a 1 × 3-inch long piece of thin DuoDerm or other protective or hydrocolloid membrane to the skin on the cheeks (A).
3. Take a 30-inch (about 2 ½-foot) piece of adhesive tape and lay it on a flat surface, sticky side up. Take another piece of tape (about 10 inches) and cover the middle portion of the tape (sticky side to sticky side) to protect the back of the patient's neck. A tongue blade on each end folded over can keep it from getting tangled or sticking prematurely.
4. Place the tape behind the patient's neck. Remove the tongue blades, and place the tape on the protective membrane up to the end of the mouth on each side. Trim the tape as needed, and split each end of the tape.
5. Take the upper part of one end of the tape and place it on the upper lip. Take the lower part of the tape and wrap it securely around the tube (B, C). Take the upper part of the other end of the tape, place it on the upper lip, and wrap the lower part securely around the tube (D, E). Do not have the tube too far to either side of the mouth, or it can cause skin breakdown in the corner of the mouth or lips.
6. The same method can be used for nasal tubes, but do not tape the tube too tightly to the nose or skin breakdown will occur on the nares (F).
7. Always tape the tube to the upper lip, never the lower. The lower jaw moves too much with attempts to speak or oral care, which will move the tube and cause irritation and discomfort for the patient. The tape should be inspected at least every shift for signs of loosening or skin irritation or breakdown, especially with increased oral secretions. Tightness of the tape should also be checked each shift if swelling in the face and neck occurs or if there is an increase in fluid retention (as in anasarca, sepsis, or adult respiratory distress syndrome).

Continued

CHART 34–8. Nursing Care Highlight: Taping an Oral and Nasal Endotracheal Tube Continued

An additional technique for securing tubing that can decrease ET tube movement and provide a fulcrum for pulling on ventilator tubing is to attach a 6-inch (50-mL) piece of flexible ventilator tubing between the ET tube adaptor and the **Y** connector of the ventilator tubing. The procedure for this technique is as follows:

1. Shave the chest or clean with alcohol a portion of the chest at right angles to the angle of Louis. Apply tincture of benzoin and allow to dry.
2. Prepare Montgomery straps by taking two 6-inch pieces of 2-inch wide adhesive tape. Double-back one end of each piece of tape, and cut a small hole in the ends that are doubled over.
3. Apply the tape to the prepared chest with the ends with the hole over each other. Take a 12-inch piece of twill (trach) tape and thread through both holes. Position the tubing with the **Y** connector over the holes and tie into place. This procedure allows all pulling on the tubing to place strain on the tape (straps) and not on the face or the tube. Caution should be taken if patients have increased partial pressure of arterial carbon dioxide retention, and end-tidal carbon dioxide monitoring may be useful when weaning.

that aggressive attempts to correct the underlying cause of the respiratory failure are always at the forefront of the management plan. If normal oxygenation, ventilation, and respiratory muscle strength are achieved, mechanical ventilation can be discontinued.

Types of Ventilators. A wide variety of ventilators are available. The ventilator selected depends on the severity of the disease process and the length of time that ventilator support is required. Two major types of ventilators are negative pressure and positive pressure.

Negative-Pressure Ventilators. This type of ventilator (Fig. 34–3) is noninvasive. The iron lung, widely used during the poliomyelitis epidemic in the 1940s, is the prototype for the negative-pressure ventilator. The client is placed in an airtight apparatus that surrounds either the chest area or the entire body and leaves the head exposed. During inspiration, with the expansion of the chest wall, negative pressure is generated in the chest cavity. Because of the pressure gradient, air rushes from the atmosphere (high pressure) into the thoracic cavity (low pressure). At a preset time, negative pressure ceases

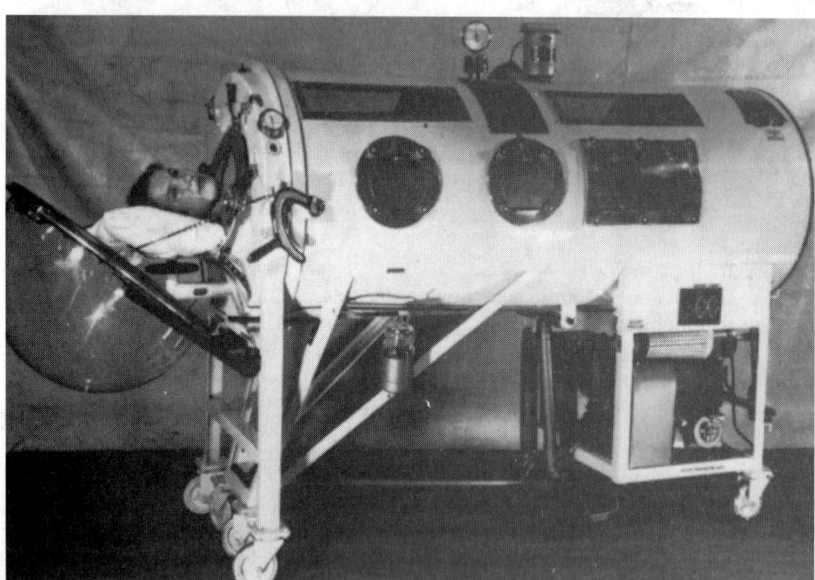
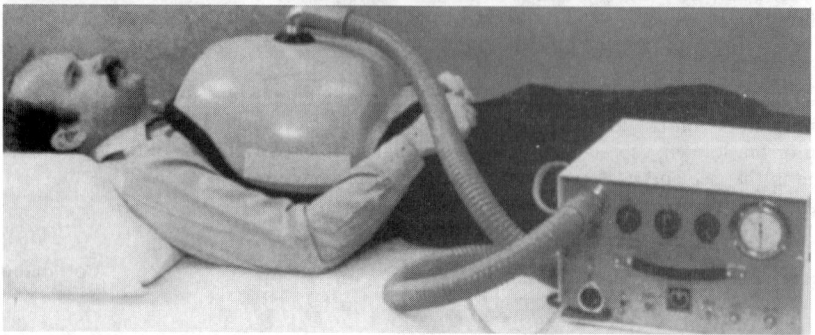

Figure 34–3. Two negative-pressure ventilators. *Top,* The Emerson iron lung. (Courtesy of J. H. Emerson Co., Cambridge, MA.) *Bottom,* Lifecare Chest Shell. (From Hill, N. [1986]. Clinical application of body ventilators. *Chest,* 90[6], 900. Used with permission.)

Nursing Care Highlight: The Client on Mechanical Ventilation

- At least once every shift check to be sure the ventilator settings are set as ordered.
- Check to be sure alarms are set (especially low pressure and low exhaled volume).
- Observe the exhaled volume digital display to be sure the client is receiving the prescribed tidal volume.
- Empty ventilator tubings when moisture collects. Never empty fluid in the tubing back into the cascade.
- Ensure adequate humidity by keeping delivered air temperature maintained at body temperature.
- If the client is on PEEP, observe the peak airway pressure dial to determine the proper level of PEEP.
- Assess the client's respiratory status each shift and as needed:
  a. Observe the client's color (especially lips and nail beds).
  b. Observe the client's chest for bilateral expansion.
  c. Auscultate the lungs for rales, rhonchi, wheezes, equal breath sounds, and decreased or absent breath sounds.
  d. Obtain pulse oximetry reading.
  e. Evaluate ABGs as ordered.
- Take vital signs at least every 4 hr.
- Be sure the tracheostomy cuff (or the endotracheal cuff) is adequately inflated to ensure tidal volume.
- Administer mouth care *at least* twice per shift.
- Observe the client's need for tracheal/oral/nasal suctioning every 2 hr. Provide adequate suctioning as needed.
- Provide tracheostomy care every shift.
- Change tracheostomy tape or endotracheal tube tape as needed. Observe the client's mouth around the endotracheal tube for pressure sores.
- Move the oral endotracheal tube to the opposite side of the mouth once every 24 hr to prevent ulcers.
- Maintain accurate intake and output records to monitor fluid balance.
- Turn the client at least every 2 hr and get the client out of bed as ordered to promote pulmonary hygiene and prevent complications of immobility.
- Schedule treatments and nursing care at intervals to provide rest.
- Explain all procedures and treatments; provide access to a call bell; visit the client frequently.
- Include the client and his or her family in care whenever possible (especially suctioning and tracheostomy care).
- Provide a letter board or pencil and paper for communication. Request consultation with a speech therapist for assistance, if necessary.
- Observe ventilated clients for gastrointestinal distress (diarrhea, constipation, tarry stools).
- Document pertinent observations in the client's medical record (chart).

PEEP = positive end-expiratory pressure; ABGs = arterial blood gases.
Courtesy of Our Lady of Lourdes Medical Center, Camden, NJ.

and expiration occurs. Thus, negative-pressure ventilators create pressure gradients that mimic normal physiologic ventilation.

Newer negative-pressure ventilators include the cuirass, poncho, and body wrap. These ventilators are used for clients with neuromuscular disease, central nervous system disorders, spinal cord injuries, and chronic airflow limitation (CAL). Clients may use negative-pressure ventilation for home nighttime ventilatory support so that their muscles can rest. Advantages are that an artificial airway is not required and the newer models are lightweight and easy to use. The enclosing ventilator makes some direct nursing care more difficult. The client must be able to clear oral secretions and must have compliant (elastic) lungs to benefit from this mode of ventilation.

Positive-Pressure Ventilators. This is the most widely used type of ventilator in the acute care setting. During inspiration, pressure is generated that pushes air into the lungs and expands the chest. In most instances, an ET tube or tracheostomy is needed. Positive-pressure ventilators are classified according to the mechanism that ends inspiration and starts expiration. Inspiration is terminated or cycled in three major ways: pressure cycled, time cycled, or volume cycled.

Pressure-Cycled Ventilators. This type of rarely used ventilator pushes air into the lungs until a preset airway pressure is reached. Tidal volumes and inspiratory time are variable. Pressure-cycled ventilators are often used for short periods, such as in the postanesthesia care unit and for respiratory therapy.

Time-Cycled Ventilators. These push air into the lungs until a preset time has elapsed. Tidal volume and pressure are variable, depending on the characteristics of the client and the ventilator. The time-cycled ventilator is used primarily in pediatric and neonatal populations.

Volume-Cycled Ventilators. This type of ventilator pushes gas into the lungs until a preset volume is delivered. A constant tidal volume is delivered regardless of the pressure needed to deliver the tidal volume. However, a pressure limit is set to prevent excessive pressure from being exerted on the lungs. The advantage of the volume-cycled ventilator is that a constant tidal volume is delivered regardless of the changing compliance of the lungs and chest wall or the airway resistance found in the client or ventilator. Examples include the Bear I, II (Fig. 34–4), and III; Puritan-Bennett MA-1, MA-2, and MA-3; and Monaghan 225/SIMV.

Microprocessor Ventilators. These are the most sophisticated of the positive-pressure ventilators. A computer or microprocessor is built into the ventilator to allow ongoing monitoring of ventilatory functions, alarms, and client parameters. The ventilator often has components of volume-, time-, and pressure-cycled ventilators. The microprocessor ventilator is more responsive to clients who have severe lung disease, who require prolonged weaning trials, and who may not be able to be ventilated on older volume-cycled ventilators. Examples include the Bear IV and V, Puritan-Bennett 7200, Erisa, and Siemens Servo C and Servo D.

Modes of Ventilation. The mode of ventilation describes the way in which the client receives breaths from the ventilator.

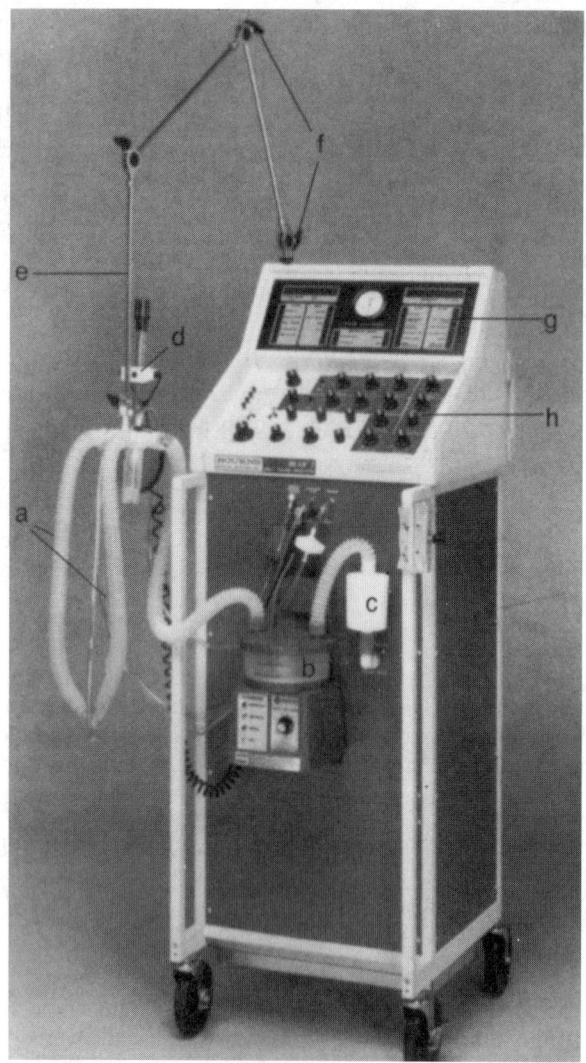

Figure 34–4. Bear II Adult Volume Ventilator. (Courtesy of Bear Medical Systems, Inc., Riverside, CA.)

Controlled Ventilation. This is the least used mode. The client receives a set tidal volume at a set rate. This mode may be used for clients who cannot initiate respiratory effort (e.g., those with polio or Guillain-Barré syndrome). It may be used for clients who are "paralyzed" as part of their medical management, such as those in status epilepticus or those with severely elevated intracranial pressure. If a client on controlled ventilation attempts to initiate a breath, the efforts are blocked by the ventilator. This maneuver may result in the client's "fighting" the ventilator.

Assist-Control Ventilation. Assist-control (AC) ventilation is the most commonly used mode. It is used mainly as a resting mode. The ventilator takes over the work of breathing for the client. Tidal volume and ventilatory rate are preset on the ventilator. If the client does not trigger spontaneous breaths, a minimal ventilatory pattern is established. The ventilator is also programmed to respond to the client's inspiratory effort if the client does initiate a breath. In this case, the ventilator delivers the preset tidal

volume while allowing the client to control the rate of breathing.

One disadvantage of the AC mode is that if the client's spontaneous ventilatory rate increases, the ventilator continues to deliver a preset tidal volume with each breath. The client may then hyperventilate, and respiratory alkalosis occurs. Causes of hyperventilation, such as pain, anxiety, or acid-base imbalances, must be corrected.

Synchronized Intermittent Mandatory Ventilation. Synchronized intermittent mandatory ventilation (SIMV) is similar to AC ventilation in that tidal volume and ventilatory rate are preset on the ventilator. Therefore, if the client does not breathe, a minimal ventilatory pattern is established. In contrast to the AC mode, SIMV allows breathing spontaneously at the client's own rate and tidal volume between the ventilator breaths. SIMV can be used as a primary ventilatory mode or as a weaning modality. When SIMV is used as a weaning mode, the number of mechanical breaths (SIMV breaths) is gradually decreased (i.e., from 12 to 2), and the client gradually resumes spontaneous breathing. The mandatory ventilator breaths are delivered when the client is ready to inspire, promoting synchrony between the ventilator and the client.

Other Modes of Ventilation. Newer modes of ventilation, such as pressure support and continuous flow (flow-by), are available only in microprocessor ventilators. Both modalities decrease the work of breathing and are often used for weaning clients from mechanical ventilation. Other modes are maximum mandatory ventilation (MMV), inverse I:E ratio, permissive hypercapnia, airway pressure release ventilation, proportional assist ventilation, high-frequency ventilation, jet ventilation, and high-frequency oscillation. Many of these modes need specialized ventilators, tubing, or airways.

Ventilator Controls and Settings. The volume-cycled ventilator is the most widely used ventilator in the acute care setting. Regardless of the type of volume-cycled ventilator used, the controls and types of settings are universal (Fig. 34–5). The physician prescribes the ventilator settings, and usually the ventilator is readied or set up by the respiratory department. The nurse assists in connecting the client to the ventilator. The nurse understands and monitors the ventilator settings as part of the nursing care for the client.

Tidal Volume. Tidal volume (V_T) is the volume of air that the client receives with each breath; it can be measured on either inspiration or expiration. The average prescribed tidal volume ranges between 7 and 15 mL/kg of body weight. Adding a zero to the weight of clients in kilograms gives an estimate of tidal volume.

Rate, or Breaths per Minute. Rate, or breaths per minute (BPM), is the number of ventilator breaths delivered per minute. The rate is usually set between 10 and 14 breaths per minute.

Fraction of Inspired Oxygen. The fraction of inspired oxygen (FIO_2) is the oxygen concentration delivered to the client. The prescribed FIO_2 is determined by the arterial blood gas value and the client's condition. Ventilators

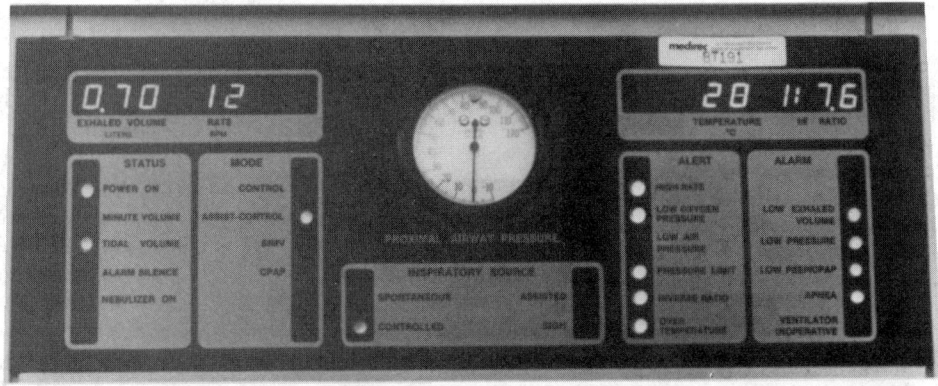

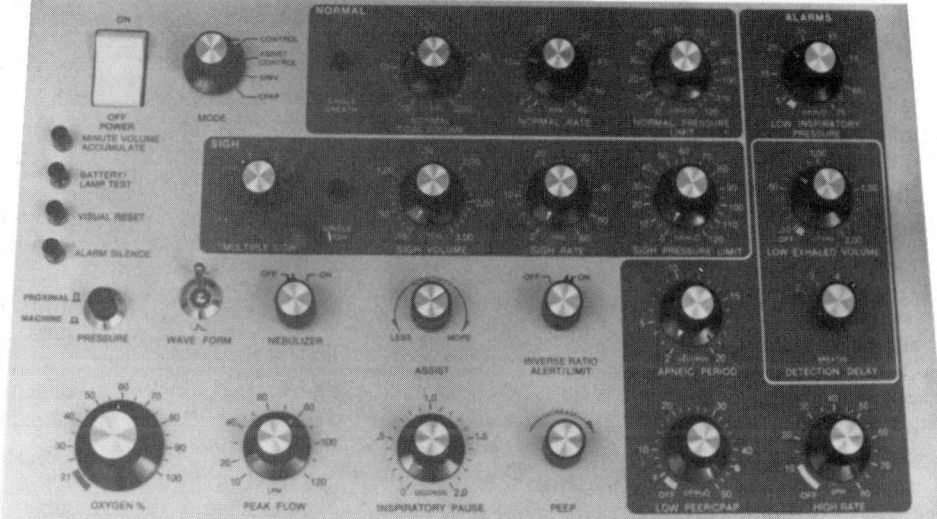

Figure 34–5. Display signals and alarms *(top)* and control panel *(bottom)* of a typical volume-cycled ventilator. (From Kersten, L. D. [1989]. *Comprehensive respiratory nursing: A decision-making approach.* Philadelphia: W. B. Saunders. Used with permission.)

can provide 21 to 100% oxygen, depending on the client's needs.

The oxygen delivered to the client is warmed to body temperature (37° C [98.6° F]) and humidified to 100%. Humidification and warming are necessary because upper air passages of the respiratory tree, which normally warm, humidify, and filter air, are bypassed by the endotracheal tube (ET) or tracheostomy tube. Humidification and warming prevent mucosal damage and facilitate clearance of secretions.

Sighs. These may be used to prevent atelectasis in special circumstances. Sighs are volumes of air that are 1½ to 2 times the set tidal volume, delivered 6 to 10 times per hour. Sighs are rarely used, however, because they can cause barotrauma (lung damage from excessive pressure) and have not been shown to be useful.

Peak Airway (Inspiratory) Pressure. Peak airway (inspiratory) pressure (PIP) indicates the pressure needed by the ventilator to deliver a set tidal volume at a given dynamic compliance. The peak airway pressure measurement appears on the digital readout or display on the front or top of the ventilator (labeled proximal airway pressure in Figure 34–5). Peak pressure is the highest pressure indicated during inspiration. Monitoring trends in PIP reflect changes in resistance of the lungs and resistance in the ventilator. An increased PIP reading means

increased airway resistance (bronchospasm, or pinched tubing), increased amount of secretions, pulmonary edema, or decreased pulmonary compliance (the lungs or chest wall are "stiffer" or harder to inflate). An upper pressure limit is set on the ventilator to prevent barotrauma. When the limit is reached, the high-pressure alarm sounds, and the remaining volume is not given.

Continuous Positive Airway Pressure. Continuous positive airway pressure (CPAP) is the application of positive airway pressure throughout the entire respiratory cycle for spontaneously breathing clients. Sedating medications should be given cautiously or not at all when a client is receiving CPAP so that respiratory effort is not suppressed. CPAP keeps the alveoli open during inspiration and prevents alveolar collapse during expiration. This process results in increased functional residual capacity (FRC), improved gas exchange, and improved oxygenation.

Continuous positive airway pressure is used primarily as a weaning modality. During CPAP, no ventilator breaths are delivered; the ventilator delivers oxygen and provides monitoring and an alarm system. The respiratory pattern is determined by the client's efforts. Normal levels of CPAP are 5 to 15 cm H_2O, adjusted to promote adequate oxygenation. If no pressure is set on the ventilator, the client receives no positive pressure. The client is essentially using the ventilator as a T piece with alarms.

Newer modifications of CPAP include nasal CPAP and BiPAP. The physician uses these modifications for select indications.

Positive End-Expiratory Pressure. Positive end-expiratory pressure (PEEP) is positive pressure exerted during the expiratory phase of ventilation. PEEP improves oxygenation by enhancing gas exchange and preventing atelectasis. It is indicated for the treatment of persistent hypoxemia that does not improve with an acceptable oxygen concentration. PEEP is often added when the PaO_2 value remains low with an FIO_2 of 50% to 70% or greater.

The need for PEEP indicates a severe gas exchange disturbance. It is important to lower the FIO_2 delivered when possible. Prolonged use of a high FIO_2 can result in lung damage from the toxic effects of oxygen. PEEP prevents alveoli from collapsing; the lungs are kept partially inflated so that alveolar-capillary gas exchange is facilitated throughout the ventilatory cycle. The effect should be an increase in arterial blood oxygenation so that the FIO_2 can be decreased.

PEEP is "dialed in" with the PEEP dial on the control panel. The amount of PEEP is often 5 to 15 cm H_2O and is read (monitored) on the peak airway pressure dial, the same dial used to read the PIP. When PEEP is added, the dial does not return to zero at the end of exhalation; rather, it returns to a baseline that has been increased from zero by the amount of PEEP applied.

Flow. Flow is how fast the ventilator delivers each breath. It is usually set at 40 L/min. If a client is agitated, restless, or has a widely fluctuating pressure reading on inspiration, or other signs of air hunger, the flow may be set too low. Increasing the flow should be tried before restraining the client chemically.

Other Settings. Other settings may be used, depending on the type of ventilator and mode of ventilation. Examples of additional settings include inspiratory and expiratory cycle, waveform, expiratory resistance, and plateau.

Nursing Management. The institution of mechanical ventilation for a client involves a complex decision-making process for both the family and the health care professionals. Both physical and psychological concerns of the client and family must be addressed. The mechanical ventilator frequently causes anxiety for the client and family. Therefore, the nurse carefully explains the purpose of the ventilator and notes that the client might feel some different sensations. The client and family are encouraged to express their concerns. The nurse acts as the coach who both physically and psychologically helps and supports the client and family through this experience. In emergencies, these explanations may not be accomplished until the emergency has been controlled. Clients undergoing mechanical ventilation in ICUs frequently experience delirium, or "ICU psychosis." Such clients require frequent, repetitive explanations and reassurance.

When caring for a ventilated client, the nurse's responsibility is to the client first and the ventilator second. It is vital that the nurse understand the reason for which the client requires mechanical ventilation. Such causes as excessive amounts of secretions, sepsis, and trauma require different interventions to facilitate ventilator independence. In addition, an appreciation of the client's chronic health problems—particularly chronic airflow limitation (CAL), left-sided heart failure, anemia, and malnutrition—is essential. These problems may impede weaning from mechanical ventilation and, therefore, warrant close monitoring and intervention.

Three nursing goals in caring for the client with mechanical ventilation are to monitor and evaluate the client's response to the ventilator, manage the ventilator system safely, and prevent complications.

Monitoring the Client's Response. The first goal of nursing care is to monitor and evaluate the client's response to the ventilator. The nurse assesses vital signs and listens to breath sounds every 30 to 60 minutes initially, monitors noninvasive respiratory parameters (e.g., capnography and pulse oximetry), and checks ABG values. Vital signs change during episodes of hypercapnia and hypoxemia. The nurse should note any precipitating causes and correct them promptly.

The nurse assesses the client's breathing pattern in relation to the ventilatory cycle to determine whether the client is fighting or tolerating the ventilator. Breath sounds are assessed and recorded, including bilateral equal breath sounds to ensure proper ET tube placement. To determine the frequency of suctioning needed, the nurse observes secretions for type, color, and amount.

The nurse assesses the area around the ET tube or tracheostomy site at least every 4 hours for color, tenderness, skin irritation, and drainage. Continuous noninvasive monitoring provides the nurse with information to guide the client's activities, such as weaning, physical or occupational therapy, and self-care. These activities can be paced so that oxygenation and ventilation are adequate. The nurse interprets ABG values to evaluate ventilation and suggests ventilator settings that help the client.

Because the nurse spends the most time with the client, he or she is most likely to be the first person to recognize slight changes in vital signs or ABG values and fatigue or distress in the client. The nurse promptly confers with the physician and implements the appropriate interventions.

While monitoring and evaluating the client's clinical status, the nurse also serves as a resource for addressing the psychological needs of the client and family. Anxiety can play a major role in the client's tolerance of mechanical ventilation. Therefore, skilled and sensitive nursing care promotes psychological well-being and facilitates synchrony with the ventilator. Because the client cannot speak, communication can be frustrating and anxiety producing. The client and family may panic because they believe the client has lost his or her voice. They must be reassured that the ET tube prevents speech but that it is temporary.

Alternative, creative methods of communication must be individualized to meet the client's needs. Magic slates, writing paper, computers, and tracheostomy tubes that permit talking are potential means of facilitating communication. Finding a successful means for communication is important because the client often feels isolated as a result of the inability to speak. Anticipation of the client's needs; easy access to frequently used belongings; visits from family, friends, and pets; and a nursing call light within reach are effective ways of giving the client a sense of control over the environment. In addition, the client can participate in self-care.

Managing the Ventilator System. The second goal of nursing care is directed toward safe management of the ventilator system. Ventilator settings are ordered by the physician and include tidal volume, respiratory rate, FIO_2, mode of ventilation (AC, SIMV), and any adjunctive modes, such as positive end-expiratory pressure (PEEP), pressure support, or continuous flow.

Nurses perform and document ventilator checks according to the standards of the unit or facility and respond promptly to emergencies as indicated by alarms. During a ventilator check, the nurse compares the ventilator settings ordered by the physician with the actual settings. The nurse checks the level of water in the humidifier and the temperature of the humidification system to ensure that they are within normal limits. Extremes in temperature cause damage to the mucosa of the airways. Any condensation in the ventilator tubing is removed by draining water into drainage collection receptacles, which should be emptied frequently. For prevention of bacterial contamination, moisture and water from the tubings are never allowed to enter the humidifier.

Mechanical ventilators have alarm systems that warn the nurse of a problem with either the client or the ventilator. Alarm systems must be activated and functional at all times. The nurse must recognize an emergency and intervene promptly so that complications are prevented. If the cause of the alarm cannot be determined, the nurse ventilates the client manually with a resuscitation bag until the problem is corrected by a second nurse, the respiratory therapist, or a physician. The two major alarms on a ventilator indicate either a high pressure or a low exhaled volume. Table 34–5 presents nursing interventions for various causes of ventilator alarms.

Ensuring proper functioning of the ventilator also includes care of the endotracheal (ET) tube or tracheostomy tube. A patent airway is maintained through suctioning only as needed. Indications for suctioning in the ventilated client include
- Presence of secretions
- Increased PIP
- Presence of rhonchi (wheezes)
- Decreased breath sounds

Careful maintenance of the ET or tracheostomy tube also ensures a patent airway. The nurse frequently assesses the tube's position, especially for the client whose airway is attached to heavy ventilator tubing that may pull on the tracheostomy or ET tube. The nurse positions the ventilator tubing in such a way that the client can move without pulling on the ET or tracheostomy tube. The ET tube can move and slip into the right mainstem bronchus. To detect minimal changes in the tube's position, the nurse marks the level at which the tube touches the client's teeth or nose. The nurse gives mouth care frequently to promote adequate oral hygiene and to prevent loosening of the tape that holds the tube.

Preventing Complications. The third goal in caring for the client receiving mechanical ventilation is to prevent complications. Most complications are due to the positive pressure from the ventilator. Nearly every body system is affected.

Cardiac Complications. Cardiac complications of mechanical ventilation include hypotension and fluid retention. Hypotension is caused by the application of positive pressure, which increases intrathoracic pressure and inhibits blood return to the heart. The decreased venous return to the right side of the heart decreases cardiac output and is clinically reflected as hypotension. Hypotension is most frequently seen in the client who is dehydrated or requires high peak airway (inspiratory) pressure (PIP) to be ventilated. The nurse instructs the client to avoid a Valsalva maneuver and plans care to prevent constipation, which could result in a Valsalva maneuver.

Fluid is retained because of decreased cardiac output. The kidneys receive less blood flow and stimulate the renin-angiotensin-aldosterone system to retain fluid. In addition, humidified air via the ventilator system can contribute to fluid retention. If humidification is not adequate, the airways become dehydrated, and the secretions solidify. The nurse monitors the client's fluid intake and output, weight, hydration, and signs of hypovolemia.

Lung Complications. The lungs experience barotrauma (damage to the lungs by positive pressure), *volutrauma* (damage to the lung by excess volume delivered to one lung over the other), and acid-base abnormalities. Barotrauma includes pneumothorax, subcutaneous emphysema, and pneumomediastinum. Clients at risk for barotrauma have diseases of chronic airflow limitation (CAL), have blebs, are on PEEP, have dynamic hyperinflation, or require high pressures to ventilate the lungs (because of decreased compliance or "stiff" lungs, as seen in ARDS). Blood gas abnormalities, another pulmonary complication of mechanical ventilation, can be corrected by appropriate ventilator changes and adjustment of fluid and electrolyte imbalances.

Gastrointestinal and Nutritional Complications. Gastrointestinal alterations result from the stress of mechanical ventilation. Stress ulcers occur in approximately 25% of clients receiving mechanical ventilation. Prophylactic antacids, sucralfate (Carafate, Sulcrate), and the histamine blockers cimetidine (Tagamet) and ranitidine (Zantac) are often instituted as soon as the client is intubated. The nurse administers these medications and suggests therapeutic strategies for stress management (see Chap. 8).

Malnutrition is a prevalent problem in clients receiving mechanical ventilation. Because many other acute or life-threatening events are occurring simultaneously, nutrition is often neglected. Malnutrition is an extreme problem for these clients and a major reason that clients cannot be weaned from the ventilator. In malnourished clients, the respiratory muscles lose their mass and strength. The diaphragm, which is the major organ of inspiration, is affected early in this process. When the diaphragm and other muscles of respiration are weakened, an ineffective

TABLE 34–5

Nursing Interventions for Various Causes of Ventilator Alarms

Cause	Interventions
High-Pressure Alarm (sounds when peak inspiratory pressure reaches the set alarm limit [usually set 10–20 mmHg above the client's baseline PIP])	
There is an increased amount of secretions in the airways or a mucous plug.	• Suction as needed.
The client coughs, gags, or bites on the oral ET.	• Insert oral airway to prevent biting on the ET tube.
The client is anxious or fights the ventilator.	• Provide emotional support to decrease anxiety. • Increase the flow rate. • Explain all procedures to the client. • Provide sedation or paralyzing agent per the physician's order.
Airway size decreases related to wheezing or bronchospasm.	• Auscultate breath sounds. • Consult with the physician for management of bronchospasm.
Pneumothorax occurs.	• Auscultate breath sounds. • Consult with the physician about a new onset of decreased breath sounds or unequal chest excursion, which may be due to pneumothorax.
The artificial airway is displaced; the ET tube may have slipped into the right mainstem bronchus.	• Assess the chest for unequal breath sounds and chest excursion. • Obtain a chest x-ray as ordered to evaluate the position of the ET tube. • After the proper position is verified, tape the tube securely in place.
Obstruction in tubing occurs because the client is lying on the tubing or there is water or a kink in the tubing.	• Assess the system, moving from the artificial airway toward the ventilator. • Empty water from the ventilator tubing and remove any kinks.
There is increased PIP associated with deliverance of a sigh.	• Consult with respiratory therapist or physician to adjust the pressure alarm.
Decreased compliance of the lung is noted; a trend of gradually increasing PIP is noted over several hours or a day.	• Evaluate the reasons for the decreased compliance of the lungs. Increased PIP occurs in ARDS, pneumonia, or any worsening of pulmonary disease.
Low Exhaled Volume (or Low-Pressure) Alarm (sounds when there is a disconnection or leak in the ventilator circuit or a leak in the client's artificial airway cuff)	
A leak in the ventilator circuit prevents breath from being delivered.	• Assess all connections and all ventilator tubings for disconnection.
The client stops spontaneous breathing in the SIMV or CPAP mode or on pressure support ventilation.	• Evaluate the client's tolerance of the mode.
A cuff leak occurs in the ET or tracheostomy tube.	• Evaluate the client for a cuff leak. A cuff leak is suspected when the client is able to talk (air escapes from the mouth) or when the pilot balloon on the artificial airway is flat (see section on tracheostomy tubes in Chapter 30).
The exhalation valve on Bear I or II is wet.	• Keep exhalation valve and flow tube vertical. • Unsnap and check the membrane for dampness. If the sensor is wet, gently dab dry and resnap.

PIP = peak inspiratory pressure; ET = endotracheal; ARDS = adult respiratory distress syndrome; CPAP = continuous positive airway pressure; SIMV = synchronized intermittent mandatory ventilation.

breathing pattern emerges, fatigue occurs, and the client cannot be weaned from the ventilator.

A balanced diet via the parenteral or enteral route is essential whenever a ventilator is used. Furthermore, nutrition for the client with CAL requires that special attention be given to the percentage of carbohydrates in the client's diet. During metabolism, carbohydrates are broken down to glucose to produce energy (adenosine triphosphate), carbon dioxide, and water. Excessive carbohydrate loads increase carbon dioxide production, which the CAL client may be unable to exhale. Hypercapnic respiratory failure results. Enteral and parenteral formulas with a higher fat content (e.g., Pulmocare, NutriVent, Intralipids) can be an alternative source of calories to combat this problem.

Another important aspect of nutritional support is electrolyte replacement. Electrolytes also have a major impact on the efficiency of respiratory muscle function. Specifically, the nurse and physician closely monitor potassium, calcium, magnesium, and phosphate levels, and the nurse replenishes deficiencies as ordered. All four electrolytes are important in respiratory muscle contraction and function and can easily be added to the nutritional regimen.

Infection. Infections are always a potential threat for the client requiring a ventilator. The ET or tracheostomy tube bypasses the body's normal process of filtering and warming air and provides bacteria direct access to the lower parts of the respiratory system. Within 48 hours, the artificial airway is usually colonized with bacteria, and an environment is established in which pneumonia can develop. In addition, aspiration of colonized fluid from the mouth or the stomach can occur and be a source of pathogens. Pneumonia is associated with prolonged hospitalization and increased morbidity. Therefore, the focus must be on prevention of infections through strict adherence to infection control, especially hand washing, during suctioning and care of the tracheostomy or ET tube. To prevent pneumonia, the nurse implements ongoing oral care and pulmonary hygiene, including chest physiotherapy, postural drainage, and turning and positioning. More information on pneumonia can be found in Chapter 33.

Muscular Complications. Overall muscle deconditioning can occur because of immobility. Getting out of bed, ambulating with assistance, and performing exercises with the nurse, physical therapist, and occupational therapist not only improve muscle tone and strength but also boost the client's morale, facilitate gas exchange, and promote oxygen delivery to all muscles.

Ventilator Dependence. The final complication of mechanical ventilation is ventilator dependence, or inability to wean. Ventilator dependence can be psychological or physiologic but more often has a physiologic basis. The longer a client uses a ventilator, the more difficult is the weaning process because the respiratory muscles fatigue and cannot assume breathing. The health care team attempts to optimize all major body systems and to exhaust every method of weaning before a client is declared unweanable.

The physician and nurse, often with a social worker or psychologist and a member of the clergy, discuss with the family and the client, as able, the client's quality of life, goals, and values. In accordance with this discussion, arrangements are made for home ventilation, nursing home placement, or withdrawal of life support (in terminal cases). Special units and facilities are available to maximize the rehabilitation and weaning of ventilator-dependent clients.

Weaning. This is the process of going from ventilatory dependence to spontaneous breathing. The weaning process can be prolonged if complications develop. Many of these complications can be avoided by skillful nursing care. For example, turning and positioning the client not only promote comfort and prevent skin breakdown but also facilitate gas exchange and prevent pulmonary complications, such as pneumonia and atelectasis. Table 34–6 summarizes various weaning techniques.

Implications for the Elderly. The older client, especially one who has smoked or who has an underlying lung dysfunction such as CAL, is at risk for ventilator dependence and failure to wean. Age-related changes that de-

TABLE 34-6

Weaning Methods

Synchronous Intermittent Mandatory Ventilation

- The client breathes between the machine's present breaths per minute rate.
- The client is initially set on a SIMV rate of 12, meaning the client receives a minimum of 12 breaths per minute by the ventilator.
- The client's respiratory rate will be a combination of ventilator breaths and spontaneous breaths.
- As the weaning process ensues, the physician orders gradual decreases in the SIMV rate, usually at a decrease of 1 to 2 breaths per minute.

T-Piece Technique

- The client is taken off the ventilator for short periods (initially 5–10 min) and allowed to breathe spontaneously.
- The ventilator is replaced with a T piece (see Chap. 30) or CPAP, which delivers humidified oxygen.
- The ordered FIO_2 may be higher for the client on the T piece than on the ventilator.
- Weaning progresses as the client is able to tolerate progressively longer periods off the ventilator.
- Nighttime weaning is not usually attempted until the client is able to maintain spontaneous respirations most of the day.

Pressure Support Ventilation

- PSV allows the client's respiratory effort to be augmented by a predetermined pressure assist from the ventilator.
- As the weaning process ensues, the amount of pressure applied to inspiration is gradually decreased.
- Another method of weaning with PSV is to maintain the pressure but gradually decrease the ventilator's preset breaths per minute rate.

SIMV = synchronized intermittent mandatory ventilation; CPAP = continuous positive airway pressure; FIO_2 = fraction of inspired oxygen; PSV = pressure support ventilation.

crease the likelihood of weaning result in ventilatory failure and include increased chest wall stiffness, reduced respiratory muscle strength, and decreased lung elasticity. Because the usual manifestations of ventilatory failure, hypoxemia and hypercapnia, may be blunted in the elderly, the nurse must use other clinical measures of oxygenation, such as a change in mental status (Thompson, 1996).

Extubation. Removal of the ET tube is termed *extubation.* The tube is removed when the indication for intubation has been resolved. Before removal, the nurse explains the procedure to the client. The nurse or respiratory therapist sets up the prescribed oxygen delivery system at the bedside and brings in the equipment for emergency reintubation. The nurse or respiratory therapist hyperoxygenates the client and thoroughly suctions the ET tube as well as the oral cavity. The cuff of the ET tube is then rapidly deflated, and the tube is removed at peak inspiration. The nurse instructs the client to take deep breaths and to cough. It is normal for large amounts of oral secretions to have accumulated in the back of the throat. The nurse or respiratory therapist administers oxygen, usually ordered to be by face mask or nasal cannula. The FIO_2 is usually ordered at 10% higher than the level that was maintained while the ET tube was in place.

Monitoring after extubation is essential. The nurse monitors the client's vital signs every hour initially, assesses the client's ventilatory pattern, and assesses for any signs or symptoms of respiratory distress. It is common for the client to experience hoarseness and a sore throat for a few days after extubation. The nurse instructs the client to

- Sit in a semi-Fowler's position
- Take deep breaths every ½ hour
- Use an incentive spirometer (see Chap. 20) every 2 hours
- Limit speaking in the immediate period after extubation

These measures facilitate gas exchange and decrease laryngeal edema and vocal cord irritation. The nurse also closely observes the client for signs or symptoms of upper airway obstruction (see Chap. 31). Early signs are mild dyspnea, coughing, and the inability to expectorate secretions. With the onset of these signs, the nurse notifies the physician, who evaluates the need for reintubation. The nurse is especially concerned if the client develops stridor, a late sign of a narrowed airway. Stridor is a high-pitched, crowing noise during inspiration caused by laryngospasm or edema above or below the glottis. Racemic epinephrine, a topical aerosol vasoconstrictor, is given, and reintubation may be performed.

Chest Trauma

Thoracic injuries are directly responsible for approximately 25% of all civilian traumatic deaths; 50% of the injured succumb before arriving at health care facilities. Only 5% to 15% of all thoracic injuries require thoracotomy. The remainder can be treated with basic resuscitation, intubation, or chest tube placement. Emergency personnel's basic and initial approach to all chest injuries is

ABC (*Airway, Breathing, Circulation*) followed by rapid assessment and treatment of potentially life-threatening conditions.

Pulmonary Contusion

Overview

Pulmonary contusion, a potentially lethal injury, is the most common chest injury seen in the United States. After a contusion, respiratory failure can develop over time rather than instantaneously. This condition most frequently follows injuries caused by rapid deceleration during vehicular accidents. Interstitial hemorrhage, which is almost invariably associated with intra-alveolar hemorrhage, is characteristic of pulmonary contusion. The resultant interstitial edema causes a decrease in pulmonary compliance and a decreased area for gas exchange. The client usually becomes hypoxemic and dyspneic. The bronchial mucosa becomes irritated, and the client has increased bronchial secretions.

Collaborative Management

 Assessment

Clients who may initially be asymptomatic can develop respiratory failure. The client presents with hemoptysis, decreased breath sounds, crackles, and wheezes. The chest x-ray of pulmonary contusion may show a hazy opacity in the lobes or parenchyma. If there is no disruption of the parenchyma, resorption of the lesion often occurs without treatment.

 Interventions

Treatment includes maintenance of ventilation and oxygenation. Central venous pressure is monitored closely, and fluid intake is restricted accordingly. The client in obvious respiratory distress may require mechanical ventilation with positive end-expiratory pressure (PEEP) to inflate the lungs and provide positive-pressure ventilation.

A vicious circle occurs in which more muscle effort is required for ventilation, and the client becomes progressively hypoxemic. Attempting to compensate causes the client to tire easily, become less efficient in breathing, and become more fatigued and hypoxemic. Flail chest may also be associated with a pulmonary contusion accompanied by parenchymal damage. The sequela to this situation is the probable development of ARDS.

Rib Fracture

Overview

After chest wall contusion, rib fractures are the next most common injury to the chest wall. Rib fractures most frequently result from direct blunt trauma to the chest, usually with involvement of the fifth through ninth ribs. Direct force applied to the ribs tends to fracture them and drive the bone ends into the thorax. Thus, there is a potential for intrathoracic injury, such as pneumothorax or pulmonary contusion. Pneumothorax is almost invariably present if ribs one through four are fractured.

Collaborative Management

The client usually experiences pain with movement and splints the chest defensively. Thoracic splinting results in impaired ventilation and inadequate clearance of tracheobronchial secretions. If the client has pre-existing pulmonary disease, the likelihood of atelectasis and pneumonia related to the rib fracture is increased. Clients with injuries to the first or second ribs, flail chest, seven or more fractured ribs, or expired volumes less than 15 mL/kg have a poor prognosis; intrathoracic injury occurs in 50% of these cases.

Treatment for uncomplicated rib fractures is nonspecific because the fractured ribs unite spontaneously. The chest is usually not splinted by tape or other materials. The primary consideration for the client is to decrease pain so that adequate ventilatory status is maintained. Intercostal nerve block may be used if pain is severe. Potent analgesia that causes respiratory depression is avoided.

Flail Chest

Overview

Flail chest (paradoxic respiration) is the inward movement of the thorax during inspiration, with outward movement during expiration. It usually involves one hemithorax (one side of the chest) and results from multiple rib fractures caused by blunt chest trauma. Flail chest is frequently associated with high-speed vehicular accidents. It is more common in older clients. It is associated with a high mortality rate (40%) and is one of the most critical chest injuries.

Flail chest occurs when a loose segment of chest wall is left because of a fracture of two or more adjacent ribs. The movement of this segment becomes paradoxic to the expansion and contraction of the rest of the chest wall. Flail chest can also occur from bilateral fracture of multiple costochondral junctions (without rib fracture) anteriorly, such as might occur during cardiopulmonary resuscitation on an elderly person. There may be associated injury to the lung tissue under the flail segment. Gas exchange is significantly impaired, as is the ability to cough and clear secretions. Defensive splinting because of the rib fracture further reduces the client's ability to exert the extra effort required for breathing, which may contribute later to failure to wean.

Collaborative Management

 Assessment

The nurse assesses the client with a flail chest for paradoxic chest movement, dyspnea, cyanosis, tachycardia, and hypotension. Anxiety is often associated with pain and dyspnea.

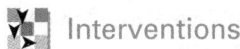 Interventions

Interventions for flail chest include
- Administration of humidified oxygen
- Pain management
- Promotion of lung expansion through deep breathing and positioning
- Secretion clearance by coughing and tracheal aspiration

The nurse gives psychosocial support to the extremely anxious client by explaining all procedures, talking slowly, and allowing the client time to verbalize feelings and concerns.

The client with a flail chest may be treated conservatively with vigilant respiratory care. The physician may prescribe mechanical ventilation if such complications as respiratory failure or shock ensue. The physician and the nurse monitor ABG values closely along with vital capacity. With severe hypoxemia and hypercapnia, the client is intubated and mechanically ventilated with PEEP. With pulmonary contusion or an underlying pulmonary disease, the potential for respiratory failure increases. Flail chest is best stabilized by positive-pressure ventilation rather than surgical intervention. Operative stabilization is reserved for extreme cases of flail chest.

The nurse monitors the client's vital signs and fluid and electrolyte balance closely so that hypovolemia or shock can be treated immediately. If the client has a pulmonary contusion, the nurse monitors central venous pressure and administers fluids as ordered. The nurse assesses the client for pain and intervenes to relieve the client's pain. The physician may order analgesic medication by the intravenous, epidural, or nerve block routes.

Pneumothorax

Overview

Any thoracic injury that allows accumulation of atmospheric air in the pleural space results in a rise in intrathoracic pressure and a reduction in vital capacity, depending on the amount of pulmonary collapse produced. Pneumothorax is often caused by blunt chest trauma and is associated with some degree of hemothorax. The pneumothorax can be open (when the pleural cavity has become exposed to the outside air, as through an open wound in the chest wall) or closed.

Collaborative Management

Assessment findings include

- Diminished breath sounds on auscultation
- Hyperresonance on percussion
- Prominence of the involved hemithorax, which moves poorly with respirations
- Deviation of the trachea away from (closed) or toward (open) the affected side

In addition, the client may have pleuritic pain, tachypnea, and subcutaneous emphysema (air under the skin in the subcutaneous tissues). A chest x-ray is used for diagnosis. Chest tubes may be indicated to allow the air to escape and the lung segment to reinflate.

Tension Pneumothorax

Overview

Tension pneumothorax, one of the most rapidly developing and life-threatening complications of blunt chest trauma, results from an air leak in the lung or chest wall. Air forced into the thoracic cavity causes complete collapse of the affected lung. Air that enters the pleural space during expiration does not exit during inspiration. As a result, air progressively accumulates under pressure, compresses the mediastinal vessels, and interferes with venous return. Because this process leads to decreased diastolic filling of the heart, cardiac output is compromised. If not promptly detected and treated, tension pneumothorax is quickly fatal. Typical causes of tension pneumothorax are

- Blunt chest trauma in which the parenchymal injury has failed to seal
- Mechanical ventilation with PEEP
- Closed chest drainage (chest tubes)
- Insertion of central venous access catheters

Collaborative Management

 Assessment

Assessment findings with tension pneumothorax include
  - Asymmetry of the thorax
  - Tracheal deviation to the unaffected side
  - Respiratory distress
  - Unilateral absence of breath sounds
  - Distended neck veins
  - Cyanosis

On percussion, there is a hypertympanic sound over the affected hemithorax. Pneumothorax is detectable on a chest x-ray. ABG assays demonstrate hypoxia and respiratory alkalosis.

 Interventions

The physician inserts a large-bore needle into the second intercostal space in the midclavicular line of the affected side as initial treatment for tension pneumothorax. After this lifesaving measure is completed, the physician places a chest tube into the fourth intercostal space of the midaxillary line and attaches the tube to a water seal drainage system until the lung reinflates.

Hemothorax

Overview

Hemothorax is one of the most common problems encountered after blunt chest trauma or penetrating injuries. A *simple* hemothorax is a blood loss of less than 1500 mL into the thoracic cavity; a *massive* hemothorax is a blood loss of more than 1500 mL.

Bleeding is frequently caused by injuries to the lung parenchyma, such as pulmonary contusions or lacerations, which are often associated with rib and sternal fractures. Massive intrathoracic bleeding in blunt chest trauma generally stems from the heart, great vessels, or major systemic arteries, such as the intercostal arteries.

Collaborative Management

 Assessment

Physical assessment findings vary with the size of the hemothorax. If the hemothorax is small, the client may be asymptomatic. If the hemothorax is larger, the client experiences respiratory distress. In addition, breath sounds are diminished on auscultation. The percussion note on the involved side is dull. Blood in the pleural space is visible on a chest x-ray and confirmed by diagnostic thoracentesis.

 Interventions

Interventions are aimed at evacuating the blood in the pleural space to normalize pulmonary function and to prevent infection related to blood accumulation. The physician inserts anterior and posterolateral chest tubes to evacuate the pleural space and to reduce the rush of clotted blood. The physician and the nurse carefully monitor the chest tube drainage, and chest x-rays are evaluated serially.

The physician considers open thoracotomy when there is initial evacuation of 1500 to 2000 mL of blood or persistent bleeding at the rate of 200 mL/hr over 3 hours. The nurse monitors the client's vital signs, blood loss, and overall intake and output; assesses the client's response to the chest tubes; and administers IV fluids and blood as ordered. Autotransfusion of the blood lost through chest drainage should be considered.

Tracheobronchial Trauma

Overview

Most tears of the tracheobronchial tree result from severe blunt trauma primarily involving the mainstem bronchi. Injuries to the cervical trachea usually occur at the junction of the trachea and cricoid cartilage. These injuries are frequently caused by striking the anterior neck against the dashboard or steering wheel during a vehicular accident. Clients with lacerations of the trachea develop massive air leaks, which produce pneumomediastinum (air in the mediastinum) and extensive subcutaneous emphysema. Upper airway obstruction may also occur and produce severe respiratory distress and inspiratory stridor. Major cervical tears are managed by cricothyroidotomy or tracheostomy below the level of injury.

Collaborative Management

The nurse assesses the client for hypoxemia by ABG assays. The nurse administers oxygen appropriately. Depending on the degree of injury, the client may require mechanical ventilation or surgical repair. Frequent assessment of vital signs is essential because the client is likely to be hypotensive and in shock. the nurse continues to assess for subcutaneous emphysema and auscultates lungs to assess for further complications every 1 to 2 hours initially. Decreased breath sounds or wheezing may indicate further obstruction, atelectasis, or pneumothorax. Care of the client with a tracheostomy is discussed in Chapter 30.

CASE STUDY for the Client with ARDS

■ H. B. is a 40-year-old man who was exposed to contents of a manure bin during a farming accident that killed three other men. He inhaled carbon dioxide, ammonia gas, hydrogen sulfide, and methane gas, and he aspirated manure. H. B. was in the bin for an unknown period and, when rescued, had no apparent respirations. A faint carotid pulse was palpated, so he was resuscitated, intubated, and transported to the hospital by helicopter, where x-ray showed bilateral diffuse infiltrates. His ABGs on 100% FIO_2 were pH 7.25; $PaCO_2$, 40 mmHg; and PaO_2, 40 mmHg. His pulmonary shunt was calculated to be 35%.

QUESTIONS:

1. What do the ABGs indicate about his oxygenation status?
2. For what treatment should you prepare?
3. He had large amounts of frothy, bloody secretions suctioned from his endotracheal tube. The colloid osmotic pressure of the secretions was 19.0 and of his serum was 14.9. What does this indicate?

BIBLIOGRAPHY

Aherns, T. S., Beattie, S., & Nienhaus, T. (1996). Experimental therapies to support the failing lung. *AACN Clinical Issues, 7*(4), 507–518.

Anderson, R. (1998). Another way to open an airway. *RN, 61*(3), 42–44.

*Arbour, R. (1993). Weaning a patient from a ventilator. *Nursing93, 23*(2), 52–56.

Baldwin-Myers, A., Geiger-Bronsky, M., Chacona, A., Ewing, L., Huiskes, B., Shiroma, J., & Gold, P. (1994). *Standards of care for the ventilator-assisted individual: A comprehensive management plan from hospital to home.* Loma Linda, CA: Loma Linda University/Respiratory Nursing Society.

Brandstetter, R., Sharma, K., DellaBadia, M., Cabreros, L., & Kabinoff, G. (1997). Adult respiratory distress syndrome: A disorder in need of improved outcome. *Heart & Lung, 26*(1), 3–14.

*Burns, S. M. (1992). A computerized assessment program for weaning patients from long-term mechanical ventilation. *Perspectives in Respiratory Nursing, 3*(6), 1, 6–8.

*Burns, S. M. (1991). Preventing diaphragm fatigue in the ventilated patient. *Dimensions of Critical Care Nursing, 10*(1), 13–20.

Burns, S. (1996). Understanding, applying, and evaluating pressure modes of ventilation. *AACN Clinical Issues: Advanced Practice in Acute Care and Critical Care, 7*(4), 495–506.

Burns, S., Clochesy, J., Goodnough-Hanneman, S., Ingersoll, G., Knebel, A., & Shekleton, M. (1995). Weaning from long-term mechanical ventilation. *American Journal of Critical Care, 4*(1), 4–22.

Carroll, P. (1997). When you WANT humidity. *RN, 60*(5), 30–35.

Carroll, P., & Milikowski, K. (1996). Getting your patient off a ventilator. *RN, 59*(6), 42–48.

Clochesy, J., Daily, B., & Montenegro, H. (1995). Weaning chronically critically ill adults from mechanical ventilatory support: A descriptive study. *American Journal of Critical Care, 4*(2), 93–99.

*Connolly, M. A., & Shekleton, M. E. (1991). Communicating with ventilator dependent patients. *Dimensions of Critical Care Nursing, 10*(2), 115–121.

*Curry, K., & Casday, L. (1992). Managing spontaneous pneumothorax. *The Nursing Spectrum, 1*(7), 12–13.

Cushinotto, N. (1997). Pharmacology update: Clinical considerations of heparinization. *Journal of the American Academy of Nurse Practitioners, 9*(6), 273–276.

Cutler, L. R. (1996). Acute respiratory distress syndrome: An overview. *Intensive and Critical Care Nursing, 12,* 316–326.

Dalen, J., & Hirsh, J. (Eds.). (1995). Fourth ACCP Consensus Conference on Antithrombotic Therapy. *Chest, 108*(3 Suppl).

*Dellenger, R. (Ed.). (1993). Adult respiratory distress syndrome: Current considerations in future directions. *New Horizons: The Science and Practice of Acute Medicine, 1*(4), 463.

*Demling, R. (1993). Acute respiratory failure. *New Horizons: The Science and Practice of Acute Medicine, 1*(3), 361.

*Demling, R. (1993). Adult respiratory distress syndrome: Current concepts. *New Horizons: The Science and Practice of Acute Medicine, 1*(3), 388–401.

*Dettenmeier, P. A., & Johnson, T. M. (1991). The art and science of mechanical ventilator adjustments. *Critical Care Nursing Clinics of North America, 3*(4), 575–583.

Ellstrom, K. (1997). Procedure for taping oral and nasal endotracheal tubes. *Perspectives in Respiratory Nursing, 8*(1), 7–8.

Enger, E. (1996). Patients with adult respiratory distress syndrome. In J. Clochesy, C. Breu, S. Cardin, A. Whittaker, & E. Rudy (Eds.), *Critical care nursing* (2nd ed., pp. 656–688). Philadelphia: W. B. Saunders

Fetzer, S. (1998). Laryngeal mask airway: Indications and management for critical-care. *Critical Care Nurse, 18*(1), 83–87.

Frederick, C. (1994). Noninvasive mechanical ventilation with the iron lung. *Critical Care Nursing Clinics of North America, 6*(4), 831–840.

Glass, C., Boling, P., & Gammon, S. (1996). Collaborative support for caregivers of individuals beginning mechanical ventilation at home. *Critical Care Nurse, 16*(4), 67–72.

Goodwin, R. S. (1996). Prevention of aspiration pneumonia: A research-based protocol. *Dimensions of Critical Care Nursing, 15*(2), 58–71.

Henneman, E. (1996). Patients with acute respiratory failure. In J. Clochesy, C. Breu, S. Cardin, A. Whittaker, & E. Rudy (Eds.), *Critical care nursing* (2nd ed., pp. 630–655). Philadelphia: W. B. Saunders.

Henneman, E., & Ellstrom, K. (1998). *Protocols for practice: Airway management.* Aliso Viejo, CA: American Association of Critical-Care Nurses.

*Hunter, F. C., & Mitchell, S. (1993). Managing ARDS. *RN, 56*(7), 52–58.

Jenny, J., & Logan, J. (1994). Promoting ventilator independence: A grounded theory perspective. *Dimensions of Critical Care Nursing, 13*(1), 29–37.

*Kelleghan, S. I., Salemi, C., & Padilla, S., et al. (1993). An effective continuous quality improvement approach to the prevention of ventilator-associated pneumonia. *American Journal of Infection Control, 21*(6), 322–330.

Kelly, M. (1996). Emergency! Acute respiratory failure. *American Journal of Nursing, 96*(12), 46.

Kite-Powell, D., Sabau, D., Ideno, K., Hargraves, D., & Dahlberg, C. (1996). Optimizing outcomes in ventilator-dependent patients: Challenging critical care practice. *Critical Care Nursing Quarterly, 19*(3), 77–90.

Knebel, A., Strider, V., & Wood, C. (1994). The art and science of caring for ventilator-assisted patients: Learning from our clinical practice. *Critical Care Nursing Clinics of North America, 6*(4), 819–830.

*Mason, S. G. (1992). When a ventilator patient is going home. *RN, 55*(10), 60–64.

Misasi, R., & Keyes, J. (1996). Matching and mismatching ventilation and perfusion in the lung. *Critical Care Nurse, 16*(3), 23–38.

Pahor, M., Guralnik, J., Havlik, R., Carbonin, P., Salive, M., Ferrucci, L.,

Corti, M., & Hennekens, C. (1996). Alcohol consumption and risk of deep vein thrombosis and pulmonary embolism in older persons. *Journal of the American Geriatrics Society, 44*(9), 1030–1037.

*Pierce, J. D., Wiggins, S. A., Plaskon, C., & Glass, C. (1993). Pressure support ventilation: Reducing the work of breathing during weaning. *Dimensions of Critical Care Nursing, 12*(6), 282–290.

Respiratory Nursing Society. (1994). *Standards and scope of respiratory nursing practice.* Washington, DC: American Nurses Publishing.

*Roberts, S. L. (1990). High-permeability pulmonary edema: Nursing assessment, diagnosis, and interventions. *Heart & Lung, 19,* 287–300.

*Roberts, S., & White, B. (1992). Common nursing diagnoses for pulmonary alveolar edema patients. *Dimensions of Critical Care Nursing, 11*(1), 13–27.

*Saul, L. (Ed.). (1991). *Activase therapy in acute myocardial infarction and acute massive pulmonary embolism.* Califon, NJ: Gardiner-Caldwell SynerMed.

Severson, A., Baldwin, L., & DeLoughery, T. (1997). International normalized ratio in anticoagulation therapy: Understanding the issues. *American Journal of Critical Care, 6*(2), 88–92.

Taggart, J. A., & Lind, M. A. (1994). Evaluating unplanned endotracheal extubations. *Dimensions of Critical Care Nursing, 13*(3), 114–122.

Thompson, L. F. (1996). Failure to wean: Exploration of the influence of age-related pulmonary changes. *Critical Care Nursing Clinics of North America, 8*(1), 7–16.

Tobin, M. J. (Ed.) (1994). *Principles and practice of mechanical ventilation.* New York: McGraw-Hill.

Vollman, K. M., & Bander, J. (1996). Improved oxygenation in patients with acute respiratory distress syndrome. *Intensive Care Medicine, 22*(10), 1105–1111.

*West, J. B. (1992). *Pulmonary pathophysiology—The essentials* (4th ed.). Baltimore, MD: Williams & Wilkins.

West, J. B. (1995). *Respiratory physiology—The essentials* (5th ed.). Baltimore, MD: Williams & Wilkins.

*White, B., & Roberts, S. (1993). Powerlessness and the pulmonary alveolar edema patient. *Dimensions of Critical Care Nursing, 12*(3), 127–137.

Wilson, D. (1996). Care of the chronic mechanically ventilated patient. In J. Clochesy, C. Breu, S. Cardin, A. Whittaker, & E. Rudy (Eds.), *Critical care nursing* (2nd ed., pp. 689–713). Philadelphia: W. B. Saunders.

SUGGESTED READINGS

Burns, S. (1996). Understanding, applying, and evaluating pressure modes of ventilation. *AACN Clinical Issues: Advanced Practice in Acute Care and Critical Care, 7*(4), 495–506.
  Earlier methods of positive-pressure mechanical ventilation involving pressure-cycled machines have been shown to increase the risk of baratrauma and other complications. Thus, their use has largely been discontinued. Newer methods of pressure ventilation are now being used successfully and show some superiority over volume-cycled ventilation. This excellent article describes and compares current pressure ventilation modes, including pressure support, pressure-controlled inverse ratio, and volume-guaranteed pressure ventilation.

Carroll, P. (1997). When you WANT humidity. *RN, 60*(5), 30–35.
  The issue of humidity and the importance of maintaining adequate humidity in clients who have artificial airways (endotracheal tube, tracheostomy tube) are discussed in clear terms. Ensuring adequate humidity in ventilated clients with artificial airways is essential to prevent complications. Different systems of humidification and their cost effectiveness are described.

Thompson, L. F. (1996). Failure to wean: Exploration of the influence of age-related pulmonary changes. *Critical Care Nursing Clinics of North America, 8*(1), 7–16.
  This excellent article discusses the age-related physiologic and anatomic changes that decrease the likelihood to wean from mechanical ventilation in the elderly. Nursing implications for evaluation of effective ventilation in the elderly are presented.

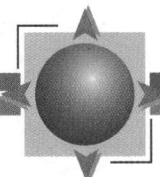

Problems of Cardiac

Output and Tissue

Perfusion: Management of

Clients with Problems of

the Cardiovascular System

Chapter 35

ASSESSMENT OF THE CARDIOVASCULAR SYSTEM

CHAPTER

HIGHLIGHTS

Since 1979, there has been a 23.4% decline in the death rate from cardiovascular disease in the United States. Despite this dramatic reduction, cardiovascular disease remains the major cause of mortality, resulting in 42% of all deaths or nearly 1 million deaths each year in the United States. Additionally, the American Heart Association (AHA) estimates that approximately one in five people has experienced, and is living with, some form of cardiovascular disease (AHA, 1996).

ANATOMY AND PHYSIOLOGY REVIEW
Heart
Structure

The human heart is a cone-shaped, hollow, muscular organ located between the lungs (Fig. 35–1). It is approximately the size of an adult fist. The heart rests on the diaphragm, tilting forward and to the left in the client's chest. This small organ must pump continuously. Each beat of the heart pumps approximately 60 mL of blood,

which is about 5 L/minute. During strenuous physical activity, the heart can double the amount of blood pumped to meet the increased oxygen needs of the peripheral tissues.

The heart is encapsulated by a protective covering called the *pericardium* (Fig. 35–2). The cardiac muscle tissue is composed of three layers: epicardium, myocardium, and endocardium. The epicardium, the outer surface, is a thin transparent tissue. The myocardium, the middle layer, is composed of striated muscle fibers interlaced into bundles. This layer is responsible for the heart's contractile force. The innermost layer, the endocardium, is composed of endothelial tissue. This tissue lines the inside of the chambers of the heart and covers the four heart valves.

Chambers of the Heart

A muscular wall, known as the septum, separates the heart into two halves: right and left. Each half has an upper chamber called an *atrium* and a lower chamber called a *ventricle* (Fig. 35–3).

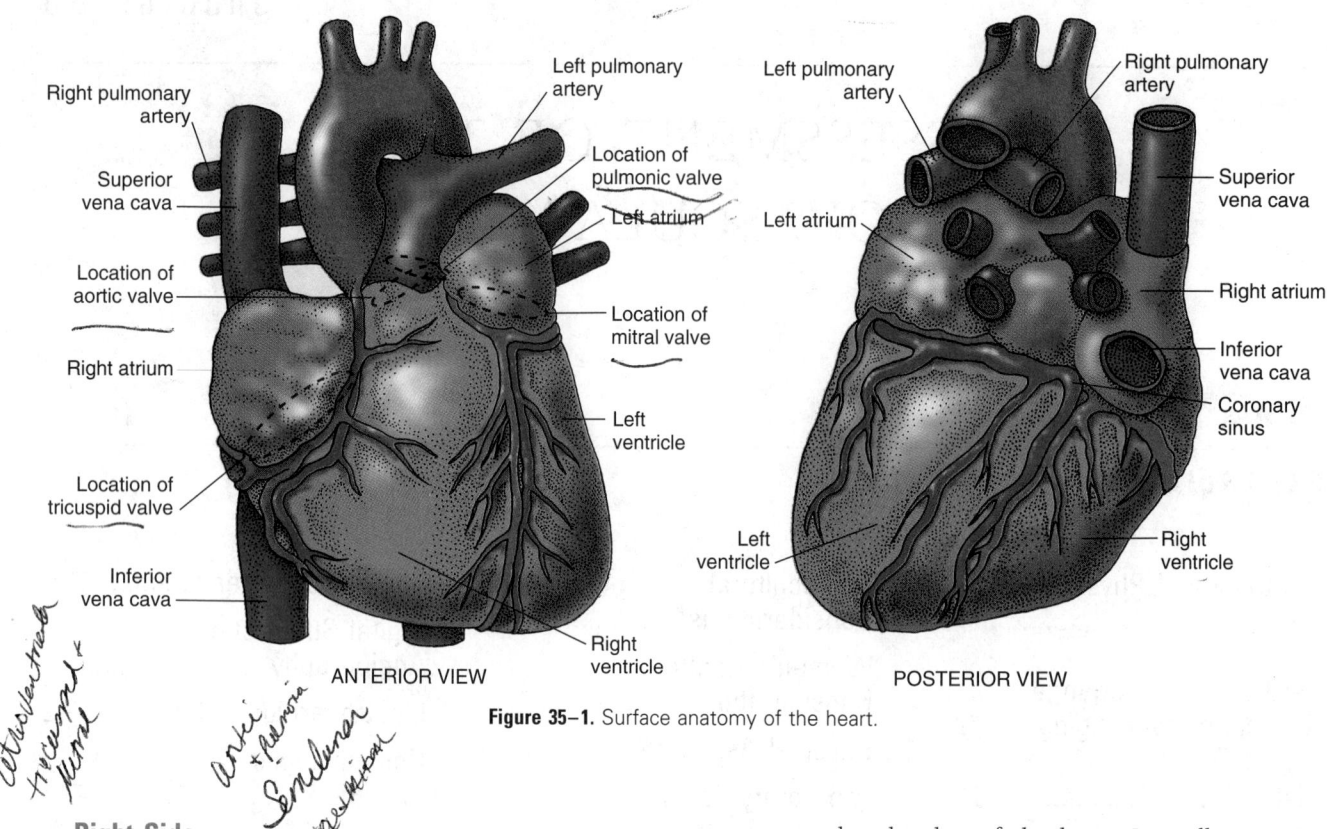

Figure 35–1. Surface anatomy of the heart.

Right Side

The right atrium is a thin-walled structure that receives deoxygenated venous blood (venous return) from all the peripheral tissues by way of the superior and inferior venae cavae and from the heart muscle by way of the coronary sinus. Most of this venous return flows passively from the right atrium through the opened tricuspid valve to the right ventricle during ventricular diastole, or filling. The remaining venous return is actively propelled by the right atrium into the right ventricle during atrial systole, or contraction.

The right ventricle is a flat muscular pump located behind the sternum. The right ventricle generates enough pressure (about 25 mmHg) to close the tricuspid valve, open the pulmonic valve, and propel blood into the pulmonary artery and the lungs. The workload of the right ventricle is light compared with that of the left ventricle because the pulmonary system is a low-pressure system, which imposes less resistance to flow.

Left Side

After blood is reoxygenated in the lungs, it flows freely from the four pulmonary veins into the left atrium. Blood then flows through an opened mitral valve into the left ventricle during ventricular diastole. When the left ventricle is almost full, the left atrium contracts, pumping the remaining blood volume into the left ventricle. Finally, with systolic contraction, the left ventricle generates enough pressure (about 120 mmHg) to close the mitral valve and open the aortic valve. Blood is propelled into the aorta and into the systemic arterial circulation. Blood flow through the heart is shown in Figure 35–2.

The left ventricle is ellipsoid and is the largest and most muscular chamber of the heart. Its wall is two to three times the thickness of the right ventricular wall. The left ventricle must generate a higher pressure than the right ventricle because it must contract against a high-pressure systemic circulation, which imposes a greater resistance to flow.

Blood is propelled from the aorta throughout the systemic circulation to the various tissues of the body; blood returns to the right atrium because of pressure differences. The pressure of blood in the aorta in a young adult averages about 100–120 mmHg, whereas the pressure of blood in the right atrium averages about 0–5 mmHg. These differences in pressure produce a pressure gradient and blood flows from an area of higher pressure to an area of lower pressure. The heart and vascular structures are responsible for maintaining these pressures.

Heart Valves

The four cardiac valves are responsible for maintaining the forward flow of blood through the chambers of the heart (see Fig. 35–2). These valves open and close passively in response to pressure and volume changes within the cardiac chambers. The cardiac valves are classified into two types: atrioventricular (AV) valves and semilunar valves.

Atrioventricular Valves

The AV valves separate the atria from the ventricles. The tricuspid valve is composed of three leaflets and separates the right atrium from the right ventricle. The mitral (bicuspid) valve is composed of two leaflets and separates the left atrium from the left ventricle.

During ventricular diastole, the valves act as funnels,

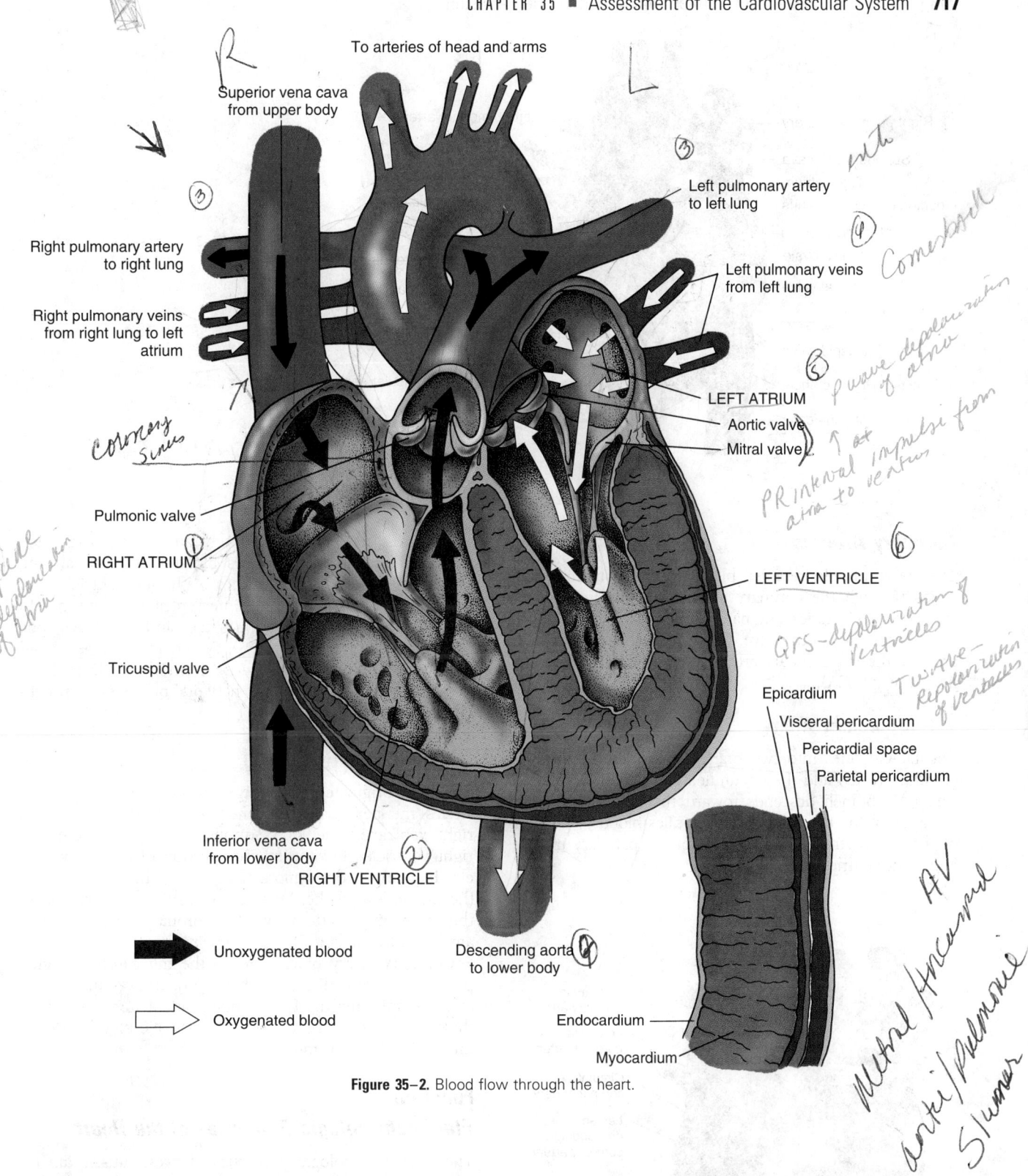

To arteries of head and arms

Superior vena cava
from upper body

Right pulmonary artery
to right lung

Left pulmonary artery
to left lung

Right pulmonary veins
from right lung to left
atrium

Left pulmonary veins
from left lung

LEFT ATRIUM

Aortic valve

Mitral valve

Pulmonic valve

RIGHT ATRIUM

LEFT VENTRICLE

Tricuspid valve

Epicardium

Visceral pericardium

Pericardial space

Parietal pericardium

Inferior vena cava
from lower body

RIGHT VENTRICLE

Descending aorta
to lower body

Endocardium

Myocardium

Unoxygenated blood

Oxygenated blood

Figure 35–2. Blood flow through the heart.

facilitating the flow of blood from the atria to the ventricles. During systole, the valves close to prevent the backflow (regurgitation) of blood into the atria.

Semilunar Valves

There are two semilunar valves: the pulmonic and the aortic valve. The pulmonic valve separates the right ven-

tricle from the pulmonary artery. The aortic valve separates the left ventricle from the aorta. Each semilunar valve consists of three cup-like cusps, or pockets, around the inside wall of the artery. These cusps prevent blood from flowing back into the ventricles during ventricular diastole. During ventricular systole, these valves are open to permit blood flow into the pulmonary artery and the aorta.

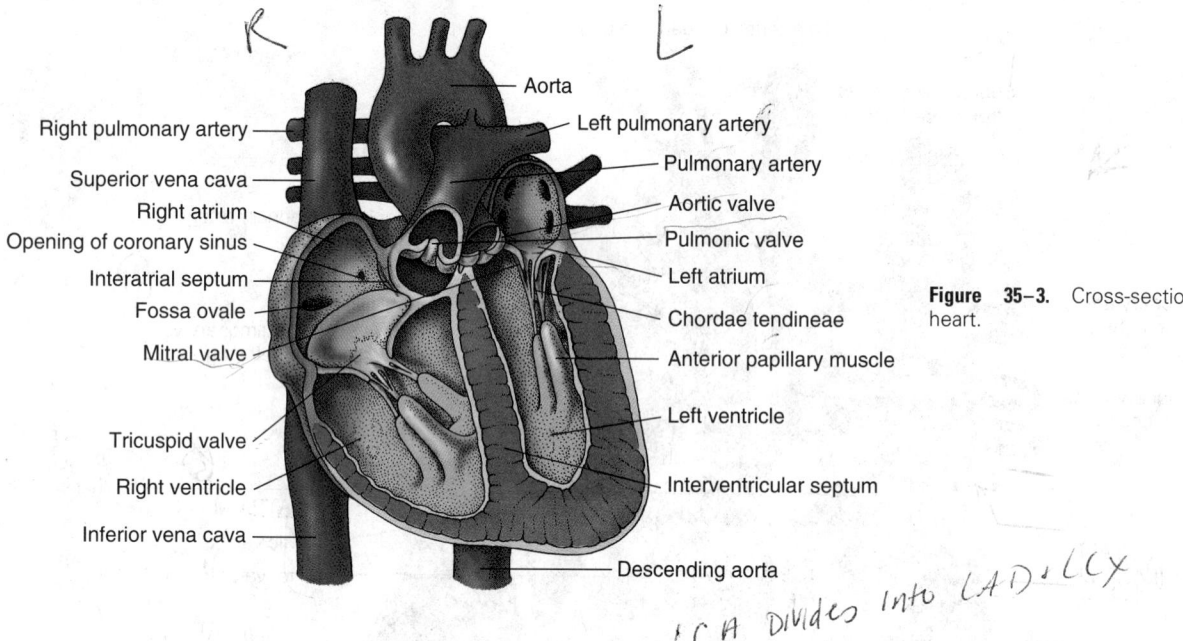

R   L

Aorta
Right pulmonary artery
Superior vena cava
Right atrium
Opening of coronary sinus
Interatrial septum
Fossa ovale
Mitral valve

Tricuspid valve
Right ventricle
Inferior vena cava

Left pulmonary artery
Pulmonary artery
Aortic valve
Pulmonic valve
Left atrium
Chordae tendineae
Anterior papillary muscle

Left ventricle

Interventricular septum

Descending aorta

Figure 35–3. Cross-section of the heart.

LCA Divides Into LAD & LCX

Coronary Arteries

The heart muscle receives blood to meet its metabolic needs through the coronary arterial system (Fig. 35–4). The coronary arteries originate from an area on the aorta just beyond the aortic valve. There are two main coronary arteries: the left coronary artery (LCA) and the right coronary artery (RCA).

Left Coronary Artery

The LCA divides into two branches: the left anterior descending (LAD) and the circumflex coronary artery (LCX). The LAD branch descends toward the anterior wall and the apex of the left ventricle. It supplies blood to portions of the left ventricle, ventricular septum, papillary muscle, and right ventricle.

The LCX descends toward the lateral wall of the left ventricle and apex. It supplies blood to the left atrium, the lateral and posterior surfaces of the left ventricle, and sometimes portions of the interventricular septum. In some people, the LCX supplies the sinoatrial (SA) node (45%) and the AV node (10%). Peripheral branches (diagonal and obtuse marginal) arise from the LAD and the LCX and form an abundant network of vessels throughout the entire myocardium.

Right Coronary Artery

The RCA originates from the right sinus of Valsalva, encircles the heart, and descends toward the apex of the right ventricle. The RCA supplies the right atrium, the right ventricle, and the inferior portion of the left ventricle. In many people (more than 50%), the RCA supplies the SA node and the AV node. Considerable variation in the branching pattern of the coronary arteries exists among individuals.

Coronary artery blood flow to the myocardium occurs primarily during diastole, when coronary vascular resistance is minimized. To maintain adequate blood flow through the coronary arteries, the diastolic blood pressure must be at least 60 mmHg.

Function
Electrophysiologic Properties of the Heart

The electrophysiologic properties of heart muscle are responsible for regulating heart rate and rhythm. Cardiac muscle cells are unique and possess the special characteristics of automaticity, excitability, conductivity, contractility, and refractoriness.

Automaticity refers to the ability of all cardiac cells to initiate an impulse spontaneously and repetitively. Excitability is the ability of the cells to respond to a stimulus by initiating an impulse (depolarization). Conductivity means that cardiac cells transmit the electrical impulses

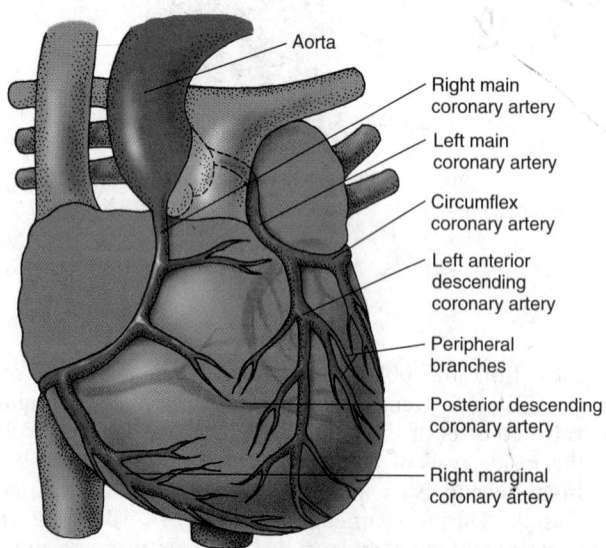

Aorta
Right main coronary artery
Left main coronary artery
Circumflex coronary artery
Left anterior descending coronary artery
Peripheral branches
Posterior descending coronary artery
Right marginal coronary artery

Figure 35–4. Coronary arterial system.

they receive. Because the cells possess the property of contractility, they also contract in response to an impulse. Refractoriness means that cardiac cells are unable to respond to a stimulus until they have repolarized from the previous stimulus. These properties are more completely described in Chapter 36.

Conduction System of the Heart

The cardiac conduction system is composed of specialized tissue capable of rhythmic electrical impulse formation (Fig. 35–5). It can conduct impulses much more rapidly than other cells located in the myocardium. The SA node, located at the junction of the right atrium and the superior vena cava, is considered the main regulator of heart rate. The SA node is composed of pacemaker cells, which spontaneously initiate impulses at a rate of 60–100 per minute, and myocardial working cells, which transmit the impulses to surrounding atrial muscle.

An impulse from the SA node initiates the process of depolarization and hence the activation of all myocardial cells. The impulse travels through both atria to the atrioventricular (AV) node located in the junctional area. After the impulse reaches the AV node, conduction of the impulse is delayed briefly. This delay allows the atria to contract completely before the ventricles are stimulated to contract. The intrinsic rate of the AV node is 40–60 beats per minute.

The bundle of His is a continuation of the AV node located in the interventricular septum. It divides into the right and left bundle branches. The bundle branches extend downward through the ventricular septum and fuse with the Purkinje fiber system. The Purkinje fibers are the terminal branches of the conduction system and are responsible for carrying the wave of depolarization to both ventricular walls. The Purkinje fibers can act as an intrinsic pacemaker, but their discharge rate is only 20–40

beats per minute. Thus, these intrinsic pacemakers seldom initiate an electrical impulse.

Sequence of Events During the Cardiac Cycle

The phases of the cardiac cycle are generally described in relation to changes in pressure and volume in the left ventricle during filling (diastole) and ventricular contraction (systole) (Fig. 35–6). Diastole, normally about two thirds of the cardiac cycle, consists of relaxation and filling of the atria and ventricles, whereas systole consists of the contraction and emptying of the atria and ventricles.

Cardiac muscle contraction results from the release of large numbers of calcium ions from the sarcoplasmic reticulum. These ions diffuse into the myofibril sarcomere (the basic contractile unit of the myocardial cell). Calcium ions promote the interaction of actin and myosin protein filaments, causing a linking and overlapping of these filaments. As the protein filaments slide over or overlap each other, cross-bridges, or linkages, are formed. These cross-bridges act as force-generating sites. The sliding of these protein filaments of multiple myofibril sarcomeres causes shortening of the sarcomeres, producing myocardial contraction.

Relaxation of the cardiac muscle occurs when calcium ions are pumped back into the sarcoplasmic reticulum, causing a decrease in the number of calcium ions around the myofibrils. This reduced number of ions causes the protein filaments to disengage or dissociate, the sarcomere to lengthen, and the muscle to relax.

Mechanical Properties of the Heart

The electrical and mechanical properties of cardiac muscle determine the function of the cardiovascular system. The heart is able to adapt to various pathophysiologic conditions (e.g., stress, infections, and hemorrhage) to maintain

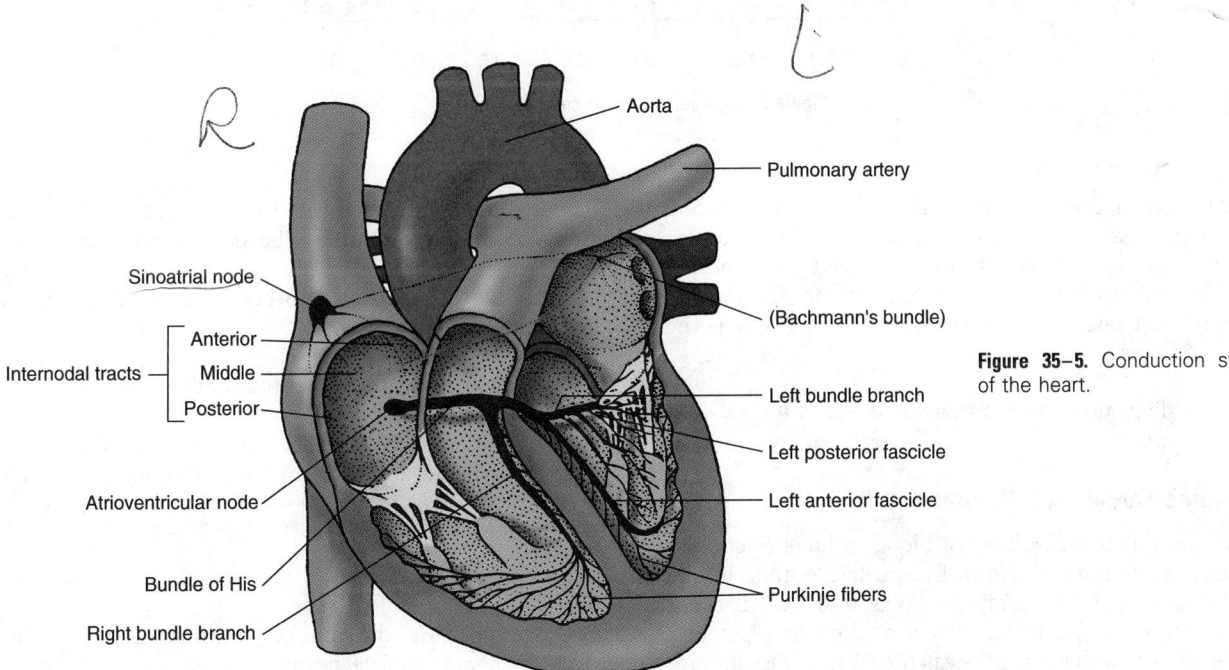

Figure 35–5. Conduction system of the heart.

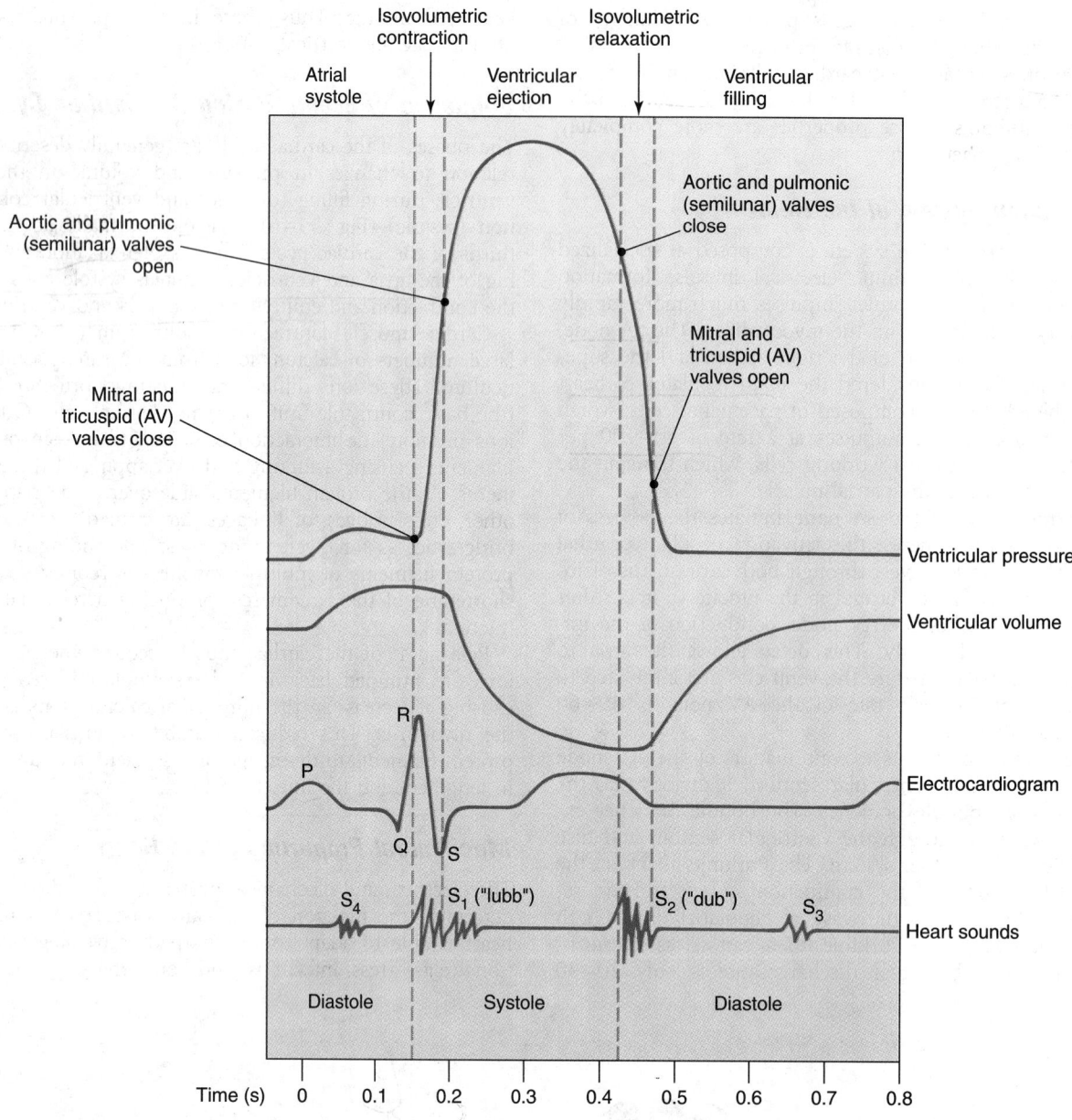

Figure 35–6. Events of the cardiac cycle.

adequate blood flow to the various body tissues. Blood flow to the tissues is measured clinically as the cardiac output (CO), the amount of blood pumped from the left ventricle each minute. CO depends on the relationship between heart rate (HR) and stroke volume (SV); it is the product of these two variables.

$$\text{Cardiac output} = \text{heart rate} \times \text{stroke volume}$$

Cardiac Output and Cardiac Index

Cardiac output is the volume of blood in liters ejected by the heart each minute. Normally, cardiac output in the adult ranges from 4–7 L/minute (Wilson, 1992). Because cardiac output requirements vary according to a person's body size, the cardiac index is calculated to adjust for size

differences. The cardiac index can be determined by dividing the cardiac output by the body surface area. The cardiac index is based on the assumption that cardiac output is more proportional to body surface area than to body mass. Therefore,

$$\text{Cardiac index} = \text{cardiac output/body surface area}$$

The normal range of cardiac index is 2.7–3.2 L/minute/m^2 of body surface area, thus adjusting for the client's body size and variability in cardiac function (Wilson, 1992).

Heart Rate

Heart rate refers to the number of times the ventricles contract per minute. The normal resting heart rate for an adult is between 60 and 100 beats per minute. Increases in heart rate increase myocardial oxygen demand. Rate is extrinsically controlled by the autonomic nervous system, which adjusts rapidly when necessary to regulate cardiac output. The parasympathetic system slows the heart rate, whereas sympathetic stimulation has an excitatory effect. An increase in circulating endogenous catecholamine, such as epinephrine and norepinephrine, usually causes an increase in heart rate, and vice versa.

Other factors, such as the central nervous system (CNS) and baroreceptor (pressoreceptor) reflexes, influence the effects of the autonomic nervous system on the heart rate. Pain, fear, and anxiety can cause an increase in heart rate. The baroreceptor reflex acts as a negative-feedback system. If a client experiences hypotension, the baroreceptors in the aortic arch sense a lessened pressure in the blood vessels. A signal is relayed to the parasympathetic system to have less inhibitory effect on the sinoatrial (SA) node, which results in a reflex increase in heart rate.

Stroke Volume

Stroke volume is the amount of blood ejected by the left ventricle during each systole. Several variables influence stroke volume and, ultimately, cardiac output (CO). These variables include heart rate, preload, afterload, and contractility.

PRELOAD. Preload refers to the degree of myocardial fiber stretch at the end of diastole just before contraction. The stretch imposed on the muscle fibers results from the volume contained within the ventricle at the end of diastole. Preload is determined by left ventricular end-diastolic (LVED) volume.

An increase in ventricular volume increases muscle fiber length and tension, thereby enhancing contraction and improving stroke volume. This statement is derived from Starling's law of the heart: the more the heart is filled during diastole (within limits), the more forcefully it contracts. However, excessive filling of the ventricles results in excessive LVED volume and pressure and decreased CO (Fig. 35–7).

AFTERLOAD. Another determinant of stroke volume is afterload. Afterload is the pressure or resistance that the ventricles must overcome to eject blood through the semilunar valves and into the peripheral blood vessels. The amount of resistance is directly related to arterial blood pressure and the diameter of the blood vessels.

Impedance, the peripheral component of afterload, is the pressure that the heart must overcome to open the aortic valve. The amount of impedance depends on aortic compliance and total peripheral vascular resistance, a combination of blood viscosity and arteriolar constriction. A decrease in stroke volume can result from an increase in afterload without the benefit of compensatory mechanisms.

CONTRACTILITY. Contractility also affects stroke volume and CO. Myocardial contractility is the force of cardiac contraction independent of preload. Contractility is

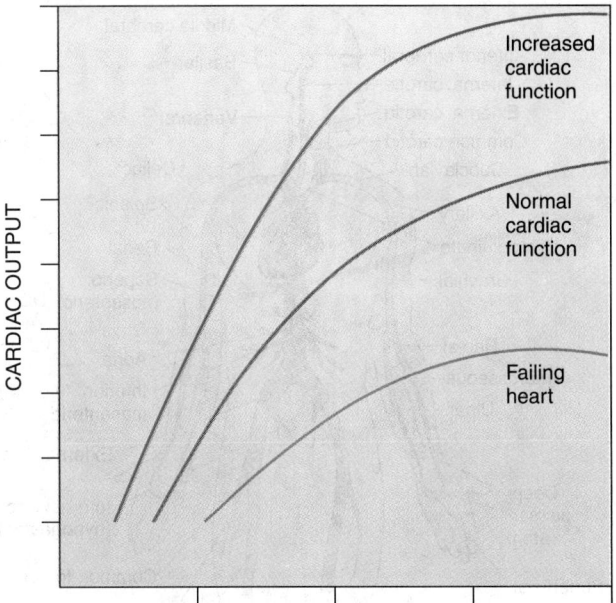

Figure 35–7. Length-tension ventricular function curves.

increased by such factors as sympathetic stimulation and calcium release. Factors such as hypoxia and acidemia decrease contractility.

Vascular System

The purpose of the vascular system is

- To provide conduits for blood to travel from the heart to nourish the various tissues of the body
- To carry away cellular wastes to the excretory organs
- To allow lymphatic flow to drain tissue fluid back into the circulation
- To return blood to the heart for recirculation

This system of conduits depends on an efficient heart and patent blood vessels to regulate and maintain systemic and regional blood flow and temperature.

The vascular system is divided into the arterial system and the venous system (Fig. 35–8). In the arterial system, blood moves from the larger conduits to a network of smaller blood vessels. In the venous system, blood travels from the capillaries to the venules and to the larger system of veins, eventually returning in the venae cavae to the heart for recirculation.

Arterial System
Structure

The high-pressure blood vessels of the arterial vascular system may be classified according to their size and wall structure. The large arteries, such as the aorta and femoral arteries, follow relatively straight routes and have few branches. Smaller arteries, such as the internal iliac and mesenteric arteries, divide from larger ones and have multiple branches.

Arteries may branch into arterioles or anastomose with

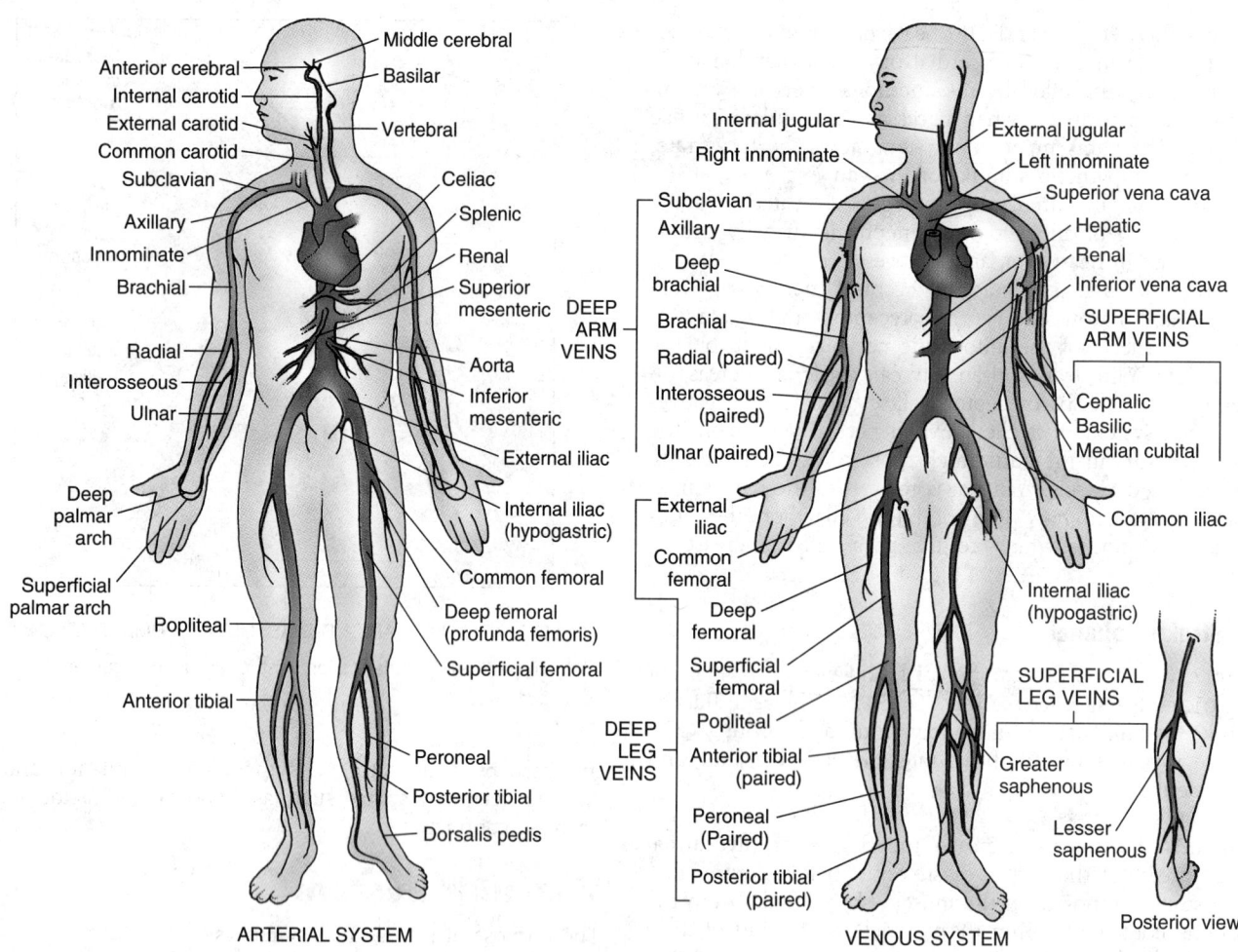

Figure 35–8. Anatomy of the arterial and venous systems.

other arteries. The arterioles branch into terminal arterioles, which join with the capillary or capillaries and ultimately with venules, forming the capillary network (Fig. 35–9). The exchange of nutrients across the capillary membrane occurs primarily by three processes: osmosis, filtration, and diffusion. (See Chapter 14 for detailed discussions of osmosis, filtration, and diffusion.)

Function

The arterial system delivers blood to various tissues for nourishment. At the tissue level, nutrients, chemicals, and body defense substances are distributed and exchanged for cellular waste products, depending on the needs of the particular tissue. The arteries transport the cellular wastes to the excretory organs, such as the kidneys and the lungs, to be reprocessed or removed. The arteries also contribute to the tissue's temperature regulation. Blood can be either directed toward the skin to promote heat loss or diverted away from the skin to conserve heat.

Blood Pressure

Blood pressure is the force of blood exerted against the vessel walls. Pressure in the larger blood vessels is greater

(about 80–100 mmHg) and decreases as blood flow reaches the capillaries (about 25 mmHg). By the time blood enters the right atrium, blood pressure is approximately 0–5 mmHg.

Indirect Measurement of Blood Pressure

The blood pressure in the arterial system is determined primarily by the quantity of blood flow or cardiac output (CO), and the resistance in the arterioles, so that

Blood pressure = CO × peripheral vascular resistance

Therefore, any factor that increases cardiac output or total peripheral vascular resistance increases blood pressure. In general, blood pressure is maintained at a relatively constant level, such that an increase or decrease in total peripheral vascular resistance is associated with a decrease or an increase in CO, respectively. Three mechanisms mediate and regulate blood pressure:

- The autonomic nervous system, which, in responding to impulses from chemoreceptors and baroreceptors, excites or inhibits sympathetic nervous system activity

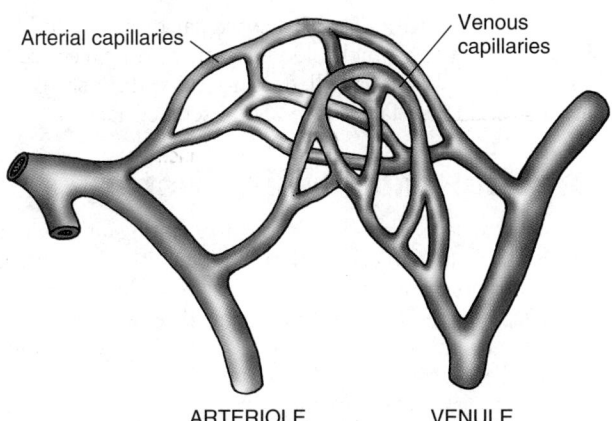

Arterial capillaries

Venous capillaries

ARTERIOLE   VENULE

Figure 35–9. Structure of the capillary bed.

- The kidneys, which sense a change in blood flow and activate the renin-angiotensin-aldosterone mechanism
- The endocrine system, which releases various hormones (e.g., catecholamine, kinins, serotonin, and histamine) to stimulate the sympathetic nervous system at the tissue level

Systolic blood pressure represents the highest pressure occurring in an artery with each contraction of the heart; diastolic blood pressure represents the lowest pressure during the relaxation phase of the heart. In the adult, systolic pressure is normally 90–135 mmHg, and diastolic pressure is normally 60–85 mmHg. Blood pressure is expressed as systolic/diastolic.

Systolic pressure is affected by a number of factors, including CO. When CO decreases, systolic pressure also decreases. Diastolic pressure is primarily determined by the amount of vasoconstriction in the periphery. An increase in peripheral vascular resistance increases diastolic pressure and cardiac workload.

Regulation of Blood Pressure

The autonomic nervous system (ANS) and the renal system are primarily responsible for regulating blood pressure, although external factors can also affect a person's blood pressure.

AUTONOMIC NERVOUS SYSTEM. Blood pressure is regulated by balancing the sympathetic and parasympathetic nervous systems of the autonomic nervous system. Changes in sympathetic and parasympathetic activity are responses to messages sent by the sensory receptors in the various tissues of the body. These receptors, including the baroreceptors, the chemoreceptors, and the stretch receptors, respond differently to biochemical and physiologic changes of the body.

Baroreceptors in the arch of the aorta and at the origin of the internal carotid arteries are stimulated when the arterial walls are stretched by an increased blood pressure. Impulses from these baroreceptors inhibit the vasomotor center, located in the pons and the medulla. Inhibition of this center results in a drop in blood pressure.

Several 1- to 2-mm collections of tissue have been identified in the bifurcations of the carotid arteries and along the aortic arch. Called the carotid and aortic bodies, respectively, they contain specialized chemoreceptors that are sensitive primarily to hypoxemia (a decrease in arterial oxygen pressure [PaO_2]). When stimulated, the carotid chemoreceptors send impulses along Hering's nerves, and the aortic chemoreceptors send impulses along the vagus nerves to activate a vasoconstrictor response.

The chemoreceptors are also stimulated by hypercapnia (an increase in arterial carbon dioxide pressure [$PaCO_2$]) and acidosis. However, the direct effect of carbon dioxide on the CNS is 10 times as strong as the effect it produces by stimulating the chemoreceptors.

Stretch receptors found in the venae cavae and the right atrium are sensitive to pressure or volume changes. When a client is hypovolemic, the stretch receptors in the blood vessels sense a reduced volume or pressure and send fewer impulses to the CNS. This reaction stimulates the sympathetic nervous system to increase heart rate and to constrict the peripheral blood vessels.

RENAL SYSTEM. The renal system also helps to regulate cardiovascular activity. When renal blood flow or pressure decreases, the kidneys retain sodium and water. Blood pressure tends to rise because of fluid retention and because of activation of the renin-angiotensin-aldosterone mechanism. Vascular volume is also regulated by the release of antidiuretic hormone (vasopressin) from the posterior pituitary gland (see Chap. 14).

EXTERNAL FACTORS. Other factors can influence the activity of the cardiovascular system. For example, emotional behaviors, such as excitement, pain, and anger, stimulate the sympathetic nervous system to increase blood pressure and heart rate. Increased physical activity such as exercise increases blood pressure and pulse rate as well. Body temperature can affect the metabolic needs of the tissues, thereby influencing the delivery of blood. In hypothermia, tissues require fewer nutrients and blood pressure falls. In hyperthermia, the metabolic requirement of the tissues is greater, and blood pressure and pulse rate rise.

Venous System

Structure

The venous system is composed of a series of veins that are located adjacent to the arterial system. In addition, a second superficial venous circulation runs parallel to the subcutaneous tissue of the extremity. These two venous systems are connected by communicating veins, which provide a means for blood to travel from the superficial veins to the deep veins. Blood flow is directed toward the deep venous circulation.

The venules collect blood from the capillaries and the terminal arterioles. Venules also serve as a location where white blood cells enter into and exit from the body tissues.

Venules branch into veins, which are low-pressure blood vessels. Veins have the ability to accommodate large shifts in volume with minimal changes in venous pressure. This flexibility allows the venous system to accommodate the administration of intravenous (IV) fluids and blood transfusions, blood loss, and dehydration. In both the superficial and deep venous systems, all veins, except for the smallest and the largest, have valves directing blood flow back to the heart, preventing retrograde flow (backflow).

Function

The primary function of the venous system is to complete the circulation of blood by returning blood from the capillaries to the right side of the heart. The venous system also acts as a reservoir for a large portion of the blood volume. In contrast to the arterial system, which consists of a high-pressure, continuous-flow system through relatively rigid conduits, the venous system consists of a low-pressure, intermittent flow system through collapsible tubes working against the effects of gravity.

Gravity exerts an increase in hydrostatic pressure (capillary blood pressure) when the client is in an upright position, which delays venous return. When the client is lying down, the hydrostatic pressure is lessened, and thus there is less hindrance of venous return to the heart.

Cardiovascular Changes Associated with Aging

A number of physiologic changes in the cardiovascular system occur with advancing age (Chart 35–1). Many of these changes result in loss of cardiac reserve. Thus, these changes are usually not evident when the older adult is resting. They become apparent only when the person is physically or emotionally stressed and the heart cannot meet the increased metabolic demands of the body.

HISTORY

The nurse obtains a thorough history, which includes demographic data, personal and family history, diet, socioeconomic status, and a functional assessment. Information relative to risk factors and symptoms of cardiovascular disease is the focus of the history.

Demographic Data

Demographic data include the client's age, sex, and ethnic origin. The incidence of conditions such as coronary artery disease (CAD) and valvular disease increases with age (Miller, 1995). The incidence of CAD also varies with the client's sex. Women who are premenopausal have a lower incidence of CAD than do men.

TRANSCULTURAL CONSIDERATIONS

Information about the client's ethnic or cultural background is important because some disease conditions may be more prevalent in specific ethnic groups. For example, African-Americans, Puerto Ricans, Cubans, and Mexican-Americans have a higher incidence of hypertension than do Caucasians (AHA, 1996; Jarvis, 1996).

Age, sex, ethnic background, and family history of cardiovascular disease are considered nonmodifiable or uncontrollable risk factors for cardiovascular disease. Modifiable risk factors (e.g., high blood pressure and excessive blood cholesterol), if controlled, can reduce the risk of heart disease. These factors are also discussed later.

Personal and Family History

The nurse reviews the client's history, noting any major illnesses, such as diabetes mellitus, renal disease, anemia, high blood pressure, stroke, bleeding disorders, connective tissue diseases, chronic pulmonary diseases, heart disease, and thrombophlebitis. These conditions can influence the client's cardiovascular status.

The nurse asks about previous treatment for cardiovascular disease, identifying previous diagnostic procedures (e.g., electrocardiography and cardiac catheterization) and requests information about any medical or invasive treatment of cardiovascular disease. It is important for the nurse to ask specifically about recurrent tonsillitis, streptococcal infections, and rheumatic fever, because these conditions may lead to valvular abnormalities of the heart. In addition, the nurse inquires about any known congenital heart defects.

The nurse questions clients in detail about their medication history beginning with any prescription or over-the-counter medications that the client is currently or has recently taken. The nurse questions clients about any known sensitivity to penicillin or any drugs that may be needed in an emergency, such as morphine. The nurse specifically asks clients whether they have recently used cocaine or any intravenous (IV) "street" drugs, because they may be associated with chest pain or endocarditis. The nurse also asks female clients whether they are taking oral contraceptives or estrogen replacement. There is an increased incidence of myocardial infarction (MI) and cerebrovascular accident (CVA) in older women who take oral contraceptives, but only if they smoke, have diabetes, or have hypertension (AHA, 1996). However, postmenopausal women who take estrogen replacement have a lower incidence of coronary artery disease (CAD).

The nurse reviews the family history, obtaining information about the age, health status, and cause of death of immediate family members. A family history of hypertension, obesity, diabetes, or sudden cardiac death is especially significant. The nurse may also ask about the extended family, including grandparents and grandchildren, and record this information in a narrative outline or as a diagram with the client's history.

Diet History

A diet history might include the client's recall of food and fluid intake during a 24-hour period, self-imposed or medically prescribed dietary restrictions or supplementations, and the amount and type of alcohol consumption. The nurse and the dietitian review the type of foods selected by the client for the amount of sodium, sugar, cholesterol, fiber, and fat. The nurse or dietitian also explores the client's attitudes toward food, knowledge level of essential and nonessential dietary elements, and willingness to make changes in the diet. Cultural beliefs and economic status can influence the client's choice of

Chart 35–1			
Nursing Focus on the Elderly: Changes in the Cardiovascular System Related to Aging			
Structure/Function	**Change**	**Nursing Implications**	**Rationale**
Cardiac valves	• Calcification and mucoid degeneration occur, especially in mitral and aortic valves.	• Assess heart sounds for murmurs. • Question clients about dyspnea.	• Murmurs may be detected before other symptoms.
Conduction system	• Pacemaker cells decrease in number. Fibrous tissue and fat in the sinoatrial node increase. • Few muscle fibers remain in the atrial myocardium and bundle of His. • Conduction time increases.	• Assess the electrocardiogram (ECG) and heart rhythm for dysrhythmias or a heart rate less than 60 beats per minute	• The SA node may lose its inherent rhythm. • Atrial dysrhythmias occur in 50–90% of elders, 80% of elders experience premature ventricular contractions (PVCs).
Left ventricle	• The size of the left ventricle increases. • The left ventricle becomes stiff and less distensible. • Fibrotic changes in the left ventricle decrease the speed of early diastolic filling by about 50%. • Conduction time increases.	• Assess the ECG for a widening QRS complex and a longer QT interval. • Assess for activity intolerance. • Assess the heart rate at rest and with activity. • Assess for activity intolerance.	• Ventricular changes result in decreased stroke volume, ejection fraction, and cardiac output during exercise; the heart is less able to meet increased oxygen demands. • Maximal heart rate with exercise is decreased. • The heart is less able to meet increased oxygen demands.
Aorta and other large arteries	• The aorta and other large arteries thicken and become stiffer and less distensible. Systolic blood pressure increases to compensate for the stiff arteries. • Systemic vascular resistance increases as a result of less distensible arteries, so the left ventricle pumps against greater resistance, contributing to left ventricular hypertrophy.	• Assess blood pressure. • Note increases in systolic, diastolic, and pulse pressures. • Assess for activity intolerance and shortness of breath. • Assess the peripheral pulses.	• Hypertension may occur, which must be treated to avoid target organ damage.
Baroreceptors	• Baroreceptors become less sensitive.	• Assess the client's blood pressure with the client lying and then sitting or standing. • Assess for dizziness when the client changes from a lying to a sitting or standing position. • Teach the client to change positions slowly.	• Orthostatic (postural) and postprandial changes occur because of ineffective baroreceptors. Changes may include decreases in blood pressure of 10 mmHg or more, dizziness, and fainting.

food items and, therefore, must be reviewed. Family members or significant others who are responsible for shopping and cooking are included in the discussion.

Socioeconomic Status

Social history includes information about the client's domestic situation, such as marital status, number of children, household members, living environment, and occupation. The nurse also identifies the client's support

systems. It is especially important for the nurse to explore the possibility that the client might have difficulty paying for medications or treatment.

The nurse asks about the client's occupation, including the type of work performed and the requirements of the specific job. For instance, does the job involve lifting of heavy objects? Is the job emotionally stressful? What does a day's work entail? Does the client's job require him or her to be outside in extreme weather conditions?

Personal habits that are risk factors for heart disease

include cigarette smoking, physical inactivity, obesity, and type A behavior. These factors are considered modifiable or controllable risk factors. The nurse queries the client about each of the following modifiable risk factors.

Cigarette Smoking

Cigarette smoking is a major risk factor for cardiovascular disease, specifically CAD and peripheral vascular disease (PVD) (AHA, 1996). According to the U. S. Department of Health and Human Services (DHHS), cigarette smoking is directly responsible for 21% of all deaths from CAD (DHHS, 1990). Three compounds in cigarette smoke (tar, nicotine, and carbon monoxide) have been implicated in the development of CAD.

The risks to the cardiovascular system from cigarette smoking appear to be dose related, noncumulative, and transient. The smoking history should include the number of cigarettes smoked daily, duration of the smoking habit, and age of the client when smoking started. A person who smokes fewer than 4 cigarettes per day has twice the risk of cardiovascular disease of a person who does not smoke; a person who smokes more than 20 cigarettes per day has four times the risk. Typically, the nurse records the smoking history in pack-years, which is the number of packs per day multiplied by the number of years that the client smoked.

The nurse should also inquire about the client's desire to quit, past attempts to quit, and the methods used. Three to four years after a client has stopped smoking, his or her cardiovascular risk appears to be similar to that of a person who has never smoked. The nurse asks clients who do not currently smoke whether they have ever smoked and when they quit.

Physical Inactivity

Sedentary lifestyle is also considered a significant risk factor in the development of heart disease. Regular physical activity promotes cardiovascular fitness and produces beneficial changes in blood pressure and levels of blood lipids and clotting factors. Unfortunately, few people in the United States engage in the recommended exercise guidelines: 30 minutes daily of light-to-moderate exercise, equivalent to a 30-minute brisk walk. According to AHA (1996), only 22% of Americans engage in this much exercise five times a week and only 10% engage in vigorous physical activity, enough to promote cardiopulmonary fitness, three times a week. This puts more people at risk for CAD from physical inactivity than any other factor. The nurse questions clients concerning the type of exercise in which they engage, the period for which they have participated in the exercise, and the frequency and the intensity of the exercise.

Obesity

Approximately 61 million Americans are 20% or more above their desirable weight (AHA, 1996). Obesity in the American population has increased 36% in the last 30 years; it is particularly a problem for African-American females and native Hawaiians (AHA, 1996). Obesity is associated with hypertension, hyperlipidemia, and diabetes; all are known contributors to cardiovascular disease.

The nurse weighs and examines the client for the pattern of obesity, also known as waist:hip ratio.

WOMEN'S HEALTH CONSIDERATIONS

Caucasian women with abdominal obesity (greater waist than hip circumference) are more likely to experience cardiovascular disease than are Caucasian women with fat distributed in their buttocks, hips, and thighs (greater hip than waist circumference). Clients with an early onset of obesity (during adolescence) and an elevated waist:hip ratio appear to be at especially high risk for cardiovascular disease (Weigle, 1992).

Type A Personality

Researchers have identified people with type A personalities as being more vulnerable to the development of heart disease (Kottke et al., 1996). Type A personalities are highly competitive, overly concerned about meeting deadlines, and often hostile or angry. The chronic anger and hostility that type A people display appear to be most closely associated with cardiovascular disease. The constant arousal of the sympathetic nervous system resulting from the anger may influence blood pressure, serum fatty acids and lipids, and clotting mechanisms. The nurse observes the client and determines the response to stressful situations.

Current Health Problems

Inquiring about the client's major concerns helps the nurse to establish priorities in nursing care and management. The nurse asks the client to describe health concerns. Then the nurse expands on the client's description by obtaining information about the onset, duration, chronology, frequency, location, quality, intensity, associated symptoms, and precipitating, aggravating, and relieving factors. Major symptoms identified by clients with cardiovascular disease include chest pain or discomfort, dyspnea, fatigue, palpitations, weight gain, syncope, and extremity pain.

Chest Pain

Chest pain or discomfort, a cardinal symptom of heart disease, can result from ischemic heart disease, pericarditis, and aortic dissection. Chest pain can also be due to noncardiac conditions, such as pleurisy, pulmonary embolus, hiatal hernia, and anxiety. Nurses must thoroughly evaluate the nature and characteristics of the client's chest pain. Because chest pain resulting from myocardial ischemia is life threatening and can lead to serious complications, the cause of chest pain should be considered ischemic (reduced or obstructed blood flow to the myocardium) until proven otherwise.

When assessing for chest pain, the nurse uses alternative terms such as "discomfort," "heaviness," and "indigestion." Often clients do not experience a true pain in the chest but instead feel discomfort or indigestion. The client may also describe the sensation as aching, choking, strangling, tingling, squeezing, constricting, or vise-like.

The nurse asks the client to identify when the pain was first noticed (onset). Did the pain begin suddenly or develop gradually (manner of onset)? How long did the pain last (duration)? If the client has repeated chest pain episodes, the nurse assesses how frequently the pain occurs (frequency). The nurse asks whether this pain is different from any other episodes of pain. The nurse asks the client to describe what activities he or she was doing at the time it first occurred (e.g., sleeping, arguing, and running) (precipitating factors). The client can be asked to point to the area where the chest pain occurred (location) and to describe how the pain spread (radiation).

In addition, the client describes how the pain feels and whether it is sharp or dull (quality). To understand how severe the pain is, the nurse asks the client to grade the pain from 0 to 10, with 0 indicating the absence of pain and 10 indicating severe pain (intensity). The client may also report other signs and symptoms that occur at the same time (associated symptoms), such as dyspnea, diaphoresis, nausea, and vomiting. Other factors that need to be addressed are those that may have made the chest

pain worse (aggravating factors) or the pain less intense (relieving factors). Chest pain may arise from a variety of sources (Table 35–1). By obtaining appropriate information from the client, the nurse may assist in identifying the source of the client's chest discomfort.

Dyspnea

Dyspnea is a symptom that can occur from both cardiac and pulmonary disease. Dyspnea is objectively described as difficult or labored breathing and is subjectively experienced as uncomfortable breathing or shortness of breath. When obtaining the client's history, the nurse ascertains what factors precipitate and relieve dyspnea, what level of activity produces dyspnea, and the client's body position when dyspnea occurred.

There are several types of dyspnea. Dyspnea that is associated with activity, such as climbing stairs, is referred to as dyspnea on exertion (DOE). This is usually an early symptom of heart failure.

The client with advanced heart disease may experience orthopnea, dyspnea that appears when the client lies flat. The client may use several pillows at night to elevate the

TABLE 35–1

Assessment of Chest Discomfort: How Various Types of Chest Pain Differ				
Source	**Onset**	**Quality and Severity**	**Location and Radiation**	**Duration and Relieving Factors**
Angina	• Sudden, usually in response to exertion, emotion, or extremes in temperature	• Squeezing, vise-like pain	• Substernal: may spread across the chest and the back and/or down the arms	• Usually lasts less than 15 min; relieved with rest, nitrate administration, or oxygen therapy
Myocardial infarction	• Sudden, without precipitating factors, often in early morning	• Intense stabbing, vise-like pain or pressure, severe	• Substernal; may spread throughout the anterior chest and to the arms, jaw, back, or neck	• Usually lasts 30 min or longer or is relieved with opioids
Pericarditis	• Sudden	• Sharp stabbing, moderate to severe	• Substernal; usually spreads to the left side or the back	• Intermittent; relieved with sitting upright, analgesia, or administration of antiinflammatory agents
Pleuropulmonary	• Variable	• Moderate ache, worse on inspiration	• Lung fields	• Continuous until the underlying condition is treated or the client has rested
Esophageal–gastric	• Variable	• Squeezing, heartburn, variable severity	• Substernal; may spread to the shoulders or the abdomen	• Variable; may be relieved with antacid administration or food intake
Anxiety	• Variable, may be in response to stress or fatigue	• Dull ache to sharp stabbing; may be associated with numbness in fingers	• Usually the left side of chest without radiation	• Usually lasts a few minutes

head and chest or sleep in a recliner to prevent nighttime breathlessness. The severity of orthopnea is measured by the number of pillows or the amount of head elevation needed to provide restful sleep. Orthopnea is usually relieved within a matter of minutes by sitting up or standing.

Paroxysmal nocturnal dyspnea occurs after the client has been recumbent for several hours. When the client is lying down, blood from the lower extremities is redistributed to the venous system, increasing venous return to the heart. A diseased heart is unable to compensate for the increased volume and is ineffective in pumping the additional fluid into the circulatory system. Therefore, pulmonary congestion results. The client awakens abruptly, often with a feeling of suffocation and panic. The client usually sits upright with the legs dangled over the bedside to relieve the dyspnea. A client may experience 20 minutes of distress before obtaining relief.

Fatigue

Fatigue may be described as the feeling of tiredness or weariness resulting from activity. The client may complain that a certain activity takes longer to complete or that he or she tires easily after activity. Although fatigue in itself is not diagnostic of heart disease, many people with heart failure are limited by leg fatigue during exercise (Sullivan, 1994). Fatigue that occurs after mild activity and exertion usually indicates an inadequate cardiac output (low stroke volume) and anaerobic metabolism in skeletal muscle.

The nurse questions the client to determine the time of day he or she experiences fatigue as well as the activities that can be performed. Fatigue resulting from decreased cardiac output is often worse in the evening. The nurse asks whether the client can perform the same activities as a year ago or the same activities as others of the same age. Often the client limits activities in response to fatigue without being aware how much less active he or she has become unless questioned.

Palpitations

A feeling of fluttering in the chest or an unpleasant awareness of the heartbeat is referred to as palpitations. Palpitations may result from a change in heart rate or rhythm or from an increase in the force of heart contractions. Rhythm disturbances that may cause palpitations include paroxysmal supraventricular tachycardia, premature contractions, and sinus tachycardia. Palpitations that occur during or after strenuous physical activity, such as running and swimming, may indicate overexertion or possibly heart disease. Some noncardiac factors that may precipitate palpitations include anxiety, stress, fatigue, insomnia, and the ingestion of caffeine, nicotine, or alcohol.

Weight Gain

A sudden increase in weight of 2.2 pounds (1 kg) can be the result of an accumulation of excessive fluid (1 L) in the interstitial spaces, commonly known as *edema*. It is possible, however, for weight gains of up to 10–15 pounds (4.5–6.8 kg, or 4–7 L of fluid) to occur before any associated edema is apparent. The nurse should in-

quire whether the client has experienced a tightness of shoes, noted indentations from socks, or noted tightness of rings.

Syncope

Syncope refers to a transient loss of consciousness. The most common cause is decreased perfusion to the brain. Any condition that suddenly reduces the cardiac output, resulting in decreased cerebral blood flow, could potentiate a syncopal episode. Conditions such as cardiac rhythm disturbances (ventricular dysrhythmias or Stokes-Adams attack) and valvular disorders (aortic stenosis) may potentiate this symptom.

ELDERLY CONSIDERATIONS

Syncope in the aging client may result from hypersensitivity of the carotid sinus bodies, located in the neck arteries. Pressure applied to the carotid arteries (e.g., during turning the head, shrugging the shoulders, shaving, or buttoning a shirt) stimulates a vagal response. A decrease in blood pressure and heart rate usually results, but an exaggerated response may produce syncope. Syncope in the older adult may also result from orthostatic (postural) or postprandial hypotension as a result of an age-affected baroreceptor response.

Near-syncope refers to dizziness with an inability to remain in an upright position. The nurse explores the circumstances that lead to dizziness or syncope.

Extremity Pain

Extremity pain may result from two conditions: ischemia from atherosclerosis and venous insufficiency of the peripheral blood vessels. Clients who report a moderate to severe cramping sensation in their legs or buttocks associated with an activity such as walking have intermittent claudication related to reduced arterial tissue perfusion. Claudication pain is usually relieved by resting or lowering the affected extremity to decrease tissue demands or to enhance arterial blood flow. Leg pain that results from prolonged standing or sitting is related to venous insufficiency from either incompetent valves or venous obstruction. This pain may be relieved by elevating the extremity.

Functional History

After obtaining the history of the client's cardiac status, the client may be classified according to the New York Heart Association's Functional Classification (Table 35–2). The four classifications (I, II, III, and IV) depend on the degree to which ordinary physical activities (routine activities of daily living [ADLs]) are affected by heart disease.

PHYSICAL ASSESSMENT

A thorough physical assessment is the foundation for the nursing data base and the formation of nursing diagnoses. Any changes noted during the client's hospital course can be compared with this initial data base. The nurse evalu-

TABLE 35–2

New York Heart Association Functional Classification of Cardiovascular Disability

Class I
- Clients with cardiac disease but without resulting limitations of physical activity
- Ordinary physical activity does not cause undue fatigue, palpitation, dyspnea, or anginal pain.

Class II
- Clients with cardiac disease resulting in slight limitation of physical activity
- They are comfortable at rest.
- Ordinary physical activity results in fatigue, palpitation, dyspnea, or anginal pain.

Class III
- Clients with cardiac disease resulting in marked limitation of physical activity
- They are comfortable at rest.
- Less than ordinary physical activity causes fatigue, palpitation, dyspnea, or anginal pain.

Class IV
- Clients with cardiac disease resulting in inability to carry on any physical activity without discomfort
- Symptoms of cardiac insufficiency or of the anginal syndrome may be present, even at rest.
- If any physical activity is undertaken, discomfort is increased.

Excerpted from *Diseases of the heart and blood vessels—nomenclature and criteria for diagnosis*, 6th edition. Boston, Little, Brown and Company, copyright 1964 by the New York Heart Association, Inc.

ates vital signs (blood pressure, pulse rate, and respiration rate) when the client is admitted to the hospital and at least every 4 hours until the client's condition improves.

General Appearance

Physical assessment begins with clients' general appearance. The nurse assesses the following areas: general build and appearance of the client as well as skin color; distress level; level of consciousness; presence of shortness of breath; position; and verbal responses.

Clients with chronic heart failure may appear malnourished, thin, and cachectic. Latent signs of severe heart failure are ascites, jaundice, and anasarca as a result of prolonged congestion of the liver. Heart failure may cause fluid retention, and clients may have engorged neck veins and generalized dependent edema.

Coronary artery disease is suspected in clients with yellow lipid-filled plaques on the upper eyelids (xanthelasma) or earlobe creases. Clients with poor cardiac output and decreased cerebral perfusion may have mental confusion, memory loss, and slowed verbal responses.

Integumentary System

Assessment and evaluation of the integumentary system are determined primarily by the color and temperature of the skin. The best areas for the nurse to assess circulation include the nail beds, the mucous membranes, and the conjunctival mucosa, because small blood vessels are located near the surface of the skin.

Skin Color

If there is normal blood flow or adequate perfusion of a given area in light-colored skin, it appears pink, perhaps rosy in color, and warm to the touch. Decreased flow is depicted as cool, pale-looking, and moist skin. Pallor is characteristic of anemia and can be seen in areas such as the nail beds, palms, and conjunctival mucous membranes.

A bluish or darkened discoloration of the skin and mucous membranes is referred to as cyanosis. Cyanosis results from an increased amount of deoxygenated hemoglobin.

In central cyanosis, there is decreased oxygenation of the arterial blood in the lungs, which manifests as a bluish tinge of the conjunctivae and the mucous membranes of the mouth and tongue. Central cyanosis may indicate impaired lung function or a right-to-left shunt found in congenital heart conditions. Because of impaired circulation, there is a marked desaturation of hemoglobin in the peripheral tissues, which produces a bluish or darkened discoloration of the nail beds, the earlobes, the lips, and the toes.

Peripheral cyanosis occurs when blood flow to the peripheral vessels is decreased by peripheral vasoconstriction. The clamping down of the peripheral blood vessels is the result of a low cardiac output or an increased extraction of oxygen from the peripheral tissues. Peripheral cyanosis localized in an extremity is usually a result of arterial or venous obstruction.

Skin Temperature

The temperature of the skin can be assessed for symmetry by touching different areas of the client's body (e.g., arms, hands, legs, and feet) with the dorsal surface of the hand or fingers. Decreased blood flow results in decreased skin temperature. The skin temperature is lowered in several clinical conditions, including heart failure, peripheral vascular disease, and shock.

Extremities

The nurse assesses the client's hands, arms, feet, and legs for skin changes, vascular changes, clubbing, capillary filling, and edema. Skin mobility and turgor are affected by the fluid status of the client. Dehydration and aging reduce skin turgor, and edema decreases skin mobility. Vascular changes of an affected extremity may include paresthesia, muscle fatigue and discomfort, numbness, pain, coolness, and loss of hair distribution from a reduced blood supply. Clubbing of the fingers and toes results from chronic oxygen deprivation in these tissue beds. Clubbing is characteristic in clients with advanced chronic pulmonary disease, congenital heart defects, and cor pulmonale. Clubbing can be identified by assessing the angle of the nail bed. The angle of the normal nail bed is 160 degrees; with clubbing, the angle of the nail bed increases to greater than 180 degrees and the base of the nail

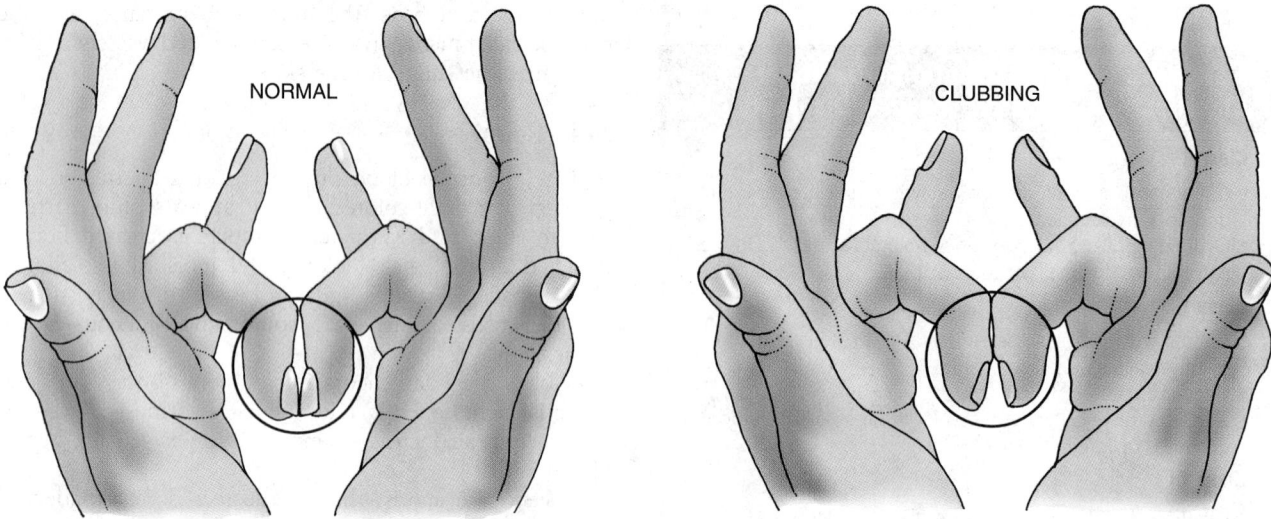

Figure 35–10. Assessment of clubbing by the Schamroth method. The client places the fingernails of the ring fingers together and holds them up to a light. If the examiner can see a diamond shape between the nails, there is no clubbing. Clubbing is identified by the absence of the diamond shape.

becomes spongy. Figure 35–10 describes the assessment of clubbing using the Schamroth method.

Capillary filling of the fingers and the toes is an indicator of peripheral circulation. Pressing or blanching the nail bed of a finger or a toe produces a whitening effect; when pressure is released, a brisk return of color should occur in the nail bed. If color returns within 3 seconds, peripheral circulation is considered intact. If the capillary refill time exceeds 3 seconds, the lack of circulation may be due to arterial insufficiency from atherosclerosis or spasm. Rubor (dusky redness) that replaces pallor in a dependent foot suggests arterial insufficiency.

Peripheral edema is a common finding in clients with cardiovascular problems. The location of edema helps the nurse to determine its potential cause. Bilateral edema of the legs may be seen in clients with heart failure or with chronic venous insufficiency. Abdominal and leg edema can be seen in clients with heart disease and cirrhosis of the liver. Localized edema in one extremity may be the result of venous obstruction (thrombosis) or lymphatic blockage of the extremity (lymphedema). Edema may also be noted in dependent areas, such as the sacrum, when a client is confined to bed.

The nurse documents the location of edema as precisely as possible (e.g., midtibial or sacral) and the number of centimeters from an anatomic landmark. Although some health care practitioners attempt to grade edema as mild, moderate, and severe or 1+, 2+, 3+, or 4+, no universal scale is used. In addition, these values are not precise and are subjective. Instead of using a grading scale, the nurse determines whether the edema is pitting (the skin can be indented) or nonpitting, the depth of the pit (in millimeters), and the amount of time the pit lasts (in seconds).

Blood Pressure Measurement

The indirect measurement of arterial blood pressure is done by sphygmomanometry (Chart 35–2). This tech-

nique of measurement is described in greater detail in nursing skills books.

The normal blood pressure in adults older than 45 years ranges from 90 to 140 mmHg for systolic pressure and from 60 to 90 mmHg for diastolic pressure (AHA, 1996). A blood pressure that exceeds 135/85 mmHg increases the workload of the left ventricle and oxygen consumption. A blood pressure less than 90/60 mmHg may be inadequate in providing proper and sufficient nutrition to the cells of the body.

In certain circumstances, such as shock, the Korotkoff sounds are less audible or absent. In such circumstances, the nurse might palpate the blood pressure, use an ultrasonic device (Doppler device), or obtain a direct measurement by arterial catheter. When a blood pressure is palpated, the diastolic pressure is usually not obtainable. More information on direct measurement of arterial pressure is available under Hemodynamic Monitoring in this chapter.

Postural Blood Pressure

Clients may report dizziness or lightheadedness when they move from a flat, supine position to a sitting or a standing position at the edge of the bed. Normally, these symptoms are transient and pass quickly; however, when these symptoms become pronounced, they may be due to orthostatic (postural) hypotension. Postural hypotension occurs when the client's blood pressure is not adequately maintained when moving from a lying to a sitting or standing position. It is defined as a decrease in blood pressure of more than 20 mmHg of the systolic pressure or a decrease of more than 10 mmHg of the diastolic pressure and a 10% to 20% increase in heart rate. The causes of postural hypotension include medications, depletion of blood volume, prolonged bed rest, and age-related changes or disorders of the autonomic nervous system.

To detect orthostatic changes in blood pressure, the

Nursing Care Highlight: Tips for Accurate Blood Pressure Measurement

- Select the proper cuff size.
  - Adult cuff size is 12- to 14-cm wide and 30-cm long.
  - Pediatric cuffs vary in width and length.
  - Larger adult cuff size is 18- to 20-cm wide.
- Ensure that equipment is properly assembled and calibrated.
  - The cuff bladder should be intact inside the cuff.
  - The sphygmomanometer should be calibrated to 0 mmHg every few months to ensure reliability.
- The cuff must be placed above the area to be auscultated (e.g., if the right arm is used, the cuff is placed above the brachial artery).
- Follow these steps to ensure correct blood pressure measurement and recording:
  - After palpating the brachial or radial pulse, inflate the cuff 30 mmHg above the level at which those pulses disappear. Release the cuff slowly to palpate the systolic pressure. Reinflate the cuff, and auscultate the systolic and diastolic pressures. The auscultated pulses are referred to as the Korotkoff sounds.
  - Record measurements on both arms to rule out dissecting aortic aneurysm, coarctation of the aorta, vascular obstruction, and possibly errors in measurement. Perform subsequent readings on the extremity with the highest pressure.
  - If the client's arms are inaccessible (after amputation or mastectomy), you can obtain readings using the client's thigh or calf. Auscultate the popliteal artery or the posterior tibial artery, respectively.
  - Obtain and record the client's blood pressure with the client in different positions, including supine, sitting, and standing positions.
  - Record the position of the client and the site used to obtain the blood pressure.

nurse first takes the client's blood pressure when the client is supine. After remaining supine for at least 3 minutes, the client changes position to sitting or standing. Normally, as the client rises, systolic pressure drops slightly or remains unchanged, whereas diastolic pressure rises slightly. After the client's change in position, a time delay of 1–5 minutes should be permitted before auscultating a blood pressure and palpating the radial pulse. The cuff should remain in the proper position on the client's arm. The nurse observes and records any signs or symptoms of distress in the client. If the client is unable to tolerate the position change, he or she is returned to the previous position of comfort.

ELDERLY CONSIDERATIONS

As a person ages, the autonomic nervous system may lose the ability to compensate rapidly for the gravitational effects of position change and may, therefore, cause postural hypotension. With autonomic insufficiency,

there is no increase in heart rate when the client moves to an upright position. Autonomic insufficiency can also occur from the effects of some cardiac drugs, including digoxin, calcium channel blockers, and beta-adrenergic blockers, that inhibit increases in heart rate. Antiparkinsonian drugs, such as levodopa (Dopar) or Sinemet, can cause severe postural hypotension as well. Some elders experience a similar phenomenon after a heavy meal (postprandial hypotension).

Paradoxical Blood Pressure

Paradoxical blood pressure is defined as an exaggerated decrease in systolic pressure by more than 10 mmHg (normal is 3–10 mmHg) during the inspiratory phase of the respiratory cycle. Certain clinical conditions, including pericardial tamponade, constrictive pericarditis, and pulmonary hypertension, that potentially alter the filling pressures in the right and left ventricles may produce a paradoxical blood pressure. During inspiration, the filling pressures normally decrease slightly. However, with decreased fluid volume in the ventricles because of these pathologic conditions, there is an exaggerated or marked reduction in cardiac output. The procedure for assessing a paradoxical blood pressure is found in Chart 37–10.

Pulse Pressure

The difference between the systolic and diastolic values is referred to as pulse pressure. A normal pulse pressure for an adult is 30–40 mmHg. This value can be used as an indirect measure of the client's cardiac output. Decreased pulse pressure is rarely normal and results from increased peripheral vascular resistance or decreased stroke volume in clients with heart failure, hypovolemia, or shock. Decreased pulse pressure can also be seen in clients who have mitral stenosis or regurgitation. An increased pulse pressure may be seen in clients with slow heart rates, aortic regurgitation, atherosclerosis, hypertension, and aging.

Ankle Brachial Index

The ankle brachial index (ABI) can be used to assess the vascular status of the lower extremities. The nurse applies a blood pressure cuff to the lower extremities just above the malleolli and measures the systolic pressure by Doppler ultrasound at both the dorsalis pedis and posterior tibial pulses. The higher of these two pressures is then divided by the higher of the two brachial pulses to obtain the ankle brachial index.

$$ABI = \frac{\text{higher systolic ankle pressure}}{\text{higher systolic brachial pressure}}$$

Normal values for ABI are 1 or higher, because blood pressure in the legs is usually higher than blood pressure in the arms. ABI values less then 0.80 usually indicate moderate vascular disease, whereas values less than 0.50 indicate severe vascular compromise.

Venous and Arterial Pulsations
Venous Pulsations

The nurse observes the venous pulsations in the neck to assess the adequacy of blood volume and central venous pressure (CVP). The nurse can assess jugular venous pressure (JVP) to estimate the filling volume and pressure on the right side of the heart (Chart 35–3). The right internal jugular vein is usually used to estimate JVP, because this vessel contains fewer valves than the left.

Jugular venous pressure is normally 3–10 cm. Increases in JVP are usually caused by right ventricular failure. Other causes include tricuspid regurgitation or stenosis, pulmonary hypertension, cardiac tamponade, constrictive pericarditis, hypervolemia, and superior vena cava obstruction.

The nurse determines hepatojugular reflux by positioning the client with the head of the bed elevated to 45 degrees and locating the internal jugular vein. The nurse compresses the right upper abdomen for 30–40 seconds. Sudden distention of the neck veins after abdominal compression is usually indicative of right-sided heart failure.

Arterial Pulsations

Assessment of arterial pulsations gives the nurse information about vascular integrity and circulation. All major peripheral pulses, including the temporal, carotid, brachial, radial, ulnar, femoral, popliteal, posterior tibial, and dorsalis pedis pulses, need to be assessed for presence or absence, amplitude, contour, rhythm, rate, and equality. The nurse examines the peripheral arteries in a head-to-toe approach with a side-to-side comparison (Fig. 35–11).

Chart 35–3

Nursing Care Highlight: Assessment of Jugular Venous Pressure and Central Venous Pressure

1. Place the client in a supine position.
2. Raise the head of the bed to approximately 30 to 45 degrees.
3. Shine a light across the client's neck (tangential lighting) to highlight the pulsations of the internal jugular vein.
4. To differentiate the internal jugular vein from the carotid artery, occlude the internal jugular vein with a fingertip at its base, then release. This maneuver easily eliminates the pulse wave in the internal jugular vein.

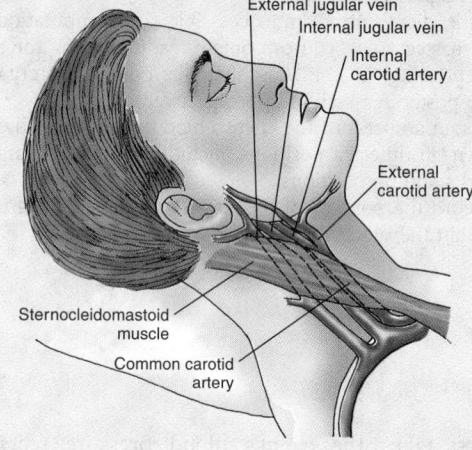

5. Locate the meniscus (the highest point at which pulsations of the internal jugular vein can be seen).
6. Locate the sternal angle (angle of Louis), which can be felt as a notch at the top of the sternum. It is roughly 4 cm above the right atrium.
7. With a centimeter rule, measure the vertical distance from the sternal angle to the meniscus of the internal jugular vein. The reading in centimeters equals the JVP, which generally does not exceed 4 cm.
8. To calculate CVP, add 4 cm to JVP.

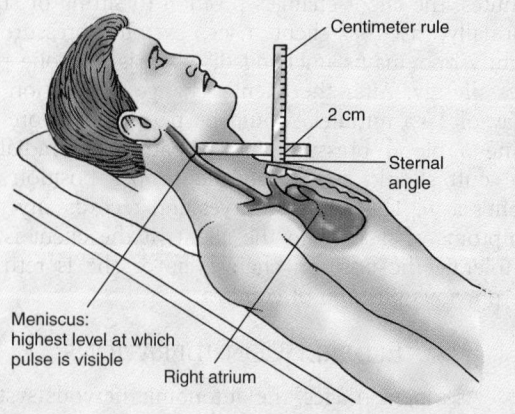

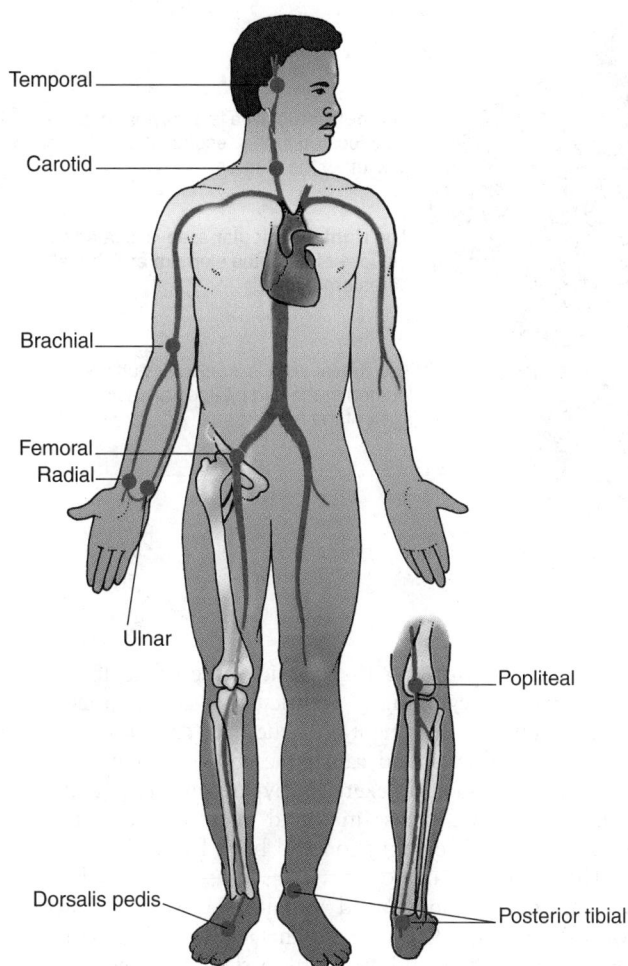

Figure 35–11. Pulse points for assessment of arterial pulses.

(labels on figure:) Temporal, Carotid, Brachial, Femoral, Radial, Ulnar, Dorsalis pedis, Popliteal, Posterior tibial

flow. A bruit may develop when the internal diameter of the vessel is narrowed by 50% or more. A bruit does not indicate the severity of disease in the carotid arteries. The severity of disease is determined by Doppler flow studies and arteriography.

Precordium

Assessment of the precordium (the area over the heart) is done by inspection, palpation, percussion, and auscultation. The nurse places the client in a supine position, with the head of the bed slightly elevated for the client's comfort. Some clients may require greater elevation of the head of the bed (to 45 degrees) for ease and comfort in breathing.

Inspection

Cardiac examination is usually done in a systematic order, beginning with inspection. The nurse inspects the chest from the side, at a right angle, and downward over areas of the precordium where vibrations are visible. Cardiac motion is of low amplitude, and sometimes the inward movements are more easily detected by the naked eye.

The nurse examines the entire precordium, focusing on the seven precordial areas (Fig. 35–12) and noting any prominent precordial pulsations. Movement over the aortic, pulmonic, and tricuspid areas is abnormal. Pulsations in the mitral area (the apex of the heart) are considered normal and are referred to as the apical impulse, or the point of maximal impulse (PMI). The PMI should be located at the left fifth intercostal space (ICS) in the midclavicular line. If the apical impulse appears in more than one intercostal space and has shifted lateral to the midclavicular line, it may indicate left ventricular hypertrophy.

Palpation

The nurse palpates with the fingers and the most sensitive part of the palm of the hand to detect precordial motion and thrills, respectively. The nurse palpates by inching his or her hand in a Z pattern along the chest, starting with the aortic area and passing through all seven areas. Turning the client on his or her left side brings the heart closer to the surface of the chest. This may be helpful for the nurse to achieve maximal tactile sensitivity.

An abnormal forceful thrust accompanied by a sustaining outward movement felt over the left anterior chest usually indicates left ventricular enlargement. An outward systolic lift along the left sternal border extending from the fourth to the fifth intercostal space represents right ventricular enlargement.

Heaves and lifts are terms found with pulsations associated with valvular diseases or pulmonary hypertension. Thrills are vibrations that are associated with abnormal heart valve function (mitral regurgitation, tricuspid regurgitation, and pulmonic stenosis). When palpating for heaves or thrills, the nurse should consider several factors, including location, amplitude, duration, distribution, and timing in relation to the cardiac cycle.

A hypokinetic pulse is a weak pulsation indicative of a narrow pulse pressure. It is seen in clients with hypovolemia, aortic stenosis, and decreased cardiac output.

A hyperkinetic pulse is a large, "bounding" pulse caused by an increased ejection of blood. It is seen in clients with a high cardiac output (with exercise or thyrotoxicosis) and in those with increased sympathetic system activity (with pain, fever, or anxiety).

In pulsus alternans, a weak pulse alternates with a strong pulse, despite a regular heart rhythm. It is seen in clients with severely depressed cardiac function. Clients may be asked to hold their breath to exclude any false readings. The nurse may palpate the brachial or radial arteries to assess this condition, but it is more accurately assessed by auscultation of blood pressure.

Auscultation of the carotid arteries is necessary to assess for bruits. Bruits are swishing sounds that may develop over narrowed carotid arteries. Using the bell of the stethoscope over the skin of the carotid artery with the client holding his or her breath, the nurse can assess for the absence or presence of sounds. Normally, there are no sounds if the carotid artery has uninterrupted blood

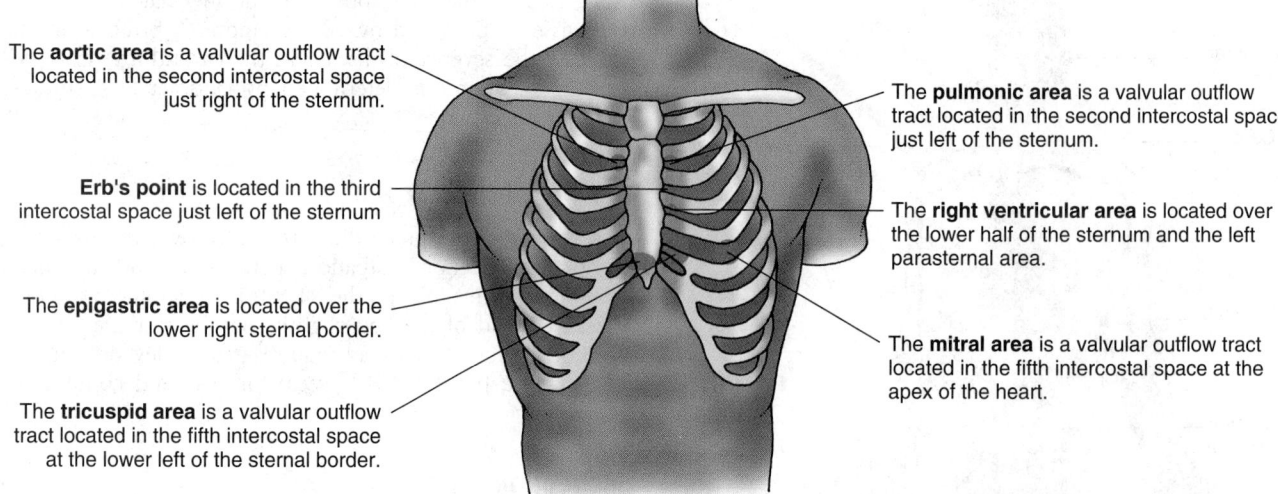

The **aortic area** is a valvular outflow tract located in the second intercostal space just right of the sternum.

Erb's point is located in the third intercostal space just left of the sternum

The **epigastric area** is located over the lower right sternal border.

The **tricuspid area** is a valvular outflow tract located in the fifth intercostal space at the lower left of the sternal border.

The **pulmonic area** is a valvular outflow tract located in the second intercostal space just left of the sternum.

The **right ventricular area** is located over the lower half of the sternum and the left parasternal area.

The **mitral area** is a valvular outflow tract located in the fifth intercostal space at the apex of the heart.

Figure 35–12. Areas for myocardial inspection, palpation, and auscultation.

Percussion

Cardiac size is determined most accurately by chest x-ray; percussion is rarely used now to determine the size of the heart. However, the size of the left ventricle should be estimated by locating the apical impulse by inspection and palpation.

Auscultation

Auscultation evaluates heart rate and rhythm, cardiac cycle (systole and diastole), and valvular function. The technique of auscultation requires a good-quality stethoscope and extensive clinical practice. The nurse evaluates heart sounds in a systematic order; examination usually begins at the aortic outflow tract area and progresses slowly to the apex of the heart, using the diaphragm of the stethoscope. The diaphragm of the stethoscope is pressed tightly against the chest to listen for high-frequency sounds and is useful in listening to the first and second heart sounds and high-frequency murmurs. The nurse then repeats the progression from the base to the apex of the heart using the bell of the stethoscope, which is held lightly against the chest. The bell is able to screen out high-frequency sounds and is useful in listening for low-frequency gallops (diastolic filling sounds) and murmurs.

The nurse auscultates by inching a stethoscope in a Z pattern across the base of the heart, down the left sternal border, then over to the apex, paying attention to the areas in Figure 35–12, except for the epigastric area. Auscultation is to check for heart rate and rhythm, murmurs, extrasystolic sounds, and rubs in the presence of a current or suspected cardiac problem.

Normal Heart Sounds

The first heart sound (S_1) is created by the closure of the mitral and tricuspid valves (AV valves) (see Fig. 35–6). When auscultated, the first heart sound is softer and longer; it is of a low pitch and is best heard at the lower left sternal border or the apex of the heart. It may be identified by palpating the carotid pulse while listening. S_1 marks the beginning of ventricular systole. On electrocardiogram, it occurs right after the QRS complex.

The first heart sound can be accentuated or intensified in conditions such as exercise, hyperthyroidism, and mitral stenosis. A decrease in sound intensity occurs in clients with mitral regurgitation and heart failure.

The second heart sound (S_2) is caused mainly by the closing of the aortic and pulmonic valves (semilunar valves) (see Fig. 35–6). S_2 is characteristically shorter. It is higher pitched and is heard best at the base of the heart at the end of ventricular systole.

Splitting of heart sounds is often difficult to differentiate from diastolic filling sounds (gallops). A splitting of S_1 (closure of the mitral valve followed by closure of the tricuspid valve) occurs physiologically because left ventricular contraction occurs slightly before right ventricular contraction. However, closure of the mitral valve is louder than closure of the tricuspid valve, so that splitting is often not heard. Normal splitting of S_2 occurs because of the longer systolic phase of the right ventricle. Splitting of S_1 and S_2 can be accentuated by inspiration (increased venous return) and narrows during expiration.

Abnormal Heart Sounds

Paradoxical Splitting

Abnormal splitting of S_2 is referred to as paradoxical splitting, which is characteristic of a wider split heard on expiration. Paradoxical splitting of S_2 is heard in clients with severe myocardial depression causing early closure of the pulmonic valve or a delay in aortic valve closure. Such conditions include myocardial infarction, left bundle branch block, aortic stenosis, aortic regurgitation, and right ventricular pacing.

Gallops and Murmurs

Gallops and murmurs are common abnormal heart sounds, which may occur when heart disease is present.

GALLOPS. Diastolic filling sounds (S_3) and (S_4) are produced when blood enters a noncompliant chamber during rapid ventricular filling. The third heart sound (S_3) is produced during the rapid passive filling phase of ventricular diastole when blood flows from the atrium to a noncompliant ventricle. The sound arises from vibrations of the valves and supporting structures. The fourth heart sound (S_4) occurs as blood enters the ventricles during the active filling phase at the end of ventricular diastole.

S_3 is termed *ventricular gallop,* and S_4 is referred to as *atrial gallop.* These sounds can be caused by decreased compliance of either or both ventricles. The nurse can best hear left ventricular diastolic filling sounds with the client on his or her left side, using the bell of the stethoscope at the apex and the left lower sternal border during expiration.

An S_3 heart sound is probably a normal finding in children or young adults up to 30 years of age. An S_3 gallop in clients older than 40 years is considered abnormal and represents a decrease in left ventricular compliance. S_3 can be detected as an early sign of heart failure, ventricular septal defect, or ruptured papillary muscle.

An atrial gallop (S_4) may be heard in clients with hypertension, anemia, ventricular hypertrophy, myocardial infarction, aortic or pulmonic stenosis, and pulmonary emboli. It may also be heard with advancing age because of a stiffened ventricle.

The auscultation of both S_3 and S_4, called a *summation,* or *quadruple gallop,* is an indication of severe heart failure. If the quadruple rhythm is present and the patient is tachycardiac (has a shortened diastole), the two sounds may actually fuse, producing a rhythm that sounds like a horse galloping.

MURMURS. Murmurs reflect turbulent blood flow through normal or abnormal valves. They are classified according to their timing in the cardiac cycle: systolic murmurs (such as aortic stenosis and mitral regurgitation) occur between S_1 and S_2, whereas diastolic murmurs (such as in mitral stenosis and aortic regurgitation) occur between S_2 and S_1. Murmurs can occur during presystole, midsystole, or late systole or diastole or last throughout both phases of the cardiac cycle. Murmurs are also graded according to their intensity, depending on their level of loudness (Table 35–3).

The nurse describes the location of a murmur by where it is best heard on auscultation. Some murmurs may transmit or radiate from their loudest point to other areas, including the neck, the back, and the axilla. The configuration of a murmur is described as crescendo (increases in intensity) or decrescendo (decreases in intensity). The quality of murmurs can be further characterized as harsh, blowing, whistling, rumbling, or squeaking. The murmur is also described by its pitch, usually high or low.

Pericardial Friction Rub

A pericardial friction rub originates from the pericardial sac and occurs with the movements of the heart during the cardiac cycle. Rubs are usually transient and are a sign of inflammation, infection, or infiltration. Pericardial friction rubs may be heard in clients with pericarditis resulting from myocardial infarction and cardiac tamponade.

The three phases of cardiac movement—atrial systole, ventricular diastole, and ventricular systole—can produce three components of a rub. Usually, only one or two components can be heard. With each movement, a short, high-pitched scratchy sound is produced; the loudest component is heard in systole. The nurse may be most able to auscultate the rubs when the client sits, leans forward, and exhales. The pericardial friction rub is better heard with the diaphragm of the stethoscope.

PSYCHOSOCIAL ASSESSMENT

To many people, the heart is the symbol of their existence and longevity. A client with a heart-related illness, whether acute or chronic, usually perceives it as a major life crisis. The client and families and significant others confront not only the possibility of death but also fears about pain, disability, lack of self-esteem, physical dependence, and changes in family role dynamics. The nurse may assess the meaning of the illness to the client and family members by asking, "What do you understand about what happened to you (or the client)?" and "What does that mean to you?" When the client or family members perceive the stressor as overwhelming, formerly adequate support systems may no longer be effective. In these circumstances, the client and family members attempt to cope to regain a sense or feeling of control.

Coping behaviors vary among clients. Those who feel helpless to meet the demands of the situation may exhibit behaviors such as disorganization, fear, and anxiety. The nurse may ask the client or family members, "Have you ever encountered such a situation before?", "How did you manage that situation?", and "To whom can you turn for help?" The answers to these questions often reassure the client that he or she has encountered difficult situations in the past and has the ability and resources to cope with them.

A common and normal response is *denial,* which is a defense mechanism to enable the client to cope with threatening circumstances. The client may deny that he or she has the current cardiovascular condition, may state that it was present but is now absent, or may be excessively cheerful. Denial of the seriousness of the illness while following the treatment regimen is a protective response. Denial becomes maladaptive only when the client

TABLE 35–3

Grading of Heart Murmurs	
• Grade I	Very faint
• Grade II	Faint, but recognizable
• Grade III	Loud, but moderate in intensity
• Grade IV	Loud and accompanied by a palpable thrill
• Grade V	Very loud, accompanied by a palpable thrill, and audible with the stethoscope partially off the client's chest
• Grade VI	Extremely loud, may be heard with the stethoscope slightly above the client's chest

is noncompliant with significant portions of medical and nursing care (see Chapter 8 on coping).

Family members and significant others of the client with heart disease may be more anxious than the client. Often they recall all the events of the illness, are unprotected by denial, and are afraid of recurrence. Disagreements frequently occur between the client and family members over compliance with appropriate follow-up care.

DIAGNOSTIC ASSESSMENT
Laboratory Tests

Assessment of the client with cardiac dysfunction includes examination of the blood for abnormalities. This is done to establish a diagnosis, detect concurrent disease, assess risk factors, and monitor response to treatment. Normal values for serum cardiac enzymes and serum lipids are listed in Chart 35–4.

Serum Cardiac Enzymes

Events leading to cellular injury cause a release of enzymes from intracellular storage, and circulating levels of these enzymes are dramatically elevated. Acute myocardial infarction (MI) can be confirmed by abnormally high levels of enzymes or isoenzymes in the serum.

Creatine Kinase

Creatine kinase (CK) is an enzyme specific to cells of the brain, myocardium, and skeletal muscle. The appearance of CK in the blood indicates tissue necrosis or injury, and CK levels follow a predictable rise and fall during a specified period of time. Cardiac specificity must be determined by measuring isoenzyme activity. There are three isoenzymes of CK: CK-MM is the predominant isoenzyme of skeletal muscle; CK-MB is found in myocardial muscle; and CK-BB occurs in the brain. CK-MB activity is most specific for MI and shows a predictable rise and fall during 3 days; a peak level occurs approximately 24 hours after the onset of chest pain.

Newer treatment modalities and shorter hospital stays require more rapid diagnosis of myocardial infarction (MI). An assay using monoclonal anti–CK-MB antibodies (stat CK) is able to detect myocardial necrosis accurately at 3 hours after emergency department admission when examined with an electrogram (ECG). Two subforms of CK-MB (CK-MB$_1$, CK-MB$_2$) have also been identified. Abnormal elevations of these CK subforms may occur as early as 2 hours after MI. These CK subforms remain elevated for up to 12 hours after MI and appear to be very sensitive and specific early diagnostic markers of MI.

Other early markers of MI are myoglobin and troponin. Myoglobin, a low-molecular-weight protein found in skeletal muscle, is an early and sensitive but nonspecific marker for myocardial injury. Troponin T and I are specific markers of myocardial injury that have a wide diagnostic time frame, making them useful for clients who present several hours after the onset of chest pain. Table 35–4 describes the characteristics of these new serum assays for myocardial damage.

Lactate Dehydrogenase

Lactate dehydrogenase (LDH) is widely distributed in the body and is found in the heart, liver, kidney, brain, and erythrocytes. LDH elevation starts within 12–24 hours after an MI, peaks between 48 and 72 hours, and falls to normal in 7 days. Because LDH is not specific to the myocardial cell, assessment of isoenzymes and patterns of elevation is necessary for confirmation of MI. There are five isoenzymes for LDH, of which LDH$_1$ and LDH$_2$ are found in the heart. If the serum level of LDH$_1$ is higher than the concentration of LDH$_2$, the pattern is said to have flipped, signifying myocardial damage.

Serum Lipids

Elevated lipid levels are considered a coronary artery disease (CAD) risk factor. Cholesterol, triglycerides, and the protein components of high-density lipoproteins (HDL) and low-density lipoproteins (LDL) are evaluated to assess a client's degree of risk for CAD. A serum cholesterol level greater than 260 mg/dL gives a client a three times greater risk of CAD than a serum level of less than 200 mg/dL.

Each of the lipoproteins contains varying proportions of cholesterol, triglyceride, protein, and phospholipid. HDL contains mainly protein and 20% cholesterol, whereas LDL is predominantly cholesterol. Elevated LDL levels are positively correlated with CAD, whereas elevated HDL levels are negatively correlated and appear to be a protective factor.

A nonfasting blood sample for the measurement of serum cholesterol levels is acceptable. However, if triglycerides are to be evaluated, the physician requests the specimen after a 12-hour fast.

Blood Coagulation Tests

Blood coagulation tests evaluate the ability of the blood to clot and are important in clients with a greater tendency to form thrombi (e.g., clients with atrial fibrillation, prosthetic valves, or infective endocarditis). They are also important for clients receiving anticoagulant therapy (e.g., during cardiac surgery, after thrombolytic therapy, and during treatment of an established thrombus).

Prothrombin Time and International Normalized Ratio

Prothrombin time (PT) and international normalized ratio (INR) are used when initiating and maintaining therapy with oral anticoagulants, such as sodium warfarin (Coumadin, Warfilone♣). They measure the activity of prothrombin, fibrinogen, and factors V, VII, and X. INR is the most reliable way to monitor anticoagulant status in warfarin therapy. Therapeutic ranges for standard anticoagulant therapy are 2.0–3.0 INR.

Partial Thromboplastin Time

Partial thromboplastin time (PTT) is assessed in clients receiving heparin (Hepalean♣). It measures deficiencies in all coagulation factors, except factors VII and XIII.

Chart 35–4

Laboratory Profile: Cardiovascular Assessment

Normal Range	Significance of Abnormal Findings
Serum Cardiac Enzymes	
Creatine kinase (CK)	• Elevations indicate possible brain, myocardial, and skeletal muscle necrosis or injury.
• Females: 10–55 U/mL, or 26–140 U/L	
• Males: 12–70 U/mL, or 38–174 U/L	
• Values higher after exercise	
CK-MM (CK_3)	• Elevations occur with muscle injury
• 95–100% of total CK	
CK-MB (CK_2)	• Elevations occur with myocardial injury or after percutaneous transluminal angioplasty and intracoronary streptokinase infusion.
• 0–5% of total CK	
CK-BB (CK_1)	• Elevations occur with brain tissue injury.
• 0%	
Lactate dehydrogenase (LDH)	• Elevation occurs with injury to heart, liver, kidney, brain, and erythrocytes.
• 140–280 U/L, or 0.4–1.7 mmol/L	
LDH_1	• Elevation occurs higher than LDH_2 with myocardial damage
• 18–33% of total LDH	
LDH_2	
• 28–40% of total LDH	
LDH_1:LDH_2 ratio	• Elevation occurs with myocardial damage.
• <1	
Serum Lipids	
Total lipids	• Elevation indicates increased risk of CAD.
• 400–1000 mg/dL	
Cholesterol	• Elevation indicates increased risk of CAD.
• 122–200 mg/dL, or 3.16–6.5 mmol/L	
• Elderly (>70 years): 144–280 mgdL, or 3.73–7.25 mmol/L	
Triglycerides	• Elevation indicates increased risk of CAD.
• Females: 39–262 mg/dL, or 0.44–2.96 mmol/L	
• Males: 37–286 mg/dL, or 0.42–3.23 mmol/L	
• Elderly (>65 years): 55–260 mg/dL, or 0.62–2.94 mmol/L	
Plasma high-density lipoproteins (HDLs)	• Elevations protect against CAD.
• Females: mean, 55–60 mg/dL	
• Males: mean, 45–50 mg/dL	
• Elderly: range increases with age	
Plasma low-density lipoproteins (LDLs)	• Elevation indicates increased risk of CAD.
• 57–197 mg/dL, or 1.48–5.10 mmol/L	
• Elderly (>65 years): 92–221 mg/dL, or 2.38–5.72 mmol/L	
HDL:LDL ratio	• Elevated ratios may protect against CAD.
• 3:1	

CAD = coronary artery disease.

Arterial Blood Gases

Arterial blood gas (ABG) determinations are frequently obtained in the client with cardiovascular disease. Determination of tissue oxygenation, carbon dioxide removal, and the acid-base status is essential to appropriate intervention and treatment. Complete discussion of ABGs can be found in Chapter 18.

Serum Electrolytes

Fluid and electrolyte balance is essential for normal cardiovascular performance. Cardiac manifestations often occur when there is an imbalance in either fluids or electrolytes in the body. For example, the cardiac effects of hypokalemia (low serum potassium level) include increased electrical instability, ventricular dysrhythmias, the

TABLE 35–4

Characteristics of New Serum Assays for Myocardial Damage				
Test	**Time to Elevation (hr)**	**Time to Peak (hr)**	**Time to Normal**	**Assay Time (min)**
Stat CK-MB	3–8	12–24	2–3 days	8–34
CK-MB subforms	1–3	5–7	24 hours	25
Myoglobin	2–3	6–9	24 hours	10–20
Troponin T & I	4–6	10–24	10–14 days	10–90

appearance of U waves on the electrocardiogram, and an increased risk of digitalis toxicity. The effects of hyperkalemia on the myocardium include slowed ventricular conduction and contraction followed by asystole (cardiac standstill).

Cardiac manifestations of hypocalcemia are ventricular dysrhythmias, prolonged QT interval, and cardiac arrest. Hypercalcemia shortens the QT interval and causes AV block, digitalis hypersensitivity, and cardiac arrest.

Serum sodium values reflect fluid balance and may be decreased, indicating a fluid excess in clients with heart failure.

Because magnesium regulates some aspects of myocardial electrical activity, hypomagnesemia has been implicated in some forms of rapid ventricular dysrhythmias. Another manifestation of hypomagnesemia is hypokalemia that is unresponsive to potassium replacement.

Complete Blood Count

The erythrocyte count is usually decreased in rheumatic fever and infective endocarditis. It is increased in heart diseases characterized by inadequate tissue oxygenation.

Decreased hematocrit and hemoglobin levels (e.g., caused by hemorrhage or hemolysis from prosthetic valves) indicate anemia and can manifest as angina or can aggravate heart failure. Vascular volume depletion with hemoconcentration (e.g., hypovolemic shock and excessive diuresis) results in an elevated hematocrit.

The leukocyte count is typically elevated after MI and in the various infectious and inflammatory diseases of the heart (e.g., infective endocarditis and pericarditis). Chapter 41 discusses the complete blood count in detail.

Radiographic Examinations
Chest Radiography

Routinely, posteroanterior and left lateral x-ray views of the chest are taken to determine the size, silhouette, and position of the heart. In acutely ill clients, a simple anteroposterior view is taken at the bedside. Cardiac enlargement, pulmonary congestion, cardiac calcifications, and placement of central venous catheters, endotracheal tubes, and hemodynamic monitoring devices are all assessed by x-ray.

Cardiac Fluoroscopy

Fluoroscopy is a simple x-ray examination that reveals the action of the heart. Continuous visual observation of the heart, the lungs, and vessel movement on a luminescent x-ray screen in a darkened room is provided. Fluoroscopy is used to place and position intracardiac catheters and IV pacemaker wires and can be helpful in identifying abnormal structures, calcifications, and tumors of the heart. In critically ill clients, fluoroscopy can be performed at the bedside for the placement of intracardiac catheters of IV pacemaker wires. Client preparation and follow-up depend on the procedure. Commonly, fluoroscopy is used in conjunction with cardiac catheterization, and the client is taken to a special cardiac catheterization room (see later discussion of cardiac catheterization).

Angiography

Angiography of arterial vessels, or arteriography, is an invasive diagnostic procedure that involves fluoroscopy and x-ray studies. This procedure is performed when an arterial obstruction, narrowing, or aneurysm is suspected. The radiologist performs selective arteriography to evaluate specific areas of the arterial system. For example, coronary arteriography, which is performed during left-sided cardiac catheterization, assesses arterial circulation within the heart (see later in this chapter). Angiography can also be performed on arteries in the extremities, the mesentery, and the cerebrum.

CLIENT PREPARATION. The radiologist explains the procedure and the risks to the client before he or she or the designated responsible party signs a consent form. Because this procedure involves injection of contrast medium (sometimes called a dye) into the arterial system, the risks are serious. They include allergic reaction, hemorrhage, thrombosis, embolism, and death. The client is told to expect a warm sensation when dye is injected during the procedure. The nurse assesses the client for any allergies to contrast medium, iodine-containing substances such as seafood, or local anesthetics. The nurse prepares the area, usually the femoral area in the groin according to the health care agency's policy and procedure. The nurse documents vital signs and marks and describes pulses distal to the puncture site in the client's medical record.

PROCEDURE. The radiologist or the technician places the client in a supine position on an x-ray table in the radiology department. A radiologist usually performs this procedure and begins by injecting a local anesthetic into the tissue surrounding the artery being catheterized. Contrast medium is injected via this catheter, and fluoroscopy and x-ray studies are done.

FOLLOW-UP CARE. After the procedure, the client is typically restricted to bed rest in the supine position for 4–6 hours. The nurse ensures that the extremity that was catheterized is not flexed during this time. A pressure dressing or bandage is kept in place over the injection site; there may be a sandbag over the dressing.

The nurse assesses the insertion site for bloody drainage or hematoma formation, assesses distal pulses, and compares skin temperature in the affected extremity with that in the opposite extremity. Vital signs are assessed at every dressing, pulse, and temperature check; the first measurement is obtained immediately after the client is transferred from the radiology department. These assessments usually continue every 15 minutes for 1 hour, then every 30 minutes for 2 hours, followed by every 4 hours or as necessary per the health care agency's protocol. The nurse notifies the radiologist immediately if bleeding, loss of pulses, or changes in vital signs occur. The nurse carefully administers the prescribed IV or oral fluids after the procedure, because the contrast medium may damage the kidneys.

Cardiac Catheterization

The most definitive, but most invasive, test in the diagnosis of heart disease is cardiac catheterization. Cardiac catheterization may include studies of the right or left side of the heart and the coronary arteries. Some of the most common indications for cardiac catheterization are listed in Table 35–5.

CLIENT PREPARATION. Many clients express anxiety and fear regarding cardiac catheterization. The nurse assesses the client's physical and psychosocial readiness and knowledge level.

TABLE 35–5

Indications for Cardiac Catheterization
• To confirm suspected heart disease, including coronary artery disease, myocardial disease, valvular disease, and valvular dysfunction
• To determine the location and extent of the disease process
• To assess
• Stable, severe angina unresponsive to medical management
• Unstable angina pectoris
• Uncontrolled heart failure, ventricular dysrhythmias, or cardiogenic shock associated with acute myocardial infarction, papillary muscle dysfunction, ventricular aneurysm, or septal perforation
• Whether cardiac surgery is necessary
• To evaluate
• Effects of medical treatment on cardiovascular function
• Percutaneous transluminal coronary angioplasty or coronary artery bypass graft patency

TABLE 35–6

Complications of Cardiac Catheterization
Right-Sided Heart Catheterization
• Thrombophlebitis
• Pulmonary embolism
• Vagal response
Left-Sided Heart Catheterization and Coronary Arteriography
• Myocardial infarction
• Cerebrovascular accident
• Arterial bleeding or thromboembolism
• Dysrhythmias
Right- or Left-Sided Heart Catheterization*
• Cardiac tamponade
• Hypovolemia
• Pulmonary edema
• Hematoma or blood loss at insertion site
• Reaction to contrast medium

*In addition to those cited for each procedure.

The nurse reviews the purpose of the procedure. The nurse informs the client how long the procedure usually takes, states who will be present while it is going on, and describes the appearance of the catheterization laboratory. The client is also informed about the sensations that may be experienced during the procedure, such as palpitations (as the catheter is passed up to the left ventricle); a feeling of heat or hot flash (as the dye is injected into either side of the heart); and a desire to cough (as the dye is injected into the right side of the heart). The nurse may use written or illustrated materials or videotapes, if available, to assist the client's understanding (Houston et al., 1996).

The risks of cardiac catheterization are usually explained by the cardiologist. The risks vary with the procedures to be performed and the client's physical status (Table 35–6). Right-sided heart catheterization is less risky than left-sided catheterization. Several complications may follow coronary arteriography, such as

- Myocardial infarction (MI)
- Cerebrovascular accident (CVA)
- Arterial bleeding
- Thromboembolism
- Lethal dysrhythmias
- Death

The cardiologist or the radiologist obtains a written informed consent from the client or the responsible party.

The client may be admitted to the hospital before the catheterization procedure. Standard preoperative tests are performed, which usually include chest x-ray, complete blood count, coagulation studies, urinalysis, and 12-lead electrocardiogram. The client receives nothing by mouth after midnight or has only a liquid breakfast if the catheterization is to take place in the afternoon. The nurse shaves the catheterization site and antiseptically prepares the skin according to the hospital's policy.

Nursing assessment before the procedure includes measurement of the client's vital signs, auscultation of the heart and the lungs, and evaluation of peripheral pulses. The nurse questions the client as to any history of allergy to iodine-containing substances (e.g., seafood and contrast agents). An antihistamine may be given to a client with a positive history. A mild sedative is given before the procedure. If the client normally takes a digitalis preparation or diuretic, it is usually withheld before the catheterization.

PROCEDURE. The client is taken to the cardiac catheterization laboratory (sometimes referred to as the "cath lab") and is placed supine on an x-ray table. The client is securely strapped to the table. The nurse informs the client that this precaution is necessary because the table turns like a cradle during the procedure. The physician injects a local anesthetic at the insertion site. The nurse in the catheterization laboratory instructs the client to report any chest pain or other symptoms to the staff.

Right-Sided Heart Catheterization. The right side of the heart is catheterized first and may be the only side examined. The cardiologist inserts a catheter through the femoral vein to the inferior vena cava or through the basilic vein to the superior vena cava. The catheter is advanced through either the inferior or the superior vena cava and, guided by fluoroscopy, is advanced through the right atrium, through the right ventricle, and, at times, into the pulmonary artery (Fig. 35–13). Intracardiac pressures (right atrial, right ventricular, pulmonary artery, and pulmonary artery wedge pressures) are obtained, and blood samples are withdrawn. Contrast dye or medium is usually injected to detect any cardiac shunts or regurgitation from the pulmonic or tricuspid valves.

Left-Sided Heart Catheterization. Left-sided heart catheterization is more risky than right-sided heart catheterization. The cardiologist advances the catheter retrogradely from the femoral or brachial artery up the aorta, across the aortic valve, and into the left ventricle (Fig. 35–14). The cardiologist may pass the catheter from the right side of the heart through the atrial septum, using a special needle to puncture the septum. Intracardiac pressures and blood samples are obtained. The pressures of the left atrium, left ventricle, and aorta as well as mitral and aortic valve status are evaluated. In addition, the cardiologist injects contrast dye into the ventricle; cineangiograms (rapidly changing films) evaluate left ventricular motion. Calculations are made of end-systolic volume, end-diastolic volume, stroke volume, and ejection fraction.

Coronary Arteriography. The technique for coronary arteriography is the same as for left-sided heart catheterization. The catheter is advanced into the aortic arch and positioned selectively in the right or left coronary artery. Injection of contrast medium permits visualization of the coronary arteries. By assessing the flow of dye through the coronary arteries, information about the site and severity of coronary lesions is obtained.

Intravascular Ultrasonography. An alternative to injecting dye into coronary arteries is intravascular ultraso-

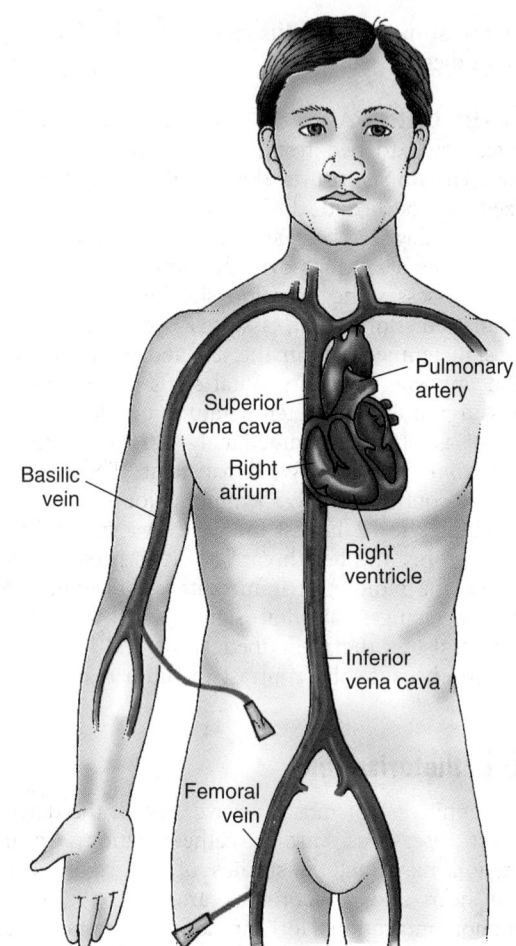

Figure 35–13. Right-sided heart catheterization. The catheter is inserted into the femoral vein and advanced through the inferior vena cava (or, if into an antecubital or basilic vein, through the superior vena cava), right atrium, and right ventricle and into the pulmonary artery.

nography (IVUS), which introduces a flexible catheter with a miniature transducer at the distal tip to visualize the coronary arteries. The transducer emits sound waves, which reflect off the plaque and the arterial wall, creating an image of the blood vessel (Strimike, 1996). IVUS is a more reliable indicator of plaque distribution and composition, arterial dissection, and degree of stenosis of the occluded artery than angiography (Strimike, 1996).

FOLLOW-UP CARE. After cardiac catheterization, the client is typically restricted to bed rest for 4–6 hours; the client is supine; the insertion site is kept extremity straight. Nursing researchers are evaluating bed rest protocols that might limit client discomfort while maintaining hemostasis (see Research Applications for Nursing).

A pressure dressing or bandage may be placed over the insertion site. A 5- or 10-pound sandbag or a C-clamp may be applied over the insertion site to ensure hemostasis. The nurse has many postcatheterization responsibilities. First, the nurse monitors vital signs every 15 minutes for 1 hour, then every 30 minutes for 2 hours or until vital signs are stable, and then every 4 hours or according

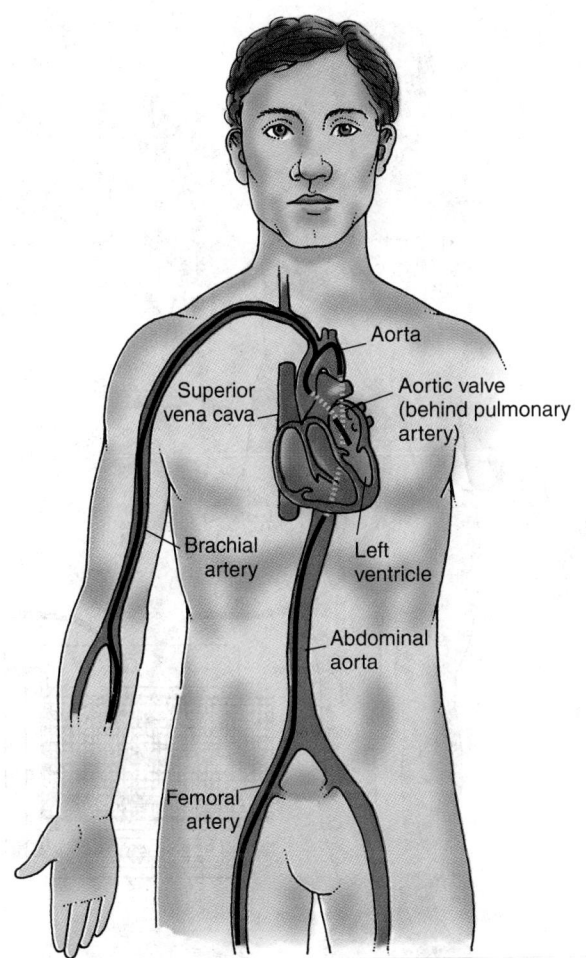

Figure 35–14. Left-sided heart catheterization. The catheter is inserted into the femoral artery or the antecubital artery. The catheter is passed through the ascending aorta, through the aortic valve, and into the left ventricle.

to the hospital's policy. The nurse observes the insertion site for bloody drainage or hematoma formation when taking vital signs. Peripheral pulses in the affected extremity as well as skin temperature and color are monitored with every vital sign check.

The nurse must be constantly vigilant for complications of cardiac catheterization (see Table 35–5). The nurse assesses the client's reports of pain and discomfort at the insertion site, chest pain, nausea, or feelings of lightheadedness. The client is often attached to a cardiac monitor. If not, the nurse auscultates the client's heart sounds, noting rhythm and rate to detect dysrhythmias. Because the contrast medium acts as an osmotic diuretic, the nurse monitors urinary output and ensures that the client receives sufficient oral and IV fluids for adequate excretion of the dye. The nurse may administer pain medication for insertion site or back discomfort, as ordered.

If the client experiences chest pain, dysrhythmias, bleeding, hematoma formation, or a dramatic change in peripheral pulses in the affected extremity, the nurse reports these findings to the physician immediately and provides prompt intervention. The nurse is also alert for neurologic changes such as visual disturbances, slurred speech, difficulty in swallowing, and extremity weakness.

Digital Subtraction Angiography

Digital subtraction angiography (DSA) combines x-ray detection methods and a computerized subtraction technique with fluoroscopy for visualization of the cardiovascular system. There is no interference from adjacent structures, such as bone and soft tissue.

CLIENT PREPARATION. Digital subtraction angiography involves the injection of dye into the venous system. Therefore, before the procedure, the nurse assesses the client for a history of allergies to contrast medium (dye), iodine, or seafood.

▷ Research Applications for Nursing

Clients May Not Need to Remain Supine for 6–12 Hours After Cardiac Catheterization.

Pooler-Lunse, C., Barkman A., & Back, B. F. (1996). Effects of modified positioning and mobilization on back pain and delayed bleeding in patients who have received heparin and undergone angiography: A pilot study. Heart and Lung, 25(2), 117–122.

This study examined the effects of early head elevation (maximum 45 degrees) and early ambulation (after 4 hours) on client perception of pain and presence of delayed bleeding after cardiac catheterization. A small sample of clients (N = 29) were randomly assigned to either the control group (6 hours of supine bedrest) or the experimental group (head of bed elevated to 45 degrees after 15 minutes, out of bed for 2 minutes to stand or urinate after 4 hours). All clients were receiving heparin before angiography.

After the procedure, both pain and presence of delayed bleeding were assessed frequently. Femoral dressings and pedal pulses were evaluated by the staff nurses, and the research assistant palpated the site for presence and size of a hematoma. Pain was evaluated using the McGill Pain Questionnaire.

There was not a significant difference between the two groups in the presence of delayed bleeding. One client in each group had sanguineous drainage through the pressure dressing. However, there was a significant difference in the presence and intensity of pain; clients in the experimental group experienced less pain overall and less intense pain.

Critique. This is a very small sample involving clients from one institution. Delayed bleeding was considered significant only if a hematoma was larger than 5 cm and occluded a pedal pulse or if there was more than 100 mL of volume lost (enough to penetrate the pressure dressing).

Possible Nursing Implications. Since clients experience considerable back discomfort and difficulty urinating while lying supine for 6–12 hours after cardiac catheterization, interventions that would reduce these without causing complications would be highly beneficial. If this pilot study's findings—that head of bed elevation to 45 degrees and early ambulation at 4 hours reduce pain and do not increase bleeding—are replicated with a larger sample and varied populations, many clients might benefit.

PROCEDURE. For a DSA, the radiologist injects dye into the venous system via the superior vena cava. As the contrast medium circulates through the heart and the arterial system, a fluoroscopic image intensifier displays the vessels and focuses the image. A computer then converts the images to numbers. The first image obtained before the injection of the dye is subtracted from the postinjection images.

FOLLOW-UP CARE. Because DSA does not involve an arterial puncture and because little contrast dye is used, nursing care after the procedure is not as extensive as that after cardiac catheterization. The nurse monitors the client for vital signs and assesses the injection site for bleeding or discomfort.

Other Diagnostic Tests
Electrocardiography

The electrocardiogram (ECG) is a routine part of every cardiovascular evaluation and is one of the most valuable diagnostic tests. Various forms are available: resting ECG, continuous ambulatory ECG (Holter monitoring), exercise ECG (stress test), and signal averaged ECG. The resting ECG provides information about cardiac dysrhythmias, myocardial ischemia, the site and extent of myocardial infarction, cardiac hypertrophy, electrolyte imbalances, and the effectiveness of cardiac drugs. The normal ECG pattern of one cardiac cycle is illustrated in Figure 35–15. Further discussion of the interpretation and evaluation of normal and abnormal patterns is found in Chapter 36.

Resting Electrocardiography

The ECG graphically records electrical current generated by the heart. This current is measured by electrodes placed on the skin and connected to an amplifier and strip chart recorder (Fig. 35–16). In the standard 12-lead ECG, five electrodes attached to the arms, legs, and chest measure current from 12 different views or leads: three bipolar limb leads (Fig. 35–17), three unipolar augmented leads (Fig. 35–18), and six unipolar precordial leads (Fig. 35–19). Placement of the leads allows the

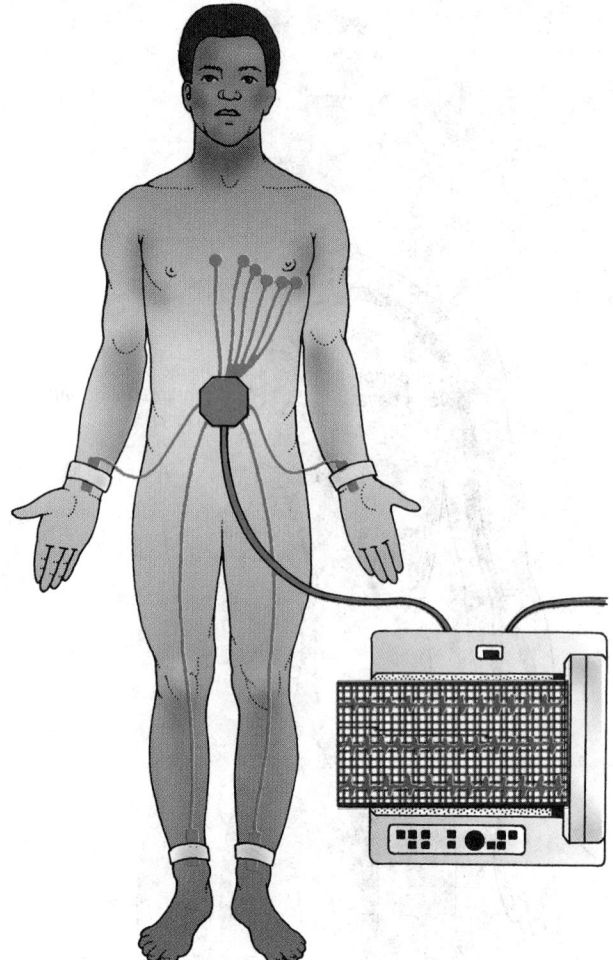

Figure 35–16. Electrode placement for a 12-lead ECG.

physician to view myocardial electrical conduction from different axes or positions, identifying sections of the heart in which electrical conduction is abnormal.

CLIENT PREPARATION. The nurse explains the purpose and procedure of the resting ECG and informs the client that the test is safe and painless. The nurse reminds the client to lie as still as possible during the test.

PROCEDURE. The ECG is performed with the client in a supine position with the chest exposed. Before applying the electrodes, the nurse or the technician washes the skin to reduce skin oils and to improve electrode contact. To ensure good contact between the skin and the electrodes for the limb leads, the electrodes should be placed on a flat surface above the wrists and the ankles. A total of 10 electrodes are used for a standard ECG and are attached to lead wires that connect to the ECG machine. The 12-lead ECG reading is obtained by selecting the indicators on the machine.

FOLLOW-UP CARE. No specific follow-up care is warranted.

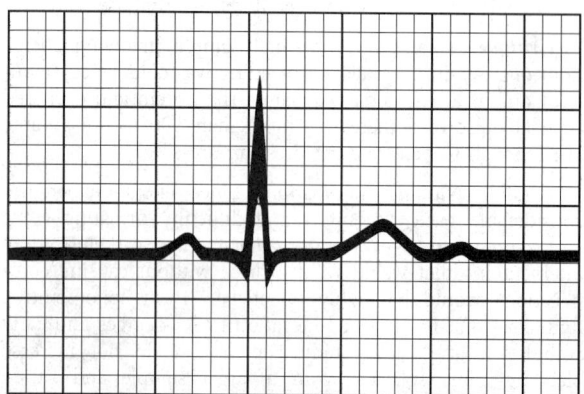

Figure 35–15. A normal ECG pattern in lead II.

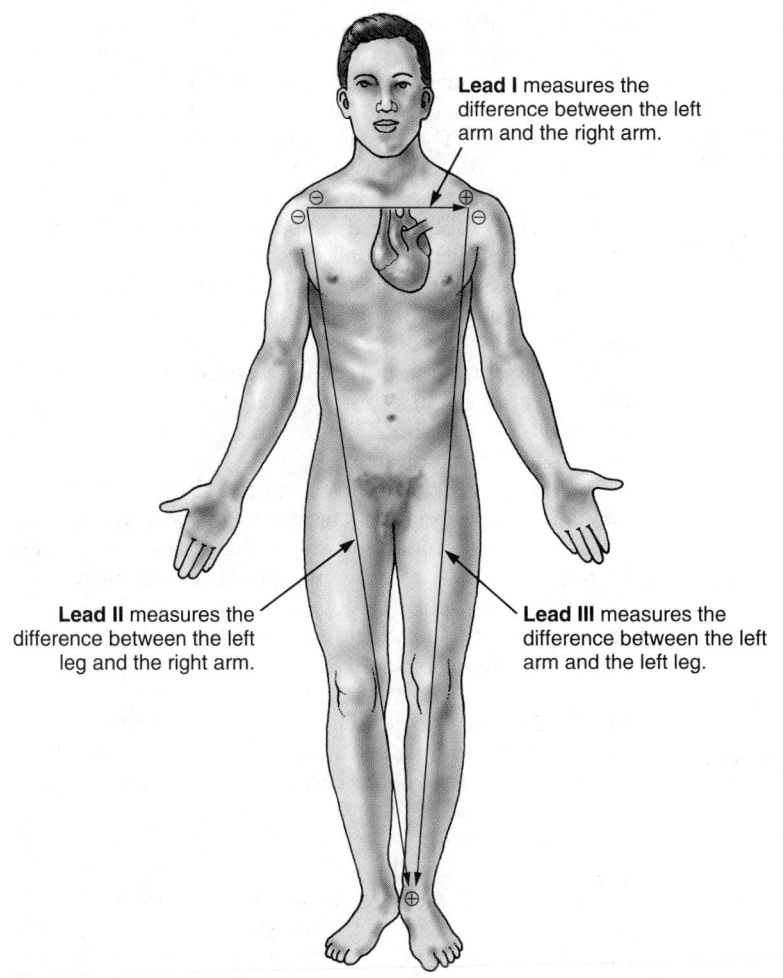

Lead I measures the difference between the left arm and the right arm.

Lead II measures the difference between the left leg and the right arm.

Lead III measures the difference between the left arm and the left leg.

Figure 35–17. Standard ECG limb leads.

Ambulatory Electrocardiography

Ambulatory ECG (also called Holter monitoring) allows continuous recording of cardiac activity during an extended period (usually 24 hours) while the client is performing the usual activities of daily living (ADLs). The ambulatory ECG allows assessment and correlation of dyspnea, chest pain, central nervous system symptoms (such as lightheadedness and syncope), and palpitations with actual cardiac events and the client's activities.

CLIENT PREPARATION. The nurse encourages the client to maintain a normal day's schedule. He or she is instructed to keep a diary, or log, in which to note the time of activities, such as eating, sleeping, walking, and working, and to record any symptoms, such as chest pain, lightheadedness, fainting, and palpitations. The nurse instructs the client to avoid operating heavy machinery, using electric shavers and hair dryers, and bathing or showering. These activities may interfere with the ECG recorder. If the client is hospitalized, the nurse may need to make the entries for the log.

PROCEDURE. The ECG technician places the electrodes on the client's chest and attaches them to the Holter monitor. The monitor is a small portable ECG tape recorder about the size of a transistor radio. The monitor is worn in a sling or holder around the client's chest or waist. After the prescribed monitoring period, the technician removes the electrodes and the monitor system. The ECG tape is analyzed by a microcomputer to allow correlation of the ECG findings with activities noted in the client's diary.

FOLLOW-UP CARE. No specific follow-up care is needed.

Exercise Electrocardiography (Stress Test)

The exercise ECG test (also known as exercise tolerance, or stress, test) assesses the cardiovascular response to an increased workload. The stress test helps to determine the heart's functional capacity and screens for asymptomatic coronary artery disease. Dysrhythmias that develop during exercise may be identified, and the effectiveness of antidysrhythmic drugs can be evaluated.

CLIENT PREPARATION. Because risks are associated with exercising, the client must be adequately informed about the purpose, procedure, and risks involved. A writ-

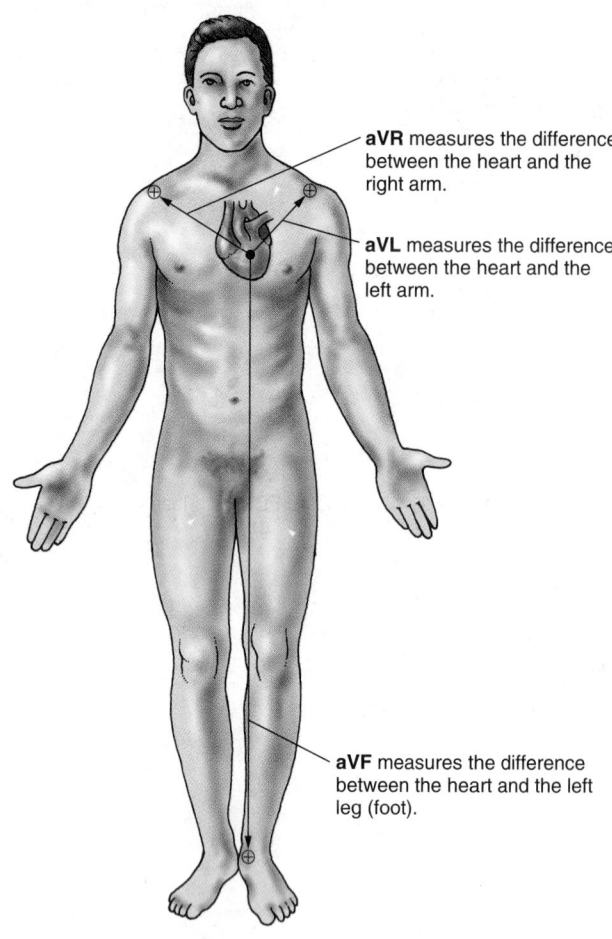

aVR measures the difference between the heart and the right arm.

aVL measures the difference between the heart and the left arm.

aVF measures the difference between the heart and the left leg (foot).

Figure 35–18. Unipolar augmented ECG leads.

ten consent must be obtained. Anxiety and fear are common before stress testing. The nurse assures the client that the procedure is performed in a controlled environment with prompt nursing and medical attention available. The nurse instructs the client to get plenty of rest the night before the procedure. The client may have a light meal 2 hours before the test and avoid smoking or drinking alcohol or caffeine-containing beverages on the day of the test. The physician decides whether the client should stop the administration of any cardiac medications. The client is advised to wear comfortable, loose clothing and rubber-soled, supportive shoes. The nurse instructs the client to tell the physician whether any symptoms, such as chest pain, dizziness, shortness of breath, and an irregular heartbeat, are experienced during the test.

Before the stress test, a resting 12-lead ECG is done, as well as cardiovascular history and physical examination, to check for any ECG abnormalities or medical factors that might contraindicate the test.

Emergency supplies such as cardiac drugs, a defibrillator, and other equipment necessary for resuscitation are available in the room in which the stress test is performed. The nurse assisting the physician during the test should be proficient in using resuscitation equipment because chest pain, dysrhythmias, and other ECG changes may occur during this test.

PROCEDURE. The technician places electrodes on the client's chest and attaches them to a multilead monitoring system. The nurse notes baseline blood pressure, heart rate, and respiratory rate. The two major modes of exercise available for stress testing are pedaling a bicycle ergometer and treadmill walking. A bicycle ergometer is a device equipped with a wheel operated by pedals that can be adjusted to increase the resistance to pedaling. The treadmill is a motorized device with an adjustable conveyor belt; it can reach speeds of 1–10 miles/hour and can also be adjusted from a flat position to a 22-degree gradient.

After the nurse shows the client how to use the bicycle or how to walk on the treadmill, the client begins to exercise. During the test, the client's blood pressure and ECG are closely monitored as the speed and incline of

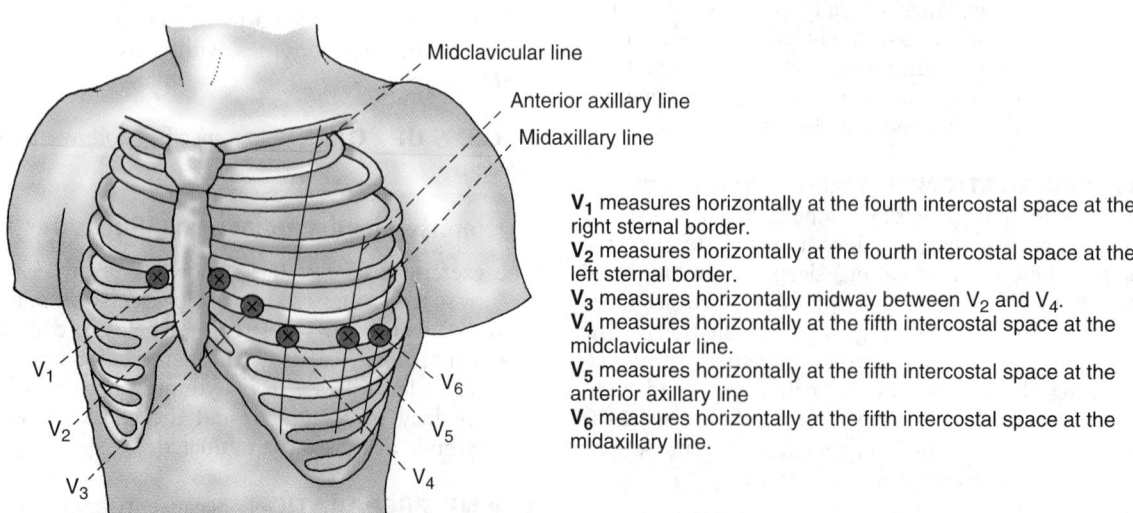

Midclavicular line

Anterior axillary line

Midaxillary line

V_1 measures horizontally at the fourth intercostal space at the right sternal border.
V_2 measures horizontally at the fourth intercostal space at the left sternal border.
V_3 measures horizontally midway between V_2 and V_4.
V_4 measures horizontally at the fifth intercostal space at the midclavicular line.
V_5 measures horizontally at the fifth intercostal space at the anterior axillary line
V_6 measures horizontally at the fifth intercostal space at the midaxillary line.

V_1
V_2
V_3
V_6
V_5
V_4

Figure 35–19. Unipolar precordial ECG leads.

the treadmill or the resistance to cycling are increased. The client exercises until one of the following occurs:

- A predetermined heart rate is reached and maintained.
- Signs and symptoms, such as chest pain, fatigue, extreme dyspnea, vertigo, hypotension, and ventricular dysrhythmias, appear.
- Significant ST-segment depression occurs.

FOLLOW-UP CARE. After the test, the nurse continues to monitor the ECG and blood pressure until the client has completely recovered. After the client has recovered, he or she can return home if the test was done on an outpatient basis. The nurse advises the client to avoid taking a hot shower for 1–2 hours after the test, because this may precipitate hypotension. If the client does not recover but continues to have chest pain or ventricular dysrhythmias or appears medically unstable, he or she is admitted to a coronary care unit for observation.

Echocardiography

As a noninvasive, risk-free test, echocardiography is easily performed at a client's bedside or on an outpatient basis. Echocardiography uses ultrasound waves to assess cardiac structure and mobility, particularly of the valves. ECGs help to assess and diagnose cardiomyopathy, valvular disorders, pericardial effusion, left ventricular function, ventricular aneurysms, and cardiac tumors.

CLIENT PREPARATION. There is no special preparation for echocardiography. The nurse informs the client that the test is painless and takes 30–60 minutes to complete. The nurse instructs the client to lie quietly during the test. The nurse assists the client to lie slightly on his or her left side with the head of the client elevated 15–20 degrees.

PROCEDURE. During an echocardiogram, a small transducer lubricated with gel to facilitate movement and conduction is placed on the client's chest at the level of the third or fourth intercostal space near the left sternal border. The transducer transmits high-frequency sound waves and receives them back from the client as they are reflected from different structures. These echoes are usually videotaped simultaneously with the client's echocardiogram and can be recorded on graph paper for a permanent copy.

Figure 35–20 is a representation of how echocardiograms examine the heart. After the images are taped, cardiac measurements that require several images can be obtained. Some routine measurements are chamber size, ejection fraction, and flow gradient across the valves.

FOLLOW-UP CARE. There is no specific follow-up care for a client having an echocardiogram.

Transesophageal Echocardiography

Echocardiograms may also be performed transesophageally. Transesophageal echocardiography examines cardiac structure and function with an ultrasound transducer placed immediately behind the heart in the esophagus or

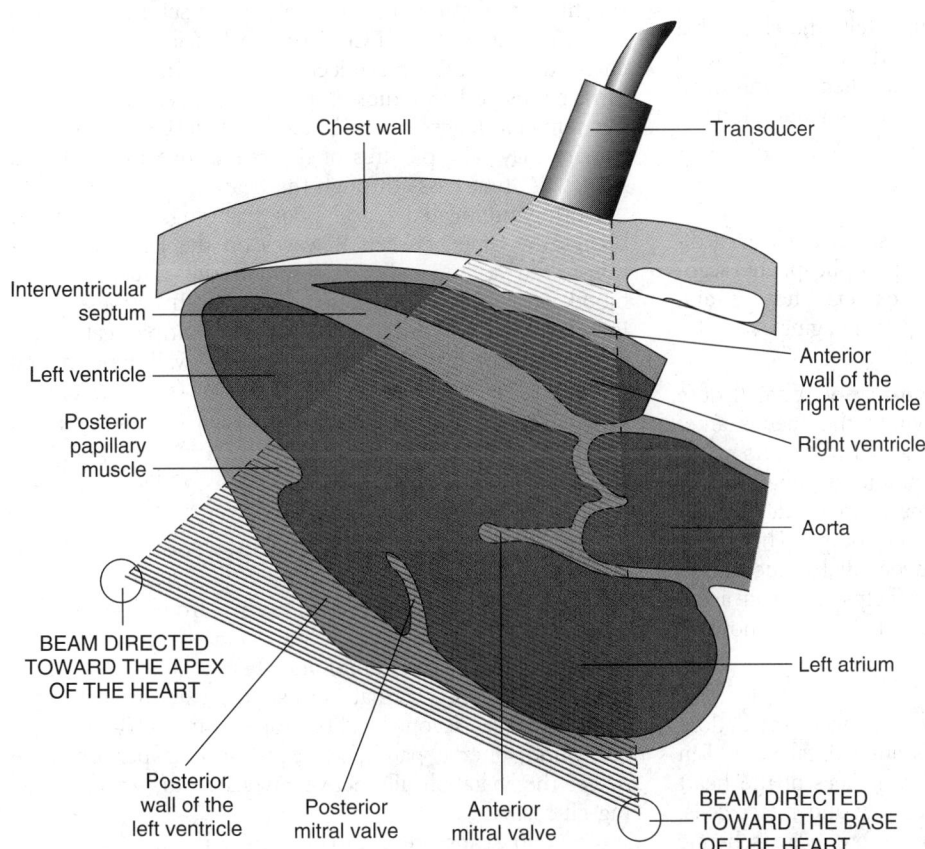

Figure 35–20. Echocardiographic imaging of the heart.

the stomach. The transducer provides especially detailed views of such posterior cardiac structures as the left atrium, the mitral valve, and the aortic arch. Preparation and follow-up are similar to those for the client having an upper gastrointestinal endoscopic examination (see Chap. 55).

Phonocardiography

Phonocardiography is the graphic recording of heart sounds during auscultation. It can be helpful in determining the exact timing and characteristics of extra heart sounds and murmurs.

A phonocardiography machine simultaneously records the pulse wave, ECG, and heart sounds. A pressure-sensitive transducer is applied to the selected pulse (e.g., apical or carotid artery), and the ECG is obtained through standard limb leads. A special microphone, used in the same manner as a stethoscope, is applied to the various areas for auscultation on the client's chest. Client preparation and follow-up care are similar to those for echocardiography (see earlier).

Nuclear Cardiography

The use of radionuclide techniques in cardiovascular assessment is called *nuclear cardiology*. Using radioactive tracer substances, cardiovascular abnormalities can be viewed, recorded, and evaluated. These studies are useful for detecting myocardial infarction (MI) and decreased myocardial blood flow and for evaluating left ventricular ejection.

CLIENT PREPARATION. The nurse tells the client that the tests are relatively noninvasive and that the radiation exposure and risks are minimal. The client is informed that the test involves the IV injection of small amounts of radioisotope. The client or responsible party must give written consent.

PROCEDURE. The most common tests in nuclear cardiology include technetium (^{99m}Tc) pyrophosphate scanning, thallium imaging, sestamibi exercise testing and scan, and multigated cardiac blood pool imaging.

Technetium Pyrophosphate Scanning. A small dose of ^{99m}Tc pyrophosphate is injected into the client's antecubital vein. The client then waits at least 2 hours while the renal system clears the unbound technetium. A gamma-scintillation camera scans the heart to identify the areas of increased uptake of the radioisotope. The radioisotope accumulates in damaged myocardial tissue and is referred to as a "hot spot." This test helps to detect acute MI and define its location and size but does not show an old infarction.

Thallium Imaging. For thallium imaging, a small dose of ^{201}Tl is injected into the client's antecubital vein. Ten minutes later, a nuclear camera takes images of the heart to detect the areas of normal blood flow and intact cells, which rapidly take up the thallium. Necrotic or ischemic

tissue does not take up the radioisotope and appears as "cold spots" on the scan. Scanning is repeated in 2–4 hours to evaluate thallium clearance.

Thallium imaging may be performed with the client at rest or during an exercise test. In the Persantine thallium test, dipyridamole (Persantine, Apo-Dipyridamole♣) is administered before the test. Dobutamine hydrochloride (Dobutrex) or Adenosine (Adenocard) may be given instead. These drugs simulate the effects of exercise and are used for clients who are unable to exercise on a bike or treadmill.

Thallium imaging performed during an exercise test may demonstrate perfusion deficits not apparent at rest. First, the stress test procedure is performed (see earlier). After the client reaches maximal activity level, a small dose of ^{201}Tl is injected IV, and the client continues to exercise for approximately 1–2 minutes. The scanning is then done.

Thallium imaging is used to assess myocardial scarring and perfusion, detect the location and extent of an acute or chronic MI, evaluate graft patency after coronary bypass surgery, and evaluate antianginal therapy, thrombolytic therapy, or balloon angioplasty.

Sestamibi (technetium-99m pertechnetate) may be used rather than thallium for exercise testing with scanning. Sestamibi more accurately identifies ischemic areas in women, and high-quality images may be obtained on the first scan.

Cardiac Blood Pool Imaging. Cardiac blood pool imaging is a noninvasive test used to evaluate cardiac motion and calculate ejection fraction. It uses a computer to synchronize pictures taken by a gamma-scintillation camera with the client's ECG. The technician attaches the client to an ECG and injects a small amount of ^{99m}Tc intravenously. The radioisotope is not taken up by tissue but remains "tagged" to red blood cells in circulation. The camera may take pictures of the radioactive material as it makes its "first pass" through the heart.

During multigated blood pool scanning, the computer breaks the time between R waves on the ECG into fractions of a second called gates, and the camera records blood flow through the heart during each of these gates. By analyzing the information from multiple gates, the computer can evaluate the ventricular wall motion and calculate the client's ejection fraction (the amount of blood the left ventricle ejects with each contraction) and ejection velocity. Areas of decreased, absent, or paradoxical movement of the left ventricle may also be identified.

Positron Emission Tomography. Positron emission scans are used to compare cardiac perfusion and metabolic function and differentiate normal from diseased myocardium. The technician administers the first radioisotope (nitrogen-13-ammonia) and then begins a 20-minute scan to detect myocardial perfusion. Next, the technician administers a second radioisotope (fluoro-18-deoxyglucose) and, after a pause, a second scan is performed to detect the metabolically active myocardium, which is using glucose.

The two scans are compared; in a normal heart, performance and metabolic function will match. In an ischemic heart, there will be a mismatch: a reduction in perfusion and increased glucose uptake by the ischemic myocardium. The scanning procedure takes 2–3 hours, and the client may be asked to use a treadmill or exercise bicycle in conjunction with the scan.

FOLLOW-UP CARE. The client may complain of fatigue, depending on which test is performed, or discomfort at the antecubital injection site. If a stress test was paired with the study, the nurse needs to be aware of the same follow-up care as for the stress test (see earlier).

Magnetic Resonance Imaging

Magnetic resonance imaging (MRI) is a noninvasive diagnostic option. An image of the heart or great vessels is produced through the interaction of magnetic fields, radio waves, and atomic nuclei showing hydrogen density. Simply put, the radio waves "bounce off" the body tissue being examined. Because each tissue has its own density, the computer image clearly differentiates between different types of tissues. MRI permits determination of cardiac wall thickness, chamber dilation, and valve and ventricular function as well as blood movement in the great vessels. Improved MRI techniques allow mapping of coronary artery blood flow with nearly the accuracy of a cardiac catheterization.

Before an MRI, the nurse determines that the client has removed all metallic objects, including watches, jewelry, clothing with metal fasteners, and hair clips. Clients with pacemakers should not have an MRI because the magnetic fields can deactivate the pacemaker. Approximately 5% of clients experience claustrophobia during the 15–60 minutes required to complete the scan.

Hemodynamic Monitoring

Hemodynamic monitoring provides quantitative information about vascular capacity, blood volume, pump effectiveness, and tissue perfusion. Hemodynamic monitoring is often referred to as direct monitoring because it involves procedures that directly measure pressures in the heart and great vessels. Usually performed for more seriously ill clients, it can provide more accurate measurements of blood pressure as well as heart function and volume status.

Informed consent is required for hemodynamic monitoring because there are significant risks, although complications are uncommon. After consent is obtained, the nurse prepares a pressure-monitoring system. The components of a pressure-monitoring system are a catheter with an infusion system, a transducer, and a monitor (Fig. 35-21). The catheter receives the pressure waves (mechanical energy) from the heart or the great vessels. The transducer converts the mechanical energy into electrical energy, which is displayed as waveforms or numbers on the monitor. To maintain patency of the catheter, the nurse prepares a heparinized solution. This solution is usually infused at 3–4 mL/hour under pressure to prevent backup of blood and occlusion of the catheter.

To prepare the transducer, the nurse must balance and calibrate it according to the equipment manufacturer's specifications and the hospital's policy. Finally, the nurse must identify the phlebostatic axis (Chart 35–5) and level the transducer to it. When the monitoring system is prepared, the physician inserts the catheter.

Right Atrial, Pulmonary Artery, and Pulmonary Wedge Pressures

A pulmonary artery catheter is a triple- or quadruple-lumen catheter with the capacity to measure right atrial and indirect left atrial pressures or pulmonary artery wedge pressure (PAWP). A cardiac output measurement may also be obtained.

CLIENT PREPARATION. The physician explains the procedure and advises the client and family members or the significant other of the risks. Then the physician obtains a written consent for the procedure. The client and the family should understand that the hemodynamic monitoring system represents an assessment tool, and, although it is used to guide therapy, it is not itself a treatment. The nurse asks the client to remain still and supine for the insertion of the catheter.

PROCEDURE. The physician inserts a balloon-tipped catheter percutaneously through a large vein and directs it to the right atrium (RA). When the catheter tip reaches the RA, the physician inflates the balloon, and the catheter advances with the flow of blood through the tricuspid valve, into the right ventricle, past the pulmonic valve, and into a branch of the pulmonary artery. The balloon is deflated after the catheter tip reaches the pulmonary artery. Waveforms visualized on the oscilloscope as the pulmonary artery catheter is advanced (Fig. 35–22) and fluoroscopy are used to determine the location of the catheter.

Right atrial pressure is measured by a pressure sensor on the catheter inside the right atrium. Normal RA pressure ranges from 1–8 mmHg. Increased RA pressures may occur with right ventricular failure, whereas low RA pressures are usually indicative of hypovolemia.

Normal pulmonary artery pressure (PAP) ranges from 15 to 28 mmHg/5 to 16 mmHg, with a mean of 15 (Daily & Kenner, 1992), and may be constantly visible on the monitor. When the balloon at the tip of the catheter is inflated, the catheter advances and wedges in a branch of the pulmonary artery. The tip of the catheter is able to sense pressures transmitted from the left atrium, which reflect left ventricular end-diastolic pressure (LVEDP). The pressure measured during balloon inflation is called the *pulmonary artery wedge pressure* (PAWP). PAWP closely approximates left atrial pressure and LVEDP in clients with normal left ventricular function, with normal heart rates, and without mitral valve disease. The PAWP is a mean pressure and is normally between 4 and 12 mmHg.

Elevated PAWP measurements may indicate left ventricular failure, hypervolemia, mitral regurgitation, or intracardiac shunt. A decreased PAWP is seen with hypovolemia or afterload reduction. Individual values may be less important than the trend in values.

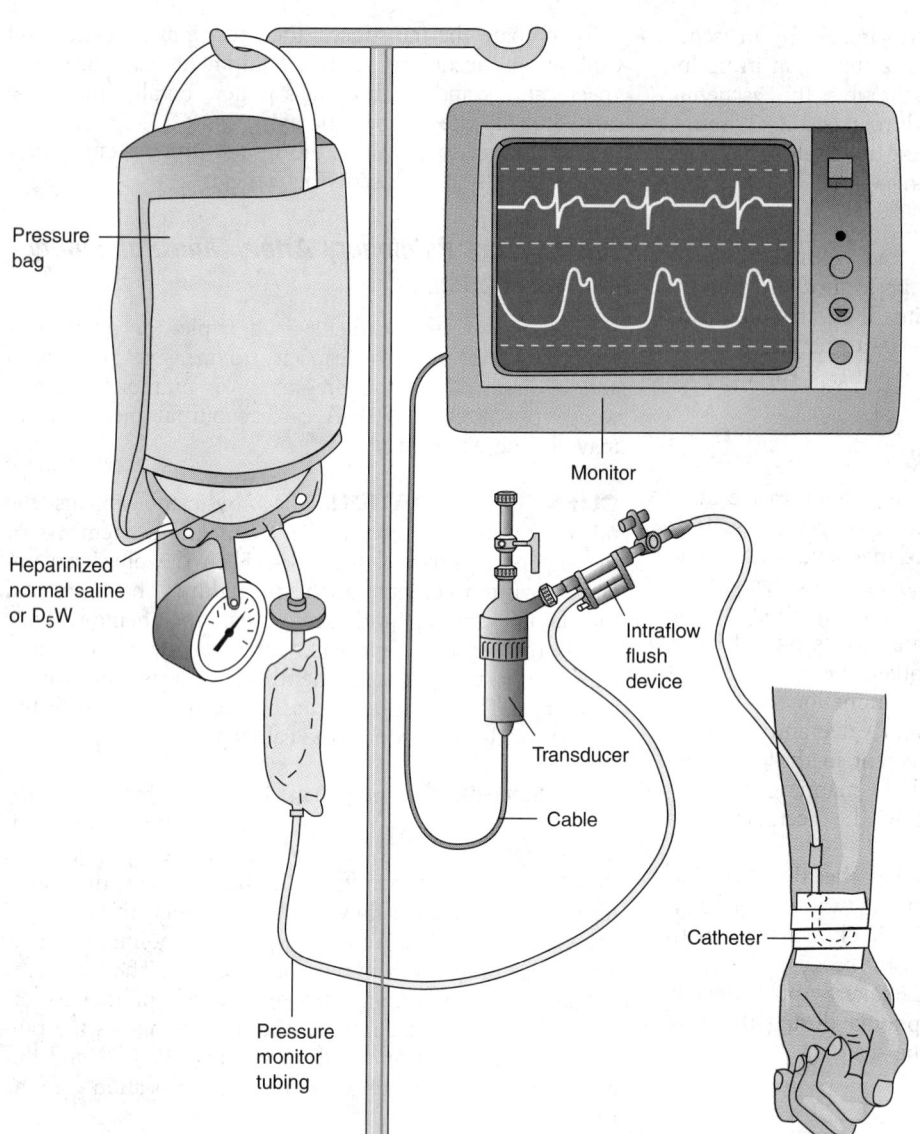

Pressure bag

Heparinized normal saline or D_5W

Monitor

Intraflow flush device

Transducer

Cable

Catheter

Pressure monitor tubing

Figure 35–21. Components of a hemodynamic monitoring system.

FOLLOW-UP CARE. The patency of the catheter is maintained with infusion of a heparinized solution under pressure. The nurse obtains and records RA pressure, pulmonary artery pressure, and PAWP at appropriate intervals (usually every 1–4 hours). The trend of these pressures helps to guide medical therapy. During pressure recording, it is important that the transducer be at the level of the phlebostatic axis and the client's position be appropriate. While PAWPs are obtained, the client is usually supine with the head elevated up to 45 degrees or turned slightly to the side. If the balloon remains in the wedge position after PAWP measurement, the nurse attempts to change the catheter's position by asking the client to cough or changing the client's position. If these methods are not successful, the nurse notifies the physician immediately.

The nurse changes the occlusive dressing over the catheter aseptically according to the hospital's policy. The nurse inspects the insertion site for redness, heat, swelling, drainage, and intactness of the sutures. Detailed dis-

cussion of the management and care of clients with pulmonary artery catheters can be found in texts on critical care nursing.

The nurse assesses for a number of complications associated with pulmonary artery catheters. For example, pulmonary infarction or pulmonary rupture may occur if the catheter remains in the wedge position. Air embolism is possible if the balloon has ruptured and repeated attempts are made to inflate it. Ventricular dysrhythmias may occur if the catheter tip slips back into the right ventricle and irritates the myocardium. Thrombus and embolus formation may occur at the catheter site. Infection may result and bleeding may be pronounced if the infusion system becomes disconnected.

Cardiac Output

Cardiac output can be measured using the thermodilution method when the patient has a pulmonary artery catheter with a thermistor. The nurse injects a specified amount (5

Nursing Care Highlight: Identification of the Phlebostatic Axis

1. Position the client supine.
2. Palpate the fourth intercostal space at the sternum.

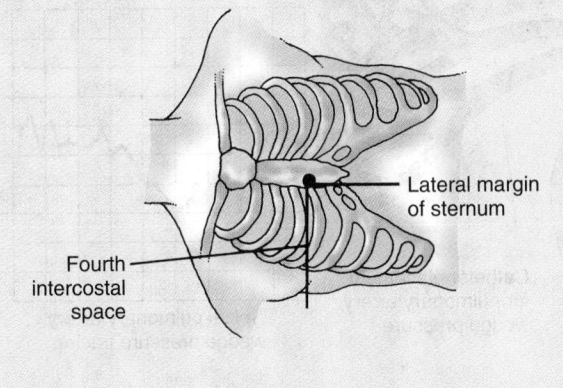

Lateral margin of sternum

Fourth intercostal space

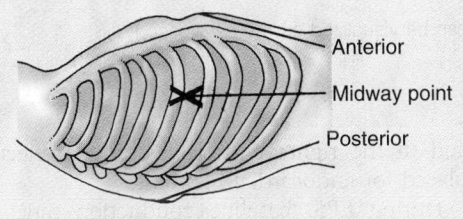

Anterior

Midway point

Posterior

3. Follow the fourth intercostal space to the side of the client's chest.
4. Determine the midway point between anterior and posterior.
5. Find the intersection between the midway point and the line from the fourth intercostal space, and mark it with an X in indelible ink. This is the phlebostatic axis.

or 10 mL) of iced or room-temperature IV solution (normal saline or dextrose in water) into the proximal port of the catheter. The solution mixes with the blood in the right atrium and travels with the flow of blood through the heart. A temperature-sensitive device located on the tip of the catheter in the pulmonary artery registers and senses the change in temperature of the blood. The information is transmitted to a cardiac output computer, which displays a digital value. The normal range of cardiac output in the adult client is 4–7 L/minute (Wilson, 1992). The cardiac index, the cardiac output adjusted for the person's size, may also be calculated.

Mixed Venous Oxygen Saturation Monitoring

Mixed venous oxygen saturation (SVO_2) reflects the balance between oxygen supply and demand. SVO_2 may be measured with a pulmonary artery catheter with fiberoptics. Light travels down one optical fiber, is reflected by the red blood cells according to the oxygen saturation of the hemoglobin, and returns to an optical module for interpretation and continuous display. Normal range for

SVO_2 is 60% to 80%. Using SVO_2 monitoring, the nurse can individualize the plan of care so the patient's SVO_2 remains in the normal range and the patient's oxygen supply and demand are in balance.

Central Venous Pressure Monitoring

If the physician desires measurement of pressures from the right atrium or central veins but a pulmonary artery catheter and pressure-monitoring system are not appropriate, pressures may be obtained with a water manometer attached to a conventional IV system. Central venous pressures (CVPs) are similar to right atrial pressures, but CVPs are measured in centimeters of water rather than millimeters of mercury. A normal CVP is 3–8 cm H_2O.

The physician inserts a catheter through the venous system into the right atrium. A chest x-ray is taken to assess placement. The nurse levels the manometer with the phlebostatic axis to ensure accurate pressure measurement (Chart 35–6).

Elevated CVPs may indicate right ventricular failure. Low CVPs may indicate hypovolemia. Caution must be used in predicting the function of the left side of the heart from a CVP reading.

Care of the site is similar to that for the pulmonary artery catheter site. Complications include pneumothorax during insertion, hemorrhage, infection, and catheter occlusion.

Systemic Intra-Arterial Monitoring

Direct measurement of arterial blood pressure is by invasive arterial catheter in critically ill clients. The physician usually inserts an intra-arterial catheter into the radial artery, but the femoral, brachial, or dorsalis pedis arteries may also be used. After the physician has inserted the catheter, the catheter is attached to pressure tubing and a heparinized solution is infused constantly under pressure to maintain the integrity of the system. A transducer attached to the tubing allows continuous direct monitoring of the arterial blood pressure. Direct measurements of blood pressure are usually 10–15 mmHg greater than indirect (cuff) measurements. The arterial catheter may also be used to obtain blood samples for arterial blood gas values and other blood tests.

Because the arterial vasculature is a high-pressure system, frequent assessment of the arterial site and infusion system is essential. The nurse notes any bleeding around the intra-arterial catheter or any loose connections and corrects the situation immediately. Collateral circulation is assessed by Doppler or Allen's tests before and during the time when an arterial catheter is in place. Color, pulse, and temperature at the insertion site should be scrupulously monitored for any early signs of circulatory compromise. Complications of systemic intra-arterial monitoring may include pain, infection, arteriospasm, obstruction at the site with potential for distal infarction, air embolism, and hemorrhage.

Electrophysiologic Studies

An electrophysiologic study (EPS) is an invasive procedure during which programmed electrical stimulation of

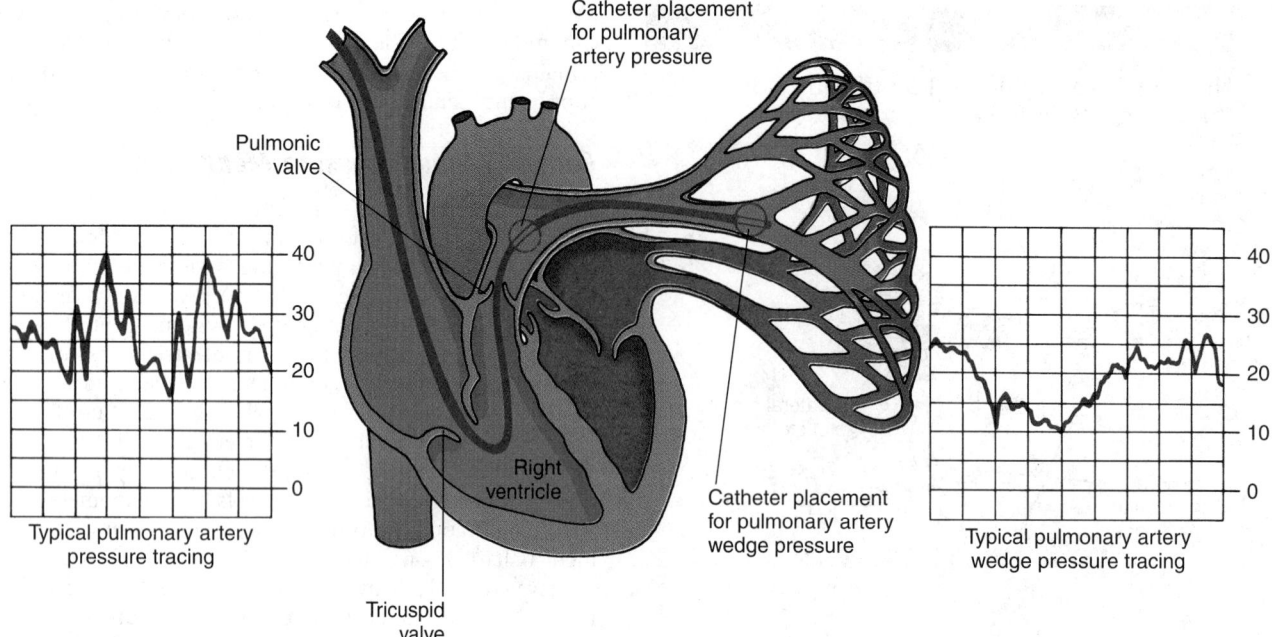

Figure 35–22. Cardiac pressure waveforms can be visualized on the oscilloscope.

the heart is used to induce and evaluate lethal dysrhythmias and conduction abnormalities. Clients who have survived cardiac arrest, have recurrent tachydysrhythmias, or experience unexplained syncopal episodes may be referred for EPS. Induction of the dysrhythmia during EPS permits accurate diagnosis of the dysrhythmia and aids in the search for an effective treatment. These procedures hold risks similar to those for cardiac catheterization and are performed in a special catheterization laboratory, where conditions are strictly controlled and immediate treatment is available for any adverse effects.

CLIENT PREPARATION. The preparation of clients for EPS parallels that of clients undergoing cardiac catheterization (see earlier). Clients may express fear or anxiety, because attempts are made to induce lethal dysrhythmias similar to those that led to the initial hospitalization or resuscitation. The nurse reassures clients that EPS is a planned, controlled event, and immediate treatment will be available for any dysrhythmia induced during the studies. An electrophysiologist (a physician who specializes in these studies) usually explains the purpose of the studies; describes the procedure, including benefits and risks; and obtains a written consent.

PROCEDURE. The client is taken to a cardiac catheterization laboratory or a similar laboratory where he or she is asked to assume a supine position on an x-ray table. Electrodes are attached for continuous ECG monitoring. Defibrillation pads are placed on the client's chest and back. After the nurse or the technician prepares the insertion site, the electrophysiologist injects a local anesthetic, and a multipolar electrode catheter is inserted. The catheter is advanced, guided by fluoroscopy, until electrodes rest in the right atrium, adjacent to the bundle of His,

and in the right ventricle. Additional electrodes may be placed for endocardial mapping.

During EPS, baseline conduction times can be measured: the AH interval (conduction time from the right atrium through the His bundle) and the HV interval (conduction time from the proximal His bundle to the ventricular myocardium). The catheter may be programmed to pace at varying rates to determine SA and AV node function, or it may be programmed to deliver premature paced stimuli in an effort to initiate and evaluate the client's tachydysrhythmia.

If the dysrhythmia is induced, it may terminate spontaneously or be treated by the physician. The physician might elect to use properly timed stimuli, rapid pacing, medications, or countershock to terminate the dysrhythmia.

The client is advised to tell the staff of any symptoms that he or she is experiencing. During rapid pacing, the client may be aware of the rapid heartbeat and state that he or she is experiencing palpitations. The client may also experience chest pain or loss of consciousness if he or she becomes hypotensive. The client often experiences back discomfort during the procedure, because he or she must remain supine for 2–6 hours. Pain may develop at the insertion site as the anesthetic wears off.

FOLLOW-UP CARE. The follow-up care is the same as that for the client who has undergone cardiac catheterization. The nurse may provide comfort measures to alleviate back discomfort, including massage and position changes. If the client lost consciousness during the procedure and received electrical cardioversion or defibrillation, the client may complain of chest discomfort over the area where the electrical current was applied. The nurse assesses the skin for any signs of redness, swelling, or burns. In addi-

Chart 35–6

Nursing Care Highlight: Obtaining a Central Venous Pressure Reading

1. Position the water manometer so that the zero mark or the air-fluid interface is at the same height as the phlebostatic axis.

2. Turn the stopcock as shown to fill the manometer with IV fluid.
3. Turn the stopcock as shown to record the CVP. With each respiration, the fluid level in the manometer should fluctuate. When the level has stabilized, read the highest level of the fluid column.
4. Return the stopcock to the position shown to resume the flow of IV fluid to the client.

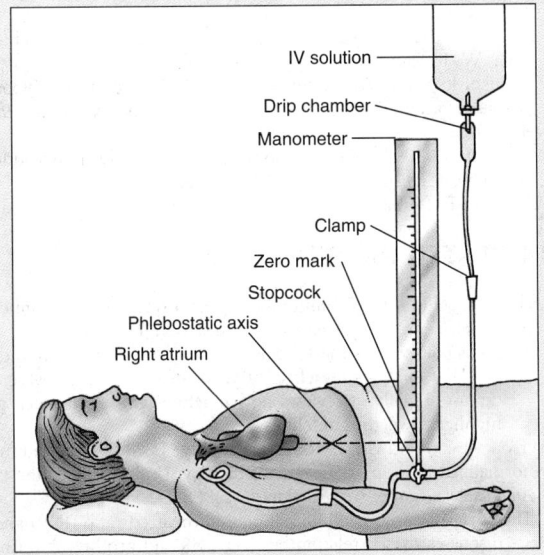

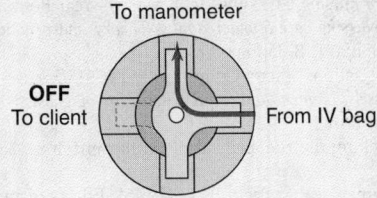

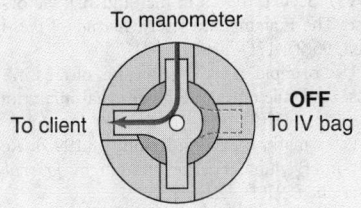

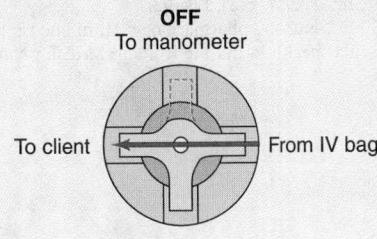

tion, the client might describe a loss of memory of the events during the procedure, and the nurse needs to provide reassurance and calmly explain the events of the procedure.

SELECTED BIBLIOGRAPHY

American Heart Association. (1996). *Heart and stroke facts: 1996 statistical supplement* (pp. 1–23). Dallas: Author.

*American Nurses' Association Division on Medical-Surgical Nursing Practice and American Heart Association Council on Cardiovascular Nursing. (1981). *Standards of cardiovascular nursing practice*. Kansas City, MO: American Nurses' Association.

Burke, M. M., & Walsh, M. B. (1997). *Gerontologic nursing: Wholistic care of the older adult* (2nd ed.). St. Louis, MO: C. V. Mosby

Chernecky, C. C., & Berger, B. J. (1997). *Laboratory tests and diagnostic procedures* (2nd ed.). Philadelphia: W. B. Saunders.

Corbett, J. V. (1996). *Laboratory tests and diagnostic procedures with nursing diagnoses* (4th ed.) Stamford, CT: Appleton & Lange.

Croft, J. B., Keenan, N. L., Sheridan, D. P., Wheeler, F., & Speers, M. (1995). Waist to hip ratio in biracial population: Measurement, implications, and cautions for using guidelines to define high risk for cardiovascular disease. *Journal of the American Dietetic Association, 95*(1), 60–64.

*Department of Health and Human Services. (1990). *Healthy people 2000: National health promotion and disease prevention objectives.* Washington, D.C.: U. S. Government Printing Office.

Gerchofsky, M. (1996). Examining the weight question: How much is too much? *Advances for Nurse Practitioners, 4*(1), 17–19.

*Hochrein, M., & Sohl, L. (1992). Heart smart: A guide to cardiac tests. *American Journal of Nursing, 92*(12), 22–25.

Hogsten, P. (1997). Hemodynamic monitoring. In P. S. Kidd (Ed.), *High acuity nursing* (pp. 227–256). Stamford, CT: Appleton & Lange.

Houston, S., Eagen, M., Freeborg, S., & Dougherty, D. (1996). A comparison of structured preheart catheterization information on mood states and coping resources. *Applied Nursing Research, 9*(4), 189–194.

Jarvis, C. (1996). *Physical examination and health assessment* (2nd ed.). Philadelphia: W. B. Saunders.

Keller, C., Fleury, J., & Bergstrom, D. L. (1995). Risk factors for coronary heart disease in African American women. *Cardiovascular Nursing, 31*(2), 9–14.

*Kirkendall, W. M., Feinleib, M. D., & Fries, E. D. (1988). *Recommendations for human blood pressure determination by sphygmomanometers.* Dallas: American Heart Association.

Kirton, C. A. (1995). Assessing normal heart sounds. *Nursing95, 25*(5), 34–35.

Kottke, T., Weidman, W., & Nguyon, Y. (1996). Prevention of coronary heart disease. In E. R. Guiliani (Ed.), *Mayo Clinic practice of cardiology* (3rd ed.). St. Louis, MO: C. V. Mosby.

Krenzer, M. E. (1995). Peripheral vascular assessment: Finding your ways through arteries and veins. *AACN Clinical Issues: Advanced Practice in Acute and Critical Care, 6*(4) 631–644.

Mahaffey, T. (1995). Cardiac catheterization. In N. Urban (Ed.), *Guidelines for critical care nursing.* St. Louis, MO: Mosby–Year Book.

Miller, C. A. (1995). *Nursing care of older adults: Theory and practice* (2nd ed.). Philadelphia: J. B. Lippincott.

*New York Heart Association Criteria Committee. (1964). *Diseases of the heart and blood vessels: Nomenclature and criteria for diagnosis* (6th ed.). Boston: Little, Brown.

Owen, A. (1995). Tracking the rise and fall of cardiac enzymes. *Nursing 95, 25*(5), 34–38.

Pooler-Lunse, C., Barkman, A., & Back, B. F. (1996). Effects of modified positioning and mobilization on back pain and delayed bleeding in patients who had received heparin and undergone angiography: A pilot study. *Heart and Lung, 25*(2), 117–122.

Posner, B. M., et al. (1995). Secular trends in diet and risk factors for cardiovascular disease: The Framingham study. *Journal of the American Dietetic Association, 95*(2), 171–179.

Puleo, P., et al. (1994). Use of rapid assay of subforms of creatine kinase MB to diagnose and rule out acute myocardial infarction. *New England Journal of Medicine, 331*(9), 561–566.

Robinson, J., Hoerr, S., Petersmark, K., & Anderson, J. (1995). Redefining success in obesity intervention: The new paradigm. *Journal of the American Dietetic Association, 95*(4) 422–423.

Scher, H. E. (1995). Chest pain: Developing rapid assessment skills. *Orthopedic Nursing, 14*(3), 30–34.

Severson, A. L., Baldwin, L. R., & Deloughty, T. G. (1996). International normalized ratio in anticoagulant therapy: Understanding the issues. *American Journal of Critical Care, 6*(2), 88–92.

Sharts-Hopro, N. C. (1995). Nursing pharmacology: Hormone replacement and cardiovascular health in midlife women. *MedSurg Nursing, 4*(4), 314–316.

Sims, L. K., D'Amico, D., Stiesmeyer, J. K., & Webster, J. A. (1995). *Health assessment in nursing.* Redwood City, CA: Addison-Wesley.

Strimike, C. (1996). New procedures: Understanding intravascular ultrasound. *American Journal of Nursing, 96*(6), 40–44.

Sullivan, M. J. (1994). New trends in cardiac rehabilitation in patients with chronic heart failure. *Progress in Cardiovascular Nursing, 9*(1), 13–21.

Swearingen, R. L., & Keen, J. L. (1995). *Manual of critical care* (3rd ed.). St. Louis, MO: Mosby Year Book.

*Thompson, E. J. (1993). Transesophageal echocardiography: A new window on the heart and great vessels. *Critical Care Nurse, 13,* 55–65.

Tietz, R. W. (1995). *Clinical guide to laboratory tests* (3rd ed.). Philadelphia: W. B. Saunders.

*Van Bushirk, M. C., & Gradman, A. H. (1993). Monitoring blood pressure in ambulatory patients. *American Journal of Nursing, 93*(6), 44–47.

*Weigle, D. S. (1992). The pathophysiology of obesity: Implications for treatment. *Clinician Reviews, 2*(5), 81–102.

*Wilson, R. F. (1992). *Critical care manual.* Philadelphia: F. A. Davis.

SUGGESTED READINGS

Gerchofsky, M. (1996). Examining the weight question: How much is too much? *Advances for Nurse Practitioners, 4*(1), 17–19.

This article examines the relationship between weight gain and early death. It explains the effect of yo-yo dieting on cardiovascular disease. Finally, it reviews how much weight is too much and highlights weight guidelines.

Severson, A. L., Baldwin, L. R., & Deloughty, T. G. (1997). International normalized ratio in anticoagulant therapy: Understanding the issues. *American Journal of Critical Care, 6*(2), 88–92.

This article defines the international normalized ratio (INR) and discusses the correlation between INR and prothrombin time (PT). It explains why it is beneficial to monitor the INR rather than the PT.

Tremko, L. (1997). Understanding diagnostic cardiac catheterization. *American Journal of Nursing, 97*(2), 16Q–16R.

This article describes the procedure of cardiac catheterization. After discussing preprocedure care and client education, it describes postprocedure care, including the prevention and control of hemorrhage.

Chapter 36

INTERVENTIONS FOR CLIENTS
WITH DYSRHYTHMIAS

Cardiac dysrhythmias are disturbances of cardiac electrical impulse formation, conduction, or both. Many diseases can affect the electrical activity of the heart, causing dysrhythmias. Although more common in the elderly, dysrhythmias may occur in infants, children, and adults. Many dysrhythmias are benign. Some cause hemodynamic instability. A few result in cardiac arrest. To understand dysrhythmias and to interpret these disturbances correctly, the nurse must understand cardiac electrophysiology, the conduction system of the heart, and the principles of electrocardiography.

REVIEW OF CARDIAC ELECTROPHYSIOLOGY
Electrophysiologic Properties

The electrophysiologic properties of cardiac cells regulate heart rate and rhythm. Specialized cardiac muscle cells possess unique properties: automaticity, excitability, conductivity, and contractility.

Automaticity

Automaticity (spontaneous depolarization) is the ability of cardiac cells to generate an electrical impulse spontaneously and repetitively. Normally, only primary pacemaker cells possess this property. Under certain conditions, such

as myocardial ischemia and infarction, however, any cardiac cell may exhibit this property, generating electrical impulses independently and creating dysrhythmias.

Excitability

Excitability is the ability of nonpacemaker cardiac cells to respond to an electrical impulse generated from pacemaker cells and to depolarize. Depolarization occurs when the normally negatively charged cells develop a positive charge.

Conductivity

Conductivity is the ability to transmit an electrical stimulus from cell membrane to cell membrane. Consequently, excitable cells depolarize in rapid succession from cell to cell until all cells have depolarized. This wave of depolarization gives rise to the deflections of the electrocardiogram (ECG) waveforms that are recognized as the P wave and the QRS complex.

Contractility

Contractility is the ability of atrial and ventricular muscle cells to shorten their fiber length in response to electrical stimulation, generating sufficient pressure to propel blood forward. This is the mechanical activity of the heart.

Action Potential

The cardiac cell membrane (sarcolemma) exhibits selective permeability to ions. This creates an electrical imbalance, known as an *action potential,* across the cell membrane.

The cardiac cell at rest has an internal negative charge, whereas the charge outside the cell is positive. This state of electrical imbalance of the resting cell is called *resting membrane potential.* Two types of cardiac cells exist: fast-response cells (myocardial and Purkinje cells) and slow-response cells (nodal, or pacemaker, cells).

Fast-Response Cells

When myocardial and Purkinje cells are at rest, they have a negative internal charge that results from a small amount of potassium, a positive ion, leaving the cells. The outside of the cell, having gained potassium, has a positive charge. Positive charged cells are ready for action. The action potential of fast-response cells consists of several phases (Fig. 36–1).

Phase 0

Phase 0 is the phase of rapid depolarization. A stimulus from an impulse generated from pacemaker cells reaches the excitable myocardial and Purkinje cells. The stimulus causes sodium, a positive ion, to diffuse rapidly into the cells. The cells now develop an internal positive charge, while the outside of the cells becomes negative. This process is called *depolarization.* As depolarization occurs from cell to cell, a wave of positive current is created. The ECG lead system senses this current and inscribes a P wave during atrial depolarization or a QRS complex during ventricular depolarization.

Phase 1

Phase 1 is the phase of early rapid repolarization. Sodium channels are inactivated. As a small amount of positive potassium ions leaves the cells and a small amount of negative chloride ions enters the cells, the internal charge becomes nearly electrically equal with the outside of the cells.

Phase 2

Phase 2 is the plateau phase. Slow calcium channels allow calcium ions to enter the cells. Sodium may also enter via slow channels. These inward currents are balanced by an outward current of potassium ions leaving the cells, thus maintaining a membrane potential that is nearly equal electrically. The calcium influx into cells triggers the initiation of muscle contraction. Phases 1 and 2 in ventricular myocardial and Purkinje cells are reflected by the ST segment on the ECG.

Phase 3

Phase 3 is the phase of rapid repolarization. The cells regain their negative charge as potassium ions leave the cells while the other channels are inactivated, allowing the cells to become negatively charged again. This process of repolarization, or electrical recovery of cells, is reflected by the T wave on the ECG.

Phase 4

During the beginning of phase 4, a sodium-potassium pump is responsible for actively pumping sodium out of the cells and potassium back into the cells, against their concentration gradients. Adenosine triphosphate (ATP)

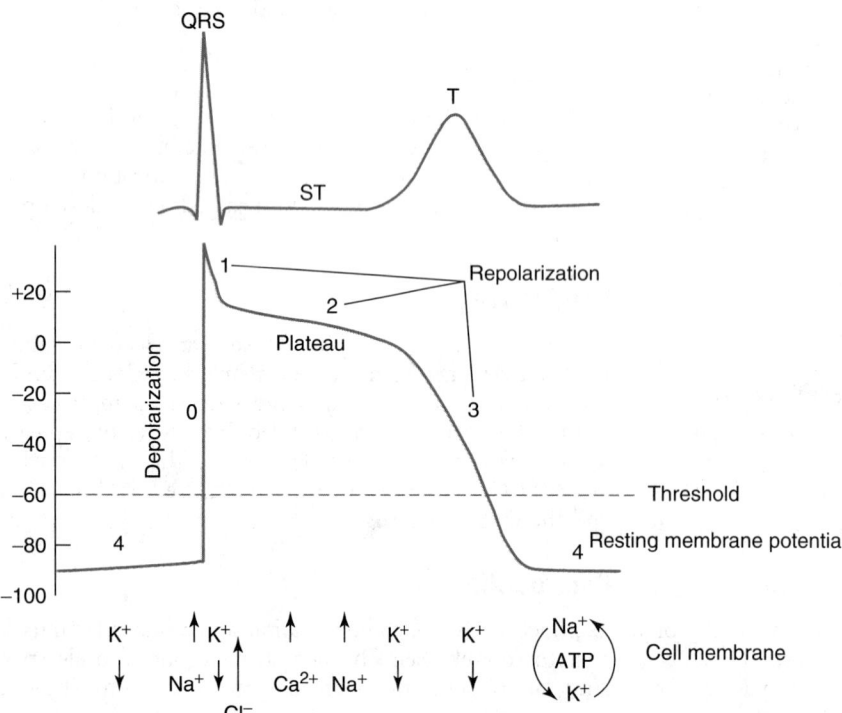

Figure 36–1. Action potential of a fast-response cell (muscle cell). Exchange of ions across the cell membrane occurs at different points of the action potential. At rest, the inside of the cardiac cell is more negatively charged than the outside of the cell, and the cell membrane is more permeable to potassium (K^+) than to sodium (Na^+) ions. With a sufficient electrical stimulus, the cell membrane becomes more permeable to Na^+. As Na^+ enters the cell, the inside becomes positively charged (Phase 0, depolarization). Sodium channels become inactivated. K^+ leaves the cell, and chloride (Cl^-) enters the cell, decreasing the positive charge (Phase 1, early repolarization). Calcium (Ca^{2+}) and Na^+ ions enter the cell while K^+ leaves the cell (Phase 2, plateau), allowing Ca^{2+} to initiate muscle contraction. K^+ leaves the cell (Phase 3, repolarization), returning the cell to its negative state. K^+ regains dominance over Na^+ diffusion and establishes equilibrium (Phase 4, resting membrane potential) before another stimulus is elicited.

provides energy. Resting membrane potential is then restored.

Slow-Response Cells

The action potential of slow-response cells (nodal, or pacemaker, cells) differs from that of fast-response cells (Fig. 36–2).

Phase 4

Phase 4 is the phase of spontaneous diastolic depolarization. It is an unstable phase, providing automaticity in pacemaker cells. This is accomplished through a slow inward current of calcium and sodium into the nodal cells. The cells thus decrease their negative charge and spontaneously reach their activation threshold, initiating an action potential. The faster the threshold is reached, the faster the heart rate becomes.

Phase 0

Phase 0, or depolarization, occurs after the cells reach their activation threshold. As calcium and sodium continue to enter the nodal cells, the electrical charge of the cells becomes less and less negative. The nodal cells then generate, or fire, an electrical impulse, which is again conducted to excitable fast-response cells.

Phase 3

Slow-response cells do not have phases 1 and 2. Slow repolarization begins (phase 3) as potassium leaves the nodal cells, causing the return of an internal negative charge (rapid repolarization). A sodium-potassium pump is then activated to return the electrolytes to their area of greatest concentration. This phase prepares the process again for the next cycle.

The sinoatrial (SA) node, which is the first structure in the heart's conduction system, is the primary pacemaker. It has the greatest number of nodal cells and conse-

quently the fastest rate of automaticity. Secondary, or subsidiary, pacemakers have fewer nodal cells and therefore a slower rate of automaticity. Subsidiary pacemakers include atrioventricular (AV) junctional cells and ventricular Purkinje cells. They can serve as "escape," or latent, pacemakers when the primary pacemaker becomes dysfunctional.

CARDIAC CONDUCTION SYSTEM

The cardiac conduction system consists of specialized cells (Fig. 36–3). It is responsible for the generation and conduction of electrical impulses that cause atrial and ventricular depolarization. The conduction system consists of the sinoatrial node, atrioventricular (AV) junctional area, and bundle branch system.

Sinoatrial Node

The conduction system begins with the sinoatrial (SA) node (also called the sinus node), located close to the epicardial surface of the right atrium near its junction with the superior vena cava. The SA node is the heart's primary pacemaker. It can spontaneously and rhythmically generate electrical impulses at a rate of 60 to 100 per minute, possessing the greatest degree of automaticity.

The SA node is richly innervated by the sympathetic and parasympathetic nervous systems, which accelerate and decelerate the rate of discharge of the sinus node, respectively. This process results in changes in the heart rate.

It is now believed that impulses from the sinus node propagate directly through atrial muscle without specialized pathways. The impulses lead to atrial depolarization and are reflected by a P wave on the ECG trace. Atrial muscle contraction should follow. Within the atrial muscle are slow and fast pathways, leading to the AV node.

Atrioventricular Junctional Area

The AV junctional area consists of a transitional cell zone, the AV node itself, and the His bundle. The AV node lies just beneath the right atrial endocardium, between the tricuspid valve and the ostium of the coronary sinus. Here, T cells (transitional cells) cause impulses to slow down or be delayed in the AV node before proceeding to the ventricles. This delay is reflected by the PR segment on the ECG. This slow conduction provides a physiologic delay, allowing the atria to contract before ventricular stimulation and contraction. Atrial contraction, known as the "atrial kick," contributes 15% to 30% of additional blood volume for a greater cardiac output. Nodal cells in the AV junctional area may occasionally demonstrate automaticity, giving rise to junctional beats or rhythms. The AV node is innervated by both the sympathetic and the parasympathetic nervous systems. The His bundle connects with the distal portion of the AV node and continues on to perforate the interventricular septum.

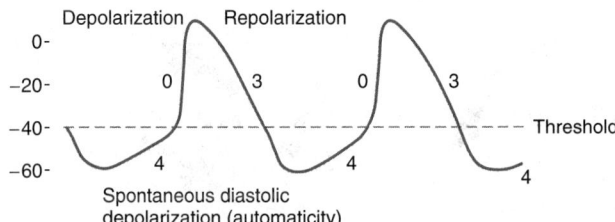

Figure 36–2. Action potential of a slow-response cell (pacemaker cell). At rest, this cell is less negative than the muscle cell. During Phase 4 (spontaneous diastolic depolarization), the pacemaker cell membrane is more permeable to Ca^{2+} and Na^+ ions than to K^+ ions. Ca^{2+} and Na^+ enter the cell, decreasing the negative charge (the property of automaticity) until threshold is reached. Ca^{2+} and Na^+ continue to enter the cell until the cell is no longer negatively charged (Phase 0, depolarization), and the cell fires an electrical stimulus. The cell is now more permeable to K^+ and less permeable to Ca^{2+} and Na^+. K^+ leaves the cell, returning the cell to its negative state (Phase 3, repolarization). The slow Ca^{2+} and Na^+ channels regain dominance over K^+, creating instability in the resting state (Phase 4), allowing the process to begin again for another cycle.

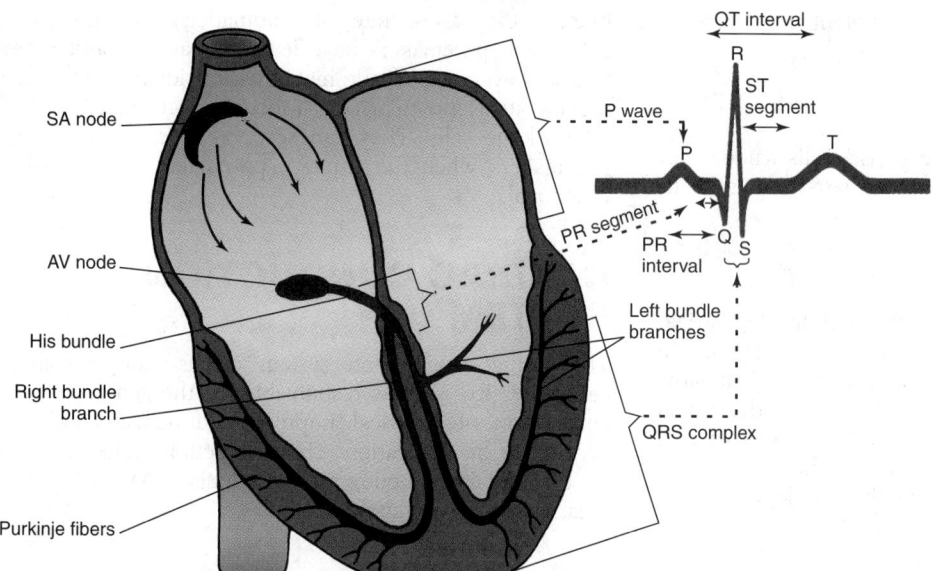

Figure 36–3. The cardiac conduction system.

Bundle Branch System

The His bundle extends as a right bundle branch down the right side of the interventricular septum to the apex of the right ventricle. On the left side, it extends as a left bundle branch, which further divides into two fascicles.

At the ends of both right and left bundle branch systems are the Purkinje fibers. These fibers are an interweaving network located on the endocardial surface of both ventricles, from apex to bases. The fibers then partially penetrate into the myocardium.

Purkinje cells make up the His bundle, bundle branches, and terminal Purkinje fibers. These cells are responsible for the rapid conduction of electrical impulses throughout the ventricles, leading to ventricular depolarization and the subsequent ventricular muscle contraction. A few nodal cells in the ventricles may also occasionally demonstrate automaticity, giving rise to ventricular beats or rhythms.

ELECTROCARDIOGRAPHY

The electrocardiogram (ECG) provides a graphic representation of cardiac electrical activity. The weak cardiac electrical currents are transmitted to the body surface. Electrodes, consisting of conductive medium on an adhesive pad, are placed on various sites on the body and attached to cables or wires connected to an ECG machine or to a monitor. The cardiac electrical current is transmitted via the electrodes and through the lead wires to the machine or monitor, which displays the cardiac electrical activity.

A lead provides one view of the heart's electrical activity. Multiple leads, or views, can be obtained. Electrode placement is the same for male and female clients.

Lead systems are made up of a positive pole and a negative pole. An imaginary line joining these two poles is called the *lead axis*. The direction of electrical current flow in the heart is the *cardiac axis*. The relationship between the cardiac axis and the lead axis is responsible for the deflections seen on the ECG pattern:

- The baseline is the isoelectric line. It occurs when there is no current flow in the heart after complete depolarization and also after complete repolarization. Positive deflections occur above this line, and negative deflections occur below it. Deflections represent depolarization and repolarization of cells.
- If the direction of electrical current flow in the heart (cardiac axis) is parallel to the lead axis with the current moving toward the positive pole, a monophasic (single-component) positive deflection is inscribed (Fig. 36–4A).
- If the cardiac axis is parallel to the lead axis but the current is moving away from the positive pole, toward

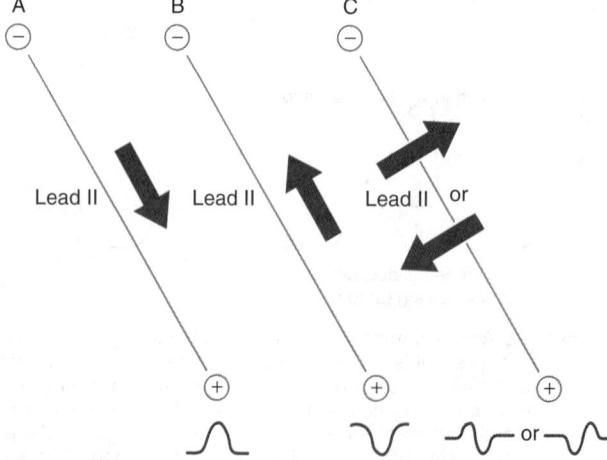

Figure 36–4. *A,* The cardiac axis (*bold arrow*) is parallel to the lead axis (the line between the negative and the positive electrodes), going toward the positive electrode; a positive deflection is inscribed. *B,* The cardiac axis is parallel to the lead axis, going toward the negative electrode; a negative deflection is inscribed. *C,* The cardiac axis is perpendicular to the lead axis, going neither toward the positive nor toward the negative electrode; a biphasic deflection is inscribed.

the negative pole, a monophasic negative deflection is inscribed (Fig. 36–4B).

- If the cardiac axis is exactly perpendicular to the lead axis, with the current crossing the lead axis, a biphasic (two-component) deflection is inscribed (Fig. 36–4C).

Lead Systems

The standard 12-lead ECG consists of 12 leads (or views) of the heart's electrical activity. Six of the leads are called limb leads because the electrodes are placed on the client's four limbs in the frontal plane. The remaining six leads are called chest (precordial) leads because the electrodes are placed on the client's chest in the horizontal plane (see Chap. 35).

Limb Leads

Standard bipolar limb leads consist of a positive and a negative electrode, which determine the lead axis, as well as a reference, or ground, electrode. Bipolar leads can be obtained by using a monitor with either three or five electrode cables, or a 12-lead ECG machine. Leads I, II, and III are bipolar leads (Table 36–1 and Chap. 35).

Unipolar limb leads consist of a positive electrode only. These leads can be obtained only by using a monitor with four or five electrode cables or a 12-lead ECG machine. The unipolar limb leads are leads aVR, aVL, and aVF, with "a" meaning augmented. "V" is a designation for a unipolar lead. The third letter denotes the positive electrode placement: "R" for right arm, "L" for left arm, and "F" for foot (left leg). The positive electrode is at one end of the lead axis. The other end is the center of the electrical field, at approximately the center of the heart (Table 36–1).

Chest Leads

Chest (precordial) leads are also unipolar, or V, leads and therefore can be obtained only from a monitor with five electrode cables or a 12-lead ECG machine, which usually has 10 electrode cables. There are six chest leads, determined by the placement of the chest electrode. The four limb electrodes are placed on the extremities, as designated on each electrode (right arm, left arm, right leg, and left leg). The fifth (chest) electrode on a monitor system is the positive, or exploring, electrode, and is placed in designated positions to obtain the desired chest lead (see Table 36–1).

TABLE 36–1

Electrode Placement for 12 Leads

Lead	Negative Electrode	Positive Electrode	Ground Electrode
I	Right arm, or under the right clavicle	Left arm, or under the left clavicle	Right leg, or lowest rib, left mid-clavicular line
II	Right arm, or under the right clavicle	Left leg, or lowest rib, left mid-clavicular line	Right leg, or under the left clavicle
III	Left arm, or under the left clavicle	Left leg, or lowest rib, left mid-clavicular line	Right leg, or under the right clavicle
aVR	Average potential of left arm (or under the left clavicle) and left leg (or lowest rib, left mid-clavicular line)	Right arm, or under the right clavicle	Right leg, or lowest rib, right mid-clavicular line
aVL	Average potential of right arm (or under the right clavicle) and left leg (or lowest rib, left mid-clavicular line)	Left arm, or under the left clavicle	Same as for aVR
aVF	Average potential of right arm (or under the right clavicle) and left arm (or under the left clavicle)	Left leg, or lowest rib, left mid-clavicular line	Same as for aVR
V_1	Average potential of right arm, left arm, and left leg	Fourth intercostal space (ICS), right sternal border	Same as for aVR
V_2	Same as for V_1	Fourth ICS, left sternal border	Same as for aVR
V_3	Same as for V_1	Midway between V_2 and V_4	Same as for aVR
V_4	Same as for V_1	Fifth ICS, left mid-clavicular line	Same as for aVR
V_5	Same as for V_1	Horizontal to V_4, left anterior axillary line	Same as for aVR
V_6	Same as for V_1	Horizontal to V_4, left mid-axillary line	Same as for aVR

The nurse instructs the female client with large breasts to displace and hold the left breast so that electrode position can be accurate.

Technicians are commonly trained to take 12-lead ECGs in all health care settings. It is imperative that the technician bring any suspected abnormality to the attention of a nurse or physician. A nurse may direct a technician to take a 12-lead ECG on a client experiencing chest pain to observe for diagnostic changes, but it is ultimately the physician's responsibility to interpret the ECG.

Continuous Electrocardiographic Monitoring

For continuous ECG monitoring, the electrodes are not placed on the client's limbs because movement of the extremities causes "noise," or motion artifact, on the ECG signal. The nurse places the electrodes on the client's trunk, a more stable area, to minimize such artifacts and to obtain a clearer signal. If the monitoring system provides five electrode cables, the nurse places the electrodes as follows:

- Right arm electrode just below the right clavicle
- Left arm electrode just below the left clavicle
- Right leg electrode on the lowest palpable rib, on the right midclavicular line
- Left leg electrode on the lowest palpable rib, on the left midclavicular line
- The fifth electrode placed to obtain one of the six chest leads

With this placement, the monitor lead select control may be changed to provide lead I, II, III, aVR, aVL, or aVF or one chest lead. The monitor automatically alters the polarity of the electrodes to provide the lead selected.

If the monitoring system provides only three electrode cables, the nurse places the right arm, the left arm, and the left leg electrodes as described. In this case, the lead select provides only lead I, II, or III.

The popular MCL$_1$ lead is a modified (M) bipolar chest (C) lead. It approximates the V$_1$ lead without requiring a five-electrode cable monitoring system because it is a bipolar lead system. To obtain MCL$_1$, the nurse places the negative electrode just below the left (L) midclavicle and the positive electrode in the V$_1$ position. The ground electrode may be placed anywhere but is usually placed under the right clavicle. The nurse uses this lead for bedside or telemetry monitoring to differentiate left from right electrical activity, such as left from right bundle branch block or left from right premature ventricular complexes (PVCs), and to differentiate certain supraventricular beats from ventricular ectopic beats. The MCL$_1$ lead provides a right-sided view of cardiac electrical activity.

Another bipolar lead, MCL$_6$, is frequently used. It can be achieved by placing the negative and ground electrodes as for MCL$_1$ and moving the positive electrode to the V$_6$ position. This approximates the V$_6$ lead and provides a left-sided view of cardiac electrical activity. It is used for the same reasons as MCL$_1$.

The clarity of continuous ECG monitor recordings is affected by skin preparation and electrode quality. To optimize signal transmission, the nurse or assistive nursing personnel (ANP) decrease skin impedance by cleaning the skin with soap and water. The nurse or ANP then shaves the area if it is hairy, wipes the electrode sites with an alcohol or other skin preparation pad, and dries the sites well. The gel on each electrode must be moist and fresh. The nurse or ANP attaches the electrode to the lead cable, rubs the skin briskly with a gauze square or a washcloth (facecloth) until the skin is slightly reddened, and then rolls the electrode onto the site for proper contact. This action rubs off surface cells and increases capillary blood flow to the area to improve transmission of electrical activity. The nurse or ANP ensures that the contact site does not have any lotion, tincture, or other substance on it that increases skin impedance. Electrodes cannot be placed on abraded or irritated skin or over scar tissue. The application of electrodes may be done by a nursing assistant under the direction of the nurse, who must determine which lead to select. The nurse assesses the quality of the ECG rhythm transmission to the monitoring system and is responsible for assessment and management of the client.

ECG cables may be attached directly to a wall-mounted monitor (a hard-wired system) if the client's activity is restricted to bed rest and sitting in a chair, as in a critical care unit. For an ambulatory client, the ECG cable is attached to a battery-operated transmitter (a telemetry system) held in a pouch worn by the client. The client's ECG is transmitted via antennae located in strategic places, usually in the ceiling, to a remote monitor. This device allows the client freedom of movement within a certain radius without losing transmission of the ECG.

In the acute care setting, some institutions employ monitor technicians. These technicians are educated in ECG rhythm interpretation and are responsible for watching a bank of monitors on a unit, printing ECG rhythm strips routinely and PRN, interpreting rhythms, and communicating with the nurse to report the client's rhythm and significant changes. This technical support is particularly helpful on a telemetry unit that does not have monitors at the bedside. The nurse is reasonably assured that the client's ECG rhythm is being monitored "continuously," though human nature dictates that some rhythms would not be observed by the technician. The nurse remains ultimately responsible for accurate ECG rhythm interpretation, as well as client assessment and management.

Some units have full-disclosure monitors, which continuously store a client's ECG rhythms in memory up to a maximum amount of time, allowing nurses and physicians to access and print these rhythms for more thorough assessment and management of clients with dysrhythmias.

Pre-hospital personnel, such as paramedics and EMTs with advanced training, frequently monitor a client's ECG rhythm at the scene and enroute to a health care facility. They function under medical direction and protocols but may also be in communication with a nurse.

Electrocardiographic Complexes, Segments, and Intervals

Complexes that make up a normal ECG consist of a P wave, a QRS complex, a T wave, and possibly a U wave. Segments include the PR segment, the ST segment, and the TP segment. Intervals include the PR interval, QRS duration, and the QT interval (Fig. 36–5).

The P Wave

The P wave is a deflection representing atrial depolarization. The morphologic configuration (shape) of the P wave may be a positive, negative, or biphasic deflection,

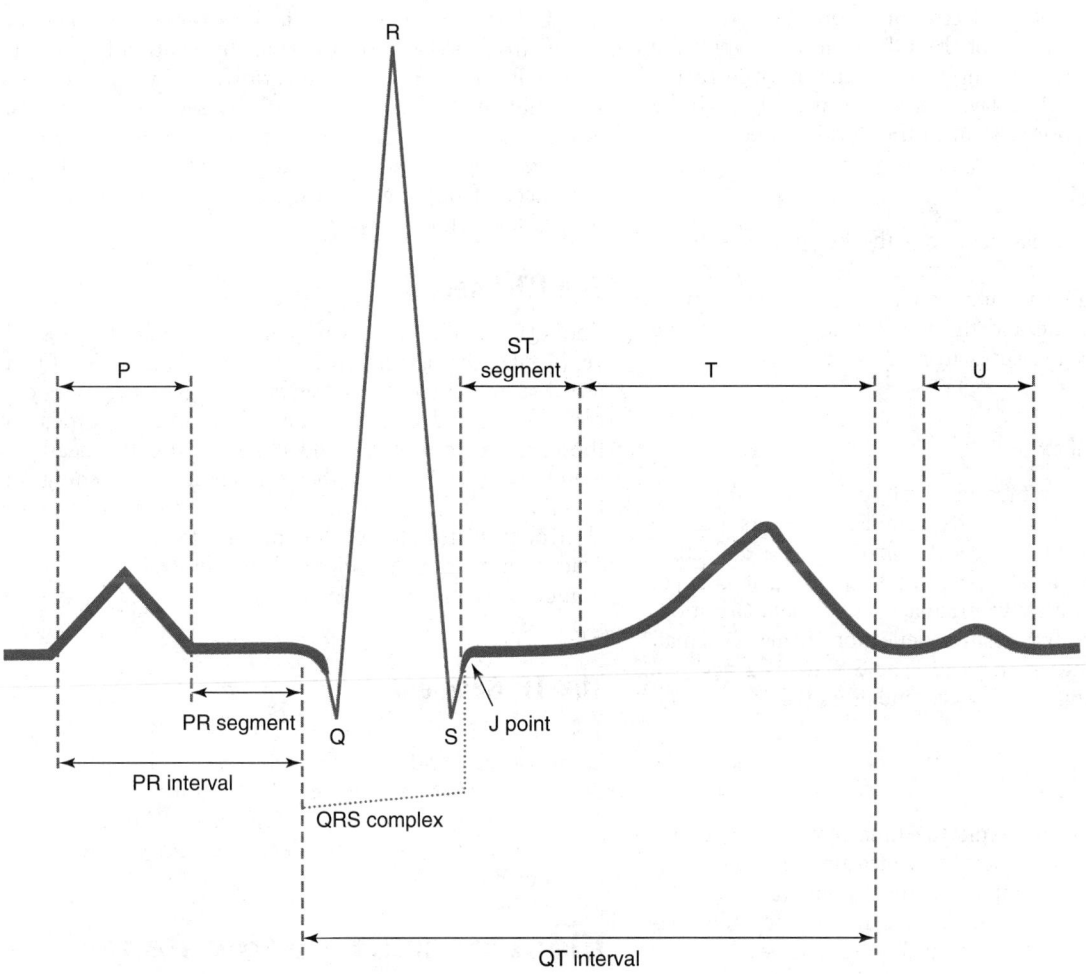

P wave:	Represents atrial depolarization.
PR segment:	Represents the time required for the impulse to travel through the AV node, where it is delayed, and through the bundle of His, bundle branches, and Purkinje fiber network, just before ventricular depolarization.
PR interval:	Represents the time required for atrial depolarization as well as impulse travel through the conduction system and Purkinje fiber network, inclusive of the P wave and PR segment. It is measured from the beginning of the P wave to the end of the PR segment.
QRS complex:	Represents ventricular depolarization and is measured from the beginning of the Q (or R) wave to the end of the S wave.
J point:	Represents the junction where the QRS complex ends and the ST segment begins.
ST segment:	Represents early ventricular repolarization.
T wave:	Represents ventricular repolarization.
U wave:	Represents late ventricular repolarization.
QT interval:	Represents the total time required for ventricular depolarization and repolarization and is measured from the beginning of the QRS complex to the end of the T wave.

Figure 36–5. The components of a normal electrocardiogram.

depending on the lead selected. When the electrical impulse is consistently generated from the SA node, the P waves have a consistent morphology in a given lead. If an impulse is then generated from a different (ectopic) focus, such as atrial tissue, the morphology of the P wave changes in that lead, indicating that an ectopic focus has fired.

The PR Segment

The PR segment is the isoelectric line from the end of the P wave to the beginning of the QRS complex, when the electrical impulse is traveling through the atrioventricular (AV) node, where it is delayed. It then travels through the ventricular conduction system to the Purkinje fibers.

The PR Interval

The PR interval is measured from the beginning of the P wave to the end of the PR segment. It represents the time required for atrial depolarization as well as the impulse delay in the AV node and the travel time to the Purkinje fibers. It normally measures from 0.12 to 0.20 second in duration.

The QRS Complex

The QRS complex represents ventricular depolarization. The morphology of the QRS complex depends on the lead selected. The Q wave is the first negative deflection and is not present in all leads. When present, it is small and represents initial ventricular septal depolarization. The R wave is the first positive deflection. It may be small or large, depending on the lead. The S wave is a negative deflection following the R wave and is not present in all leads.

The QRS Duration

The QRS duration represents the time required for depolarization of both ventricles. It is measured from the beginning of the QRS complex to the J-point (the junction where the QRS complex ends and the ST segment begins). It normally measures from 0.04 to 0.10 second.

The ST Segment

The ST segment is normally an isoelectric line and represents early ventricular repolarization. It occurs from the J-point to the beginning of the T wave. Its length varies with changes in the heart rate, the administration of medications, and electrolyte disturbances. It is normally not elevated more than 1 mm or depressed more than 0.5 mm from the isoelectric line as seen in the TP segment. Its amplitude is measured at a point 1.5 to 2 mm after the J-point. It is affected by myocardial ischemia or infarction, conduction abnormalities, and the administration of medications.

The T Wave

The T wave follows the ST segment and represents ventricular repolarization. It is usually positive, rounded, and slightly asymmetric. If an ectopic stimulus excites the ventricles during this time, it may cause ventricular irritability and possible cardiac arrest in the vulnerable heart. This is known as the *R-on-T phenomenon*. T waves may become tall and peaked, inverted (negative), or flat as a result of myocardial ischemia, potassium or calcium imbalances, administered medications, or autonomic nervous system effects.

The U Wave

The U wave, when present, follows the T wave and may result from slow repolarization of ventricular Purkinje fibers. It is of the same polarity as T waves, although generally smaller. It is not normally seen in all leads and is more common in lead V_3. Abnormal prominence of the U wave suggests an electrolyte abnormality or other disturbance. Identifying it correctly is important so that it is not mistaken for a P wave.

The QT Interval

The QT interval represents the total time required for ventricular depolarization and repolarization. The QT interval is measured from the beginning of the QRS complex to the end of the T wave. This interval varies with the client's age and sex and changes with the heart rate; lengthening with slower heart rates and shortening with faster rates. It may be prolonged by certain medications, electrolyte disturbances, Prinzmetal's angina, or subarachnoid hemorrhage. A prolonged QT interval may lead to a unique type of ventricular tachycardia called torsades de pointes.

The TP Segment

The TP segment is the isoelectric line following the T (or U) wave and ending with the next P wave. During this time, all cardiac cells are at their resting membrane potential, and there is no current flow. The TP segment lengthens as the heart rate decreases and shortens as the rate increases.

Electrocardiographic Paper

The ECG strip is printed on graph paper (Fig. 36–6), with each small block measuring 1 mm in height and width. ECG recorders and monitors are standardized at a speed of 25 mm/second. Time is measured on the horizontal axis. At this speed, each small block represents 0.04 second. Five small blocks make up one large block, defined by darker bold lines and representing 0.20 second. Five large blocks represent 1 second, whereas 30 large blocks represent 6 seconds. Vertical lines in the top margin of the graph paper are usually 15 large blocks apart, representing 3-second segments (Fig. 36–7).

Determination of Heart Rate

The heart rate may be estimated by counting the number of P-P intervals (atrial rate) or R-R intervals (ventricular rate) in 6 seconds and multiplying that number by 10 to calculate the rate for a full minute (Fig. 36–8). For accuracy, timing should begin on the P wave or the QRS

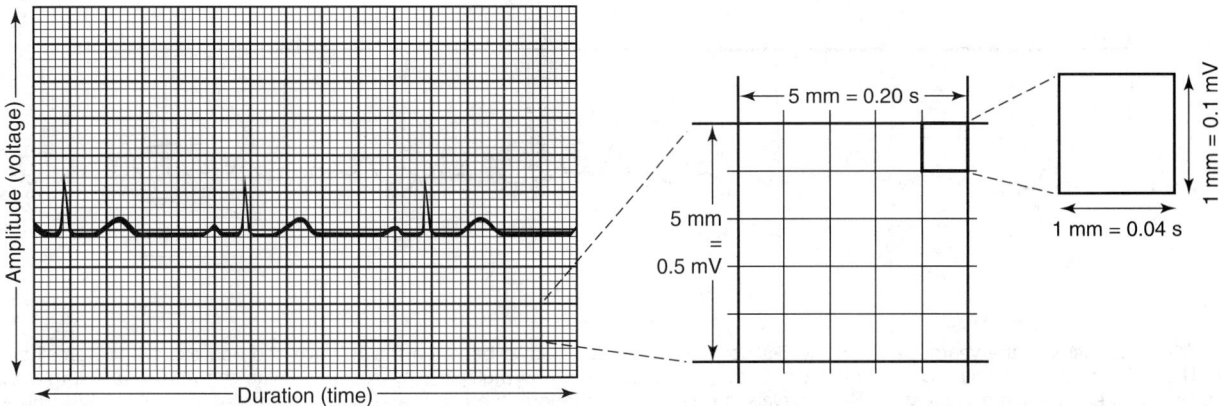

Figure 36–6. ECG waveforms are measured in amplitude (voltage) and duration (time).

complex and end exactly 30 large blocks (150 small blocks) later. The initial complex is the reference point and counts as zero. Subsequent complexes are counted until the end of 6 seconds, to include a fraction of the last interval: for example, if there are exactly seven R-R intervals, the heart rate is 70 beats per minute; if there are 9½ intervals, the heart rate is 95 beats per minute. This method may be used for both regular and irregular rhythms. It is called the 6-second strip method.

Another method, which may be used *only* if the rhythm is regular, relies on either of the following mathematic calculations:

- Count the number of small blocks in a P-P or R-R interval and divide into 1500 (the number of small blocks in 1 minute). For example, 20 small blocks equals a heart rate of 75 beats per minute (1500/20 = 75).
- Count the number of large blocks in an interval and divide into 300 (the number of large blocks in 1 minute). For example, three large blocks equals a heart rate of 100 beats per minute (300/3 = 100).

Commercially prepared ECG rate rulers are based on these calculations and may be used for regular rhythms.

Electrocardiographic Rhythm Analysis

Analysis of an ECG rhythm strip requires a systematic approach and is facilitated by the use of an ECG caliper (Chart 36–1):

1. *Analyze the P waves.* The nurse checks that the P wave morphology (shape) is consistent throughout the strip, indicating that atrial depolarization is occurring from impulses originating from one focus, normally the sinoatrial (SA) node. The nurse determines whether there is one P wave occurring before each QRS complex, establishing that a relationship exists between the P wave and the QRS complex. This relationship indicates that impulses from one focus are responsible for both atrial and ventricular depolarization. The nurse may observe more than one P wave shape, or more P waves than QRS

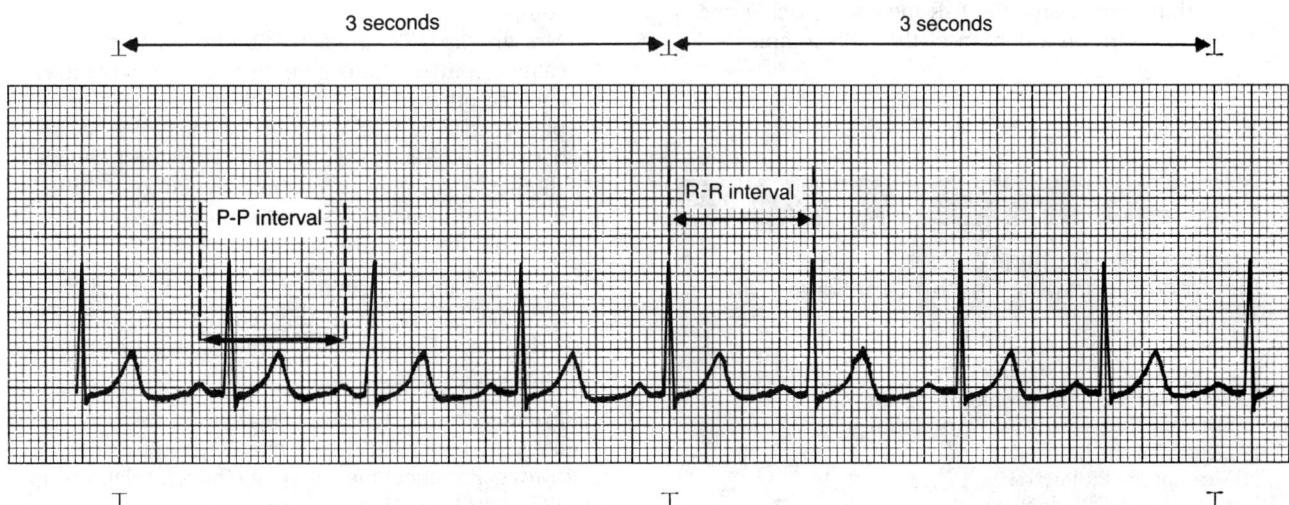

Figure 36–7. Each segment between the dark lines (above the monitor strip) represents 3 seconds, when the monitor is set at a speed of 25 mm/second.

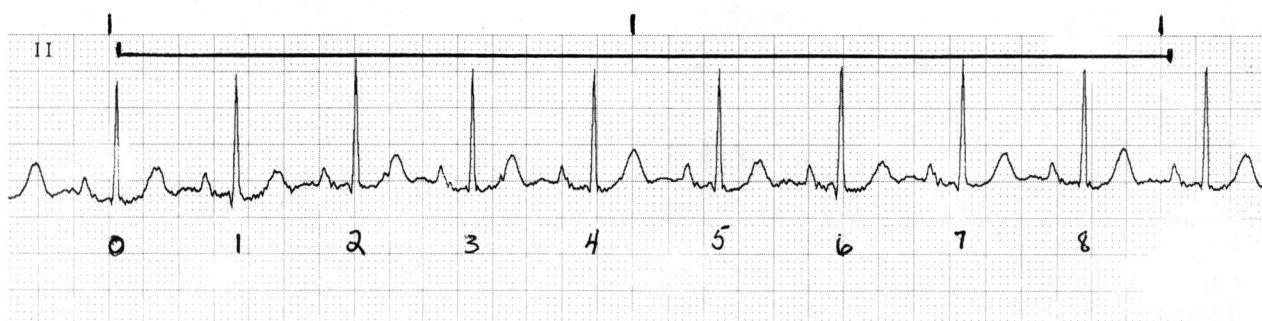

Figure 36–8. To estimate the ventricular rate, the 6-second timing is adjusted to begin on the R wave and end exactly 150 small blocks later. The R-R intervals are counted in the 6-second strip, and that number is multiplied by 10 to estimate the rate for a full minute. In this example, there are approximately 8¾ R-R intervals in 6 seconds. Therefore, the heart rate can be estimated to be 87 or 88/minute.

complexes, or absent P waves, or P waves coming after the QRS, each indicating that a dysrhythmia exists.

2. *Analyze the QRS complexes.* The nurse checks that the QRS complex morphology is consistent throughout the strip. The nurse may observe more than one QRS complex morphologic pattern or occasionally missing QRS complexes, indicating a dysrhythmia.

3. *Determine the atrial rhythm or regularity.* The nurse checks the regularity of the atrial rhythm by assessing the P-P intervals, placing one caliper point on a P wave and the other point on the next P wave. Then the caliper is moved from P wave to P wave along the entire strip ("walking out" the P waves) to determine the regularity of the rhythm. P waves of a different morphology (ectopic waves), if present, create an irregularity and do not walk out with the other P waves. A slight irregularity in the P-P intervals, varying no more than three small blocks, is considered essentially regular if the P waves are all of the same morphology.

4. *Determine the ventricular rhythm or regularity.* The nurse checks the regularity of the ventricular rhythm by assessing the R-R intervals, placing one caliper point on a portion of the QRS complex

(usually the most prominent portion of the deflection) and the other point on the same portion of the next QRS complex. The caliper is then moved from QRS complex to QRS complex along the entire strip (walking out the QRS complexes) to determine the regularity of the rhythm. QRS complexes of a different morphology (ectopic QRS complexes), if present, create an irregularity and do not walk out with the other QRS complexes. A slight irregularity of no more than three small blocks between intervals is considered essentially regular if the QRS complexes are all of the same morphology.

5. *Determine the heart rate.* If the atrial and ventricular rhythms are regular, the nurse may use any of the methods previously described to calculate the heart rate. If the rhythms are irregular, the nurse must use the 6-second strip method for accuracy.

6. *Measure the PR interval.* The nurse places one caliper point at the beginning of the P wave and the other point at the end of the PR segment. The PR interval normally measures between 0.12 and 0.20 second. The measurement should be constant throughout the strip. It cannot be measured if there are no P waves or if P waves occur after the QRS complex.

7. *Measure the QRS duration.* The nurse places one caliper point at the beginning of the QRS complex and the other at the J-point, where the QRS complex ends. The QRS duration normally measures between 0.04 and 0.10 second. The measurement should be constant throughout the entire strip.

8. *Interpret the rhythm.* Using accepted rules, the nurse can now interpret the cardiac rhythm.

These steps can be reorganized and formatted as the basis for rules or criteria to differentiate normal and abnormal rhythms. The following format is used to describe electrocardiographic criteria:

> *Rhythm:* Atrial and ventricular rhythms
> *Rate:* Atrial and ventricular rates
> *P waves:* Presence, morphology (shape), relationship to QRS complexes
> *PR interval:* Measurement and constancy
> *QRS duration:* Measurement and constancy

Chart 36–1

Nursing Care Highlight:
Electrocardiographic Rhythm Analysis

1. Analyze the P waves.
2. Analyze the QRS complexes.
3. Determine the atrial rhythm or regularity.
4. Determine the ventricular rhythm or regularity.
5. Determine the heart rate.
6. Measure the PR interval.
7. Measure the QRS duration.
8. Interpret the rhythm.

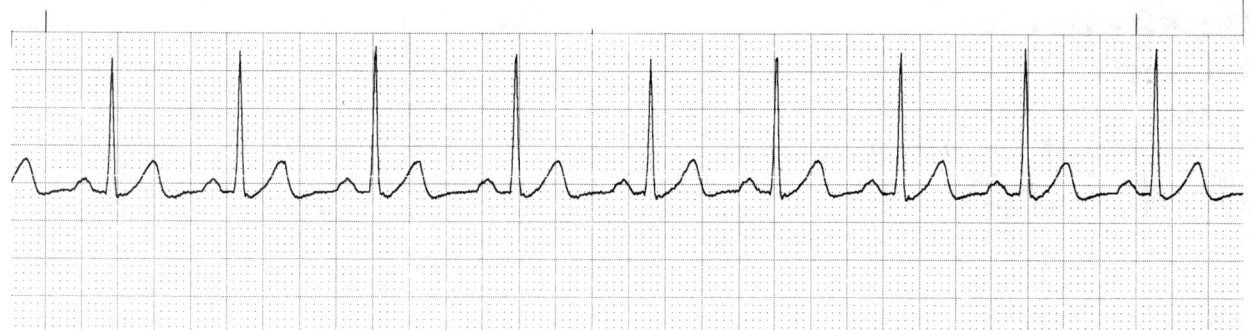

Figure 36–9. Normal sinus rhythm (NSR). Both atrial and ventricular rhythms are essentially regular (a slight variation in rhythm is normal). Atrial and ventricular rates are both 83/minute. There is one P wave before each QRS complex, and all the P waves are of a consistent morphology or shape. The PR interval measures 0.18 second and is constant; the QRS complex measures 0.06 second and is constant.

NORMAL RHYTHMS
Normal Sinus Rhythm

Normal sinus rhythm (NSR) is the rhythm originating from the sinoatrial node (dominant pacemaker) that meets the following electrocardiographic (ECG) criteria (Fig. 36–9):

Rhythm: Atrial and ventricular rhythms regular

Rate: Atrial and ventricular rates 60 to 100 beats per minute

P waves: Present, consistent morphologic configuration, one P wave before each QRS complex

PR interval: 0.12 to 0.20 second and constant

QRS duration: 0.04 to 0.10 second and constant

Sinus Arrhythmia

Sinus arrhythmia is a variant of normal sinus rhythm. It results from changes in intrathoracic pressure during breathing. In this context, the term *arrhythmia* does not denote an absence of rhythm, as the term suggests. Instead, the heart rate increases slightly during inspiration and decreases slightly during expiration. This irregular rhythm is frequently observed in healthy children as well as adults.

Sinus arrhythmia has all the characteristics of normal sinus rhythm, except for its irregularity. The P-P and R-R intervals vary, with the difference between the shortest and the longest intervals greater than 0.12 second (three small blocks) (Fig. 36-10):

Rhythm: Atrial and ventricular rhythms irregular, with the shortest P-P or R-R interval varying at least 0.12 second from the longest P-P or R-R interval

Rate: Atrial and ventricular rates normal or less than 60 beats per minute

P waves: One P wave before each QRS complex, consistent morphologic configuration

PR interval: Normal, constant

QRS duration: Normal, constant

Sinus arrhythmias may occasionally be due to nonrespiratory causes, such as the administration of digitalis or morphine. These drugs enhance vagal tone and cause decreased heart rate and irregularity unrelated to the respiratory cycle.

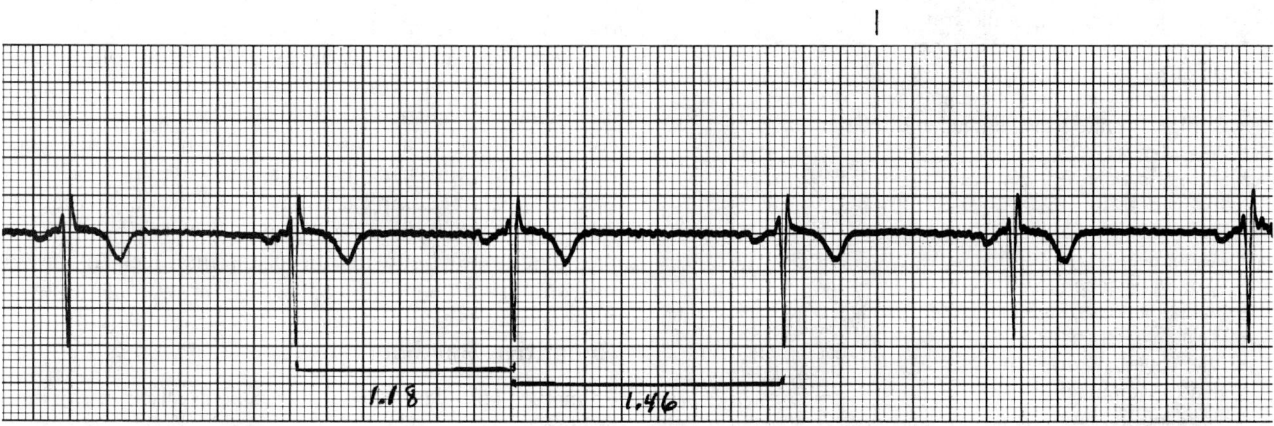

Figure 36–10. Sinus arrhythmia, considered normal, with sinus bradycardia, heart rate 46/minute. All the P waves have the same morphology, indicating that they are all from the sinus node. The rhythm is irregular, with the shortest RR interval (1.18 seconds) varying more than 0.12 second from the longest RR interval (1.46 seconds).

DYSRHYTHMIAS
Overview

Any disorder of the heartbeat is termed "dysrhythmia." Historically, the term "arrhythmia" has been used in the literature; however, it means an absence of cardiac rhythm. Although the terms are often used interchangeably, dysrhythmia, which means a disturbance in cardiac rhythm, is more accurate.

Dysrhythmias result from a disturbance in impulse formation (either from an abnormal rate or from an ectopic focus), from a disturbance in impulse conduction (delays and blocks), or from both mechanisms. Although many dysrhythmias have no clinical manifestations, many others have serious consequences. A summary is provided in Chart 36–2.

Dysrhythmia Terminology
Tachydysrhythmias

Tachydysrhythmias are heart rates greater than 100 beats per minute (BPM) in adults and older children or above the normal range for heart rates in infants and young children. These rhythms may have serious hemodynamic consequences in the adult client with coronary artery disease (CAD). Coronary artery blood flow occurs predominantly during diastole, when the aortic valve is closed, and is determined by diastolic time and blood pressure in the root of the aorta. The nurse must understand three important points to appreciate the seriousness of tachydysrhythmias in adults:

- Tachydysrhythmias shorten the diastolic time and therefore the coronary perfusion time (the amount of time

available for blood to flow through the coronary arteries to the myocardium).
- Tachydysrhythmias initially increase cardiac output and blood pressure. However, a continued rise in heart rate decreases the ventricular filling time because of a shortened diastole, decreasing the stroke volume. Consequently, at some point, cardiac output and blood pressure begin to decrease, reducing aortic pressure and therefore coronary perfusion pressure.
- Tachydysrhythmias increase the work of the heart, increasing myocardial oxygen demand.

The adult client with a tachydysrhythmia could present with palpitations, chest discomfort, pressure or pain from myocardial ischemia or infarction, restlessness, anxiety, and syncope from hypotension, along with pale, cool skin. Tachydysrhythmias may also lead to heart failure in adults, children, or infants. The client may present with dyspnea, orthopnea, pulmonary crackles, distended neck veins, fatigue, and weakness.

Bradydysrhythmias

Bradydysrhythmias are heart rates less than 60 beats per minute in adults and older children or below the normal range for heart rates in infants and young children. These rhythms can have serious hemodynamic consequences. The nurse considers the following three points:

- Coronary perfusion time is adequate because of a prolonged diastole. This is desirable.
- Coronary perfusion pressure may decrease if the heart rate is too slow to provide adequate cardiac output and blood pressure. This is a serious consequence.
- Myocardial oxygen demand is reduced from the slow heart rate. This is beneficial.

Therefore, the client may tolerate the bradydysrhythmia well if the blood pressure is adequate. If the blood pressure is not adequate, symptomatic bradydysrhythmias may lead to myocardial ischemia or infarction, dysrhythmias, hypotension, and heart failure.

Premature Complexes

Premature complexes are early complexes. They occur when a cardiac tissue, other than the sinoatrial node, becomes irritable and fires an impulse prematurely before the next sinus impulse is generated. This abnormal focus is called an *ectopic focus* and may be generated by atrial, junctional, or ventricular tissue. Following the premature complex, there is a pause before the next normal complex, creating an irregularity in the rhythm. The client with premature complexes may be unaware of them or may feel palpitations or a "skipping" of the heartbeat. If palpitations are frequent, the client may feel anxious or concerned.

Repetitive Rhythms

Premature complexes may occur repetitively in a rhythmic fashion.

- *Bigeminy* exists when normal complexes and premature complexes occur alternately in a repetitive two-beat pat-

---

Chart 36–2

Key Features of Sustained Tachydysrhythmias and Bradydysrhythmias

- Chest discomfort, pressure, or pain, which may radiate to the jaw, the back, or the arm
- Restlessness, anxiety, nervousness, confusion
- Dizziness, syncope
- Palpitations (in tachydysrhythmias)
- Change in pulse strength, rate, and rhythm
- Pulse deficit
- Shortness of breath, dyspnea
- Tachypnea
- Pulmonary crackles
- Orthopnea
- S_2 or S_4 heart sounds
- Jugular venous distention
- Weakness, fatigue
- Pale, cool skin; diaphoresis
- Nausea, vomiting
- Decreased urinary output
- Delayed capillary refill
- Hypotension

tern, with a pause occurring after each premature complex so that complexes occur in pairs.

- *Trigeminy* is a repetitive three-beat pattern, usually occurring as two sequential normal complexes followed by a premature complex and a pause, with the same pattern repeating itself in triplets.
- *Quadrigeminy* is a repetitive four-beat pattern, usually occurring as three sequential normal complexes followed by a premature complex and a pause, with the same pattern repeating itself in a four-beat pattern.

Such patterns may occur with atrial, junctional, or ventricular premature complexes. Clients may be unaware of the premature beats or may feel palpitations.

Escape Complexes and Rhythms

Escape complexes or escape rhythms may occur when the sinoatrial (SA) node fails to discharge or is blocked or when a sinus impulse fails to depolarize the ventricles because of an atrioventricular (AV) nodal block. Escape complexes or rhythms serve as a subsidiary or escape pacemaker and are seen after a pause. Such impulses may originate from AV junctional or ventricular tissue. They cease when the SA node or the AV node regains the ability to function normally. If there are pauses followed by escape beats or rhythms, clients may feel lightheaded, dizzy, or faint during the pause.

Classification of Dysrhythmias

Dysrhythmias are classified according to their site of origin. The sites include sinus, atrial, junctional, ventricular, and AV nodal tissue. Dysrhythmias may be caused by a disturbance in impulse formation or by conduction delays or blocks. The incidence and the prevalence of dysrhythmias are not precisely known because they usually result from an underlying condition, such as heart disease. The incidence of dysrhythmias increases with age. A summary of the common dysrhythmias and their treatment is provided in Table 36–2.

Sinus Dysrhythmias

The sinus node is the pacemaker in all sinus dysrhythmias. Sympathetic and parasympathetic nerve fibers are distributed to the SA node. Innervation from these two systems is normally in balance to ensure a normal sinus rhythm. An imbalance increases or decreases the rate of SA node discharge either as a normal response to activity or physiologic changes or as a pathologic response to illness.

Sinus Tachycardia

Pathophysiology

Dominant sympathetic nervous system stimulation of the heart or vagal inhibition results in an increased rate of SA node discharge, which increases the heart rate (positive chronotropic effect).

When the rate of SA node discharge exceeds 100 beats per minute, the rhythm is called sinus tachycardia (Fig. 36–11A). Sinus tachycardia is normal in infants and chil-

dren, with the rate gradually decreasing until age 10 years. From 10 years to adulthood, the resting rate normally does not exceed 100 beats per minute except in response to activity and then usually does not exceed 160. Rarely, the resting rate may reach 180 beats per minute. Heart rates in infants and young children may reach 200 to 220 beats per minute. Sinus tachycardia initially enhances cardiac output and blood pressure. However, excessive increases in heart rate decrease coronary perfusion time and coronary perfusion pressure, while increasing myocardial oxygen demand.

Electrocardiographic criteria include

> *Rhythm:* Atrial and ventricular rhythms regular
> *Rate:* Atrial and ventricular rates 100 to 180 beats per minute in adults and up to 220 beats per minute in infants and young children
> *P waves:* One P wave before each QRS complex, consistent morphologic configuration. P waves may encroach on preceding T waves
> *PR interval:* Normal, constant
> *QRS duration:* Normal, constant

Etiology

Increased sympathetic stimulation is a normal response to physical activity but may also be caused by anxiety, pain, stress, fear, fever, anemia, hypoxemia, hyperthyroidism, pulmonary embolus, and the administration of drugs such as catecholamines, atropine, caffeine, alcohol, nicotine, aminophylline, and thyroid drugs. Sinus tachycardia may also be a compensatory response to decreased cardiac output or blood pressure, as occurs in hypovolemia, shock, myocardial infarction, and heart failure. Common causes in infants and children include fever, anxiety, pain, anemia, and dehydration.

Physical Assessment/Clinical Manifestations

The client may be asymptomatic except for the increased pulse rate. However, if the rhythm is not well tolerated, the client may become symptomatic. The nurse assesses the client for fatigue, weakness, shortness of breath, orthopnea, neck vein distention, decreased oxygen saturation, and decreased blood pressure. The nurse also assesses for restlessness and anxiety from decreased cerebral perfusion and for decreased urinary output from decreased renal perfusion. The adult client may experience anginal pain. The electrocardiographic (ECG) pattern may show T-wave inversion or ST-segment elevation or depression in response to myocardial ischemia. During sinus tachycardia, the TP segment shortens.

Interventions

The nurse and the physician collaborate to identify the cause of sinus tachycardia and select the appropriate treatment. The goal is to decrease the heart rate to normal levels by treating the underlying cause. For example, if the client has angina, the nurse administers oxygen, assists the client to rest, and administers nitroglycerin or morphine as prescribed. The nurse administers diuretics and inotropic agents to the client in heart failure, initiates intravascular volume replacement for the hypovolemic cli-

TABLE 36–2

Common Dysrhythmias and Their Treatment

Dysrhythmia	Treatment*	Dysrhythmia	Treatment*
Sinus tachycardia	• Correction of the underlying problem (e.g., fever, hypovolemia, pain, anxiety, and CHF) • Beta-adrenergic blockade if increased catecholamine secretion is the underlying problem	**Premature Beats and Ectopic Rhythms** *Continued*	• Digitalis • Propranolol • Esmolol • Quinidine • Procainamide • Vagal stimulation with carotid massage • Valsalva maneuvers • Overdrive atrial pacing • Synchronized cardioversion if the above measures are unsuccessful

Sinus bradycardia	• Treatment necessary only if the client is symptomatic (has hypotension, diaphoresis, chest discomfort or pain, pulmonary congestion, or altered level of consciousness);
	  • Atropine
	  • Pacemaker
	  • Avoidance of parasympathetic stimulation, such as prolonged suctioning and stimulation of the gag reflex
		Premature ventricular complexes and ventricular tachycardia (not sustained)	• Correction of any underlying problem (e.g., infection, electrolyte imbalance, effects of drugs, myocardial infarction, CHF, stress, fatigue, and nicotine)
			• Medication administration
			  • Lidocaine bolus and infusion
			  • Procainamide bolus and infusion
			  • Bretylium tosylate bolus and infusion
			  • Magnesium sulfate infusion
			  • Class I and II antidysrhythmics
			  • Amiodarone
			• Restoration of electrolyte balance

Premature Beats and Ectopic Rhythms			

Supraventricular beats (PACs, PJCs)	• Correction of any underlying problem (e.g., anxiety, stress, caffeine and nicotine intake, CFH, effects of drugs, and CAL)
	• Medication administration
	  • Quinidine
	  • Procainamide
	  • Digitalis
	  • Propranolol
	  • Sedatives		

Supraventricular rhythms	• Correction of any underlying problem (e.g., CHF, CAL, stress, and drugs)
	• Medication administration
	  • Verapamil
	  • Diltiazem
	  • Adenosine
		Atrial flutter	• Medication administration
			  • Diltiazem
			  • Verapamil
			  • Digitalis
			  • Propranolol

ent, administers antipyretics and antibiotics to the client with fever and infection, or provides comfort measures and administers analgesics or opioids to the client with noncardiac pain.

The nurse collaborates with the respiratory therapist when indicated to oxygenate and suction the client with hypoxemia from excessive airway secretions. The nurse administers beta-adrenergic–blocking agents when prescribed for the client with inappropriate sympathetic nervous system stimulation. The nurse provides emotional support and relevant teaching to the client and family and administers antianxiety agents for clients who are anxious.

Sinus Bradycardia

Pathophysiology

Dominance of the parasympathetic nervous system, with excessive vagal stimulation to the heart, causes a de-

creased rate of sinus node discharge. This slows the heart rate and decreases the speed of conduction through the AV node and conduction system. When the rate of sinus node discharge is less than 60 beats per minute in adults or below the normal range in infants and children, the rhythm is called *sinus bradycardia* (see Fig. 36–11B). Sinus bradycardia increases coronary perfusion time but may decrease coronary perfusion pressure. However, myocardial oxygen demand is decreased. Sinus bradycardia is not normal in infants and young children and may be an ominous sign.

Electrocardiographic criteria include

Rhythm: Atrial and ventricular rhythms regular
Rate: Atrial and ventricular rates less than 60 beats per minute in adults or less than the normal range in infants and children
P waves: One P wave before each QRS complex, consistent morphologic configuration

TABLE 36-2

Common Dysrhythmias and Their Treatment *Continued*

Dysrhythmia	Treatment*	Dysrhythmia	Treatment*
Premature Beats and Ectopic Rhythms *Continued*		**Conduction Delays** *Continued*	
	• Esmolol • Quinidine • Procainamide • Atrial overdrive pacing • Cardioversion • Catheter or surgical ablation	Second-degree AV block type II	• Pacemaker • Isoproterenol administration if pacemaker unavailable

Atrial fibrillation	• Medication administration
	  • Digitalis
	  • Diltiazem
	  • Verapamil
	  • Quinidine
	  • Procainamide
	• Anticoagulation
	• Atrial overdrive pacing
	• Cardioversion
	• Surgery
		Third-degree AV block	• Pacemaker
			• Isoproterenol administration if pacemaker unavailable

		Life-Threatening Dysrhythmias	

		Sustained ventricular tachycardia	• Medication administration
			  • Lidocaine bolus and infusion
			  • Procainamide bolus and infusion
			  • Bretylium tosylate bolus and infusion
			  • Magnesium sulfate infusion
			• If unstable: synchronized cardioversion
			• If pulseless: defibrillation, CPR

Escape beats and rhythms	• Correction of the underlying cause if the client is symptomatic
	• Atropine administration
	• Pacemaker
	• Isoproterenol administration if pacemaker unavailable
		Ventricular fibrillation	• Defibrillation
			• CPR
			• Medication administration
			  • Epinephrine
			  • Lidocaine
			  • Bretylium tosylate
			  • Procainamide
			  • Magnesium sulfate

Conduction Delays			

First-degree AV block	• Treatment necessary only if the client is symptomatic
	• Withhold digitalis (if the cause)
	• Atropine administration if block is associated with symptomatic bradycardia
		Ventricular asystole	• CPR
			• Medication administration
			  • Epinephrine
			  • Atropine
			  • Pacemaker

Second-degree AV block type I	• Same as for first-degree AV block		

*CHF, congestive heart failure; CAL, chronic airway limitation.

PR interval: Normal, constant
QRS duration: Normal, constant

Etiology

Increased parasympathetic stimulation of the heart by the vagus nerve is a normal response to decreased physical activity. It also often occurs in well-conditioned athletes because the strong heart muscle is extremely efficient in providing an adequate stroke volume while not requiring a higher heart rate for a normal cardiac output. Excessive vagal stimulation may result from carotid sinus massage, vomiting, suctioning, Valsalva maneuvers such as bearing down for a bowel movement or gagging, inferior myocardial infarction, ocular pressure, pain, and hypothyroidism. Sinus bradycardia may also result from the administration of drugs such as beta-adrenergic–blocking agents, calcium channel blockers, and digitalis. In infants and children, sinus bradycardia may be due to hypervagal tone but may also occur with cardiac disease or as a late response to hypoxia, acidosis, and hypotension, when it may be an ominous sign.

Physical Assessment/Clinical Manifestations

The client may be asymptomatic, except for the decreased pulse rate. However, at times the rhythm may not be well tolerated. The nurse assesses the client for dizziness, weakness, syncope, confusion, hypotension, diaphoresis, shortness of breath, and ventricular ectopy. Infants and children may become listless and lethargic. The adult client may experience anginal pain; T-wave inversion or ST-segment elevation or depression may occur in response to myocardial ischemia.

Interventions

In the adult, the treatment of choice for the client with a symptomatic sinus bradycardia is atropine administration. The nurse administers oxygen and atropine as prescribed to increase the client's heart rate to approximately 60 beats per minute. If the heart rate does not increase sufficiently, the nurse may apply a noninvasive pacemaker to increase the heart rate and notifies the physician. However, if atropine administration succeeds in achieving an

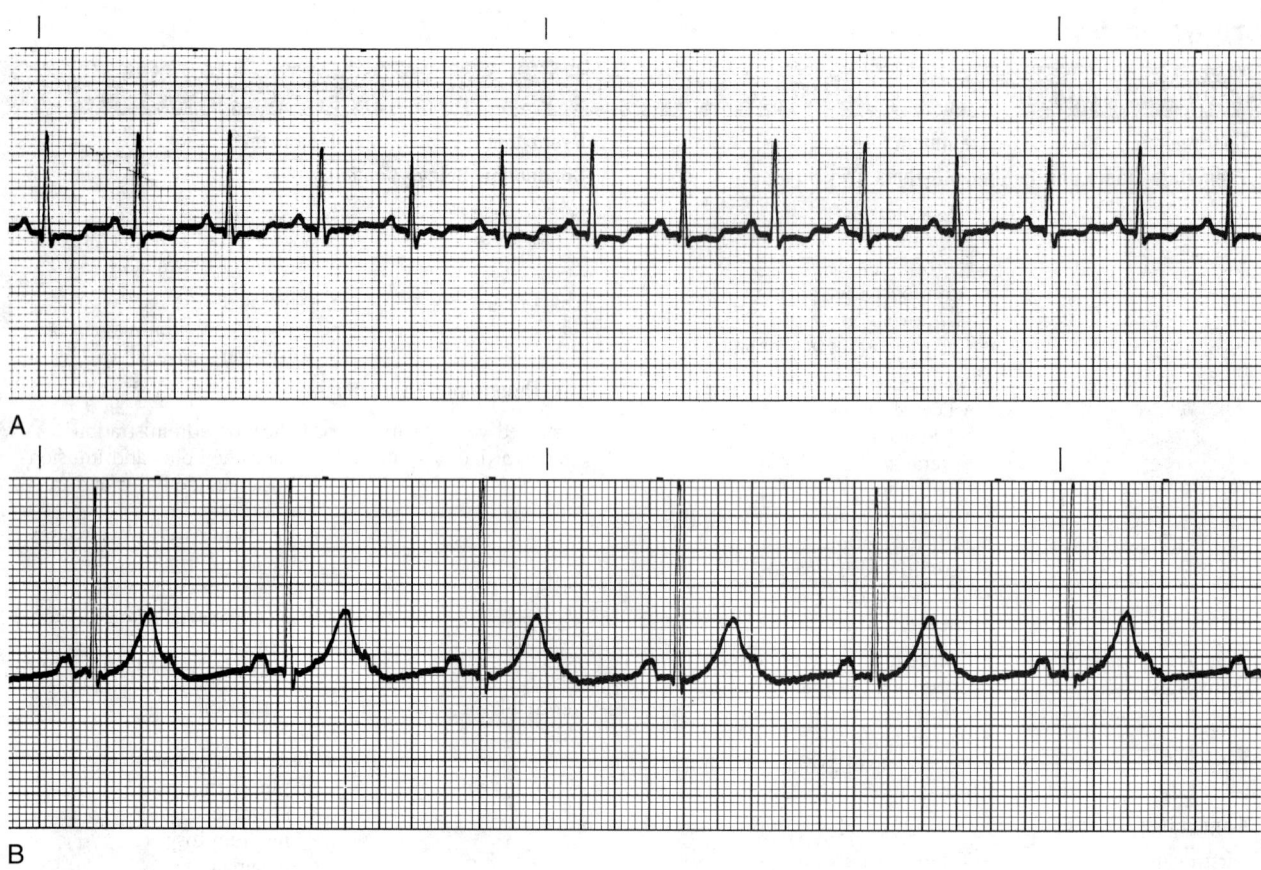

Figure 36–11. Sinus rhythms. *A*, Sinus tachycardia (HR = 110/minute, PR = 0.12 second, QRS = 0.08 second). *B*, Sinus bradycardia (HR = 52/minute, PR = 0.18 second, QRS = 0.08 second).

adequate heart rate but the client remains hypotensive, the nurse initiates intravascular volume replacement as ordered rather than administering another dose of atropine, because excessive atropine may induce tachycardia. If an offending drug is determined to be the cause, the nurse withholds the drug and notifies the physician for an order to discontinue the drug temporarily or permanently. Sinus bradycardia in infants and children may respond to oxygen administration and correction of acidosis and hypovolemia. Administration of atropine may be warranted for hypervagal tone.

Atrial Dysrhythmias

With atrial dysrhythmias, the focus of impulse generation has shifted away from the sinus node to the atrial tissue, which now acts as an ectopic pacemaker, for one or more beats. This shift changes the axis (direction) of atrial depolarization, resulting in a P-wave morphology that differs from that of P waves from sinus node origin.

Premature Atrial Complexes

Pathophysiology

A premature atrial complex (PAC or APC) occurs when atrial tissue becomes irritable, and this ectopic focus fires an impulse before the next sinus impulse is due, thus

usurping the sinus pacemaker (Fig. 36–12). The premature P wave from the atrial focus is early and has a morphology different from the P waves generated from the sinus focus. The premature P wave may not always be clearly visible, as it is often hidden in the preceding T wave. The T wave must be closely examined for any change in shape and compared with other T waves, to reveal a hidden P wave.

Electrocardiographic criteria include

Rhythm: The underlying sinus rhythm usually regular, unless sinus arrhythmia is present. Atrial and ventricular rhythms become irregular because of the early beat. There is a pause after the PAC

Rate: May be any rate, depending on underlying sinus rhythm. Atrial and ventricular rates are usually equal

P waves: One P wave before each QRS complex. Sinus P waves have one consistent morphologic pattern. The premature atrial P wave is early with a different morphologic configuration

PR interval: Normal and constant for sinus beats, normal or prolonged for PAC

QRS duration: Usually normal and constant

Etiology

The causes of atrial irritability include stress; fatigue; anxiety; inflammation; infection; intake of caffeine, nicotine,

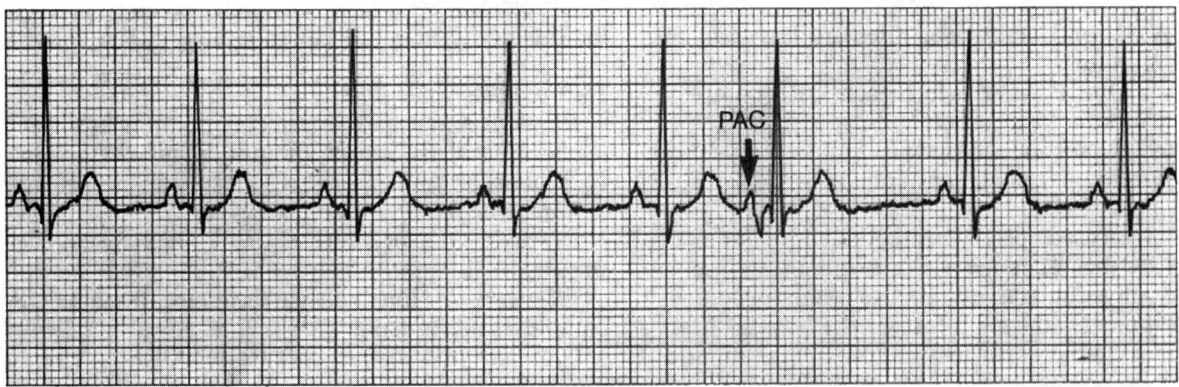

Figure 36–12. Atrial dysrhythmias. Normal sinus rhythm (NSR) with a premature atrial complex (PAC) at arrow.

and alcohol; and the administration of drugs such as digitalis, catecholamines, sympathomimetics, amphetamines, and anesthetic agents. PACs may also result from myocardial ischemia, hypermetabolic states, electrolyte imbalance, or atrial stretch, as may occur with congestive heart failure, valvular disease, and pulmonary hypertension with cor pulmonale.

Physical Assessment/Clinical Manifestations

The client is usually asymptomatic, except for possible heart palpitations, because PACs usually have no hemodynamic consequences.

Interventions

No intervention is usually needed except to treat the cause, such as heart failure or valvular disease. If PACs occur frequently, they may herald the onset of more serious atrial tachydysrhythmias and therefore may warrant treatment. The nurse administers prescribed type IA antidysrhythmics, such as quinidine and procainamide, or other drugs such as digitalis and propranolol. The nurse also initiates measures to reduce the client's stress and teaches the client to avoid substances known to increase atrial irritability.

Supraventricular Tachycardia

Pathophysiology

Supraventricular tachycardia (SVT) involves the rapid stimulation of atrial tissue at a rate of 100 to 280 beats per minute, with a mean of 170 beats per minute in adults (Fig. 36–13) and 200 to 300 beats per minute in children. SVT is most often due to a re-entry mechanism in which one impulse circulates repeatedly in a circuitous atrial pathway, restimulating the atrial tissue repetitively at a rapid rate. The term *paroxysmal supraventricular tachycardia* is used when the rhythm is intermittent, initiated suddenly by a premature complex such as a PAC, and terminated suddenly with or without intervention.

During SVT the P waves have a morphology different from that of sinus P waves. The P waves are usually not seen, however, if there is a 1:1 conduction with rapid rates because the P waves are obscured in the preceding T wave.

Electrocardiographic criteria include

Rhythm: Atrial and ventricular rhythms regular or nearly regular

Rate: Atrial and ventricular rates 100 to 280 beats per minute (mean 170 beats per minute) in adults and 200 to 300 beats per minute in children

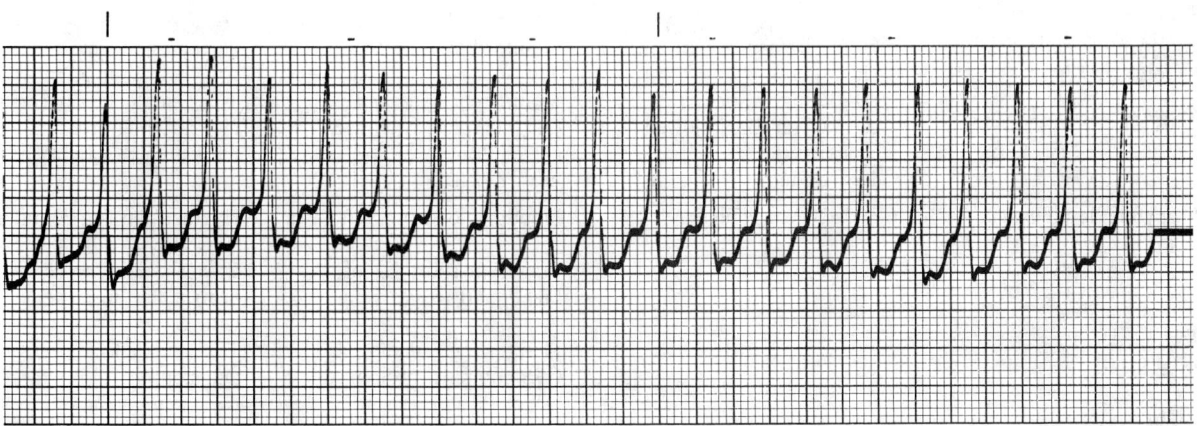

Figure 36–13. Atrial dysrhythmias. Sustained supraventricular tachycardia (SVT) in a client with Wolff-Parkinson-White syndrome. Heart rate is 200/minute.

P waves: Morphologic pattern of the first P (PAC) different from that of sinus P waves. Subsequent P waves are seldom visible, being buried in preceding T waves

PR interval: The PR interval prolonged with the first P (PAC); thereafter, not measurable

QRS duration: Usually normal and constant

Etiology

The causes of supraventricular tachycardia are the same as those for PACs. SVT may occur in healthy young people without evidence of heart disease, usually women under 40 years of age, and is also common in children. The condition commonly occurs in clients with a pre-excitation syndrome, such as Wolff-Parkinson-White syndrome.

Physical Assessment/Clinical Manifestations

The clinical manifestations depend on the duration of the SVT and the rate of the ventricular response. In clients with a sustained rapid ventricular response, the nurse assesses for palpitations, weakness, fatigue, shortness of breath, nervousness, anxiety, and syncope. Hemodynamic deterioration may occur in the client with cardiac disease, causing angina, heart failure, and shock. The infant or young child may demonstrate poor feeding, extreme irri-

tability, and pallor. With a nonsustained or slower ventricular response, the client may be asymptomatic except for transient palpitations.

Interventions

If SVT occurs in a healthy person and terminates spontaneously, no intervention is necessary other than eliminating identified causative factors. If it is recurrent, the client should be studied in the electrophysiology laboratory. The preferred treatment for recurrent SVT is radiofrequency catheter ablation (Bubien et al., 1995). In sustained supraventricular tachycardia with a rapid ventricular response, the goals of treatment are to decrease the ventricular response, convert the dysrhythmia to a sinus rhythm, and treat the cause. Vagal stimulation may be successful, but often only transiently, and must be performed only by a physician.

The nurse administers oxygen and prescribed antidysrhythmic drugs, which slow the ventricular rate by increasing the AV block. These drugs include adenosine, verapamil, diltiazem, digitalis, esmolol, and propranolol (see Chart 36–3). Some may also succeed in converting the dysrhythmia.

Text continued on page 776

Chart 36–3

Drug Therapy for Dysrhythmias

Drug	Usual Dosage	Nursing Interventions	Rationale
Class I Drugs			
Type IA			
Quinidine sulfate (Quinidine, Apo-Quinidine✶)	• 300–600 mg q8–12h PO • 6–10 mg/kg IV slowly, may be given IM	• Monitor blood pressure. • Watch for diarrhea, nausea, or vomiting and administer with food if these occur. • Monitor for widening QRS complex, prolonged QT interval, heart block, and onset or increase in number of PVCs.	• Hypotension is a common side effect. • Diarrhea is common during early therapy. Diarrhea and other gastrointestinal symptoms often decrease when quinidine is administered with food. • Toxic side effects necessitate stopping quinidine administration.
Procainamide hydrochloride (Pronestyl)	• 50 mg/kg/day PO in 4 divided doses • 20–30 mg IV, not to exceed 17 mg/kg, followed by infusion of 1–4 mg/min	• Monitor blood pressure. • Monitor for widening QRS complex, prolonged QT or PR interval, or heart block.	• Hypotension warrants drug discontinuation. • Toxic side effects necessitate stopping procainamide administration.
Disopyramide phosphate (Norpace)	• 100–200 mg q6h PO	• Monitor blood pressure. • Watch for shortness of breath and weight gain. • Monitor for widening QRS complex, prolonged QT or PR interval, or heart block	• Hypotension is a common side effect. • Disopyramide can cause heart failure in a client with CAD. • Toxic side effects necessitate stopping disopyramide administration.

Chart 36–3. Drug Therapy for Dysrhythmias   Continued

Drug	Usual Dosage	Nursing Interventions	Rationale
Class I Drugs			
Type IB			
Lidocaine (Xylocaine)	• 1–1.5 mg/kg IV bolus, then 0.5–0.75 mg/kg IV boluses q5–10min to a loading dose of 3 mg/kg, followed by 2–4 mg/min infusion • For VF or pulseless VT: 1–1.5 mg/kg IV bolus q3–5 min to a loading dose of 3 mg/kg, followed by 2–4 mg/min infusion	• Watch for confusion, paresthesias, slurring of speech, drowsiness, or seizure activity.	• CNS adverse effects predominate; they may require a decrease in dosage or discontinuation of the infusion.
Mexiletine hydrochloride (Mexitil)	• 200–300 mg q8h PO with food • 125–250 mg IV bolus for 5–10 min • 0.5–1.5 mg/min infusion	• Monitor blood pressure and heart rate. • Assess for tremors, blurred vision, dizziness, ataxia, or confusion.	• Hypotension and bradycardia may occur. • CNS adverse reactions predominate.
Tocainide hydrochloride (Tonocard)	• 400 mg q8h PO initially • 400–800 mg q8h PO • Maximum of 2.4 g/day • Take with food.	• Watch for tremors. • Monitor heart rate and blood pressure. • Teach the client to report shortness of breath, wheezing, chest pain, or cough, as well as dyspnea and distended neck veins or swelling of the extremities	• Tremors indicate that the maximum dose is being approached. • Bradycardia and hypotension may occur. • Pulmonary fibrosis is a serious side effect, which necessitates discontinuation of the drug; the drug also may cause CHF.
Type IC			
Flecainide acetate (Tambocor)	• 100 mg bid PO • Maximum dose of 400 mg/day	• Monitor for an increase in frequency and severity of dysrhythmias. • Monitor heart rate and blood pressure. • Monitor for CHF, dizziness, visual disturbances, paresthesias, and tremors.	• Flecainide can induce dysrhythmias. • Bradycardia and hypotension may occur. • Side effects may require a decrease in dosage or discontinuation of the drug.
Propafenone hydrochloride (Rythmol)	• 150–300 mg q8h PO	• Monitor for an increase in dysrhythmias. • Monitor heart rate and blood pressure. • Monitor for CNS effects, dizziness, anxiety, ataxia, insomnia, confusion, and seizures, as well as CHF and gastrointestinal distress.	• Propafenone can induce dysrhythmias. • Bradycardia and hypotension may occur. • Side effects may require a decrease in dosage or discontinuation of the drug.
Moricizine hydrochloride (Ethmozine)	• 200–300 mg q8H PO	• Monitor for an increase in dysrhythmias. • Monitor heart rate and blood pressure. • Monitor for dizziness, hyperesthesias, anxiety, ataxia, insomnia, confusion, and seizures.	• Drug can induce dysrhythmias. • Bradycardia and hypotension may occur. • Side effects may require a decrease in dosage or discontinuation of the drug.

Continued

Chart 36–3. Drug Therapy for Dysrhythmias Continued

Drug	Usual Dosage	Nursing Interventions	Rationale
Class II Drugs			
Propranolol hydrochloride (Inderal, Apo-Propranolol✢)	• 10–80 mg qid PO before meals • 0.1 mg/kg slow IV bolus divided in 3 equal doses given at 2–3 min intervals, at rate of 1 mg/min	• Monitor heart rate and blood pressure. • Assess for shortness of breath or wheezing. • Assess for insomnia, fatigue, and dizziness.	• Bradycardia and decreased blood pressure are expected effects. • Beta$_2$-blocking effects on the lungs can cause bronchospasm. • Side effects may require decrease in dosage or discontinuation of the drug.
Acebutolol hydrochloride (Sectral)	• 600–1200 mg daily PO	• Monitor heart rate and blood pressure. • Assess for shortness of breath or wheezing. • Assess for insomnia, fatigue, and dizziness.	• Bradycardia and decreased blood pressure are expected effects. • Beta$_2$-blocking effects on the lungs can cause bronchospasm. • Side effects may require a decrease in dosage or discontinuation of the drug.
Esmolol hydrochloride (Brevibloc)	• Initially, 500 μg/kg/min for 1 min, then 50 μg/kg/min for 4 min IV • Titrate up, if necessary.	• Monitor heart rate and blood pressure. • Assess for shortness of breath or wheezing. • Assess for insomnia, fatigue, and seizures.	• Bradycardia and decreased blood pressure are expected effects. • Beta$_2$-blocking effects on the lungs can cause bronchospasm. • Side effects may require a decrease in dosage or discontinuation of the drug.
Sotalol hydrochloride (Beta-pace)	• Initial dose of 80 mg PO bid • Dosage may be increased every 2–3 days to 240–320 mg/day in 2–3 divided doses, if necessary	• Assess ECG rhythm for torsades de pointes and other serious new ventricular dysrhythmias. • Assess for fatigue, bradycardia, dyspnea, CHF, chest pain, hypotension, dizziness, hypoglycemia, nausea, and vomiting. • Sotalol should not be administered to clients with hypokalemia or hypomagnesemia before correction of these imbalances. • Sotalol is contraindicated in clients with bronchial asthma, sinus bradycardia, or second- and third-degree AV block (unless a functioning pacemaker is present), prolonged QT syndrome, cardiogenic shock, and CHF.	• Sotalol may have proarrhythmic effects. • Adverse reactions may warrant drug discontinuation. • Hypokalemia or hypomagnesemia may prolong the QT interval and cause torsades de pointes. • Sotalol has beta-blocking (class II) effects and class III effects.

Chart 36-3. Drug Therapy for Dysrhythmias   Continued

Drug	Usual Dosage	Nursing Interventions	Rationale
Class III Drugs			
Bretylium tosylate (Bretylol, Bretylate✱)	• 5–10 mg/kg, diluted in 50 mL IV, for 8–10 min, may repeat in 1–2 hr; maximum of 30–35 mg/kg • 1–2 mg/min infusion • For VF or pulseless VT: 5 mg/kg IV undiluted, IV bolus, followed by defibrillation; may give 10 mg/kg IV bolus, followed by defibrillation, and repeat q5min to maximum of 30–35 mg/kg	• Observe cardiac monitor for PVCs, increased heart rate, and other dysrhythmias. • Monitor blood pressure. • Maintain the client in a supine position for up to 8 hr. • When the client begins to sit up or get out of bed, raise the head of the bed slowly and advise the client to make position changes slowly. • Anticipate vomiting during drug administration. Except in cardiac arrest, the drug must be diluted and given slowly.	• PVCs and increased heart rate commonly occur within 30 min. • Hypertension may occur in the first hour, followed by significant hypotension. • Orthostatic hypotension is a significant problem until tolerance to the drug develops. • The client could become dizzy and faint. • Vomiting is a common side effect.
Amiodarone hydrochloride (Cordarone)	• 800–1600 mg qd PO in divided doses for 1–3 wk, then 600–800 mg qd for 1 mo, then 200–600 mg qd (average of 400 mg qd) • Rapid loading dose: 150 mg IV over first 10 min (15 mg/min); slow loading dose: 360 mg IV over next 6 hr (1 mg/min); maintenance infusion: 540 mg IV over next 18 hr (0.5 mg/min), then 720 mg/24 hr (0.5 mg/min)	• Administer IV dose diluted in D_5W in glass bottle; use volumetric infusion pump and PVC tubing with in-line filter and infuse via central line. • Rapid loading IV dose must not be administered faster than 10 min. Must stay with client and monitor heart rate and BP. • Continually monitor ECG rhythm during IV infusion; measure QT and QT_c. • Assess the client's knowledge of the treatment regimen and side effects. • Monitor heart rate, blood pressure, and cardiac rhythm when initiating therapy. • Teach clients to report any muscle weakness, tremors, or difficulty with ambulation.	• Drug is irritating to peripheral vasculature; drug is more stable in glass bottle. • Hypotension may occur. It should be treated by slowing the infusion and other standard therapy. Cordarone should not be discontinued unless necessary. • Bradycardia and AV block may occur and are treated by slowing the infusion rate and pacemaker therapy, if necessary. May cause a worsening of ventricular dysrhythmias. • Drug has major side effects, which make noncompliance a problem; clients may take the drug for 1½–3 mo before full clinical effects are apparent. • Bradycardia, hypotension, and worsening dysrhythmia can occur. • Muscle-related side effects usually develop during the first week of treatment.

Continued

Chart 36–3. Drug Therapy for Dysrhythmias   Continued

Drug	Usual Dosage	Nursing Interventions	Rationale
Class III Drugs			
		• Teach clients to report shortness of breath, cough, pleuritic pain, or fever. • Teach clients to report any visual disturbances and to wear sunglasses outdoors in the daytime if they have photophobia. • Teach clients to use barrier sunscreens. • Teach clients to report any signs of thyroid problems or hepatotoxicity.	• Pulmonary side effects may indicate drug-induced pulmonary toxicity. • Corneal pigmentation occurs in most clients but generally does not interfere with vision; if it does, the dosage is decreased. • Photosensitivity reactions may occur. • Thyroid problems or hepatotoxicity may occur, necessitating a decrease in dosage or discontinuation of the drug.
Ibutilide fumarate (Covert)	• 1 mg IV over 10 min for clients >60 kg; 0.01 mg/kg over 10 min for clients <60 kg • May repeat dose 10 min after completion of first infusion if necessary	• Stop infusion as soon as arrhythmia is terminated, or in event of sustained or nonsustained VT, or marked prolongation of QT or QT$_c$. • Observe clients with continuous ECG monitoring and measure QT or QT$_c$ for at least 4 hr following infusion or until QT$_c$ has returned to baseline. • Clients with atrial fibrillation of >2–3 days' duration must be adequately anticoagulated for at least 2 wk. • Hypokalemia and hypomagnesemia must be corrected before Covert infusion.	• Drug may cause potentially fatal dysrhythmias. • Acute ventricular dysrhythmias must be promptly identified and treated. Client may develop heart blocks. • Atrial fibrillation is associated with formation of thrombi in atrial chambers. • This is important to reduce potential for proarrhythmia effects.
Class IV Drugs			
Verapamil hydrochloride (Calan, Isoptin✱)	• 2.5–5 mg IV, for 1–2 min for narrow-complex SVT or PSVT; after 15–30 min may give 5–10 mg IV for 1–2 min if necessary, and repeat to a maximum of 20 mg • 80–120 mg q6–8h PO	• Monitor heart rate and blood pressure. • Teach clients to remain recumbent for at least 1 hr after IV administration. • Teach clients to change positions slowly when receiving oral therapy. • Teach clients to report dyspnea, orthopnea, distended neck veins, or swelling of the extremities.	• Bradycardia and hypotension are common side effects. • Hypotension may occur; may be reversed with calcium chloride (CaCl$_2$), 0.5–1 g slow IV. • Dizziness and orthostatic hypotension often occur until tolerance develops. • Heart failure may occur, necessitating a decrease in dosage or discontinuation of the drug.
Diltiazem hydrochloride (Cardizem)	• 0.25 mg/kg IV for 2 min • After 15 min, give 0.35 mg/kg IV for 2 min • 5–15 mg/hr IV infusion	• Monitor heart rate and blood pressure. • Teach clients to remain recumbent for at least 1 hr after IV administration. • Teach clients to report dyspnea, orthopnea, distended neck veins, or swelling of the extremities.	• Bradycardia and hypotension are common side effects. • Hypotension may occur. • Heart failure may occur, necessitating a decrease in dosage or discontinuation of the drug.

Chart 36-3. Drug Therapy for Dysrhythmias   Continued

Drug	Usual Dosage	Nursing Interventions	Rationale
Other Drugs			
Digoxin (Lanoxin, Novodigoxin✦)	• Rapid digitalization: 0.5–1 mg PO or IV initially; 0.125–0.5 mg PO or IV q6h until a total of 1–1.5 mg is reached • Maintenance: 0.125–0.25 mg qd or qod PO or IV (may be less for elderly)	• Assess apical heart rate for 1 min before each dose; withhold the dose if the heart rate is less than 60 beats per min. • Assess for sudden increase of heart rate and change of rhythm from regular to irregular, or irregular to regular. • Teach clients to report anorexia, nausea, vomiting, diarrhea, paresthesias, confusion, or visual disturbances. • Monitor serum potassium levels. • Monitor serum creatinine levels	• Decreased heart rate is an expected response, but bradycardia may indicate toxicity. • Changes in heart rate or rhythm may indicate toxicity. • Side effect can indicate toxicity. • Hypokalemia increases the risk of toxicity and ventricular dysrhythmias. • Impaired renal function can cause toxicity; the dosage is altered if this occurs.
Atropine sulfate	• 0.5–1 mg IV bolus may be repeated q3–5 min, if necessary, to a maximum of 0.04 mg/kg • For asystole, PEA, or EMD: 1 mg IV bolus q3–5min to a total of 0.04 mg/kg, if necessary	• Monitor heart rate and rhythm after administration. • Assess for chest pain after administration. • Assess for urinary retention and dry mouth after administration. • Avoid using in clients with angle-closure glaucoma.	• Increased heart rate is expected. • Increased heart rate may cause ischemia in client with CAD. • Atropine is an anticholinergic agent. • Atropine increases intraocular pressure.
Adenosine (Adenocard)	• 6 mg IV for 1–3 sec followed by 20-mL saline flush; may repeat in 1–2 min, if necessary, at 12 mg IV for 1–3 sec with 20-mL flush; may repeat 12 mg IV after 1–2 min, if necessary	• Monitor heart rate and rhythm after administration. • Assess clients for facial flushing, shortness of breath, dyspnea, and chest pain. • Assess clients for recurrence of PSVT or ventricular ectopy.	• A short period of asystole is common after administration; bradycardia and hypotension may occur. • These side effects commonly occur. • Recurrence of PSVT is common; PVCs may occur.
Magnesium sulfate	• 1–2 g diluted in 100 mL of D$_5$W administered for 1–2 min for VF or VT • 1–2 g in 50–100 mL of D$_5$W for 5–60 min for loading dose; 0.5–1 g/hr for 24 hr for supplementation	• Assess ECG rhythm for conversion to sinus rhythm. • Assess clients for facial flushing, hypotension, and respiratory and CNS depression.	• Hypomagnesemia may precipitate refractory VF. • Magnesium sulfate causes vasodilation and respiratory and CNS depression.

VF, ventricular fibrillation; VT, ventricular tachycardia; SVT, supraventricular tachycardia; PSVT, premature supraventricular tachycardia; PEA, pulseless electrical activity; EMD, electromechanical dissociation; PVC, premature ventricular contraction; CHF, congestive heart failure; CNS, central nervous system; CAD, coronary artery disease.

In the severely compromised client, the nurse may assist the physician to attempt atrial overdrive pacing or to deliver a synchronized electrical shock (cardioversion) to re-establish an organized rhythm and regain hemodynamic stability.

Atrial Flutter

Pathophysiology

Atrial flutter is rapid atrial depolarization occurring at a rate of 250 to 350 times per minute. The most common rate is approximately 300 times per minute. An AV block limits the number of impulses that reach the ventricles as a protective mechanism (Fig. 36–14A). When untreated, atrial flutter typically has a 2:1 block (Fig. 36–14B). In general, when a client's ventricular rate is 150 beats per minute, the nurse should suspect atrial flutter with 2:1 block and carefully scrutinize the ECG baseline for evidence of atrial flutter waves.

Electrocardiographic criteria include

Rhythm: Atrial rhythm regular. Ventricular rhythm regular if block is consistent; ventricular rhythm irregular if block is variable

Rate: Atrial rate 250 to 350 beats per minute. Ventricular rate variable, depending on block; usually rapid without treatment

P waves: Flutter (F) waves seen in a regular pattern, with a sawtooth or "picket fence" configuration and lack of an isoelectric segment between flutter waves. Some flutter waves may be partially hidden in QRS complexes

PR interval: Actually FR interval, may be constant or variable. Usually not measured

QRS duration: Usually normal and constant

Etiology

Atrial flutter may be caused by rheumatic or ischemic heart disease, congestive heart failure, AV valve disease, pre-excitation syndromes, septal defects, pulmonary emboli, thyrotoxicosis, alcoholism, or pericarditis. The condition commonly occurs after cardiac surgery.

Physical Assessment/Clinical Manifestations

The clinical manifestations depend on the rate of ventricular response. The nurse assesses the client for palpitations, weakness, fatigue, shortness of breath, nervousness, anxiety, syncope, and evidence of hemodynamic deterioration such as angina, heart failure, and shock. Carotid sinus massage transiently increases the AV block to facilitate rhythm interpretation but can be performed only by the physician. The client with a normal ventricular rate is usually asymptomatic.

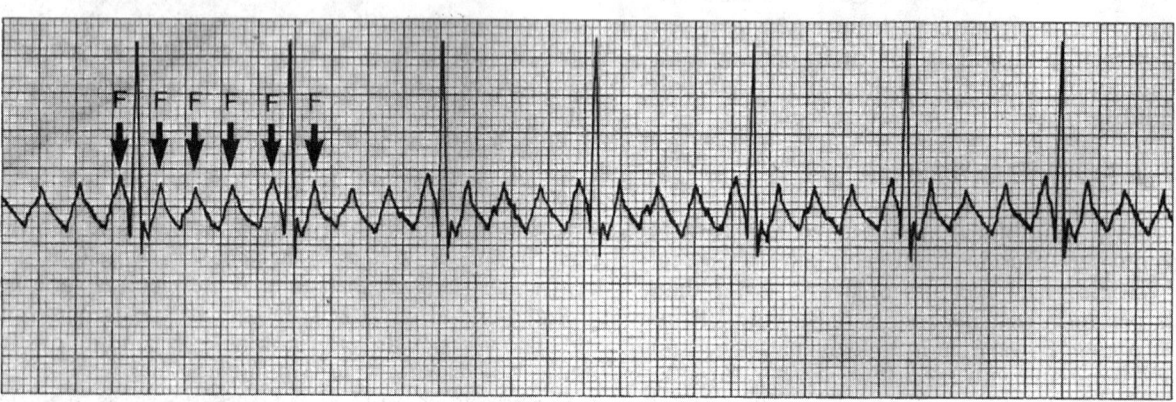

Figure 36–14. Atrial dysrhythmias. *A,* Atrial flutter (F) with 4:1 block. The atrial rate is 280/minute; the ventricular rate is 70/minute. *B,* Atrial flutter with 4:1 conduction, then an 11-beat run with 2:1 conduction.

Interventions

The treatment goals are the same as those for supraventricular tachycardia. The nurse administers oxygen and prescribed drugs, such as ibutilide, amiodarone, diltiazem, verapamil, propranolol, esmolol, and digoxin, to slow the rapid ventricular response. Quinidine or procainamide must not be administered unless one of the above agents has slowed the ventricular response. Both drugs slow the atrial rate and may increase AV conduction, which could cause a 1:1 conduction with an increase in ventricular rate and hemodynamic deterioration.

The nurse assists the physician to attempt rapid atrial overdrive pacing or to achieve cardioversion if the client is hemodynamically compromised. If the client is medically refractory, the physician may recommend radiofrequency catheter ablation to abolish the irritable focus in some types of atrial flutter. If the His bundle is ablated, the client is usually in a third-degree heart block and requires permanent pacemaker therapy.

Atrial Fibrillation

Pathophysiology

Multiple, rapid impulses from many foci, at a rate of 350–600 times per minute, depolarize the atria in a totally disorganized manner. The result is chaos, with no P waves, no atrial contractions, loss of the atrial kick, and an irregular ventricular response (Fig. 36–15). The atria merely quiver in fibrillation (commonly called "A fib"), which may lead to the formation of mural thrombi (within the cardiac wall) and potential embolic events.

Electrocardiographic criteria include

> *Rhythm:* Atrial rhythm consisting of an irregular undulating baseline. Ventricular rhythm totally irregular
> *Rate:* Atrial rate that cannot be counted because there are no P waves. The ventricular rate is usually 100 to 160 beats per minute or faster when untreated (uncontrolled "A fib"). The ventricular rate is 60 to 100 beats per minute when treated (controlled "A fib"). The ventricular rate may be less than 60 beats per minute when excessive AV nodal block occurs with drug treatment, such as with digoxin ("A fib" with high-grade AV block)

> *P waves:* P waves absent. Irregular fibrillatory (f) waves vary in amplitude and morphologic features in baseline
> *PR interval:* None
> *QRS duration:* Usually normal and constant

Etiology

Atrial fibrillation occurs most commonly in clients with systemic hypertension and is frequently seen in the elderly. It may also occur in clients with

- Myocardial infarction
- Rheumatic heart disease with mitral stenosis
- Atrial septal defect
- Congestive heart failure
- Cardiomyopathy
- Hyperthyroidism
- Pulmonary emboli
- Wolff-Parkinson-White syndrome
- Congenital heart disease
- Chronic constrictive pericarditis

Atrial fibrillation commonly occurs following cardiac surgery, in which case it is most often transient and usually responds well to treatment.

Physical Assessment/Clinical Manifestations

Atrial fibrillation may be intermittent or chronic. Symptoms depend on the ventricular rate. If the ventricular rate is rapid, the client may present as described for supraventricular tachycardia. Because of loss of the atrial kick, however, the client in uncontrolled atrial fibrillation is at greater risk for an inadequate cardiac output. The nurse assesses the client for the presence of a pulse deficit, fatigue, weakness, shortness of breath, distended neck veins, dizziness, decreased exercise tolerance, anxiety, syncope, palpitations, chest discomfort or pain, and hypotension.

In addition, the client is at risk for systemic emboli, particularly an embolic stroke, which may cause permanent severe neurologic impairment or death. Because approximately one-third of clients with atrial fibrillation have thromboemboli, the nurse must be astute in assessing the client for evidence of embolic events. The nurse

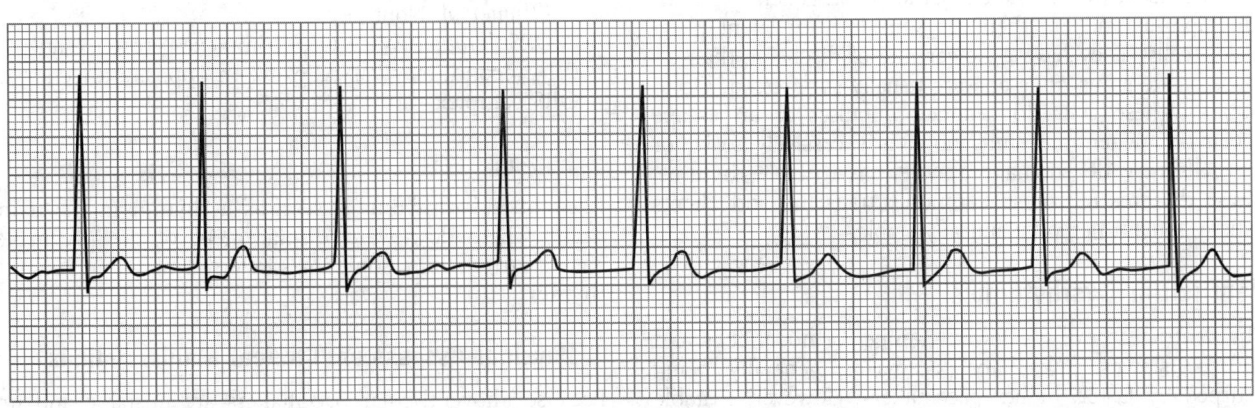

Figure 36–15. Atrial dysrhythmias. Atrial fibrillation, controlled, with a ventricular rate of approximately 80/minute.

particularly notes changes in mentation, speech, sensory function, and motor function and reports these to the physician immediately. Clients with atrial fibrillation who have valvular disease are particularly at risk for thromboemboli.

Interventions

Treatment is the same as for atrial flutter. In addition, the nurse may administer anticoagulants, such as heparin and sodium warfarin, as prescribed by the physician for clients considered to be at high risk for emboli. Prior to elective cardioversion, the nurse must initiate anticoagulation therapy for 4 to 5 weeks as prescribed to prevent a thromboembolic event if the rhythm is successfully converted. To assess for the presence of atrial clots, a contraindication for cardioversion in the hemodynamically compromised client, the physician may order a transesophageal echocardiogram prior to attempting emergency cardioversion. Atrial fibrillation of greater than 12 months duration is not likely to respond to attempts at conversion to sinus rhythm by drug therapies and may fail to respond to cardioversion.

Clients with recurring, symptomatic atrial fibrillation resistant to medical therapies may be treated with radiofrequency catheter ablation to the His bundle to interrupt all conduction between the atria and the ventricles. However, this requires implantation of a permanent ventricular pacemaker and does not stop the atria from fibrillating. The atrial kick is not restored, and patients remain at risk for embolic events.

Clients may benefit from the "maze" procedure, an open heart surgical technique (Futterman and Lemberg, 1994). In this procedure, the nurse first prepares the client for electrophysiologic mapping studies for confirmation of the diagnosis of atrial fibrillation. The nurse then prepares the client for surgery. The surgeon places a maze of sutures in strategic places in the atrial myocardium to prevent electrical circuits from developing and perpetuating atrial fibrillation. Sinus impulses can then depolarize the atria before reaching the AV node and preserve the atrial kick. The postoperative care of the client is similar to that after other open heart surgical procedures (see Chap. 40).

Junctional Dysrhythmias

Nodal cells in the AV junctional area can generate electrical impulses and are therefore subsidiary or latent pacemaker cells. They have a slower rate of discharge than do those of the sinus node and are usually suppressed. Occasionally, these cells do generate impulses as an escape pacemaker when the sinus node is excessively slow, or the cells may do so inappropriately as irritable rhythms. These rhythms are most commonly transient, and clients usually remain hemodynamically stable.

Ventricular Dysrhythmias

The ventricles have the fewest number of nodal cells and are the slowest subsidiary pacemaker, generally being usurped by faster, higher pacemakers. However, irritable ventricular cells may generate electrical impulses and fire

prematurely. Because the impulse originates in and depolarizes one ventricle first, then spreads to depolarize the other, the resultant QRS complex is wide, usually measuring greater than 0.12 second. The QRS complex is bizarre or odd in shape, looking different from the normal QRS complexes. The repolarization sequence is also deranged so that the T wave is large and occurs in a direction opposite to the largest deflection of the QRS complex. The impulse most commonly is blocked in the AV node and cannot proceed further with retrograde conduction so that the atria and the SA node are usually not affected by the ventricular impulse. The atrial rhythm typically remains regular, unless the underlying rhythm is sinus arrhythmia.

A sinus P wave may sometimes be seen immediately preceding a wide QRS complex, or the sinus P wave may occur immediately after the QRS complex. Often, the sinus P wave is obscured by the QRS complex. In each case, the P-P interval remains regular in normal sinus rhythm but irregular in sinus arrhythmia. These P waves are not related to and are independent of the QRS complex; that is, the sinus impulse does not proceed forward to depolarize the ventricles. The ventricles are stimulated by an independent ventricular impulse. This is known as *AV dissociation*, meaning that a sinus impulse depolarizes the atria, and a separate ventricular impulse depolarizes the ventricles, so that the two impulses are not related.

Idioventricular Rhythm (Ventricular Escape Rhythm)

Pathophysiology

During idioventricular rhythm (ventricular escape rhythm), the ventricular nodal cells pace the ventricles. Because their inherent rate of firing is slow, the rate is usually less than 40 beats per minute (Fig. 36–16). If P waves are seen, they are independent of the QRS complexes and not related (AV dissociation).

Electrocardiographic criteria include

Rhythm: Atrial rhythm is usually absent because of downward displacement of the pacemaker with atrial standstill. Ventricular rhythm may be regular; often becomes irregular

Rate: No atrial rate. Ventricular rate usually less than 40 beats per minute

P waves: Usually absent

PR interval: None

QRS duration: Wide QRS complexes greater than 0.14 second, may vary; T wave in opposite direction of QRS complex

Etiology

Idioventricular rhythm is seen as a rhythm in the dying heart, where downward displacement of the pacemaker has occurred. It is sometimes referred to as an "agonal" rhythm.

Physical Assessment/Clinical Manifestations

Because idioventricular pacemakers are unstable and unreliable, the client is hypotensive and in shock or, most

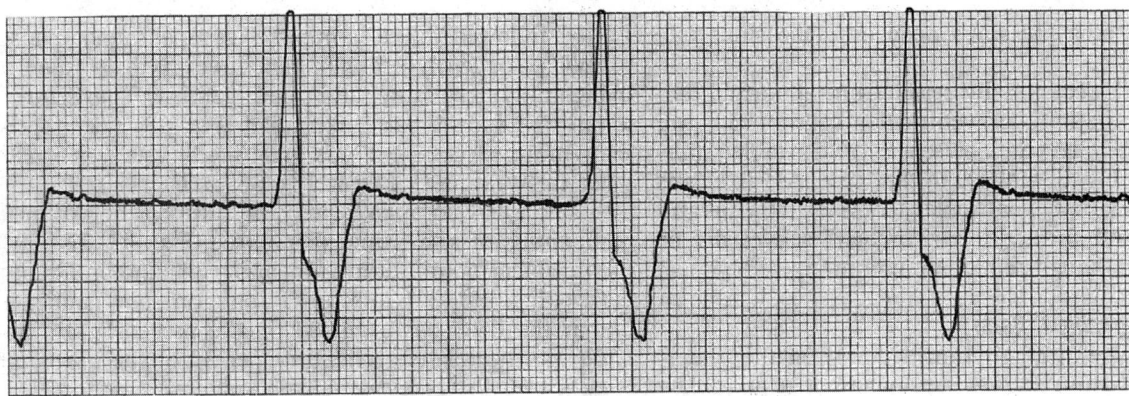

Figure 36-16. Ventricular dysrhythmias. Idioventricular rhythm with a rate of 35/minute.

typically, is pulseless and therefore in cardiac arrest. The nurse assesses the client's pulse, respirations, blood pressure, level of consciousness, and pupil response.

Interventions

Usually, idioventricular rhythms require immediate resuscitation measures, unless there is a DNR order. The nurse initiates cardiopulmonary resuscitation (CPR) and summons assistance. The team may initiate advanced cardiac life support (ACLS) measures, including epinephrine administration, intravascular volume replacement, and other measures, which tend to be unsuccessful. The physician may attempt pacemaker therapy or discontinue resuscitation efforts.

Premature Ventricular Complexes

Pathophysiology

Premature ventricular complexes (PVCs), also called ventricular premature beats (VPBs), result from increased irritability of ventricular cells. PVCs are early ventricular complexes, followed by a pause. When multiple PVCs are present, the QRS complexes may be unifocal or uniform, meaning of the same shape (Fig. 36–17A), or multifocal or multiform, meaning of different shapes (see Fig. 36–17B). PVCs frequently occur in repetitive rhythms, such as bigeminy, trigeminy, and quadrigeminy. Two sequential PVCs are a pair, or couplet. Three or more successive PVCs are usually called nonsustained ventricular tachycardia (NSVT) (see Fig. 36–17C).

R-on-T phenomenon indicates that the PVC has occurred on the preceding T wave, which is considered the vulnerable period. This may precipitate ventricular fibrillation.

Electrocardiographic criteria include

Rhythm: Underlying rhythm regular or irregular. PVC creates an irregularity, followed by a pause

Rate: Rate dependent on the underlying rhythm. PVCs can occur with any rate

P wave: With an underlying sinus rhythm, one P wave before each normal QRS complex. Sinus P waves are not related to PVC (AV dissociation); P waves may occur anywhere relative to PVCs. The underlying rhythm may be atrial flutter or atrial fibrillation

PR interval: PR interval not measured with the PVC because of AV dissociation

QRS duration: QRS duration normal in sinus rhythm. In PVC, it is wider than 0.14 second and may vary; the T wave condition occurs in the opposite direction

Etiology

PVCs are common, and their frequency increases with age. PVCs may be insignificant or may occur with myocardial ischemia or infarction; congestive heart failure; hypokalemia; hypomagnesemia; the administration of catecholamines, sympathomimetic drugs, and digitalis; acidosis; anesthesia; stress; nicotine intake; ingestion of caffeine and alcohol; infection; trauma; or surgery.

Physical Assessment/Clinical Manifestations

The client may be asymptomatic or may experience palpitations or chest discomfort caused by increased stroke volume of the normal beat after the pause. Peripheral pulses may be diminished or absent with the PVCs themselves because the decreased stroke volume of the premature beats may decrease peripheral perfusion. With acute myocardial infarction, PVCs may be considered warning dysrhythmias, possibly heralding the onset of VT or VF. For a client with chest discomfort or pain, the nurse reports to the physician whether PVCs increase in frequency, are multiform, are R-on-T phenomena, or occur in runs of VT.

Interventions

If there is no underlying heart disease, PVCs are not usually treated other than by eliminating any contributing cause (e.g., caffeine, stress). With acute myocardial ischemia or infarction, the nurse treats significant PVCs by administering oxygen and lidocaine as prescribed. Lidocaine is considered the drug of choice. The nurse may administer other drugs as ordered, including procainamide, bretylium, magnesium sulfate, propranolol, quinidine, mexiletine, tocainide, sotalol, and amiodarone (see

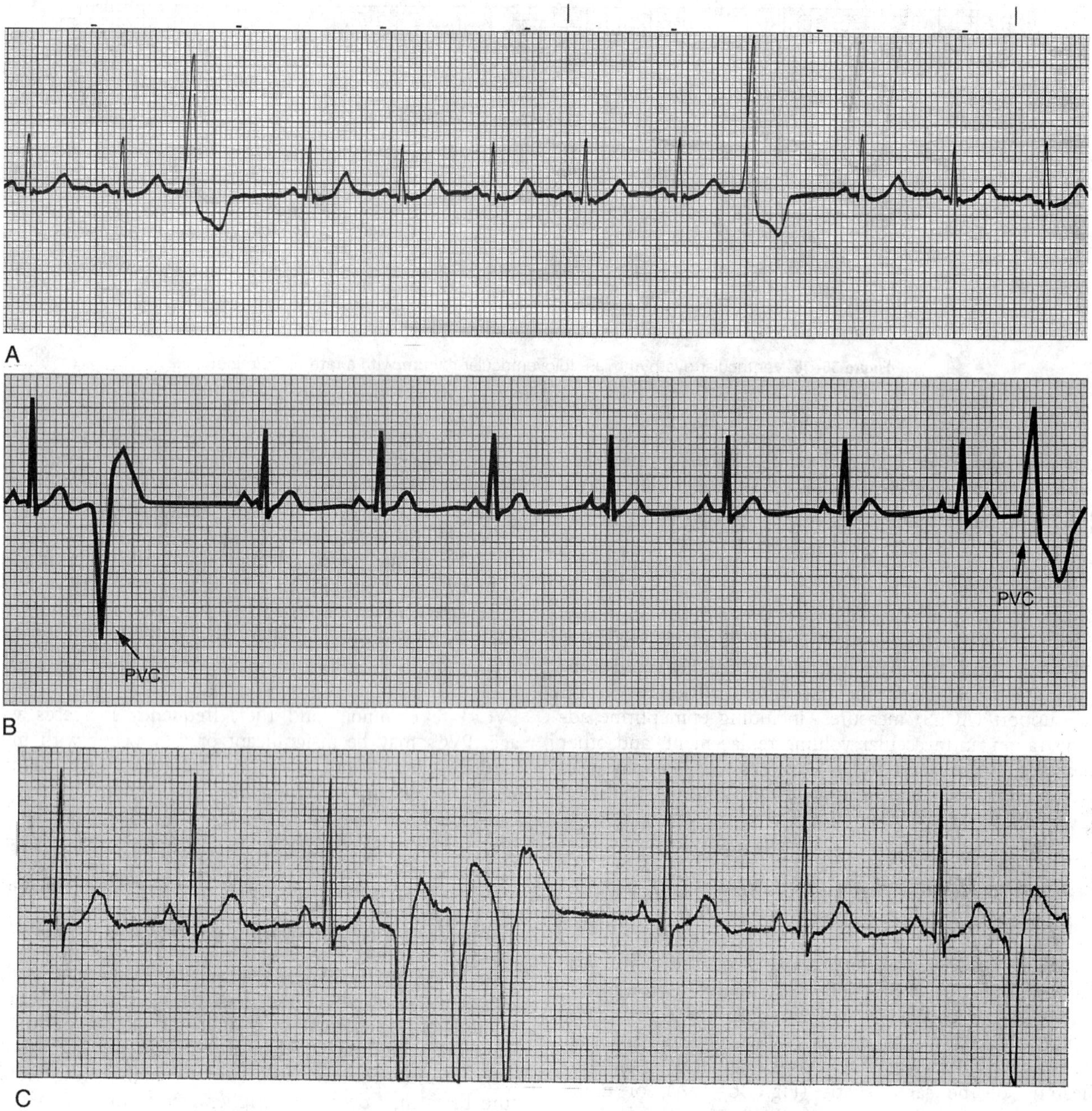

Figure 36–17. Ventricular dysrhythmias. *A,* Normal sinus rhythm (NSR) with unifocal premature ventricular complexes (PVCs). *B,* Normal sinus rhythm with multifocal PVCs (one negative and the other positive). *C,* Normal sinus rhythm with three consecutive PVCs (nonsustained ventricular tachycardia) and another unifocal PVC.

Chart 36–3). The nurse administers potassium as ordered for replacement therapy if hypokalemia is the cause.

Ventricular Tachycardia

Pathophysiology

Ventricular tachycardia (VT) (sometimes referred to as "V tach") occurs with repetitive firing of an irritable ventricular ectopic focus usually at a rate of 140 to 180 beats per minute or more (Fig. 36–18). VT may result from increased automaticity or a re-entry mechanism. VT may

present as a paroxysm of three or more self-limiting beats (nonsustained VT) or as a sustained rhythm (lasting longer than 15 to 30 seconds). The sinus node continues to discharge independently, depolarizing the atria but not the ventricles (AV dissociation), although P waves are seldom seen in sustained VT.

Electrocardiographic criteria include

Rhythm: Usually not possible to determine the atrial rhythm. Ventricular rhythm usually regular or nearly regular

Rate: Not possible to determine the atrial rate. Ven-

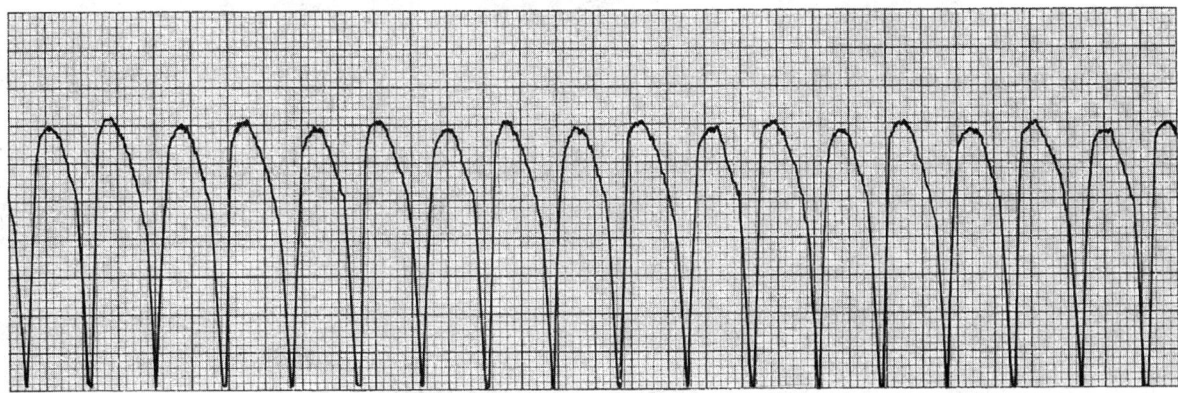

Figure 36–18. Ventricular dysrhythmias. Sustained ventricular tachycardia at a rate of 166/minute.

tricular rate can range from 100 to 250 beats per minute but most commonly 140 to 180 beats per minute

P waves: P waves usually not visible and obscured in QRS complexes. AV dissociation

PR interval: Not measured because of AV dissociation

QRS duration: Wide, greater than 0.14 second, may vary

Etiology

VT may occur in clients with ischemic heart disease, myocardial infarction, cardiomyopathy, hypokalemia, hypomagnesemia, valvular heart disease, heart failure, drug toxicity, hypotension, or ventricular aneurysm. In clients who go into cardiac arrest, VT is commonly the initial rhythm before deteriorating into ventricular fibrillation as the terminal rhythm. VT is not common in infants and children unless they have cardiac disease.

Physical Assessment/Clinical Manifestations

Clinical manifestations of sustained VT partially depend on the ventricular rate. Slower rates are better tolerated. Clients may be hemodynamically compromised if the cardiac output decreases because of the shortened ventricular filling time and loss of the atrial kick. In some clients, VT causes cardiac arrest. The nurse assesses the client's pulse, respirations, blood pressure, level of consciousness, and pupil response.

Interventions

For the stable client with sustained VT, the nurse administers oxygen and lidocaine as prescribed. If this is not successful, procainamide, bretylium, or magnesium sulfate may be given. The physician may prescribe an oral antidysrhythmic agent, such as procainamide, mexiletine, or sotalol.

For the client with unstable VT, the nurse assists the physician to attempt emergency cardioversion followed by oxygen and antidysrhythmic therapy (Chart 36–4). The nurse may instruct the client to perform cough CPR if prescribed, telling the client to inhale deeply and cough hard every 1 to 3 seconds. Cough CPR is sometimes

successful in either terminating the VT or at least briefly sustaining cerebral and coronary perfusion until other measures can be initiated. The physician may attempt rapid atrial or ventricular overdrive pacing if the VT is related to a significant bradydysrhythmia.

A precordial thump is sometimes successful in terminating VT, at least transiently. The physician or the ACLS-qualified nurse may administer a precordial thump to a client with unstable VT only if a defibrillator and pacemaker are immediately available (Cummins et al., 1994).

For the client with pulseless VT, the physician or ACLS-qualified nurse or other health care provider must *immediately* defibrillate the client or initiate cardiopulmonary resuscitation (CPR) and defibrillate as soon as possible. A precordial thump may be administered initially, though it is frequently not successful in terminating VT. If the patient remains pulseless, the nurse or other health care provider must resume CPR and full resuscitative measures following defibrillation. This includes airway management and administration of oxygen, epinephrine, and antidysrhythmic therapy with lidocaine, bretylium, magnesium sulfate, and procainamide.

Chart 36–4

Nursing Care Highlight: The Client with Unstable Ventricular Tachycardia

- Assist the physician with cardioversion.
- Provide oxygen and antidysrhythmic drugs as ordered.
- Teach the client how to perform cough cardiopulmonary resuscitation (CPR), if ordered.
- Assist with or provide defibrillation (if you are qualified in advanced cardiac life support [ACLS]).
- Initiate CPR if the client does not respond to the above measures.
- Maintain a patent airway at all times.
- Monitor the client for premature ventricular complexes (PVCs) and the recurrence of VT.
- Assess for signs and symptoms of myocardial infarction, hypokalemia, or hypomagnesemia.

If the rhythm has been successfully converted, attention is given to treating reversible causes of VT, such as myocardial ischemia, hypokalemia, and hypomagnesemia. The nurse ensures that oxygen therapy and antidysrhythmic agent administration are continued, and the client is closely monitored for PVCs and the recurrence of VT. The client with recurrent, medically refractory VT should be studied in the electrophysiology lab and may benefit from radiofrequency catheter ablation. Some forms of VT may require surgical intervention, such as coronary artery bypass graft (CABG) surgery, implantation of a cardioverter/defibrillator, aneurysmectomy, encircling endocardial ventriculotomy, cryosurgery, or endocardial resection (see Chap. 40).

Ventricular Fibrillation

Pathophysiology

Ventricular fibrillation (VF) (sometimes called "V fib") is the result of electrical chaos in the ventricles. Impulses from many irritable foci fire in a totally disorganized manner so that ventricular contraction cannot occur. There are no recognizable deflections. Instead, there are irregular undulations of varying amplitudes, from coarse to fine (Fig. 36–19A). The ventricles merely quiver, consuming a tremendous amount of oxygen. There is no cardiac output, therefore no cerebral, myocardial, or systemic perfusion. This rhythm is *rapidly fatal* if not successfully terminated within 3 to 5 minutes.

Electrocardiographic criteria include

Rhythm: Irregular, chaotic undulations of varying amplitudes in baseline
Rate: Not measurable
P waves: Not visible
PR interval: Not measurable
QRS duration: None. Fibrillatory waves may be coarse or fine

Etiology

VF may be the first manifestation of coronary artery disease. Clients with myocardial infarction are at great risk for VF. VF may also occur in clients with myocardial ischemia, hypokalemia, hypomagnesemia, antidysrhythmic therapy, rapid supraventricular tachydysrhythmias, shock, asynchronous pacing with competition, or severe metabolic derangements. VF also occurs following surgery or trauma.

Physical Assessment/Clinical Manifestations

On initiation of VF, the client becomes faint, immediately loses consciousness, and becomes pulseless and apneic. There is no blood pressure, and heart sounds are absent. Respiratory and metabolic acidosis develop. Seizures may occur. Within minutes, the pupils become fixed and dilated, and the skin becomes cold and mottled. Death

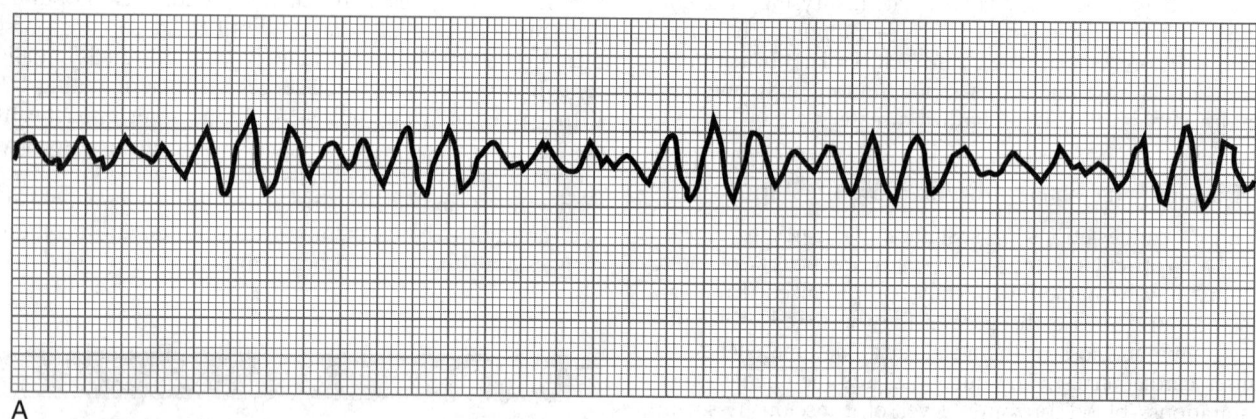

A

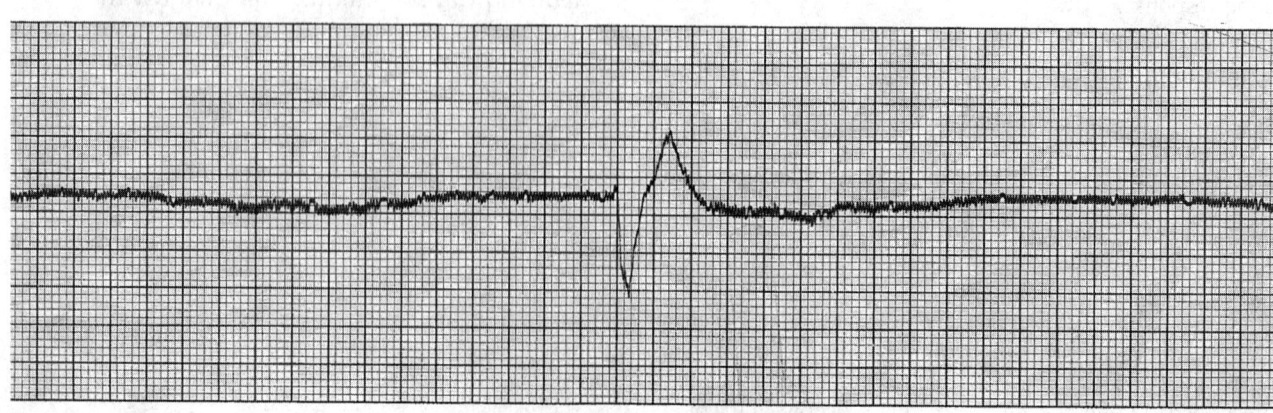

B

Figure 36–19. Ventricular dysrhythmias. *A,* Coarse ventricular fibrillation. *B,* Ventricular asystole with one idioventricular complex.

ensues without prompt restoration of an organized rhythm and cardiac output.

Interventions

The goals of treatment are to terminate VF promptly and to convert it to an organized rhythm. The physician or the advanced cardiac life support (ACLS)–qualified nurse or other health care provider must immediately defibrillate the client to accomplish this goal. This is the management priority. If a defibrillator is not readily available, a precordial thump may be delivered. CPR must be continued until the defibrillator arrives.

If the VF does not terminate after three rapid successive shocks of increasing energy, the nurse and resuscitation team resume CPR and provide airway management. They also administer oxygen, epinephrine, and antidysrhythmic therapy with lidocaine, bretylium, magnesium sulfate, and procainamide, along with attempting defibrillation frequently. Cough CPR may be successful in terminating the VF or at least in briefly sustaining cerebral and coronary perfusion until definitive treatment can be initiated if the client coughs vigorously before losing consciousness. If VF is successfully converted to an organized rhythm, the nurse continues supportive therapy and assists the physician to treat potential causes of VF and to prevent its recurrence.

Ventricular Asystole

Pathophysiology

Ventricular asystole, sometimes called *ventricular standstill,* is the complete absence of any ventricular rhythm (see Fig. 36–19B). There are no electrical impulses in the ventricles and therefore *no* ventricular depolarization, no QRS complex, no contraction, no cardiac output, and no pulse, respirations, or blood pressure. The client is in full cardiac arrest. The sinoatrial (SA) node, in some cases, may continue to fire and depolarize the atria, with only P waves seen on the electrocardiogram (ECG), but the sinus impulses do not conduct to the ventricles, and QRS complexes remain absent. In most cases, the entire conduction system is electrically silent, with no P waves seen on the ECG. There is only a mildly undulating line on the ECG. Fine VF may resemble asystole in some leads. Because treatment of these two rhythms differs significantly, the nurse must assess two ECG leads for an accurate rhythm interpretation.

Electrocardiographic criteria include

Rhythm: Atrial rhythm usually absent. If P waves present, atrial rhythm may be regular. Ventricular rhythm absent
Rate: No ventricular rate
P waves: P waves usually absent. Occasionally, regular P waves if the SA node continues to function
PR interval: None
QRS duration: QRS complexes absent

Etiology

Ventricular asystole usually results from myocardial hypoxia, which may be a consequence of advanced heart

failure. It may also be caused by severe hyperkalemia and acidosis. If P waves are seen, asystole is likely because of severe ventricular conduction blocks. Rarely, excessive vagal stimulation may cause asystole.

Physical Assessment/Clinical Manifestations

Clients are in full cardiac arrest with loss of consciousness and absence of pulse, respirations, and blood pressure. Ventricular asystole is often fatal, unresponsive to resuscitation measures.

Interventions

The goal of treatment is to restore cardiac electrical activity. The nurse or other health care provider initiates CPR immediately and summons assistance. The nurse must assess another ECG lead to ensure that the rhythm is asystole and not fine VF, which warrants immediate defibrillation. When in doubt, the client should be defibrillated. The nurse and resuscitation team manage the airway and administer oxygen, epinephrine, and atropine. The nurse assists the physician with the initiation of noninvasive pacing or invasive transvenous or epicardial pacing, although pacemaker therapy is generally not effective. An isoproterenol infusion may also be tried. The prognosis for clients with asystole is poor.

Atrioventricular Blocks

Atrioventricular blocks (AV blocks) exist when supraventricular impulses are excessively delayed or totally blocked in the AV node or intraventricular conduction system. Conduction may be transiently or permanently abnormal for a number of reasons. The SA node continues to function normally, and atrial depolarizations and P waves occur regularly. Because of the conduction dysfunction, ventricular depolarizations and QRS complexes are either delayed or blocked.

There are different degrees of heart blocks, as follows:

- In first-degree AV block, all sinus impulses eventually reach the ventricles.
- In second-degree heart block, some sinus impulses reach the ventricles, but others do not because they are blocked.
- In third-degree heart block (complete heart block), none of the sinus impulses reach the ventricles. The ventricles, therefore, are depolarized by a second, independent pacemaker.

AV blocks are differentiated by their PR intervals.

First-Degree Atrioventricular Block

Pathophysiology

First-degree AV block is actually a conduction delay rather than a block. AV node conduction is slow, prolonging the PR interval to greater than 0.20 second. However, all sinus impulses eventually reach the ventricles. The underlying rhythm must still be identified (e.g., sinus tachycardia with first-degree AV block) (Fig. 36–20A).

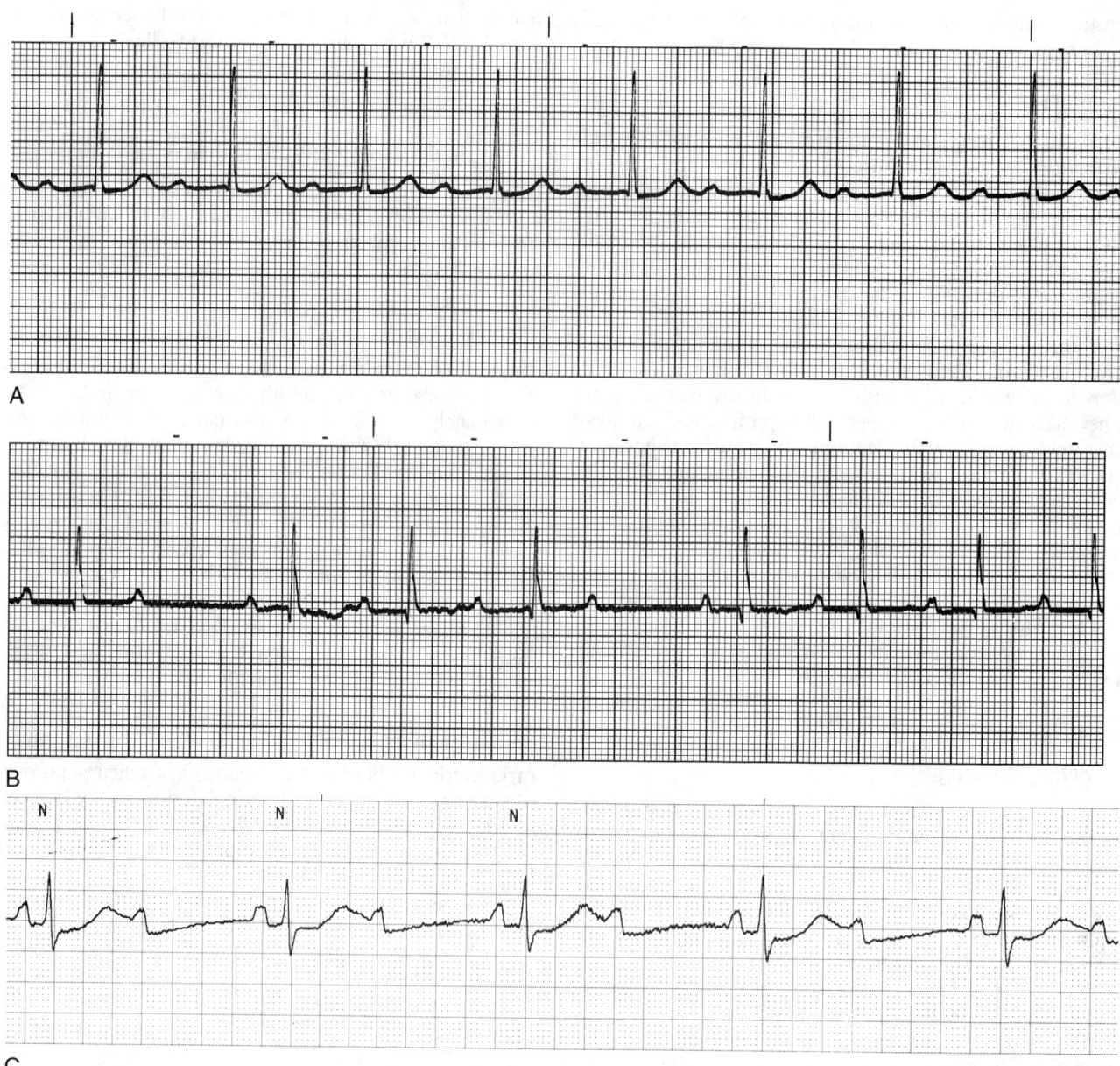

Figure 36–20. AV blocks. *A,* Normal sinus rhythm (NSR) with first-degree AV block (PR interval 0.36 second). *B,* Second-degree AV block type I (Wenckebach AV) with an irregular rhythm, grouped beating, and progressive prolongation of the PR interval until a P wave is completely blocked and not followed by a QRS complex. *C,* Second-degree AV block type II (Mobitz II) with 2:1 conduction, a constant PR interval, and wide QRS complex.

Electrocardiographic criteria include

Rhythm: Atrial and ventricular rhythms usually regular unless sinus arrhythmia is present

Rate: Depends on the underlying rhythm. Atrial and ventricular rates are equal

P waves: One P wave preceding each QRS complex. Constant morphologic pattern

PR interval: PR interval prolonged, greater than 0.20 second. It usually does not exceed 0.40 second

QRS duration: Normal, constant

Etiology

First-degree AV block may be due to AV nodal ischemia from occlusion of the right coronary artery, as with an inferior or posterior myocardial infarction. It may also result from hypokalemia or hyperkalemia; the administration of digitalis, beta-adrenergic blockers, calcium channel blockers; excessive vagal stimulation; or degenerative AV nodal disease. In children, it may occur following cardiac surgery as a result of edema in the AV nodal area and usually resolves without treatment.

Physical Assessment/Clinical Manifestations

First-degree AV block has no hemodynamic consequences and produces no symptoms. Any symptoms are the result of the underlying rhythm (e.g., sinus bradycardia). First-degree AV block may be insignificant and transient or may progress to more severe AV blocks, although this is uncommon.

Interventions

In the stable client, no treatment is needed. If the first-degree AV block is due to drug therapy, the nurse must withhold the offending drug and notify the physician. If the PR interval is particularly long or is getting progressively longer, the nurse must notify the physician. When first-degree AV block is associated with symptomatic bradycardia, the nurse administers oxygen and atropine as prescribed to accelerate AV conduction.

Second-Degree Atrioventricular Block Type I (AV Wenckebach or Mobitz Type I)

Pathophysiology

In second-degree AV block type I, each successive sinus impulse takes a little longer to conduct through the impaired AV node, until one impulse is completely blocked and fails to depolarize the ventricles because the AV node has become completely refractory. This block results in a nonconducted or dropped beat (missing QRS complex). There is progressive prolongation of the PR interval, followed by a dropped beat and a pause (the most characteristic feature of this rhythm). The pause allows sufficient time for the AV node to recover so that the next beat is conducted with a shorter PR interval and the Wenckebach sequence is repeated. Although the atrial rhythm is usually regular, the ventricular rhythm is irregular, with an appearance of grouped beats separated by pauses. Group size (conduction ratios) may be constant or may vary. Because of the dropped QRS complex, each group normally has one more P wave than QRS complexes (see Fig. 36–20B).

Electrocardiographic criteria include

Rhythm: Atrial rhythm usually regular. Ventricular rhythm irregular, with grouped beating and shortening R-R intervals in the group
Rate: Atrial rate dependent on the underlying sinus rhythm, which may be normal or slow. Because of dropped beats, ventricular rate always less than atrial rate
P waves: P waves normal, with constant morphologic pattern. Some P waves not conducted to the ventricles and not followed by a QRS complex
PR interval: Progressive lengthening of PR intervals until a dropped beat, which is followed by a pause. A new sequence then begins
QRS duration: QRS duration usually normal and constant. One QRS complex is missing in each grouped sequence

Etiology

The causes of AV Wenckebach are the same as for first-degree AV block. It is often a transient rhythm and may revert to first-degree AV block or even a normal sinus rhythm. Second-degree AV block type I is also seen with rheumatic fever and digitalis administration. AV Wenckebach may occur in a child following cardiac surgery and is usually transient.

Physical Assessment/Clinical Manifestations

The client is usually asymptomatic if the frequency of dropped beats and the overall ventricular rate do not decrease the cardiac output. If the ventricular rate is too slow, decreasing the cardiac output, the client presents with symptoms of a symptomatic bradydysrhythmia. This rhythm is usually transient and terminates spontaneously.

Interventions

No intervention is required in the stable client, because this rhythm rarely progresses to a more severe block. In the symptomatic client, the nurse administers oxygen and atropine as prescribed. If atropine is not successful in speeding AV nodal conduction time and increasing the heart rate, the nurse initiates pacemaker therapy as ordered and notifies the physician.

Second-Degree Heart Block Type II (Mobitz Type II)

Pathophysiology

In Mobitz type II block, the block is actually infranodal, occurring below the His bundle. It involves a constant block in one of the bundle branches, resulting in a wide QRS complex in conducted beats, and an intermittent block in the other bundle branch, resulting in dropped beats because both bundles are blocked. (P waves are not followed by a QRS complex.) Because the block is not in the AV node, sinus impulses that conduct to the ventricles always do so with a constant PR interval. Impulses may be blocked randomly, making the ventricular rhythm irregular. Alternatively, the impulses may be blocked at regular intervals, such as in 2:1 block, in which case the ventricular rhythm is regular (see Fig. 36–20C).

Electrocardiographic criteria include

Rhythm: Atrial rhythm usually regular. Ventricular rhythm regular or irregular, depending on the block
Rate: Atrial rate dependent on the underlying sinus rhythm. May be normal or slightly fast. Because of dropped beats, the ventricular rate is less than the atrial rate. This rate may be slow
P waves: P waves normal, with a constant morphologic pattern. One or more P waves not conducted to the ventricles
PR interval: Constant in conducted beats
QRS duration: Usually wide, indicating that the block is infranodal in one of the bundle branches, with missing QRS complexes because of intermittent block of the other bundle branch

Etiology

Second-degree AV block type II is less common than type I. It may occur in the adult with anterior myocardial infarctions and results from severe ischemic damage to the conduction system. It may also be caused by rheumatic heart disease or degenerative disease of the conduction system. It is a serious block that may progress suddenly to a third-degree AV block (complete heart block) and an ominous prognosis. Mobitz II may occur in children following cardiac surgery or, less frequently, children with congenital AV block.

Physical Assessment/Clinical Manifestations

Symptoms depend on the frequency of dropped beats and the overall ventricular rate. If the cardiac output is inadequate, the client presents with a symptomatic bradydysrhythmia.

Interventions

In the asymptomatic client, the nurse may assist the physician to initiate prophylactic pacing to avert the threat of sudden third-degree AV block. If slow ventricular rates are present, the nurse administers oxygen and atropine as prescribed. Atropine is usually ineffective because it does not reverse the infranodal block. An isoproterenol (Isuprel) infusion may be administered with caution but may be dangerous in adults with ischemic heart disease. Noninvasive or invasive pacing is preferred. A permanent pacemaker may be required in adults and children with recurrent or medically refractory Mobitz type II.

Third-Degree Heart Block (Complete Heart Block)

Pathophysiology

In third-degree heart block, none of the sinus impulses conducts to the ventricles. The SA node is usually the pacemaker for the atria, producing P waves at a normal or even accelerated rate. A separate, independent pacemaker paces the ventricles. Thus, AV dissociation exists. If the block is in the AV node, a junctional escape focus paces the ventricles, producing normal QRS complexes at a rate of 40 to 60 beats per minute (Fig. 36–21A). If the block is below the bundle of His (infranodal), a ventricular escape focus paces the ventricles, producing wide QRS complexes at a rate usually less than 40 beats per minute (see Fig. 36–21B). In either case, the atrial and ventricular rhythms are usually regular but independent of each other, with more P waves than QRS complexes.

Because the P waves and the QRS complexes are totally independent and bear no relationship to each other, the PR interval is inconstant, which is the most characteristic feature of this rhythm. The ventricular escape pacemaker is the least stable, least dependable pacemaker. It may abruptly fail, causing ventricular asystole, or it may predispose to irritability in the form of premature ventricular complexes (PVCs), ventricular tachycardia (VT), or ventricular fibrillation (VF).

Electrocardiographic criteria include

Rhythm: Atrial and ventricular rhythms usually regular, but independent of each other because of AV dissociation

Rate: Atrial rate dependent on the underlying sinus rhythm. May be normal or slightly fast. If paced by a junctional escape rhythm, the ventricular rate is 40 to 60 beats per minute. If paced by a ventricular escape rhythm, the ventricular rate is usually less than 40 beats per minute.

P waves: Normal, constant morphologic pattern, but not related to QRS complexes (AV dissociation); more P waves than QRS complexes

PR interval: Inconstant because of AV dissociation

QRS duration: With a junctional escape pacemaker, QRS complexes normal and constant. With a ventricular escape pacemaker, QRS complexes wide (greater than 0.14 second) and constant

Etiology

Third-degree heart block in the adult may occur from ischemic injury with coronary artery disease or myocardial infarction, degenerative disease of the conduction system, or calcific aortic stenosis. In adults and children, third-degree heart block may occur with congenital heart disease, the effects of drugs or electrolyte disturbances, or cardiac surgery.

Physical Assessment/Clinical Manifestations

Clinical manifestations depend on the overall ventricular rate and cardiac output. Transient third-degree heart block may be well tolerated, particularly when the block is in the AV node. If the block is infranodal, if may have serious hemodynamic consequences. If cerebral perfusion is inadequate, clients may be confused and lightheaded or may experience episodes of syncope with or without seizures (Stokes-Adams attacks). Inadequate cardiac output may cause myocardial ischemia or infarction, heart failure, and hypotension. Third-degree heart block may predispose to cardiac arrest, causing VT, VF, or asystole. Therefore, it is regarded as a dangerous rhythm.

Interventions

Third-degree AV block with a junctional escape pacemaker is often transient and well tolerated. If the client is symptomatic, the nurse administers oxygen and atropine as prescribed. Clients with third-degree heart block with a ventricular escape pacemaker are frequently symptomatic. The nurse administers oxygen and assists the physician to initiate prophylactic pacing to avert the threat of cardiac arrest. Atropine is usually not successful in infranodal blocks with wide QRS complexes. Cautious use of isoproterenol (Isuprel) infusions may be necessary as a temporary measure while awaiting pacemaker therapy but is dangerous in clients with acute myocardial infarction. Implantation of a permanent pacemaker may be required in patients with recurrent or medically refractory third-degree infranodal block.

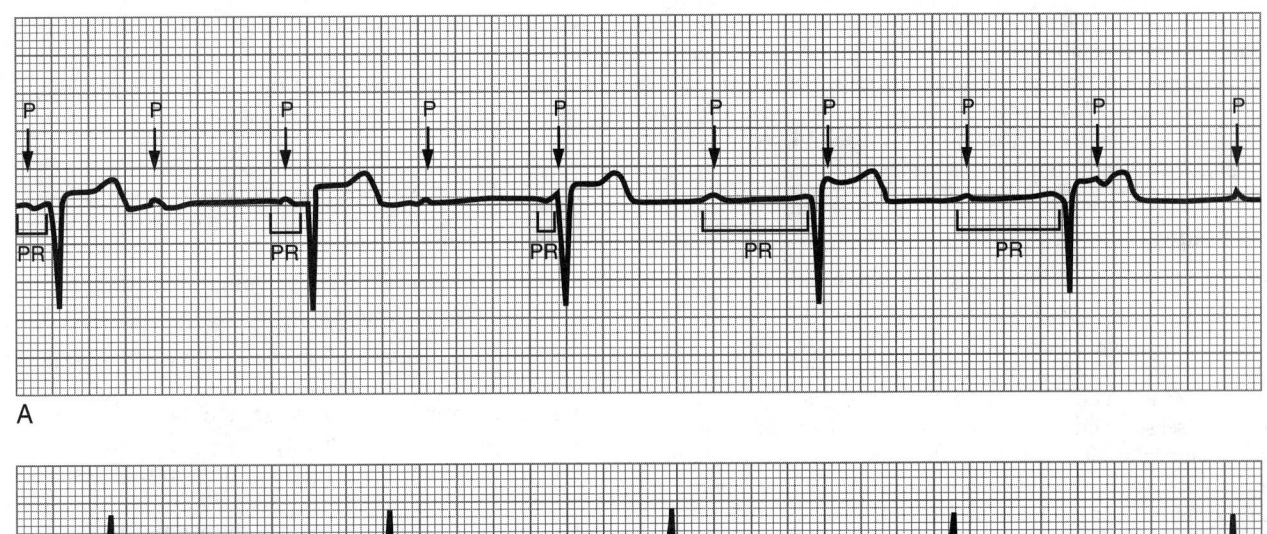

A

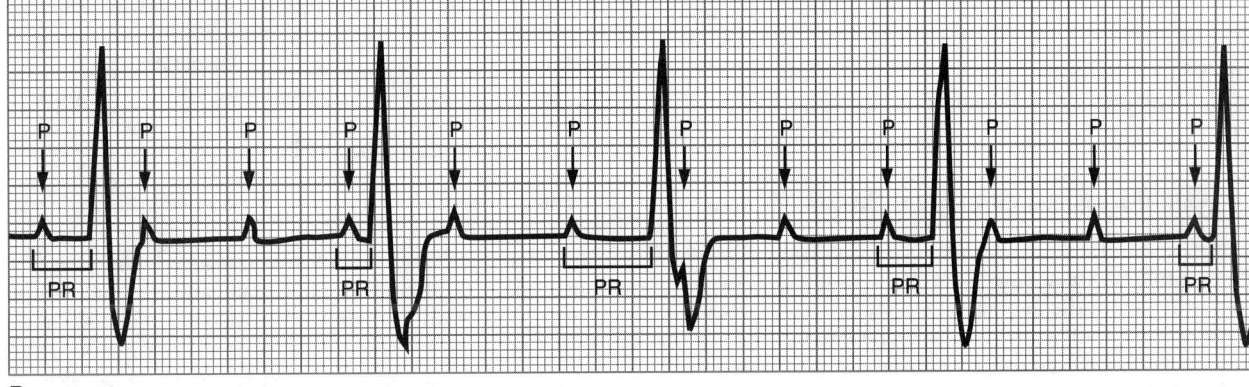

B

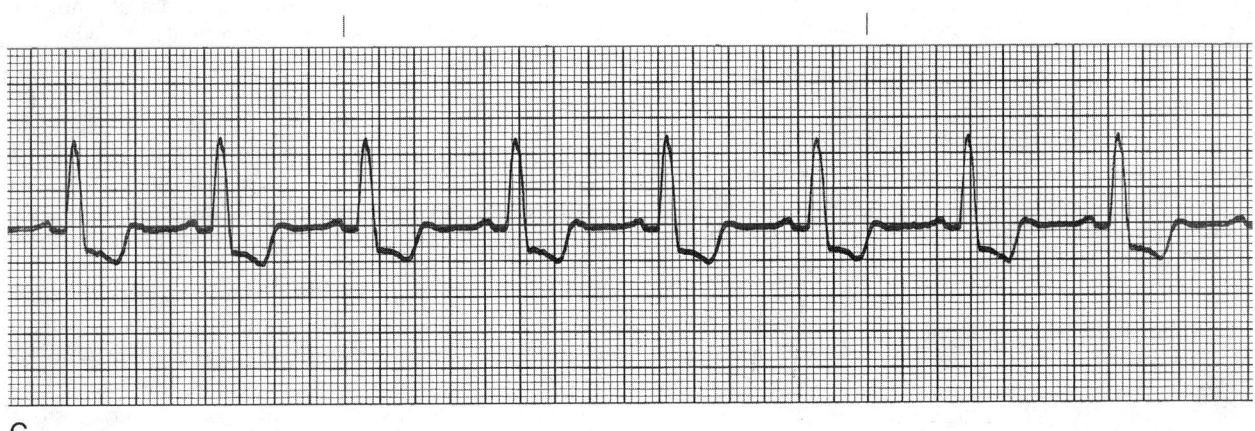

C

Figure 36-21. AV blocks. *A,* Third-degree AV block (complete heart block) with regular atrial and ventricular rhythms, inconstant PR intervals (AV dissociation), and a junctional escape focus (normal QRS complexes) pacing the ventricles at a rate of 44/minute. *B,* Third-degree AV block with regular atrial and ventricular rhythms, inconstant PR intervals (AV dissociation), and a ventricular escape focus pacing the ventricles at a rate of 38/minute, with wide QRS complexes. *C,* Normal sinus rhythm (NSR) with bundle branch block (wide QRS complexes measuring 0.12 second).

Bundle Branch Blocks

Pathophysiology

Bundle branch block is a conduction delay or block within one of the two main bundle branches below the bifurcation of the His bundle. When one bundle branch is blocked, the supraventricular impulse is able to descend only down the normal bundle branch and to depolarize that ventricle. The other ventricle is depolarized afterward, as the wave of depolarization from the first ventricle proceeds from cell to cell to the other ventricle. Such slow depolarization prolongs the QRS duration to 0.12 second or longer. The underlying rhythm is usually sinus in origin (e.g., sinus rhythm with bundle branch block) (see Fig. 36-21C).

Electrocardiographic criteria include

Rhythm: Atrial and ventricular rhythms usually regular

Rate: Atrial and ventricular rates equal. Bundle branch block may occur at any rate

P waves: One P wave before each QRS complex, with a constant morphologic pattern

PR interval: May be normal or may be prolonged (first-degree AV block)

QRS duration: Wide, usually 0.12 to 0.14 second and usually constant, but may vary slightly

Etiology

Bundle branch block may be a temporary or a permanent conduction disorder. Right or left bundle branch blocks may occasionally be seen in clients with normal hearts. More commonly, they are seen in clients with cardiovascular disease, such as congenital heart disease, rheumatic heart disease, ventricular hypertrophy, cardiomyopathy, severe aortic stenosis, chronic degenerative disease of the conduction system, and fibrotic scarring of the conduction system. Transient bundle branch block may be seen with acute conditions such as coronary insufficiency, myocardial infarction, and heart failure; during right-sided heart catheterization; or with rapid supraventricular rates.

Physical Assessment/Clinical Manifestations

There are no clinical manifestations specifically related to bundle branch block. The nurse must notify the physician when a new bundle branch block develops, especially in the client with an acute myocardial infarction. The conduction disorder may deteriorate to a more significant block requiring pacemaker therapy.

Interventions

No interventions are specifically related to bundle branch block. The nurse ensures that the client is resting and has adequate ventilation and oxygenation. The nurse assesses the client during alterations in heart rate for symptoms of hemodynamic compromise. The nurse reports symptoms to the physician and assists the physician in treating any underlying disorder.

Collaborative Management

 Analysis

➤ *Common Nursing Diagnoses and Collaborative Problems*

The most common nursing diagnoses pertinent to the client with dysrhythmias are
1. Decreased Cardiac Output related to electrical and mechanical dysfunction
2. Altered Tissue Perfusion related to decreased cardiac output

➤ *Additional Nursing Diagnoses and Collaborative Problems*

In addition to the common nursing diagnoses, some clients have one or more of the following:
- Impaired Gas Exchange related to altered oxygen supply

- Ineffective Individual Coping related to fear of death
- Activity Intolerance

The additional collaborative problem is Potential for Pulmonary Edema.

 Planning and Implementation

➤ *Decreased Cardiac Output and Altered Tissue Perfusion*

Planning: Expected Outcomes. The client is expected to
- Have a normal, regular pulse rate
- Have normal mental acuity
- Have a normal rate, rhythm, and depth of respiration
- Have normal skin color and temperature
- Perform activities of daily living without dyspnea or excess fatigue
- Be free of pulmonary edema

Interventions. The nurse or assistive nursing personnel monitors the client's ECG rhythm and/or assesses the client for signs and symptoms associated with dysrhythmias, such as abnormal pulse rate and rhythm, palpitations, chest pain, syncope, decreased oxygen saturation, decreased blood pressure, dyspnea, pulmonary congestion, neck vein distention, anxiety, restlessness, skin pallor, and poor capillary refill.

The nurse may assess the client's apical and radial pulses for a full minute for any irregularity, which may occur with premature beats, escape beats, atrial fibrillation, or second-degree heart blocks. If the apical pulse rate differs from the radial pulse rate, a pulse deficit exists and suggests that not all beats are perfusing. Clinical manifestations of sustained tachydysrhythmias and bradydysrhythmias are summarized in Chart 36–2.

In an acute care setting, if the client has a pulmonary artery catheter and an arterial line, the nurse assesses the client's hemodynamic profile to determine the physiologic effects of the dysrhythmia. The nurse must also assess the psychosocial impact of dysrhythmias on clients and families and the effectiveness of their coping mechanisms.

Assessment of the client's past and current history is essential because dysrhythmias are associated with both acute and chronic disorders and also with medical and surgical therapies. The nurse should also review the interpretation of the client's 12-lead ECG and other electrocardiographic diagnostic tests, such as the Holter monitor, event monitor, or signal-averaged ECG. The nurse must identify the client who is at risk for serious consequences from dysrhythmias.

Interventions are specific to the type of dysrhythmia, the cause, the effect it has on the client's cardiac output, and the risk it presents to the client. Interventions for specific dysrhythmias are summarized in Table 36–2.

Nonsurgical Management. Nonsurgical management of dysrhythmias includes drug therapy, vagal maneuvers, temporary pacing, cardioversion, cardiopulmonary resuscitation (CPR), defibrillation, and catheter ablation.

Drug Therapy. Pharmacologic therapy administered for the control of dysrhythmias often includes drugs from one or more classes of antidysrhythmic agents (see Chart 36–3). The Vaughn-Williams classification is commonly used to classify drugs according to their effects on the action potential of cardiac cells. Other drugs also have antidysrhythmic effects but do not fit the Vaughn-Williams classification.

Vaughn-Williams Classification. Class I antidysrhythmics are membrane-stabilizing agents, stabilizing phase 4 to decrease automaticity. There are three subclassifications in this group. Type IA drugs moderately slow conduction and prolong repolarization, prolonging the QT interval. These drugs are used to treat or to prevent supraventricular and ventricular premature beats and tachydysrhythmias. Examples include quinidine sulfate and procainamide hydrochloride (Pronestyl). Type IB drugs shorten repolarization. These drugs are used to treat or prevent ventricular premature beats, ventricular tachycardia (VT), and ventricular fibrillation (VF). Examples include lidocaine and mexiletine hydrochloride (Mexitil). Type IC drugs markedly slow conduction and widen the QRS complex. These drugs are used primarily to treat or to prevent recurrent, life-threatening ventricular premature beats, VT, and VF. Examples include flecainide acetate (Tambocor) and propafenone hydrochloride (Rythmol).

Class II antidysrhythmics control dysrhythmias associated with excessive beta-adrenergic stimulation by competing for receptor sites and thereby decreasing heart rate and conduction velocity. Beta-adrenergic–blocking agents, such as propranolol hydrochloride (Inderal) and esmolol hydrochloride (Brevibloc), are class II drugs. They are used to treat or to prevent supraventricular and ventricular premature beats and tachydysrhythmias. Sotalol hydrochloride (Betapace) is an antidysrhythmic agent with both noncardioselective beta-adrenergic–blocking effects (class II) and action potential duration prolongation properties (class III). It is an oral agent recommended for the treatment of documented ventricular dysrhythmias, such as VT, that are life-threatening.

Class III antidysrhythmics lengthen the absolute refractory period and prolong repolarization and the action potential duration of ischemic cells. They decrease the disparity with normal cells to prevent a re-entry response. Class III drugs include bretylium tosylate (Bretylol, Bretylate✴), amiodarone hydrochloride (Cordarone), and ibutilide fumarate (Corvert) and are used to treat or prevent ventricular premature beats, VT, and VF.

Class IV antidysrhythmics impede the flow of calcium into the cell during depolarization, thereby depressing automaticity of the sinoatrial (SA) and atrioventricular (AV) nodes, decreasing heart rate, and prolonging AV nodal refractoriness and conduction. Calcium channel blockers, such as verapamil hydrochloride (Calan, Isoptin✴) and diltiazem hydrochloride (Cardizem), are class IV drugs. They are used to treat supraventricular tachycardia (SVT), atrial flutter, and atrial fibrillation to slow down the ventricular response.

Other Antidysrhythmic Drugs. Other drugs, such as digoxin, atropine, adenosine, and magnesium sulfate, are frequently used to treat dysrhythmias. Digoxin increases vagal tone, slowing AV nodal conduction. It is useful in treating supraventricular tachydysrhythmias, particularly chronic atrial fibrillation, by controlling the rate of ventricular response. Atropine is a parasympatholytic or vagolytic agent. It is used to treat vagally induced symptomatic bradydysrhythmias. Adenosine is an endogenous nucleoside that slows AV nodal conduction to interrupt re-entry pathways. It is effective in terminating paroxysmal supraventricular tachycardia, a re-entrant tachydysrhythmia. Magnesium sulfate is an electrolyte administered to treat refractory VT or VF because these clients may be hypomagnesemic, with increased ventricular irritability.

Emergency Cardiac Drugs. In addition to antidysrhythmics, several other drugs are used during cardiac arrest (Chart 36–5). Epinephrine (Adrenalin) is a first-line agent in all cardiac arrests. It is given predominantly for its alpha-adrenergic effects to increase vasomotor tone for myocardial and cerebral perfusion. Its beta-adrenergic effects may stimulate the heart and increase myocardial contractility to improve cardiac output. Dopamine hydrochloride (Intropin) is generally used for its beta-adrenergic effects after cardiac arrest but may be used for its alpha-adrenergic effects during resuscitation. Dobutamine hydrochloride (Dobutrex) is a beta-adrenergic agent used to improve myocardial contractility and increase cardiac output.

Norepinephrine may be used for its alpha-adrenergic effects to increase vasomotor tone and increase perfusion pressure. Sodium bicarbonate is administered during cardiac arrest for clients who are hyperkalemic. It may also be used, if necessary, to treat a bicarbonate metabolic acidosis, as occurs in diabetic ketoacidosis or tricyclic antidepressant overdose. Isoproterenol (Isuprel), a beta-adrenergic agent, is rarely used to increase heart rate in an atropine-refractory, symptomatic bradydysrhythmia. Isoproterenol is indicated to increase the heart rate in heart transplant patients. Pacing is preferred. Calcium chloride, which increases myocardial contractility, is also rarely indicated. It is reserved for clients with hyperkalemia, hypocalcemia, or calcium channel–blocker toxicity because it may cause cell damage and cerebrovascular vasospasm.

Vagal Maneuvers. Vagal maneuvers induce vagal stimulation of the cardiac conduction system, specifically the SA and AV nodes. Vagal maneuvers are used to terminate supraventricular tachydysrhythmias. They include carotid sinus massage and Valsalva maneuvers.

Carotid Sinus Massage. The physician massages over the carotid artery for a few seconds, observing for a change in cardiac rhythm. Massaging the carotid sinus causes vagal stimulation, slowing SA nodal and AV nodal conduction. The nurse prepares the client for this procedure, instructs the client to turn the head slightly away from the side to be massaged, and observes the cardiac monitor for a change in rhythm. The nurse records an ECG rhythm strip before, during, and after the procedure. The nurse then assesses the client's vital signs and level of consciousness. Complications include bradydysrhythmias, asystole, ventricular fibrillation, and cerebral damage. Ca-

Drug Therapy for Cardiac Arrest

Drug	Usual Dosage	Nursing Interventions	Rationale
Epinephrine (Adrenalin)	• 1-mg IV bolus followed by 20-mL saline flush q3–5 min • If this fails, may consider: 2–5 mg IV bolus q3–5 min; 1-mg, 3-mg, and 5-mg IV bolus (3 min apart); or 0.1 mg/kg IV bolus q3–5 min • If necessary, may give endotracheally with dose at least 2–2½ times IV dose	• Monitor for return of rhythm and pulse when used for asystole or VF. • Assess for tachycardia, dysrhythmias, or hypertension. • Assess for the development of coarse VF when given during fine VF.	• Return of rhythm and pulse is the expected response. • Adverse reactions can occur with a dramatic response. • This may improve the response to defibrillation.
Dopamine hydrochloride (Intropin)	• 2.5–5 μg/kg/min IV infusion; titrate to desired clinical response • 1–2 μg/kg/min for renal and mesenteric vasodilation • 2–10 μg/kg/min for beta-adrenergic effects • 10–20 μg/kg/min for alpha-adrenergic effects	• Assess clients for increased blood pressure. • Monitor for tachycardia, dysrhythmias, or hypertension. • Monitor the IV site for infiltration. • Assess for urinary output <30 mL/hr, or pallor, cyanosis, pain, or numbness in the extremities.	• Increased blood pressure is the expected response. • Adverse reactions may occur. • Extravasation of drug can occur, causing necrosis. • Dosages >10 μg/kg/min cause vasoconstriction of renal and peripheral blood vessels; dosages of 2–5 μg/kg/min may improve urinary output by causing renal vasodilation and improving renal blood flow.
Dobutamine hydrochloride (Dobutrex)	• 2–20 μg/kg/min IV infusion	• Assess for increased blood pressure. • Assess for hypertension and dysrhythmias.	• Increased blood pressure is the expected response. • Adverse reactions may occur.
Norepinephrine (Levophed)	• 0.5–1 μg/min IV infusion, titrate to desired effect, up to 8–30 μg/min	• Assess for increased blood pressure. • Monitor for bradycardia.	• Increased blood pressure is the expected response. • Reflex bradycardia may occur with a rise in blood pressure.

rotid sinus massage is contraindicated in clients with cerebral arteriosclerosis and carotid bruits. A defibrillator and resuscitative equipment must be immediately available during the procedure.

Valsalva Maneuvers. To stimulate a vagal reflex, the health care provider instructs the client to bear down as if straining to have a bowel movement or induces the gag reflex in the client. The nurse prepares the client for the procedure; assesses the client's heart rate, heart rhythm, and blood pressure; observes the cardiac monitor; and records an ECG rhythm strip before, during, and after the procedure to determine the effect of therapy. If gagging is induced, the nurse provides an emesis basin and oral hygiene if the client vomits and takes measures to prevent aspiration.

Unintended vagal stimulation may sometimes occur, and the nurse must be cautious when performing procedures that may inadvertently cause vagal stimulation. For example, tracheal suctioning, enema administration, and rectal temperature checks can stimulate the vagus nerve and decrease the heart rate inappropriately. The nurse administers stool softeners as prescribed. The nurse instructs the client not to strain during bowel movements and to avoid constipation through proper diet and exercise. The client is also told to avoid inducing gagging during oral hygiene, which triggers a vagal response. The nurse assesses the heart rate and rhythm of a client who is vomiting, which may induce a vagal reflex. Some clients experience a vagal response when raising their arms above their head and must be instructed to avoid this movement.

Chart 36–5. Drug Therapy for Cardiac Arrest   Continued

Drug	Usual Dosage	Nursing Interventions	Rationale
		• Monitor for hypertension and dysrhythmias.	• Adverse reactions may occur with a dramatic response.
		• Monitor the IV site for infiltration.	• Extravasation can occur, which necessitates immediate treatment with phentolamine injected at the site.
		• Assess for urinary output <30 mL/hr or pallor, cyanosis, pain, or numbness in the extremities.	• Norepinephrine is a powerful vasoconstrictor.
		• Assess for chest pain after resuscitation.	• Norepinephrine increases myocardial oxygen demand.
Sodium bicarbonate	• 1 mEq/kg IV bolus given after the first 10 min of cardiac arrest if necessary • 0.5 mEq/kg IV bolus q10min thereafter, if necessary	• Assess arterial blood gas values for metabolic acidosis.	• Administration without evidence of metabolic acidosis can result in alkalosis, which can hinder resuscitation efforts.
Isoproterenol (Isuprel)	• 2–10 μg/min IV infusion; titrate to desired clinical response	• Assess for increased heart rate. • Assess for tachycardia, hypotension, or hypertension. • Assess for chest pain after resuscitation. • Monitor for ventricular dysrhythmias.	• Increased heart rate is the expected response. • Adverse reactions may occur with a dramatic response. • Isoproterenol increases myocardial oxygen demand. • Isoproterenol increases ventricular irritability, especially in clients who are hypokalemic or who are receiving digitalis.
Calcium chloride (CaCl$_2$)	• 2–4 mg/kg IV slowly, may repeat, if necessary, q10min	• Calcium chloride is indicated only for cardiac arrest associated with hyperkalemia, hypocalcemia, or calcium channel blocker toxicity.	• Calcium chloride may cause cellular damage and cerebrovascular spasm.

VF, ventricular fibrillation.

Temporary Pacing. Temporary pacing is a nonsurgical intervention that provides a timed electrical stimulus to the heart when either the impulse initiation or the intrinsic conduction system of the heart is defective. The electrical stimulus then spreads throughout the heart to depolarize the cells, which should be followed by contraction and cardiac output. Electrical stimuli may be delivered to the right atrium or right ventricle (single-chamber pacemakers) or to both (dual-chamber pacemakers).

When a pacing stimulus is delivered to the heart, a spike (or pacemaker artifact) is seen on the monitor or ECG strip. The spike should be followed by evidence of depolarization (i.e., a P wave indicating atrial depolarization or a QRS complex indicating ventricular depolarization). This pattern is referred to as *capture,* indicating that the pacemaker successfully depolarized, or captured, the chamber.

Temporary pacing is generally initiated in clients with symptomatic, atropine-refractory bradydysrhythmias, particularly second-degree heart block type II and third-degree heart block, or in clients with asystole. Temporary pacing may also be initiated prophylactically in hemodynamically stable clients with left bundle branch block in certain situations, such as insertion of a pulmonary artery catheter.

A different type of pacing may be used to terminate symptomatic tachydysrhythmias. Occasionally, atrial overdrive pacing is attempted to terminate atrial tachydysrhythmias, such as atrial flutter or atrial fibrillation. Overdrive pacing is accomplished by rapidly pacing the atrium to capture the heart and control depolarization, followed by no pacing, in the hope that the sinus node will regain control of the heart. Ventricular overdrive pacing may be done to terminate ventricular tachydysrhythmias in much the same way. Overdrive pacing is usually performed by the physician or the physician's assistant. The nurse must

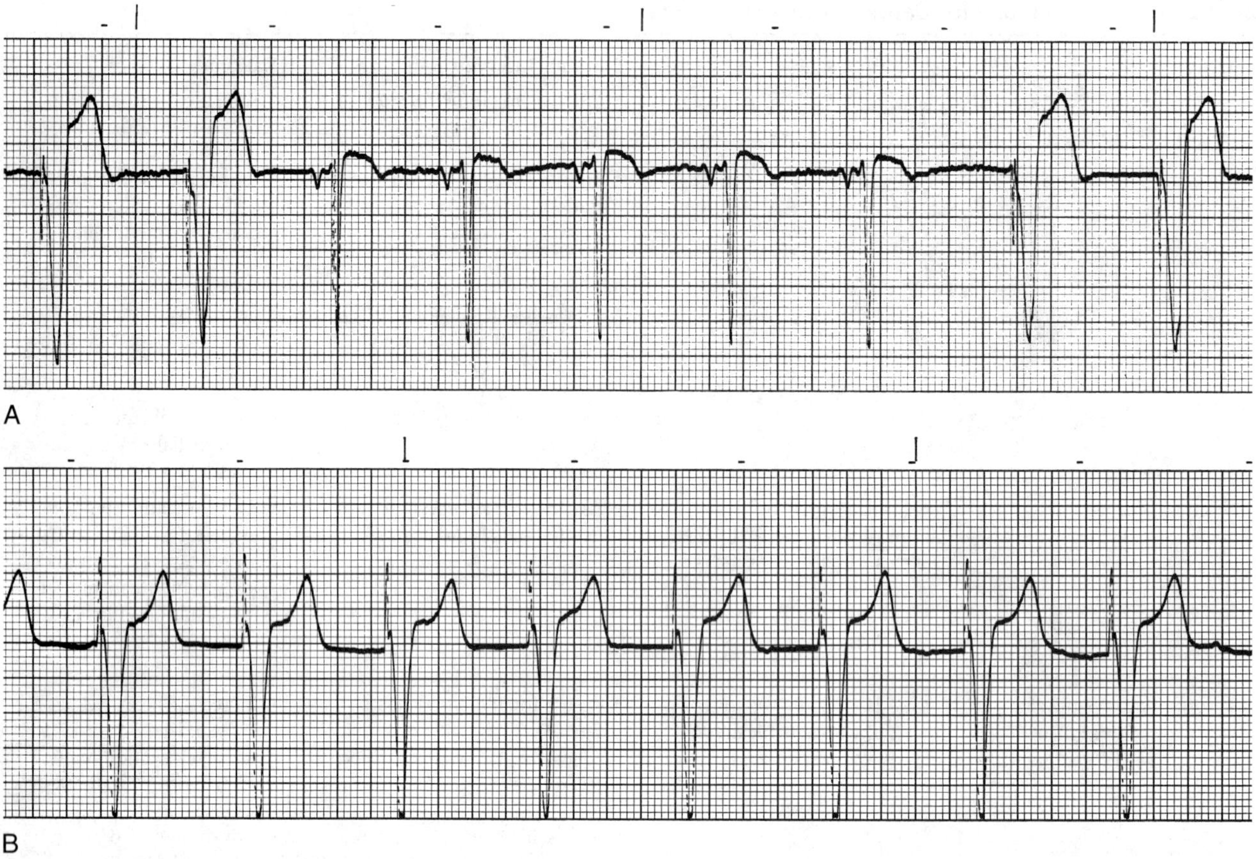

Figure 36–22. Modes of pacing. *A,* Synchronous (demand) ventricular pacing (VVI). *B,* Asynchronous (fixed-rate) ventricular pacing at a rate of 70 beats/minute (VOO).

have emergency equipment available in case the client becomes more unstable or goes into cardiac arrest.

Modes of Pacing. There are two basic modes of pacing: synchronous (demand) pacing and asynchronous (fixed-rate) pacing.

Synchronous (Demand) Pacing. Temporary pacing is most commonly done in the demand mode. The pacemaker's sensitivity is set to sense the client's own beats. When the client's intrinsic rate is above the rate set on the pulse generator, the pacemaker is inhibited from firing. When the client's rate is below that set on the generator, the pacemaker fires electrical impulses to stimulate depolarization (Fig. 36–22A).

Asynchronous (Fixed-Rate) Pacing. The asynchronous mode is used when the client is asystolic or profoundly bradycardiac, as may occur after open heart surgery. When the pulse generator is set in an asynchronous mode, it does not sense any intrinsic beats of the client. The pacemaker continues to fire at a fixed rate as set on the generator, regardless of the client's intrinsic rhythm. This continued firing is not a problem as long as the client remains asystolic or has a rate slower than the pacemaker rate, because all beats come from the pacemaker and there is no competition from the client's beats (see Fig. 36–22B). However, if the client's rate increases and equals or exceeds the pacemaker rate, competition (undersensing) is noted. The danger is that a pacemaker

stimulus may reach the heart during the vulnerable period of repolarization (R-on-T phenomenon, with the pacer spike falling on the T wave) and possibly induce ventricular fibrillation. The nurse must observe for pacemaker competition and set the pacemaker to a synchronous mode to avert potential problems.

Universal Pacemaker Code. In 1974, the Intersociety Commission for Heart Disease established a three-position pacemaker code (ICHD code) to standardize the description of pacemaker systems (Woods et al., 1995).

- The first letter of the code represents the chamber being paced: "A" for atrium, "V" for ventricle, "D" for dual (both atrium and ventricle), and "O" for none.
- The second letter represents the chamber being sensed, using the same three letters. This indicates a demand-pacing mode. If the pacemaker is asynchronous, the second letter is "O," because no chamber is sensed.
- The third letter represents the mode of response: "I" for inhibited, when the pacemaker senses an intrinsic depolarization and inhibits the pacemaker output; "T" for triggered, when the pacemaker senses an intrinsic depolarization and discharges an electrical stimulus along with the intrinsic one; "O" for no mode of response, when the pacemaker is asynchronous and therefore discharges electrical stimuli at a set rate; and "D" for dual mode of response, when sensed events may result in pacemaker inhibition or

TABLE 36-3

The Five-Position Pacemaker Code*

I Chamber(s) Paced	II Chamber(s) Sensed	III Mode of Response	IV Programmability, Rate Modulation	V Antitachycardia Function(s)
A = Atrium	A = Atrium	I = Inhibited	P = Simple programmable	P = Pacing
V = Ventricle	V = Ventricle	T = Triggered	M = Multiprogrammable	S = Shock

D = Dual (atrium
  and ventricle)
	D = Dual (atrium
	  and ventricle)
		D = Atrial triggered
		  and ventricular
		  inhibited
			C = Communicating
			R = Rate modulation
				D = Dual (pacing
				  and shock)

O = None	O = None	O = None	O = None	O = None

From Bernstein, A. D., et al. (1987). The NASPE/BPEG pacemaker code. *PACE, 10*(4), 794.
*The North American Society for Pacing and Electrophysiology (NASPE) and the British Pacing and Electrophysiology Group (BPEG) code (the NASPE/BPEG generic [NBG] code).

triggering so that a sensed atrial event initiates a pacemaker ventricular output unless an intrinsic ventricular event is sensed before a predetermined delay.

This code is used universally and makes it easier to identify quickly the primary functions of the pacemaker. AAI denotes an atrial demand pacemaker. AOO denotes an asynchronous atrial pacemaker. VVI denotes a ventricular demand pacemaker. VOO refers to an asynchronous ventricular pacemaker. DVI denotes a demand AV sequential pacemaker that can pace both chambers but senses only the ventricular chamber. DOO indicates an asynchronous dual-chamber pacemaker. DDD denotes a demand dual-chamber pacemaker that paces and senses both chambers and has a dual mode of response.

The code was expanded to five positions for standardization of multiprogrammable pacemakers and tachydysrhythmia functions, incorporating the original three-position code. This code was designed by the North American Society for Pacing and Electrophysiology (NASPE) and the British Pacing and Electrophysiology Group (BPEG). The code is referred to as the NASPE/BPEG generic (or NBG) code (Table 36–3).

There are two basic types of temporary pacing: noninvasive temporary pacing and invasive temporary pacing.

Noninvasive Temporary Pacing. Noninvasive temporary pacing (NTP) is accomplished through the application of two large patch electrodes. The electrodes are attached to

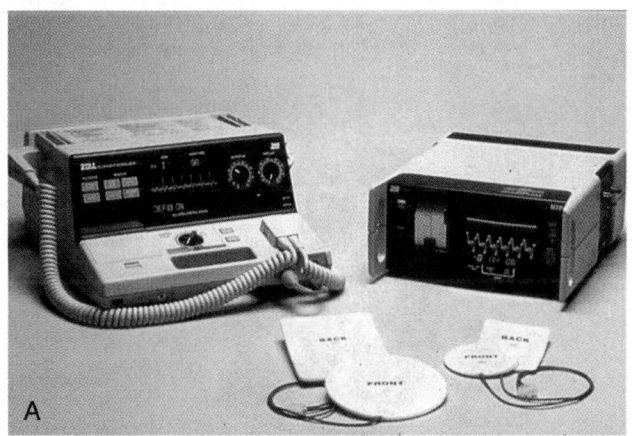
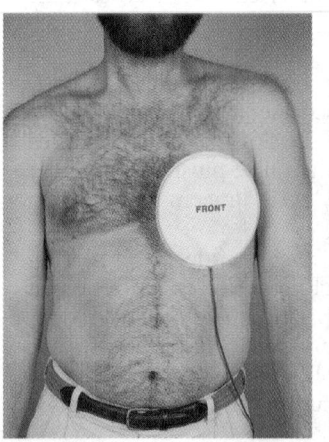
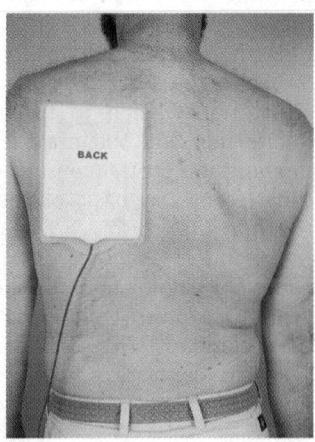
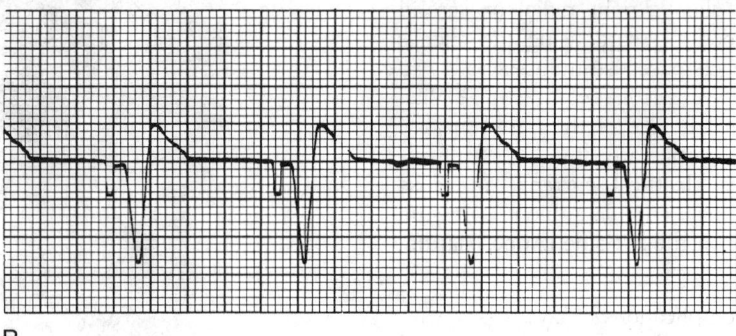

Figure 36–23. *A,* Equipment and electrode placement for transcutaneous external pacing. *B,* ECG rhythm strip showing wide pacing spikes. (*A,* courtesy of Zoll Medical Corporation, Burlington, MA.)

an external pulse generator, which can operate on alternating current (AC) or battery power (Fig. 36–23). The generator emits electrical pulses, which are transmitted through the cutaneous patches and then transcutaneously to stimulate ventricular depolarization when the client's heart rate is slower than the rate set on the pacemaker. Electrical currents of 60 milliamperes (mA) or more are usually required to achieve ventricular depolarization. The current is applied for 20 to 40 milliseconds (msec), producing a pacing stimulus, or spike, that occupies 0.02 to 0.04 second on the ECG paper.

NTP is used as an emergency measure to provide demand ventricular pacing in a profoundly bradycardiac or asystolic client until invasive pacing can be instituted or the client's intrinsic rate returns to normal. It may be used prophylactically when performing procedures or transporting clients at risk for bradydysrhythmias.

Procedure. The nurse explains NTP to the client and prepares the equipment. The nurse washes the client's skin with soap and water. To prevent skin abrasion, the skin must not be shaved. The nurse should not rub the skin or apply alcohol or tinctures on the skin, because electrical current flows from the patches through the skin and causes some discomfort. The nurse then applies the large posterior electrode on the client's back, between the spine and the left scapula, behind the heart. The electrode should not be placed higher over bone because bone is a poor conductor of electrical current. The anterior electrode is then applied on the client's chest, between the V_2 and the V_5 positions, over the heart. The electrode cannot be placed over female breast tissue. The nurse must displace the breast and position the electrode underneath the breast, avoiding a lower position that paces the diaphragm and causes discomfort and possible dyspnea.

The high electrical pacing current distorts the ECG signal transmission to the bedside monitor. To reduce interference and obtain a clear ECG signal on the bedside monitor and central console, the nurse must attach a filter cable from the back of the NTP unit to the bedside monitor.

The nurse sets the pacing rate as ordered and establishes the stimulation threshold, the lowest current that achieves capture with each pacing spike followed by a QRS complex. The QRS complex is wide because one ventricle depolarizes first, followed by the other. The nurse then sets the electrical current 10% above threshold levels.

The nurse palpates the client's right radial or carotid pulse and assesses the blood pressure using the client's right arm, ensuring that each paced stimulus is followed by a mechanical response (ventricular contraction). Vital signs are not taken on the left side of the body because they may not be accurate, particularly if a high milliamperage is used. This large electrical current can cause muscle twitching, which may stimulate blood pressure sounds or simulate a pulse on the left side (Appel-Hardin, 1992).

Complications. Three complications may arise with NTP. The first includes discomfort from cutaneous and muscle stimulation and skin irritation and diaphoresis from the patch electrodes. The nurse must ensure that the electrodes are in good contact with the skin and in the best location to achieve the lowest threshold for consistent capture. The nurse also administers prescribed analgesics or sedatives and provides comfort and support.

The second problem is loss of capture, when the pacing spike is not followed by a QRS complex. The nurse ensures that the electrodes are in good contact with the skin and, if necessary, increases the current until capture is regained; however, higher currents cause more discomfort for the client.

The third problem is inappropriate pacing, when the pacemaker does not sense the client's intrinsic QRS complex and therefore fires impulses at its preset rate, competing with the client's rhythm. The nurse must assess electrode contact and the effect of the client's position on pacemaker function. The client may have to avoid lying on the left side. If diaphoresis has caused poor contact and the electrodes must be replaced, the nurse must first turn the pacing function off to avoid receiving electrical shocks when touching the gel side of the electrodes.

Invasive Temporary Pacing. An invasive temporary pacemaker system consists of an external, battery-operated pulse generator (Fig. 36–24) and pacing electrodes, or lead wires. These wires attach to the generator on one end and are in contact with the heart on the other end. Electrical pulses, or stimuli, are emitted from the negative terminal of the generator, flow through a lead wire, and stimulate the myocardial cells to depolarize. The current seeks ground by returning through the other lead wire to the positive terminal of the generator, thus completing a circuitous route. The intensity of electrical current is set by selecting the appropriate current output, measured in milliamperes.

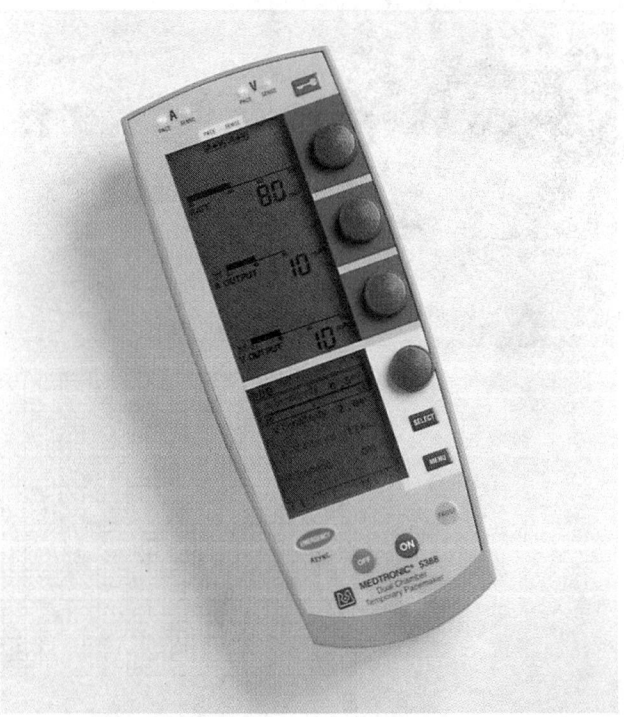

Figure 36–24. Temporary dual-chamber pacemaker. (Courtesy of Medtronic, Inc., Minneapolis, MN.)

The client does not usually feel invasive pacemaker stimuli; however, clients occasionally feel an uncomfortable sensation from the stimuli if strong electrical currents (high milliamperage) are delivered by the pacemaker. The discomfort may be alleviated by decreasing the current if possible.

The two types of invasive temporary pacing are transvenous pacing and epicardial pacing.

Transvenous Pacing. Transvenous ventricular pacing involves the use of fluoroscopy to thread a sterile catheter, containing two lead wires, percutaneously through a vein to the right ventricle for temporary pacing. The catheter electrode tip (negative electrode) is in contact with the endocardial surface of the ventricle, where it fixates for stability (Fig. 36–25A). The positive electrode is located just proximal to the tip of the catheter. The bifurcated

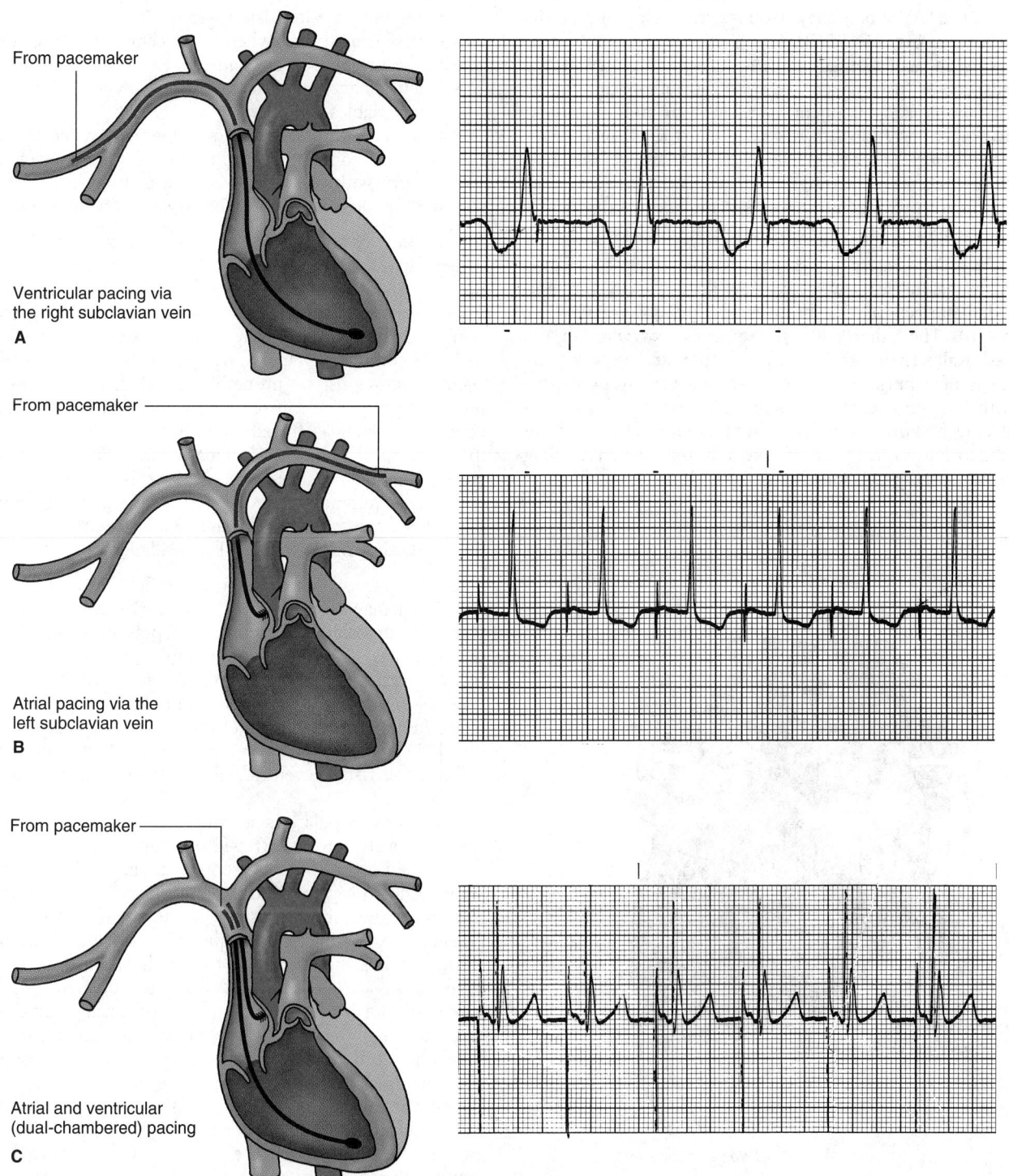

Figure 36–25. Pacemaker catheter electrode placement and corresponding ECG patterns in temporary transvenous pacing. *A,* Ventricular pacing at a rate of 72/minute. *B,* Atrial pacing at a rate of 88/minute, with intrinsic QRS complexes. *C,* AV pacing at a rate of 80/minute.

external end of the catheter is attached to the negative and positive terminals of a battery-operated pulse generator. The generator provides the electrical current to stimulate the myocardial cells to depolarize.

If the client needs the atrial kick from atrial contractions, a temporary dual-chamber pacemaker is used, with one catheter tip in the right atrium and the other in the right ventricle (see Fig. 36–25B). This preserves the normal synchrony of atrial contraction preceding ventricular contraction. Some clients with a dysfunctional sinus node but intact AV node may require only temporary atrial pacing (see Fig. 36–25C).

Nursing management of the client after temporary transvenous pacemaker insertion includes continuous ECG monitoring, frequent assessment of vital signs and pacemaker insertion site, restriction of the client's movement to prevent lead wire displacement, and documentation of pacemaker settings. The qualified nurse or other health care provider must assess stimulation and sensitivity thresholds according to institutional protocols.

Epicardial Pacing. Epicardial pacing is accomplished with separate lead wires loosely threaded on the epicardial surface of the heart after cardiac surgery (Fig. 36–26). The other ends of the wires exit through the chest wall. They attach to the negative and positive terminals of a pulse generator. There are usually two wires on the atrium and two wires on the ventricle. The electrical current flows from epicardium to endocardium, from right to left. Nursing management of the client following cardiac surgery is detailed in Chapter 40.

Complications. Complications of invasive temporary pacing may be serious and include

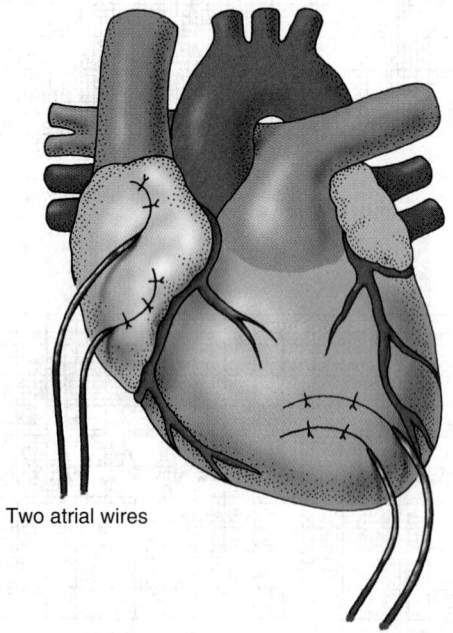

Figure 36–26. Lead wire placement for epicardial pacing after cardiac surgery. Two wires are sutured on the right atrium and two on the right ventricle.

Two atrial wires

Two ventricular wires

- Infection or hematoma at the pacemaker wire insertion site
- Ectopic complexes (usually premature ventricular complexes), caused by irritability from the pacing wire in the ventricle, use of high current, or undersensing with pacemaker competition
- Loss of capture, noted by the presence of a pacing stimulus or spike but no depolarization
- Undersensing or pacemaker competition, noted when pacing stimuli occur at a fixed rate in the presence of an adequate intrinsic rhythm
- Oversensing, noted when the pacemaker fails to fire in the presence of an inadequate intrinsic rhythm
- Electromagnetic interference, noted by altered generator variables
- Stimulation of chest wall or diaphragm, noted by rhythmic contraction of the chest wall muscles or hiccups with use of high current or from lead wire perforation, which could cause cardiac tamponade

Prevention of Microshock. When the metal external ends of lead wires are not attached to a pulse generator, the nurse must insulate the wire ends to prevent microshock. The fingertips of rubber gloves work well for this purpose, and the wire ends may then be looped and covered with nonconductive tape. All electrical equipment in the client's room must be properly grounded, using a three-pronged plug. The nurse must report faulty electrical equipment, such as frayed or broken electrical wires, to the biomedical engineering department. The nurse must ensure that neither the client nor the bed is in contact with such equipment. The risk is that ungrounded electrical current may conduct through the lead wire, stimulate the heart, and induce ventricular fibrillation.

Cardioversion. Cardioversion is a synchronized countershock that may be performed in emergencies for hemodynamically unstable ventricular or supraventricular tachydysrhythmias or electively for stable tachydysrhythmias that are resistant to medical therapies. If the client has been taking digitalis, the nurse withholds the drug for up to 48 hours preceding an elective cardioversion, as ordered. Digitalis increases ventricular irritability and puts the client at risk for ventricular fibrillation after the countershock.

The shock depolarizes a critical mass of myocardium simultaneously during intrinsic depolarization. The shock is intended to stop the re-entry circuit and allow the sinus node to regain control of the heart. The physician and skilled personnel must be in attendance during this procedure, with emergency equipment at hand. The physician explains the procedure to the client and assists the client to sign a consent form unless the procedure is an emergency for a life-threatening dysrhythmia. Because the client is usually conscious, the nurse must administer IV sedation as ordered. An anesthesiologist may administer a short-acting anesthetic agent.

The nurse examines the client's skin to ensure that no ECG electrodes and no topical nitroglycerin preparations are on the sites where the paddles will be placed. If present, they must be removed and the skin cleaned and dried. The physician or advanced cardiac life support (ACLS)–qualified nurse places conductive pads, one on

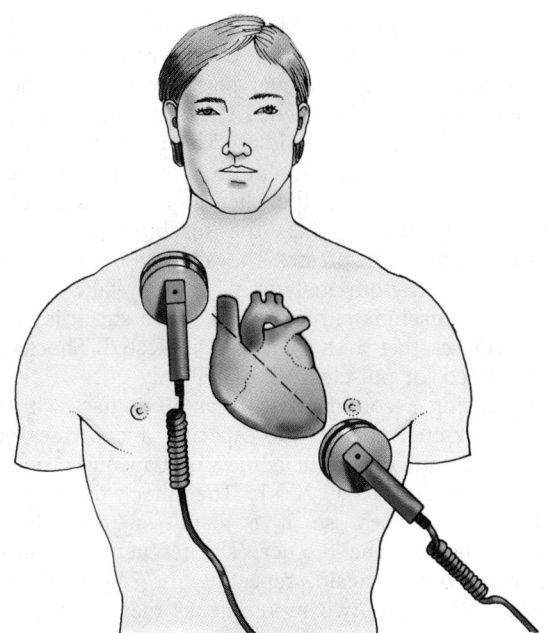

Figure 36–27. Standard electrode paddle placement for cardioversion or defibrillation.

the client's upper right chest below the clavicle and the other left of the nipple with the center in the mid–axillary line (Cummins et al., 1994). The nurse places the electrode paddles over the pads (Fig. 36–27), applying firm pressure.

The ECG electrodes from the monitor-defibrillator are applied for continuous monitoring. The nurse ensures that the defibrillator is synchronized to the client's R wave. This avoids discharging the shock during the vulnerable period (T wave), which may increase ventricular irritability, causing ventricular fibrillation. The nurse charges the capacitor on the defibrillator to the energy ordered by the physician, usually starting at 50–100 J. The nurse ensures that the oxygen delivery device has been removed and turned away from the client. Oxygen supports combustion, and a fire may result if there is arcing from the paddles. Arcing is usually due to improper paddle contact on the chest. The nurse then loudly and clearly commands all personnel to clear contact with the client and the bed, as required for electrical safety. The nurse ensures compliance of all personnel before delivering the shock. While the client is exhaling, the nurse discharges both paddles simultaneously to deliver the shock at end-expiration, when the heart is closer to the chest wall, so that more current flow can reach the heart for a better chance of success. This procedure may also be performed by a physician's assistant, paramedic, or other qualified health care provider following medical protocols.

After cardioversion, the nurse assesses the client's response and heart rhythm. Therapy is repeated as ordered, if necessary, until the desired result is obtained or alternative therapies are considered. If the client goes into ventricular fibrillation after cardioversion, the nurse must ensure that the synchronizer is turned off and then immediately defibrillate the client.

Nursing care after cardioversion includes
- Maintaining a patent airway
- Administering oxygen
- Assessing the client's vital signs and level of consciousness
- Administering antidysrhythmic drug therapy
- Monitoring for dysrhythmias
- Assessing for chest burns from paddle edges that may not have been on the conductive pad
- Providing emotional support for the client

Cardiopulmonary Resuscitation. Management of the client in cardiac arrest depends on prompt recognition and therapeutic interventions for successful reversal of a potentially fatal event.

When cardiac arrest occurs, cardiac output ceases. The underlying rhythm is usually ventricular tachycardia, ventricular fibrillation, or asystole. In rare instances, cardiac arrest occurs in the presence of an organized electrocardiographic (ECG) rhythm, but with no effectual mechanical response, a condition referred to as PEA (pulseless electrical activity) (Cummins et al., 1994). Without a cardiac output, the client is pulseless and becomes unconscious because of inadequate cerebral perfusion. Shortly after cardiac arrest, respiratory arrest occurs.

CPR must be initiated immediately to help prevent brain damage and death. The nurse, finding an unresponsive client, calls out loudly for help while initiating CPR. The initial priorities are
- Maintenance of a patent airway
- Ventilation with a mouth-to-mask device
- Chest compressions

As soon as help arrives, a board is placed under a client who is not on a firm surface. To make room for the resuscitation team and the crash cart, the nurse commands that the area be cleared of movable items and unnecessary personnel.

Complications of CPR include rib fractures, fracture of the sternum, costochondral separation, lacerations of the liver and spleen, pneumothorax, hemothorax, cardiac tamponade, lung contusions, and fat emboli. The goal of resuscitation is the rapid return of a pulse, blood pressure, and consciousness in the client. This is rarely achieved by CPR and basic measures alone. More definitive therapy must be initiated as soon as possible with ACLS measures, including defibrillation, if warranted.

Advanced Cardiac Life Support. When the crash cart arrives, the nurse applies ECG electrodes to the client's chest and turns on the monitor, directing the team to continue CPR. If the client is found to be in ventricular fibrillation or pulseless ventricular tachycardia, the immediate priority is to defibrillate the client. Following defibrillation, CPR is resumed. An oropharyngeal airway is inserted in the client to facilitate proper ventilation. A manual resuscitation bag (MRB) with mask is attached to an oxygen flowmeter, running at 10 to 15 L/minute. The nurse directs that the person managing the airway now ventilate the client with the MRB, maintaining the proper head-tilt, chin-lift position of the client. Nurses initiate two intravenous (IV) lines if the client does not have any, infusing normal saline. These lines provide access for emergency drug administration. Suction equipment is also set up, with a tonsillar suction tube for suctioning vomitus and a suction catheter for endotracheal suctioning. Carotid or femoral pulse checks, during chest compressions and without chest compressions, blood pressure measurements, and pupil assessments are done at frequent intervals. A nurse documents all assessments and findings, therapeutic measures, and the client's responses throughout the resuscitation.

Additional measures include endotracheal intubation with ventilation and oxygenation, IV administration of emergency cardiac drugs, and, occasionally, pacing. Chest compressions are continued as long as the client remains pulseless or until a physician decides to terminate resuscitation attempts.

Defibrillation. Defibrillation, an asynchronous countershock, depolarizes a critical mass of myocardium simultaneously to stop the re-entry circuit and to allow the sinus node to regain control of the heart. Early defibrillation is critical to terminate pulseless ventricular tachycardia (VT) or ventricular fibrillation (VF). It must not be delayed for any reason after the equipment and skilled personnel are present. The earlier defibrillation is performed, the greater the chance of survival.

If a defibrillator is not immediately available, an ACLS-qualified nurse may deliver a precordial thump to a pulseless client in VF. There is a slight chance that it may succeed in terminating the VF (Cummins et al., 1994). A precordial thump is performed by striking the lower half of the sternum with a closed fist from a height of 8 to 12 inches (12 to 30 cm) above the sternum. If the client remains in VF, CPR is resumed and the nurse prepares the client's chest for defibrillation.

The physician or the ACLS-qualified nurse places conductive gel pads, one on the client's upper right chest below the clavicle and the other to the left of the nipple with the center in the mid–axillary line (Cummins et al., 1994). The nurse places the electrode paddles over the pads (see Fig. 36–27), applies firm pressure, and charges the capacitor on the defibrillator to an initial energy of 200 J. The nurse ensures that the oxygen delivery device has been removed and turned away from the client. If the client is already intubated, the MRB may be left attached. The nurse loudly and clearly commands all personnel to clear contact with the client and the bed and ensures their compliance before delivering the shock.

After defibrillation, the nurse maintains paddle position while assessing the client's heart rhythm. If the first shock was unsuccessful, the nurse immediately delivers a second shock at 200 to 300 J, followed by a third shock at 360 J, if necessary. The shocks are given in rapid succession. Successive shocks decrease transthoracic impedance, allowing more current flow to reach the heart for a better chance of success. If defibrillation is successful, the nurse and team members maintain a patent airway, provide oxygen and ventilatory support, assess vital signs frequently, and continuously monitor the client for the recurrence of dysrhythmias. IV access, hemodynamic support, and antidysrhythmic medications are also essential.

Automatic External Defibrillation. The American Heart Association promotes the use of automatic external defibrillators (AEDs) for use by lay persons and health care

providers responding to cardiac arrest emergencies (Cummins et al., 1994). The client in cardiac arrest must be on a firm, dry surface. The rescuer places two large adhesive patch electrodes on the client's chest, in the same positions as for defibrillator paddles. The rescuer stops CPR and commands anyone present to move away, ensuring that no one is touching the client. This measure eliminates motion artifact when the machine analyzes the rhythm. The rescuer presses the analyze button on the machine. After rhythm analysis, which may take up to 30 seconds, the machine either advises that a shock is necessary or advises that a shock is not indicated. Shocks are recommended for pulseless VF or VT only.

After issuing a command to clear all contact with the client, the rescuer charges the capacitor and presses both discharge buttons on the machine simultaneously, delivering the first shock at 200 J. The shock is delivered through the patches, so it is hands-off defibrillation, which is safer for the rescuer. The rescuer then presses the analyze button again, repeating the sequence. With sustained VF or VT, two more shocks may be delivered, with the third at 360 J. If the client remains in cardiac arrest, CPR is performed for 1 minute, and then another series of three shocks may be delivered, each at 360 J. It is imperative that ACLS be provided as soon as possible. Use of AEDs results in earlier defibrillation of clients and therefore a greater chance of successful rhythm conversion and survival.

Current-Based Defibrillation. Research is being conducted on the use of current-based defibrillation. Defibrillators in use deliver energy, measured in joules. It is not known what the optimal energy for defibrillation is or whether energy selected may be too low, which may be ineffective, or too high, which could result in myocardial damage. These problems would be avoided by the use of electrical current, measured in amperes, as it would take into account transthoracic impedance. Optimal defibrillation current has been found to be 30 to 40 mA (Cummins et al., 1994). Such defibrillators are under investigation.

Radiofrequency Catheter Ablation. Radiofrequency catheter ablation is an invasive procedure that may be used to abolish an irritable focus causing a supraventricular or ventricular tachydysrhythmia. The client must undergo electrophysiologic studies and mapping procedures to locate the focus. Then radiofrequency waves are delivered to abolish the irritable focus. When ablation is performed in the AV nodal or His bundle area, damage may also occur to the normal conduction system, causing heart blocks, requiring implantation of a permanent pacemaker.

Surgical Management. Clients who experience life-threatening dysrhythmias may require surgical treatment for long-term management. The type of treatment depends on the nature of the dysrhythmia. Procedures include permanent pacing, coronary artery bypass grafting, aneurysmectomy, insertion of an implantable cardioverter/defibrillator, and open-chest cardiac massage.

Permanent Pacing. Permanent pacemaker insertion is performed for the resolution of conduction disorders that are not temporary, including complete heart block and sick sinus syndrome. Permanent pacemakers are usually powered by a lithium battery and have an average life span of 10 years. After the battery power is depleted, the generator must be replaced, a procedure done under local anesthesia. Some pacemakers are nuclear powered and have a life span of 20 years or longer. Other pacemakers can be recharged externally.

Types of Pacemakers. Pacemakers may be single chambered or dual chambered. With single-chamber pacemakers, a lead wire is positioned in the chamber to be paced, most commonly the right ventricle. Occasionally, it is positioned in the right atrium for bradydysrhythmias originating from SA node disease with an intact atrioventricular (AV) conduction system.

Dual-chamber pacemakers have lead wires placed in the right atrium and the right ventricle (Fig. 36–28A,B) for a more physiologic effect, preserving the atrial kick. A programmed AV interval, which closely relates to the PR interval, ensures a ventricular response shortly after atrial depolarization. The DDD pacemaker is commonly implanted. It is able to sense both atrial and ventricular intrinsic activity and pace both the atrium and the ventricle. It allows sinus control of the ventricular rate to meet increased metabolic demands when the sinus node is functioning well. If the client's sinus rate drops below the lower rate set, the generator paces both the atrium and the ventricle.

Another feature of many pacemakers is rate responsiveness. To allow faster pacing rates to meet increased body demands, the generator changes pacing rate in response to a detected change in a physiologic variable, such as muscle movement within the client with impaired sinus or atrial function. Hysteresis, on the other hand, is a feature that allows the client's rate to slow to 10 to 20 beats lower than the generator's pre-set rate before the generator paces the client. The slower pace allows a more normal physiologic slowing response during rest or sleep.

Surgical Procedures. For both single-chamber and dual-chamber pacemakers, the surgeon most commonly implants the pulse generator in a surgically made subcutaneous pocket at the shoulder in the right or left subclavicular area. The leads are introduced transvenously via the cephalic or the subclavian vein to the endocardium on the right side of the heart. After the procedure, the nurse monitors the client's ECG rhythm to ensure that the pacemaker is functioning correctly. The nurse also assesses the implantation site for evidence of bleeding, swelling, redness, tenderness, and infection. The dressing over the site should remain clean and dry, and the client should be afebrile and have stable vital signs. The physician orders activity restrictions to enhance lead fixation. After 24 hours, activity is gradually increased. Complications of permanent pacemakers are similar to those for temporary invasive pacing.

Pacemaker checks are done on an outpatient basis at regular intervals. Reprogramming may be warranted if there are pacemaker problems. The pulse generator is interrogated using an electronic device to determine the pacemaker settings and battery life (Fig. 36–29).

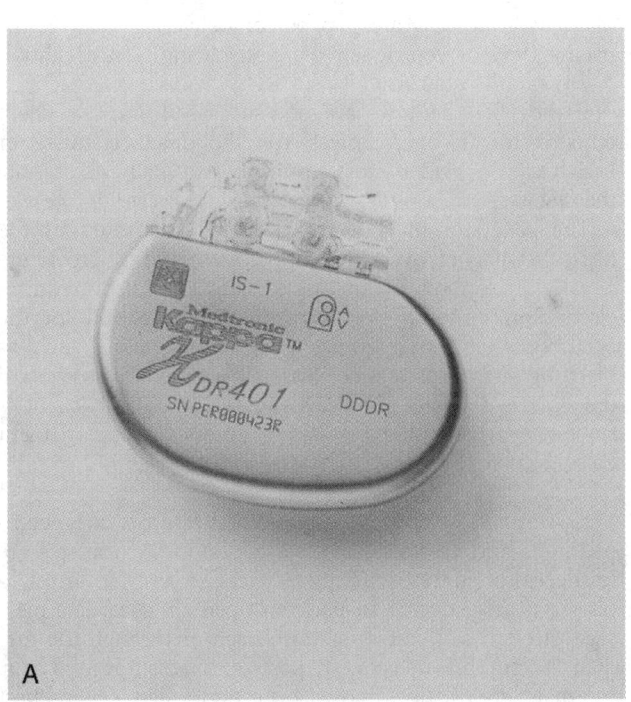

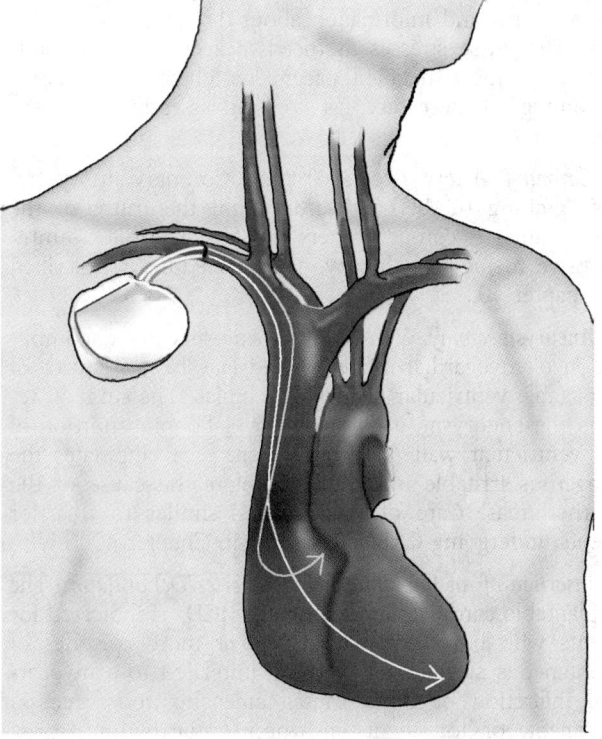

Figure 36–28. *A,* Permanent dual-chamber pacemaker. *B,* Implanted permanent dual-chamber pacemaker with endocardial leads introduced via the right subclavian vein into the right atrium and right ventricle. (Courtesy of Medtronic, Inc., Minneapolis, MN.)

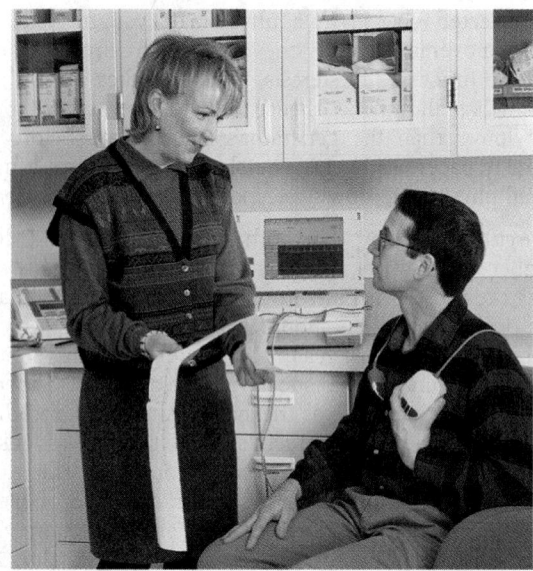

Figure 36-29. Permanent pacemaker check. The "head" of the device (shown being held in the client's left hand) is placed over the pulse generator to interrogate the pacemaker and reprogram it if necessary. (Courtesy of Medtronic, Inc., Minneapolis, MN.)

For clients who live far from the pacemaker clinic or physician's office, pacemaker information can be sent via transtelephonic transmission of data. The client attaches ECG electrodes to the wrists and places the telephone receiver in a transmitting unit. The sound signals are relayed via telephone lines to the clinic or office, where they are converted and recorded as the client's ECG rhythm strip and information about the pacemaker variables. The nurse stresses the need to keep clinic appointments for more detailed pacemaker checks and reprogramming, if necessary, as well as assessment of the client.

Coronary Artery Bypass Grafting. Coronary artery bypass grafting (CABG) is performed if the cause of the dysrhythmia is coronary artery insufficiency that is unresponsive to medical therapy. This procedure is described in Chapter 40.

Aneurysmectomy. Ventricular aneurysms are a complication of myocardial infarction and may be the source of intractable ventricular tachydysrhythmias. The surgeon resects the aneurysm, a dyskinetic or ballooning portion of the ventricular wall. Resection of the area eliminates the dangerous irritable focus and therefore the cause of the dysrhythmias. Care of the client is similar to that for clients undergoing CABG, described in Chapter 40.

Insertion of an Implantable Cardioverter/Defibrillator. The implantable cardioverter/defibrillator (ICD) is indicated for clients who have experienced one or more episodes of spontaneous sustained VT or VF, unrelated to a myocardial infarction or other causes amenable to correction treatment, or for clients in whom antiarrhythmic drug therapy to control life-threatening dysrhythmias has not been successful or is limited by drug intolerance or noncompliance. Clients undergo electrophysiologic studies to assess the inducibility of ventricular tachydysrhythmias and their response to medication. If the dysrhythmias can be induced despite medical therapy, the client is considered a candidate for ICD implantation. A psychological profile is done to determine whether the client will be able to cope with the discomfort and fear associated with internal defibrillation from the ICD.

In the past, a median sternotomy or left thoracotomy approach for implanting the leads of the device was used, and the generator was implanted in a paraumbilical pocket. This procedure was performed in an operating suite. Currently, the leads are introduced percutaneously, and the generator is implanted in the left pectoral area, similar to a permanent pacemaker insertion procedure. This procedure is performed in the electrophysiology laboratory.

The electronic pulse generator is designed to monitor and to deliver therapy for ventricular tachycardia or ventricular fibrillation. The generator is powered by a lithium battery and is connected to a transvenous endocardial lead. The ends of the lead are tunneled under the skin to attach to the generator. The sensing lead transmits electrical signals from the heart to the generator, which continuously monitors the heart rhythm. If the client's heart rate exceeds the generator's programmed rate (rate cutoff), such as with ventricular tachycardia, the generator takes a few seconds to sense the cardiac electrical activity and then delivers a burst of antitachycardia pacing (ATP) to overdrive pace the rhythm. A programmed number of ATP therapies may be delivered. If the client's rate continues to exceed the rate cutoff, the device can deliver a programmed number of low-energy and high-energy cardioversion shocks. In response to ventricular fibrillation, the device delivers defibrillation shocks. Following such therapy, the client may develop a transient bradycardia. Many ICD devices are capable of delivering bradycardia pacing (VVI or ventricular demand pacing). This technology is rapidly changing.

If the ICD therapies are not successful and the client remains in VF or pulseless VT, the qualified nurse or health care provider must promptly externally defibrillate the client.

The generator may be activated or deactivated by the use of a magnet over the implantation site, a procedure usually performed by the physician. The client requires close monitoring in the postimplantation period for the occurrence of dysrhythmias and complications such as bleeding and cardiac tamponade. The nurse must know if the ICD is activated or deactivated. Care of the client is similar to that following implantation of a permanent pacemaker.

Open-Chest Cardiac Massage. When external chest compressions and advanced cardiac life support measures are unsuccessful in resuscitating a client in cardiac arrest, a physician may decide to perform open-chest cardiac massage through a thoracotomy approach or through the median sternotomy incision in post-cardiac surgery clients. Internal defibrillation may also be performed. Open-chest cardiac massage is usually reserved for the cardiac surgical client who goes into cardiac arrest, often because of cardiac tamponade. It may also be beneficial but is rarely indicated for clients with hypothermia, crushing or penetrating chest injuries, penetrating abdominal trauma, or chest deformities prohibiting external chest compressions.

 ## Continuing Care

For many clients, dysrhythmias are a chronic disorder resulting from chronic cardiac and pulmonary diseases. Clients may be cared for in a variety of settings, including the acute care hospital, subacute unit, traditional nursing home, or their own homes. Clients are admitted to the hospital when they experience life-threatening or potentially life-threatening dysrhythmias, often associated with an acute disorder. Other clients can be managed with office or clinic visits or in other settings.

Clients discharged from the hospital may have considerable needs, often more related to their underlying chronic diseases than to their dysrhythmias, which should be essentially controlled by drug or device therapy. A case manager or care coordinator can assess the client's needs for health care resources and coordinate access to needed services.

➤ *Health Teaching*

Prevention of Recurrence. Clients who have experienced a dysrhythmia associated with an acute disorder, such as electrolyte imbalance or ischemia related to a myocardial infarction, are instructed in the prevention, early recognition, and management of that disorder. The nurse teaches the client and family about lifestyle modifications designed to prevent, decrease, or control the occurrence of dysrhythmias, as outlined in Chart 36–6. This teaching may be provided in the acute care setting, physician's office, health care clinic, or home setting.

Drug Therapy. Clients and the parents of children receiving antidysrhythmic drugs must have a thorough understanding of their medications. Pharmacies provide written instructions about antidysrhythmic agents prescribed for the client. The nurse teaches clients and families the generic and trade names of their drugs, as well as their purposes, using basic terms that are easily understood. The nurse must provide clear instructions on dosage schedules and common side effects (see Chart 36–3). The nurse emphasizes the importance of reporting these side effects and any dizziness, nausea, vomiting, chest discomfort, or shortness of breath to the health care provider. Chart 36–7 highlights special considerations for elderly clients receiving antidysrhythmic therapy.

Pulse Check. The nurse teaches all clients and their significant others or family members how to take the client's pulse. The nurse instructs them to report any signs of a change in heart rhythm, such as a significant decrease in pulse rate, a rate greater than 100 beats per minute, or increased irregularity.

Pacemaker. Clients and parents of children who have a permanent pacemaker are given written and verbal information about the type and settings of their pacemaker. The nurse teaches them to report any pulse rate lower than that set on the pacemaker or lower than the hystere-

---

Chart 36–6

Education Guide: How to Prevent or Decrease Dysrhythmias

For Clients at Risk for Vasovagal Attacks Causing Bradydysrhythmias

- Avoid doing things that stimulate the vagus nerve, such as raising your arms above your head, applying pressure over your carotid artery, applying pressure on your eyes, bearing down or straining during a bowel movement, and stimulating a gag reflex when brushing your teeth or putting objects in your mouth.

For Clients with Premature Beats and Ectopic Rhythms

- Take the medications that have been prescribed for you, and report any adverse effects to your physician.
- Stop smoking, avoid caffeinated beverages as much as possible, and drink alcohol only in moderation.
- Learn ways to manage stress and avoid getting too tired.

For Clients with Ischemic Heart Disease

- If you have an angina attack, treat it promptly with rest and nitroglycerin administration as prescribed by your physician. This decreases your chances of experiencing a dysrhythmia.
- If chest pain is not relieved after taking the amount of nitroglycerin that has been prescribed for you, seek medical attention promptly. Also, seek prompt medical attention if the pain becomes more severe or you experience other symptoms, such as sweating, nausea, weakness, and palpitations.

For Clients at Risk for Potassium Imbalance

- Know the symptoms of decreased potassium levels, such as muscle weakness and cardiac irregularity.
- Eat foods high in potassium, such as tomatoes, beans, prunes, avocados, bananas, strawberries, and lettuce.
- Take the potassium supplements that have been prescribed for you.

---

sis rate. The nurse teaches the client the proper care of the pacemaker insertion site and the importance of reporting any fever or any redness, swelling, or drainage at the pacemaker insertion site. If the surgical incision is near either shoulder, the nurse teaches and demonstrates range-of-motion exercises for the client to perform to prevent shoulder stiffness. The nurse instructs the client to keep hand-held cellular phones at least 6 inches away from the generator, with the handset on the ear opposite the side of the generator. The nurse also teaches clients with pacemakers to avoid sources of strong electromagnetic fields, such as magnets and telecommunications transmitters. These may cause interference and could change the pacemaker settings, causing a malfunction. Magnetic resonance imaging is contraindicated for clients with pacemakers. The nurse instructs the client to carry a pacemaker identification card and to wear a medical alert (Medic-Alert) bracelet. Chart 36–8 outlines the major points for client and family teaching after the insertion of a permanent pacemaker.

Nursing Focus on the Elderly: Dysrhythmias

Elderly clients are at increased risk for dysrhythmias because of changes in their cardiac conduction system. The sinoatrial node has fewer pacemaker cells. There is a loss of fibers in the bundle branch system. Therefore, elderly clients are at risk for sinus node dysfunction and may require pacemaker therapy. The most common dysrhythmias in the elderly are premature atrial contractions, premature ventricular contractions, and atrial fibrillation. Dysrhythmias tend to be more serious in elderly clients because of underlying heart disease, causing cardiac decompensation. Consequently, blood flow to organs, which may already be decreased because of the aging process, is further compromised, leading to multisystem organ dysfunction. The following are special nursing considerations for the elderly client with dysrhythmias:

- Evaluate the client with dysrhythmias immediately for the presence of a life-threatening dysrhythmia or hemodynamic deterioration.
- Assess the client with a dysrhythmia for angina, hypotension, heart failure, and decreased cerebral and renal perfusion.
- Consider the following causes of dysrhythmias when taking the client's history: hypoxia, drug toxicity, electrolyte imbalances, heart failure, and myocardial ischemia or infarction.
- Assess the client's level of education, hearing, learning style, and ability to understand and recall instructions to determine the best approaches for teaching.

- Assess the client's ability to read written instructions.
- Teach the client the generic and trade names of prescribed antidysrhythmic drugs, as well as their purposes, dosage, side effects, and special instructions for their use.
- Provide clear, written instructions in basic language and easy-to-read print.
- Provide a written drug dosage schedule for the client, taking into account all the medications the client is taking and possible drug interactions.
- Assess the client for possible side effects or adverse reactions to drugs, considering the client's age and health status.
- Teach the client to take his or her pulse and to report significant changes in heart rate or rhythm to the physician.
- Inform the client of available resources for blood pressure and pulse checks, such as blood pressure clinics, home health agencies, and cardiac rehabilitation programs.
- Instruct the client on the importance of keeping follow-up visit appointments with the physician and of reporting symptoms promptly.
- Include the client's family members or significant other in all teaching whenever possible.
- Instruct the client to avoid drinking caffeinated beverages, to stop smoking, to drink alcohol only in moderation, and to follow his or her prescribed diet.

Implantable Cardioverter/Defibrillator. Clients with an implantable cardioverter/defibrillator (ICD) usually continue to receive antidysrhythmic drugs after discharge from the hospital. The nurse stresses the importance of continuing to take these medications as prescribed. The nurse provides clear instructions about the purposes of the medications, the dosage schedules, special instructions for taking the medications, and side effects to report. The nurse teaches clients that if they experience an internal defibrillator shock, they must sit or lie down immediately and must notify the physician. Some clients describe the experience of a shock as a quick thud or kick in the chest, whereas other clients relate severe pain similar to that of external defibrillation. The nurse informs family members that they may feel an electrical shock if they are touching the client during delivery of the shock, but it is not harmful. The nurse provides instructions to the client and family members on how to access the emergency medical services (EMS) system in their community. The nurse also recommends resources for the family to learn how to perform CPR.

The nurse teaches clients with an ICD to avoid sources of strong electromagnetic fields, such as large electrical generators and radio or television transmitters. These may inhibit tachydysrhythmia detection and therapy or may cause inadvertent antitachycardia pacing or shocks. Mag-

netic resonance imaging is contraindicated for clients with ICDs. Hand-held cellular phones must be at least 6 inches away from the generator, with the handset to the ear opposite the side of the ICD. The nurse stresses that if the pulse generator emits a beeping sound or provides some other indicator, the client must move away from the area as quickly as possible to prevent deactivation of the device. The nurse instructs the client with an ICD to carry an ICD identification card and to wear a medical alert (Medic-Alert) bracelet. Chart 36–9 highlights the important points for teaching clients and family members and significant others.

➤ Home Care Management

The focus of the home care nurse's interventions is assessment and health teaching. Clients and families often fear recurrence of a life-threatening dysrhythmia. Clients with an ICD may dread or fear the activation of the ICD. The continuing care nurse provides the client and family members with the opportunity to verbalize their concerns and fears. The nurse provides emotional support, as well as information about support groups in the community, and makes appropriate referrals. The nurse assesses the client for possible side effects from antidysrhythmic agents or complications from a pacemaker or ICD and communicates concerns and problems to the client's

---

Chart 36-8

Education Guide: Permanent Pacemakers

- Follow the instructions for pacemaker site skin care that have been specifically prepared for you. Report any fever or redness, swelling, or drainage from the incision site to your physician.
- Keep your pacemaker identification card in your wallet and wear a medical alert (MedicAlert) bracelet.
- Take your pulse for one full minute at the same time each day and record the rate in your pacemaker diary. Take your pulse any time you feel symptoms of a possible pacemaker failure and report your heart rate and symptoms to your physician.
- Know the rate at which your pacemaker is set and the basic functioning of your pacemaker. Know what rate changes to report to your physician.
- Do not apply pressure over your generator. Avoid tight clothing or belts.
- You may take baths or showers without concern for your pacemaker.
- Inform other physicians and dentists that you have a pacemaker. Certain tests they may wish to perform (such as magnetic resonance imaging) could affect or damage your pacemaker.
- Know the indications of battery failure for your pacemaker as you were instructed, and report these findings to your physician if they occur.
- Do not operate electrical appliances directly over your pacemaker site, because this may cause your pacemaker to malfunction.
- Do not lean over electrical or gasoline engines or motors. Be sure that electrical appliances or motors are properly grounded.

- Avoid all transmitter towers for radio, television, and radar. Radio, television, other home appliances, and antennas do not pose a hazard.
- Be aware that antitheft devices in stores may cause temporary pacemaker malfunction. If symptoms develop, move away from the device.
- Inform airport personnel of your pacemaker before passing through a metal detector and show them your pacemaker identification card. The metal in your pacemaker will trigger the alarm in the metal detector device.
- Stay away from any arc welding equipment.
- Be aware that it is safe to operate a microwave oven unless it does not have proper shielding (old microwave ovens) or is defective.
- Report any of the following symptoms to your physician if you experience them: difficulty breathing, dizziness, fainting, prolonged weakness or fatigue, swelling of arms or legs, chest pain, weight gain, and prolonged hiccupping. If you have any of these symptoms, check your pulse rate and call your physician.
- If you feel symptoms when near any device, move 5 to 10 feet away from it and then check your pulse. Your pulse rate should return to normal.
- Keep all your physician and pacemaker clinic appointments.
- Take all medications prescribed for you as instructed.
- Follow your prescribed diet.
- Follow instructions on restrictions on physical activity, such as no sudden, jerky movement for 8 weeks to allow the pacemaker to settle in place.

---

health care provider or assists the client to access health care resources.

➤ Health Care Resources

The cardiac rehabilitation department nurse typically provides written and oral information about dysrhythmias, antidysrhythmic drugs, pacemakers, and ICDs, as well as information about cardiac exercise programs, educational classes, and support groups. The office or clinic nurse may also provide information about resources. The nurse instructs the client on how to contact the local affiliate of the American Heart Association or the provincial affiliate of the Heart and Stroke Foundation in Canada for information about dysrhythmias, pacemakers, and CPR training.

Manufacturers of pacemakers and ICDs provide helpful booklets and videotapes to assist clients and their families to better understand these therapies. Clients with pacemakers may have transtelephonic systems for transmission of their rhythms to a clinic or health care provider's office. The nurse teaches clients how to use these systems. The nurse stresses the importance of keeping ap-

pointments scheduled for office visits with the cardiologist and pacemaker or ICD clinic. The nurse instructs clients with an ICD to contact the local ambulance or paramedic services and emergency facilities to inform them that they have these devices implanted. The client and family are encouraged to attend pacemaker or ICD support groups.

 Evaluation

On the basis of the identified nursing diagnoses and collaborative problems, the nurse evaluates the care of the client with dysrhythmias. Outcomes include that the client is expected to

- Have a normal, regular pulse rate
- Have normal mental acuity
- Have a normal rate, rhythm, and depth of respiration
- Have normal skin color and temperature
- Perform activities of daily living without dyspnea or excess fatigue
- Be free of pulmonary edema

Chart 36-9

Education Guide: Implantable Cardioverter/Defibrillator (ICD)

- Follow the instructions for ICD site skin care that have been specifically prepared for you.
- Report to your physician any fever or redness, swelling, soreness, or drainage from your incision site.
- Do not wear tight clothing or belts that could cause irritation over the ICD generator.
- Avoid activities that involve rough contact with the ICD implantation site.
- Keep your ICD identification card in your wallet and consider wearing a medical alert (Medic-Alert) bracelet.
- Know the basic functioning of your ICD device and its rate cutoff, as well as the number of consecutive shocks it can deliver.
- Avoid magnets directly over your ICD because they can inactivate the device. If beeping tones are coming from the ICD, move away from the electromagnetic field immediately (within 30 sec) before the inactivation sequence is completed, and notify your physician.
- Inform all physicians and dentists caring for you that you have an ICD implanted, because certain diagnostic tests and procedures must be avoided to prevent ICD malfunction. These include diathermy, electrocautery, and nuclear magnetic resonance tests.
- Avoid other sources of electromagnetic interference, such as devices emitting microwaves (not microwave ovens); transformers; radio, television, and radar transmitters; large electrical generators; metal detectors, including hand-held security devices at airports; antitheft devices; arc welding equipment; and sources of 60-cycle (Hz) interference. Also avoid leaning directly over the alternator of a running motor of a car or boat.
- Report to your physician symptoms such as fainting, nausea, weakness, blackout, and rapid pulse rates.
- Take all medications prescribed for you as instructed.
- Follow instructions on restrictions on physical activity, such as not swimming, driving motor vehicles, or operating dangerous equipment.
- Follow your prescribed diet.
- Keep all physician and ICD clinic appointments.
- Sit or lie down immediately if you feel dizzy or faint to avoid falling if the ICD discharges.
- Post emergency telephone numbers.
- Know how to contact the local emergency medical services (EMS) systems in your community. Inform them in advance that you have an ICD so that they can be prepared if they need to respond to an emergency call for you.
- Know how to perform cough CPR as instructed.
- Encourage family members to learn how to perform CPR. Family members should know that, if they are touching you when the device discharges, they may feel a slight shock but that this is not harmful to them.
- Follow instructions on what to do if the ICD successfully discharges, after which you feel well. This may include maintaining a diary of the date, the time, activity preceding the shock, symptoms, the number of shocks delivered, and how you feel after the shock. The physician may wish to be notified each time the device discharges.
- Avoid strenuous activities that may cause your heart rate to meet or exceed the rate cutoff of your ICD, because this causes the device to discharge inappropriately.
- Notify your physician if you are leaving town or are relocating for information regarding access to health care.

CASE STUDY for the Client with a Dysrhythmia

■ A 78-year-old woman is a client admitted to a telemetry unit directly from a physician's office for evaluation and management of congestive heart failure. She has a history of systemic hypertension and chronic moderate mitral regurgitation. Her medication orders include Lasix 80 mg PO qid, digoxin 0.125 mg PO qd, and Cardizem 60 mg PO tid.

Your initial assessment of the client reveals a pulse rate that is rapid and very irregular. The client is restless, and her skin is pale and cool. Her blood pressure is 106/88. She is short of breath and anxious. Her ECG monitor pattern shows uncontrolled atrial fibrillation, with a rate ranging from 150 to 170 beats per minute. Her oxygen saturation level is 90%.

Q U E S T I O N S :

1. Given the above assessment findings, what should you do first?
2. What additional physical assessment techniques would you perform?
3. Because it is not known how long she has been in atrial fibrillation, what potential problem should be evaluated before attempts to convert the rhythm are implemented?

SELECTED BIBLIOGRAPHY

Alton, R. (1994). Arrhythmias associated with cardiopulmonary arrest. *Nursing Times, 90*(19), 42–44.

*Appel-Hardin, S. (1992). The role of the critical care nurse in noninvasive temporary pacing. *Critical Care Nurse, 12*(3):10–16, 18–19.

Aronow, W. S. (1995). Treatment of ventricular arrhythmias in older adults. *Journal of the American Geriatrics Society, 43*(6), 688–695.

Bashford, C. W. (1994). When a patient survives sudden cardiac death. *RN, 57*(4), 34–37.

Boisvert, J. T., et al. (1995). Overview of pediatric arrhythmias. *Nursing Clinics of North America, 30*(2), 365–379.

Bubien, R. S., et al. (1995). Radiofrequency catheter ablation: Concepts and nursing implications. *Cardiovascular Nursing, 31*(3), 17–23.

Bush, D. E. (1994). Permanent cardiac pacemakers in the elderly. *Journal of the American Geriatrics Society, 42*(3), 326–334.

Cerrato, P. L. (1996). What's new in drugs. A new option for ventricular arrhythmias . . . amiodarone (Cordarone IV). *RN, 59*(2), 79.

Conover, M. B. (1996). *Understanding electrocardiography: Arrhythmias and the 12-lead ECG* (7th ed.). St. Louis: Mosby-Year Book.

Crowley, A. (1997). Emergency! Paroxysmal supraventricular tachycardia. *AJN, 97*(1), 53.

Cummins, R. O., et al. (1994). *Textbook of advanced cardiac life support.* Dallas, TX: American Heart Association.

Cunningham, C. A. (1995). Skills primer: ICD and AED defibrillation. *Emergency, 27*(2), 23–25.

Davenport, J. & Morton, P. G. (1997). Identifying nonischemic causes of life-threatening arrhythmias. *AJN, 97*(11), 50–56.

Dougherty, C. M. (1995). Psychological reactions and family adjustment in shock versus no shock groups after implantation of internal cardioverter defibrillator. *Heart & Lung, 24*(4), 282–292.

Dougherty, C. M., & Shaver, J. F. (1995). Psychophysiological responses after sudden cardiac arrest during hospitalization. *Applied Nursing Research, 8*(4), 160–168.

Dracup, K. (1995). *Meltzer's intensive coronary care* (5th ed.). Stamford, CT: Appleton & Lange.

Dunbar, S. B., et al. (1996). Mood disturbance in patients with recurrent ventricular dysrhythmia before insertion of implantable cardioverter defibrillator. *Heart & Lung: Journal of Acute and Critical Care, 25*(4), 253–261.

Elder, A. N. (1994a). Sinus bradycardia: Elevating a slow heart rate. *Nursing, 24*(11), 48–50.

Elder, A. N. (1994b). Sinus tachycardia: Lowering a high heart rate. *Nursing, 24*(12), 62–64.

Elder, A. N. (1996). Adenosine: Putting the brakes on SVT. *Nursing (Critical Care), 26*(10), 32aa–bb.

*Eorgan, P. A., & Greer, J. L. (1992). Cough CPR: A consideration for high-risk cardiac patient discharge teaching. *Critical Care Nurse, 12*(6), 21–27.

Fiore, L. D. (1996). Anticoagulation: Risks and benefits in atrial fibrillation. *Geriatrics, 51*(6), 22–24.

Flanders, A. (1994). A detailed explanation of defibrillation. *Nursing Times, 90*(18), 37–39.

Futterman, L. G., & Lemberg, L. (1994). An alternative to pharmacologic management of atrial fibrillation: The maze procedure. *American Journal of Critical Care, 3*(3), 238–242.

Goldberger, A. L. & Goldberger, E. (1994). *Clinical electrocardiography: A simplified approach* (5th ed.). St. Louis: Mosby-Year Book.

Gomes, J. A., et al. (1994). Atrial fibrillation: Common—and ominous. *Patient Care, 28*(16), 96–99.

Guaglianone, D. M., & Tyndall, A. (1995). Comfort issues in patients undergoing radiofrequency catheter ablation. *Critical Care Nurse, 15*(1), 47–50.

Hasemeier, C. S. (1996). Clinical snapshot. Permanent pacemaker. *American Journal of Nursing, 96*(2), 30–31.

Hayes, D. D. (1997). Bradycardia: Keeping the current flowing. *Nursing97, 27*(6), 50–56.

Hoffman, R. S. (1995). Lidocaine. *Emergency Medicine, 26*(4), 86, 88.

Holcomb, S. S. (1995). Sotalol. New weapon against ventricular tachycardia. *Nursing, 25*(12), 240–24P, 24R.

Holcomb, S. S. (1996). When beta-blockers aren't the drug of choice. *Nursing (Critical Care), 26*(10), 32dd, 32ff–gg.

Horwood, L., et al. (1995). Antitachycardia pacing: An overview. *American Journal of Critical Care, 4*(5), 397–404.

Huszar, R. J. (1994). *Basic dysrhythmias: Interpretation and management.* St. Louis: Mosby-Year Book.

Ide, B. (1995). Bedside electrocardiographic assessment. *Journal of Cardiovascular Nursing, 9*(4):10–23.

Karnes, N. (1995). Adenosine: A quick fix for PSVT . . . paroxysmal supraventricular tachycardia. *Nursing, 25*(7), 55–56.

Kastor, J. A. (1994). *Arrhythmias.* Philadelphia: W. B. Saunders.

Kishore, A. B., & Camm, A. J. (1995). Guidelines for the use of propafenone in treating supraventricular arrhythmias. *Drugs, 50*(2), 250–262.

Klein, L. S., & Miles, W. M. (1995). Ablative therapy for ventricular arrhythmias. *Progress in Cardiovascular Diseases, 37*(4), 225–242.

Lascelles, K. (1995). Permanent pacemakers. *Nursing Standard, 9*(20), 52–53.

Lenhart, R. C. (1995). Pacemaker assessment and care plans in long-term care. *Geriatric Nursing–American Journal of Care for the Aging, 16*(6):276–280.

Levine, J. H., et al. (1996). Implantable cardioverter defibrillator: Use in patients with no symptoms and at high risk. *American Heart Journal, 131*(1), 59–65.

Lewandowski, D. M., et al. (1995). AV blocks: Are you up to date? *American Journal of Nursing, 95*(12), 26–33.

Mancini, M. E., Richards, N., & Kaye, W. (1997). Saving lives with automated external defibrillators. *Nursing97, 27*(10), 42–43.

Nattel, S. (1995). Newer developments in the management of atrial fibrillation. *American Heart Journal, 130*(5), 1094–1106.

Nicolai, C. (1995). Ventricular dysrhythmias in ischemic heart disease. *AACN Clinical Issues: Advanced Practice in Acute & Critical Care, 6*(3), 452–463.

Norman, E. M. (1994). Identifying risks for atrial fibrillation. *American Journal of Nursing, 94*(10), 48N.

Perez, A. (1995). EKG electrode placement: A refresher course. *RN, 59*(9), 29–31.

Petrosky-Pacini, A. J. (1996). The automatic implantable cardioverter defibrillator in home care. *Home Healthcare Nurse, 14*(4), 238–243.

Pill, M. W., & McCloskey, W. W. (1995). Sotalol: What the emergency nurse needs to know. *Journal of Emergency Nursing, 21*(3), 229–231.

Robinson, B., et al. (1994). A primer on pediatric ECGs. *Contemporary Pediatrics, 11*(4), 69–72, 77–78, 80+.

Ruppert, S. D., et al. (1996). *Dolan's critical care nursing: Clinical management through the nursing process* (2nd ed.) Philadelphia: F. A. Davis.

Sbaih, L. (1995). Ventricular fibrillation in adults. *Emergency Nursing, 3*(2), 10–15.

Schneiderman, H., et al. (1995). What's your diagnosis . . . Wenckebach block (Mobitz type I second-degree atrioventricular block). *Consultant, 35*(4), 519–520, 522.

Searle, C., & Jeffrey, J. (1994). Uncertainty and quality of life of adults hospitalized with life-threatening ventricular arrhythmias. *Canadian Journal of Cardiovascular Nursing, 5*(3), 15–22.

Sims, J. M., & Miracle, V. (1997). Ventricular tachycardia. *Nursing97, 27*(11), 47.

Smith, L. F., & Fish, F. H. (1995). *Pure practice ECGs*. St. Louis: Mosby-Year Book.

Stahl, L. (1995). How to manage common arrhythmias in medical patients. *American Journal of Nursing, 95*(3), 36–41.

Vitale, M. B., & Funk, M. (1995). Quality of life in younger persons with an implantable cardioverter defibrillator. *Education Dimension, 14*(2):100–111.

Wagner, G. S. (1994). *Marriott's practical electrocardiography* (9th ed.). Baltimore: Williams & Wilkins.

Wood, K. (1995). Mechanisms and clinical manifestations of supraventricular tachycardias. *Progress in Cardiovascular Nursing, 10*(2):3–14.

Woods, S. L., et al. (1995). *Cardiac nursing* (3rd ed.). Philadelphia: J. B. Lippincott.

Yacone-Morton, L. A. (1995). Cardiovascular drugs: Antiarrhythmics. *RN, 58*(4):26–31, 33–36.

SUGGESTED READINGS

Aronow, W. S. (1995). Treatment of ventricular arrhythmias in older adults. *Journal of the American Geriatrics Society, 43*(6), 688–695.
This article summarizes the findings of studies and reports from available data in published articles on the treatment of ventricular arrhythmias in older adults. It provides guidelines for the use of class I antiarrhythmic agents, beta blockers, amiodarone, and angiotensin-converting enzyme inhibitors, all of which are commonly prescribed for elderly patients.

Davenport, J., & Morton, P. G. (1997). Identifying nonischemic causes of life-threatening arrhythmias. *AJN, 97*(11), 50–56.
This excellent article describes noncardiac health problems that can cause life-threatening dysrhythmias. The authors discuss electrolyte imbalances, metabolic disorders, drugs, and aging changes that can lead to cardiac irregularities. A CEU quiz follows the article.

Hayes, D. D. (1997). Bradycardia: Keeping the current flowing. *Nursing97, 27*(6), 50–56.
The author describes four categories of bradycardia and illustrates the electrocardiographic findings for each type. A case study is used to discuss treatment that focuses on drug therapy. The article concludes with a CEU quiz.

Chapter 37

INTERVENTIONS FOR CLIENTS WITH CARDIAC PROBLEMS

Primary cardiac dysfunction may have a number of causes, including impaired cardiac muscle function, structural cardiac defects, infections within the heart, and inflammatory conditions of the heart. Although most Americans do not consider heart disease an incurable illness, more people die of heart disease than of any other disorder. Five-year mortality rates range between 25% and 50% (Pratt, 1995). Moderately severe heart failure and dilated cardiomyopathy have 2-year survival rates of only 50%.

Long-term survival of clients with heart disease depends on a coordinated interdisciplinary approach to ensure the best management of the illness and the highest possible quality of life. Therefore, these high-risk clients are often targeted for case management to coordinate their care through the health care continuum, as described in Chapter 3.

HEART FAILURE

Overview

Heart failure, also called *cardiac failure* or *pump failure,* is the inability of the heart to pump sufficient blood to meet the demands of the body. Because fluid excess is not always present, the term *congestive heart failure* may not be applicable. Heart failure may be due to either increased cellular demands or, more commonly, impaired pumping of the heart. When the heart fails, cardiac output is diminished, and peripheral tissue is not adequately perfused. Congestion of the lungs and periphery may also develop.

Pathophysiology

Compensatory Mechanisms

When cardiac output is insufficient to meet the demands of the body, compensatory mechanisms operate to improve cardiac output. Although the compensatory mechanisms may initially increase cardiac output, they eventually have a damaging effect on pump function. Compensatory mechanisms include

- Increased heart rate
- Improved stroke volume
- Arterial vasoconstriction
- Sodium and water retention
- Myocardial hypertrophy

In heart failure, stimulation of the sympathetic nervous system represents the most immediate compensatory mechanism. Stimulation of the adrenergic receptors causes an increase in heart rate and vasoconstriction.

INCREASED HEART RATE. Because cardiac output equals heart rate times stroke volume, an increase in heart rate results in an immediate increase in cardiac output. The increase in heart rate is limited in its ability to compensate for decreased cardiac output. If the heart rate becomes too rapid, diastolic filling time is limited and cardiac output may start to fall.

IMPROVED STROKE VOLUME. Stroke volume is also improved by sympathetic stimulation. With sympathetic stimulation, there is increased venous return to the heart, which stretches the myocardial fibers further. This increased stretch is referred to as *preload*. In accordance with Starling's law of the heart, increased myocardial stretch results in more forceful contraction, increasing stroke volume and cardiac output. However, after a critical point is reached, further volume and stretch reduce the force of contraction and cardiac output.

ARTERIAL VASOCONSTRICTION. Sympathetic stimulation also results in arterial vasoconstriction. Constriction of arteries has the beneficial effect of maintaining blood pressure and improving tissue perfusion in low-output states. However, constriction of arteries increases *afterload,* the resistance against which the heart must pump. Afterload is the major determinant of myocardial oxygen requirements. As afterload increases, the left ventricle requires more energy to eject its contents and stroke volume may decline.

RETENTION OF SODIUM AND WATER. Reduced blood flow to the kidneys, a common occurrence in low-output states, results in the activation of the renin-angiotensin-aldosterone mechanism. Vasoconstriction becomes more pronounced in response to angiotensin, while aldosterone secretion causes sodium and water retention. The volume of blood returning to the left ventricle is further increased by activation of this mechanism.

MYOCARDIAL HYPERTROPHY. Myocardial hypertrophy, with or without chamber dilation, is the final compensatory mechanism. A thickening of the walls of the heart occurs, providing more muscle mass, resulting in more forceful contractions, and further increasing cardiac output. However, cardiac muscle may hypertrophy more rapidly than collateral circulation can provide adequate blood supply to the muscle. Often, a hypertrophied heart is slightly oxygen deprived.

These mechanisms of compensation act primarily to restore cardiac output to near-normal levels. However, when these cardiac and peripheral circulatory adjustments become excessive, they may decrease pump function. All of them contribute to an increase in myocardial oxygen consumption. When this occurs and myocardial reserve has been exhausted, clinical manifestations of heart failure develop.

Classification of Heart Failure

Heart failure can be classified in many ways. Several important categories are discussed here.

Systolic Versus Diastolic Dysfunction

Systolic dysfunction results when the heart is unable to contract forcefully enough during systole to eject adequate amounts of blood into the circulation. The ejection fraction (the percentage of blood ejected from the heart during systole) drops from a normal of 50% to 70% to below 40%. As the ejection fraction decreases, tissue perfusion diminishes and the blood accumulates in the pulmonary vasculature. Symptoms of systolic dysfunction may be symptoms of inadequate tissue perfusion or pulmonary and systemic congestion.

In contrast, diastolic failure occurs when the left ventricle is unable to relax adequately during diastole. Inadequate relaxation prevents the ventricle from filling with sufficient blood to ensure an adequate cardiac output. Diastolic failure may represent 20% to 40% of all heart failure, primarily occurring in older adults and women following a myocardial infarction (Redfield, 1996). Symptoms of diastolic failure are similar to those of systolic. However, treatment is not clearly established and is not discussed in this text.

Left Versus Right Ventricular Failure

Because the two ventricles of the heart represent two separate pumping systems, it is possible for one to fail alone for a short period. Most heart failure begins with failure of the left ventricle and progresses to failure of both ventricles. Typical causes of left ventricular failure include hypertensive disease, coronary artery disease, and valvular disease (involving the mitral or aortic valve).

Decreased tissue perfusion from poor cardiac output and pulmonary congestion from increased pressure in the pulmonary vessels indicate left ventricular failure.

Right ventricular failure may be caused by left ventricular failure, right ventricular myocardial infarction, or pulmonary hypertension.

In right ventricular failure, the right ventricle is unable to empty completely, increased volume and pressure develop in the systemic veins, and systemic venous congestion and peripheral edema develop. Figure 37–1 illustrates the pathophysiology of heart failure.

Low-Output Versus High-Output Syndrome

Low-output syndrome, the more common type of heart failure, occurs when the heart fails as a pump, resulting in impaired peripheral circulation and peripheral vasoconstriction. When cardiac output remains normal or above normal but the metabolic needs of the body are not met, high-output syndrome is present. It may be caused by increased metabolic needs (hyperthyroidism, fever, pregnancy) or hyperkinetic conditions (arteriovenous fistulas, Paget's disease).

Functional Status

Heart failure may also be categorized by its effect on the client's functional status. Table 35–2 summarizes the New York Heart Association (NYHA) categories.

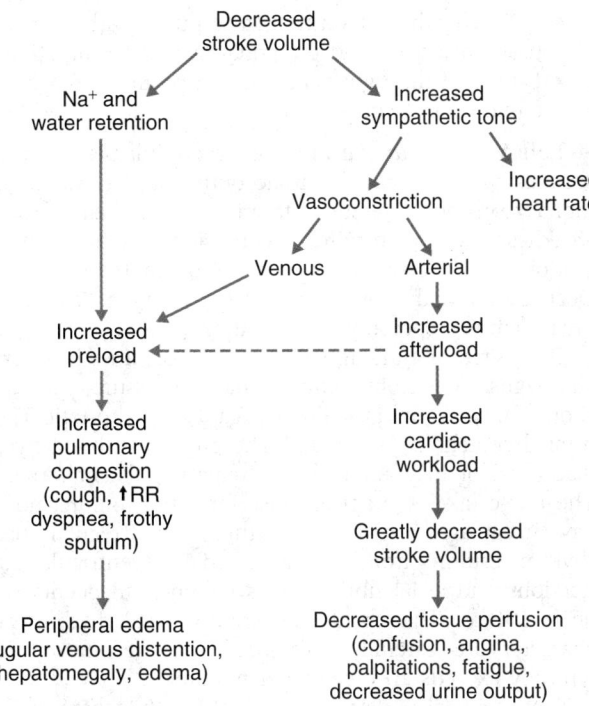

Figure 37–1. Pathophysiology of heart failure.

Etiology

The most common cause of heart failure is myocardial infarction. The next most common causes are conditions such as systemic hypertension and pulmonary stenosis, which cause pressure or volume overload on the heart. Other direct causes of heart failure are myocardial dysfunction, filling disorders, and increased metabolic demand. Some of the conditions capable of causing heart failure are listed in Table 37–1.

Incidence/Prevalence

More than 4.5 million people in the United States are living with heart failure (American Heart Association [AHA], 1996), with about 400,000 new cases occurring each year. Treatment and care for clients with heart failure costs over $10 billion every year (Konstam et al., 1994).

ELDERLY CONSIDERATIONS

Heart failure occurs most commonly in older adults, and its prevalence increases with age; 75% of clients with heart failure are older than 60 years. Heart failure is the most frequent cause of hospitalization for adults older than 65 (AHA, 1996). The prevalence of heart failure steadily increases with aging; heart failure occurs in 3% of people 45 to 64 years old, 6% of people 65 and older, and 10% of people older than 75 (Jensen and Miller, 1995). Heart failure is more common in men than women at all ages.

Collaborative Management

 Assessment

Manifestations of heart failure depend on the type of failure, the ventricle involved, and the underlying cause. Impaired tissue perfusion, pulmonary congestion, and edema dominate the picture of left ventricular failure. Systemic venous congestion and peripheral edema are associated with right ventricular failure.

➤ History

When taking a history, the nurse should keep in mind the many conditions that can lead to heart failure. The nurse carefully questions the client about past medical history, including a history of high blood pressure, angina, myocardial infarction, rheumatic heart disease, valvular disorders, endocarditis, and pericarditis.

The nurse asks about the client's perception of his or her activity tolerance, breathing pattern, urinary pattern, and fluid volume status and the client's knowledge about heart failure.

Left Ventricular Failure. With left ventricular systolic dysfunction, the cardiac output is diminished, impaired tissue perfusion results, anaerobic metabolism occurs, and the client often reports unusual fatigue. The nurse assesses the client's activity tolerance by asking if the client can perform normal activities of daily living (ADLs) or climb flights of stairs without fatigue or dyspnea. Many clients with heart failure experience weakness or fatigue with activity as a feeling of heaviness in their arms or legs. Clients should be asked about their ability to perform simultaneous arm and leg work (e.g., walking while carrying a bag of groceries). Such activity may place an unacceptable demand on the failing heart. The nurse should ask clients to name their most strenuous activity in the past week. Many clients unconsciously limit their activities in response to fatigue or dyspnea and may not realize how limited they have become.

Perfusion to the myocardium is often impaired, especially if cardiac muscle has hypertrophied. The client may report chest discomfort or may describe palpitations, skipped beats, or a fast heartbeat.

As the amount of blood ejected from the left ventricle diminishes, pressure builds in the pulmonary venous sys-

TABLE 37–1

Predisposing Factors to Systolic Heart Failure
Hypertension
Coronary artery disease
Cardiomyopathy
Alcohol
Valvular disease
Congenital defects

tem resulting in fluid-filled alveoli and pulmonary congestion. Thus, cough is often an early manifestation of heart failure. The client in early heart failure describes the *cough* as irritating, nocturnal, and usually nonproductive. As heart failure becomes more severe, the client may begin expectorating frothy pink-tinged sputum, a sign of pulmonary edema.

Dyspnea also results from rising pulmonary venous pressure and pulmonary congestion. The nurse carefully questions the client about the presence of dyspnea and when and how it developed. The client may refer to dyspnea as "trouble in catching one's breath," "breathlessness," or "difficulty in breathing."

As exertional dyspnea develops, the client often discontinues previously tolerated levels of activity owing to shortness of breath. Dyspnea at rest in the recumbent position is known as *orthopnea*. The nurse asks how many pillows the client usually uses to sleep or if the client sleeps in an upright position in a bed or a chair.

Clients who describe sudden awakening with a feeling of breathlessness 2 to 5 hours after falling asleep have paroxysmal nocturnal dyspnea (PND). Sitting upright, dangling their feet, or walking usually relieves this condition.

ELDERLY CONSIDERATIONS

Decreased cerebral perfusion resulting from low cardiac output leads to changes in mental status. Confusion may occur with even mild or moderate heart failure in the very old client. The nurse asks the client and his or her family members if any lapses in memory or periods of disorientation have occurred.

Right Ventricular Failure. Signs of systemic congestion occur as the right ventricle fails, fluid is retained, and pressure builds in the venous system. Edema develops in the lower legs and ascends to the thighs and the abdominal wall. Clients may note that shoes fit more tightly, or indentations may develop on their swollen feet from shoes or socks. Clients may indicate that they have removed their rings because of swelling in their fingers and hands. The nurse asks the client about weight gain. An adult may retain 4 to 7 L of fluid (10–15 pounds [4.5–6.8 kg]) before pitting edema occurs.

Gastrointestinal complaints of nausea and anorexia may be a direct consequence of the liver engorgement due to fluid retention. Another finding related to fluid retention is diuresis at rest. At rest, edema fluid is mobilized and excreted so the client describes frequent awakening at night to urinate.

The nurse or dietitian takes a careful nutritional history, questioning the client about the use of salt and the types of food consumed. The nurse also questions the client concerning daily fluid intake. Clients in heart failure may experience increased thirst and take in excessive fluid (4000–5000 mL) because of aldosterone secretion.

► *Physical Assessment/Clinical Manifestations*

The signs and symptoms of heart failure can be considered in the context of these components of the syndrome:

- Failure of the left ventricle as a pump with decreased tissue perfusion and pulmonary venous congestion
- Failure of the right ventricle as a pump with systemic venous congestion

Left Ventricular Failure. Left ventricular failure is associated with decreased cardiac output and elevated pulmonary venous pressure. It may appear clinically as weakness, fatigue, dizziness, confusion, pulmonary congestion, breathlessness, oliguria, or death (Chart 37–1). Decreased blood flow to major body organs can cause organ failure, especially renal failure.

The nurse or nursing staff member obtains the client's vital signs. When obtaining the blood pressure, the nurse should note if an auscultatory gap or orthostatic (postural) hypotension is present. The pulse may be tachycardiac (fast) or may alternate in strength (pulsus alternans). The nurse takes the apical pulse for a full minute, noting any irregularity in heart rhythm. An irregular heart rhythm resulting from premature atrial or ventricular contractions and atrial fibrillation is common in clients with heart failure. The client's respiratory rate, rhythm, and character are carefully monitored. The respiratory rate typically exceeds 20 breaths per minute.

The nurse also determines whether the client is oriented to person, place, and time. If there are concerns about orientation, a short mental status examination may be used (see Chap. 43). Objective data are important because many people are skillful at covering up memory losses in daily conversation.

The nurse palpates the precordium. Increased heart size is common, with a displacement of the apical impulse to the left. On auscultation, the nurse may hear a third heart sound (S_3) gallop, an early diastolic filling sound indicating an increase in left ventricular pressure. A fourth heart sound (S_4) can also occur, although it is not a sign of failure but a reflection of decreased ventricular compliance.

Chart 37–1

Key Features of Left-Sided Heart Failure

Decreased Cardiac Output
- Fatigue
- Weakness
- Oliguria during the day
- Angina
- Confusion, restlessness
- Dizziness
- Tachycardia, palpitations
- Pallor
- Weak peripheral pulses
- Cool extremities

Pulmonary Congestion
- Hacking cough, worse at night
- Dyspnea/breathlessness
- Crackles or wheezes in lungs
- Frothy pink-tinged sputum
- Tachypnea

When the nurse auscultates the lungs, crackles and wheezes may be present. Late inspiratory crackles and fine profuse crackles that repeat themselves from breath to breath and do not diminish with coughing indicate heart failure. Crackles are produced by intra-alveolar fluid and are frequently noted first in the dependent areas of the lungs. Usually, crackles develop in the bases and spread upward as the condition worsens. The nurse identifies precisely the location of the crackles. Wheezes indicate narrowing of the bronchial lumen caused by engorged pulmonary vessels.

Right Ventricular Failure. Right ventricular failure is associated with increased systemic venous pressures. Signs and symptoms are listed in Chart 37–2.

On inspection, the nurse assesses the neck veins for distention (see Chap. 35). The nurse also measures the client's abdominal girth and assesses for the presence of hepatomegaly (liver engorgement), hepatojugular reflux (see Chap. 35), and ascites. The collection of fluid in the abdomen (ascites) can reach volumes of more than 10 L.

In addition, the nurse examines the client for dependent edema. In the ambulatory client, edema is normally located in the ankles and legs. However, when the client is restricted to bed rest, the sacrum is dependent and edema accumulates there. Edema is an extremely unreliable sign of heart failure so accurate daily weights are needed to document fluid retention. Weight is the most reliable indicator of fluid gain or loss.

► Psychosocial Assessment

Acute episodes of heart failure may be precipitated in susceptible people by stressful life situations. Acute exacerbations of heart failure may result from feelings of rejection, insecurity, frustration, or rage. The nurse needs to question clients sensitively about any recent stressors in their lives. The nurse asks clients to rate their current level of stress and describe any significant recent life changes.

Many clients with heart failure have symptoms that are not well controlled. These clients may have anxiety and frustrations related to dealing with a chronic illness. The nurse assesses clients and their families for fears, anxieties, and frustrations and also assesses their usual methods of coping (see Chap. 8).

Chart 37–2

Key Features of Right-Sided Heart Failure

- Jugular (neck vein) distention
- Enlarged liver and spleen
- Anorexia and nausea
- Dependent edema (legs and sacrum)
- Distended abdomen
- Swollen hands and fingers
- Polyuria at night
- Weight gain
- Increased blood pressure (from excess volume) or decreased blood pressure (from failure)

Hope is a major determinant of well-being for clients in heart failure. Clients who are hopeful tend to feel better and to be more socially involved. The nurse might ask clients what activities they engage in, who the significant people are in their life, and how often they are able to interact with them.

► Laboratory Assessment

Electrolyte imbalance in heart failure may occur from complications of failure or as side effects of drug therapy, especially diuretic therapy. It is essential that regular evaluations of a client's serum electrolytes be done, including sodium, potassium, magnesium, calcium, and chloride. Any impairment of renal function may be reflected by elevated blood urea nitrogen, serum creatinine, and creatinine clearance levels. Urinalysis may reveal proteinuria and high specific gravity. Hemoglobin and hematocrit tests should be performed to identify heart failure resulting from anemia.

Arterial blood gas values often reveal hypoxia (low oxygen level) because oxygen does not diffuse easily through fluid-filled alveoli. Respiratory alkalosis may occur because of hyperventilation; respiratory acidosis may occur because of carbon dioxide retention. Metabolic acidosis may indicate lactic acid accumulation.

ELDERLY CONSIDERATIONS

In clients who are over 65 years, have atrial fibrillation, or have evidence of thyroid disease, thyroxine (T_4) and thyroid-stimulating hormone (TSH) levels should be determined (Konstam et al., 1994). Heart failure may be due to or aggravated by hypo- or hyperthyroidism.

► Radiographic Assessment

Chest x-rays can be helpful in diagnosing left ventricular failure. Typically, the heart is enlarged (cardiomegaly), representing hypertrophy or dilation. Pleural effusions develop less often and generally reflect biventricular failure.

► Other Diagnostic Assessment

In addition to a chest x-ray, an electrocardiogram (ECG) is performed. The ECG may demonstrate ventricular hypertrophy, dysrhythmias, and any degree of myocardial ischemia, injury, or infarction. It is not helpful in determining the presence or extent of heart failure.

Echocardiography is useful in diagnosing cardiac valvular changes, pericardial effusion, chamber enlargement, and ventricular hypertrophy. Radionuclide studies (thallium imaging or technetium pyrophosphate scanning) can also indicate the presence and cause of heart failure. Multigated angiographic (MUGA) scans provide information about left ventricular ejection fraction and velocity, which is typically low in clients with heart failure.

Pulmonary artery catheters allow assessment of cardiac function and volume status in acutely ill clients. These measurements can confirm the diagnosis and guide the management of heart failure. The right atrial pressure may be normal or elevated in left ventricular failure and is elevated in right ventricular failure. Pulmonary artery pressure and pulmonary artery wedge pressure (PAWP) are elevated in left-sided heart failure because volumes and pressures are increased in the left ventricle. (See Chapter 35 for a more detailed description of the pulmonary artery catheter.)

 Analysis

> *Common Nursing Diagnoses and Collaborative Problems*

The most common nursing diagnoses pertinent to the client with heart failure are

1. Impaired Gas Exchange related to altered oxygen supply
2. Decreased Cardiac Output related to a reduction in stroke volume as a result of mechanical malfunctions
3. Activity Intolerance related to an imbalance between oxygen supply and demand, fatigue, or an electrolyte imbalance

The primary collaborative problem is Potential for Pulmonary Edema.

> *Additional Nursing Diagnoses and Collaborative Problems*

Some clients have one or more of the following:

- Ineffective Management of Therapeutic Regime related to failed social support systems, inadequate follow-up, inadequate discharge planning, or knowledge deficit
- Ineffective Individual Coping related to physical inactivity, major changes in lifestyle, loss of control over body function, or fear of death
- Altered Thought Processes related to impaired gas exchange or fear of the unknown
- Impaired Physical Mobility related to fatigue and activity intolerance

Some clients are also at risk for the following collaborative problems:

- Potential for Pneumonia
- Potential for Dysrhythmias

 Planning and Implementation

> *Impaired Gas Exchange*

Planning: Expected Outcomes. The client is expected to have a normal rate, rhythm, and depth of respiration and to have an O_2 saturation greater than 92%.

Interventions. The nurse or assistive nursing personnel monitors the client's respiratory rate, rhythm, and character every 1 to 4 hours and auscultates breath sounds. If clients are experiencing pulmonary congestion, the oxygen content of their blood is often markedly reduced. The nurse may titrate the amount of supplemental oxygen delivered to the client within a range prescribed by the health care provider to maintain the client's oxygen saturation at 92% or greater.

If the client experiences respiratory difficulty, the nurse or assistive nursing personnel places the client in a high Fowler's position with pillows under each arm to maximize chest expansion and improve oxygenation. Repositioning the client and having the client perform coughing and deep breathing exercises every 2 hours helps to improve oxygenation and to prevent atelectasis.

> *Decreased Cardiac Output*

Planning: Expected Outcomes. The primary outcome is that the client is expected to resume and maintain an adequate cardiac output.

Interventions. Interventions are aimed at improving cardiac output. A critical pathway for congestive heart failure that reflects an interdisciplinary approach to client care is included in this chapter. Therapy may be directed toward optimizing the two major components of cardiac output: stroke volume (determined by preload, afterload, and contractility) and heart rate.

Interventions to optimize stroke volume include reducing afterload, reducing preload, and improving cardiac muscle contractility.

Reducing Afterload. By relaxing arterioles, arterial vasodilators can reduce impedance to left ventricular ejection (afterload) and improve cardiac output. In the strictest sense, these drugs do not act as vasodilators but reverse some of the inappropriate or excessive vasoconstriction that is common in heart failure.

Clients with even mild heart failure due to left ventricular dysfunction should be given a trial of angiotensin-converting enzyme (ACE) inhibitors. ACE inhibitors, a group of arterial vasodilators such as enalapril (Vasotec), moexipril (Univasc), and captopril (Capoten), generally prolong and improve the quality of life of clients in heart failure (see Chart 37–3). Studies have shown that these drugs enhance functional status, with 40% to 80% of clients showing an improvement in NYHA class (Baker et al., 1994).

ACE inhibitors suppress the renin-angiotensin-aldosterone system, which is activated in response to decreased renal blood flow. ACE inhibitors benefit clients by reducing arterial resistance, decreasing pulmonary artery wedge pressure, and increasing stroke volume and cardiac output.

The health care provider usually starts ACE inhibitor doses slowly and cautiously. The first dose of an ACE inhibitor has been associated with a rapid drop in blood pressure in some clients. Clients at risk for hypotension following ACE inhibitor administration have initial systolic blood pressures less than 100, are older than 75 years, have a serum sodium level less than 135, or are volume depleted (Baker et al., 1994). After the initial dose and each increased dose, the nurse monitors the client's blood pressure for several hours.

The nurse clarifies with the health care provider the guidelines for administering the vasodilator. For example, many clinicians maintain clients in heart failure at systolic blood pressures ranging from 90 to 110 mmHg. When such a blood pressure is the client's maintenance level, the nurse assesses the client for orthostatic hypotension, confusion, poor peripheral perfusion, and reduced urinary output. While the client is receiving ACE inhibitors, the

OUR LADY OF LOURDES MEDICAL CENTER
CRITICAL PATHWAY
CONGESTIVE HEART FAILURE DUE TO LEFT VENTRICULAR DYSFUNCTION NOT REQUIRING ADMISSION TO A CRITICAL CARE UNIT

	DAY #1 DATE_____	DAY #2 DATE_____	DAY #3 DATE_____	DAY #4 DATE_____
LOCATION OF PATIENT	CARDIOLOGY FLOOR (PREFERRED) OR MED-SURG FLOOR	CARDIOLOGY FLOOR (PREFERRED) OR MED-SURG FLOOR	CARDIOLOGY FLOOR (PREFERRED) OR MED-SURG FLOOR	CARDIAC FLOOR (PREFERRED) OR MED-SURG FLOOR
RESPONSIBLE SERVICE	INTERNAL MEDICINE, FAMILY PRACTICE, OR CARDIOLOGY	INTERNAL MEDICINE, FAMILY PRACTICE, OR CARDIOLOGY	INTERNAL MEDICINE, FAMILY PRACTICE, OR CARDIOLOGY	INTERNAL MED, FAMILY PRACTICE, OR CARDIOLOGY
CONSULTS	CARDIOLOGY, DIETARY AND PATIENT EDUCATION, AS NECESSARY. CARDIAC REHAB	CARDIOLOGY, DIETARY AND PATIENT EDUCATION, AS NECESSARY. CARDIAC REHAB	CARDIOLOGY, DIETARY AND PATIENT EDUCATION, AS NECESSARY. CARDIAC REHAB	CARDIOLOGY, DIETARY AND PATIENT EDUCATION, AS NECESSARY. CARDIAC REHAB
LAB	BUN, CREATININE, LYTES, BLOOD GLUCOSE, ALBUMIN, URIC ACID, CBC, URINALYSIS. IF ACUTE MI IS BEING EXCLUDED, CK ON ADMISSION AND Q8H X3. CK-MB IF TOTAL CK ELEVATED	BUN, CREATININE, LYTES	BUN, CREATININE, LYTES, DIGOXIN LEVEL.	NONE
RADIOLOGY	CHEST X-RAY, PA AND LATERAL	NONE	CHEST X-RAY, PA AND LATERAL	NONE
OTHER TESTS	EKG ON ADMISSION AND FOR ANGINA AS PER PROTOCOL - CHEST LEAD LOCATIONS MARKED WITH PEN. CARDIAC ECHO - DOPPLER ORDERED FOR DAY 1 OR DAY 2. PULSE OXIMETRY.	ECHO - DOPPLER HEART IF NOT DONE DAY 1	NONE	NONE
ACTIVITY	BED REST, DANGLE TID, OR OUT OF BED, AS TOLERATED	AMBULATE AS TOLERATED	AMBULATE AD LIB	AMBULATE AD LIB
NURSING CARE	CHECK AND RECORD BP, HEART RATE, AND RESPIRATORY RATE ON ADMISSION, 1 HR AFTER ADMISSION AND Q 2 HRS UNTIL STABLE. AFTER STABLE, RECORD BP, HR, AND RR Q 4 H. CHECK AND RECORD TEMPERATURE ON ADMISSION AND Q 8 H THEREAFTER. WEIGH PATIENT ON ADMISSION (USE BED OR CHAIR SCALE IF NECESSARY: ESTIMATED WEIGHT NOT ALLOWED) I&O. ARRHYTHMIA AND ANGINA CARE PER PROTOCOLS.	RECORD I&O. MEASURE AND RECORD BP, HR, RR, AND TEMP EVERY 8 HOURS. RECORD AND EVALUATE RHYTHM STRIPS IF PATIENT ON TELEMETRY. WEIGH DAILY IN AM (POST-VOID, PRE-PRANDIAL). ARRHYTHMIA AND ANGINA CARE PER PROTOCOLS.	MEASURE AND RECORD BP, HEART RATE, RESP RATE Q 4 H. RECORD TEMP Q 8 H. WEIGH DAILY (POST-VOID), PRE-PRANDIAL.	ENCOURAGE AMBULATION
LINES, MONITORS, AND TUBES	TELEMETRIC MONITORING IF INDICATED. TEXAS OR FOLEY CATHETER AS INDICATED. PRN ADAPTER. SUPPLEMENTAL O2 PRN SOB, CHEST PAIN, OR O2 SAT<93%.	PRN ADAPTER. TELEMETRIC EKG MONITOR IF INDICATED. REMOVE TEXAS OR FOLEY CATHETER. O2, PRN SOB, CHEST PAIN, OR O2 SAT<93%.	DISCONTINUE TELEMETRIC MONITORING. REMOVE PRN ADAPTER AFTER TELEMETRY D/C'D. D/C O2 SUPPLEMENT.	NONE
MEDS	INTRAVENOUS DIURETICS. LOW DOSE ORAL ACE INHIBITOR. DIGOXIN LOAD, IF APPROPRIATE. ORAL OR CUTANEOUS NITRATES. MOM PRN. MAALOX, MYLANTA PRN. TYLENOL PRN. DAYTIME SEDATIVE PRN. HS SEDATIVE PRN. HEPARIN 5000 U SC Q 12 H WHILE PATIENT IS NON-AMBULATORY. COLACE 100 MG BID.	IV DIURETIC; SWITCH TO ORAL DIURETIC IF DIURESIS ADEQUATE. CONTINUE ORAL OR CUTANEOUS NITRATE AS INDICATED. ACE INHIBITOR; INCREASE DOSE AS TOLERATED. DIGOXIN, MAINTENANCE DOSE. MOM PRN. MAALOX, MYLANTA PRN. TYLENOL PRN. DAYTIME SEDATIVE PRN. HS SEDATIVE PRN. D/C S.C. HEPARIN WHEN PATIENT AMBULATORY.	ORAL DIURETIC; ADJUST DOSAGE AS INDICATED. ORAL OR CUTANEOUS NITRATE. ACE INHIBITOR; INCREASE DOSE AS TOLERATED. DIGOXIN. MOM PRN. MAALOX, MYLANTA PRN. TYLENOL PRN. DAYTIME SEDATIVE PRN. HS SEDATIVE PRN.	ORAL DIURETIC. ORAL OR CUTANEOUS NITRATE. ACE INHIBITOR. DIGOXIN. MOM PRN. MAALOX, MYLANTA PRN. TYLENOL PRN.
DIET	CARDIAC DIET (3 GM SODIUM, LOW CHOLESTEROL) AS TOLERATED.	CARDIAC DIET	CARDIAC DIET	CARDIAC DIET
PATIENT AND FAMILY EDUCATION	UNIT AND ROOM ORIENTATION. EXPLANATION OF MEDS. INTRODUCTION TO CRITICAL PATHWAY. EXPLAIN ADVANCED DIRECTIVES.	EXPLANATION OF MEDS TO PATIENT AND FAMILY. REHAB TEACHING AS PER PROTOCOL.	EXPLANATION OF MEDS TO PATIENT AND FAMILY. REHAB TEACHING AS PER PROTOCOL. DIET INSTRUCTIONS.	FINAL REVIEW OF MEDICATIONS, DIET, AND DISCHARGE INSTRUCTIONS.
DISCHARGE PLANNING	SOCIAL SERVICES CONSULT AS INDICATED. HOME HEALTH SERVICES CONSULT AS INDICATED.		REMIND PATIENT THAT DISCHARGE IS PLANNED FOR AM OF DAY 4. NOTIFY FAMILY OF PLANNED DISCHARGE AND MAKE TRANSPORTATION ARRANGEMENTS. SOCIAL SERVICES RE-EVALUATION. CONFIRM ARRANGEMENTS FOR HOME HEALTH.	ASSIST PATIENT IN PREPARING TO LEAVE HOSPITAL AND WITH TRANSPORTATION ARRANGEMENTS. PATIENT DISCHARGED TO HOME.

THIS CRITICAL PATHWAY HAS BEEN DEVELOPED TO SERVE AS A GUIDELINE FOR THE "OPTIMAL" MANAGEMENT OF PATIENTS HOSPITALIZED PRIMARILY FOR THE ABOVE NOTED DIAGNOSIS OR PROCEDURE WITHOUT COMPLICATING COMORBIDITIES.

Chart 37–3

Drug Therapy for Cardiac Failure

Drug	Usual Dosage	Nursing Interventions	Rationale
Drugs Used Primarily to Reduce Afterload			
Angiotensin-Converting Enzyme Inhibitors Captopril (Capoten)	• To start: 6.25–12.5 mg PO tid • May increase to 50–100 mg PO tid	• Monitor the client's blood pressure closely for several hours after the first dose. Consult with the physician to determine the desired range for blood pressure. • Monitor the serum creatinine and potassium levels carefully. • Report fever and sore throat to the physician. Monitor the results of the complete blood count. • Report cough to the health care provider	• Hypotension may occur as a first-dose effect. It is most common in Na⁺- or volume-depleted clients. • Clients with impaired renal function may develop hyperkalemia. • Neutropenia, although rare, can be a hazardous complication. • Cough is a side effect of the drug.
Enalapril maleate (Vasotec)	• To start: 2.5–5 mg/day • May increase to 10–40 mg/day as a single dose or divided doses.	• Administer 1 hr before or 2 hr after meals. • Enalapril is similar to captopril but may be administered less frequently.	• Administration on an empty stomach enhances absorption. • Enalapril has a longer half-life than captopril.
Drugs Used Primarily To Reduce Preload			
Loop Diuretics Furosemide (Lasix, Furoside♣)	• 40 mg qd or bid PO • 40 mg qd IV push (may increase to 80 mg and repeat × 1 in 30 min in acute situations) • **Elderly:** Older adults may be more sensitive to the effects of the usual adult dose.	• Administer once daily when the client arises. • Assess the client for adequate diuresis. Obtain daily weights. Note changes in breath sounds and edema. • Monitor the client's serum electrolytes (especially K⁺, Na⁺, and Cl⁻). Provide K⁺ supplementation if prescribed. • Monitor the client for signs of dehydration (hypotension, dry mucous membranes, poor skin turgor, thirst, and oliguria). • Note any report of ringing in the ears.	• The volume and frequency of urination increase for 6–8 hr after an oral dose. • Weight is one of the most accurate noninvasive measurements of volume status. • Loop diuretics may produce excessive loss of these electrolytes. • Loop diuretics continue to cause diuresis even after the excessive fluid has been removed. • Tinnitus may indicate toxicity.
Nitrates Isosorbide dinitrate (Isodil, Sorbitrate, Coronex♣, Novosorbide♣)	• PO (tablet) 15–30 mg q6h • PO (sustained release) 40 mg q6–12h	• Observe the client for postural hypotension. Supervise ambulation until the dose response is determined.	• Relaxation of venous smooth muscle causes blood to pool in the veins when the client stands.
Nitroglycerin (Nitro-Dur)	• Transdermal ointment: starting dose of ½ inch q4–8h increasing to 2 inches q4–8h	• Assess the client for headache. Inform the physician and provide relief.	• Headache diminishes with tolerance. Mild analgesics and administration with food should provide relief until then.

Continued

CHART 37–3. Drug Therapy for Cardiac Failure   Continued

Drug	Usual Dosage	Nursing Interventions	Rationale
Nitroglycerin (Nitrodisc)	• Transdermal patch: 2.5–15 mg/12–18 hr	• Administer PO dose 30 min before or 2 hr after meals. Make sure the client does not chew. • Administer the ointment on a hairless part of the body in a uniform layer using an applicator. • If so prescribed, allow an 8–12-hr nitrate-free period at night. • Rotate the skin sites of transdermal nitrate administration. • Remove transdermal nitrates before defibrillation.	• Oral nitrates are most rapidly absorbed from an empty stomach. • Proper administration ensures consistent dose administration. • A nitrate-free period prevents the development of tolerance to the vasodilating effect of nitrates. • Nitrates cause skin irritation. • Skin burns have occurred, and explosion is possible.
Cardiac Glycosides Digoxin (Lanoxin, Novodigoxin✻)	• Loading dose of 1 mg divided over 24 hr. • Then maintenance 0.125–0.5 mg PO qd • Usually 0.25–0.375 mg IV qd	• Ask the client about previous use of digitalis; provide the preparation previously taken. (Do not substitute one preparation for another.)	• Dosages, absorption rates, and duration of effects differ among drugs.

Digitoxin (Crystodigin) (infrequently used)	• Loading dose of 1.2–1.6 mg divided during 24 hr
	• Then 0.1 mg daily IV or PO
		• Be alert for the following:
		  • Myocardial infarction
		  • Hypokalemia
		  • Renal or hepatic disorders
		  • Diuretic therapy
		  • Diarrhea
		  • Advanced age
		  • Metabolic alkalosis
		• Monitor serum potassium levels and electrocardiograms.
		
		• Take the apical pulse or check the cardiac monitor pattern before administering each dose of digitalis.
		• Monitor serum levels of digitalis. Therapeutic digoxin level is 0.9–1.2 ng/mL.
		
		• Observe for signs of digitalis toxicity and notify the physician if any occur:
		  • Confusion
		  • Dysrhythmias
		  • Anorexia
		  • Fatigue
		  • Muscle weakness
			• Any of these factors may result in an increased sensitivity to digitalis and increase the risk of toxicity.
			
			• Hypokalemia is often associated with digitalis toxicity and dysrhythmias.
			• Changes in pulse rate and rhythm may signify digitalis toxicity.
			• There is a narrow margin between therapeutic and toxic doses of digitalis. Toxicity occurs in approximately 10%–20% of clients receiving digitalis.

nurse monitors serum potassium levels for hyperkalemia, serum creatinine for renal dysfunction, and the client for development of a cough. Table 37–2 compares the effects of selected agents that reduce the preload and the afterload. (Intravenous medications used to decrease preload and afterload are described in Chapter 40.)

Reducing Preload. When ventricular fibers are overstretched, as in the failing heart, they contract less forcefully. Interventions aimed at preload reduction attempt to decrease volume and pressure in the left ventricle, optimizing ventricular muscle stretch and contraction. Preload reduction is appropriate for clients in heart failure who

TABLE 37–2

Effects of Vasodilators*		
Drug	**Preload Reduction (Vasodilates Peripheral Veins)**	**Afterload Reduction (Vasodilates Arterioles)**
Nitrates (nitroglycerin, isosorbide dinitrate)	+++	+
Hydralazine hydrochloride (Apresoline)	0	+++
Nifedipine (Procardia)	0	++
Sodium nitroprusside (Nitropress)	+++	+++
Captopril (Capoten)	+	++
Prazosin (Minipress)	++	+

*0, no effect; +, mild effect; ++, moderate effect; +++, maximal effect.

have congestion with total body sodium and water overload.

Diet Therapy. In heart failure, diet therapy is aimed at reducing sodium and water retention.

Sodium Restriction. In collaboration with the dietitian, the health care provider may restrict sodium intake in an attempt to decrease fluid retention. Many clients with heart failure need to omit only table salt (ingest no added salt) from their diet, thus reducing the sodium intake to 2 to 3 g/day. If salt intake must be reduced further, the client may need to eliminate all salt in cooking, thus reducing sodium intake to 1.2 to 2.0 g/day. The dietitian helps the client select foods that meet the prescribed therapeutic diet. Table 14–6 lists the sodium contents of some common foods.

Fluid Volume Restriction. Few clients are placed on severe fluid restrictions. However, because clients with excessive aldosterone secretion may experience thirst and drink 3 to 5 L of fluid each day, their fluid intake may be limited to a more normal 2 L/day. Compliance with these simple strategies may be high, especially if the client experiences relief of any of the symptoms of volume excess. When a fluid restriction is imposed on the hospitalized client, the nurse adjusts oral and intravenous therapy accordingly.

The nurse or assistive nursing personnel weighs the client daily (1 kg of weight gain or loss equals 1 L of retained or lost fluid, respectively) and keeps accurate records of fluid intake and output. The same scale should be used every morning before breakfast for the most accurate assessment of weight.

Drug Therapy. Common drugs prescribed to reduce preload are diuretics and venous vasodilators.

Diuretics. The health care provider adds diuretics to the regimen when diet and fluid restriction have not been effective in the management of symptoms of systemic or pulmonary congestion associated with heart failure. Diuretics enhance renal excretion of sodium and water

by reducing the circulating blood volume, decreasing preload, and reducing systemic and pulmonary congestion.

The type and dosage of diuretic prescribed depend on the degree of heart failure and renal function. The high-ceiling (loop) diuretics, such as furosemide (Lasix, Furoside✦), torsemide (Demadex), and ethacrynic acid (Edecrin), are most effective for treating fluid volume overload. However, the practitioner may initially use a thiazide diuretic, such as hydrochlorothiazide (Hydro-DIURIL, Urozide✦) and metolazone (Zaroxolyn), for elderly clients with mild volume overload. The action of thiazide diuretics is self-limiting (i.e., diuresis decreases after edema fluid is lost), so the excessive diuresis and dehydration that may occur with loop diuretics are uncommon. Clients often prefer thiazide diuretics because of the gradual onset of diuresis. However, for many clients in heart failure, loop diuretics are needed to ensure effective diuresis.

The nurse also needs to monitor for and prevent potassium deficiency (hypokalemia) from diuretic therapy. The signs of hypokalemia are nonspecific neurologic and muscular complaints, such as generalized weakness, depressed reflexes, and irregular heart rate. Therefore, to accurately identify hypokalemia, the physician, nurse, and dietitian monitor serum potassium levels.

If the client's serum potassium level is less than 4.0 mEq/L, the health care provider has several alternatives:

- Adding a potassium-sparing diuretic to the regimen
- Requesting that clients increase their dietary intake of potassium-rich foods
- Prescribing a potassium supplement

Clients being treated simultaneously with ACE inhibitors and diuretics may not experience hypokalemia. If their kidneys are not functioning well, they may develop hyperkalemia, an elevated serum potassium level. The nurse should review the client's serum creatinine level; if the creatinine is greater than 1.8, the nurse should notify the health care provider before administering supplemental potassium.

ELDERLY CONSIDERATIONS

Elderly clients receiving loop diuretics are very prone to dehydration, especially those with type 2 diabetes mellitus. The nurse must check orthostatic blood pressures in the elderly client receiving loop diuretics to detect volume depletion. The nurse also examines the client for flat neck veins when the client is supine, a loss of skin turgor, and a slow progressive weight loss despite an adequate diet. All of these signs, plus disorientation in the very old client, may indicate excessive diuresis and volume depletion (Chart 37–4).

Venous Vasodilators. The health care provider may prescribe venous vasodilators. (e.g., nitrates) for the client in heart failure with persistent dyspnea. To compensate for the client's reduced cardiac output, significant constriction of venous and arterial blood vessels occurs, reducing the volume of fluid that the vascular bed can hold and increasing the preload. Venous vasodilators may benefit clients by

- Returning the venous vasculature to a more normal capacity
- Decreasing the volume of blood returning to the heart
- Improving left ventricular function

Some of the most common vasodilators are summarized in Chart 37–3.

Nitrates may be administered intravenously, orally, or topically. These drugs cause primarily venous vasodilation but also a significant amount of arteriolar vasodilation. It is essential for the nurse to monitor the client's blood pressure when initiating nitrate therapy or increasing the dosage. Clients may initially report headache. The nurse should assure clients that they will develop a toler-ance to this effect and that the headache will cease or diminish.

Unfortunately, when nitrates are uniformly administered during 24 hours, clients may develop tolerance to the vasodilating effects. To prevent such tolerance, the health care provider may order at least one 12-hour nitrate-free period out of every 24 hours, usually overnight. However, clients whose major complaint is nocturnal dyspnea may experience relief when nitroglycerine ointment is applied at bedtime and removed during the day.

Digitalis. Digoxin (Lanoxin), a cardiac glycoside, has been demonstrated to provide benefits for clients in heart failure with sinus rhythm and atrial fibrillation. "Dig" therapy reduces exacerbations of heart failure and hospitalizations, resulting in an estimated savings of $406 million annually. When added to a regimen of ACE inhibitors and diuretics, digoxin increases functional capacity and improves hemodynamic parameters in clients with NYHA class III and IV heart failure due to left systolic dysfunction (Redfield, 1996).

The potential benefits of digitalis derivatives include an increase in contractility, reduction in heart rate, slowing of conduction through the atrioventricular node, and inhibition of sympathetic activity while enhancing parasympathetic activity. Digitalis also may have a mild diuretic effect. At toxic digitalis levels, increased automaticity occurs, and ectopic beats (premature ventricular contractions [PVCs]) may result.

The most commonly prescribed cardiac glycoside is digoxin (Lanoxin, Novodigoxin✱). Digoxin is erratically absorbed from the gastrointestinal tract. Many medications, especially antacids, interfere with its absorption. It is eliminated primarily by renal excretion.

ELDERLY CONSIDERATIONS

The half-life of digoxin in middle-aged adults is 36 hours; in older adults, who typically have diminished renal function, the half-life may be 48 hours. Thus, elderly clients are particularly susceptible to digoxin toxicity. Toxicity occurs in 10% to 20% of all clients taking digoxin, more commonly in older clients and clients with hypokalemia. Toxicity in older, hypokalemic clients may be fatal.

Digitalis Toxicity. The presentation of digitalis toxicity may be vague and nonspecific. Toxicity may cause nearly any dysrhythmia, but PVCs are most commonly noted. The nurse or nursing staff member carefully monitors the apical pulse rate and heart rhythm of clients receiving digoxin. The nurse must identify and report to the health care provider when the resting heart rate is less than 60 beats per minute or greater than 100 beats per minute and when there is a significant change in rhythm or rate. It is equally important to report the development of an irregular rhythm in a client with a previously regular rhythm and a regular rhythm in a client with a previously irregular one. The nurse also monitors serum digoxin and potassium levels to identify toxicity. Chart 37–3 presents information about selected cardiac glycosides.

Any medication that increases the workload of the fail-

Chart 37–4

Nursing Focus on the Elderly: Heart Failure

- Assess older clients with confusion for indications of heart failure. People older than 80 years often present with restlessness or confusion as the initial manifestation of heart failure.
- Auscultate the lungs carefully, recognizing that dependent crackles may not be an indication of heart failure in the older adult.
- Do not expect crackles to clear rapidly after treatment. Crackles may persist in the lung bases of older adults for an extended period after pulmonary congestion has decreased.
- Be especially alert for the signs of digitalis toxicity in the elderly client because it occurs frequently.
- If loop diuretics are used for diuresis, monitor the client closely for signs of excessive diuresis, dehydration, and hypokalemia.
- In older clients receiving drug therapy for heart failure, monitor for orthostatic hypotension. Cardiovascular changes associated with aging make this likely to develop.

ing heart also increases its oxygen requirement. The nurse should be alert for the possibility that the client may experience angina (chest pain) in response to digoxin. Intravenous medications that increase contractility are described in Chapter 40.

➤ *Activity Intolerance*

Planning: Expected Outcomes. The client is expected to perform activities of daily living and walk at least two blocks without dyspnea or excessive fatigue.

Interventions. Initially, the client in severe heart failure requires physical and emotional rest. On the first day of hospitalization, clients may sit up in a chair for meals and do basic leg exercises while up. Nursing care should be organized to allow periods of rest. The interdisciplinary team observes and documents the client's physiologic response to activity.

As the client's condition improves, the nurse or physical therapist (PT) initiates ambulation, usually on hospital day 2. The nurse checks the client's blood pressure, pulse, and oxygen saturation before and after the activity. A blood pressure change of more than 20 mmHg or a pulse increase of more than 20 beats per minute may indicate that the activity is too stressful. Other indications that the client cannot tolerate the activity include dyspnea, fatigue, and chest pain. If a client displays any of these symptoms, he or she is asked to rate how hard he or she has been working on a scale of 1 to 20, with 20 being maximum perceived exertion. If the client rates the exertion higher then 12, the nurse counsels the client to slow down. If the client tolerates the activity, the nurse or PT steadily increases the client's activity level until the client is ambulating 200 to 400 feet several times a day.

If the client is able, the nurse or assistive nursing personnel might time the client for 6 minutes while walking at a comfortable pace. The distance the client can walk can be used to determine the client's functional level and activity plan.

➤ *Potential for Pulmonary Edema*

Planning: Expected Outcomes. The client is expected to be free of pulmonary edema.

Interventions. The nurse monitors clients for acute pulmonary edema, a life-threatening event that can result from severe heart failure. In pulmonary edema, the left ventricle fails to eject sufficient blood, and pressure increases in the lungs because of the accumulated blood. The increased pressure causes fluid to leak across the pulmonary capillaries and into the pulmonary interstitium.

The nurse assesses for early signs and symptoms of pulmonary edema, such as crackles in the lung bases, disorientation, and confusion, especially in the elderly client. Documentation of the precise location of the crackles is crucial, as the level of the fluid ascends as the pulmonary edema worsens. The client in pulmonary edema is also extremely anxious, tachycardic, and struggling for air. He or she may have a moist cough productive of frothy, blood-tinged sputum, and the client's skin may be cold, clammy, or cyanotic.

The client diagnosed with pulmonary edema is admitted to the acute care hospital. The physician prescribes rapid-acting diuretics, such as furosemide (Lasix, Furoside✶). Furosemide is given intravenously over 1 to 2 minutes, usually at a starting dose of 40 mg and another 40 mg repeated if needed in 30 minutes (Booker & Ignatavicius, 1996).

Oxygen is always ordered, and the client is placed in a high-Fowler's position. IV morphine sulfate may be prescribed, 1 to 2 mg at a time, to reduce venous return (preload), but the nurse should monitor respiratory rate and blood pressure closely. Vasodilators, such as nitroglycerin (Tridil) and sodium nitroprusside (Nitropress), may be administered via continuous infusion pumps. Low dosages of these drugs must be given initially and increased slowly to avoid severe hypotension.

Once commonly used to decrease preload, rotating tourniquets and phlebotomy are now used rarely during the wait for these medications to be effective.

The nurse or assistive personnel inserts a Foley catheter, if ordered, to assess the client's urinary output after diuretic administration and to minimize exertion related to voiding. Diuresis normally begins within 5 minutes of the administration of IV furosemide and peaks at 30 minutes. Chart 37–5 summarizes the care of the client with acute pulmonary edema.

Clients often respond dramatically and quickly to these interventions, but their condition can also deteriorate rapidly because of pulmonary congestion and severe hypoxemia. Clients occasionally require Bipap or intubation and ventilation to survive the acute episode. A skilled nurse is needed to assist with intubation. (Management of the client who is critically ill with heart failure is detailed in Chapter 40.)

Chart 37–5

Nursing Care Highlight: Care of the Client with Pulmonary Edema

- Identify the client's chief complaint.
- If the client's blood pressure is adequate, place the client in a high-Fowler's position.
- Auscultate the client's lungs briefly (posterior assessment).
- Ensure that vascular access is present and check for patency.
- Provide oxygen as ordered.
- Provide IV diuretic (usually furosemide) as prescribed.
- Anticipate urinary output in 5–15 min after diuretic administration; catheterize if ordered.
- Monitor blood pressure, respiratory rate, pulse oximetry, pulse, and cardiac rhythm, and the client's subjective feelings of ability to breathe.
- Provide additional medications as prescribed (usually morphine sulfate or nitroglycerin).
- Provide comfort measures and reassurance.
- Notify the physician if the client does not have a rapid improvement and diuresis.

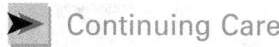 Continuing Care

➤ Case Management

Clients who have not been adequately prepared for discharge or who do not have good community support and follow-up are at high risk for recurrent hospital admissions for heart failure (Dracup et al., 1995). In a case management system, the case manager or care coordinator assesses the client's needs for health care resources and facilitates appropriate placement. It is imperative that the case manager assess the available social supports because inability to obtain help in such activities as food shopping and obtaining medications is a major contributor to hospital readmission (Dracup et al., 1995). If home support is available, the client may be discharged home in the care of a family member or other caregiver. Home care nurses may direct the care, while aides may provide assistance with ADLs.

If the client has multiple health problems or has been severely compromised by heart disease, he or she may require admission to a subacute unit or traditional nursing home for either transitional or long-term care. Home care services cost about $125 per nursing visit compared with $150 to $300 per day in a traditional nursing home and up to $1,000 per day for hospital care.

➤ Health Teaching

Activity Schedule. Medicare usually provides reimbursement for client assessment and teaching so that a home care care nurse can continue teaching and assessment when the client returns home. The nurse encourages clients with heart failure to stay as active as possible and to develop a regular exercise regimen. Clients who are more active appear to have better outcomes (Dracup et al., 1995). The goal for clients with heart failure is development of a regular exercise routine, probably a home walking program, several times a week. Medicare and third-party payers do not reimburse for cardiac rehabilitation for heart failure clients, and paying for a cardiac rehabilitation program out of pocket would cost a client approximately $1,620 (Newkirk & Leeper, 1996).

Although most clients with heart failure appear to benefit from exercise programs, clients with persistent crackles and uncontrolled edema despite medical therapy are not encouraged to exercise until their heart failure is stabilized (Sullivan, 1994). When exercise is indicated, the nurse teaches the client to begin walking 200 to 400 ft/day. At home, the client should slowly increase the amount of time walked (perhaps 2 minutes a week) over several months, trying to walk at least three times a week. If the client experiences chest pain or pronounced dyspnea while exercising or fatigue the next day, he or she is probably advancing the activity too quickly and should slow down. The nurse encourages the client to keep an exercise diary that documents the time and duration of each exercise session as well as the client's heart rate and any symptoms occurring with exercise.

Twenty percent of clients who are readmitted to hospitals for treatment of heart failure fail to seek medical attention promptly when symptoms reoccur (Dracup et al., 1995). The nurse instructs the client and caregiver to immediately report the occurrence of any of the following symptoms of worsening heart failure to his or her health care provider:

- Rapid weight gain (3 pounds in a week)
- Decrease in exercise tolerance lasting 2 to 3 days
- Cold symptoms (cough) lasting more than 3 to 5 days
- Excessive awakening at night to urinate
- Development of dyspnea or angina at rest

Drug Therapy. The nurse or pharmacist provides oral and written instructions about the medication regimen. If the client is taking digoxin, the caregiver and the client are taught how to count a pulse rate. The nurse assesses the client's ability to accurately take and record his or her pulse rate. Chart 37–6 lists instructions for the client taking digoxin at home.

The nurse advises clients taking diuretics to take them in the morning to avoid waking during the night for voiding. After determining if the client has a weight scale and can use it, the nurse instructs the client to take his or her weight each morning. Daily weights indicate whether the client is losing or retaining fluid. Some motivated clients are taught to use a sliding scale to adjust their daily diuretic dose depending on their daily weight, similar to the way a diabetic adjusts an insulin dose based on the capillary glucose level. The home care nurse may reliably assess a client's volume status by checking the pattern of daily weights and noting jugular venous distention and hepatojugular reflux (see Chap. 35).

Clients receiving angiotensin-converting enzyme (ACE) inhibitors should be taught to move slowly when changing positions, especially from a lying to a sitting position. Dizziness, lightheadedness, and cough need to be reported to the health care provider.

Clients taking diuretics and ACE inhibitors require

Chart 37–6

Education Guide: Digoxin Therapy

- Noon is the best time of day to take this medication if you can remember to take it then.
- Continue administration of this medication unless you are told to stop it by your health care provider.
- Do not take digoxin at the same time as antacids or cathartics (laxatives).
- Take your pulse rate before taking each dose of digoxin. Notify your health care provider of a change in pulse rate (60–100 beats per minute is normal) or rhythm as well as increasing fatigue, muscle weakness, confusion, or loss of appetite (signs of digitalis toxicity).
- If you forget to take a dose, it may be delayed a few hours. However, if you do not remember it until the next day, you should take only your usual daily dose.
- Report for scheduled laboratory test (such as potassium and digoxin levels).
- If potassium supplements are prescribed, continue the dose until told to stop by your health care provider.

their serum potassium level and renal function to be monitored at least every few months. Diuretics, especially loop diuretics like furosemide, deplete potassium and often cause hypokalemia. Conversely, ACE inhibitors may result in potassium retention. If potassium levels drop below 4.0 mEq/L, the primary care physician may prescribe potassium supplementation or a potassium-sparing diuretic. A dietician may be consulted to provide the client with information about potassium-rich foods to include in the diet.

Diet Therapy. Clients with chronic heart failure are advised to restrict their dietary sodium. The dietitian provides written instructions on low- or restricted-sodium diets. For mild or moderate failure, a 3-g sodium diet is recommended. Clients usually find this diet palatable and fairly easy to follow. They are asked to avoid salty foods and table salt. For clients with severe heart failure, a 2-g sodium diet may be attempted. These clients are told not to add salt during or after meal preparation, to avoid milk and milk products, and to use few canned or prepared foods. The home care nurse or dietitian should assess the client for compliance with this diet because it is unpalatable and for many clients the cost of low-sodium foods can be a financial burden.

Clients are also instructed to confer with their health care provider if they want to use commercial salt substitutes. Most salt substitutes contain potassium, and the client's renal status and serum potassium level need to be considered before one can recommend these products. To enhance the flavor of low-salt foods, clients may use lemon, garlic, and herbs.

Advance Directives. Approximately 50% of deaths from heart failure are sudden, many without any warning or worsening of symptoms (Dracup et al., 1995). Because the majority of these deaths occur at home, it is important for the primary care provider or home care nurse to discuss advance directives with the client and family. The family should be prepared to act in accordance with the client's wishes in the event of cardiac arrest. If the client desires resuscitation to be attempted, the family should know how to activate the EMS system and how to provide CPR until an ambulance arrives. If the client does not wish to have CPR, the client, family, and nurse should plan how the family will respond.

➤ Home Care Management

The focus of the home care nurse's interventions is assessment and health teaching, which are reimbursable by Medicare and other third-party payers. Chart 37–7 lists major areas of assessment that the home care nurse performs.

Clients with chronic heart failure must make many adjustments in their lifestyles (Research Applications for Nursing). They must adhere to a medical regimen that includes dietary restrictions, activity prescriptions, and drug therapy. Clients need careful, concise explanations of the treatment plan. The continuing care nurse in any setting encourages the client to verbalize fears and concerns about his or her illness and assists the client

Chart 37–7

Focused Assessment for Home Care Clients with Heart Failure

- Assess for signs of heart failure, including
  - Changes in vital signs (heart rate >100 bpm at rest, new atrial fibrillation, BP <90 or >150 systolic)
  - Indications of poor tissue perfusion
    Fatigue
    Angina
    Activity intolerance
    Changes in mental status
    Pallor or cyanosis
  - Indications of congestion
    Presence of cough or dyspnea
    Weight gain
    Jugular venous distention and peripheral edema
- Assess functional ability, including
  - Performance of activities of daily living
  - Mobility and ambulation (review frequency and duration of walking, development of symptoms, and pulse rate)
  - Cognitive ability
- Assess nutritional status, including
  - Food and fluid intake
  - Intake of sodium-rich foods
  - Alcohol consumption
  - Skin turgor
- Assess home environment, including
  - Safety hazards, especially related to oxygen therapy
  - Structural barriers affecting functional ability
- Assess client's compliance and understanding of illness and its treatment, including
  - Signs and symptoms to report to health care provider
  - Dosages, effects, and side or toxic effects of medications
  - When to report for lab and health care provider visits
  - Ability to accurately weigh self on scale
  - Presence of advanced directive
  - Use of home oxygen, if appropriate
- Assess client and caregiver coping skills

in exploring appropriate coping skills. Clients' participation in treatment can help alleviate and control symptoms.

➤ Health Care Resources

A home care nurse may be needed to assess the client's adherence to medication and diet therapy and to monitor for worsening heart failure. Clients with activity limitations benefit from the services of a home care aide. A dietitian might be consulted to assist with menu planning and teaching. Although clients have been demonstrated to benefit from participation in structured cardiac rehabilitation programs, referral to such programs is not widespread because coverage is usually not provided by third-party payers.

In addition to home care support, other resources are available for client education and family support. The American Heart Association is an excellent community

Martensson, J., Karlsson, J. E., & Fridlund, B. (1997). *Male patients with congestive heart failure and their conception of the life situation.* Journal of Advanced Nursing, 25, 579–586.

Research Applications for Nursing

This qualitative study examined the experiences of 12 male Swedish clients with heart failure during the first 2 months to 2 years following diagnosis. Clients ranged from NYHA classification II (5) to IV (2), and most were married.

Six categories emerged that described how clients with heart failure perceived of their situation. Six men described feeling a belief in the future. These more hopeful men were more engaged in daily activities, possibly ignoring certain aspects of their illness. Eight men mentioned gaining awareness of their bodies' signals, changing their lifestyles, and adapting to heart failure. All of the men indicated that support from their environment affected their ability to function. Unfortunately, all of them expressed negative feelings about their relationship with their family and friends. Ten men identified feeling physically restricted by heart failure. Seven men identified a lack of physical and emotional energy or no energy at all. Finally, four men described being resigned, accepting that nothing could be done for them and passively awaiting death.

Critique. This is a qualitative study done on a small sample of 12 Swedish men; the size might limit its generalizability to others with heart failure. Because a saturation of the concepts was reached before data collection was completed, the results may be more trustworthy. In addition, a comparative study with women is currently in progress.

The study is a phenomenographic study that attempts to describe how people conceive of something. These conceptions are thought to be the basis on which opinions rest. It is different from a phenomenologic study, which attempts to explore what the person is experiencing.

Possible Nursing Implications. Additional studies to validate these six categories and relate them to other variables (such as NYHA classification or duration of heart failure) could assist nurses to further understand heart failure. Nursing interventions that focus on helping clients feel more positive are needed to prevent the negative feelings that these male subjects experienced.

resource for pamphlets, books, cookbooks, and videotapes related to heart failure and heart disease. The organization also provides referrals to various local support groups for clients and their caregivers in the community.

For equipment needs, such as home oxygen therapy or a hospital bed, medical supply companies provide set-up and maintenance services. A detailed description of home oxygen therapy is found in Chapter 30.

 Evaluation

On the basis of the identified nursing diagnoses and collaborative problems, the nurse evaluates the care of the client with heart failure. Outcomes include that the client will

- Have a normal rate, rhythm, and depth of respiration
- Have an O_2 saturation greater than 92%
- Resume and maintain an adequate cardiac output
- Perform activities of daily living without dyspnea or excessive fatigue
- Be free of pulmonary edema

VALVULAR HEART DISEASE

Valvular heart disease occurs when the heart valves cannot open fully (valvular stenosis) or close completely (valvular insufficiency or regurgitation). Acquired valvular dysfunctions most often involve the left side of the heart, especially the mitral valve. Acquired valvular dysfunctions, in rank order of occurrence, are mitral stenosis, mitral regurgitation, mitral valve prolapse, aortic stenosis, and aortic regurgitation.

The tricuspid valve is involved infrequently, and the pulmonic valve is affected rarely. Often, stenosis and regurgitation occur simultaneously in a defect called a mixed lesion.

Mitral Stenosis

Mitral stenosis usually results from rheumatic carditis, which can cause valve thickening by fibrosis and calcification. The valve leaflets fuse and become stiff, while the chordae tendineae contract and shorten. The valvular orifice narrows, preventing normal blood flow from the left atrium to the left ventricle. As a result of these changes, the left atrial pressure rises, the left atrium dilates, pulmonary artery pressures increase, and the right ventricle hypertrophies.

Initially, pulmonary congestion and right-sided heart failure occur. Later, when the left ventricle receives insufficient blood volume, the preload is decreased, and the cardiac output falls.

Clients with mild mitral stenosis are usually asymptomatic. As the valvular orifice narrows, and pressure in the lungs increases, the client experiences dyspnea on exertion, orthopnea, paroxysmal nocturnal dyspnea (sudden dyspnea at night), and dry cough. As the pulmonary hypertension and congestion progress, hemoptysis and pulmonary edema appear. Right-sided heart failure can cause hepatomegaly, neck vein distention, and pitting edema late in the disorder.

The pulse may be normal on palpation, tachycardiac, or irregularly irregular, as in atrial fibrillation. Because the development of atrial fibrillation indicates that the client may decompensate, the physician should be notified immediately. On auscultation, the nurse notes a rumbling, apical diastolic murmur.

Rheumatic fever is the most common cause of mitral stenosis. Nonrheumatic causes include atrial myxoma (tumor), calcium accumulation, and thrombus formation.

WOMEN'S HEALTH CONSIDERATIONS

Two-thirds to three-fourths of all clients with mitral stenosis are women. About two-thirds of the women with rheumatic mitral stenosis are younger than 45 years.

Mitral Regurgitation (Insufficiency)

The fibrotic and calcific changes occurring in mitral regurgitation prevent the mitral valve from closing completely during *systole*. Incomplete closure of the valve allows backflow of blood into the left atrium when the left ventricle contracts. During *diastole,* regurgitant output is returned with the normal blood flow from the left atrium to the left ventricle, increasing the volume that must be ejected during the next systole. To compensate for the increased volume and pressure, the left atrium and ventricle dilate and hypertrophy.

Mitral insufficiency usually progresses slowly; clients may remain symptom free for decades. Symptoms begin to occur when the left ventricle fails in response to increased blood volumes. The client most often reports fatigue and chronic weakness as a result of reduced cardiac output. Dyspnea on exertion and orthopnea develop later. A significant number of clients complain of anxiety, atypical chest pains, and palpitations.

Nursing assessment may reveal normal blood pressure, atrial fibrillation (an irregularly irregular rhythm occurring in 75% of clients), or changes in respirations characteristic of left ventricular failure.

When right-sided heart failure develops, the neck veins become distended, the liver enlarges (hepatomegaly), and pitting edema is noted. On auscultation, the nurse hears a high-pitched systolic murmur at the apex, with radiation to the left axilla. Severe regurgitation often exhibits a third heart sound.

Rheumatic heart disease is the predominant cause of mitral insufficiency. When mitral insufficiency results from rheumatic heart disease, it usually co-exists with some degree of mitral stenosis. Nonrheumatic causes include papillary muscle dysfunction or rupture due to ischemic heart disease, infective endocarditis, and a congenital anomaly.

Mitral regurgitation resulting from rheumatic heart disease is more common in women than in men. Mitral regurgitation of a nonrheumatic etiology occurs more often in men.

Mitral Valve Prolapse

Mitral valve prolapse occurs because the valvular leaflets enlarge and prolapse into the left atrium during systole. Usually this is a benign abnormality, but it may progress to pronounced mitral regurgitation.

Most clients with mitral valve prolapse are asymptomatic. However, clients may report chest pain, palpitations, or exercise intolerance. Chest pain is usually atypical, with clients describing a sharp pain localized to the left side of the chest. Dizziness, syncope, and palpitations may be associated with atrial or ventricular dysrhythmias.

On physical examination, the nurse usually finds a normal heart rate and blood pressure. A midsystolic click and a late systolic murmur may be audible at the apex.

The etiology of mitral valve prolapse is variable; it has been associated with such conditions as Marfan's syndrome and other cardiac defects. However, most of the time no other cardiac abnormality is found. A familial occurrence is well established.

Mitral valve prolapse affects 5% to 10% of people. Although it is present in all age groups, it is most common in women between the ages of 20 and 54 years.

Aortic Stenosis

In people with aortic stenosis, the aortic valve orifice narrows, obstructing left ventricular outflow during systole. This increased resistance to ejection or afterload results in ventricular hypertrophy. As the stenosis progresses, the cardiac output becomes fixed, unable to increase to meet the demands of the body during exertion, and symptoms develop. Eventually the left ventricle fails, volume backs up in the left atrium, and the pulmonary system becomes congested. Late in the disease process, right-sided heart failure can occur.

The classic symptoms of aortic stenosis result from the fixed cardiac output. They are dyspnea, angina, and syncope occurring on exertion. When cardiac output falls in the late stages of the disease, the client has marked fatigue, debilitation, and peripheral cyanosis. A narrow pulse pressure is noted when the blood pressure is examined. A diamond-shaped systolic crescendo-decrescendo murmur is usually noted on auscultation.

Congenital valvular disease or malformation is the predominant etiologic factor in aortic stenosis. Bicuspid or unicuspid aortic valves are the primary reason for aortic stenosis in clients younger than 30 years and account for about 50% of the disease in clients 30 to 70 years. Rheumatic aortic stenosis is always concomitant with rheumatic disease of the mitral valve. It develops in clients between the ages of 30 and 70. Atherosclerosis and degenerative calcification of the aortic valve are the predominant factors in people older than age 70. Aortic stenosis has become the most common valvular disorder in countries with aging populations. Of clients with aortic stenosis, 80% are men.

Aortic Regurgitation (Insufficiency)

In clients with aortic regurgitation, the aortic valve leaflets do not close properly during diastole, and the annulus (the valve ring that attaches to the leaflets) may be dilated, loose, or deformed. This allows regurgitation of blood from the aorta back into the left ventricle during diastole. The left ventricle, in compensation, dilates to accommodate the greater blood volume and eventually hypertrophies.

Clients with aortic regurgitation remain asymptomatic for many years because of the compensatory mechanisms of the left ventricle. As the disease progresses and left ventricular failure occurs, the principal concerns of the client are exertional dyspnea, orthopnea, and paroxysmal nocturnal dyspnea. The client with severe disease may note palpitations, especially while lying on the left side. Many clients with aortic regurgitation experience nocturnal angina with diaphoresis.

On palpation, the nurse notes a "bounding" arterial pulse. The pulse pressure is usually widened, with an elevated systolic pressure and diminished diastolic pressure. The classic auscultatory finding is a high-pitched, blowing, decrescendo diastolic murmur.

Aortic insufficiency is usual in nonrheumatic conditions such as infective endocarditis, congenital anatomic aortic valvular abnormalities, hypertension, and Marfan's syndrome (a rare, generalized, systemic disease of connective tissue). Approximately 75% of clients with aortic regurgitation are men.

Collaborative Management

 Assessment

A client with valvular disease may suddenly become ill or may slowly develop symptoms over the course of many years. The nurse collects information on the client's family health history, including valvular or other forms of heart disease to which the client may be genetically predisposed. The nurse questions the client about attacks of rheumatic fever, the specific dates when these occurred, and the use of antibiotic prophylaxis against recurrence of rheumatic fever. The client's fatigue level, the level of activity that is tolerated, the presence of angina or dyspnea, and the occurrence of palpitations, if present, are also discussed.

As part of physical assessment, the nurse obtains the client's vital signs, inspects the client for signs of edema, palpates and auscultates the client's heart and lungs, and palpates the client's peripheral pulses. Findings consistent with valvular malformation are summarized in Chart 37–8.

In clients with mitral stenosis, the chest x-ray shows left atrial enlargement, prominent pulmonary arteries, and an enlarged right ventricle. In those with mitral regurgitation, the chest x-ray reveals an increased cardiac shadow, indicating left ventricular and left atrial enlargement.

In the later stages of aortic stenosis, the chest x-ray may show left ventricular enlargement and pulmonary congestion. In clients with aortic *insufficiency,* left atrial and left ventricular dilation appear on the chest x-ray. If heart failure is present, pulmonary venous congestion is also evident.

For clients with valvular heart disease, echocardiography is usually indicated because it is an excellent noninvasive tool for defining cardiac structure, movement of the valve leaflets, and size and function of the cardiac chambers. Exercise tolerance testing (ETT) is sometimes performed to evaluate symptomatic response, to assess functional capacity, and to enhance auscultatory findings. In clients with either mitral or aortic stenosis, cardiac catheterization is frequently indicated to assess the severity of the stenosis and its other effects on the heart.

The health care provider also orders an electrocardiogram (ECG) to assess abnormalities such as left ventricular hypertrophy, as seen with mitral regurgitation and aortic regurgitation, or right ventricular hypertrophy, as seen in severe mitral stenosis. Atrial fibrillation is a common finding in both mitral stenosis and mitral regurgitation.

 Interventions

Management of valvular heart disease depends on which valve is affected and the degree of valve impairment. Some clients can be managed with yearly monitoring and medications, but other clients require invasive procedures or heart surgery.

➤ Nonsurgical Management

Nonsurgical management focuses on drug therapy and rest. During the course of valvular disease, clients may

---

Chart 37–8

Key Features of Valvular Heart Disease

Mitral Stenosis	Mitral Insufficiency	Mitral Valve Prolapse	Aortic Stenosis	Aortic Insufficiency
• Fatigue	• Fatigue	• Atypical chest pain	• Dyspnea on exertion	• Palpitations
• Dyspnea on exertion	• Dyspnea on exertion	• Dizziness, syncope	• Angina	• Dyspnea
• Orthopnea	• Orthopnea	• Palpitations	• Syncope on exertion	• Orthopnea
• Paroxysmal nocturnal dyspnea	• Palpitations	• Atrial tachycardia	• Fatigue	• Paroxysmal nocturnal dyspnea
• Hemoptysis	• Atrial fibrillation	• Ventricular tachycardia	• Orthopnea	• Fatigue
• Hepatomegaly	• Neck vein distention	• Systolic click	• Paroxysmal nocturnal dyspnea	• Angina
• Neck vein distention	• Pitting edema		• Harsh, systolic crescendo-decrescendo murmur	• Sinus tachycardia
• Pitting edema	• High-pitched holosystolic murmur			• Blowing, decrescendo diastolic murmur
• Atrial fibrillation				
• Rumbling, apical diastolic murmur				

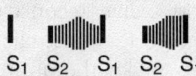
S_1 S_2 S_1 S_2 S_1

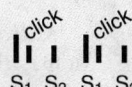
S_1 S_2S_3 S_1 S_2S_3

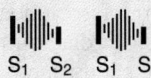
click   click
S_1 S_2 S_1 S_2

S_1 S_2 S_1 S_2

S_1 S_2 S_1 S_2 S_1

develop left ventricular failure with pulmonary or systemic congestion. Diuretics, digoxin, and oxygen are often administered to improve the symptoms of heart failure (see earlier). Nitrates are administered cautiously to clients with aortic stenosis because of the potential for syncope associated with a reduction in left ventricular volume (preload). Vasodilators such as nifedipine (Adalat, Procardia) may be used to reduce the regurgitant flow for clients with aortic or mitral stenosis.

Prophylactic antibiotic therapy is required for all clients with valve disease before any invasive procedure. Procedures for which clients require antibiotic coverage include bronchoscopy, endoscopy, sigmoidoscopy, colonoscopy, genitourinary instrumentations, surgery, and dental procedures of any type.

A major concern in valvular heart disease is maintaining cardiac output should atrial fibrillation develop. Atrial fibrillation occurs frequently in both mitral stenosis and mitral regurgitation because of distention of the atria. With mitral valvular disease, left ventricular filling is especially dependent on atrial contraction. When atrial fibrillation develops, there is no longer a single, coordinated atrial contraction. Cardiac output can decrease by 25% to 30%, and heart failure may occur. Ineffective atrial contraction may also lead to stasis of blood and thrombosis in the left atrium. The nurse monitors the client for the development of an irregularly irregular rhythm and notifies the primary care provider should it develop.

The primary care provider will usually institute therapy to restore normal sinus rhythm or, if that is unsuccessful, to slow the ventricular rate. The physician might elect to convert a client from atrial fibrillation to sinus rhythm using intravenous diltiazem (Cardiazem). The client should be on a unit where nurses are able to monitor the client's cardiac rhythm and blood pressure closely. If atrial fibrillation is rapid and the client is unresponsive to medical treatment, synchronized countershock (cardioversion) may be attempted (see Chap. 36).

Whether the client is converted to sinus rhythm or remains in an atrial fibrillation, digoxin is often prescribed to slow the ventricular rate and increase the force of contraction. If atrial fibrillation does not resolve, quinidine gluconate (Quinaglute, Quinate♣) or procainamide hydrochloride (Pronestyl hydrochloride, Procanbid) may be added to the regimen. A beta-blocking agent, such as propranolol hydrochloride (Inderal, Apo-Propranolol♣), or a calcium channel blocker, such as verapamil hydrochloride (Calan), may also be considered.

When a client has valvular heart disease and chronic atrial fibrillation, anticoagulation with sodium warfarin (Coumadin, Warfilone♣) is usually a part of the medical treatment plan to prevent thrombus formation. Thrombi may form in the atria or on defective valve segments, resulting in systemic emboli. As a result, clients may experience one or more cerebrovascular accidents (CVAs). Therefore, the nurse assesses the client's baseline neurologic status and regularly reassesses the client for neurologic changes.

Rest is often an important part of treatment. Activity may be limited because the client's cardiac output cannot meet the increased metabolic demands, and angina or heart failure can result.

➤ Surgical Management

Surgical repair or replacement of heart valves has a major effect on the prognosis of valvular heart disease. Correct timing is crucial. Repair or replacement of the valve is usually performed after symptoms of left ventricular failure have developed but before irreversible dysfunction occurs. Surgical therapy is the only definitive treatment of aortic stenosis and is recommended when angina, syncope, or dyspnea on exertion develop.

Reparative Procedures. Reparative procedures are gaining in popularity because of continuing problems with thrombi, endocarditis, and left ventricular dysfunction after valvular replacement. Reparative procedures do not result in a normal valve, but they usually "turn back the clock," resulting in a more functional valve and an improvement in cardiac output. Turbulent blood flow through the valve may persist, and degeneration of the repaired valve is possible.

Balloon Valvuloplasty. Balloon valvuloplasty, an invasive nonsurgical procedure, is possible for stenotic mitral and aortic valves. Careful selection of clients is necessary. For people with noncalcified, mobile, mitral valves, valvuloplasty may be the initial treatment of choice. Many clients selected for aortic valvuloplasty are older and are at high risk for surgical complications or have refused operative treatment. However, young adults with noncalcified congenital aortic stenosis may also benefit.

When performing mitral valvuloplasty, the physician passes a balloon catheter from the femoral vein through the atrial septum and to the mitral valve. The balloon is inflated, enlarging the mitral orifice. For aortic valvuloplasty, the physician inserts the catheter through the femoral artery and advances it to the aortic valve, where it is inflated, enlarging the orifice. Valvuloplasty usually offers immediate relief of symptoms because the balloon has dilated the orifice and improved leaflet mobility. The results are comparable with those of surgical commissurotomy for appropriately selected clients.

After the procedure, the nurse observes the client closely for bleeding from the catheter insertion site and institutes precautions for arterial puncture if appropriate. Bleeding is likely after valvuloplasty because of the large size of the catheter. The nurse also observes the client for signs of a regurgitant valve by closely monitoring the client's heart sounds, cardiac output, and heart rhythm. Because vegetations (thrombi) may have been dislodged from the valve, the nurse observes for any indication of systemic emboli (see Infective Endocarditis later in this chapter).

Direct, or Open, Commissurotomy. Direct commissurotomy is accomplished with cardiopulmonary bypass during open heart surgery. The surgeon visualizes the valve, removes thrombi from the atria, incises the fused commissures (leaflets), and debrides calcium from the leaflets, widening the orifice.

Mitral Valve Reconstruction. Mitral valve reconstruction is the reparative procedure of choice for most clients with acquired mitral insufficiency. To make the annulus (the valve ring that attaches to and supports the leaflets)

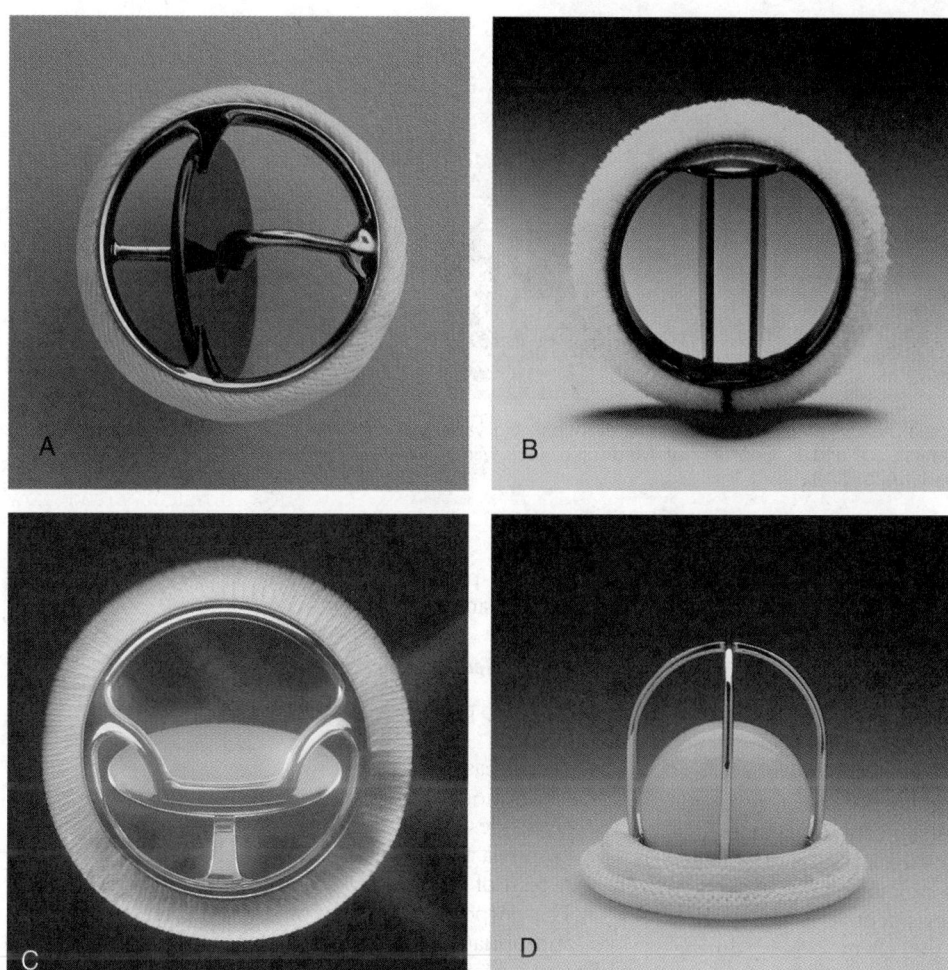

Figure 37–2. Examples of prosthetic (synthetic) heart valves. *A,* Medtronic Hall, a tilting-disk valve. *B,* St. Jude Medical mechanical heart valve. *C,* Monostrat mechanical heart valve. *D,* Starr-Edwards Silastic ball valve. (*A,* Courtesy of Medtronic, Inc., Minneapolis, MN; *B,* Courtesy of St. Jude Medical, Inc. All rights reserved. St. Jude Medical is a registered trademark of St. Jude Medical, Inc.; *C,* Courtesy of Alliance Medical Products, Irvine, CA; *D,* Courtesy of Baxter Healthcare Corporation, Edwards CVS Division, Santa Ana, CA.)

smaller, the physician may suture the leaflets to an annuloplasty ring or take tucks in the client's annulus. Leaflet repair is frequently performed at the same time. Elongated leaflets may be shortened; shortened leaflets may be repaired by lengthening the chordae that bind them in place; and perforated leaflets may be patched with synthetic grafts.

Annuloplasty and leaflet repair result in an annulus of the appropriate size and leaflets that can close completely. Thus, regurgitation is eliminated or markedly reduced.

Replacement Procedures. The development of prosthetic (synthetic) and biological (tissue) valves has improved the surgical therapy and prognosis of valvular heart disease. Prosthetic valves come in a wide variety (Fig. 37–2). Although prosthetic valves are very durable, all clients must receive oral anticoagulation for the rest of their lives because of the possibility of clot formation.

Biological valves may be xenograft (valves from other species), such as a porcine valve (from a pig) (Fig. 37–3) or a bovine valve (from a cow). Because tissue valves are associated with little risk of clot formation, long-term anticoagulation is not indicated. However, xenografts are not as durable as prosthetic valves and usually must be replaced every 7 to 10 years. A xenograft's durability is related to the age of the recipient. Calcium in the blood, present in larger quantities in younger patients, breaks down the valves. The older the patient, the longer the xenograft will last. Valves donated from human cadavers and pulmonary autographs (the client's own pulmonary valve relocated to the aortic position) are also being used for valve replacement, especially in younger clients.

The mitral valve should be replaced if the leaflets are calcified and immobile. The surgeon excises the valve during cardiopulmonary bypass surgery, and the new valve, either biological or prosthetic, is sutured into place.

An aortic valve is replaced for most symptomatic adults with aortic stenosis and aortic insufficiency. As with mitral valve replacement, the surgeon excises the aortic valve during cardiopulmonary bypass surgery and sutures the new valve into place.

Preoperative Care. Clients undergoing valve surgery have open heart surgery similar to the procedure for clients undergoing a coronary artery bypass graft (CABG) (see Chap. 40). Ideally, surgery is an elective, planned procedure. Therefore, the nurse can assist in preparing the client by instructing the client and family members or a significant other about the management of postoperative pain, incision care, and strategies to prevent respiratory complications (see Chaps. 20 and 22).

The nurse may also introduce the client and the family

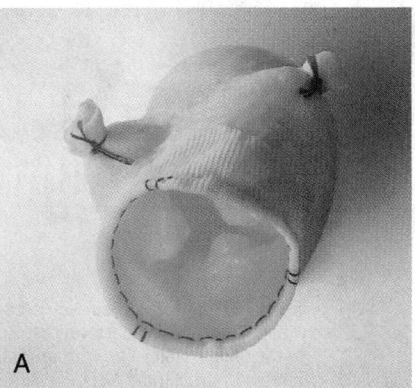 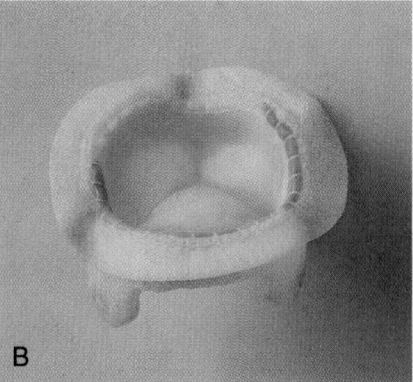 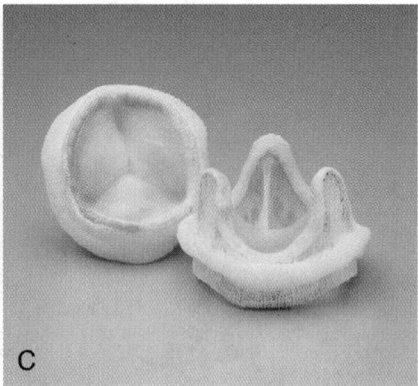

Figure 37–3. Examples of biologic (tissue) heart valves. *A,* Freestyle, a stentless pig valve with no frame. *B,* Hancock II, a stented pig valve. *C,* Carpentier-Edwards bioprosthesis. (*A* and *B,* Courtesy of Medtronic, Inc., Minneapolis, MN; *C,* Courtesy of Baxter Healthcare Corporation, Edwards CVS Division, Santa Ana, CA.)

or the significant other to the staff and the environment of the surgical critical care unit where the client will be transferred after surgery. Clients receiving oral anticoagulants stop taking these medications at least 72 hours before the procedure.

Postoperative Care. Nursing interventions for clients undergoing open heart surgery for valve disorders are similar to those for clients undergoing a CABG (see Chap. 40). However, there are a few significant differences depending in part on the type of valvular surgery. Clients with mitral stenosis often have pulmonary hypertension and stiff lungs. The nurse must be attentive to the client's respiratory status and monitor the client closely during weaning from the ventilator. Clients undergoing aortic valve replacements may be at a higher risk for postoperative hemorrhage, and the nurse is especially vigilant for indications of bleeding.

Clients with valve replacements are also more likely to have significant reductions in cardiac output postoperatively, especially those with aortic stenosis or left ventricular failure from mitral valve disease. The nurse is particularly attentive to monitoring the client's cardiac output and identifying any indications of pump failure. High filling pressures (pulmonary artery wedge pressure greater than 18 mmHg) may be required to maintain an acceptable cardiac output in the immediate postoperative period. The physician may prescribe digoxin (Lanoxin, Novodigoxin✦) for 3 to 6 months postoperatively to maintain cardiac output and to prevent atrial fibrillation. Clients who have had valve replacements with prosthetic valves require lifetime prophylactic anticoagulation therapy to prevent thrombus formation.

➤ Continuing Care

The client with valvular heart disease may be discharged home on medical therapy or postoperatively after valve repair or replacement. Because fatigue is a common problem for clients with valve disorders, the nurse helps the client and family ensure that the home environment is conducive to providing rest. Older clients with aortic stenosis may reside in long-term care.

➤ Health Teaching

The teaching plan for the client with valvular heart disease includes

- The disease process
- Medications, including diuretics, vasodilators, cardiac glycosides, antibiotics, and anticoagulants
- Prophylactic use of antibiotics
- A plan of work, activity, and rest to conserve energy
- The purpose and nature of surgical intervention, if appropriate

Because clients with defective or repaired valves are at risk for infective endocarditis, the nurse teaches them to adhere to the precautions described for the client with endocarditis. The nurse instructs clients to inform all health care providers of the valvular heart disease history; the clients are also told that they require antibiotic administration before all invasive procedures and tests. Instructions for the client are described in (Chart 37–9.)

Chart 37–9

Education Guide: Valvular Heart Disease

- Notify all of your health care providers that you have a defective heart valve.
- Remind the health care provider of your valvular problem when you have any dental work (cleaning, filling, or extraction), any examination by instrument (cystoscopy, endoscopy, or sigmoidoscopy), or any other invasive procedure (arteriogram, surgery).
- Request antibiotic prophylaxis before and after these procedures if the health care provider does not offer it.
- Clean all wounds and apply antibiotic ointment to prevent infection.
- Notify your health care provider immediately if you experience fever, petechiae (pinpoint red dots on your skin), or shortness of breath.

The nurse teaches clients taking anticoagulants how to manage their drug therapy successfully and to prevent bleeding. For example, the client should use an electric razor to avoid skin cuts. The client should report any bleeding or excessive bruising to the health care provider. (For more information on anticoagulants, see Chapter 38.)

The nurse teaches clients who have undergone valve surgery how to care for the sternal incision. The nurse instructs clients to watch for and report any fever or drainage or redness at the site. Clients can usually return to normal activity after 6 weeks but should avoid heavy physical labor with their upper extremities for 3 to 6 months to allow healing of the sternotomy incision. Clients who have had valvular surgery should also avoid any dental procedures for 6 months.

Clients with valvular heart disease may have complicated medication schedules as well as long-term antibiotic or anticoagulant therapy. These circumstances may potentially lead to noncompliance. The nurse ensures that the client is an active participant in care decisions. The nurse also provides clear, concise instructions about medication schedules.

The psychological response to valve surgery is similar to that after coronary artery bypass surgery. Clients may experience an altered self-image as a result of the changes required in lifestyle or the visible medial sternotomy incision. In addition, clients with prosthetic valves may have to adjust to a soft but audible clicking sound of the prosthetic valve. The nurse encourages clients to verbalize their feelings about the sternotomy incision and the prosthetic heart valve.

➤ Home Care Management

A home care nurse may be needed to help the client adhere to medication and activity schedules and to detect any problems, particularly with anticoagulant therapy. Clients who have undergone surgery may also require a nurse for assistance with incision care. A home care aide may assist clients with activities of daily living.

➤ Health Care Resources

The American Heart Association is a community resource that provides information to clients about valvular heart disease. A wallet-sized card can be obtained for the client that identifies him or her as needing prophylactic antibiotics. The nurse advises clients receiving anticoagulants to obtain an identification bracelet stating the name of the drug they are taking.

INFLAMMATIONS AND INFECTIONS

Inflammations and infections of the heart frequently follow systemic infections. Recovery from these infections is often prolonged, and clients are at great risk for future heart problems. Inflammation and infection may involve the endocardium (endocarditis), the pericardium (pericarditis), or the entire heart (rheumatic carditis).

Infective Endocarditis
Overview
Pathophysiology

Infective endocarditis (previously called *bacterial endocarditis*) refers to a microbial infection involving the endocardium. The client's own defective valve or a prosthetic valve is most commonly affected, but infection may also occur on apparently healthy endocardium or in septal defects. Current classification of infective endocarditis is by site of involvement, type of pathogen, and definitiveness of diagnosis.

Etiology

Infective endocarditis occurs primarily in clients who are intravenous drug abusers or who have had valve replacements or have structural cardiac defects.

In a client with a cardiac defect, blood may flow rapidly from a high-pressure area to a low-pressure zone, eroding a section of endocardium. Platelets and fibrin adhere to the denuded endocardium, forming a vegetative lesion. During bacteremia, bacteria become trapped in the low-pressure "sinkhole" and are deposited in the vegetation. Additional platelets and fibrin are deposited, causing the vegetative lesion to grow, and the endocardium and valve are destroyed. When the lesion interferes with normal alignment of the valve, valvular insufficiency may result, or, if vegetations become so large that blood flow through the valve is obstructed, the valve appears stenotic.

Possible ports of entry for infecting organisms include

- The oral cavity (especially if dental procedures have been performed)
- Skin rashes, lesions, or abscesses
- Infections (cutaneous, genitourinary, or gastrointestinal)
- Surgery or invasive procedures, including IV line placement

Incidence/Prevalence

The incidence of infective endocarditis is estimated to be 5:100,000 (Matthews, 1994). Men have a higher incidence then women. Mortality rates for infective endocarditis have remained high at 15% to 40% despite antibiotic therapy (Matthews, 1994).

Collaborative Management

 Assessment

Because mortality remains high, early detection of infective endocarditis is essential. Unfortunately, many clients, especially older adults, are misdiagnosed (Matthews, 1994). Clinical manifestations usually occur within 2 weeks of a bacteremia (Chart 37–10).

Assessment usually reveals recurrent fever. Most clients have temperatures from 37.2° to 39.4° C (99° to 103° F). However, many older adults remain afebrile. The severity

Chart 37–10

Key Features of Infective Endocarditis

- Fever associated with chills, night sweats, malaise, and fatigue
- Anorexia and weight loss
- Cardiac murmur (newly developed or change in existing)
- Development of heart failure
- Evidence of systemic embolization
- Petechiae
- Splinter hemorrhages
- Osler's nodes
- Janeway's lesions

of the symptoms may depend on the virulence of the infecting organism.

➤ Cardiovascular Manifestations

The nurse assesses the client's cardiovascular status. More than 90% of clients with infective endocarditis develop murmurs. The nurse carefully auscultates the precordium, noting and documenting any new murmurs (usually regurgitant in nature) or any changes in the intensity or quality of an old murmur. An S_3 or S_4 heart sound may also be heard.

Heart failure is the most common complication of infective endocarditis. The nurse assesses for right-sided heart failure (as evidenced by peripheral edema, weight gain, and anorexia), as well as left-sided heart failure (as evidenced by fatigue, shortness of breath, and crackles on auscultation of breath sounds).

➤ Embolic Complications

Arterial embolization is a major complication in up to 50% of clients with infective endocarditis. Fragments of vegetation break loose and travel randomly through the circulation. When the left side of the heart is involved, vegetation fragments are carried to the spleen, the kidneys, the gastrointestinal (GI) tract, the brain, and the extremities. When the right side of the heart is involved, emboli enter the pulmonary circulation.

Clients with splenic infarction describe sudden abdominal pain with radiation to the left shoulder. When performing an abdominal assessment, the nurse notes rebound tenderness on palpation. The classic pain described by the client with renal infarction is flank pain with radiation to the groin, accompanied by hematuria or pyuria.

Emboli to the central nervous system cause either transient ischemic attacks (TIAs) or a cerebrovascular accident (CVA). The client may appear confused, have reduced concentration and aphasia, or have dysphagia. Pleuritic chest pain, dyspnea, and cough are often described by the client who is experiencing pulmonary infarction related to embolization.

➤ Peripheral Manifestations

Petechiae (pinpoint red spots) occur in up to 40% of clients with endocarditis. The nurse examines the mucous membranes, the palate, the conjunctivae, and the skin above the clavicles for small red, flat lesions. The nurse also examines the distal third of the nail bed for the black longitudinal lines or small red streaks called *splinter hemorrhages* (Fig. 37–4).

Osler's nodes and Janeway's lesions are also considered classic manifestations of endocarditis, although they may occur with other conditions. The nurse inspects the pads of the fingers, hands, and toes for Osler's nodes, which are reddish tender lesions with a white center. Janeway's lesions (Fig. 37–5) are nontender hemorrhagic lesions found on the fingers, toes, nose, or earlobes. Splenomegaly and clubbing of the fingers may occur in clients who have had infective endocarditis for longer than 6 weeks.

➤ Diagnostic Assessment

A positive blood culture is of prime diagnostic and therapeutic importance. Both aerobic and anaerobic specimens are obtained for culture. Some slow-growing organisms may take 3 weeks and require a specialized medium to isolate. So, cultures should be monitored by the lab for 3 to 4 weeks. Low hemoglobin and hematocrit levels may also be found.

Echocardiography has improved the ability to accurately diagnose infective endocarditis. Transesophageal echocardiography (TEE) allows visualization of cardiac structures that are difficult to see with transthoracic echocardiography (TTE). TEE provides good resolution and is very sensitive for discovering valvular abnormalities, ena-

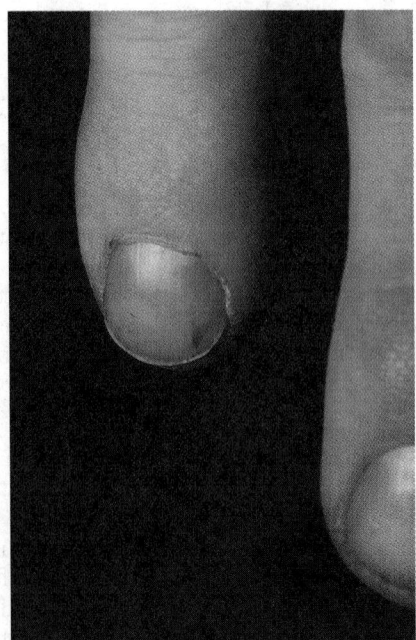

Figure 37–4. Splinter hemorrhage lesions in endocarditis. (From Callen, J. P., et al. [1993]. *Color atlas of dermatology.* Philadelphia: W. B. Saunders.)

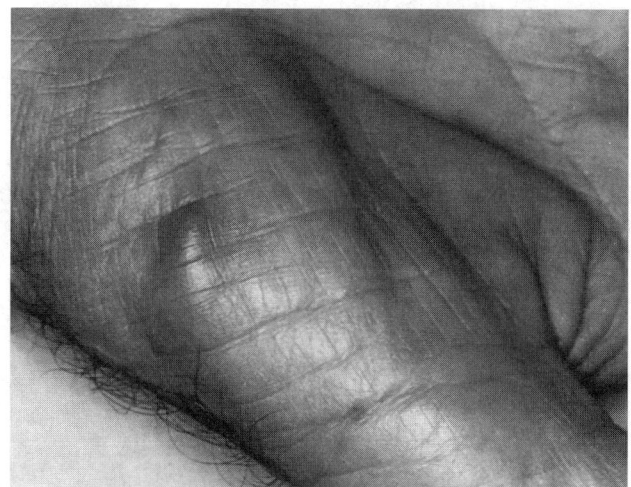

Figure 37–5. Janeway's lesions on the palm. (From Braverman, I. M. [1998]. *Skin signs of systemic disease* [3rd ed.]. Philadelphia: W. B. Saunders.)

bling the clinician to diagnose infective endocarditis more accurately (see Chap. 35).

The most reliable criteria for diagnosing endocarditis include positive blood cultures, a new regurgitant murmur, and evidence of endocardial involvement by echocardiography (Durack, 1995).

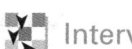 Interventions

Care of the client with endocarditis usually includes antibiotics, rest, and supportive therapy for heart failure. If these interventions are successful, then surgery is usually not required.

➤ *Nonsurgical Management*

The major component of treatment for endocarditis is drug therapy. Other interventions help to prevent the life-threatening complications.

Drug Therapy. Antibiotics are the mainstay of treatment, with the choice of antibiotics depending on the specific organism involved. Because vegetations surround and protect the bacteria, an appropriate antibiotic must be given in a sufficiently high dose to ensure a bactericidal effect. Antibiotics are most often given intravenously, with the course of treatment lasting 4 to 6 weeks. In most cases, the ideal antibiotic is one of the penicillins.

Until recently, clients with endocarditis were hospitalized for up to 6 weeks for intravenous (IV) antibiotic therapy. Now clients are hospitalized for 5 to 7 days to institute IV therapy and then are discharged for continued IV therapy at home. During hospitalization, the nurse assesses the client's response to therapy. Clients are responding to antimicrobial therapy and may be considered for home therapy when they are afebrile, have negative blood cultures, and have no signs of heart failure or embolization.

Anticoagulants are of no value in preventing emboliza-

tion from vegetations. They are avoided unless they are required to retard thrombus formation on a prosthetic valve because they may result in bleeding.

Other Interventions. Complete bed rest need not be enforced unless clients have fever or signs of heart failure. However, the nurse carefully monitors activities to allow adequate rest. The nurse explains proper oral and general body hygiene and consistently uses appropriate aseptic technique when caring for the client to protect the client from contact with potentially infective organisms. Nursing assessment for signs of heart failure (including rapid pulse, fatigue, cough, and dyspnea; new heart murmurs; and early signs of embolization) continues throughout the client's antibiotic regimen.

➤ *Surgical Management*

The cardiac surgeon may be consulted if antibiotic therapy is ineffective in sterilizing a valve, refractory heart failure develops secondary to a defective valve, large valvular vegetations are present, or multiple embolic events occur. Current surgical interventions for infective endocarditis include
- Removing the infected valve (either biological or prosthetic)
- Removing congenital shunts
- Repairing injured valves and chordae tendineae
- Draining abscesses in the heart or elsewhere

Preoperative and postoperative care of clients having surgery involving the valves is similar to that described earlier for clients undergoing a valve replacement.

 Continuing Care

Continuing care for clients with infective endocarditis is essential to resolve the problem and avoid complications. Clients and families involved in the treatment need to be motivated and have the knowledge, physical ability, and resources to administer IV antibiotics at home. The home health nurse may be contacted to complete teaching started in the acute care institution and to monitor client compliance and health status.

The home care nurse and pharmacist arrange for appropriate supplies to be available to the client at home. Supplies include the prepared antibiotic, IV tubing, alcohol wipes, IV access device, normal saline solution, and heparin or saline lock flush solution drawn up in syringes. A heparin or saline lock or central catheter is positioned at a new venous site that is easily accessible to the client or a family member.

The nurse teaches the client, family members, or a significant other how to administer the antibiotic and care for the infusion site while maintaining aseptic technique. The client or a family member demonstrates this technique before the client is discharged from the hospital. The nurse emphasizes the importance of maintaining a blood level of the antibiotic by administering the antibiotics as scheduled.

The nurse encourages the client to maintain proper hygiene, particularly oral hygiene. Clients are advised to use a soft toothbrush, to brush their teeth at least twice a day, and to rinse the mouth with water after brushing. Clients should not use irrigation devices or floss the teeth because bacteremia may result. The nurse instructs clients to wash lacerations well and apply an antibiotic ointment.

Clients must remind health care providers, including their dentists, of their endocarditis and request prophylactic antibiotic coverage for every invasive procedure, including dental care (Table 37–3). This is essential because studies have documented low compliance with prophylaxis regimens by health care providers (Guzzetta, 1992).

The nurse teaches the client self-monitoring for the manifestations of endocarditis, including the complications of heart failure and embolic phenomena. The client is instructed to monitor his or her temperature daily and record it for up to 6 weeks. Clients are also taught to report fever, chills, malaise, weight loss, increase in fatigue, or dyspnea to their primary care provider.

Pericarditis

Overview

Pericarditis is an inflammation or alteration of the pericardium, the membranous sac that encloses the heart. There are two general types of pericarditis: acute pericarditis and chronic constrictive pericarditis.

Acute pericarditis may be fibrous, serous, hemorrhagic, purulent, or neoplastic. Acute pericarditis is most commonly associated with

- Malignant neoplasms
- Idiopathic causes
- Infective organisms (bacteria, viruses, or fungi)
- Post–myocardial infarction (MI) syndrome (Dressler's syndrome)
- Postpericardiotomy syndrome
- Systemic connective tissue disease

The cause of the pericarditis determines its presentation. Acute viral pericarditis commonly follows a respiratory infection and is more common in men aged 20 to 50 years. Dressler's syndrome occurs in 5% to 15% of clients who experience an MI from 1 to 12 weeks after infarction. Postpericardotomy syndrome occurs in 10% to 40% of clients after cardiac surgery.

Chronic constrictive pericarditis occurs when chronic pericardial inflammation causes a fibrous thickening of the pericardium. It is caused by tuberculosis, radiation therapy, trauma, renal failure, or metastatic cancer. In chronic constrictive pericarditis, the pericardium becomes rigid, preventing adequate filling of the ventricles and eventually resulting in cardiac failure.

Collaborative Management

 Assessment

Assessment findings include substernal precordial pain that radiates to the left side of the neck, the shoulder, or the back. Pain is classically grating and oppressive and is aggravated by breathing (mainly on inspiration), coughing, and swallowing. The pain is worse when the client is in the supine position and may be relieved by the client's sitting up and leaning forward. The nurse asks all of the questions to evaluate chest discomfort (see Chap. 35) because it is important that the pain of pericarditis be differentiated from that of acute myocardial infarction.

The nurse may hear a pericardial friction rub with the diaphragm of the stethoscope positioned at the left lower sternal border. This is a scratchy, high-pitched sound; it is produced when the inflamed, roughened pericardial layers create friction as their surfaces rub together.

Clients with acute pericarditis may have an elevated white blood cell count and ECG changes consisting of ST-T wave elevation in all leads, with a T-wave inversion occurring after ST segments return to baseline. Clients with infectious pericarditis usually have fever. Blood specimens for culture may be obtained to assess for possible

TABLE 37–3

Antibiotic Prophylaxis* for Clients Susceptible to Infective Endocarditis		
Procedure	**Standard Regimen**	**For Clients Allergic to Penicillin**
Dental, oral, upper respiratory tract, or esophageal procedures and surgery	One of the following: Amoxicillin 2 g PO Ampicillin 2 g IM or IV	One of the following: Clindamycin (Cleocin) 600 mg PO or IV Cephalexin (Keflex) 2 g PO Azithromycin (Zithromax) 500 mg PO Clarithromycin (Biaxin) 500 mg PO Cefazolin (Ancef) 1 g IM or IV
Genitourinary tract and gastrointestinal tract surgery or instrumentation	One of the following: Ampicillin (2 g IM or IV) plus gentamicin (1.5 mg/kg—not to exceed 120 mg—IM or IV) 30 min before the procedure. Then, ampicillin 1 g IM/IV or amoxicillin 1 g PO 6 hr later. Ampicillin 2 g IM or IV Amoxicillin 2 g PO	One of the following: Vancomycin 1 g IV given over 1–2 hr plus gentamicin (1.5 mg/kg—not to exceed 120 mg—IM or IV) Vancomycin (as above) without the gentamicin

*PO doses are given 1 hr prior to the procedure; IM or IV doses are given or completed 30 min prior to the procedure.

bacterial infection. Echocardiograms may demonstrate a pleural effusion.

Clients with chronic constrictive pericarditis show signs of right-sided heart failure, elevated systemic venous pressure with jugular distention, hepatic engorgement, and dependent edema. The client usually complains of exertional fatigue and dyspnea. These clients may have thickening of the pericardium on echocardiography or computed tomography (CT) scan. ECG changes include inverted or flat T waves. Atrial fibrillation is common.

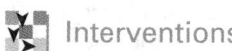 Interventions

➤ Medical Therapy

The client with acute pericarditis may be hospitalized for diagnostic evaluation, observation for complications, and symptom relief. The health care provider usually prescribes nonsteroidal anti-inflammatory drugs for the relief of pain. Clients who do not obtain pain relief within 24 to 48 hours and who do not have bacterial pericarditis may receive corticosteroid therapy. The nurse assesses for pain relief and assists the client to assume positions of comfort, usually sitting upright and leaning slightly forward. If the pain is not relieved within 24 to 48 hours, the nurse notifies the primary care provider.

The various causes of pericarditis require specific therapies. For example, bacterial pericarditis (acute) usually requires antibiotics and pericardial drainage. The usual clinical course of acute pericarditis is short term, from 2 to 6 weeks; however, episodes may recur. Chronic pericarditis caused by malignant disease may be treated with radiation or chemotherapy, while uremic pericarditis is treated by hemodialysis.

The definitive treatment for chronic constrictive pericarditis is surgical excision of the pericardium (pericardiectomy).

➤ Monitoring for Complications of Pericarditis

A significant complication of pericarditis is pericardial effusion, which occurs when the space between the parietal and visceral layers of the pericardium fills with fluid. Pericardial effusion puts the client at risk for cardiac tamponade, excessive fluid within the pericardial cavity. Tamponade restricts diastolic ventricular filling, and cardiac output drops. Findings of cardiac tamponade include
- Jugular venous distention
- Paradoxical pulse, a systolic blood pressure 10 mmHg higher or more on expiration than on inspiration (Chart 37–11)
- Decreased cardiac output
- Muffled heart sounds

➤ Management of Acute Cardiac Tamponade

Acute tamponade may occur when small volumes (20 to 50 mL) of fluid accumulate in the pericardium. The nurse reports any suspicion of this complication to the physician immediately. The physician may initially manage the decreased cardiac output with increased fluid volume administration while awaiting a chest x-ray or echocardiogram to confirm the diagnosis. Unfortunately, these tests

---

Chart 37–11

Nursing Care Highlight: Care of the Client with Pericarditis

- Assess the nature of the client's chest discomfort. (Pericardial pain is typically substernal; it is worse on inspiration and decreases when the client leans forward.)
- Auscultate for a pericardial friction rub.
- Assist the client to a position of comfort.
- Provide anti-inflammatory agents as prescribed.
- Explain that anti-inflammatory agents usually decrease the pain within 48 hr.
- Avoid the administration of aspirin and anticoagulants because these may increase the possibility of tamponade.
- Auscultate the blood pressure carefully to detect paradoxical blood pressure (pulsus paradoxus), a sign of tamponade:
  - Palpate the blood pressure and inflate the cuff above the systolic pressure.
  - Deflate the cuff gradually, and note when sounds are first audible on expiration.
  - Identify when sounds are also audible on inspiration.
  - Subtract the inspiratory pressure from the expiratory pressure to determine the amount of pulsus paradoxus (>10 mmHg is an indication of tamponade).
- Inspect for other indications of tamponade, including jugular venous distention with clear lungs, muffled heart sounds, and decreased cardiac output.
- Notify the physician if tamponade is suspected.

---

are not always helpful because the fluid volume around the heart may be too small to visualize. Hemodynamic monitoring in a specialized critical care unit usually demonstrates compression of the heart, with all pressures (right atrial, pulmonary artery, and wedge) being similar and elevated (plateau pressures).

The physician may elect to perform a pericardiocentesis to relieve the pressure on the heart. Under echocardiographic or fluoroscopic and hemodynamic monitoring, the cardiologist inserts an 8-inch (20.3-cm) long 16- or 18-gauge pericardial needle into the pericardial space. The physician and the nurse monitor the needle's position, recognizing that ST- and T-wave changes indicate myocardial injury, and the needle must be withdrawn slightly. When the needle is properly positioned, a catheter is inserted, and all available pericardial fluid is withdrawn. The nurse monitors the pulmonary artery, wedge, and right atrial pressures during the procedure. The pressures should return to normal as the fluid compressing the heart is removed.

After the pericardiocentesis, the nurse closely monitors the client for the recurrence of tamponade. Often, pericardiocentesis alone does not resolve acute tamponade. The nurse should be prepared to provide adequate fluid volumes to increase cardiac output and to prepare the client for emergency sternotomy if tamponade recurs.

If the client experiences a recurrence of tamponade or recurrent effusions or adhesions from chronic pericarditis, a portion or all of the pericardium may need to be removed to allow adequate ventricular filling and contraction. The surgeon may perform a pericardial window, the removal of a portion of the pericardium permitting the excessive pericardial fluid to drain into the pleural space. In more severe cases, pericardiectomy, removal of the toughened encasing pericardium, may be necessary.

Rheumatic Carditis

Overview

Rheumatic carditis occurs in about 40% of clients with rheumatic fever and affects more than 1 million Americans. It is a sensitivity response that develops after an upper respiratory tract infection with group A beta-hemolytic streptococci. The precise mechanism by which the infection causes inflammatory lesions in the heart is not established. However, inflammation is evident in all layers of the heart. The inflammation results in impaired contractile function of the myocardium, thickening of the pericardium, and valvular damage.

Rheumatic myocarditis is characterized by the formation of Aschoff's bodies, small nodules in the myocardium that are replaced by scar tissue. A diffuse cellular infiltrate also develops and appears to be responsible for the heart failure. The pericardium becomes thickened and covered with exudate, and a serosanguineous pleural effusion may develop. However, the most serious damage occurs to the endocardium, with inflammation of the valve leaflets developing. Hemorrhagic and fibrous lesions form along the inflamed surfaces of the valves, resulting in stenosis or regurgitation primarily of the mitral and aortic valves.

Rheumatic fever may be a complication of 3% of group A beta-hemolytic throat infections. Although the primary attacks occur most often in childhood, rheumatic fever may occur in adulthood. The incidence of rheumatic carditis had been decreasing consistently until the mid-1980s. At that time, a resurgence of rheumatic fever began in both the United States and Europe.

Collaborative Management

Rheumatic carditis is one of the major indicators of rheumatic fever. Common clinical manifestations are
- Tachycardia
- Cardiomegaly
- Development of a new murmur or a change in an existing murmur
- A pericardial friction rub
- Precordial pain
- Changes in the ECG (prolonged PR interval)
- Indications of heart failure
- Evidence of an existing streptococcal infection

Primary prevention is extremely important. The nurse teaches all clients to consult their health care providers and receive appropriate antibiotic therapy if they develop the following indications of streptococcal pharyngitis: moderate to high fever, abrupt onset of a sore throat, a reddened throat with exudate, and enlarged tender lymph nodes. Penicillin is the antibiotic of choice for treatment. Erythromycin (ERYC, Erythromid✦) is the alternative for penicillin-sensitive clients.

The signs of rheumatic carditis must be recognized

promptly, and antibiotic therapy must be instituted immediately for secondary prevention. The client is urged to continue the antibiotic administration for the full 10 days to prevent reinfection. The nurse suggests ways to manage the fever, such as maintaining hydration and administering antipyretics. The nurse encourages the client to obtain adequate rest.

The nurse emphasizes tertiary prevention in client education, explaining that a recurrence of rheumatic carditis is probable with reinfection by a streptococcal organism. Thus, antibiotic therapy is essential for streptococcal infection. The nurse also informs the client that antibiotic prophylaxis is necessary for the rest of the client's life to prevent infective endocarditis (see earlier).

Cardiomyopathy

Overview

Cardiomyopathy is a subacute or chronic disorder of cardiac muscle. It is not common, occurring in only 10 to 20 per 100,000 population. The cause is usually unknown.

Treatment is usually palliative, not curative; approximately 50% of clients die within 2 years of symptom onset. Clients have to deal with a shortened life span along with numerous changes in lifestyle.

Cardiomyopathies are classified into three categories on the basis of abnormalities in structure and function: dilated cardiomyopathy, hypertrophic cardiomyopathy, and restrictive cardiomyopathy (Table 37–4).

Dilated Cardiomyopathy

In 87% of cardiomyopathy, dilated cardiomyopathy (DCM) is the structural abnormality. In DCM, there is extensive damage to the myofibrils and interference with myocardial metabolism. There is normal ventricular wall thickness but dilation of both ventricles and impairment of systolic function. Decreased cardiac output from the inadequate pumping of the heart causes the client to experience dyspnea on exertion, decreased exercise capacity, fatigue, and palpitations. DCM is twice as common in men as in women and occurs most often in middle age.

Hypertrophic Cardiomyopathy

The cardinal features of hypertrophic cardiomyopathy (HCM), are asymmetric ventricular hypertrophy of the left ventricle and disarray of the myocardial fibers. The left ventricular hypertrophy leads to a hypercontractile left ventricle with rigid ventricular walls. Obstruction in the left ventricular outflow tract is seen in 75% to 80% of clients with HCM. The abnormal stiffness of the ventricle in HCM results in diastolic filling abnormalities. In approximately 50% of clients, HCM is transmitted as a single-gene autosomal dominant trait.

Restrictive Cardiomyopathy

Restrictive cardiomyopathy, the rarest of the three cardiomyopathies, results in restriction of filling of the ventricles. It is caused by endocardial and/or myocardial disease

TABLE 37–4

Pathophysiology, Signs and Symptoms, and Treatment of Cardiomyopathies

	Hypertrophic Cardiomyopathy		
Dilated Cardiomyopathy	**Nonobstructed**	**Obstructed**	**Restrictive Cardiomyopathy**
Pathophysiology			
Fibrosis of myocardium and endocardium Dilated chambers Mural wall thrombi prevalent	Hypertrophy of all walls Hypertrophied septum Relatively small chamber size	Same as for nonobstructed except for obstruction of left ventricular outflow tract associated with the hypertrophied septum and mitral valve incompetence	Mimics constrictive pericarditis Fibrosed walls cannot expand or contract Chambers narrowed; emboli common

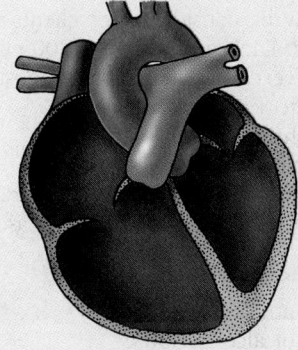 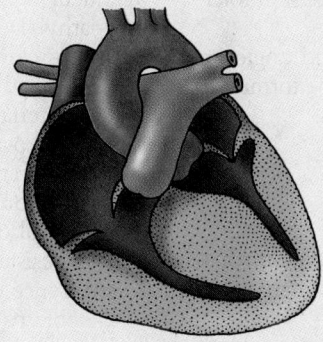 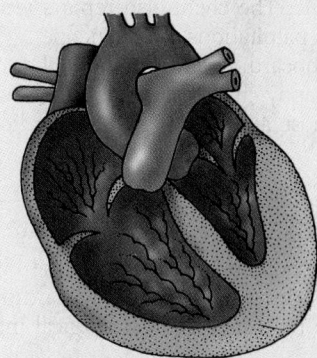

Signs and Symptoms			
Fatigue and weakness Heart failure (left side) Dysrhythmias or heart block Systemic or pulmonary emboli S_3 and S_4 gallops Moderate to severe cardiomegaly	Dyspnea Angina Fatigue, syncope, palpitations Mild cardiomegaly S_4 gallop Ventricular dysrhythmias Sudden death common Heart failure	Same as for nonobstructed except with mitral regurgitation murmur Atrial fibrillation	Dyspnea and fatigue Heart failure (right-sided) Mild to moderate cardiomegaly S_3 and S_4 gallops Heart block Emboli
Treatment			

Symptomatic treatment of heart failure
Vasodilators
Control of dysrhythmias
Surgery: heart transplant
	For both:
	  Symptomatic treatment
	  Beta-blockers
	  Conversion of atrial fibrillation
	  Surgery: ventriculomyotomy or muscle resection with mitral valve replacement
	  Digitalis, nitrates, and other vasodilators **contraindicated** with the obstructed form
			Supportive treatment of symptoms
			Treatment of hypertension
			Conversion from dysrhythmias
			Exercise restrictions
			Emergency treatment of acute pulmonary edema

Data from Wynne, J., & Braunwald, E. (1992). The cardiomyopathies and myocarditis. In E. Braunwald (Ed.), *Heart disease: A textbook of cardiovascular medicine* (3rd ed.). Philadelphia: W. B. Saunders.

and produces a clinical picture similar to that of constrictive pericarditis.

Collaborative Management

 Assessment

Findings in cardiomyopathy depend on the structural and functional abnormalities. Left ventricular or biventricular failure is characteristic of *dilated* cardiomyopathy (DCM). Some clients with DCM are asymptomatic for months to years and have left ventricular dilation identified on x-ray. Other clients experience sudden, pronounced symptoms of left ventricular failure such as progressive dyspnea on exertion, orthopnea, palpitations, and activity intolerance. Right-sided heart failure develops late in the disease and is associated with a poor prognosis. Atrial fibrillation occurs in 25% of clients and is associated with embolism.

The clinical picture of *hypertrophic* cardiomyopathy

(HCM) results from the hypertrophied septum, which in 80% of cases causes a mechanical obstruction and thereby reduces stroke volume and cardiac output. Most clients are asymptomatic until late adolescence or early adulthood. The primary symptoms of HCM are exertional dyspnea (90% of clients), angina (75% of clients), and syncope. The chest pain is atypical in that it usually occurs at rest, is prolonged, has no relation to exertion, and is not relieved by the administration of nitrates. A high incidence of ventricular dysrhythmias is associated with HCM. Sudden death occurs and may be the first manifestation of the disease.

The earliest clinical finding in *restrictive* cardiomyopathy is exertional dyspnea. Cardiac output cannot increase during periods of exertion because of the fixed ventricular volume. The client also reports weakness, exercise intolerance, palpitations, and syncope.

Echocardiography, radionuclide imaging, and angiocardiography during cardiac catheterization are performed to diagnose and to differentiate cardiomyopathies.

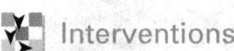 Interventions

The treatment of choice for the client with cardiomyopathy varies with the type of cardiomyopathy and may include both medical and surgical interventions.

➤ *Nonsurgical Management*

The care of clients with dilated or restrictive cardiomyopathy is initially the same as for clients with heart failure. Drug therapy includes the use of diuretics, vasodilating agents, and cardiac glycosides to increase cardiac output. Because clients are at risk for sudden death, the nurse urges them to report any palpitations, dizziness, or fainting, which might indicate a dysrhythmia. Antidysrhythmic drugs or implantable cardiac defibrillators may be used to control life-threatening dysrhythmias. Beta-blockers (e.g., metoprolol) are used experimentally for clients with excessive sympathetic stimulation and resting tachycardia. If cardiomyopathy has developed in response to a toxin, clients are instructed to avoid further exposure. The nurse teaches all clients with cardiomyopathy to abstain from alcohol ingestion because of its cardiac depressant effects.

Management of obstructive hypertrophic cardiomyopathy (HCM) includes administration of negative inotropic agents such as beta-adrenergic blocking agents and calcium antagonists. They decrease the outflow obstruction that accompanies exercise and decrease heart rate, resulting in less angina, dyspnea, and syncope. Vasodilators and cardiac glycosides are contraindicated in clients with obstructive HCM because vasodilating and positive inotropic effects may augment the obstruction.

➤ *Surgical Management*

The type of surgery performed depends on the type of cardiomyopathy.

Excision of Hypertrophied Septum. When clients with obstructive HCM do not respond to medical therapy, surgery may be considered. The most commonly used surgical treatment (ventriculomyomectomy) includes ex-

cising a portion of the hypertrophied ventricular septum resulting in a widened outflow tract. Surgery results in long-term improvement in exercise tolerance in most clients with HCM.

Cardiomyoplasty. Cardiomyoplasty is used for some clients with DCM who cannot undergo cardiac transplantation and are asymptomatic at rest. The latissimus dorsum muscle is dissected free of its distal insertion and wrapped around the heart. For the next 2 months, the muscle is stimulated with increasing frequency until it can contract in synchrony with each heartbeat. Six months after surgery, the client should begin to feel the effects of an enhanced cardiac output.

Heart Transplantation. Heart transplantation is the treatment of choice for clients with severe dilated cardiomyopathy (DCM) and may be considered for clients with restrictive cardiomyopathy. Each year, about 2,300 clients in the United States receive cardiac transplants, most for DCM. Criteria for candidate selection include
- Life expectancy less than 1 year
- Age generally less than 65 years
- New York Heart Association (NYHA) class III or IV
- Normal or only slightly increased pulmonary vascular resistance
- Absence of active infection
- Stable psychosocial status
- No evidence of drug or alcohol abuse

The surgeon transplants a heart from a donor with a comparable body weight and ABO compatibility into a recipient less than 6 hours after procurement. In the most common procedure (*orthotopic transplantation*), the surgeon removes the diseased heart, leaving the posterior walls of the client's atria. The remnant atria serve as the anchor for the donor heart; anastomoses are made between the recipient and donor atria, aorta, and pulmonary arteries (Fig. 37–6). Because the remaining remnant of the recipient's atria contains the sinoatrial node, two unrelated P waves are visible on ECG.

The postoperative care of the heart transplant recipient is similar to that of the conventional cardiac surgery client (UNOS, 1996). However, the nurse must be especially vigilant to identify occult bleeding into the pericardial sac with the potential for tamponade. The recipient's pericardium has usually stretched considerably to accommodate the diseased, hypertrophied heart. This predisposes the client to concealed postoperative bleeding (UNOS, 1996).

The transplanted heart is denervated, unresponsive to vagal stimulation. The client's heart rate approximates 100 beats per minute, responding slowly with increases in heart rate, contractility, and cardiac output to exercise, stress, or position change. In the early postoperative phase, the nurse may titrate isoproterenol (Isuprel) to support the heart rate and maintain cardiac output. Atropine, digitalis, and carotid sinus pressure are not used because they do not have their usual effects on the heart because of denervation. Denervation of the heart may cause pronounced orthostatic hypotension in the immediate postoperative phase, and the nurse cautions the client to change position slowly.

To suppress natural defense mechanisms and prevent transplant rejection, clients require immunosuppressant

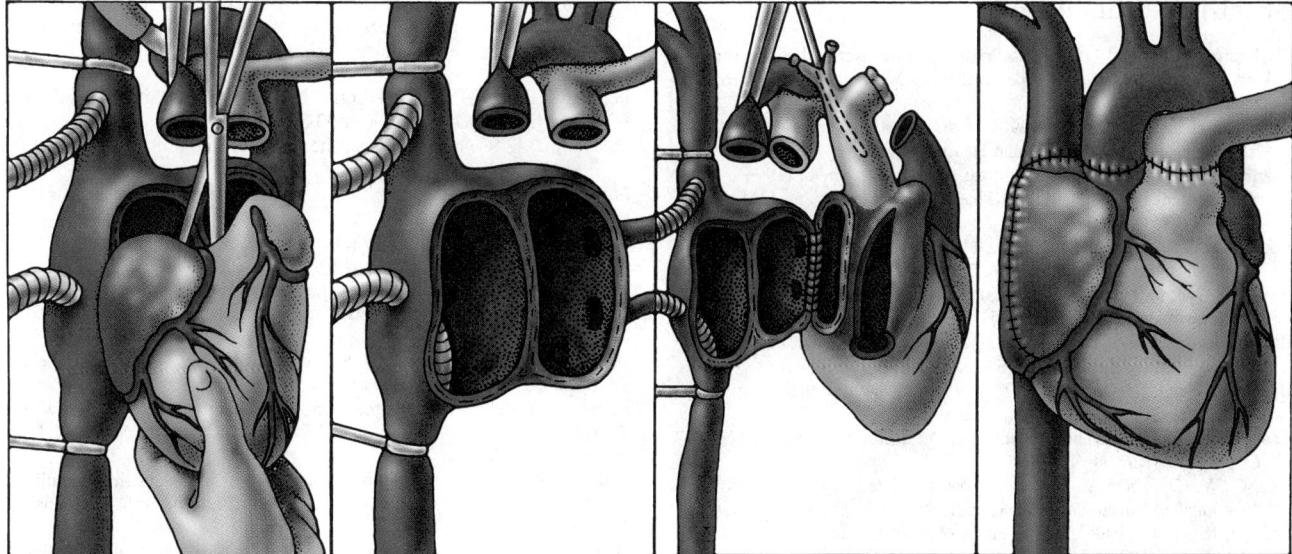

1. After the recipient is placed on cardiopulmonary bypass, the heart is removed.

2. The posterior walls of the recipient's left and right atria are left intact.

3. The left atrium of the donor heart is anastomosed to the recipient's residual posterior atrial walls, and the other atrial walls, the atrial septum, and the great vessels are joined.

POSTOPERATIVE RESULT

Figure 37–6. Heart transplantation.

therapy for the rest of their lives. Most commonly, the physician prescribes therapy with cyclosporine (Sandimmune) and azathioprine (Imuran). Nurses must be vigilant about handwashng and aseptic technique because clients are immunosuppressed and infection is the major cause of death, usually developing in the immediate post-transplant period or during treatment for acute rejection.

Most clients experience their initial episode of acute rejection of the transplanted heart in the first 3 months after transplantation. Symptoms of rejection of the heart are nonspecific, occurring late in the rejection process. They include cardiac dysrhythmias (especially atrial dysrhythmias), hypotension, weakness, fatigue, and dizziness. To detect rejection, the surgeon performs right endomyocardial biopsies at regularly scheduled intervals and whenever symptoms occur.

Approximately 75% of clients survive 3 years after transplantation; most return to NYHA class I or II status (UNOS, 1996). Five years after transplantation, many of the surviving clients (20% to 40%) have evidence of coronary artery disease (CAD) presenting as diffuse plaque in the arteries of the donor heart. Because the heart is denervated, clients do not usually experience angina and regularly scheduled exercise tolerance tests and angiography are required to identify CAD.

To delay the development of CAD, clients are encouraged to follow a prudent lifestyle similar to the client with CAD (see Chap. 40). The physician may prescribe a calcium channel blocker such as diltiazem (Cardizem) to decrease the rate of coronary artery narrowing. The nurse stresses the importance of compliance with dietary modifications and medication regimens. The client is encour-

aged to participate in a regular exercise program but cautioned to allow at least 10 minutes of warm up and cool down for the denervated heart to adjust to changes in activity level.

🔹 CASE STUDY for the Client with Heart Failure

■ An 85-year-old woman is one of your nursing home residents. She has a long history of heart failure, myocardial infarction, pulmonary emphysema, hypertension, and degenerative joint disease. Her medications include Lasix 20 mg qd, Vasotec 5 mg qd, digoxin 0.125 mg qd, KCl 40 mEq qd, and Motrin 200 mg qd.

Today the resident complains that she "just doesn't feel right." The nursing assistant reports that her pulse is weak and irregular at 116 bpm, and her skin feels cooler than usual. You go to her room for further assessment.

QUESTIONS:

1. When taking a history from this client, what important questions would you ask?
2. What physical assessments techniques would you perform?
3. During the assessment, you find that she is dyspneic at rest, has a respiratory rate of 32, a blood pressure of 180/95, is very anxious, and has crackles in the bases of her lungs. What should you do first?

SELECTED BIBLIOGRAPHY

Abelmann, W. H. (Ed.). (1995). *Atlas of heart diseases: Volume II. Cardiomyopathies, myocarditis, and pericardial disease.* Philadelphia: Current Medicine.

American Heart Association. (1996). *Heart and stroke facts: 1996 statistical supplement.* Dallas: American Heart Association.

Baker, D. W., Konstam, M. A., Bottorff, M., & Bertram, B. (1994). Management of heart failure: I. Pharmacologic treatment. *JAMA, 272*(17), 1361–1365.

Booker, M. F., & Ignatavicius, D. D. (1996). *Infusion therapy: Techniques and medications.* Philadelphia: W. B. Saunders.

Bove, L. A., et al. (1995). Nursing care of patients undergoing dynamic cardiomyoplasty. *Critical Care Nurse, 15*(3), 96–104.

Braunwald, E. (1997). *Heart disease: A textbook of cardiovascular medicine* (5th ed.). Philadelphia: W. B. Saunders.

Byers, J. F., & Goshorn, J. (1995). How to manage diuretic therapy. *AJN, 95*(2), 38–43.

Cash, A. (1996). Heart failure from diastolic dysfunction. *Dimensions of Critical Care Nursing, 15*(4), 171–177.

Dec, G. W., & Fuster, V. (1994). Idiopathic dilated cardiomyopathy. *New England Journal of Medicine, 331*(23), 1564–1573.

Dracup, K., et. al. (1994). Management of heart failure: II. Counseling, education and lifestyle modifications. *JAMA, 272*(18), 1442–1445.

Dracup, K., Dunbar, S., & Baker, D. W. (1995). Rethinking heart failure. *AJN, 95*(7), 23–27.

Durack, D. T. (1995) Prevention of infective endocarditis. *New England Journal of Medicine, 332*(1), 38–44.

Fowler, N. (1995). Pericardial disease. In W. H. Abelmann (Ed.), *Atlas of heart disease: Volume II. Cardiomyopathies, myocarditis, and pericardial disease* (pp. 13.1–13.15). St. Louis: C. V. Mosby.

Funk, M., & Krumholtz, H. M. (1996). Epidemiologic and economic impact of advanced heart failure. *Journal of Cardiovascular Nursing, 10*(2), 11–28.

*Guzzetta, C. (1992). Infective endocarditis. In B. Dossey (Ed.), *Critical care nursing: Body-mind-spirit* (3rd ed., p. 523). Philadelphia: J. B. Lippincott.

Hawthorne, M. H., & Hixon, M. E. (1994). Functional status, quality of life and mood disturbance in patients with heart failure. *Progress in Cardiovascular Nursing, 9*(1), 22–32.

Hixon, M. E. (1994). Aging and heart failure. *Progress in Cardiovascular Nursing, 9*(1), 4–12.

Jaarsma, T., Dracup, K., Walden, J., et al. (1996). Sexual function in patients with advanced heart failure. *Heart and Lung, 25*(4), 262–270.

Jensen, G. A., & Miller, D. S. (1995). The heart of aging: Special challenges of cardiac ischemic disease and failure in the elderly. *AACN Clinical Issues, 6*(3), 471–481.

Kayser, S. R. (1994). Management of chronic congestive heart failure: Part II—Selection of treatment. *Progress in Cardiovascular Nursing, 9*(2), 30–37.

Konick-McMahon, J. (1997). Discharged with dobutamine. *RN, 60*(4), 24–28.

Konstam, M., Dracup, K., Baker, D., et al. (1994). *Heart failure: Evaluation and treatment of patients with left ventricular systolic dysfunction.* Clinical practice guideline No. 11. Rockville, MD: U.S. Department of Health and Human Services, Public Health Service, Agency for Health Care Policy and Research. AHCPR Pub. No. 94-0612.

Korzeniowski, O., & Kaye, D. (1992). Infective endocarditis. In E. Braunwald (Ed.), *Heart disease: A textbook of cardiovascular medicine* (4th ed., pp. 1078–1105). Philadelphia: W. B. Saunders.

Martens, K. H., & Mellor, S. D. (1997). A study of the relationship between home care services and hospital readmission of patients with congestive heart failure. *Home Healthcare Nurse, 15*(2), 123–129.

Matthews, D. (1994). The prevention and diagnosis of infective endocarditis. *Nurse Practitioner, 19*(8), 53–59.

McGrath, D. (1997). Clinical snapshot: Mitral valve prolapse. *AJN, 97*(5), 40–41.

Miner, P. D. (1994). Infective endocarditis. *Nursing Clinics of North America, 29*(2), 269–283.

Moser, D. K. (1996). Maximizing therapy in the advanced heart failure patient. *Journal of Cardiovascular Nursing, 10*(2), 29–46.

Newkirk, T., & Leeper, B. (1996). Congestive heart failure: Mapping the way to quality outcomes. *AJN: Critical Care Issues Supplement, 96*(5), 25–28.

Pratt, N. G. (1995). Pathophysiology of heart failure: Neuroendocrine response. *Critical Care Nursing Quarterly, 18*(1), 22–31.

Recker, D. (1994). Patient perception of preoperative cardiac surgical teaching—Done pre- and postadmission. *Critical Care Nurse, 14*(1), 52–58.

Redfield, M. (1996). Evaluation of congestive heart failure. In E. Guiliani (Ed.), *Mayo Clinic practice of cardiology* (3rd ed., p. 569). St. Louis: C. V. Mosby.

Schwabauer, N. J. (1996). Retarding progression of heart failure: Nursing actions. *Dimensions of Critical Care Nursing, 15*(6), 307–317.

Shine, L., & Howland-Gradman, J. (1996). Aortic stenosis in elderly: Valvuolplasty versus surgery. *AJN: Critical Care Issues Supplement.* May, pp. 7–11.

Sullivan, M. J. (1994). New trends in cardiac rehabilitation in patients with chronic heart failure. *Progress in Cardiovascular Nursing, 9*(1), 13–21.

Swearubgen, P. L., & Keen, J. H. (Eds.). (1995). *Manual of critical care* (3rd ed.). St. Louis: Mosby–Year Book.

UNOS. (1996). *Donation and transplantation: Nursing curriculum.* UNOS.

U.S. Department of Health and Human Services, Agency for Health Care Policy and Research. (1994). *Heart failure: Evaluation and care of patients with left-ventricular systolic dysfunction.* Rockville, MD: U.S. Department of Health and Human Services.

SUGGESTED READINGS

Cash, A. (1996). Heart failure from diastolic dysfunction. *Dimensions of Critical Care Nursing. 15*(4), 171–177.

This article presents a detailed explanation of the pathophysiology of diastolic heart failure. It describes tests to differentiate diastolic from systolic heart failure and describes possible management strategies for diastolic heart failure.

Konick-McMahon, J. (1997). Discharged with dobutamine. *RN, 60*(4), 24–28.

This article describes clients who might benefit from home dobutamine therapy for heart failure, and discusses the cost of therapy and insurance criteria for coverage. Finally, it describes education essential for the client and caregiver for the home dobutamine therapy to be effective.

Schwabauer, N. J. (1996). Retarding progression of heart failure: Nursing actions. *Dimensions of Critical Care Nursing. 15*(6), 307–317.

This article describes tests that evaluate myocardial performance, monitor neurohormonal activity, and assess functional status of the patient with heart failure. Nursing actions to enhance myocardial performance and functional status are described.

Chapter 38

INTERVENTIONS FOR CLIENTS WITH VASCULAR PROBLEMS

CHAPTER
HIGHLIGHTS

Disorders of the vascular (blood vessel) system cause many problems and may lead to complete shutdown of all body organs or eventually death. Each year, vascular disorders result in disability or death, and the financial impact is overwhelming.

Although vascular disease can affect any portion of the human body, such as the heart, brain, and kidneys, the peripheral vascular system and its associated diseases are described here.

Arteriosclerosis and Atherosclerosis

Overview

Arteriosclerosis is a thickening, or hardening, of the arterial wall. Atherosclerosis, a type of arteriosclerosis, involves the formation of plaque within the arterial wall. Atherosclerosis is the most common cause of arterial obstruction. The process of atherosclerosis can lead to cardiovascular diseases, such as coronary artery disease (CAD), cerebrovascular disease, and peripheral vascular disease (PVD). Cardiovascular disease is the primary cause of death in the United States. Over 1 million people die of heart and blood vessel disease each year (American Heart Association, 1995).

Pathophysiology

The exact pathophysiology of atherosclerosis is not known, but it is thought to occur in the following way (Fig. 38–1). A fatty streak appears on the intimal surface (inner lining) of the artery. At this stage, the fatty streak may appear flattened or elevated, but it generally does not affect the integrity of the arterial wall.

Next, a fibrous plaque develops. This plaque is described as a white, glistening, fibrous elevation that covers a lipid core. At this stage, the plaque is elevated enough to partially or completely occlude the blood flow of an artery.

In the final stage, the fibrous lesions become calcified, hemorrhagic, ulcerated, or thrombosed. The rate of progression of this process may be influenced by genetic factors; certain chronic diseases, such as diabetes mellitus; and lifestyle habits, including smoking, eating habits, and level of exercise.

Etiology

Theories

The exact etiology of atherosclerosis is unknown, but several theories attempt to explain its cause. It is believed

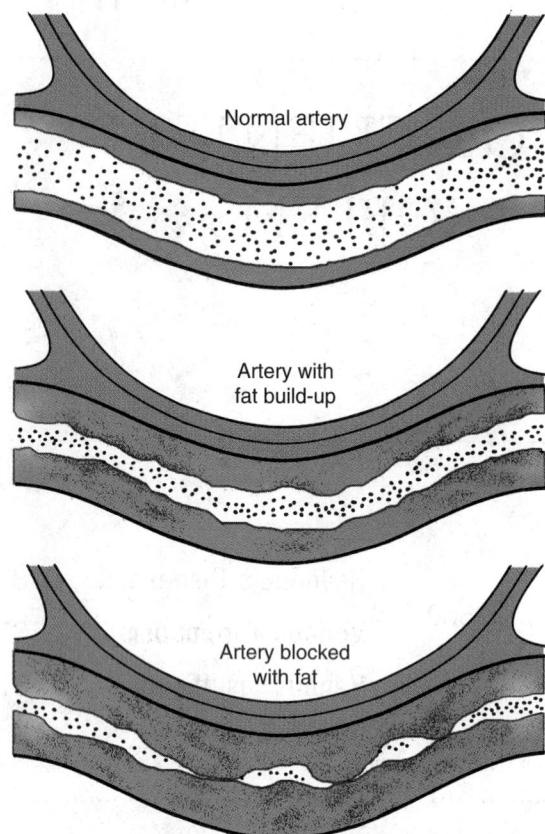

Figure 38–1. Pathophysiology of atherosclerosis.

that an injury to the intimal layer of the artery may initiate the development of atherosclerosis. One popular theory (*platelet aggregation*) is that, after the intimal injury has occurred, platelets form a cluster at the arterial wall and produce a peptide that stimulates the proliferation of the smooth muscle cells of the intima. Eventually, this proliferation can narrow the artery enough to compromise the flow of blood or completely occlude arterial blood flow.

Another theory, the *lipid hypothesis,* assumes that, after an intimal injury, a group of blood lipids (fats) accumulate. Again, this accumulation can partially or completely occlude arterial blood flow. The principal lipids involved are cholesterol and triglyceride.

Many theorists believe that a combination of these two events is the most appropriate view of the atherosclerotic process and that this can occur in any arterial wall of the body. Usually, the disease affects the larger arteries, such as the coronary arterial beds, the major branches of the aorta, the visceral branches of the aorta, the terminal abdominal aorta, the carotid and vertebral arteries, or any combination of these.

Factors Causing Arterial Injury

Intimal injury of the major arteries of the body can be attributed to many factors. Hypertension can cause a mechanical injury, whereas elevated levels of low-density lipoproteins (LDLs) and decreased levels of high-density lip-

oproteins (HDLs) can cause chemical injuries to the intimal wall. Chemical injury can also be caused by elevated levels of toxins in the bloodstream, which may occur with renal failure, or by circulating carbon monoxide in the bloodstream from cigarette smoking. The intimal wall can be weakened by the natural process of aging or by physiologic disorders, such as diabetes.

Genetic predisposition and diabetes have a fairly direct effect on the development of atherosclerosis. Some families demonstrate inherited hyperlipidemia, an elevation in levels of blood lipids. In these people, the liver makes excessive cholesterol, which accounts for the development of atherosclerosis. In some people with hereditary atherosclerosis, however, the blood cholesterol level is normal. The reason for the development and progression of plaque in these people is not understood.

People with severe diabetes mellitus frequently have premature and severe atherosclerosis, often involving the microvasculature. This occurs because diabetes promotes an increase in LDL in plasma. In addition, intimal arterial damage may result from the effect of hyperglycemia.

Factors indirectly related to atherosclerosis include obesity, a sedentary lifestyle, and stress. Clients who are obese are at greater risk, most often because of concomitant elevations in cholesterol levels. Long-term physical activity is important in maintaining ideal body weight; it is also thought to help in maintaining optimal blood pressure and cholesterol levels and improved glucose tolerance. The effect of stress may be due to its effect on the sympathetic and parasympathetic release of catecholamines and an acute rise in blood pressure.

Incidence/Prevalence

It is not known exactly how many people have atherosclerosis, but small plaques are almost always present in the arteries of young adults. The incidence can be better quantified by assessing diseases that result from this process.

WOMEN'S HEALTH CONSIDERATIONS

 Although the process of atherosclerosis does not appear to differ between men and women, coronary artery disease (CAD) is much less common in premenopausal women than in age-matched men because of the lipid-lowering effect of estrogen. Postmenopausal women have similar rates of CAD as men in the same age group. People in the United States have a higher incidence of CAD related to atherosclerosis than in other industrialized nations (American Heart Association, 1995).

Collaborative Management

◆ Assessment

➤ *Vital Signs*

Because of the high incidence of hypertension in clients with atherosclerosis, the nurse assesses the blood pressure in both arms. The heart is also thoroughly assessed because concomitant cardiac disease is often present.

The nurse palpates pulses at all of the major sites on

the body and notes any differences. Carotid arteries are palpated separately because of the risk of inadequate cerebral perfusion. The nurse also palpates for temperature differences in the lower extremities and checks capillary filling. Prolonged capillary filling (>3 seconds in young to middle-aged adults; >5 seconds in older adults) generally indicates poor circulation. An extremity with significant atherosclerotic disease may be cool or cold, with a diminished or absent pulse.

> ➤ *Assessment for Bruits*

After palpating the pulses, the nurse auscultates each large artery from the carotid to the dorsalis pedis with a stethoscope or a Doppler probe. Many clients with vascular disease have a bruit in the larger arteries. A bruit is described as a turbulent, swishing sound, which can be soft or loud in pitch. The mere existence of a bruit is considered abnormal, but the role it plays in indicating the severity of vascular disease is not understood. The nurse should document the location of bruits. They often occur in the carotid, aortic, femoral, and popliteal arteries and usually indicate some degree of narrowing of the arterial wall. The rate and intensity of the pulse in each artery during auscultation is also noted. A decrease in intensity and audibility or a complete loss of a pulse may indicate an arterial occlusion. The nurse records at which point the pulse intensity changes and reports these findings immediately to the health care provider.

> ➤ *Laboratory Assessment*

Serum cholesterol levels are often elevated in clients with atherosclerosis. It is recommended that clients keep their cholesterol levels below 200 mg/dL. The National Cholesterol Education Program has recommended screening guidelines based on three classifications of cholesterol levels (Table 38–1).

Elevated cholesterol levels must be validated by low-density lipoprotein (LDL) and high-density lipoprotein (HDL) determinations. Elevated LDL levels indicate that a person is at an increased risk for atherosclerosis. Low or normal levels of HDL also indicate an increased risk. A desirable LDL cholesterol level is one below 130 mg/dL, whereas a desirable HDL cholesterol level is 35 mg/dL or above. In some people, particularly women, an elevated cholesterol level may be due to an elevated HDL level, which is not considered a risk.

Triglyceride levels may also be elevated with atherosclerosis. A level of 200 mg/dL or above indicates hypertriglyceridemia. Elevated triglyceride levels may not cause atherosclerosis, but an elevated triglyceride level is often associated with the condition.

 Interventions

Atherosclerosis progresses for years before clinical manifestations are evident. Clients with or at risk for atherosclerosis can often be identified by cholesterol screening. Because of the high incidence of atherosclerosis in the United States, all people 20 years of age and older are advised to have their serum cholesterol level evaluated.

Diet Therapy. Clients with LDL values of 130–159 mg/dL are advised to follow a fat-modified diet. In collaboration with the dietitian, the nurse instructs clients with LDLs of 160 mg/dL or greater to follow a more structured diet aimed at decreasing saturated fat and cholesterol and, if appropriate, promoting weight loss. A decrease in fat, particularly saturated fat, is considered more important than simply decreasing the cholesterol number because saturated fat is one of the main determinants of cholesterol synthesis in the body.

In the United States, 37% of the total caloric intake in the diets of many people is made up of fat, and this over consumption of fat and cholesterol leads to hypercholesterolemia—an elevated total blood cholesterol level (Whitney et al., 1994). Elevated cholesterol levels, however, can often be decreased if fat in the diet is limited to no more than 30% of the caloric intake.

TABLE 38–1

Classification of Serum Cholesterol Levels		
Serum Cholesterol Level (mg/dL)	**Classification**	**Intervention**
<200	• Optimal level	• Provide dietary information • Determine cholesterol levels again within 5 years
200–239 with *no* CAD or risks for CAD	• Borderline high blood cholesterol	• Provide dietary information • Determine cholesterol level again within 1 year
200–239 *with* CAD or risks for CAD 240 or higher, with or without CAD or risks for CAD	• High blood cholesterol	• Obtain serum LDL and HDL cholesterol levels • If LDL is 130–159, advise client to follow fat-modified diet, and repeat LDL annually • If LDL is 160 or higher, provide dietary therapy and frequent monitoring

CAD, coronary artery disease; LDL, low-density lipoprotein; HDL, high-density lipoprotein.

To assess what 30% of the caloric intake is, clients first need to determine their ideal daily caloric intake. They can then calculate their fat limit in grams (see Table 38–2). In addition to tracking fat in grams, people need to assess the fatty acid content of foods.

Step One Diet. The Step One American Heart Association diet, which is often recommended to decrease serum cholesterol level, calls for a total fat intake of less than 30%, with less than 10% of total caloric intake coming from saturated fat, up to 10% of total calories coming from polyunsaturated fat, and 10% to 15% coming from monounsaturated fat. Cholesterol intake with this diet is limited to less than 300 mg daily.

In collaboration with the dietitian, the nurse educates the client about the fat content of foods in terms of the total degree of fat (Table 38–2) and saturation. Meats and eggs contain mostly saturated fats. Because canola (rapeseed) oil is rich in monounsaturated fat and safflower and sunflower oil are rich in polyunsaturated oils, they are recommended over highly saturated oils, such as palm or coconut oil. Cholesterol is found only in animal sources, such as meat and eggs, which are also high in saturated fats.

Step Two Diet. The client's serum cholesterol levels are retested 6 and 12 weeks after the initial dietary intervention. If the cholesterol level has not significantly decreased, the client may be referred to a registered dietitian for instruction on a more restricted diet, such as the Step Two Diet. The Step Two Diet limits saturated fat to less than 7% of total calories and cholesterol to less than 200 mg/day.

In addition to elevated LDLs, other variations of hyperlipidemias put clients at risk for atherosclerosis. A low-fat, low-cholesterol diet, however, can play a significant role in improving a lipid profile, regardless of the lipid alteration.

Smoking Cessation. Cigarette smoking lowers levels of HDL cholesterol and dramatically increases the rate of progression of atherosclerosis.

The nurse advises all clients who smoke to stop smoking and all clients to avoid secondhand smoke. The nurse describes the relationship of smoking to atherosclerosis and assesses the client's willingness to change this behavior. Nurses and other health care providers can refer to the Agency on Health Care Policy and Research's Practice Guidelines on Smoking Cessation. This reference provides

TABLE 38–2

Fat Content of Selected Foods

Food	Fat (g)	Calories	Food	Fat (g)	Calories
Beef (3 oz with removable fat trimmed)			**Poultry** *Continued*		
Corned beef	16	213	Chicken drumstick, meat only, 1 average	2	76
Eye of round (roasted)	5	151	Turkey, light meat with skin	7	168
London broil, braised (choice)	12	208	Turkey, light meat only	3	133
T-bone steak, broiled (choice)	9	182	Turkey, dark meat with skin	10	188
Luncheon Meats (1 slice)			Turkey, dark meat only	6	160
Louis Rich 96% fat-free turkey pastrami	0	25	**Eggs**		
			1 large	5	75
Oscar Mayer bologna	4	50	Fleischmann's Egg Beaters, ¼ c	0	60
Weaver Chicken Frank with cheese	12	140	Morningstar Scramblers, ¼ c	3	60
Seafood (3 oz cooked unless otherwise indicated)			**Milk and Other Dairy Products**		
			Milk (1 c)		
Haddock	1	95	Whole	8	150
Lobster	1	83	2% fat	5	120
Swordfish	4	132	1% fat	3	100
Tuna, canned in oil and drained	7	158	Skim	0	90
Tuna, canned in water and drained	0	111	**Cream (1 tbsp)**		
			Half and half	2	20
Shrimp	1	84	Heavy whipping cream	6	52
Shrimp, breaded and fried	10	206	Sour cream	3	27
Poultry (3 oz roasted unless otherwise indicated)			**Cheese**		
			American, 1 oz	9	106
Chicken breast, meat with skin	7	165	Cheddar, 1 oz	9	114
Chicken breast, meat only	3	142	Cottage cheese, creamed, 1 c	9	217
Chicken drumstick, meat with skin, batter dipped and fried, 1 average	11	193	Cottage cheese, 1% fat, 1 c	2	164
			Cream cheese, 1 oz	10	99
			Ricotta, ½ c	16	216
			Ricotta, part-skim, ¼ c	10	171
			Swiss, 1 oz	8	107

strategies to assist clients to quit smoking. A smoking cessation group, such as the American Cancer Society's "Fresh Start," may help the client with this difficult process. Most formal programs encourage people to stop smoking "cold turkey."

Johns Hopkins Hospital has developed a "stage of readiness" model that classifies clients into one of six stages (Stillman, 1995). The nurse can assess the client's readiness to stop smoking using this model (Table 38–3).

Clients may also consider using the nicotine patch (Nicoderm, Habitrol, ProStep), which helps relieve nicotine withdrawal symptoms. The patch is about 50% effective in helping clients to stop smoking and is available over the counter. The dose is determined by the client's weight and the extent to which he or she smokes. Clients are urged to stop smoking completely when the nicotine patch is initiated. The nurse informs clients that if they continue to smoke while using the patch, their risks for adverse effects are increased because the peak levels of nicotine are higher than those experienced from smoking alone. Serious cardiovascular effects, such as angina and dysrhythmias, may result from the patch, although the most common side effect is skin irritation. Patches cost approximately $100 a month, or a total of $300 over 3 months. Many health insurance programs will not cover the costs associated with nicotine patches unless the client is enrolled in a smoking cessation program.

Nicotine gum (Nicorette) is necessary if a client feels the need to smoke. Clients should not chew more than 30 pieces of gum per day (Schlafer, 1993).

TRANSCULTURAL CONSIDERATIONS

African-Americans have a higher prevalence of smoking than other ethnic groups. African-American women are less likely to stop smoking than Caucasian women. The reason for this difference is not known (Allen & Phillips, 1997).

Exercise. Regular exercise is recommended to promote optimal lipid levels, and it can actually prevent atherosclerosis. Exercise can also lead to regression of atherosclerotic plaque and the building of collateral circulation in people with atherosclerosis. The level of exercise required to provide protection from atherosclerotic dis-

TABLE 38–2

Fat Content of Selected Foods *Continued*

Food	Fat (g)	Calories	Food	Fat (g)	Calories
Milk and Other Dairy Products *Continued*			**Spreads and Oils** *Continued*		
Weight Watchers American Pasteurized Process Cheese Product, 1 slice	2	45	Margarine, 1 tsp	4	34
			Diet margarine, 1 tsp	2	17
Yogurt			Vegetable oil (corn, safflower, olive, peanut, soybean, sunflower, and sesame), 1 tbsp	14	120
Colombo, plain, 8 oz	7	150	Vegetable oil, spray, 2.5-sec spray	1	6
Colombo, plain, nonfat lite, 8 oz	0	110	**Salad Dressings**		
Breads			Blue cheese, 1 tbsp	8	77
Bagel, 1	1	163	French, 1 tbsp	6	67
English muffin, 1	1	135	Italian, 1 tbsp	7	69
Whole-wheat bread, 1 slice	1	61	Russian, 1 tbsp	8	76
Other Grains			Thousand Island, 1 tbsp	6	59
Pasta, 1 c cooked	1	159	**Sweets**		
White rice, 1 c cooked	1	223	Apple pie, ⅛	12	282
Pancakes, 4-in plain	2	62	Cheesecake, ⅛	13	278
Waffles, 7-in plain	8	206	Chocolate pudding, 1 c	12	385
French toast, 1 slice	7	153	Chocolate syrup, 2 tbsp	1	92
Fruits and Vegetables			Fudge topping, 2 tbsp	5	124
Apple, 1 medium	1	81	Ice cream, Sealtest, vanilla, chocolate, or strawberry, ½ c	6	140
Banana, 1 medium	1	105			
Orange, 1 medium	1	65	Orange sherbet, ½ c	3	92
Raisins, ⅓ c	1	150	Popsicle ice pop	0	50
Avocado, ½ medium	15	153	**Snack Foods**		
Broccoli, ½ c cooked	0	23	Lay's Bar-B-Q Flavored Potato Chips, 1 oz	9	150
Carrot, raw, 1 medium	0	31	Orville Redenbacher's Natural Microwave Popping Corn, 4 c popped	7	110
Corn, canned, ½ c	1	66			
Green beans, ½ c cooked	0	22			
Peas, ½ c cooked	0	67	Popcorn, air-popped, 1 c	0	23
Spreads and Oils			Pringle's Light Potato Chips, 1 oz	8	150
Butter, 1 tsp	4	36			

TABLE 38–3

Stage-of-Readiness Model for Smoking Cessation

Stage	Description of Stage	Nursing Strategies
Precontemplation	Clients have no desire to quit smoking	Teach negative effects of smoking; reassure client that feelings are part of addiction process; deliver a "fear" message related to poor health consequences
Contemplation	Clients have thought about smoking cessation but have taken no action	Provide specific examples of how smoking is affecting the client; stress health benefits if client quits smoking
Preparation	Client has taken some steps to quit smoking	Provide behavioral reinforcement; help the client identify cues that lead to smoking, such as after eating; help the client identify coping strategies
Action	Client quits smoking	Provide positive reinforcement to prevent relapse
Maintenance	Client has not smoked for 6 months	Continue with positive reinforcement

Information from Stillman, F. A. (1995). Smoking cessation for the hospitalized cardiac patient: Rationale for and report of a model program. *Journal of Cardiovascular Nursing, 9,* 25–36.

ease has not been established. The nurse instructs clients at risk for or with atherosclerosis—when it results from hyperlipidemia, hypertension, or diabetes—to undergo an exercise tolerance (treadmill or stress) test before undertaking an exercise program, such as aerobics, walking, or running.

Drug Therapy. Clients with elevated total and LDL cholesterol levels that do not respond adequately to dietary intervention are started on lipid-lowering agents (Chart 38–1). Drug choice is dependent on the triglyceride levels. Because most of these drugs can produce major side effects, they are generally given only when nonpharmacologic management has been unsuccessful. Bile acid-binding resins, such as cholestyramine (Questran) or colestipol (Colestid), may be recommended initially because of their low toxicity. Medications such as lovastatin (Mevacor), simvastatin (Zocor), and fluvastatin (Lescol) lower both LDL and triglyceride levels. These statins are contraindicated in active liver disease and pregnancy as they can cause muscle myopathies and marked increases in liver functions. Nicotinic acid lowers LDL and VLDL cholesterol levels and increases HDL cholesterol level. It is used as a single agent or in combination with an acid-binding

Chart 38–1

Drug Therapy for Hyperlipidemia

Drug	Usual Dosage	Nursing Interventions	Rationale
Bile acid sequestrants, e.g., cholestyramine Questran Colestipol (Colestid)	• 12–24 g/day • 30 g/day	• Encourage clients to increase fluid intake and consider stool softeners/psyllium if needed	• Chloestyramine is constipating
Nicotinic acid (Nicobid, Nicolar, Nia-Bid [niacin])	• 1.5–3 g/day • Maximum dose 6 g/day	• Encourage clients to take with meals • Increase dose gradually	• Flushing of skin and pruritus are common side effects, which can be minimized when drug is taken with meals
Fibric acid, usually derivatives, e.g., gemfibrozil (Lopid)	• 600 mg bid • 1–2 mg	• Instruct clients to take with meals if nausea or gastrointestinal discomfort occurs	• Although well tolerated, nausea and gastrointestinal discomfort may occur and can be prevented if taken with meals
HMG-CoA reductase inhibitors, e.g., Lovastatin (Mevacor) Simvastatin (Zocor) Fluvastatin (Lescol)	• Starting dose 20 mg; increased to 40–80 mg • 10–40 mg/day • 20–40 mg/day	• Instruct clients to report muscle tenderness	• Although rare, myopathy has occured as a side effect

resin drug or a statin. Low doses (1.0–1.5 g/day) are generally well tolerated, but higher doses can result in an elevation of hepatic enzymes and various other side effects. Gemfibrozil (Lopid) raises HDL and lowers triglyceride and VLDL cholesterol levels, but is not as effective in lowering LDL.

Hypertension

Overview

Hypertension is generally defined as a systolic blood pressure greater than or equal to 130 mmHg and/or a diastolic blood pressure greater than or equal to 85 mmHg (Joint National Committee, 1993). Generally, hypertension is determined by three separate readings unless the systolic pressure is 210 mmHg or higher and the diastolic pressure is 120 mmHg or more.

Hypertension has been classified into four stages (Table 38–4). The significance of this disease is that it is a major risk factor for coronary, cerebral, renal, and peripheral vascular disease. However, control of hypertension has resulted in significant decreases in cardiovascular morbidity and mortality.

Although mortality rates have declined over the last 20 years, hypertension costs over $500 million per year and accounts for the largest number of health care provider visits per year, as well as the largest consumption of prescription drugs (Eaton et al., 1996). To achieve the Healthy People 2000 objective of increased blood pressure control among clients with hypertension, nurses must be able to assess and intervene appropriately in the care of these clients.

Pathophysiology

The systemic arterial pressure is a product of the cardiac output and the total peripheral resistance (Fig. 38–2). Cardiac output is determined by stroke volume and heart rate. Control of peripheral resistance is maintained by the autonomic nervous system and circulating hormones, such as norepinephrine and epinephrine. Consequently, any factor producing an alteration in peripheral resistance, heart rate, or stroke volume affects the systemic arterial pressure.

TABLE 38–4

Stages of Hypertension		
Stage 1	Systolic, 140–159 mmHg	Diastolic, 90–99 mmHg
Stage 2	Systolic, 160–179 mmHg	Diastolic, 100–109 mmHg
Stage 3	Systolic, 180–209 mmHg	Diastolic, 110–119 mmHg
Stage 4	Systolic, ≥210 mmHg	Diastolic, ≥120 mmHg

From U.S. Department of Health and Human Services. (1993). *The Fifth Report of the Joint National Committee on Detection, Evaluation, and Treatment of High Blood Pressure* (NIH Publication). Washington, DC: U.S. Government Printing Office.

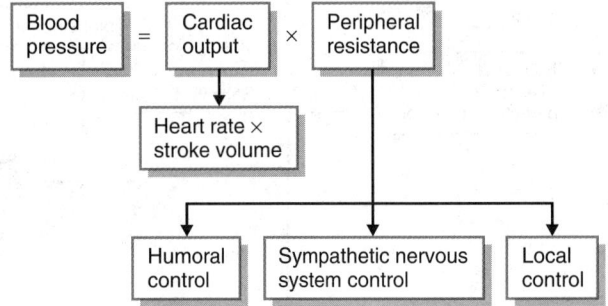

Figure 38–2. The components of blood pressure.

Regulation of Blood Pressure

Stabilizing mechanisms exist in the body to exert an overall regulation of systemic arterial pressure and to prevent circulatory collapse. Four control systems play a major role in maintaining blood pressure: the arterial baroreceptor system, regulation of body fluid volume, the renin-angiotensin-aldosterone system, and vascular autoregulation.

Arterial Baroreceptors

The arterial baroreceptors are found primarily in the carotid sinus but also in the aorta and the wall of the left ventricle. These baroreceptors monitor the level of arterial pressure. The baroreceptor system counteracts a rise in arterial pressure through vagally mediated cardiac slowing and vasodilation with decreased sympathetic tone. Therefore, reflex control of circulation elevates the systemic arterial pressure when it falls and lowers it when it rises. Why this control fails in hypertension is unknown. There is evidence for upward resetting of baroreceptor sensitivity so that pressure rises are inadequately sensed even though pressure decreases are not.

Regulation of Body Fluid Volume

Changes in fluid volume also affect the systemic arterial pressure. If there is an excess of salt and water in a person's body, the blood pressure rises through complex physiologic mechanisms that change the venous return to the heart, producing a rise in cardiac output. If the kidneys are functioning adequately, a rise in systemic arterial pressure produces diuresis and a fall in pressure. Pathologic conditions that change the pressure threshold at which the kidneys excrete salt and water alter the systemic arterial pressure.

Renin-Angiotensin-Aldosterone System

Renin, angiotensin, and aldosterone also regulate blood pressure (Fig. 38–3) (see also Chap. 14). The kidney produces renin, an enzyme that acts on a plasma protein substrate to split off angiotensin I, which is removed by a converting enzyme in the lung to form angiotensin II, then angiotensin III. Angiotensins II and III have strong vasoconstrictor action on blood vessels and are the controlling mechanism for aldosterone release. The signifi-

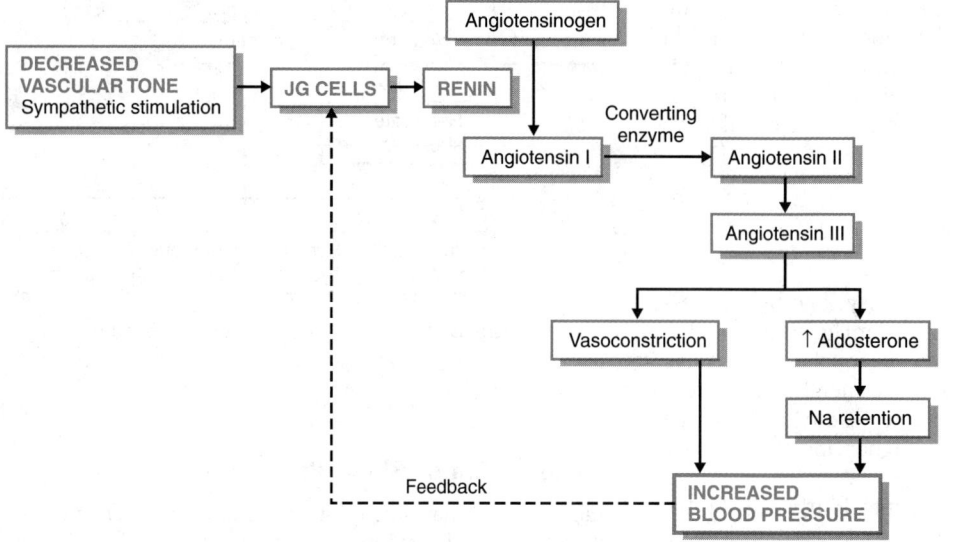

Figure 38–3. The effect of the renin-angiotensin system on blood pressure control. (From Copstead, L. E. C. [1995]. *Perspectives on Pathophysiology*. Philadelphia, W. B. Saunders.)

cance of aldosterone in hypertension is most evident in primary aldosteronism. By increasing the activity of the sympathetic nervous system, angiotensins II and III also appear to inhibit sodium excretion, resulting in an elevation in blood pressure.

Inappropriate secretion of renin may cause increased peripheral vascular resistance in essential (primary) hypertension. In high blood pressure, renin levels should be expected to fall because the increased renal arteriolar pressure should inhibit renin secretion. In most people with essential hypertension, however, renin levels are normal.

Vascular Autoregulation

The process of vascular autoregulation, which keeps perfusion of tissues in the body relatively constant, appears to be important in causing hypertension accompanying salt and water overload. This mechanism is poorly understood.

Complications of Hypertension

Sustained blood pressure elevation in clients with essential (primary) hypertension results in damage to blood vessels in vital organs. Essential hypertension produces medial hyperplasia (thickening) of the arterioles. As the blood vessels thicken and perfusion decreases, body organs are damaged; these changes can result in myocardial infarctions, cerebrovascular accidents, peripheral vascular disease, or renal failure.

Malignant hypertension is a severe type of elevated blood pressure that is rapidly progressive. A person with malignant hypertension usually has symptoms such as morning headaches, blurred vision, and dyspnea and/or symptoms of uremia (accumulation in the blood of substances ordinarily eliminated in the urine). Clients are often in their 30s, 40s, or 50s. The diastolic blood pressure is greater than 110 mmHg and frequently much higher, ranging from 130 to 170 mmHg. Unless intervention occurs promptly, a client with malignant hypertension may experience renal failure, left ventricular failure, or stroke.

Etiology

Hypertension can be essential (primary) or secondary (Table 38–5). Essential hypertension accounts for 95% of all cases (Massie, 1995).

TABLE 38–5

Etiology of Hypertension

Essential (Primary)
- No known cause
- Associated risk factors
  - Family history of hypertension
  - High sodium intake
  - Excessive calorie consumption
  - Physical inactivity
  - Excessive alcohol intake
  - Low potassium intake

Secondary
- Renal vascular and renal parenchymal disease
- Primary aldosteronism
- Pheochromocytoma
- Cushing's disease
- Coarctation of the aorta
- Brain tumors
- Encephalitis
- Psychiatric disturbances
- Pregnancy
- Medications
  - Estrogen (e.g., oral contraceptives)
  - Glucocorticoids
  - Mineralocorticoids
  - Sympathomimetics

Essential Hypertension

Although there is no known cause for essential hypertension, several associated risk factors have been discovered on the basis of common characteristics of people with this disease:

- A family history of hypertension
- High sodium intake
- Excessive calorie consumption
- Physical inactivity
- Excessive alcohol intake
- Low potassium intake

A family history of hypertension is a major risk factor. In families with hypertension, there may be a defect in renal secretion of sodium or a heightened sympathetic nervous response to stress.

Secondary Hypertension

Specific disease states and medications can increase a person's susceptibility to hypertension; a person with this type of elevation in blood pressure has secondary hypertension.

Diseases

Renal vascular and renal parenchymal diseases are two of the most common causes of secondary hypertension. Hypertension can develop when there is any sudden damage to the kidneys. Renovascular hypertension is associated with narrowing of one or more of the main arteries carrying blood directly to the kidneys. Renal parenchymal diseases are related to infection, inflammation, and changes in kidney structure and function.

Dysfunction of the adrenal medulla or the adrenal cortex can cause secondary hypertension. Adrenal-mediated hypertension is due to primary excesses of aldosterone, cortisol, and catecholamines. In *primary aldosteronism,* excessive aldosterone causes hypertension and hypokalemia (low potassium levels). Primary aldosteronism usually arises from benign adenomas of the adrenal cortex. *Pheochromocytomas* originate most commonly in the adrenal medulla and result in excessive secretion of catecholamines. In *Cushing's syndrome,* excessive glucocorticoids are excreted from the adrenal cortex. The cause of Cushing's syndrome may be either adrenocortical hyperplasia or adrenocortical adenoma (see Chap. 66).

Coarctation of the aorta is a congenital narrowing of the aorta that may cause hypertension. Occurring at any level of the thoracic or abdominal aorta, the narrowing restricts blood flow through the aortic arch, resulting in an elevated blood pressure above the constriction. After surgical repair, the elevation in blood pressure eventually subsides.

Secondary hypertension is also associated with other neurogenic disturbances, such as brain tumors, encephalitis, and psychiatric disturbances.

Medications

Medications that can cause secondary hypertension include estrogen, glucocorticoids, mineralocorticoids, sympathomimetics, cyclosporine, and erythropoietin. The use of estrogen-containing oral contraceptives is probably the most common cause of secondary hypertension in women. Discontinuation of medications capable of causing hypertension often reverses this problem.

Incidence/Prevalence

It is estimated that 50 million Americans, or 1 in every 4 adults, have high blood pressure or are currently being treated for hypertension.

ELDERLY CONSIDERATIONS

As adults age they are more likely to develop hypertension (Massie, 1995). In fact, the most prevalent cardiovascular disease in the elderly is hypertension, which is a significant risk factor for death in that population (Matteson et al., 1997).

TRANSCULTURAL CONSIDERATIONS

In the United States, the incidence of hypertension among African-Americans is two times greater than that for Caucasians. Hypertension is more prevalent in African-Americans and Caucasians living in the southeastern United States than in African-Americans and Caucasians living in other parts of the country.

WOMEN'S HEALTH CONSIDERATIONS

African-American women have a higher incidence of hypertension than Caucasian women, Hispanic, women, Caucasian men, and African-American men. Studies are beginning to show that hypertension is being found in African-American teenage girls, especially those who are obese (Allen & Phillips, 1997).

Collaborative Management

Assessment

➤ History

When obtaining the history, the nurse considers a client's risk factors for hypertension. The nurse ascertains the client's age; ethnic origin or race; family history of hypertension; average dietary intake of calories, sodium- and potassium-containing foods, and alcohol; and exercise habits. Past and present history of renal or cardiovascular disease and current use of medications are also assessed.

➤ Physical Assessment/Clinical Manifestations

When a diagnosis of hypertension is made, most clients have no symptoms; however, they may experience headaches, dizziness, or fainting as a result of the elevated blood pressure. The nurse obtains blood pressure readings in both of the client's arms. Two or more readings are taken at each visit, with the average reading obtained used as the value for the visit. To detect postural (orthostatic) changes, the nurse should also take readings with the client in the supine (lying) or sitting position and at least 2 minutes later with the client standing.

Funduscopic examination of the eyes is done by a skilled practitioner to observe vascular changes in the retina. The appearance of the retina can be a reliable index of the severity and prognosis of hypertension. The Keith-Wagener (KW) classification of retinal changes in hypertension is commonly used to stage changes:

- Stage I is characterized by minimal arteriolar narrowing.
- Stage II involves more marked narrowing of arterioles and arteriovenous nicking (changes at the arteriovenous crossings).
- Stage III shows circular or flame-shaped hemorrhages, fluffy "cotton wool" exudates.
- Stage IV, the most severe, is the same as stage III but with the addition of papilledema (malignant hypertension is always associated with papilledema).

Physical assessment is helpful in diagnosing several conditions that produce secondary hypertension. The presence of abdominal bruits is typical of clients with renovascular disease. Tachycardia, sweating, and pallor suggest pheochromocytoma or adrenal medulla tumor. Coarctation of the aorta is often characterized by elevation of blood pressure in the arms, with normal or low blood pressure in the lower extremities. Femoral pulses are also delayed or absent.

➤ Psychosocial Assessment

The nurse assesses for psychosocial stressors that can worsen the client's hypertension and that may affect the client's ability to collaborate in a treatment. Job-related, economic, and other life stressors are evaluated, as well as the client's response to these stressors.

Some clients may have difficulty coping with the lifestyle changes needed to control hypertension. The nurse assesses the coping strategies that the client has used in the past (see Chap. 8).

➤ Laboratory Assessment

Although no laboratory tests are diagnostic of essential hypertension, several laboratory tests can assess possible causes of secondary hypertension. The presence of protein, red blood cells, pus cells, and casts in the urine; elevated levels of blood urea nitrogen (BUN); and elevated serum creatinine levels indicate renal disease. In clients with a pheochromocytoma, a urinary test for the presence of catecholamines is positive. An elevation in levels of serum corticoids and 17-ketosteroids in the urine is diagnostic of Cushing's disease.

➤ Radiographic Assessment

No specific x-rays can diagnose hypertension. Routine chest radiography may be of assistance in recognizing left ventricular hypertrophy that results from hypertension.

Intravenous pyelography (IVP) is performed when clinical findings suggest renovascular hypertension. Renal arteriography is undertaken to establish the exact location and the extent of any lesions, the degree of obstruction, and the basic pathologic change in the renal arteries.

➤ Other Diagnostic Assessment

An electrocardiogram (ECG) is of value in determining the degree of cardiac involvement. Left atrial abnormality is the first electrocardiographic sign of cardiac involvement resulting from hypertension.

 Analysis

➤ Common Nursing Diagnoses and Collaborative Problems

Common nursing diagnoses for a client with hypertension include
1. Knowledge Deficit related to information misinterpretation or unfamiliarity with information resources
2. Risk for Ineffective Management of Therapeutic Regime

➤ Additional Nursing Diagnoses and Collaborative Problems

The client may also have one or more of the following diagnoses:
- Altered Tissue Perfusion (renal, cerebral, cardiopulmonary, and peripheral) related to decreased blood flow
- Altered Nutrition: Risk for More than Body Requirements related to learned eating behaviors, ethnic and cultural values, lack of social support for weight loss, and/or imbalance between activity level and caloric intake
- Fatigue related to altered body chemistry (medications)
- Altered Sexuality Patterns related to effects of medical treatment (drugs)
- Ineffective Individual Coping related to effects of chronic illness and major changes in lifestyle
- Risk of Noncompliance with treatment regimen

The following collaborative problems may also occur in some clients with hypertension:
- Potential for Cerebrovascular Hemorrhage
- Potential for Retinal Hemorrhage

 Planning and Implementation

➤ Knowledge Deficit

Planning: Expected Outcomes. The client is expected to verbalize an understanding of the management of hypertension.

Interventions. For the client with essential hypertension, the nurse initially recommends the following lifestyle modifications:
- Sodium restriction
- Weight reduction
- Moderation of alcohol intake
- Exercise
- Relaxation techniques
- Tobacco avoidance

These modifications are considered the foundation of hypertension control. If these modifications are unsuccessful, the health care provider considers the use of antihypertensive drugs.

There is no surgical treatment for essential hypertension. However, surgery may be indicated for certain causes of secondary hypertension, such as renal vascular disease, coarctation of the aorta, and pheochromocytoma.

Sodium Restriction. In collaboration and consultation with the dietitian, the nurse advises all clients with hypertension to decrease their sodium chloride intake from the average of 150 mmol/L (150 mEq/L) to less than 100 mmol/L (100 mEq/L) each day (less than 2.3 g of sodium). To accomplish this goal, clients should avoid adding salt at the table, avoid cooking with salt, avoid adding seasonings that contain sodium, and limit eating canned, frozen, or other processed foods.

The dietitian reviews a 3-day dietary recall with the client to identify whether sodium intake has been excessive. In collaboration with the dietitian, the nurse suggests spices, herbs, fruits, and other non-salt-containing substances, such as powdered garlic and onion, to enhance the flavor of meat, chicken, seafood, and snacks. The nurse and dietitian instruct clients to read the labels on processed foods and to avoid those that are high in sodium. Salt substitutes are an alternative to salt, but the client needs a physician's order to use them. This order is necessary because salt substitutes are high in potassium, and the client may have hyperkalemia (high potassium levels) associated with a concomitant problem, such as renal impairment. Although hyperkalemia is unusual, it can also occur in clients who are taking potassium-sparing diuretics.

While salt is restricted, the client should include recommended daily allowances of potassium, calcium, and magnesium in the diet. Studies are not conclusive, but data suggest that low levels of these electrolytes are associated with high blood pressure.

Weight Reduction. If a client's weight is more than 10% above ideal, the nurse encourages the client to lose weight. The nurse discusses the rationale for reducing or maintaining weight and plans a weight-reducing diet with the dietitian and client. The nurse may then refer the client to a group or organization for weight reduction.

Because of the relationship of saturated fat and cholesterol to weight, a weight-reduction plan is formulated with the following limits:
- Total fat, less than 30% of daily caloric intake
- Saturated fat, less than 10%
- Cholesterol, less than 300 mg/day

Table 38–6 describes how to calculate grams of fat.

Moderation of Alcohol Intake. The nurse instructs clients to limit alcohol intake to no more than 1 oz of ethanol (2 oz of liquor, 8 oz of wine, 24 oz of beer) daily. The client is taught that alcohol consumption may elevate arterial blood pressure and can add "empty" calories.

Exercise. With the physician's approval and in collaboration with the physical therapist, the nurse can help the client develop a regular exercise program. The therapist usually recommends that the client perform regular aerobic exercise, such as brisk walking, running, cycling, swimming, or stair climbing, 30–45 minutes three to five times a week. The client should initiate exercise gradually and should stop and notify the physician if severe short-

TABLE 38–6

How to Determine Dietary Fat Limits	
Procedure	**Example**
1. Begin with the number of calories consumed in a day	• 1800 kcal
2. Multiply the number of calories by 0.3 (30% of total calories) to determine the maximal number of calories that should be obtained from fat	• 1800 × 0.30 = 540 kcal/day from fat
3. Divide by 9 (1 g of fat contains 9 kcal) to determine the maximal number of grams of fat in the diet per day	• 540 ÷ 9 = 60 g/day of fat. To limit fat intake to no more than 30% of calories, the client must take in no more than 60 g of fat daily

ness of breath, fainting, or chest pain occurs. Clients should avoid muscle-building isometric exercise (weight lifting, wrestling, rowing) because it may raise blood pressure to dangerous levels.

Tobacco Avoidance. Although cigarette smoking is unrelated to hypertension, it is a major risk factor for cardiovascular disease. Therefore, the client who smokes is strongly urged to stop. With input from the nurse and physician, the client plans a smoking cessation program that best fits into his or her lifestyle. The nurse explains the nicotine patch and smoking cessation programs and implements follow-up to assess the client's plans for quitting (see earlier discussion of smoking cessation under Arteriosclerosis and Atherosclerosis).

Drug Therapy. Drug therapy is individualized for each client, with consideration given to the client's culture, age, concomitant illness, severity of blood pressure elevation, and cost of drugs and follow-up. Therapy may not be instituted for clients with diastolic readings between 90 and 94 mmHg because there is controversy about the advantage of treatment in this group.

Treatment of hypertension generally begins with a single drug. Once-a-day drug therapy is best, because the more doses required each day, the higher the risk that a client will not follow the treatment regimen. Several classifications of medications are available to control hypertension. Examples of commonly used drugs are listed in Chart 38–2.

Diuretics. Three basic types of diuretics are used to decrease blood volume and lower blood pressure:
- Thiazide diuretics, such as hydrochlorothiazide (HydroDIURIL, Urozide*), prevent sodium and water reabsorption in the distal tubules while promoting potassium excretion.
- Loop (high-ceiling) diuretics, such as furosemide (Lasix, Furoside*), depress sodium reabsorption in the ascending loop of Henle and promote potassium excretion

---

Chart 38–2

Drug Therapy for Hypertension

Drug	Usual Dosage	Nursing Interventions	Rationale
Diuretics			
Thiazides			
Chlorothiazide (Diuril)	• 125–500 mg/day	• Monitor potassium levels and watch for muscle weakness or irregular pulse.	• Hypokalemia is a common occurrence.
Hydrochlorothiazide (Esidrix, HydroDIURIL)	• 12.5–50 mg/day	• Encourage intake of foods high in potassium (e.g., bananas and orange juice).	• Depleted potassium needs to be replaced.
Loop Diuretics			
Furosemide (Lasix, Furoside♣)	• 20–40 mg/day	• Same as for thiazide diuretics.	• Same as for chlorothiazide.
Ethacrynic acid (Edecrin)	• 25–100 mg/day		
Potassium-Sparing Diuretics			
Spironolactone (Aldactone)	• 25–100 mg/day	• Monitor potassium levels and watch for muscle weakness or irregular pulse.	• Hypokalemia or hyperkalemia may occur.
Triamterone (Dyrenium)	• 50–100 mg/day		
Beta-Blocking Agents			
Propranolol (Inderal, Apo-Propranolol♣)	• 40–240 mg/day	• Monitor pulse rate.	• A drop in pulse is expected, and bradycardia may occur.
Atenolol (Tenormin)	• 25–100 mg once a day		
Nadolol (Cogard)	• 20–240 mg/day	• Watch for shortness of breath or cough.	• Bronchospasm caused by blockage of beta-receptors in the lungs may occur.
Metoprolol (Lopressor)	• 50–200 mg/day	• Instruct client to report any difficulty in sexual function, fatigue, weakness, or depression.	• Although these are common side effects, newer beta-blocking agents may be more "selective" in terms of side effects.
		• Instruct clients with diabetes to monitor blood glucose levels.	• Hypoglycemic symptoms may be blocked in clients taking beta-blocking agents.
Calcium Channel Blockers			
Nifedipine (Procardia, Adalat)	• 10–30 mg tid	• Monitor blood pressure. • Assess for dizziness.	• A drop in blood pressure occurs within 30 min after oral administration.
		• Assess lower extremities.	• Pedal edema can occur as a result of peripheral vasodilation.

▪ Potassium-sparing diuretics, such as spironolactone (Aldactone, Norospiroton♣), act on the distal tubule to inhibit reabsorption of sodium ions in exchange for potassium, thereby retaining potassium.

Diuretics are the drugs of choice for clients who have asthma, chronic airway limitation, and chronic renal disease and for selected clients with congestive heart failure. They are particularly effective for African-American clients.

Diuretics are relatively inexpensive, and adherence to the medication regimen is enhanced because the drug can

usually be prescribed on a once-a-day or, at most, a twice-a-day schedule. However, the frequent voiding that occurs after a person takes a diuretic may interfere with one's daily activities. The most frequent side effect associated with diuretics is hypokalemia (low potassium levels). The nurse monitors the client's serum potassium level and assesses for signs and symptoms of irregular pulse and muscle weakness, which may indicate hypokalemia. The nurse advises clients receiving potassium-depleting diuretics to eat foods high in potassium, such as bananas and orange juice. However, the client may need a potas-

Chart 38–2. Drug Therapy for Hypertension Continued

Drug	Usual Dosage	Nursing Interventions	Rationale
Verapamil (Calan, Isoptin)	• 40–80 mg q8h, 240 mg SR once a day	• Monitor blood pressure and pulse. • Encourage intake of foods high in fiber.	• Hypotension and decreased heart rate may occur. • Constipation is a common side effect.
Diltiazem hydrochloride (Cardizem)	• 30–60 mg q8h	• Monitor blood pressure and pulse.	• Hypotension and decreased heart rate may occur.
Angiotension-Converting-Enzyme Inhibitors			
Captopril (Capoten)	• 6.25 mg tid initially, increased to 50 mg tid	• Instruct client to stay in bed for 3 hr after the first dose.	• Severe hypotension may follow the first dose.
Enalapril (Vasotec)	• 2.5 mg/d initially, increased to 10–40 mg/day	• Monitor blood pressure.	• Hypotension needs to be detected promptly.
Lisinopril/Zestil (Prinvil)	• 5 mg/d initially, increased to 10–40 mg/day	• Monitor renal function tests.	
Central Alpha Agonists			
Clonidine hydrochloride (Catapres)	• 0.1–1.2 mg h.s. or 0.1–0.3 mg once a week transdermally	• Administer at bedtime. • Instruct client to report rash associated with transdermal route.	• Sedation is a common side effect. • Bothersome skin rashes occur in about 25% of clients using transdermal patch.
Methyldopa (Aldomet)	• 250–500 mg qid	• Instruct client to sit on the side of the bed for several minutes before arising and to avoid changing position suddenly. • Warn clients that sedation can occur when drug is initiated and dose is increased. • Instruct male clients to report any difficulty in sexual functions.	• Postural hypotension is a common complication. • This information can assist clients in planning activity and rest periods. • Impotence is a common side effect.
Vasodilators			
Hydralazine (Apresoline)	• 10–50 mg qid	• Monitor pulse rate.	• Tachycardia may occur as a result of reflex increase in sympathetic activity.
Alpha$_1$-receptor blockers Doxazosin (Cardura)	• 1.0–16 mg/day	• Monitor blood pressure.	• A drop in blood pressure can occur between 2 and 6 h after initial dose or dose increases.
Terazosin (Hytrin)	• 1.0–20 mg/day	• Assess for dizziness.	• Give first dose at bedtime to avoid postural hypotension.

sium supplement to maintain adequate serum potassium levels (see Chap. 16). The nurse assesses clients taking potassium-sparing diuretics for hypokalemia and hyperkalemia. Both of these electrolyte disturbances are characterized by weakness and irregular pulse.

Beta-Adrenergic Blocking Agents. Beta-blockers lower blood pressure by blocking beta-receptors in the heart and peripheral vessels, reducing cardiac rate and output. By blocking beta-adrenergic receptors in the heart, beta-blockers cause a decrease in heart rate and decreased contractility. Bradycardia (slow heart rate) and heart fail-

ure may result. Beta-blockers can also prohibit bronchodilation by blocking beta-receptors in the lungs. Therefore, clients with a history of asthma or bronchospasm are generally not given these drugs, and all clients taking these drugs must be monitored for shortness of breath and wheezing.

Common side effects of beta-blockers include fatigue, weakness, depression, and sexual dysfunction, although the potential for side effects depends on the "selective" blocking effects of the drug. A variety of beta-blockers are available, and they differ from each other in terms of their cardioselectivity (primarily beta$_1$ effects, with less beta$_2$ effects), lipid solubility, and sympathomimetic activity throughout the body.

Diabetic clients who take beta-blockers may not have the usual signs and symptoms of hypoglycemia because the sympathetic nervous system is blocked. Counterregulatory responses to hypoglycemia, such as gluconeogenesis, may also be inhibited by certain beta-blockers.

Calcium Channel-Blocking Agents. Calcium channel blockers, such as verapamil hydrochloride (Calan), nifedipine (Procardia, Adalat), and diltiazem (Cardizem), lower blood pressure by interfering with the transmembrane flux of calcium ions, resulting in reduced vasoconstriction.

TRANSCULTURAL CONSIDERATIONS

 These medications are thought to be particularly effective for elderly and African-American clients.

Verapamil and diltiazem can affect atrial-ventricular conduction and often lower the heart rate. Oral nifedipine can reduce blood pressure quickly, often decreasing blood pressure by 25% within 30 minutes. Sublingual administration of nifedipine, given by puncturing the capsule and placing the liquid contents under the tongue, acts within 10–15 minutes.

Angiotensin-Converting Enzyme Inhibitors. Angiotensin-converting enzyme (ACE) inhibitors are also used as single or combination agents in the treatment of hypertension. The angiotensin-converting enzyme converts angiotensin I to angiotensin II, one of the most powerful vasoconstrictors in the body. ACE inhibitors include captopril (Capoten), enalapril (Vasotec), and lisinopril (Prinivil).

The client receiving an ACE inhibitor for the first time is instructed to stay in bed for 3–4 hours to avoid the severe hypotensive effect that can occur with initial use. The nurse monitors the client's blood pressure every 15 minutes after this first dose. *Postural (orthostatic) hypotension* may occur with subsequent doses, but it is less severe. The nurse checks for postural hypotension by taking the blood pressure when the client is lying, sitting, and standing. If there is a significant decrease in the systolic blood pressure (< 20 mmHg), the nurse notifies the physician.

ELDERLY CONSIDERATIONS

The elderly client is at the greatest risk for postural hypotension because of the cardiovascular changes associated with aging (Chart 38–3).

TRANSCULTURAL CONSIDERATIONS

ACE inhibitors are most effective in young Caucasian adults. They are less effective in African-American clients or older adults.

Central Alpha Agonists. Central alpha agonists act on the central nervous system, preventing reuptake of norepinephrine, resulting in a lowering of peripheral vascular resistance and blood pressure. Common central alpha agonists include clonidine (Catapres) and methyldopa (Aldomet, Apo-Methyldopa✦). Methyldopa can cause unique side effects, such as hemolytic anemia and inflammatory disorders of the liver, although they happen rarely. Because of this potential, clonidine is the more commonly used central alpha agonist. Clonidine can also be given as a transdermal patch, providing control of blood pressure for as long as 7 days. Side effects common to clonidine and methyldopa include sedation, postural hypotension, and impotence.

Vasodilators. Vasodilators lower blood pressure by relaxing vascular smooth muscle tone, thus reducing total peripheral resistance. Vasodilators include minoxidil (Loniten), nitroglycerin (Nitro-Bid), and nitroprusside (Nitropress).

Alpha-Adrenergic Receptor Agonists. Alpha-adrenergic agonists, such as prazosin (Minipress), dilate the arterioles and veins. These drugs can lower blood pressure quickly, but their use is limited because of frequent and bothersome side effects.

The Joint National Committee on Detection, Evaluation, and Treatment of High Blood Pressure (1993) has recommended that initial therapy for hypertension include either a thiazide diuretic or a beta-blocker unless these drugs are contraindicated or ineffective or there are special indications for agents such as calcium antagonists or ACE inhibitors. If after 1–3 months a client's blood pressure does not decrease adequately in response to initial therapy, the health care provider may increase the dose of the drug, substitute a drug from another class of antihypertensives, or add a second drug from another class.

Chart 38–3

Nursing Care Highlights: Assessment and Interventions for Hypertensive Crisis

Assess

- Severe headache
- Extremely high blood pressure
- Dizziness
- Blurred vision
- Disorientation

Intervene

- Place client in a semi-Fowler's position
- Administer oxygen
- Administer IV nitroprusside (Nitropress) or other infusion drug as ordered (for nitroprusside, cover infusion bag to prevent drug breakdown by light)
- Monitor the blood pressure every 5 to 15 minutes until the diastolic pressure is also below 90 and not less than 75; then monitor blood pressure every 30 minutes
- Observe for neurologic or cardiovascular complications, such as seizures; numbness, weakness, or tingling of extremities; dysrhythmias; or chest pain

Because of changes in recommendations and the availability of more drug options and more information on drug tolerance, the nurse sees a variety of drug protocols used by the health care provider to meet the individual needs of clients with hypertension.

➤ Risk for Ineffective Management of Therapeutic Regimen

Planning: Expected Outcomes. The client is expected to adhere to the therapeutic regimen, thus minimizing the risk of target organ damage.

Interventions. Clients who require pharmacologic treatment to control essential hypertension usually need to take medication for the rest of their lives. Frequently, though, clients stop taking antihypertensive medications because they have no symptoms. They may also discontinue medication because of cost or side effects.

In collaboration with the pharmacist, the nurse and client discuss the goals of therapy, including potential side effects, to help the client identify potential problems. The nurse then assists the client in tailoring the therapeutic regimen to the client's activities of daily living

Clients who do not comply with antihypertensive treatment are at great risk for target organ damage and hypertensive crisis (malignant hypertension). Clients in hypertensive crisis are admitted to critical care units, where they receive intravenous antihypertensive therapy such as nitroprusside (Nitropress), nitroglycerin (Nitro-Bid, Tridil IV), labetalol (Normodyne), diazoxide (Hyperstat), or sublingual nifedipine (Procardia, Adalat) (Chart 38–4). Hospitalization for complications of hypertension can be financially costly in both medical expenses and lost income.

 ## Continuing Care

Clients who require pharmacologic treatment to control essential hypertension usually need to take medication for the rest of their lives. Studies have shown that within the first year of therapy, over 50% of clients discontinue their treatment (Eaton et al., 1996). Frequently, clients stop taking antihypertensive medications, assuming that because they have no symptoms the hypertension is under control. Clients may assume that if their blood pressure returns to normal levels with antihypertensives, they no longer need them. Clients may also stop taking antihypertensives because of adverse side effects or cost.

➤ Home Care Management

If possible, the client should obtain a blood pressure monitor for use at home so that the pressure can be checked periodically. The nurse evaluates the client's ability to learn how to check his or her blood pressure. If the client cannot monitor blood pressure, a family member or significant other may be taught how to perform this procedure.

If weight reduction is a goal, the nurse suggests that the client have a scale in the home for weight monitoring.

➤ Health Teaching

The nurse instructs the client about sodium restriction, weight maintenance or reduction, alcohol restriction, stress management, and exercise (see earlier discussion). If necessary, the nurse also explains about the need to stop smoking. The elderly can also benefit from lifestyle modifications (Matteson et al., 1997) (see Chart 38–4).

For clients taking medication for hypertension, the nurse provides oral and written information about the indications, dosage, times of administration, side effects, and drug interactions (see Chart 38–2). The nurse stresses that the medication must be taken as prescribed and that, when all of it has been consumed, the prescription must be renewed on a continual basis. Abrupt discontinuation of medications, such as beta-blockers, can result in angina (chest pain) or myocardial infarction.

The nurse also urges clients to report unpleasant side effects, such as sexual dysfunction. In many instances, an alternative medication can be prescribed to minimize certain side effects.

Hypertension is a chronic illness, and clients may not be prepared to accept this fact. The nurse allows clients to verbalize feelings about this disease and its treatment. Clients are advised that their involvement in the treatment can lead to control of this disease and can prevent complications.

➤ Health Care Resources

A home health nurse may be needed for follow-up to monitor blood pressure. The nurse evaluates the ability of the client or the family to obtain accurate blood pressure measurements and assesses their compliance with treatment. If clients cannot purchase equipment to monitor

---

Chart 38–4

Nursing Focus on the Elderly: Hypertension

- Before initiating drug therapy, obtain blood pressure measurements with the client lying, sitting, and standing to assess for postural changes.
- Monitor the client's standing blood pressure during treatment.
- Instruct the client to avoid caffeine and nicotine for 1 hour before blood pressure measurements to obtain accurate readings.
- Teach the client that dizziness is a symptom of hypotension that should be reported.
- Instruct clients how to avoid orthostatic (postural) hypotension by avoiding sudden changes in position. Clients should arise from bed in three stages: sit in bed for 1 minute; sit on the side of the bed with legs dangling for 1 minute; stand, holding onto a nonmovable object for 1 minute before walking. Clients should also be cautious about heat exposure (hot tub), alcohol intake, and exercise, which can lead to orthostatic hypotension.

blood pressure, the nurse may suggest the American Heart Association, the Red Cross, or a local pharmacy for free blood pressure checks.

Evaluation

On the basis of the identified nursing diagnoses and collaborative problems, the nurse evaluates the care of the hypertensive client. The expected outcomes are that the client will:

- Explain the rationale for treatment of hypertension
- Maintain blood pressure of less than 130/85 mmHg
- Demonstrate no signs or symptoms of target organ damage, such as renal or heart disease

Peripheral Arterial Disease

Overview

Peripheral vascular disease (PVD) includes disorders that alter the natural flow of blood through the arteries and veins of the peripheral circulation. PVD affects the lower extremities much more frequently than the upper extremities. Generally, a client with a diagnosis of PVD has arterial disease (peripheral arterial disease) rather than venous involvement. Some clients have both arterial and venous disease.

Pathophysiology

Peripheral arterial disease (PAD) is a chronic condition in which partial or total arterial occlusion deprives the lower extremities of oxygen and nutrients. PAD of the lower extremities is sometimes referred to as lower extremity arterial disease (LEAD). Body tissues cannot live without an adequate oxygen and nutrient supply, and tissue eventually dies. Atherosclerosis is the most common cause of chronic altered blood flow. Fatty substances accumulate at the site of vessel wall injury and alter or totally occlude blood flow within the arteries. Tissue damage generally occurs below the arterial obstruction.

Obstructions are classified as inflow or outflow, according to the arteries involved and their relationship to the inguinal ligament (Fig. 38–4). *Inflow* obstructions involve the distal end of the aorta and the common, internal, and external iliac arteries. They are located above the inguinal ligament. *Outflow* obstructions involve infrainguinal arterial segments (the femoral, popliteal, and tibial arteries) and are below the superficial femoral artery (SFA). Gradual inflow occlusions may not cause significant tissue damage; gradual outflow occlusions typically do.

Etiology

Because atherosclerosis is the most common cause of chronic arterial obstruction, the risk factors for atherosclerosis apply to peripheral arterial disease as well. These

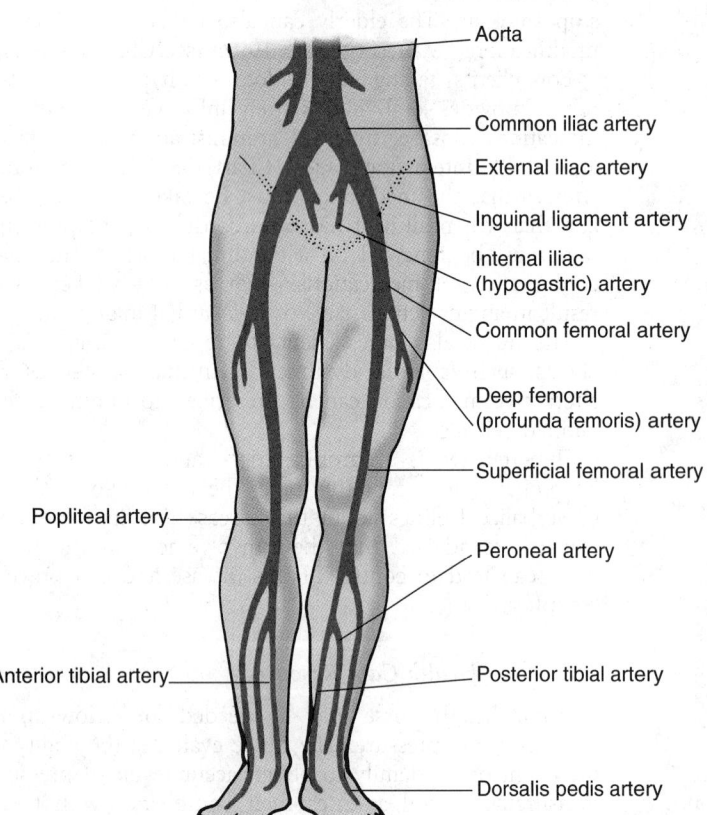

Figure 38–4. Common locations of inflow and outflow lesion.

include hypertension, hyperlipidemia, diabetes mellitus, cigarette smoking, obesity, and familial predisposition. Advancing age also increases the risk of disease related to atherosclerosis.

Incidence/Prevalence

In the United States, at least 10% of people over age 70 years and 1%–2% of people aged 37–69 years have symptomatic, chronic peripheral arterial disease (American Heart Association, 1995). PAD generally occurs in men older than age 45 years and in postmenopausal women.

Collaborative Management

 Assessment

➤ *History*

The clinical course of chronic peripheral arterial disease (PAD) can be divided into four stages (Chart 38–5). Clients do not experience symptoms in the early stages of disease.

Pain Assessment. Most clients initially seek treatment for a characteristic leg pain known as *intermittent claudication* (a term derived from a word meaning "to limp"). Usually, clients can walk only a certain distance before a cramping, burning muscle discomfort or pain forces them

---

Chart 38–5
Key Features of Chronic Peripheral Arterial Disease

Stage I: Asymptomatic
- No claudication is present.
- Bruit or aneurysm may be present.
- Pedal pulses are decreased or absent.

Stage II: Claudication
- Muscle pain, cramping, or burning occurs with exercise and is relieved with rest.
- Symptoms are reproducible with exercise.

Stage III: Rest Pain
- Pain while resting commonly awakens the client at night.
- Pain is described as numbness, burning, toothache-type pain.
- Pain usually occurs in the distal portion of the extremity—toes, arch, forefoot, or heel—rarely in the calf or the ankle.
- Pain is relieved by placing the extremity in a dependent position.

Stage IV: Necrosis/Gangrene
- Ulcers and blackened tissue occur on the toes, the forefoot, and the heel.
- Distinctive gangrenous odor is present.

---

to stop. The pain subsides after rest. When clients resume walking, they can walk the same distance before the pain returns. The pain is thus considered reproducible. As the disease progresses, clients can walk only shorter and shorter distances before pain recurs. Ultimately, pain may occur even while clients are at rest. The nurse questions the client about the nature and characteristics of leg pain to determine whether the client may be experiencing intermittent claudication.

Rest pain, which may begin while the disease is still primarily in the stage of intermittent claudication, is a numbness or burning, often described as feeling like a toothache, that is severe enough to awaken clients at night. It is usually located in the distal portion of the extremities—in the toes, the foot arches, the forefeet, and the heels—rarely in the calves or ankles. Clients can sometimes achieve pain relief by keeping the limb in a dependent position. Clients with rest pain have advanced disease that may result in limb loss.

Inflow and Outflow Disease. Clients with *inflow* disease experience discomfort in the lower back, buttocks, or thighs. Lower back or buttock discomfort indicates obstruction at or above the common iliac artery or abdominal aorta. Thigh discomfort indicates obstruction at or above the profunda femoris artery.

Clients with *mild* inflow disease experience discomfort after walking about two blocks. This discomfort is not severe but causes the client to stop walking. It is relieved with rest.

Clients with *moderate* inflow disease experience pain in these areas after walking about one or two blocks. The discomfort is described more like pain, but it subsides with rest most of the time.

Severe inflow disease causes the client severe pain after walking less than one block. These clients usually have rest pain.

Clients with *outflow* disease describe burning or cramping in the calves, ankles, feet, and toes. Calf discomfort usually indicates arterial obstruction at or below the superficial femoral or popliteal artery. Instep or foot discomfort indicates an obstruction below the popliteal artery.

The nurse asks specific questions about when the pain occurs and whether it occurs at rest.

Clients with *mild* outflow disease experience discomfort after walking about five blocks. This discomfort is relieved by rest.

Clients with *moderate* outflow disease have pain after walking about two blocks. Intermittent rest pain may be present.

Clients with *severe* outflow disease are usually unable to walk more than one-half block and usually experience rest pain. They may hang their feet off the bed at night for comfort.

Clients with outflow disease complain more frequently of rest pain than do clients with inflow disease.

WOMEN'S HEALTH CONSIDERATIONS

 Women suffer serious problems related to peripheral vascular disease of the lower extremities after menopause. In fact, 25% of women aged 55–74 years develop peripheral vascular disease (Gerhard et al., 1995). The major risk factors for women with PVD are cigarette smoking, diabetes mellitus, hypertension, hyperlipidemia, and menopause.

Conservative treatment for women includes exercise training and quitting smoking. Estrogen replacement therapy and cholesterol-lowering drugs may slow the development of arteriosclerosis in the lower extremities in women. Women appear to be at higher risk for amputation than men and should be encouraged to adhere to conservative therapy recommendations to prevent progression of the disease.

➤ Physical Assessment/Clinical Manifestations

Specific findings for peripheral arterial disease (PAD) depend on the severity of the disease. The nurse may observe loss of hair on the lower calf, ankle, and foot; dry, scaly, dusky, pale, or mottled skin; and thickened toenails. With severe arterial disease, the extremity is cold and gray-blue (cyanotic) or darkened. The nurse may also note elevational pallor and dependent rubor. Muscle atrophy can accompany prolonged chronic arterial disease.

The nurse palpates all pulses in both legs. The most sensitive and specific indicator of arterial function is the quality of the posterior tibial pulse. The pedal pulse is not palpable in a small percentage of people. The strength of the pulse should be compared bilaterally. Several scales are available for grading pulse strength. A popular system is presented in Table 38–7.

The nurse may also note early signs of ulcer formation or complete ulcer formation, a complication of peripheral arterial disease. The nurse must differentiate arterial and venous stasis ulcers from diabetic ulcers, which may have a different cause (Chart 38–6).

Initally, *arterial* ulcers are painful and develop on the toes (often the great toe), between the toes, or on the upper aspect of the foot. With prolonged occlusion, the toe(s) can become gangrenous. *Diabetic* ulcers develop on the plantar surface of the foot, over the metatarsal heads, and on the heel—anywhere that pressure is exerted. Diabetic ulcers may not be painful because of diabetic neuropathy. *Venous stasis* ulcers cause minimal pain and occur in the ankle area. The foot is warm, and distal pulses are palpable. The nurse notes discoloration of the lower extremity at the ulcer site. (Skin lesions are discussed in further detail in Chapter 70.)

TRANSCULTURAL CONSIDERATIONS

In clients with dark skin, the soles of the feet and the toenails enable the nurse to detect cyanosis or duskiness in the lower extremities because these areas are less pigmented.

➤ Radiographic Assessment

The most common x-ray for peripheral arterial disease is arteriography of the lower extremities. Because arteriography involves injecting contrast medium into the arterial system, the risks, which include hemorrhage, thrombosis, embolus, and death, are serious. Arteriography is often performed before surgery to pinpoint the exact location of the occlusion. The nurse prepares the client for the procedure and carefully implements follow-up care (see Chap. 35).

➤ Other Diagnostic Assessment

The advent of noninvasive evaluation of arterial disease has become a popular method of diagnosis. Noninvasive testing provides information about the arterial system with minimal risk to the client.

Segmental Systolic Blood Pressure Measurements. Segmental systolic blood pressure measurements of the lower extremities at the thigh, calf, and ankle are a noninvasive method of assessing peripheral arterial disease (PAD). Normally, blood pressure readings in the thigh and calf are higher than those in the upper extremities. With the presence of arterial disease, these pressures are lower than the brachial pressure.

With *inflow* disease, pressures taken at the thigh level indicate the severity of disease. Mild inflow disease may cause a difference of only 10–30 mmHg in pressure on the affected side compared with the brachial pressure. Severe inflow disease can cause a pressure difference of greater than 40–50 mmHg. The ankle pressure is normally equal to or greater than the brachial pressure.

To evaluate *outflow* disease, the nurse compares ankle pressure with the brachial pressure, which provides a ratio known as the *ankle/brachial index* (ABI). This value can be derived by dividing the ankle blood pressure by the brachial blood pressure.

With mild outflow disease, the client has an ankle/brachial index of 0.8–1.0; pressures are decreased by about 10 to 30 mmHg. The client with moderate outflow disease has an ankle/brachial index of 0.5–0.8, with pressure differences of 20–40 mmHg. An ankle/brachial index less than 0.5 indicates severe outflow disease.

Exercise Tolerance Testing. Exercise tolerance testing (by stress test or treadmill) may give valuable information

TABLE 38–7

Pulse Grading Scale	
Value	**Characteristic**
0	No detectable pulse (0/4)
1	Pulse thready, weak, difficult to detect; may fade in and out, easily obliterated by pressure (1/4)
2	Pulse difficult to palpate, hypokinetic, and may be obliterated by pressure; light palpation recommended (2/4)
3	Pulse easily palpable, not easily obliterated by pressure; considered normal in volume (3/4)
4	Pulse strong, bounding, hyperkinetic, easily palpated, not obliterated by pressure; may be pathologic if aortic regurgitation is present (4/4)

Chart 38–6

Key Features of Lower Extremity Ulcers

Feature	Arterial Ulcers	Venous Ulcers	Diabetic Ulcers
History	Client complains of claudication after walking approximately 1–2 blocks Rest pain usually present Pain at ulcer site Two or three risk factors present	Chronic nonhealing ulcer No claudication or rest pain Moderate ulcer discomfort Client complains about ankle or leg swelling	Diabetes Peripheral neuropathy No complaints of claudication
Ulcer location and appearance	End of the toes Between the toes Deep Ulcer bed pale, with even edges Little granulation tissue	Ankle area Brown pigmentation Ulcer bed pink Usually superficial, with uneven edges Granulation tissue present	Plantar area of foot Metatarsal heads Pressure points on feet Deep Pale, with even edges Little granulation tissue
	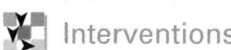		
Other assessment findings	Cool or cold foot Decreased or absent pulses Atrophy of skin Hair loss Pallor with elevation Dependent rubor Possible gangrene When acute, neurologic deficits noted	Ankle discoloration and edema Full veins when leg slightly dependent No neurologic deficit Pulses present May have scarring from previous ulcers	Pulses usually present Cool or warm foot Painless
Treatment	Treat underlying cause (surgical, revascularization) Prevent trauma and infection Client education, stressing foot care	Long-term wound care (Unna boot, damp-to-dry dressings) Elevate extremity Client education Prevent infection	Rule out major arterial disease Control diabetes Client education regarding foot care Prevent infection

Photographs of arterial ulcer and diabetic ulcer from Callen, J. P., Greer, K. E., Hood, A. F., Paller, A. S., & Swinyer, L. J. (1993). *Color atlas of dermatology: Slide set.* Philadelphia: W. B. Saunders.

about clients who are experiencing claudication (muscle pain) without rest pain. The nurse or technician obtains resting pulse volume recordings and has the client walk on a treadmill until the symptoms are reproduced. At the time of symptom onset or after approximately 5 minutes, the nurse or technician obtains another pulse volume recording. Normally, there may be an increased waveform with minimal, if any, drop in the ankle pressures. In clients with arterial disease, the waveforms are decreased (dampened) and there is a decrease in the ankle pressure of the affected limb of 40–60 mmHg for 20–30 seconds. If the return to normal pressure is delayed (longer than 10 minutes), the results suggest abnormal arterial flow in the affected limb.

Plethysmography. Plethysmography can also be performed to evaluate arterial flow in the lower extremities. This measurement provides graph or tracing readings of arterial flow in the limb. If an occlusion is present, the waveforms are dampened to flattened, depending on the degree of occlusion.

Interventions

The nurse first determines whether the altered tissue perfusion is of arterial or venous origin. An accurate assessment often provides this information, but in some people both conditions may exist. In this case, each disease must be considered separately when appropriate interventions are planned.

➤ *Nonsurgical Management*

The interventions of exercise, position changes, promotion of vasodilation, drug therapy, and invasive nonsurgical procedures are used to increase arterial flow to the affected limb.

Exercise. Exercise may improve arterial blood flow to the affected limb through build up of the *collateral* circulation. (Collateral circulation provides blood to the affected area through smaller vessels that develop and compensate for the occluded vessels.) Exercise is individualized for each client, but people with severe rest pain, venous ulcers, or gangrene should not participate. Other clients with peripheral arterial disease (PAD) can benefit from exercise that is initiated gradually and is slowly increased; an excellent exercise for these clients is walking. The nurse instructs the client to walk until the point of claudication, stop and rest, then walk a little farther. Eventually, clients are able to walk longer distances as collateral circulation develops. The nurse collaborates with the health care provider and physical therapist in determining an appropriate exercise program.

Positioning. Positioning of the client to promote circulation has been somewhat controversial. Some clients have swelling in their extremities. Because swelling prevents arterial flow, these clients should elevate their feet at rest, but the nurse teaches clients to refrain from raising their legs above the heart level. Extreme elevation *slows* arterial blood flow to the feet.

In severe cases, clients with PAD and swelling may sleep with the affected limb hanging from the bed, or they may sit upright in a chair for comfort. The nurse instructs all clients with PAD to avoid crossing their legs, which may interfere with blood flow.

Promoting Vasodilation. Vasodilation can be achieved by providing warmth to the affected extremity and preventing long periods of exposure to cold. The nurse encourages the client to maintain a warm environment at home and to wear socks or insulated shoes at all times. The client is cautioned *never* to apply direct heat to the limb, such as with the use of heating pads or extremely hot water. Sensitivity is decreased in the affected limb, and the client may get burned without feeling it.

The nurse encourages clients to prevent exposure of the affected limb to the cold because cold temperatures cause vasoconstriction (decreasing of the diameter of the blood vessels) and therefore decrease arterial blood flow. Emotional stress, caffeine, and nicotine also can cause vasoconstriction. The nurse emphasizes that complete abstinence from smoking or chewing tobacco is the most effective method of preventing vasoconstriction. The vasoconstrictive effects of each cigarette may last up to 1 hour after the cigarette is smoked.

Drug Therapy. For clients with chronic peripheral arterial disease (PAD), prescribed drugs include hemorrheologic and antiplatelet agents. Pentoxifylline (Trental) is a hemorrheologic agent that increases the flexibility of red blood cells; it decreases blood viscosity by inhibiting platelet aggregation and decreasing fibrinogen and thus increases blood flow in the extremities. Many clients report limited improvement in their daily lives after taking pentoxifylline. Moreover, clients with extremely limited endurance for walking have reported improvement to the point that they can perform some activities (e.g., walk to the mailbox or dining room) that were previously impossible.

Two commonly used drugs for clients with PAD are the antiplatelet agents, such as aspirin (acetylsalicylic acid, Ancasal✦), and dipyridamole (Persantine, Apo-Dipyridamole✦). Aspirin, 325 mg/day, is typically recommended for life for all clients with chronic PAD.

Controlling hypertension can improve tissue perfusion by maintaining pressures that are adequate to perfuse the periphery but not vasoconstrict the vessels. Nurses should make clients aware of the effect of blood pressure on the circulation and should instruct clients in methods of control. For example, clients taking beta-blockers may experience drug-related claudication or an exacerbation of their symptoms. The physician, Nurse Practitioner, and/or nurse closely monitor clients with PAD who are receiving beta-blockers.

Percutaneous Transluminal Angioplasty. Another nonsurgical but invasive method of improving arterial flow is percutaneous transluminal balloon angioplasty (PTBA) (Fig. 38–5). One or more arteries are dilated with a balloon catheter advanced through a cannula, which is inserted into or above an occluded or stenosed artery. When the procedure is successful, it opens the vessel lumen and improves arterial blood flow, creating a smooth inner vessel surface. Clients who are candidates for PTBA must have occlusions or stenoses that are accessible to the catheter. The physician often uses PTA for

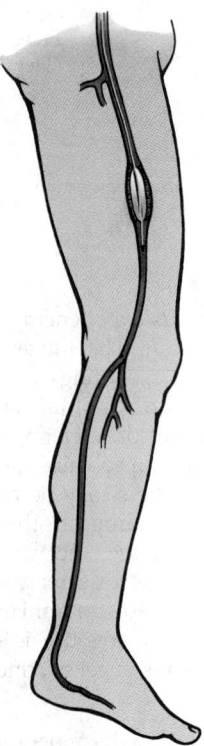

Figure 38–5. Percutaneous transluminal balloon angioplasty.

clients who are poor surgical candidates who cannot withstand general anesthesia or for whom amputation may be inevitable. Clients can experience reocclusion after this procedure, and the procedure may be repeated. Some clients have been occlusion free for up to 3–5 years, whereas others experience reocclusion within a year of PTBA.

During percutaneous transluminal angioplasty, intravascular stents may be placed to ensure adequate blood flow in a stenosed vessel. Candidates for this type of procedure are individuals with stenosis of the common or external iliac arteries. This type of procedure is cost effective and results in shorter hospital stays and earlier recoveries.

Laser-Assisted Angioplasty. Another invasive procedure is laser-assisted angioplasty. A laser probe is advanced through a cannula similar to that used for percutaneous transluminal angioplasty (PTA). Laser-assisted angioplasty is usually reserved for clients with smaller occlusions in the distal superficial femoral, proximal popliteal, and common iliac arteries. Heat from the laser vaporizes the arteriosclerotic plaque to open the occluded or stenosed artery. If significant stenosis remains after the artery is opened, a PTA balloon catheter may be inserted to further dilate the artery.

Preparation of the client for PTA or laser-assisted angioplasty is similar to that for diagnostic angiography. The client must have nothing by mouth (NPO) after midnight. The surgeon may require that the client scrub the groin area with an antiseptic solution.

Post-procedure nursing care involves observing for bleeding at the puncture site. The nurse or assistive nursing personnel closely observes vital signs and frequently checks the distal pulses in both limbs. These clients are typically restricted to bed rest, with the limb straight for approximately 6–8 hours before ambulation. Many of these clients receive anticoagulant therapy, such as heparin (Heplean♦), for approximately 3 days and then dipyridamole (Persantine, Apo-Dipyridamole♦) for 3–6 months at home. Clients usually take aspirin on a permanent basis.

Atherectomy. The technique of mechanical rotational abrasive atherectomy is used to improve blood flow to ischemic limbs in people with peripheral arterial disease. The rotational atherectomy device (Rotablator) is a high-speed rotary, metal bur ranging in size from 1.25 to 4.5 mm in diameter. The distal half of the bur is embedded with fine abrasive bits, which at rotational speeds of 100,000–120,000 rotations per minute result in fine-particle destruction of tissue. The Rotablator is designed to preferentially scrape "hard" surfaces (such as plaque) while minimizing damage to the vessel surface.

➤ Surgical Management

Clients with severe rest pain or claudication that interferes with the ability to work or threatens loss of a limb become surgical candidates. Arterial revascularization is the surgical procedure most commonly used to increase arterial blood flow in an affected limb.

Surgical procedures are classified as inflow or outflow. Inflow procedures involve bypassing arterial occlusions above the superficial femoral arteries (SFAs). Outflow procedures involve surgical bypassing of arterial occlusions at or below the superficial femoral arteries. For clients who have both inflow and outflow problems, the inflow procedure (for larger arteries) is done before the outflow repair.

Inflow procedures include aortoiliac, aortofemoral, and axillofemoral bypasses. Outflow procedures include femoropopliteal and femorotibial bypasses. Inflow procedures are more successful, with less chance of reocclusion or postoperative ischemia. Outflow procedures are less successful in relieving ischemic pain and are associated with a higher incidence of reocclusion.

Graft materials for the bypasses are selected on an individual basis. For outflow procedures, the preferred graft material is an autogenous saphenous vein. However, these clients can experience systemic vascular disease and may need this vein for coronary artery bypass. When the saphenous vein is not usable, the client's cephalic or basilic arm veins may be used.

Grafts made of synthetic materials, such as polytetrafluoroethylene, Gore-Tex, and Dacron, have also been used when autogenous veins were not available. Although synthetic grafts have achieved adequate patency in arteries above the knee, they have failed to achieve satisfactory results in infrapopliteal outflow vessels. In addition, autogenous veins are often not long enough for use in these vessels. Composite grafts constructed from multiple vein segments offer even better patency to arteries below the knee.

Preoperative Care. Preparing the client for surgery is similar to that described for the client having general or epidural anesthesia (see Chap. 20). Documentation of vital signs and peripheral pulses provides a baseline of information for comparison during the postoperative phase. Depending on the surgical procedure, the client may have an intravenous (IV) line, urinary catheter, central venous catheter, and/or arterial line. To prevent postoperative infection, clients typically receive antibiotic therapy before the procedure.

Operative Procedures. The anesthesiologist or nurse anesthetist places the client under general, epidural, or spinal anesthesia. Epidural or spinal induction is preferred for older adults to decrease the risk of cardiopulmonary complications in this group. If arterial bypass is to be accomplished by autogenous grafts, the surgeon excises the appropriate veins through an incision. The occluded artery is then exposed through an incision, and the conduit veins or synthetic graft material is sutured above and below the occlusion to facilitate blood flow around the occlusion.

For *aortoiliac* and *aortofemoral* bypass surgery, the surgeon makes a midline incision into the abdominal cavity to expose the abdominal aorta, with additional incisions into each groin (Fig. 38–6). Graft material is tunneled from the aorta to the groin incisions, where it is sutured in place.

In an *axillofemoral* bypass (Fig. 38–7), the surgeon makes an incision beneath the clavicle and tunnels graft material subcutaneously with a catheter from the chest to the iliac crest, into a groin incision, where it is sutured in place. Neither the thoracic nor the abdominal cavity is entered. For this reason, the axillofemoral bypass is used for high-risk clients who cannot tolerate a procedure requiring abdominal surgery.

Postoperative Care. Graft occlusion often occurs within the first 24 hours. Therefore, astute nursing care is crucial. The Client Care Plan highlights the most important aspects of postoperative care.

Assessment for Graft Occlusion. The nurse monitors the patency of the graft by checking the extremity every 15 minutes for the first hour, then hourly for changes in color, temperature, and pulse intensity. Warmth, redness, and edema of the affected extremity are often expected outcomes of surgery as a result of increased blood flow. Immediately postoperatively, the operating room or post-anesthesia unit (PACU) nurse marks the site where the distal (dorsalis pedis or posterior tibial) pulse is best palpated or heard by Doppler ultrasonography. The nurse communicates this information to the nursing staff on the unit where the client will go.

Pain is frequently the first indicator of postoperative graft occlusion. Many people experience a throbbing pain owing to the increased blood flow to the extremity. This sensation is different from ischemic pain, and the nurse must assess the type of pain that the client is experiencing. If graft occlusion occurs, the client will experience a sharp increase in ischemic pain, described as similar to the pain felt before surgery. The nurse reports severe pain to the surgeon immediately.

Promotion of Graft Patency. To promote graft patency, the nurse monitors the client's blood pressure and notifies the surgeon if the pressure increases or decreases beyond normal limits. Hypotension may indicate hypovolemia, which can increase the risk of clotting. Range of motion of the affected limb is usually limited, with bending of the hip and knee contraindicated. The nurse consults with the surgeon on a case-by-case basis regarding

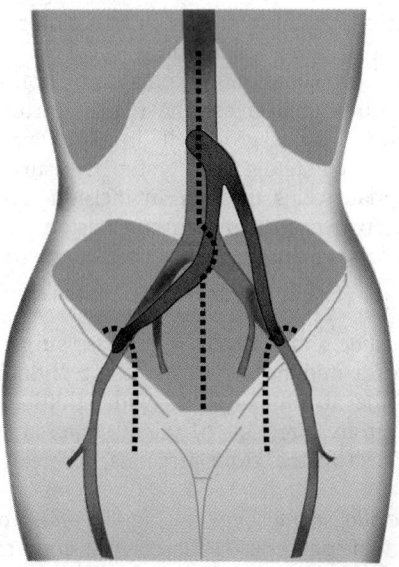

Figure 38–6. In aortoiliac and aortofemoral bypass surgery, a midline incision into the abdominal cavity is required, with an additional incision in each groin.

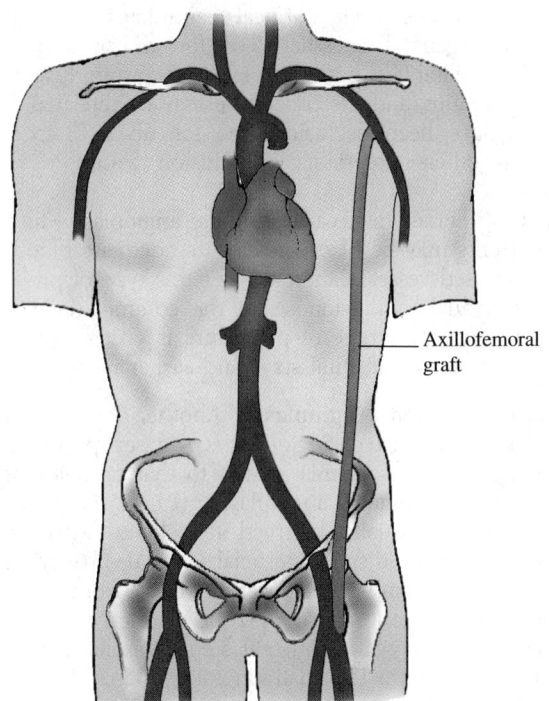

Figure 38–7. An axillofemoral bypass graft.

limitations of movement, including turning. Clients are restricted to bed rest for at least 24 hours postoperatively.

The nurse instructs all clients to cough and deep breathe every 1–2 hours and to use an incentive spirometer. Clients who have had aortoiliac or aortofemoral bypass are allowed nothing by mouth (NPO) for at least 1 day postoperatively. Clients who have undergone bypass surgery of the lower extremities not involving the aorta or abdominal wall (femoropopliteal or femorotibial bypass) may be on NPO status the night of surgery but are often allowed clear liquids the morning after surgery.

Treatment of Graft Occlusion. If manifestations of graft occlusion occur, the nurse notifies the surgeon immediately. Perfusion through the graft must be resolved promptly to avoid ischemic injury to the limb. Emergency *thrombectomy* (removal of the clot), which the surgeon may perform at the bedside, is the most common treatment for acute graft occlusion. Thrombectomy is associated with excellent results in prosthetic grafts but variable results in autogenous vein grafts, which often necessitate graft revision and even replacement.

Local intra-arterial *thrombolytic therapy* with urokinase (Abbokinase) may be used for acute graft occlusions in selected clients in settings where health providers are experts on its use. The physician considers thrombolytic therapy when the surgical alternative (e.g., thrombectomy with or without graft revision or replacement) carries high morbidity or mortality or when surgery for this type of occlusion has traditionally yielded poor results. When the physician uses urokinase, the nurse closely assesses the client for signs and symptoms of bleeding.

Monitoring for Compartment Syndrome. Compartment syndrome occurs when tissue pressure within a

Client Care Plan

The Client Having Peripheral Arterial Revascularization (Bypass) Surgery

Nursing Diagnosis No. 1: Altered Tissue Perfusion (Peripheral)

Expected Outcomes	Nursing Interventions	Rationale
The client will retain and maintain an increase in arterial blood flow to an extremity previously deprived of arterial blood flow.	■ Assess color, temperature, and pulse intensity of the affected extremity hourly. Notify the surgeon of a significant change.	■ Color, temperature, and pulse intensity immediately postoperatively indicate optimal arterial flow achieved with revascularization. Any increase in pallor or cyanosis or decrease in temperature or pulse intensity indicates postoperative graft occlusion.
	■ Assess the client for pain in the affected extremity, and report, if described, as "severe, similar to the pain before surgery."	■ Severe pain, similar to the pain felt before surgery, is frequently the first indicator of postoperative graft occlusion.
	■ Monitor the client's blood pressure, and report if it is increased or decreased beyond the client's normal limits.	■ Hypotension may indicate hypovolemia, which can increase the risk of clotting. Hypertension may put stress on the graft.
	■ Instruct the client to keep the affected extremity straight, limit movement, and avoid flexion of the knee and hip. Consult with the surgeon about turning the client.	■ Pressure on the graft can facilitate clot formation.
	■ Assess the incision for drainage, edema, and temperature.	■ Edema of the affected extremity is an expected outcome, but excessive edema should be reported.
		■ A small amount of bloody drainage is expected, but excessive bleeding is abnormal.
		■ Warmth, erythema, or a hard, tender area around the incision may indicate infection.

confined body space becomes elevated and restricts blood flow. The resultant ischemia can lead to tissue damage and eventually tissue death. The nurse assesses the client's motor and sensory function of the affected extremity. The extremity should also be assessed for worsening pain, fullness, swelling, and tenseness. These symptoms should be reported to the health care provider immediately. When compartment syndrome is suspected, the nurse continues to assess the extremity and removes or loosens the dressings and places the extremity at the level of the heart.

Assessment of Infection. Graft or wound infections can be life threatening and can endanger the client's limb. The nurse uses sterile technique when in contact with the incision and observes for symptoms of infection at or around the graft and incision sites. If the area over the graft becomes hard, tender, red, or warm, the client may have an infection. The nurse notifies the surgeon if any of these symptoms occurs.

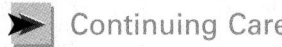

➤ Continuing Care

➤ *Case Management*

Peripheral arterial disease is a chronic, long-term problem with frequent complications. PAD may benefit from a case manager who can follow the client across the continuum of care. The goal is to maintain the client in the home environment.

➤ *Home Care Management*

Managing the client at home often requires an interdisciplinary team approach. Chart 38–7 outlines the assessment highlights for home care clients with peripheral vascular disease. The clinical guide in Figure 38–8 shows how one home care agency documents care for homebound clients with PAD.

➤ *Health Teaching*

The nurse instructs all clients on methods to promote vasodilation. Clients are taught to avoid raising their legs above the level of the heart unless they also have venous stasis. The nurse provides written and oral instructions on foot care and methods to prevent injury and ulcer development for all clients (Chart 38–8).

The nurse teaches clients receiving pentoxifylline (Trental) to take the drug as prescribed, whether or not they notice improvement, because the drug may take 6–8 weeks to be effective and the effect may not be apparent. Pentoxifylline should be taken with meals to prevent side effects of nausea and vomiting.

Clients receiving dipyridamole (Persantine) are instructed to take the medication 1 hour before meals to promote optimal absorption. The nurse advises clients taking aspirin to take the drug with meals or milk and crackers and to report any nausea or vomiting.

Clients who have had surgery require additional instruction on incision care (see Chap. 22). The nurse encourages all clients to avoid smoking and to limit dietary fat intake to less than 30% of the total daily calories.

The client with chronic arterial obstruction may fear recurrent occlusion or further narrowing of the artery. Clients often fear that they might lose a limb or become debilitated in other ways. Indeed, chronic peripheral arterial disease (PAD) may worsen, especially in clients with diabetes mellitus. The nurse, however, reassures clients that their participation in prescribed exercise, diet, and pharmacologic therapy, along with cessation of smoking, can limit further formation of atherosclerotic plaques.

ELDERLY CONSIDERATIONS

Older clients with peripheral vascular disease may have visual or mobility problems that impede their ability to effectively provide foot care. The nurse can suggest using magnifying mirrors to check the feet and toes for cracks or blisters. Prior to washing the feet with mild soap and warm water, the temperature of the water should be tested with a thermometer or elbow, not the hand. Older adults may be at increased risk for trauma or self-inflicted injury. They should be advised never to go barefoot, to wear cotton socks, and to wear protective shoes. They should be advised to see a podiatrist to trim their toenails and manage corns or calluses.

➤ *Health Care Resources*

Clients with arterial compromise may need assistance with activities of daily living (ADLs) if activity is limited by pain. The client may need to limit or avoid stair climbing depending on the severity of disease. Clients who have undergone surgery usually need temporary help with activities of daily living.

Clients who must limit activity because of peripheral arterial disease may benefit from the assistance of a home health aide. The client who has undergone surgery may require a home health nurse to assist with incision care. The nurse or case manager arranges for home care resources before the client is discharged.

Acute Peripheral Arterial Occlusion

Overview

Although chronic peripheral arterial disease (PAD) progresses slowly, the onset of acute arterial occlusions may be sudden and dramatic. An embolus is the most common cause of peripheral occlusions, although a local

---

Chart 38–7

Focused Assessment for Home Care: Clients with Peripheral Vascular Disease

- Assess tissue perfusion to affected extremity(ies), including
  - Distal circulation, sensation, and motion
  - Presence of pain, pallor, paresthesias, pulselessness, paralysis, poikilothermia (coolness)
  - Ankle/brachial index
- Assess adherence to therapeutic regime, including
  - Following foot care instructions
  - Quitting smoking
  - Maintaining dietary restrictions
  - Participating in exercise regime
  - Avoiding exposure to cold and constrictive clothing
- Assess ability to manage wound care and prevent further injury, including
  - Use of compression stockings or compression pumps as directed
  - Use of various dressing materials
  - Signs and symptoms to report to nurse
- Assess coping ability of client and family members
- Assess home environment, including
  - Safety hazards, especially related to falls

Multidisciplinary Clinical Guide
Visit Summary

Instructions: Associate Nurse or Practitioner of an Associated Discipline, please complete this visit summary and transmit to the Nursing Case Manager within 24 hours of the completion of each visit.

Date: _____   Name of Patient: _____   and/or Caregiver: _____

Medical Diagnoses: _____

Discipline of Professional Making Visit: _____

Discharge Planning Started: _____

Discipline-Specific Diagnoses Treated at this visit:

_____

_____

Discipline-Specific Goals: (Note any change in goal(s) with reason for change)

_____

_____

Assessment Changes to Be Noted by Case Manager:

_____

_____

Variances from POC Detected: (use key numbers and explain if needed)

_____

_____

_____

Note follow-up care needed or plan for discharge:

_____

_____

Physician Contacted: _____

New Orders: _____

Signature: _____   Date: _____

Variances:

Key
1. Psychosocial
2. Environment
3. Physiological
4. Health-related behaviors
5. Other

Figure 38–8. Multidisciplinary clinical guide visit summary. (From Wills, E. M., & Sloan, H. L. [1996]. Assessing peripheral arterial disorders in the home: A multidisciplinary clinical guide. *Home Health Care Nurse, 14*(9), 670–674.)

thrombus may be the cause. Occlusion may affect the upper extremities, but it is more common in the lower extremities. Emboli originating from the heart are the most common cause of acute arterial occlusions. Most clients with an embolic occlusion have had an acute myocardial infarction and/or atrial fibrillation within the preceding weeks.

Collaborative Management

 Assessment

Clients with acute arterial occlusion describe severe pain below the level of the occlusion that occurs even at rest.

Criterion		Admission Date:	V	V	V	V	V
KNOWLEDGE	**Assessment Data Key:** 1 = none; 2 = minimal; 3 = basic; 4 = adequate; 5 = superior						
Patient/family	General knowledge about PAD (include smoking)						
Caregiver able to:	1. Inspect daily: blisters, itching, cuts, lesions, redness, pain, swelling, heat, dryness, calluses, corns 2. Administer hygiene: 　a. Wash daily with warm water 　b. Dry carefully between toes 　c. Change socks, shoes daily						
Selecting footwear	1. Shoes (leather, avoids synthetic) 　a. Style (wide toe, avoids sandals) 　b. Inside condition (no foreign objects, nail points, lining intact, no rough areas) 　c. Wears shoes in- and outdoors 　d. Correctly breaks in new shoes (wear for 20–30 minutes daily)						
Skin care	1. Corn/callus care 　a. No chemical products used 　b. Pumice stone if sensitive 2. Dry skin care 　a. Uses superfatted soap 　b. Water temp 90–105°F 　c. Emollient to dry areas before drying skin (none between toes)						
Professional care	1. Identifies need for care 2. Reports problems (skin breakdown, edema, ingrown toenails, inability to trim nails safely, shoe problems, rest or night pain) 3. Has routine foot assessment quarterly						
Medications	1. Identifies name and dose 2. Verbalizes reason for use 3. Avoids over-the-counter drugs (interactions with prescriptions)						
Monitors pain and complications	1. Degree and type of pain 2. Identifies one complication (ulcer, gangrene, amputation, functional limitations)						
Exercise/rest	1. Exercise patterns 2. Control of symptoms						
Diet	Knows diet. Type: Activate teaching plan if necessary						

Figure 38–8. *Continued*

The affected extremity is cool or cold, pulseless, and mottled. Minute areas on the toes may be blackened or gangrenous. Clients with acute arterial insufficiency often present with the "six Ps" of ischemia: pain, pallor, pulselessness, paresthesia, paralysis, and poikilothermia (coolness) of the involved extremity.

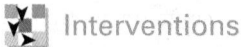 Interventions

The health care provider must initiate treatment promptly to avoid permanent damage or loss of an extremity. Anticoagulant therapy with heparin (Hepalean♦) is usually the first intervention to prevent further clot formation. A bo-

Criterion		Admission Date:	V	V	V	V	V
KNOWLEDGE *(continued)*	**Assessment Data Key:** 1 = none; 2 = minimal; 3 = basic; 4 = adequate; 5 = superior						
Discipline-specific diagnoses and goal dates:	1. Goal date: Met? (y/n)						
Discipline: Specifiy							
Goal achieved (y/n) Variances: Key 1. Psychosocial 2. Environment 3. Physiological 4. Health-related behaviors 5. Other							
Comments							
BEHAVIOR	**Behavior displayed is appropriate: Key:** 1 = not; 2 = rarely; 3 = inconsistently; 4 = usually; 5 = consistently						
Diet	Type of diet: Follows diet:						
Smoking	Changes in smoking behavior:						
Medications List:	Medications taken correctly						
Problem solving	Identifies preferences, assists nurse to individualize plan of care (POC)						
Community resources	Needs referrals for: a. Meal preparation d. Healthcare funding b. Transportation e. Support groups c. Personal care f. Shoe fitting, care						
Coping skills	Identifies ways to deal with pain, loss of function						
Beliefs/self-efficacy	a. Identifies beliefs about ability to follow POC b. Beliefs about insensitive feet 1. no pain = no problem 2. no pain means no care is required c. Nurse may have to reinterpret signs and symptoms for client						
Motivation	Client/family motivation to follow POC?						
Diagnoses and goal dates:	1. Goal date: Met? (y/n)						

Figure 38–8. *Continued*

Criterion		Admission Date:	V	V	V	V	V
BEHAVIOR (continued)	**Behavior displayed is appropriate:** **Key:** 1 = not; 2 = rarely; 3 = inconsistently; 4 = usually; 5 = consistently						
Discipline(s): Specify with diagnosis							
Goal achieved (y/n) Variances: Key 1. Psychosocial 2. Environment 3. Physiological 4. Health-related behaviors 5. Other							
Comments							
STATUS	**Assessment Data Key: Signs & Symptoms:** 1 = extreme; 2 = severe; 3 = moderate; 4 = minimal; 5 = none						
Foot assessment Nails Hygiene Footwear	Inspection: 1. Nails cut straight across or slightly rounded 2. Rate hygiene good, fair, poor 3. Footwear adequate or inadequate a. Socks (materials: cotton, wool, polyester blend) Cautions: nonrestricting fit, no circular garters or constricting clothes, no knee-highs b. Shoes (Check type, fit, condition)						
Skin	1. Color (rubor, pallor, cyanosis, blackened areas) 2. Temperature (check both extremities, note differences) 3. Edema (pitting/nonpitting Grade [1−4]/4)						
Atrophy	Skin (shiny, pale, translucent)						
Changes to foot	1. Toenails (label as thickened, discolored, deformed) 2. Corns/calluses (describe location, size) 3. Deformities (describe in nurse's note; presence of hammer toes, claw toes, bunions)						
Vital signs Post, tibial pulse Blood pressure	Grade pulse (Use 0−4/4 [0 = not palpable, 1 = easily obliterated, 2 = easily palpable, 3 = not easily obliterated, 4 = strong, bounding]) Both arms and do orthostatic if possible						
Ulcerations (location)	Describe completely in nurse's notes and on wound flow sheet						

Figure 38–8. Continued

Criterion		Admission Date:	V	V	V	V	V
STATUS (continued)	**Assessment Data Key: Signs & Symptoms:** 1 = extreme; 2 = severe; 3 = moderate; 4 = minimal; 5 = none						
Complication potential (Evaluate on admission and every 60 days)	Ulcer, ischemia gangrene, functional limitations						
ABI on admission (Reassess if post-tibial pulse changes)	1. Blood pressure at brachial and ankle locations bilaterally 2. Use Doppler if possible 3. Calculate index from highest readings (A/B = ABI)						
Protective sensation	Measure with Semmes/Weinstein Monofilament. (10 g/0.5). Apply to feet and ankles and random areas (present or not).						
Discipline-specific diagnoses and goal dates:	1. Goal date: Met? (y/n)						
Discipline: Specify							
Goal achieved (y/n) Variances: Key 1. Psychosocial 2. Environment 3. Physiological 4. Health-related behaviors 5. Other							
Comments							

Figure 38–8. *Continued*

Education Guide: Foot Care for the Client with Peripheral Vascular Disease

- Keep your feet clean by washing them with a mild soap in room-temperature water.
- Keep your feet dry, especially between the toes and ankles.
- Avoid injury to your feet and ankles. Wear comfortable, well-fitting shoes. Never go without shoes.
- Keep your toenails clean and filed. Have someone cut them if you cannot see them clearly. Cut your toenails straight across.
- To prevent dry, cracked skin, apply a lubricating lotion to your feet.
- Prevent exposure to extreme heat or cold. Never use a heating pad on your feet.
- Avoid constricting garments.
- If a problem develops, see a podiatrist or physician.
- Avoid extended pressure on your feet or ankles, such as occurs when you lean against something.

lus up to 10,000 U may be ordered. The client may also undergo angiography.

A surgical thrombectomy or embolectomy with local anesthesia may be performed to remove the occlusion. The physician makes an incision, followed by an arteriotomy (a surgical opening into an artery). The physician then inserts a Fogarty catheter into the artery and retrieves the embolus. It may be necessary to close the artery with a patch graft.

Postoperatively, the nurse monitors the affected extremity for improvement in color, temperature, and pulse, as well as other extremities for signs and symptoms of new thrombi or emboli. Pain should significantly diminish after the surgical procedure, although mild incisional pain remains. The nurse watches closely for complications caused by reperfusing the artery after thrombectomy or embolectomy, which include spasms and swelling of the skeletal muscle. Swelling of the skeletal muscles is characterized by edema, pain on passive movement, poor capillary refill, numbness, and muscle tenseness. Fasciotomy (surgical opening into the tissues) may be necessary to prevent further injury and save the limb.

The use of systemic thrombolytic therapy for acute arterial occlusions has been disappointing because bleeding complications have outweighed the benefits obtained. Local intra-arterial thrombolytic therapy with urokinase (Abbokinase) has emerged as an alternative to surgical treatment in selected clients in settings where health providers are familiar with its use and its complications. When urokinase is given, the nurse monitors the client for signs and symptoms of bleeding, bruising, or hematoma. If any of these complications occurs, the nurse notifies the physician immediately.

Aneurysms

Overview

An aneurysm is a permanent localized dilation of an artery, which enlarges the artery to at least two times its normal diameter.

Types of Aneurysms

An aneurysm may be described as *fusiform* (a diffuse dilation affecting the entire circumference of the artery) or *saccular* (an out pouching affecting only a distinct portion of the artery). Aneurysms may also be described as true or false. In true aneurysms the arterial wall is weakened by congenital or acquired problems. False aneurysms occur as the result of vessel injury or trauma to all three layers of the arterial wall.

Dissecting hematomas, traditionally called *dissecting aneurysms,* are more accurately described as *aortic dissections* (see later). Aortic dissections differ from aneurysms in that they are formed when blood accumulates in the wall of an artery.

Aneurysms tend to occur at specific anatomic sites (Fig. 38–9), most commonly in the abdominal aorta. Aneurysms often occur at a point where the artery is not supported by skeletal muscles or on the lines of curves or flexion in the arterial tree.

Pathophysiologic Process

An aneurysm forms when the middle layer (media) of the artery is weakened, producing a stretching effect in the inner layer (intima) and outer layers (adventitia) of the artery. As the artery widens, tension in the wall increases and further widening occurs, thus enlarging the aneurysm. Hypertension (high blood pressure) produces more tension and enlargement within the artery. As the aneurysm grows, the risk of arterial rupture increases.

Abdominal aortic aneurysms account for approximately 75% of all aneurysms. Most of these aneurysms are located between the renal arteries and the aortic bifurcation. Of all abdominal aortic aneurysms greater than 6 cm in diameter, 50% rupture within 1 year; of those aneurysms smaller than 6 cm in diameter, 15%–20% rupture.

Thoracic aneurysms account for approximately 25% of all aneurysms. They commonly develop between the origin of the left subclavian artery and the diaphragm. They are located in the descending, ascending, and transverse sections of the aorta.

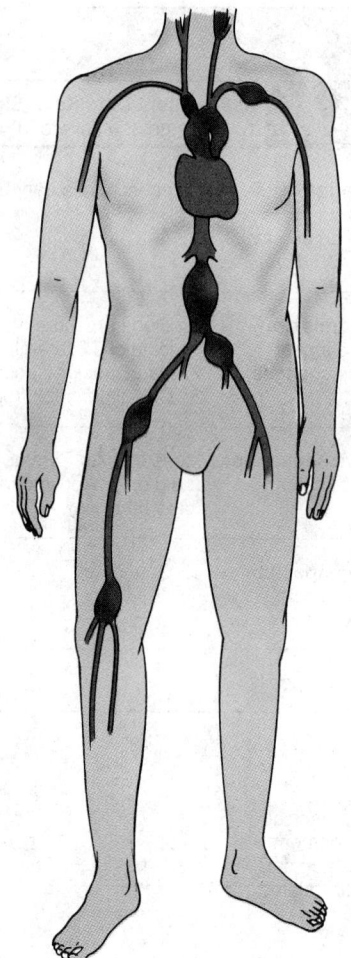

Figure 38–9. Common anatomic sites of arterial aneurysms.

Aneurysms can cause symptoms by exerting pressure on surrounding structures or by rupturing. Rupture of an aneurysm is the most frequent complication and is life threatening because abrupt and massive hemorrhagic shock occurs with the rupture. Thrombi within the wall of an aneurysm can also be the source of emboli in distal arteries below the aneurysm.

Atherosclerosis is the most common cause of all aneurysms, with hypertension and cigarette smoking being contributing factors. Syphilis and Ehlers-Danlos syndrome are other causes of abdominal aortic aneurysms, and there may be a familial risk.

The incidence of abdominal aortic aneurysms, estimated to be between 30 and 66 per 1000 people, is increasing in the Western world. Approximately 15,000 people in the United States die annually from abdominal aneurysms, making it the 13th leading cause of death in the United States. Thoracic aneurysms occur most often in older adults.

Abdominal aortic aneurysms are more common in men than women (with a ratio of 4:1). Approximately 10% of aortic aneurysms are thoracic (Tierney, 1995).

Collaborative Management

 Assessment

Most clients with abdominal aortic or thoracic aneurysms are asymptomatic when their aneurysms are first discovered by routine examination or during radiographic study performed for another reason.

➤ *Abdominal Aortic Aneurysms*

Because clients may have symptoms, the nurse assesses clients with known or suspected abdominal aortic aneurysm for abdominal, flank, or back pain. Pain related to an abdominal aortic aneurysm is usually steady, with a gnawing quality, unaffected by movement, and may last for hours or days.

The nurse observes for a pulsation in the upper abdomen slightly to the left of the midline between the xiphoid process and the umbilicus. A detectable aneurysm is at least 5 cm in size. The nurse then auscultates for a bruit over the mass but avoids palpating the mass because it may be tender and there is a risk of rupture.

Although some clients have symptoms when the aneurysm is intact, many clients are asymptomatic until the time of rupture. If expansion and impending rupture of an abdominal aortic aneurysm is suspected, the nurse assesses for severe pain of sudden onset in the back or lower abdomen, which may radiate to the groin, buttocks, or legs.

Clients with a rupturing abdominal aortic aneurysm are critically ill in hemorrhagic (hypovolemic) shock. Signs include hypotension, diaphoresis, mental obtundation, oliguria, and dysrhythmias. Retroperitoneal hemorrhage is manifested by hematomas in the flanks. Rupture into the abdominal cavity causes abdominal distention.

➤ *Thoracic Aneurysms*

When a thoracic aneurysm is suspected, the nurse assesses the client for back pain and manifestations of compression of the aneurysm on adjacent structures. Signs include shortness of breath, hoarseness, and difficulty swallowing.

Thoracic aneurysms are not often detected by physical assessment, but occasionally a mass may be visible above the suprasternal notch.

The client with suspected rupture of a thoracic aneurysm is assessed for sudden and excruciating back or chest pain. Rupture of a thoracic aneurysm is also indicated by hemorrhagic shock (see Chap. 39).

➤ *Radiographic Assessment*

An abdominal x-ray or lateral film of the spine often shows an abdominal aortic aneurysm. The "eggshell" appearance of the aneurysm is essentially diagnostic.

Computed tomographic (CT) scanning is the standard tool for assessing the size and location of an aortic aneurysm. A thoracic aneurysm can be diagnosed by chest x-ray. A CT scan is used to assess size and location. Aortic arteriography is performed for all clients who are to undergo surgical repair of a thoracic aneurysm.

➤ *Other Diagnostic Assessment*

Ultrasonography is a noninvasive technique that provides an accurate diagnosis as well as information about the size and location of an abdominal aortic aneurysm.

 Interventions

The size of the aneurysm and the presence of symptoms are the most important parameters in the determination of treatment.

➤ *Nonsurgical Management*

The goal of nonsurgical management is to maintain the blood pressure at a normal level to decrease the risk of rupture and monitor the growth of the aneurysm.

Because elevated blood pressure can increase the rate of aneurysmal enlargement, hypertension is an important risk factor for rupture. Clients with hypertension are treated with antihypertensives to decrease the rate of enlargement and the risk for early rupture.

For clients with small or asymptomatic aneurysms, frequent CT scans are necessary to monitor the growth of the aneurysm. The nurse emphasizes the importance of following through with scheduled tests to monitor the growth. The nurse also explains the clinical manifestations of aneurysms that need to be promptly reported.

➤ *Surgical Management*

Surgical management of an aneurysm may be an elective or an emergency procedure. For all clients with either a rupturing abdominal aortic or a thoracic aneurysm, emergency surgery is performed.

Clients with an abdominal aortic aneurysm 6 cm in diameter or wider undergo elective surgery. Some surgeons favor surgical treatment for clients with aneurysms 4–6 cm in diameter if the client is in good health. Clients in good health with aneurysms smaller than 4 cm and clients in poor health with aneurysms 4–6 cm in diameter undergo nonsurgical treatment until the aneurysm reaches 6 cm.

Clients with thoracic aneurysms measuring 7 cm or more in diameter and clients with smaller aneurysms that are producing symptoms are advised to have elective surgery. Clients with aneurysms smaller than 7 cm in diameter that are not causing symptoms are treated nonsurgically until symptoms occur or the aneurysm enlarges to 7 cm.

The most common procedure performed for clients with an abdominal aortic aneurysm is an abdominal aortic aneurysm (AAA) resection or repair (aneurysmectomy). The mortality rate for elective AAA resection is 2%–5%. The mortality rate for emergency surgery for expanding abdominal aortic aneurysms is 5%–15% and 50% for those that have ruptured.

The major surgery for clients with a thoracic aneurysm is a thoracic aneurysm repair. Elective resection of these aneurysms is associated with a 10% mortality rate.

Abdominal Aortic Aneurysm Resection. In an abdominal aortic aneurysm resection, the physician excises the aneurysm from the abdominal aorta to prevent or repair its rupture. The goal is to secure stable aortic integrity and tissue perfusion throughout the body.

Preoperative Care. Interventions are similar to those for clients undergoing surgery with general anesthesia (see Chap. 20). A bowel preparation and emphasis on coughing and deep breathing are very important. Because a significant blood loss often occurs during AAA resection, clients planning elective surgery may be advised to bank their blood for autologous (self) transfusions postoperatively.

The nurse assesses all peripheral pulses to serve as a baseline for comparison postoperatively. The nurse may mark where the pulse is palpated or heard by Doppler ultrasonography to facilitate locating the pulse postoperatively.

Clients with ruptured aneurysms are brought to the operating suite directly from the emergency department. Preoperative care of clients with ruptured aneurysms involves administration of large volumes of intravenous (IV) fluids to maintain tissue perfusion.

Operative Procedure. The surgeon makes a midline abdominal incision from the xiphoid process to the symphysis pubis, or a wide transverse incision from flank to flank, to expose the aneurysm. Clamps are applied just above the aneurysm and below it, the aneurysm is excised, and a preclotted Dacron graft is sutured in an end-to-end fashion (Fig. 38–10).

Postoperative Care. Immediately postoperatively, the client is typically admitted to a critical care unit for 24 to 48 hours, depending on the age and condition of the client. In addition to providing the routine postoperative care discussed in Chapter 22, the nurse assesses for and

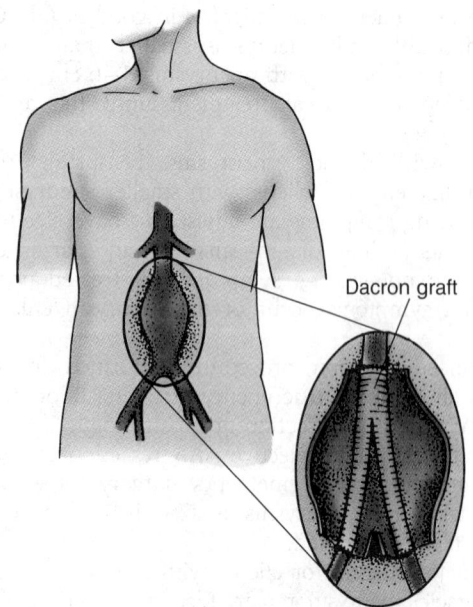

Figure 38–10. Surgical repair of abdominal aortic aneurysm with a woven Dacron graft.

assists in the prevention of the postoperative complications that can occur after an AAA repair. These complications include myocardial infarction, graft occlusion or rupture causing hemorrhage, hypovolemia and/or renal failure, respiratory distress, and paralytic ileus.

Myocardial Infarction. During the immediate postoperative period, the client's blood pressure will be monitored with an arterial catheter. Continuous cardiac monitoring will be used to detect any dysrhythmias. Using hemodynamic monitoring, the nurse monitors for low cardiac output and other findings consistent with acute myocardial infarction. The nurse also assesses for other signs of myocardial infarction, including chest pain, shortness of breath, complaints of dyspnea, diaphoresis, anxiety, and restlessness.

Graft Occlusion or Rupture. The nurse or assistive nursing personnel assesses vital signs and circulation every 15 minutes for the first hour, then hourly with assessment of pulses distal to the graft site (including posterior tibial and dorsalis pedis). The nurse reports any signs of graft occlusion or rupture, including

- Changes in pulses
- Cool to cold extremities below the graft
- White or blue extremities or flanks
- Severe pain
- Abdominal distention

The nurse limits elevation of the head of the bed to 45 degrees to avoid flexion of the graft.

Hypovolemia or Renal Failure. Hypovolemia and renal failure occur because there is often a large blood loss during surgery or before if rupture occurred. The nurse assesses urine output via Foley catheter hourly. If urine output is less than 50 mL/hour, the nurse notifies the surgeon. Although advances in surgical technique have decreased the risk of renal failure after clamping during surgery, renal failure may occur. Renal failure caused by acute tubular necrosis is more common after emergency surgery. In addition to monitoring urine output, the nurse and physician monitor serum creatinine and blood urea nitrogen levels daily.

Respiratory Distress. The nurse or assistive nursing personnel assesses the client's respiratory rate and depth every hour and auscultates breath sounds every 4 hours to monitor for respiratory complications. Often, the client is maintained on a ventilator at least overnight to facilitate respiratory exchange. The nurse administers opioids for pain, as ordered, and turns and suctions the client according to protocol. The nurse ensures firm abdominal support of the incision with a pillow or bath blanket, while the client is coughing, to prevent the incision from separating. After the client is extubated, the nurse or assistive nursing personnel assesses that the client turns, coughs, and deep breathes every 1 to 2 hours and increases his or her mobility as ordered.

Paralytic Ileus. Paralytic ileus after AAA repair is expected for 2–3 days. Clients have a nasogastric tube to low suction until bowel sounds return. The nurse listens for bowel sounds every 8 hours and reports their return to the physician. The nurse assesses for prolonged absence of bowel sounds and distention, which may indicate a prolonged ileus or a bowel infarction.

Thoracic Aneurysm Repair. Repair of thoracic aneurysms is tailored to each client; the procedure depends on the type and location of the aneurysm. Total cardiopulmonary bypass (CPB) is necessary for excision of aneurysms in the ascending aorta, and partial bypass is often used during excision of aneurysms in the descending aorta.

Preoperative Care. The care of the client undergoing thoracic aneurysm resection is similar to that provided for the client having thoracic surgery (see Chap. 34). Clients undergoing cardiopulmonary bypass receive care similar to that described in Chapter 40.

Operative Procedure. The surgeon uses either a thoracotomy or a median sternotomy approach to enter the thoracic cavity. The surgeon exposes the aneurysm and excises it. After excising the aneurysm, the surgeon usually sews a Dacron graft or prosthesis onto the aorta. Saccular aneurysms, which have an out pouching from a distinct portion of the arterial wall, can sometimes be removed without resection of the aorta.

Postoperative Care. The care of a client who has undergone thoracic aneurysm repair is similar to that after other chest surgery. Clients undergoing cardiopulmonary bypass receive care similar to that described in Chapter 40. The nurse assesses for and assists in the prevention of postoperative complications that can occur after a thoracic aneurysm repair. These complications include hemorrhage, ischemic colitis, spinal cord ischemia resulting in paraplegia, respiratory distress, and cardiac dysrhythmias.

Hemorrhage. The nurse assesses vital signs at least hourly, reporting any signs of hemorrhage (a drop in blood pressure, an increase in pulse rate, rapid respirations, diaphoresis) to the physician immediately. The nurse assesses for bleeding or separation at the graft site by noting significant increases in chest drainage from the chest tubes.

Paraplegia. Inadvertent interruption of the blood supply to the spinal cord during thoracic aneurysm repair can result in paraplegia. The nurse assesses the client hourly for sensation and motion in all extremities and reports deficits immediately.

Respiratory Distress. After thoracic aneurysm repair, clients are especially susceptible to respiratory distress from atelectasis or pneumonia. This problem occurs as a result of both cardiopulmonary bypass and incisional discomfort. Both atelectasis and pneumonia may cause shallow breathing and poor cough effort. These clients are often maintained on a ventilator, at least overnight, after surgery. For clients with a median sternotomy, the surgeon firmly splints the incision to prevent separation of the sternum.

Cardiac Dysrhythmias. The nurse assesses all clients recovering from thoracic aneurysm repair for cardiac dysrhythmias. The stress of the thoracic surgery, added to the increased incidence of arteriosclerosis in this group, may predispose these clients to a myocardial infarction, cardiac dysrhythmias, or heart failure.

 Continuing Care

Most clients after aneurysm repair are discharged home. In rare instances, the postoperative client may be discharged to an extended (long-term) care facility for rehabilitation in the absence of family or other support systems.

▶ *Home Care Management*

If discharged to home, the client must follow the instructions provided by the nurse regarding activity level and incisional care. Because stair climbing may be restricted initially, the client may need a bedside commode if the bathroom is inaccessible.

▶ *Health Teaching*

For clients who have not undergone surgical aneurysm repair, the teaching plan emphasizes the importance of compliance with the schedule of computed tomography (CT) scanning to monitor the size of the aneurysm. The nurse educates the client receiving treatment for hypertension about the importance of continuing to take prescribed medication. The client and family or significant other are instructed about signs and symptoms that they must promptly report to their health care provider:

- Clients with abdominal aortic aneurysms must report abdominal fullness or pain or back pain.
- Clients with thoracic aneurysms must report chest or back pain, shortness of breath, difficulty swallowing, or hoarseness.

The nurse teaches the client who has undergone repair of the aneurysm about activity restrictions, wound care, and pain management. Clients may not engage in activities that involve lifting heavy objects (usually more than 15–20 pounds, or 6.8–9.1 kg) for 6–12 weeks postoperatively. The nurse advises the client to use discretion in activities that involve pulling, pushing, or straining, such as vacuuming, changing bed linens, moving furniture, mopping or sweeping, raking leaves, mowing grass, and chopping wood. Clients should temporarily avoid such hobbies as tennis, swimming, horseback riding, and golf, although putting practice is allowed. Because of postoperative weakness, the client is usually restricted from driving a car for several weeks after discharge.

Clients who have not undergone aneurysm repair may fear rupture and subsequent death. The nurse assesses for the client's and family's perceptions of this potential situation. The nurse reinforces the rationales for CT monitoring of aneurysmal size and for controlling hypertension and encourages clients to verbalize their fears.

▶ *Health Care Resources*

In collaboration with the discharge planner, the nurse assesses the availability of transportation to and from appointments for clients needing CT monitoring. If transportation is a problem, the nurse consults the social worker to assist in arranging this service.

Clients who have undergone surgery may require the services of a home health nurse for assistance with dressing changes. A home health aide may be needed to assist with activities of daily living.

Aneurysms of the Peripheral Arteries

Overview

Although femoral and popliteal aneurysms are relatively uncommon, they are often associated with an aneurysm in another location of the arterial tree. To detect a popliteal aneurysm, the nurse palpates a pulsating mass in the popliteal space. To detect a femoral aneurysm, the nurse palpates a pulsatile mass over the femoral artery. The nurse evaluates both extremities because more than one femoral or popliteal aneurysm may be present.

Collaborative Management

The client may exhibit symptoms of limb ischemia, and the nurse assesses for diminished or absent pulses, cool to cold skin, and pain. Pain may also be present if an adjacent nerve is compressed. The recommended treatment for either type of aneurysm, regardless of the size, is surgery because of the risk of thromboembolic complications associated with their presence.

To treat a femoral aneurysm, the physician excises the aneurysm and restores circulation using a Dacron graft or an autogenous saphenous vein graft. Most surgeons prefer to bypass rather than resect a popliteal aneurysm.

Postoperatively, the nurse monitors for lower limb ischemia. The nurse palpates pulses below the graft to assess graft patency. Often, Doppler ultrasonography is necessary to assess blood flow when pulses are not palpable. Sudden development of pain or discoloration of the extremity is reported immediately to the physician because it may indicate graft occlusion.

Aortic Dissection

Overview

Aortic dissection has traditionally been referred to as a "dissecting aneurysm." However, because this condition is more accurately described as a dissecting hematoma, the term aortic dissection has gained favor.

Aortic dissection is thought to be caused by a sudden tear in the aortic intima, opening the way for blood to enter the aortic wall. Degeneration of the aortic media might be a prerequisite for this condition, with hypertension an important contributing factor.

Aortic dissection is a relatively common event, occurring in at least 2000 people in the United States annually. It is frequently associated with connective tissue disorders such as Marfan's syndrome. It also occurs in older people, peaking in adults in their 50s and 60s and in women in their third trimester of pregnancy.

Because the circulation of any major artery arising from the aorta can be impaired in clients with aortic dissection, this condition is highly lethal and represents an emergency situation.

Dissections are classified in various ways. Debakey's classification contains three groups:

- Type 1: Characterized by an intimal tear in the ascending (proximal) aorta, with extension of the dissection into the descending (distal) aorta
- Type 2: Originates in and is limited to the ascending (proximal) aorta
- Type 3: Arises within the descending (distal) thoracic aorta and often progresses distally

Proximal dissections occur almost twice as often as distal dissections. Although the ascending aorta and descending thoracic aorta are the most common sites, dissection can also occur in the abdominal aorta and other arteries.

Collaborative Management

The most common presenting symptom of aortic aneurysm is pain, with painless dissection occurring rarely. The pain is described as "tearing," "ripping," and "stabbing" and tends to move from its point of origin. Depending on the site of dissection, the client may feel pain in the anterior chest, back, neck, throat, jaw, or teeth.

Diaphoresis, nausea, vomiting, faintness, and apprehension are also common. Blood pressure is usually elevated unless complications, such as cardiac tamponade or rupture, have occurred. A decrease or absence of peripheral pulses is common, as is aortic regurgitation, characterized by a musical murmur heard better along the right sternal border. Neurologic deficits, such as altered level of consciousness, paraparesis, and cerebrovascular accidents, can also occur.

Chest x-ray, Doppler echocardiogram, computed tomography (CT), and aortic angiography are commonly used to confirm the diagnosis.

The goals of emergency treatment include
- The elimination of pain
- A reduction of blood pressure to 100 to 120 mmHg
- A decrease in the velocity of left ventricular ejection

The physician prescribes intravenous (IV) sodium nitroprusside (Nitropress) by continuous drip initially to lower the blood pressure. If this regimen is ineffective, nicardipine hydrochloride (Cardene) may be used. Propranolol (Inderal, Apo-Propranolol✦) is given in increments of 1 mg IV to decrease left ventricular ejection.

Subsequent treatment depends on the location of the dissection. Generally, clients receive continued medical treatment for uncomplicated distal dissections and surgical treatment for proximal dissections.

For clients receiving long-term medical treatment, the systolic blood pressure must be maintained at or below 130–140 mmHg. Beta-blockers (propranolol) and calcium channel antagonists are indicated.

Clients receiving surgical intervention for a proximal dissection always require total cardiopulmonary bypass (see Chap. 40). The surgeon excises the intimal tear and obliterates entry in the false opening by suturing edges of the dissected aorta. Usually, a prosthetic graft is used.

Buerger's Disease

Overview

Buerger's disease (thromboangiitis obliterans) is a relatively uncommon occlusive disease limited to the medium and small arteries and veins. The distal upper and lower limbs are the most frequently affected. Typically, Buerger's disease is identified in young adult males who smoke. Larger arteries, such as the femoral and brachial, become involved in the late stages of the disease. The veins are less commonly involved.

The disease often extends into the perivascular tissues, resulting in fibrosis and scarring that binds the artery, vein, and nerve firmly together. For people who have this disease, cessation of cigarette smoking usually arrests the disease process, but persistence in smoking causes occlusion in the more proximal vessels.

The cause of Buerger's disease is unknown, although there is a strong association with tobacco smoking. A familial or genetic predisposition and autoimmune etiologic factors are also possible.

Collaborative Management

 ### Assessment

The first clinical manifestation of Buerger's disease is usually claudication (pain in the muscles resulting from an inadequate blood supply) of the arch of the foot. Intermittent claudication may occur in the lower extremities. The pain may be ischemic, occurring in the digits while the client is at rest. Often, there is an aching pain that is more severe at night. Paroxysmal shock–like pain can be the result of ischemic neuropathy. Clients often experience increased sensitivity to cold and complain of coldness and numbness. On physical examination, the nurse notes that the pulses are often diminished in the distal extremities, and the extremities are cool and red or cyanotic in the dependent position.

A diagnosis of Buerger's disease is commonly based on a physical finding of peripheral ischemia, often in association with migratory superficial phlebitis. Ulcerations and gangrene may be seen in the digits. The ulcerations are usually sharply demarcated. The gangrenous lesion can be small or can affect the entire digit.

Arteriograms can be useful in delineating the degree of disease in the arteries. Commonly, arteriography reveals multiple segmental occlusions in the smaller arteries of the forearm, hand, leg, and foot. Plethysmographic studies of the fingers or toes may be diagnostic of the disease in the early stages. These studies can also be useful in following the progression of the disease in more proximal arteries.

 ### Interventions

Nursing interventions are directed at
- Preventing the progression of the disease
- Avoiding vasoconstriction
- Promoting vasodilation
- Relieving pain
- Treating ulceration and gangrene

To prevent progression of Buerger's disease, complete abstinence from tobacco in all forms is essential. The client is instructed to prevent extreme or prolonged exposure to cold to prevent vasoconstriction. The nurse instructs the client about medications that are prescribed for vasodilation, such as nifedipine (Procardia, Adalat). (See Chapter 9 for interventions and nursing management for pain relief.)

The treatment of clients with Buerger's disease is similar to that of clients with peripheral arterial disease (see earlier).

Subclavian Steal
Overview

Subclavian steal occurs in the upper extremities from a subclavian artery occlusion or stenosis. The result is altered blood flow and ischemia in the arm. Subclavian steal can occur in people at any age but is more common in those with risk factors for atherosclerosis. Symptoms include tiredness in the arm with exertion, paresthesias, dizziness, and exercise-induced pain in the forearm when the arms are elevated.

Collaborative Management

Physical examination usually reveals a significant difference in the blood pressures between the arms. A difference greater than 20 mmHg is considered significant. Another important finding is a subclavian bruit, which can occur on the affected side. The subclavian pulse may be decreased on the occluded side compared with the opposite side. The client's arm may also be discolored or cyanotic; however, this finding generally occurs only in severe cases.

Surgery is the recommended intervention when a client has cyanosis or pain. One of three procedures may be used: endarterectomy of the subclavian artery, carotidsubclavian bypass, or dilation of the subclavian artery.

Nursing care encompasses postoperative care of the client and monitoring the arterial flow in the affected arm. The nurse should check brachial and radial pulses frequently and observe for ischemic changes. The nurse also observes the arm for edema, redness, or any other signs.

Thoracic Outlet Syndrome
Overview

Thoracic outlet syndrome is a compression of the subclavian artery at the thoracic outlet by anatomic structures, such as a rib or muscle. The arterial wall may be damaged, producing thrombosis or embolization to distal arteries of the arms. The three common sites of compression in the thoracic outlet are

- The interscalene triangle
- Between the coracoid process of the scapula and the pectoralis minor tendon
- Most commonly, the costoclavicular space

Collaborative Management

Thoracic outlet syndrome is more common in females and in people whose occupations require holding their arms up or leaning over, such as baseball players, golfers, or swimmers. It is also seen in clients who have had trauma such as whiplash or after clavicular fracture. Clients generally complain of neck, shoulder, and arm pain that may be intermittent. The client may also have numbness and moderate edema of the extremity. The pain and numbness are worse when the arm is placed in certain positions, such as over the client's head or out to the side. The client may have overdeveloped neck and shoulder muscles, and the affected arm may appear cyanotic.

Treatment includes physical therapy, exercises, and avoiding aggravating positions, such as elevating the arms. Surgical treatment involves resection of the anatomic structure that is compressing the artery. Surgery is performed only if a client has severe pain, has lost hand function, or is responding poorly to conservative treatment.

Raynaud's Phenomenon

Overview

Raynaud's phenomenon is caused by vasospasm of the arterioles and arteries of the upper and lower extremities, usually unilaterally. *Raynaud's disease* occurs bilaterally. The two terms are sometimes used interchangeably, but, although they are related, there are some differences. Raynaud's phenomenon usually occurs in people older than 30 years; Raynaud's disease can occur between the ages of 17 and 50 years. Raynaud's phenomenon can occur in either sex, but Raynaud's disease is more common in women.

The pathophysiology is the same for both entities. The etiology is unknown. Clients often have an associated systemic connective tissue disease, such as systemic lupus erythematosus or progressive systemic sclerosis (see Chap. 24).

As a result of vasospasm, the cutaneous vessels are constricted and blanching of the extremity occurs, followed by cyanosis. When the vasospasm is relieved, the tissue becomes reddened or hyperemic. The client's extremities are numb and cold, and the client may complain of pain and swelling. Ulcers may also be present. These attacks are intermittent and can be aggravated by cold or stress. In severe cases, the attack lasts longer and gangrene of the digits can occur.

Collaborative Management

Treatment involves relieving or preventing the vasoconstriction by drug therapy. Commonly prescribed drugs are nifedipine (Procardia), cyclandelate (Cyclospasmol), and phenoxybenzamine (Dibenzyline). These vasodilating agents may help to relieve the symptoms, but they can cause uncomfortable side effects, such as facial flushing, headaches, hypotension, and dizziness.

For severe symptoms that cannot be alleviated by drugs, a lumbar sympathectomy can be performed. The physician cuts the sympathetic nerve fibers that cause vasoconstriction of blood vessels in the lower extremities. This method is effective when clients are experiencing foot symptoms. For the upper extremities, a similar procedure—sympathetic ganglionectomy—may provide symptom relief. The long-term effectiveness of these treatments is questionable.

Education of the client is important in prevention of complications. The nurse explains methods to prevent vasoconstriction, such as minimizing exposure to cold and decreasing stress. The client is instructed to wear warm clothes, socks, or gloves when exposed to cool or cold temperatures. Clients should keep their homes at a comfortably warm temperature. The nurse helps the client to identify stressors and provides suggestions for reducing them.

Popliteal Entrapment

Popliteal entrapment causes ischemic symptoms in the affected leg or foot because of anatomic compression of the popliteal artery. Popliteal entrapment occurs in young people, most often in men complaining of intermittent claudication of one or both extremities.

Physical examination may reveal ischemic changes of the affected extremity, with normal function of the unaffected limb. When the client is at rest, the nurse may note diminished distal pulses, although this is a rare finding.

Diagnosis of popliteal entrapment is possible only after an accurate client history, physical examination, and arteriography.

The recommended treatment is surgical repair of the anatomic compression. Reconstruction of the popliteal artery may be necessary to restore arterial blood flow to the limb.

Nursing care involves preventing general postoperative complications and evaluating the patency of the graft or artery postoperatively. The nurse observes for ischemic changes and evaluates distal pulses frequently postoperatively.

Peripheral Venous Disease

To function properly, veins must be patent (unobstructed) with competent valves. Vein function also necessitates the assistance of the surrounding muscle beds to help pump blood toward the heart. If one or more veins are not operating efficiently, they become distended and clinical manifestations occur.

Two distinct phenomena alter the blood flow in veins:

- Thrombus formation (*venous thrombosis*) can lead to pulmonary embolism, a life-threatening complication (see Chap. 34).
- Defective valves lead to *venous insufficiency* and *varicose veins,* which are not life-threatening but are problematic.

Venous Thrombosis

Overview

Thrombus formation constitutes one of health care's greatest challenges. A thrombus (also called a thrombosis) is a blood clot believed to result from an endothelial injury, venous stasis, or hypercoagulability. However, the thrombosis may not be specifically attributable to one element, or it may involve all three elements. Thrombosis is often associated with an inflammatory process. When a thrombus develops, inflammation can occur around the thrombus, thickening the vein wall and consequently leading to embolization (the formation of an embolus).

Thrombophlebitis refers to a thrombus that is associated with inflammation; *phlebothrombosis* is a thrombus without inflammation. Thrombophlebitis can occur in superficial veins; however, it most frequently occurs in the deep veins of the lower extremities.

Deep venous (vein) thrombophlebitis, commonly referred to as *deep venous thrombosis* (DVT), not only is more common but also is more serious than superficial thrombophlebitis because it presents a greater risk for *pulmonary embolism,* in which a dislodged blood clot travels to the pulmonary artery.

Thrombus formation has been associated with stasis of blood flow, endothelial injury, and/or hypercoagulability, known as Virchow's triad. The precise cause of these events remains unknown; however, a few predisposing factors have been identified (see Research Applications for Nursing). Thrombosis has commonly occurred in people undergoing certain surgical procedures. The highest incidence of clot formation occurs in clients who have undergone hip surgery or open prostate surgery. Other conditions that seem to promote thrombus formation are pregnancy, ulcerative colitis, and heart failure.

Immobility can predispose a person to thrombosis. This can occur during prolonged bed rest, such as when a client is confined to bed during the perioperative period. *Phlebitis* (vein inflammation) associated with invasive procedures, such as intravenous therapy, can predispose cli-

---

▷ Research Applications for Nursing

A Nursing Assessment Tool for Deep Vein Thrombosis Shows Promise

Autar, R. (1996). Nursing assessment of clients at risk for deep vein thrombosis (DVT): The Autar DVT scale. Journal of Advanced Nursing, 23, 763–770.

This study examined the effectiveness of using the Autar DVT scale to predict the development of deep vein thrombosis (DVT). This scale includes seven risk factors: age, build and body mass index, immobility, special DVT risk, trauma, surgery, and high-risk disease. Studying 21 subjects on two clinical units, the scale was evaluated for reliability, sensitivity, and specificity.

In this study group, the sensitivity of the scale was 100%, and the specificity was 81.2%. The reliability of the scale was reported at 0.98 and had an 83% predicted accuracy.

Critique. The researcher attempted to develop a reliable and valid tool to assess DVT risk. This scale provides a comprehensive nursing assessment to predict individuals at risk for DVT. This study cannot be generalized due to the limited small sample size and to the fact that the subjects were all orthopedic clients. The scale may be helpful in other populations and should be tested in a number of settings and with a number of client groups.

Possible Nursing Implications. This study shows the need to question and validate some of the assessments that nurses have routinely performed without a scientific basis. It clearly raises questions about exploring the various factors that may contribute to the development of DVT.

---

ents to thrombosis. Severe infections, systemic lupus erythematosus, polycythemia vera, oral contraceptives, and trauma have also been linked to thrombosis.

Collaborative Management

Assessment

The classic signs and symptoms of deep vein thrombosis (DVT) are calf or groin tenderness and pain, with or without leg swelling. Pain in the calf on dorsiflexion of the foot (Homan's sign) is another possible indicator of DVT, although the reliability of this assessment finding is controversial. The nurse examines the area that the client describes as painful, comparing this site with the contralateral limb. The nurse gently palpates the site, observing for warmth and edema. Signs and symptoms, however, may be absent with thrombophlebitis. Because there are often silent clinical findings, the nurse must have a high index of suspicion for this disorder when caring for clients at high risk.

Localized edema in one extremity may suggest thrombophlebitis. The nurse can measure and compare right and left calf and thigh circumferences for changes over time as an indicator of DVT or venous insufficiency. However, serial leg measurements may not be the most reliable indicator of DVT.

Although diagnostic tests for DVT are available, physical examination findings are often adequate for diagnosis. If a definitive diagnosis is lacking from physical examination alone, other diagnostic tests may be performed, such as venography, Doppler studies, and impedance phlebography.

Venography with contrast medium visualizes clot formation in approximately 95% of people with DVT. However, this study is generally not performed because it may precipitate thrombosis and is very painful.

Duplex ultrasonographic scanning, a noninvasive test, is the preferred diagnostic test for DVT if a definitive diagnosis cannot be made by physical examination. Doppler ultrasonography is also useful in the diagnosis of deep vein thrombosis. Normal venous circulation is characterized by audible signals, whereas thrombosed veins produce little or no flow.

Interventions

The focus of treatment for thrombophlebitis is to prevent complications, such as pulmonary emboli, and to prevent an increase in size of the thrombus. Deep venous thrombophlebitis (thrombosis) is the most common type of thrombophlebitis. All clients with DVT are hospitalized for treatment.

> ➤ *Nonsurgical Management*

Deep vein thrombosis (DVT) is most often treated medically, using a combination of rest, drug therapy, and preventive measures.

Rest. Supportive therapy for DVT includes bed rest and elevation of the extremity. Some health care providers order intermittent or continuous warm, moist soaks to the affected area. All clients are evaluated for signs and symptoms of pulmonary embolus (PE), which include shortness of breath and chest pain. Emboli may also travel to the brain or heart, but these complications are not as common as PE (see Chap. 34).

Drug Therapy. Anticoagulants are the drugs of choice for a client with DVT and for clients at risk for DVT. Heparin is used when immediate anticoagulation is indicated, but other agents, such as aspirin or warfarin, may be used for clot prevention.

Heparin Therapy. Most clients with a confirmed diagnosis of an existing blood clot are started on a regimen of intravenous (IV) heparin (Hepalean✲) therapy. Heparin is an anticoagulant agent that, at low doses, interacts with antithrombin III to produce selective inhibition of clotting factor X. At higher doses, heparin inhibits practically all clotting factors. The ultimate result is inhibition of fibrin formation (Pinnell, 1996). Heparin does nothing to the existing clot. The physician prescribes heparin to prevent the formation of other clots, which often develop in the presence of an existing clot, and to prevent enlargement of the existing clot. Over a long period of time, the existing clot is slowly absorbed by the body.

Heparin is initially given by a bolus IV dose of approximately 100 U/kg, followed by constant infusion. The infusion is regulated by a reliable electronic infusion device that protects against accidental free flow of solution. The physician or clinical pharmacist orders concentrations of heparin (in 5% dextrose in water) and the number of units or milliliters per hour to maintain a therapeutic activated partial thromboplastin time (APTT). APTTs are obtained daily, or more frequently, and are reported to the health care provider as soon as the results are available to allow adjustment of heparin dosage. Therapeutic levels of APTTs are usually one to two times normal control levels. The nurse assesses clients for signs and symptoms of bleeding, which include hematuria, frank or occult blood in the stool, ecchymosis, petechiae, an altered level of consciousness, or pain.

Heparin can also decrease platelet counts. Mild reductions are common and are resolved with continued heparin therapy. Severe platelet reductions, although rare, result from the development of antiplatelet bodies between 6 and 14 days into treatment. Platelets aggregate into "white clots" that can cause thrombosis, usually an acute arterial occlusion (Simko & Lockhart, 1996). The provider discontinues heparin administration if severe heparin-induced thrombocytopenia and thrombosis (HITT) (>100,000 mm³) occurs. An oral anticoagulant may then be substituted for heparin, if necessary.

The nurse also ensures that protamine sulfate, the antidote for heparin, is available, if needed, for excessive bleeding. Chart 38–9 highlights information important to nursing care and client education associated with anticoagulant therapy.

To prevent DVT, heparin may be given in low doses subcutaneously. The health care provider usually orders a dose of 5000 U every 8–12 hours for high-risk clients, especially after orthopedic surgery. Other pharmacologic agents that may be used for prophylaxis are
- Low-molecular-weight heparin (e.g., enoxaparin)

Chart 38–9

Nursing Care Highlight: The Client Receiving Anticoagulant Therapy

- Carefully check the dosage of anticoagulant to be administered, even if the pharmacy prepared the medication.
- Monitor the client for signs and symptoms of bleeding, including hematuria, frank or occult blood in the stool, ecchymosis, petechiae, altered mental status (indicating possible cranial bleeding), or pain (especially abdominal pain, which could indicate abdominal bleeding).
- Monitor vital signs frequently for decreased blood pressure and increased pulse (indicating possible internal bleeding).
- Have antidotes available as needed, e.g., protamine sulfate for heparin and vitamin K for warfarin (Coumadin, Warfilone✲).
- Monitor activated partial thromboplastin time (APTT) for clients receiving heparin; monitor prothrombin time (PT) or International Normalized Ratio (INR) for clients receiving warfarin.
- Apply prolonged pressure over venipuncture sites and injection sites.
- When administering *subcutaneous* heparin, apply pressure over the site and do not massage.
- Teach the client going home on an anticoagulant to
- Use only an electric razor.
- Take precautions to avoid injury, for example, do not use tools like hammers or saws, where accidents commonly occur.
- Report signs and symptoms of bleeding, such as blood in the urine or stool, nosebleeds, ecchymosis, or altered mental status.
- Take the prescribed dosage of medication at the precise time that it was ordered to be given.
- Not stop taking the medication abruptly; the physician usually tapers the anticoagulant gradually.

- Dextran, an intravenous plasma expander
- Dihydroergotamine (DHE)
- Warfarin (Coumadin, Warfilone✲)
- Aspirin

Warfarin Therapy. After treatment for deep vein thrombosis (DVT) with heparin therapy, and after the signs and symptoms of DVT have greatly resolved, the client is usually started on oral warfarin sodium. Warfarin works in the liver to inhibit synthesis of the four vitamin K–dependent clotting factors. It takes 3–4 days before warfarin can exert therapeutic anticoagulation. For this reason, warfarin administration is started while the intravenous (IV) heparin is being infused. The heparin continues to provide therapeutic anticoagulation until this effect is achieved with warfarin. IV heparin is discontinued at that time.

Therapeutic levels of warfarin are monitored by measuring prothrombin time (PT) and the International Normalized Ratio (INR). Because prothrombin times are often inconsistent and misleading, the INR was developed. Most laboratories report both results. Most clients on warfarin for DVT should have an INR between 2.0 and 3.0 (Coyne, 1997).

The initial dosage of warfarin is usually 10–15 mg daily for 1–2 days. Maintenance therapy generally ranges from 2.5 to 7.5 mg given once a day in the evening. Clients usually receive warfarin for up to 6 months after an episode of DVT.

Nursing assessment for bleeding is similar to that described for clients receiving heparin. The nurse ensures that vitamin K, the antidote for warfarin, is available in case of excessive bleeding (see Chart 38–9).

Thrombolytic Therapy. The use of systemic thrombolytic therapy for deep vein thrombosis (DVT) is effective in dissolving thrombi quickly and completely. The greatest advantage is thought to be the prevention of valvular damage and consequential venous insufficiency, or "postphlebitic syndrome." However, thrombolytic therapy is contraindicated postoperatively, during pregnancy, and after childbirth, trauma, cerebrovascular accidents, or spinal injuries. To be most effective, thrombolytic therapy must be initiated within 5 days after the onset of symptoms.

Tissue plasminogen activator (t-PA) is the thrombolytic that has been studied the most for DVT. It should be used for at least 3 days but not more than 5. The nurse caring for clients receiving t-PA must monitor closely for signs and symptoms of bleeding (see also Chap. 40).

Prevention and Treatment of Peripheral Edema. The client's legs should be elevated when in bed and when in the chair. To help prevent chronic venous insufficiency, clients with active and resolving deep vein thrombosis are often instructed to wear knee or thigh-high compression or elastic stockings.

➤ *Surgical Management*

A deep venous thrombus is rarely removed surgically unless there is a massive occlusion that does not respond to medical treatment and the thrombus is of recent (1 to 2 days) onset. *Thrombectomy* is the most common surgical procedure for removing the thrombus. Preoperative and postoperative care of clients undergoing thrombectomy are similar to that for clients undergoing arterial surgery (see earlier).

Inferior Vena Caval Interruption. For clients with recurrent deep vein thrombosis or pulmonary emboli that do not respond to medical treatment and for clients who cannot tolerate anticoagulation, inferior vena caval interruption may be indicated to prevent pulmonary emboli.

Preoperative care is similar to that provided for clients receiving local anesthesia (see Chap. 20). If clients have recently been taking anticoagulants, such as warfarin (Coumadin, Warfilone♣) or heparin (Hepalean♣), the nurse consults with the physician about interrupting this therapy in the preoperative period to avoid hemorrhage.

The surgeon inserts a filter device, or "umbrella," percutaneously into the inferior vena cava (Fig. 38–11). The device is meant to trap emboli in the inferior vena cava before they progress to the lungs. Holes in the device allow blood to pass through, thus not significantly interfering with the return of blood to the heart. Popular IVC

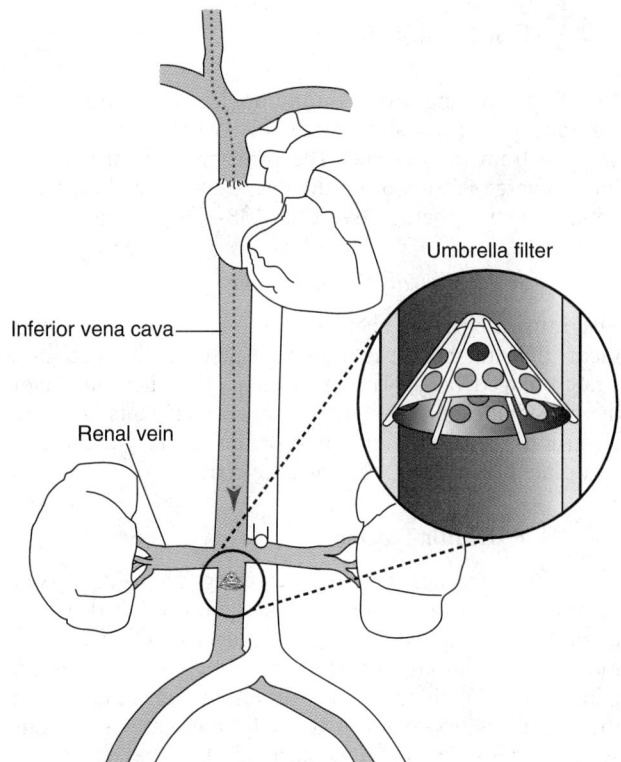

Figure 38–11. An inferior vena caval (IVC) filter.

filters include the bird's-nest filter and the Greenfield filter.

Postoperatively, the nurse inspects the incision on the right side of the chest for bleeding and signs or symptoms of infection. Other postoperative nursing care is similar to that for any client having surgery (see Chap. 22).

Ligation or External Clips. If an inferior vena cava (IVC) filter is not successful in preventing pulmonary emboli or if the filter becomes blocked with thrombi, the surgeon may perform ligation or insert external clips on the inferior vena cava to prevent pulmonary emboli.

Preoperative care for clients undergoing ligation of the vena cava or placement of an external clip is similar to that for clients undergoing abdominal laparotomy. If the client is receiving anticoagulation therapy, the nurse consults with the surgeon about temporary interruption of therapy.

Ligation and insertion of external clips in the inferior vena cava are often performed by means of an abdominal laparotomy. In a ligation, the surgeon ties off the inferior vena cava to block emboli. Application of an external clip, such as the Adams-DeWeese, narrows the inferior vena cava to four serrated transverse slits, 3–5 mm in diameter. If laparotomy is performed, the external clip procedure is preferred because there are fewer hemodynamic and venous complications and a low frequency of recurrent pulmonary emboli associated with its use.

Postoperative care for the client with IVC ligation or external clip placement is similar to that for the client after an abdominal laparotomy.

Continuing Care

Clients recovering from thrombophlebitis or deep vein thrombosis are usually ambulatory when they are discharged from the hospital. The primary focus of planning for discharge is to educate the client about the hazards of anticoagulation therapy (see Chart 38–9).

► Home Care Management

The nurse helps the client identify situations and equipment that might cause trauma, such as the use of a straight-edged razor. The nurse helps the client and family or significant others to make arrangements to avoid hazardous situations and to procure alternative types of equipment, if needed, such as an electric razor.

► Health Teaching

The nurse teaches clients recovering from deep vein thrombosis to stop or avoid smoking and to avoid the use of oral contraceptives to decrease the risk of recurrence. Most clients are discharged on a regimen of warfarin (Coumadin, Warfilone♣). The nurse instructs clients and their families to avoid potentially traumatic situations, such as participation in contact sports. The nurse provides all clients with written and oral information about the signs and symptoms of bleeding (see earlier). The client must report any of these manifestations to the health care provider immediately.

The anticoagulant effect of warfarin may be reversed by the omission of one or two doses of the drug or by the administration of vitamin K. In case of injury, clients are directed to apply pressure to bleeding wounds and to seek medical assistance immediately. The nurse encourages clients to carry an identification card or wear a medical alert (Medic-Alert) bracelet that states that they are taking warfarin.

The nurse also instructs clients to inform their dentist and other health care providers that they are taking warfarin before receiving treatment or prescriptions. Prothrombin times are affected by many prescription and over-the-counter medications, such as antacids, antihistamines, aspirin, mineral oil, oral contraceptives, and large doses of vitamin C. The action of warfarin is also affected by high-fat and vitamin K–rich foods, such as cabbage, cauliflower, broccoli, asparagus, lettuce, turnips, spinach, kale, fish, liver, and coffee. Clients are therefore instructed to eat a well-balanced diet and to avoid taking additional medications without consulting a health care provider. The nurse arranges for clients to have determinations of prothrombin time 1–2 weeks after discharge.

ELDERLY CONSIDERATIONS

Warfarin is used with caution with older adults or debilitated patients. A reduced dose is often recommended in an effort to prevent spontaneous intracranial bleeding or excessive bleeding related to trauma. Many older adults may have reduced kidney or liver function and a decreased ability to metabolize and excrete the drug. For this reason, it is usually used only when the benefits outweigh the risks. The older adult may have problems adhering to the routine laboratory tests required to monitor the medication's effectiveness.

If the health care provider prescribes antiembolism stockings, the nurse teaches clients how and when to apply them.

Clients who have experienced deep vein thrombosis (DVT) may fear recurrence of a thrombus and may also be concerned about treatment with warfarin and the risk for bleeding. The nurse assures such clients that participation in the prescribed treatment frequently helps in resolving this problem and that ongoing assessment of prothrombin levels and INRs should minimize the risks of bleeding.

► Health Care Resources

Clients discharged on warfarin need access to a pharmacy to renew prescriptions and, if feasible, to obtain a Medic-Alert bracelet. Clients also need access to a laboratory for frequent monitoring of prothrombin times and INRs.

Venous Insufficiency

Overview

Venous insufficiency occurs as a result of prolonged venous hypertension, which stretches the veins and damages the valves. This can lead to a back-up of blood and further venous hypertension, resulting in edema. Edema occurs as the by-products of red blood cell break down and infiltrate the surrounding tissues. Because the client cannot eliminate waste products, they accumulate within the tissues. With time, this stasis (stoppage) results in venous stasis ulcers, swelling, and cellulitis.

Venous efficiency is altered when thrombosis occurs or when valves are not functioning correctly. Defective valves can result from prolonged venous hypertension, which stretches the veins and damages valves. This can occur in people who stand or sit in one position for long periods, such as teachers and office personnel. Pregnancy and obesity can also cause chronically distended veins, which lead to damaged valves. Thrombus formation can contribute to valve destruction. Chronic venous insufficiency often occurs in clients who have had thrombophlebitis.

Collaborative Management

 Assessment

Clients with venous insufficiency may have edema in both extremities. There may be *stasis dermatitis* or discoloration along the ankles, extending up to the calf. In people with long-term venous insufficiency or stasis, *ulcers* often form. Ulcer formation can result from the edema or from minor injury to the limb. Venous ulcers typically occur over the malleolus, more often medially than laterally. The ulcer usually has irregular borders. Generally, these ulcers are chronic and difficult to heal (see Chart 38–6). Many clients live with ulcers for years, and recurrence is common. Some clients may lose one or both limbs if ulcers are not controlled.

⬛ Interventions

The focus of treating venous insufficiency is to decrease edema and promote venous return from the affected extremity. Clients are not usually hospitalized for venous insufficiency alone unless it is complicated by an ulcer or another disorder is occurring simultaneously.

➤ Nonsurgical Management

Treatment of chronic venous insufficiency is primarily nonsurgical, unless it is complicated by a venous stasis ulcer that requires surgical debridement. The goal of managing venous stasis ulcers is twofold: to heal the ulcer and to prevent stasis with recurrence of ulcer formation.

Treatment of Edema. Clients with chronic venous insufficiency wear elastic or compression stockings, which fit from the middle of the foot to just below the knee or to the thigh. Clients should wear the stockings during the day and evening. The nurse instructs clients to elevate their legs for at least 20 minutes four or five times per day but to avoid long periods of sitting or standing in place. When the client is in bed, the legs should be elevated above the level of the heart (Chart 38–10).

The nurse and physician should also confer about the use of intermittent sequential pneumatic compression of the lower extremities for clients with past or present ve-

---

Chart 38–10

Education Guide: Venous Insufficiency

Elastic Stockings
- Wear elastic stockings as prescribed, usually during the day and evening.
- Put the stockings on upon awakening and before getting out of bed.
- When applying the stockings, do not "bunch up" and apply like socks. Instead, place your hand inside the stocking and pull out the heel. Then place the foot of the stocking over your foot and slide the rest of the stocking up. Be sure that rough seams on the stocking are on the outside, not next to your skin.
- Do not push stockings down for comfort because they may function like a tourniquet and further impair venous return.
- Put on a clean pair of stockings each day. Wash them by hand (not in a washing machine) in a gentle detergent and warm water.
- If the stockings seem to be "stretched out," replace them with a new pair.

Do's and Don'ts
- Elevate your legs for at least 20 minutes four or five times a day. When in bed, elevate your legs above the level of your heart.
- Avoid prolonged sitting or standing.
- Do not cross your legs; crossing at the ankles is acceptable for short periods of time.
- Do not wear tight, restrictive pants; avoid girdles and garters.

---

nous stasis ulcers. If the client is being treated for an open venous ulcer, the device is applied over a dressing such as an Unna boot. The nurse instructs the client to apply the pump as directed during the period of healing. Because of the high incidence of venous ulcer recurrence, clients with chronic venous insufficiency whose ulcers have healed are encouraged to continue compression therapy for life.

Treatment of Venous Stasis Ulcers. Venous stasis ulcers are slightly more manageable than ulcers resulting from arterial disease. They are chronic in nature, with some clients manifesting the same ulcer for years. Ulcers often heal, only to reoccur later in the same area. The client may have simultaneous ulcers for several years.

Dressings. Two types of occlusive dressings are used for venous stasis ulcers: oxygen permeable and oxygen impermeable. Because the role of atmospheric oxygen in wound healing is controversial, opinions vary with regard to which type of dressing is preferred. The oxygen-permeable polyethylene film (e.g., Op Site) and an oxygen-impermeable hydrocolloid dressing (e.g., DuoDerm) are common. Hydrocolloid dressings are left in place for a minimum of 3–5 days for best effect.

Implications for the Elderly. A potential problem is that some occlusive dressings stick to the skin and can cause more damage to friable skin, especially in older clients. Newer dressings have calcium alginate (e.g., Sorbsan), which prevents maceration of healthy tissue.

If the client is ambulatory, an Unna boot may be used. This dressing is constructed of gauze that has been moistened with zinc oxide. The health care provider applies the boot to the affected limb, from the toes to the knee, after the ulcer has been cleaned with normal saline solution. Povidone-iodine (Betadine) and hydrogen peroxide are not used because they destroy granulation tissue. The Unna boot is then covered with an elastic wrap and hardens like a cast; this promotes venous return and prevents stasis. The Unna boot also forms a sterile environment for the ulcer. The physician should change the boot approximately once a week. The nurse instructs the client about what to look for if arterial occlusion should occur from an Unna boot that is too tight.

Drug Therapy. The provider may prescribe topical agents to chemically debride the ulcer, eliminating necrotic tissue and promoting healing. Fibrinolysin and desoxyribonuclease (Elase) are most effective after dry eschar (outer) tissue has been surgically removed. Because these agents can injure healthy tissue, the nurse protects the surrounding skin with an oil-based agent such as petroleum jelly (Vaseline). Injury to healthy tissue can prolong healing time.

If an infection occurs or cellulitis develops, systemic antibiotics are more effective than local ointments. Ointments are not well absorbed in the presence of edema. They may also inhibit the ulcer's healing by occluding the ulcer and prohibiting the needed interactions with air.

Surgical Management. Surgery for chronic venous insufficiency is not usually performed because historically it has not been successful. Attempts at transplanting vein valves have had limited success. Surgical debridement of venous ulcers is similar to that performed for arterial ulcers (see earlier).

 Continuing Care

The goal for the client with chronic venous insufficiency is to manage the client in the home. For clients with frequent acute complications and repeated hospital admissions, case management can help to meet appropriate clinical and cost outcomes.

➤ Home Care Management

The nurse helps clients with chronic venous insufficiency to plan for opportunities and facilities that allow for elevation of the lower extremities in and outside the home. In addition, clients with venous stasis ulcers need to plan for care of the ulcers.

➤ Health Teaching

The nurse instructs clients with chronic venous stasis to
- Avoid standing still if possible
- Elevate their legs when sitting
- Avoid crossing their legs
- Avoid wearing tight girdles, tight pants, and narrow-banded knee-high socks

The physician prescribes support hose or antiembolism stockings. The nurse teaches clients to apply these stockings before they get out of bed in the morning and to remove them just before going to bed at night (see Chart 38–10). The nurse also advises clients that they will probably need to wear these stockings for the rest of their lives.

To improve circulation and aid in weight reduction, the nurse prescribes an exercise program on an individual basis with the health care provider input. The nurse encourages all clients to maintain an optimal weight and may consult with the dietitian to plan a weight-reducing diet. The nurse instructs clients with venous stasis ulcers how to care for the ulcers at home.

Clients with venous stasis disease, especially those with venous stasis ulcers, may require long-term emotional support to assist them in meeting chronic needs. They may also need assistance in coping with necessary lifestyle adjustments, such as changes in occupation.

➤ Health Care Resources

Clients with venous stasis ulcers may need the assistance of a home health nurse to perform dressing changes. Clients with Unna boots will need weekly transportation to their health provider for dressing changes. The nurse will need to arrange for a sequential compression device in the home if the health care provider prescribes one.

Varicose Veins

Overview

Varicose veins are distended, protruding veins that appear darkened and tortuous. They can occur in anyone, but they are common in clients older than 30 years whose occupations require prolonged standing. Varicose veins are also frequently seen in pregnant women, clients with systemic problems, such as heart disease, obese clients, and clients with a family history of varicose veins.

As the vein wall weakens and dilates, venous pressure increases and the valves become incompetent (defective). The incompetent valves enhance the vessel dilation, and the veins become tortuous and distended. The client may complain of pain, especially after standing, and may experience a fullness in the legs. Nursing assessment reveals distended protruding veins.

The Trendelenburg test assists with the diagnosis. The client is placed in a supine position with elevated legs. As the client sits up, the veins would normally fill from the distal end; however, if there are varicosities, the veins fill from the proximal end.

Collaborative Management

Conservative measures are the treatment of choice. These involve wearing elastic stockings and elevating the extremities as much as possible. Clients who continue to have pain or unsightly veins, despite this treatment, may opt for either sclerotherapy or surgical removal of the vein.

Sclerotherapy is performed on small or a limited number of varicosities. The physician injects a solution, such as sodium tetradecyl, directly into the vein. A pressure dressing is applied over the sclerosed vein to keep vessels free of blood for 24–72 hours. The surgeon performs an incision and drainage of trapped blood in the sclerosed vein 14–21 days after injection, followed by application of a second pressure dressing for 12–18 hours.

Varicose veins are surgically removed when they are larger than 4 mm in diameter or are in clusters. The surgeon may use the stab avulsion technique if the saphenous veins are competent. The surgeon exposes varices through 2- to 3-mm stab incisions, grasping the veins with hooks, and dividing and avulsing each vein.

The surgeon may need to strip (remove) affected veins if the saphenous vein is incompetent. The surgeon threads a long wire through an incision above an affected vein, pulling it down through the vein and out through an incision below the vein. After this procedure, the client's legs are bandaged with firm elastic (Ace) bandages.

Postoperatively, the nurse assesses the groin and entire leg for bleeding through the elastic bandage. The nurse instructs the client to keep the legs elevated and to perform range-of-motion exercises of the legs at least hourly. Clients are ambulatory and are often discharged from the hospital by the first postoperative day. At this time, the nurse instructs clients to continue to wear elastic stockings, walk, limit sitting, avoid standing in one place, and elevate their legs when sitting.

Phlebitis

Phlebitis is an inflammation of the superficial veins caused by an irritation, such as intravenous therapy (also see Chap. 17). The client has a reddened, warm area radiating up an extremity, commonly an arm. The client may also experience pain, soreness, and swelling of the extremity.

Treatment involves application of warm, moist soaks, which dilate the vein and promote circulation. Sometimes a heating unit is used to keep the soaks warm. Rarely, ice packs are used. The nurse applies the soaks, making sure that the temperature is not warm enough to burn the client, and assesses for complications, such as tissue necrosis, infection, or pulmonary embolus. After a few days of conservative therapy, the inflammation usually subsides.

Vascular Trauma

Overview

Many types of trauma can result in vascular injury. Injuries to the blood vessels in the upper and lower extremities account for approximately 70% of all vascular injuries to the human body. Vascular injuries to the blood vessels include punctures, lacerations, and transections. Acute blunt or penetrating trauma may result in a false aneurysm or hematoma. Arteriovenous fistulas may be seen after penetrating injuries. The more common causes of penetrating injuries to the blood vessels are gunshot and knife wounds.

Blunt trauma, which is less common, can result from high-speed automobile accidents as a result of the shearing force of rapid deceleration. Vascular trauma can also occur during arterial puncture for arteriographic or hemodynamic studies in which a dissection, hematoma, or occlusive lesion occurs.

Collaborative Management

The history and physical examination aid in establishing the diagnosis in the client with vascular injury. The nurse questions the client or family about the mechanism of injury, the site of injury, the amount of blood loss, and symptoms present after the injury.

The nurse assesses for circulatory, sensory, or motor impairment but is aware that, despite significant trauma, impairment may not be apparent, especially if deep vessels have been injured. Arteriography provides essential information about the vascular injury. Emergency or urgent surgical intervention is warranted for clients with ischemia to maximize successful revascularization.

Management of vascular injuries is often initiated in a hospital emergency department. Careful triage by the nurse is crucial. Snyder and associates (1989) suggest three types of vascular injuries, with variations in the time at which definitive treatment is essential:

- Category I: These injuries expose clients to immediate threats of survival and must be treated immediately (e.g., tension pneumothorax, cardiac tamponade, exsanguinating hemorrhage).
- Category II: These injuries are serious but not quite as severe, allowing time for more extensive evaluation before treatment is initiated (e.g., major fractures, abdominal trauma in the presence of stable vital signs, genitourinary trauma).

- Category III: These injuries permit management of the injury at a more leisurely pace (e.g., lacerations, simple lacerations, contusions).

The most important principles in the management of vascular trauma are establishment of a patent airway, control of bleeding, and restoration of blood flow.

The method of repair varies with the type of vascular injury. Techniques include vein bypass grafting, lateral suture repair, thrombectomy (excision of blood clot), resection with end-to-end anastomosis, and vein patch grafting.

SELECTED BIBLIOGRAPHY

Allen, K. M., & Phillips, J. M. (1997). *Women's health across the lifespan.* Philadelphia: J. B. Lippincott.

Allen, S. L. (1995). Perioperative nursing interventions for intravascular stent placement. *AORN, 61* (4), 689–709.

American Heart Association. (1995). *Heart and stroke facts.* Chicago: American Heart Association.

Autar, R. (1996). Nursing assessment of clients at risk of deep vein thrombosis (DVT): The Autar DVT scale. *Journal of Advanced Nursing, 23,* 763–770.

*Bickerstaff, L. K., Hollier, L. H., Van Peenen, H. J., et al. (1984). Abdominal aortic aneurysm: The changing natural history. *Journal of Vascular Surgery, 1,* 6–12.

Bunt, T. J. (1995). Revascularization versus amputation for elderly patient. *AORN Journal, 62* (3), 433–435.

Cahall, E., & Spence, R. K. (1995). Practical nursing measures for vascular compromise in the lower leg. *Ostomy and Wound Management, 41* (9), 16–32.

Calhoun, D. A., & Oparil, S. (1995). Racial differences in the pathogenisis of hypertension. *American Journal of the Medical Sciences, 310,* 586–590.

Carlson, K. J., & Eisenstat, S. A. (1995). *Primary care of women.* St. Louis: C. V. Mosby.

Clagett, G. P., & Krupski, W. C. (1995). Antithrombotic therapy in peripheral arterial occlusive disease. *Chest, 108* (4), 431S–443S.

Cookingham, A. (1995). Peripheral vascular disease: Education concerns for patients with a chronic disease in the changing health-care environment. *AACN Clinical Issues, 6* (4), 670–676.

Coyne, N. (1997). Current concepts in anticoagulant therapy. *The Journal of Care Management, 3* (4), 28–46, 73.

Dorgan, M. B., Birke, J. A., Moretto, J. A., Patout, C. A., & Rehm, K. B. (1995, November). Performing foot screening for diabetic patients. *American Journal of Nursing, 95,* 32–36.

Dumas, M. A. S. (1995). Intermittent claudication. *American Journal of Nursing, 95* (12), 34.

Eaton, L. E., Buck, E. A., & Catanzaro, J. E. (1996). The nurse's role in facilitating compliance in clients with hypertension. *MEDSURG Nursing, 5,* 339–345, 359.

Fahey, V. A. (1994). *Vascular nursing* (2nd ed.). Philadelphia: W. B. Saunders.

Freis, E. D. (1995). The efficacy and safety of diuretics in treating hypertension. *Annals of Internal Medicine, 122* (3), 223–226.

Gerhard, M., Baum, P., & Raby, K. E. (1995). Peripheral arterial-vascular disease in women: Prevalence, prognosis, and treatment. *Cardiology, 86,* 349–355.

Harris, A. H., Brown-Etris, M., & Troyer-Caudle, J. (1996, January). Managing vascular leg ulcers part I: Assessment. *American Journal of Nursing, 96,* 38–43.

Harris, A. H., Brown-Etris, M., & Troyer-Caudle, J. (1996, February). Managing vascular leg ulcers part II: Treatment. *American Journal of Nursing, 96,* 40–46.

Hatton, D. C., Yue, Q., & McCarron, D. A. (1995). Mechanisms of calcium's effects on blood pressure. *Seminars in Nephrology, 15,* 593–602.

Henderson, L. J., & Kirkland, J. S. (1995). Angioplasty with stent placement in peripheral arterial occlusive disease. *AORN Journal, 61* (4), 671–685.

Hill, E. M. (1995). Perioperative management of patients with vascular disease. *AACN Clinical Issues, 6* (4), 547–561.

Hulley, S. B., & Newman, T. B. (1994). Cholesterol in the elderly. Is it important? *Journal of American Medical Association, 272,* 1372–1373.

*Joint National Committee. (1993). The fifth report of the Joint National Committee on detection, evaluation, and treatment of high blood pressure. *Archives of Internal Medicine, 153,* 154–183.

Kannel, W. B., & Wilson, P. W. (1995). An update of coronary risk factors. *Medical Clinics of North America, 79,* 951–971.

Karch, A. M. (1995). Pain, pills, and possibilities: Drug therapy in peripheral vascular disease. *AACN Clinical Issues, 6* (4), 614–630.

Krenzer, M. E. (1995). Peripheral vascular assessment: Finding your way through arteries and veins. *AACN Clinical Issues, 6* (4), 631–644.

Krikorian, R. K., & Vacek, J. L. (1995). Peripheral arterial disease. *Postgraduate Medicine, 97* (6), 109–119.

Kuncl, N., & Nelson, K. M. (1997). Antihypertensive drugs: Balancing risks and benefits. *Nursing 97, 27* (8), 46–49.

LaPalio, L. R. (1995). Hypertension in the elderly. *American Family Physician, 52,* 1161–1165.

Lewis, C. E. (1996). Characteristics and treatment of hypertension in women: A review of the literature. *American Journal of Medical Sciences, 311,* 193–199.

Littenberg, B. (1995). A practice guideline revisited: Screening for hypertension. *Annals of Internal Medicine, 122,* 937–939.

Lowe, G. D. O., Reid, A. W., & Leiberman, D. P. (1994). Management of thrombosis in peripheral arterial disease. *British Medical Bulletin, 50* (4), 923–935.

Manolio, T. A., Cutler, J. A., Furber, C. D., Psaty, B. M., Whelton, P. K., & Applegate, W. B. (1995). Trends in pharmacologic management of hypertension in the United States. *Archives of Internal Medicine, 15* (5), 829–837.

Massie, B. M. (1995). Systemic hypertension. In L. M. Tierney, S. J. McPhee, & M. A. Papadakis (Eds.), *Current therapy* (pp. 373–390). Norwalk, CT: Appleton & Lange.

Matteson, M. A., McConnell, E. S., & Linton, A. D. (1997). *Gerontological nursing: Concepts and practice* (2nd ed.). Philadelphia: W. B. Saunders.

McKenney, J. M., Proctor, J. D., Harris, S., & Chinchili, V. M. (1994). A comparison of the efficacy and toxic effects of sustained- vs immediate-release niacin in hypercholesterolemic patients. *Journal of American Medical Association, 271,* 672–677.

*National Cholesterol Education Program. (1993). Summary of the second report of the national cholesterol education program. *Journal of American Medical Association, 269,* 3015–3023.

Nunnelee, J. D. (1995, December). Minimize the risk of DVT. *RN,* 28–31.

Pinnell, N. L. (1996). *Nursing pharmacology.* Philadelphia: W. B. Saunders.

Schaefer, E. J., Lamon-Fava, S., Jenner, J. L., McNamara, J. R., Ordovas, J. M., Davis, E., Abolafia, J. M., Lippel, K., & Levey, R. I. (1994). Lipoprotein(a) levels and risk of coronary heart disease in men. *Journal of American Medical Association, 271,* 999–1003.

*Schlafer, M. (1993). *The nurse, pharmacology, and drug therapy: A prototype approach* (2nd ed.). Redwood City, CA: Addison-Wesley.

Schwartz, L. B. (1998). Conventional and alternative therapies for acute deep vein thrombosis. *The Journal of Care Management, 4* (suppl), 9–13.

Simko, L. C., & Lockhart, J. S. (1996). Action stat: Heparin-induced thrombocytopenia and thrombosis. *Nursing 96, 26* (3), 33.

*Snyder, W. H., Thal, E. R., & Perry, M. O. (1989). Vascular injuries of the extremities. In R. B. Rutherford (Ed.), *Vascular surgery* (3rd ed., pp. 613–637). Philadelphia: W. B. Saunders.

Sparks, K. S. (1996). Are you up to date on weight-based heparin dosing? *American Journal of Nursing, 96,* (4) 33–36.

Stillman, F. A. (1995). Smoking cessation for the hospitalized cardiac patient: Rationale for and report of a model program. *Journal of Cardiovascular Nursing, 9,* 25–36.

Tierney, L. M. (1995). Blood vessels and lymphatics. In L. M. Tierney, S. J. McPhee, & M. A. Papadakis (Eds.), *Current therapy* (pp. 391–422). Norwalk, CT: Appleton & Lange.

Warbinek, E., & Wyness, A. (1994). Caring for patients with complications after elective abdominal aortic aneurysm surgery: A case study. *Journal of Vascular Nursing, 12* (3), 73–79.

Wheeler, E. C., & Brenner, Z. R. (1995). Peripheral vascular anatomy, physiology, and pathophysiology. *AACN Clinical Issues, 6* (4), 505–514.

Whitney, E. N., Cataldo, C. B., & Rolfes, S. R. (1994). *Understanding normal and clinical nutrition.* St. Paul: West Publishing Co.

Wills, E. M., & Sloan, H. L. (1996). Assessing peripheral arterial disorders in the home: A multidisciplinary clinical guide. *Home Healthcare Nurse, 14,* 669–682.

Wilson, R. F. (1994). Pre-existing peripheral arterial disease in trauma. *Critical Care Clinics, 10* (3), 567–593.

SUGGESTED READINGS

Cahall, E., & Spence, R. K. (1995). Practical nursing measures for vascular compromise in the lower leg. *Ostomy and Wound Management, 41* (9), 16–32.

This article presents the resources for patient education and treatment for individuals with peripheral vascular disease of the lower extremity. It presents the nursing measures for individuals with chronic venous insufficiency and strategies to improve compliance. Tables that define food label claims, differentiate venous and arterial ulcers, and describe compression devices provide helpful information to nurses.

Kuncl, N., & Nelson, K. M. (1997). Antihypertensive drugs: Balancing risks and benefits. *Nursing 97, 27* (8), 46–49.

This article reviews the major classifications of drugs used for hypertensive clients. The primary focus of the discussion is on health teaching, with an emphasis on how the nurse can teach clients to minimize drug side effects.

Wills, E. M., & Sloan, H. L. (1996). Assessing peripheral arterial disorders in the home: A multidisciplinary clinical guide. *Home Healthcare Nurse, 14,* 669–682.

This article presents a comprehensive approach to care of the client with PAD at home. In addition to the clinical guide presented, the authors discuss the interdisciplinary health problems and interventions that are needed for PAD. A continuing education (CE) test at the end of the article allows the reader to apply for CE credit.

INTERVENTIONS FOR CLIENTS IN SHOCK

The syndrome of shock is a common occurrence in acute care settings, although conditions leading to shock can occur anywhere. Shock is a whole body response to any situation that causes poor oxygenation of tissues and organs. Multisystem organ failure (MOF) and death can result if conditions causing shock are not treated. Nurses can play a vital role in the prevention of shock and its complications by initiating appropriate early interventions. Table 39–1 lists important concepts related to shock.

Overview

Body organs, tissues, and cells need a continuous supply of oxygen for proper metabolism and function. The cardiovascular system delivers oxygen to all tissues and removes cellular wastes. The components of the cardiovascular system are the blood, blood vessels, and heart. When any component of the cardiovascular system does not function properly for any reason, the syndrome of shock can result.

Shock is a pathologic condition rather than a disease state. It is initiated by abnormal cellular metabolism that occurs when insufficient oxygen is delivered to the tissues (Guyton & Hall, 1996). Shock was previously classified as hypovolemic, cardiogenic, vasogenic, or septic, indicating the site of origin of the problem causing shock. The condition, now classified by the specific functional impairment manifested, consists of *hypovolemic shock*, *cardiogenic shock*, *distributive shock*, and *obstructive shock* (Effron & Chernow, 1992). Table 39–2 compares the old and new classification systems and common conditions causing each category of shock. Because the functional classification is used by researchers and guides clinicians, it is used in this chapter.

Many clinical manifestations of shock are similar, regardless of the cause or specific impairment. Common findings are due to physiologic compensatory mechanisms. Manifestations unique to any type of shock are due to specific tissue dysfunction. The common clinical features of shock are listed in Chart 39–1.

TABLE 39-1

Key Concepts Related to Shock

- Shock results when too little oxygen reaches cells and tissues.
- Anyone is susceptible to shock.
- Shock progresses in a predictable, orderly fashion.
- Shock is reversible when the compensatory mechanisms are supported and the underlying causes are eliminated.
- Most clinical manifestations of shock are related to the body's compensatory responses to shock and not the cause of shock.
- The nurse always considers the possibility and probability of shock development.
- Subtle changes in heart rate, level of consciousness, and behavior may herald the onset of shock.
- Clients experiencing the early phase of sepsis-induced distributive shock may be warm and pink with a high cardiac output.
- Oxygen administration is an appropriate therapy for any type of shock.
- Changes in systolic blood pressure are not reliable indicators of initial and nonprogressive stages of shock.

Physiology Review

Oxygenation of any organ or tissue depends on how much oxygenated arterial blood perfuses (moves into and through) the organ or tissue. Organ perfusion is related to mean arterial pressure (MAP). Because the cardiovascular system is a closed but continuous circuit, the factors that influence MAP include

- Total blood volume
- Cardiac output
- Size of the vascular bed

Total blood volume and cardiac output are directly related to MAP, so that increases in either total blood volume or cardiac output usually raise MAP. Decreases in either total blood volume or cardiac output eventually lower MAP.

The size of the vascular bed is inversely related to MAP, so that increases in the size of the vascular bed lower MAP and decreases raise MAP (Fig. 39-1). The blood vessels, especially those connected directly to capillaries (arterioles and venules), can increase in size by relaxing the smooth muscle in vessel walls or decrease by

TABLE 39-2

Comparison of New and Old Shock Classification Systems

Classification by Functional Impairment

Hypovolemic	Cardiogenic	Distributive	Obstructive
• Total body fluid decreased (in all fluid compartments)	• Direct pump failure	• Fluid shifted from central vascular space	• Cardiac function decreased by noncardiac factors
• Hemorrhage	• Fluid volume not affected	• Total body fluid volume normal or increased	• Total body fluid volume not affected
• Dehydration	• Myocardial infarction Valvular problems Stenosis Incompentence	• Neural-induced loss of vascular tone	• Central volume decreased
	• Myopathies	• Chemical-induced loss of vascular tone	• Pulmonary hypertension
	• Dysrhythmias	Sepsis	• Tension pneumothorax
	• Cardiac arrest	Anaphylaxis	• Pericarditis
		Capillary leak	• Thoracic tumor
			• Tamponade

Classification by Site of Origin

Hypovolemic	Cardiogenic	Vasogenic	Septic
• Central vascular volume decreased	• Direct pump failure	• Loss of vascular tone	• Loss of vascular tone
• Total body fluid may or may not be decreased	• Indirect pump failure	• Total body fluid not decreased	• Eventual reduced cardiac output
• Hemorrhage	• Decreased cardiac output	• Neurogenic	• Seen as a more intense type of vasogenic shock
• Dehydration	• Total body fluid not decreased	Head trauma	• Infection
• Fluid shifts	• Valvular problems	Vasovagal response	
Trauma	Stenosis	• Vessel dilation	
Burns	Incompetence	Anaphylaxis	
Anaphylaxis	• Myocardial infarction	Inflammation	
	• Myopathies		
	• Dysrhythmias		
	• Cardiac arrest		
	• Tamponade		
	• Pericarditis		
	• Pulmonary hypertension		
	• Pulmonary emboli		

Chart 39–1

Key Features of Shock

Cardiovascular
- Decreased cardiac output
- Increased pulse rate
- Thready pulse quality
- Decreased blood pressure
- Narrowed pulse pressure
- Postural hypotension
- Low central venous pressure
- Flat neck and hand veins in dependent positions
- Slow capillary refill in nail beds
- Diminished peripheral pulses

Respiratory
- Increased respiratory rate
- Shallow depth of respirations
- Decreased arterial $PaCO_2$
- Decreased arterial PaO_2
- Cyanosis, especially around lips and nail beds

Neuromuscular
- Early
  - Anxiety
  - Restlessness
- Late
  - Decreased central nervous system activity (lethargy to coma)
  - Generalized muscle weakness
  - Diminished or absent deep tendon reflexes
  - Sluggish pupillary response to light

Renal
- Decreased urinary output
- Increased specific gravity
- Sugar and acetone present in urine

Integumentary
- Cool to cold
- Pale to mottled to cyanotic
- Moist, clammy
- Mouth dry, paste-like coating present

Gastrointestinal
- Decreased motility
- Diminished or absent bowel sounds
- Nausea and vomiting
- Constipation
- Increased thirst

contracting the muscle. When blood vessels dilate but the total blood volume remains the same, blood pressure decreases, and blood flow is slower. When blood vessels constrict but the total blood volume remains the same, blood pressure increases, and blood flow is faster.

Blood vessels contain nerves from the sympathetic division of the autonomic nervous system. Some nerves continuously stimulate vascular smooth muscle, so that the blood vessels are normally partially constricted. This state of variable blood vessel constriction is called *sympathetic tone*. An increase in sympathetic stimulation causes the

vascular smooth muscle to constrict further, raising MAP; a decrease in sympathetic stimulation causes the vascular smooth muscle to dilate, lowering MAP.

Blood flow to body organs varies to adjust to changes in tissue oxygen needs. The body can selectively increase blood flow to some areas while reducing blood flow to others. Some organs, such as the skin and skeletal muscles, can tolerate low levels of oxygen for hours without dying or becoming damaged. Other organs, such as the heart, brain, and liver, tolerate hypoxic conditions (low levels of tissue oxygenation) poorly, and even just a few minutes without adequate oxygen results in serious or permanent damage.

Pathophysiology

The underlying problems common to all types of shock, regardless of cause, are the effects of anaerobic cellular metabolism (metabolism without oxygen), which result from inadequate tissue oxygenation (Shoemaker, 1994). These effects cause adverse changes in tissue function. The body then begins to compensate in an attempt to maintain or restore tissue perfusion and oxygenation even while the triggering events of shock are still present.

When the conditions that cause shock remain uncorrected, shock progresses in a predictable sequence consisting of

1. Initial stage
2. Nonprogressive stage
3. Progressive stage
4. Refractory stage

The stages of shock are identified on the basis of

- How well the client's compensatory mechanisms are working
- The severity of the clinical manifestations
- The reversibility of tissue damage

The main triggering event leading to the recognizable picture of shock is a sustained decrease in mean arterial pressure (MAP) that results from decreased cardiac output, decreased circulating blood volume, or expansion of the vascular bed. A decrease in MAP of 5 to 10 mmHg below the client's baseline value is immediately detected by pressure-sensitive nerve receptors (baroreceptors) located in the aortic arch and the carotid sinus (Guyton & Hall, 1996). This information is transmitted to brain centers, stimulating compensatory mechanisms, which in turn ensure continued blood flow and oxygen delivery to vital organs while limiting blood flow to less vital areas. This moving of blood into selected areas while bypassing others (shunting) leads to the physiologic changes and clinical manifestations of shock.

If the events that caused the initial decrease in MAP are halted at this point, the compensatory mechanisms can return the body to a normal perfused and oxygenated state, even without outside intervention. If the initiating events continue and MAP decreases further, some tissues perform metabolic activities under anaerobic conditions, creating an increase in lactic acid and other harmful me-

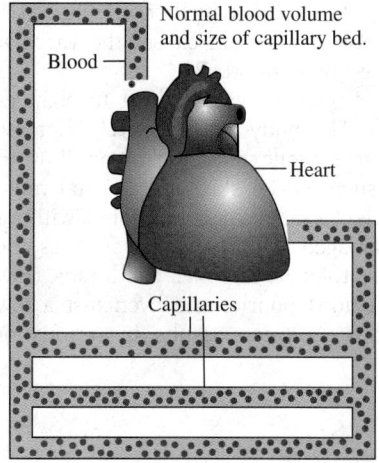

Normal blood volume and size of capillary bed.

Blood

Heart

Capillaries

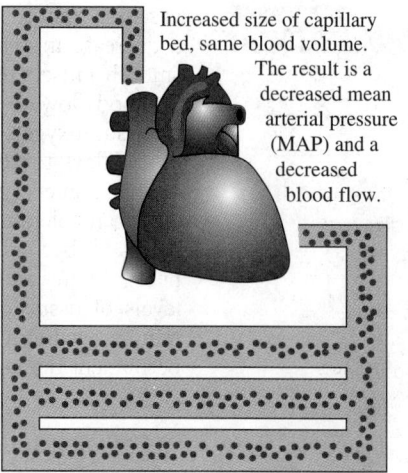

Increased size of capillary bed, same blood volume. The result is a decreased mean arterial pressure (MAP) and a decreased blood flow.

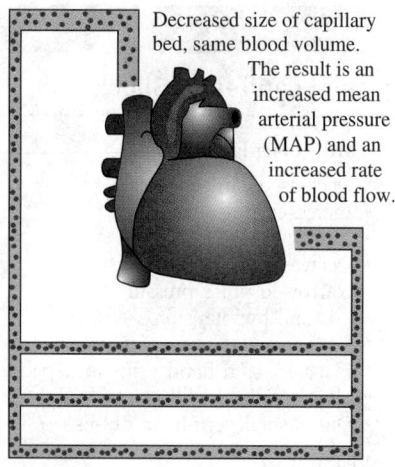

Decreased size of capillary bed, same blood volume. The result is an increased mean arterial pressure (MAP) and an increased rate of blood flow.

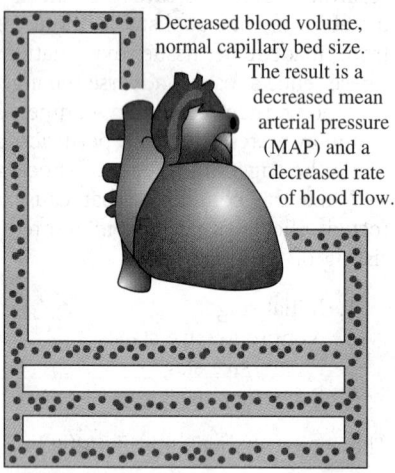

Decreased blood volume, normal capillary bed size. The result is a decreased mean arterial pressure (MAP) and a decreased rate of blood flow.

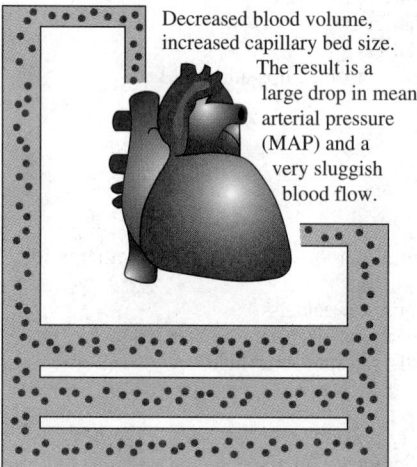

Decreased blood volume, increased capillary bed size. The result is a large drop in mean arterial pressure (MAP) and a very sluggish blood flow.

Figure 39–1. Interaction of blood volume and the size of the capillary bed affecting mean arterial pressure.

tabolites (such as degradative enzymes and oxygen radicals). These substances cause electrolyte and acid-base imbalances that have generalized, tissue-damaging effects and depress cardiac activity. Such effects are temporary and reversible if the cause of shock is corrected within 1 to 2 hours after onset. When conditions causing shock continue for longer periods without interventions, the resulting acid-base imbalance, electrolyte imbalances, and increased levels of toxic metabolites so damage the cells in vital organs that full recovery from shock is no longer possible. Table 39–3 summarizes the progression of shock.

Initial Stage of Shock (Early Shock)

The initial, or early, stage of shock is present when any condition causes MAP to decrease from the client's baseline level by less than 10 mmHg. During this stage, activated compensatory mechanisms are so effective at returning MAP to normal levels that oxygenated blood flow to all vital organs is maintained. Cellular changes in this stage are a decrease in aerobic metabolism and an increase in anaerobic metabolism with production of lactic acid (although overall cellular metabolism is still aerobic).

Compensation, by vascular constriction and heart rate increase, is relatively complete, and both cardiac output and MAP are maintained within the normal range. Because vital organ function is not disrupted, however, the signs and symptoms of shock are subtle and difficult to detect. A heart rate increase from the client's baseline level may be the only manifestation of this early stage of shock.

Nonprogressive Stage of Shock (Compensatory Stage)

The nonprogressive, or compensatory, stage of shock is observed when conditions have caused a 10- to 15-mmHg drop in MAP from baseline level. Renal and chemical compensatory mechanisms are activated because cardiovascular compensation alone is not enough to maintain MAP and to supply needed oxygen to vital organs.

The kidneys and baroreceptors sense a sustained decrease in MAP, resulting in the release of renin, antidiuretic hormone (ADH), aldosterone, and the catecholamines epinephrine and norepinephrine. Renal compensation occurs through the actions of renin, aldosterone, and ADH (see Chap. 14). Renin, secreted by the kidney, starts the reactions that eventually cause de-

TABLE 39–3

Physiologic Events During Shock

Stage of Shock	Physiologic Event
Initial stage	• Decrease in baseline mean arterial pressure (MAP) of 5–10 mmHg • Increased sympathetic stimulation • Mild vasoconstriction • Increase in heart rate
Nonprogressive stage	• Decrease in MAP of 10–15 mmHg from the client's baseline value • Continued sympathetic stimulation • Moderate vasoconstriction • Increased heart rate • Decreased pulse pressure • Chemical compensation • Renin, aldosterone, and antidiuretic hormone secretion • Increased vasoconstriction • Decreased urinary output • Stimulation of the thirst reflex • Some anaerobic metabolism in nonvital organs • Mild acidosis • Mild hyperkalemia
Progressive stage	• Decrease in MAP of >20 mmHg from the client's baseline value • Anoxia of nonvital organs • Hypoxia of vital organs • Overall metabolism is anaerobic • Moderate acidosis • Moderate hyperkalemia • Tissue ischemia
Refractory stage	• Severe tissue hypoxia with ischemia and necrosis • Release of myocardial depressant factor from pancreas • Build-up of toxic metabolites

creased urine output, increased reabsorption of sodium, and systemic vasoconstriction (see Chap. 14, Fig. 14–8). ADH is secreted by the posterior pituitary gland. The activity of ADH both increases reabsorption of water in the kidney and causes blood vessel constriction in the skin and other less vital tissue areas. Together, these actions attempt to compensate for shock by maintaining the volume in the central blood vessels (Guyton & Hall, 1996).

Tissue hypoxia is present in nonvital organs and in the kidney but is not great enough to cause severe symptoms or permanent damage. Because some metabolism is anaerobic, acid-base and electrolyte changes occur in response to the build-up of metabolites. Changes include acidosis and hyperkalemia (see Chaps. 16 and 19).

If the client's condition is stable and compensatory mechanisms are supported by medical and nursing interventions, the client can remain in this stage for hours without sustaining permanent damage. Halting the conditions that have caused shock and providing supportive interventions will prevent progression of shock, so that the effects of the nonprogressive stage are reversible.

Progressive Stage of Shock (Intermediate Stage)

The progressive stage of shock, sometimes called the intermediate stage, is characterized by a sustained decrease in MAP of greater than 20 mmHg from baseline level. In this stage, compensatory mechanisms are functioning but no longer able to maintain sufficient oxygen supply, even to vital organs. Compensatory mechanisms require heavy use of oxygen in certain tissues, so that the problem of general inadequate oxygenation becomes even worse. Vital organs develop hypoxia, and less vital organs experience anoxia and ischemia. As a result of inadequate oxygenation and a build-up of toxic metabolites, some tissues develop extensive cell damage and experience cell death.

The progressive stage of shock is a life-threatening emergency. Vital organs can tolerate this situation for only a short time before being permanently damaged. Immediate interventions are required to reverse the effects of this stage of shock. Tolerance of this stage is highly individual and depends greatly on the client's pre-existing health. Usually the client's life can be saved if precipitating conditions are corrected within an hour after the onset of the progressive stage.

Refractory Stage of Shock (Irreversible Stage)

The refractory stage of shock, once called the irreversible stage, is reached when too much cell death and tissue damage have occurred because of too little oxygen getting to the tissues. Vital organs then experience overwhelming changes. This stage is termed refractory because the body is unable to respond effectively to interventions, and the syndrome of shock continues. The remaining cells perform metabolic functions anaerobically. Therapy is ineffective in saving the client's life, even if the underlying cause of shock is corrected and MAP temporarily returns to normal. So much tissue damage has occurred, causing systemic release of toxic metabolites and destructive enzymes, that cellular deterioration of vital organs continues.

This sequence of damage is termed *multisystem organ failure* (MOF), or *multiple organ dysfunction syndrome* (MODS). Once the damage has started, the sequence becomes a vicious cycle as ischemic cells break open and release more harmful metabolites. The metabolites lead to the formation of small clots, disrupting tissue oxygenation, damaging more cells, and thus continuing the devastating cycle. The most profound ongoing change is deterioration of the myocardium. One contributing factor is the release of myocardial depressant factor (MDF) from the ischemic pancreas (Wilson, 1992).

Etiology

Because shock is a manifestation of a pathologic condition rather than a disease state, the causes of shock vary. Specific conditions leading to hypovolemic, cardiogenic, distributive, and obstructive shock are listed in Table 39–4. More than one type of shock can be present at the same time. For example, trauma caused by an automobile accident may trigger both hemorrhage, leading to hypovo-

TABLE 39–4

Types and Causes of Shock

Shock Type	Overall Cause	Specific Cause or Risk Factors

Hypovolemic shock	• Body fluid depletion	• Hemorrhage
		  • Trauma
		  • Gastrointestinal ulcer
		  • Surgery
		  • Inadequate clotting
		    • Hemophilia
		    • Liver disease
		    • Malnutrition
		    • Bone marrow suppression
		    • Cancer
		    • Anticoagulation therapy
		• Dehydration
		  • Vomiting
		  • Diarrhea
		  • Heavy diaphoresis
		  • Diuretic therapy
		  • Nasogastric suction
		  • Diabetes insipidus
		  • Hyperglycemia

Cardiogenic shock	• Direct pump failure	• Myocardial infarction
		• Cardiac arrest
		• Ventricular dysrhythmias
		  • Fibrillation
		  • Tachycardia
		• Cardiac amyloidosis
		• Cardiomyopathies
		  • Viral
		  • Toxic
		• Myocardial degeneration

Distributive shock	• Decreased vascular volume or tone	• Neural-induced
		  • Pain
		  • Anesthesia
		  • Stress
		  • Spinal cord injury
		  • Head trauma
		• Chemical-induced
		  • Anaphylaxis
		  • Sepsis
		  • Capillary leak
		    • Burns
		    • Extensive trauma
		    • Hepatic dysfunction
		    • Hypoproteinemia

Obstructive shock	• Indirect pump failure	• Cardiac tamponade • Arterial stenosis • Pulmonary embolus • Pulmonary hypertension • Constrictive pericarditis • Thoracic tumors • Tension pneumothorax

lemic shock, and a myocardial infarction (MI), leading to cardiogenic shock.

Hypovolemic Shock

Hypovolemic shock occurs when too little circulating (intravascular) fluid volume causes a MAP decrease, so that the body's total need for tissue oxygenation is not met. The most common conditions leading to hypovolemic shock are hemorrhage (external or internal) and dehydration.

Hypovolemic shock caused by external hemorrhage is associated with soft-tissue trauma, wounds, and surgery. Hypovolemic shock caused by internal hemorrhage is associated with blunt trauma, gastrointestinal (GI) ulcers, and poor surgical hemostasis. In addition, external and internal hemorrhage can be caused by any health problem that results in inadequate levels of coagulation factors (see Table 39–4).

Hypovolemia as a result of dehydration can be caused by any condition that decreases fluid intake or increases renal and insensible fluid loss (see Table 39–4).

Cardiogenic Shock

Cardiogenic shock occurs when the actual heart muscle is unhealthy and contractility is directly impaired. Table 39–4 lists common causes of direct pump failure. These conditions decrease cardiac output and afterload, thus reducing MAP. (Chapter 40 provides an in-depth discussion of cardiogenic shock resulting from myocardial infarction.)

Distributive Shock

Distributive shock is characterized by a loss of sympathetic tone, vasodilation, pooling of blood in venous and capillary beds, and increased vascular permeability. All of these factors contribute to decreased mean arterial pressure (MAP) and may be induced either neurogenically or chemically.

Neural-Induced Distributive Shock

Neural-induced loss of MAP occurs when sympathetic stimulation of nerves regulating the vascular smooth muscle is inhibited and the smooth muscles of blood vessels relax, causing vasodilation. Neural-induced vasodilation can be a normal local response to injury, but shock results when the vasodilation is systemic. Common conditions that can cause a systemic loss of sympathetic tone are listed in Table 39–4.

Chemical-Induced Distributive Shock

Chemical-induced distributive shock has three common origins: anaphylaxis, sepsis, and capillary leak syndrome. Chemical-induced distributive shock occurs when certain chemicals or foreign substances within the blood and blood vessels stimulate widespread changes in blood vessel walls. Usually, the chemicals are exogenous (come from outside the body), but this type of shock can be induced by substances normally found in the body.

ANAPHYLAXIS. Anaphylaxis is one result of type I hypersensitivity immune reactions (see Chap. 25). Although it usually begins within seconds to minutes after exposure to a specific allergen, this reaction is termed *delayed* because the person rarely has this type of reaction the first time the allergen is encountered. Rather, anaphylaxis occurs on repeated exposure to the same allergen (Guyton & Hall, 1996). Table 25–8 lists common allergens that can cause anaphylaxis.

Anaphylaxis is due to an antigen-antibody reaction occurring systemically in response to contact with a substance to which the person has a severe hypersensitivity (allergy). The widespread antigen-antibody reaction involves the interaction of the allergen, immunoglobulin E (IgE), basophils, and mast cells. The reaction occurs within the walls of blood vessels, myocardial cells, and bronchial epithelium (see Chaps. 23 and 25). Anaphylaxis damages cells and causes the release of large amounts of histamine and other vasoactive amines. These substances are distributed rapidly throughout the circulatory system, causing massive vasodilation and increased capillary permeability, which result in profound hypovolemia and vascular collapse. Decreased cardiac contractility and dysrhythmias occur during anaphylaxis. These symptoms may be direct results of myocardial changes induced by the antigen-antibody reaction, or may be due to the profound hypovolemia. Antigen-antibody reactions in bronchial tissues cause severe edema and pulmonary obstruction, which greatly reduce pulmonary gas exchange. The pulmonary problems, together with inadequate circulation, cause the person to experience extreme hypoxia. Without intervention, this condition results in death.

SEPSIS. Sepsis leading to distributive shock occurs when microorganisms are present in the blood and other normally sterile areas of the body. Often, sepsis is associated with disseminated intravascular coagulation (DIC). Although distributive shock has been reported among clients with viral and yeast sepsis, it is more commonly associated with bacteremia. Organisms often causing sepsis include gram-negative bacteria (*Pseudomonas aeruginosa, Escherichia coli,* and *Klebsiella pneumoniae*) and gram-positive bacteria (*Staphylococcus* and *Streptococcus*) (Beam, 1994; Hazinski, 1994; Lawler, 1994). Table 39–5 lists some of the conditions that predispose clients to sepsis-induced distributive shock.

Sepsis-induced distributive shock results from the large amounts of toxins and endotoxins produced by the bacteria and secreted into the blood, causing a whole body inflammatory reaction. The bacteria-produced toxins and endotoxins react with blood vessels and cell membranes. The resulting reactions, through white blood cell activity, stimulate a variety of inflammatory and immune events known as the *systemic inflammatory response syndrome* (SIRS). These toxin-host interactions stimulate systemic complement activation, altered microcirculation within vascular organs (including selective coagulation and thrombus formation), increased capillary permeability, cell

TABLE 39–5

Conditions That Predispose to Sepsis-Induced Distributive Shock

- Malnutrition
- Immunosuppression
- Large open wounds
- Mucous membrane fissures in prolonged contact with bloody or drainage-soaked packing
- Gastrointestinal ischemia
- Loss of gastrointestinal integrity
- Exposure to invasive procedures
- Malignancy

injury, and increased cellular metabolism (in combination with an inability of some cells to take up necessary oxygen). Metabolism becomes anaerobic because of decreased MAP, clot formation in capillaries, and poor cellular uptake of oxygen. Although bacterial toxins are generally implicated in initiating these events, some evidence indicates that the bacteria in the extracellular fluid, as well as the toxins, can start the SIRS and cause shock.

CAPILLARY LEAK SYNDROME. Capillary leak syndrome leading to distributive shock occurs when there is a shift of fluid from the vascular space to the interstitial space. Such shifts are caused by increased capillary permeability, loss of plasma osmolarity, and increased vascular hydrostatic pressure. Specific conditions associated with fluid shifts include severe burns, bullous skin disease, liver disorders, abdominal ascites, acute peritonitis, paralytic ileus, severe malnutrition, surgical wounds, hyperglycemia, renal disease, hypoproteinemia, and trauma.

Obstructive Shock

Obstructive shock results from conditions that affect the ability of the normal heart muscle to pump effectively. The heart itself is normal, but conditions outside the heart prevent either adequate filling of the heart or adequate contraction of the healthy heart muscle. Some causes of obstructive shock (Effron & Chernow, 1992; Wilson, 1992) are listed in Table 39–4.

Incidence/Prevalence

Because it is a secondary response rather than a separate disease entity, the exact incidence of shock is not known. However, some degree of shock is a common complication among hospitalized clients. Hypovolemic shock is the most common type experienced by clients in emergency departments and after surgery or procedures that involve invasion of a major artery. Cardiogenic shock is the most frequent complication of myocardial infarction, occurring in an estimated 15% of clients who experience damage to 40% or more of the myocardium (Effron & Chernow, 1992). The frequency of distributive shock as a result of sepsis, which ranges in mortality from 40% to 85%, is increasing among clients who are immunocompromised or who have infections (Ackerman, 1994; Clochesy, 1996).

This chapter presents the collaborative management of clients experiencing hypovolemic shock caused by hemorrhage and distributive shock caused by sepsis. Chapter 25 discusses interventions for anaphylaxis, and Chapter 40 discusses care of the client experiencing cardiogenic shock as a result of myocardial infarction.

Collaborative Management

 Assessment

➤ *History*

The nurse collects data on risk factors, as well as causative factors, related to hypovolemic shock. Age is impor-

tant because hypovolemic shock associated with trauma is more frequently seen in young adults, whereas sepsis is more common among the elderly. Clients are asked specific questions about recent illness, trauma, procedures, or chronic conditions that may lead to the development of shock. Such conditions include GI ulcers, general surgery, hemophilia, liver disorders, prolonged vomiting, and prolonged diarrhea. The use of such medications as aspirin, diuretics, and antacids may directly cause changes leading to hypovolemic shock or may indicate the presence of a disease or a problem that can contribute to hypovolemic shock.

The nurse inquires about the client's fluid intake and output during the previous 24 hours. Information about urine output is especially critical because the initial and nonprogressive stages of shock are characterized by a reduced urine output, even when fluid intake is normal.

The nurse assesses the client and the immediate environment for obvious signs of factors leading to shock. Areas to examine for signs of hemorrhage include the gums, wounds, and sites of dressings, drains, and vascular access. The nurse observes for any swelling, skin discoloration, or visible manifestations of pain that may indicate internal hemorrhage.

➤ *Physical Assessment/Clinical Manifestations*

Most of the observable manifestations of hypovolemic shock result from the physiologic changes that accompany compensatory efforts. Manifestations of shock are first evident as changes in cardiovascular function. As shock progresses, changes in the renal, pulmonary, integumentary, musculoskeletal, and central nervous systems become evident.

Cardiovascular Manifestations

Because shock involves a decrease of mean arterial pressure (MAP) and the resulting early compensatory mechanisms are cardiovascular, the earliest clinical manifestations of hypovolemic shock are also cardiovascular.

Pulse. The nurse or other assistive personnel assesses the central and peripheral pulses for rate and quality. In the initial stage of hypovolemic shock, the pulse rate increases to maintain cardiac output and MAP at normal levels, although the actual stroke volume per beat is usually decreased. Because the cardiac output is decreased, the distal peripheral pulses are more difficult to palpate and are easily blocked with minimal pressure. As hypovolemic shock progresses, superficial peripheral pulses may be absent.

Blood Pressure. Changes in blood pressure are not always present in the initial stage of hypovolemic shock. When assessing the blood pressure of a client at risk for shock, the nurse considers his or her normal baseline blood pressure level. Although a blood pressure measurement of 90/50 may indicate severe shock in one person, it may represent the normal blood pressure value for another healthy, but slightly built adult.

When compensatory efforts include vasoconstriction, the result is an increased diastolic pressure, whereas the systolic pressure remains the same. As a result, the pulse pressure, or the difference between the systolic and diastolic pressure measurements, is smaller. Nursing personnel monitor the client's blood pressure for changes from baseline levels and changes from the previous measurement. For accuracy, the same equipment is used on the same extremity. When the client's condition permits, the nurse measures the blood pressure with the client in the lying, sitting, and standing positions.

As hypovolemic shock progresses and cardiac output changes, the systolic pressure level decreases, reducing the pulse pressure even further. When hypovolemic shock continues and interventions are not adequate, compensation fails, and both the systolic and diastolic pressures decrease. At this stage, blood pressure is difficult to hear. Palpation or a Doppler device may be needed to detect the systolic blood pressure.

Oxygen Saturation. The nurse assesses peripheral oxygen saturation through pulse oximetry. Hemoglobin oxygen saturation values between 90% and 95% are associated with the nonprogressive stage of shock, and values between 75% and 80% are associated with the progressive stage of shock. Any value below 70% is considered a life-threatening emergency and may signal the refractory stage of shock.

Integumentary Manifestations

In hypovolemic shock, the skin is affected by altered perfusion. Because the skin can tolerate low oxygen levels and other vital organs cannot, an early compensatory mechanism for hypovolemic shock is vasoconstriction in the skin and superficial tissues to the extent that perfusion of these tissues is minimal or absent.

The nurse assesses the skin for temperature, color, and degree of moisture. The skin feels cool or cold to the touch, and the color is pale to cyanotic. Color changes are first evident in mucous membranes and in the skin around the mouth. Because pallor or cyanosis may be difficult to observe in many areas in dark-skinned clients, the nurse particularly assesses color changes in oral mucous membranes. As hypovolemic shock progresses, color changes in clients with lighter skin are noted in the extremities and then in the central trunk area. The skin also feels clammy or moist to the touch, not because sweating increases but because the normal fluid lost through the skin does not evaporate quickly on cold skin.

The nurse evaluates capillary refill time by pressing on a fingernail until it blanches and then observing how fast the nail bed resumes color when pressure is released. Normally, the nail bed capillaries resume color as soon as pressure is released. Capillary refill in clients experiencing hypovolemic shock is usually slow and sometimes absent.

Respiratory Manifestations

The nurse assesses the rate, depth, and ease of respiration and also auscultates the lungs for abnormal breath sounds. Respiratory rate increases during hypovolemic shock. This increase is a compensatory mechanism to provide adequate oxygenation to critical tissues. When shock has progressed to the stage at which lactic acidosis is present, the depth of respiration also increases.

Renal/Urinary Manifestations

The renal system compensates for the decreased MAP during hypovolemic shock by conserving body water through decreasing glomerular filtration and increasing the reabsorption of filtrate. The nurse or assistive personnel measures urine output every hour. Urine is assessed for color, specific gravity, and the presence of blood or protein. Urine output is decreased (compared with fluid intake) or even absent in severe shock. Of the four vital organs (heart, brain, liver, and kidney), only the kidney can tolerate hypoxia and anoxia for up to an hour without permanent damage. When hypoxic or anoxic conditions persist beyond this time, clients are at grave risk for acute tubular necrosis and renal failure.

Central Nervous System Manifestations

Clients who have hypovolemic shock are thirsty. This sensation is caused by stimulation of the osmoreceptors in the brain in response to the decreased blood volume (see Chapter 14).

The nurse assesses clients' level of consciousness (LOC) and orientation to person, time, and place. Most causes of hypovolemic shock do not interfere with nerve impulse transmission. Rather, central nervous system manifestations of hypovolemic shock are associated with cerebral hypoxia. In the initial and nonprogressive stages, clients may be restless or agitated and may experience anxiety or a feeling of impending doom that has no obvious cause. As hypoxia progresses, clients become confused and lethargic. Lethargy progresses to somnolence and loss of consciousness as cerebral hypoxia intensifies.

Musculoskeletal Manifestations

Tissue hypoxia, anaerobic metabolism, and lactic acidosis cause skeletal muscle weakness and pain. This weakness is generalized, with no specific pattern of presentation. The accompanying electrolyte disturbances in progressive and refractory stages of shock compound this muscle weakness by interfering with the generation and transmission of action potentials. In this situation, deep tendon reflexes are decreased or absent.

The nurse assesses muscle strength by having the client squeeze the nurse's hand and try to keep the arms flexed while the nurse pulls downward on the lower arms. The nurse assesses deep tendon reflexes by lightly tapping the patellar tendons and Achilles tendons with a reflex hammer and observing the degree of reflexive movement.

➤ Psychosocial Assessment

Changes in mental status and behavior may be early indicators of hypovolemic shock. The nurse observes the client closely and documents behavior. The nurse assesses current mental status by evaluating LOC. The nurse notes whether the client is asleep or awake. If the client is asleep, the nurse attempts to awaken the client and documents the ease with which the client is aroused. If the client is awake, the nurse establishes whether the client is oriented to person, time, and place. The nurse avoids asking questions that can be answered with a "yes" or a "no" response. The nurse documents the manner in

Chart 39–2

Laboratory Profile: Hypovolemic Shock

Test	Normal Range for Adults	Significance of Abnormal Findings
pH (arterial)	7.35–7.45	Decreased: insufficient tissue oxygenation causing anaerobic metabolism and acidosis
PaO_2	83–100 mmHg	Decreased: anaerobic metabolism
$PaCO_2$	Females: 32–45 mmHg Males: 35–48 mmHg	Increased: anaerobic metabolism
Lactic acid (venous)	0.9–1.7 mmol/L	Increased: anaerobic metabolism with build-up of metabolites
Hematocrit	Females: 35–47% Males: 39–50%	Increased: fluid shift, dehydration Decreased: hemorrhage
Hemoglobin	Females: 11.7–16 g/dL Males: 13.1–17.2 g/dL	Increased: fluid shift, dehydration Decreased: hemorrhage
Potassium	3.5–4.5 mEq/L or mmol/L	Increased: dehydration, acidosis

PaO_2 = arterial partial pressure of oxygen; $PaCO_2$ = arterial partial pressure of carbon dioxide.
Data from Tietz, N. W. (1995). *Clinical guide to laboratory tests* (3rd ed.). Philadelphia: W. B. Saunders.

which the client responds to the questions. The following points are considered during evaluation:

- Is it necessary to repeat questions to obtain a response?
- Does the response answer the question asked?
- Does the client have difficulty with word choices during the responses?
- Is the client irritated or upset by the questions?
- Can the client concentrate on a question long enough to provide an appropriate response, or is attention span limited?

If possible, the nurse questions family members or a significant other to determine whether the behavior and mental status are typical of this client.

➤ Laboratory Assessment

No single laboratory finding confirms or rules out the presence of shock, although changes in laboratory data may support the diagnosis of hypovolemic shock. (Chart 39–2 lists the common laboratory findings associated with hypovolemic shock.) As shock progresses, arterial blood gas values become abnormal. Most commonly, the pH decreases, the arterial partial pressure of oxygen (PaO_2) decreases, and the arterial partial pressure of carbon dioxide ($PaCO_2$) increases. Changes in other laboratory values may be associated with specific causes of hypovolemic shock.

Hematocrit and hemoglobin concentrations decrease with hypovolemic shock caused by hemorrhage. When hypovolemic shock is the result of dehydration or fluid shift, the hematocrit and hemoglobin values are elevated.

Interventions

Interventions for clients who have hypovolemic shock are focused on reversing the shock, restoring fluid volume, and preventing ischemic complications through support-

ive and drug therapies. Surgery may be necessary to correct the underlying problem leading to hypovolemic shock. Chart 39–3 summarizes nursing care priorities for clients experiencing hypovolemic shock.

➤ Nonsurgical Management

Interventions are aimed at maintaining tissue oxygenation, increasing the body fluid compartment volumes to achieve normal ranges, and supporting the client's operating compensatory mechanisms. Oxygen therapy, intravenous (IV) therapy, fluid replacement therapy, and drug therapies are the management choices for this problem.

Oxygen Therapy

Oxygen therapy is useful whenever shock is present. Oxygen can be administered by mask, hood, nasal cannula, nasopharyngeal tube, endotracheal tube, and tracheostomy tube. Usually, masks and nasal cannulas are used to

Chart 39–3

Nursing Care Highlight: The Client in Hypovolemic Shock

- Ensure a patent airway.
- Start an intravenous (IV) catheter or maintain an established catheter.
- Administer oxygen.
- Elevate the client's feet, keeping his or her head flat or elevated to a 30-degree angle.
- Examine the client for overt bleeding.
- If overt bleeding is present, apply direct pressure to the site.
- Take the client's vital signs every 5 minutes until stable.
- Administer medications as ordered.
- Increase the rate of IV fluid delivery.
- Do not leave the client.

provide oxygen to clients in shock. The nurse gives oxygen to the client in liters per minute (for administration via cannula) or concentration by percentage (for administration by mask), as specified by the physician's or nurse practitioner's order.

Intravenous Therapy

The two types of fluids commonly used for volume replacement during hemorrhagic hypovolemia are colloids and crystalloids. Colloids contain large molecules (usually composed of proteins or starches); IV colloid solutions are used to restore plasma volume and colloidal osmotic pressure (see Chap. 14). IV crystalloid solutions are administered for fluid and electrolyte replacement; they contain nonprotein substances, such as minerals, salts, and

▷ Research Applications for Nursing

Rapid Infusion of Intravenous Fluids During Hemorrhagic Shock May Increase Bleeding

Matsuoka, T., Hildreth, J., & Wisner, D. (1996). Uncontrolled hemorrhage from parenchymal injury: Is resuscitation helpful? Journal of Trauma, 40(6), 915–922.

A routine intervention for hypovolemic shock is the rapid infusion of crystalloidal and colloidal intravenous fluids in an attempt to increase mean arterial pressure (MAP). The investigators hypothesized that increasing MAP by rapid infusion of intravenous fluid before the cause of hemorrhage is identified and corrected could result in an increased rate of bleeding.

The investigators used an animal model to test this theory. After inflicting a standardized injury to the livers of 120 rats resulting in abdominal hemorrhage, the rats were assigned to one of four interventions groups: no resuscitation, small-volume infusion of isotonic fluid (4 mL/kg), large-volume infusion of isotonic fluid (24 mL/kg), and small-volume infusion of hypertonic saline (HS 4 mL/kg). The variables of blood pressure, intraperitoneal blood volume, and mortality rates were measured. Rats receiving large-volume infusions had higher blood pressures with greater mortality rates and significantly greater intraperitoneal blood volumes than did those receiving small-volume infusions of either fluid. Overall, the best outcomes were seen among the rats receiving small-volume infusions of hypertonic normal saline.

Critique. The study was well controlled and conducted under ideal laboratory conditions; all rat subjects were as similar as possible for most variables. Although animal models have been used successfully to mimic human responses to trauma and interventions for trauma, a major limitation of the study is the size of the animal model. Replication of the study using a larger animal model more comparable to humans is warranted.

Possible Nursing Implications. The results of this study indicate that, although intravenous access and infusion should be a mainstay of intervention for clients with hypovolemic shock, when hemorrhage is suspected, the infusion rate should not be excessive. It is imperative that the health care provider assess all indicators of hemorrhage for response to the infusion therapy.

sugars. A current controversy involves the infusion rate of fluids when hypovolemia is a result of hemorrhage but control of the hemorrhage has not yet been achieved. A consideration is that rapid infusion of IV fluids can increase blood pressure and may increase the rate of blood loss (see Research Application for Nursing).

Colloid Fluid Replacement. Protein-containing colloid fluids are good for restoring vascular osmotic pressure as well as fluid volume. Blood and blood products are frequently used for this purpose and are the treatment of choice when hypovolemia is caused by blood loss. These products include whole blood, packed red blood cells, and plasma.

Whole blood and packed red blood cells increase the hematocrit and hemoglobin concentrations as well as vascular fluid volume. Whole blood is used to replace large volumes of blood loss because it provides increased intravascular volume while improving the oxygen-carrying capacity of the blood. Packed red cells are given for moderate blood loss because they replenish the red cell deficit and improve the oxygen-carrying capacity without adding excessive fluid volume. (Chapter 42 discusses nursing care issues in blood and blood product administration.)

Human plasma, an acellular blood product containing some clotting factors, is given to correct plasma deficits and restore osmotic pressure when the hematocrit and hemoglobin levels are within normal ranges. Plasma protein fractions (such as Plasmanate) and synthetic plasma expanders, such as hetastarch (hydroxyethyl starch, Hespan), increase plasma volume and are frequently used as early treatment for hypovolemic shock before a cause is established.

Crystalloid Fluid Replacement. Crystalloid solutions are given to help establish and maintain an adequate fluid and electrolyte balance. Two common crystalloid solutions are Ringer's lactate and normal saline. Ringer's lactate contains physiologic concentrations of sodium, chloride, calcium, potassium, and lactate in water. This isotonic solution is a good volume expander, and the lactate is a buffer in the presence of acidosis. Normal saline (0.9% sodium chloride in water) is a fluid replacement used to increase the plasma volume when there has been no loss of red blood cells.

Drug Therapy

If the volume deficit is severe and the client does not respond sufficiently to the replacement of fluid volume and blood products, the administration of medications may increase venous return, improve cardiac contractility, or ensure adequate cardiac perfusion through dilation of coronary vessels. Chart 39–4 lists drugs commonly used to treat hypovolemic shock.

Vasoconstricting Agents. A variety of drugs stimulate venous return by causing vasoconstriction and decreasing venous pooling of blood. These actions increase cardiac output and mean arterial pressure (MAP), helping to improve tissue perfusion and oxygenation. Most of these drugs produce serious side effects, and their dosages must be carefully calculated on the basis of the client's size and degree of response (see Chart 39–4).

Chart 39–4

Drug Therapy for Hypovolemic Shock

Drug	Usual Dosage	Nursing Interventions	Rationale
Vasoconstrictors			
Dopamine hydrochloride (Intropin, Revimine✦)	• 5–30 μg/kg/min IV (for hypotension) • 2–5 μg/kg/min IV (for renal perfusion)	• Assess the client for chest pain. • Monitor urinary output hourly. • Assess blood pressure every 15 minutes. • Assess the client for headache.	• Dopamine increases myocardial oxygen consumption. • Higher doses decrease renal perfusion and urinary output. • Hypertension is a symptom of overdose. • Headache is an early symptom of drug excess.
Epinephrine (Adrenalin)	• 0.5–1 mg IV initially, followed by 0.5 mg every 5 minutes • May also be given by intracardiac injection	• Monitor the client for dysrhythmias. • Assess the client for chest pain.	• Epinephrine may cause ventricular tachyarrhythmias. • Vasoconstriction may impair cardiac oxygenation.
Norepinephrine (Levophed)	• 0.5–1.0 μg/kg/min continuous IV infusion to maintain blood pressure at 90–100 mmHg	• Assess for extravasation. • Observe the client's extremities for color and perfusion.	• Norepinephrine can cause severe tissue damage and necrosis. • Norepinephrine can cause such vasoconstriction that peripheral ischemia may result.
Phenylephrine (Neo-Synephrine)	• 80–200 μg/min IV	• Assess for chest pain.	• Vasoconstriction may impair cardiac oxygenation.
Agents Enhancing Contractility			
Amrinone (Inocor)	• 0.75–1.5 mg/kg bolus • 5–20 μg/kg/min continuous IV infusion	• Assess blood pressure every 15 minutes. • Do not administer through the same tubing as furosemide.	• Hypertension is a symptom of overdose. • Amrinone and furosemide form a precipitate.
Atropine sulfate	• 0.5–1 mg IV every 5 minutes, up to a total of 2 mg	• Take pulse every 5 minutes. • Monitor urinary output every 30 minutes. • Administer cautiously to clients with glaucoma.	• Atropine sulfate may cause a rebound tachycardia. • Atropine sulfate may cause urinary retention. • Atropine sulfate may precipitate an episode of acute angle-closure glaucoma.
Dobutamine hydrochloride (Dobutrex)	• 2.5–20 μg/kg/min continuous IV infusion	• Assess the client for chest pain. • Assess blood pressure every 15 minutes.	• Dobutamine increases myocardial oxygen consumption. • Hypertension is a symptom of overdose.
Agents Enhancing Myocardial Perfusion			
Sodium nitroprusside (Nitropress, Nipride✦)	• 0.5–10 μg/kg/min continuous IV infusion	• Assess blood pressure every 15 minutes.	• Hypotension may result from the systemic dilation of veins and arteries.

Agents Enhancing Myocardial Contractility. Some drugs directly stimulate adrenergic receptor sites on the myocardium (especially beta$_1$-receptors) and increase the contraction of the cardiac muscle cells. Other agents enhance cardiac contractility by slowing the heart rate through altering electrical conduction and allowing the left ventricle a longer filling time. When the filling time is increased, more blood enters the left ventricle and stretches the myocardial fibers. Thus, greater recoil is achieved, and more blood leaves the left ventricle during contraction. Some of these drugs also stimulate the ventricles at the same time. Agents with these types of actions include digoxin (Lanoxin) and dobutamine (Dobutrex).

Agents Enhancing Myocardial Perfusion. The treatment of shock includes giving agents that cause systemic vasoconstriction to help enhance venous return and increase MAP. However, it is important to ensure that the heart is well perfused so that aerobic metabolism is maintained in the cardiac cells and maximum contractility can be achieved. Agents that dilate coronary blood vessels while causing minimal systemic vasodilation are used for this purpose. Care is taken because higher dosages can cause some systemic vasodilation and increase shock.

Monitoring

A major nursing responsibility in caring for the client in hypovolemic shock is monitoring vital signs and level of consciousness (LOC). On the acute nursing unit, the nurse monitors the client's

- Pulse
- Blood pressure
- Pulse pressure
- Central venous pressure
- Respiratory rate
- Skin and mucosal color
- Pulse oximetry values

The nurse performs these assessments at least every 15 minutes until the shock is under control and the client's condition improves. More extensive monitoring of cardiac output (hemodynamic monitoring), including intra-arterial monitoring, mixed venous oxygen saturation (SvO_2), and pulmonary artery wedge pressures, is done in critical care settings.

Clients with shock who require more invasive monitoring, such as central venous pressure (CVP), pulmonary artery pressure (PAP), and pulmonary artery wedge pressure (PAWP), should be transported to a critical care unit. Table 39–6 compares changes seen in hemodynamic patterns with different types of shock.

Insertion of a CVP catheter allows monitoring of the client's right atrial or superior vena cava pressure while providing venous access. Changes in CVP reflect the syndrome of hypovolemic shock. As the circulating volume decreases, the amount of blood returning to the right atrium also decreases, causing the CVP to decrease from baseline levels.

Intra-arterial catheter placement provides a means of monitoring blood pressure continuously and serves as an access for arterial blood sampling. Intra-arterial catheters are inserted into an artery (radial, brachial, femoral, or dorsalis pedis artery). The arterial catheter is attached to pressure tubing and a transducer. The transducer converts the pressure in the artery (mechanical energy) into an electrical signal that is expressed as a visible waveform on an oscilloscope, and a digital numeric value is displayed.

➤ Surgical Management

The nurse monitors the client's fluid loss and uses the nonsurgical interventions described earlier to stabilize the client's hemodynamic status. After a cause has been established, surgical intervention may be necessary to correct the underlying problem. Such interventions include vascular repair or revision, surgical hemostasis of major wounds, oversewing of bleeding ulcers, and chemical scarring (chemosclerosis) of varicosities.

Collaborative Management

 Assessment

Distributive shock caused by sepsis does not resemble other types of shock in that it has two distinctive phases (Figure 39–2). The first phase is relatively long, frequently lasting from hours to a day or longer. The clinical manifestations during this phase are subtle. However, when the client is recognized to be in the first phase of sepsis-induced distributive shock and the appropriate interventions are made, there is a good chance for recovery. The second phase of sepsis-induced distributive shock has a sudden onset and a rapid downhill course. If sepsis-induced distributive shock progresses without intervention to the second phase, chances for the client's recovery are slim. Identification of the first phase of sepsis-induced distributive shock can make the greatest difference in survival among affected clients.

TABLE 39–6

Hemodynamic Pattern Changes Associated with Different Types of Shock				
Type of Shock	Cardiac Output (CO)	Central Venous Pressure (CVP)	Pulmonary Artery Pressure (PAP)	Pulmonary Capillary Wedge Pressure (PCWP)
Hypovolemic	↓	↓	↓	↓
Cardiac	↓	↑	↑	↑
Obstructive	↓	↑	↑	↑
Distributive				
Anaphylactic	↓	↓	↓	↓
Sepsis (early)	↑	∅	∅ or ↑	∅ or ↑
Sepsis (late)	↓	↓	↓	↓

↑ = increased; ↓ = decreased; ∅ = normal or unchanged.
Data from Jones, K. (1996). Shock. In J. Clochesy, C. Breu, S. Cardin, A. Whittaker, & E. Rudy (Eds.), *Critical care nursing* (2nd ed., pp. 1371–1318). Philadelphia: W. B. Saunders.

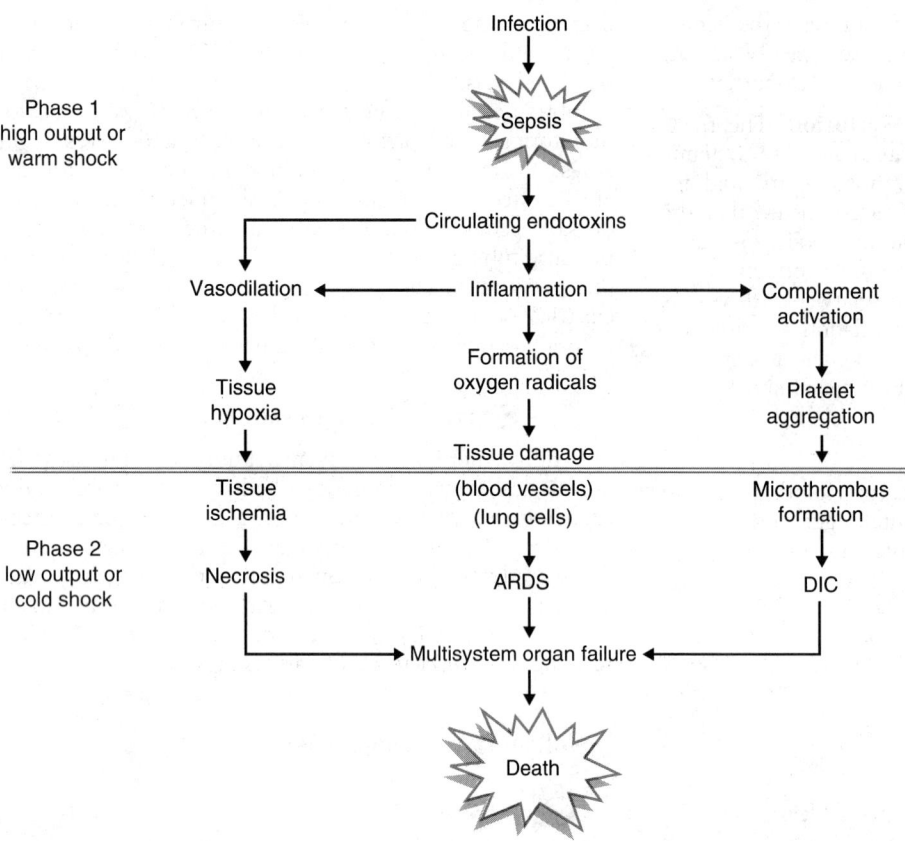

Figure 39–2. The sequence of sepsis-induced distributive shock. (ARDS = adult respiratory distress syndrome; DIC = disseminated intravascular coagulation.)

➤ History

The nurse collects data about risk factors, as well as causative factors, related to sepsis-induced distributive shock. Age is important because sepsis-induced distributive shock can develop more easily among elderly, debilitated people with any degree of immunosuppression. Chart 39–5 lists some of the factors that increase the elderly person's risk for shock. Clients are asked specific questions about recent illness, trauma, or procedures or chronic conditions that may lead to sepsis and distributive shock. The use of some medications may directly cause changes leading to shock. A medication regimen may also indicate a disease or a problem that can contribute to sepsis-induced distributive shock. Such medications include aspirin and aspirin-containing drugs, antibiotics, and chemotherapeutic agents.

➤ Physical Assessment/Clinical Manifestations

Many of the clinical manifestations of the first phase are unique to sepsis-induced distributive shock and, frequently, opposite from those associated with all other types of shock. Chart 39–6 summarizes the clinical manifestations of the first phase of sepsis-induced distributive shock. These findings, affecting the cardiovascular, integumentary, and pulmonary systems, result from the body's reaction to the presence of endotoxins.

Cardiovascular Manifestations

Endotoxins in the client's blood and other extracellular fluids interact with leukocytes as well as blood vessel walls and trigger an inflammatory reaction. In addition, some endotoxins appear to stimulate myocardial tissue directly. As a result, cardiac output is actually increased during the first phase of sepsis-induced distributive shock. This phase also may be called the *high-output* or

---

Chart 39–5

Nursing Focus on the Elderly: Risk Factors for Shock

Type of Shock	Specific Risk Factor
Hypovolemic shock	• Diuretic therapy • Diminished thirst reflex • Immobility
Cardiogenic shock	• Diabetes mellitus • Presence of cardiomyopathies
Distributive shock	• Diminished immune response • Reduced skin integrity • Presence of cancer • Peripheral neuropathy • Cerebrovascular accidents • Institutionalization (hospital or extended care facility) • Malnutrition • Anemia
Obstructive shock	• Pulmonary hypertension • Presence of cancer

---

Chart 39–6

Key Features of Phase 1 Sepsis-Induced Distributive Shock

Assessment	Findings
General	
Assess the mental status and level of consciousness.	• Irritability, restlessness, lethargy, disorientation, and inappropriate euphoria
Check the oral temperature.	• Normal, subnormal, or elevated temperature
Cardiovascular System	
Check the pulse and blood pressure. Document the pulse pressure with each blood pressure reading.	• Tachycardia: normal mean arterial blood pressure; widening pulse pressure
Check peripheral pulses.	• "Bounding" peripheral pulses
Auscultate heart sounds at four valvular sites, and record the onset of murmur or gallop.	• No murmur or gallop
Respiratory System	
Observe the rate, rhythm, and effort of breathing. Observe the symmetry of chest expansion.	• Tachypnea, hyperventilation
Percuss and auscultate the lungs. Note the onset of adventitious sounds.	• Crackles and decreased breath sounds
Check blood gas levels.	• Respiratory alkalosis
Integumentary System	
Inspect and palpate the skin. Note color, vascularity, moisture, temperature, texture, thickness, mobility, and turgor. Assess the oral mucosa.	• Warm flushed skin and peripheral edema

---

warm-shock phase. The increased cardiac output is reflected by tachycardia, increased stroke volume, a normal-to-elevated systolic blood pressure, and a normal CVP. The increased cardiac output causes good perfusion of the skin, so that the skin may appear to be normal in color with pink mucous membranes and may feel warm to the touch. This situation is temporary, and eventually the cardiac output greatly diminishes in clients experiencing sepsis-induced distributive shock.

As sepsis-induced distributive shock progresses, disseminated intravascular coagulation (DIC) may accompany it. The presence of the endotoxins and the inflammatory reactions stimulate complement activation (see Chap. 23). These actions cause thousands of small clots to form in the tiny capillaries of vascular organs (e.g., liver, kidney, brain, spleen, and heart). These small clots interfere with the oxygenation in those organs, causing hypoxia and ischemia and making overall metabolism anaerobic. The enormous number of small clots use clotting factors and fibrinogen faster than they can be regenerated by the liver, making clients much more susceptible to hemorrhage. These occurrences mark the beginning of the second phase of sepsis-induced distributive shock. Because some of the blood has already clotted, most of the clotting factors are gone, and blood vessels are dilated; clients are hypovolemic in this phase of distributive shock. The cardiac output now decreases dramatically, as do systolic blood pressure and pulse pressure. This phase is called the *low-output,* or *cold-shock*, phase of sepsis-induced distributive shock, and the clinical manifestations resemble those of the later stages of all forms of shock.

Respiratory Manifestations

In the high-output phase of sepsis-induced distributive shock, respiratory rate and depth are increased. Often, clients experience a respiratory alkalosis.

When sepsis-induced distributive shock progresses to the low-output phase, the possible life-threatening pulmonary complication of adult respiratory distress syndrome (ARDS) may occur. Although this complication has many causes, ARDS in cases of sepsis is thought to be related to the formation of oxygen-free radicals, which damage the pulmonary cells (Wilson, 1992). Oxygen-free radicals can form as a result of oxygen therapy and in response to cellular destruction and subsequent release of oxidizing enzymes. The presence of ARDS in a client who has sepsis-induced distributive shock is an ominous clinical sign associated with a high mortality rate.

Integumentary Manifestations

Often, clients in the early phase of sepsis-induced distributive shock are not recognized as having a problem because the appearance of the skin and mucous membranes leads health care professionals to believe that circulation is unimpaired. Clients feel warm to the touch, and their lips and mucous membranes appear well oxygenated.

When sepsis-induced distributive shock progresses so that circulation is compromised, the skin is cool and clammy with pallor or cyanosis present. In clients with disseminated intravascular coagulation (DIC), petechiae and ecchymoses occur anywhere. Blood may ooze from gums, other mucous membranes, venipuncture sites, and around IV catheters.

➤ *Psychosocial Assessment*

Often, the indicator that all is not well with clients at the beginning of sepsis-induced distributive shock is a change in affect or behavior. The nurse compares their presenting behavior, verbal responses, and general affect with those assessed earlier in the day or the day before and notes changes. Clients may seem just slightly different in their reactions to greetings, comments, or jokes. They may be less patient than usual or act restless or fidgety. Clients may verbalize feelings, such as "I feel as if something is wrong, but I don't know what." If this behavior represents a change from prior assessments, the nurse always considers the possibility of sepsis and shock.

➤ *Laboratory Assessment*

The presence of bacteria in blood and other extracellular fluids supports the diagnosis of sepsis. The nurse obtains specimens of urine, blood, sputum, and any drainage for culture to identify the causative organisms for both diagnostic and therapeutic purposes. Other abnormal laboratory findings associated with sepsis-induced distributive shock include changes in the white blood cell count; the differential leukocyte count may demonstrate a left shift (see Chap. 23). Changes in hematocrit and hemoglobin levels usually are not evident until late in septic shock when the client is hemorrhaging. At that point, the hematocrit and hemoglobin concentrations are low, as are the fibrinogen levels and the platelet count.

 Analysis

A common collaborative problem for clients with sepsis-induced distributive shock is the potential for multisystem organ failure (MOF), also called multiple organ dysfunction syndrome (MODS).

 Planning and Implementation

➤ *Planning: Expected Outcomes*

The client is expected to
- Have normal arterial blood gases
- Maintain a urine output of at least 20 mL/hour
- Have a mean arterial blood pressure within 10 mmHg of baseline

➤ *Interventions*

Interventions for the client experiencing sepsis-induced distributive shock focus on correcting the conditions causing shock and on preventing complications. Chart 39–7 summarizes the nursing care priorities for clients experiencing sepsis-induced distributive shock.

Control of fluid volume deficit associated with sepsis-induced distributive shock is accomplished through supportive and drug therapies. IV therapy is the same as for hypovolemic shock.

Oxygen Therapy. Oxygen therapy is useful whenever inadequate tissue perfusion and inadequate oxygenation

are present, such as during distributive shock. Oxygen therapy for sepsis-induced distributive shock is administered in the same ways as for hypovolemic shock (see p. 390).

Drug Therapy. The same agents used to enhance cardiac output and restore vascular volume in hypovolemic shock are used for sepsis-induced distributive shock. A major focus is the administration of antibiotics to combat sepsis. In addition, agents to counteract disseminated intravascular coagulation (DIC) may be required. Sepsis-induced distributive shock and DIC have two distinctly different phases, and drug therapies for each phase of sepsis-induced distributive shock are different. Drug therapy in the first phase is aimed at preventing coagulation and usually consists of heparin administration. Drug therapy in the second, late phase of sepsis-induced distributive shock is aimed at increasing the blood's ability to clot and usually consists of clotting factor administration.

Antibiotics. Although sepsis and distributive shock can be caused by any microorganism, the most common agents are gram-negative bacteria. When blood cultures have identified specific bacteria, IV antibiotics with known activity against the bacteria are administered. When the causative agent is not known, multiple agents with wide activity are prescribed. A common "triple-antibiotic" regimen includes vancomycin, one of the aminoglycosides, and a systemic penicillin derivative.

Antibodies. Antibodies against the body's mediators for inflammation are being tested for their effectiveness against sepsis-induced distributive shock. Antibodies have been developed against different substances that white blood cells produce to stimulate the inflammatory response. The mediators thought to start the inflammatory

---

Chart 39–7

Nursing Care Highlight: The Client in Sepsis-Induced Distributive Shock

- Ensure a patent airway.
- Start or maintain an established intravenous (IV) catheter.
- Administer oxygen.
- Administer antibiotics.
- Obtain specimens of blood, urine, wound drainage, and sputum for culture.
- Increase the rate of IV fluid delivery.
- Use aseptic technique for any invasive procedure.
- Handle the client gently.
- Examine the client for overt bleeding, especially of gums, injection sites, and IV sites.
- Elevate the client's feet, keeping his or her head flat or elevated to a 30-degree angle.
- Take the client's vital signs every 5 minutes until they are stable.
- Administer medications as ordered:
  - Heparin during phase 1
  - Clotting factors during phase 2
- Do not leave the client.

responses in blood vessels and lead to the cascade of sepsis-induced distributive shock are interleukin-1 (IL-1), interleukin-6 (IL-6), and tumor necrosis factor (TNF). This experimental therapy shows promise in reducing the extensive mortality associated with sepsis-induced distributive shock (Clochesy, 1996; Workman, 1995).

Anticoagulants. When clients are identified as being in the early phase of sepsis-induced distributive shock and are beginning to form numerous small clots, heparin is given to limit unnecessary clotting and to prevent the consumption of clotting factors.

Clotting Factors. When sepsis-induced distributive shock progresses to the point that small clots have formed to such an extent that the client no longer has sufficient clotting factors to prevent hemorrhage, clotting factors are given intravenously. These factors are obtained from pooled human serum. Administration of fresh frozen plasma also helps to replace clotting factors.

Providing a Safe Environment

Primary prevention is possible for some types of shock by identifying clients at risk for conditions and complications leading to sepsis and preventing those complications. Strict adherence to aseptic technique during invasive procedures and during the manipulation of nonintact skin and mucous membranes of clients who are immunocompromised to any degree can help to prevent or limit sepsis and sepsis-induced distributive shock.

Early detection of the clinical manifestations of shock is a major nursing responsibility. Because shock is a common complication of many conditions found among clients in acute care settings, the nurse always considers the possibility of sepsis-induced distributive shock. For early detection, the nurse continuously assesses vital signs for specific changes from normal values or from baseline levels. After distributive shock is recognized, health care providers rapidly take action to halt or change the conditions contributing to shock, to support the client's physiologic compensatory mechanisms, and to prevent life-threatening complications.

➤ Continuing Care

For most clients, shock is a complication of another condition and is resolved before discharge from an emergency department or acute care setting. However, with more clients receiving treatment on an outpatient basis and with earlier discharge from acute care settings, more clients at home are at increased risk for infection and sepsis-induced distributive shock.

➤ *Health Teaching*

Protecting vulnerable clients from infection and sepsis at home is an important nursing function. The nurse instructs clients about the importance of self-care strategies, such as good hygiene, hand washing, balanced rest and exercise, skin care, and mouth care. If clients or family members do not know how to take a temperature or read

---

> ## Chart 39–8
>
> ### Education Guide: Infection Precautions
>
> - Avoid crowds and other large gatherings of people, who might be ill.
> - Do not share eating utensils or personal toilet articles, such as toothbrushes, toothpaste, washcloths, or deodorant sticks, with others.
> - If possible, bathe daily.
> - Wash the armpits, groin, genitals, and anal area at least twice a day with an antimicrobial soap.
> - Clean your toothbrush daily by either running it through the dishwasher or rinsing it in liquid laundry bleach.
> - Wash your hands thoroughly with an antimicrobial soap before you eat or drink, after touching a pet, after shaking hands with anyone, as soon as you come home from any outing, and after using the toilet.
> - Wash dishes between use with hot, sudsy water, or use a dishwasher.
> - Do not drink water that has been standing for longer than 15 minutes.
> - Do not reuse cups and glasses without washing.
> - Do not change pet litter boxes.
> - Take your temperature at least once a day.
> - Refrigerate and prepare food appropriately. Do not eat raw or undercooked meat, fish, poultry, or eggs.
> - Report any of the following signs or symptoms of infection to your physician immediately:
>   - Temperature greater than 100°F (38°C)
>   - Persistent cough (with or without sputum)
>   - Pus or foul-smelling drainage from any open skin area or normal body opening
>   - Presence of a boil or abscess
>   - Urine that is cloudy or foul-smelling or that causes burning on urination
> - Do not dig in the garden or work with houseplants.
> - Use antibacterial cleansers to clean kitchen and bathroom surfaces at least twice each week. If you clean these areas yourself, wear rubber or vinyl work gloves while cleaning.
> - Use a condom when having sex.
> - Take all prescribed medications as the physician ordered.

a thermometer, the nurse provides instruction and obtains a return demonstration. Clients are instructed to avoid crowds or other people with known illnesses and to notify the health care provider immediately upon experiencing any fever or other sign of infection. Specific recommendations for infection precautions are listed in Chart 39–8.

➤ *Home Care Management*

The nurse or home health aide evaluates the home environment for safety regarding infection hazards. General cleanliness is noted, and particular attention is paid to the kitchen and bathrooms. Chart 39–9 lists focused client and environmental assessment data to obtain during a home visit.

Chart 39-9

Focused Assessment for Home Care Clients at Risk for Sepsis

- Assess the client for any clinical manifestations of infection including:
  - Temperature, pulse, respiration, and blood pressure
  - Color of skin and mucous membranes
  - The mouth and perianal area for fissures or lesions
  - Any nonintact skin area for the presence of exudates, redness, increased warmth, swelling
  - Any pain, tenderness, or other discomfort anywhere
  - Cough or any other symptoms of a cold or the flu
  - Urine; or ask client whether urine is dark or cloudy; has an odor; or causes pain or burning during urination
- Assess client's and caregiver's compliance with and understanding of infection prevention techniques
- Assess home environment, including
  - General cleanliness
  - Kitchen and bathroom facilities, including refrigeration
  - Availability and type of soap for hand washing
  - Presence of pets, especially cats, rodents, or reptiles

CASE STUDY for the Client with Hypovolemic Shock

■ A 38-year-old woman has returned to the post-anesthesia recovery area 2 hours ago, after having a tubal ligation by colposcopy (through the back wall of the vagina behind the cervix). Her last documented vital signs, taken 30 minutes ago, were as follows: BP, 102/80; pulse, 88; and respirations, 22. You now note that her face is pale, and the skin around her lips has a bluish cast. Her current vital signs are BP, 90/76; pulse, 98; and respirations, 28.

QUESTIONS:

1. What additional assessment techniques would you perform?
2. Where would you look for hemorrhage?
3. What other data would you gather?
4. When you reassess her in 15 minutes, you find her vital signs are now BP, 88/70; pulse, 102; and respirations, 30. She wakens when you shake her arm and complains of back pain and thirst. Given these findings, what are your action priorities?
5. What expected outcomes would be specific to this situation?

SELECTED BIBLIOGRAPHY

Ackerman, M. (1994). The systemic inflammatory response, sepsis and multiple organ dysfunction: New definitions for an old problem. *Critical Care Clinics of North America, 6*(2), 243–250.

Beam, T. (1994). Anti-infective drugs in the prevention and treatment of sepsis syndrome. *Critical Care Clinics of North America, 6*(2), 275–294.

Brown, K. (1994a). Septic shock: How to stop the deadly cascade, part 1. *American Journal of Nursing, 94*(9), 20–27.

Brown, K. (1994b). Septic shock: Critical interventions, part 2. *American Journal of Nursing, 94*(10), 20–26.

Chernow, B. (1996). New advances in the pharmacologic approach to circulatory shock. *Journal of Clinical Anesthesiology, 8*(Suppl. 3), 67s–69s.

Clochesy, J. (1996). Patients with systemic inflammatory response syndrome. In J. Clochesy, C. Breu, S. Cardin, A. Whittaker, & E. Rudy (Eds.), *Critical care nursing* (2nd ed., pp. 1359–1370). Philadelphia: W. B. Saunders.

Cotran, R., Kumar, V., & Robbins, S. (1994). *Robbins pathologic basis of disease* (5th ed.). Philadelphia: W. B. Saunders.

*Effron, M., & Chernow, B. (1992). Shock. In E. Rubenstein & D. Federman (Eds.), *Scientific American: Medicine* (pp. I card III Shock 1-12). New York: Scientific American.

Flavell, C. (1994). Combating hemorrhagic shock. *RN, 57*(12), 26–31.

Grap, M. (1998). Pulse oximetry. *Critical-Care Nurse, 18*(1), 94–99.

Grap, M., Glass, C., & Constatino, S. (1994). Accurate assessment of ventilation and oxygenation. *Medsurg Nursing, 3*(6), 435–443.

Guyton, A., & Hall, J. (1996). *Textbook of medical physiology* (9th ed.). Philadelphia: W. B. Saunders.

Hazinski, M. (1994). Mediator-specific therapies for the systemic inflammatory response syndrome, sepsis, severe sepsis, and septic shock: Present and future approaches. *Critical Care Clinics of North America, 6*(2), 309–319.

Headley, J. (1995). Analyzing normal hemodynamic waveforms. *Nursing95, 25*(3), 32AA–32DD.

Jones, K. (1996). Shock. In J. Clochesy, C. Breu, S. Cardin, A. Whittaker, & E. Rudy (Eds.), *Critical care nursing* (2nd ed., p. 1371). Philadelphia: W. B. Saunders.

Lawler, D. (1994). Hormonal response in sepsis. *Critical Care Clinics of North America, 6*(2), 265–274.

Martin, J. (1995). The Trendelenburg position: A review of current slants about head down tilt. *American Association of Nurse Anesthetists Journal, 63*(1), 29–36.

Matsuoka, T., Hildreth, J., & Wisner, D. (1996). Uncontrolled hemorrhage from parenchymal injury: Is resuscitation helpful? *Journal of Trauma, 40*(6), 915–922.

Mattice, C. (1996). It's not always obvious when a patient's in shock. *RN, 59*(3), 61–62.

Miller, L. (1996). Hemodynamic monitoring. In J. Clochesy, C. Breu, S. Cardin, A. Whittaker, & E. Rudy (Eds.), *Critical care nursing* (2nd ed., pp. 203–234). Philadelphia: W. B. Saunders.

Nawas, Y., & Balk, R. (1994). General approach to shock. *Clinics in Geriatric Medicine, 10*(1), 185–196.

O'Neal, P. (1994). How to spot early signs of cardiogenic shock. *American Journal of Nursing, 94*(5), 36–40.

Price, C. (1994). Acute renal failure: A sequela of sepsis. *Critical Care Clinics of North America, 6*(2), 359–372.

Raimer, F. (1995). Identifying abnormal hemodynamic waveforms. *Nursing95, 25*(4), 32MM–32QQ.

Russell, S. (1994a). Hypovolemic shock: Is your patient at risk? *Nursing94, 24*(4), 34–39.

Russell, S. (1994b). Septic shock: Can you recognize the clues? *Nursing94, 24*(4), 40–48.

Shelton, B. (1994). Disorders of hemostasis in sepsis. *Critical Care Nursing Clinics of North America, 6*(2), 373–387.

Shoemaker, W. (1994). Pathophysiology, monitoring and therapy of acute circulatory problems. *Critical Care Clinics of North America, 6*(2), 295–307.

Stengle, J., & Dries, D. (1994). Sepsis in the elderly. *Critical Care Nursing Clinics of North America, 6*(2), 421–427.

Tangredi, M. (1998). Clinical snapshot: Septic shock. *American Journal of Nursing, 98*(3), 46–47.

Vollman, K. (1994). Adult respiratory distress syndrome. *Critical Care Clinics of North America, 6*(2), 341–358.

*Wilson, R. (1992). *Critical care manual: Applied physiology and principles and therapy* (2nd ed.). Philadelphia: F. A. Davis.

Workman, M. L. (1995). Essential concepts of inflammation and immunity. *Critical Care Clinics of North America, 7*(4), 601–615.

SUGGESTED READINGS

Brown, K. (1994a). Septic shock: How to stop the deadly cascade, part 1. *American Journal of Nursing, 94*(9), 20–27.

Using a case study approach, the author presents the pathophysiology, assessment data, and initial care needs for people with sepsis-induced distributive shock. Self-assessment/CEU questions are included at the end of the article.

Martin, J. (1995). The Trendelenburg position: A review of current slants about head down tilt. *American Association of Nurse Anesthetists Journal, 63*(1), 29–36.

The author reviews current and historical practice-based research literature about the value of the Trendelenburg position in different clinical situations. The consensus reached for modern techniques is that, although the Trendelenburg position may have some value in specific clinical situations, it is not useful for clients in shock or with head injuries.

Stengle, J., & Dries, D. (1994). Sepsis in the elderly. *Critical Care Nursing Clinics of North America, 6*(2), 421–427.

This excellent article compares the clinical manifestations of sepsis in elderly people with those considered "classic for the adult population," emphasizing the subtle changes that can be easily overlooked in an elderly client. In addition, the authors describe risk factors, usual clinical course, and treatment.

Chapter 40

INTERVENTIONS FOR CRITICALLY ILL CLIENTS WITH CORONARY ARTERY DISEASE

Since the 1960s, deaths from myocardial infarction (MI) have decreased approximately 30% (American Heart Association [AHA], 1996). This reduction is partly due to improved health promotion, but management of the client with coronary artery disease (CAD) has also changed dramatically.

Most deaths today from MI occur because of dysrhythmias before the client reaches the hospital. During the past 10 years, in-hospital mortality from MI has dropped from 15% to 5%. Advances in cardiac care, especially new strategies for opening and maintaining the patency of obstructed coronary vessels, contributed to this decline.

Overview

Coronary artery disease is the leading cause of death in the United States. This disease affects the arteries that provide blood, oxygen, and nutrients to the myocardium. When blood flow through the coronary arteries is par-

tially or completely blocked, ischemia and infarction (necrosis) of the myocardium may result. Ischemia occurs when insufficient oxygen is supplied to meet the requirements of the myocardium. Infarction occurs when severe ischemia is prolonged and irreversible damage to tissue results.

Pathophysiology

Atherosclerosis is the leading contributor to CAD and death in Western civilizations. Three basic processes occur in atherosclerosis:

- Overgrowth of intimal smooth muscle cells with accumulation of macrophages and T cells
- Formation of a connective tissue matrix in the vessel intima
- Accumulation of lipids, especially cholesterol, in the connective tissue

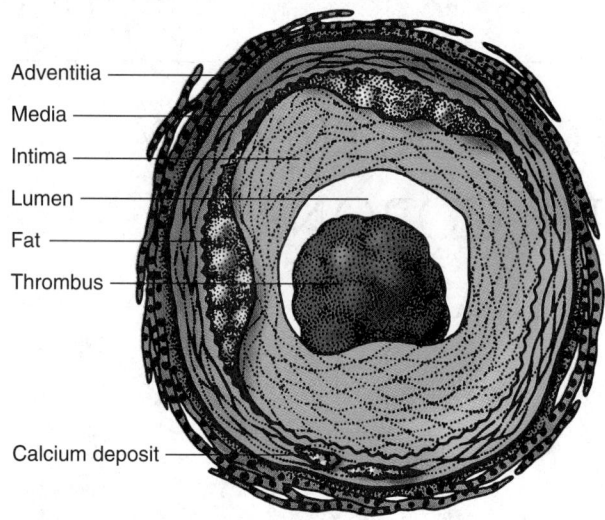

Adventitia
Media
Intima
Lumen
Fat
Thrombus
Calcium deposit

Figure 40–1. A cross-section of an atherosclerotic coronary artery.

These processes narrow the vessel lumen (Fig. 40–1). Blood flow through the restricted lumen may be adequate to perfuse myocardial tissue when the client is at rest.

At rest, the heart extracts a larger amount of oxygen (75%) from its blood flow than does any other major organ in the body. When additional oxygen is needed to meet increased tissue demands, an increase in coronary artery blood flow is required. Once the lumen of a coronary artery is obstructed by more than 70%, blood flow may not be able to increase in response to tissue demands. Increases in myocardial oxygen requirements (e.g., exercise or aortic stenosis) or transient reductions in blood flow (e.g., hypotension or coronary spasm) may result in inadequate oxygen supply to and ischemia of the myocardium. Ischemic myocardium is oxygen-deprived myocardium, and the client typically experiences angina.

Angina Pectoris

Angina pectoris, a name derived from a Latin phrase, means "strangling of the chest." Angina is a temporary imbalance between the coronary arteries' ability to supply oxygen and the cardiac muscle's demand for oxygen. Ischemia that occurs with angina is limited in duration, and it does not cause permanent damage of myocardial tissue.

Angina may be of two predominant types. *Stable angina* is chest discomfort occurring with moderate to prolonged exertion in a pattern that is familiar to the client; frequency, duration, and intensity of symptoms have not increased over the past several months. Stable angina results in only slight limitation of activity. This condition is usually associated with a stable atherosclerotic plaque.

Unstable angina is chest pain or discomfort that occurs at rest or with minimal exertion and causes marked limitation of activity. An increase in the number of attacks and an increase in the intensity of the pain characterize unstable angina. The pain may last longer than 15 minutes or be poorly relieved by rest or nitroglycerin. Unstable angina describes a broad spectrum of disorders, including *new-onset angina, variant (Prinzmetal's) angina, preinfarction angina,* and *crescendo angina.*

The atherosclerotic plaque may rupture in unstable angina, with resultant platelet aggregation, thrombus formation, and vasoconstriction. The incidence of MI (10–30% per year) and death from MI (29% in 5 years) are higher for clients with unstable angina than for those with stable angina (Matrisciano, 1992).

WOMEN'S HEALTH CONSIDERATIONS

Many women experience atypical angina; they may describe angina as a choking sensation that occurs with exertion. Angina is more likely to be the primary presenting symptom of CAD in women (56%) than in men (46%) and is twice as common as MI in women. For 86% of women, compared with 56% of men, angina does not progress to MI.

Myocardial Infarction

Myocardial infarction occurs when myocardial tissue is abruptly and severely deprived of oxygen. When blood flow is acutely reduced by 80%–90%, ischemia develops. Ischemia can lead to necrosis of myocardial tissue if blood flow is not restored. Most MIs are the result of atherosclerosis of a coronary artery, rupture of the plaque, subsequent thrombosis, and occlusion of blood flow. However, other factors may be implicated, such as coronary artery spasm, platelet aggregation, and emboli from mural thrombi (thrombi lining the walls of the cardiac chambers).

Myocardial infarctions often begin with infarction (necrosis) of the subendocardial layer of cardiac muscle. This layer has the longest myofibrils in the heart, the greatest oxygen demand, and the poorest oxygen supply.

Around the initial area of infarction in the subendocardium are two zones: (1) the zone of injury, tissue that is injured but not necrotic; (2) the zone of ischemia, tissue that is oxygen deprived. This pattern is illustrated in Figure 40–2.

Process of Infarction

Infarction is a dynamic process. It does not occur instantly; rather, it evolves over several hours. Hypoxia from ischemia may lead to local vasodilation of blood vessels and acidosis. Imbalances of potassium, calcium, and magnesium as well as acidosis at the cellular level may lead to suppression of normal pacemaker and contractile functions. Automaticity and ectopy are enhanced. Catecholamines released in response to hypoxia and pain may increase the heart's rate and force of contraction. These factors increase oxygen requirements in tissue that is already oxygen deprived. The area of infarction may extend into the zones of injury and ischemia.

The actual extent of the zone of infarction depends on three factors: collateral circulation, anaerobic metabolism, and workload demands on the myocardium.

The infarction may involve only the subendocardium (called a subendocardial MI), or it may spread to the epicardium or to all three layers of cardiac muscle. When all three layers are involved, the MI is termed *transmural.* Subendocardial MIs have less effect on wall motion and cardiac output than transmural infarctions do.

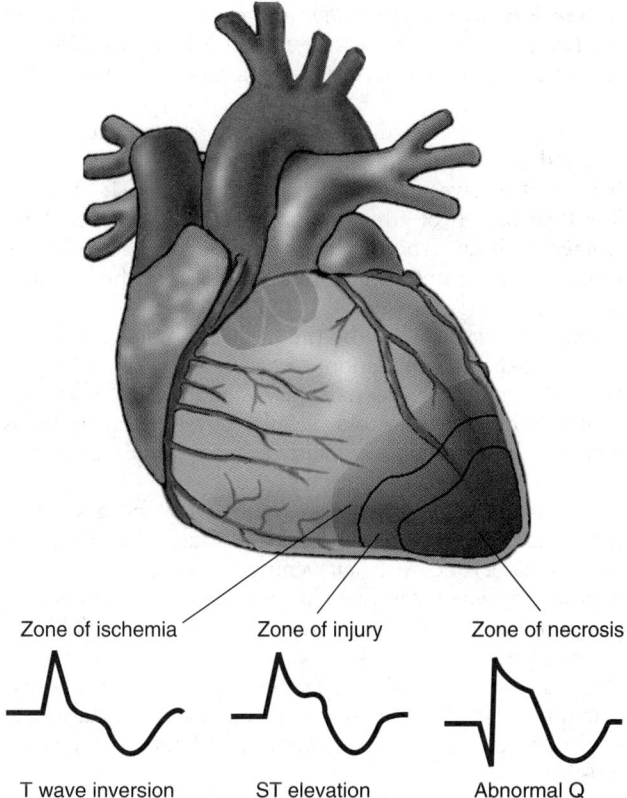

Figure 40–2. Electrocardiogram changes seen in myocardial infarction.

Zone of ischemia — T wave inversion

Zone of injury — ST elevation

Zone of necrosis — Abnormal Q

Physiologic Response to the Infarction

Obvious physical changes do not occur in the heart until 6 hours after the infarction, when the infarcted region appears blue and swollen. After 48 hours, the infarct turns gray with yellow streaks as neutrophils invade the tissue and begin to remove the necrotic cells. By 8–10 days after infarction, granulation tissue forms at the edges of the necrotic tissue. Over 2–3 months, the necrotic area eventually develops into a shrunken, thin, firm scar (Pasternak et al., 1992). Scar tissue permanently changes the size and shape of the entire left ventricle (ventricular remodeling). Remodeling may decrease left ventricular function, cause heart failure, and increase morbidity and mortality.

Classification of Myocardial Infarction by Location

The client's response to an MI also depends on which coronary artery or arteries were obstructed and which part of the left ventricle wall was damaged: anterior, lateral, septal, inferior, or posterior. Figure 40–3 details the major coronary arteries, and Table 40–1 describes the structures they perfuse.

Clients with obstruction of the left anterior descending (LAD) artery usually have anterior or septal MIs because the LAD artery perfuses the anterior wall and most of the septal wall of the left ventricle. Anterior wall MIs account for 25% of all MIs and, at 25%, have the highest mortal-

ity rate. Clients with anterior MIs are most likely to experience left ventricular heart failure and ventricular dysrhythmias, because a large segment of the left ventricle wall may have been damaged.

The circumflex artery supplies the lateral wall of the left ventricle and possibly portions of the posterior wall or the sinoatrial (SA) and atrioventricular (AV) nodes. Clients with obstruction of the circumflex artery may experience posterior wall MI (2% of MIs) or lateral wall MI (3% of MIs) and sinus dysrhythmias.

In most people, the right coronary artery perfuses the SA and AV nodes as well as the inferior or diaphragmatic portion of the left ventricle. Clients with obstruction of the right coronary artery often have inferior MIs. Inferior wall MIs account for approximately 17% of all MIs and have a mortality rate of about 10%. Clients are most likely to experience bradydysrhythmias or AV conduction defects, especially transient second-degree heart blocks. About one third of clients with inferior MIs have right ventricular MI and right ventricular failure (Braunwald, 1992).

WOMEN'S HEALTH CONSIDERATIONS

Women have higher morbidity and mortality rates after MI than men in part because, when an MI occurs, women are older and sicker and are more likely to have pre-existing diabetes and heart failure. Women also delay longer, an average of 5 hours, before seeking medical assistance for chest pain. These factors often make women ineligible for interventions to reperfuse coronary arteries (Arnstein, Buselli, & Rankin, 1996).

Etiology

Atherosclerosis is the primary factor in the development of coronary artery disease (CAD). Numerous risk factors contribute to atherosclerosis (see Chap. 38). Risk factors are classified as nonmodifiable and modifiable.

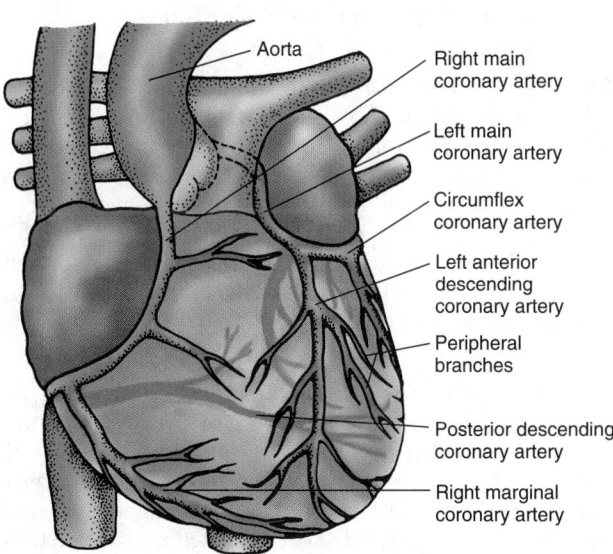

Aorta

Right main coronary artery

Left main coronary artery

Circumflex coronary artery

Left anterior descending coronary artery

Peripheral branches

Posterior descending coronary artery

Right marginal coronary artery

Figure 40–3. Coronary arterial system.

TABLE 40–1

Major Coronary Vessels and the Structures They Perfuse

Left Anterior Descending Coronary Artery
- Most of the left ventricular muscle mass and septum

Left Circumflex Coronary Artery
- Posterior wall of the left ventricle
- SA node in 39% of clients
- AV node in 12% of clients
- Left ventricular muscle in 10% of clients

Right Coronary Artery
- Right ventricle
- Inferior portion of the left ventricle
- SA node in 59% of clients
- AV node in 88% of clients

SA = sinoatrial; AV = atrioventricular.

Nonmodifiable Risk Factors

Nonmodifiable risk factors are personal elements that cannot be altered or controlled. These risk factors, which interact with each other, include age, gender, family history, and ethnic background. The risk of CAD increases with age; 55% of clients who experience an MI are 65 years or older (AHA, 1996).

Premenopausal women have a lower incidence of MI than men do. However, for postmenopausal women in their 70s, the incidence of MI equals that of men. Family history is also a risk factor; people whose parents had CAD are more susceptible.

Modifiable Risk Factors

Modifiable risk factors include elevated serum cholesterol levels, cigarette smoking, hypertension, impaired glucose tolerance, obesity, physical inactivity, and stress. Viagra, a drug to treat impotence, has recently been identified as a risk factor for clients who take nitroglycerin for CAD.

Elevated Serum Cholesterol Levels. The risk of CAD rises as serum cholesterol levels increase. The AHA estimates that 52% of Americans have serum cholesterol levels greater than 200 mg/dL and 20% have levels above 240, putting them at risk for CAD. A 1% reduction in serum cholesterol has been associated with a 2% reduction in CAD. Elevated levels of low-density lipoprotein (LDL) with low levels of high-density lipoprotein (HDL) increase the risk further.

Cigarette Smoking. Cigarette smokers have twice the risk of MI that nonsmokers have and two to four times the risk of sudden cardiac death (AHA, 1996). An estimated 27.5% of men and 22.7% of women in the United States are smokers (AHA, 1996). Reducing the tar and nicotine content of the cigarettes smoked does not reduce the risk of CAD.

Other Factors. *Hypertension* increases the workload of the heart, which increases the risk of MI. *Impaired glucose tolerance* (e.g., diabetes) seriously increases the risks, especially in women.

Obesity is associated with increased serum cholesterol, elevated blood pressure, and abnormal glucose tolerance. It may also have an independent effect on risk of CAD. The distribution of adipose tissue seems to be important; women with fat deposited about the waist rather than the hips often have unfavorable lipid profiles and higher rates of CAD.

Physical inactivity may be the most important risk factor for the general population, because between 40% and 60% of Americans are sedentary, and physical inactivity relates to other risk factors. Regular physical activity helps maintain body weight and muscle mass while optimizing blood pressure and lipid values.

The individual's response to stress may be associated with heart disease. Some evidence indicates that job stress may be associated with left ventricular hypertrophy. *Type A behavior,* when described as hostility in response to a stressful event, has been associated with a twofold increase in angina.

Clients with several risk factors (hypertension, obesity, smoking, high cholesterol levels, and diabetes) have several times the risk of CAD as those without these characteristics.

Although many factors place a client at risk for heart disease, there are well-documented, effective ways of promoting cardiovascular health. Some of these methods are described in Chart 40–1.

TRANSCULTURAL CONSIDERATIONS

Modifiable risk factors vary for people of differing race and ethnic backgrounds. African-Americans do not have significantly higher overall heart disease rates than other groups. However, among African-Americans the incidence of diabetes is 33% higher, and hypertension develops at an earlier age and is more severe at every decade of life. Obesity is significantly more common in African-American women than in the corresponding Caucasian-American populations (U.S. Department of Health and Human Services [DHHS], 1990).

Hispanics have lower death rates from heart disease than non-Hispanics. However, smoking continues in 43% of Hispanic men (higher than in other American populations) (DHHS, 1990). Above-normal weight is more of a problem for Hispanic women, especially Mexican-American women (AHA, 1996) and may be associated with less-than-average physical activity.

Tremendous diversity among the Asian and Pacific Island American populations makes generalizations difficult. However, Filipino-Americans seem to have an increased incidence of hypertension, and more than 60% of native Hawaiians are overweight.

The major modifiable cardiovascular risk factors for Native Americans seem to be obesity and diabetes. The increase in obesity in Native Americans has paralleled the increase in diabetes (DHHS, 1990). In many tribes, more than 20% of the members have diabetes.

Health Promotion Guide: Prevention of Coronary Artery Disease

Smoking
• If you smoke, quit.
• If you don't smoke, don't start.

Diet
• Follow a prudent daily diet:
• Consume sufficient calories for your body: you must obtain
  • 50–55% of your calories from carbohydrates.
  • 30–35% of your calories from complex carbohydrates.
  • 10% of your calories from simple sugars.
  • Less than 30% of your calories from fat.
  • 15% of your calories from monounsaturated fat.
  • 10% of your calories from polyunsaturated fat.
  • The remainder of your calories (5–10%) from saturated fat.
  • 12–20% of your calories from protein.
• Limit your cholesterol intake to less than 300 mg daily.
• Limit your sodium intake to less than 130 mEq daily.

Cholesterol
• Have your cholesterol and low-density lipoprotein (LDL) levels checked regularly.
• If your cholesterol and LDLs are elevated, follow your health care provider's advice.

Physical Activity
• If you are middle aged or older or have a history of medical problems, check with your health care provider before starting an exercise program.
• Appropriate exercise should be enjoyable; burn 400 calories/session, and sustain a heart rate of 120–150 beats per minute, depending on your age.
• Exercise moderately at least three times each week, preferably five.
• Exercise periods should be at least 20–30 minutes long with 10-minute warm-up and 5-minute cool-down periods.
• If you are unable to exercise moderately three to five times each week, walk daily for 30 minutes at a comfortable pace.
• If you are unable to walk 30 minutes daily, walk any distance you can (e.g., park further away from a site than necessary; use the stairs, not the elevator, to go one floor up or two floors down).

Diabetes
• Manage your diabetes with your health care provider.

Blood Pressure
• Have your blood pressure checked regularly.
• If your blood pressure is elevated, follow your health care provider's advice.
• Continue to monitor your blood pressure at regular intervals.

Obesity
• Avoid severely restricted or fad diets.
• Consider a restriction in intake of saturated fats, simple sugars, and cholesterol-rich foods.
• Increase your physical activity.

Incidence/Prevalence

Approximately 1,500,000 MIs occur each year in the United States, and about one third of these people die (AHA, 1996). MI is the single largest cause of death for both men and women. Approximately half of deaths from MI occur in the first hour before reaching the hospital.

Approximately 350,000 people experience angina for the first time each year, and 750,000 people are hospitalized yearly with the diagnosis of unstable angina (Matrisciano, 1992). The AHA estimates that more than 7 million people who have experienced angina or MI are still living (AHA, 1996). The estimated cost of caring for people with CAD is slightly less then $150 billion yearly.

Collaborative Management

 Assessment

➤ History

If chest discomfort is present at the time of the interview, the nurse delays collection of historical data until interventions for pain, vital sign instability, and dysrhythmias are initiated and the discomfort resolves. The nurse obtains information about how the client has managed the current episode of chest discomfort and which medications the client is taking. When the client is *pain-free,* the nurse obtains information about family history and modifiable risk factors, including eating habits, lifestyle, and physical activity levels.

➤ Physical Assessment/Clinical Manifestations

The nurse asks clients to describe the immediate concern. The nurse notes the presence of chest, epigastric, jaw, back, or arm discomfort and asks clients to rate the discomfort on a scale of 0–10, with 10 being the highest level of discomfort. Clients often describe the discomfort as tightness, a burning sensation, pressure, or indigestion. The nurse asks clients what they have already done to try to relieve the pain.

➤ Pain Assessment

The nurse rapidly yet completely assesses the client with ongoing chest pain. Because chest discomfort may occur from a variety of causes (see Table 35–1), it is important to differentiate among the types of chest pain and to identify the source. Both the physician and nurse may question the client to determine the characteristics of the discomfort. Appropriate questions for the nurse to ask concerning the discomfort include onset, location, radiation, intensity, duration, and precipitating and relieving factors.

Chart 40–2 compares and contrasts anginal and infarction pain. Because anginal pain is ischemic pain, it usually improves when the disparity between oxygen supply and demand is resolved. For example, rest reduces tissue demands, and nitroglycerin improves oxygen supply. Discomfort from an MI does not usually resolve with such simple measures. The nurse also notes the presence of any associated symptoms, including nausea, vomiting, di-

Chart 40-2

Key Features of Angina and Myocardial Infarction

Angina
Substernal chest discomfort
- Radiating to the left arm
- Precipitated by exertion or stress
- Relieved by nitroglycerin or rest
- Lasting <15 min
- Few associated symptoms

Myocardial Infarction
Substernal chest pressure
- Radiating to the left arm, back, or jaw
- Occurring without cause, primarily early in the morning
- Relieved only by opioids
- Lasting 30 min or more
- Frequent associated symptoms:
  - Nausea
  - Diaphoresis
  - Dyspnea
  - Feelings of fear and anxiety
  - Dysrhythmias

aphoresis, dizziness, weakness, palpitations, and shortness of breath.

WOMEN'S HEALTH CONSIDERATIONS

Chest discomfort is often not the initial symptom reported by women experiencing an MI. Women are more likely to have initially atypical symptoms such as heart "flutters" without pain, shortness of breath, fatigue, or depression (Hahn, 1995).

TRANSCULTURAL CONSIDERATIONS

African-Americans have experienced longer delays in seeking treatment for MI and higher mortality rates than Caucasians. One factor thought to contribute to this delay is a greater incidence of dyspnea as an acute symptom of MI among male and female African-Americans rather than the more classic chest discomfort (Lee, 1997).

ELDERLY CONSIDERATIONS

The presence of the associated symptoms without chest discomfort is also significant. In 15%–25% of all clients with MI, primarily older adults and diabetics, chest pain or discomfort may be mild or absent, and clients may complain primarily of the associated symptoms. Twenty-five percent of older adults experiencing MI complain only of shortness of breath (Jensen & Miller, 1995). Clients older then 80 may display disorientation or confusion as a result of poor cardiac output as the major manifestation of MI.

► Cardiovascular Assessment

The nurse immediately obtains a blood pressure measurement, determines the heart rate, interprets the cardiac

rhythm, and assesses for dysrhythmias. Sinus tachycardia with premature ventricular contractions (PVC) frequently occurs in the first few hours after MI. If an intravenous (IV) access is available, the nurse ensures that it is patent because the client will most likely receive IV fluids and medications. If an access is not available, the nurse initiates one or contacts the appropriate person to establish an IV route as quickly as possible. The nurse may administer oxygen, titrating the fraction of inspired oxygen (FIO_2) to the client's oxygen (O_2) saturation according to protocols or the physician's order.

Next, the nurse assesses distal peripheral pulses and skin temperature. The skin should be warm, with all pulses palpable. In the client with unstable angina or MI, poor cardiac output may be manifested by cool, diaphoretic skin and diminished or absent pulses.

The nurse auscultates for an S_3 gallop, which often indicates heart failure, a serious and common complication of MI. The nurse also assesses respiratory rate and breath sounds for signs of heart failure. An increased respiratory rate is common because of anxiety and pain, but crackles or wheezes may indicate heart failure. Auscultation of an S_4 heart sound is a common finding in the client who has had a previous MI or hypertension.

The client with MI may experience a temperature elevation for several days after infarction. Temperatures as high as 102° F (38.9° C) may occur in response to myocardial necrosis.

► Psychosocial Assessment

Denial is a common early reaction to chest discomfort associated with angina or MI. On average, the client with acute MI waits more than 2 hours before seeking medical attention. Often the client rationalizes that symptoms are due to indigestion or overexertion. In some situations, denial is a normal part of adapting to a stressful event. However, denial that interferes with identification of a symptom, such as chest discomfort, can be harmful to the client. The nurse explains the significance of reporting any discomfort, emphasizing that health care provisions attempt to relieve the discomfort immediately.

Fear, anxiety, and anger are other common reactions of clients and families. Nursing assessment focuses on assisting the client and family members in identifying these feelings. The nurse allows the client and family time to explain their understanding of the event and clarifies any misconceptions.

► Laboratory Assessment

Cardiac Enzymes. An MI can be confirmed by abnormally high blood levels of cardiac enzymes and isoenzymes. Of all the cardiac enzymes, creatine kinase (CK) is considered the most sensitive and reliable indicator for diagnosis of MI. Total CK levels rise within 3 hours after the onset of chest pain and peak within 24 hours after damage and death of cardiac tissue. Because total CK also rises with brain or muscle injury, an elevation is not specific for myocardial damage.

When cardiac muscle tissue dies, the CK specific to myocardial cells—CK-MB isoenzyme—enters the bloodstream (serum does not normally contain CK-MB isoenzymes). Peak elevation occurs approximately 12–24 hours after the onset of chest pain; levels return to normal 48–72 hours later. Confirmation of myocardial damage within 2 hours of emergency room admission is possible with the use of stat-CKs and CK subforms. These are gaining popularity as a result of the need to confirm or rule out MI rapidly.

The physician may also use serum measurement of lactate dehydrogenase (LDH) to confirm MI. However, identification of LDH is not as reliable as that of CK-MB. LDH levels start to rise within 12–24 hours after MI, peak between 48 and 72 hours, and fall to normal in 7 days. Thus, they may be useful in diagnosing an MI in a client who has delayed seeking medical help for several days after the onset of chest discomfort. Serum levels of LDH_1 isoenzyme rise higher than serum levels of LDH_2 in the presence of MI. (See Chapter 35 for a more detailed discussion of cardiac enzymes.)

No laboratory test can confirm the diagnosis of angina. Serum enzyme determinations are not useful in assessing the presence of angina. However, serum enzymes remaining within normal limits are an indication that the client has not had an acute MI.

Other Laboratory Tests. The finding of an elevated white blood cell count (10,000–20,000 cells/mm³) helps in the diagnosis of MI. It typically appears on the second day and lasts up to a week.

➤ Radiographic Assessment

Unless there is associated cardiac dysfunction (e.g., valvular disease) or heart failure, the chest x-ray is not diagnostic for angina or MI.

➤ Other Diagnostic Assessment

Electrocardiography. Twelve-lead electrocardiograms (ECG) allow the health care provider to examine the heart from varying perspectives and note both the occurrence and the location of ischemia (angina) or necrosis (infarction).

Ischemic myocardium does not repolarize normally. Thus, 12-lead ECGs obtained during an anginal episode reveal ST depression, T-wave inversion, or both. *Variant angina,* caused by coronary spasm, usually causes elevation of the ST segment during anginal attacks. These ST and T wave changes usually subside when the ischemia is resolved and the pain is relieved. However, the T wave may remain flat or inverted for a period of time. If the client is not experiencing angina at the moment of the test, the ECG for the client with angina is usually normal.

When infarction occurs, three ECG changes are usually observed: ST-segment elevation, T-wave inversion, and an abnormal Q wave (wider than 0.04 seconds or more than one third the height of the QRS complex). Figure 40–2 displays the ECG changes seen in MI.

The Q wave develops because necrotic cells do not conduct electrical stimuli. Hours to days after the MI, the ST- and T-wave changes will return to normal, but the Q wave usually remains permanently. By identifying the lead in which the ECG changes are occurring, the health care provider can identify the extent and location of the infarction.

Stress Test. The health care provider often orders an *exercise tolerance test* (stress test) after the acute stages of an anginal episode or MI to assess for ECG changes consistent with ischemia, evaluate medical therapy, and identify clients who might benefit from referral for invasive therapy.

Scans. *Thallium scans* use radioisotope imaging to assess for ischemia or necrotic muscle tissue related to angina or MI. Areas of decreased or absent perfusion, referred to as cold spots, identify ischemia or infarction. *Multigated acquisition* (MUGA) scans may be used to evaluate left ventricular function.

Cardiac Catheterization. This procedure may be performed to determine the extent and location of obstructions of the coronary arteries. Cardiac catheterization, the "gatekeeper" to invasive management, allows the cardiologist and cardiac surgeon to identify clients who might benefit from percutaneous transluminal angioplasty (PCTA) or coronary artery bypass grafting (CABG). (Chapter 35 describes each of these tests in detail.)

 Analysis

➤ Common Nursing Diagnoses and Collaborative Problems

The client with coronary artery disease (CAD) may have either angina or myocardial infarction (MI). If MI is suspected or cannot be completely ruled out, the client is admitted to a coronary or critical care unit for continuous monitoring. On the basis of the assessment data, the nurse often identifies the following common diagnoses for the client with CAD:

1. Pain related to imbalance between myocardial oxygen supply and demand
2. Altered Tissue Perfusion (cardiopulmonary) related to interruption of blood flow
3. Activity Intolerance related to imbalance between oxygen supply and demand
4. Ineffective Individual Coping related to effects of acute illness, major changes in lifestyle, or loss of control over a body part

For the client experiencing an MI, the most important collaborative problems are

1. Potential for dysrhythmias
2. Potential for heart failure
3. Potential for recurrent chest discomfort and extension of injury

➤ Additional Nursing Diagnoses and Collaborative Problems

Clients with CAD may also experience one or more of the following diagnoses:

- Fear related to threat of death
- Altered Sexuality Patterns related to pain and effects of illness
- Impaired Physical Mobility related to pain or fear of movement

Planning and Implementation

Pain

Planning: Expected Outcomes. The client is expected to state that chest discomfort is alleviated.

Interventions. The objective of management is to eliminate chest discomfort by providing pain relief, decreasing myocardial oxygen demand, and increasing myocardial oxygen supply. Chart 40–3 summarizes appropriate interventions for the client with chest discomfort.

Drug Therapy. The nurse evaluates the chest pain, obtains the client's vital signs, ensures the patency of an intravenous (IV) access, and notifies the physician of the client's condition. If appropriate, the nurse may administer the prescribed pain medication. One of the initial medications prescribed for chest pain is usually sublingual nitroglycerin (Chart 40–4). Aspirin, 325 mg po (chewed), also may be administered immediately.

Nitroglycerin. Nitroglycerin, a nitrate often referred to as "nitro," increases collateral blood flow, redistributes blood flow toward the subendocardium, and causes dilation of the coronary arteries. The nurse instructs the client to hold the tablet under the tongue and provides 5 mL of water, if necessary, to allow the tablet to dissolve. Pain relief should begin within 1 or 2 minutes and be

clearly evident in 3–5 minutes. After 5 minutes, the nurse rechecks the client's pain intensity and vital signs. If the client's blood pressure is less than 100 systolic or 25 mmHg lower than the previous reading, the nurse

---

Chart 40–3

Nursing Care Highlight: The Client with Chest Discomfort

- Obtain the client's description of the chest discomfort.
- Obtain the client's vital signs (blood pressure, pulse, respiration).
- Assess the client's vascular access.
- Consult standing orders or notify the physician for specific intervention.
- Obtain a 12-lead electrocardiogram, if indicated.
- Provide pain relief medication and ASA as ordered.
- Administer oxygen therapy as prescribed.
- Remain calm; stay with the client if possible.
- Assess the client's vital signs and intensity of pain 5 min after administration of medication.
- Remedicate (if vital signs remain stable), and check the client every 5 min.
- Notify the physician if vital signs deteriorate or pain is not relieved after three doses of nitroglycerin.

Chart 40–4

Drug Therapy for Coronary Artery Disease

Drug	Usual Dosage	Nursing Interventions	Rationale
Nitrates			
Nitroglycerin (Nitrostat, Tridil)	• 0.3–0.4 mg q5min sublingually, up to three tablets	• Instruct the client to lie down with the head of the bed at a level of comfort when taking the sublingual form.	• Hypotension can be dramatic, immediate, and intensified by the upright position.
		• Monitor blood pressure. Pay attention to orthostatic changes.	• A decrease in blood pressure occurs with vasodilation.
		• Instruct the client to allow the sublingual tablet to dissolve and to avoid swallowing the tablet.	• The sublingual dose is absorbed through the sublingual mucous membranes.
		• Check the expiration date on sublingual tablets. Tablets should be replaced every 3–5 mo.	• The efficacy of the tablets decreases with time.
		• Determine whether pain is relieved.	• Additional medication may be required to relieve pain.
		• Monitor for headache.	• Vasodilation is generalized.
Isosorbide dinitrate (Isordil, Iso-Bid)	• 2.5 mg q4–6h sublingually • 5–30 mg qid PO	• Instruct the client taking sublingual forms to lie down before administration.	• The hypotensive effect can be dramatic and immediate with sublingual administration.
	• 40-mg sustained-release tablet 2–3 times daily	• Monitor blood pressure and assess for dizziness.	• A decrease in blood pressure occurs with vasodilation.

Chart 40–4. Drug Therapy for Coronary Artery Disease   Continued

Drug	Usual Dosage	Nursing Interventions	Rationale
Isosorbide mononitrate	• 60 mg extended release tab qd	• Schedule sustained-release form with an 8–12 h dose-free interval.	• Tolerance may develop.
Nitroglycerin patch (Nitro-bid Patch)	• Transdermally started at 5 mg/24 hr (10 cm² system)	• Remove the patch from the client before defibrillation. • Rotate application sites. • Apply the patch to a clean, dry, hairless area. • Remove patch for 8–12 hours each day.	• The client may develop a burn. • Rotation prevents skin irritation. • The drug is better absorbed when the skin is clean, dry, and hairless. • Tolerance will develop.
Beta-Blockers Propranolol (Inderal)	• 10–80 mg bid–qid to 240 mg/day PO • 1–3 mg at rate not to exceed 1 mg/min IV	• Assess heart rate before administration. • Monitor blood pressure. • Observe for signs of heart failure. • Assess for shortness of breath and wheezing.	• Beta-blocking effects cause a decrease in heart rate. • The hypotensive effect is due to a decrease in cardiac output, suppressed renin activity, and beta-blocking effects. • Heart failure may occur as a result of a decrease in cardiac output. • Beta$_2$-blocking effects in the lungs can cause bronchoconstriction.
Metoprolol (Lopressor, Betaloc✦), a cardio-selective beta-adrenergic blocker	• 100–450 mg/day PO • 5 mg IV over 2 min may be repeated twice for a total of 15 mg	• Assess heart rate before administration; do not administer if heart rate <50. • Monitor BP and hold for systolic <90. • Assess client for cough, shortness of breath, edema, and weight gain.	• Beta-blockers may cause further decreases in heart rate. • Decreased blood pressure is an anticipated effect. • These are indications of heart failure.
Calcium Channel Blockers Nifedipine (Procardia, Adalat)	• 10–30 mg tid PO or sublingually	• Monitor blood pressure and assess for dizziness. • Assess for headache and edema of the lower extremities.	• Vasodilation can cause dramatic hypotension, which occurs within minutes, especially after sublingual administration. • These are common side effects.
Verapamil hydrochloride (Calan, Isoptin)	• 40–80 mg qid PO or 120–240 mg sustained-release tablet once a day • 5–10 mg over 2 min IV	• Monitor heart rate. • Monitor blood pressure and assess for dizziness. • Assess for constipation.	• This agent slows SA and AV node conduction. • Vasodilation decreases blood pressure. • This is a common side effect.
Diltiazem hydrochloride (Cardizem)	• 30–60 mg qid PO or 120–480 mg sustained-release tablet once a day; increase dose slowly	• Monitor blood pressure and assess for dizziness. • Monitor heart rate.	• Vasodilation decreases blood pressure. • This drug slows SA and AV node conduction, but the decrease is not as great as that which occurs with verapamil.

Continued

Chart 40–4. Drug Therapy for Coronary Artery Disease   Continued

Drug	Usual Dosage	Nursing Interventions	Rationale
Antiplatelet Agents Aspirin (Empirin, Apoasa✽)	• 80–325 mg PO	• Suggest that the client take the daily dose with food. • Question the client about ringing in the ears. • Emphasize to the client that aspirin is an important cardiac medication and should be continued unless the client is told to stop.	• Gastric irritation may occur. • Tinnitus may occur with aspirin toxicity. • Studies document significantly better survival rates for clients with coronary artery disease receiving aspirin.

SA = sinoatrial; AV = atrioventricular

lowers the head of the client's bed and notifies the physician. If the client is experiencing some but not complete relief and vital signs remain stable, another nitroglycerin tablet may be used. A total of three tablets may be administered in an attempt to relieve anginal pain.

Angina usually responds to nitroglycerin. The client typically states that the pain is relieved or markedly diminished. When simple measures, such as three repeated sublingual nitroglycerin tablets, do not relieve chest discomfort, the client may be experiencing MI. The nurse should inform the physician immediately and prepare the client for transfer to a specialized unit where the client can be closely monitored and appropriately managed.

In a specialized unit, the physician may prescribe IV nitroglycerin for management of the chest pain. The nurse begins the nitroglycerin infusion slowly, checking the client's blood pressure and pain level every 3–5 minutes. The nitroglycerin dose is increased until the pain is relieved, the blood pressure falls excessively, or the maximal prescribed dose is reached. The nurse continues to monitor the blood pressure frequently (Chart 40–5).

Morphine Sulfate. The physician may prescribe morphine sulfate (MS) to relieve chest discomfort that is unresponsive to nitroglycerin. Morphine relieves MI pain, decreases myocardial oxygen demand, and reduces circulating catecholamines. It is usually administered in 2- to 5-mg increments intravenously every 5–15 minutes until the maximal prescribed dose is reached or until the client experiences relief or signs of toxicity. Signs of morphine toxicity include respiratory depression, hypotension, and severe vomiting.

The nurse monitors the client's vital signs and cardiac rhythm every few minutes. These strategies are often enough to relieve the client's pain. If these methods are not adequate, additional interventions, identified later under Altered Tissue Perfusion (Cardiopulmonary), may be attempted.

Other Interventions. Several interventions may assist in relieving chest pain. Supplemental oxygen may increase the amount of oxygen available to myocardial tissue. Therefore, oxygen is often prescribed and administered at 2–4 L/min by nasal cannula titrated to maintain an oxy-

gen saturation greater then 92%. If the client's blood pressure is stable, the nurse may assist the client in assuming any position of comfort. Placing the client in semi-Fowler's position often enhances comfort and tissue oxygenation. A quiet, calm environment and explanations of interventions often reduce the client's anxiety and assist in relief of chest pain.

When the pain has subsided and the client is stabilized, the physician may change the client's medication to an oral or topical nitrate. During administration of long-term oral and topical nitrates, a 12-hour nitrate-free period should be maintained to prevent tolerance. The client may complain initially of headache. The physician may prescribe acetaminophen (Tylenol, Exdol) before the nitrate to prevent some of this discomfort.

Altered Tissue Perfusion (Cardiopulmonary)

Planning: Expected Outcomes. The client is expected to exhibit (1) relief of chest discomfort, (2) resolution of ST- and T-wave changes, (3) sinus rhythm (or normal rhythm for the client) rate of approximately 60, and (4) blood pressure within an acceptable range.

Interventions. Because myocardial infarction (MI) is a dynamic process, restoration of perfusion to the injured area often reduces infarct size and improves left ventricular function. Complete, sustained reperfusion of coronary arteries in the first few hours after MI has decreased mortality in MI patients.

Thrombolytic Therapy. Thrombolytic agents are used to dissolve thrombi in the coronary arteries and restore myocardial blood flow. Examples include streptokinase (Kabikinase), tissue plasminogen activator (t-PA, Activase), anisoylated plasminogen-streptokinase activator complex (APSAC), reteplase (Retavase), and urokinase. The physician may order administration of thrombolytics intravenously or by the intracoronary route during cardiac catheterization. Thrombolytic agents are most effective when administered within the first 6 hours of the coronary event. Thrombolytics are underused nationwide in men and women, young and old (Clem, 1995).

Thrombolytic therapy should be given in a unit where the client can be continuously monitored. It is indicated

Chart 40–5

Drug Therapy with Intravenous Vasodilators and Inotropes

Drug	Usual Dosage	Nursing Interventions	Rationale
Nitroprusside sodium (Nipride, Nitropress)	• IV only by infusion device • Begin with 0.2 μg/kg/min • May increase gradually to 10 μg/kg/min	• Monitor BP q2–5 min when initiating therapy. If BP drops excessively, elevate the legs, decrease the dose, and increase fluids per unit policies. • Monitor PAWP, SVR, BP, heart rate, and urine output frequently. • Titrate medication to obtain the desired effect. • Protect from light. • Maintain dose at less than 3 μg/min if possible. • In clients requiring doses >3 μg/min for >24–36 hr, monitor for metabolic acidosis, confusion, or hyperreflexia. Examine blood thiocyanate level.	• This agent is a potent, rapidly reversible vasodilator acting on both peripheral venous and arterial musculature. BP may drop in 2 min. • This agent is light sensitive. • Doses >3 μg/min are associated with thiocyanate or cyanide toxicity. • These are indications of the toxic effects of cyanide.
Nitroglycerin (Tridil)	• IV only by infusion device started at 0.3 μg/min and gradually increased in increments of 3 μg/min until maximum of 20 μg/min	• Monitor BP q1–3 min when initiating therapy. If BP drops excessively, elevate the legs and decrease the dose according to unit policies. • Monitor RAP, PAWP, SVR, BP, heart rate, and urine output frequently. • Titrate medication to obtain the desired effect. • Intermittent administration of IV nitroglycerin should be considered. • Monitor the client for headache.	• This agent dilates coronary arteries. It is a more potent systemic venodilator than an arterial vasodilator. BP may drop in 1 min. • Tolerance may develop rapidly to nitroglycerin administered by continuous IV. • Headache is a frequent side effect of initial nitroglycerin therapy.
Sympathomimetics Dopamine (Intropin)	• IV only by infusion device • Starting dose 2–5 μg/kg/min • Titrate up to 20 μg/kg/min	• Determine the reason for use and the expected result. • Observe the client's heart rate, ECG, BP, PAWP, SVR, CO, and urine output q5min to q1h. • Titrate the dose carefully to maintain the dose range and obtain the desired effect. • Infuse through a central catheter. • Monitor the client for ectopy and angina.	• This agent is a dose-dependent activator of alpha, beta, and dopaminergic receptors. • 2–5 μg/kg/min stimulates dopaminergic receptors, which promotes renal and mesenteric blood flow. • 5 μg/kg/min stimulates beta-receptors. This increases heart rate and contractility. • >10–15 μg/kg/min, alpha effects predominate. This causes peripheral constriction. • Extravasation can cause tissue necrosis and sloughing. • These are adverse effects.

Continued

Chart 40–5. Drug Therapy with Intravenous Vasodilators and Inotropes   Continued

Drug	Usual Dosage	Nursing Interventions	Rationale
Dobutamine (Dobutrex)	• IV only by infusion device, 2–10 μg/kg/min	• Observe the client continuously during administration. • Titrate the drug on the basis of heart rate, ECG findings, BP, PAWP, CO, SVR, and urine output. • Monitor for atrial and ventricular ectopy.	• This agent is a very strong beta₁-receptor activator and a moderately strong beta₂-activator. • Dysrhythmias are an adverse effect.

PAWP = pulmonary artery wedge pressure; SVR = systemic vascular resistance; BP = blood pressure; RAP = right atrial pressure; ECG = electrocardiogram; CO = cardiac output.

for clients who have chest pain of greater than 30 minutes duration unrelieved by nitroglycerin with indications of transmural ischemia and injury as shown by the ECG. Contraindications include recent abdominal surgery or cerebrovascular accident (CVA), because bleeding may occur when fresh clots are lysed. Table 40–2 lists the current contraindications to thrombolytic therapy.

Before thrombolytic administration, the nurse may need to apply pressure dressings to IV puncture sites or wounds to limit bleeding. Clients who weigh less than 65 kg should have their dose of thrombolytic weight adjusted to lessen the likelihood of bleeding. During administration, the nurse immediately reports any indications of bleeding to the physician. After administration, the nurse observes for signs of bleeding by

- Documenting the client's neurologic status
- Observing all IV sites
- Monitoring clotting studies
- Observing for signs of internal bleeding (watching hemoglobin and hematocrit)
- Testing stools, urine, and emesis for occult blood

Some concerns in thrombolytic administration are associated with the specific thrombolytic. *Streptokinase,* a first-generation thrombolytic agent, is not fibrin specific; thus, it may create systemic bleeding problems. Because it is a bacteria protein, streptokinase can cause a hypersensitivity

reaction in the client who has had previous exposure. Therefore, the nurse questions the client about streptococcal infections or doses of streptokinase within the past year. To prevent an allergic reaction, the physician may prescribe steroids or antihistamines before the administration of streptokinase. During administration, the nurse observes the client closely for hives and shivering, the most common responses. The half-life of the drug is 16 minutes.

Second-generation thrombolytics include tissue plasminogen activator (t-PA, Activase), anisoylated plasminogen-streptokinase activator complex (APSAC, Eminase), and reteplase (Retavase). t-PA is fibrin specific, has a short half-life (3–5 minutes), and lacks antigenicity. Because some studies have associated t-PA with a more frequent occurrence of cerebrovascular bleeding, the nurse carefully documents neurologic findings. t-PA is much more expensive than streptokinase.

APSAC is a streptokinase derivative; it has a longer half-life (90–105 minutes) than streptokinase but has the same antigenic properties.

Identification of Coronary Artery Reperfusion. The nurse monitors the client for indications that the clot has been lysed and the artery reperfused. These indications include

- Abrupt cessation of chest pain
- Sudden onset of ventricular dysrhythmias
- Resolution of ST-segment depression
- A peak at 12 hours of CK-MB

After clot lysis with thrombolytics, large amounts of thrombin are released into the system, increasing the risk of vessel re-occlusion. To maintain the patency of the coronary artery after thrombolytic therapy, the physician usually prescribes aspirin and IV heparin. The nurse monitors the activated partial thromboplastin time (aPTT; the usual appropriate range is 1½–2½ times control) and maintains the heparin infusion for 3–5 days, as prescribed.

Drug Therapy. Clients who have had an MI, whether receiving thrombolytics or not, should begin aspirin therapy unless contraindicated. Clients may receive a chewable aspirin immediately and then an enteric-coated aspirin (Ancasal, Ecotrin), 80–325 mg daily or every other day, to prevent platelet aggregation at the site of the obstruction.

TABLE 40–2

Contraindications to Thrombolytic Therapy

Absolute
- Active internal bleeding
- Cerebrovascular processes
  - Recent cerebrovascular accident (within 2 mo)
  - Recent spinal or cerebral surgery
  - Cranial neoplasm
- Prolonged cardiopulmonary resuscitation (CPR)

Relative
- Endocarditis or pericarditis
- Hemostatic defects
- Severe uncontrolled hypertension
- Pregnancy or recent delivery
- Trauma within last 10 days
- Surgery within last 10 days

Beta-adrenergic blocking agents (e.g., metoprolol [Lopressor, Betaloc]) decrease infarction size, ventricular dysrhythmias, and mortality rates in clients with MI. The physician usually prescribes a cardioselective beta-blocking agent within the first 24 hours after MI. Beta-blockers slow the heart rate and decrease the force of cardiac contraction. Thus, these agents prolong the period of diastole and increase myocardial perfusion while reducing the force of myocardial contraction. With beta-blockade, the heart is capable of performing 25% to 30% more work without ischemia. During beta-blocker therapy, the nurse

- Monitors the heart rate (bradycardia is common)
- Checks the BP
- Measures the PR interval
- Checks the client's level of consciousness
- Monitors for any chest discomfort

The nurse assesses the client's lungs for crackles (indicative of heart failure) and wheezes (indicative of bronchospasm). Hypoglycemia, depression, nightmares, and forgetfulness are also problems with beta-blockade, especially in older clients (see Chart 40–4).

Physicians frequently prescribe angiotensin-converting enzyme (ACE) inhibitors within 48 hours of an MI to prevent ventricular remodeling and the development of heart failure. ACE inhibitors have been demonstrated to increase survival after MI (Connors & Lamas, 1995). The nurse monitors the client for hypotension, cough, and changes in serum potassium, creatinine, and blood urea nitrogen. (See Chapter 37 for a more detailed discussion of ACE inhibitors.)

For clients with angina, the health care provider may prescribe calcium channel blockers to enhance vasodilation and myocardial perfusion. Calcium channel blockers are indicated for clients with variant angina or for clients who are hypertensive and continue to have angina despite beta-blocker therapy. They are not indicated for clients after MI. The nurse monitors the client receiving calcium channel blockers for hypotension and headaches, and reviews the frequency of anginal episodes.

Activity Intolerance

Planning: Expected Outcomes. The client is expected to walk at least 200 feet four times a day without chest discomfort or shortness of breath.

Interventions. Activity intolerance is reduced by a planned program of cardiac rehabilitation implemented primarily by the nurse and physical therapist. Cardiac rehabilitation is a process of actively assisting the client with cardiac disease to achieve and maintain a vital and productive life while remaining within the heart's ability to respond to increases in activity and stress. Cardiac rehabilitation can be divided into three phases. *Phase 1* begins with the acute illness and ends up with discharge from the hospital. *Phase 2* begins after discharge and continues through convalescence at home. *Phase 3* refers to long-term conditioning.

In the acute phase (phase 1), the nurse promotes rest and yet ensures some limited mobility. The nurse assists with some activities of daily living (ADL), such as bathing and toileting. Clients progress at their own rate to in-

creasing activity levels, depending on their clinical status, age, and physical capabilities. For example, for the first 24 hours, the client may be maintained on bed rest but allowed to stand to void or to use the bedside commode. The second day, the client may be out of bed sitting in a chair as tolerated, usually for 30 minutes three times a day.

The next step in phase 1 is ambulation of the client in the room and to the bathroom. Finally, the nurse encourages progressive ambulation in the hallway, usually 50, 100, and then 200 feet three times a day. In addition, the client may begin showering for 5 or 10 minutes with warm water; a stool should be available for the client to sit on if necessary.

The nurse assesses the client's heart rate, blood pressure, respiratory rate, and level of fatigue with each level of activity. Decreases in systolic blood pressure greater than 20 mmHg, changes in pulse rate of 20 beats/minute, and complaints of dyspnea or chest pain indicate intolerance of activity. When such signs and symptoms develop, the nurse notifies the physician and does not advance the client to the next level. Older adults with CAD often have needs and concerns different from those of younger adults (Chart 40–6).

Ineffective Individual Coping

Planning: Expected Outcomes. The client is expected to indicate a reduction in anxiety and indicate the beginning of control over life.

Interventions. The nurse assesses the client's level of anxiety while allowing the client to express any anxiety

---

Chart 40–6

Nursing Focus on the Elderly: Coronary Artery Disease

- Recognize that chest pain may not be evident in the older client; associated symptoms, such as dyspnea and confusion, may prevail.
- Although older adults have a greater reduction in mortality from myocardial infarction (MI) with the use of thrombolytics, they also have the most severe side effects. Monitor older clients receiving thrombolytics extremely carefully.
- Dysrhythmia may be a normal age-related change rather than a complication of MI. Determine whether the dysrhythmia is causing significant symptoms, then notify the physician.
- If beta-blockers are used, assess the client carefully for the development of side effects. Exacerbation of the depression already present in older adults is a significant problem with beta-blockade.
- Plan slow, steady increases in activity. Older adults with minimal previous exercise show particular benefit from a gradual increase in activity.
- Older adults should plan longer warm-up and cooldown periods when participating in an exercise program. Their pulse rates may not return to baseline until 30 minutes or longer after exercise.

and attempt to define its origin. Simple, repeated explanations of therapies, expectations, and surroundings may help the client. During the acute phase of illness, the physician may prescribe anxiolytic (antianxiety) medications, such as alprazolam (Xanax). The nurse identifies the client's current coping mechanisms; the most common are denial, anger, and depression.

Denial allows the client to minimize a threat and use problem-focused coping mechanisms. The client may avoid discussing what has happened yet comply with treatment regimens. This type of denial decreases the client's anxiety, and the nurse should not discourage it. However, denial that results in a client's "acting out" and refusing to follow treatment regimens can be harmful. Because this behavior is usually due to extreme anxiety or fear, threats only worsen the behavior. The nurse remains calm and avoids confronting the client but clearly indicates when a behavior is not acceptable and is potentially harmful.

Anger may represent an attempt to regain control of life. The nurse encourages the client to verbalize the source of frustration and provides the client with opportunities for decision-making and control.

Depression may be a client's response to grief and loss of function. The nurse listens as the client verbalizes feelings of loss, being careful not to offer false or general reassurances. The nurse acknowledges that the client is depressed but expects the client to perform activities of daily living (ADL) and other activities within restrictions. The nurse identifies all improvements in the client's condition and shares them with the client. (Chapter 8 describes interventions and positive coping strategies.)

Potential for Dysrhythmias

Planning: Expected Outcomes. The client is expected to resume a normal sinus or normal rhythm for the client and be hemodynamically stable.

Interventions. Dysrhythmias are the cause of death in most clients with myocardial infarction (MI) who die before they can be hospitalized. Even in the early hospitalization period, 70% to 90% of MI clients experience some abnormality of cardiac rhythm. Whenever a dysrhythmia develops in a client with coronary artery disease (CAD), the nurse
- Identifies the dysrhythmia
- Assesses the client's hemodynamic status
- Evaluates the client for chest discomfort

Dysrhythmias are treated when they are causing hemodynamic compromise, are increasing myocardial oxygen requirements, or predispose to lethal ventricular dysrhythmias.

Inferior MI. Typical dysrhythmias for a client with an inferior MI are bradycardias and second-degree AV blocks resulting from ischemia of the AV node. These rhythms tend to be transient. The nurse monitors the client's cardiac rhythm and rate and hemodynamic status. If the client becomes hemodynamically unstable, a temporary pacemaker may be necessary.

Anterior MI. Clients with *anterior* MIs are likely to exhibit ventricular irritability (premature ventricular contractions [PVCs]). Third-degree or bundle branch block is a serious complication in the client with an anterior MI, because it indicates that a large portion of the left ventricle is involved. The physician may insert a pacemaker. The nurse should observe the client closely to detect the development of heart failure. (Appropriate interventions for dysrhythmias are described in Chapter 36.)

Potential for Heart Failure

Planning: Expected Outcomes. The client is expected to regain hemodynamic stability as evidenced by
- Blood pressure and pulse rate within the client's acceptable range
- Adequate urine output
- Mental alertness
- Clear lungs on auscultation
- Palpable peripheral pulses

Interventions. Decreased cardiac output related to heart failure is a relatively common complication after MI. After MI, the client may experience heart failure as a result of left ventricular dysfunction, rupture of the intraventricular septum, papillary muscle rupture with valvular dysfunction, or right ventricular infarction. The most severe form of heart failure, *cardiogenic shock,* accounts for most in-hospital deaths after MI. The type of management used to increase cardiac output depends on the location of the MI and the type of heart failure that resulted from the infarction.

Managing Left Ventricular Failure. When a client with MI experiences damage to the left ventricle, rupture of the intraventricular septum, or tear of a papillary muscle, a reduction occurs in the amount of blood that the heart can eject. This reduction in ejection fraction results in a decreased cardiac output and greater left ventricular residual volumes. Volume and pressure increase first in the left ventricle but eventually in the pulmonary vasculature. When volume and pressure are markedly increased in the pulmonary vasculature, pulmonary complications develop.

Nursing Assessment and Monitoring. The nurse assesses for the development of left ventricular failure and pulmonary edema by auscultating for crackles and identifying their location in the lung fields. Wheezing, tachypnea, and frothy sputum may also occur with pulmonary edema. The nurse auscultates the heart, paying particular attention to the presence of an S_3 heart sound. The nurse monitors for the following signs of poor organ perfusion that may result from decreased cardiac output:
- A change in the client's orientation or mental status
- Urine output less than 30 mL/hr
- Cool, clammy extremities with decreased or absent pulses
- Unusual fatigue
- Recurrent chest pain

In specialized units, hemodynamic monitoring may be instituted to assess the client's preload, afterload, and cardiac output. Hemodynamic monitoring requires the insertion of a pulmonary artery catheter (see Chap. 35). The nurse obtains and records hemodynamic measurements, which include right atrial (RA) pressure, pulmonary artery (PA) systolic and diastolic pressures, pulmonary artery wedge pressure (PAWP) (a measure of preload), systemic vascular resistance (SVR) (a measure of afterload), cardiac output (CO), and cardiac index (CI). Single values of these measurements are less significant than the trend of values combined with the client's clinical manifestations. These measurements help both the nurse and the physician to identify heart failure and guide the administration of fluids and vasoactive drugs.

Classification of Post-myocardial Infarction Heart Failure. Killip categorized heart failure after MI into four classes based on prognosis (Table 40–3).

Class I. Clients with class I heart failure often respond well to reduction in preload with IV diuretics. The nurse monitors the urine output hourly, checks the client's vital signs hourly, continues to assess for signs of heart failure, and reviews the serum potassium level.

Classes II and III. Clients with class II and class III failure may require diuresis and more aggressive medical intervention, such as reduction of afterload or enhancement of contractility. Intravenous nitroprusside or nitroglycerin may be used to decrease both preload and afterload. These drugs are administered as continuous infusions in specialized units where the PAWP and blood pressure can be closely monitored. The client's blood pressure can drop in response to excessive vasodilation (see Chart 40–5).

Positive inotropes, such as dopamine (Intropin), dobutamine (Dobutrex), and amrinone (Inocor), increase the force of cardiac contraction. They are administered by continuous IV infusion. The effects of these drugs on the vasculature and heart rate vary and may be dose dependent. The nurse must understand the anticipated effect of the drug and the desired dosage range. The nurse titrates the infusions to optimize cardiac output. The nurse must use caution when administering these drugs because of the potential risk of increasing myocardial oxygen consumption and further decreasing cardiac output. The nurse continues to assess the client, paying particular attention to the development of chest pain.

TABLE 40–3

The Killip Classification of Heart Failure	
Class	**Description**
I	Absent crackles and S_3
II	Crackles in the lower half of the lung fields and possible S_3
III	Crackles more than halfway up the lung fields and frequent pulmonary edema
IV	Cardiogenic shock

Class IV: Cardiogenic Shock. Killip class IV is cardiogenic shock. In cardiogenic shock, necrosis of more than 40% of the left ventricle has occurred. Most clients have a stuttering pattern of chest pain, resulting in piecemeal extension of the MI. Manifestations of cardiogenic shock include

- Tachycardia
- Hypotension
- Blood pressure less than 90 or 30 mmHg less than the client's baseline
- Urine output less than 30 mL/hr
- Cold, clammy skin with poor peripheral pulses
- Agitation, restlessness, or confusion
- Pulmonary congestion
- Tachypnea
- Continuing chest discomfort

Early detection is essential because established cardiogenic shock has a mortality rate of 65% to 100%.

Medical Management. Medical interventions aim to relieve pain and decrease myocardial oxygen requirements through preload and possibly afterload reduction (see Chart 40–5). The physician orders IV morphine, which is used to decrease pulmonary congestion and relieve pain. Oxygen is administered; intubation and ventilation may be necessary. The nurse uses the information gained from hemodynamic monitoring to titrate drug therapy. Preload reduction may be cautiously attempted with diuretics, nitroglycerin, or nitroprusside, as described with Killip class III clients. Because vasodilation may result in a further decline in blood pressure, the nurse monitors systolic pressure constantly. Vasopressors and positive inotropes may be used to maintain organ perfusion, but such drugs increase myocardial oxygen consumption and can worsen ischemia.

Use of an Intra-aortic Balloon Pump. When clients do not respond to drug therapy with improved tissue perfusion, decreased workload of the heart, and increased cardiac contractility, an intra-aortic balloon pump (IABP) may be inserted. Insertion of an intra-aortic counterpulsation device, such as the IABP, is an invasive intervention that is used to improve myocardial perfusion during an acute MI, reduce afterload, and facilitate left ventricular emptying.

The physician can insert an IABP percutaneously or through surgical cutdown. Inflation of the IABP during diastole increases the client's diastolic pressure and improves coronary perfusion. Deflation of the balloon just before systole reduces afterload at the time of systolic contraction. This facilitates emptying of the left ventricle and improves cardiac output. The balloon catheter is attached to a pump console, which is triggered by an ECG tracing and arterial waveform (Fig. 40–4).

Immediate Reperfusion. Immediate reperfusion is an invasive intervention that shows some promise for clients with cardiogenic shock (Pasternak et al., 1992). The client is taken to the cardiac catheterization laboratory and an emergency left-sided heart catheterization is performed. If the client has a treatable lesion or lesions, the surgeon

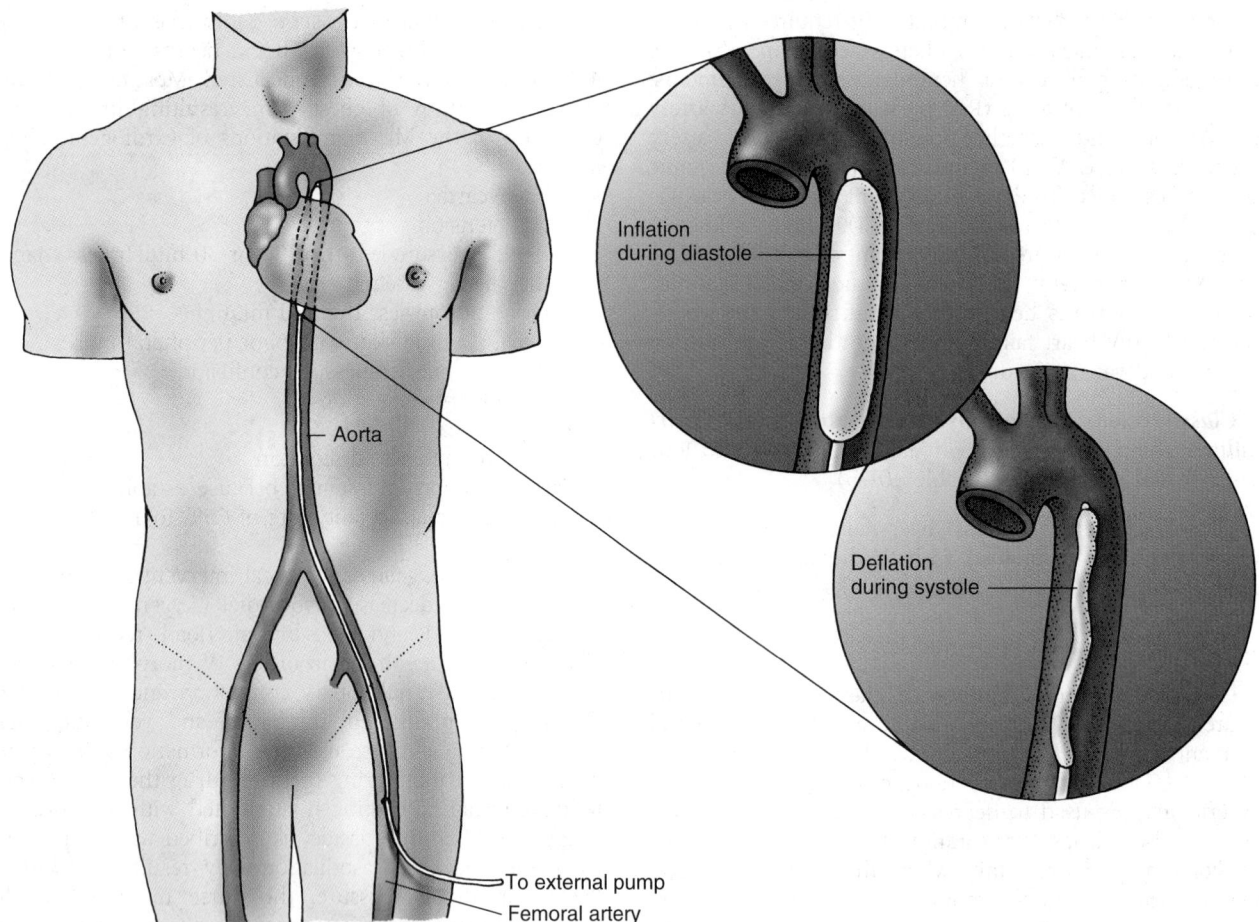

Inflation
during diastole

Deflation
during systole

Aorta

To external pump
Femoral artery

Figure 40-4. Intra-aortic balloon pumping. An intra-aortic balloon catheter is inserted into the femoral artery and advanced into the descending aorta. The polyethylene balloon lies just distal to the left subclavian artery. Immediately after it is inserted, the catheter is connected to the external pump.

performs an immediate percutaneous transluminal coronary angioplasty (PTCA) in the catheterization laboratory, or the client is transferred to the operating suite for coronary artery bypass graft (CABG).

Managing Right Ventricular Failure. Conditions other than left ventricular failure may result in decreased cardiac output after MI. In approximately 30% of clients with inferior MIs, right ventricular infarction and failure develop. In this instance, the right ventricle fails independently of the left. Decreased cardiac output with a paradoxical pulse, clear lungs, and jugular venous distention results when the client is in semi-Fowler's position.

A right ventricular MI may be documented by echocardiography and by an ECG using right-sided precordial leads. The goal of medical management is to improve right ventricular stroke volume by increasing right ventricular fiber stretch or preload. To enhance right ventricular preload, the nurse administers sufficient fluids (as much as 200 mL/hr) to increase right atrial (RA) pressure to 20 mmHg, as ordered. The nurse monitors the pulmonary artery wedge pressure (PAWP) (attempting to maintain it below 15-20 mmHg) and auscultates the lungs to

ensure that left-sided failure is not developing. The nurse monitors the client's cardiac output to ensure that fluid administration is having the desired effect.

Potential for Recurrent Chest Discomfort and Extension of Injury

Planning: Expected Outcomes. The client is expected to experience minimal angina while engaging in ADLs and an exercise program.

Interventions. Recurrent chest discomfort despite medical therapy is one of the major indications for surgical management of coronary artery disease (CAD). Clients who continue to have chest discomfort despite medical therapy may require invasive correction by percutaneous transluminal angioplasty or coronary artery bypass graft (CABG) to resolve angina or prevent MI. Before invasive treatment, a left-sided cardiac catheterization with coronary angiogram (see Chap. 35) is performed to document that the client's lesions are correctable and that left ventricular pump function is adequate.

Percutaneous Transluminal Coronary Angioplasty. Percutaneous transluminal coronary angioplasty (PTCA) is

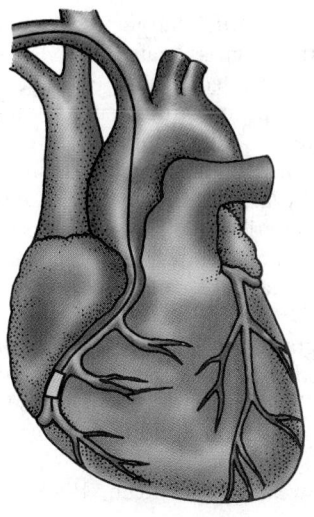 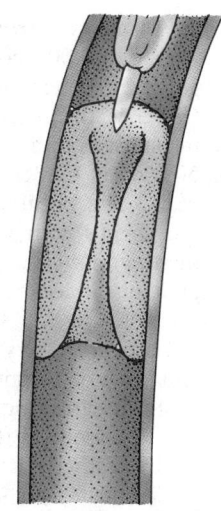 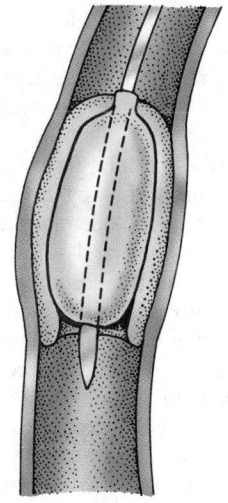 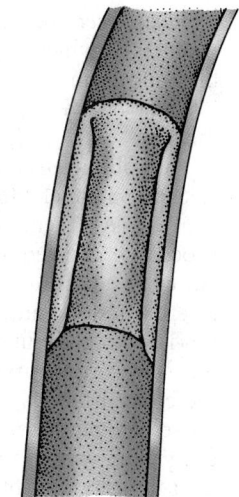

1. The balloon-tipped catheter is positioned in the artery.

2. The uninflated balloon is centered in the obstruction.

3. The balloon is inflated, which flattens plaque against the artery wall.

4. The balloon is removed, and the artery is left unoccluded.

Figure 40–5. Percutaneous transluminal coronary angioplasty.

an invasive but technically nonsurgical technique. It is performed to reduce the frequency and severity of chest discomfort for clients with angina. The risk of complications is not significant.

Indications. Clients who are most likely to benefit from PTCA have single- or double-vessel disease with discrete, proximal, noncalcified lesions. When identifying which lesions are treatable with PTCA, the cardiologist considers the lesion's complexity and location as well as the amount of myocardium at risk. PTCA often will not open complex lesions. Treating lesions located in the left main artery would place a large amount of myocardial tissue at risk should the vessel close acutely; therefore, these lesions are rarely treated with PTCA.

Percutaneous transluminal coronary angioplasty may also be used for the client with an evolving acute MI, either alone or in conjunction with thrombolytic therapy, to reperfuse the damaged myocardium. Approximately 50% of clients needing revascularization are initially treated with PTCA.

Procedure. The physician performs PTCA under fluoroscopic guidance in the cardiac catheterization laboratory. A balloon-tipped catheter is introduced through a guide wire to the occlusion in the coronary vessel. The physician activates a compressor that inflates the balloon at 4–

14 atmospheres of pressure. This process compresses the plaque against the vessel wall and reduces or eliminates the occluding lesion (Fig. 40–5). Balloon inflation may be repeated until angiography indicates decrease of the stenosis (narrowing) to less than 50% of the vessel's diameter.

Intravenous heparin is administered in a continuous infusion to prevent thrombus formation; IV or intracoronary nitroglycerin or sublingual nifedipine is given to prevent coronary spasm. PTCA initially reopens the vessel in more than 90% of appropriately selected clients. However, restenosis occurs in a large number of these clients.

Techniques being used to ensure continued patency of the vessel are laser angioplasty, arthrectomy, and stents. Lasers may be used alone to remove atherosclerotic material from coronary arteries, or they may be used in conjunction with balloon angioplasty to create a smooth lumen about the size of the balloon. Arthrectomy devices can either excise and retrieve plaque or emulsify it. One of the advantages of arthrectomy is that it creates a less bulky vessel with better elastic recoil. Stents are used to maintain the patent lumen obtained by angioplasty or arthrectomy. By providing a supportive scaffold, stents prevent acute closure of the vessel from arterial dissection or vasospasm (Forsha, 1997). Figure 40–6 depicts a stent positioned in a coronary artery.

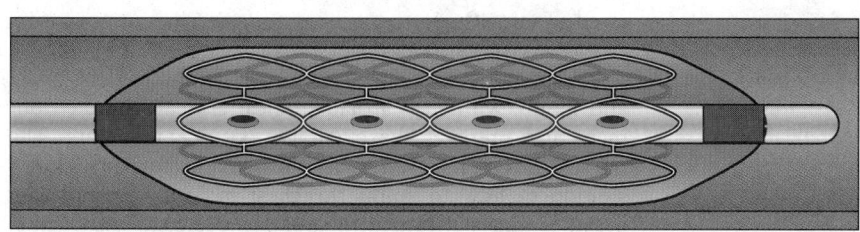

Figure 40–6. A coronary stent open after balloon inflation.

Postprocedure Care. The nurse monitors for potential problems, which include acute closure of the vessel, bleeding from the insertion site, reaction to the dye used in angiography, hypotension, hypokalemia, and dysrhythmias.

The physician usually prescribes a long-term nitrate, calcium channel blocker, and aspirin therapy for clients after PTCA. Clients may experience hypokalemia after the procedure and require careful monitoring and supplementation of potassium. Clients who have intracoronary stents inserted require anticoagulation with warfarin (Coumadin) for 1–3 months until an endothelial covering is laid over the stent. The nursing interventions for clients receiving these medications are described in Chart 40–4. The nurse provides the client with careful explanations of drug therapy and any recommended lifestyle changes. Patient perceptions of PTCA are described in a study by Gulanich and colleagues (1997) (see Research Applications for Nursing).

▷ Research Applications for Nursing

Clients Appreciate Supportive Environment in Angioplasty Laboratory But Experience Postprocedure Discomfort

Gulanich, M., Billey, A., Perino, B., & Keough, V. (1997). Patients' responses to the angioplasty experience: A qualitative study. American Journal of Critical Care, 6(1), 25–32.

This qualitative study examined clients' emotional responses to percutaneous transluminal coronary angioplasty (PTCA). Seven focus group interviews were conducted about the PTCA experience from 45 clients (26 men and 19 women) who had undergone PTCA 3 to 18 months earlier. Most participants described positive experiences during and after PTCA. The most frequent emerging theme was supportive care before, during, and after the procedure. Clients indicated that emotional support and educational preparation for the procedures were very important. However, anger over unmet needs for emotional support and physical comfort was evident. Some clients felt alone during long waits for "tentatively" scheduled procedures. Others complained of back and leg pain from lying flat during and after the procedure. Clients also described discomfort from distended bladders and uncertainty about being allowed to urinate.

Critique. This sample population was drawn from one institution; therefore, generalization to client experiences elsewhere is limited. The interviews were conducted in a group setting. Although investigators encouraged "disagreement" with participants' statements, members of a focus group may be influenced by each other.

Possible Nursing Implications. Because clients move rapidly through health care systems and are awake and aware during PTCA, it is imperative that nurses know what information and interventions clients find most helpful and supportive. This study supports the need for continuing nursing research on comfort measures during and after PTCA as well as on effective methods to educate clients about procedures when time constraints are severe.

Coronary Artery Bypass Graft Surgery. Approximately 490,000 coronary artery bypass graft (CABG) surgeries are performed in the United States each year. CABG is the most common type of cardiac surgery and the most common procedure for older adults; more than 50% of all CABGs are performed on clients older than 65 years. The occluded coronary arteries are bypassed with the client's own venous or arterial blood vessels or synthetic grafts. The internal mammary artery is the current graft of choice because it has a 90% patency rate at 12 years.

Coronary artery bypass grafting is indicated when clients do not respond to medical management of CAD or when disease progression is evident. The decision for surgery is based on the client's symptoms and the results of cardiac catheterization.

Candidates for surgery (Swearingen & Keen, 1995) are clients who have

- Angina with greater than 50% occlusion of the left main coronary artery
- Unstable angina with severe two-vessel or moderate three-vessel disease
- Ischemia with heart failure
- Acute MI
- Signs of ischemia or impending MI after angiography or PTCA

The vessels to be bypassed should have proximal lesions occluding more than 70% of the vessel's diameter but good distal run-off. Bypass of less occluded vessels may result in poor perfusion through the graft and early obstruction. CABG is most effective when good ventricular function remains and the ejection fraction is more than 40%–50%. Clients with lower ejection fractions are poorer risks.

For most clients, the risk is low and the benefits of bypass surgery are clear. Surgical treatment of CAD does not appear to affect the client's life span. Early mortality rates are 1% to 2%. Left ventricular function is the most important long-term indicator of survival. CABG does improve quality of life for most clients; 80%–90% of clients are pain free 1 year after CABG, and 70% remain pain free at 5 years. The percentage of clients experiencing some pain increases sharply after 5 years.

Preoperative Care. CABG surgery may be planned as an elective procedure or performed on an emergency basis. Clients for elective surgery are often admitted the morning of surgery. Preoperative preparations and teaching are completed during prehospitalization interviews. Clients must understand that some medication will need to be adjusted because of the surgery. The nurse ensures that appropriate medications have been discontinued preoperatively and that the necessary ones have been administered (Table 40–4).

Prehospital Preparation. The nurse familiarizes the client and family with the cardiac surgical critical care environment and prepares the client for postoperative care. The nurse demonstrates and has the client return a demonstration of how to splint the chest incision, cough, deep breathe, and perform arm and leg exercises (see Chap. 20). The nurse stresses the following:

TABLE 40-4

Medication Administration Before Coronary Artery Bypass Graft Surgery

Medications Often Discontinued
- Digitalis 12 hr before surgery
- Diuretics 2–3 days before surgery
- Aspirin and anticoagulants 1 week before surgery

Medications Often Administered
- Potassium chloride to maintain potassium between 3.5 and 4.0
- Scheduled beta-blockers
- Scheduled calcium channel blockers
- Scheduled antidysrhythmics
- Scheduled antihypertensives
- Prophylactic antibiotic 20–30 min before surgery

- The client should identify any pain to the nursing staff
- Most of the pain will be in the sternal incision
- Pain medication will be available

The nurse explains that the client should expect to have a sternal incision, possibly a leg incision, one or two chest tubes, a Foley catheter, and several IV fluid catheters postoperatively. An endotracheal tube will be connected to a ventilator for 6–24 hours postoperatively. The client and family must understand that the client will not be able to talk while the endotracheal tube is in place. The client should breathe with the ventilator and not fight it. When describing the postoperative course, the nurse emphasizes that close monitoring and the use of sophisticated equipment are standard treatment.

Psychosocial Preparation. Preoperative anxiety is common. Clients often wait 1–6 weeks for CABG surgery to be scheduled and performed. As the length of the wait increases, anxiety may increase. An appropriate nursing assessment should identify the level of anxiety and the coping methods clients have used successfully in the past. Some clients may find it helpful to define their fears. Common sources of fear include fear of the unknown, fear of bodily harm, and fear of death.

Clients may benefit from detailed information about the surgery, or they may feel overwhelmed by so much material. Some clients need to discuss their feelings in detail or describe the experiences of people they know who have undergone CABG. The nurse assesses clients' anxiety level and helps them to cope. Preoperative anxiety has been positively associated with postpericardiotomy delirium.

Operative Procedure. Coronary artery bypass surgery is performed with the client under general anesthesia and undergoing cardiopulmonary bypass (CPB). The anesthesiologist or nurse anesthetist administers anesthesia and intubates the client. Once the client is anesthetized, one surgical team may begin harvesting the saphenous vein if it is to be used for the graft. The cardiac surgical team begins the procedure with a median sternotomy incision and visualization of the heart and great vessels.

Cardiopulmonary bypass is accomplished by cannulation of the inferior and superior venae cavae. The purpose of CPB is to provide oxygenation, circulation, and hypothermia during induced cardiac arrest. Blood is diverted from the heart to the bypass machine, where it is heparinized, oxygenated, and returned to the circulation through a cannula placed in the ascending aortic arch or femoral artery (Fig. 40–7). During bypass, the client's core temperature is cooled to 82.6°–89.6° F (28–32° C). Cooling decreases the rate of metabolism and demand for oxygen. The heart is perfused with a cardioplegic solution containing potassium, which decreases myocardial oxygen consumption and causes the heart to stop during diastole. This process ensures a still operative field and prevents myocardial ischemia.

Once the heart is arrested, the grafting procedure can begin. The surgeon uses the internal mammary artery (IMA) or a saphenous vein, or both, to bypass lesions in the coronary arteries (Fig. 40–8). The distal end of the IMA is dissected and attached below the lesion on the coronary artery. If the surgeon uses a venous graft, it is anastomosed (sutured) proximally to the aorta and distally to the coronary artery just beyond the occlusion. Thus, myocardial perfusion is improved. After flow rates through the grafts are measured, the heart is rewarmed slowly. The cardioplegic solution is flushed from the heart. The heart regains its rate and rhythm, or it may be defibrillated to return it to a normal rhythm. When the procedure is completed, the client is rewarmed by CPB and weaned from the bypass machine while the grafts are observed for patency and leakage. The surgeon then places atrial and ventricular pacemaker wires and mediastinal chest tubes. Finally, the surgeon closes the sternum with wire sutures.

Postoperative Care. After surgery, the client is transported to a post–open heart surgery unit. There the client undergoes mechanical ventilation for 6–24 hours. The client requires highly skilled nursing care from a nurse qualified to care for clients after cardiac surgery. The nurse connects mediastinal tubes to water seal drainage systems and grounds the epicardial pacer wires and tapes them to the client. The nurse monitors pulmonary artery and arterial pressures and the client's heart rate and rhythm, which are displayed on a monitor. See accompanying clinical pathway for postoperative clients having CABG surgery.

The nurse closely assesses the client for dysrhythmias, such as ventricular ectopic rhythms, bradydysrhythmias, or heart block. The nurse treats symptomatic dysrhythmias according to unit protocols or the physician's order. If the client has symptomatic bradydysrhythmias or heart block, the nurse connects the pacer wires to a pacemaker box and sets the appropriate rate as ordered (see Chap. 36). The nurse also monitors for other complications of CABG surgery, including fluid and electrolyte imbalance, hypotension, hypothermia, hypertension, bleeding, cardiac tamponade, and altered cerebral perfusion. Table 40–5 lists some of the possible postoperative complications of CABG.

Management of Fluid and Electrolyte Imbalance. Assessing fluid and electrolyte balance is a high priority in the

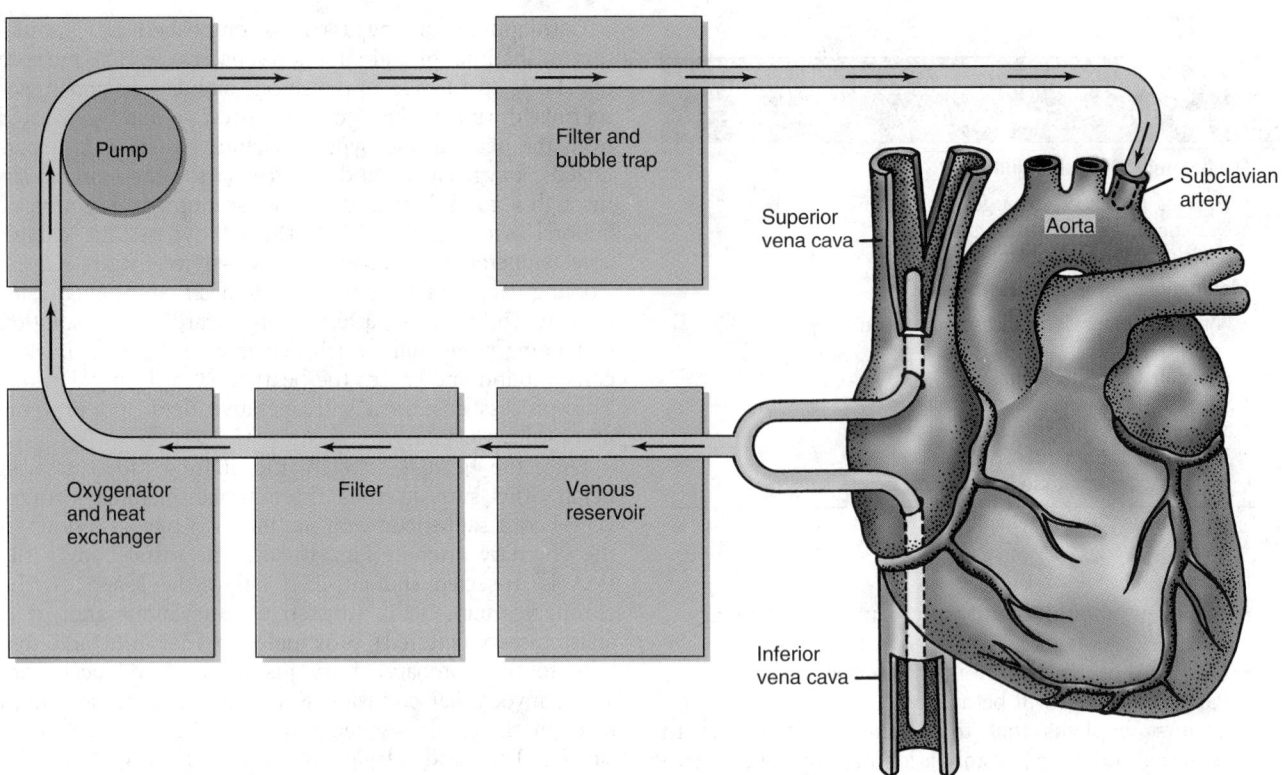

Figure 40–7. Heart-lung bypass circuitry used during cardiopulmonary bypass.

early postoperative period. Clients usually have edema, and fluids may be limited to 1500–2000 mL. However, decisions concerning fluid administration are made on the basis of the client's blood pressure, pulmonary artery wedge pressure (PAWP), right atrial pressure, cardiac output, cardiac index, systemic vascular resistance, and urine output. An experienced nurse interprets assessment findings and adjusts fluid administration on the basis of

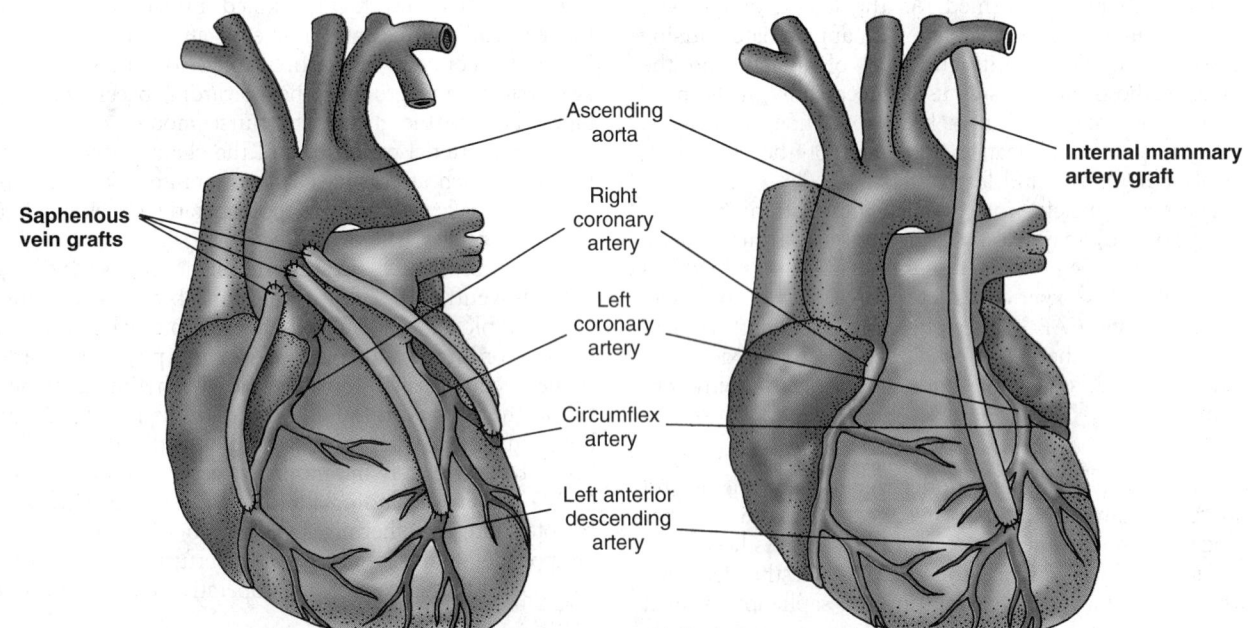

Figure 40–8. Two methods of coronary artery bypass grafting. The procedure used depends on the nature of the coronary artery disease, the condition of the vessels available for grafting, and the client's health status.

TABLE 40-5

Some Possible Postoperative Complications of Coronary Artery Bypass Graft Surgery

Decreased Cardiac Output
- Reduced preload
  - Hypovolemia
  - Hemorrhage
- Increased preload
  - Heart failure
  - Cardiogenic shock
- Increased afterload
  - Hypothermia
  - Increased sympathetic activity
- Dysrhythmias
  - Bradydysrhythmias
  - Conduction defects
  - Tachydysrhythmias
- Myocardial infarction

Pulmonary Dysfunction
- Atelectasis
- Pneumonia
- Pulmonary edema
- Hemothorax/pneumothorax

Neurologic Dysfunction
- Transient neurologic deficits
- Postpericardiotomy delirium
- Cerebrovascular accident

Acute Renal Failure

Gastrointestinal Dysfunction
- Stress ulcer
- Paralytic ileus

Infection

standing unit policies or specific orders from the physician.

Serum electrolytes (especially calcium, magnesium, and phosphorus) may be reduced postoperatively and are monitored carefully by both the physician and the nurse. Because the serum potassium level can fluctuate dramatically, electrolyte levels are checked frequently. Potassium depletion is common and may result from hemodilution, diuretic therapy, and nasogastric suction. To prevent dysrhythmias, potassium concentrations are maintained between 4 and 5mEq/L.

If the serum potassium level is depleted, the physician may order IV potassium replacement. The dose of potassium administered exceeds the usual recommended level of no more than 20 mEq of potassium per hour. For a potassium bolus, as much as 40–80 mEq may be mixed in 100 mL of IV solution and given at a rate as high as 40 mEq/hr. The drug must be given through a central catheter and the rate of administration controlled by an infusion pump. The client must be on a cardiac monitor for extremely careful observation.

Management of Hypotension. Hypotension (systolic blood pressure less than 90 mmHg) is a significant problem because it may result in the collapse of a vein graft. The nurse reviews the assessment parameters to identify what might be causing the hypotension. Decreased preload (decreased PAWP) can result from hypovolemia or vasodilation. If the client is hypovolemic, it might be appropriate to increase fluid administration or administer blood. The physician may treat the client with a low PAWP, decreased systemic vascular resistance, and vasodilation with vasopressor therapy to increase the blood pressure. However, if hypotension is the result of left ventricular failure (increased PAWP), IV inotropes might be necessary.

Management of Hypothermia. Although the client is rewarmed to 98.6° F (37° C) before being removed from bypass, it is not uncommon for the temperature to drift downward after the client leaves the surgical suite. The nurse monitors the client's body temperature and institutes rewarming procedures should the temperature drop below 96.8° F (36° C). Rewarming may be accomplished with warm blankets, rewarming lights, or thermal blankets. The danger of rewarming a client too quickly is that the client may begin shivering, resulting in metabolic acidosis and hypoxia. To prevent shivering, rewarming should proceed no faster than 1.8° F (1° C) per hour. The nurse discontinues rewarming when the client's temperature approaches 98.6° F (37° C) and the client's extremities feel warm.

Management of Hypertension. Hypothermia is a significant risk for the client undergoing coronary artery bypass graft (CABG) surgery because it promotes vasoconstriction and hypertension. Other factors contributing to hypertension in the CABG client include CPB, medications, and the client's own sympathetic activity.

When hypertension is defined as a systolic blood pressure greater than 140–150 mmHg, most CABG clients experience hypertension. Hypertension is dangerous because increased pressure promotes leakage from suture lines and may cause bleeding. To return the blood pressure to acceptable limits, the nurse titrates IV nitroprusside or nitroglycerin (see Chart 40–5).

Management of Bleeding. Bleeding occurs to a limited extent postoperatively in all clients. The nurse measures the mediastinal and chest tube drainage at least hourly and reports drainage exceeding 150 mL/hr to the surgeon. Clients with IMA grafts may have more chest drainage. The nurse may autotransfuse the chest drainage to assist with volume management when 500 mL have accumulated or 4 hours have elapsed, depending on the clinical pathway or physician's order. The nurse must maintain the patency of the mediastinal and chest tubes. One effective way of promoting chest tube drainage is to prevent a dependent loop from forming in the tubing.

Management of Cardiac Tamponade. If the client is bleeding and the mediastinal tubes are not kept patent, blood may accumulate around the heart. The myocardium is compressed, and cardiac tamponade results. The fluid accumulating around the heart compresses the atria and ventricles, prevents them from filling adequately, and reduces cardiac output. Hallmarks of cardiac tamponade include

- Sudden cessation of previously heavy mediastinal drainage

Text continued on page 926

University Hospitals
of Cleveland

CARE PATH NAME: CABG/VALVE (SICU)

SICU ELOS: 24 Hours

TOTAL ELOS: 5 Days (Anticipated Discharge on POD 4)

Expected Disposition: Telemetry Unit

Pre-Op Weight: _____ kg.

Collaborative Problem List
1. Home maintenance management
2. Potential for decreased cardiac output
3. Potential for fluid overdrive
4.
5.
6.

Focus	DAY OF SURG.: 1st 15 min.	DAY OF SURG.: 15 min. to 2 hrs.	DAY OF SURG.: 2 hrs to 6 am	POST-OP DAY 1: 6 am to Time of Transfer
Laboratory Tests/ Procedures	• ABG, CBC/diff, Chem 7, ionized Ca++, Mg++, PT/PTT, surgical isoenzymes • Dextrose stick • Pulse oximetry	• EKG, chest x-ray • Dextrose stick as ordered	• Labs q 8 h: CBC (no diff), Chem 7, Ionized Ca++, Mg++, Surg. isoenzymes, ABG after extubation • Others as ordered	• EKG and chest x-ray
Consults	• Respiratory Care Consultant	• Notify Surgical Cardiologist on call		• Order PT Consult on transfer orders for all patients ≥ 75 years old or if in SICU > 48 hours
Physical Assessment	• Complete assessment • Continuous cardiac monitoring • Hemodynamic monitoring q 15 min. & prn • I & O	• Ongoing physical and hemodynamic assessment • Vital signs q 15 min • Wean vent as tolerated and extubate per algorithm.	• Ongoing physical assessment q 4 h • VS/Hemodynamic evaluation q 1-2 h • Weight in AM • Assess bowel sounds • After extubation, O2 at 40-50% VM or nasal cannula and wean O2 as tolerated to Sat. ≥ 92	• VS/Hemodynamic evaluation q 2-4 h
Activity	• Bedrest	• Bedrest: turn q 2 h	• Bedrest: turn q 2 h • Dangle at bedside or sit in cardiac chair 2 h after extubation • In chair at bedside before 5 am	• Sit in chair for breakfast • OOB tid
Diet	• NPO		• Clear liquids after extubation • Assess needs for metoclopramide (Reglan)	• Clear liquids • Advance to low cholesterol diet as tolerated
Medications	• IV: D5 1/4 NS with _____ meq. KCL/L • Antibiotics • MS 2-12 mg IV q 1 h prn • Medications as ordered: Titrate drips according to ordered parameters • Insulin coverage per orders • Other: consider pre-admission meds			• Enteric coated ASA • Dipyridamole (DVH only)

Treatments	• Insert NG/OG tube to low continuous suction • Connect to Vent/mode IMV • CT: autotransfusion - 30 cm suction or H2O seal • Document initial CT output • Blood replacement: autotransfuse to IL • Blood products as ordered • IABP/Pacer: stand by • Foley	• CT/MSCT output q 15 min • Warming light or Bair hugger for temp < 35.5° C • Isolate epicardial wires (using 3 cc syringe with syringe cannula)	• D/C NG tube when extubated if bowel sounds present • CT/MSCT output q 1 h. D/C CTs by 6 am • Change epicardial wire dressing when MSCT D/C • Incentive spirometry Q 1 h WA • Encourage C&DB • O2 at 40-50% VM or nasal cannula • Wean as tolerated to keep O2 > 90%	• D/C foley prior to transfer if urine output adequate • D/C Swan Ganz if hemodynamically stable • D/C A-line • D/C Chest tubes • O2 per nasal cannula; Wean as tolerated to keep O2 Sat. > 90%
Discharge Planning		• Assess and document discharge needs when family in to visit to facilitate early D/C planning		• Make referral to Home Care or Social Work if needs are known
Teaching/ Learning		• Discuss "usual post-op" course with family, including anticipated D/C home on POD 4		
Intermediate Outcomes		• Adequate oxygenation/ventilation • Hemodynamically stable	• Extubate with 4 h post-op • Hemodynamically stable without pharmacological support • CT output ≤ 75 cc/h • Neurologically intact	• Extubate with adequate oxygenation/ventilation • Hemodynamically stable without pharmacological support • Neurologically intact • Swan Ganz and arterial line discontinued • Transferred to telemetry unit on ___/___/___ at _____ hours
Intermediate Outcomes		☐ Met ☐ Not Met (see progress notes)	☐ Met ☐ Not Met (see progress notes)	☐ Met ☐ Not Met (see progress notes)
Date				
RN Signature				

University Hospital's carepaths have been developed to assist clinicians in patient management and clinical decision-making. The carepaths are intended to meet the needs of patients in most circumstances. They are not intended to replace a clinician's judgment or establish a protocol for all patients with this diagnosis.
SP-9339 (01/23/97)

University Hospitals
of Cleveland

CARE PATH NAME: CABG/VALVE (TELEMETRY)
ELOS: 4 Days
Expected Disposition: Home
Pre-Op Weight: _____

Collaborative Problem List
1. Home maintenance management
2. Potential for decreased cardiac output
3. Potential for fluid overdrive
4. Potential for activity intolerance
5.
6.

Focus	POST-OP DAY 1: Time of Transfer to 7:00 AM	POST-OP DAY 2	POST-OP DAY 3	POST-OP DAY 4
Laboratory Tests/ Procedures	• Dextrose stick AC and HS (Diabetics) → • Pulse ox q shift and prn while on O2 → • Telemetry until discontinued →	• PT/PTT q d (valve) • EKG • CBC, Chem 7	• Dextrose stick bid (Diabetics) → • Pulse ox prn → • CBC, Chem 23 • CXR, EKG	
Consults	• Cardiology consult established in SICU • Respiratory care consult established in SICU • PT evaluation for all patients > 75 years old or with SICU LOS > 48 h and for other patients, if ordered • OT consult and evaluation if ordered • Cardiac rehab. referral • Nutrition Screen (see "Diet") • Home Care Consult if applicable Social Work Consult today if: • Patient is expected to need short or long term placement • Patient lives alone and/or has inadequate caregiver and is anticipated to have new functional impairment at discharge • Patient currently resides in an extended care facility • Patient has dementia • Patient and family have a conflictual or difficult relationship • Patient has no insurance • Not meeting carepath ambulation criteria		Social Work Consult Today If: • Patient not previously referred and is expected to need short or long term placement • Patient expresses concerns re: obtaining medications at discharge • Patient requires equipment/supplies/home oxygen at discharge • Patient not previously referred and is now expected to require community agency involvement • Patient was being followed by homecare or community agency prior to admission • Other concerns as identified by team	
Physical Assessment	• Nursing assessment q shift → • Vital signs q 4 h → • Arrhythmia management protocol as needed → • I&O q shift, weight qd →	• Assess bowel status and medicate as necessary	• Vital signs q shift →	
Activity	• OOB tid → • Ambulate to bathroom → • Ambulate to door (Appx. 20 ft) → • Activity participates in ADL → • Performs UE and LE exercises on handouts: 5 reps	• OOB to chair for all meals → • Ambulate at least 50 ft qid → • 5-10 reps	• Ambulate at least 100 ft tid → • Independently performs ADLs → • 10-15 reps	• Up ad lib • Ambulate at least 150 ft tid • Climb up/down stairs (Same # as at home) • 20 reps
Diet	• Advance as tolerated to low cholesterol diet → • Nutrition Screen: Assess need for diet instruction and consult for nutrition education if indicated → • Assess need for metoclopramide (Regan) →			

Focus	POST-OP DAY 1: Time of Transfer to 7:00 AM	POST-OP DAY 2	POST-OP DAY 3	POST-OP DAY 4
Treatments	• Check isolated epicardial wires at time of transfer • Temporary pacemaker as ordered • Heparin lock/IVF. D/C IVF when tolerating PO • O2 per NC. Wean as tolerated • D/C O2 when room air pulse ox ≥ 90% • Incentive spirometry q 1 h WA • Encourage C+DB • Arrhythmia management protocol as needed	• Maintain electrical isolation • Evaluate need for temporary pacer. D/C as appropriate • Change CT, graft, epicardial wires, DSGs	• Evaluate possibility of pulling epicardial wires in PM	• D/C epicardial wires; if not already done, apply bandaids • D/C heparin lock
Medications	• Medications as ordered • Beta blocker as ordered • Consider pre-admission meds	• Continue with all medications as ordered • Consider changing IV medications to oral dose		

Discharge Planning/ Teaching	• Orient to Lerner Tower 3 at transfer
	• Assess home care needs
	• Review meds while administering
	• Review activity, incisional care, diet
	• Initiate GRF, if applicable
		• Assess home care needs
		• Review meds while administering
		• Review activity, incisional care, diet
		• Initiate Gold Referral Form (GRF) if applicable
			• Refer to Ambulatory Nutrition Practice or other outpatient nutrition program if further nutrition education identified
			• Review medications, activity, incisional care, diet
			• Update GRF if applicable
			• Initiate D/C folder:
			  Med schedule
			  Med cards
			  PI sheets
			  CTS booklet
			• Cardiac rehab pamphlet
			• Offer videos, PI sheets
				• F/U appts (if known) Final Review:
				• Referral(s) to appropriate agencies
				• Confirm arrangements for equipment
				• Finalize GRF
				• D/C folder
				• Cardiac rehab pamphlet
				• F/U appts

Intermediate Outcomes	• Hemodynamically stable • Pain controlled • Bowel sounds x 4 quads • Ambulates 20 ft with pulse ox ≥ 90% • Home situation assessed and home health services determined • Social Work Consult ordered if indicated by criteria	• Hemodynamically stable • Pain controlled • Ambulates 50 ft and participate in ADLs with pulse ox ≥ 90% • D/C plans discussed with patient/family; plan D/C by 11 AM on Day 4	• Hemodynamically stable • Pain controlled • Ambulates 100 ft and perform ADLs with pulse ox ≥ 90% • No arrhythmias • No signs of hypoxia • Bowel movement x 1 • D/C planning continuing • D/C orders/prescriptions written in evening	• Hemodynamically stable • Pain controlled • Ambulates 150 ft and independently performs ADLs • No arrhythmias • No signs of hypoxia • Bowel movement x 1 • Epicardial wires and graft site sutures D/C'd • D/C plans confirmed • Social Work Consult ordered if indicated by criteria • See discharge outcomes sheet
Intermediate Outcomes	☐ Met ☐ Not Met	☐ Met ☐ Not Met	☐ Met ☐ Not Met	☐ Met ☐ Not Met
Date				
RN Signature				

Discharge Outcomes

Discharge Outcomes	Met	Not Met	Comments	Date/Initials
Patient/family will verbalize understanding of: a. Medications, Incisional care, Signs/symptoms of infection, Activity progression, Diet, Physician follow-up b. Epicardial wires removed c. No signs of bleeding, PT level < 24 d. Arrhythmia free for 24 hours, or controlled arrhythmia e. Telemetry off f. No heart failure or treated heart failure g. Adequate urine output h. O2 Sat. greater than or equal to 90% i. CBC, Chem-23, EKG, within normal limits j. PT/INR within accepted therapeutic range (valve only) k. Free of uncontrolled infection l. Adequate bowel movement Pain controlled Able to ambulate 150 ft, and/or increasing ability to perform ADLs Heparin lock out				

SP-9345 (01/23/97)

- Jugular venous distention but clear lung sounds
- Pulsus paradoxus (blood pressure greater than 10 mmHg higher on expiration than on inspiration)
- An equalizing of PAWP and right atrial pressure

Tamponade can be confirmed by echocardiogram or chest x-ray. Pericardiocentesis (see Chap. 37) may not be appropriate for tamponade after CABG because the blood in the pericardium may have clotted. Volume expansion and emergency sternotomy with drainage are then the treatments of choice.

Management of Altered Levels of Consciousness. The client may demonstrate changes in the level of consciousness, which may be permanent or transient. Transient changes related to anesthesia, CPB, or hypothermia occur in as many as 75% of clients. Transient neurologic deficits may include slowness to arouse, memory loss, and confusion.

Clients with transient neurologic deficits usually return to baseline neurologic status over 4–8 hours. Permanent deficits may be associated with a cerebrovascular accident (CVA) during surgery. The client may demonstrate
- Abnormal pupillary response
- Failure to awaken from anesthesia
- Seizures
- Absence of sensory or motor function

The nurse checks the client's neurologic status every 30–60 minutes until the client has awakened from anesthesia; then the nurse checks every 2–4 hours.

Pain Management. The nurse must differentiate between sternotomy pain, which is expected after CABG, and anginal pain, which might indicate graft failure. Typical sternotomy pain is localized, does not radiate, and often becomes worse when the client coughs or breathes deeply. The client may describe the pain as sharp, aching, or burning. Pain may stimulate the client's sympathetic nervous system, which increases the client's heart rate and vascular resistance while decreasing cardiac output. The nurse administers the prescribed medication, in adequate doses, frequently enough to limit pain. However, during the process of weaning the client from mechanical ventilation, it may be necessary to limit pain medication because of the respiratory depressant effects of analgesia.

Transfer from the Special Care Unit. Ventilation is usually provided for 6–24 hours postoperatively, until the client is breathing adequately and is hemodynamically stable. During the first 2 days, the client usually is weaned from the ventilator; has pacer wires, hemodynamic monitoring lines, and mediastinal tubes removed; and is transferred to an intermediate care unit. All CABG clients, but especially those with IMA grafts, are at high risk for atelectasis, so the nurse encourages the client to splint, cough, turn, and deep breathe to raise secretions. The nurse guides the client in a gradual resumption of activity (see clinical pathway). The nurse continues to monitor the client for decreased cardiac output, pain, dysrhythmias, and infection.

Approximately one third of clients with CABG and two thirds of clients with valve replacements experience supraventricular dysrhythmias (especially atrial fibrillation) during the postoperative period, most commonly on the second or third postoperative day. The nurse examines the monitor pattern for atrial fibrillation. When auscultating the heart, the nurse listens for an irregular rhythm. (See Chapter 36 for interventions for atrial fibrillation.)

Sternal wound infections develop between 5 days and several weeks postoperatively in about 2% of clients and represent a significant complication (Hussey & Leeper, 1998). The nurse is alerted to the presence of *mediastinitis* by
- Fever continuing beyond the first 4 days after CABG
- Instability (bogginess or stepping) of the sternum
- Redness or purulent drainage from suture sites
- An increased white blood cell count

The physician may perform a needle biopsy to confirm a sternal infection. Surgical debridement, antibiotic wound irrigation, and IV antibiotics are usually indicated. Four to 6 weeks of IV antibiotics are required if sternal osteomyelitis has developed.

Postpericardiotomy syndrome is a source of chest discomfort in 10% to 40% of postcardiac surgery clients. The syndrome is characterized by pericardial and pleural pain, pericarditis, a friction rub, elevated temperature and white blood cell count, and dysrhythmias. Postpericardiotomy syndrome may occur days to weeks after surgery and seems to be associated with blood remaining in the pericardial sac. The nurse observes the client for the development of pericardial or pleural pain. For most clients, the syndrome is mild and self-limiting. However, the client may require treatment similar to that for pericarditis. The nurse should be prepared to detect pericardial tamponade (see Chap. 37).

Older adults may have different needs and experience slightly different problems after CABG. Nursing concerns related to the older CABG client are detailed in Chart 40–7.

*** Minimally Invasive Direct Coronary Arterial Bypass.*** The minimally invasive direct coronary arterial bypass (MIDCAB) may be indicated for clients with a lesion of the left anterior descending artery (LAD). After a 2-inch left thoracotomy incision is made and the fourth rib removed, the left internal mammary artery (IMA) is dissected and attached to the still-beating heart below the level of the lesion in the LAD. Cardiopulmonary bypass (CPB) is not required. Nurses must assess the client postoperatively for chest pain and ECG changes because occlusion of the IMA graft occurs acutely in 10% of clients. Because they have a thoracotomy incision and a chest tube, clients are encouraged to cough and deep breathe. Most clients spend less than 6 hours in a critical care unit and are discharged in 2–3 days.

*** Transmyocardial Laser Revascularization.*** Transmyocardial laser revascularization is an experimental procedure for clients with unstable angina and inoperable CAD but areas of reversible myocardial ischemia. After a single-lung intubation, a left anterior thoracotomy is performed and the heart is visualized. A laser is used to create 20–24 long, narrow channels through the left ventricular muscle to the left ventricle. These channels will eventually allow oxygenated blood to flow during diastole from the left ventricle to nourish the muscle. After the surgery, the client is transported to a critical care unit, where the nurse institutes hemodynamic monitoring and monitors for anginal episodes and bleeding disturbances.

 Continuing Care

➤ Case Management

Case management is most appropriate for clients who meet high-cost, high-volume, and high-risk criteria (Kegel, 1996). Clients with CAD clearly meet all these criteria. Clinical pathways and case management programs for clients who have CAD are in effect in most U.S. hospitals. By focusing on cardiovascular risk reduction and improving the continuity of care, the length and cost of hospital stays have been reduced. Posthospital case management should reduce hospital readmission rates and improve client health.

➤ Home Care Management

Clients who have experienced myocardial infarction (MI), angina, or coronary artery bypass graft (CABG) surgery are usually discharged to home or to a subacute care setting with pharmacologic therapy and specific activity prescriptions. Hospital stays are approximately 5–7 days for MI and CABG clients and only 2 days for percutaneous transluminal coronary angioplasty (PTCA) clients; therefore, clients are still recovering when they are discharged. Clients may require a home health nurse for assessment and teaching postdischarge and an aide for assistance with ADLs if they are older or weaker (Chart 40–8). Additionally, women, who tend to be older and more frequently living alone when coronary events occur,

may have a greater need for home assistance after CABG surgery (see Research Applications for Nursing). Clients who were residents in long-term care may be returned there after hospitalization for unstable angina, MI, or CABG surgery.

Cardiac rehabilitation is available in many communities for clients after MI or CABG surgery, but only 10% to 30% of clients participate in structured rehabilitation programs. The most frequently cited reasons for nonparticipation are lack of insurance coverage, physicians' directive that it is unnecessary, and client decision that it was not necessary. Clients who participate in structured rehabilitation programs report greater improvement in exercise tolerance and improved ability to control stress. However, there is no difference in clients' return to work.

➤ Health Teaching

Because hospital stays are short and clients are quite ill during hospitalization, most in-hospital education programs concentrate on survival skills after discharge. As part of home visits or a cardiac rehabilitation program, the nurse identifies the additional educational needs of

Moore, S. M. (1995). *A comparison of women's and men's symptoms during home recovery after coronary artery bypass surgery.* Heart & Lung, 24(6), 495–501.

➤ Research Applications for Nursing

Gender Differences in Concerns After Coronary Artery Bypass Graft Surgery

The purpose of this descriptive, comparative study was to determine whether men and women differed in their physical and emotional symptoms during the recovery period after coronary artery bypass graft (CABG) surgery. Secondary analysis was performed on interview data obtained from 40 clients (20 women and 20 men) at three time points within the first 4 weeks after surgery. Questions were asked about specific symptoms experienced as well as recovery concerns, difficulties, and problems. Results showed clear demographic and recovery-specific differences. The women in this study tended to be older, unemployed, and living alone more frequently than the men. Although both men and women reported physical discomfort, men experienced more incisional pain and fatigue and women experienced more physical discomfort associated with their breasts. The most common worry among the men was related to physical recovery. The most common worry among the women was who would assist in their care during home recovery.

Critique. This excellent study points out some gender differences with recovery issues after coronary artery bypass surgery. Although the sample size was small, its composition reflected the national demographics regarding people undergoing CABG.

Possible Nursing Implications. Gender differences are known to exist regarding age at onset, severity of disease, mortality, and time to treatment between men and women experiencing coronary artery disease and myocardial infarction. This is the first study examining possible differences in the postoperative recovery period. The increased age of the women, coupled with the fact that the majority lived alone, has relevance for changes for discharge planning. Additionally, the breast symptoms experienced by the women should be considered for inclusion in home-going information.

the client and family as well as their readiness to learn. The nurse then develops a teaching plan, which usually includes education about the normal anatomy and physiology of the heart, the pathophysiology of angina and MI, risk factor modification, activity and exercise protocols, cardiac medications, and the time to seek medical assistance.

The nurse informs the client about the normal function of the heart and coronary arteries and explains angina and MI. Clients are taught that after MI myocardial healing begins early and is usually complete in 6–8 weeks. Clients who have undergone CABG are told that the sternotomy heals in about 6–8 weeks.

Clients who have undergone CABG require instruction on incisional care for the sternum and the graft site. Clients should inspect the incisions daily for any redness, swelling, or drainage. The leg of a saphenous vein donor site is often edematous. The nurse instructs clients to avoid crossing legs, to wear elastic stockings until the edema subsides, and to elevate the surgical limb when sitting in a chair.

➤ Risk Factor Modification

Modification of risk factors is a necessary part of a client's management and involves changing the client's health maintenance patterns. Such modifications may include smoking cessation, altered dietary habits, regular exercise, blood pressure control, and blood glucose control.

Smoking Cessation. For clients who smoke, the nurse explains the detrimental effects on the cardiovascular system of smoking tobacco, especially cigarettes. Many clients spontaneously quit smoking soon after an MI. By encouraging all clients who have smoked to participate in smoking cessation and relapse programs, the nurse ensures that an additional 17%–26% of clients will cease smoking. One effective model uses nurse-managed behavioral intervention with biochemical verification of smoking status (Wenger et al., 1995).

Cholesterol Control. The mainstays of cholesterol control are diet therapy and administration of antihyperlipidemic agents.

Diet Therapy. The nurse collaborates with the dietitian to encourage the client to follow a prudent diet. Less than 30% of the calories in the diet should be from fat, and the fat consumed should be primarily monounsaturated or polyunsaturated. Clients should avoid saturated fats and foods rich in cholesterol. The nurse or dietitian also instructs the client not to add salt at the table. Booklets and cookbooks that can assist the client in learning to cook with reduction of fats, oils, and salt are available from the American Heart Association (AHA).

Weight reduction can normalize plasma lipid and lipoprotein levels in overweight clients. The cardiac rehabilitation nurse collaborates with the dietitian and physical therapist to provide multifactorial rehabilitation, including nutrition education, counseling, behavior modification, and exercise training to assist the overweight client to lose weight permanently (Wenger et al., 1995).

Antihyperlipidemic Agents. Cholesterol reduction with antihyperlipidemic agents, such as pravastatin (Pravacol), has been demonstrated to reduce significantly the risk of further CAD, including recurrent MI, death from CAD, and need for revascularization procedures. Thus, many clients with both normal and high cholesterol levels are encouraged to take these agents after CAD develops.

An area of controversy is the use of antioxidants (such as vitamin E). Some researchers report that the use of such agents counteracts the adverse effects of oxygen free radicals (derived from high cholesterol levels) on blood vessels and protects arteries. Other reports point out that excessive vitamin E increases the risk for liver damage and that the long-term effects of antioxidants are not known.

Physical Activity. The nurse collaborates with the physical therapist to establish an activity and exercise schedule as part of client rehabilitation. The nurse instructs the client to remain near home during the first week after discharge and to continue a walking program. The client may engage in light housework or any activity done sitting that does not precipitate angina. During the second week, the client is encouraged to increase social activities and possibly to return to work part time. By the third week, the client may begin to lift objects as heavy as 15 pounds (such as 2 gallons of milk), but should avoid lifting or pulling heavier objects for the first 6–8 weeks. Chart 40–9 lists suggested instructions for exercise.

The client may begin a simple walking program by walking 400 feet twice a day at the rate of 1 mile/hour the first week after discharge and increasing the distance and rate as tolerated, usually weekly, until the client can walk 2 miles at 3–4 miles/hour. The nurse instructs the client to take a pulse reading before, halfway through, and after exercise. The client should stop exercising if the target pulse rate is exceeded or if dyspnea or angina develops.

After a limited exercise tolerance test, the physical therapist or nurse encourages the client to join a formal exercise program, ideally one that assists the client in monitoring cardiovascular progress. The program should include 5- to 7-minute warm-up and cool-down periods as well as 30 minutes of aerobic exercise. The client should engage in aerobic exercise a minimum of three, but preferably five, times a week.

Complementary Therapies. Complementary therapies can aid in reducing a client's anxiety about progressive activity both in the immediate postoperative period and during the rehabilitation phase. Such techniques as progressive muscle relaxation, guided imagery, and music therapy have been shown to decrease anxiety, reduce depression, and increase client compliance with activity/exercise regimens after CABG (Barnason, Zimmerman, & Nieveen, 1995; Collins & Rice, 1997).

Sexual Activity. Sexual activity is often of great concern to clients and their partners. The nurse informs the client and partner that engaging in their usual sexual activity is unlikely to cause any damage to the client's heart. Clients can resume sexual intercourse on the advice of the physician, usually after exercise tolerance is assessed. The client who can walk one block or climb two flights of stairs without symptoms can usually safely resume sexual activity.

The nurse suggests that initially clients schedule intercourse after a period of rest. Clients might try having intercourse in the morning when they are well rested or wait 1½ hours after exercise or a heavy meal. They may take nitroglycerin before intercourse as a prophylactic measure. The position selected should be comfortable for both the client and his or her partner (e.g., side-lying) so that no undue stress is placed on the heart or suture line.

Blood Pressure Control. The nurse may make arrangements for the client to have blood pressure measured at regular intervals and collaborates with the primary care provider to establish parameters for reporting the blood pressure to the provider. Lifestyle modifications such as weight reduction, physical activity, and reduced sodium diets may assist in the management of hypertension. If the client is taking medication, the nurse assesses the client's compliance with the medication regimen.

Blood Glucose Control. Clients with diabetes mellitus are assessed for their participation in efforts to control hyperglycemia. The nurse reviews the prescribed dosage of insulin or oral hypoglycemic agents with the client and family. The client should demonstrate accurate testing of blood for glucose levels.

Cardiac Medications. The nurse assists the client in understanding the type of cardiac medications prescribed, the benefit of each drug, potential side effects to watch for, and the correct dosage and time of day to take each drug. Medication regimens vary considerably from client to client. However, many clients with angina are discharged taking aspirin, a beta-blocker, a calcium channel blocker, an antihyperlipidemic agent, and a nitrate. Clients who have experienced a myocardial infarction (MI) may require aspirin, a beta-blocker, an antihyperlipidemic agent, and an angiotensin-converting enzyme (ACE) inhibitor. The regimen can be complex. The nurse must determine that the client can comply with the instructions.

Use of sublingual nitroglycerin deserves special attention. The nurse instructs the client to carry nitroglycerin tablets at all times and to keep the tablets in a light-resistant container. Nitroglycerin tablets should be replaced every 3–5 months before they lose their potency and stop tingling when the client places one under the tongue. Chart 40–10 gives instructions for clients about management of chest discomfort at home.

Seeking Medical Assistance. Clients are encouraged to notify their health care provider if they experience

■ Heart rate remaining less than 50 after arising
■ Wheezing or difficulty breathing
■ Weight gain of 3 pounds in 1 week
■ Slow persistent increase in nitroglycerin use
■ Dizziness, faintness, or shortness of breath with activity

Chart 40–9

Education Guide: Activity for the Client with Coronary Artery Disease

- Begin by walking the same distance at home as in the hospital (usually 400 feet) three times each day.
- Carry nitroglycerin with you.
- Check your pulse before, during, and after the exercise.
- Stop the activity for a pulse increase of more than 20 beats per minute, shortness of breath, angina, or dizziness.
- Exercise outdoors when the weather is good.
- Gradually increase the walking until the distance is ¼ mile twice daily (usually the end of the second week).
- After an exercise tolerance test and with your physician's approval, walk at least three times each week, increasing the distance by ½ mile every other week, until the total distance is 2 miles.
- Avoid straining (lifting, pushups, pull-ups, and straining at bowel movements).

Chart 40-10

Education Guide: Management of Chest Pain at Home

- Keep fresh nitroglycerin available for immediate use.
- At the first indication of chest discomfort, cease activity and sit or lie down.
- Place one nitroglycerin tablet under your tongue and allow it to dissolve.
- Wait 5 minutes for relief.
- If no relief results, repeat the nitroglycerin and wait 5 more minutes.
- If there is no relief, repeat and wait 5 more minutes.
- If there is still no relief, call for transportation to a health care facility.

Clients are encouraged to call for transportation to the hospital if they experience

- Chest discomfort that does not improve after 20 minutes or 3 nitroglycerin tablets
- Extremely severe chest discomfort with weakness, nausea, or fainting.

WOMEN'S HEALTH CONSIDERATIONS

 Women with CAD report requiring more assistance from friends and extended family than men. Male spouses of clients with CAD may be unaccustomed to assuming a caregiving role and the older, widowed or divorced woman may live alone. If a woman is able to develop two or more sources of emotional support, her chance of surviving 5 years is three times higher than if she remains isolated and alone (Arnstein, Buselli, & Rankin, 1996). The cardiac rehabilitation nurse should assess the emotional support available to women with CAD. If there is not adequate support available, the nurse should provide it or arrange for the client to participate in a support group.

Women are less likely to enroll and stay in structured cardiac rehabilitation programs or participate in home walking programs than men. Most cite family and domestic responsibilities for not participating. Although housework is important to the role satisfaction of many older women, it is a poor choice for cardiovascular activity. The home health or cardiac rehabilitation nurse should assess the activity level of the woman with CAD and encourage her to participate in an appropriate exercise program.

➤ *Health Care Resources*

The American Heart Association (AHA) is an excellent source for booklets, films, video cassettes, cookbooks, and professional service referrals for the client with coronary artery disease (CAD). Many local affiliates have their own cardiac rehabilitation programs for clients to join.

Within the community, cardiac rehabilitation programs may be affiliated with local hospitals, community centers, or other facilities, such as clinics. Many shopping malls open before shopping hours to allow a measured walking

program indoors; this is particularly popular with elderly clients and also provides a good support group.

Mended Hearts is a nationwide program with local chapters that provides education and support to CABG clients and their families. Smoking cessation programs and clinics as well as weight reduction programs are found within the community. Many hospitals sponsor health fairs, blood pressure screening, and risk factor modification programs as well.

⬇ Evaluation

The nurse evaluates the client on the basis of the identified nursing diagnoses and collaborative problems. The expected outcomes are that the client will

- State that the chest discomfort is alleviated, appear comfortable, and have resolution of ST- and T-wave changes.
- Remain hemodynamically stable: maintain a normal sinus rhythm or normal rhythm for the client at a rate of approximately 60; maintain blood pressure within an acceptable range, adequate urine output, mental alertness, palpable pedal pulses, and clear lungs on auscultation.
- Walk 200 feet four times a day without chest discomfort or shortness of breath
- Indicate decreased anxiety
- Indicate a sense of having some control over life
- Experience minimal angina while engaging in ADLs or an exercise program.

🔵 CASE STUDY for the Client After CABG

■ **You are making the first home visit to a 76-year-old man who has been home for 2 days after a 12-day hospitalization for left main coronary artery bypass surgery. His hospital stay was complicated by angina, anxiety, and constipation. He was discharged home taking furosemide (Lasix), 40 mg every day; acetylsalicylic acid (aspirin), 1 tablet every day; metoprolol (Lopressor), 100 mg every day; Metamucil, 1 packet every morning; and allopurinol, 100 mg three times a day. He lives alone in a four-room house; his brother and sister-in-law live next door.**

Q U E S T I O N S :

1. What initial information is most important for you to obtain?
2. The client will only answer you in monosyllables. He says he is having trouble sleeping because of shortness of breath and nightmares. What should you do?
3. The client also says his left leg is sore where they removed the saphenous vein. He has been sitting in the chair with his leg dependent all day. What should you do?
4. The client's brother and sister-in-law are extremely worried. They say the client is eating and drinking very little and is leaking liquid stool. The client says he is constipated. What do you think is happening?

SELECTED BIBLIOGRAPHY

American Heart Association. (1996). *1992 Heart and Stroke Facts: 1996 statistical supplement.* Dallas, TX: Author.

Arnstein, P. M., Buselli, E. F., & Rankin, S. H. (1996). Women and heart attacks: Prevention, diagnosis and care. *Nurse Practitioner, 21*(5), 57–69.

Barnason, S., Zimmerman, L., & Nieveen, J. (1995). The effects of music interventions on anxiety in the patient after coronary artery bypass grafting. *Heart & Lung, 24*(2), 124–132.

Beach, E., Smith, A., Luthringer, L., Utz, A., Ahrens, S., & Whitmire, V. (1996). Self-care limitations of persons after acute myocardial infarction. *Applied Nursing Research, 9*(1), 24–28.

Bernat, J. (1997). Smoothing the CABG patient's road to recovery. *American Journal of Nursing, 97*(2), 23–27.

*Braunwald, E. (Ed.). (1992). *Heart disease: A textbook of cardiovascular medicine* (4th ed.). Philadelphia: W. B. Saunders.

Braunwald, E., Mark, D. B., Jones, R. H., et al. (1994). *Diagnosing and managing unstable angina. Quick reference guide for clinicians, #10* (AHCPR Publication No. 94-0603). Rockville, MD: U.S. Department of Health and Human Services.

Bruce, S. L., & Grove, S. K. (1994). The effect of a coronary artery risk evaluation program on serum lipid values and cardiovascular risk levels. *Applied Nursing Research, 7*(2), 67–74.

Carroll, D. (1995). The importance of self-efficacy expectations in elderly patients recovering from coronary artery bypass surgery. *Heart & Lung, 24*(1), 50–59.

Clem, J. R. (1995). Pharmacology of ischemic disease. *AACN Clinical Issues, 6*(3) 404–417.

Collins, J., & Rice, V. (1997). Effects of relaxation intervention in phase II cardiac rehabilitation: Replication and extension. *Heart & Lung, 26*(1), 31–44.

Connors, K. F., & Lamas, G. A. (1995). Postmyocardial infarction patients: Experience from the SAVE trial. *American Journal of Critical Care, 4*(1), 23–28.

Fleury, J., Keller, C., & Murdaugh, C. (1996). Patients with coronary artery disease. In J. Clochesy, C. Breu, S. Cardin, A. Whittaker, & E. Rudy (Eds.), *Critical care nursing* (2nd ed., pp. 336–353). Philadelphia: W. B. Saunders.

Forsha, B. (1997). Scaffolding the coronary arteries: Intracoronary stenting. *Home Healthcare Nurse, 15*(4), 247–255.

Futterman, L. G., Corea, L. F., & Lemberg, L. (1996). Thrombolysis or primary angioplasty? An ongoing controversy in the management of acute myocardial infarction. *American Journal of Critical Care, 5*(2), 160–167.

Futterman, L. G., & Lemberg, L. (1996). Cardiomyoplasty: A potential alternative to cardiac transplantation. *American Journal of Critical Care, 5*(1), 80–86.

Gaw-Ens, B. (1994). Informational support for families immediately after CABG surgery. *Critical Care Nurse, 14*(1), 41–49.

*Gortner, S. R., Dirks, J., & Wolfe, M. M. (1992). The road to recovery for elders after CABG. *American Journal of Nursing, 92*(8), 44–49.

Gulanich, M., Billey, A., Perino, B., & Keough, V. (1997). Patients' responses to the angioplasty experience: A qualitative study. *American Journal of Critical Care, 6*(1), 25–32.

Hahn, M. (1995). Matters of the heart: Women and cardiac disease. *Advance for Nurse Practitioners, 3*(9), 13–19.

Hawthorne, M. H. (1994). Gender differences in recovery after coronary artery surgery. *IMAGE: Journal of Nursing Scholarship, 26*(1), 75–80.

Huerta-Torres, V. (1998). Preparing patients for early discharge after CABG. *American Journal of Nursing, 98*(5), 49–51.

Hussey, L., & Leeper, B. (1998). Sternal wound infection: A case study of a devastating postoperative complication. *Critical Care Nurse, 18*(1), 31–39.

Jarvis, C. (1996). *Physical examination and health assessment* (2nd ed.). Philadelphia: W. B. Saunders.

Jensen, G. A., & Miller, D. S.(1995). The heart of aging: Special challenges of cardiac ischemia and failure in the elderly. *AACN Clinical Issues, 6*(3), 471–481.

Jensen, L., & King, K. (1997). Women and heart disease. *Critical Care Nurse, 17*(2), 45–52.

Kegel, L. M. (1996). Case management, critical pathways, and myocardial infarction. *Critical Care Nurse, 16*(2), 97–111.

Lee, H. O. (1997). Typical and atypical clinical signs and symptoms of myocardial infarction and delayed seeking of professional care among Blacks. *American Journal of Critical Care, 6*(1), 7–13.

Lee, S. (1996). Hospital-home care critical pathways in disease management: Improving case management and patient outcomes in postoperative cardiothoracic surgical patients. *The Journal of Care Management, 2*(3), 42–53.

*Matrisciano, L. (1992). Unstable angina: An overview. *Critical Care Nurse, 12*(8), 30–38.

Meluch, F., & Mitchell, S. (1997). Decreasing intracoronary stent complications. *Dimensions of Critical Care Nursing, 16*(3), 114–121.

Moore, S. M. (1995). A comparison of women's and men's symptoms during home recovery after coronary artery bypass surgery. *Heart & Lung, 24*(6), 495–501.

Moser, D. (1997). Correcting misconceptions about women and heart disease. *American Journal of Nursing, 97*(4), 26–33.

Norris, S. O. (1995). Sternal wound infection. In N. Urban (Ed.), *Guidelines for critical care nursing* (pp. 240–249). St. Louis, MO: C. V. Mosby.

O'Neal, P. V. (1994). How to spot early signs of cardiogenic shock. *American Journal of Nursing, 94*(5), 36–41.

*Pasternak, R., Braunwald, E., & Sobel B. (1992). Acute myocardial infarction. In E. Braunwald (Ed.), *Heart disease: A textbook of cardiovascular medicine* (4th ed., pp. 1200–1291). Philadelphia: W. B. Saunders.

Ray, G. L. (1994) Decisions, decisions: Which thrombolytic is best for your patient? *American Journal of Nursing, 94*(Suppl.), 11–15.

Redeker, N., Mason, D., Wykpisz, E., & Glica, B. (1996). Sleep patterns in women after coronary artery bypass surgery. *Applied Nursing Research, 9*(3), 115–122.

Redeker, N. S., & Sadowski, A. (1995). Update on cardiovascular drugs and elders. *American Journal of Nursing, 95*(9), 34–41.

Riegel, B. (1996). Myocardial infarction. In J. Clochesy, C. Breu, S. Cardin, A. Whittaker, & E. Rudy (Eds.), *Critical care nursing* (2nd ed., pp. 354–379). Philadelphia: W. B. Saunders.

Romeo, K. C. (1995). The female heart: Physiologic aspects of cardiovascular disease in women. *Dimensions of Critical Care, 14*(4), 170–175.

Shuster, P., Wright, C., & Tomish, P. (1995). Gender differences in outcomes of participants in home care programs compared to those in structured cardiac rehabilitation programs. *Rehabilitiation Nursing, 20*(2), 96–100.

Strimike, C. L. (1995). Caring for a patient with an intracoronary stent. *American Journal of Nursing, 95*(1), 40–46.

Swearingen, P. L., & Keen, J. H. (1995). *Manual of critical care: Applying nursing diagnoses to adult critical illness* (2nd ed.). St. Louis, MO: Mosby Year Book.

Tsunoda, D. (1996). Clinical snapshot: Acute myocardial infarction. *American Journal of Nursing, 96*(5), 38–39.

Turner, L., Linden, W., van der Wal, R., & Schamberger, W. (1995). Stress management for patients with heart disease: A pilot study. *Heart and Lung, 24*(2), 145–153.

*U.S. Department of Health and Human Services. (1990). *Healthy people 2000: National health promotion and disease prevention objectives.* Washington, DC: U.S. Government Printing Office.

Valle, B. K., & Lember, L. (1994). Estrogen replacement therapy in women: Prevention and treatment of coronary artery disease. *American Journal of Critical Care, 3*(5), 398–401.

Villaire, M. (1996). Early heart attack care—The critical paradigm shift toward prevention. *Critical Care Nurse, 16*(1), 79–85.

Wenger, N. K., Froelicher, E. S., & Smith, L. K., et al. (1995). *Cardiac rehabilitation as secondary prevention: clinical practice guideline* (quick reference guide for clinicians no. 17, AHCPR publication no. 96-0673). Rockville, MD: U.S. Department of Health and Human Services, Public Health Service, Agency for Health Care Policy and Research and National Heart, Lung, and Blood Institute.

Wright, J. (1995). Pharmacologic management of congestive heart failure. *Critical Care Nursing Quarterly, 18*(1), 32–44.

Workman, M. L. (1994). Anticoagulants and thrombolytics: What's the difference? *AACN Clinical Issues in Critical Care Nursing, 5*(1), 26–34.

SUGGESTED READINGS

Bernat, J. (1997). Smoothing the CABG patient's road to recovery. *American Journal of Nursing, 97*(2), 23–27.
Recent advances in the care of clients undergoing coronary artery bypass graft surgery are identified. The changing client profile

and surgical procedure are described. Risks to vulnerable body systems are detailed specifically.

Hussey, L., & Leeper, B. (1998). Sternal wound infection: A case study of a devastating postoperative complication. *Critical Care Nurse,* *18*(1), 31–39.

This excellent article describes the phenomenon of sternal wound infection comprehensively and concisely. The nursing care needs are outlined, and a teaching guide for clients with sternal incisions is included.

Jensen, L., & King, K. (1997). Women and heart disease. *Critical Care Nurse,* *17*(2), 45–52.

The influence of gender on cardiovascular anatomy and physiology is discussed. Differences between men's and women's risk factors, diagnoses, and treatment for coronary artery disease are explained. Strategies for prevention, diagnosis, and treatment of CAD in women are detailed.

Meluch, F., & Mitchell, S. (1997). Decreasing intracoronary stent complications. *Dimensions of Critical Care Nursing, 16*(3), 114–121.

The primary focus of this comprehensive article is the nursing management of clients after intracoronary stent implantation. Detailed medication guides are included. Focused assessment techniques are highlighted for the prevention of complications.

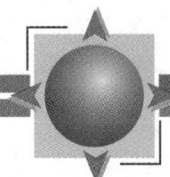

Management of Clients

with Problems of the

Hematologic System

ASSESSMENT OF THE HEMATOLOGIC SYSTEM

The hematologic system is made up of lymphatic fluid, blood, cellular elements in blood, and blood-forming organs. Blood and lymph circulate through all body tissues and organs, and the functions of the hematologic system influence the health and well-being of all body systems. This chapter and Chapter 23 (Concepts of Inflammation and the Immune Response) review the normal physiology of the hematologic system and the skills necessary to accurately assess the client's hematologic status.

ANATOMY AND PHYSIOLOGY REVIEW
Bone Marrow

Bone marrow is the blood-forming (hematopoietic) organ. It produces most of the cellular elements of the blood, including red blood cells (RBCs), white blood cells (WBCs), and platelets. Bone marrow also is involved in some aspects of the immune response (see Chapter 23).

Each day, the bone marrow in a healthy adult produces and releases about 2.5 billion RBCs, 2.5 billion platelets, and 1 billion granulocytes per kilogram of body weight (Williams et al., 1995).

In the fetus, blood components are formed in the liver and spleen and, by the last trimester, the bone marrow. At birth, blood-producing marrow is present in every bone. The flat bones (sternum, skull, pelvic and shoulder girdles) contain active blood-producing marrow throughout life. In small, irregularly shaped bones and in the long bones, the amount of functional bone marrow decreases as a person ages, until by age 18, blood production is limited to the ends of the long bones. During adulthood, fatty tissue replaces inactive bone marrow. In elderly people, the proportion of fatty marrow increases to about one half of the marrow found in the sternum and ribs, and only a relatively small portion of the remaining marrow continues active blood production.

The bone marrow produces all blood cells, initially producing stem cells. Bone marrow contains *pluripotent stem cells*, immature and undifferentiated cells capable of maturing into any one of several lines of blood cells—an RBC, WBC, or platelet line, depending on the body's needs (see Fig. 23–3).

The next stage in cell development is the committed stem cell (also called the precursor cell or the unipotent stem cell). A committed stem cell has one specific maturational pathway and matures or differentiates into only one cell type. Committed stem cells are in the active phase of growth but require the presence of a sp

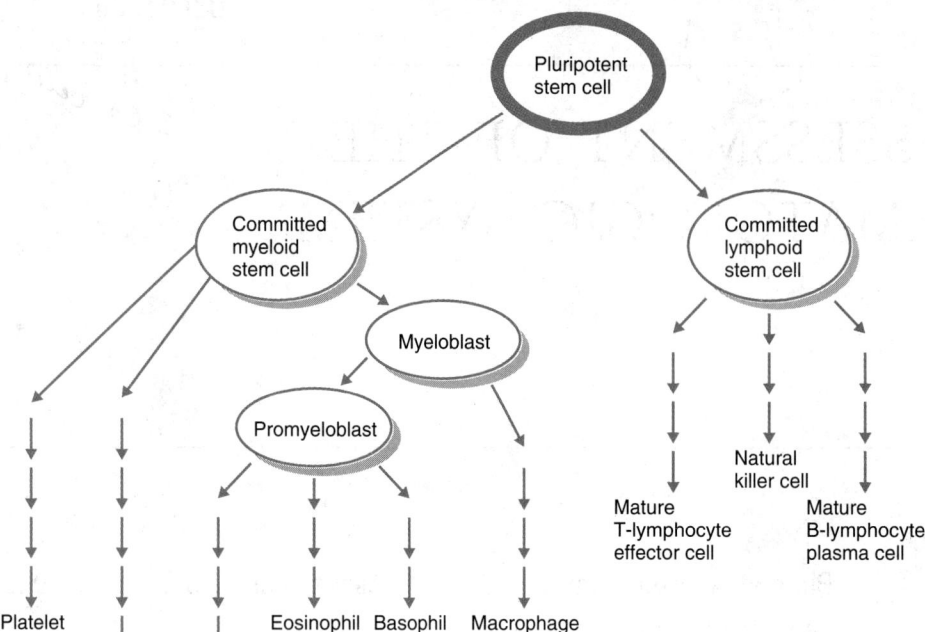

Figure 41–1. Bone marrow cell differentiation and maturational pathways.

growth factor for further development and maturation. For example, erythropoietin is a growth factor made in the kidneys that is specific for the red blood cell line. A variety of other growth factors influence white blood cell and platelet maturation (see Chaps. 23, 27, and 42).

Blood Components

Blood is composed of plasma and cellular elements. Plasma, part of the extracellular fluid of the body, is similar to the interstitial fluid found between tissue cells; however, plasma contains about three to four times more protein than does interstitial fluid. There are three major types of plasma proteins: albumin, globulins, and fibrinogen.

The primary function of albumin is to increase osmotic pressure of the blood, preventing the plasma from leaking into the tissues (see Chap. 14). Globulins perform many functions, such as transporting other substances and protecting the body against infection. Globulins are also the main component of antibodies. Fibrinogen is a protein molecule that can be activated to form a molecule of fibrin. Individual molecules of fibrin assemble to form large structures important in the blood clotting process.

The cellular components of the blood include RBCs, WBCs, and platelets. These blood components differ in structure, site of maturation, and function.

Red Blood Cells (Erythrocytes)

blood cells, or erythrocytes, make up the largest ortion of blood cells. Mature RBCs have no nucleus ve a biconcave disk shape. This feature, together flexible membrane, allows RBCs to change their thout breaking as they pass through narrow,

winding capillaries. The number of RBCs a person has varies according to gender, age, and general health, but the normal range is from 4,400,000 to 5,500,000/mm³.

As shown in Figures 41–1 and 41–2, RBCs start out as pluripotent stem cells, enter the myeloid pathway, and progress in stages to the mature RBC, the erythrocyte. Healthy mature RBCs have a life span of approximately 120 days after being released into circulation from the bone marrow. As RBCs age, their membranes become more fragile. These old cells are trapped and destroyed by fixed macrophages in the tissues, the spleen, and the liver. Some intracellular parts of destroyed RBCs, such as iron, are recycled and used in the formation of new RBCs.

Red blood cells are responsible for the formation of hemoglobin (Hgb). Each normal mature RBC contains many thousands of hemoglobin molecules (Guyton & Hall, 1996). The heme portion of each hemoglobin molecule requires a molecule of iron. Only when the heme molecule is complete with iron can it transport up to four molecules of oxygen. Therefore, iron is a critical component of hemoglobin. The globin portion of the hemoglobin molecule carries carbon dioxide. RBCs also serve as a buffer and help maintain acid-base balance.

The most important feature of the hemoglobin molecule is its ability to combine loosely with oxygen. With only a small drop in oxygen tension at the tissue level, a considerable increase in the transfer of oxygen from hemoglobin to tissues occurs. This transfer is also known as *oxygen dissociation*. Some pathologic conditions can alter the speed and quantity of oxygen release to the tissues.

The total number of RBCs a person has is carefully regulated through *erythropoiesis* (selective maturation of stem cells into mature erythrocytes). Regulation ensures

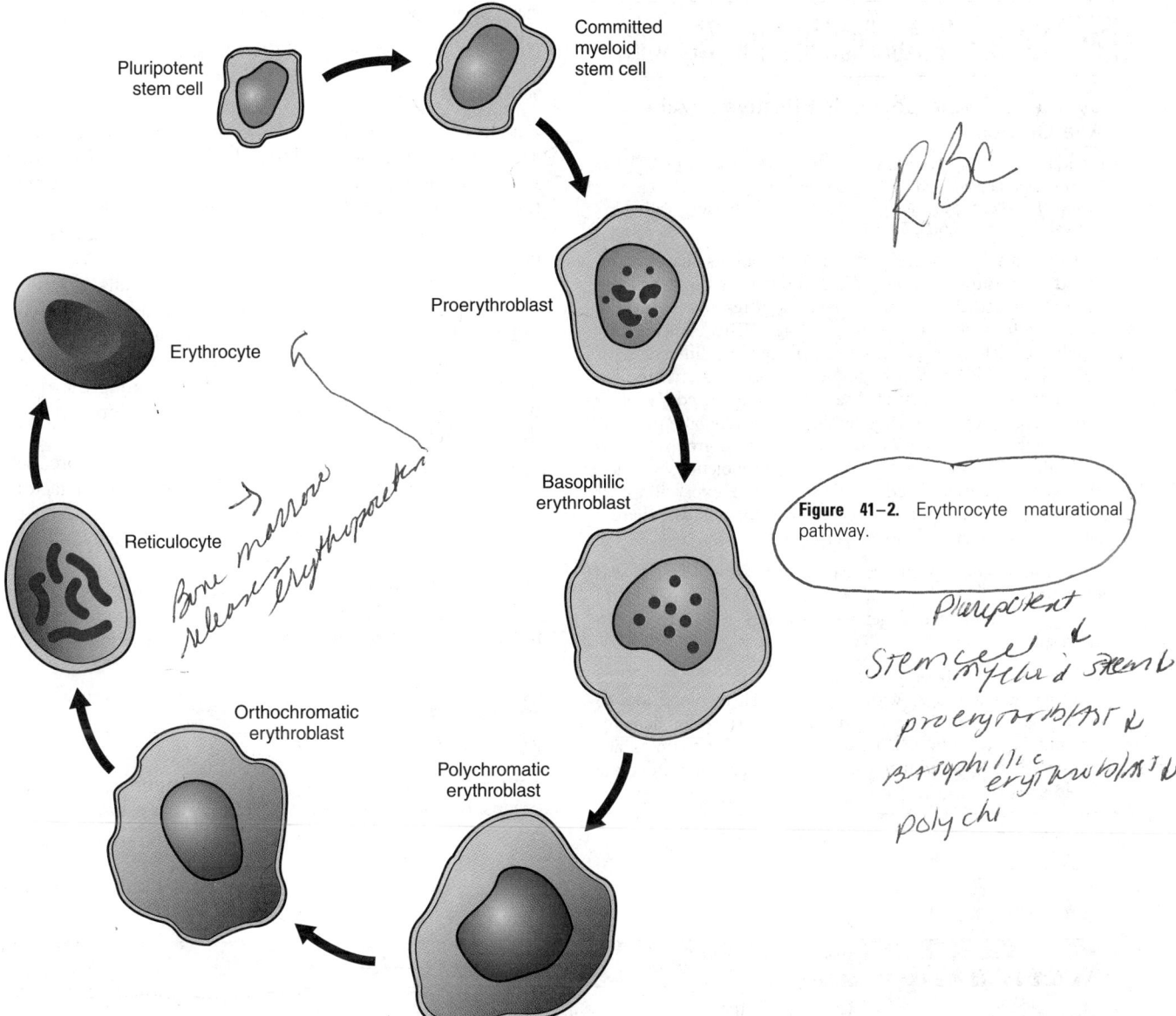

Figure 41-2. Erythrocyte maturational pathway.

that enough RBCs are present for good oxygenation without having an overconcentration, which causes hypercellularity. The trigger for control of erythropoiesis is tissue oxygenation. The kidney produces the RBC growth factor (erythropoietin) at a rate consistent with RBC destruction to maintain a constant normal level of circulating RBCs. When tissue oxygenation is less than normal (*hypoxia*), the kidney increases the production and release of erythropoietin. This growth factor then stimulates the bone marrow to increase RBC production. When tissue oxygenation is excessive, the kidney decreases erythropoietin production, inhibiting RBC production. Synthetic erythropoietin is now available and appears to have the same effect on bone marrow as the naturally occurring erythropoietin in all age groups (see the Research Applications for Nursing box).

Many substances are essential to form hemoglobin and RBCs, including iron, vitamin B_{12}, folic acid, copper, pyridoxine, cobalt, and nickel. A lack of any of these substances can lead to anemia. Anemia is a feature of any of a variety of conditions in which either the function or the number of erythrocytes is insufficient to meet tissue oxygen demands (see Chap. 42).

White Blood Cells (Leukocytes)

White blood cells, or leukocytes, are the second category of blood cells. There are multiple types of leukocytes, each type performing at least one specific function critical to inflammation or immunity (Table 41–1). Most WBCs are formed in the bone marrow and therefore are considered part of the hematopoietic system. However, because leukocytes provide immunity and protect people from the effects of invasion, infection, and injury, a detailed di

▷ Research Applications for Nursing

Synthetic Erythropoietin Is Effective in All Age Groups

Goodnough, L., Price, T., & Parvin, C. (1995). The endogenous erythropoietin response and the erythropoietic response to blood loss anemia: The effects of age and gender. Journal of Laboratory and Clinical Medicine, 126(1), 57–64.

Clinicians have speculated that older adults may not respond to erythropoietin as younger individuals do. It has also been postulated that gender differences in responses to exogenous erythropoietin may exist at all ages. This clinical study sought to determine whether actual gender differences or age-related differences in response to exogenous erythropoietin stimulation are present. The study randomized 71 older and younger adults undergoing aggressive phlebotomy therapy to either a placebo group or one of three groups receiving different doses of recombinant erythropoietin six times. Responses in terms of red blood cell volume expansion over time were not different for men or women, nor was there a difference in older versus younger people.

Critique. The descriptive, comparative study design was appropriate for the research questions. Use of a control group to determine endogenous responses adds strength to the results.

Possible Nursing Applications. Nurses can expect clients of all genders and ages with anemia related to blood loss to respond at a known rate of percentage increase for hematocrit and hemoglobin when exogenous erythropoietin is administered. Dosage adjustments solely for age or gender are unnecessary.

sion of leukocyte anatomy and function is presented in Chapter 23.

Platelets

Platelets are the third cellular component of blood. They are the smallest of the formed elements of the blood, fragments of a giant precursor cell in the bone marrow, the megakaryocyte. Figure 41–1 shows the overall blood cell developmental pathway, and Figure 41–3 shows specific platelet development.

Platelets stick to injured blood vessel walls and form platelet plugs that can stop the flow of blood from the injured site. Platelets also produce substances called *phospholipids,* important to coagulation. Platelets are thought to maintain blood vessel integrity by beginning the repair of damage to small blood vessels. They perform most of their functions by aggregation (clumping).

Platelet production in the bone marrow also is precisely regulated by general and platelet-specific growth factors. After platelets leave the bone marrow, they are taken up by the spleen for storage and are released slowly, according to the body's needs. Normally, 80% of platelets circulate and 20% are stored in the spleen. Each platelet has a life span of 1 to 2 weeks, after which it is gradually used up or destroyed during normal clotting activities.

Accessory Organs of Hematopoiesis

Both the spleen and the liver are important accessory organs of the hematopoietic system. They have roles in

TABLE 41–1

Functions of Specific Leukocytes		
	Leukocyte	**Function**
Inflammation	Neutrophil	• Nonspecific ingestion and phagocytosis of microorganisms and foreign protein
	Macrophage	• Nonspecific recognition of foreign proteins and microorganisms; ingestion and phagocytosis
	Monocyte	• Destruction of bacteria and cellular debris; matures into macrophage
	Eosinophil	• Weak phagocytic action; releases vasoactive amines during allergic reactions
	Basophil	• Releases histamine and heparin in areas of tissue damage
Antibody-mediated immunity	B lymphocyte	• Becomes sensitized to foreign cells and proteins
	Plasma cell	• Secretes immunoglobulins in response to the presence of a specific antigen
	Memory cell	• Remains sensitized to a specific antigen and can secrete increased amounts of immunoglobulins specific to the antigen
Cell-mediated immunity	T lymphocyte helper/inducer T cell	• Enhances immune activity through secretion of various factors, cytokines, and lymphokines
	Cytotoxic-cytolytic T cell	• Selectively attacks and destroys non-self cells, including virally infected cells, grafts, and transplanted organs
	Natural killer cell	• Nonselectively attacks non-self cells, especially body cells that have undergone mutation and become malignant; also attacks grafts and transplanted organs

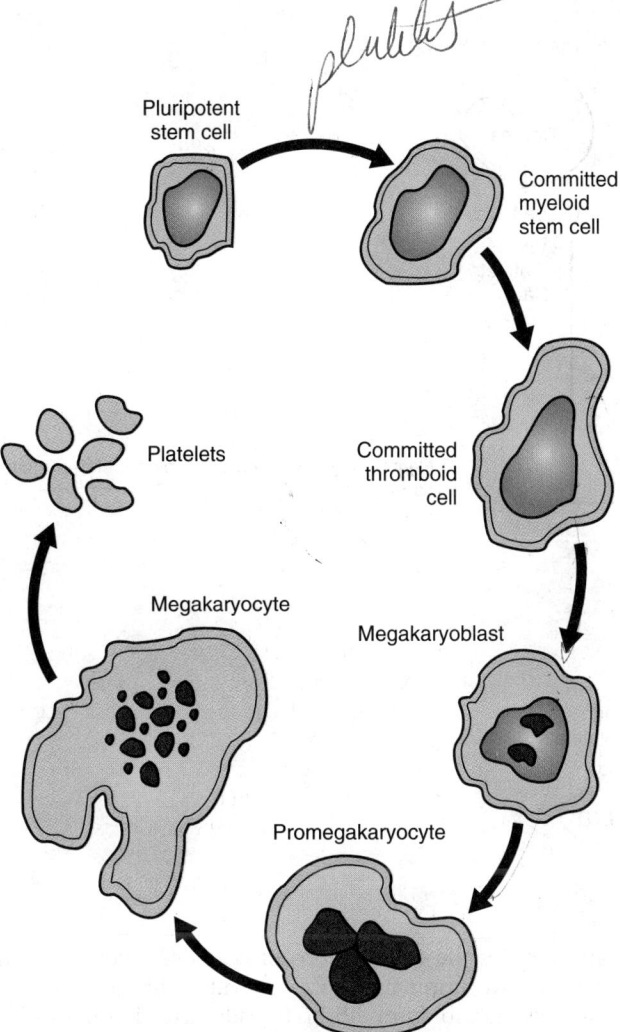

Figure 41-3. Platelet maturational pathway.

the regulation and maturation of blood cells to help maintain hematologic homeostasis.

Spleen

The spleen is located under the diaphragm to the left of the stomach. It contains three types of tissue: white pulp, red pulp, and marginal pulp, which all help balance blood cell production and destruction and assist with immunologic defensive mechanisms. White pulp is filled with lymphocytes and macrophages, filtering the circulating blood and removing unwanted cells (such as bacteria and old RBCs). Red pulp is composed of vascular sinuses that are storage sites for erythrocytes and platelets. Marginal pulp contains the termination sites of many arteries and other blood vessels.

During blood formation, the spleen destroys aged or imperfect RBCs through phagocytosis and mechanical deformation, assists in iron metabolism by breaking down the hemoglobin released from these destroyed cells, stores platelets, and filters antigens. A client who has undergone splenectomy has impairment of some immune functions. As a result, a splenectomized client's body is not efficient at ridding the body of many bloodborne

pathogenic microorganisms and is at a greatly increased risk for infection and sepsis (Workman et al., 1993).

Liver

The liver, important for normal erythropoiesis, is the primary production site for most of the blood clotting factors and prothrombin. In addition, proper liver function, including bile production, is critical to the formation of vitamin K in the intestinal tract. (Vitamin K is essential in the formation of blood clotting factors VII, IX, and X and prothrombin.) Large quantities of whole blood and blood cells can be stored in the liver. The liver also converts bilirubin (one end-product of hemoglobin breakdown) to bile and stores extra iron within a storage protein called ferritin. Small amounts of erythropoietin are synthesized in the liver.

HEMOSTASIS

In hemostasis, selective localized blood clotting occurs in damaged blood vessels while blood circulation to all other areas is maintained. It is a complex process that balances the production of clotting and dissolving factors. Hemostasis begins with the formation of a platelet plug and continues with a series of events that eventually cause the formation of a fibrin clot. Intrinsic and extrinsic factors are involved in fibrin clot formation and blood coagulation.

Platelet Aggregation

Platelets normally circulate as individual cell-like structures. They are not attracted to each other until activated or until the presence of other substances causes platelet membranes to become sticky, allowing aggregation to occur. When platelets become activated and aggregate, they form large, semisolid plugs within the lumens and walls of blood vessels and disrupt blood flow. Some of the substances capable of causing platelets to aggregate include adenosine diphosphate (ADP), calcium, thromboxane A_2, and collagen. Platelets themselves can be stimulated to secrete some of these substances, whereas other substances causing platelet aggregation are exogenous. Formation of a platelet plug can start the cascade reaction that ultimately causes blood coagulation to occur through the formation of a fibrin clot.

The Blood Clotting Cascade

The beginning of the blood clotting cascade is rapidly amplified or enhanced. That is, the final result is much larger than the triggering event. Cascades work like a landslide: A few small pebbles rolling down a steep hillside can dislodge large rocks and pieces of soil, causing a final enormous movement of earth. Just like landslides, cascade reactions are hard to stop once set into motion. Platelet plug formation starting the clotting cascade can result from intrinsic or extrinsic factors.

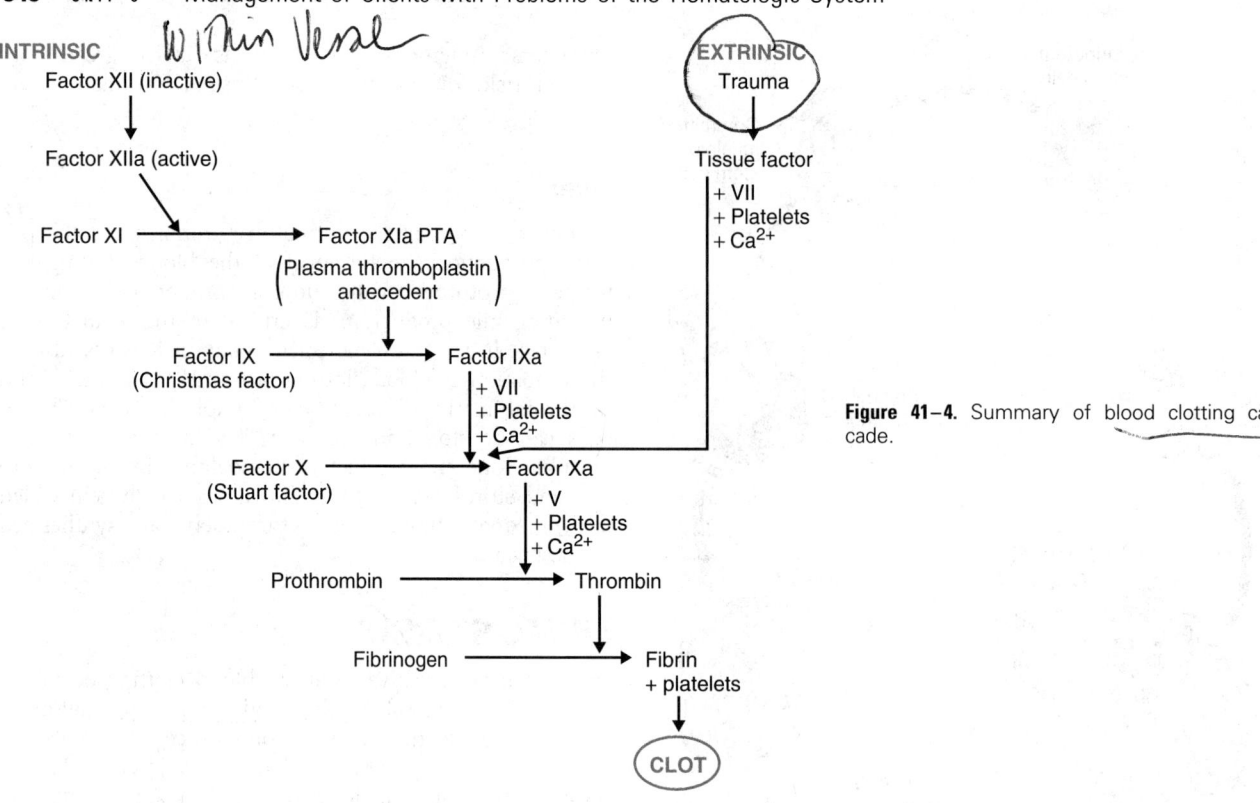

Figure 41–4. Summary of blood clotting cascade.

Intrinsic Factors

Platelet plugs begin to form when changes occur inside blood vessels. Trauma to the blood cells or exposure of the blood to collagen in the linings of blood vessels can cause platelet aggregation, the formation of a platelet plug, and the beginning of the clotting cascade (Fig. 41–4; see also Fig. 42–4). Other intrinsic events stimulating platelet aggregation include antigen-antibody reactions, circulating debris, prolonged venous stasis, and bacterial endotoxins. Having the cascade continue to the point of fibrin clot formation depends on the presence of sufficient amounts of all the various clotting factors and cofactors, presented in Table 41–2.

Extrinsic Factors

Platelet plugs can begin to form due to changes external to the blood vessels. The most common extrinsic events starting the clotting cascade are trauma to tissues and damage to blood vessels. The platelet plug is formed within seconds of the trauma, causing the blood clotting cascade to be started sooner than by the intrinsic pathway, because some of the steps of the intrinsic pathway are bypassed.

Whether initiated by intrinsic or extrinsic factors, the result is the same—the formation of a fibrin clot and coagulation.

Fibrin Clot Formation

Fibrinogen is a large, inactive protein molecule made in the liver and secreted into the blood. An enzyme, throm-bin, removes the end portions of fibrinogen, converting it to the active fibrin molecule. Individual fibrin molecules link together to form fibrin threads. The fibrin threads make a lattice-like meshwork that forms the base of a blood clot (Fig. 41–5).

After the fibrin mesh is formed, a stabilizing factor (clotting factor XIII) tightens up the mesh, making it more dense. Platelets stick to the threads of the mesh and attract other blood cells and proteins to form an actual blood clot. As this clot retracts, the serum (plasma without the clotting factors) is extruded, and clot formation is complete.

Fibrinolysis

Because blood coagulation occurs through a rapid cascade process, whenever the cascade is set into motion, in theory it keeps forming fibrin clots until all blood throughout the entire body has coagulated. Such widespread coagulation is not compatible with life. Therefore, whenever the blood clotting cascade is started, counterclotting or anticoagulant forces are also started to limit clot formation just to damaged areas, and normal blood flow is maintained everywhere else. When blood clotting and anticlotting actions are appropriately balanced, coagulation occurs only where it is needed and normal circulation is maintained.

The fibrinolytic system dissolves the fibrin clot with special enzymes (Fig. 41–6). The central event of fibrinolysis is the conversion of plasminogen to plasmin. Plasmin, an active enzyme, then digests fibrin, fibrinogen, prothrombin, and factors V, VIII, and XII, thus breaking down the fibrin clot (Colman et al., 1994).

TABLE 41–2

The Coagulation Factors

Factor	Action
I: Fibrinogen	• Factor I is converted to fibrin by the enzyme thrombin. Individual fibrin molecules form fibrin threads, which are the scaffold for clot formation and wound healing.
II: Prothrombin	• Factor II is the inactive precursor of thrombin. Prothrombin is activated to thrombin by coagulation factor X (Stuart-Prower factor). After it is activated, thrombin converts fibrinogen (coagulation factor I) into fibrin and activates factors V and VIII. • Synthesis is vitamin K–dependent.
III: Tissue thromboplastin	• Factor III interacts with factor VII to initiate the extrinsic clotting cascade.
IV: Calcium	• Calcium (Ca^{2+}), a divalent cation, is a cofactor for most of the enzyme-activated processes required in blood coagulation. • Calcium also enhances platelet aggregation and makes red blood cells clump together.
V: Proaccelerin	• Factor V is a cofactor for activated factor X, which is essential for converting prothrombin to thrombin.
VI: Discovered to be an artifact	• No factor VI is involved in blood coagulation.
VII: Proconvertin	• Factor VII activates factors IX and X, which are essential in converting prothrombin to thrombin. • Synthesis is vitamin K–dependent.
VIII: Antihemophilic factor	• Factor VIII together with activated factor IX enzymatically activates factor X. In addition, factor VIII combines with another protein (von Willebrand's factor) to help platelets adhere to capillary walls in areas of tissue injury. • A lack of factor VIII is the basis for classic hemophilia (hemophilia A).
IX: Plasma thromboplastin component (Christmas factor)	• Factor IX, when activated, activates factor X to convert prothrombin to thrombin. • This factor is essential in the common pathway between the intrinsic and extrinsic clotting cascades. • A lack of factor IX is the basis for hemophilia B. • Synthesis is vitamin K–dependent.
X: Stuart-Prower factor	• Factor X, when activated, converts prothrombin into thrombin. • Synthesis is vitamin K–dependent.
XI: Plasma thromboplastin antecedent	• Factor XI, when activated, assists in the activation of factor IX. However, a similar factor must exist in tissues. People who are deficient in factor XI have mild bleeding problems after surgery but do not bleed excessively as a result of trauma.
XII: Hageman factor	• Factor XII is critically important in the intrinsic pathway for the activation of factor XI.
XIII: Fibrin-stabilizing factor	• Factor XIII assists in forming crosslinks among the fibrin threads to form a strong fibrin clot.

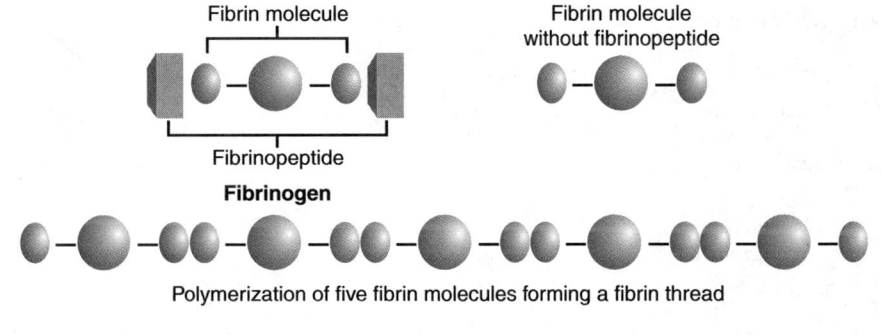

Polymerization of five fibrin molecules forming a fibrin thread

Figure 41–5. Activation and polymerization of fibrin to form fibrin clot.

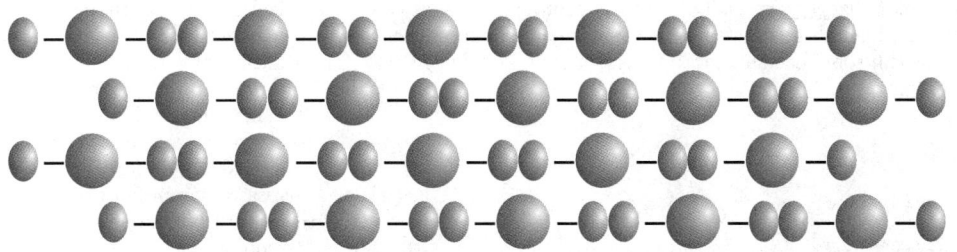

Meshwork of fibrin threads forming scaffold of fibrin clot

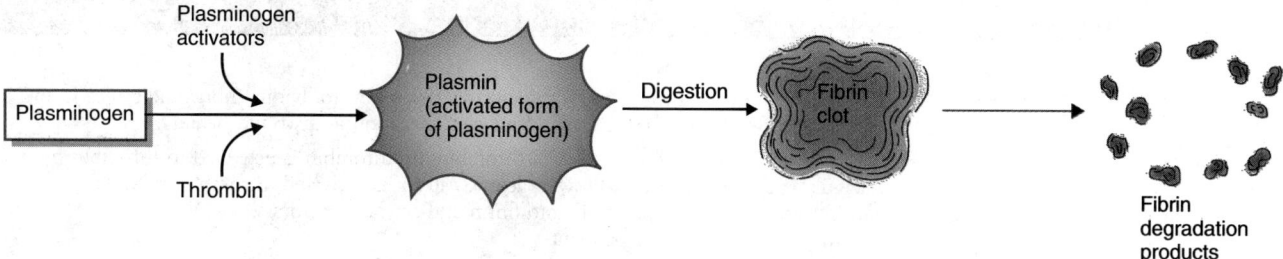

Figure 41–6. The process of fibrinolysis.

Hematologic Changes Associated with Aging

Aging changes the cellular and plasma components of blood, making accurate assessment of the hematologic system in elderly people more difficult. Chart 41–1 lists assessment tips for this population. Several factors cause a decreased blood volume in elderly people. Total body water is decreased among elderly clients. In addition, elderly people tend to have a lower concentration of plasma proteins and decreased plasma osmotic pressure (possibly related to a decreased dietary intake of proteins), which also causes some loss of blood volume into the interstitial space.

As bone marrow ages, it produces fewer blood cells. Total RBC and WBC counts (especially lymphocyte counts) are lower among elderly people, although platelet counts do not appear to change with age. Lymphocytes become less reactive to antigens and have a loss of immune function. Antibody levels and responses are lower in older adults. The leukocyte count does not rise as high in response to infection in elderly people as in young people (Workman et al., 1993).

Hemoglobin levels also change with age. Hemoglobin levels in men and women fall after middle age. Iron-deficient diets may play a role in this phenomenon.

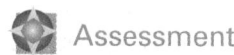 ## Assessment

➤ History

Demographic Data

Age and gender are important variables to obtain in assessments of the client's hematologic status. Bone marrow and immune activity diminish with age.

Chart 41–1

Focus on the Elderly: Hematologic Assessment

Assessment Area	Findings in Hematologic Disorders	Normal Changes in the Elderly	Significance/Alternatives
Nail beds (for capillary refill)	• Pallor or cyanosis may indicate a hematologic disorder	• Thickened or discolored nails make visualization of skin color beneath the nails impossible	• Use another body area, such as the lip, to assess central capillary refill
Hair distribution	• Thin or absent hair on the trunk or extremities may indicate poor circulation to a particular area	• Progressive loss of body hair is a normal facet of aging	• A relatively even pattern of hair loss that has occurred over an extended period is not significant
Skin moisture	• Skin dryness may indicate any of a number of hematologic disorders	• Skin dryness is a normal result of aging	• Skin moisture is not usually a reliable indicator of an underlying pathologic condition in the elderly
Skin color	• Skin color changes, especially pallor and jaundice, are associated with some hematologic disorders	• Pigment loss and skin yellowing are common changes associated with aging	• Pallor in an elderly person may not be a reliable indicator of anemia; laboratory testing is required. • Yellow-tinged skin in an elderly person may not be a reliable indicator of increased serum bilirubin levels; laboratory testing is required

WOMEN'S HEALTH CONSIDERATIONS

At all ages, women have lower blood cell counts than do men, but this difference is more profound during menstrual years. This gender difference may be related to a dilutional effect of female hormones, which cause an increased volume of vascular fluid, or to differences in bone marrow activity.

It is also important for the nurse to collect information on occupation, hobbies, and the location of housing. This information may indicate exposure to agents or chemicals that affect bone marrow growth and hematologic function.

Personal and Family History

Because many types of bleeding disorders are inherited, the nurse obtains an accurate family history. The nurse asks whether anyone in the family has had hemophilia, frequent nosebleeds, postpartum hemorrhages, excessive bleeding after dental extractions, or continuous heavy bruising in response to relatively mild trauma. Familial information about sickle cell disease or sickle cell trait also is obtained. Although sickle cell disease is seen primarily among African-Americans, anyone may have the trait.

Personal factors to be included in the hematologic assessment are liver function, the presence of known immunologic or hematologic disorders, and current medication use. Because liver function is important in the synthesis of clotting factors, the nurse also asks about jaundice, anemia, and gallstones.

The nurse questions the client about use of blood "thinners" such as sodium warfarin (Coumadin, Warfilone*) and aspirin. A person who takes aspirin on a daily basis may have bleeding problems, and many over-the-counter medications contain aspirin or other salicylates that disrupt platelet aggregation. The nurse determines all medications that the client is using or has used in the past 3 weeks. Clients are also asked about the use of antibiotics, because prolonged antibiotic therapy can lead to coagulopathies or bone marrow depression. Table 41–3 lists drugs known to alter hematologic function. Previous radiation therapy, especially if marrow-forming bones were in the radiation path, may result in some permanent impairment of hematologic function.

Diet History

Dietary pattern can alter cell quality and blood coagulation. The nurse asks clients to record everything eaten during the previous week. This information is helpful in determining the causes of anemias, as well as deficiencies of proteins, minerals, or vitamins. Diets high in fat and carbohydrates and low in protein, iron, and vitamins can cause many types of anemia as well as a decrease in the functions of all blood cells.

The nurse also asks the client about alcohol consumption. Chronic alcoholism is associated with nutritional deficiencies and liver impairment, both of which can adversely affect the hematologic system.

Some dietary habits can enhance blood clotting. Diets high in vitamin K may increase the rate of blood coagulation. The nurse assesses the amount of raw, leafy green vegetables that the client consumes and whether the client routinely takes supplemental vitamins. The nurse also assesses the amount of calcium consumed within the diet or in supplements.

Socioeconomic Status

The nurse assesses the client's ability to understand and follow instructions related to proper diet, specific procedures and tests, and therapeutic regimens. The nurse also determines the client's personal resources, such as finances and social support. A person with a marginal income may have a diet low in iron and protein. The nurse also notes the client's occupation and asks about potential exposure to chemicals.

Current Health Problem

The nurse determines whether the client has had swelling of lymph nodes or excessive bruising or bleeding and whether the bleeding was spontaneous or induced by trauma. The nurse also inquires about the amount and duration of bleeding after routine dental work. Women are asked about the presence of menorrhagia, or excessive menstrual flow. These clients are asked to estimate the number of pads or tampons used during the most recent menstrual cycle and whether this amount represents a change from the client's usual pattern of menstrual flow. The nurse asks whether clots are present in menstrual blood. The client is asked to estimate clot size using coins or fruit for comparison ("clots are dime-sized" or "clots are the size of lemons").

The nurse determines whether the client experiences dyspnea on exertion, palpitations, frequent infections, fevers, recent weight loss, headaches, or paresthesias. Any or all of these symptoms may accompany hematologic disease.

The single most common symptom of anemia is fatigue. The nurse questions the client about feeling tired, needing more rest, or losing endurance during normal activities. Clients are asked to compare the extent and intensity of their activities during the past month with those of the same month a year ago. The nurse asks about other symptoms associated with anemia, such as vertigo, tinnitus, anorexia, dysphagia, and a sore tongue.

▶ Physical Assessment

The nurse performs a comprehensive physical assessment because hematologic dysfunction affects the whole body. Certain problems are specific for hematologic assessment in elderly clients, as noted in Chart 41–1.

Assessment of the Integumentary System

The nurse inspects the color of the skin for pallor or jaundice and of the mucous membranes and nail beds for pallor or cyanosis. Pallor of the gums, conjunctivae, and palmar creases indicates decreased hemoglobin levels. The

TABLE 41–3

Drugs Impairing the Hematologic System	
Generic Name	**Common Trade Names**
Drugs Causing Bone Marrow Suppression	
Altretamine	Hexalen, Hexastat✱
Amphotericin B	Fungizone
Azathioprine	Imuran
Chemotherapeutic agents*	
Chloramphenicol	Chloromycetin, Novochlorocap✱
Chromic phosphate	Phosphocol
Colchicine	(Generic only)
Didanosine	Videx
Eflornithine	Ornidyl
Foscarnet sodium	Foscavir
Ganciclovir	Cytovene
Interferon alfa	Actimmune, Alferon, Intron-A, Roferon-A, Wellferon-A✱
Pentamidine	Pentam 300, NebuPent, Pentacarinat✱
Sodium iodide	Iodopen
Zalcitabine	Hivid
Zidovudine	AZT, Retrovir, Novo-AZT✱
Drugs Causing Hemolysis	
Acetohydroxamic acid	Lithostat
Chlorpropamide	Diabinese, Glucamide, Novopropamide✱
Doxapram	Dopram
Glyburide	Diabeta, Micronase, Euglucon✱
Mefenamic acid	Ponstel, Ponstan✱
Menadiol diphosphate	Synkayvite
Methyldopa	Aldomet, Dopamet✱
Nitrofurantoin	Macrodantin, Novofuran✱
Amoxicillin	Amoxil, Augmentin, Apo-Amoxi✱
Penicillin G benzathine	Bicillin, Crystapen
Penicillin V	Pen Vee K, Pen Vee, Nu-Pen-VK✱
Primaquine	(Generic only)
Procainamide hydrochloride	Procan-SR, Promide, Pronestyl hydrochloride
Quinidine polygalacturonate	Cardioquin, Quinalan, Novoquinidin✱
Quinine	Legatrin, Quindan
Sulfonamides	Sulfamethoxazole (Gantanol), sulfisoxazole (Gantrisin, Novosoxazole✱)
Tolbutamide	Oramide, Orinase, Apo-Tolbutamide✱, Mobenol✱
Vitamin K	AquaMEPHYTON, Konakion
Drugs Disrupting Platelet Action	
Aspirin	Anacin, Ascriptin, Bufferin, Ecotrin, Entrophen✱, Riphen✱, Triaphen✱
Carbenicillin	Geopen, Pyopen✱
Carindacillin	Geocillin
Dipyridamole	Persantine, Apo-Dipyridamole✱, Novodipiradol✱
Moxalactam	Moxam
Pentoxifylline	Trental
Sulfinpyrazone	Anturane, Antazone✱, Novopyrazone✱
Ticarcillin	Ticar
Ticlopidine	Ticlid
Valproic acid	Dalpro, Depakene, Epvil✱

Data from United States Pharmacopeial Convention, Inc. (1998). *Volume I: Drug information for the health care professional* (18th ed.). Taunton, MA: World Color Book Services.
*General categories of chemotherapeutic agents include alkylating agents, antimitotics, antitumor antibiotics, and antimetabolites.

gums are also assessed for active bleeding in response to light pressure or brushing the teeth with a soft-bristled brush, and any lesions or draining areas are noted. The nurse assesses for signs of bleeding in the form of petechiae and large bruises (ecchymoses). Petechiae are pinpoint hemorrhagic lesions in the skin. Bruises may be confluent or clustered. For hospitalized clients, the nurse determines whether the client is bleeding from sites such as nasogastric tubes, endotracheal tubes, central lines, peripheral intravenous sites, or Foley catheters. The nurse also notes skin turgor and itching, because dry skin or intense itching can indicate hematologic disease.

TRANSCULTURAL CONSIDERATIONS

The nurse may have difficulty assessing people with darker skin for pallor, jaundice, petechiae, and bruising. The oral mucous membranes and the conjunctiva of the eye are areas where pallor and cyanosis are more easily detected, and the roof of the mouth is an area where jaundice can be seen more easily. Petechiae may be visible only on the palms of the hands or the soles of the feet. Bruises can be seen as darker areas of skin and palpated as slight swellings or irregular skin surfaces. The nurse asks the client about pain when skin surfaces are touched lightly or palpated. (Chapter 69 provides additional information on accurate assessment techniques for darker skin.)

Assessment of the Head and Neck

The nurse notes pallor or ulceration of the oral mucosa. The tongue may be completely smooth in pernicious anemia and iron deficiency anemia or smooth and red in nutritional deficiencies. These manifestations may be accompanied by fissures at the corners of the mouth. The nurse also observes for jaundice of the sclera.

All lymph node areas are inspected and palpated. The nurse documents any lymph node enlargement, noting whether palpation of the enlarged node causes pain. In addition, the nurse determines whether the enlarged node moves or remains fixed with palpation.

Assessment of the Respiratory System

The nurse measures the rate and depth of respiration while the client is at rest, and during and after mild physical activity (such as walking 20 steps in 10 seconds). The nurse notes whether the client can complete a ten-word sentence without stopping for a breath. The nurse determines whether the client is fatigued easily, experiences shortness of breath at rest or on exertion, or requires additional pillows to sleep comfortably at night. Many anemias cause these symptoms.

Assessment of the Cardiovascular System

The nurse observes for heaves, distended neck veins, edema, or signs of phlebitis. The nurse auscultates for murmurs, gallops, irregular rhythms, and abnormal blood pressure. In clients with anemia, systolic blood pressure tends to be lower than normal. In conditions of hypercellularity, blood pressure is greater than normal. Severe anemias cause right ventricular hypertrophy and heart disease.

Assessment of the Renal/Urinary System

Because the kidneys are extremely vascular, bleeding problems may manifest as overt or occult hematuria (blood in the urine). The nurse inspects a voided sample of urine for color. Hematuria may be detected by grossly, bloody red or dark brownish-gold urine. Because blood contains significant amounts of proteins, the nurse tests the urine for proteins with a urine test dipstick. The urine sample also is tested for occult blood (Hemoccult test).

Assessment of the Musculoskeletal System

Increased rib or sternal tenderness is an important sign of hematologic malignancy. The nurse examines the superficial surfaces of all bones by applying intermittent firm pressure with the fingertips. The nurse also assesses the client's range of joint motion and notes any swelling or joint pain.

Assessment of the Abdomen

The normal adult spleen is usually not palpable. Enlarged spleens may be detected by percussion, although palpation is more reliable. The spleen lies just beneath the abdominal wall and is identified by its movement during respiration. During palpation, the client lies in a relaxed, supine position while the nurse, standing on the client's right, palpates the left upper quadrant. The nurse palpates gently and cautiously because an enlarged spleen may be tender and easily ruptured.

Palpating the edge of the liver in the right upper quadrant of the abdomen can detect hepatic enlargement. The normal liver may be palpable as much as 4 to 5 cm below the right costal margin but is usually not palpable in the epigastrium. Both the liver and the spleen may be enlarged in hematologic disease.

A common cause of anemia among older adults is a chronically bleeding gastrointestinal lesion. If the lesion is located in the stomach or the small intestine, obvious blood may not be visible in the stool, or such a small amount is passed each day that the client is not aware of it. Therefore, the nurse obtains and tests a stool specimen for occult blood.

Assessment of the Central Nervous System

A thorough examination of cranial nerves and neurologic function is necessary in many clients with hematologic disease. Vitamin B_{12} deficiency impairs cerebral, olfactory, spinal cord, and peripheral nerve function, and severe chronic deficiency may lead to irreversible neurologic degeneration. A variety of neurologic abnormalities may develop in clients who have hematologic malignancies as a consequence of bleeding, infection, or tumor spread. When the client has a known or suspected bleeding disorder and has experienced any head trauma, the nurse expands the physical assessment to include frequent neurologic checks and mental status examinations (see Chap. 43).

Other important signs and symptoms associated with impaired hematologic function include fever, chills, and night sweats.

➤ *Psychosocial Assessment*

The person with hematologic abnormalities may have a chronic illness, such as hemophilia or cancer, or an acute exacerbation of a chronic disease, such as pernicious anemia. In either instance, each person brings his or her own coping style to the illness. After developing a rapport with the client, the nurse can learn what coping mechanisms the client has used successfully during past illness or crises.

The nurse also asks the client and family members about social support networks, community resources, and financial health. A problem in any of these areas can interfere with the client's compliance with therapy and, ultimately, recovery.

➤ DIAGNOSTIC ASSESSMENT

Laboratory Tests

In hematologic disease, the most definitive signs are often the laboratory test results. Chart 41–2 lists laboratory data associated with hematologic function.

Tests of Cell Number and Function

Complete Blood Count. A complete blood count (CBC) includes a number of studies: red blood cell (RBC) count, white blood cell (WBC) count, hematocrit, and hemoglobin level. The RBC count measures circulating RBCs in 1 mm^3 of venous blood, and the WBC count measures all leukocytes present in 1 mm^3 of venous blood. To determine the percentages of different kinds of leukocytes circulating in the blood, a WBC count with differential leukocyte count is performed (Chap. 23). The hemoglobin level represents the total amount of he-

---

Chart 41–2

Laboratory Profile: Hematologic Assessment

Test	Reference Range		International Reference Units	Significance of Abnormal Findings
Red blood cell (RBC) count	18–44 yr	F: 3.8–5.1 million/μL M: 4.3–5.7 millon/μL	3.8–5.1 × 10^{12} cells/L 4.3–5.7 × 10^{12} cells/L	• *Decreased levels* indicate possible anemia or hemorrhage
	45–64 yr	F: 3.8–5.3 millon/μL M: 4.2–5.6 millon/μL	3.8–5.3 × 10^{12} cells/L 4.2–5.6 × 10^{12} cells/L	• *Increased levels* indicate possible chronic anoxia or polycythemia vera
	> 64 yr	F: 3.8–5.2 millon/μL M: 3.8–5.8 millon/μL	3.8–5.2 × 10^{12} cells/L 3.8–5.8 × 10^{12} cells/L	
Hemoglobin (Hgb)	18–44 yr	F: 11.7–15.5 g/dL M: 13.2–17.3 g/dL	117–155 g/L 132–173 g/L	• Same as for RBC
	45–64 yr	F: 11.7–16.0 g/dL M: 13.1–17.2 g/dL	117–160 g/L 131–172 g/L	
	> 65 yr	F: 11.7–16.1 g/dL M: 12.6–17.4 g/dL	117–161 g/L 126–174 g/L	
Hematocrit	18–44 yr	F: 34–45% M: 39–49%	0.34–0.45 fraction 0.39–0.49 fraction	• Same as for RBC
	45–64 yr	F: 35–47% M: 39–50%	0.35–0.47 fraction 0.39–0.50 fraction	
	> 65 yr	F: 35–47% M: 37–51%	0.35–0.47 fraction 0.37–0.51 fraction	
Mean cell volume (MCV)	80–100 fL (fL = femtoliter)		Same as reference range	• *Increased levels* indicate macrocytic cells, possible anemia • *Decreased levels* indicate microcytic cells, possible iron deficiency anemia
Mean cell hemoglobin (MCH)	26–35 pg/cell (pg = picogram)		Same as reference range	• Same as for MCV
Mean cell hemoglobin concentration (MCHC)	31–37 g/dL cells		310–370 g/L	• *Increased levels* may indicate spherocytosis or anemia • *Decreased levels* may indicate iron deficiency anemia or a hemaglobinopathy
White blood cell count (WBC)	4500–11,000/μL		4.5–11.0 × 10^9 cells/L	• *Increased levels* are associated with infection, inflammation, autoimmune disorders, and leukemia • *Decreased levels* may indicate prolonged infection or bone marrow suppression
Reticulocyte count	0.5%–1.5% of RBCs		0.005–0.015 fraction	• *Increased levels* may indicate chronic blood loss • *Decreased levels* indicate possible inadequate RBC production

Continued

moglobin in peripheral blood. The hematocrit (Hct) is calculated as the percentage of red blood cells in the total blood volume.

Complete blood cell studies can also measure other variables of the circulating cells, including the mean corpuscular volume (MCV), the mean corpuscular hemoglobin (MCH), and the mean corpuscular hemoglobin concentration (MCHC). The MCV measures the average

volume or size of a single RBC and is useful for classifying anemias. When the MCV is elevated, the cell is said to be macrocytic, or abnormally large, as seen in megaloblastic anemias. When the MCV is decreased, the cell is abnormally small, or microcytic, as seen in iron deficiency anemia. The MCH is the average amount of hemoglobin in a single RBC. The MCHC measures the average concentration of hemoglobin in a single RBC. When the

MCHC - Average hgb conc. in RBC [handwritten]

CHART 41–2. Laboratory Profile: Hematologic Assessment Continued

Test	Reference Range	International Reference Units	Significance of Abnormal Findings
Total iron binding capacity (TIBC)	250–425 µg/dL	44.8–76.1 µmol/L	• *Increased levels* indicate iron deficiency • *Decreased levels* may indicate anemia, hemorrhage, hemolysis
Serum haptoglobin	40–240 mg/dL	0.4–2.5 g/L	• *Increased levels* indicate possible inflammatory disease • *Decreased levels* may indicate liver disease or hemolytic disease
Iron (Fe)	F: 50–170 µg/dL M: 65–175 µg/dL	9.0–30.4 µmol/L 11.6–31.3 µmol/L	• *Increased levels* indicate iron excess, hemochromocytosis, liver disorders, megaloblastic anemia • *Decreased levels* indicate possible iron deficiency anemia, hemorrhage
Serum ferritin	F: 10–120 ng/mL M: 20–250 ng/mL	Same as reference range	• Same as for iron
Platelet count	150,000–400,000/µL	150–400 × 10⁹/L	• *Increased levels* may indicate polycythemia vera or malignancy • *Decreased levels* may indicate bone marrow suppression, autoimmune disease, hypersplenism
Hemoglobin electrophoresis	Hgb A₁: > 95% Hgb A₂: 1.5–3.7% Hgb F: < 2% Hgb S: 0% Hgb C: 0%	> 0.95 fraction 0.015–0.037 fraction < 0.02 fraction 0.0 fraction 0.0 fraction	• *Variations* indicate hemoglobinopathies
Direct Coombs' and indirect Coombs' test	Negative	Negative	• *Positive findings* indicate antibodies to RBCs
Prothrombin time (PT)	11–15 sec	Patient PT/normal/PT (INR) (INR = International Normalized Ratio)	• *Increased time* indicates possible deficiency of clotting factors V and VII • *Decreased time* may indicate vitamin K excess
Bleeding time	2–7 min	Same as reference range	• *Increased time* may indicate inadequate platelet function or number, clotting factor deficiencies
Euglobin lysis time	2–4 hr	Same as reference range	• *Decreased time* may indicate possible fibrinolysis
Fibrin degradation products	< 10 µg/mL	< 10 mg/L	• *Increased levels* may indicate disseminated intravascular coagulation or fibrinolysis

Data from Tietz, N. (1995). *Clinical guide to laboratory tests* (3rd ed.), Philadelphia: W. B. Saunders.
F = female; M = male.

MCHC is decreased, the cell has a hemoglobin deficiency and is hypochromic, as in iron deficiency anemia.

Reticulocyte Count. Another hematologic test helpful in determining bone marrow function is the reticulocyte count. A reticulocyte is an immature RBC, and an elevated reticulocyte count indicates increased RBC production by the bone marrow. Normally, about 2% of circulating RBCs are reticulocytes. An elevated reticulocyte count is desirable in an anemic client or after hemorrhage, when an elevation indicates that the bone marrow is responding appropriately to a decrease in the total RBC mass. An elevated reticulocyte count without a precipitating cause may indicate pathologic conditions, such as polycythemia vera.

Hemoglobin Electrophoresis. Hemoglobin electrophoresis detects abnormal forms of hemoglobin, such as hemoglobin S in sickle cell disease. Hemoglobin A is the major component of hemoglobin in the normal RBC.

Leukocyte Alkaline Phosphatase. Leukocyte alkaline phosphatase (LAP) is an enzyme produced by normal mature neutrophils. Elevated LAP levels occur during episodes of infection or stress. An elevated neutrophil count without an accompanying elevation in LAP level is associated with chronic myelogenous leukemia.

Coombs' Test. The two Coombs' tests (direct and indirect) are used for blood typing. The direct test detects the presence of antibodies (also called antiglobulins) against RBCs that may be attached to a person's RBCs. Although healthy people can make these antibodies, certain diseases, such as systemic lupus erythematosus, mononucleosis, and lymphomas, are associated with the production of antibodies directed against the client's own RBCs. The presence of these antibodies usually causes a hemolytic anemia.

The indirect Coombs' test detects the presence of circulating antiglobulins. The test is used to determine whether the client has serum antibodies to the type of RBCs that he or she is about to receive by blood transfusion.

Serum Ferritin, Transferrin, and Total Iron-Binding Capacity. Serum ferritin, transferrin, and the total iron-binding capacity (TIBC) tests measure iron levels. Abnormal levels of iron and TIBC are characteristic of many diseases, including iron deficiency anemia.

The serum ferritin test measures the quantity of iron present as free iron in the plasma. Because the amount of serum ferritin is proportionally related to the amount of intracellular iron, representing 1% of the total body iron stores, the serum ferritin level provides a means to assess a person's total iron stores. People who have serum ferritin levels within 10 g of the normal range for their gender have adequate iron stores; people with levels 10 g or more lower than the normal range have inadequate iron stores and have difficulty recovering from any hemorrhagic event.

Transferrin is a protein that transports iron from the gastrointestinal tract to the intracellular storage sites. Because the amount of transferrin cannot be easily measured, measuring the amount of iron that can be bound to serum transferrin indirectly determines whether an adequate amount of transferrin is present. This test is the TIBC test. In healthy people, only about 30% of the transferrin is bound to iron in the blood. TIBC is measured by taking a sample of blood and adding measured amounts of iron to it. When the blood no longer binds the iron but allows it to precipitate, the TIBC can be calculated. TIBC increases when a person is deficient in serum iron and stored iron levels. Such a value indicates that an adequate amount of transferrin is present but less than 30% of it is bound to serum iron.

Tests Measuring Bleeding and Coagulation

Capillary Fragility Test. The capillary fragility test, or Rumpel-Leede test, measures vascular hemostatic function by increasing intracapillary pressure in the arm by occluding venous outflow or by applying controlled negative pressure to a skin area. Usually, a blood pressure cuff is inflated to a pressure halfway between the systolic and diastolic pressures and maintained for 5 minutes. The petechiae that appear distal to the cuff are counted. Normally, five to ten petechiae appear. The capillary fragility test can help determine whether excessive bleeding or bruising results from increased capillary fragility or impaired platelet action.

Bleeding Time Test. The bleeding time test evaluates vascular and platelet activity during hemostasis. A small incision (using a special spring-loaded lancet that ensures uniform wound depth) is made in the forearm while a blood pressure cuff remains inflated at 40 mmHg. Blood is blotted from the site at 30-second intervals, and the time required for the bleeding to stop is recorded. Normal bleeding time ranges from 1 to 9 minutes.

Prothrombin Time. The prothrombin time (PT) evaluates the adequacy of the extrinsic coagulation cascade. PT is prolonged when factors II, V, VII, and X are deficient or when liver disease is present. Sodium warfarin (Coumadin, Warfilone✦) therapy is monitored using PT levels. Appropriate warfarin therapy prolongs the PT by one and a half to two times the client's normal PT value. The PT test results are given in seconds, along with a control value. A normal PT is nearly equal to the control value.

Partial Thromboplastin Time. The partial thromboplastin time (PTT) assesses the intrinsic coagulation cascade. It evaluates the presence of factors II, V, VIII, IX, XI, and XII. When any of these factors is deficient, as in hemophilia or disseminated intravascular coagulation (DIC), the PTT is prolonged. Because factors II, IX, and X are vitamin K–dependent and are produced in the liver, liver disease can decrease their concentration and prolong the PTT. Heparin (Calciparin, Liquémin, Hepalean✦) therapy is monitored by PTT. Desired ranges for therapeutic anticoagulation are one and a half to two and a half times normal values.

Platelet Agglutination/Aggregation. Platelet aggregation, or the ability to clump, can be tested by mixing the client's plasma with a substance called ristocetin. The degree of aggregation is noted. Aggregation can be impaired in von Willebrand's disease and during the use of drugs such as aspirin, anti-inflammatory agents, and psychotropic agents.

➤ Radiographic Examinations

Assessment of the client with a suspected hematologic abnormality can include radioisotopic imaging. Isotopes are used to evaluate the bone marrow for sites of active erythropoiesis and sites of iron storage. Radioactive colloids are routinely used to determine organ size and liver and spleen function.

The client is given a radioactive isotope intravenously about 3 hours before the procedure. The client is then taken to the nuclear medicine department for the scan, where he or she must lie still for about an hour. No special client preparation or follow-up care is needed for these tests.

Standard x-rays may be used to diagnose some hematologic disorders. For example, multiple myeloma causes characteristic bone destruction, with a "Swiss cheese" appearance on x-ray.

➤ Bone Marrow Aspiration and Biopsy

Bone marrow aspiration or biopsy is frequently done to evaluate the client's hematologic status when other tests show persistent abnormal findings. Results can provide important information about bone marrow function, including RBC, WBC, and platelet production. Bone marrow aspiration and bone marrow biopsy are similar procedures. In a bone marrow aspiration, cells and fluids are suctioned from the bone marrow. In a bone marrow biopsy, solid tissue and cells are obtained by coring out an area of bone marrow with a large-bore needle.

A physician's order and a signed, informed consent are obtained from the client before a bone marrow aspiration or biopsy is done. Bone marrow aspiration may be performed by a physician, a sanctioned clinical nurse specialist, a nurse practitioner, or a physician assistant, depending on the agency's policy and regional law. The procedure may be performed at the client's bedside, in an examination room, in a laboratory, or in a clinic setting.

On learning what specific tests will be performed on the marrow, the nurse consults the facility's procedure manual and its hematology laboratory to determine how to handle the specimen. Some tests necessitate the addition of heparin or other special solutions to the specimen.

Client Preparation

Most clients experience anxiety or fear before a bone marrow aspiration. Clients who have experienced a bone marrow aspiration may have less or more anxiety, depending on how the previous experience was perceived. The nurse can help reduce anxiety and allay fears by providing accurate information and continuous emotional support. Some clients like to have their hand held during the procedure; other clients may want the nurse to hug or hold their entire upper body.

The nurse explains the procedure to the client and says that he or she will stay with the client during the entire procedure. Occasionally, a friend or family member is permitted to be present to hold the client's hand and provide additional emotional support. If a local anesthetic is to be used, the nurse tells the client that the injection will feel like a stinging or burning sensation. The nurse tells the client to expect a heavy sensation of pressure and pushing while the needle is being inserted. Some clients also can hear a crunching sound or feel a scraping sensation as the needle punctures the bone. The nurse explains that as the marrow is being aspirated by mild suction in the syringe, a brief sensation of painful pulling will be experienced. If a biopsy is performed, the client may feel more pressure and discomfort as the needle is rotated into the bone.

The client is assisted onto an examining table, and the site is exposed, most commonly the iliac crest. If this site is not available or if more marrow is needed, the sternum can be used. If the iliac crest is the site, the client is usually placed in the prone position or, occasionally, in the side-lying position. Depending on the tests to be performed on the specimen, a laboratory technician may also be present to ensure appropriate handling of the specimen.

Procedure

The procedure usually lasts from 5 to 15 minutes. Clients may be uncomfortable and may experience pain. The type and the amount of anesthesia or sedation depend on the physician's preference, the client's preference and previous experience with bone marrow aspiration and biopsy, and the setting.

A local anesthetic solution might be injected into the skin around the site. The client may also receive a mild tranquilizer or a rapid-acting sedative, such as midazolam hydrochloride (Versed) or lorazepam (Ativan, Apo-Lorazepam✲, Novolorazem✲). Some clients do well with guided imagery or autohypnosis.

The procedure for either aspiration or biopsy is invasive, and sterile precautions are observed. The skin over the site is cleaned with a disinfectant solution. For an aspiration, the needle is inserted with a twisting motion and the marrow is aspirated by pulling back on the plunger of the syringe. When sufficient marrow has been aspirated to ensure accurate analysis, the needle is carefully and rapidly withdrawn while the tissues are supported at the site. For a biopsy, a small skin incision is made and the biopsy needle is inserted through the skin opening. Pressure and several twisting motions are performed to ensure coring and loosening of an adequate amount of marrow tissue. External pressure is applied to the site until hemostasis is ensured. A pressure dressing or sandbags may be applied to minimize bleeding at the site.

Follow-Up Care

The site is covered with a dressing after hemostasis is achieved. The site of the aspiration is observed closely for 24 hours for signs of bleeding and infection. A mild analgesic (aspirin-free) is prescribed for discomfort, and ice packs are applied over the aspiration site to limit bruising. The nurse instructs the client to inspect the site every 2 hours for the first 24 hours and to note the presence of active bleeding or bruising. The nurse advises the client not to engage in contact sports or any other activity that might result in trauma to the site for 48 hours.

Information obtained from bone marrow aspiration or biopsy reflects the degree and quality of bone marrow activity present. The counts made on a marrow specimen can indicate whether stem cells, blast cells, committed cells, and more mature cell forms are present in the expected quantities and proportions. In addition, bone marrow aspiration or biopsy can confirm the spread of cancer cells from other tumor sites.

SELECTED BIBLIOGRAPHY

Abboud, C., & Lichtman, M. (1995). Structure of the marrow. In E. Beutler, M. Lichtman, B. Coller, & T. Kipps (Eds.), *William's hematology* (5th ed., pp. 25–38). New York: McGraw-Hill.

Colman, R., Hirsch, J., Marder, V., & Salzman, E. (1994). *Hemostasis and thrombosis: Basic principles and clinical practice* (3rd ed.). Philadelphia: J. B. Lippincott.

Frizzell, J. (1998). Avoiding lab test pitfalls. *American Journal of Nursing, 98*(2), 34–38.

Goodnough, L., Price, T., & Parvin, C. (1995). The endogenous erythropoietin response and the erythropoietic response to blood loss anemia: The effects of age and gender. *Journal of Laboratory and Clinical Medicine, 126*(1), 57–64.

Guyton, A., & Hall, J. (1996). *Textbook of medical physiology* (9th ed.). Philadelphia: W. B. Saunders.

*Hays, K. (1990). Physiology of normal bone marrow. *Seminars in Oncology Nursing, 6*(1), 3–8.

Higgins, C. (1995). Haematology blood testing for anaemia. *British Journal of Nursing, 4*(5), 248–253.

Malaguarnera, M., Bentivegna, P., Giugno, I., DeFazio, I., Motta, M., & Trovato, B. (1996). Erythropoietin in healthy elder subjects. *Archives of Gerontology and Geriatrics, 22*(2), 131–135.

Pitler, L. (1996). Hematopoietic growth factors in clinical practice. *Seminars in Oncology Nursing, 12*(2), 115–129.

Tietz, N. (1995). *Clinical guide to laboratory tests* (3rd ed). Philadelphia: W. B. Saunders.

United States Pharmacopeial Convention, Inc. (1998). *Volume I: Drug information for the health care professional* (18th ed.). Taunton, MA: World Color Book Services.

Williams, W. (1995). Hematology in the aged. In E. Beutler, M. Lichtman, B. Coller, & T. Kipps (Eds.). *Williams hematology* (5th ed., pp. 72–77). New York: McGraw-Hill.

Williams, W., Morris, M., & Nelson, D. (1995). Examination of the blood. In E. Beutler, M. Lichtman, B. Coller, & T. Kipps (Eds.). *Williams hematology* (5th ed., pp. 8–15). New York: McGraw-Hill.

Williams, W., & Nelson, D. (1995). Examination of the marrow. In E. Beutler, M. Lichtman, B. Coller, & T. Kipps (Eds.). *William's hematology* (5th ed., pp. 15–22). New York: McGraw-Hill.

*Workman, M., Ellerhorst-Ryan, J., & Koertge, V. (1993). *Nursing care of the immunocompromised patient*. Philadelphia: W. B. Saunders.

SUGGESTED READINGS

*Hays, K. (1990). Physiology of normal bone marrow. *Seminars in Oncology Nursing, 6*(1), 3–8.

   Although several years old, this excellent article provides useful information on the blood-forming functions of bone marrow. Terms are explained simply and concisely. The reference list contains both informational and research-based sources.

Pitler, L. (1996). Hematopoietic growth factors in clinical practice. *Seminars in Oncology Nursing, 12*(2), 115–129.

   This clinically focused article explains the mechanisms of action and clinical uses of a variety of hematopoietic growth factors. Side effects, precautions, and nursing responsibilities also are addressed.

Chapter 42

INTERVENTIONS FOR CLIENTS WITH HEMATOLOGIC PROBLEMS

CHAPTER

HIGHLIGHTS

Hematologic system disorders can occur in the synthesis, function, or normal destruction of any type of blood cell. The impact of hematologic disorders on the client's well-being depends on the type, degree, and rate of onset of the specific disorder. This chapter discusses hematologic conditions that minimally disrupt activities of daily living (ADLs) as well as potentially life-threatening conditions such as sickle cell disease and leukemia.

RED BLOOD CELL DISORDERS

The major cellular population of the blood is red blood cells (RBCs), or erythrocytes. Physiologic function depends on maintaining the circulating volume of RBCs within the normal range for the person's age and gender and ensuring that the erythrocytes can perform their normal functions. RBC disorders include problems in production, function, and destruction. These problems may result in an insufficient number or function of RBCs (anemia) or an excess of RBCs (polycythemia).

Anemia

Anemia is a reduction in either the number of RBCs, the quantity of hemoglobin, or the hematocrit (the volume of packed RBCs per deciliter of blood). Anemia is a clinical sign, not a diagnosis, because it is a manifestation of a number of abnormal conditions. Anemia can result from dietary deficiency, hereditary disorders, bone marrow disease, and bleeding.

There are many types and causes of anemia. Some anemias arise from a deficiency in one or more of the components needed to make fully functional RBCs. Such anemias can be caused by deficiencies of iron, vitamin B$_{12}$, folic acid, or intrinsic factor. Additional causes include decreased development of the RBC line precursors, decreased rate of erythrocyte production, and increased destruction of RBCs. Table 42–1 lists common causes of various types of anemia. Despite the many causes of anemia, the effects of anemia on the client (Chart 42–1) and the corresponding nursing care are similar for all types of anemia.

Anemias Resulting from Increased Destruction of Red Blood Cells

Sickle Cell Disease

Overview

Sickle cell disease is a condition in which chronic anemia is one of many client problems leading to discomfort,

TABLE 42–1

Common Causes of Anemia

Type of Anemia	Common Causes
Sickle cell disease	• Autosomal recessive inheritance of two defective genes for hemoglobin synthesis
G6PD deficiency anemia	• X-linked recessive inherited deficiency of the enzyme glucose-6-phosphate dehydrogenase.
Autoimmune hemolytic anemia	• Abnormal immune function in which a person's immune reactive cells fail to recognize his or her own red blood cells as self cells

Iron deficiency anemia	• Inadequate iron intake caused by
	  • Iron-deficient diet
	  • Chronic alcoholism
	  • Malabsorption syndromes
	  • Partial gastrectomy
	• Rapid metabolic (anabolic) activity caused by
	  • Pregnancy
	  • Adolescence
	  • Infection

Vitamin B$_{12}$ deficiency anemia	• Dietary deficiency
	• Failure to absorb vitamin B$_{12}$ from intestinal tract as a result of
	  • Partial gastrectomy
	  • Pernicious anemia

Folic acid deficiency anemia	• Dietary deficiency
	• Malabsorption syndromes
	• Drugs
	  • Oral contraceptives
	  • Anticonvulsants
	  • Methotrexate

Aplastic anemia	• Exposure to myelotoxic agents
	  • Radiation
	  • Benzene
	  • Chloromycetin
	  • Alkylating agents
	  • Antimetabolites
	  • Sulfonamides
	  • Insecticides
	• Viral infection (unproven)
	  • Epstein-Barr virus
	  • Hepatitis B
	  • Cytomegalovirus

disability, increased risk for disease, and early death. Once considered a childhood disorder, clients with sickle cell disease who receive appropriate supportive care may live into their 30s and 40s. In addition, there is great individual variation in the severity of the disease and the onset of complications.

Pathophysiology

The primary problem in this hereditary disorder is the formation of abnormal beta chains in the hemoglobin molecule. The hemoglobin molecule of adults is composed of several different substances partially held together by a protein (globin), consisting of two alpha chains and two beta chains of amino acids. This normal adult hemoglobin is called hemoglobin A (HbA). The total hemoglobin of normal healthy adults is usually composed of 98% to 99% HbA with a small percentage of a fetal form of hemoglobin (HbF).

In clients who have sickle cell disease, at least 40% of their total hemoglobin contains an abnormality of the beta chains, hemoglobin S (HbS). HbS is sensitive to changes in the oxygen content of the RBC. When RBCs containing large amounts of HbS are exposed to conditions of decreased oxygen, the abnormal beta chains contract and pile together within the cell, distorting the overall shape of the RBC. These cells assume a sickle shape, become rigid, clump together, and form clusters that obstruct capillary blood flow (Fig. 42–1). Capillary obstruction leads to further tissue hypoxia (reduced oxygen supply) and more sickling, causing blood vessel obstructions and infarctions in the locally affected tissues. Situations that precipitate sickling include hypoxia, dehydration, infections, vascular stasis, low environmental or body temperatures, acidosis, strenuous exercise, and anesthesia.

Usually, sickled cells resume a normal shape when the precipitating condition is removed and proper oxygenation occurs. However, although the outward appearance of the RBCs is normal, at least some of the hemoglobin remains twisted, decreasing cell flexibility. The membranes of the cells become damaged over time, and cells

Chart 42–1

Key Features of Anemia

Integumentary Manifestations

• Pallor, especially of the ears, the nail beds, the palmar creases, the conjunctiva, and around the mouth
• Cool to the touch
• Intolerance of cold temperatures
• Nails become brittle and may lose the normal convex shape; over time, nails become concave and fingers assume club-like appearance

Cardiovascular Manifestations

• Tachycardia at basal activity levels, increasing with activity and during and immediately after meals
• Murmurs and gallops heard on auscultation when anemia is severe
• Orthostatic hypotension

Respiratory Manifestations

• Dyspnea on exertion
• Decreased oxygen saturation levels

Neurologic Manifestations

• Increased somnolence and fatigue
• Headache

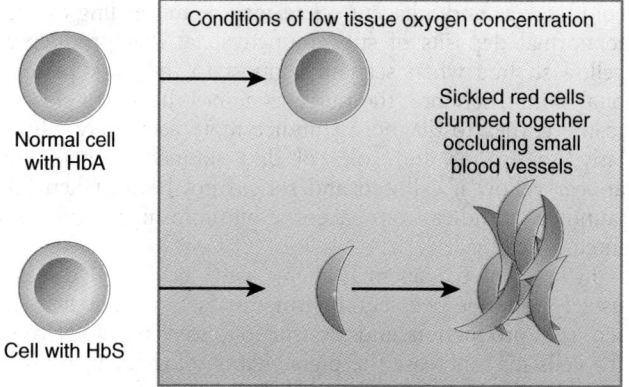

Figure 42–1. Red blood cell actions under conditions of low tissue oxygenation. (HbS = hemoglobin S; HbA = hemoglobin A.)

become irreversibly sickled. Additionally, the altered membranes of cells with HbS make them more fragile and more easily destroyed in the spleen and in other organs that have long, twisted capillary pathways. The average life span of an RBC containing 40% or more of HbS is approximately 20 days, considerably less than the 120-day life span of RBCs containing only HbA. This reduced life span is responsible for hemolytic anemia in clients with sickle cell disease.

The client with sickle cell disease experiences periodic episodes of extensive cellular sickling, or *crises*. The crises have a sudden onset and can occur as frequently as weekly or as seldom as once a year. Many clients are in good health much of the time, with crises occurring sporadically in response to precipitating conditions that stimulate local or systemic hypoxemia (deficient oxygen in the blood).

Repeated occlusions of progressively larger blood vessels have long-term negative effects on tissues and organs (Chart 42–2). Most effects are thought to occur as a result of capillary and blood vessel occlusion leading to tissue hypoxia, anoxia, ischemia, and cell death. Tissues and organs begin to have small infarcted areas that eventually destroy all healthy cells and lead to organ failure. Tissues and organs most commonly affected in this way are the spleen, liver, heart, kidney, brain, bones, and retina.

Etiology

Sickle cell disease is a genetic disorder with an autosomal recessive pattern of inheritance. The formation of the beta chains of the hemoglobin molecule is dependent on a pair of genes. A mutation leads to the formation of HbS instead of HbA. When the client inherits one abnormal gene of this pair, the condition is called *sickle cell trait*. The client can pass the condition on to offspring but has only mild manifestations of the disease under severe precipitating conditions because less than about 30% of the person's hemoglobin is abnormal. When the client inherits two abnormal genes, the condition is called *sickle cell disease* (formerly sickle cell anemia), and the

client has severe manifestations of the disease even under relatively mild precipitating conditions. In addition, if the client has children, each child will inherit one of the two abnormal genes and at least have sickle cell trait.

Incidence/Prevalence

Sickle cell trait and different forms of sickle cell disease occur in people of all races and ethnicities but infrequently among Caucasians.

TRANSCULTURAL CONSIDERATIONS

Sickle cell disease occurs most frequently in African-Americans as well as in African, Mediterranean, Caribbean, Middle Eastern, and Central American populations. Approximately 1 of every 12 African-Americans has the sickle cell trait. One of every 375 African-American infants inherits two abnormal genes (one from each parent) and has overt sickle cell disease (Agency for Health Care Policy and Research, 1993).

Chart 42–2

Key Features of Sickle Cell Disease

Hematologic Manifestations
- Fragile red blood cells that sickle and clump under conditions of low tissue oxygenation, venous stasis, lower environmental or body temperature
  - Anemia
- Tissue hypoxia and ischemia
  - Pain
  - Hardened, enlarged spleen

Respiratory Manifestations
- Pulmonary infarcts
  - Chest pain
  - Pneumonia

Genitourinary Manifestations
- Renal ischemia
  - Decreased urine concentration
- Priapism

Cardiovascular Manifestations
- Cardiac ischemia
  - Myocardial infarctions
  - Chest pain
  - Congestive heart failure
- Cerebrovascular accidents

Musculoskeletal Manifestations
- Necrosis of femur head
- Pain in extremities with moderate physical exercise
- Delayed growth—small stature

Integumentary Manifestations
- Leg ulcers
- Pale, cyanotic skin

Collaborative Management

 Assessment

► History

An adult with sickle cell disease has a long-standing diagnosis of the disorder. However, an adult who has sickle cell trait may have had such mild clinical manifestations that he or she is unaware of the problem until it is diagnosed with an accompanying disorder or when anesthesia is administered.

The nurse asks the client about previous crises, including precipitating events, severity, and usual treatments. Recent activities and situations are explored with the client to determine the probable precipitating condition or event. The nurse also reviews all activities and events during the previous 24 hours, including food and fluid intake, exposure to temperature extremes, types of clothing worn, medications taken, exercise, trauma, stress, and ingestion of alcohol or other recreational drugs. This activity review provides the nurse with important information about fatigue, activity tolerance, and participation in activities of daily living (ADLs).

The nurse also asks about changes in sleep and rest patterns, ability to climb stairs, and any activity that induces shortness of breath. Obtaining a subjective baseline assessment of the individual's perceived energy level using a scale ranging from 1 to 10 (1 = not tired with plenty of energy; 10 = total exhaustion) can be useful in evaluating the degree of fatigue and the effectiveness of later treatments.

► Physical Assessment/Clinical Manifestations

Pain is the most common symptom experienced during sickle cell crisis. Jaundice may also be present as a result of increased RBC destruction and release of bilirubin. Other clinical manifestations vary with the site of tissue damage.

Cardiovascular Assessment. The nurse assesses the client's cardiovascular and peripheral vascular status by comparing peripheral pulses, temperature, and capillary refill in all extremities. Extremities distal to blood vessel occlusion are cool to the touch with slow capillary refill and may have diminished or absent pulses. Heart rate may be rapid and blood pressure low to average, with a decreased pulse pressure because lysing of red blood cells (RBCs) leads to anemia.

Integumentary Assessment. The skin may be pale or cyanotic as a result of decreased perfusion and anemia. The nurse examines the lips, tongue, nail beds, conjunctivae, palms, and soles at regular intervals for subtle color changes. With cyanosis, the lips and tongue are gray, and the palms, soles, conjunctivae, and nail beds have a bluish tinge.

Another skin manifestation associated with sickle cell disease is jaundice. Bilirubin, a major component of RBCs, is released when fragile cells are damaged, leading to jaundice. The nurse assesses for jaundice in clients with darker skin by inspecting the oral mucosa, especially the hard palate, for yellow discoloration. Inspection of the conjunctivae and adjacent sclera may be misleading owing to normal deposits of subconjunctival fat that produce a yellowish hue when seen in contrast to the dark periorbital skin. Therefore, the nurse examines the sclera closest to the cornea to diagnose jaundice more accurately. Similarly, the palms and soles of dark-skinned clients may appear yellow if callused and should not be mistaken for jaundice. Jaundice from excessive bilirubin may also cause intense itching.

In spite of the anemia, clients with sickle cell disease usually are not deficient in iron. In fact, with increased red cell production and destruction, iron released from the cells may increase the pigmentation of the skin.

Adult clients with sickle cell disease may present with stasis ulcers or pressure ulcers on the lower extremities. The ulcers usually occur on the lateral or medial aspect of the ankle or on the shin (Blaylock, 1996). The nurse inspects the legs and feet for open lesions or darkened areas that may indicate necrotic tissue.

Abdominal Assessment. Abdominal organs are usually the first to be damaged as a result of multiple episodes of hypoxia and ischemia. The nurse inspects the abdomen for asymmetry or bulging areas, gently palpating it. Affected organs, such as the liver or spleen, may be firm and enlarged with a nodular texture in later stages of the disease.

Musculoskeletal Assessment. Extremities are a common site of vascular occlusion among clients who have sickle cell disease. In addition, joints may be damaged from frequent hypoxic episodes and undergo necrotic degeneration. The nurse inspects the extremities for symmetry and notes any areas of swelling or color difference. Clients are asked to move all joints, and the nurse notes the range of motion and any accompanying pain.

Central Nervous System Assessment. Changes in central nervous system (CNS) function may occur directly or indirectly in clients with sickle cell disease. During crises, clients may have low-grade fever. If the CNS sustains infarcts or repeated episodes of hypoxia, clients may have seizure activity or clinical manifestations of a stroke. Handgrasps are assessed bilaterally. The nurse assesses gait and coordination in those clients who are permitted to walk.

► Psychosocial Assessment

Psychosocial assessment is important because behavioral changes may be the first observable clinical manifestations of cerebral hypoxia. The nurse observes the clients and documents presenting behavior. Family members and significant others are questioned to determine whether the presenting behavior and mental status are typical.

Sickle cell disease represents a chronic, painful, life-limiting disorder that can be passed on to one's children. The nurse assesses clients' psychosocial needs in terms of new factors, established support systems, previous and current coping patterns, and disease progression. The nurse also asks clients how they view the disease and what adjustments in lifestyle have been made to accommodate limitations.

➤ Laboratory Assessment

The primary laboratory finding associated with sickle cell disease is the large percentage of HbS present on electrophoresis. A person who has sickle cell trait usually expresses less than 40% HbS, but one with sickle cell disease may express 85% to 95% HbS. This percentage does not change during crises. Another indicator of sickle cell disease is the percentage of RBCs showing irreversible sickling. This value is less than 1% among people who do not have sickle cell disease, is 5% to 50% among people with sickle cell trait, and may exceed 90% among people with sickle cell disease.

A variety of other laboratory tests reflect the problems associated with sickle cell disease, especially during crises. The hematocrit of clients with sickle cell disease is usually low (between 20% and 30%). This value decreases even more dramatically during vascular occlusive crises or aplastic crisis, when the bone marrow temporarily fails to produce cells during physiologically stressful periods (such as infection). The reticulocyte count is elevated, indicating anemia of long duration. Often the mean corpuscular hemoglobin concentration (MCHC) and total bilirubin level are elevated in clients who have sickle cell disease.

The total white blood cell (WBC) count is usually above normal among clients who have sickle cell disease. It is thought that this elevation is related to chronic inflammation resulting from tissue hypoxia and ischemia.

➤ Radiographic Assessment

Bone changes occur as a result of chronically stimulated marrow and hypoxic bone tissue. The skull may show radiographic changes resulting from chronic bone surface resorption and regeneration, giving the skull a "crew cut" appearance. Joint necrosis and degeneration also are obvious on x-ray.

➤ Other Diagnostic Assessment

Electrocardiographic (ECG) changes document cardiac infarcts and tissue damage. Specific ECG changes are related to the area of the myocardium sustaining the damage. Ultrasonography, computed tomography (CT), positron emission tomography (PET), and magnetic resonance imaging (MRI) may reveal soft tissue and organ degenerative changes resulting from inadequate oxygenation and chronic inflammation.

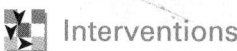 Interventions

The most common health problems for clients with sickle cell disease are pain and the potential complications of sepsis and multiple organ dysfunction. Interventions are aimed at reducing or preventing these problems.

➤ Pain

Pain associated with sickle cell crisis is the result of ischemic tissue injury caused by obstructed blood flow. The pain is often severe enough to require hospitalization and large doses of opioid analgesics (Miller, 1994). Pain is chronic with acute episodes and can occur anywhere in the body, often where circulation is impaired. It is sudden in nature and frequently described as gnawing or throbbing. Subjective reports of pain may be the only evidence, because the chronic nature of the pain may make physiologic changes less obvious.

The subjective nature of the pain, racial prejudice, and concern for addiction often cause these clients to be labeled as difficult (Marchiondo & Thompson, 1996). Health care providers must be aware of their own attitudes when caring for this population, and realize that lack of knowledge and concern for addiction often prevent proper pain management of sickle cell patients. Use of a pain rating scale by all nursing personnel can promote proper pain management. The nurse asks the client to rate pain on a scale ranging from 1 to 10 and evaluates the effectiveness of interventions based on the client's ratings. Use of pain-control contracts can also be useful.

Clients in acute sickle cell crisis often require at least 48 hours of parenteral analgesics. (Chart 42–3 lists specific priorities for nursing care of the client in sickle cell crisis.) Meperidine (Demerol), morphine, and hydromorphone (Dilaudid) are the medications most frequently ordered, administered intravenously (IV) on a routine schedule. Once relief is obtained, the dose can be tapered by 10% to 20% daily (Marchiondo & Thompson, 1996). As needed (PRN) schedules are discouraged because they do not provide adequate relief, and intramuscular (IM) injections are avoided because frequent injections lead to sclerosing of tissue, and absorption may be impaired by poor circulation. Moderate pain may be treated with oral doses of codeine, morphine sulfate, or nonsteroidal anti-inflammatory drugs (NSAIDs). See Chapter 9 for more information on pain management.

➤ Complementary Therapies

Complementary therapies and other nonpharmacologic measures such as keeping the room warm, using distrac-

---

Chart 42–3

Nursing Care Highlight: The Client in Sickle Cell Crisis

- Administer oxygen.
- Administer pain medication as ordered.
- Hydrate the client with normal saline intravenously and with beverages of choice (without caffeine) orally.
- Remove any constrictive clothing.
- Encourage the client to keep extremities extended to promote venous return.
- Do not raise the knee gatch of the bed.
- Elevate the head of the bed no more than 30 degrees.
- Keep room temperature at or above 72° F.
- Avoid taking blood pressure with external cuff.
- Check circulation in extremities every hour.
  - Pulse oximetry of fingers and toes
  - Capillary refill
  - Peripheral pulses
  - Toe temperature

tion and relaxation techniques, proper positioning with support for painful areas, aroma therapy, therapeutic touch, and warm soaks or compresses have all been useful in decreasing pain. However, the nurse must not assume that these methods alone will provide adequate pain relief. Analgesics are required to treat sickle cell pain.

➤ Potential for Sepsis

The client with sickle cell disease is more susceptible to blood-borne infections and infection by encapsulated microorganisms, such as *Streptococcus pneumoniae* and *Haemophilus influenzae*, as a result of decreased spleen function.

Interventions aim at preventing or halting the infection processes, controlling infection, and initiating early, effective treatment regimens for specific infections.

Prevention/Early Detection. A major objective is to protect the client in sickle cell crisis from infection. Frequent, thorough hand washing is of the utmost importance. Any person with an upper respiratory tract infection who must enter the client's room wears a mask. Strict aseptic technique is used for all invasive procedures.

The nurse continually assesses the client for the presence of infection, monitoring daily CBC with differential WBC count. The oral mucosa is inspected during every nursing shift for lesions indicating fungal or viral infection. Lung sounds are auscultated every 8 hours for crackles, wheezes, or diminished breath sounds. Each time the client voids, assistive nursing personnel inspect the urine for odor and cloudiness, and the client is asked about any sensation of urgency, burning, or pain during urination. The client's vital signs are taken at least every 4 hours to assess for fever.

Drug Therapy. Drug therapy is a primary defense against the infections that develop in the client with sickle cell disease. Prophylactic therapy with twice-daily administration of oral penicillin in the penicillin-tolerant client has resulted in dramatic reductions of pneumonia and other streptococcal infections. Drug therapy for an actual infection can control infection and prevent complications associated with sepsis. Agents used depend on the sensitivity of the specific organism causing the infection as well as the extent of the infection.

➤ Potential for Multiple Organ Dysfunction

The threat of multiple organ dysfunction arises from continued vascular occlusions after clumping of sickled cells. Management of sickle cell disease focuses on prevention of vascular occlusion and promotion of adequate oxygenation.

The client in sickle cell crisis is admitted to the acute care hospital. The nurse assesses the client for adequacy of circulation to all body areas. Restrictive clothing is removed, and the client is instructed to avoid keeping the hips or knees in a flexed position.

Dehydration perpetuates cell sickling and must be avoided. Nursing personnel assist the client in maintaining an adequate hydration status. An oral or parenteral intake of at least 200 mL hourly is desired for the client in crisis.

Oxygen is ordered, and the nurse ensures that oxygen therapy is delivered appropriately, including nebulization to prevent dehydration. Transfusion therapy has been used to decrease the incidence of organ dysfunction and stroke (Miller, 1994). RBC transfusions are therapeutic because levels of HbA are sustained while diluting levels of HbS. Transfusions also suppress erythropoiesis, thereby decreasing the production of sickle cells. Transfusions may be administered either in the acute care or clinic setting by a registered nurse. The nurse monitors the client closely for complications of transfusion therapy, discussed later in this chapter.

In some treatment centers, bone marrow transplantation is being performed to correct abnormal hemoglobin permanently. Because bone marrow transplantation is expensive and may result in chronic and life-threatening complications, its risks and benefits need to be seriously considered for each client.

➤ Continuing Care

Sickle cell disease is a progressive disorder with periods of varying degrees of exacerbation. Rarely is there a true remission, although crisis episodes may be infrequent. Care focuses on prevention of complications, an ongoing daily necessity for the client with sickle cell disease. The client with sickle cell disease may be cared for in a variety of settings, including acute care, subacute care, extended or assistive care, and home care.

➤ Health Teaching

Clients are taught to avoid specific activities that lead to hypoxia and hypoxemia. In addition, they are taught to recognize the early signs and symptoms of crisis, so that appropriate treatment can be initiated early to prevent undue pain, complications, and permanent tissue damage. Clients are often given opioid analgesics for self-management of sickle cell crises at home; the nurse teaches clients and families about the correct administration. Additionally, clients are counseled about the hereditary aspects of sickle cell disease, and information concerning prenatal diagnosis, birth control methods, and pregnancy options is offered.

WOMEN'S HEALTH CONSIDERATIONS

 Pregnancy in women with sickle cell disease presents special physiologic challenges and may be life threatening. Clients who show evidence of damage to vital organs are advised against becoming pregnant. Usually, barrier methods of contraception (cervical cap, diaphragm, or condoms with or without spermicides) are recommended for women with sickle cell disease. The use of oral contraceptives among these women is controversial, however. Oral contraceptives may increase susceptibility to occlusion by increasing clot formation, especially among smokers. However, the use of oral contraceptives also can reduce menstrual blood loss, thus decreasing the

TABLE 42–2

Indications for Treatment with Blood Components			
Component	**Volume**	**Infusion Time**	**Indications**
Packed red blood cells (PRBCs)	• 200–250 mL	• 2–4 hour	• Anemia, hemoglobin <8
Washed red blood cells (WBC-poor PRBCs)	• 200 mL	• 2–4 hour	• History of allergic transfusion reactions • Bone marrow transplant clients
Platelets Pooled	• Approx. 300 mL	• 15–30 minutes	• Thrombocytopenia platelet count <20,000 • Clients who are actively bleeding with a platelet count <80,000
Platelets Single donor	• 200 mL	• 30 minutes	• History of febrile or allergic reactions
Fresh frozen plasma	• 200 mL	• 15–30 minutes	• Deficiency in plasma coagulation factors
Cryoprecipitate	• 10–20 mL/U	• 15–30 minutes	• Hemophilia VIII or von Willebrand's disease
White blood cells (WBCs)	• 400 mL	• 1 hour	• Sepsis, neutropenic infection not responding to antibiotic therapy

degree of anemia. Therefore, the determination of risks versus benefits of oral contraceptives must be individualized.

Glucose-6-Phosphate Dehydrogenase Deficiency Anemia

Overview

Many forms of congenital hemolytic anemia result from defects or deficiencies of one or more enzymes within the red blood cell (RBC). More than 200 such disorders have been identified. Most of these enzymes are needed to complete some critical step in intracellular energy production. The most common type of congenital hemolytic anemia is associated with a deficiency of the enzyme glucose-6-phosphate dehydrogenase (G6PD). This disease is inherited as an X-linked recessive disorder and affects about 10% of all African-Americans (Cotran et al., 1994).

G6PD stimulates critical reactions in the glycolytic pathway. RBCs contain no mitochondria (sites of high-efficiency production of the energy compound adenosine triphosphate [ATP]), so active glycolysis is essential for energy metabolism. Newly produced RBCs from clients with G6PD deficiency have relatively sufficient quantities of G6PD; however, as the cells age, the concentration diminishes drastically. Cells that have reduced amounts of G6PD are more susceptible to hemolysis during exposure to specific drugs (e.g., phenacetin, sulfonamides, aspirin [acetylsalicylic acid], quinine derivatives, thiazide diuretics, and vitamin K derivatives) and toxins.

After exposure to any of these agents, clients experience acute intravascular hemolysis lasting from 7 to 12 days. During this acute phase, anemia and jaundice develop. The hemolytic reaction is self-limited because only older erythrocytes, containing less G6PD, are destroyed.

Collaborative Management

It is imperative that the precipitating drug or the agent responsible for the hemolytic reaction be identified and

totally removed. People should be screened for this deficiency before donating blood, because administration of cells deficient in G6PD can be hazardous for the recipient.

During and immediately after an episode of hemolysis, adequate hydration is essential to prevent precipitation of cellular debris and hemoglobin in the kidney tubules, which can lead to acute tubular necrosis. Osmotic diuretics, such as mannitol (Osmitrol✦), may assist in preventing this complication. Transfusion therapy is indicated when anemia is present and kidney function is normal. Table 42–2 lists indications for transfusion with various types of blood components.

Immunohemolytic Anemia

Overview

Increased RBC destruction through hemolysis can occur in response to many situations, including mechanical trauma, infection (especially malarial infections), and autoimmune reactions. All increase the rate at which RBCs are destroyed by causing lysis (disintegration) of the RBC membrane. The most common types of hemolytic anemias in industrialized countries are the immunohemolytic anemias, also referred to as autoimmune hemolytic anemias (Cotran et al., 1994).

In clients with immunohemolytic anemia, immune system components attack their own RBCs. The exact mechanism that causes immune components to no longer recognize blood cells as self and to initiate destructive processes against RBCs is not known. Some hemolytic anemias are present with other autoimmune disorders (such as systemic lupus erythematosus) or lymphoproliferative disorders. Regardless of the cause, the RBC is viewed as non-self by the immune system and is destroyed.

There are two types of immunohemolytic anemia: warm and cold antibody. The *warm antibody* type is usually associated with immunoglobulin G (IgG) antibody excess. These antibodies are most active at 37° C (98° F) and may be stimulated by drugs, chemicals, or other autoimmune problems. The *cold antibody* type is associated with fixation of complement proteins on immunoglobulin M (IgM), occurs best at 30° C (86° F), and is commonly associated with a Raynaud-like response in which the arteries in the distal extremities constrict profoundly in response to cold temperatures or stress.

Collaborative Management

Treatment depends on clinical severity. Steroid therapy for mild to moderate immunosuppression is the first line of treatment and is temporarily effective in most clients. Splenectomy and more intensive immunosuppressive therapy with cyclophosphamide (Cytoxan, Procytox✣) and azathioprine (Imuran) may be instituted if steroid therapy fails. Plasma exchange therapy to remove attacking antibodies is effective for clients who do not respond to immunosuppressive therapy.

Anemias Resulting from Decreased Production of Red Blood Cells

Anemias associated with decreased RBC production can result from pathologic alterations in any of a variety of physiologic mechanisms. Some anemias arise from failure or inability of the bone marrow to properly synthesize RBCs, others because the body cannot synthesize or absorb a specific component necessary for RBC production.

ELDERLY CONSIDERATIONS

Elderly clients often have restricted diets and may be unable to consume enough meat because of poor dentition or economic reasons, and thus are at risk for iron deficiency anemia (Cotran et al., 1994). The nurse should ask about a family history of anemia. B₁₂ deficiency anemia often occurs in individuals 50 to 80 years of age and may be genetically transmitted.

Iron Deficiency Anemia

Overview

The adult body contains between 2 and 6 g of iron, depending on the size of the person and the amount of hemoglobin in the cells. Approximately two thirds of this iron is contained in hemoglobin; the other third is stored in the bone marrow, spleen, liver, and muscle (see Chap. 41). If a person has an iron deficiency, the iron stores are depleted first followed by the hemoglobin stores. As a result, RBCs are small (microcytic), and the client has relatively mild manifestations of anemia, including weakness and pallor. In iron deficiency anemia, serum ferritin values are less than 12 μg/L.

Iron deficiency anemia is the most common type of anemia and can result from blood loss, increased metabolic energy demands, gastrointestinal malabsorption, and dietary inadequacy. The basic problem of iron deficiency anemia is a decreased supply of iron for the developing RBC. Iron deficiency anemia can occur at any age but is

TABLE 42–3

Common Food Sources of Iron, Vitamin B₁₂, and Folic Acid	
Essential Element	**Common Food Source**
Iron	• Liver (especially pork and lamb) • Red meat • Organ meats • Kidney beans • Whole wheat breads and cereals • Leafy green vegetables • Carrots • Egg yolks • Raisins
Vitamin B₁₂	• Liver • Organ meats • Dried beans • Nuts • Green leafy vegetables • Citrus fruit • Brewer's yeast
Folic acid	• Liver • Organ meats • Eggs • Cabbage • Broccoli • Brussels sprouts

Data from Pennington, J. (1994). *Bowe's and Church's food values of portions commonly used* (16th ed.). Philadelphia: J. B. Lippincott.

more frequent in women, the elderly, and people with poor diets.

Collaborative Management

The primary treatment of clients with iron deficiency anemia is to increase the oral intake of iron, from common food sources, listed in Table 42–3. An adequate diet supplies a person with about 10 to 15 mg of iron per day, of which only 5% to 10% is absorbed (Higgins, 1995). This amount is sufficient to meet the needs of healthy men and healthy women after childbearing age, but is not sufficient to supply the greater needs of menstruating women and adolescents during growth spurts. Fortunately, if iron intake is inadequate or if bleeding or pregnancy occurs, the gastrointestinal (GI) tract is capable of increasing the absorption of iron to about 20% to 30% of the total daily intake (Cotran et al., 1994).

When iron deficiency anemia is severe, iron preparations can be administered intramuscularly. Such preparations are administered using the Z-track method outlined in Chart 42–4.

Vitamin B₁₂ Deficiency Anemia

Overview

Proper production of red blood cells (RBCs) depends on adequate deoxyribonucleic acid (DNA) synthesis in the precursor cells, so mitosis and further maturation into

pins + needles

sias (abnormal sensations) in the feet and the hands and disturbances of balance and gait (Chart 42–5).

Collaborative Management

When anemia is the result of a dietary deficiency, clients must increase their intake of foods rich in vitamin B_{12} (animal proteins, eggs, dairy products). Vitamin supplements may be prescribed when anemia is severe. For clients who have anemia as a result of a deficiency of intrinsic factor, vitamin B_{12} must be administered parenterally on a regular schedule (usually weekly for initial treatment, then monthly for maintenance).

Folic Acid Deficiency Anemia

Overview

Primary folic acid deficiency can also cause megaloblastic anemia. Clinical manifestations are similar to those of vitamin B_{12} deficiency without the accompanying nervous system manifestations, because folic acid does not appear to affect neuronal function. The absence of neurologic problems is an important diagnostic finding to differentiate folic acid deficiency from vitamin B_{12} deficiency. The disease develops slowly, and symptoms may be attributed to other coexisting diseases.

The three common causes of folic acid deficiency are poor nutrition, malabsorption, and drugs. Poor nutrition, especially a diet lacking green leafy vegetables, liver, yeast, citrus fruits, dried beans, and nuts, is the most common cause. Chronic alcohol abuse and parenteral alimentation without folic acid supplement are other dietary causes. Malabsorption syndromes, such as Crohn's disease, are the second most common cause.

Specific drugs impede the absorption and conversion of folic acid to its active form (tetrahydrofolate) and can also lead to folic acid deficiency and anemia. Such drugs include methotrexate, some anticonvulsants, and oral contraceptives.

Collaborative Management

Folic acid deficiency anemia prevention is aimed at identifying high-risk clients, such as the older, debilitated alcoholic; others prone to malnutrition; and those with increased folic acid requirements. A diet high in folic acid

---

Chart 42–4

Nursing Care Highlight: Administering Intramuscular Medications by the Z-Track Method

- Draw medication up into the syringe using aseptic technique.
- Add 0.25 mL of air to the syringe.
- Discard the needle used to draw up the medication.
- Place a new needle (22-gauge, 2–3 inches long) on syringe.
- Make certain that the injection site is in a bright light.
- *Select the dorsal gluteal site only.*
- Identify appropriate landmarks for administration into the upper, outer quadrant.
- Once the site is selected, pull the skin and subcutaneous tissues sideways away from the muscle.
- Clean the site while holding the skin and subcutaneous tissues off to the side.
- Insert the needle deeply into the muscle tissue.
- Aspirate to determine needle placement.
- Iron dextran is black; look very closely to determine whether or not blood is being aspirated into the syringe.
- If blood is aspirated, withdraw needle and begin procedure again from the first step.
- If no blood is aspirated, inject medication slowly, followed by injection of the air-bubble.
- Quickly withdraw the needle.
- Release the skin and subcutaneous tissue.
- *Do not massage the injection site.*

---

functional erythrocytes occur. All DNA synthesis requires adequate amounts of folic acid (folate) to ensure the availability of the nucleotide thymidine, which stimulates DNA synthesis. One function of vitamin B_{12} is to serve as an essential cofactor to activate the enzyme system responsible for transporting folic acid from the extracellular fluid into the cell, where DNA synthesis occurs. Thus, a deficiency of vitamin B_{12} indirectly causes anemia by inhibiting folic acid transportation and limiting DNA synthesis in RBC precursor cells. These precursor cells then undergo improper DNA synthesis and mitosis and increase in size. Only a few are released from the bone marrow. This type of anemia is called *megaloblastic* (macrocytic) because of the large size of these abnormal cells.

Vitamin B_{12} deficiency can result from either inadequate intake (dietary deficiency) or poor absorption from the intestinal tract. Anemia caused by failure to absorb vitamin B_{12} (*pernicious* anemia) results from a deficiency of intrinsic factor (normally secreted by the gastric mucosa) necessary for intestinal absorption of vitamin B_{12}.

Vitamin B_{12} deficiency anemia may be mild or severe, usually develops slowly, and produces few symptoms. Clients usually have severe pallor and slight jaundice. Clients also have glossitis (a smooth, beefy-red tongue), fatigue, and weight loss. Because vitamin B_{12} also is necessary for normal nervous system functioning, especially of the peripheral nerves, clients with pernicious anemia may also have neurologic abnormalities, such as paresthe-

---

Chart 42–5

Key Features of Vitamin B_{12} Deficiency Anemia

- Severe pallor
- Slight jaundice
- Smooth, beefy-red tongue
- Fatigue
- Weight loss
- Paresthesias of the hands and feet — *pins + needles*
- Difficulty with gait

and vitamin B_{12} prevents a deficiency (see Table 42–3). By routinely including assessment of dietary habits in a health history, the nurse can determine which clients are at risk for diet-induced anemias and provide appropriate follow-up.

Aplastic Anemia

Overview

Aplastic anemia is a deficiency of circulating erythrocytes resulting from arrested development of RBCs within the bone marrow. It is caused by an injury to the hematopoietic precursor cell, the pluripotent stem cell. Although aplastic anemia sometimes occurs alone, it is usually accompanied by agranulocytopenia (a reduction in leukocytes) and thrombocytopenia (a reduction in platelets). These three problems occur simultaneously because the bone marrow produces not only RBCs but also white blood cells (WBCs) and platelets. Consequently, if the bone marrow is abnormal for any reason or if it has been exposed to a myelotoxin (any substance toxic and damaging to bone marrow), production of erythrocytes, leukocytes, and thrombocytes slows greatly. Pancytopenia (a deficiency of all three cell types) is common in aplastic anemia. The onset of aplastic anemia may be insidious or rapid.

The development of aplastic anemia, although relatively rare, is associated with chronic exposure to several myelotoxic agents (see Table 41–3).

In about 50% of cases, the cause of aplastic anemia is unknown. Aplastic anemia may occur as a sequela of viral infection (Cotran et al., 1994), but the mechanism of bone marrow damage is unknown.

Collaborative Management

Blood transfusions are the mainstay of treatment for clients with aplastic anemia. Transfusion is indicated only when the anemia causes real disability or when bleeding is life threatening because of thrombocytopenia. Unnecessary transfusion, however, increases the opportunity for the development of immune reactions to platelets, shortens the life span of the transfused cell, and may increase the rate of rejection of transplanted marrow cells. Transfusions are thus discontinued as soon as the bone marrow begins to produce RBCs.

Because clients with some types of aplastic anemia have a disease course consistent with that of autoimmune problems, immunosuppressive therapy may be helpful. Agents that selectively suppress lymphocyte activity, such as antilymphocyte globulin (ALG), antithymocyte globulin (ATG), and cyclosporine (Sandimmune) have brought about partial or complete remissions. In more severe cases, general immunosuppressive agents, such as prednisone and cyclophosphamide (Cytoxan, Procytox◆), have been effective.

Splenectomy is considered in clients with an enlarged spleen that is either destroying normal RBCs or suppressing their development. Bone marrow transplantation in which defective stem cells are replaced has also resulted in a cure for some clients (Cotran et al., 1994). Cost,

availability, and complications limit this technique for treatment of aplastic anemia, however.

Polycythemia

In polycythemia, the number of RBCs in whole blood is greater than normal. Polycythemia is characterized by hyperviscosity, or increased blood thickness. The problem may be transitory, subsequent to other conditions, or chronic. One type of polycythemia, polycythemia vera (PV), is fatal if left untreated.

Polycythemia Vera

Overview

Polycythemia vera is characterized by a sustained increase in blood hemoglobin concentration to 18 g/dL, a red blood cell (RBC) count of 6 million/mm^3, or a hematocrit increase to 55% or greater. PV is an RBC malignancy with three major hallmarks: unrestrained production of massive numbers of RBCs, excessive leukocyte production, and overproduction of thrombocytes. As described in Chart 42–6, extreme hypercellularity of the peripheral blood occurs in people with PV. The skin, especially facial, and mucous membranes have a dark, flushed (plethoric) appearance. These areas may appear purplish or cyanotic because the blood in these tissues is incompletely oxygenated. Most clients experience intense itching related to vasodilation and variation in tissue oxygenation. Blood viscosity is also greatly increased, causing a corresponding increase in vascular friction and peripheral resistance. Superficial veins are visibly distended. Blood moves more slowly through all tissues and thus places increased demands on the pumping action of the heart, resulting in hypertension. In some highly vascular areas, blood flow may become so slow that vascular stasis occurs. Vascular stasis causes thrombosis within the smaller vessels to the extent that the vessels are occluded and the surrounding tissues experience hypoxia, progressing to anoxia and further to infarction and necrosis. Tissues

---

Chart 42–6

Key Features of Polycythemia Vera

- Persistently elevated hematocrit value (>55%)
- Hypertension
- Dark, flushed appearance of the hands and face
- Distention of superficial veins
- Weight loss
- Fatigue
- Intense itching
- Enlarged hemorrhoids
- Swollen, painful joints
- Enlarged, firm spleen
- Infarctions of the heart
  - Chest pain
  - Congestive heart failure
- Cerebrovascular accidents
- Bleeding tendency

most prone to this complication are the heart, spleen, and kidneys, although infarction with loss of tissue and organ function can occur in any organ or tissue.

Because the actual number of cells in the blood is greatly increased and the cells are not completely normal, individual cell life spans are shorter. The shorter life spans, coupled with increased cell production, result in a rapid turnover of peripheral blood cells. This rapid turnover increases the amount of intracellular products (released when cells die) in the blood, adding to the general "sludging" of the blood. These products include uric acid and potassium, which can cause the associated symptoms of gout and hyperkalemia.

Later clinical manifestations of PV are related to abnormal blood cells. Even though the number of circulating erythrocytes is greatly increased, their oxygen-binding capacity is impaired, and clients experience severe generalized hypoxia. In spite of the RBC excess, most clients with PV are susceptible to bleeding problems because of an apparent associated platelet dysfunction (Cotran et al., 1994).

Collaborative Management

Polycythemia vera is a malignant disease that progresses in severity over time. If left untreated, few people with PV live longer than 2 years. Conservative management with repeated phlebotomies (two to five times per week) can prolong life for 5 to 10 years. (Phlebotomy is the routine collection of the client's RBCs to decrease the number of RBCs and diminish blood viscosity.) Maintaining adequate hydration and promoting venous return are essential to prevent thrombus formation. Therapy aims to prevent clot formation and includes the use of anticoagulants. Chart 42–7 lists preventive tips for clients with PV.

As the disease progresses, clients need more intensive therapies that suppress bone marrow activity, including oral alkylating agents and/or irradiation with injections of radioactive phosphorus. Allogeneic bone marrow trans-

---

Chart 42–7

Education Guide: Polycythemia Vera

- Drink at least 3 L of liquids each day.
- Avoid tight or constrictive clothing, especially garters or girdles.
- Wear gloves when outdoors in temperatures lower than 50° F.
- Keep all health care–related appointments.
- Contact your physician at the first sign of infection.
- Take anticoagulants as ordered.
- Wear support hose or stockings while you are awake and up.
- Elevate your feet whenever you are seated.
- Exercise slowly and only on the advice of your physician.
- Stop activity at the first sign of chest pain.
- Use an electric razor, not a manual one.
- Use a soft-bristled toothbrush to brush your teeth.
- Do not floss between your teeth.

---

plantation, an experimental treatment, is promising, but the results are too limited to determine its application to PV.

WHITE BLOOD CELL DISORDERS

As discussed in Chapter 23, white blood cells (WBCs or leukocytes) provide protection from invading non-self cells and cancer cells in several ways. These protective functions depend on maintaining normal numbers and ratios of many specific mature, circulating leukocytes. When any one type of WBC is present in either abnormally high or low amounts, hematopoietic function and immune function may be altered to some degree, placing clients at risk for specific complications. This section covers the pathologic changes and nursing care requirements for clients with disorders characterized by overgrowth of specific types of WBCs. (See Chapter 25 for the pathologic alterations and care requirements for clients with leukocyte-related problems of immunodeficiency, allergy, and autoimmune disorders.)

Leukemia

Overview

The leukemias are a group of malignant disorders involving abnormal overproduction of a specific WBC type, usually at an immature stage, in the bone marrow. Leukemia may be acute, with a sudden onset and short duration, or chronic, with a slow onset and persistent symptoms over a period of years.

Leukemias are categorized by the specific maturational pathway from which the abnormal cells arose (Devine & Larson, 1994). Leukemias in which the abnormal cells arise from within the committed lymphoid maturational pathways (see Figure 23–3) are lymphocytic or lymphoblastic. Leukemias in which the abnormal cells arise within the committed myeloid maturational pathways are myelocytic or myelogenous. Several subtypes exist for each of these diseases, classified by the degree of maturity of the abnormal cell and the specific cell type involved (Table 42–4).

Pathophysiology

The basic pathologic defect in leukemia is a malignant transformation of the stem cells or early committed precursor leukocyte cells, causing an abnormal proliferation of a specific type of leukocyte. The functionally and structurally abnormal immature leukocytes, produced in excessive quantities in the bone marrow, essentially shut down normal bone marrow production of erythrocytes, platelets, and other functionally mature leukocytes. This situation leads to anemia, thrombocytopenia, and leukopenia of the unaffected WBC types, even though the number of immature, abnormal WBCs in the circulation is greatly elevated. Unless treatment is instituted, clients usually die from infection or hemorrhage. For clients with acute leukemias, these pathologic changes occur rapidly and without intervention, progress quickly to death. Chro

TABLE 42–4

Differentiating Characteristics of the Four Types of Leukemia

Leukemia Type	Age at Onset (yr)	Gender Predilection	Racial Predilection	Cell of Origin	Specific Markers	Comments
Acute lymphocytic (ALL)	• <15	• Males	• Caucasian	• B cell	• CALLA+ • Hyperdiploidy • TDT+	• Prognosis poorer for adults than for children • Prognosis better than in AML • Curable in children
Acute myelogenous (AML)	• 15–39	• Equal incidence	• None	• Myeloblast • Myelocyte • Promyelocyte • Myelomonocyte	• TDT– • t(9;22) • t(15;17)	• Prognosis generally poor • Heterogeneous tumor cell populations • Best prognosis with bone marrow transplant
Chronic myelogenous (CML)	• >50	• Males	• None	• Myeloid cell	• Ph¹ chromosome	• Prognosis generally poor; worse if no Ph¹ chromosome • No blockage of maturation of nonmalignant leukocytes • Blastic crisis indicative of more acute disease
Chronic lymphocytic (CLL)	• >50	• Males	• Caucasian	• B cell	• Trisomy 12	• Prognosis poor • Long (4–10 yr) course with rare conversion to acute form • Only leukemia with a possible genetic predisposition

leukemia may be present for many years before overt pathologic changes occur.

Etiology

Epidemiologic studies suggest that many different genetic and environmental factors may be involved in the development of leukemia. Although only a few of these factors have been definitely identified, the basic mechanism appears to involve gene damage of cells, leading to transformation of those cells from a normal to a malignant state. The following constitute possible risk factors: ionizing radiation, chemicals and drugs, marrow hypoplasia, environmental interactions, genetic factors, viral factors, immunologic factors, and the interaction of these factors (Callaghan, 1996).

Ionizing radiation exposure in large quantities appears to be a major risk factor. Exposures ranging from therapeutic irradiation (for such diseases as ankylosing spondylitis and Hodgkin's lymphoma) to environmental irradiation (such as the atomic bomb at Hiroshima or the nuclear accident at Chernobyl) are associated with leukemia.

Chemicals and drugs have been linked to the development of leukemia. Table 41–3 lists many common offenders.

Marrow hypoplasia can increase the risk of leukemia. A reduction or alteration in the production of hematopoietic cells may be responsible. Examples of conditions associated with the later development of leukemia include Fanconi's syndrome, paroxysmal nocturnal hemoglobinuria during its aplastic phase, and myelodysplastic syndromes (Callaghan, 1996).

Genetic factors are suspected as a cause of leukemia because of the increased frequency of leukemia in the following populations: identical twins of clients with leukemia and people with Down syndrome, Bloom syndrome, Fanconi's syndrome, and Klinefelter's syndrome. Chromosomal aberration may be an important factor in these syndromes.

Immunologic factors, especially immune deficiencies, may also favor the development of leukemia. Leukemia among immunodeficient people may be a result of immunosurveillance failure, or the pathologic mechanisms that cause the immune deficiency may also trigger malignant transformation of leukopoietic cells.

Interaction of multiple host and environmental factors may result in leukemia. Because each person tolerates the interaction of these factors differently, it is difficult to determine the origin of any specific leukemia.

Incidence/Prevalence

The leukemias account for 2% of all newly diagnosed cases of cancer and 4% of all cancer deaths (American Cancer Society, 1998). The incidence and frequency of leukemia depend on many factors, including the type of WBC affected, age, gender, race, and geographic locale.

In the United States, an estimated 28,700 new cases of leukemia were projected for 1998 (American Cancer Society, 1998). In this country, leukemia is categorized into any one of four basic types based on the cell type affected and the rate of progression of the leukemia. Characteris-

tics and risk factors associated with these four types of leukemia are presented in Table 42–4.

1. *Acute myelogenous leukemia* (AML) occurs with similar frequency in all ages and is the most common form of leukemia in adults.
2. *Acute lymphocytic leukemia* (ALL) constitutes about 10% of adult leukemias but is most common in children.
3. *Chronic myelogenous leukemia* (CML) constitutes about 20% of adult leukemias, occurring more frequently in people older than 50 years.
4. *Chronic lymphocytic leukemia* (CLL) is the rarest type of leukemia, occurring primarily in people older than 50 years.

Collaborative Management

 Assessment

> ### History

The nurse asks the client about risk factors and causative factors. Age is important because the incidence of adult leukemia increases with age. The client's occupation and hobbies may also reveal specific environmental exposures that increase the risk of leukemia. Previous illnesses and medical history may indicate exposure to ionizing radiation or medications that increase risk as well.

Because of leukemia-related alterations of immune function, the risk for infection is increased in the client with leukemia. The nurse asks the client about the frequency and severity of infectious processes (such as colds, influenza, pneumonia, bronchitis, and unexplained episodes of fever) during the preceding 6 months.

Because platelet function may be diminished in people with leukemia, the nurse questions the client about any overt or hidden excessive bleeding episodes, such as

- A tendency to bruise easily
- Nosebleeds
- Increased menstrual flow
- Bleeding from the gums
- Rectal bleeding
- Hematuria (blood in the urine)
- Prolonged bleeding after minor abrasions or lacerations

If the client has experienced such an episode, the nurse asks whether this type and extent of bleeding constitute the client's usual response to injury or represent a change.

The client with leukemia frequently experiences weakness and fatigue resulting from anemia and increased metabolic and energy demands of the leukemic cells. The nurse asks the client whether he or she has experienced any of the following:

- Headaches
- Behavior changes
- Increased somnolence
- Decreased alertness
- Decreased attention span
- Lethargy, muscle weakness
- Diminished appetite

■ Weight loss
■ Increased fatigue

Listing activities in the previous 24 hours may disclose additional information about activity intolerance, changes in behavior, and unexplained fatigue. The nurse determines how long the client has had any of these debilitating symptoms.

➤ *Physical Assessment/Clinical Manifestations*

Because leukemia affects all blood cells, and blood influences the health and functional capacity of all organs and systems, many areas remote from the actual site of origin of malignant cells may be affected (Chart 42–8). The following clinical manifestations are associated with the acute leukemias (Cotran et al., 1994). Some of these findings may also be present in the client with chronic leukemia in the blast phase.

Cardiovascular Manifestations. These are usually related to anemia. The client's heart rate may be increased and blood pressure decreased. Murmurs and bruits may be present. Capillary filling time is increased.

Respiratory Manifestations. These are primarily associated with anemia and infectious complications. The cli-

---

Chart 42–8

Key Features of Acute Leukemia

Integumentary Manifestations

• Ecchymoses
• Petechiae
• Open infected lesions
• Pallor of the conjunctiva, nail beds, and palmar creases and around the mouth

Gastrointestinal Manifestations

• Bleeding gums
• Anorexia
• Weight loss
• Enlarged liver and spleen

Renal Manifestations

• Hematuria

Cardiovascular Manifestations

• Tachycardia at basal activity levels
• Orthostatic hypotension
• Palpitations

Respiratory Manifestations

• Dyspnea on exertion

Neurologic Manifestations

• Fatigue
• Headache
• Fever

Musculoskeletal Manifestations

• Bone pain
• Joint swelling and pain

---

ent's respiratory rate increases as the degree of anemia becomes greater. If respiratory tract infections are present, the client may experience signs and symptoms of pneumonia, including cough and shortness of breath. Abnormal breath sounds are present on auscultation.

Integumentary Manifestations. The client's skin and mucous membranes may manifest abnormalities. The skin may be pale and cool to the touch as a result of accompanying anemia. Pallor is especially evident on the face, around the mouth, and in the nail beds. The conjunctiva of the eye also is pale, as are the creases on the palmar surface of the hand (most evident when the skin over the palm of the hand is stretched). Petechiae (raised red spots) may be present on any area of skin surface, especially the lower extremities. The petechiae may be unrelated to any obvious trauma. The nurse carefully inspects for any skin infections or traumatized areas that have failed to heal. The nurse also inspects the client's mouth for evidence of bleeding from the gums and any sore or lesion of the oral cavity indicating infection.

Gastrointestinal Manifestations. Gastrointestinal manifestations may be related to increased bleeding tendency and to fatigue. Weight loss, nausea, and anorexia are common. The nurse examines the rectal area for fissures and tests the stool for occult blood. Many clients with leukemia have diminished bowel sounds and constipation. Enlargement of the liver and spleen and abdominal tenderness also may be present from leukemic infiltration of abdominal viscera.

Central Nervous System Manifestations. Cranial nerve disturbances, headache, and papilledema as a result of leukemic infiltration of the meninges or central nervous system (CNS) and, in advanced cases, seizure activity and coma may occur. Although clients often have fever, this manifestation may be more a response to infection than to malignant changes in the CNS.

Miscellaneous Manifestations. Other manifestations include bone and joint tenderness as a result of marrow involvement and bone resorption. Leukemic cell growth or infiltration may produce enlarged lymph nodes or masses.

➤ *Psychosocial Assessment*

The client with newly diagnosed leukemia is extremely anxious, because the average layperson equates a diagnosis of any cancer with a death sentence. Current therapies have greatly improved the prognoses of most cancers, yet the public is largely unaware of these advances. The nurse spends time with the client and family to ascertain what the diagnosis means to them and what they expect from the future. Without knowing the client's expectations and feelings, the nurse cannot educate and provide support in an individualized manner or develop a meaningful plan of care.

A diagnosis of leukemia has dramatic implications for a client's lifestyle. Hospitalization for initial treatment often lasts several weeks, and clients become bored, lonely, and isolated. The nurse assesses the client's coping patterns, including activities that the client finds enjoyable and methods that help the client to relax. A care plan to prevent diversional activity deficit is particularly beneficial for such clients. After initial therapy, the client may be able to resume work, depending on the occupation. However, the client often must make adjustments to accommodate changes in functional status. Repeated hospitalizations may also be necessary.

➤ Laboratory Assessment

The client with acute leukemia usually has decreased hemoglobin and hematocrit levels, a decreased platelet count, and an altered white blood cell (WBC) count. The WBC count may be low, normal, or elevated but usually is quite elevated; counts of 20,000 to 100,000 are common. The client with a higher WBC count on diagnosis has a poorer prognosis (Callaghan, 1996).

The definitive test for leukemia includes various examinations of cells obtained from bone marrow aspiration and biopsy. The bone marrow is full of leukemic blast phase cells. The composition of various cell surface proteins (antigens) on the leukemic cells helps diagnose the type of leukemia (Devine & Larson, 1994). Such markers include the T-11 protein, the enzyme terminal deoxynucleotidyl transferase (TDT), and the common acute lymphoblastic leukemia antigen (CALLA). These markers also indicate prognosis.

Coagulation variables are usually abnormal for the client with acute leukemia. Reduced levels of fibrinogen and other coagulation factors are typical. Whole blood clotting time (Lee-White clotting test) is increased, as is the activated partial thromboplastin time (PTT).

Chromosomal analysis of the malignant bone marrow cells may identify specific marker chromosomes to assist in the diagnosis of leukemia type, predict prognosis, and determine the effectiveness of therapy.

➤ Radiographic Assessment

Specific symptoms determine the feasibility of specific tests. For instance, a client with dyspnea needs chest radiography to determine whether leukemic infiltrates are present in the lung. Skeletal x-rays may help to determine the degree of bone reabsorption present with subperiosteal involvement.

 Analysis

➤ Common Nursing Diagnoses and Collaborative Problems

The following nursing diagnoses are commonly seen in adult clients with acute myelogenous leukemia (AML), the most common type of adult leukemia:
1. Risk for Infection related to decreased immune response
2. Risk for Injury related to thrombocytopenia
3. Fatigue related to decreased tissue oxygenation and increased energy demands

The primary collaborative problem is Potential for Antineoplastic Therapy Adverse Effects.

➤ Additional Nursing Diagnoses and Collaborative Problems

In addition, many clients with AML have one or more of the following nursing diagnoses:
- Impaired Skin Integrity related to prolonged immobility
- Altered Oral Mucous Membrane related to effects of chemotherapy and pancytopenia
- Total Self-Care Deficit related to progressive debilitation and weakness
- Altered Nutrition: Less than Body Requirements related to anorexia, nausea, and vomiting
- Anxiety related to fear of death
- Powerlessness related to an inability to control disease progression
- Altered Family Processes related to acute, life-threatening illness of a family member
- Altered Role Performance related to perceived inability to fulfill parental and other family roles and prolonged hospitalization
- Diversional Activity Deficit related to prolonged hospitalizations.

 Planning and Implementation

Risk for Infection

Planning: Expected Outcomes. After intervention, the client is expected to
- Remain free from cross-contamination–induced infection
- Remain free of autocontamination-induced infection
- Not experience sepsis

Interventions. Infection is a major cause of death in the immunosuppressed client, and septicemia is a common sequela. Infection of the client with leukemia occurs through both *autocontamination* (the client's normal flora overgrows and penetrates the internal environment) and *cross-contamination* (microorganisms from another person or the environment are transmitted to the client). The three most common sites of infection are the skin, respiratory tract, and gastrointestinal tract.

Gram-negative bacteria frequently cause infection, although gram-positive and fungal infections do occur (Dean, Haeuber, & Rivera, 1996). Interventions aim to interrupt or halt the infection processes and control specific infections early. Chart 42–9 emphasizes the importance of thorough assessment for the client at risk for infection. The accompanying client care plan outlines specific interventions for the client with AML.

Drug Therapy for Leukemia. Drug therapy for clients with AML is divided into three distinctive phases: induction, consolidation, and maintenance.

Induction Therapy. This is intensive and consists of combination chemotherapy initiated at the time of diagnosis. This therapy is aimed at achieving a rapid, complete remission of all manifestations of disease (Wujcik, 1996). Institutions and physicians differ in agents used

---

Chart 42–9

Focused Assessment for Hospitalized or Home Care Clients with Potential or Actual Risk for Infection

General Condition

Age, fatigue, malaise
History of allergies
History of chemotherapy, radiation therapy, or other immunosuppressive therapies such as steroid use
Chronic diseases
History of febrile neutropenia and associated symptoms
Nutritional status
Functional status—problems with immobility
Tobacco use—cigarettes, pipe, cigars, oral
Recreational drug use
Alcohol use
Prescribed and over-the-counter medication use
Baseline and ongoing vital signs—blood pressure, heart rate, respiratory rate, and temperature

Skin and Mucous Membranes

Thorough inspection of all skin surfaces with special attention to axilla, perineum (particularly the anorectal area), and under breasts. Inspect skin for color, vascularity, bleeding, lesions, edema, moist areas, excoriation, irritation, erythema. General condition of hair and nails, pressure areas, swelling, pain, tenderness, biopsy or surgical sites, wounds, enlarged lymph nodes, catheters, or other devices
Inspect the oral cavity, including lips, tongue, mucous membranes, gingiva, teeth, and throat—color, moisture, bleeding, ulcerations, lesions, exudate, mucositis, stomatitis, placque, swelling, pain, tenderness, taste changes, amount and character of saliva, ability to swallow, changes in voice, dental caries, client's oral hygiene routine
History of current skin disorders or problems with the mucous membranes

Head, Eyes, Ears, Nose

Pain, tenderness, exudate, crusting, enlarged lymph nodes

Cardiopulmonary

Respiratory rate and pattern, breath sounds (presence/absence, adventitious sounds), quantity and characteristics of sputum, shortness of breath, use of accessory muscles, dysphagia, diminished gag reflex, tachycardia, blood pressure

Gastrointestinal

Pain, diarrhea, bowel sounds, character and frequency of bowel movements, constipation, rectal bleeding, hemorrhoids, change in bowel habits, sexual practices, erythema, ulceration

Genitourinary

Dysuria, frequency, urgency, hematuria, pruritus, pain, vaginal or penile discharge, vaginal bleeding, burning, lesions, ulcerations, characteristics of urine

Central Nervous System

Cognition, level of consciousness, personality, behavior

Musculoskeletal

Tenderness, pain, loss of function

Modified from Dean, G. E., Haeuber, D., & Rivera, L. M. (1996). Infection. In R. McCorkle, M. Grant, M. Frank-Stromborg, & S. Baird (Eds.), *Cancer nursing: A comprehensive textbook* (2nd ed., p. 975). Philadelphia: W. B. Saunders. Used with permission.

---

and the treatment schedule, but a typical course of aggressive chemotherapy includes intravenous (IV) administration of cytosine arabinoside (at 100–200 mg/m² of body surface area per day) for 7 days with concomitant administration of daunorubicin (45 mg/m²/per day) for the first 3 days (Devine & Larson, 1994).

A major side effect of these agents is severe bone marrow suppression. As a result, the client becomes even more vulnerable to infection than before the treatment started. Prolonged hospitalizations are common while the client is immunosuppressed. Recovery of hematopoiesis requires at least 2 to 3 weeks, during which time the

client must be protected from life-threatening infections. Other adverse reactions include nausea, vomiting, diarrhea, alopecia (hair loss), stomatitis, renal toxicity, hepatic toxicity, and cardiac toxicity. For information on nursing management of adverse reactions to antineoplastic agents, refer to Chapter 27.

Consolidation Therapy. This usually consists of another course of either the same agents used for induction at a different dosage or a different combination of chemotherapeutic agents. This treatment occurs early in remission, and its intent is to cure (Ong & Larson, 1995). At

Text continued on page 971

Client Care Plan

The Client with Acute Myelogenous Leukemia

Nursing Diagnosis No. 1: Risk for Infection related to decreased immune response

Expected Outcomes	Nursing Interventions	Rationale
The client is expected to remain free from cross-contamination–induced infection. ■ Limits close contact with other people ■ Maintains a core body temperature of <100° F (38° C) ■ Does not have pathogenic organisms in cultures of blood, urine, or wound drainage	■ Initiate protective isolation procedures according to institutional policy (e.g., thorough hand washing between clients, reverse isolation, private room, wear masks). ■ Keep supplies for the client (e.g., paper cups, straws, dressing materials, gloves) separate from supplies for other clients. ■ Limit the number of care personnel entering the client's room. ■ Have the client maintained in a private room. ■ Limit visitors to healthy adults.	■ These procedures reduce the number of vector-transmissible microorganisms. ■ Separation of these supplies limits the potential for cross-contamination infection. ■ This precaution decreases the client's exposure to non-self microorganisms. ■ Isolation reduces traffic and exposure to non-self microorganisms. ■ This precaution prevents transmission of microorganisms by small children, who may incubate microorganisms and inadvertently transmit them to the client by not adhering to infection control procedures.
	■ Reduce exposure to environmental microorganisms by eliminating raw fruits and vegetables in the client's diet and by not having standing water in the client's room (e.g., remove vases, humidifiers, and water games). ■ Clean the client's room at least once per day.	■ These measures prevent contact with potentially harmful microorganisms. ■ A clean environment inhibits proliferation of environmental microorganisms.
The client is expected to remain free from auto-contamination–induced infection. ■ Complies with prescribed hygiene measures ■ Maintains a core body temperature of <100° F (38° C) ■ Does not have pathogenic organisms in cultures of blood, urine, or wound drainage	■ Instruct or assist the client with daily bathing using antimicrobial soap. ■ Touch the client gently to avoid injuring the skin. ■ Instruct and assist the client to perform oral hygiene every 4 hours, including the use of antimicrobial rinses, mouth swabs, and moisturizing rinses. ■ Change IV tubing every 48 hours.	■ Antisepsis reduces microorganisms on skin surfaces. ■ Keeping the skin intact prevents new portals of entry for microorganisms. ■ Proper hygiene reduces the number of oral tract microorganisms. ■ Fresh tubing reduces the risk for contamination.

(Continued)

Client Care Plan

Nursing Diagnosis No. 1: Risk for Infection related to decreased immune response

Expected Outcomes	Nursing Interventions	Rationale
	■ Prevent rectal trauma by initiating a bowel program, including stool softeners and laxatives and sitz baths.	■ Preventing constipation reduces intestinal stasis and bacterial overgrowth.
	■ Change wound dressings daily, teaching the client or performing central venous catheter site care per institutional protocol.	■ Fresh dressings reduce the number of colony-forming microorganisms at the site of a portal of entry and allow inspection of the site for signs and symptoms of infection.
	■ Teach client to identify signs and symptoms of infections and instruct him or her to inform a health care professional should any new symptom occur.	■ Often clients are more in touch with subtle changes that occur to their own person. Involving the client can help with early detection of infection.
	■ Avoid invasive procedures, such as injections, rectal temperatures, and urinary catheterization.	■ Invasive procedures and trauma can disrupt mucosal linings and skin, resulting in a portal of entry for infectious organisms.
	■ Encourage the client to cough and deep breathe; counsel regarding smoking cessation.	■ These measures help to prevent respiratory infection.
The client is expected to not experience septicemia.	■ Assess the client for signs and symptoms of infection.	■ These assessments identify the infectious process early so that appropriate interventions can be initiated.
■ Does not experience a "left shift" in white blood cell (WBC) populations	■ Measure oral temperature q4h.	
■ Maintains a core body temperature of < 100° F (38° C)	■ Inspect wound areas for redness, swelling, or drainage q8h.	
■ Does not have pathogenic organisms in cultures of blood, urine, or wound drainage	■ Auscultate lungs q8h.	
	■ Check urine for odor and cloudiness.	
■ Maintains a pulse rate and blood pressure (BP) within normal limits	■ Monitor pulse and BP q4h.	
	■ Monitor the differential WBC, especially the absolute neutrophil count (ANC).	■ These values determine the client's risk for infection and indicate a return of immune function.
	■ If symptoms of infection are present, notify the physician immediately and be prepared to	■ Appropriate treatment can be instituted:
	■ Obtain blood specimens through the venous access device and the peripheral vein before antibiotic therapy is initiated.	■ It is important to determine whether microorganisms are present in the blood and whether the venous access device is the source of contamination.

Client Care Plan

Nursing Diagnosis No. 1: Risk for Infection related to decreased immune response

Expected Outcomes	Nursing Interventions	Rationale
	■ Obtain specimens for culture of open lesions, urine, and sputum.	■ It is important to determine the origin of the infection and to identify the infecting organism.
	■ Administer prescribed antibiotic, antifungal, and/or antiviral therapy.	■ These therapeutic measures limit proliferation of microorganisms within the client and prevent progression to sepsis.
The client is expected to not experience injury. ■ Has intact skin and mucous membranes ■ Manifests no bruising or petechiae ■ Does not participate in activities that increase the risk for falls and other injuries	■ Handle the client gently. ■ Use soft-bristle toothbrush or sponge tooth cleaners. Avoid dental floss. ■ Avoid intravenous, intramuscular, and subcutaneous injections. ■ Apply firm but gentle pressure to a needlestick site for at least 10 minutes after removal of the needle. ■ Offer soft foods cool to warm in temperature. ■ Permit the client to use only an electric razor for shaving. ■ Pad side rails and sharp corners of bed. ■ Remove extra furniture from the client's room.	■ Gentle handling prevents trauma to sensitive tissues. ■ It is important to prevent damage to oral mucous membranes. ■ Avoiding injections prevents trauma to the skin and bleeding. ■ Gentle pressure prevents excessive capillary blood loss. ■ These dietary measures avoid mucous membrane injury. ■ Electric razors reduce the risk for abrasions or lacerations. ■ Padding reduces the risk of contusion injuries. ■ Removing extra furniture increases the client's space and reduces the risk of bumping into environmental objects and becoming injured.
	■ Discourage the client from engaging in activities involving the use of sharp objects (e.g., hand sewing, whittling). ■ Use soft cloths, mild soap, and a light touch when bathing the client. ■ Avoid dressing the client in clothing that is tight or rubs. ■ Avoid taking blood pressures with a standard, external, inflatable cuff. ■ Instruct the client to avoid blowing or picking the nose. ■ Avoid rectal suppositories, enemas, and rectal thermometers.	■ Eliminating sharp objects in hobbies reduces the risk of injury. ■ These measures prevent abrasion injury. ■ Loose clothing reduces risk for abrasion injury. ■ It is important to prevent skin injury from cuff pressure. ■ It is important to minimize the risk of trauma to nasal mucous membranes. ■ Rectal mucosa bleeds easily; avoiding these items prevents rectal trauma.

(Continued)

Client Care Plan

Nursing Diagnosis No. 1: Risk for Infection related to decreased immune response

Expected Outcomes	Nursing Interventions	Rationale

The client is expected to not experience significant blood loss.
■ Has normal hematocrit and hemoglobin values
■ Has no manifestation of overt bleeding from wounds or body orifices
	■ Examine the client q4h for signs and symptoms of bleeding, including
	  ■ Increase in abdominal girth
	  ■ Presence of petechiae
	  ■ Oozing from mucous membranes
		■ These measures help determine sites and extent of bleeding.

Nursing Diagnosis No. 2: Risk for Injury related to excessive bleeding secondary to thrombocytopenia

Expected Outcomes	Nursing Interventions	Rationale

■ Maintains pulse rate and BP within normal limits	■ Increase in bruise size
	■ Drainage on dressings and around IV sites
	■ Scleral hemorrhage
	■ Persistent headaches
	■ Vaginal or rectal bleeding
	■ Epistaxis
	■ Examine all body fluids and excrement for the presence of overt or occult blood.
	  ■ Vomitus
	  ■ Urine
	  ■ Stool
	■ Administer ice and topical agents (e.g., Gelfoam, thrombin) to wound sites.
	■ When the client is menstruating, count the number of pads or tampons used and weigh each before and after use.
	
	■ Administer oral medications to stop menses.
	■ Instruct the client in the signs and symptoms of overt and occult hemorrhage.
	
	■ Instruct the client to avoid drug products that contain aspirin and nonsteroidal antiinflammatory drugs (NSAIDs).
	■ Monitor laboratory values (e.g., platelet count, hematocrit, coagulation studies).
	
	■ Administer blood products as ordered.
		
		■ Ice and topical agents promote blood clotting at the wound site.
		■ Noting the number of pads and tampons used during menstruation can help determine the rate and amount of blood loss.
		■ Interrupting menstruation prevents excessive blood loss.
		■ If clients know the signs and symptoms of overt hemorrhage, they can participate in self-care and accept responsibility in health maintenance.
		■ Aspirin and NSAIDs may trigger bleeding episodes. Limiting their use can prevent excess bleeding.
		■ Laboratory findings can pinpoint potential and actual blood loss and help to determine the need for blood product replacement therapy.
		■ This will provide cells necessary for coagulation and tissue oxygenation.

(Continued)

Client Care Plan

Nursing Diagnosis No. 3: Fatigue related to anemia and increased energy demands

Expected Outcomes	Nursing Interventions	Rationale
The client is expected to be able to participate in some self-care activities without becoming excessively fatigued. ■ Verbalizes symptoms of mild fatigue ■ Performs self-care activities within limitations ■ Identifies alternative means of performing daily activities that require less energy than normal	■ Assist the client in selecting food items high in protein and calories. ■ Provide small meals that require little chewing. ■ Administer blood products as ordered. ■ Assist the client in turning and self-care activities. ■ Allow the client to rest between nursing interventions. ■ Cancel activities not essential to the client's immediate well-being.	■ High-protein and high-calorie foods restore nutritional balance and increase available energy substrates. ■ Small meals prevent the client from becoming fatigued while eating. ■ Blood products replace red blood cells and hemoglobin, ameliorating anemia and decreasing fatigue. ■ These measures conserve the client's energy. ■ Rest conserves the client's energy. ■ Eliminating nonessential activities conserves the client's energy.

some institutions, consolidation therapy is a single course of chemotherapy; at others, it involves regularly scheduled, repeated courses of chemotherapy over 1 to 2 years.

Maintenance Therapy. This may be prescribed for months to years after successful induction and consolidation therapies. The purpose is to maintain the remission achieved through induction and consolidation. Maintenance agents are milder and are often given orally for 2 to 5 years. There are conflicting data regarding the effectiveness of maintenance therapy. Future research will help to determine the benefit of different maintenance protocols on the various types of leukemia (Callaghan, 1996).

WOMEN'S HEALTH CONSIDERATIONS

Pregnancy may increase a woman's risk of developing leukemia, although the current data are inconclusive. The diagnosis of acute leukemia during pregnancy forces a woman to face a difficult ethical dilemma regarding treatment. AML is fatal for the mother if not treated aggressively with chemotherapeutic agents, many of which are harmful and potentially lethal to the fetus. A review of the current literature suggests the following findings regarding chemotherapy treatment for AML during pregnancy:

■ Certain chemotherapeutic and supportive agents may be used judiciously in pregnant women.

■ First-trimester treatment can cause severe fetal malformation or miscarriage.
■ Normal live births to mothers treated after the first trimester are well documented.
■ Infants born to mothers treated during the second and third trimesters did not differ from those born to healthy mothers.
■ Side effects experienced by the mother, such as malnutrition, infection, and death, may harm the fetus.

Nursing care for the pregnant client with leukemia focuses on prevention of infection, bleeding, injury, and premature delivery. The nurse assists the client to maintain adequate nutrition and provides resources to help cope with a diagnosis that can be fatal to both the mother and fetus (Ramirez-Smiley & Ingle, 1995).

Drug Therapy for Infection. Drug therapy is the primary defense against infections that develop in clients undergoing therapy for AML. Agents used depend on the sensitivity of the specific organism causing the infection and the extent of the infection, and are categorized by specificity as antibacterial, antiviral, or antifungal. Figure 42–2 outlines pharmacologic management of the febrile neutropenic client.

Antibiotic and Antibacterial Agents. These agents used for prophylaxis or treatment of infection in clients with AML usually include at least one of the aminoglycosides (amikacin, gentamicin, and tobramycin) and a sys-

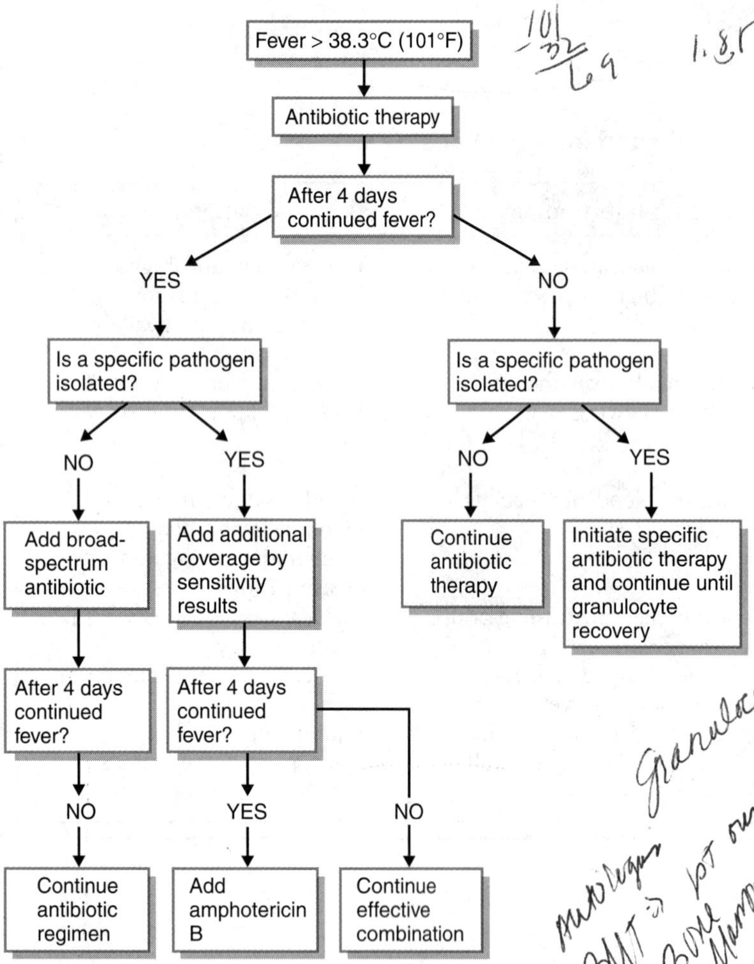

```
                    ┌─────────────────────────┐
                    │ Fever > 38.3°C (101°F)  │
                    └─────────────────────────┘
                                │
                    ┌─────────────────────────┐
                    │   Antibiotic therapy    │
                    └─────────────────────────┘
                                │
                    ┌─────────────────────────┐
                    │      After 4 days       │
                    │   continued fever?      │
                    └─────────────────────────┘
                      │                      │
                    YES                      NO
                      │                      │
        ┌──────────────────────┐   ┌──────────────────────┐
        │ Is a specific pathogen│   │ Is a specific pathogen│
        │      isolated?        │   │      isolated?        │
        └──────────────────────┘   └──────────────────────┘
           │            │              │             │
          NO           YES            NO            YES
           │            │              │             │
  ┌──────────┐  ┌──────────────┐  ┌──────────┐  ┌──────────────┐
  │Add broad-│  │Add additional│  │Continue  │  │Initiate      │
  │spectrum  │  │coverage by   │  │antibiotic│  │specific      │
  │antibiotic│  │sensitivity   │  │therapy   │  │antibiotic    │
  │          │  │results       │  │          │  │therapy       │
  └──────────┘  └──────────────┘  └──────────┘  │and continue  │
       │             │                          │until         │
       │             │                          │granulocyte   │
       │             │                          │recovery      │
       │             │                          └──────────────┘
  ┌──────────┐  ┌──────────────┐
  │After 4   │  │After 4 days  │
  │days      │  │continued     │──────────┐
  │continued │  │fever?        │          │
  │fever?    │  │              │          │
  └──────────┘  └──────────────┘          │
       │             │                    │
      NO            YES                   NO
       │             │                    │
  ┌──────────┐  ┌──────────┐  ┌──────────────┐
  │Continue  │  │Add       │  │Continue      │
  │antibiotic│  │amphoteri-│  │effective     │
  │regimen   │  │cin B     │  │combination   │
  └──────────┘  └──────────┘  └──────────────┘
```

Figure 42–2. Example of antibiotic management for fever in the neutropenic patient.

temic penicillin. Additional, powerful antibiotics used may include vancomycin and drugs from the tetracycline and third-generation cephalosporin classes.

Antifungal Agents. Systemic antifungal agents, used when a fungal infection has been diagnosed or is strongly suggested, include amphotericin B, ketoconazole (Nizoral), and nystatin (Mycostatin, Nadostine✽, Nilstat). In neutropenic clients, antifungal creams such as miconazole nitrate are administered intravaginally to prevent yeast infections.

Antiviral Agents. These are commonly used in clients with leukemia to prevent and treat viral infections. Acyclovir is administered either orally or parenterally before the initiation of antineoplastic agents, especially in clients who are cytomegalovirus positive. If a viral infection is suspected or diagnosed with positive cultures, pharmacologic treatments may include ganciclovir, foscarnet, or steroids (Dean et al., 1996).

The antivirals, although helpful in combating severe infections, are associated with a wide range of serious adverse effects, especially ototoxicity and nephrotoxicity. The nurse carefully monitors the client treated with such drugs for signs of hearing impairment and renal insufficiency.

Infection Control. A major objective in caring for the leukemic client is protection from infection. Nurses and all assistive personnel must use extreme care during all nursing procedures. Frequent, thorough hand washing is of the utmost importance. Anyone with an upper respiratory tract infection who must enter the client's room must wear a mask. Nurses must also observe strict procedures when performing dressing changes or when assisting a physician insert a central venous catheter. The nurse maintains strict aseptic technique in the care of these catheters at all times.

If possible, the nurse ensures that a client is in a private room to minimize cross-contamination. Because infection in the immunosuppressed person is most commonly caused by normal body microorganisms, protective (reverse) isolation has been eliminated from the Centers for Disease Control and Prevention (CDC) guidelines for infection control. However, other environmental precautions are heeded, such as allowing no standing collections of water in vases, denture cups, or humidifiers in the client's room, because they are excellent breeding grounds for microorganisms.

Some institutions prescribe a "minimal bacteria diet" for the client during the neutropenic period. Any uncooked foods, such as raw fruit and vegetables, and pepper are eliminated from the diet because they contain large numbers of microorganisms. Whether clients benefit from this diet is controversial.

In some institutions, the immunosuppressed client is placed in a room with a high-efficiency particulate air (HEPA) filtration or laminar airflow system. These systems decrease the number of airborne pathogens. Again, whether these restrictions benefit clients is debatable.

The nurse continually assesses the client for the presence of infection. This task is difficult because manifestations of infection may not be obvious in the client with leukopenia. The development of fever and the formation of pus (both common indicators of infection) depend on the presence of leukocytes. Therefore, the leukopenic client may have severe infections without pus and with relatively low fevers.

The nurse monitors the client's daily complete blood count (CBC) with differential white blood cell (WBC) count. The nurse inspects the oral mucosa during every nursing shift for lesions indicating fungal or viral infection. The nurse also auscultates the client's lung sounds every 8 hours for crackles, wheezes, or diminished breath sounds. Each time the client voids, the nurse inspects the urine for odor and cloudiness, and then asks the client about any urgency, burning, or pain present on urination.

The nurse takes the client's vital signs at least every 4 hours to assess for fever. A temperature elevation of even 0.5° F or C above baseline is significant for a leukopenic client and indicates infection until proven otherwise.

Many hospital units that specialize in the care of the neutropenic client have specific protocols for antibiotic therapy if infection is suspected. Usually, physicians are notified immediately, and specific specimens are obtained for culture. Blood for bacterial and fungal cultures is obtained from peripheral sites and from the central venous catheter. Urine specimens, sputum specimens, and specimens from open lesions are taken for culture, and chest x-rays taken. After the specimens are obtained, the client begins a regimen of IV antibiotics.

Skin Care. This is important for preventing infection in the leukemic client. The skin may be the client's only intact defense. The nurse teaches the ambulatory client thorough hygiene care and encourages daily bathing. If the client is immobile, turning is necessary every hour and skin lubricants are applied.

Respiratory Care. Respiratory care, including pulmonary hygiene, is performed every 2 to 4 hours. The nurse auscultates the lungs for crackles, wheezes, or diminished breath sounds. The nurse encourages the client to cough and deep breathe or to perform sustained maximal inhalations every hour while awake.

Transplantation. This is now considered a standard treatment for the client with leukemia. This treatment modality began with allogeneic bone marrow transplantation (BMT) (transplantation of human leukocyte antigen [HLA]–identical bone marrow from a sibling) and has advanced to the use of HLA-matched marrow from unrelated donors (Viele, 1996). During the 1980s, autologous BMT was introduced. In this procedure, the donor's own marrow is harvested during a period of remission, frozen, and stored for transplant at a later date. All of these transplant procedures use stem cells harvested from bone marrow.

The newest type of transplantation, peripheral blood stem cell (PBSC) or peripheral blood progenitor cell (PBPC) transplantation, was introduced in the past decade. It involves use of stem cells obtained from the blood rather than the bone marrow (Ford et al., 1996). Multiple pheresis (removal of cells from the plasma) harvests stem cells from the client.

Advances in the field of transplantation have been remarkable. Even as recently as the late 1980s, the client undergoing transplantation would have been seen only in major medical centers. Today, transplant units are becoming commonplace, even in community hospital settings. With long-term survival after transplantation increasing, nurses can expect to be caring for these people if not during the actual transplantation or recovery period, then during the post-transplant period in a variety of health care settings.

Bone marrow transplantation is the treatment of choice for the client with leukemia who has a closely matched donor and who is experiencing temporary remission with induction therapy. Because of BMT success in the client with leukemia, this therapy is now being used for clients with lymphoma, aplastic anemia, inborn errors of metabolism, and many solid tumors (Ford et al., 1996).

For many malignant disorders, the dose-limiting toxicity of treatments is bone marrow suppression. The aim of BMT or PBSC transplantation is to rid the client of all leukemic or other malignant cells through high doses of chemotherapy, often in conjunction with whole body irradiation. These treatments are lethal to the bone marrow and, without replacement of bone marrow function through transplantation of progenitor cells of the hematopoietic system, the client would die of infection or hemorrhage.

The bone marrow is the actual site of production of leukemic cells. Because it can be difficult to ensure that all leukemic cells have been eradicated during induction therapy, the goal is for extremely high doses of chemotherapy to destroy all the affected marrow. The new, healthy marrow then begins the process of hematopoiesis, which results in normal, properly functioning cells and, it is hoped, a permanent cure.

Although marrow donated from a person whose human leukocyte antigens (HLA) match the those of the client is assumed to be disease free, autologous marrow, even if harvested during remission, may contain abnormal cells. In some centers, the harvested autologous marrow is "purged" with chemotherapy or monoclonal antibody treatments to remove any residual leukemia cells. It is not known whether clients who receive purged marrow have better long-term responses than those who receive untreated marrow (Viele, 1996).

Transplantation procedures have five phases: stem cell procurement, conditioning regimen, transplantation, engraftment, and post-transplantation recovery.

Obtaining Stem Cells. Stem cells for transplantation are obtained either by harvest of bone marrow or by pheresis for peripheral blood stem cells. Bone marrow is harvested either from the client directly (autologous marrow) or from an HLA-matched person (allogeneic marrow). For allogeneic marrow, a suitable donor is selected after family members are tested for HLA types. The most preferred transplantations are those between HLA-identical siblings, but transplantation can also be successful between those with closely matched HLA types. The chance of matching with any given sibling is 25%. Several donor registries have been formed that keep records of people willing to donate marrow to provide marrow for clients who do not have a family member HLA match.

After a suitable donor is identified by tissue typing, the donor is taken to the operating room, where sufficient marrow for transplant is harvested through multiple aspirations from the iliac crests. About 500 to 1000 mL of marrow is aspirated, approximately 3% to 5% of the donor's marrow supply (Whedon, 1991). The marrow is then filtered and may be further processed to purge the autologous marrow of any residual cancer cells or to deplete the allogeneic marrow of T cells, which may later cause graft-versus-host disease (GVHD) (described later). Allogeneic marrow is transfused into the recipient immediately; autologous marrow is frozen for later use.

The nurse monitors the donor for signs and symptoms of fluid loss, assesses for complications of anesthesia, and manages postoperative pain. During surgery, donors may lose a significant amount of fluid in addition to the volume of marrow donated. Donors are often hydrated with saline infusions before and immediately after surgery. Occasionally, the donor may require an infusion of packed RBCs.

The nurse assesses the harvest sites to ensure that the dressings are dry and intact and that the donor is not bleeding excessively. Donors often experience pain at the harvest sites (hip), usually managed effectively with oral non–aspirin-containing analgesics. Individual differences do occur, however. Some donors refuse pain medication, but others require opioid analgesics.

There are three phases to obtaining peripheral blood stem cells: mobilization, collection, and reinfusion. During the mobilization phase, chemotherapy or hematopoietic growth factors are administered to the client (Viele, 1996). These agents cause stem cells to circulate in the peripheral blood and the number of WBCs to increase. The stem cells are then collected by pheresis (Ford et al., 1996). Four to seven pheresis procedures, each lasting 2 to 4 hours, are usually required to obtain enough stem cells for PBSC transplantation (Jassak & Riley, 1994). The stem cells are then frozen and stored for reinfusion after the conditioning regimen.

The nurse must monitor the patient closely during pheresis. Common complications include catheter clotting, which may delay pheresis, or hypocalcemia caused by anticoagulants. The client with hypocalcemia may experience chills, paresthesia, abdominal or muscle cramping, or chest pain, and the nurse may need to administer oral calcium supplements to manage these symptoms. The nurse must also monitor vital signs frequently. The client may experience hypotension as a result of fluid volume changes during the procedure.

Conditioning Regimen. Figure 42–3 outlines the timing and steps typically involved in bone marrow transplantation. The day the client receives the bone marrow is considered day T-0. Pretransplantation conditioning days are counted in reverse chronologic order from T-0, just like a rocket countdown. Post-transplantation days are counted in chronologic order from day of transplantation to discharge.

The client must first undergo a conditioning regimen, which varies with the diagnosis and type of transplant to be received. The conditioning regimen serves two purposes: to obliterate, or "wipe out," the client's own bone marrow, thus preparing the client for optimal graft take, and to give higher than normal doses of chemotherapy and/or radiotherapy to obliterate, or wipe out, a malignancy, such as breast cancer. Usually, anywhere from 5 to 10 days is required. The conditioning regimen always includes intensive chemotherapy and sometimes includes radiotherapy, usually total body irradiation (TBI). Each conditioning regimen is individually tailored with the client's specific disease, overall health, and previous treatment taken into account.

A typical conditioning regimen for an adult client receiving an allogenic bone marrow transplant for treatment of acute myelogenous leukemia (AML) is as follows (Workman et al., 1993):

1. Days T-7 through T-5: high-dose chemotherapy to obliterate the client's own bone marrow cells and to eradicate any remaining leukemic cells. Specific agents include busulfan, carmustine, cyclophosphamide, cytosine arabinoside, etoposide, and melphalan. The dosages are many times higher than those used for normal chemotherapy (Ford et al., 1996).

2. Days T-4 through T-2: delivery of fractionated TBI (smaller doses of radiation given over a period of time instead of one larger dose). The typical radia-

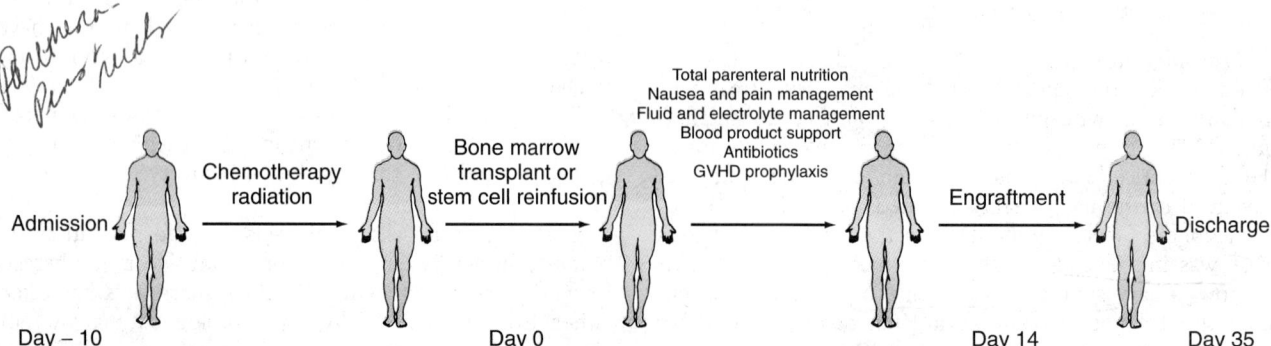

Figure 42–3. Timing and steps of allogeneic bone marrow transplantation. (GVHD = graft-versus-host disease.)

tion dose for TBI is 1200 rad. The client usually receives no cell-killing treatment on day T-1. During conditioning, bone marrow and normal tissues begin to respond immediately to the chemotherapy and radiotherapy. The client experiences all the expected side effects associated with both therapies. Because the chemotherapy is administered in such high doses, these side effects are much more intense than those seen with either normal chemotherapy or radiation. These side effects include severe nausea and vomiting, mucositis, capillary leak syndrome, diarrhea, and bone marrow suppression.

Late effects from the conditioning regimen are also common, occurring as late as 3 to 10 years after transplantation, and include veno-occlusive disease (VOD), skin toxicities, cataracts, fibrotic pulmonary disease, secondary malignancies, cardiomyopathy, endocrine complications, and neurologic complications.

Transplantation. Day T-0, transplantation day, is separated from the chemotherapy conditioning by at least 2 days to ensure that the chemotherapeutic agent has cleared and will not exert any cytotoxic effects on the transplanted stem cells. The client should have few, if any, circulating WBCs at this point, indicating successful conditioning.

The transplantation itself is very simple. Frozen marrow or PBSCs are thawed in a warm water bath (37°–40° C [99°–102° F]) (Jassak & Riley, 1994). The bone marrow is administered through the client's central catheter like an ordinary blood transfusion but not using blood administration tubing. Usually, the marrow is infused over a 30-minute period, although it may also be administered by IV push directly into the central catheter with syringes.

Side effects of BMT and PBSC transfusion are similar. The client may experience fever and hypertension as a result of a reaction to dimethylsulfoxide (DMSO), the preservative used for storage of stem cells (Ford et al., 1996). To prevent these reactions, the nurse administers acetaminophen, hydrocortisone, and diphenhydramine before the transfusion. Antihypertensives or diuretics may also be required to treat fluid volume changes (Jassak & Riley, 1994). The client may experience red urine secondary to hemolysis of erythrocytes in the infused product.

Engraftment. The transfused PBSCs and marrow cells circulate only briefly in the peripheral blood. Most of the cells, especially the stems cells, find their way to the marrow-forming sites of the recipient's bones and establish residency there. The mechanism by which the donated marrow cells "home in" on the appropriate sites is not yet understood.

Engraftment is the key to the whole transplantation process. In order for the donated marrow or PBSCs to "rescue" the client after large doses of chemotherapy and/or radiotherapy wipe out his or her own bone marrow, the transfused stem cells must survive and grow in the clients' bone marrow sites. When successful, the engraftment process takes 2 to 5 weeks, when the client's WBC, erythrocyte, and platelet counts begin to rise.

Prevention of Complications. The post-transplantation period is difficult. Because the client remains without any natural immunity until the transfused stem cells begin to

proliferate and engraftment occurs, infection and severe thrombocytopenia are major problems. The nursing care requirements for this client are virtually identical to those for the client undergoing aggressive induction therapy for AML. Helping the client to maintain hope through this long recovery period is difficult (Larson, 1995). Complications are often severe and life threatening. The nurse should try to encourage the client to maintain a positive attitude and be involved in his or her own recovery (Research Applications for Nursing).

In addition to the problems related to the period of pancytopenia (too few circulating blood cells), other immediate hazards associated with BMT include failure to engraft, development of GVHD, and VOD.

Failure to Engraft. Sometimes the donated marrow or PBSCs fail to engraft. This possibility is discussed in advance with the client and the donor. Failure to engraft occurs more frequently among allogeneic trans-

► Research Applications for Nursing

What Are the Client's Perceptions of Needs After Bone Marrow Transplantation?

Larson, P. J. (1995). Perceptions of the needs of hospitalized patients undergoing bone marrow transplantation. Cancer Practice, 3(3), 173–179.

This qualitative descriptive study identified patient needs during the first 4 weeks after bone marrow transplant (BMT). A sample of 30 patients were interviewed four times during their hospital stay at approximately 1-week intervals. A constant comparative analysis suggested the following care needs: week 1, team effort of cure; week 2, management of symptoms and side effects; week 3, getting better; week 4, recovery and returning home. Patients perceived that they, as well as physicians, nurses, and family, were responsible for meeting these needs.

Other findings included that patients viewed physicians as in charge of planning and monitoring medical care and verifying that progress was satisfactory. Nurses were perceived as "responsible for carrying out medical orders, managing symptoms, and keeping things in order." The patients wanted family members to be emotionally supportive and to take care of nonmedical needs. Patients perceived their own role as maintaining a positive attitude and participating in their recovery.

Critique. The study was an excellent attempt to capture patients' perceptions of care needs during hospitalization for BMT. The small sample size and the fact that interviews were only conducted at two West Coast BMT centers limited the generalizability of the results. This study further limited its scope to the short-term needs of hospitalized BMT patients. Additional studies are needed to assess patient needs over longer periods of time.

Possible Nursing Implications. Nurses can discuss with patients expectations of their care needs throughout the hospital stay. Helping patients maintain realistic self-expectations and hope is important. Nurses can also monitor emotionally and physically labile periods, which often occur at week 3 or 4, when providing support and managing symptoms is critical.

plant recipients than among autologous marrow or PBSC transplant recipients. The causes may be related to insufficient numbers of cells transplanted, attack or rejection of donor cells by residual immunologically competent recipient cells, infection of transplanted cells, and unknown biological factors. If the transplanted marrow or PBSCs fail to engraft, the client will die unless another transplantation is successful.

Graft-Versus-Host Disease. GVHD is an immunologic event that occurs if the recipient is not immunocompetent and the donor tissue has active leukocytes, especially effector T cells and T-cell precursors. Because the recipient is totally immunosuppressed, the recipient cannot recognize the donated bone marrow cells as foreign or non-self. Instead, the immunocompetent cells of the donated marrow recognize the client's (recipient) cells, tissues, and organs as foreign and mount an immune offense against them. The graft is actually trying to attack the host.

Although all host tissues can be attacked and harmed, the tissues most commonly damaged are the skin, gastrointestinal tract, and liver. Approximately 30% to 70% of all allogeneic BMT recipients experience some degree of GVHD, and more than 15% of the clients who experience GVHD die from its complications (Whedon, 1991). The presence of GVHD indicates that the transplanted cells are competent and have successfully engrafted.

Clients with GVHD are managed with immunosuppressive agents and support of the systems sustaining the heaviest damage. Care is taken to avoid suppressing the new immune system to the extent that either the client becomes more susceptible to infection or the transplanted cells stop engrafting.

Veno-Occlusive Disease. VOD involves occlusion of the hepatic venules by thrombosis and phlebitis. This condition occurs in up to 20% of clients who receive a BMT, and symptoms usually occur within the first 30 days after transplantation. Clients who have received high doses of chemotherapy, especially alkylating agents, are at risk for life-threatening hepatic complications. Clinical signs include jaundice, pain in the right upper quadrant, ascites, weight gain, and liver enlargement.

Because there is no known way of opening the hepatic vessels, treatment is supportive. Early detection enhances the chances of client survival. Fluid management is also crucial. The nurse assesses the client daily for weight gain, fluid accumulation, increases in abdominal girth, and hepatomegaly (Ford et al., 1996).

Risk for Injury

Because normal bone marrow production is severely limited in the client with AML, the number of circulating platelets is severely diminished, creating thrombocytopenia. This condition puts the client with AML at a greatly increased risk for excessive bleeding in response to minimal trauma.

Planning: Expected Outcomes. After intervention, the client is expected to remain free from bleeding.

Interventions. As a result of chemotherapy-induced pancytopenia, the client's platelet count is decreased. During the period of greatest bone marrow suppression (the nadir), the platelet count may be extremely low ($<10,000/mm^3$). The client is at great risk for bleeding once the platelet count falls below $50,000/mm^3$, and spontaneous bleeding frequently occurs when the platelet count is lower than 20,000 (Lin & Beddar, 1996). The nurse's major objectives are to protect the client from situations that could lead to bleeding and to closely monitor any bleeding that does occur.

The nurse assesses the client frequently for evidence of bleeding: oozing, confluent ecchymoses, petechiae, or purpura. All stools, urine, nasogastric drainage, and vomitus are examined visually for blood and tested for occult blood. The nurse measures any blood loss as accurately as possible and measures the client's abdominal girth during every nursing shift. Increases in abdominal girth can indicate internal hemorrhage. Bleeding precautions are instituted (Chart 42–10).

The nurse also monitors laboratory values daily. CBC results are reviewed daily to determine the client's risk for bleeding as well as actual blood loss. The client with a platelet count below $20,000/mm^3$ may need a platelet transfusion. For the client with severe blood loss, packed RBCs may be ordered (see Transfusion Therapy later).

Chart 42–10

Nursing Care Highlight: Bleeding Precautions

- Handle the client gently.
- Use a lift sheet when moving and positioning in bed.
- Avoid intramuscular injections and venipunctures.
- When injections or venipunctures are necessary, use the smallest gauge needle for the task.
- Apply firm pressure to the needlestick site for 10 minutes or until the site no longer oozes blood.
- Apply ice to areas of trauma.
- Test all urine and stool for the presence of occult blood.
- Observe IV sites every 2 hours for bleeding.
- Avoid trauma to rectal tissues:
  - Do not take temperatures rectally.
  - Do not give enemas.
  - Administer well-lubricated suppositories with caution.
  - Advise client not to have anal intercourse.
- Measure abdominal girth daily.
- Teach the client to use an electric razor.
- Teach the client to avoid mouth trauma:
  - Use soft-bristled toothbrush or tooth sponges.
  - Do not floss between teeth.
  - Avoid dental work, especially extractions.
  - Avoid hard foods.
  - Make sure that dentures fit and do not rub.
- Encourage the client not to blow the nose or insert objects into the nose.
- Teach the client to avoid contact sports.
- Teach client to wear shoes with firm soles whenever ambulating.

Fatigue

Because normal bone marrow production is severely limited in clients with AML, the number of circulating erythrocytes is severely diminished, creating a condition of anemia, leading in turn to fatigue. Because leukemic cells tend to have higher rates of metabolism and greater utilization of oxygen, the anemic client with leukemia is at risk for severe fatigue.

Planning: Expected Outcomes. After appropriate intervention, the client is expected to
- Experience no increase in fatigue
- Recognize symptoms of fatigue and alter activity before fatigue becomes excessive

Interventions. These are aimed at decreasing the effects of anemia and conserving the client's energy expenditure.

Diet Therapy. Diet therapy is indirectly related to fatigue and subsequent activity intolerance. The client must ingest enough calories to meet at least basal energy requirements, but increasing dietary intake can be difficult when the client is extremely fatigued. The nurse thus provides small, frequent meals high in protein and carbohydrates. Food items that are liquid or easy to chew also require less effort to eat.

Blood Replacement Therapy. Blood transfusions are sometimes indicated for the client with fatigue. Transfusions increase the blood's oxygen-carrying capacity and replace missing RBCs and some coagulation factors (see Table 42-3). For the leukemic client experiencing fatigue related to anemia, packed RBCs are usually the blood component of choice. (See Transfusion Therapy for a discussion of nursing care during transfusions.)

Drug Therapy. Clients may receive subcutaneous injections of epoetin alfa (Epogen or Procrit) 50 to 100 U/kg three times per week (DeLaPena et al., 1996). This growth factor is naturally secreted by the kidney and boosts the production of RBCs. Epoetin alfa has previously been used in anemia associated with chronic renal failure and human immunodeficiency virus (HIV) clients receiving zidovudine and is now approved for use in anemia associated with chemotherapy (Rieger & Haeuber, 1995).

The nurse administers injections three times a week and assesses for side effects such as hypertension, headaches, fever, myalgia, and rashes (DeLaPena et al., 1996). For more information on hematopoietic growth factors, see Chapter 27.

Conservation of Energy. The nurse examines the hospitalized client's schedule of prescribed and routine activities. Those activities that do not have a direct positive effect on the client's condition are assessed in terms of their usefulness to the client. If the actual or potential benefit of an activity is less than its actual or potential worsening of the client's fatigue, the nurse consults with other members of the health care team about eliminating or postponing it. Candidates for cancellation or postpone-

ment include hair washing, physical therapy, and certain invasive diagnostic tests not required for assessment or treatment of current problems.

 Continuing Care

The leukemic client is discharged after induction chemotherapy or transplantation. Follow-up care is provided on an outpatient basis.

➤ *Home Care Management*

Planning for home care for the client with leukemia begins as soon as a client achieves remission. The client will need assistance at home until the condition improves. The nurse assesses the available support mechanisms. Many clients require the services of a visiting nurse to assist with dressing changes for central venous catheters, to assist with hyperalimentation infusions, to transfuse platelets, and to answer questions. Occasionally, the client may require home transfusion therapy for one or more blood components as well (Randolph et al., 1995).

➤ *Health Teaching*

The client and the family need to be educated about the importance of continuing therapy and appropriate medical follow-up, despite the unpleasant side effects of therapy. Many clients go home with a central venous catheter in place and require instructions about its care and maintenance. Chart 42-11 lists general guidelines for central venous catheter care at home. These guidelines may be altered depending on the home setting, assistance available, and agency policy.

Protecting the client from infection after discharge from the hospital is just as important as when the client was

---

Chart 42-11

Education Guide: Home Care of the Central Venous Catheter

- To maintain patency, flush the catheter briskly with heparinized saline (10 U/mL) once a day and after completing infusions.
- Change the Luer-lok cap on each catheter lumen weekly.
- Change the dressing every other day:
  - Use clean technique with thorough hand washing.
  - Clean the exit site with alcohol and povidone-iodine (Betadine).
  - Apply antibacterial ointment to the site.
  - Cover the site with dry sterile gauze dressing, taped securely, or with transparent adherent dressing.
- To prevent tension, always tape the catheter to yourself.
- Look for and report any signs of infection (redness, swelling, or drainage at the exit site).
- In case of a break or puncture in the catheter lumen, immediately clamp the catheter between yourself and the opening. *Notify your physician immediately.*

hospitalized. (See Chart 42–9 for focused assessment for the client at risk for infection.) The nurse urges the client to use proper hygiene and avoid crowds or others with infections. Neither the client nor any household member should receive live virus immunization (poliomyelitis, measles, or rubella) for 1 year after transplantation. The client should continue mouth care regimens at home. The nurse emphasizes that the client should immediately notify the physician if he or she experiences any fever or other sign of infection.

Because platelet recovery is usually slower than that of white blood cells (WBCs), many clients return home still at risk for bleeding. The nurse reinforces the safety and bleeding precautions initiated in the hospital, emphasizing that the client follow these precautions until the platelet count is above 50,000. The nurse also instructs the client and family to assess for petechiae, avoid trauma and sharp objects, apply pressure to wounds for 10 minutes, and report any unusual symptoms, including blood in the stool or urine, or headache that does not respond to acetaminophen.

Psychosocial Preparation

The nurse's responsibility in psychosocial preparation of the client before discharge is very important. A diagnosis of leukemia threatens the client's self-esteem and family role (Larson, 1995). The client is confronted with the reality of death, and treatment causes major adjustments in self-image. The client and family also experience changes in the client's body image, level of independence, and lifestyle. Some clients feel threatened by their environment, seeing everything as potentially infectious. The nurse helps the client and family redefine priorities, understand the illness and its treatment, and find hope. The nurse makes referrals to support groups sponsored by organizations such as the American Cancer Society ("I Can Cope" and "Make Today Count"), which can be enormously beneficial to both the client and the family.

➤ Health Care Resources

The client with limited social support may need assistance at home until strength and energy return. A home care aide may suffice for some clients, whereas a visiting nurse may be needed for other clients to reinforce teaching. The client may also need equipment to facilitate ADLs and ambulation. Financial resources are assessed. Treatment of cancer is expensive, and the nurse works closely with the local social services department to ensure that insurance is adequate. If the client is uninsured, other sources, such as drug-company sponsored compassionate aid programs, are explored. The Leukemia Society of America, Inc., offers limited financial assistance for clients with leukemia, sponsors support groups, and provides publications for clients and health care providers.

Prolonged outpatient contact and follow-up will be necessary, and clients will need transportation to the outpatient facility. Many local divisions of the American Cancer Society offer free transportation to clients with cancer, including leukemia.

 Evaluation

The nurse evaluates the care of the client with leukemia based on the identified nursing diagnoses. The expected outcomes include that the client will

- Remain free from cross-contamination–induced infection
- Remain free of autocontamination-induced infection
- Not experience sepsis
- Remain free from episodes of bleeding
- Not experience an increase in fatigue
- Recognize symptoms of fatigue and alter activity before fatigue becomes excessive

Malignant Lymphoma

Malignant lymphomas reflect abnormal proliferation of one type of leukocyte (lymphocytes), but differ from the leukemias in the degree of differentiation of the affected cells and the location of cell production. Lymphomas are malignancies characterized by a proliferation of committed lymphocytes rather than stem cell precursors (as in leukemia). This proliferation occurs not in bone marrow but in other lymphoid tissues scattered throughout the body, especially the lymph nodes and spleen. Lymphomas are actually solid tumors rather than cellular suspensions within the blood and bone marrow, and fall into two major categories among adults: Hodgkin's and non-Hodgkin's.

Hodgkin's Lymphoma
Overview

Hodgkin's lymphoma is a cancer that can affect any age group, although incidence peaks first in people in their mid-to-late 20s and then in people older than 50. Men and women are affected equally in the first group, but the disease is more prevalent in men in the older group (Carson, 1996).

Factors implicated as possible causes of Hodgkin's lymphoma include viral infections and previous exposure to alkylating chemical agents. This cancer usually originates in a single lymph node or a single chain of nodes. The lymphoid tissues within the node undergo malignant transformation, usually initiating some inflammatory processes. These nodes contain a specific transformed cell type, the Reed-Sternberg cell, a characteristic marker of Hodgkin's lymphoma. The disease first metastasizes (spreads) to other adjacent lymphoid structures and eventually invades nonlymphoid tissues.

Collaborative Management

Assessment most often reveals a greatly enlarged but painless lymph node or nodes, usually the earliest manifestation of Hodgkin's lymphoma. The client also often experiences fever, malaise, and night sweats (Table 42–5). More specific clinical manifestations depend on the site (or sites) of malignancy and the extent of disease.

Diagnosis and grade are established when biopsy of a node or mass reveals Reed-Sternberg cells. The client then

TABLE 42-5

Manifestations and Staging Criteria for Hodgkin's Lymphoma	
Stage	**Manifestations**
Stage Ia	• Disease is confined to a single lymph node region or only one extranodal site.
Stage Ib	• Disease is confined to a single lymph node region or only one extranodal site. The client also experiences some or all of the following systemic symptoms: persistent fever, night sweats, and significant weight loss (>10%).
Stage IIa	• Disease is confined to either two or more lymph node regions on the same side of the diaphragm or contiguous extranodal sites on the same side of the diaphragm.
Stage IIb	• Disease is confined to either two or more lymph node regions on the same side of the diaphragm or contiguous extranodal sites on the same side of the diaphragm. Client also experiences some or all of the following systemic symptoms: persistent fever, night sweats, and significant weight loss (>10%).
Stage IIIa	• Disease extends to lymph node regions on both sides of the diaphragm.
Stage IIIb	• Disease extends to lymph node regions on both sides of the diaphragm. The client also experiences some or all of the following systemic symptoms: persistent fever, night sweats, and significant weight loss (>10%).
Stage IIIc	• Disease extends to lymph node regions on both sides of the diaphragm. The client also experiences some or all of the following systemic symptoms: persistent fever, night sweats, and significant weight loss (>10%). The spleen is also involved in disease.
Stage IV	• Disease has widely disseminated foci of involvement, including one or more extranodal tissues and organs.

undergoes extensive staging procedures to determine the exact extent of disease (see Table 42-5). Staging must be detailed and accurate because the treatment regimen is determined by the extent of disease. Staging procedures for Hodgkin's lymphoma include biopsies of distant lymph nodes, lymphangiography, computed tomography (CT) of the thorax and the abdomen, CBC, liver function studies, and bilateral bone marrow biopsies.

Such great progress has been made in treatment regimens that Hodgkin's lymphoma is now one of the most curable types of cancer. Generally, for stage I and II disease without mediastinal node involvement, the treatment of choice is extensive external radiation of involved lymph node regions. With more extensive disease, radiation coupled with an aggressive multiagent chemotherapy

regimen is most effective in achieving a cure. (See Chapter 27 on general care of clients receiving radiation and/or chemotherapy.)

Specific nursing management of the client undergoing treatment for Hodgkin's lymphoma focuses on the side effects of therapy, especially

- Drug-induced pancytopenia, which results in increased risk for infection, bleeding, and anemia
- Severe nausea and vomiting
- Skin irritation and breakdown at the site of radiation
- Impaired hepatic function either by metastasis to the liver or by the multiagent chemotherapy
- Permanent sterility for male clients receiving radiation in an inverted-Y pattern to the abdominopelvic region along with specific chemotherapeutic agents (client should be informed of this side effect and given the option to store sperm in a sperm bank before treatment)

Non-Hodgkin's Lymphoma

Overview

Non-Hodgkin's lymphoma is the classification for all cancers originating from lymphoid tissues that are not diagnosed as Hodgkin's lymphoma. There are more than 12 subtypes of non-Hodgkin's lymphoma, including low grade, intermediate, and high grade.

The low-grade lymphomas usually arise from B-cell lymphocytes and progress slowly. Although clients with low-grade lymphomas have longer survival rates, the diseases are less responsive to treatment, and consequently, cures are rare.

At the other end of the spectrum are the high-grade lymphomas, which are aggressive tumors of usually mixed cellularity with rapid doubling times. High-grade lymphomas are more responsive to chemotherapy, and the chances for a long-term cure are greater.

Most non-Hodgkin's lymphomas arise from lymph nodes but can originate in virtually any tissue or organ. A low-grade lymphoma also can convert to a higher grade lymphoma. Most non-Hodgkin's lymphomas occur among older adults. Definitive causes are unknown, but viral infection, exposure to ionizing radiation, and exposure to toxic chemicals have all been implicated.

Collaborative Management

Because lymphomas may arise from lymphoid cells in any tissue and because the malignancy can spread to any organ, assessment reveals no specific clinical manifestations other than lymphadenopathy common to all types of lymphoma. Diagnosis is made from the histologic features apparent on biopsy of any suspicious node or mass. Classification of specific lymphoma subtype is based on a complex grading of surface markers, cytogenetic features, cell size, and expression of viral antigens. Staging is similar to that for Hodgkin's lymphoma (see Table 42-5).

Depending on the cell type, prognosis ranges from excellent to poor. Overall, however, clients with non-

Hodgkin's lymphomas have a poorer prognosis than those with Hodgkin's lymphoma. Some types of non-Hodgkin's lymphoma run a protracted course, extending over many years, and are not treated in the early phases. However, for most types of non-Hodgkin's lymphoma, death ensues rapidly if clients are not treated. Treatment consists of radiation therapy and multiagent chemotherapy. Nursing care needs are similar to those for clients with Hodgkin's lymphoma, with additional organ-specific problems taken into account if the disease is widely disseminated.

COAGULATION DISORDERS

Coagulation disorders are synonymous with bleeding disorders, and are characterized by abnormal or increased bleeding resulting from defects in one or more components regulating hemostasis. Bleeding disorders may be spontaneous or traumatic, localized or generalized, life-long or acquired. They can originate from a defect in the hemostatic processes at the vascular, platelet, or clotting

factor level. Figure 42–4 outlines blood clotting cascades and sites where specific defects and drugs disrupt the hemostatic processes.

Platelet Disorders

Platelets play a vital role in hemostasis. For both the intrinsic and extrinsic pathways, coagulation starts with platelet adhesion and formation of a platelet plug. Any condition that either diminishes the number of platelets or interferes with their ability to adhere (to one another, blood vessel walls, collagen, or fibrin threads) can be manifested as increased bleeding. Platelet disorders can be inherited, acquired, or temporarily induced by the ingestion of substances that limit platelet production or inhibit aggregation.

A drop in the number of platelets below the level needed for normal coagulation is called *thrombocytopenia* (Lapka et al., 1994). Thrombocytopenia may occur as a result of other conditions or treatments that suppress gen-

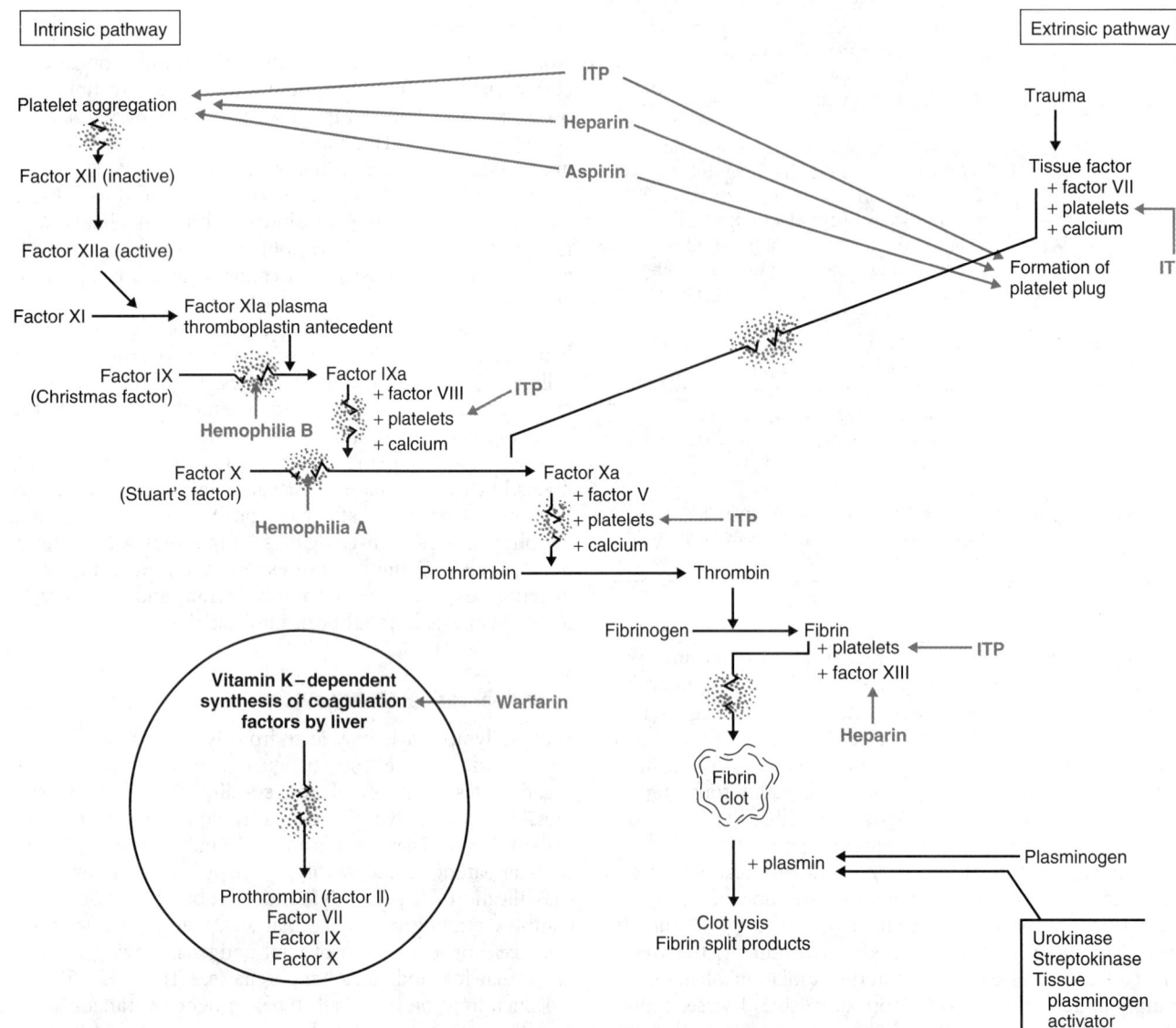

Figure 42–4. Sites of disruption of the coagulation mechanisms by drugs and disease. (ITP = idiopathic thrombocytopenic purpura.)

eral bone marrow activity. It also can occur through processes that specifically limit platelet formation or increase the rate of platelet destruction. The two thrombocytopenic conditions affecting adults are autoimmune thrombocytopenic purpura and thrombotic thrombocytopenic purpura.

Autoimmune Thrombocytopenic Purpura

Overview

Before the underlying cause of autoimmune thrombocytopenic purpura was identified, this condition was known as idiopathic thrombocytopenic purpura (ITP). Although the cause is now thought to be an autoimmune reaction, the condition is still commonly known as ITP. The total number of circulating platelets is greatly diminished in ITP, even though platelet production in the bone marrow is normal.

Clients with idiopathic thrombocytopenic purpura make an antibody directed against the surface of their own platelets (an antiplatelet antibody). This antibody coats the surface of the platelets, making them more susceptible to attraction and destruction by phagocytic leukocytes, especially macrophages (see the discussion of opsonization in Chapter 23). Because the spleen contains a large concentration of fixed macrophages and because the blood vessels of the spleen are long and tortuous, antibody-coated platelets are destroyed primarily in the spleen. When the rate of platelet destruction exceeds that of production, the number of circulating platelets decreases and blood clotting slows.

Although the cause of this disorder appears to be autoimmune, the exact mechanism initiating the production of autoantibodies is unknown. ITP is most common among women between the ages of 20 and 40 and among people with a pre-existing autoimmune condition, such as systemic lupus erythematosus (Cotran et al., 1994).

Collaborative Management
Clinical Manifestations

Clinical manifestations associated with ITP are generally limited to the skin and mucous membranes: large ecchymoses (bruises) on the arms, legs, upper chest, and neck or a petechial rash. Mucosal bleeding occurs easily. If the client has experienced significant blood loss, signs of anemia may also be present.

A rare complication is an intracranial bleeding–induced cerebrovascular accident. The nurse assesses the client for neurologic function and mental status (see Chap. 43). The nurse asks family members or significant others if the client's behavior and responses to the mental status examination are typical or represent a change from usual reactions.

Diagnosis

Idiopathic thrombocytopenic purpura is diagnosed by a decreased platelet count and large numbers of megakaryocytes in the bone marrow. Antiplatelet antibodies may be present in detectable levels in peripheral blood. If the client experiences any episodes of bleeding, hematocrit and hemoglobin levels also are low.

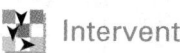 Interventions

➤ *Nonsurgical Management*

As a result of the decreased platelet count, the client is at great risk for bleeding. Interventions include therapy for the underlying condition as well as protection of the client from trauma-induced bleeding episodes.

Drug Therapy. Agents used to control ITP include drugs that suppress immune function to some degree. The premise for the use of agents such as corticosteroids and azathioprine is to inhibit immune system synthesis of antiplatelet autoantibodies. More aggressive therapy can include low doses of chemotherapeutic agents, such as the antimitotic agents and cyclophosphamide.

Blood Replacement Therapy. For the client with a platelet count of less than $20,000/mm^3$ who is experiencing an acute life-threatening bleeding episode, a platelet transfusion may be required. Platelet transfusions are not performed routinely because the donated platelets are just as rapidly destroyed by the spleen as the client's own platelets (see Transfusion Therapy later).

Maintaining a Safe Environment. The nurse's major objectives are to protect the client from situations that can lead to bleeding and to closely monitor the amount of bleeding that is occurring. (For nursing care actions, see the earlier nursing diagnosis Risk for Injury under Leukemia.)

➤ *Surgical Management*

For the client who does not respond to drug therapy, splenectomy may be the treatment of choice. Because the leukocytes in the spleen perform many different immunodefensive functions, the client who has a splenectomy is at increased risk for infection.

Thrombotic Thrombocytopenic Purpura
Overview

Thrombotic thrombocytopenic purpura (TTP) is a rare disorder in which platelets clump together inappropriately in the microcirculation, and insufficient platelets remain in systemic circulation. The client experiences inappropriate clotting; yet the blood fails to coagulate properly when trauma occurs. The clinical picture is similar to that of disseminated intravascular coagulation (DIC) but is not initiated by the same factors. The underlying cause of TTP appears to be an autoimmune reaction in blood vessel cells (endothelial cells) that makes platelets aggregate in the microcirculation.

Collaborative Management

Treatment for the client with TTP focuses on inhibiting the inappropriate platelet aggregation and disrupting the underlying autoimmune process. Immunosuppressive therapy reduces the intensity of this disorder. Interventions to inhibit platelet aggregation include plasma exchange therapy and the administration of platelet aggregation inhibitors, such as aspirin, alprostadil (Prostin), and plicamycin.

Clotting Factor Disorders

Coagulation or bleeding disorders can result from a clotting factor defect, including the inability to produce a specific clotting factor, or production of insufficient quantities, or a less active form of a clotting factor.

Most clotting factor disorders are congenitally transmitted gene abnormalities of one clotting factor. The few acquired clotting factor disorders are related to an inability to synthesize many clotting factors at the same time as a result of liver damage or an insufficiency of clotting cofactors and precursor products. Common congenital disorders that result in defects at the clotting factor level include hemophilias A and B and von Willebrand's disease. DIC may be considered an acquired clotting disorder but is more closely associated with sepsis-induced distributive shock (see Chap. 39).

Hemophilia

Overview

Hemophilia comprises two hereditary bleeding disorders resulting from deficiencies of specific clotting factors. Hemophilia A (classic hemophilia) results from a deficiency of factor VIII and accounts for 80% of hemophilia cases. Hemophilia B (Christmas disease) is a deficiency of factor IX and accounts for 20% of cases.

The incidence of both is 1 in 10,000. Hemophilia is an X-linked recessive trait. Female carriers risk transmitting the gene for hemophilia to half of their daughters (who then are carriers) and half their sons (who will have overt hemophilia). Hemophilia A is, with rare exceptions, a disease affecting males, none of whose sons will have the gene for hemophilia and all of whose daughters will be obligatory carriers. In about 30% of clients with hemophilia, there is no family history, and it is presumed that their disease is the result of a new mutation (Cotran et al., 1994).

The bleeding disorder associated with hemophilia A is so severe that, before blood transfusions were available, hemophiliacs rarely survived past age 3 years. With the availability of blood transfusion and factor VIII therapy, mean survival time has increased so greatly that hemophilia now is commonly seen among adult clients.

The clinical pictures of hemophilia A and B are identical. The client has abnormal bleeding in response to any trauma because of an absence or deficiency of the specific clotting factor. Hemophiliacs form platelet plugs at the bleeding site, but the clotting factor deficiency impairs the hemostatic response and the capacity to form a stable fibrin clot. This produces abnormal bleeding, which may be mild, moderate, or severe, depending on the degree of factor deficiency.

Collaborative Management

Assessment of the client with hemophilia reveals

- Excessive hemorrhage from minor cuts or abrasions caused by abnormal platelet function
- Joint and muscle hemorrhages that lead to disabling long-term sequelae
- A tendency to bruise easily
- Prolonged and potentially fatal postoperative hemorrhage

The laboratory test results for a true hemophiliac demonstrate a prolonged partial thromboplastin time (PTT), a normal bleeding time, and a normal prothrombin time (PT) (Cotran et al., 1994). The most common health problem associated with hemophilia is degenerating joint function resulting from chronic bleeding into the joints, especially at the hip and knee.

The bleeding problems of hemophilia A can be well managed by either regularly scheduled IV administration of factor VIII cryoprecipitate or intermittent administration as needed, depending on activity level and injury probability (see Transfusion Therapy). However, the cost of cryoprecipitate is prohibitive for many people with hemophilia. In addition, because the precipitated clotting factors are derived from pooled human serum, a risk of viral contamination remains (even with the use of heat-inactivated serum). Major complications of hemophilia therapy during the 1980s were infection with hepatitis B virus, cytomegalovirus, and human immunodeficiency virus (HIV). Although heat-inactivated serum and the elimination of HIV-positive donors have reduced these risks, they have not yet been eliminated. New techniques for producing synthetic factor VIII will lead to uncontaminated and less expensive sources of this vital substance.

TRANSFUSION THERAPY

Any blood component may be removed from a donor and transfused to benefit a recipient. Components may be transfused individually or collectively, with varying degrees of benefit to the recipient.

Pretransfusion Responsibilities

Nursing actions during transfusions aim largely at prevention or early recognition of adverse transfusion reactions. Preparation of the client for transfusion therapy is imperative, and institutional blood product administration procedures should be carefully followed. Before administering any blood product to a client, the nurse reviews the agency's policies and procedures (Chart 42–12 presents a general guideline).

Legally, a physician's order is needed to administer blood or its components. The order specifies the type of component to be delivered, the volume to be transfused, and any special conditions the physician judges to be important. The nurse verifies the order for accuracy and completeness. The nurse also evaluates the need for transfusion, considering both the client's clinical condition and the laboratory values. In many hospitals, a separate con-

Chart 42–12

Nursing Care Highlight: Guidelines for Transfusion Therapy

Nursing Actions	Rationale
Before Infusion	
1. Assess laboratory values.	• Many institutions have specific guidelines for blood product transfusions (i.e., platelet count <20,000 or hemoglobin <8.0).
2. Verify the medical order.	• Legally, a physician's order is required for transfusions. The order should state the type of product, dose, and transfusion time.
3. Assess the client's vital signs, urine output, skin color, and history of transfusion reactions.	• Determine whether the client can tolerate infusion. Baseline information may be needed to help identify transfusion reactions.
4. Obtain venous access. Use a central catheter or 19-gauge needle, if possible.	• The larger bore needle allows cells to flow more easily without occluding the lumen of the catheter.
5. Obtain blood products from a blood bank. Transfuse immediately.	• Once a blood product has been released from the blood bank, the product should be transfused as soon as possible (e.g., red blood cell transfusions should be completed within 4 hours of removal from refrigeration).
6. With another registered nurse, verify the client by name and number, check blood compatibility, and note expiration time.	• Human error is the most common cause of ABO incompatibility reactions.
7. Administer the blood product using the appropriate filtered tubing.	• Filters are needed to remove aggregates and possible contaminants.
8. If the blood product needs to be diluted, use *only* normal saline solution.	• Hemolysis occurs if any other intravenous solution is used.
9. Remain with the client during the first 15–30 minutes of the infusion.	• Hemolytic reactions occur most often within the first 50 mL of the infusion.
10. Infuse the blood product at the ordered rate.	• Fluid overload is a potential complication of rapid infusion.
11. Monitor vital signs.	• Vital sign changes often indicate transfusion reactions.
12. When the transfusion is completed, discontinue infusion and dispose of the bag and tubing properly.	• Bloodborne pathogens may be spread inadvertently through improper disposal.
13. Document.	• The client record should indicate type of product infused, product number, volume infused, time of infusion, and any adverse reactions.

sent form must be obtained for the administration of blood products before a transfusion is performed.

A blood specimen is obtained for cross-matching (the testing of the donor's blood and the recipient's blood for compatibility). The procedure and responsibility for obtaining this specimen are specified by hospital policy. In most hospitals, a new cross-matching specimen is required at least every 48 hours.

Because of the viscosity of blood components, a 19-gauge needle or larger is used, whenever possible, for venous access. Both Y tubes and straight tubing sets are available for blood component administration. A blood filter (approximately 170 μ) to remove aggregates from the stored blood products is included with component administration equipment and must be used to transfuse all blood products. In massive transfusion, a microaggregate filter (20–40 μ) may be used (Kefer et al., 1996).

Normal saline is the solution of choice for administration. Ringer's lactate and dextrose in water are contraindicated for administration with blood or blood products because they cause clotting or hemolysis of blood cells

(Bradbury & Cruickshank, 1995). *Medications are never added to blood products.*

Before the transfusion is initiated, it is essential to determine that the blood component delivered is correct. Two registered nurses simultaneously check the physician's order, the client's identity, and whether the hospital identification band name and number are identical to those on the blood component tag. The blood bag label, the attached tag, and the requisition slip are examined to ensure that the ABO and Rh types are compatible. The expiration date is also checked, and the product is inspected for discoloration, gas bubbles, or cloudiness, indicators of bacterial growth or hemolysis (Huston, 1996).

Transfusion Responsibilities

The nurse takes the client's vital signs, including temperature, immediately before initiating the transfusion. Infusion begins slowly. A nurse remains with the client for the first 15 to 30 minutes. Any severe reaction usually occurs with administration of the first 50 mL of blood. The nurse assesses vital signs 15 minutes after initiation

Nursing Focus on the Elderly: Transfusion Therapy

- Assess the client's circulatory, renal, and fluid status before initiating the transfusion.
- Use no larger than a 19-gauge needle.
- Try to use blood that is less than 1 week old. (Older blood cell membranes are more fragile, break easily, and release potassium into the circulation.)
- Take vital signs (especially pulse, blood pressure, and respiratory rate) every 15 minutes throughout the transfusion. Changes in these parameters can indicate fluid overload and may also be the only indicators of adverse transfusion reactions.

Overload
- Rapid bounding pulse
- Hypertension
- Swollen superficial veins

Transfusion reaction
  - Rapid thready pulse
  - Hypotension
  - Increased pallor, cyanosis
- Administer blood slowly, taking 3–4 hours for each unit of whole blood, packed red blood cells, or plasma.
- Avoid concurrent fluid administration into any other intravenous site.
- If possible, allow 2 full hours after the administration of 1 unit of blood before administering the next unit.

of the transfusion to detect signs of a reaction. If there are none, the infusion rate can be increased to transfuse 1 unit in about 2 hours (depending on the client's cardiovascular status). The nurse takes the client's vital signs every hour throughout the transfusion or as specified by agency policy.

Blood components without large amounts of RBCs can be infused more quickly. The identification checks are the same as for RBC transfusions. Physiologic changes in elderly clients may necessitate that blood products be transfused at a slower rate. See Chart 42–13 for other nursing care needs of older clients undergoing transfusion therapy.

Types of Transfusions

Red Blood Cell Transfusions

Red blood cells are administered to replace erythrocytes lost as a result of trauma or surgical interventions. Clients with clinical conditions that result in the destruction or abnormal maturation of RBCs may also benefit from RBC transfusions. Packed RBCs, supplied in 250-mL bags, are a concentrated source of RBCs and are the most common component administered to RBC-deficient clients.

Blood transfusions are actually transplantations of tissue from one person to another. The donor and recipient blood must thus be carefully checked for compatibility to prevent potentially lethal reactions (Table 42–6). Com-

patibility is determined by two different types of antigen systems (cell surface proteins): the ABO system antigens and the Rh antigen, present on the membrane surface of RBCs.

Red blood cell antigens are inherited. For the ABO antigen system, a person inherits one of the following:

- A antigen (type A blood)
- B antigen (type B blood)
- Both A and B antigens (type AB blood)
- No antigens (type O blood)

Within the first few years of a child's life, circulating antibodies develop against the blood type antigens that were not inherited. For example, a child with type A blood will form antigens against type B blood. A child with type O blood has not inherited either A or B antigens and will form antibodies against RBCs that contain either A or B antigens. If erythrocytes that contain a foreign antigen are infused into a recipient, the donated tissue can be recognized by the immune system of the recipient as non-self, and the client may have a reaction to the transfused products (Kefer et al., 1996).

The mechanism of the Rh antigen system is slightly different. An Rh-negative person is born without the antigen and does not form antibodies unless he or she is specifically sensitized to the it. Sensitization can occur with RBC transfusions from an Rh-positive person or from exposure during pregnancy and birth. Once an Rh-negative person has been sensitized and antibody development has occurred, any exposure to Rh-positive blood can cause a transfusion reaction. Antibody development can be prevented by administration of Rh-immune globulin as soon as exposure to the Rh antigen is suspected. People who have Rh-positive blood can receive an RBC transfusion from an Rh-negative donor, but Rh-negative people must never receive Rh-positive blood (Bradbury & Cruickshank, 1995).

Platelet Transfusions

Platelets are administered to clients with platelet counts below 20,000 mm³ and to thrombocytopenic clients who are actively bleeding or scheduled for an invasive procedure (Kefer et al., 1996). Platelet transfusions are usually pooled from as many as 10 donors, and do not have to be of the same blood type as the client. For clients who are candidates for bone marrow transplant (BMT) or who

TABLE 42–6

Compatibility Chart for Red Blood Cell Transfusions				
	Recipient			
Donor	A	B	AB	O
A	X		X	
B		X	X	
AB			X	
O	X	X	X	X

require multiple platelet transfusions, single-donor platelets may be ordered. Single-donor platelets are obtained from one person and decrease the amount of antigen exposure to the recipient, helping prevent the formation of platelet antibodies. The chances of allergic transfusion reactions to future platelet transfusions are thus reduced.

Platelet infusion bags usually contain 300 mL for pooled platelets and 200 mL for single-donor platelets. Because the platelet is a fragile cell, platelet transfusions are administered rapidly after being brought to the client's room, usually over 15 to 30 minutes. A special transfusion set with a smaller filter and shorter tubing is used.

Standard transfusion sets are not used with platelets because the filter traps the platelets, and the longer tubing increases platelet adherence to the lumen. Additional platelet filters help remove WBCs in the platelet concentrate. These filters are connected directly to the platelet transfusion set and are used for clients who have a history of febrile reactions or who will require multiple platelet transfusions.

The nurse takes the client's vital signs before the infusion, 15 minutes after infusion is initiated, and at its completion. The client may be premedicated with meperidine or hydrocortisone to minimize the chances of a reaction. The client can become febrile and experience rigors (severe chills) during transfusion, but these symptoms are not considered a true transfusion reaction. IV administration of amphotericin B, an antifungal agent given to many leukemic clients, is discontinued during platelet transfusion and not resumed for at least 1 hour after transfusion. Amphotericin B can cause severe allergic reactions that are difficult to distinguish from transfusion reactions.

Plasma Transfusions

Historically, plasma infusions have been administered to replace blood volume, and they are occasionally still used for this purpose. It is more common for plasma to be immediately frozen after donation. Freezing preserves the clotting factors, and the plasma can then be used for clients with clotting disorders. Fresh frozen plasma (FFP) is infused immediately after thawing while the clotting factors are still viable.

ABO compatibility is required for transfusion of plasma products. The volume of the infusion bag is approximately 200 mL. The infusion takes place as rapidly as the client can tolerate, generally over 30 to 60 minutes, through a regular Y-set or straight-filtered tubing.

Cryoprecipitate

Cryoprecipitate is a product derived from plasma. Clotting factors VIII and XIII, von Willebrand's factor, fibronectin, and fibrinogen are precipitated from pooled plasma to produce cryoprecipitate. This highly concentrated blood product is administered to clients with clotting factor disorders at a volume of 10 to 15 mL/unit. Although cryoprecipitate can be infused, it usually is given by IV push within 3 minutes. Dosages are individualized, and it is best if the cryoprecipitate is ABO compatible.

Granulocyte Transfusions

At some centers, neutropenic clients with infections receive granulocyte transfusions for WBC replacement. However, this practice is highly controversial because the potential benefit to the client must be weighed against the potential severe reactions that often accompany granulocyte transfusions (Kefer et al., 1996). The surface of granulocytes contains numerous antigens that can cause severe antibody-antigen reactions when infused into a recipient whose immune system recognizes these antigens as nonself. In addition, transfused granulocytes have a very short life span and are probably of minimal benefit to the client (see Chap. 23). There is some evidence that treatment with antibiotics alone results in better survival rates.

Granulocytes are suspended in 400 mL of plasma and should be transfused over 45 to 60 minutes (Kefer et al., 1996). Institutional policies often require more stringent monitoring of clients receiving granulocytes. A physician may need to be present on the hospital unit and vital signs taken every 15 minutes throughout the transfusion. Administration of amphotericin B and granulocyte transfusions should be separated by 4 to 6 hours (Kefer et al., 1996).

Transcultural Considerations

Although transfusion with blood products is relatively common in acute care settings, the nurse remains sensitive to those clients who view receiving blood or blood products of others as repugnant, even sinful. Approximately 800,000 Jehovah's Witnesses live in the United States (Marelli, 1994). The tenets of this religion include that receiving human or animal blood is the same as "consuming" blood, an act specifically prohibited in the Old Testament. Devout Jehovah's Witnesses believe that to receive blood condemns them to eternal damnation. When possible, transfusion therapy with human blood products is avoided for this group. When clients are transfused with blood products against their will, the nurse shows respect for the client's distress and religious beliefs.

Some of the newer therapies for clients with anemia or hypovolemia may reduce the need for transfusion of human or animal blood products. One such therapy is the increasing use of hemoglobin substitutes, also known as "artificial blood." These agents increase the oxygen-carrying and oxygen-releasing power of the client's own blood.

Transfusion Reactions

Clients can experience any of the following transfusion reactions: hemolytic, allergic, febrile, bacterial, circulatory overload, and transfusion-associated graft-versus-host disease. The nurse is vigilant to prevent serious complications through early detection and initiation of appropriate treatment.

Hemolytic Transfusion Reactions

Hemolytic transfusion reactions are caused by blood type or Rh incompatibility. When blood containing antibodies against the recipient's blood is infused, antigen-antibody complexes are formed and released into the circulation. These complexes can destroy the transfused cells and initiate inflammatory responses in the recipient's blood vessel walls and organs (Huston, 1996). The ensuing reaction may be mild, with fever and chills, or severe, with disseminated intravascular coagulation (DIC) and circulatory collapse. Other clinical signs include

- Apprehension
- Headache
- Chest pain
- Low back pain
- Tachycardia
- Tachypnea
- Hypotension
- Hemoglobinuria
- A sense of impending doom

The onset of this type of reaction may be immediate or may not occur until subsequent units have been transfused.

Allergic Transfusion Reactions

Allergic transfusion reactions are most often seen in the client with a history of allergy. The client may have urticaria, itching, bronchospasm, or occasionally anaphylaxis. Onset of this type of reaction usually occurs during or up to 24 hours after the transfusion. The client with a history of allergy can be given buffy coat–poor or washed RBCs in which the WBCs and plasma are removed. This procedure minimizes the possibility of an allergic reaction.

Febrile Transfusion Reactions

Febrile transfusion reactions occur most commonly in the client with anti-WBC antibodies, a situation seen after multiple transfusions (Bradbury & Cruickshank, 1995). The recipient experiences

- Sensations of cold
- Tachycardia
- Fever
- Hypotension
- Tachypnea

Again, the physician can order buffy coat–poor RBCs or single-donor HLA-matched platelets. Leukocyte filters may also be used to trap WBCs and prevent their transfusion into the client.

Bacterial Transfusion Reactions

Bacterial transfusion reactions are seen after transfusion of contaminated blood products. Usually, a gram-negative organism is the source because these bacteria grow rapidly in blood stored under refrigeration. Symptoms include

- Tachycardia
- Hypotension
- Fever

- Chills
- Shock

Onset is rapid. (See Chapter 39 for care of the client experiencing sepsis-induced distributive shock.)

Circulatory Overload

Circulatory overload can occur when a blood product is administered too quickly. This complication is most common with whole blood transfusions or when the client requires multiple transfusions. The elderly are most at risk for this condition. See Chart 42–13. Symptoms include

- Hypertension
- Bounding pulse
- Distended jugular veins
- Dyspnea
- Restlessness
- Confusion

The nurse can both manage and prevent this complication by monitoring intake and output, transfusing blood products more slowly, and administering diuretics. See Chapter 15 for management of clients with fluid overload.

Transfusion-Associated Graft-Versus-Host Disease

Transfusion-associated graft-versus-host disease (TA-GVHD) is an infrequent but life-threatening complication that can occur in both immunosuppressed and immunocompetent clients. Its cause in immunosuppressed clients is similar to that of GVHD associated with allogeneic BMT, discussed earlier in this chapter, in which donor T-cell lymphocytes attack host tissues.

The cause of TA-GVHD in immunocompetent hosts is uncertain. Reactions are more common when the host and donor share similar human leukocyte antigens (HLAs), such as in first-degree relatives or individuals with similar ethnic background (Spector, 1995). Symptoms typically occur within 1 to 2 weeks and include thrombocytopenia, anorexia, nausea, vomiting, chronic hepatitis, weight loss, and recurrent infection.

Transfusion-associated GVHD has a 90% mortality rate, but can be prevented by transfusing irradiated blood products, thus preventing TA-GVHD by destroying T cells and their cytokine products (Spector, 1995).

Autologous Blood Transfusion

Autologous blood transfusions involve collection and transfusion of the client's own blood. Advantages of this type of transfusion are guaranteed compatibility and elimination of the risk of transmitting diseases such as hepatitis or HIV (Smith et al., 1995). The four types of autologous blood transfusions are preoperative autologous blood donation, acute normovolemic hemodilution, intraoperative autologous transfusion, and postoperative blood salvage.

Preoperative autologous blood donation, the most common type of autologous blood transfusion, involves collection of whole blood from the client, division into components, and then storage for later use (such as after a scheduled surgical procedure). As long as hematocrit and hemoglobin levels are within a safe range, client-donors donate blood on a weekly basis until the prescribed amount of blood is obtained. Fresh packed RBCs may be stored for 42 days. For individuals with rare blood types, blood may be frozen for up to 10 years. Platelets and plasma may be collected via pheresis (Gerber, 1994). Some cardiovascular problems and bacteremia are contraindications for autologous blood donation.

Acute normovolemic hemodilution involves withdrawal of a client's RBCs and volume replacement just before a surgical procedure. The goal is to decrease RBC loss during surgery. The blood is stored at room temperature for up to 6 hours and reinfused after surgery. This type of autologous transfusion is appropriate for healthy clients, but is contraindicated for individuals who are anemic or who have poor renal function (Gerber, 1994).

Intraoperative autologous transfusion and *postoperative blood salvage* involve the recovery and reinfusion of a client's own blood, collected either from an operative field or postoperatively from a wound. Several commercial products are available that collect, filter, and drain the blood into a transfusion bag (Smith et al., 1995). This autologous blood is often used for trauma or surgical clients with severe blood loss and must be reinfused within 6 hours.

The nurse transfuses autologous blood products using the guidelines previously mentioned. Although the client receiving autologous blood is not at risk for most types of transfusion reactions, the nurse must still assess for circulatory overload or bacterial transfusion reactions that can occur as a result of contamination.

CASE STUDY for the Client with Hematologic Complications

■ A 25-year-old woman is hospitalized on your unit for acute myelogenous leukemia. She completed induction chemotherapy 4 days ago, and today her major complaint is feeling tired and weak. Last night she reports waking up with epistaxis after an episode of coughing. Today's CBC with differential indicates an absolute neutrophil count of 180, a platelet count of 8000, and a hematocrit of 19.4.

QUESTIONS:

1. Given the treatment and laboratory values, what other type of symptoms might you expect?
2. What type of transfusions might be ordered?
3. What nursing interventions would help protect this client from infection?

SELECTED BIBLIOGRAPHY

*Agency for Health Care Policy and Research. (1993). *Sickle cell disease: Screening, diagnosis, management, and counseling in newborns and infants.* Rockville, MD: Author.

American Cancer Society. (1998). *Cancer facts and figures 1998.* 98–300M–No. 5008.98. Atlanta, GA: Author.

Blaylock, B. (1996). Sickle cell ulcers. *MedSurg Nursing, 5*(1), 41–43.

Bradbury, M., & Cruickshank, J. P. (1995). Blood and blood transfusion reactions: 2. *British Journal of Nursing, 4*(15), 861–868.

Callaghan, M. (1996). Leukemia. In R. McCorkle, M. Grant, M. Frank-Stromborg, & S. Baird (Eds.), *Cancer nursing: A comprehensive textbook* (2nd ed., pp. 752–772). Philadelphia: W. B. Saunders.

Carson, C.(1996). Hodgkin's disease and non-Hodgkin's lymphoma. In R. McCorkle, M. Grant, M. Frank-Stromborg, & S. Baird (Eds.), *Cancer nursing: A comprehensive textbook* (2nd ed., pp. 729–751). Philadelphia: W. B. Saunders.

Chernow, B., Jackson, E., Miller, J., & Wiese, J. (1996). Blood conservation in acute care and critical care. *AACN Clinical Issues: Advanced Practice in Acute and Critical Care, 7*(2), 191–197.

Cotran, R., Kumar, V., & Robbins, S. (1994). *Robbins pathologic basis of disease* (5th ed.). Philadelphia: W. B. Saunders.

D'Andrea, B., Belliveau, D., Birmingham, J., & Cooper, D. (1997). High-dose chemotherapy followed by stem cell transplant: The clinical/home care experience. *Journal of Care Management, 3*(2), 46–58, 80–85.

Dean, G. E., Haeuber, D., & Rivera, L. M. (1996). Infection. In R. McCorkle, M. Grant, M. Frank-Stromborg, & S. Baird (Eds.), *Cancer nursing: A comprehensive textbook* (2nd ed., pp. 963–978). Philadelphia: W. B. Saunders.

DeLaPena, L., Woolery-Antill, M., Tomaszewski, J. G., Gantz, S., Bernato, D. L., DiLorenzo, K., Molenda, J., & Kryk, J. A. (1996). Hematopoietic growth factors. *Cancer Nursing, 19*(2), 135–150.

Devine, S. M., & Larson, R. A. (1994). Acute leukemia in adults: Recent developments in diagnosis and treatment. *CA: A Cancer Journal for Clinicians, 44,* 326–352.

Eisenberg, D. (1997). Advising patients who seek alternative medical therapies. *Annals of Internal Medicine, 127*(1), 61–69.

*Ford, R. (1991). Bone marrow transplantation. In S. Baird, R. McCorkle, & M. Grant (Eds.), *Cancer nursing: A comprehensive textbook* (pp. 385–406). Philadelphia: W. B. Saunders.

Ford, R., McDonald, J., Mitchell-Supplee, K. J., & Jagels, B. A. (1996). Marrow transplant and peripheral blood stem cell transplantation. In R. McCorkle, M. Grant, M. Frank-Stromborg, & S. Baird (Eds.), *Cancer nursing: A comprehensive textbook* (2nd ed., pp. 505–530). Philadelphia: W. B. Saunders.

Gerber, L. (1994). Autologous blood transfusion: Why and how. *Journal of Intravenous Nursing, 17*(2), 65–69.

Higgins, C. (1995). Haematology blood testing for anaemia. *British Journal of Nursing, 4*(5), 248–253.

Hurley, C. (1997). Ambulatory care after bone marrow or peripheral blood stem cell transplantation. *Clinical Journal of Oncology Nursing, 1*(1), 19–21.

Huston, C. J. (1996). Hemolytic transfusion reaction. *American Journal of Nursing, 96*(3), 47.

Jacobs, L. A., & Piper, B. F. (1996). The phenomenon of fatigue and the cancer patient. In R. McCorkle, M. Grant, M. Frank-Stromborg, & S. Baird (Eds.), *Cancer nursing: A comprehensive textbook* (2nd ed., pp. 1193–1210). Philadelphia: W. B. Saunders.

Jassak, P. F., & Riley, M. B. (1994). Autologous stem cell transplant: An overview. *Cancer Practice, 2*(2), 141–145.

Kefer, C. A., Godwin, J., & Jassak, P. F. (1996). Blood component therapy. In R. McCorkle, M. Grant, M. Frank-Stromborg, & S. Baird (Eds.), *Cancer nursing: A comprehensive textbook* (2nd ed., pp. 485–503). Philadelphia: W. B. Saunders.

Lapka, D. M. V., Wild, L. D., & Barbour, L. A. (1994). Heparin-induced thrombocytopenia and thrombosis: A case study and clinical overview. *Oncology Nursing Forum, 21*(5), 871–876.

Larson, P. J. (1995). Perceptions of the needs of hospitalized patients undergoing bone marrow transplantation. *Cancer Practice, 3*(3), 173–179.

Lin, E. M., & Beddar, S. M. (1996). Abnormalities in hemostasis and hemorrhage. In R. McCorkle, M. Grant, M. Frank-Stromborg, & S. Baird (Eds.), *Cancer nursing: A comprehensive textbook* (2nd ed., pp. 979–1008). Philadelphia: W. B. Saunders.

Marchiondo, K., & Thompson, A. (1996). Pain management in sickle cell disease. *MedSurg Nursing, 5*(1), 29–33.

Marelli, T. (1994). Use of a hemoglobin substitute in the anemic Jehovah's Witness patient. *Critical Care Nurse, 14*(1), 31–38.

McBrien, N. (1997). Thrombotic thrombocytopenic purpura. *American Journal of Nursing, 97*(2), 28–29.

Miller, C. (1994). The role of transfusion therapy in treatment of sickle cell disease. *Journal of Intravenous Nursing, 17*(2), 70–73.

Morrison, V. A. (1994). Chronic leukemias. *CA: A Cancer Journal for Clinicians, 44,* 353–377.

Ong, S. T., & Larson, R. A. (1995). Current management of acute lymphoblastic leukemia in adults. *Oncology, 9*(5), 433–442.

Poliquin, C. (1997). Overview of bone marrow and peripheral blood stem cell transplantation. *Clinical Journal of Oncology Nursing, 1*(1), 11–17.

Ramirez-Smiley, M., & Ingle, B. (1995). Leukemia during pregnancy. *Oncology Nursing Forum, 22*(9), 1363–1367.

Randolph, S. R., Kelley, C. H., & McBride, L. H. (1995). Discharge planning for bone marrow recipients. *Journal of Care Management, 1*(4), 13, 14, 29–33.

Richardson, A., Ream, E., Wilson-Barnett, J. (1998). Fatigue in patients receiving chemotherapy: Patterns of change. *Cancer Nursing, 21*(1), 17–30.

Rieger, P. T., & Haeuber, D. (1995). A new approach to managing chemotherapy-related anemia: Nursing implications of epoetin alpha. *Oncology Nursing Forum, 22*(1), 71–81.

Smith, R. N., Fallentine, J., Kessel, S., & Maloney, M. (1995). Autotransfusion. *Nursing95, 25*(3), 52–55.

Spector, D. (1995). Transfusion-associated graft-versus-host disease: An overview and two case reports. *Oncology Nursing Forum, 22*(8), 97–101.

Vernon, S., & Pfeifer, G. (1997). Are you ready for bloodless surgery? *American Journal of Nursing, 97*(9), 40–46.

Viele, C. S. (1996). Chronic myelogenous leukemia and acute promyelocytic leukemia: New bone marrow transplantation options. *Oncology Nursing Forum, 23*(3), 488–502.

Walker, F., Roethke, S. K., & Martin, G. (1994). An overview of the rationale, process, and nursing implications of peripheral blood stem cell transplantation. *Cancer Nursing, 17*(2), 141–148.

*Whedon, M. B. (1991). *Bone marrow transplantation principles, practice and nursing insights.* Boston: Jones and Bartlett.

*Workman, M. L., Ellerhorst-Ryan, J., & Koertge, V. (1993). *Nursing care of the immunocompromised patient.* Philadelphia: W. B. Saunders.

Wujcik, D. (1996). Update on the diagnosis of and therapy for acute promyelocytic leukemia and chronic myelogenous leukemia. *Oncology Nursing Forum, 23*(3), 478–486.

SUGGESTED READINGS

Bradbury, M., & Cruickshank, J. P. (1995). Blood and blood transfusion reactions: 2. *British Journal of Nursing, 4*(15), 861–868.

This article describes different types of transfusion reactions, their etiology, and presenting symptoms. Detailed guidelines for nursing management of hemolytic, febrile, urticarial, septic, and anaphylactic transfusion reactions are provided in a tabular format.

Gerber, L. (1994). Autologous blood transfusion: Why and how. *Journal of Intravenous Nursing, 17*(2), 65–69.

The author describes the four different types of autologous blood transfusions: preoperative blood donation, acute normovolemic hemodilution, intraoperative blood recovery, and postoperative blood salvage. Patient eligibility, indications, and contraindications for each modality are also explained.

Jassak, P. F., & Riley, M. B. (1994). Autologous stem cell transplant: An overview. *Cancer Practice, 2*(2), 141–145.

This informational article helps the reader understand the rationale for bone marrow transplantation, with a complete description of the transplantation process. The authors highlight supportive care issues, particularly those required after the client goes home.

Marelli, T. (1994). Use of a hemoglobin substitute in the anemic Jehovah's Witness patient. *Critical Care Nurse, 14*(1), 31–38.

The author uses a case report approach to present the clinical applications and limitations of Fluosol DA, a hemoglobin substitute used to treat anemia. Jehovah's Witness views on blood transfusion are presented, with historic and physiologic information about Fluosol DA. Specific nursing needs for clients receiving hemoglobin substitutes are addressed.

Wujcik, D. (1996). Update on the diagnosis of and therapy for acute promyelocytic leukemia and chronic myelogenous leukemia. *Oncology Nursing Forum, 23*(3), 478–486.

The diagnosis and treatment of these leukemias are the focus of this article, with pathophysiology, diagnostic parameters, and common treatments discussed in detail. This is a valuable article for students who have clinical experience caring for clients with leukemia or who are considering this setting for employment.

Index

Note: Page numbers in *italics* indicate illustrations; those followed by t, b, and c indicate tables, boxed material, and charts, respectively.

CONTENTS IN BRIEF